W9-DEU-809

Pediatric Dosage Handbook

including

Neonatal Dosing, Drug Administration,
& Extemporaneous Preparations

7th Edition *2000-2001*

lexi-comp

APhA

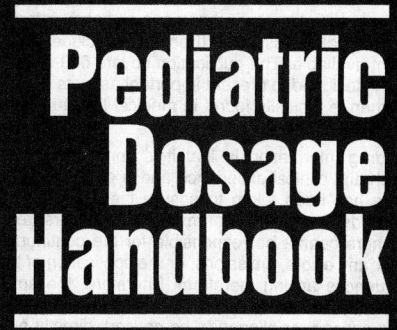

Pediatric Dosage Handbook

including
Neonatal Dosing, Drug Administration, & Extemporaneous Preparations

7th Edition | **2000-2001**

Carol K. Taketomo, PharmD
Pharmacy Manager
Children's Hospital of Los Angeles
Los Angeles, California

Jane Hurlburt Hodding, PharmD
Supervisor, Children's Pharmacy
Memorial Miller Children's Hospital
Long Beach, California

Donna M. Kraus, PharmD
Associate Professor of Pharmacy Practice
Departments of Pharmacy Practice and Pediatrics
Pediatric Clinical Pharmacist
University of Illinois at Chicago
Chicago, Illinois

LEXI-COMP INC
Hudson (Cleveland)

AMERICAN PHARMACEUTICAL ASSOCIATION APhA

NOTICE

This handbook is intended to serve the user as a handy reference and not as a complete drug information resource. It does not include information on every therapeutic agent available. The publication covers 659 commonly used drugs and is specifically designed to present important aspects of drug data in a more concise format than is typically found in medical literature or product material supplied by manufacturers.

The nature of drug information is that it is constantly evolving because of ongoing research and clinical experience and is often subject to interpretation. While great care has been taken to ensure the accuracy of the information presented, the reader is advised that the authors, editors, reviewers, contributors, and publishers cannot be responsible for the continued currency of the information or for any errors, omissions, or the application of this information, or for any consequences arising therefrom. Therefore, the author(s) and/or the publisher shall have no liability to any person or entity with regard to claims, loss, or damage caused, or alleged to be caused, directly or indirectly, by the use of information contained herein. Because of the dynamic nature of drug information, readers are advised that decisions regarding drug therapy must be based on the independent judgment of the clinician, changing information about a drug (eg, as reflected in the literature and manufacturer's most current product information), and changing medical practices. The editors are not responsible for any inaccuracy of quotation or for any false or misleading implication that may arise due to the text or formulas as used or due to the quotation of revisions no longer official.

The authors, editors, and contributors have written this book in their private capacities. No official support or endorsement by any federal or state agency or pharmaceutical company is intended or inferred.

The publishers have made every effort to trace the copyright holders for borrowed material. If they have inadvertently overlooked any, they will be pleased to make the necessary arrangements at the first opportunity.

If you have any suggestions or questions regarding any information presented in this handbook, please contact our drug information pharmacist at

1-877-837-LEXI (5394)

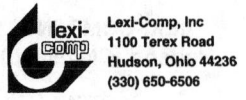

lexi-comp
Lexi-Comp, Inc
1100 Terex Road
Hudson, Ohio 44236
(330) 650-6506

ISBN 1-930598-34-3 (Domestic Edition)

ISBN 1-930598-36-X (International Edition)

TABLE OF CONTENTS

TABLE OF CONTENTS *(Continued)*

PREFACE

This seventh edition of the *Pediatric Dosage Handbook* is designed to be a practical and convenient guide to the dosing and usage of medications in children. The pediatric population is a dynamic group, with major changes in pharmacokinetics and pharmacodynamics taking place throughout infancy and childhood. Therefore, the need for the evaluation and establishment of medication dosing regimens in children of different ages is great.

Special considerations must be taken into account when dosing medications in pediatric patients. Unfortunately, due to a lack of appropriate studies, most medications commonly used in children do not have FDA approved labeling for use in pediatric patients. Only 30% of drugs used in children in a 1988 survey carried FDA approval in their labeling. Seventy-five percent of medications listed in the *1990 Physicians Desk Reference* carry some type of precaution or disclaimer statement for use in children.[1]

Both the FDA Modernization Act of 1997 and the 1998 Pediatric Final Rule will help to increase pediatric drugs studies. The FDA Modernization Act of 1997 was signed into law on November 21, 1997 (Section 111, Public Law 105-115, 105th Congress). This bill **encourages** pharmaceutical companies to conduct pediatric drug studies by allowing 6 months of market exclusivity to certain designated drugs. A list of drugs, for which additional pediatric information may produce pediatric healthcare benefits, was required by this law to be developed by the U.S. Department of Health and Human Services (HHS), with input from the American Academy of Pediatrics, the Pediatric Pharmacology Research Unit Network,[2] and the U.S. Pharmacopoeia. To date, the FDA has received 184 proposals from pharmaceutical companies to conduct pediatric drug studies under this Act and has approved 153 proposals. If these pediatric studies are completed as the FDA has specified, then these 153 medications will qualify for the 6 month patent extension or additional market exclusivity. Twenty-three products have already had their marketing patents extended by this law[3]. The 1998 Pediatric Final Rule is an FDA regulation, "Regulations Requiring Manufacturers to Assess the Safety and Effectiveness of New Drugs and Biological Products in Pediatric Patients; Final Rule,"[4] which became effective April 1, 1999. This important regulation **requires** that manufacturers conduct pediatric studies for certain new and marketed drugs and biological products. This requirement is mandatory, and its scope includes new drugs (ie, new chemical entities, new dosage forms, new indications, new routes of administration, and new dosing regimens) and certain marketed drugs (ie where the drug product offers meaningful therapeutic benefit or has substantial use in pediatric patients, AND the absence of pediatric labeling poses a risk). This important law and FDA regulation, plus other FDA regulations, such as the recent FDA labeling changes[5] that require expanded information in the Pediatric Use section of the package insert for all prescription drugs, will certainly help to increase and disseminate pediatric drug information.

Currently, however, most commonly used pharmacy references do not include information regarding pediatric dosing, drug administration, or special pediatric concerns. It is, therefore, not surprising that in order to obtain pediatric dosing information, oftentimes the pediatric clinician is faced with extensive literature searches to arrive at a logical dose. This handbook was developed with the intent to serve as a compilation of recommended pediatric doses found in the literature and to provide relevant clinical information regarding the use of drugs in children.

This new edition incorporates additions and revisions in a format which we hope the user will find beneficial. As with each edition, drug monographs have been updated and revised. Twenty-three new medications have been added. Four medications (astemizole, idoxuridine, rotavirus vaccine, and terfenadine) that were withdrawn from the U.S. market have been deleted. This brings the total number of drug monographs to 659. New monographs added to this edition include: Aldesleukin, amiloride, amprenavir, botulinum toxin type A, cyanide antidote kit, cyclopentolate and phenylephrine, dextroamphetamine and

PREFACE *(Continued)*

amphetamine, dextrose, ephedrine, etanercept, ethyl alcohol, ferric gluconate, fomepizole, hydroxocobalamin, imiglucerase, lamivudine and zidovudine, levalbuterol, metaraminol, metoprolol, oxcarbazepine, pirbuterol, poractant alfa, and quinpristin / dalopristin.

A new feature of this edition is the running header at the top of the drug monograph section. Very similar to the headers at the top of a page in a dictionary, the name of the drug that begins or ends a page, now appears at the top of the page. This header should help the user to find a drug monograph more quickly. For select drugs that have demonstrated involvement with cytochrome P-450 enzymes, the initial line of the drug interaction field now identifies the drug as a substrate, inducer, or inhibitor of the specific isoenzyme (eg, CYP1A2). In addition, 27 new extemporaneous preparations have been added to this edition, including 13 new extemporaneous preparations for drugs that did not previously have one. This brings the total number of drug monographs with extemporaneous preparations to 64 and the total number of "recipes" to 80.

Several new tables have been added to the appendix including: Cytochrome P-450 and Drug Metabolism; the new CDC 2000 Growth Charts; Compatibility of Chemotherapy and Related Supportive Care Medications; Pediatric, and Adult and Adolescent HIV Treatment Guidelines; and Commonly Used Antidotes for Acute Overdoses. Appendix material has been updated to include the 2000 Childhood Immunization Schedule and the 90th and 95th Percentile Blood Pressure Measurements by Percentiles of Height. The following tables were also updated or revised: Multiple Vitamin Products, Pediatric OTC Cough & Cold Preparations, Extravasation Treatment, Burn Management, Infant Enteral Nutritional Product Formulary, Composition of Frequently Used Oral Replacement Solutions, Parenteral Nutrition, Emetogenic Potential of Single Chemotherapeutic Agents, Management of Tumor Lysis Syndrome, Hotline Numbers, and Overdose and Toxicology.

We hope this edition continues to be a valuable and practical source of clinical drug information for the pediatric healthcare professional. We welcome comments to further improve future editions.

Footnotes

1. Food and Drug Letter, Washington Business Information, Inc. November 23, 1990.

2. "NIH Funds Network of Centers for Pediatric Drug Research," *Am J Hosp Pharm*, 1994, 51:2546.

3. Center for Drug Evaluation and Research, U.S. Food and Drug Administration," Approved Active Moieties to Which FDA has Granted Exclusivity for Pediatric Studies Under Section 505A of the Federal Food, Drug, and Cosmetic Act," http://www.fda.gov/cder/pediatric/exgrant.htm

4. Department of Health and Human Services, Food and Drug Administration, 21CFR Parts 201, 312, 314, and 601, Regulations Requiring Manufacturers to Assess the Safety and Effectiveness of New Drugs and Biological Products in Pediatric Patients; Final Rule,' *Fed Regist* 1998, 63(231):66631-72.

5. "Pediatric Use Drug Labeling NDA Supplements Due by December 1996 - FDA Final Rule; Agency Establishing Pediatric Subcommittee to Track Implementation," *F-D-C Reports - The Pink Sheet*, Wallace Werble Jr, Publisher, December 19, 1994.

ACKNOWLEDGMENTS

The *Pediatric Dosage Handbook* exists in its present form as the result of the concerted efforts of the following individuals: Robert D. Kerscher, publisher and president of Lexi-Comp Inc; Lynn D. Coppinger, managing editor; Barbara F. Kerscher, production manager; Mark F Bonfiglio, BS, PharmD, RPh, director of pharmacotherapy resources; Elizabeth Tomsik, BS, PharmD, pharmacotherapy specialist; Joni L. Stahura, BS, PharmD, pharmacotherapy specialist; Matthew Fuller, PharmD, clinical pharmacy specialist, psychiatry (VA Medical Center, Brecksville, OH); Leonard L. Lance, RPh, BSPharm, pharmacist; David C. Marcus, director of information systems; Leslie J. Ruggles, project manager; and Julian I. Graubart, American Pharmaceutical Association (APhA), Director of Books and Electronic Products.

Special acknowledgment goes to all Lexi-Comp staff for their contributions to this handbook.

Special thanks goes to Chris Lomax, PharmD, director of pharmacy, Children's Hospital, Los Angeles, who played a significant role in bringing APhA and Lexi-Comp together.

Some of the material contained in the book was a result of pediatric pharmacy contributors throughout the United States and Canada. Lexi-Comp has assisted many pediatric medical institutions to develop hospital-specific formulary manuals that contain clinical drug information as well as dosing. Working with these pediatric clinical pharmacists, pediatric hospital pharmacy and therapeutics committees, and hospital drug information centers, Lexi-Comp has developed an evolutionary drug database that reflects the practice of pediatric pharmacy in these major pediatric institutions.

The authors wish to thank their families, friends, and colleagues who supported them in their efforts to complete this handbook.

In addition, Dr Taketomo would like to thank Robert Taketomo, PharmD, MBA and Chris Lomax, PharmD for their professional guidance and continued support, and the pharmacy staff at Childrens Hospital, Los Angeles for their assistance.

Dr Kraus would like to especially thank Keith A. Rodvold, PharmD, for his ongoing professional and personal support.

Dr Hodding would like to thank Glenn Hodding, PharmD, Carl Kildoo, PharmD, and the pediatric pharmacists at Miller Children's Hospital for their continued professional and personal support.

EDITORIAL ADVISORY PANEL

EDITORIAL ADVISORY PANEL *(Continued)*

Bradley G. Phillips, PharmD, BCPS
Assistant Professor
University of Iowa College of Pharmacy
Clinical Pharmacist
Veterans Affairs Medical Center
Iowa City, Iowa

Martha Sajatovic, MD
Assistant Professor of Psychiatry
Case Western Reserve University
Cleveland, Ohio

Todd P. Semla, PharmD
Associate Director of the Psychopharmacology Clinical and Research Center
Department of Psychiatry and Behavioral Sciences
Evanston Northwestern Healthcare
Evanston, Illinois
Clinical Assistant Professor of Pharmacy Practice in Medicine,
Section of Geriatric Medicine
University of Illinois at Chicago
Chicago, Illinois

Dominic A. Solimando, Jr, MA
Oncology Pharmacist
Director of Oncology Drug Information
cancereducation.com
Arlington, VA

Virend K. Somers, MD, DPhil
Consultant in Hypertension and in Cardiovascular Disease
Mayo Clinic
Professor
Mayo Medical School
Rochester, MN

Lowell L. Tilzer, MD
Associate Medical Director
Community Blood Center of Greater Kansas City
Kansas City, Missouri

Beatrice B. Turkoski, RN, PhD
Professor, Advanced Pharmacology and Applied Therapeutics
Kent State University School of Nursing
Kent, Ohio

Richard L. Wynn, PhD
Professor and Chairman of Pharmacology
Baltimore College of Dental Surgery
Dental School
University of Maryland at Baltimore
Baltimore, Maryland

ABOUT THE AUTHORS

Carol K. Taketomo, PharmD

Dr Taketomo received her doctorate from the University of Southern California School of Pharmacy. Subsequently, she completed a clinical pharmacy residency at the University of California Medical Center in San Diego. With over 23 years of clinical experience at one of the largest pediatric teaching hospitals in the nation, she is an acknowledged expert in the practical aspects of pediatric drug distribution and clinical pharmacy practice.

In her current capacity as Pharmacy Manager at Children's Hospital of Los Angeles, Dr Taketomo plays an active role in the education and training of the medical, pharmacy, and nursing staff. She coordinates the Pharmacy Department's quality assurance and drug use evaluation programs; maintains the hospital's strict formulary program; and is the editor of the house staff manual. Her particular interests are strategies to influence physician prescribing patterns and methods to decrease medication errors in the pediatric setting. She has been the author of numerous publications, and is an active presenter at professional meetings. She currently holds an appointment with the University of Southern California School of Pharmacy.

Dr Taketomo is a member of the American Pharmaceutical Association (APhA), American Society of Health-System Pharmacists (ASHP), California Society of Hospital Pharmacists (CSHP), and Southern California Pediatric Pharmacy Group.

Jane Hurlburt Hodding, PharmD

Dr Hodding earned a doctorate and completed her pharmacy residency at the University of California School of Pharmacy in San Francisco. She has held teaching positions as Assistant Clinical Professor of Pharmacy at UCSF as well as Assistant Clinical Professor of Pharmacy Practice at the University of Southern California in Los Angeles. Currently, Dr Hodding is the Supervisor of Children's Pharmacy at Miller Children's Hospital at Long Beach Memorial in Long Beach, California.

Throughout her 23 years of pediatric pharmacy practice, Dr Hodding has actively pursued methods to improve neonatal intensive care, pediatric intensive care, and parenteral nutrition. She has published numerous articles covering neonatal medication administration and aminoglycoside and theophylline clearance in premature infants.

Dr Hodding is a member of the American Pharmaceutical Association (APhA), American Society of Health-System Pharmacists (ASHP), California Society of Hospital Pharmacists (CSHP), Children's Oncology Group, and Southern California Pediatric Pharmacy Group. She is frequently an invited speaker on the topics of Monitoring Drug Therapy in the NICU, Fluid and Electrolyte Therapy in Children, Drug Therapy Considerations in Children, and Parenteral Nutrition in the Premature Infant.

Donna M. Kraus, PharmD

Dr Kraus received her Bachelor of Science in Pharmacy from the University of Illinois at Chicago (UIC). She worked for several years as a hospital pediatric/obstetric satellite pharmacist before earning her doctorate degree at the UIC. Dr Kraus then completed a postdoctoral pediatric specialty residency at the University of Texas Health Science Center in San Antonio. She has served as a pediatric intensive care clinical pharmacist for 15 years and currently is an ambulatory care pediatric clinical pharmacist, specializing in pediatric HIV pharmacotherapy and patient/parent medication adherence. Dr Kraus has also served as a clinical pharmacist consultant to a pediatric long-term care facility for over 15 years. She currently holds the appointment of Associate Professor of Pharmacy Practice in both the Departments of Pharmacy Practice and Pediatrics at the University of Illinois in Chicago.

In her 23 years of active pharmacy experience, Dr Kraus has dealt with pediatric pharmacy issues and pharmacotherapy problems. She is an active educator and has been a guest lecturer in China, Thailand, and Hong Kong. Dr Kraus has played a leading role in the advanced training of postgraduate pharmacists and has been the Director of the UIC (ASHP accredited) Pediatric Residency and Fellowship Program for 13 years. Dr Kraus' research areas include pediatric drug dosing and developmental pharmacokinetics and pharmacodynamics. She has published a number of articles on various issues of pediatric pharmacy and pharmacotherapy.

Dr Kraus has been an active member of numerous professional associations including the American Pharmaceutical Association (APhA), American Society of Health-System Pharmacists (ASHP), Illinois Pharmacists Association (IPhA), American College of Clinical Pharmacy (ACCP), Illinois College of Clinical Pharmacy (ICCP), and the Pediatric Pharmacy Advocacy Group (PPAG). She served as Chairperson of the ASHP Commission on Therapeutics, and was an APhA, Academy of Pharmaceutical Research and Science, Member-at-Large. Currently, Dr. Kraus serves as an Editorial Board member of the *American Journal of Health-System Pharmacy* and the *Journal of Pediatric Pharmacy Practice*. She is also the APhA designated author for this handbook.

DESCRIPTION OF SECTIONS AND FIELDS USED IN THIS HANDBOOK

The *Pediatric Dosage Handbook, 7th Edition* is organized into a drug information section, an appendix, and a therapeutic category & key word index.

Drug information is presented in a consistent format and provides the following:

Generic Name	U.S. adopted name
Pronunciation Guide	Phonetic listing of generic name
Related Information	Cross-reference to other pertinent drug information found in the Appendix
Brand Names	Common trade names used in the U.S. and Canada
Available Salts	Lists the various salt forms of the drug
Synonyms	Other names or accepted abbreviations for the generic drug
Therapeutic Category	Unique systematic classification of medications
Generic Available	Indicated by a "Yes" or "No" as to whether a generic form of the drug is available
Use	Information pertaining to appropriate indications or use of the drug
Restrictions	Drug Enforcement Agency (DEA) classification for federally scheduled controlled substances
Pregnancy Risk Factor	Five categories established by the FDA to indicate the potential of a systemically absorbed drug for causing birth defects
Contraindications	Information pertaining to inappropriate use of the drug, or disease states and patient populations in which the drug should not be used
Warnings	Hazardous conditions related to use of the drug
Precautions	Disease states or patient populations in which the drug should be cautiously used
Adverse Reactions	Side effects are grouped by body system
Drug Interactions	For select drugs that have demonstrated involvement with cytochrome P-450 enzymes, the initial line of this field identifies the drug as a substrate, inducer, or inhibitor of specific isoenzymes (eg, CYP1A2). A summary of this information can also be found in a tabular format within the appendix. The remainder of the field presents a description of common or significant interactions between the drug listed in the monograph and other drugs or drug classes that are commonly used in pediatric patients. Due to space limitations, the reader is advised to read the drug interaction field of both drugs involved in the interaction.
Food Interactions	Possible interactions between the drug listed in the monograph and certain foods and/or nutritional substances
Stability	Storage, refrigeration, and compatibility information
Mechanism of Action	How the drug works in the body to elicit a response
Pharmacodynamics	Dose-response relationships including onset of action, time of peak action, and duration of action

Pharmacokinetics	Drug movement through the body over time. Pharmacokinetics deals with absorption, distribution, protein binding, metabolism, bioavailability, half-life, time to peak concentration, elimination, and clearance of drugs. Pharmacokinetic parameters help predict drug concentration and dosage requirements.
Usual Dosage	The amount of the drug to be typically given or taken during therapy

Please note that doses for neonates are often listed by postnatal age (PNA) (eg, PNA ≤ 7 days) and/or by body weight (eg, 1200-2000 g)

When both milligram and milligram per kilogram doses are listed, the milligram per kilogram dosing method is preferred. If using a milligram dosing guideline according to age, special care and lower doses should be used in children who have a low weight for their age. When ranges of doses are listed, initiate therapy at the lower end of the range and titrate the dose accordingly. References are listed at the end of drug monographs to support doses listed when little dosing information exists.

For select drugs, the dosing adjustment in renal impairment or dosing interval in renal impairment is given according to creatinine clearance (Cl_{cr}). Since most studies that recommend dosing guidelines in renal dysfunction are conducted in adult patients, Cl_{cr} is usually expressed in units of mL/minute. However, in order to extrapolate the adult information to the pediatric population, one must assume that the adults studied were of standard surface area (ie, 1.73 m^2). Therefore, although the value of Cl_{cr} listed for dosing adjustment in renal impairment or dosing interval in renal impairment may be expressed in mL/minute, it is assumed to be equal to the same value in mL/minute/1.73 m^2.

To calculate the dose in a pediatric patient with renal dysfunction, first calculate the normal dose (ie, the dose for a patient without renal dysfunction), then use the guidelines to adjust the dose. For example, the normal piperacillin dose for a 20 kg child is 200-300 mg/kg/day divided every 4-6 hours. If one selected 300 mg/kg/day divided every 6 hours, the dose would be 1.5 g every 6 hours in normal renal function. If Cl_{cr} was 20-40 mL/minute/1.73 m^2, the dose would be 1.5 g every 8 hours and if Cl_{cr} was <20 mL/minute/1.73 m^2, the dose would be 1.5 g every 12 hours.

Administration	Information regarding the recommended final concentrations and rates for administration of parenteral drugs are listed when appropriate, along with pertinent oral, ophthalmic, and topical administration information.
Monitoring Parameters	Laboratory tests and patient physical parameters that should be monitored for safety and efficacy of drug therapy are listed when appropriate.
Reference Range	Therapeutic and toxic serum concentrations are listed when appropriate
Test Interactions	Listing of assay interferences when relevant; (S) = Serum; (U) = Urine

DESCRIPTION OF SECTIONS AND FIELDS USED IN THIS HANDBOOK *(Continued)*

Patient Information	Advice, warnings, precautions, and other information of which the patient should be informed
Nursing Implications	Comments regarding nursing care of the patient are offered when appropriate
Additional Information	Other data and facts about the drug are offered when appropriate
Dosage Forms	Information with regard to form, strength, and availability of the drug
Extemporaneous Preparations	Directions for preparing liquid formulations from solid drug products. May include stability information and references (listed when appropriate).
References	Bibliographic information referring to specific pediatric literature findings, especially doses

Appendix

The appendix offers a compilation of tables, guidelines, and conversion information which can often be helpful when considering patient care. This section is broken down into various sections for ease of use.

Therapeutic Category & Key Word Index

This index provides a useful listing by an easy-to-use therapeutic classification system. Also listed are controlled substances, preservative free, sugar free, and alcohol free medications.

DEFINITION OF AGE GROUP TERMINOLOGY

Information in this handbook is listed according to specific age or by age group. The following are definitions of age groups and age-related terminologies. These definitions should be used unless otherwise specified in the monograph.

Gestational age (GA)	The time from conception until birth. More specifically, gestational age is defined as the number of weeks from the first day of the mother's last menstrual period (LMP) until the birth of the baby. Gestational age at birth is assessed by the date of the LMP and by physical exam (Dubowitz score).
Postnatal age (PNA)	Chronological age since birth
Postconceptional age (PCA)	Age since conception. Postconceptional age is calculated as gestational age plus postnatal age (PCA = GA + PNA).
Neonate	A full-term newborn 0-4 weeks postnatal age. This term may also be applied to a premature neonate whose postconceptional age (PCA) is 42-46 weeks.
Premature neonate	Neonate born at <38 weeks gestational age
Full-term neonate	Neonate born at 38-42 weeks (average ~40 weeks) gestational age
Infant	1 month to 1 year of age
Child/Children	1-12 years of age
Adolescent	13-18 years of age
Adult	>18 years of age

FDA PREGNANCY CATEGORIES

Throughout this book there is a field labeled Pregnancy Risk Factor and the letter A, B, C, D, or X immediately following which signifies a category. The FDA has established these five categories to indicate the potential of a systemically absorbed drug for causing birth defects. The key differentiation among the categories rests upon the reliability of documentation and the risk:benefit ratio. Pregnancy Category X is particularly notable in that if any data exists that may implicate a drug as a teratogen and the risk:benefit ratio is clearly negative, the drug is contraindicated during pregnancy.

These categories are summarized as follows:

A   Controlled studies in pregnant women fail to demonstrate a risk to the fetus in the first trimester with no evidence of risk in later trimesters. The possibility of fetal harm appears remote.

B   Either animal-reproduction studies have not demonstrated a fetal risk but there are no controlled studies in pregnant women, or animal-reproduction studies have shown an adverse effect (other than a decrease in fertility) that was not confirmed in controlled studies in women in the first trimester and there is no evidence of a risk in later trimesters.

C   Either studies in animals have revealed adverse effects on the fetus (teratogenic or embryocidal effects or other) and there are no controlled studies in women, or studies in women and animals are not available. Drugs should be given only if the potential benefits justify the potential risk to the fetus.

D   There is positive evidence of human fetal risk, but the benefits from use in pregnant women may be acceptable despite the risk (eg, if the drug is needed in a life-threatening situation or for a serious disease for which safer drugs cannot be used or are ineffective).

X   Studies in animals or human beings have demonstrated fetal abnormalities or there is evidence of fetal risk based on human experience, or both, and the risk of the use of the drug in pregnant women clearly outweighs any possible benefit. The drug is contraindicated in women who are or may become pregnant.

SYMBOLS & ABBREVIATIONS USED IN THIS HANDBOOK*

°C	degrees Celsius (Centigrade)
<	less than
>	greater than
≤	less than or equal to
≥	greater than or equal to
µg	microgram
µmol	micromole
AAP	American Academy of Pediatrics
AAPC	antibiotic associated pseudomembranous colitis
ABG	arterial blood gas
ABMT	autologous bone marrow transplant
ACE	angiotensin-converting enzyme
ACLS	advanced cardiac life support
ADH	antidiuretic hormone
AED	antiepileptic drug
AIDS	acquired immunodeficiency syndrome
ALL	acute lymphoblastic leukemia
ALT	alanine aminotransferase (formerly called SGPT)
AML	acute myeloblastic leukemia
ANA	antinuclear antibodies
ANC	absolute neutrophil count
ANLL	acute nonlymphoblastic leukemia
APTT	activated partial thromboplastin time
ARDS	adult respiratory distress syndrome
ASA (class I-IV)	American Society of Anesthesiology physical status classification of surgical patients according to their baseline health
	ASA I: Normal healthy patients
	ASA II: Patients having controlled disease states (eg, controlled hypertension)
	ASA III: Patients having a disease which compromises their organ function (eg, decompensated CHF, end stage renal failure)
	ASA IV: Patients who are extremely critically ill
AST	aspartate aminotransferase (formerly called SGOT)
ATP	adenosine triphosphate
AUC	area under the curve (area under the serum concentration-time curve)
A-V	atrial-ventricular
BMT	bone marrow transplant
BPD	bronchopulmonary disease
BUN	blood urea nitrogen
cAMP	cyclic adenosine monophosphate
CBC	complete blood count
CDC	center for Disease Control and Prevention
CF	cystic fibrosis
CHF	congestive heart failure
CI	cardiac index

SYMBOLS & ABBREVIATIONS USED IN THIS HANDBOOK* *(Continued)*

Cl_{cr}	creatinine clearance
CML	chronic myelogenous leukemia
CMV	cytomegalovirus
CNS	central nervous system
COPD	chronic obstructive pulmonary disease
CRF	chronic renal failure
CSF	cerebrospinal fluid
CT	computed tomography
CVA	cerebral vascular accident
CVP	central venous pressure
d	day
D_5/LR	dextrose 5% in lactated Ringer's
D_5/NS	dextrose 5% in sodium chloride 0.9%
D_5W	dextrose 5% in water
$D_5/^1/_4$ NS	dextrose 5% in sodium chloride 0.2%
$D_5/^1/_2$ NS	dextrose 5% in sodium chloride 0.45%
$D_{10}W$	dextrose 10% in water
DIC	disseminated intravascular coagulation
DL_{co}	pulmonary diffusion capacity for carbon monoxide
DNA	deoxyribonucleic acid
DVT	deep vein thrombosis
ECHO	echocardiogram
ECMO	extracorporeal membrane oxygenation
EEG	electroencephalogram
EKG	electrocardiogram
ESR	erythrocyte sedimentation rate
ESRD	end stage renal disease
E.T.	endotracheal
FDA	Food and Drug Administration (United States)
FEV_1	forced expiratory volume exhaled after 1 second
FSH	follicle-stimulating hormone
FVC	forced vital capacity
g	gram
G-6-PD	glucose-6-phosphate dehydrogenase
GA	gestational age
GABA	gamma-aminobutyric acid
GE	gastroesophageal
GERD	gastroesophageal reflux disease
GI	gastrointestinal
GVHD	graft versus host diease
GU	genitourinary
h	hour
Hct	hematocrit
Hgb	hemoglobin
HIV	human immunodeficiency virus
HPLC	high performance liquid chromatography
HSV	herpes simplex virus
ICP	intracranial pressure

IgG	immune globulin G
I.M.	intramuscular
INR	international normalized ratio
I.O.	intraosseous
I & O	input and output
IOP	intraocular pressure
I.T.	intrathecal
I.V.	intravenous
IVH	intraventricular hemorrhage
IVP	intravenous push
JRA	juvenile rheumatoid arthritis
kg	kilogram
L	liter
LDH	lactate dehydrogenase
LE	lupus erythematosus
LH	luteinizing hormone
LP	lumbar puncture
LR	lactated Ringer's
M	molar
MAC	*Mycobacterium avium* complex
MAO	monoamine oxidase
MAP	mean arterial pressure
mcg	microgram
mg	milligram
MI	myocardial infarction
min	minute
mL	milliliter
mM	millimole
mo	month
MOPP	mustargen (mechlorethamine), Oncovin® (vincristine), procarbazine, and prednisone
mOsm	milliosmoles
MRI	magnetic resonance image
MRSA	methicillin-resistant *Staphylococcus aureus*
NCI	National Cancer Institute
ND	nasoduodenal
ng	nanogram
NG	nasogastric
NMDA	n-methyl-d-aspartate
nmol	nanomole
NPO	nothing per os (nothing by mouth)
NS	normal saline (0.9% sodium chloride)
½NS	0.45% sodium chloride
NSAID	nonsteroidal anti-inflammatory drug
O.R.	operating room
OTC	over-the-counter (nonprescription)
PABA	para-aminobenzoic acid
PALS	pediatric advanced life support
PCA	postconceptional age
PCP	*Pneumocystis carinii* pneumonia
PCWP	pulmonary capillary wedge pressure

SYMBOLS & ABBREVIATIONS USED IN THIS HANDBOOK* *(Continued)*

PDA	patent ductus arteriosus
PICU	Pediatric Intensive Care Unit
PIP	peak inspiratory pressure
PNA	postnatal age
PSVT	paroxysmal supraventricular tachycardia
PT	prothrombin time
PTT	partial thromboplastin time
PUD	peptic ulcer disease
PVC	premature ventricular contraction
PVR	peripheral vascular resistance
qsad	add an amount sufficient to equal
RAP	right arterial pressure
RDA	recommended daily allowance
RIA	radioimmunoassay
RNA	ribonucleic acid
RSV	respiratory syncytial virus
S-A	sino-atrial
S.C.	subcutaneous
S_{cr}	serum creatinine
SIADH	syndrome of inappropriate antidiuretic hormone
S.L.	sublingual
SLE	systemic lupus erythematosus
STD	sexually-transmitted disease
SVR	systemic vascular resistance
SVT	supraventricular tachycardia
SWI	sterile water for injection
T_3	triiodothyronine
T_4	thyroxine
TIA	transient ischemic attack
TIBC	total iron binding capacity
TPN	total parenteral nutrition
TSH	thyroid stimulating hormone
TT	thrombin time
UA	urine analysis
UTI	urinary tract infection
V_d	volume of distribution
V_{dss}	volume of distribution at steady-state
VMA	vanillylmandelic acid
VZV	varicella zoster virus
w/v	weight for volume
w/w	weight for weight
y	year

*Other than drug synonyms

SAFE WRITING

Health professionals and their support personnel frequently produce handwritten copies of information they see in print; therefore, such information is subjected to even greater possibilities for error or misinterpretation on the part of others. Thus, particular care must be given to how drug names and strengths are expressed when creating written health-care documents.

The following are a few examples of safe writing rules suggested by the Institute for Safe Medication Practices, Inc.*

1. There should be a space between a number and its units as it is easier to read. There should be no periods after the abbreviations mg or mL.

Correct	Incorrect
10 mg	10mg
100 mg	100mg

2. Never place a decimal and a zero after a whole number (2 mg is correct and 2.0 mg is **incorrect**). If the decimal point is not seen because it falls on a line or because individuals are working from copies where the decimal point is not seen, this causes a tenfold overdose.

3. Just the opposite is true for numbers less than one. Always place a zero before a naked decimal (0.5 mL is correct, .5 mL is **incorrect**).

4. Never abbreviate the word unit. The handwritten U or u, looks like a 0 (zero), and may cause a tenfold overdose error to be made.

5. IU is not a safe abbreviation for international units. The handwritten IU looks like IV. Write out international units or use int. units.

6. Q.D. is not a safe abbreviation for once daily, as when the Q is followed by a sloppy dot, it looks like QID which means four times daily.

7. O.D. is not a safe abbreviation for once daily, as it is properly interpreted as meaning "right eye" and has caused liquid medications such as saturated solution of potassium iodide and Lugol's solution to be administered incorrectly. There is no safe abbreviation for once daily. It must be written out in full.

8. Do not use chemical names such as 6-mercaptopurine or 6-thioguanine, as sixfold overdoses have been given when these were not recognized as chemical names. The proper names of these drugs are mercaptopurine or thioguanine.

9. Do not abbreviate drug names (5FC, 6MP, 5-ASA, MTX, HCTZ, CPZ, PBZ, etc) as they are misinterpreted and cause error.

10. Do not use the apothecary system or symbols.

11. Do not abbreviate microgram as µg; instead use mcg as there is less likelihood of misinterpretation.

12. When writing an outpatient prescription, write a complete prescription. A complete prescription can prevent the prescriber, the pharmacist, and/or the patient from making a mistake and can eliminate the need for further clarification. The legible prescriptions should contain:

    a. patient's full name

    b. for pediatric or geriatric patients: their age (or weight where applicable)

    c. drug name, dosage form and strength; if a drug is new or rarely prescribed, print this information

    d. number or amount to be dispensed

    e. complete instructions for the patient, including the purpose of the medication

    f. when there are recognized contraindications for a prescribed drug, indicate to the pharmacist that you are aware of this fact (ie, when prescribing a potassium salt for a patient receiving an ACE inhibitor, write "K serum leveling being monitored")

*From "Safe Writing" by Davis NM, PharmD and Cohen MR, MS, Lecturers and Consultants for Safe Medication Practices, 1143 Wright Drive, Huntington Valley, PA 19006. Phone: (215) 947-7566.

SELECTED REFERENCES

Dorr RT and Von Hoff DD, *Cancer Chemotherapy Handbook*, 2nd ed, Norwalk, CT: Appleton & Lange, 1994.

Drug Interaction Facts, St Louis, MO: J.B. Lippincott Co (Facts and Comparisons Division), 1999.

Facts and Comparisons, St Louis, MO: J.B. Lippincott Co (Facts and Comparisons Division), 1999.

Feigin RD and Cherry JD, *Textbook of Pediatric Infectious Diseases,* 4th ed, Philadelphia, PA: WB Saunders Company, 1997.

Hale T, *Medications and Mother's Milk*, 8th ed, Amarillo, TX: Pharmasoft Medical Publishing, 1999.

Handbook on Extemporaneous Formulations, Bethesda, MD: American Society of Health-System Pharmacists, 1987.

Handbook of Nonprescription Drugs, 12th ed, Washington, DC: American Pharmaceutical Association, 1998.

Jacobs DS, DeMott WR, Grady HJ, et al, *Laboratory Test Handbook with Key Word Index*, 4th ed, Hudson, OH: Lexi-Comp Inc, 1996.

Jenson HB and Baltimore RS, *Pediatric Infectious Diseases - Principles and Practice*, Norwalk, CT: Appleton & Lange, 1995.

Lacy CF, Armstrong LL, Goldman MP, et al, *Drug Information Handbook*, 8th ed, Hudson, OH: Lexi-Comp, Inc, 2000.

Mandell GL, Bennett JE, and Dolin R, *Principles and Practice of Infectious Diseases*, 4th ed, New York, NY: Churchill Livingstone, 1995.

McEvoy GK and Litvak K, *AHFS Drug Information*, 42nd ed, Bethesda, MD: American Society of Health-System Pharmacists, 2000.

Nahata MC and Hipple TF, *Pediatric Drug Formulations,* 3rd ed, Cincinnati, OH: Harvey Whitney Books Company, 1997.

Nelson JD and Bradley JS, *Nelson's Pocket Book of Pediatric Antimicrobial Therapy*, 14th ed, Philadelphia, PA: Lippincott Williams & Wilkins, 2000.

PDR® Generics™, 2nd ed, Montvale, New Jersey: Medical Economics Co, 1996.

Phelps SJ and Hak EB, *Guidelines for Administration of Intravenous Medications to Pediatric Patients,* 5th ed, Bethesda, MD: American Society of Health-System Pharmacists, 1996.

Physician's Desk Reference, 54th ed, Montvale, NJ: Medical Economics Co, 2000.

Pickering LK, ed, *2000 Red Book, Report of the Committee on Infectious Diseases*, 25th ed, Elk Grove Village IL: American Academy of Pediatrics, 2000.

Pizzo PA and Poplack DG, *Principles and Practice of Pediatric Oncology*, 3rd ed, Philadelphia, PA: Lippincott Raven Publishers, 1996.

Pronsky ZM, *Powers and Moore's Food Medication Interactions*, 11th ed, Pottstown, PA: Food Medication Interactions, 2000.

Radde IC and MacLead SM, *Pediatric Pharmacology and Therapeutics*, St. Louis, MO: Mosby, 1993.

Rogers MC and Helfaer MA, *Handbook of Pediatric Intensive Care*, 2nd ed, Baltimore, MD: Williams & Wilkins, 1995.

Rogers MC and Nichols DG, *Textbook of Pediatric Intensive Care*, 3rd ed, Baltimore, MD: Williams & Wilkins, 1996.

Rudolph AM, *Rudolph's Pediatrics*, 20th ed, Norwalk, CT: Appleton & Lange, 1996.

Toro-Figueroa LO, Levin DL, and Morriss FC, *Essentials of Pediatric Intensive Care Manual,* St Louis, MO: Quality Medical Pub, Inc, 1992.

Trissel L, *Handbook of Injectable Drugs*, 10th ed, Bethesda, MD: American Society of Health-System Pharmacists, 1998.

Trissel LA, *Trissel's Stability of Compounded Formulations*, Washington, DC: American Pharmaceutical Association, 1996.

United States Pharmacopeia Dispensing Information (USP DI), 20th ed, Englewood, CO: Micromedex, Inc, 2000.

Yaffe SJ and Aranda JV, *Pediatric Pharmacology: Therapeutic Principles in Practice*, Philadelphia, PA: WB Saunders Company, 1992.

ALPHABETICAL LISTING OF DRUGS

♦ **A-ase** *see* Asparaginase *on page 98*

Abacavir (uh BACK ah veer)
Related Information
  Adult and Adolescent HIV *on page 1133*
  Pediatric HIV *on page 1129*
Brand Names Ziagen®
Available Salts Abacavir Sulfate
Therapeutic Category Antiretroviral Agent; HIV Agents (Anti-HIV Agents); Nucleoside Reverse Transcriptase Inhibitor (NRTI)
Generic Available No
Use Treatment of HIV-1 infection in combination with other antiretroviral agents. (**Note:** HIV regimens consisting of **three** antiretroviral agents are strongly recommended)
Pregnancy Risk Factor C
Contraindications Hypersensitivity to abacavir or any component; **do not rechallenge** patients who have experienced hypersensitivity to abacavir
Warnings Fatal hypersensitivity reactions may occur; discontinue therapy immediately in patients who show signs or symptoms of hypersensitivity reaction such as fever, fatigue, skin rash, respiratory symptoms (cough, dyspnea, pharyngitis), and GI symptoms (nausea, vomiting, diarrhea, or abdominal pain); carefully consider the diagnosis of hypersensitivity reaction in patients who present with acute onset respiratory symptoms, even if other diagnoses, such as bronchitis, flu-like illness, pharyngitis, or pneumonia, are possible; skin rash may be maculopapular or urticarial, but hypersensitivity reaction may occur without a rash; other symptoms may include edema, lethargy, malaise, arthralgia, myalgia, paresthesia, shortness of breath, mouth ulcerations, conjunctivitis, and lymphadenopathy; laboratory abnormalities include increase in liver function tests, creatine phosphokinase, creatinine, and lymphopenia; **do not restart** abacavir after a hypersensitivity reaction occurs; more severe symptoms can recur within hours and can include life-threatening hypotension and death; hypersensitivity reactions occur in ~5% of adult and pediatric patients; most hypersensitivity reactions occur within the first 6 weeks of therapy, but can occur at any time; call the Abacavir Hypersensitivity Reaction Registry at 1-800-270-0425 to facilitate reporting and collection of information on patients experiencing abacavir hypersensitivity reactions

Cases of lactic acidosis, severe hepatomegaly with steatosis and death have been reported; prolonged nucleoside use, obesity, and prior liver disease may be risk factors; use with extreme caution in patients with other risk factors for liver disease; discontinue abacavir in patients who develop laboratory or clinical evidence of lactic acidosis or pronounced hepatotoxicity
Precautions Always use abacavir in combination with other antiretroviral agents; do not add abacavir as a single agent to antiretroviral regimens that are failing; resistance to abacavir develops relatively slowly, but cross resistance between abacavir and other nucleoside reverse transcriptase inhibitors (NRTIs) may occur; limited response may be seen in patients with HIV isolates containing multiple mutations conferring resistance to NRTIs or in patients with a prolonged prior NRTI exposure
Adverse Reactions
  Central nervous system: Insomnia, fever, headache, malaise, fatigue
  Dermatologic: Rash
  Endocrine & metabolic: Mild elevations of blood glucose, hypertriglyceridemia, lactic acidosis
  Gastrointestinal: Nausea, vomiting, diarrhea, anorexia
  Hepatic: Hepatomegaly with steatosis
  Neuromuscular & skeletal: Asthenia
  Miscellaneous: Hypersensitivity reaction (see Warnings)
  Respiratory: Cough
Drug Interactions Use with ethanol increases abacavir AUC by 41% and prolongs half-life by 26%
Food Interactions Food does not significantly affect AUC
Stability Store tablets and oral solution at room temperature; oral solution may be refrigerated; do not freeze
Mechanism of Action A carbocyclic analogue that is converted within cells to the active metabolite carbovir triphosphate; carbovir triphosphate serves as an alternative substrate to deoxyguanosine-5'-triphosphate (dGTP), a natural substrate for cellular DNA polymerase and reverse transcriptase; carbovir triphosphate inhibits HIV viral reverse transcriptase by competing with natural dGTP and by becoming incorporated into viral DNA causing chain termination

Pharmacokinetics
Absorption: Rapid and extensive

Distribution: Apparent V_d: Adults: 0.86 ± 0.15 L/kg
CSF to plasma AUC ratio: 27% to 33%

Protein binding: 50%

Metabolism: In the liver by alcohol dehydrogenase and glucuronyl transferase to inactive carboxylate and glucuronide metabolites; not significantly metabolized by cytochrome P-450 enzymes

Bioavailability: Tablet: 83%; solution and tablet provide comparable AUCs

Half-life:
Children 3 months to 13 years: 1-1.5 hours (range)
Adults: 1.54 ± 0.63 hours

Time to peak concentration: Children 3 months to 13 years: Within 1.5 hours

Clearance (apparent): Single dose 8 mg/kg:
Children 3 months to 13 years: 17.84 mL/minute/kg
Adults: 10.14 mL/minute/kg

Elimination: ~83% of dose excreted in the urine as unchanged drug (1.2%) and metabolites (30% as 5'-carboxylic acid metabolite, 36% as the glucuronide, and 15% as other metabolites); 16% eliminated in feces

Usual Dosage Oral (use in combination with other antiretroviral agents):
Neonates: Not approved for use

Infants 1-3 months: Not approved for use; doses of 8 mg/kg twice daily are being studied

Infants ≥3 months, Children, and Adolescents: 8 mg/kg twice daily (maximum: 300 mg twice daily)

Adults: 300 mg twice daily

Administration Oral: May be administered without regard to food

Monitoring Parameters Signs and symptoms of hypersensitivity reaction; serum glucose and triglycerides, viral load, CD4 counts

Patient Information Abacavir is not a cure for HIV. Stop taking abacavir and notify physician immediately if skin rash or 2 or more of the following sets of symptoms occur: Fever, GI symptoms (nausea, vomiting, diarrhea or abdominal pain), flu-like symptoms (severe tiredness, achiness, or generally ill feeling), or respiratory symptoms (sore throat, shortness of breath, cough). If you experience an allergic (hypersensitivity) reaction to abacavir, **never** take the medication again. Take abacavir everyday as prescribed; do not change dose or discontinue without physician's advice; if a dose is missed, take it as soon as possible, then return to normal dosing schedule; if a dose is skipped, do **not** double the next dose

Nursing Implications Inform patients of the possibility of a fatal hypersensitivity reaction and the signs and symptoms (see Warnings)

Additional Information The patient Medication Guide, which includes written manufacturer information, should be dispensed to the patient with each new prescription and refill; the Warning Card describing the hypersensitivity reaction should be given to the patient to carry with them; oral solution contains methylparaben and propylparaben (preservatives) and propylene glycol

Dosage Forms Available as abacavir sulfate; mg strength refers to abacavir sulfate equivalent of abacavir free base
Oral solution (strawberry-banana flavor): 20 mg/mL
Tablet: 300 mg

References
Foster RH and Faulds D, "Abacavir," *Drugs*, 1998, 55(5):729-36.

Hughes W, McDowell JA, Shenep J, et al, "Safety and Single-Dose Pharmacokinetics of Abacavir (1592U89) in Human Immunodeficiency Virus Type 1-Infected Children," *Antimicrob Agents Chemother*, 1999, 43(3):609-15.

Kline MW, Blanchard S, Fletcher CV, et al, "A Phase I Study of Abacavir (1592U89) Alone and in Combination With Other Antiretroviral Agents in Infants and Children With Human Immunodeficiency Virus Infection," *Pediatrics*, 1999, 103(4):e47; http://www.pediatrics.org/cgi/content/full/103/4/e47.

Panel on Clinical Practices for Treatment of HIV Infection, "Guidelines for the Use of Antiretroviral Agents in HIV-Infected Adults and Adolescents," January 28, 2000, http://www.hivatis.org.

Working Group on Antiretroviral Therapy and Medical Management of HIV-Infected Children, "Guidelines for the Use of Antiretroviral Agents in Pediatric HIV Infection," January 7, 2000, http://www.hivatis.org.

- **Absorbine Jr.® Antifungal [OTC]** see Tolnaftate *on page 936*
- **A-Caine® Rectal [OTC]** see Hemorrhoidal Preparations *on page 470*
- **Accolate®** see Zafirlukast *on page 987*
- **Accurbron®** see Theophylline *on page 910*
- **Accutane®** see Isotretinoin *on page 537*
- **Acephen® [OTC]** see Acetaminophen *on page 26*
- **Aceta® [OTC]** see Acetaminophen *on page 26*

Acetaminophen (a seet a MIN oh fen)

Related Information
Acetaminophen Toxicity Nomogram *on page 1207*
Carbohydrate and Alcohol Content of Liquid Medications for Use in Patients Receiving Ketogenic Diets *on page 1228*
OTC Cough & Cold Preparations, Pediatric *on page 1037*
Overdose and Toxicology *on page 1191*

Brand Names Abenol® (Canada); Acephen® [OTC]; Aceta® [OTC]; AF® (Canada); Apacet® [OTC]; Atasol® (Canada); Dapa® [OTC]; Dapacin® [OTC]; Dorcol® [OTC]; Feverall™ [OTC]; Genapap® [OTC]; Genebs® [OTC]; Liquiprin® [OTC]; Mapap® [OTC]; Maranox® [OTC]; Meda-Cap® [OTC]; Meda® Tab [OTC]; Myapap® [OTC]; Neopap® [OTC]; Panadol® [OTC]; Pediatrix® (Canada); Redutemp® [OTC]; Ridenol® [OTC]; Silapap® [OTC]; Snaplets-FR® Granules [OTC]; Tantaphen® (Canada); Tapanol® [OTC]; Tempra® [OTC]; Tylenol® [OTC]; Ty-Pap [OTC]; Uni-Ace® [OTC]

Synonyms APAP; N-Acetyl-P-Aminophenol; Paracetamol

Therapeutic Category Analgesic, Non-narcotic; Antipyretic

Generic Available Yes

Use Treatment of mild to moderate pain and fever; does not have antirheumatic or systemic anti-inflammatory effects

Pregnancy Risk Factor B

Contraindications Hypersensitivity to acetaminophen or any component

Warnings May cause severe hepatic toxicity with overdose

Precautions Some products (eg, Children's Tylenol® chewable tablets) contain aspartame; aspartame is metabolized to phenylalanine and must be avoided or used with caution in patients with phenylketonuria

G-6-PD deficiency: Although several case reports of acetaminophen-associated hemolytic anemia have been reported in patients with G-6-PD deficiency, a direct cause and effect relationship has not been well established (concurrent illnesses such as fever or infection may precipitate hemolytic anemia in patients with G-6-PD deficiency); therefore, acetaminophen is generally thought to be safe when given in therapeutic doses to patients with G-6-PD deficiency.

Adverse Reactions
Dermatologic: Rash
Hematologic: Blood dyscrasias (neutropenia, pancytopenia, leukopenia)
Hepatic: Hepatic necrosis with overdose
Renal: Renal injury with chronic use
Miscellaneous: Hypersensitivity reactions (rare)

Drug Interactions Cytochrome P-450 isoenzyme CYP1A2 substrate (minor), CYP2E1 and CYP3A3/4 isoenzyme substrate
Enzyme inducers (barbiturates, carbamazepine, phenytoin), carmustine (with high dose acetaminophen), alcohol (especially chronic use) can increase hepatotoxicity; rifampin may decrease acetaminophen's therapeutic effect; anticholinergic agents (scopolamine) may effect GI absorption; acetaminophen may increase the clearance of lamotrigine; acetaminophen may increase zidovudine concentration and toxicity

Food Interactions Rate of absorption may be decreased when given with food high in carbohydrates

Mechanism of Action Inhibits the synthesis of prostaglandins in the central nervous system and peripherally blocks pain impulse generation; produces antipyresis from inhibition of hypothalamic heat-regulating center

Pharmacokinetics
Protein binding: 20% to 50%
Metabolism: At normal therapeutic dosages the parent compound is metabolized in the liver to sulfate and glucuronide metabolites, while a small amount is metabolized by microsomal mixed function oxidases to a highly reactive intermediate (N-acetyl-imidoquinone) which is conjugated with glutathione and inactivated; at toxic doses (as little as 4 g in a single day) glutathione can become depleted, and conjugation becomes insufficient to meet the metabolic demand causing an

increase in N-acetyl-imidoquinone concentration, which is thought to cause hepatic cell necrosis.

Half-life:
Neonates: 2-5 hours
Adults: 1-3 hours

Time to peak serum concentration: 10-60 minutes after normal oral doses, but may be delayed in acute overdoses

Usual Dosage Oral, rectal:
Neonates: 10-15 mg/kg/dose every 6-8 hours as needed
Infants and Children: 10-15 mg/kg/dose every 4-6 hours as needed; do **not** exceed 5 doses in 24 hours; alternatively, the following doses may be used. See table.

Acetaminophen Dosing

Age	Dosage (mg)	Age	Dosage (mg)
0-3 mo	40	4-5 y	240
4-11 mo	80	6-8 y	320
1-2 y	120	9-10 y	400
2-3 y	160	11 y	480

Children ≥12 years and Adults: 325-650 mg every 4-6 hours or 1000 mg 3-4 times/day; do **not** exceed 4 g/day

Administration Oral: Administer with food to decrease GI upset; shake suspension well before use; do not crush or chew extended release products

Reference Range Acute ingestions: Toxic concentration with probable hepatotoxicity: >200 µg/mL at 4 hours or 50 µg/mL at 12 hours after ingestion of overdose

Patient Information Avoid alcohol; do not take longer than 10 days without physician's advice

Additional Information Some elixir preparations contain sodium benzoate; drops contain saccharin

Acetaminophen (15 mg/kg/dose given orally every 6 hours for 24 hours) did **not** relieve the intraoperative or the immediate postoperative pain associated with neonatal circumcision; some benefit was seen 6 hours after circumcision (see Howard, 1994).

There is currently no scientific evidence to support alternating acetaminophen with ibuprofen in the treatment of fever (see Mayoral, 2000).

Dosage Forms Most commonly available concentrations for nonsolid dosage forms are **bolded**
Caplet: 160 mg, 325 mg, 500 mg
Caplet, extended: 650 mg
Capsule: 325 mg, 500 mg
Drops: 80 mg/1.66 mL (30 mL); **100 mg/mL** (15 mL); 120 mg/2.5 mL (35 mL)
Elixir: 80 mg/2.5 mL (237 mL); 80 mg/5 mL (120 mL); 120 mg/5 mL (27 mL, 120 mL); **160 mg/5 mL** (5 mL, 10 mL, 20 mL, 120 mL, 240 mL, 500 mL, 3780 mL); **325 mg/5 mL** (480 mL, 3780 mL)
Gelcap: 500 mg
Granules, premeasured packs: 80 mg (32s)
Liquid, oral: **160 mg/5 mL** (2.5 mL, 5 mL, 60 mL, 120 mL, 240 mL, 480 mL); 500 mg/15 mL (240 mL)
Powder, in capsules: 80 mg, 160 mg
Suppository, rectal: 80 mg, 120 mg, 125 mg, 300 mg, 325 mg, 650 mg
Suspension, oral: **160 mg/5 mL**
Suspension, oral drops: 100 mg/mL
Tablet: 160 mg, 325 mg, 500 mg, 650 mg
Tablet, chewable: 80 mg, 160 mg
Tablet, extended release: 650 mg

References
Howard CR, Howard FM, and Weitzman ML, "Acetaminophen Analgesia in Neonatal Circumcision: The Effect on Pain," *Pediatrics*, 1994, 93(4):641-646.
Mayoral CE, Marino RV, Rosenfeld W, et al, "Alternating Antipyretics: Is This An Alternative?" *Pediatrics*, 2000, 105(5):1009-12.

Acetaminophen and Codeine (a seet a MIN oh fen & KOE deen)
Related Information
Carbohydrate and Alcohol Content of Liquid Medications for Use in Patients Receiving Ketogenic Diets *on page 1228*
Overdose and Toxicology *on page 1191*
(Continued)

Acetaminophen and Codeine *(Continued)*

Brand Names Atasol® 8, 15, 30 W/ Caffeine (Canada); Capital® and Codeine; Empracet®-30, -60 (Canada); Emtec-30® (Canada); Lenoltec® No.1, 2, 3, 4 (Canada); Novo-Gesic-C8® (Canada); Novo-Gesic-C15® (Canada); Novo-Gesic-C30® (Canada); Phenaphen® With Codeine; Tylenol® With Codeine

Available Salts Acetaminophen and Codeine Phosphate

Synonyms Codeine and Acetaminophen

Therapeutic Category Analgesic, Narcotic

Generic Available Yes

Use Relief of mild to moderate pain

Restrictions C-III; C-V

Pregnancy Risk Factor C

Contraindications Hypersensitivity to acetaminophen, codeine phosphate, or any component

Warnings Tablets contain metabisulfite which may cause allergic reactions

Precautions Use with caution in patients with hypersensitivity reactions to other phenanthrene derivative opioid agonists (morphine, hydrocodone, hydromorphone, levorphanol, oxycodone, oxymorphone) or respiratory disease/compromise.

G-6-PD deficiency: Although several case reports of acetaminophen-associated hemolytic anemia have been reported in patients with G-6-PD deficiency, a direct cause and effect relationship has not been well established (concurrent illnesses such as fever or infection may precipitate hemolytic anemia in patients with G-6-PD deficiency); therefore, acetaminophen is generally thought to be safe when given in therapeutic doses to patients with G-6-PD deficiency.

Adverse Reactions

Acetaminophen:

Dermatologic: Rash

Hematologic: Blood dyscrasias (neutropenia, pancytopenia, leukopenia)

Hepatic: Hepatic necrosis with overdose

Renal: Renal injury with chronic use

Miscellaneous: Hypersensitivity reactions (rare)

Codeine:

Cardiovascular: Palpitations, hypotension, bradycardia, peripheral vasodilation

Central nervous system: CNS depression, dizziness, drowsiness, sedation, increased intracranial pressure

Dermatologic: Pruritus

Endocrine & metabolic: Antidiuretic hormone release

Gastrointestinal: Nausea, vomiting, constipation, biliary tract spasm

Genitourinary: Urinary retention

Ocular: Miosis

Respiratory: Respiratory depression

Miscellaneous: Histamine release, physical and psychological dependence with prolonged use

Drug Interactions See Acetaminophen *on page 26* and Codeine *on page 249*

Food Interactions Rate of absorption of acetaminophen may be decreased when given with food high in carbohydrates

Mechanism of Action See individual monographs for Acetaminophen *on page 26* and Codeine *on page 249*

Pharmacokinetics See individual monographs for Acetaminophen *on page 26* and Codeine *on page 249*

Usual Dosage Oral (doses should be titrated to appropriate analgesic effect):

Children: Analgesic: 0.5-1 mg codeine/kg/dose every 4-6 hours

3-6 years: 5 mL 3-4 times/day as needed

7-12 years: 10 mL 3-4 times/day as needed

>12 years: 15 mL every 4 hours as needed

Adults: 1-2 tablets every 4 hours; maximum dose: 12 tablets/24 hours

Administration Oral: Administer with food to decrease GI upset; shake suspension well before use

Patient Information Codeine may be habit-forming; avoid abrupt discontinuation after prolonged use; may cause drowsiness and impair ability to perform activities requiring mental alertness or coordination; avoid alcohol

Nursing Implications Observe patient for excessive sedation, respiratory depression

Additional Information Tylenol® With Codeine elixir contains sodium benzoate and saccharin

Dosage Forms
Capsule:
#2: Acetaminophen 325 mg and codeine phosphate 15 mg (C-III)
#3: Acetaminophen 325 mg and codeine phosphate 30 mg (C-III)
#4: Acetaminophen 325 mg and codeine phosphate 60 mg (C-III)
Elixir: Acetaminophen 120 mg and codeine phosphate 12 mg per 5 mL with alcohol 7% (C-V)
Suspension, oral, alcohol free: Acetaminophen 120 mg and codeine phosphate 12 mg per 5 mL (C-V)
Tablet: Acetaminophen 500 mg and codeine phosphate 30 mg (C-III); acetaminophen 650 mg and codeine phosphate 30 mg (C-III)
Tablet:
#1: Acetaminophen 300 mg and codeine phosphate 7.5 mg (C-III)
#2: Acetaminophen 300 mg and codeine phosphate 15 mg (C-III)
#3: Acetaminophen 300 mg and codeine phosphate 30 mg (C-III)
#4: Acetaminophen 300 mg and codeine phosphate 60 mg (C-III)

- ◆ **Acetaminophen and Codeine Phosphate** see Acetaminophen and Codeine on page 27
- ◆ **Acetaminophen and Hydrocodone** see Hydrocodone and Acetaminophen on page 485
- ◆ **Acetaminophen and Oxycodone** see Oxycodone and Acetaminophen on page 716
- ◆ **Acetaminophen and Propoxyphene** see Propoxyphene and Acetaminophen on page 815
- ◆ **Acetaminophen Toxicity Nomogram** see page 1207
- ◆ **Acetazolam® (Canada)** see Acetazolamide on page 29

Acetazolamide (a set a ZOLE a mide)
Related Information
Antiepileptic Drugs on page 1176
Brand Names Acetazolam® (Canada); Apo®-Acetazolamide (Canada); Diamox®; Diamox Sequels®; Novo-Zolamide® (Canada)
Therapeutic Category Anticonvulsant, Miscellaneous; Carbonic Anhydrase Inhibitor; Diuretic, Carbonic Anhydrase Inhibitor
Generic Available Yes
Use Reduce elevated intraocular pressure in glaucoma; diuretic; adjunct to the treatment of refractory seizures; prevent acute altitude sickness; treatment of centrencephalic epilepsies
Pregnancy Risk Factor C
Contraindications Hypersensitivity to acetazolamide, any component, or other sulfonamides; patients with hepatic disease or insufficiency; decreased serum sodium and/or potassium; adrenocortical insufficiency; hyperchloremic acidosis; or severe renal disease
Warnings Tolerance to antiepileptic effects may require dosage adjustment
Precautions Use with caution in patients with respiratory acidosis, COPD, diabetes mellitus, and gout
Adverse Reactions
Cardiovascular: Cyanosis
Central nervous system: Drowsiness, fatigue, vertigo, fever, seizures, dizziness, depression, malaise
Dermatologic: Rash, erythema multiforme, photosensitivity, Stevens-Johnson syndrome
Endocrine & metabolic: Hypokalemia, hyperchloremic metabolic acidosis, hyperglycemia
Gastrointestinal: GI irritation, anorexia, nausea, vomiting, xerostomia, melena, dysgeusia, metallic taste, black stools
Genitourinary: Dysuria, polyuria
Hematologic: Bone marrow suppression, thrombocytopenia, hemolytic anemia, pancytopenia, agranulocytosis
Hepatic: Hepatic insufficiency
Neuromuscular & skeletal: Paresthesia, muscle weakness
Ocular: Myopia
Renal: Renal calculi, phosphaturia, renal colic
Respiratory: Hyperpnea
Drug Interactions Increases lithium excretion; may decrease the rate of excretion of other drugs such as procainamide, flecainide, quinidine, and tricyclic antidepressants; may increase the excretion of salicylates and phenobarbital; may inactivate methenamine in the urine; may increase cyclosporine levels; may increase the risk
(Continued)

Acetazolamide *(Continued)*

of developing osteomalacia in patients receiving phenytoin or phenobarbital; topiramate may increase risk of nephrolithiasis and paresthesia; salicylates increase acetazolamide serum levels resulting in CNS toxicity; ammonium chloride increases plasma concentration of nonionized acetazolamide; increased toxicity with propofol (cardiorespiratory instability)

Food Interactions Avoid natural licorice (causes sodium and water retention and increases potassium loss)

Stability After reconstitution, acetazolamide injection is stable for 12 hours at room temperature and for 1 week when refrigerated; physically incompatible with parenteral multivitamins

Mechanism of Action Competitive, reversible inhibition of the enzyme carbonic anhydrase resulting in increased renal excretion of sodium, potassium, bicarbonate, and water and decreased formation of aqueous humor; also inhibits carbonic anhydrase in central nervous system to retard abnormal and excessive discharge from CNS neurons

Pharmacodynamics

Onset of action:
 Capsule, extended release: 2 hours
 Tablet: 1-1.5 hours
 I.V.: 2 minutes
Peak effect:
 Capsule, extended release: 3-6 hours
 Tablet: 1-4 hours
 I.V.: 15 minutes
Duration:
 Capsule, extended release: 18-24 hours
 Tablet: 8-12 hours
 I.V.: 4-5 hours

Pharmacokinetics

Distribution: Into erythrocytes, kidneys, and breast milk (breast milk to plasma ratio of 0.25 has been reported); crosses the blood-brain barrier and the placenta;
Protein binding: 95%
Half-life: 2.4-5.8 hours
Elimination: 70% to 100% of an I.V. or tablet dose and 47% of an extended release capsule excreted unchanged in urine within 24 hours

Usual Dosage

Neonates and Infants: Hydrocephalus: To slow the progression of hydrocephalus in neonates and infants who may not be good candidates for surgery, acetazolamide I.V. or oral doses of 5 mg/kg/dose every 6 hours increased by 25 mg/kg/day to a maximum of 100 mg/kg/day, if tolerated, have been used. Furosemide was used in combination with acetazolamide.

Children:
 Glaucoma:
  Oral: 8-30 mg/kg/day or 300-900 mg/m^2/day divided every 8 hours
  I.V.: 20-40 mg/kg/day divided every 6 hours, not to exceed 1 g/day
 Edema: Oral, I.V.: 5 mg/kg/dose or 150 mg/m^2/dose once daily
 Epilepsy: Oral: 8-30 mg/kg/day in 1-4 divided doses, not to exceed 1 g/day; **extended release capsule is not recommended for treatment of epilepsy**

Adults:
 Glaucoma:
  Chronic simple (open-angle): Oral: 250 mg 1-4 times/day or 500 mg sustained release capsule twice daily
  Secondary, acute (closed-angle): I.V.: 250-500 mg, may repeat in 2-4 hours to a maximum of 1 g/day
 Edema: Oral, I.V.: 250-375 mg/day
 Epilepsy: Oral: 8-30 mg/kg/day in 1-4 divided doses, not to exceed 1 g/day; **extended release capsule is not recommended for treatment of epilepsy**
 Altitude sickness: Oral: 250 mg every 8-12 hours or 500 mg extended release capsules every 12-24 hours; therapy should begin 24-48 hours before and continued during ascent and for at least 48 hours after arrival at the high altitude
 Urine alkalinization: Oral: 5 mg/kg/dose repeated 2-3 times over 24 hours

Dosing interval in renal impairment: Children and Adults:
 Cl$_{cr}$ 10-50 mL/minute: Administer every 12 hours
 Cl$_{cr}$ <10 mL/minute: Avoid use

Administration

Oral: Administer with food to decrease GI upset; tablet may be crushed and suspended in cherry or chocolate syrup to disguise the bitter taste of the drug (See Extemporaneous Preparations)

Parenteral:

I.V.: Reconstitute with at least 5 mL sterile water to provide a solution containing not more than 100 mg/mL; maximum concentration: 100 mg/mL; maximum rate of I.V. infusion: 500 mg/minute

I.M.: I.M. administration is not generally recommended as the drug's alkaline pH makes it very painful

Monitoring Parameters Serum electrolytes, periodic hematologic determinations

Test Interactions May cause false-positive results for urinary protein with Albustix®, Labstix®, Albutest®, Bumintest®

Patient Information Do not crush or chew long-acting capsule

Additional Information Sodium content of 500 mg injection: 2.049 mEq

Extended release capsules are indicated only for use for the adjunctive treatment of open-angle or secondary glaucoma and the prevention of high altitude sickness; avoid using extended release capsules for anticonvulsant or diuretic therapy

Dosage Forms

Capsule, sustained release: 500 mg

Injection: 500 mg/5 mL

Tablet: 125 mg, 250 mg

Extemporaneous Preparations A 25 mg/mL suspension may be made by crushing tablets and mixing with either a 1:4 cherry syrup concentrate:simple syrup mixture or a 1:1 mixture of Ora-Sweet® and Ora-Plus® or a 1:1 mixture of Ora-Sweet® SF and Ora-Plus®. The resulting suspension is stable for 60 days at room temperature or refrigerated.

Allen LV and Erickson MA, "Stability of Acetazolamide, Allopurinol, Azathioprine, Clonazepam, and Flucytosine in Extemporaneously Compounded Oral Liquids," *Am J Health Sys Pharm*, 1996, 53:1944-9.

References

Shinnar S, Gammon K, Bergman EW Jr, et al, "Management of Hydrocephalus in Infancy: Use of Acetazolamide and Furosemide to Avoid Cerebrospinal Fluid Shunts," *J Pediatr*, 1985, 107(1):31-7.

♦ **Acetoxyl® (Canada)** *see* Benzoyl Peroxide *on page 126*

♦ **Acetoxymethylprogesterone** *see* Medroxyprogesterone *on page 599*

Acetylcholine (a se teel KOE leen)

Brand Names Miochol-E®

Available Salts Acetylcholine Chloride

Therapeutic Category Cholinergic Agent, Ophthalmic; Ophthalmic Agent, Miotic

Generic Available No

Use Produces complete miosis in cataract surgery, keratoplasty, iridectomy and other anterior segment surgery where rapid miosis is required

Pregnancy Risk Factor C

Contraindications Hypersensitivity to acetylcholine chloride or any component; acute iritis and acute inflammatory disease of the anterior chamber

Warnings Open under aseptic conditions only

Precautions Systemic effects rarely occur, but can cause problems for patients with acute CHF, bronchial asthma, peptic ulcer, hyperthyroidism, GI spasm, and urinary tract obstruction

Adverse Reactions

Cardiovascular: Transient bradycardia and hypotension

Central nervous system: Headache

Ocular: Iris atrophy, temporary lens opacities (attributed to osmotic effect of 5% mannitol present in preparation)

Respiratory: Dyspnea

Miscellaneous: Diaphoresis

Drug Interactions Flurbiprofen decreases effectiveness; sodium nitrate antagonizes acetylcholine's effects

Stability Prepare solution immediately before use; do not use solution which is not clear and colorless

Mechanism of Action Causes contraction of the sphincter muscles of the iris, resulting in miosis and contraction of the ciliary muscle, leading to accommodation

Pharmacodynamics

Onset of action: Miosis occurs promptly

Duration: ~10-20 minutes

(Continued)

Acetylcholine *(Continued)*

Usual Dosage Adults: 0.5-2 mL of 1% injection (5-20 mg)

Administration Ophthalmic: Instill into anterior chamber before or after securing one or more sutures; instillation should be gentle and parallel to the iris face and tangential to the pupil border; in cataract surgery, acetylcholine should be used only after delivery of the lens

Dosage Forms Powder, intraocular, as chloride: 1% 1:100 [10 mg/mL] (2 mL, 15 mL)

♦ **Acetylcholine Chloride** *see Acetylcholine on page 31*

Acetylcysteine *(a se teel SIS teen)*

Brand Names Mucomyst®; Mucosil™; Parvolex® (Canada)

Available Salts Acetylcysteine Sodium

Synonyms *N*-Acetylcysteine; *N*-Acetyl-L-Cysteine

Therapeutic Category Antidote, Acetaminophen; Mucolytic Agent

Generic Available Yes

Use Adjunctive therapy in patients with abnormal or viscid mucous secretions in bronchopulmonary diseases, pulmonary complications of surgery, and cystic fibrosis; diagnostic bronchial studies; antidote for acute acetaminophen toxicity; enema to treat bowel obstruction due to meconium ileus or its equivalent

Pregnancy Risk Factor B

Contraindications Hypersensitivity to acetylcysteine or any component

Warnings Since increased bronchial secretions may develop after inhalation, percussion, postural drainage and suctioning should follow

Precautions If bronchospasm occurs, administer a bronchodilator; discontinue acetylcysteine if bronchospasm progresses

Adverse Reactions
Cardiovascular: Tachycardia, hypotension, hypertension (after large oral doses)
Central nervous system: Drowsiness, chills
Dermatologic: Generalized urticaria, rash
Gastrointestinal: Stomatitis, nausea, vomiting, hemoptysis
Hepatic: Mild increases in liver function tests have occurred after oral therapy
Respiratory: Bronchospasm, rhinorrhea
Miscellaneous: Unpleasant odor during administration

Drug Interactions May potentiate the effects of nitrates; adsorbed by activated charcoal

Stability Store opened vials in the refrigerator; use within 96 hours; contact with rubber, copper, iron, and cork may inactivate the drug; the light purple color of solution does **not** affect its activity

Mechanism of Action Exerts mucolytic action through its free sulfhydryl group which opens up the disulfide bonds in the mucoproteins thus lowering the viscosity. The exact mechanism of action in acetaminophen toxicity is unknown. It may act by maintaining or restoring glutathione levels or by acting as an alternative substrate for conjugation with the toxic metabolite.

Pharmacodynamics
Onset of action: Upon inhalation, mucus liquefaction occurs maximally within 5-10 minutes
Duration of mucus liquefaction: More than 1 hour

Pharmacokinetics
Protein binding: ~50%
Half-life:
  Reduced acetylcysteine: 2 hours
  Total acetylcysteine: 5.5 hours
Time to peak serum concentration: 1-2 hours

Usual Dosage
Acetaminophen poisoning: Children and Adults: Oral: 140 mg/kg; followed by 17 doses of 70 mg/kg every 4 hours; repeat dose if emesis occurs within 1 hour of administration; therapy should continue until all doses are administered even though the acetaminophen plasma level has dropped below the toxic range
Inhalation:
  Infants: 1-2 mL of 20% solution or 2-4 mL of 10% solution until nebulized, given 3-4 times/day
  Children: 3-5 mL of 20% solution or 6-10 mL of 10% solution until nebulized, given 3-4 times/day
  Adolescents: 5-10 mL of 10% to 20% solution until nebulized, given 3-4 times/day

Note: Patients should receive an aerosolized bronchodilator 10-15 minutes prior to acetylcysteine

Intratracheal: Children and Adults: 1-2 mL of 10% to 20% solution every 1-4 hours as needed

Meconium ileus equivalent: Children and Adults (varying regimens have been reported): Oral, Rectal Irrigation: 5-30 mL of 10% to 20% solution 3-6 times/day for at least 24 hours and symptom improvement

Administration
Oral: For treatment of acetaminophen overdosage, administer as a 5% solution; dilute the 20% solution 1:3 with a cola, orange juice, or other soft drink; use within 1 hour of preparation

Oral inhalation: May be administered either undiluted (both 10% and 20%) or diluted in NS

Monitoring Parameters When used in acetaminophen overdose, determine acetaminophen level as soon as possible, but no sooner than 4 hours after ingestion (to ensure peak levels have been obtained); liver function tests

Patient Information Clear airway by coughing deeply before aerosol treatment

Nursing Implications Assess patient for nausea, vomiting, and skin rash following oral administration for treatment of acetaminophen poisoning; intermittent aerosol treatments are commonly given when patient arises, before meals, and just before retiring at bedtime

Additional Information I.V. route is investigational in the U.S.; contact a poison control center for more information

Dosage Forms Solution, as sodium: 10% [100 mg/mL] (4 mL, 10 mL, 30 mL); 20% [200 mg/mL] (4 mL, 10 mL, 30 mL, 100 mL)

References
Hanly JG and Fitzgerald MX, "Meconium Ileus Equivalent in Older Patients With Cystic Fibrosis," *Br Med J (Clin Res Ed)*, 1983, 286(6375):1411-3.

Walson PD and Groth JF Jr, "Acetaminophen Hepatotoxicity After Prolonged Ingestion," *Pediatrics*, 1993, 91(5):1021-2.

♦ **Acetylcysteine Sodium** *see* Acetylcysteine *on page 32*
♦ **Acetylsalicylic Acid** *see* Aspirin *on page 99*
♦ **Aches-N-Pain® [OTC]** *see* Ibuprofen *on page 501*
♦ **Achromycin® Ophthalmic** *see* Tetracycline *on page 908*
♦ **Achromycin® Topical** *see* Tetracycline *on page 908*
♦ **Achromycin® V Oral** *see* Tetracycline *on page 908*
♦ **Aciclovir** *see* Acyclovir *on page 34*
♦ **Acid Mantle® [OTC]** *see* Aluminum Acetate *on page 53*
♦ **Acidulated Phosphate Fluoride** *see* Fluoride *on page 427*
♦ **Acilac (Canada)** *see* Lactulose *on page 550*
♦ **Acnex® (Canada)** *see* Salicylic Acid *on page 854*
♦ **Acnomel® B.P.5 (Canada)** *see* Benzoyl Peroxide *on page 126*
♦ **Acnomel® (Canada)** *see* Salicylic Acid *on page 854*
♦ **ACRobafen® AC** *see* Guaifenesin and Codeine *on page 465*
♦ **ACT** *see* Dactinomycin *on page 281*
♦ **ACT® [OTC]** *see* Fluoride *on page 427*
♦ **Actagen® [OTC]** *see* Triprolidine and Pseudoephedrine *on page 957*
♦ **Act-D** *see* Dactinomycin *on page 281*
♦ **ACTH** *see* Corticotropin *on page 254*
♦ **Acticort® Topical** *see* Hydrocortisone *on page 486*
♦ **Actidose-Aqua® [OTC]** *see* Charcoal *on page 202*
♦ **Actidose® With Sorbitol [OTC]** *see* Charcoal *on page 202*
♦ **Actifed® [OTC]** *see* Triprolidine and Pseudoephedrine *on page 957*
♦ **Actifed® Allergy Tablet (Day) [OTC]** *see* Pseudoephedrine *on page 822*
♦ **Actigall™** *see* Ursodiol *on page 965*
♦ **Actinomycin D** *see* Dactinomycin *on page 281*
♦ **Actiprofen® (Canada)** *see* Ibuprofen *on page 501*
♦ **Actiq®** *see* Fentanyl *on page 406*
♦ **Activated Carbon** *see* Charcoal *on page 202*
♦ **Activated Charcoal** *see* Charcoal *on page 202*
♦ **Activated Dimethicone** *see* Simethicone *on page 868*
♦ **Activated Ergosterol** *see* Ergocalciferol *on page 377*
♦ **Activated Methylpolysiloxane** *see* Simethicone *on page 868*
♦ **Acular® Ophthalmic** *see* Ketorolac *on page 544*

- ◆ **Acutrim® Precision Release® [OTC]** *see* Phenylpropanolamine *on page 761*
- ◆ **ACV** *see* Acyclovir *on page 34*
- ◆ **Acycloguanosine** *see* Acyclovir *on page 34*

Acyclovir (ay SYE kloe veer)
Related Information
Carbohydrate and Alcohol Content of Liquid Medications for Use in Patients Receiving Ketogenic Diets *on page 1228*
Brand Names Avirax™ (Canada); Zovirax®
Synonyms Aciclovir; ACV; Acycloguanosine
Therapeutic Category Antiviral Agent, Oral; Antiviral Agent, Parenteral; Antiviral Agent, Topical
Generic Available Yes; Capsule
Use Treatment of initial and prophylaxis of recurrent mucosal and cutaneous herpes simplex (HSV 1 and HSV 2) infections; herpes simplex encephalitis; herpes zoster infections; varicella-zoster infections in healthy, nonpregnant persons >13 years of age, children >12 months of age who have a chronic skin or lung disorder or are receiving long-term aspirin therapy, and immunocompromised patients
Pregnancy Risk Factor C
Contraindications Hypersensitivity to acyclovir, valacyclovir, or any component
Warnings HSV and VZV with reduced susceptibility to acyclovir have been isolated from immunocompromised patients, especially with advanced HIV infection; renal failure, in some cases resulting in death, has occurred with acyclovir
Precautions Use with caution in patients with renal disease, dehydration, underlying neurologic disease, and in patients with hypoxia, hepatic, or electrolyte abnormalities; dosage should be reduced in patients with renal impairment
Adverse Reactions
Central nervous system: Headache, lethargy, delirium, coma, dizziness, seizures, pain, insomnia, fever, hallucinations
Dermatologic: Skin rash, pruritus, alopecia, erythema multiforme, urticaria, photosensitivity, Stevens-Johnson syndrome
Gastrointestinal: Nausea, vomiting, diarrhea
Hematologic: Bone marrow suppression, thrombotic thrombocytopenic purpura/hemolytic uremic syndrome
Hepatic: Elevated liver enzymes, hepatitis, jaundice
Local: Phlebitis at injection site, local pain and stinging with topical use
Neuromuscular & skeletal: Tremulousness, myalgia, paresthesia
Renal: Nephrotoxicity, hematuria, elevated BUN and serum creatinine
Respiratory: Sore throat
Miscellaneous: Diaphoresis, anaphylaxis
Drug Interactions Zidovudine (neurotoxicity); probenecid decreases renal clearance of acyclovir
Food Interactions Food does not appear to affect absorption
Stability Incompatible with blood products and protein-containing solutions; reconstituted 50 mg/mL solution should be used within 12 hours; do not refrigerate reconstituted solutions as they may precipitate
Mechanism of Action Inhibits DNA synthesis and viral replication by competing with deoxyguanosine triphosphate for viral DNA polymerase and by incorporation into viral DNA
Pharmacokinetics
Absorption: Oral: 15% to 30%
Distribution: Widely distributed throughout the body including brain, kidney, lungs, liver, spleen, muscle, uterus, vagina, and the CSF; CSF acyclovir concentration is 50% of serum concentration; crosses the placenta; excreted into breast milk; V_d:
Neonates to 3 months of age: 28.8 L/1.73 m^2
Children 1-2 years: 31.6 L/1.73 m^2
Children 2-7 years: 42 L/1.73 m^2
Protein binding: <30%
Half-life, terminal phase:
Neonates: 4 hours
Children 1-12 years: 2-3 hours
Adults: 2-3.5 hours (with normal renal function)
Time to peak serum concentration: Oral: Within 1.5-2 hours
Elimination: Primary route is the kidney with 30% to 90% of a dose excreted unchanged in the urine; requires dosage adjustment with renal impairment; hemodialysis removes ~60% of a dose while removal by peritoneal dialysis is to a much lesser extent; supplemental dose recommended after hemodialysis

Usual Dosage

Children and Adults: Oral:

Genital herpes simplex virus (HSV), first infection: 1000 mg/day in 5 divided doses **or** 1200 mg/day in 3 divided doses for 7-10 days; maximum dose in children: 80 mg/kg/day in 3-5 divided doses

Genital HSV infection recurrence: 1000 mg/day in 5 divided doses **or** 1200 mg/day in 3 divided doses or 1600 mg/day in 2 divided doses for 5 days; maximum dose in children: 80 mg/kg/day in 2-5 divided doses

Recurrent genital HSV: Chronic suppressive therapy for frequent recurrences: 800-1000 mg/day in 2-5 divided doses; maximum dose in children: 80 mg/kg/day in 2-5 divided doses

HSV in immunocompromised host: 1000 mg/day in 3-5 divided doses for 7-14 days; maximum dose in children: 80 mg/kg/day in 3-5 divided doses

Prophylaxis of HSV in immunocompromised HSV-seropositive patient: 600-1000 mg/day in 3-5 divided doses during risk period; maximum dose in children: 80 mg/kg/day in 3-5 divided doses

Zoster in immunocompetent host: 4000 mg/day in 5 divided doses for 5-7 days; maximum dose in children: 80 mg/kg/day in 5 divided doses

Herpes zoster in immunocompromised patients:

Children: 250-600 mg/m^2/dose 4-5 times/day

Adults: 800 mg every 4 hours (5 times/day) for 7-10 days; prophylaxis: 400 mg 5 times/day

Varicella zoster (chickenpox) in immunocompetent host: 80 mg/kg/day in 4 divided doses for 5 days; maximum daily dose: 3200 mg/day; start treatment within the first 24 hours of rash onset

Prophylaxis of CMV infection in immunocompromised host: 800-3200 mg/day in 1-4 divided doses during risk period; maximum dose in children: 80 mg/kg/day in 3-4 divided doses

Premature neonates: HSV infection: I.V.: 20 mg/kg/day divided every 12 hours for 14-21 days

Neonates: HSV infection: I.V.: 1500 mg/m^2/day divided every 8 hours **or** 30 mg/kg/day divided every 8 hours for 14-21 days. Doses as high as 45-60 mg/kg/day divided every 8 hours have been used in term infants with normal renal function.

Children and Adults: I.V. (dosage for obese patients should be based on ideal body weight):

HSV infection: 750 mg/m^2/day divided every 8 hours **or** 15 mg/kg/day divided every 8 hours for 5-7 days

HSV in immunocompromised host:

Children <1 year: 15-30 mg/kg/day divided every 8 hours for 7-14 days

Children ≥1 year: 750-1500 mg/m^2/day divided every 8 hours or 15-30 mg/kg/day divided every 8 hours for 7-14 days

Prophylaxis of HSV in immunocompromised HSV-seropositive patients: 750 mg/m^2/day divided every 8 hours during risk period

HSV encephalitis: 1500 mg/m^2/day divided every 8 hours **or** 30 mg/kg/day divided every 8 hours for 14-21 days

Varicella or zoster in immunocompromised host or zoster in immunocompetent host:

Children <1 year (some experts also recommend this dose for children ≥1 year): 30 mg/kg/day divided every 8 hours for 7-10 days

Children ≥1 year: 1500 mg/m^2/day divided every 8 hours or 30 mg/kg/day divided every 8 hours for 7-10 days

Prophylaxis of CMV infection in immunocompromised host: 1500 mg/m^2/day divided every 8 hours during risk period

Prophylaxis of bone marrow transplant recipients:

Autologous patients who are HSV-seropositive: 250 mg/m^2/dose every 8 hours

Autologous patients who are CMV seropositive: 500 mg/m^2/dose every 8 hours; for clinically symptomatic CMV infection, consider replacing acyclovir with ganciclovir

Children and Adults: Topical: Apply ½" ribbon of ointment for a 4" square surface area every 3 hours (6 times/day) for 7 days

Dosing interval in renal impairment: Children ≥6 months and Adults:

Oral:

Usual Dose	Creatinine Clearance	Adjusted Dose
200 mg 5 times/day	Cl$_{cr}$ <10 mL/minute	Administer 200 mg q12h
800 mg 5 times/day	Cl$_{cr}$ 10-25 mL/minute	Administer 800 mg q8h
800 mg 5 times/day	Cl$_{cr}$ <10 mL/minute	Administer 800 mg q12h

(Continued)

Acyclovir *(Continued)*

I.V.:
Cl_{cr} 25-50 mL/minute: Administer normal dose every 12 hours
Cl_{cr} 10-25 mL/minute: Administer normal dose every 24 hours
Cl_{cr} <10 mL/minute: 50% decrease in dose, administer every 24 hours

Administration
Oral: May administer with food; shake suspension well before use
Parenteral: Reconstitute vial for injection with paraben-free sterile water; administer by slow I.V. infusion over at least 1 hour at a final concentration not to exceed 7 mg/mL since rapid infusions can cause nephrotoxicity with crystalluria and renal tubular damage; in patients who require fluid restriction, a concentration of up to 10 mg/mL has been infused; concentration >10 mg/mL increases the risk of phlebitis

Monitoring Parameters Urinalysis, BUN, serum creatinine, I & O; liver enzymes, CBC

Nursing Implications Maintain adequate hydration and urine output the first 2 hours after I.V. infusion to decrease the risk of nephrotoxicity; check infusion site for phlebitis

Additional Information Sodium content of 1 g: 4.2 mEq

Dosage Forms
Capsule: 200 mg
Injection: 500 mg (10 mL); 1000 mg (20 mL)
Ointment, topical: 5% (3 g, 15 g)
Suspension, oral (banana flavor): 200 mg/5 mL (473 mL)
Tablet: 400 mg, 800 mg

References
American Academy of Pediatrics Committee on Infectious Diseases, "The Use of Oral Acyclovir in Otherwise Healthy Children With Varicella," *Pediatrics*, 1993, 91(3):674-6.
Dunkle LM, Arvin AM, Whitley RJ, et al, "A Controlled Trial of Acyclovir for Chickenpox in Normal Children," *N Engl J Med*, 1991, 325(22):1539-44.
Englund JA, Fletcher CV, and Balfour HH Jr, "Acyclovir Therapy in Neonates," *J Pediatr*, 1991, 119(1 Pt 1):129-35.
Meyers JD, Reed EC, Shepp DH, et al, "Acyclovir for Prevention of Cytomegalovirus Infection and Disease After Allogenic Marrow Transplantation," *N Engl J Med*, 1988, 318(2):70-5.
Novelli VM, Marshall WC, Yeo J, et al, "High-Dose Oral Acyclovir for Children at Risk of Disseminated Herpes Virus Infections," *J Infect Dis*, 1985, 151(2):372.

♦ **Adalat®** *see* Nifedipine *on page 687*
♦ **Adalat® CC** *see* Nifedipine *on page 687*
♦ **Adalat PA® (Canada)** *see* Nifedipine *on page 687*
♦ **Adamantanamine** *see* Amantadine *on page 53*
♦ **Adapin® Oral** *see* Doxepin *on page 345*
♦ **Adderall®** *see* Dextroamphetamine and Amphetamine *on page 302*
♦ **Adek®** *see page 1034*
♦ **Adenine Arabinoside** *see* Vidarabine *on page 977*
♦ **Adenocard®** *see* Adenosine *on page 36*

Adenosine *(a DEN oh seen)*

Related Information
Adult ACLS Algorithm, Tachycardia *on page 1010*

Brand Names Adenocard®

Synonyms 9-Beta-D-ribofuranosyladenine

Therapeutic Category Antiarrhythmic Agent, Miscellaneous

Generic Available No

Use Treatment of paroxysmal supraventricular tachycardia (PSVT); investigationally used as a continuous infusion for the treatment of primary pulmonary hypertension in adults and persistent pulmonary hypertension of the newborn (see Konduri, 1996)

Pregnancy Risk Factor C

Contraindications Hypersensitivity to adenosine or any component; second and third degree A-V block or sick sinus syndrome unless pacemaker placed

Warnings Heart block, including transient or prolonged asystole may occur as well as other arrhythmias; episodes of asystole or other arrhythmias may be fatal; if arrhythmia is not due to re-entry pathway through A-V node or sinus node (ie, atrial fibrillation, flutter, or tachycardia or ventricular tachycardia), adenosine will not terminate the arrhythmia but can produce transient ventriculoatrial or A-V block; possible mutagenic effects

Precautions Bronchoconstriction may occur in asthmatics (avoid use in patients with bronchospasm or bronchoconstriction); use with caution in patients with underlying dysfunction of sinus or A-V node, obstructive lung disease, and those taking digoxin or verapamil; initial adenosine dose should be significantly decreased in patients receiving dipyridamole

Adverse Reactions
Cardiovascular: Flushing, arrhythmias, palpitations, chest pain, bradycardia, heart block, minimal hemodynamic disturbances, hypotension (<1%)
Central nervous system: Irritability, headaches, lightheadedness, dizziness
Gastrointestinal: Nausea, metallic taste
Respiratory: Dyspnea, hyperventilation, bronchoconstriction in asthmatics

Drug Interactions Dipyridamole potentiates effects of adenosine (dose of adenosine should be significantly reduced); methylxanthines (aminophylline, theophylline, caffeine) antagonize adenosine's effects so that larger doses of adenosine or an alternative agent may be required; carbamazepine may increase heart block; digoxin and verapamil may cause ventricular fibrillation (rare cases reported)

Stability Do **not** refrigerate, precipitation may occur; contains no preservatives, discard unused portion

Mechanism of Action Slows conduction time through the A-V node, interrupting the re-entry pathways through the A-V node, restoring normal sinus rhythm

Pharmacodynamics
Onset of action: Rapid
Duration: Very brief

Pharmacokinetics
Metabolism: Removed from systemic circulation primarily by vascular endothelial cells and erythrocytes (by cellular uptake); rapidly metabolized intracellularly; phosphorylated by adenosine kinase to adenosine monophosphate (AMP) which is then incorporated into high-energy pool; intracellular adenosine is also deaminated by adenosine deaminase to inosine; inosine can be metabolized to hypoxanthine, then xanthine and finally to uric acid.
Half-life: <10 seconds

Usual Dosage Rapid I.V. (via **peripheral line**):
Note: Adequate controlled studies in pediatric patients have not been conducted.
Manufacturer's recommendations:
Neonates, Infants, Children, and Adolescents weighing <50 kg: Initial dose: 0.05-0.1 mg/kg; if not effective within 1-2 minutes, increase dose by 0.05-0.1 mg/kg increments every 1-2 minutes to a maximum single dose of 0.3 mg/kg or until termination of PSVT
Children and Adolescents weighing ≥50 kg and Adults: 6 mg, if not effective within 1-2 minutes, 12 mg may be given; may repeat 12 mg bolus if needed

Alternative pediatric dosing:
Neonates: Initial dose: 0.05 mg/kg; if not effective within 2 minutes, increase dose by 0.05 mg/kg increments every 2 minutes to a maximum dose of 0.25 mg/kg or until termination of PSVT; do not exceed 12 mg/dose
Infants and Children: PALS dose for treatment of SVT: 0.1 mg/kg; if not effective, give 0.2 mg/kg; maximum single dose: 12 mg
Alternatively: Initial dose: 0.05 mg/kg; if not effective within 2 minutes, increase dose by 0.05 mg/kg increments every 2 minutes to a maximum dose of 0.25 mg/kg or until termination of PSVT; median dose required: 0.15 mg/kg; do not exceed 12 mg/dose

Administration Parenteral: For rapid bolus I.V. use only, administer over 1-2 seconds at peripheral I.V. site closest to patient; follow each bolus with NS flush; to administer doses <600 mcg (0.2 mL of commercial product), a dilution with NS (final concentration: 300 mcg/mL) may be made. **Note:** Preliminary results in adults suggest adenosine may be administered via a **central line** at lower doses (eg, Adults: Initial dose: 3 mg); FDA approved labeling for pediatric patients weighing <50 kg states that doses listed may be administered either peripherally or centrally (further studies are needed)

Monitoring Parameters Continuous EKG, heart rate, blood pressure, respirations

Nursing Implications Be alert for dyspnea, shortness of breath, and possible exacerbation of asthma

Additional Information Not effective in atrial flutter, atrial fibrillation, or ventricular tachycardia; short action an advantage as adverse effects are usually rapidly self-limiting. Individualize treatment of prolonged adverse effects: Give I.V. fluids for hypotension, aminophylline/theophylline may antagonize effects.

Dosage Forms Injection, preservative free: 3 mg/mL (2 mL, 5 mL)

References
Emergency Cardiac Care Committee and Subcommittees, American Heart Association, "Guidelines for Cardiopulmonary Resuscitation and Emergency Cardiac Care, III: Adult Advanced Cardiac Life Support" and "VI: Pediatric Advanced Life Support," *JAMA*, 1992, 268(16):2199-241 and 2262-75.
(Continued)

Adenosine *(Continued)*

Eubanks AP and Artman M, "Administration of Adenosine to a Newborn of 26 Weeks' Gestation," *Pediatr Cardiol*, 1994, 15(3):157-8.

Konduri GG, Garcia DC, Kazzi NJ, et al, "Adenosine Infusion Improves Oxygenation in Term Infants With Respiratory Failure," *Pediatrics*, 1996, 97(3):295-300.

McIntosh-Yellin NL, Drew BJ, and Scheinman MM, "Safety and Efficacy of Central Intravenous Bolus Administration of Adenosine for Termination of Supraventricular Tachycardia," *J Am Coll Cardiol*, 1993, 22(3):741-5.

Till J, Shinebourne EA, Rigby ML, et al, "Efficacy and Safety in the Treatment of Supraventricular Tachycardia in Infants and Children," *Br Heart J*, 1989, 62(3):204-11.

Zeigler V, "Adenosine in the Pediatric Population: Nursing Implications," *Pediatr Nurs*, 1991, 17(6):600-2.

- ◆ **ADH** *see* Vasopressin *on page 971*
- ◆ **Adlone® Injection** *see* Methylprednisolone *on page 629*
- ◆ **ADR** *see* Doxorubicin *on page 346*
- ◆ **Adrenalin® Chloride** *see* Epinephrine *on page 371*
- ◆ **Adrenaline** *see* Epinephrine *on page 371*
- ◆ **Adrenocorticotropic Hormone** *see* Corticotropin *on page 254*
- ◆ **Adriamycin PFS™** *see* Doxorubicin *on page 346*
- ◆ **Adriamycin RDF™** *see* Doxorubicin *on page 346*
- ◆ **Adrucil® Injection** *see* Fluorouracil *on page 430*
- ◆ **Adsorbent Charcoal** *see* Charcoal *on page 202*
- ◆ **Adsorbocarpine® Ophthalmic** *see* Pilocarpine *on page 770*
- ◆ **Adsorbonac® Ophthalmic [OTC]** *see* Sodium Chloride *on page 871*
- ◆ **Adult ACLS Algorithm, Asystole** *see page 1008*
- ◆ **Adult ACLS Algorithm, Bradycardia** *see page 1012*
- ◆ **Adult ACLS Algorithm, Electrical Conversion** *see page 1014*
- ◆ **Adult ACLS Algorithm, Hypotension, Shock** *see page 1016*
- ◆ **Adult ACLS Algorithm, Pulseless Electrical Activity** *see page 1006*
- ◆ **Adult ACLS Algorithm, Tachycardia** *see page 1010*
- ◆ **Adult ACLS Algorithm, V. Fib and Pulseless V. Tach** *see page 1004*
- ◆ **Adult and Adolescent HIV** *see page 1133*
- ◆ **Advanced Formula Oxy® Sensitive Gel [OTC]** *see* Benzoyl Peroxide *on page 126*
- ◆ **Advil® [OTC]** *see* Ibuprofen *on page 501*
- ◆ **Advil® Migraine Liqui-Gels** *see* Ibuprofen *on page 501*
- ◆ **AeroBid®-M Oral Aerosol Inhaler** *see* Flunisolide *on page 423*
- ◆ **AeroBid® Oral Aerosol Inhaler** *see* Flunisolide *on page 423*
- ◆ **Aerolate III®** *see* Theophylline *on page 910*
- ◆ **Aerolate JR®** *see* Theophylline *on page 910*
- ◆ **Aerolate SR® S** *see* Theophylline *on page 910*
- ◆ **Aeroseb-Dex® Topical Aerosol** *see* Dexamethasone *on page 294*
- ◆ **Aeroseb-HC® Topical** *see* Hydrocortisone *on page 486*
- ◆ **Aerosporin® Injection** *see* Polymyxin B *on page 782*
- ◆ **AF® (Canada)** *see* Acetaminophen *on page 26*
- ◆ **Afrin® Allergy Nasal Spray** *see* Phenylephrine *on page 758*
- ◆ **Afrin® Children's Nose Drops [OTC]** *see* Oxymetazoline *on page 718*
- ◆ **Afrin® Nasal Decongestant Children's Pump Mist** *see* Phenylephrine *on page 758*
- ◆ **Afrin® Nasal Solution [OTC]** *see* Oxymetazoline *on page 718*
- ◆ **Afrinol® [OTC]** *see* Pseudoephedrine *on page 822*
- ◆ **Afrin® Saline Mist [OTC]** *see* Sodium Chloride *on page 871*
- ◆ **Aftate® [OTC]** *see* Tolnaftate *on page 936*
- ◆ **Agenerase®** *see* Amprenavir *on page 82*
- ◆ **Agoral® Plain [OTC]** *see* Mineral Oil *on page 649*
- ◆ **AHD 2000®** *see* Ethyl Alcohol *on page 394*
- ◆ **AHF** *see* Antihemophilic Factor (Human) *on page 89*
- ◆ **AHG** *see* Antihemophilic Factor (Human) *on page 89*
- ◆ **A-hydroCort® Injection** *see* Hydrocortisone *on page 486*
- ◆ **Airet®** *see* Albuterol *on page 40*
- ◆ **Akarpine® Ophthalmic** *see* Pilocarpine *on page 770*
- ◆ **AKBeta® Ophthalmic** *see* Levobunolol *on page 564*
- ◆ **AK-Chlor® Ophthalmic** *see* Chloramphenicol *on page 207*

♦ **AK-Con® Ophthalmic** *see* Naphazoline *on page 671*

♦ **AK-Dex® Ophthalmic** *see* Dexamethasone *on page 294*

♦ **AK-Dilate® Ophthalmic Solution** *see* Phenylephrine *on page 758*

♦ **AK-Homatropine®** *see* Homatropine *on page 477*

♦ **AK-Mycin®** *see* Erythromycin *on page 379*

♦ **AK-NaCl® [OTC]** *see* Sodium Chloride *on page 871*

♦ **AK-Nefrin® Ophthalmic Solution** *see* Phenylephrine *on page 758*

♦ **Akne-Mycin®** *see* Erythromycin *on page 379*

♦ **AK-Pentolate®** *see* Cyclopentolate *on page 266*

♦ **AK-Poly-Bac® Ophthalmic** *see* Bacitracin and Polymyxin B *on page 119*

♦ **AK-Pred® Ophthalmic** *see* Prednisolone *on page 791*

♦ **AK-Spore H.C.® Otic** *see* Neomycin, (Bacitracin) Polymyxin B, and Hydrocortisone *on page 679*

♦ **AK-Spore® Ophthalmic Ointment** *see* Neomycin, Polymyxin B, and Bacitracin *on page 680*

♦ **AK-Sulf®** *see* Sulfacetamide *on page 888*

♦ **AK-Taine®** *see* Proparacaine *on page 811*

♦ **AKTob® Ophthalmic** *see* Tobramycin *on page 931*

♦ **AK-Tracin® Ophthalmic** *see* Bacitracin *on page 117*

♦ **AK-Trol® Ophthalmic** *see* Dexamethasone, Neomycin, and Polymyxin B *on page 297*

♦ **Ala-Cort® Topical** *see* Hydrocortisone *on page 486*

♦ **Ala-Scalp® Topical** *see* Hydrocortisone *on page 486*

♦ **Alazide®** *see* Hydrochlorothiazide and Spironolactone *on page 484*

♦ **Albalon® Liquifilm® Ophthalmic** *see* Naphazoline *on page 671*

♦ **Albert® Docusate (Canada)** *see* Docusate *on page 336*

Albumin (al BYOO min)

Related Information
CPR Pediatric Drug Dosages *on page 999*

Brand Names Albuminar®; Albumisol®; Albutein®; Buminate®; Plasbumin®

Synonyms Albumin Human; Normal Human Serum Albumin; Normal Serum Albumin (Human); Salt Poor Albumin

Therapeutic Category Blood Product Derivative; Plasma Volume Expander

Generic Available Yes

Use Treatment of hypovolemia; plasma volume expansion and maintenance of cardiac output in the treatment of certain types of shock or impending shock; hypoproteinemia resulting in generalized edema or decreased intravascular volume (eg, hypoproteinemia associated with acute nephrotic syndrome, premature neonates)

Pregnancy Risk Factor C

Contraindications Patients with severe anemia or cardiac failure; hypersensitivity to albumin or any component

Warnings Avoid 25% concentration in preterm neonates due to risk of IVH

Precautions Rapid infusion of albumin solutions may cause vascular overload. Do not administer albumin to burn patients for the first 24 hours after the burn (capillary exudation of albumin will occur); use with caution in patients with hepatic or renal failure (added protein load) and in patients who require sodium restriction; monitor for signs of hypervolemia

Due to the occasional shortage of 5% human albumin, 5% solutions may at times be prepared by diluting 25% human albumin with NS or with D_5W (if sodium load is a concern); however, **do not use sterile water** to dilute albumin solutions, as this may result in hypotonic-associated hemolysis which can be fatal

Adverse Reactions
Cardiovascular: Precipitation of CHF or pulmonary edema, hypertension, tachycardia, hypervolemia, hypotension due to hypersensitivity reaction
Central nervous system: Fever, chills
Dermatologic: Rash
Gastrointestinal: Nausea, vomiting

Stability Use within 4 hours after opening vial, do not use if turbid or contains a deposit; do not use sterile water to dilute albumin (see Precautions)

Mechanism of Action Provides increase in intravascular oncotic pressure and causes mobilization of fluids from interstitial into intravascular space

Pharmacodynamics Duration of volume expansion: ~24 hours

Pharmacokinetics Half-life: 21 days

(Continued)

39

Albumin *(Continued)*

Usual Dosage 5% should be used in hypovolemic or intravascularly depleted patients; 25% should be used in patients with fluid or sodium restrictions (eg, patients with hypoproteinemia and generalized edema). Dose depends on condition of patient. I.V.:

Hypoproteinemia: Neonates, Infants, Children: 0.5-1 g/kg/dose; may repeat every 1-2 days; see Administration

Hypovolemia:

Neonates: Usual dose: 0.5 g/kg/dose; range: 0.25-0.5 g/kg/dose

Infants and Children: 0.5-1 g/kg/dose; may repeat as needed; maximum dose: 6 g/kg/day; see Administration

Adults: 25 g; no more than 250 g should be administered within 48 hours

Administration Parenteral: I.V.: Administer through a 5-micron filter or larger, do **not** give through 0.22 micron filter; too rapid infusion may result in vascular overload

Hypoproteinemia: Infuse over 2-4 hours; for neonates, dose may be added to hyperalimentation fluid and infused over 24 hours

Hypovolemia: Rate of infusion depends on severity of hypovolemia and patient's symptoms; usually infuse dose over 30-60 minutes (faster infusion rates may be clinically necessary)

Maximum rates of I.V. infusion after initial volume replacement:

5%: 2-4 mL/minute

25%: 1 mL/minute

Monitoring Parameters Observe for signs of hypervolemia, pulmonary edema, and cardiac failure

Nursing Implications Albumin administration must be completed within 6 hours after entering container, provided that administration is begun within 4 hours of entering the container

Additional Information In certain conditions (eg, hypoproteinemia with generalized edema, nephrotic syndrome), doses of albumin may be followed with I.V. furosemide: 0.5-1 mg/kg/dose. Both 5% and 25% albumin contain 130-160 mEq of sodium/L; osmolarity: 5% albumin = 300 mOsm/L; 25% albumin = 1500 mOsm/L

Dosage Forms Injection, as human: 5% [50 mg/mL] (50 mL, 250 mL, 500 mL, 1000 mL); 25% [250 mg/mL] (10 mL, 20 mL, 50 mL, 100 mL)

♦ **Albuminar®** *see Albumin on page 39*

♦ **Albumin Human** *see Albumin on page 39*

♦ **Albumisol®** *see Albumin on page 39*

♦ **Albutein®** *see Albumin on page 39*

Albuterol *(al BYOO ter ole)*

Related Information

Asthma Guidelines *on page 1178*

Carbohydrate and Alcohol Content of Liquid Medications for Use in Patients Receiving Ketogenic Diets *on page 1228*

Brand Names Airet®; Apo®-Salvent (Canada); Novo-Salmol® (Canada); Proventil®; Proventil® HFA; Sabulin® (Canada); Ventolin®; Ventolin® Rotocaps®; Volmax®; Volmax® (Canada)

Available Salts Albuterol Sulfate

Synonyms Salbutamol

Therapeutic Category Adrenergic Agonist Agent; Antiasthmatic; Beta$_2$-Adrenergic Agonist Agent; Bronchodilator; Sympathomimetic

Generic Available Yes

Use Prevention and relief of bronchospasm in patients with reversible airway obstruction due to asthma or COPD; prevention of exercise-induced bronchospasm

Pregnancy Risk Factor C

Contraindications Hypersensitivity to albuterol, any component, or adrenergic amine

Precautions Use with caution in patients with hyperthyroidism, diabetes mellitus; cardiovascular disorders including coronary insufficiency or hypertension; excessive or prolonged use can lead to tolerance

Adverse Reactions

Cardiovascular: Tachycardia, palpitations, hypertension, chest pain

Central nervous system: Nervousness, CNS stimulation, hyperactivity and insomnia occur more frequently in younger children than adults; dizziness, lightheadedness, drowsiness, headache

Dermatologic: Angioedema, urticaria

Endocrine & metabolic: Hypokalemia

Gastrointestinal: GI upset, xerostomia, heartburn, vomiting, nausea, unusual taste, hoarseness (inhalation only)

Genitourinary: Dysuria

Neuromuscular & skeletal: Tremor, weakness, muscle cramping

Respiratory: Irritation of oropharynx, coughing, paradoxical bronchospasm (oral inhalation only)

Miscellaneous: Diaphoresis (increased)

Drug Interactions Action of albuterol is antagonized by beta-adrenergic blocking agents such as propranolol; cardiovascular effects are potentiated in patients also receiving MAO inhibitors or tricyclic antidepressants; concomitant administration of sympathomimetics may result in enhanced cardiovascular effects

Food Interactions Caffeinated beverages may increase side effects of albuterol

Stability Liquid, tablets, Rotocaps®, and oral inhalation solutions are stable at room temperature; Nebules® should be refrigerated, but may be kept at room temperature for 2 weeks; compatible with cromolyn and ipratropium nebulizer solutions

Mechanism of Action Relaxes bronchial smooth muscle by action on beta$_2$-receptors with little effect on heart rate

Pharmacodynamics

Nebulization/oral inhalation:

Peak bronchodilation: Within 0.5-2 hours nebulization

Duration: 2-5 hours

Oral:

Peak bronchodilatation: 2-3 hours

Duration: 4-6 hours

Extended release tablets: Duration: Up to 12 hours

Pharmacokinetics

Metabolism: By the liver to an inactive sulfate

Half-life:

Oral: 2.7-5 hours

Inhalation: 3.8 hours

Elimination: 30% appears in urine as unchanged drug

Usual Dosage

Oral:

Children 2-6 years: 0.1-0.2 mg/kg/dose 3 times/day; maximum dose not to exceed 4 mg 3 times/day

Children 6-12 years: 2 mg/dose 3-4 times/day; Repetabs®: 4 mg 2 times/day (maximum daily dosage: 24 mg)

Children >12 years to Adults: 2-4 mg/dose 3-4 times/day; Repetabs®: 4-8 mg 2 times/day (maximum daily dosage: 32 mg)

Inhalation: MDI: 90 mcg/spray:

Children <12 years: 1-2 inhalations 4 times/day

Children ≥12 years to Adults: 1-2 inhalations every 4-6 hours; maximum 12 inhalations/day

Exercise-induced bronchospasm: Children ≥12 years to Adults: 2 inhalations 30 minutes before exercising

Inhalation: Children and Adults: Nebulization: See dosage table; administer every 4-6 hours

Albuterol Nebulization Dosage

Age	Dose (by weight)	0.5% Solution (mL/kg)	0.083% Solution (mL/kg)
Children <12 y	0.15-0.25 mg/kg (maximum: 5 mg)*	0.01-0.05 (maximum: 1 mL)*	0.06-0.3 (maximum 6 mL)*
Children 12 y - Adults	2.5 mg	0.5 mL	3 mL

*Doses >2.5 mg have been associated with a higher frequency of adverse systemic effects.

Intensive care patients may require more frequent administration; continuous nebulized albuterol at 0.3 mg/kg/hour has been used safely in the treatment of severe status asthmaticus in children; continuous nebulized doses of 3 mg/kg/hour ± 2.2 mg/kg/hour (Katz, et al) in children whose mean age was 20.7 months resulted in no cardiotoxicity; the optimal dosage for continuous nebulization remains to be determined

Oral inhalation (Rotahaler®): Children >4 years and Adults: 200-400 mcg every 4-6 hours

(Continued)

Albuterol *(Continued)*

Administration

Inhalation: Nebulization: Using 0.5% solution, dilute dosage in 1-2 mL NS (0.083% solution does not require further dilution); adjust nebulizer flow to deliver dosage over 5-15 minutes

Oral: Administer with food; do not crush or chew extended release tablets (Repetabs® or Volmax®)

Oral inhalation: It is recommended to prime the inhaler (before first use or if it has not been used for more than 2 weeks) by releasing 4 test sprays into the air away from the face; shake well before use; use spacer for children <8 years of age

Monitoring Parameters Serum potassium, heart rate, pulmonary function tests, respiratory rate; arterial or capillary blood gases (if patient's condition warrants)

Patient Information Do not exceed recommended dosage; rinse mouth with water following each inhalation to help with dry throat and mouth; if more than one inhalation is necessary, wait at least 1 full minute between inhalations; notify physician if palpitations, tachycardia, chest pain, muscle tremors, dizziness, headache, flushing, or if breathing difficulty persists; limit caffeinated beverages

Dosage Forms

Aerosol, chlorofluorocarbon free (Proventil® HFA): 90 mcg/dose (17 g)

Aerosol, oral: 90 mcg/spray [200 inhalations] (17 g)

Capsule, microfine, for inhalation, as sulfate (Rotacaps®): 200 mcg [to be used with Rotahaler® inhalation device]

Solution, inhalation, as sulfate: 0.083% [0.83 mg/mL] (3 mL); 0.5% [5 mg/mL] (20 mL)

Nebules®: 0.083% [0.83 mg/mL] (3 mL)

Syrup, alcohol and sugar free, as sulfate (strawberry flavor): 2 mg/5 mL (480 mL)

Tablet, as sulfate: 2 mg, 4 mg

Tablet, extended release, as sulfate: Proventil®, Repetabs®: 4 mg; Volmax®: 4 mg, 8 mg

References

Katz RW, Kelly HW, Crowley MR, et al, "Safety of Continuous Nebulized Albuterol for Bronchospasm in Infants and Children," *Pediatrics*, 1993, 92(5):666-69.

O'Callaghan C, Milner AD, and Swarbrick A, "Nebulized Salbutamol Does Have a Protective Effect on Airways in Children Under One Year Old," *Arch Dis Child*, 1988, 63(5):479-83.

Papo MC, Frank J, and Thompson AE, "A Prospective, Randomized Study of Continuous Versus Intermittent Nebulized Albuterol for Severe Status Asthmaticus in Children," *Crit Care Med*, 1993, 21(10):1479-86.

Rachelefsky GS and Siegel SC, "Asthma in Infants and Children - Treatment of Childhood Asthma: Part II," *J Allergy Clin Immunol*, 1985, 76(3):409-25.

Schuh S, Parkin P, Rajan A, et al, "High- Versus Low-Dose, Frequently Administered, Nebulized Albuterol in Children With Severe, Acute Asthma," *Pediatrics*, 1989, 83(4):513-8.

Schuh S, Reider MJ, Canny G, et al, "Nebulized Albuterol in Acute Childhood Asthma: Comparison of Two Doses," *Pediatrics*, 1990, 86(4):509-13.

♦ **Albuterol Sulfate** *see* Albuterol *on page 40*

♦ **Alcaine®** *see* Proparacaine *on page 811*

♦ **Alcohol** *see* Ethyl Alcohol *on page 394*

♦ **Alconefrin® Nasal Solution [OTC]** *see* Phenylephrine *on page 758*

♦ **Aldactazide®** *see* Hydrochlorothiazide and Spironolactone *on page 484*

♦ **Aldactone®** *see* Spironolactone *on page 877*

Aldesleukin *(al des LOO kin)*

Brand Names Proleukin®

Synonyms Epidermal Thymocyte Activating Factor; ETAF; IL-2; Interleukin-2; Lymphocyte Mitogenic Factor; NSC-373364; T-Cell Growth Factor; TCGF; Thymocyte Stimulating Factor

Therapeutic Category Antineoplastic Agent, Miscellaneous; Biological Response Modulator

Generic Available No

Use Treatment of metastatic renal cell carcinoma and metastatic melanoma; for investigational use in tumors known to have a response to immunotherapy such as colorectal cancer and non-Hodgkin's lymphoma (alone or in combination with lymphokine-activated killer cells); investigational treatment of Kaposi's sarcoma in combination with zidovudine and acute myelogenous leukemia (AML)

Pregnancy Risk Factor C

Contraindications Hypersensitivity to aldesleukin or any component; abnormal thallium stress test or pulmonary function tests; organ allografts (due to increased risk of rejection); **retreatment** in patients who have experienced sustained ventricular tachycardia (≥5 beats), cardiac rhythm disturbances not controlled or unresponsive to management, recurrent chest pain with EKG changes (consistent with angina or myocardial infarction), intubation required >72 hours, pericardial tamponade; renal dysfunction requiring dialysis >72 hours, coma or toxic psychosis lasting >48 hours, repetitive or difficult to control seizures, bowel ischemia/perforation, and GI bleeding requiring surgery

Warnings High-dose aldesleukin therapy is associated with capillary leak syndrome (CLS) resulting in hypotension and reduced organ perfusion (occurring within 2-12 hours after start of treatment) which may be severe and fatal; CLS may be associated with cardiac arrhythmias, angina, MI, respiratory insufficiency requiring intubation, GI bleeding or infarction, renal insufficiency, edema, and mental status changes; therapy should be restricted to patients with normal cardiac and pulmonary functions as defined by thallium stress and formal pulmonary function testing; hold aldesleukin administration in patients developing moderate to severe lethargy or somnolence as continued administration may result in coma; may exacerbate disease symptoms in patients with clinically unrecognized or untreated CNS metastases; thoroughly evaluate and treat all patients with CNS metastases prior to therapy

Precautions Use with extreme caution in patients with normal thallium stress tests and pulmonary functions tests who have a history of prior cardiac or pulmonary disease; intensive aldesleukin treatment is associated with impaired neutrophil function (reduced chemotaxis) and with an increased risk of disseminated infection (particularly with *Staphylococcus aureus*) including sepsis and bacterial endocarditis; patients with indwelling central lines are particularly at increased risk of infection; treat pre-existing bacterial infections prior to initiation of aldesleukin therapy; standard supportive care during high-dose aldesleukin treatment includes acetaminophen to relieve fever and chills and an H_2 antagonist to reduce the risk of GI ulceration and/or bleeding; aldesleukin may exacerbate autoimmune disease; closely monitor for thyroid abnormalities or other potentially autoimmune phenomena; use with caution in patients with known seizure disorders

Adverse Reactions Many adverse effects of aldesleukin are dosage and schedule dependent; greater toxicity occurs with high dose, bolus administration and the least toxicity with low dose, subcutaneous administration

Cardiovascular: Hypotension (dose-limiting, possibly fatal), sinus tachycardia, arrhythmias, edema, angina, MI, CHF, capillary leak syndrome

Central nervous system: Confusion, drowsiness, transient memory loss, dizziness, cognitive changes, fatigue, chills, malaise, somnolence, disorientation, headaches, insomnia, paranoid delusion, seizures, coma, fever, pain

Dermatologic: Macular erythematous rash, pruritus, erythema, exfoliative dermatitis, dry skin, alopecia, petechiae, purpura, vitiligo

Endocrine & metabolic: Hypomagnesemia, hypocalcemia, hypokalemia, hypophosphatemia, hyponatremia, hypoglycemia, hyperglycemia, hypermagnesemia, hypercalcemia, hyperkalemia. hyperphosphatemia, hypernatremia, thyroid dysfunction

Gastrointestinal: Nausea, vomiting, diarrhea, stomatitis, GI bleeding, anorexia, weight gain, pancreatitis

Hematologic: Anemia, thrombocytopenia, leukopenia, eosinophilia

Hepatic: Transient elevations of bilirubin and liver enzymes, jaundice, ascites, decreased clotting factors

Neuromuscular & skeletal: Weakness, rigors, arthralgia, myalgia

Renal: Oliguria, proteinuria, transient increase in BUN, hematuria

Respiratory: Congestion, dyspnea, pleural effusion, pulmonary edema

Miscellaneous: Allergic reactions

Drug Interactions Corticosteroids may decrease efficacy; increased CNS depression when administered concomitantly with other sedating agents; increased toxicity when administered concomitantly with other potentially nephrotoxic, myelotoxic, cardiotoxic, or hepatotoxic agents; increased hypotensive effects with antihypertensives or beta-blocking agents; acute reactions including fever, chills, nausea, vomiting, pruritus, rash, diarrhea, hypotension, edema, and oliguria with iodinated contrast media (may occur within 4 weeks to several months after aldesleukin administration); hypersensitivity reactions have been reported when combined with dacarbazine, cis-platinum, tamoxifen, and interferon-alfa; exacerbation of autoimmune and inflammatory disorders and myocardial injury when used in combination with interferon-alfa

Stability Store in refrigerator; do not freeze; reconstituted solution is stable 48 hours in refrigerator or at room temperature; since aldesleukin contains no preservatives, refrigerated storage of the reconstituted solution is preferred; compatible **only** with (Continued)

Aldesleukin *(Continued)*

D$_5$W; incompatible with sodium chloride solutions; do not mix with other medications

Final Dilution Concentration (mcg/mL)	Final Dilution Concentration (10^6 international units/mL)	Stability
<30	<0.49	Albumin must be added to bag **prior to addition** of aldesleukin at a final concentration of 0.1% (1 mg/mL) albumin; stable at room temperature for 6 days*
≥30 - ≤70	≥0.49 - ≤1.1	Stable at room temperature for 6 days*
71-99	1.2-1.6	Unstable; avoid use
100-500	1.7-8.2	Unstable at room temperature; avoid use; stable at ≥32°C (89°F) for 6 days*†

*These solutions do not contain a preservative; use for more than 24 hours may not be advisable.

†Continuous infusion via CADD pump or similar infusion device raises aldesleukin to this temperature.

Mechanism of Action Aldesleukin, a human recombinant interleukin-2 product, promotes proliferation, differentiation, and recruitment of T and B cells, natural killer cells, and thymocytes; it also causes cytolytic activity in some lymphocytes and subsequent interactions between lymphokine-activated killer cells and tumor-infiltrating lymphocytes; causes multiple immunological effects including activation of cellular immunity with lymphocytosis, eosinophilia, and thrombocytopenia; production of cytokines (including tumor necrosis factor, interleukin-1), and inhibition of tumor growth

Pharmacokinetics

Absorption: Oral: Not absorbed

Distribution: Primarily into plasma, lymphocytes, lungs, liver, kidney, and spleen

V$_d$: Adults: 4-7 L

Metabolism: Metabolized to amino acids in the cells lining the proximal convoluted tubules of the kidney

Bioavailability: I.M.: 30% to 37%

Half-life:

Children:

Distribution: 14 ± 6 minutes

Elimination: 51 ± 11 minutes

Adults:

Distribution: 6-27 minutes

Elimination: 85 minutes

Time to peak concentration: S.C.: 2-3 hours

Clearance: Adults: 7.2-16.1 L/hour

Usual Dosage A wide variety of dosages have been or are currently under investigation (refer to individual protocols):

AML: Children: (Investigational use only, Sievers, 1998): Continuous I.V. infusion: 9 million international units (9 x 10^6 international units) daily for 4 days; repeat 4 days later with 1.6 million international units (1.6 x 10^6 international units) daily for 10 days

Metastatic renal cell carcinoma and metastatic melanoma: Adults:

I.V.:

Initial: Treatment consists of two 5-day treatment cycles separated by a rest period: 600,000 international units/kg (0.037 mg/kg) every 8 hours for a total of 14 doses; followed by a rest period of 9 days, then repeat the 14-dose regimen; these two cycles constitute one course of therapy

Retreatment: Each treatment course should be separated by a rest period of at least 7 weeks from the date of completion; patients should be evaluated for response approximately 4 weeks after completion of a course of therapy and again immediately prior to the scheduled start of the next treatment course

S.C.: (Investigational): 11 million international units (11 x 10^6 international units) daily for 4 days per week for 4 consecutive weeks; repeat every 6 weeks, or alternatively, 18 million international units (18 x 10^6 international units) daily for 5 days followed by a 2-day rest period, then 9 million international units (9 x

10⁶ international units) for 2 days, followed by 18 million international units (18 x 10⁶ international units) daily for 3 days

Dosage modification for toxicity: In high-dose therapy, see manufacturer's guidelines (or refer to specific protocol for recommendations) for holding and restarting therapy; hold or interrupt a dose, **do not dose reduce**

Administration Parenteral:

I.V.: Reconstitute with 1.2 mL sterile water for injection (swirl, do not shake); resulting concentration is 1.1 mg/mL [18 million (18 x 10⁶) international units/mL]; further dilute dosage in D_5W to a final concentration between 30-70 mcg/mL (0.49-1.1 million international units/mL) and infuse over 15 minutes; for continuous infusions, dilute in D_5W maintaining the same final concentration; final dilutions <30 mcg/mL or >70 mcg/mL have shown increased variability in drug stability and bioactivity; addition of albumin has been used to improve stability if final dilution concentrations <30 mcg/mL are necessary; when continuous infusion is via devices which expose aldesleukin to temperatures higher than room temperature (≥32°C/89.6°F) (eg, CADD pump or similar infusion device), drug stability is also altered; see Stability for more detailed information; do not use in-line filter when administering

S.C.: Reconstituted solution may be administered subcutaneously without further dilution (**Note:** Subcutaneous administration is a non-FDA approved route)

Monitoring Parameters Baseline chest x-ray, pulmonary function tests and thallium stress study; CBC with differential, platelet counts, electrolytes, BUN, serum creatinine, hepatic enzymes, vital signs, weight, pulse oximetry, arterial blood gases (if pulmonary symptoms), fluid intake and output

Nursing Implications See Warnings and Precautions

Additional Information

1 Cetus Unit = 6 international units

1 Roche Unit (Teceleukin) = 3 international units

1.1 mg = 18 x 10⁶ international units or 3 x 10⁶ Cetus units

Dosage Forms Powder for injection, lyophilized: 22 x 10⁶ international units (1.3 mg) [18 x 10⁶ international units/mL] [1.1 mg/mL]

References

Sievers EL, Lange BJ, Sondel PM, et al, "Feasibility, Toxicity, and Biologic Response of Interleukin-2 After Consolidation Chemotherapy for Acute Myelogenous Leukemia: A Report From the Children's Cancer Group," *J Clin Oncol*, 1998, 16(3):914-9.

Whittington R and Faulds D, "Interleukin-2: A Review of Its Pharmacological Properties and Therapeutic Use in Patients With Cancer," *Drugs*, 1993, 46(3):446-514.

♦ **Aldomet®** *see* Methyldopa *on page 625*

♦ **Aleve® [OTC]** *see* Naproxen *on page 672*

♦ **Alfenta® (Canada)** *see* Alfentanil *on page 45*

♦ **Alfenta® Injection** *see* Alfentanil *on page 45*

Alfentanil (al FEN ta nil)

Related Information

Narcotic Analgesics Comparison *on page 1035*

Overdose and Toxicology *on page 1191*

Brand Names Alfenta® (Canada); Alfenta® Injection

Available Salts Alfentanil Hydrochloride

Therapeutic Category Analgesic, Narcotic; General Anesthetic

Generic Available Yes

Use Analgesia; analgesia adjunct; anesthetic agent

Restrictions C-II

Pregnancy Risk Factor C

Contraindications Hypersensitivity to alfentanil hydrochloride or any component; increased intracranial pressure; severe respiratory depression

Warnings Rapid I.V. infusion may result in skeletal muscle and chest wall rigidity → impaired ventilation → respiratory distress/arrest; inject slowly over 3-5 minutes; nondepolarizing skeletal muscle relaxant may be required

Precautions Use with caution in patients with bradycardia

Adverse Reactions

Cardiovascular: Bradycardia, peripheral vasodilation, hypotension

Central nervous system: Drowsiness, dizziness, sedation, CNS depression, increased intracranial pressure

Dermatologic: Pruritus

Endocrine & metabolic: Antidiuretic hormone release

Gastrointestinal: Nausea, vomiting, constipation, biliary tract spasm

Genitourinary: Urinary tract spasm

(Continued)

Alfentanil (Continued)

Neuromuscular & skeletal: Skeletal muscle and chest wall rigidity especially following rapid I.V. administration

Ocular: Miosis

Respiratory: Respiratory depression, apnea, respiratory arrest

Miscellaneous: Histamine release, physical and psychological dependence with prolonged use

Drug Interactions Cytochrome P-450 isoenzyme CYP3A3/4 substrate

CNS depressants, phenothiazines, tricyclic antidepressants may potentiate the adverse effects of opiate agonists; erythromycin may significantly decrease alfentanil clearance; chronic beta-blocker therapy may potentiate alfentanil-induced bradycardia; propofol may increase serum concentrations of alfentanil

Mechanism of Action Binds with stereospecific receptors at many sites within the CNS, increases pain threshold, alters pain reception, inhibits ascending pain pathways

Pharmacodynamics

Onset: Within 5 minutes

Duration: <15-20 minutes

Pharmacokinetics

Distribution: V_d beta:

Newborns, premature: 1 L/kg

Children: 0.163-0.48 L/kg

Adults: 0.46 L/kg

Protein binding:

Neonates: 67%

Adults: 88% to 92%

Bound to alpha$_1$-acid glycoprotein

Metabolism: Hepatic

Half-life, elimination:

Newborns, premature: 320-525 minutes

Children: 40-60 minutes

Adults: 83-97 minutes

Usual Dosage Doses should be titrated to appropriate effects; wide range of doses is dependent upon desired degree of analgesia/anesthesia

Neonates, Infants, and Children <12 years: Dose not established; A high percent of newborn infants receiving alfentanil (prior to procedures) at doses of 9-15 mcg/kg (mean dose: 11.7 mcg/kg) developed chest wall rigidity; 9 out of 20 newborns (45%) developed mild or moderate rigidity that did not affect ventilation, while 4 out of 20 (20%) had severe rigidity interfering with respiration for ~5-10 minutes;

Alfentanil: Adult Dosing

Indication	Approximate Duration of Anesthesia (min)	Induction Period (Initial Dose) (mcg/kg)	Maintenance Period (Increments/ Infusion)	Total Dose (mcg/kg)	Effects
Incremental injection	≤30	8-20	3-5 mcg/kg or 0.5-1 mcg/kg/min	8-40	Spontaneously breathing or assisted ventilation when required.
	30-60	20-50	5-15 mcg/kg	Up to 75	Assisted or controlled ventilation required. Attenuation of response to laryngoscopy and intubation.
Continuous infusion	>45	50-75	0.5-3 mcg/kg/min; average infusion rate: 1-1.5 mcg/kg/min	Dependent on duration of procedure	Assisted or controlled ventilation required. Some attenuation of response to intubation and incision, with intraoperative stability.
Anesthetic induction	>45	130-245	0.5-1.5 mcg/kg/min or general anesthetic	Dependent on duration of procedure	Assisted or controlled ventilation required. Administer slowly (over 3 minutes). Concentration of inhalation agents reduced by 30% to 50% for initial hour.

use of a skeletal muscle relaxant to prevent chest wall rigidity is recommended; however, smaller alfentanil doses may be required in newborns. Further studies are needed to determine appropriate doses of alfentanil in pediatric patients.

Adults: Use lean body weight for patients who weigh >20% over ideal body weight; see **Alfentanil: Adult Dosing** table on previous page.

Administration Parenteral: I.V.: Inject slowly over 3-5 minutes or by I.V. continuous infusion

Monitoring Parameters Respiratory rate, blood pressure, heart rate, neurological status (for degree of analgesia/anesthesia)

Nursing Implications Alfentanil may produce more hypotension compared to fentanyl, therefore, be sure to administer slowly and ensure patient has adequate hydration

Dosage Forms Injection, preservative free, as hydrochloride: 500 mcg/mL (2 mL, 5 mL, 10 mL, 20 mL)

References

Davis PJ, Killian A, Stiller RL, et al, "Pharmacokinetics of Alfentanil in Newborn Premature Infants and Older Children," *Dev Pharmacol Ther*, 1989, 13(1):21-7.

Marlow N, Weindling AM, Van Peer A, et al, "Alfentanil Pharmacokinetics in Preterm Infants," *Arch Dis Child*, 1990, 65(4 Spec No):349-51.

Meistelman C, Saint-Maurice C, Lepaul M, et al, "A Comparison of Alfentanil Pharmacokinetics in Children and Adults," *Anesthesiology*, 1987, 66(1):13-6.

Pokela ML, Ryhanen PT, Koivisto ME, et al, "Alfentanil-Induced Rigidity in Newborn Infants," *Anesth Analg*, 1992, 75(2):252-7.

♦ **Alfentanil Hydrochloride** see Alfentanil on page 45

Alglucerase (al GLOO ser ase)

Brand Names Ceredase® Injection

Synonyms Glucocerebrosidase

Therapeutic Category Enzyme, Glucocerebrosidase; Gaucher's Disease, Treatment Agent

Generic Available No

Use Long-term enzyme replacement in patients with confirmed Type I Gaucher's disease who exhibit one or more of the following conditions: Moderate to severe anemia; thrombocytopenia and bleeding tendencies; bone disease; hepatomegaly or splenomegaly

Pregnancy Risk Factor C

Contraindications Hypersensitivity to alglucerase or any component

Precautions Alglucerase is prepared from pooled human placental tissue that may contain the causative agents of some viral diseases; the risk of contamination from slowly active or latent viruses is believed to be remote due to steps taken in the manufacturing process; observe for signs of early virilization in males <10 years of age

Adverse Reactions

Central nervous system: Fever, chills, fatigue

Gastrointestinal: Abdominal discomfort, nausea, vomiting, diarrhea, oral ulcerations

Local: Discomfort, burning, and edema at the site of injection

Neuromuscular: Weakness, backache

Miscellaneous: Hypersensitivity reactions

Drug Interactions No information available at this time

Stability When diluted to 100-200 mL with NS, resultant solution is stable up to 18 hours when stored at 2°C to 8°C

Mechanism of Action Glucocerebrosidase is an enzyme prepared from human placental tissue. Gaucher's disease is an inherited metabolic disorder caused by the defective activity of beta-glucosidase and the resultant accumulation of glucosyl ceramide laden macrophages in the liver, bone, and spleen. The disease affects an estimated 10,000-15,000 people in the United States, primarily of Eastern European Jewish descent, with up to 5000 being symptomatic and requiring treatment. Alglucerase acts by replacing the missing enzyme associated with Gaucher's disease.

Pharmacodynamics

Onset of significant improvement in symptoms:

Hepatosplenomegaly and hematologic abnormalities: Occurs within 6 months

Improvement in bone mineralization: Noted at 80-104 weeks of therapy

Pharmacokinetics

Distribution: V_d: 0.05-0.28 L/kg

Half-life, elimination: ~4-10 minutes

Usual Dosage Children and Adults: I.V. infusion: Dosage varies with the severity of disease; the recommended dosage ranges from 1.15 units/kg 3 times/week to 60

(Continued)

Alglucerase *(Continued)*

units/kg administered as frequently as once weekly or as infrequently as every 4 weeks; a common low-dose high-frequency protocol is 30 units/kg/month divided into 3 infusions weekly; after a response is firmly established, the dosage may be progressively lowered at periods of 3-6 months

Administration Parenteral: Dilute to a final volume of 100-200 mL NS and infuse I.V. over 1-2 hours; an in-line filter should be used; do not shake solution as it denatures the enzyme

Monitoring Parameters CBC, platelets, liver function tests

Dosage Forms Injection: 10 units/mL (5 mL); 80 units/mL (5 mL)

References

Barton NW, Brady RO, Dambrosia JM, et al, "Replacement Therapy for Inherited Enzyme Deficiency - Macrophage-Targeted Glucocerebrosidase for Gaucher's Disease," *N Engl J Med*, 1991, 324(21):1464-70.

♦ **Alkaban-AQ®** *see* Vinblastine *on page 978*

♦ **Alka-Mints® [OTC]** *see* Calcium Supplements *on page 157*

♦ **Alkeran®** *see* Melphalan *on page 600*

♦ **Aller-Chlor® Oral [OTC]** *see* Chlorpheniramine *on page 214*

♦ **Allercon® [OTC]** *see* Triprolidine and Pseudoephedrine *on page 957*

♦ **Allerdryl® (Canada)** *see* Diphenhydramine *on page 327*

♦ **Allerest® 12 Hour Nasal Solution [OTC]** *see* Oxymetazoline *on page 718*

♦ **Allerest® Eye Drops [OTC]** *see* Naphazoline *on page 671*

♦ **Allerfrin® [OTC]** *see* Triprolidine and Pseudoephedrine *on page 957*

♦ **Allergen® Ear Drops** *see* Antipyrine and Benzocaine *on page 90*

♦ **AllerMax® Oral [OTC]** *see* Diphenhydramine *on page 327*

♦ **Allernix® (Canada)** *see* Diphenhydramine *on page 327*

♦ **Allerphed® [OTC]** *see* Triprolidine and Pseudoephedrine *on page 957*

Allopurinol (al oh PURE i nole)

Related Information

Tumor Lysis Syndrome, Management *on page 1125*

Brand Names Aloprim™; Apo®-Allopurinol (Canada); Novo-purol® (Canada); Purinol® (Canada); Zyloprim®

Therapeutic Category Antigout Agent; Uric Acid Lowering Agent

Generic Available Yes (oral forms only)

Use Prevention of attacks of gouty arthritis and nephropathy; also used in treatment of secondary hyperuricemia which may occur during treatment of tumors or leukemia; prevention of recurrent calcium oxalate calculi

Pregnancy Risk Factor C

Contraindications Hypersensitivity to allopurinol or any component

Warnings Do not treat asymptomatic hyperuricemia; monitor liver function and complete blood counts before initiating therapy and periodically

Precautions Reduce dosage in renal impairment; discontinue drug at the first sign of rash; risk of skin rash may be increased in patients receiving amoxicillin or ampicillin; risk of hypersensitivity may be increased in patients receiving thiazides and possibly ACE inhibitors

Adverse Reactions

Cardiovascular: (reported with I.V. administration) Hypotension, flushing, hypertension, bradycardia, heart failure

Central nervous system: Drowsiness, fever, headache, chills, somnolence, agitation

Dermatologic: Pruritic maculopapular rash, exfoliative dermatitis, erythema multiforme, alopecia

Gastrointestinal: GI irritation, dyspepsia, nausea, vomiting, diarrhea, abdominal pain, gastritis

Genitourinary: Hematuria

Hematologic: Leukocytosis, leukopenia, thrombocytopenia, eosinophilia, bone marrow suppression

Hepatic: Hepatitis, elevated liver enzymes, hepatomegaly, hyperbilirubinemia, jaundice

Local: Local injection site reaction

Neuromuscular & skeletal: Peripheral neuropathy, paresthesia, neuritis, arthralgia, myoclonus

Ocular: Cataracts, optic neuritis

Renal: Renal impairment

Respiratory: Epistaxis; (reported with I.V. administration) apnea, hyperpnea, ARDS

Vascular: Necrotizing angiitis, vasculitis

Drug Interactions Inhibits metabolism of azathioprine and mercaptopurine; use with ampicillin or amoxicillin may increase the incidence of skin rash; may increase myelosuppressive effects of cyclophosphamide; large doses may decrease theophylline clearance; increased risk of hypersensitivity reactions when coadministered with ACE inhibitors and thiazide diuretics; decreased allopurinol effectiveness when coadministered with uricosuric agents; increases kidney stone formation when taken with large doses of vitamin C; aluminum hydroxide antacids decrease allopurinol's absorption; increased chlorpropamide effects; may increase risk of osteomalacia in patients receiving phenytoin or phenobarbital; prolongs the half-life of oral anticoagulants; may increase cyclosporine serum levels

Stability Reconstituted parenteral solution should be stored at room temperature; do not refrigerate; use within 10 hours of preparation; physically **incompatible** when mixed with or infused through the same line with the following: Amikacin, amphotericin B, carmustine, cefotaxime, chlorpromazine, cimetidine, clindamycin, cytarabine, dacarbazine, daunorubicin, diphenhydramine, doxorubicin, doxycycline, droperidol, floxuridine, gentamicin, haloperidol, hydroxyzine, idarubicin, imipenem-cilastatin, mechlorethamine, meperidine, metoclopramide, methylprednisolone sodium succinate, minocycline, nalbuphine, netilmicin, ondansetron, prochlorperazine, promethazine, sodium bicarbonate, streptozocin, tobramycin, vinorelbine

Mechanism of Action Decreases the production of uric acid by inhibiting the action of xanthine oxidase, an enzyme that converts hypoxanthine to xanthine and xanthine to uric acid

Pharmacodynamics Decrease in serum uric acid occurs in 1-2 days with a nadir achieved in 1-3 weeks

Pharmacokinetics

Absorption: Oral: ~80% from the GI tract

Distribution: Into breast milk; breast milk to plasma ratio: 0.9-1.4

Protein binding: <1%

Metabolism: ~75% of drug metabolized to active metabolites, chiefly oxypurinol

Half-life:

Parent: 1-3 hours

Oxypurinol metabolite: 18-30 hours in patients with normal renal function

Time to peak serum concentration: Within 2-6 hours

Allopurinol and oxypurinol are dialyzable

Usual Dosage

Prevention of acute uric acid nephropathy in myeloproliferative neoplastic disorders (beginning 1-2 days before chemotherapy): Daily doses >300 mg should be administered in divided doses:

Children ≤10 years:

I.V.: 200 mg/m^2/day in 1-3 divided doses; maximum dose: 600 mg/day

Oral: 10 mg/kg/day in 2-3 divided doses or 200-300 mg/m^2/day in 2-4 divided doses; maximum dose: 800 mg/day

Alternative:

<6 years: 150 mg/day in 3 divided doses

6-10 years: 300 mg/day in 2-3 divided doses

Children >10 years and Adults:

I.V.: 200-400 mg/m^2/day in 1-3 divided doses; maximum: 600 mg/day

Oral: 600-800 mg/day in 2-3 divided doses

Gout: Children >10 years and Adults: Oral:

Mild: 200-300 mg/day

Severe: 400-600 mg/day

Recurrent calcium oxalate stones: Children >10 years and Adults: Oral: 200-300 mg daily in divided or single daily dosage

Dosing adjustment in renal impairment:

Cl$_{cr}$ >50 mL/minute: No dosage change

Cl$_{cr}$ 10-50 mL/minute: Reduce dosage to 50% of recommended

Cl$_{cr}$ <10 mL/minute: Reduce dosage to 30% of recommended

Administration

Oral: Administer after meals with plenty of fluid

Parenteral: Reconstitute 500 mg vial with 25 mL sterile water; prior to administration, further dilute with D$_5$W or NS to a maximum concentration of 6 mg/mL; rate of infusion is dependent upon the volume of infusate (in research studies, 100-300 mg doses were infused over 30 minutes)

Monitoring Parameters CBC, liver function tests, renal function, serum uric acid; 24-hour urinary urate (when treating calcium oxalate stones)

(Continued)

Allopurinol *(Continued)*

Reference Range
Uric acid: Male: 3.0-7.0 mg/dL; Female: 2.0-6.0 mg/dL
Urinary urate excretion: Male: <800 mg/day; Female: <750 mg/day

Patient Information Report any skin rash, painful urination, blood in urine, irritation of the eyes, or swelling of lips or mouth; avoid alcohol; drink plenty of fluids; may produce drowsiness; use with caution when performing hazardous activities which require mental alertness or physical coordination

Dosage Forms
Injection: 500 mg
Tablet: 100 mg, 300 mg

Extemporaneous Preparations A 20 mg/mL suspension may be made by crushing tablets and mixing with either a 1:4 cherry syrup concentrate:simple syrup mixture or a 1:1 mixture of Ora-Sweet® and Ora-Plus® or a 1:1 mixture of Ora-Sweet® SF and Ora-Plus®. The resulting suspension is stable for 60 days at room temperature or refrigerated.

Allen LV and Erickson MA, "Stability of Acetazolamide, Allopurinol, Azathioprine, Clonazepam, and Flucytosine in Extemporaneously Compounded Oral Liquids," *Am J Health Sys Pharm*, 1996, 53:1944-9.

References
Bennett WM, Aronoff GR, Golper TA, et al, *Drug Prescribing in Renal Failure*, Philadelphia, PA: American College of Physicians, 1987.
Krakoff IH and Murphy ML, "Hyperuricemia in Neoplastic Disease in Children: Prevention With Allopurinol, A Xanthine Oxidase Inhibitor" *Pediatrics*, 1968, 41(1):52-6.

♦ **Almora®** *see* Magnesium Supplements *on page 588*
♦ **Alocril™** *see* Nedocromil *on page 674*
♦ **Aloprim™** *see* Allopurinol *on page 48*
♦ **Alpha-Baclofen® (Canada)** *see* Baclofen *on page 119*
♦ **Alphamul® [OTC]** *see* Castor Oil *on page 175*
♦ **Alphanate®** *see* Antihemophilic Factor (Human) *on page 89*
♦ **Alphatrex® Topical** *see* Betamethasone *on page 130*

Alprazolam (al PRAY zoe lam)

Related Information
Carbohydrate and Alcohol Content of Liquid Medications for Use in Patients Receiving Ketogenic Diets *on page 1228*
Overdose and Toxicology *on page 1191*
Serotonin Syndrome *on page 1217*

Brand Names Alprazolam Intensol®; Apo®-Alpraz (Canada); Novo-Aloprazol® (Canada); Nu-Alprax® (Canada); Xanax®

Therapeutic Category Antianxiety Agent; Benzodiazepine

Generic Available Yes

Use Treatment of generalized anxiety disorder (GAD); symptoms of anxiety (short-term treatment); anxiety associated with depression; management of panic attacks

Restrictions C-IV

Pregnancy Risk Factor D

Contraindications Hypersensitivity to alprazolam, any component, or other benzodiazepines; severe uncontrolled pain, narrow-angle glaucoma, severe respiratory depression, pre-existing CNS depression; not to be used in pregnancy or lactation or in patients taking certain medications (see Drug Interactions)

Warnings Withdrawal symptoms including seizures have occurred 18 hours to 3 days after abrupt discontinuation; when discontinuing therapy, decrease daily dose by no more than 0.5 mg every 3 days; reduce dose in patients with significant hepatic disease

Precautions Safety and effectiveness have not been established in children <18 years of age

Adverse Reactions
Central nervous system: Drowsiness, dizziness, confusion, sedation, headache, ataxia
Gastrointestinal: Xerostomia, constipation, diarrhea, nausea, vomiting
Ocular: Blurred vision
Miscellaneous: Physical and psychological dependence with prolonged use

Drug Interactions Cytochrome P-450 isoenzyme CYP3A3/4 substrate
Enzyme inducers may increase metabolism of alprazolam; CNS depressants including alcohol may enhance CNS effects; cimetidine, fluvoxamine, fluoxetine, propoxyphene, and oral contraceptives may decrease the metabolism of alprazolam; delavirdine, ritonavir, ketoconazole, or itraconazole may decrease the

metabolism of alprazolam and significantly increase alprazolam levels; concurrent use of delavirdine, ritonavir, ketoconazole, or itraconazole with alprazolam is not recommended

Mechanism of Action Depresses all levels of the CNS, including the limbic and reticular formation, by binding to the benzodiazepine site on the gamma-aminobutyric acid (GABA) receptor complex and modulating GABA, which is a major inhibitory neurotransmitter in the brain

Pharmacokinetics
Absorption: Oral: Rapidly and well absorbed
Distribution: 0.9-1.2 L/kg; distributes into breast milk
Protein binding: 80%
Metabolism: Extensive in the liver; major metabolites: alpha-hydroxy-alprazolam (about half as active as alprazolam) and a benzophenone metabolite (inactive)
Half-life: Adults: 6.3-26.9 hours; mean: 11.2 hours
Time to peak serum concentration: Within 1-2 hours
Elimination: Excretion of metabolites and parent compound in urine

Usual Dosage Oral:
Children <18 years: Dose not established; investigationally in children 7-16 years of age (n=13), initial doses of 0.005 mg/kg or 0.125 mg/dose were given 3 times/day for situational anxiety and increments of 0.125-0.25 mg were used to increase doses to maximum of 0.02 mg/kg/dose or 0.06 mg/kg/day; a range of 0.375-3 mg/day was needed. **Note:** A more recent study in 17 children (8-17 years of age) with overanxious disorder or avoidant disorders used initial daily doses of 0.25 mg for children <40 kg and 0.5 mg for those >40 kg. The dose was titrated at 2-day intervals to a maximum of 0.04 mg/kg/day. Required doses ranged from 0.5-3.5 mg/day with a mean of 1.6 mg/day. Based on clinical global ratings, alprazolam appeared to be better than placebo, however, this difference was **not** statistically significant; further studies are needed.
Adults: 0.25-0.5 mg 2-3 times/day, titrate dose upward; maximum dose: 4 mg/day (antianxiety); 10 mg/day (antipanic)

Administration Oral: Administer with food to decrease GI upset

Monitoring Parameters CNS status, respiratory rate

Patient Information May cause drowsiness and impair ability to perform activities requiring mental alertness or coordination; may be habit-forming; avoid abrupt discontinuation after prolonged use; avoid alcohol

Nursing Implications Assist with ambulation during beginning of therapy; allow patient to rise slowly to avoid fainting

Dosage Forms
Solution, oral: 1 mg/mL (30 mL); 0.5 mg/5 mL (500 mL)
Tablet: 0.25 mg, 0.5 mg, 1 mg, 2 mg

References
Bernstein GA, Garfinkel BD, and Borchardt CM, "Comparative Studies of Pharmacotherapy for School Refusal," J Am Acad Child Adolesc Psychiatry, 1990, 29(5):773-81.
Pfefferbaum B, Overall JE, Boren HA, et al, "Alprazolam in the Treatment of Anticipatory and Acute Situational Anxiety in Children With Cancer," J Am Acad Child Adolesc Psychiatry, 1987, 26(4):532-5.
Simeon JG and Ferguson HB, "Alprazolam Effects in Children With Anxiety Disorders," Can J Psychiatry, 1987, 32(7):570-4.
Simeon JG, Ferguson HB, Knott V, et al, "Clinical, Cognitive, and Neurophysiological Effects of Alprazolam in Children and Adolescents With Overanxious and Avoidant Disorders," J Am Acad Child Adolesc Psychiatry, 1992, 31(1):29-33.

♦ **Alprazolam Intensol®** see Alprazolam on page 50

Alprostadil (al PROS ta dill)

Brand Names Caverject® Injection; Edex® Injection; Muse® Pellet; Prostin VR Pediatric® Injection

Synonyms PGE₁; Prostaglandin E₁

Therapeutic Category Prostaglandin

Generic Available Yes: Injection (500 mcg/mL)

Use Temporary maintenance of patency of ductus arteriosus in neonates with ductal-dependent congenital heart disease until surgery can be performed. These defects include cyanotic (eg, pulmonary atresia, pulmonary stenosis, tricuspid atresia, Fallot's tetralogy, transposition of the great vessels) and acyanotic (eg, interruption of aortic arch, coarctation of aorta, hypoplastic left ventricle) heart disease.

Investigationally used for the treatment of pulmonary hypertension in infants and children with congenital heart defects with left-to-right shunts
Adult males: Diagnosis and treatment of erectile dysfunction

Pregnancy Risk Factor X
(Continued)

Alprostadil *(Continued)*

Contraindications Respiratory distress syndrome or persistent fetal circulation

Warnings Apnea occurs in 10% to 12% of neonates with congenital heart defects (especially in those weighing <2 kg at birth) and usually appears during the first hour of drug infusion

Precautions Use cautiously in neonates with bleeding tendencies; if hypotension or pyrexia occurs, the infusion rate should be reduced until symptoms subside; severe hypotension, apnea, or bradycardia requires drug discontinuation with cautious reinstitution at a lower dose

Adverse Reactions

Cardiovascular: Systemic hypotension, flushing, bradycardia, rhythm disturbances, tachycardia

Central nervous system: Seizure-like activity, fever

Endocrine & metabolic: Hypocalcemia, hypoglycemia; cortical proliferation of long bones (cortical hyperostosis) has been seen with long-term infusions (incidence and severity are related to duration of therapy and cumulative dose)

Gastrointestinal: Diarrhea, gastric-outlet obstruction secondary to antral hyperplasia (occurrence related to duration of therapy and cumulative dose)

Hematologic: Inhibition of platelet aggregation

Respiratory: Respiratory depression, apnea

Stability Compatible in D_5W, $D_{10}W$, and saline solutions; refrigerate ampuls at 2°C to 8°C

Mechanism of Action Causes vasodilation by means of direct effect on vascular and ductus arteriosus smooth muscle

Pharmacodynamics

Maximum effect:

Acyanotic congenital heart disease: Usual: 1.5-3 hours; range: 15 minutes to 11 hours

Cyanotic congenital heart disease: Usual: ~30 minutes

Duration: Ductus arteriosus will begin to close within 1-2 hours after drug is stopped

Pharmacokinetics

Metabolism: ~70% to 80% metabolized by oxidation during a single pass through the lungs; metabolite (13,14 dihydro-PGE_1) is active and has been identified in neonates

Half-life: 5-10 minutes; since the half-life is so short, the drug must be administered by continuous infusion

Elimination: Metabolites excreted in urine

Usual Dosage Neonates and Infants: 0.05-0.1 mcg/kg/minute; with therapeutic response, rate is reduced to lowest effective dosage; with unsatisfactory response, rate is increased gradually; maintenance: 0.01-0.4 mcg/kg/minute

PGE_1 is usually given at an infusion rate of 0.1 mcg/kg/minute; but it is often possible to reduce the dosage to ½ or even $\frac{1}{10}$ without losing the therapeutic effect. The mixing schedule is shown in the table.

Add 1 Ampul (500 mcg) to:	Concentration (mcg/mL)	Infusion Rate to Deliver 0.1 mcg/kg/min		
		mL/kg/min	mL/kg/h	mL/kg/24 h
250 mL	2	0.05	3	72
100 mL	5	0.02	1.2	28.8
50 mL	10	0.01	0.6	14.4
25 mL	20	0.005	0.3	7.2

Administration Parenteral: I.V. continuous infusion into a large vein or alternatively through an umbilical artery catheter placed at the ductal opening; maximum concentration listed (per package insert) for I.V. infusion: 20 mcg/mL; has also been administered via continuous infusion into the right pulmonary artery for investigational treatment of pulmonary hypertension in infants and children with congenital heart defects with left-to-right shunts; rate of infusion (mL/hour) = dose (mcg/kg/minute) x weight (kg) x 60 minutes/hour divided by the concentration (mcg/mL)

Monitoring Parameters Arterial pressure, respiratory rate, heart rate, temperature, pO_2; monitor for gastric obstruction in patients receiving PGE_1 for longer than 120 hours; x-rays may be needed to assess cortical hyperostosis in patients receiving prolonged PGE_1 therapy

Nursing Implications Prepare fresh solution every 24 hours; flushing of arm or face may indicate misplacement of intra-arterial catheter and infusion of drug into subclavian or carotid artery; reposition catheter

Additional Information Therapeutic response is indicated by an increase in systemic blood pressure and pH in those with restricted systemic blood flow and acidosis, or by an increase in oxygenation (pO_2) in those with restricted pulmonary blood flow; cortical hyperostosis resolves over 6-12 months after stopping PGE_1 therapy

Dosage Forms
Injection:
Caverject®: 5 mcg, 10 mcg, 20 mcg
Edex® Injection: 5 mcg, 10 mcg, 20 mcg, 40 mcg
Prostin VR Pediatric®: 500 mcg/mL (1 mL)
Pellet, urethral: 125 mcg, 250 mcg, 500 mcg, 1000 mcg

References
Peled N, Dagan O, Babyn P, et al, "Gastric-Outlet Obstruction Induced by Prostaglandin Therapy in Neonates," *N Engl J Med*, 1992, 327(8):505-10.
Weesner KM, "Hemodynamic Effects of Prostaglandin E₁ in Patients With Congenital Heart Disease and Pulmonary Hypertension," *Cathet Cardiovasc Diagn*, 1991, 24(1):10-5.
Woo K, Emery J, and Peabody J, "Cortical Hyperostosis: A Complication of Prolonged Prostaglandin Infusion in Infants Awaiting Cardiac Transplantation," *Pediatrics*, 1994, 93(3):417-20.

♦ **AL-Rr® Oral [OTC]** *see* Chlorpheniramine *on page 214*

Aluminum Acetate (a LOO mi num AS e tate)

Brand Names Acid Mantle® [OTC]; Bluboro® [OTC]; Boropak®; Domeboro® [OTC]; Pedi-Boro® [OTC]
Synonyms Burow's Solution
Therapeutic Category Topical Skin Product
Generic Available Yes
Use Astringent wet dressing for relief of inflammatory conditions of the skin and to reduce weeping that may occur in dermatitis
Pregnancy Risk Factor C
Contraindications Use with topical collagenase
Precautions Do not use plastic or other impervious material to prevent evaporation
Adverse Reactions Local: Irritation
Usual Dosage Children and Adults: Topical: Soak the affected area in the solution 2-4 times/day for 15-30 minutes or apply wet dressing soaked in the solution 2-4 times/day for 30-minute treatment periods; rewet dressing with solution every few minutes to keep it moist
Administration Topical: Keep away from eyes, external use only; one tablet dissolved in a pint of water makes a modified Burow's solution equivalent to a 1:40 dilution, 2 tablets: 1:20 dilution, 4 tablets: 1:10 dilution; one powder packet dissolved in a pint of water makes a modified Burow's solution equivalent to a 1:40 dilution
Dosage Forms
Powder, to make topical solution: 1 packet/pint of water = 1:40 solution
Tablet: 1 tablet/pint = 1:40 dilution

♦ **Aluminum Carbonate** *see* Antacid Preparations *on page 86*
♦ **Aluminum Carbonate Gel** *see* Antacid Preparations *on page 86*
♦ **Aluminum Hydroxide** *see* Antacid Preparations *on page 86*
♦ **Aluminum Hydroxide and Magnesium Carbonate** *see* Antacid Preparations *on page 86*
♦ **Aluminum Hydroxide and Magnesium Hydroxide** *see* Antacid Preparations *on page 86*
♦ **Aluminum Hydroxide and Magnesium Trisilicate** *see* Antacid Preparations *on page 86*
♦ **Aluminum Hydroxide Gel** *see* Antacid Preparations *on page 86*
♦ **Aluminum Hydroxide, Magnesium Hydroxide, and Simethicone** *see* Antacid Preparations *on page 86*
♦ **Aluminum Sucrose Sulfate, Basic** *see* Sucralfate *on page 886*
♦ **Alupent®** *see* Metaproterenol *on page 611*

Amantadine (a MAN ta deen)

Brand Names Endantadine™ (Canada); PMS-Amantadine (Canada); Symadine®; Symmetrel®
Available Salts Amantadine Hydrochloride
Synonyms Adamantanamine
Therapeutic Category Anti-Parkinson's Agent; Antiviral Agent, Oral
Generic Available Yes
(Continued)

Amantadine *(Continued)*

Use Prophylaxis and treatment of influenza A viral infection; symptomatic and adjunct treatment of parkinsonism

Pregnancy Risk Factor C

Contraindications Hypersensitivity to amantadine hydrochloride or any component

Precautions Use with caution in patients with liver disease, epilepsy, history of recurrent eczematoid dermatitis, uncontrolled psychosis, and in patients receiving CNS stimulant drugs; may increase seizure activity or EEG disturbances in patients with pre-existing seizure disorders; modify dosage in patients with renal impairment and in patients with active seizure disorders

Adverse Reactions

Cardiovascular: Orthostatic hypotension, edema

Central nervous system: Dizziness, confusion, headache, insomnia, difficulty in concentrating, anxiety, restlessness, irritability, hallucinations, seizures

Dermatologic: Livedo reticularis

Gastrointestinal: Nausea, vomiting, xerostomia

Genitourinary: Urinary retention

Drug Interactions Additive anticholinergic effects in patients receiving drugs with anticholinergic activity; additive CNS stimulant effect with CNS stimulants

Mechanism of Action As an antiviral, blocks the uncoating of influenza A virus preventing penetration of virus into host and inhibits M_2 protein in the assembly of progeny virions; antiparkinsonian activity may be due to its blocking the reuptake of dopamine into presynaptic neurons and causing direct stimulation of postsynaptic receptors

Pharmacokinetics

Absorption: Well absorbed from the GI tract

Half-life, patients with normal renal function: 10-28 hours

Time to peak serum concentration: 1-4 hours

Elimination: 80% to 90% excreted unchanged in the urine by glomerular filtration and tubular secretion

0% to 5% removed by hemodialysis; no supplemental dose needed after hemodialysis or peritoneal dialysis

Usual Dosage Oral:

Children: Influenza A prophylaxis and treatment:

1-9 years: 5 mg/kg/day in 1-2 divided doses; maximum dose: 150 mg/day

≥10-12 years: 5 mg/kg/day in 1-2 divided doses; maximum dose: 200 mg/day

Note: After first influenza A virus vaccine dose, amantadine prophylaxis may be administered for up to 6 weeks, or until 2 weeks after the second dose of vaccine; administer a 10-day course of therapy following exposure; for symptomatic treatment, administer within 24-48 hours of symptom onset with usual duration of therapy between 2-5 days or for 24-48 hours after patient becomes asymptomatic

Alternative dosage for influenza A prophylaxis: Children >20 kg and Adults: 100 mg/day in 1-2 divided doses

Adults:

Parkinson's disease: 100 mg twice daily

Influenza A viral infection: 200 mg/day in 1-2 divided doses

Prophylaxis: Minimum 10-day course of therapy following exposure, or continue for 2-3 weeks after influenza A virus vaccine is given

Dosing interval in renal impairment: Adults:

Cl_{cr} 30-50 mL/minute: Administer 100 mg/day

Cl_{cr} 15-29 mL/minute: Administer 100 mg every other day

Cl_{cr} <15 mL/minute: Administer 200 mg every 7 days

Monitoring Parameters Renal function; monitor for signs of neurotoxicity

Patient Information Causes drowsiness and may impair ability to perform activities requiring mental alertness or coordination; do not abruptly discontinue therapy, may precipitate a parkinsonian crisis; avoid alcohol

Nursing Implications If insomnia occurs, the last daily dose should be taken several hours before retiring

Dosage Forms

Capsule, as hydrochloride: 100 mg

Syrup, as hydrochloride: 50 mg/5 mL (480 mL)

References

Strong DK, Eisenstat DD, Bryson SM, et al, "Amantadine Neurotoxicity in a Pediatric Patient With Renal Insufficiency," *DICP*, 1991, 25(11):1175-7.

♦ **Amantadine Hydrochloride** *see* Amantadine *on page 53*

♦ **Ambi 10® [OTC]** see Benzoyl Peroxide *on page 126*
♦ **AmBisome®** see Amphotericin B Liposome *on page 77*
♦ **AMCA** see Tranexamic Acid *on page 943*
♦ **Amcort® Injection** see Triamcinolone *on page 946*
♦ **Amen® Oral** see Medroxyprogesterone *on page 599*
♦ **Americaine® [OTC]** see Benzocaine *on page 124*
♦ **A-methaPred® Injection** see Methylprednisolone *on page 629*
♦ **Amethocaine** see Tetracaine *on page 907*
♦ **Amethopterin** see Methotrexate *on page 621*
♦ **Amicar®** see Aminocaproic Acid *on page 60*

Amifostine (am i FOS teen)

Brand Names Ethyol®

Therapeutic Category Antidote, Cisplatin; Cytoprotective Agent

Use Cytoprotective agent which scavenges free radicals and binds to reactive drug derivatives due to radiation therapy, cisplatin, carboplatin, cyclophosphamide, ifosfamide, carmustine, melphalan, and mechlorethamine to selectively protect normal tissues against toxicity due to these agents; reduction of moderate to severe xerostomia from radiation treatment of the head and neck where the radiation port includes a substantial portion of the parotid glands

Pregnancy Risk Factor C

Contraindications Hypersensitivity to amifostine, aminothiol compounds, or any component; patients who are hypotensive or dehydrated

Warnings Due to limited experience and the possibility of amifostine interference with antineoplastic efficacy, amifostine should not be administered to patients in settings where chemotherapy can produce a significant survival benefit or cure, except in the context of a clinical study. Monitor serum calcium levels in patients at risk of hypocalcemia (eg, those patients receiving multiple doses of amifostine, patients with nephrotic syndrome).

Precautions Use with caution in patients with pre-existing cardiovascular or cerebrovascular conditions such as ischemic heart disease, arrhythmias, CHF, history of stroke or transient ischemic attacks; may cause hypotension; use special caution in situations where concomitant antihypertensive therapy cannot be interrupted 24 hours prior to starting amifostine or in patients in whom the adverse effects of nausea/vomiting may be more likely to have serious consequences

Adverse Reactions
Cardiovascular: Transient hypotension (62%; incidence is higher in patients with head and neck cancer, esophageal cancer, non-small cell lung cancer, prior neck irradiation, or hypercalcemia), flushing, warm sensation
Central nervous system: Chills, fever, dizziness, somnolence, hiccups, anxiety, malaise
Dermatologic: Rash
Endocrine & metabolic: Hypocalcemia, hypomagnesemia
Gastrointestinal: Nausea, vomiting, metallic taste in mouth
Genitourinary: Urinary retention (reversible)
Respiratory: Sneezing

Drug Interactions Antihypertensive agents may potentiate the hypotensive effects of amifostine

Stability When 500 mg amifostine is reconstituted with 9.7 mL of NS, the resultant solution is stable for 5 hours at room temperature or up to 24 hours if refrigerated; amifostine solutions diluted to 5-40 mg/mL in NS are chemically stable for 5 hours at room temperature or 24 hours if refrigerated; decreased stability in low pH conditions; incompatible with acyclovir, amphotericin B, chlorpromazine, cisplatin, ganciclovir, hydroxyzine, prochlorperazine

Mechanism of Action Amifostine is a prodrug that is converted by the plasma membrane-bound enzyme alkaline phosphatase to the active free sulfhydryl compound WR-1065 which is further oxidized to a symmetrical disulfide (WR-33278) or to mixed disulfides. The active drug scavenges free radicals, donates hydrogen ions to free radicals, and binds to active derivatives of antineoplastic agents, thus preventing the alkylation of nucleic acid. Selective protection of normal tissue is demonstrated by:
  1) decreased alkaline phosphatase activity in tumor cells,
  2) decreased vascularity of tumors, and
  3) lower pH in tumor tissues due to the predominance of anaerobic metabolism (WR-1065 requires a pH in the range of 6.6-8.2 for uptake into tissues)
(Continued)

AMIKACIN

Amifostine *(Continued)*

Pharmacokinetics
Distribution: V_d: Adults: 6.4 L; unmetabolized prodrug is largely confined to the intravascular compartment; active metabolite is distributed into normal tissues with high concentrations in bone marrow, GI mucosa, skin, liver, and salivary glands
Protein binding: 4%
Metabolism: Amifostine (phosphorylated prodrug) is hydrolyzed by alkaline phosphatase to an active free sulfhydryl compound (WR-1065)
Half-life: 8 minutes (amifostine)
Elimination: Metabolites excreted in urine

Usual Dosage I.V. (refer to individual protocols):
Children: Limited data available on use in pediatric patients; dosing based on a prior clinical phase I trial and single case reports: 740 mg/m² once daily administered 30 minutes prior to chemotherapy; doses as high as 1650 mg/m² administered 30 minutes prior to melphalan have been used in phase II trials; repeat amifostine doses may be required when using a cytotoxic agent with a long half-life or long infusion time
Adults: 910 mg/m² once daily administered 30 minutes prior to chemotherapy; reduce dose to 740 mg/m² in patients who have a higher incidence of hypotension
Reduction of moderate to severe xerostomia from radiation of the head and neck: 200 mg/m² once daily starting 15-30 minutes prior to standard fraction radiation therapy

Administration Parenteral: I.V.: Reconstituted amifostine dose must be further diluted with NS to a final volume of 50 mL (adults) or a final concentration of 5-40 mg/mL (children). Administer amifostine doses >740 mg/m² as an I.V. intermittent infusion over 15 minutes since the 15-minute infusion is better tolerated than a more prolonged infusion. Administer 200 mg/m² dose as a 3-minute infusion. Amifostine should be interrupted if the blood pressure decreases significantly from baseline or if the patient develops symptoms related to decreased cerebral or cardiovascular perfusion. Patients experiencing decreased blood pressure should receive a rapid infusion of NS and be kept supine or placed in the Trendelenburg position. Amifostine can be restarted if the blood pressure returns to the baseline level.

Monitoring Parameters Baseline blood pressure followed by a blood pressure reading every 3-5 minutes during the 15-minute infusion; monitor electrolytes, urinalysis, serum calcium, serum magnesium; monitor I & O

Nursing Implications Pretreat patient with antiemetics; patients should be well hydrated prior to amifostine infusion; patients taking antihypertensive medications should discontinue therapy 24 hours before administration of amifostine; begin chemotherapy or radiation therapy 15 minutes after completion of amifostine

Dosage Forms Injection: 500 mg vial

References
Adamson PC, Balis FM, Belasco JE, et al, "A Phase I Trial of Amifostine (WR-2721) and Melphalan in Children With Refractory Cancer," *Cancer Res*, 1995, 55(18): 4069-72.
Bukowski R, "Cytoprotection in the Treatment of Pediatric Cancer: Review of Current Strategies in Adults and Their Application to Children," *Med Pediatr Oncol*, 1999, 32(2):124-34.
Schuchter LM, "Guidelines for the Administration of Amifostine," *Semin Oncol*, 1996, 23(4 Suppl 8):40-3.
Shaw LM, Bonner H, and Lieberman R, "Pharmacokinetic Profile of Amifostine," *Semin Oncol*, 1996, 23(4 Suppl 8):18-22.

Amikacin *(am i KAY sin)*

Related Information
Blood Level Sampling Time Guidelines *on page 1189*
Overdose and Toxicology *on page 1191*

Brand Names Amikin® (Canada); Amikin® Injection
Available Salts Amikacin Sulfate
Therapeutic Category Antibiotic, Aminoglycoside
Generic Available Yes
Use Treatment of documented gram-negative enteric infection resistant to gentamicin and tobramycin; documented infection of mycobacterial organisms susceptible to amikacin
Pregnancy Risk Factor D
Contraindications Hypersensitivity to amikacin sulfate or any component; cross-sensitivity may exist with other aminoglycosides
Warnings Aminoglycosides are associated with significant nephrotoxicity or ototoxicity; the ototoxicity is directly proportional to the amount of drug given and the

duration of treatment. Tinnitus or vertigo are indications of vestibular injury and impending bilateral irreversible deafness. Risk of nephrotoxicity increases when used concurrently with other potentially nephrotoxic drugs; renal damage is usually reversible. Aminoglycosides can cause fetal harm when administered to a pregnant woman, and have been associated with several reports of total irreversible bilateral congenital deafness in pediatric patients exposed *in utero.*

Precautions Use with caution in neonates (due to renal immaturity that results in a prolonged half-life); patients with pre-existing renal impairment, auditory or vestibular impairment, hypocalcemia, myasthenia gravis, and in conditions which depress neuromuscular transmission; dose and/or frequency of administration must be modified in patients with renal impairment

Adverse Reactions

Central nervous system: Fever, headache, dizziness, drowsiness, ataxia, vertigo

Dermatologic: Rash

Gastrointestinal: Nausea, vomiting

Hematologic: Eosinophilia, anemia, leukopenia

Neuromuscular & skeletal: Neuromuscular blockade, tremor, paresthesia, weakness, gait instability

Otic: Ototoxicity

Renal: Nephrotoxicity

Drug Interactions Extended-spectrum penicillins (decrease serum amikacin concentration in patients with renal failure); loop diuretics may potentiate the ototoxicity of the aminoglycosides; amphotericin, vancomycin, acyclovir, cisplatin, or cephalosporins may increase nephrotoxicity; may potentiate the effects of neuromuscular blocking agents and general anesthetics; indomethacin may increase serum amikacin concentrations

Mechanism of Action Inhibits protein synthesis in susceptible bacteria by binding to ribosomal subunits

Pharmacokinetics

Distribution: Primarily into extracellular fluid (highly hydrophilic); 12% of serum concentration penetrates into bronchial secretions; poor penetration into the blood-brain barrier even when meninges are inflamed; V_d is increased in neonates and patients with edema, ascites, fluid overload; V_d is decreased in patients with dehydration; crosses the placenta

Half-life:

Infants:

Low birth weight, 1-3 days of age: 7 hours

Full-term >7 days: 4-5 hours

Children: 1.6-2.5 hours

Adolescents: 1.5 ± 1 hour

Adults: 2-3 hours

Anuria: 28-86 hours; half-life and clearance are dependent on renal function

Time to peak serum concentration:

I.M.: Within 45-120 minutes

I.V.: Within 30 minutes following a 30-minute infusion

Elimination: 94% to 98% is excreted unchanged in the urine via glomerular filtration within 24 hours

Dialyzable (50% to 100%); supplemental dose recommended after hemodialysis or peritoneal dialysis

Usual Dosage I.M., I.V. (dosage should be based on an estimate of ideal body weight except in neonates; neonatal dosage should be based on actual weight unless the patient has hydrocephalus or hydrops fetalis):

Neonates:

0-4 weeks, <1200 g: 7.5 mg/kg/dose every 18-24 hours

Postnatal age ≤7 days:

1200-2000 g: 7.5 mg/kg/dose every 12 hours

>2000 g: 7.5-10 mg/kg/dose every 12 hours

Postnatal age >7 days:

1200-2000 g: 7.5-10 mg/kg/dose every 8-12 hours

>2000 g: 10 mg/kg/dose every 8 hours

Infants and Children: 15-22.5 mg/kg/day divided every 8 hours; some consultants recommend initial doses of 30 mg/kg/day divided every 8 hours in patients who may require larger doses; see Note

Treatment for nontuberculous mycobacterial infection: 15-30 mg/kg/day divided every 12-24 hours as part of a multiple drug regimen; maximum dose: 1.5 g/day

Adults: 15 mg/kg/day divided every 8-12 hours; maximum: 1.5 g/day

(Continued)

Amikacin *(Continued)*

Treatment of *M. avium* complex infection: 7.5-15 mg/kg/day divided every 12-24 hours as part of a multiple drug regimen

Dosing interval in renal impairment: Loading dose: 5-7.5 mg/kg; subsequent dosages and frequency of administration are best determined by measurement of serum levels and assessment of renal insufficiency

Note: Some patients may require larger or more frequent doses if serum levels document the need (ie, cystic fibrosis or febrile granulocytopenic patients)

Administration Parenteral: Administer by intermittent I.V. infusion over 30 minutes at a final concentration not to exceed 5 mg amikacin/mL

Monitoring Parameters Urinalysis, urine output, BUN, serum creatinine, peak and trough serum amikacin concentrations; be alert to ototoxicity

Not all infants and children who receive aminoglycosides require monitoring of serum aminoglycoside concentrations. Indications for use of aminoglycoside serum concentration monitoring include:

- treatment course >5 days
- patients with decreased or changing renal function
- patients with poor therapeutic response
- infants <3 months of age
- atypical body constituency (obesity, expanded extracellular fluid volume)
- clinical need for higher doses or shorter intervals (eg, cystic fibrosis, burns, endocarditis, meningitis, critically ill patients, relatively resistant organisms)
- patients on hemodialysis or chronic ambulatory peritoneal dialysis
- signs of nephrotoxicity or ototoxicity
- concomitant use of other nephrotoxic agents

Reference Range

Peak: 20-30 µg/mL

Trough: <10 µg/mL

Patient Information Report loss of hearing, ringing or roaring in the ears, or feeling of fullness in head

Nursing Implications Aminoglycoside levels measured from blood taken from Silastic® central catheters can sometimes give falsely elevated readings; peak serum levels should be drawn 30 minutes after the end of a 30-minute infusion; trough levels are drawn within 30 minutes before the next dose; provide optimal patient hydration

Dosage Forms Injection, as sulfate: 50 mg/mL (2 mL); 250 mg/mL (2 mL, 4 mL)

References

Kenyon CF, Knoppert DC, Lee SK, et al, "Amikacin Pharmacokinetics and Suggested Dosage Modifications for the Preterm Infant," *Antimicrob Agents Chemother*, 1990, 34(2):265-8.

Public Health Service Task Force on Prophylaxis and Therapy for *Mycobacterium avium* Complex, "Recommendations on Prophylaxis and Therapy for Disseminated *Mycobacterium avium* Complex Disease in Patients Infected With the Human Immunodeficiency Virus," *N Engl J Med*, 1993, 329(12):898-904.

Starke JR and Correa AG, "Management of Mycobacterial Infection and Disease in Children," *Pediatr Infect Dis J*, 1995, 14(6):455-69.

Vogelstein B, Kowarski A, and Lietman PS, "The Pharmacokinetics of Amikacin in Children," *J Pediatr*, 1977, 91(2):333-9.

♦ **Amikacin Sulfate** *see* Amikacin *on page 56*

♦ **Amikin® (Canada)** *see* Amikacin *on page 56*

♦ **Amikin® Injection** *see* Amikacin *on page 56*

Amiloride *(a MIL oh ride)*

Brand Names Midamor®

Available Salts Amiloride Hydrochloride

Therapeutic Category Antihypertensive Agent; Diuretic, Potassium Sparing

Generic Available Yes

Use Management of edema associated with CHF, hepatic cirrhosis, and hyperaldosteronism; hypertension; primary hyperaldosteronism; hypokalemia induced by kaliuretic diuretics

Pregnancy Risk Factor B

Contraindications Hypersensitivity to amiloride or any component; hyperkalemia; anuria

Warnings Due to potential severe hyperkalemia, amiloride should be discontinued in diabetic patients for at least 3 days prior to glucose tolerance testing; discontinue if serum potassium >6.5 mEq/L

Precautions Use with caution in patients with dehydration, electrolyte imbalance, metabolic or respiratory acidosis, diabetes (particularly those with nephropathy), hyponatremia, impaired renal function, or hepatic dysfunction; patients receiving potassium or other potassium-sparing diuretics

Adverse Reactions

Cardiovascular: Angina, orthostatic hypotension, arrhythmia, palpitations

Central nervous system: Headache, dizziness, encephalopathy, vertigo, nervousness, mental confusion, insomnia, depression, somnolence

Dermatologic: Skin rash, pruritus, alopecia

Endocrine & metabolic: Hyperkalemia, hyperchloremic metabolic acidosis, dehydration, hyponatremia, gynecomastia

Gastrointestinal: Nausea, anorexia, diarrhea, vomiting, abdominal pain, appetite changes, constipation, GI bleeding, xerostomia, heartburn, flatulence, dyspepsia

Genitourinary: Impotence, dysuria, urinary frequency, bladder spasms

Hematologic: Aplastic anemia, neutropenia

Hepatic: Abnormal liver function

Neuromuscular & skeletal: Weakness, muscle cramps, joint and back pain, paresthesia, tremors

Ophthalmic: Visual disturbances, increased intraocular pressure

Otic: Tinnitus

Renal: Polyuria

Respiratory: Cough, dyspnea, nasal congestion, shortness of breath

Drug Interactions Potassium, other potassium-sparing diuretics, and ACE inhibitors (eg, captopril) may additively increase the serum potassium; may decrease digoxin clearance and attenuate its inotropic effect; decreases lithium clearance; decreased diuresis and antihypertensive effects with concomitant NSAID use

Food Interactions Avoid natural licorice (causes sodium and water retention and increases potassium loss) and salt substitutes; food decreases absorption to ~30%

Mechanism of Action Acts directly on the distal renal tubule to inhibit sodium-potassium ion exchange; decreases sodium reabsorption in the distal tubule by inhibiting cellular sodium transport mechanisms such as the conductive sodium influx pathway and possibly the sodium-hydrogen ion exchange system; also inhibits hydrogen ion secretion; its diuretic activity is **independent** of aldosterone.

Pharmacodynamics

Onset of action: 2 hours

Peak effect: 6-10 hours

Duration: 24 hours

Pharmacokinetics

Absorption: 50%

Distribution: Adults: V_d: 350-380 L

Metabolism: No active metabolites

Half-life: Adults:

Normal renal function: 6-9 hours

End stage renal disease: 21-144 hours

Elimination: Unchanged drug, equally in urine and feces

Usual Dosage Oral:

Children 6-20 kg: 0.625 mg/kg/day once daily; maximum dose: 10 mg/day

Children >20 kg and Adults: 5-10 mg/day; maximum dose: 20 mg/day

Dosing adjustment in renal impairment:

Cl_{cr} 10-50 mL/minute: Administer at 50% of normal dose

Cl_{cr} <10 mL/minute: Avoid use

Administration Oral: Administer with food or milk

Monitoring Parameters Serum potassium, sodium, creatinine, BUN, blood pressure, fluid balance

Test Interactions May falsely elevate serum digoxin levels done by radioimmunoassay

Patient Information Report to your physician any muscle cramps, weakness, nausea, or dizziness; may cause drowsiness and impair ability to perform hazardous tasks which require mental alertness or physical coordination

Additional Information Studies utilizing aerosolized amiloride (5 mmol/L in 0.3% saline) in adult cystic fibrosis patients (Tomkiewicz, 1993) have suggested that inhaled amiloride is capable of improving the rheologic properties of the abnormally thickened mucus by increasing mucus sodium content

Dosage Forms Tablet, as hydrochloride: 5 mg

Extemporaneous Preparations A 1 mg/mL oral liquid may be prepared from crushed tablets added to a small quantity of sterile water to which glycerin (final concentration of 40% w/v) is added; sterile water is then added in sufficient quantity to make the desired volume; stable 21 days when refrigerated

(Continued)

Amiloride *(Continued)*

Fawcett JP, Woods DJ, Ferry DG, et al, "Stability of Amiloride Hydrochloride Oral Liquids Prepared From Tablets and Powder," *Aust J Hosp Pharm*, 1995, 25:10-23.

References
Tomkiewicz RP, App, EM, Zayas JG, et al, "Amiloride Inhalation Therapy in Cystic Fibrosis. Influence on Ion Content, Hydration, and Rheology of Sputum," *Am Rev Resp Dis*, 1993, 148:1002-7.

♦ **Amiloride Hydrochloride** *see Amiloride on page 58*
♦ **2-Amino-6-mercaptopurine** *see Thioguanine on page 918*
♦ **Aminobenzylpenicillin** *see Ampicillin on page 78*

Aminocaproic Acid (a mee noe ka PROE ik AS id)

Related Information
Carbohydrate and Alcohol Content of Liquid Medications for Use in Patients Receiving Ketogenic Diets *on page 1228*

Brand Names Amicar®

Therapeutic Category Hemostatic Agent

Generic Available Yes: Injection

Use Treatment of excessive bleeding resulting from systemic hyperfibrinolysis, urinary fibrinolysis, or traumatic ocular hyphema

Pregnancy Risk Factor C

Contraindications Disseminated intravascular coagulation; evidence of an intravascular clotting process; injectable product contains benzyl alcohol; avoid use in newborns; use of factor IX concentrate or anti-inhibitor coagulant concentrate

Warnings Aminocaproic acid may accumulate in patients with decreased renal function; intrarenal obstruction may occur secondary to glomerular capillary thrombosis or clots in the renal pelvis and ureters; do not use in hematuria of upper urinary tract origin unless benefits outweigh potential risks; inhibition of fibrinolysis may promote clotting or thrombosis

Precautions Use with caution in patients with cardiac, renal or hepatic disease; use with caution in patients at risk for veno-occlusive disease of the liver

Adverse Reactions

Cardiovascular: Hypotension, bradycardia and arrhythmias (following rapid I.V. administration)

Central nervous system: Dizziness, headache, malaise, seizures, confusion

Dermatologic: Rash

Endocrine & metabolic: Hyperkalemia

Gastrointestinal: GI irritation, nausea, cramps, diarrhea

Hematologic: Decreased platelet function, agranulocytosis, leukopenia

Neuromuscular & skeletal: Myopathy, acute rhabdomyolysis, weakness

Ocular: Glaucoma, watery eyes

Otic: Tinnitus, deafness

Renal: Renal failure

Respiratory: Nasal congestion, dyspnea, pulmonary embolism

Drug Interactions Increased risk of thrombosis with oral contraceptives, estrogens, and factor IX

Mechanism of Action Competitively inhibits activation of plasminogen thereby reducing fibrinolysin, without inhibiting lysis of clot

Pharmacodynamics Onset of action: Fibrinolysis: Within 1-72 hours (onset shortened substantially if loading dose is used)

Pharmacokinetics

Distribution: Widely distributes through intravascular and extravascular compartments

Metabolism: Hepatic metabolism is minimal

Bioavailability: Oral: 100%

Half-life: 1-2 hours

Elimination: 40% to 60% excreted as unchanged drug in the urine within 12 hours

Usual Dosage

Children:

Oral, I.V.: Loading dose: 100-200 mg/kg; maintenance: 100 mg/kg/dose every 6 hours; maximum daily dose: 30 g

or as an alternative: I.V. loading dose: 100 mg/kg or 3 g/m² followed by a continuous infusion of 33.3 mg/kg/hour or 1 g/m²/hour; total dosage should not exceed 18 g/m²/day

Traumatic hyphema: Oral, I.V.: 100 mg/kg/dose every 4 hours (maximum dose: 5 g/dose; maximum daily dose: 30 g/day)

Adults:
　　Oral: For the treatment of acute bleeding syndromes due to elevated fibrinolytic activity, give 5 g during first hour, followed by 1-1.25 g/hour for about 8 hours or until bleeding stops; daily dose should not exceed 30 g
　　I.V.: Give 4-5 g during first hour followed by continuous infusion at the rate of 1-1.25 g/hour, continue for 8 hours or until bleeding stops
Dosing adjustment in renal impairment: Oliguria or ESRD: Reduce dose to 25% of normal

Administration
Oral: May administer without regard to food
Parenteral: Maximum concentration for I.V. administration: 20 mg/mL; administer single doses over at least 1 hour

Monitoring Parameters Fibrinogen, fibrin split products, serum creatinine kinase (long-term therapy); serum potassium (may be elevated by aminocaproic acid, especially if the patient has impaired renal function)

Reference Range Therapeutic concentration: >130 μg/mL (concentration necessary for inhibition of fibrinolysis)

Nursing Implications Rapid I.V. injection (IVP) should be avoided since hypotension, bradycardia, and arrhythmias may result

Dosage Forms
Injection: 250 mg/mL (20 mL, 96 mL, 100 mL)
Syrup (raspberry flavor): 250 mg/mL (480 mL)
Tablet: 500 mg

References
McGetrick JJ, Jampol LM, Goldberg MP, et al, "Aminocaproic Acid Decreases Secondary Hemorrhage After Traumatic Hyphema," *Arch Ophthalmol*, 1983, 101(7):1031-3.

◆ **Aminohydroxypropylidene Diphosphonate** *see* Pamidronate *on page 722*
◆ **Amino-Opti-E® [OTC]** *see* Vitamin E *on page 982*
◆ **Aminophyllin™** *see* Aminophylline *on page 61*

Aminophylline (am in OFF i lin)

Related Information
Adult ACLS Algorithm, Hypotension, Shock *on page 1016*
Asthma Guidelines *on page 1178*
Overdose and Toxicology *on page 1191*
Theophylline *on page 910*

Brand Names Aminophyllin™; Phyllocontin®; Somophyllin®; Truphylline®
Synonyms Theophylline Ethylenediamine
Therapeutic Category Antiasthmatic; Bronchodilator; Respiratory Stimulant; Theophylline Derivative
Generic Available Yes
Use Bronchodilator in reversible airway obstruction due to asthma or COPD; increase diaphragmatic contractility; neonatal idiopathic apnea of prematurity
Pregnancy Risk Factor C
Contraindications Uncontrolled arrhythmias
Warnings Some commercial products may contain sulfites which may produce hypersensitivity reactions in sensitive individuals
Adverse Reactions See Theophylline *on page 910*

Clinical Factors Reported to Affect Theophylline Clearance

Decreased Theophylline Level	Increased Theophylline Level
Smoking (cigarettes, marijuana)	Acute pulmonary edema
High protein/low carbohydrate diet	Cessation of smoking (after chronic use)
Charcoal broiled beef	Cor pulmonale
	Congestive heart failure
	Hypothyroidism
	Fever (≥102° for 24 hours or more, or lesser temperature elevations for longer periods)
	Hepatic cirrhosis/acute hepatitis
	Renal failure in infants <3 mo of age
	Sepsis with multisystem organ failure
	Shock
	Viral illness

(Continued)

Aminophylline *(Continued)*

Drug Interactions Decreases adenosine, benzodiazepines, and pancuronium effects; decreases zafirlukast serum levels; increases lithium clearance; increases central nervous system side effects with ephedrine; increases risk of cardiac arrhythmias with halothane; for medications which change aminophylline (theophylline) clearance, see tables on pages 61 and 62.

Medications Affecting Theophylline Clearance Resulting in Either Increased or Decreased Serum Levels

Decreased Theophylline Level	Increased Theophylline Level
Aminoglutethimide	Alcohol
Carbamazepine	Allopurinol (>600 mg/day)
Isoproterenol (I.V.)	Beta-blockers
Isoniazid*	Calcium channel blockers
Ketoconazole	Cimetidine
Loop diuretics*	Ciprofloxacin
Nevirapine	Clarithromycin
Phenobarbital	Corticosteroids
Phenytoin	Disulfiram
Rifampin	Ephedrine
Ritonavir	Erythromycin
Sulfinpyrazone	Esmolol
Sympathomimetics	Influenza virus vaccine
	Interferon, human recombinant alpha 2-a and 2-b
	Isoniazid*
	Loop diuretics*
	Methotrexate
	Mexiletine
	Oral contraceptives
	Propafenone
	Propranolol
	Tacrine
	Thiabendazole
	Thyroid hormones
	Troleandomycin (TAO®)
	Verapamil
	Zileuton

*Both increased and decreased theophylline levels have been reported.

Food Interactions Food does not appreciably affect absorption; avoid extremes of dietary protein and carbohydrate intake; limit charcoal-broiled foods and caffeinated beverages

Mechanism of Action See Theophylline *on page 910*

Pharmacokinetics Aminophylline is the ethylenediamine salt of theophylline, pharmacokinetic parameters are those of **theophylline**; fraction available: 80% (eg, 100 mg aminophylline = 80 mg theophylline); see Theophylline *on page 910*

Usual Dosage All dosages based upon **aminophylline**

Neonates:

Apnea of prematurity: Oral, I.V.:

Loading dose: 5 mg/kg

Maintenance: Initial: 5 mg/kg/day every 12 hours; increased dosages may be indicated as liver metabolism matures (usually >30 days of life); monitor serum levels to determine appropriate dosages

Theophylline levels should be initially drawn after 3 days of therapy; repeat levels are indicated 3 days after each increase in dosage or weekly if on a stabilized dosage

Infants, Children, and Adults: Treatment of acute bronchospasm: I.V.: Loading dose (in patients not currently receiving aminophylline or theophylline): 6 mg/kg (based on aminophylline) given I.V. over 20-30 minutes

Approximate I.V. maintenance dosages are based upon **continuous infusions**; intermittent dosing (often used in children <6 months of age) may be determined by multiplying the hourly infusion rate by 24 hours and dividing by the desired number of doses/day (usually in 3-4 doses/day)

6 weeks to 6 months: 0.5 mg/kg/hour

6 months to 1 year: 0.6-0.7 mg/kg/hour

1-9 years: 1-1.2 mg/kg/hour

9-12 years and young adult smokers: 0.9 mg/kg/hour

12-16 years: 0.7 mg/kg/hour

Adults (healthy, nonsmoking): 0.7 mg/kg/hour

Older patients and patients with cor pulmonale, patients with congestive heart failure or liver failure: 0.25 mg/kg/hour

Oral dose: See Theophylline *on page 910*, (consider mg theophylline available when using aminophylline products)

Dosage should be adjusted according to serum level measurements during the first 12- to 24-hour period. Avoid using suppositories due to erratic, unreliable absorption. See table.

Guidelines for Drawing Theophylline Serum Levels

Dosage Form	Time to Draw Level*
I.V. bolus	30 min after end of 30-min infusion
I.V. continuous infusion	12-24 h after initiation of infusion
P.O. liquid, fast-release formulation	Peak: 1 h postdose after at least 1 day of therapy Trough: Just before a dose after at least 1 day of therapy
P.O. slow-release formulation	Peak: 4 h postdose after at least 1 day of therapy Trough: Just before a dose after at least 1 day of therapy

*The time to achieve steady-state serum levels is prolonged in patients with longer half-lives (eg, premature neonates, infants, and adults with cardiac or liver failure (see theophylline half-life table). In these patients, serum theophylline levels should be drawn after 48-72 hours of therapy; serum levels may need to be done prior to steady-state to assess the patients current progress or evaluate potential toxicity.

Administration

Oral: Sustained release preparations should be administered with a full glass of water, whole or cut by half only; do not crush; sustained release capsule forms may be opened and sprinkled on soft foods; do not chew or crush beads

Parenteral: Dilute with I.V. fluid to a concentration of 1 mg/mL and infuse over 20-30 minutes; maximum concentration: 25 mg/mL; maximum rate of infusion: 0.36 mg/kg/minute, and no greater than 25 mg/minute

Monitoring Parameters Serum theophylline levels, heart rate, respiratory rate, number and severity of apnea spells (when used for apnea of prematurity); arterial or capillary blood gases (if applicable); pulmonary function tests

Reference Range Therapeutic: For asthma 10-20 µg/mL; for neonatal apnea 6-13 µg/mL (serum levels are reduced for neonatal apnea due to decreased binding of theophylline to fetal albumin resulting in a greater amount of free "active" theophylline)

Dosage Forms Theophylline (anhydrous) equivalent listed in brackets

Injection, I.V. (Aminophyllin™): 25 mg/mL [19.7 mg/mL] (10 mL, 20 mL)

Liquid, oral: 105 mg/5 mL [90 mg/5 mL] (240 mL)

Suppository, rectal (Truphylline®): 250 mg [197.5 mg], 500 mg [395 mg]

Tablet (Aminophyllin™): 100 mg [79 mg], 200 mg [158 mg]

Tablet, controlled release [12 hours] (Phyllocontin®): 225 mg [178 mg]

♦ **5-Aminosalicylic Acid** *see* Mesalamine *on page 608*

Amiodarone (a MEE oh da rone)

Brand Names Cordarone®; Pacerone®

Available Salts Amiodarone Hydrochloride

Therapeutic Category Antiarrhythmic Agent, Class III

Generic Available Yes

Use Management of resistant, life-threatening ventricular arrhythmias (eg, recurrent ventricular fibrillation or hemodynamically unstable ventricular tachycardia) unresponsive to conventional therapy with less toxic agents; treatment of supraventricular arrhythmias unresponsive to conventional therapy

Note: A benzyl alcohol-free injectable product is available from the manufacturer via orphan drug status or compassionate use for acute treatment and prophylaxis of life-threatening ventricular tachycardia or ventricular fibrillation (see Dosage Forms)

Pregnancy Risk Factor D

Contraindications Hypersensitivity to amiodarone or any component; severe sinus node dysfunction; marked sinus bradycardia, second and third degree A-V block; (Continued)

Amiodarone *(Continued)*

cardiogenic shock; bradycardia-induced syncope, except if pacemaker is placed; thyroid disease

Warnings Not considered first-line antiarrhythmic due to high incidence of toxicity; 75% of patients experience adverse effects with large doses. Discontinuation is required in 5% to 20% of patients. Pulmonary and hepatic toxicities may be fatal; reserve for use in life-threatening arrhythmias refractory to other therapy. Optic neuropathy and/or optic neuritis resulting in visual impairment may occur at any time and can progress to permanent blindness; prompt ophthalmic exam is recommended if visual impairment occurs; re-evaluate amiodarone therapy if optic neuropathy or neuritis occurs. Hypotension with I.V. product occurs in about 16% of patients and may be associated with infusion rate. Bradycardia and AV block may occur; temporary pacemaker should be available when I.V. product is used in patients with known predisposition to bradycardia or AV block. Patients should be hospitalized for initiation of therapy and loading dose administration.

Precautions Amiodarone HCl contains 37% iodine by weight; avoid use during pregnancy and while breast-feeding (fetal/neonatal goiters, hypothyroidism, and possible cerebral damage may occur); when possible, hypokalemia and hypomagnesemia should be corrected prior to I.V. amiodarone use due to increased risk for torsade de pointes; use with caution in neonates as injectable product (Cordarone®) contains benzyl alcohol (benzyl alcohol has been associated with neonatal toxicities) and polysorbate (Tween®) 80

Adverse Reactions

Cardiovascular: Proarrhythmia (including torsade de pointes), atropine-resistant bradycardia, heart block, sinus arrest, myocardial depression, CHF, paroxysmal ventricular tachycardia, cardiogenic shock, hypotension (**Note:** In adults, I.V. daily doses >2100 mg are associated with a greater risk of hypotension.)

Central nervous system (20% to 40% incidence): Lack of coordination, fatigue, malaise, abnormal gait, dizziness, headache, insomnia, nightmares, ataxia, behavioral changes, fever

Dermatologic: Discoloration of skin (slate blue), photosensitivity, rash, angioedema

Endocrine & metabolic: Hypothyroidism (or less commonly hyperthyroidism), hyperglycemia, increased triglycerides

Gastrointestinal: Nausea, vomiting, anorexia, constipation

Hematologic: Coagulation abnormalities, thrombocytopenia

Hepatic: Increased liver enzymes, severe hepatic toxicity (potentially fatal), increased bilirubin, increased serum ammonia

Local: Phlebitis (with I.V. formulation; concentration dependent)

Neuromuscular & skeletal: Paresthesia, tremor, peripheral neuropathy (rare)

Ocular: Corneal microdeposits, halos or blurred vision (10% incidence), photophobia, optic neuropathy, optic neuritis, visual impairment, permanent blindness (**Note:** Asymptomatic corneal microdeposits alone do not require dose reduction or discontinuation)

Respiratory (potentially fatal): Interstitial pneumonitis, hypersensitivity pneumonitis, pulmonary fibrosis (may present with cough, fever, dyspnea, malaise, chest x-ray changes); adult respiratory distress syndrome following surgery

Drug Interactions Cytochrome P-450 isoenzyme CYP3A3/4 substrate; isoenzyme CYP2C9, CYP2D6, and CYP3A3/4 inhibitor

Amiodarone inhibits P-450 enzymes and may increase plasma concentrations of digoxin, cyclosporine, flecainide, lidocaine, methotrexate, theophylline, procainamide, quinidine, warfarin, and phenytoin resulting in toxicities. **Note:** Dosage reduction of these agents and follow-up serum concentration monitoring are recommended (eg, a 50% dosage reduction in digoxin, 30% dosage reduction in flecainide, and a 30% to 50% dosage reduction in warfarin have been recommended). Combined use with beta-blockers, digitalis glycosides, or calcium channel blockers may result in bradycardia, sinus arrest; use with class I antiarrhythmics may cause ventricular arrhythmias; amiodarone and general anesthetics may result in bradycardia, hypotension, heart block; phenytoin and cholestyramine may decrease and cimetidine may increase amiodarone serum levels. Concurrent use of amiodarone with ritonavir or nelfinavir is not recommended.

Food Interactions Food increases rate and extent of oral absorption (high fat meal increased AUC by a mean of 2.3 times)

Stability

Storage: Tablets and I.V. product should be kept at room temperature and protected from light during storage; injection should also be protected from excessive heat; there is no need to protect diluted solutions from light during I.V. administration

Compatibility: Injection is compatible in D_5W at concentrations of 1-6 mg/mL for 24 hours in glass or polyolefin bottles and for 2 hours in polyvinyl chloride bags; although amiodarone adsorbs to polyvinyl chloride tubing, all clinical studies used polyvinyl chloride tubing and the recommended doses take adsorption into account, therefore, polyvinyl chloride tubing is recommended; amiodarone I.V. in D_5W is **not** compatible with aminophylline, cefamandole, cefazolin, mezlocillin, heparin, or sodium bicarbonate when administered together at the Y-site (a precipitate will occur)

Mechanism of Action A class III antiarrhythmic agent which inhibits adrenergic stimulation, prolongs the action potential and refractory period in myocardial tissue; decreases A-V conduction and sinus node function

Pharmacodynamics

Onset of effect: Oral: 2-3 days to 1-3 weeks after starting therapy; I.V.: (electrophysiologic effects) within hours; antiarrhythmic effects: 2-3 days to 1-3 weeks; mean onset of effect may be shorter in children vs adults and in patients receiving I.V. loading doses

Maximum effect: Oral: 1 week to 5 months

Duration of effects after discontinuation of oral therapy: Variable, 2 weeks to months: Children: less than a few weeks; adults: several months

Pharmacokinetics

Absorption: Oral: Slow and incomplete

Distribution: Amiodarone and its active metabolite cross the placenta; both distribute to breast milk in concentrations higher than maternal plasma concentrations

  I.V.: Rapid redistribution with a decrease to 10% of peak values within 30-45 minutes after completion of infusion

  V_{dss}: I.V. single dose in adults: Mean range: 40-84 L/kg

  V_d: Oral dose in adults: 66 L/kg: range: 18-148 L/kg

Protein binding: 96%

Metabolism: In the liver and possibly the GI tract via cytochrome P-450 enzymes; the major metabolite N-desethylamiodarone is active

Bioavailability: Oral: ~50% (range: 35% to 65%)

Half-life:

  Amiodarone:

    Single dose in adults: Mean: 58 days (range 15-142 days)

    Oral chronic therapy in adults: Mean range: 40-55 days (range: 26-107 days)

    I.V. single dose in adults: Mean range: 20-47 days

    Half-life is shortened in children vs adults

  N-desethylamiodarone (active metabolite):

    Single dose in adults: Mean: 36 days (range 14-75 days)

    Oral chronic therapy in adults: Mean: 61 days

Elimination: Via biliary excretion; possible enterohepatic recirculation; <1% excreted unchanged in urine

Nondialyzable (parent and metabolite)

Usual Dosage

Infants and Children:

  Oral: **Note:** Calculate dose using body surface area for children <1 year of age: Loading dose: 10-15 mg/kg/day or 600-800 mg/$1.73 \, m^2$/day in 1-2 divided doses/day for 4-14 days or until adequate control of arrhythmia or prominent adverse effects occur; dosage should then be reduced to 5 mg/kg/day or 200-400 mg/$1.73 \, m^2$/day given once daily for several weeks; if arrhythmia does not recur, reduce to lowest effective dosage possible; usual daily minimal dose: 2.5 mg/kg; maintenance doses may be given for 5 of 7 days/week.

  I.V.: Limited data is available. Three retrospective studies (Figa, 1994; Raja, 1994; Soult, 1995) used I.V. loading doses of 5 mg/kg. Loading doses were administered over 1 hour in two of these studies to treat various life-threatening tachyarrhythmias including junctional ectopic tachycardia after cardiac surgery (in conjunction with atrial pacing). Soult 1995 used I.V. amiodarone for short-term treatment of paroxysmal supraventricular tachycardia (PSVT) and administered the loading dose via slow I.V. bolus over 5 minutes. For continuous infusion, Figa 1994 used initial maintenance doses of 5 mcg/kg/minute (7.2 mg/kg/day) and increased incrementally until the desired effect was seen or a maximum dose of 15 mcg/kg/minute (21.6 mg/kg/day) was reached. The mean effective dose in the study (n=30) was 9.5 mcg/kg/minute (13.7 mg/kg/day).

    A recent multicenter study (Perry, 1996; n=40; mean age 5.4 years with 24 of 40 children <2 years of age) used an I.V. loading dose of 5 mg/kg that was divided into five 1 mg/kg aliquots, with each aliquot given over 5-10 minutes.

    Additional 1-5 mg/kg doses could be administered 30 minutes later in a

(Continued)

Amiodarone *(Continued)*

similar fashion if needed. The mean loading dose was 6.3 mg/kg. A maintenance dose (continuous infusion of 10-15 mg/kg/day) was administered to 21 of the 40 patients. Further studies are needed.

Adults:

Ventricular arrhythmias:

Oral: Loading dose: 800-1600 mg/day divided in 1-2 doses/day for 1-3 weeks, then 600-800 mg/day in 1-2 doses for 1 month; maintenance: 400 mg/day; lower doses are recommended for supraventricular arrhythmias.

I.V.: Loading dose: 150 mg given over 10 minutes (at a rate of 15 mg/minute) followed by 360 mg given over 6 hours (at a rate of 1 mg/minute); follow with maintenance dose: 540 mg given over the next 18 hours (at a rate of 0.5 mg/minute); after the first 24 hours the maintenance dose is continued at 0.5 mg/minute; additional supplemental bolus doses of 150 mg infused over 10 minutes may be given for breakthrough VF or hemodynamically unstable VT; maintenance dose infusion may be increased to control arrhythmia

Atrial fibrillation (see Goldschlager, 2000):

Oral: Loading dose: 600-800 mg/day divided in 2 doses/day for 2-4 weeks, then 400 mg/day; at 3-6 months, dose may be reduced further to 100-300 mg/day based on clinical efficacy and adverse effects; usual maintenance: 200 mg/day; **Note:** some patients may require higher maintenance doses or increased maintenance doses for short periods of time for breakthrough arrhythmias; some patients can be maintained with 200 mg/day given for 5 of 7 days/week

Dosing adjustment in renal impairment: No adjustment necessary

Administration

Oral: Administer at same time in relation to meals

I.V.: Injection must be diluted before I.V. use; administer via central venous catheter, if possible; increased phlebitis may occur with peripheral infusions >3 mg/mL in D_5W, but concentrations ≤2.5 mg/mL may be less irritating; the use of a central venous catheter with concentrations >2 mg/mL for infusions >1 hour is recommended; use glass or polyolefin bottles for infusions >2 hours; the use of polyvinyl chloride tubing is recommended (see Stability); must be infused via volumetric infusion device; drop size of I.V. solution may be reduced and underdosage may occur if drop counter infusion sets are used; use in-line filter during administration; adults: Do not exceed 30 mg/minute initial infusion rate; infants and children: See Usual Dosage I.V.

Monitoring Parameters Heart rate and rhythm, blood pressure, EKG, chest x-ray, pulmonary function tests, thyroid function tests, liver enzymes, ophthalmologic exams including fundoscopy and slit-lamp examinations, physical signs and symptoms of thyroid dysfunction (lethargy, edema of hands and feet, weight gain or loss), and pulmonary toxicity (dyspnea, cough)

Reference Range Therapeutic: Chronic oral dosing: 1-2.5 mg/L (SI: 2-4 µmol/L) (parent); desethyl metabolite (active) is present in equal concentration to parent drug; serum levels may not be of great value for predicting toxicity and efficacy; toxicity may occur even at therapeutic concentrations

Patient Information Avoid exposure to sunlight; use sunscreen and sunglasses; may discolor skin to a slate blue color; notify physician if persistent dry cough, shortness of breath, or decreased vision occurs

Nursing Implications Ambulation of patient may be impaired due to adverse effects; due to possible infusion rate-related hypotension, the I.V. infusion rate should be carefully monitored

Additional Information Intoxication with amiodarone necessitates EKG monitoring; bradycardia may be atropine resistant, I.V. isoproterenol or cardiac pacemaker may be required; hypotension, cardiogenic shock, heart block, Q-T prolongation and hepatotoxicity may also be seen; patients should be monitored for several days following overdose due to long half-life

I.V. product is used for acute treatment; the duration of I.V. treatment is usually 48-96 hours, however, in adults, infusions may be used cautiously for 2-3 weeks; there is limited experience with administering infusions for >3 weeks

Thyroid function tests: Amiodarone partially inhibits the peripheral conversion of thyroxine (T_4) to triiodothyronine (T_3); serum T_4 and reverse triiodothyronine (RT_3) concentrations may be increased and serum T_3 may be decreased; most patients remain clinically euthyroid, however, clinical hypothyroidism or hyperthyroidism may occur

Dosage Forms
Injection, as hydrochloride: 50 mg/mL (3 mL); Cordarone® contains benzyl alcohol and polysorbate (Tween®) 80

Injection, as hydrochloride, benzyl alcohol-free and polysorbate-free: 15 mg/mL (10 mL); Amio-Aqueous® contains an aqueous acetate buffer; available via orphan drug status or compassionate use from the manufacturer Academic Pharmaceuticals, Inc (847) 735-1170

Tablet, scored, as hydrochloride: 200 mg

Extemporaneous Preparations
A 5 mg/mL oral suspension can be made from tablets; two stability studies using different vehicles exist; a 5 mg/mL oral suspension made with simple syrup NF containing methylcellulose 1% (50:50, v/v) was stable for 42 days at room temperature (25°C) and 91 days under refrigeration (4°C) in both glass and plastic prescription bottles (Nahata, 1997); label "shake well" and "protect from light"

Five 200 mg tablets were crushed in a mortar; the vehicle (either a 1:1 mixture of Ora-Sweet® and Ora-Plus® or a 1:1 mixture of Ora-Sweet® SF and Ora-Plus®) was adjusted to a pH between 6-7 using a sodium bicarbonate solution (5 g/100 mL of distilled water). A small amount of the vehicle was added to the mortar to make a uniform paste; geometric amounts of the vehicle were added while mixing to **almost** the desired volume; suspension was transferred to a graduate and qsad to 200 mL while mixing. Suspensions prepared in both vehicles were stable for 42 days at room temperature (25°C) and 91 days under refrigeration (4°C) in plastic prescription bottles (Nahata 1999); label "shake well" and "protect from light"

Neither of these 2 studies determined microbial growth; extended storage under refrigeration is recommended

Nahata MC, "Stability of Amiodarone in an Oral Suspension Stored Under Refrigeration and at Room Temperature," *Ann Pharmacother*, 1997, 31(7-8):851-2.

Nahata MC, Morosco RS, and Hipple TF, "Stability of Amiodarone in Extemporaneous Oral Suspensions Prepared From Commercially Available Vehicles," *J Ped Pharmacy Practice*, 1999, 4(4):186-9.

References
Coumel P and Fidelle J, "Amiodarone in the Treatment of Cardiac Arrhythmias in Children: One Hundred Thirty-Five Cases," *Am Heart J*, 1980, 100(6 Pt 2):1063-9.

Figa FH, Gow RM, Hamilton RM, et al, "Clinical Efficacy and Safety of Intravenous Amiodarone in Infants and Children," *Am J Cardiol*, 1994, 74(6):573-7.

Garson A Jr, Gillette PC, McVey P, et al, "Amiodarone Treatment of Critical Arrhythmias in Children and Young Adults," *J Am Coll Cardiol*, 1984, 4(4):749-55.

Goldschlager N, Epstein AE, Naccarelli G, et al, "Practical Guidelines for Clinicians Who Treat Patients With Amiodarone," *Arch Intern Med*, 2000, 160(12):1741-8.

Paul T and Guccione P, "New Antiarrhythmic Drugs in Pediatric Use: Amiodarone," *Pediatr Cardiol*, 1994, 15(3):132-8.

Perry JC, Fenrich AL, Hulse JE, et al, "Pediatric Use of Intravenous Amiodarone: Efficacy and Safety in Critically Ill Patients From a Multicenter Protocol," *J Am Coll Cardiol*, 1996, 27(5):1246-50.

Raja P, Hawker RE, Chaikitpinyo A, et al, "Amiodarone Management of Junctional Ectopic Tachycardia After Cardiac Surgery in Children," *Br Heart J*, 1994, 72(3):261-5.

Shahar E, Barzilay Z, Frand M, et al, "Amiodarone in Control of Sustained Tachyarrhythmias in Children With Wolff-Parkinson-White Syndrome," *Pediatrics*, 1983, 72(6):813-6.

Shuler CO, Case CL, and Gillette PC, "Efficacy and Safety of Amiodarone in Infants," *Am Heart J*, 1993, 125(5 Pt 1):1430-2.

Soult JA, Munoz M, Lopez JD, et al, "Efficacy and Safety of Intravenous Amiodarone for Short-Term Treatment of Paroxysmal Supraventricular Tachycardia in Children," *Pediatr Cardiol*, 1995, 16(1):16-9.

♦ **Amiodarone Hydrochloride** *see* Amiodarone *on page 63*

♦ **Amitone® [OTC]** *see* Calcium Supplements *on page 157*

Amitriptyline (a mee TRIP ti leen)
Related Information
Comparison of Adverse Effects of Antidepressants *on page 1030*

Comparison of Usual Adult Dosage and Mechanism of Action of Antidepressants *on page 1029*

Drugs and Breast-Feeding *on page 1213*

Overdose and Toxicology *on page 1191*

Serotonin Syndrome *on page 1217*

Brand Names Apo®-Amitriptyline (Canada); Elavil®; Enovil®; Levate® (Canada); Novo-Tryptin® (Canada)

Available Salts Amitriptyline Hydrochloride

Therapeutic Category Antidepressant, Tricyclic; Antimigraine Agent

Generic Available Yes

Use Treatment of various forms of depression, often in conjunction with psychotherapy; analgesic for certain chronic and neuropathic pain; migraine prophylaxis
(Continued)

Amitriptyline *(Continued)*

Pregnancy Risk Factor D

Contraindications Hypersensitivity to amitriptyline (cross-sensitivity with other tricyclics may occur) or any component; narrow-angle glaucoma; patients receiving MAO inhibitors within past 14 days

Warnings Do not discontinue abruptly in patients receiving high doses chronically

Precautions Use with caution in patients with cardiac conduction disturbances, cardiovascular disease, seizure disorders, narrow-angle glaucoma, history of urinary retention or bowel obstruction, hepatic or renal dysfunction, hyperthyroidism or those receiving thyroid hormone replacement; degree of sedation, anticholinergic effects, and risk of orthostatic hypotension are very high relative to other antidepressants

Adverse Reactions Anticholinergic effects may be pronounced; moderate to marked sedation can occur (tolerance to these effects usually occurs)

Cardiovascular: Postural hypotension, arrhythmias, tachycardia, sudden death

Central nervous system: Sedation, fatigue, anxiety, confusion, insomnia, impaired cognitive function, seizures; extrapyramidal symptoms are possible

Dermatologic: Photosensitivity, urticaria, rash

Endocrine & metabolic: Rarely SIADH

Gastrointestinal: Xerostomia, constipation, decrease of lower esophageal sphincter tone, GE reflux, increased appetite, weight gain

Genitourinary: Urinary retention, discoloration of urine (blue-green)

Hematologic: Rarely agranulocytosis, leukopenia, eosinophilia

Hepatic: Increased liver enzymes, cholestatic jaundice

Neuromuscular & skeletal: Tremor, weakness

Ocular: Blurred vision, increased intraocular pressure

Miscellaneous: Allergic reactions

Drug Interactions Cytochrome P-450 isoenzyme CYP1A2, CYP2C9, CYP2C19, CYP2D6 and CYP3A3/4 substrate

Amitriptyline may decrease the effects of clonidine and guanethidine; with clonidine, hypertensive crisis may occur following discontinuation of clonidine; amitriptyline may increase the effects of CNS depressants (including alcohol), adrenergic agents (epinephrine, isoproterenol), anticholinergic agents and warfarin. With MAO inhibitors, hyperpyrexia, tachycardia, hypertension, confusion, seizures, and death have been reported. Cimetidine, fluoxetine, and methylphenidate may decrease the metabolism and phenobarbital, carbamazepine, and rifampin may increase the metabolism of amitriptyline; amitriptyline may potentiate the cardiac effects of cisapride (do not administer concurrently)

Food Interactions Riboflavin dietary requirements may be increased

Stability Protect injection and Elavil® 10 mg tablets from light; store injection at <40°C (preferably 15°C to 30°C)

Mechanism of Action Increases the synaptic concentration of serotonin and/or norepinephrine in the central nervous system by inhibition of their reuptake by the presynaptic neuronal membrane

Pharmacodynamics Onset of action: Therapeutic antidepressant effects begin in 7-21 days; maximum effects may not occur for ≥2 weeks and as long as 4-6 weeks

Pharmacokinetics

Absorption: Oral: Rapid, well absorbed

Distribution: Crosses placenta; enters breast milk

Protein binding: >90%

Metabolism: In the liver to nortriptyline (active), hydroxy derivatives and conjugated derivatives

Half-life, adults: 9-25 hours (15-hour average)

Time to peak serum concentration: Within 4 hours

Elimination: Renal excretion of 18% as unchanged drug; small amounts eliminated in feces by bile

Nondialyzable

Usual Dosage

Chronic pain management: Children: Oral: Initial: 0.1 mg/kg at bedtime, may advance as tolerated over 2-3 weeks to 0.5-2 mg/kg at bedtime

Depressive disorders: Oral:

Children: Investigationally initial doses of 1 mg/kg/day given in 3 divided doses with increases to 1.5 mg/kg/day have been reported in a small number of children (n=9) 9-12 years of age; clinically, doses up to 3 mg/kg/day (5 mg/kg/day if monitored closely) have been proposed

Adolescents: Initial: 25-50 mg/day; may give in divided doses; increase gradually to 100 mg/day in divided doses; maximum dose: 200 mg/day

Adults:
  Oral: 30-100 mg/day single dose at bedtime or in divided doses; dose may be
    gradually increased up to 300 mg/day; once symptoms are controlled,
    decrease gradually to lowest effective dose
  I.M.: 20-30 mg 4 times/day

Administration
  Oral: May administer with food to decrease GI upset
  Parenteral: Administer by I.M. route only; do not administer I.V.

Monitoring Parameters Heart rate, blood pressure, mental status, weight

Reference Range Note: Plasma levels do not always correlate with clinical effec-
tiveness
  Therapeutic:
    Amitriptyline plus nortriptyline (active metabolite): 100-250 ng/mL (SI: 360-900
      nmol/L)
    Nortriptyline 50-150 ng/mL (SI: 190-570 nmol/L)
  Toxic: >500 ng/mL (SI: >1800 nmol/L)

Patient Information Avoid alcohol; limit caffeine intake; may cause drowsiness
and impair ability to perform activities requiring mental alertness or coordination;
may cause dry mouth; do not discontinue abruptly; may discolor urine to a blue-
green color

Additional Information Due to promotion of weight gain with amitriptyline, other
antidepressants (ie, imipramine or desipramine) may be preferred in heavy or
obese children and adolescents

Dosage Forms
  Injection, as hydrochloride: 10 mg/mL (10 mL)
  Tablet, as hydrochloride: 10 mg, 25 mg, 50 mg, 75 mg, 100 mg, 150 mg

References
Elser JM and Woody RC, "Migraine Headache in the Infant and Young Child," *Headache*, 1990,
  30(6):366-8.
Kashani JH, Shekim WO, and Reid JC, "Amitriptyline in Children With Major Depressive Disorder: A
  Double-Blind Crossover Pilot Study," *J Am Acad Child Psychiatry*, 1984, 23(3):348-51.
Levy HB, Harper CR, and Weinberg WA, "A Practical Approach to Children Failing in School," *Pediatr
  Clin North Am*, 1992, 39(4):895-928.

♦ **Amitriptyline Hydrochloride** *see* Amitriptyline *on page 67*
♦ **Ammonapse** *see* Sodium Phenylbutyrate *on page 873*

Ammonium Chloride (a MOE nee um KLOR ide)

Synonyms NH_4Cl

Therapeutic Category Metabolic Alkalosis Agent; Urinary Acidifying Agent

Generic Available Yes

Use Diuretic or systemic and urinary acidifying agent; treatment of hypochloremic
states

Pregnancy Risk Factor C

Contraindications Severe hepatic and renal dysfunction; patients with primary
respiratory acidosis

Adverse Reactions
  Cardiovascular: Bradycardia
  Central nervous system: Mental confusion, coma, headache
  Dermatologic: Rash
  Endocrine & metabolic: Metabolic acidosis secondary to hyperchloremia
  Gastrointestinal: GI irritation
  Local: Pain at site of injection
  Respiratory: Hyperventilation

Drug Interactions Chlorpropamide's effects may be enhanced due to decreased
urinary excretion; may decrease flecainide levels due to increased urinary excretion; systemic acidosis may occur when used with spironolactone

Mechanism of Action Its dissociation to ammonium and chloride ions increases
acidity by increasing free hydrogen ion concentration which combines with bicarbonate ion to form CO_2 and water; the net result is the replacement of bicarbonate
ions by chloride ions

Pharmacokinetics
  Absorption: Rapid from the GI tract with absorption being complete in 3-6 hours
  Metabolism: In the liver
  Elimination: In urine

Usual Dosage Children and Adults: I.V.: The following equations represent different
methods of chloride or alkalosis correction utilizing either the serum HCO_3^-, the
serum Cl^- or the base excess
  (Continued)

Ammonium Chloride *(Continued)*

Correction of refractory hypochloremic metabolic alkalosis: mEq NH_4Cl = 0.5 L/kg x wt in kg x [serum HCO_3^- - 24] mEq/L; give $^1/_2$ to $^2/_3$ of the calculated dose, then re-evaluate

Correction of hypochloremia: mEq NH_4Cl = 0.2 L/kg x wt in kg x [103 - serum Cl^-] mEq/L, give $^1/_2$ to $^2/_3$ of calculated dose, then re-evaluate

Correction of alkalosis via base excess method: mEq NH_4Cl = 0.3 L/kg x wt in kg x base excess (mEq/L), give $^1/_2$ to $^2/_3$ of calculated dose, then re-evaluate

Children: Oral, I.V.: 75 mg/kg/day in 4 divided doses for urinary acidification; maximum daily dose: 6 g

Adults:
Oral: 2-3 g every 6 hours; maximum daily dose: 12 g
I.V.: 1.5 g/dose every 6 hours

Administration
Oral: Administer dose after meals
Parenteral: Dilute to 0.2 mEq/mL and infuse I.V. over 3 hours; maximum concentration: 0.4 mEq/mL; maximum rate of infusion: 1 mEq/kg/hour

Monitoring Parameters Serum electrolytes, serum ammonia

Nursing Implications Rapid I.V. injection may increase the likelihood of ammonia toxicity

Dosage Forms
Injection: 26.75% [5 mEq/mL] (20 mL)
Tablet: 500 mg
Tablet, enteric coated: 500 mg

♦ **Ammonium Molybdate** *see* Trace Metals *on page 940*

Amoxicillin (a moks i SIL in)

Related Information
Carbohydrate and Alcohol Content of Liquid Medications for Use in Patients Receiving Ketogenic Diets *on page 1228*
Endocarditis Prophylaxis *on page 1127*

Brand Names Amoxil®; Apo®-Amoxi (Canada); Biomox®; Novamoxin® (Canada); Nu-Amoxi® (Canada); Polymox®; Pro-Amox® (Canada); Trimox®; Wymox®

Synonyms Amoxycillin; *p*-Hydroxyampicillin

Therapeutic Category Antibiotic, Penicillin

Generic Available Yes

Use Treatment of otitis media, sinusitis, and infections involving the respiratory tract, skin, and urinary tract due to susceptible *H. influenzae*, *N. gonorrhoeae*, *E. coli*, *P. mirabilis*, *E. faecalis*, streptococci, and nonpenicillinase-producing staphylococci; treatment of Lyme disease in children <8 years of age; prophylaxis of bacterial endocarditis

Pregnancy Risk Factor B

Contraindications Hypersensitivity to amoxicillin, penicillin, or any component

Warnings Epstein-Barr virus infection, acute lymphocytic leukemia or cytomegalovirus infection increases risk for amoxicillin-induced maculopapular rash

Precautions In patients with renal dysfunction, doses and/or frequency of administration should be modified in response to the degree of renal impairment; use with caution in patients with history of cephalosporin allergy

Adverse Reactions
Central nervous system: Fever
Dermatologic: Rash, exfoliative dermatitis, Stevens-Johnson syndrome, urticaria
Gastrointestinal: Diarrhea, nausea, vomiting, pseudomembranous colitis
Hematologic: Anemia, neutropenia, eosinophilia, thrombocytopenia, prolongation of bleeding time
Miscellaneous: Superinfection, hypersensitivity reactions, serum sickness, vasculitis, anaphylaxis

Drug Interactions Probenecid (increases serum amoxicillin concentration); allopurinol may increase frequency for amoxicillin rash; decreases oral contraceptive efficacy

Food Interactions Food does not interfere with absorption

Stability Suspensions are stable for 14 days at room temperature or if refrigerated; refrigeration is preferred

Mechanism of Action Interferes with bacterial cell wall synthesis during active multiplication by binding to one or more of the penicillin-binding proteins, causing cell wall death and resultant bactericidal activity against susceptible bacteria

Pharmacokinetics
Absorption: Oral: Rapid and nearly complete

Distribution: Into liver, lungs, prostate, muscle, middle ear effusions, maxillary sinus secretions, bile, and into ascitic and synovial fluids; excreted into breast milk

Protein binding: 17% to 20%, lower in neonates

Half-life:

Neonates, full-term: 3.7 hours

Infants and children: 1-2 hours

Adults with normal renal function: 0.7-1.4 hours

Patients with Cl_{cr} <10 mL/minute: 7-21 hours

Metabolism: Partial

Time to peak serum concentration:

Capsule: Within 2 hours

Suspension: Neonates: 3-4.5 hours; children: 1 hour

Elimination: Renal excretion (80% unchanged drug)

Moderately dialyzable (20% to 50%); ~30% removed by 3-hour hemodialysis; supplemental dose is recommended after hemodialysis

Usual Dosage Oral:

Neonates and Infants: ≤3 months: 20-30 mg/kg/day in divided doses every 12 hours

Infants >3 months and Children: 25-50 mg/kg/day in divided doses every 8 hours or 25-50 mg/kg/day in divided doses every 12 hours; doses as high as 80-90 mg/kg/day divided every 12 hours have been used to treat acute otitis media due to highly resistant strains of S. pneumoniae

Uncomplicated gonorrhea:

<2 years, probenecid is contraindicated in this age group

≥2 years: 50 mg/kg plus probenecid 25 mg/kg as a single dose

Endocarditis prophylaxis: 50 mg/kg 1 hour before procedure, not to exceed adult dose

Adults: 250-500 mg every 8 hours or 500-875 mg tablets twice daily; maximum dose: 2-3 g/day

Uncomplicated gonorrhea: 3 g plus probenecid 1 g as a single dose

Endocarditis prophylaxis: 2 g 1 hour before procedure

Dosing interval in renal impairment:

Cl_{cr} 10-30 mL/minute: Administer every 12 hours

Cl_{cr} <10 mL/minute: Administer every 24 hours

Administration Oral: May be administered on an empty or full stomach; may be mixed with formula, milk, or juice; shake suspension well before use

Monitoring Parameters With prolonged therapy, monitor renal, hepatic, and hematologic function periodically; monitor for diarrhea

Additional Information Appearance of a rash should be carefully evaluated to differentiate a nonallergic amoxicillin rash from a hypersensitivity reaction. Rash occurs in 5% to 10% of children receiving amoxicillin and is a generalized dull, red, maculopapular rash, generally appearing 3-14 days after the start of therapy. It normally begins on the trunk and spreads over most of the body. It may be most intense at pressure areas, elbows, and knees. Incidence of rash is higher in patients with viral infections, cytomegalovirus infections, infectious mononucleosis, lymphocytic leukemia, or patients with hyperuricemia who are receiving allopurinol.

Dosage Forms

Capsule, as trihydrate: 250 mg, 500 mg

Powder for oral suspension, as trihydrate: 125 mg/5 mL (80 mL, 100 mL, 150 mL, 200 mL); 200 mg/5 mL (5 mL, 50 mL, 75 mL, 100 mL); 250 mg/5 mL (80 mL, 100 mL, 150 mL, 200 mL); 400 mg/5 mL (5 mL, 50 mL, 75 mL, 100 mL)

Powder for oral suspension, drops, as trihydrate: 50 mg/mL (15 mL, 30 mL)

Tablet, chewable, as trihydrate: 125 mg, 200 mg, 250 mg, 400 mg

Tablet, film coated, as trihydrate: 500 mg, 875 mg

References

Boguniewicz M and Leung DY, "Hypersensitivity Reactions to Antibiotics Commonly Used in Children," Pediatr Infect Dis J, 1995, 14(3):221-31.

Canafax, DM, Yuan Z, Chonmaitree T, et al, "Amoxicillin Middle Ear Fluid Penetration and Pharmacokinetics in Children with Acute Otitis Media," Pediatr Infect Dis J, 1998, 17(2):149-56.

Dajani AS, Taubert KA, Wilson WW, et al, "Prevention of Bacterial Endocarditis. Recommendations by the American Heart Association," JAMA, 1997, 277(22):1794-1801.

Amoxicillin and Clavulanic Acid

(a moks i SIL in & klav yoo LAN ic AS id)

Related Information

Carbohydrate and Alcohol Content of Liquid Medications for Use in Patients Receiving Ketogenic Diets on page 1228

Brand Names Augmentin®; Clavulin® (Canada)

Available Salts Amoxicillin Trihydrate and Clavulanate Potassium

(Continued)

Amoxicillin and Clavulanic Acid *(Continued)*

Synonyms Clavulanic Acid and Amoxicillin

Therapeutic Category Antibiotic, Beta-lactam and Beta-lactamase Combination; Antibiotic, Penicillin

Generic Available No

Use Infections caused by susceptible organisms involving the lower respiratory tract, otitis media, sinusitis, skin and skin structure, and urinary tract; spectrum same as amoxicillin in addition to beta-lactamase producing *M. catarrhalis, H. influenzae, N. gonorrhoeae,* and *S. aureus* (not MRSA)

Pregnancy Risk Factor B

Contraindications Hypersensitivity to amoxicillin, clavulanic acid, penicillins, or any component; concomitant use of disulfiram; history of amoxicillin/clavulanic acid-associated cholestatic jaundice or hepatic dysfunction

Warnings Epstein-Barr virus infection, acute lymphocytic leukemia or cytomegalovirus infection increase the risk for amoxicillin-induced maculopapular rash

Precautions Use with caution in patients with history of cephalosporin hypersensitivity; in patients with renal dysfunction, doses and/or frequency of administration should be modified in response to the degree of renal impairment; avoid using the "BID" formulation in patients with phenylketonuria since it contains phenylalanine

Adverse Reactions

Central nervous system: Headache

Dermatologic: Rash, urticaria, exfoliative dermatitis, Stevens-Johnson syndrome

Gastrointestinal: Nausea, vomiting, pseudomembranous colitis; incidence of diarrhea (9%) is higher than with amoxicillin alone

Genitourinary: Vaginal candidiasis

Hepatic: Elevated AST, ALT, alkaline phosphatase, and bilirubin

Miscellaneous: Superinfection, hypersensitivity reactions, serum sickness, vasculitis, anaphylaxis

Drug Interactions Probenecid (increases serum amoxicillin concentration), allopurinol, disulfiram

Stability Reconstituted oral suspension should be refrigerated; discard unused suspension after 10 days

Mechanism of Action Clavulanic acid binds and inhibits beta-lactamases that inactivate amoxicillin resulting in amoxicillin having an expanded spectrum of activity; amoxicillin interferes with bacterial cell wall synthesis by binding to one or more of the penicillin-binding proteins and causing cell wall death

Pharmacokinetics

Absorption: Both amoxicillin and clavulanate are well absorbed

Distribution: Both widely distributed into lungs, pleural, peritoneal, synovial, and ascitic fluid as well as bone, gynecologic tissue, and middle ear fluid; crosses the placenta; excreted in breast milk

Metabolism: Clavulanic acid: Metabolized in the liver

Half-life of both agents in adults with normal renal function: ~1 hour; amoxicillin pharmacokinetics are not affected by clavulanic acid

Time to peak serum concentration: Within 2 hours

Elimination: Amoxicillin: Excreted primarily unchanged in the urine

Dialysis: ~30% of amoxicillin removed by 3-hour hemodialysis; supplemental dose recommended after hemodialysis

Usual Dosage Oral (dosing based on amoxicillin component):

Neonates and Infants <3 months: 30 mg/kg/day divided every 12 hours using the 125 mg/5 mL suspension

Children <40 kg: 20-40 mg (amoxicillin component)/kg/day in divided doses every 8 hours **or** 25-45 mg (amoxicillin component)/kg/day divided every 12 hours using either 200 mg/5 mL or 400 mg/5 mL suspension, or 200 mg, 400 mg chewable tablet formulation; 80-90 mg/kg/day divided every 12 hours has been used for multidrug-resistant pneumococcal otitis media (use a 7:1, "BID" formulation)

Adults:

Less severe infection: 250 mg every 8 hours or 500 mg every 12 hours

More severe infections and respiratory tract infections: 500 mg every 8 hours or 875 mg every 12 hours

Dosing interval in renal impairment:

Cl_{cr} 10-30 mL/minute: Administer 250-500 mg every 12 hours; do not administer the 875 mg tablet

Cl_{cr} <10 mL/minute: Administer 250-500 mg every 24 hours

Administration Oral: Administer at the start of a meal to decrease the frequency or severity of GI side effects; may mix with milk, formula, or juice; shake suspension well before use

Monitoring Parameters With prolonged therapy, monitor renal, hepatic, and hematologic function periodically

Test Interactions May interfere with urinary glucose determinations using Clinitest®

Patient Information Adverse GI effects may occur less frequently if taken with food

Additional Information Potassium content: 0.16 mEq of potassium per 31.25 mg of clavulanic acid; since both the 250 mg and 500 mg tablets contain the same amount of clavulanic acid, two 250 mg tablets are not equivalent to one 500 mg tablet; the "q12h" chewable tablet and oral suspension (200 mg, 400 mg) formulations contain phenylalanine

Appearance of a rash should be carefully evaluated to differentiate a nonallergic amoxicillin rash from a hypersensitivity reaction. Rash occurs in 5% to 10% of children receiving amoxicillin and is a generalized dull, red, maculopapular rash, generally appearing 3-14 days after the start of therapy. It normally begins on the trunk and spreads over most of the body. It may be most intense at pressure areas, elbows, and knees. Incidence of rash is higher in patients with viral infections, *Salmonella* infections, lymphocytic leukemia, or patients with hyperuricemia who are receiving allopurinol.

Dosage Forms

Suspension, oral (banana flavor):

   125: Amoxicillin, as trihydrate, 125 mg and clavulanic potassium 31.25 mg per 5 mL (75 mL, 150 mL)

   200: Amoxicillin, as trihydrate, 200 mg and clavulanic potassium 28.5 mg per 5 mL (50 mL, 75 mL, 100 mL) ["BID" formulation]

   250: Amoxicillin, as trihydrate, 250 mg and clavulanic potassium 62.5 mg per 5 mL (75 mL, 150 mL)

   400: Amoxicillin, as trihydrate, 400 mg and clavulanic potassium 57 mg per 5 mL (50 mL, 75 mL, 100 mL) ["BID" formulation]

Tablet:

   250: Amoxicillin, as trihydrate, 250 mg and clavulanic potassium 125 mg

   500: Amoxicillin, as trihydrate, 500 mg and clavulanic potassium 125 mg

   875: Amoxicillin, as trihydrate, 875 mg and clavulanic potassium 125 mg: ["BID" formulation]

Tablet, chewable:

   125: Amoxicillin, as trihydrate, 125 mg and clavulanic potassium 31.25 mg

   200: Amoxicillin, as trihydrate, 200 mg and clavulanic potassium 28.5 mg: ["BID" formulation]

   250: Amoxicillin, as trihydrate, 250 mg and clavulanic potassium 62.5 mg

   400: Amoxicillin, as trihydrate, 400 mg and clavulanic potassium 57 mg: ["BID" formulation]

References

Gan VN, Kusmiesz H, Shelton S, et al, "Comparative Evaluation of Loracarbef and Amoxicillin-Clavulanate for Acute Otitis Media," *Antimicrob Agents Chemother*, 1991, 35(5):967-71.

Hoberman A, Paradise JL, Burch DJ, et al, "Equivalent Efficiency and Reduced Occurrence of Diarrhea From a New Formulation of Amoxicillin/Clavulanate Potassium (Augmentin®) for Treatment of Acute Otitis Media in Children," *Pediatr Infect Dis J*, 1997, 16(5):463-70.

Reed MD, "Clinical Pharmacokinetics of Amoxicillin and Clavulanate," *Pediatr Infect Dis J*, 1996, 15(10):949-54.

Thoene DE and Johnson CE, "Pharmacotherapy of Otitis Media," *Pharmacotherapy*, 1991, 11(3):212-21.

Todd PA and Benfield P, "Amoxicillin/Clavulanic Acid. An Update of Its Antibacterial Activity, Pharmacokinetic Properties and Therapeutic Use," *Drugs*, 1990, 39(2):264-307.

♦ **Amoxicillin Trihydrate and Clavulanate Potassium** *see* Amoxicillin and Clavulanic Acid *on page 71*

♦ **Amoxil®** *see* Amoxicillin *on page 70*

♦ **Amoxycillin** *see* Amoxicillin *on page 70*

♦ **Amphetamine and Dextroamphetamine** *see* Dextroamphetamine and Amphetamine *on page 302*

♦ **Amphetamine Aspartate, Amphetamine Sulfate, Dextroamphetamine Saccharate, and Dextroamphetamine Sulfate** *see* Dextroamphetamine and Amphetamine *on page 302*

♦ **Amphojel® [OTC]** *see* Antacid Preparations *on page 86*

Amphotericin B, Conventional

(am foe TER i sin bee con VEN sha nal)

Brand Names Fungizone®

Therapeutic Category Antifungal Agent, Systemic; Antifungal Agent, Topical

Generic Available Yes

Use Treatment of severe systemic infections and meningitis caused by susceptible fungi such as *Candida* species, *Histoplasma capsulatum*, *Cryptococcus neoformans*, *Aspergillus* species, *Mucor* species, *Blastomyces dermatitidis*, *Torulopsis glabrata*, *Sporothrix schenckii*, *Paracoccidioides brasiliensis*, and *Coccidioides immitis*; fungal peritonitis; irrigant for bladder fungal infections; treatment of amebic meningoencephalitis caused by *Naegleria fouleri*; topically for cutaneous and mucocutaneous candidal infections

Pregnancy Risk Factor B

Contraindications Hypersensitivity to amphotericin or any component

Warnings I.V. amphotericin is used primarily for the treatment of patients with progressive and potentially fatal fungal infections; not to be used for common clinically inapparent forms of fungal disease; anaphylaxis has been reported with amphotericin B-containing drugs; facilities for cardiopulmonary resuscitation should be available during administration due to the possibility of anaphylactic reaction

Precautions Due to the nephrotoxic potential of amphotericin, other nephrotoxic drugs should be avoided

Adverse Reactions

Cardiovascular: Hypotension, hypertension, cardiac arrhythmias, flushing

Central nervous system: Fever, chills, and headache are the most common adverse effects reported with amphotericin B infusion; delirium, seizures, malaise

Endocrine & metabolic: Hypokalemia, hypomagnesemia

Gastrointestinal: Anorexia, nausea, vomiting, steatorrhea, weight loss

Hematologic: Anemia, leukopenia, thrombocytopenia

Hepatic: Acute hepatic failure, jaundice

Local: Phlebitis

Renal: Renal tubular acidosis, renal failure (oliguria, azotemia, elevated serum creatinine)

Respiratory: Wheezing, hypoxemia

Miscellaneous: Anaphylactoid reaction

Adverse effects due to intrathecal amphotericin:

Central nervous system: Headache, pain along lumbar nerves, arachnoiditis

Gastrointestinal: Nausea, vomiting

Genitourinary: Urinary retention

Neuromuscular & skeletal: Paresthesia, leg and back pain, foot drop

Ocular: Vision changes

Drug Interactions Nephrotoxic drugs may cause additive toxic effects; corticosteroids may increase potassium depletion caused by amphotericin; may predispose patients receiving cardiac glycosides or skeletal muscle relaxants to toxicity secondary to hypokalemia; imidazole derivatives (eg, miconazole, fluconazole, ketoconazole) may antagonize the effect and induce fungal resistance to amphotericin; may increase toxicity of flucytosine by increasing cellular uptake and/or impairing its renal excretion; may potentiate renal toxicity, bronchospasm, and hypotension of antineoplastic agents

Stability Reconstitute only with sterile water without preservatives, not bacteriostatic water; benzyl alcohol, sodium chloride, or other electrolyte solutions may cause precipitation; can be diluted in D_5W, $D_{10}W$, up to $D_{20}W$; for I.V. infusion, an in-line filter (>1 micron mean pore diameter) may be used; irrigating solutions should be diluted in sterile water; short-term exposure (<24 hours) to light during I.V. infusion does **not** appreciably affect potency

Mechanism of Action Binds to ergosterol altering cell membrane permeability in susceptible fungi and causing leakage of cell components with subsequent cell death

Pharmacokinetics

Absorption: Poor oral absorption

Distribution: Minimal amounts enter the aqueous humor, bile, amniotic fluid, pericardial fluid, pleural fluid, and synovial fluid; poor CSF penetration

Protein binding: 90%

Half-life: Increased in small neonates and young infants

Initial: 15-48 hours

Terminal phase: 15 days

Elimination: 2% to 4% of dose eliminated in urine unchanged; ~40% eliminated over 7-day period and may be detected in urine for up to 8 weeks after discontinued use

Poorly dialyzed

Usual Dosage Medication errors, including deaths, have resulted from confusion between lipid-based forms of amphotericin (Abelcet™, Amphotec®, AmBisome®) and conventional amphotericin B for injection; conventional amphotericin B for injection doses should not exceed 1.5 mg/kg/day

Neonates, Infants, and Children:

I.V.: Test dose: 0.1 mg/kg/dose to a maximum of 1 mg; infuse over 20-60 minutes; an alternative method to the 0.1 mg/kg test dose is to initiate therapy with 0.25 mg/kg amphotericin administered over 6 hours; frequent observation of the patient and assessment of vital signs during the first several hours of the infusion is recommended

Initial therapeutic dose: If the 0.1 mg/kg test dose is tolerated without the occurrence of serious adverse effects, a therapeutic dose of 0.4 mg/kg can be given the same day as the test dose

The daily dose can then be gradually increased, usually in 0.25 mg/kg increments on each subsequent day until the desired daily dose is reached; in critically ill patients, more rapid dosage acceleration (up to 0.5 mg/kg increments on each subsequent day) may be warranted

Maintenance dose: 0.25-1 mg/kg/day given once daily; infuse over 2-6 hours; rapidly progressing disease may require short-term use of doses to 1.5 mg/kg/day; once therapy has been established, amphotericin B can be administered on an every-other-day basis at 1-1.5 mg/kg/dose

Intrathecal, intraventricular, or intracisternal (preferably into the lateral ventricles through a cisternal Ommaya reservoir): 25-100 mcg every 48-72 hours; increase to 500 mcg as tolerated

Adults:

I.V.: Test dose: 1 mg infused over 20-30 minutes

Initial therapeutic dose (if the test dose is tolerated): 0.25 mg/kg

The daily dose can then be gradually increased, usually in 0.25 mg/kg increments on each subsequent day until the desired daily dose is reached

Maintenance dose: 0.25-1 mg/kg/day once daily, infuse over 2-6 hours; or 1-1.5 mg/kg/dose every other day; do not exceed 1.5 mg/kg/day

Intrathecal, intraventricular, or intracisternal (preferably into the lateral ventricles through a cisternal Ommaya reservoir): 25-100 mcg every 48-72 hours; increase to 500 mcg as tolerated

Children and Adults:

Bladder irrigation: 5-15 mg amphotericin/100 mL of sterile water irrigation solution at 100-300 mL/day. Fluid is instilled into the bladder; the catheter is clamped for 60-120 minutes and the bladder drained. Perform irrigation 3-4 times/day for 2-5 days.

Dialysate: 1-4 mg/L of peritoneal dialysis fluid either with or without low-dose I.V. amphotericin B therapy

Topical: Apply to affected areas 2-4 times/day

Note: Amphotericin B has been administered intranasally to reduce the frequency of invasive aspergillosis in neutropenic patients; 7 mg amphotericin B in 7 mL sterile water was placed in a De Vilbiss atomizer and the aerosolized solution was instilled intranasally to each nostril 4 times/day delivering an average of 5 mg amphotericin/day

Dosing adjustment in renal impairment: Dosage adjustments are not necessary with pre-existing renal impairment; if decreased renal function is due to amphotericin, the daily dose can be decreased by 50% or the dose can be given every other day. Therapy may be held until serum creatinine concentrations begin to decline.

Administration Parenteral: Amphotericin is administered by I.V. infusion over 2-3 hours (range: 1-6 hours) at a final concentration not to exceed 0.1 mg/mL through a peripheral venous catheter; in patients unable to tolerate a large fluid volume, amphotericin B at a final concentration not to exceed 0.5 mg/mL in D_5W or $D_{10}W$ may be administered through a central venous catheter

Monitoring Parameters BUN and serum creatinine levels should be determined every other day while therapy is increased and at least weekly thereafter; serum potassium and magnesium should be monitored closely; monitor electrolytes, liver function, hematocrit, CBC regularly; monitor input and output; monitor for signs of hypokalemia (muscle weakness, cramping, drowsiness, EKG changes, etc); blood pressure, temperature, pulse, respiration

(Continued)

Amphotericin B, Conventional *(Continued)*

Patient Information Amphotericin cream may slightly discolor skin and stain clothing; personal hygiene is very important to help reduce the spread and recurrence of lesions; avoid covering topical applications with occlusive bandages; most skin lesions require 1-3 weeks of therapy

Nursing Implications Cardiovascular collapse has been reported after rapid amphotericin injection; may premedicate patients who experience mild adverse reactions with acetaminophen and diphenhydramine 30 minutes prior to the amphotericin infusion. Meperidine and ibuprofen may help to reduce fevers and chills. Hydrocortisone can be added to the infusion solution to reduce febrile and other systemic reactions.

Additional Information Amphotericin B-induced nephrotoxicity may be minimized by sodium loading with 10-15 mL/kg of NS infused prior to each amphotericin B dose or pentoxifylline, and avoiding use of other nephrotoxic agents

Dosage Forms
Cream: 3% (20 g)
Lotion: 3% (30 mL)
Ointment, topical: 3% (20 g)
Powder for injection, lyophilized: 50 mg

References

The Ad Hoc Advisory Panel on Peritonitis Management. "Continuous Ambulatory Peritoneal Dialysis (CAPD) Peritonitis Treatment Recommendations: 1989 Update," *Perit Dial Int*, 1989, 9(4):247-56.

Benson JM and Nahata MC, "Pharmacokinetics of Amphotericin B in Children," *Antimicrob Agents Chemother*, 1989, 33(11):1989-93.

Bianco JA, Almgren J, Kern DL, et al, "Evidence That Oral Pentoxifylline Reverses Acute Renal Dysfunction in Bone Marrow Transplant Recipients Receiving Amphotericin B and Cyclosporine," *Transplantation*, 1991, 51(4):925-7.

Branch RA, "Prevention of Amphotericin B-Induced Renal Impairment. A Review on the Use of Sodium Supplementation," *Arch Intern Med*, 1988, 148(11):2389-94.

Jeffery GM, Beard ME, Ikram RB, et al, "Intranasal Amphotericin B Reduces the Frequency of Invasive Aspergillosis in Neutropenic Patients," *Am J Med*, 1991, 90(6):685-92.

Kintzel PE and Smith GH, "Practical Guidelines for Preparing and Administering Amphotericin B," *Am J Hosp Pharm*, 1992, 49(5):1156-64.

Koren G, Lau A, Klein J, et al, "Pharmacokinetics and Adverse Effects of Amphotericin B in Infants and Children," *J Pediatr*, 1988, 113(3):559-63.

Amphotericin B Lipid Complex

(am foe TER i sin bee LIP id KOM pleks)

Brand Names Abelcet™

Synonyms ABLC

Therapeutic Category Antifungal Agent, Systemic

Generic Available No

Use Treatment of aspergillosis or invasive fungal infections in patients who are refractory to or intolerant of conventional amphotericin B therapy (refractory to or intolerant is defined as renal dysfunction with a serum creatinine ≥1.5 mg/dL that develops during therapy, or disease progression after a total dose of conventional amphotericin B of at least 10 mg/kg). This indication is primarily based on results of emergency studies for the treatment of aspergillosis; may be useful in the treatment of hepatosplenic candidiasis and cryptococcal meningitis.

Pregnancy Risk Factor B

Contraindications Hypersensitivity to amphotericin B, dimyristoylphosphatidylcholine (DMPC) and dimyristoylphosphatidylglycerol (DMPG) which are two phospholipids in the formulation, or any component

Warnings Anaphylaxis has been reported with amphotericin B-containing drugs; facilities for cardiopulmonary resuscitation should be available during administration due to the possibility of anaphylactic reaction

Precautions Due to the nephrotoxic potential of amphotericin B, other nephrotoxic drugs should be avoided

Adverse Reactions
Cardiovascular: Hypotension, cardiac arrest, arrhythmias, flushing
Central nervous system: Headache; transient chills and fever and during infusion of the drug are the most common effects reported with ABLC
Dermatologic: Rash, pruritus
Endocrine & metabolic: Hypokalemia, bilirubinemia, hypomagnesemia
Gastrointestinal: Diarrhea, abdominal pain
Hematologic: Thrombocytopenia, leukopenia, anemia
Renal: Renal tubular acidosis, elevated serum creatinine (occurs to a lesser degree than with conventional amphotericin B), azotemia, oliguria
Respiratory: Dyspnea, respiratory failure
Miscellaneous: Anaphylactoid and other allergic reactions

Drug Interactions Nephrotoxic drugs may cause additive nephrotoxic effects; corticosteroids may increase potassium depletion caused by amphotericin; may predispose patients receiving cardiac glycosides or skeletal muscle relaxants to toxicity secondary to hypokalemia; may increase myelotoxicity and nephrotoxicity of zidovudine; imidazole derivatives (eg, miconazole, fluconazole, ketoconazole) may antagonize the effect and induce fungal resistance to amphotericin; may increase toxicity of flucytosine by increasing cellular uptake and/or impairing its renal excretion; may potentiate renal toxicity, bronchospasm, and hypotension of antineoplastic agents

Stability Prior to admixture, refrigerate vial and protect from light; diluted ABLC infusion solution is stable up to 15 hours refrigerated and an additional 6 hours at room temperature. Do not freeze. Do not dilute with saline solutions or mix with other drugs or electrolytes.

Mechanism of Action Binds to ergosterol altering cell membrane permeability in susceptible fungi and causing leakage of cell components with subsequent cell death

Pharmacokinetics Exhibits nonlinear kinetics; volume of distribution and clearance from blood increases with increasing dose
Distribution: High tissue concentration found in the liver, spleen, and lung
Half-life, terminal: 173 hours
Elimination: 0.9% of dose excreted in urine over 24 hours; effects of hepatic and renal impairment on drug disposition are unknown
ABLC is not hemodialyzable

Usual Dosage Children and Adults: I.V.: 2.5-5 mg/kg given as a once daily infusion
Dosing adjustment in renal failure: Renal toxicity is dose dependent; there are no firm guidelines for dose adjustment based on lab test results (serum creatinine levels).

Administration Parenteral: I.V.: Prior to administration, assure serum potassium is >3.2 mEq/L; do not use an in-line filter less than 5 microns; administer at a rate of 2.5 mg/kg/hour (over 2 hours) at a final concentration of 1 mg/mL in D_5W. A maximum concentration of 2 mg/mL may be used in fluid-restricted patients

Monitoring Parameters BUN, serum creatinine, liver function tests, serum electrolytes, CBC; vital signs, I & O; monitor for signs of hypokalemia (muscle weakness, cramping, drowsiness, EKG changes, etc)

Nursing Implications If infusion time exceeds 2 hours, mix the contents by gently rotating the infusion bag every 2 hours.

Additional Information Management of side effects is similar to conventional amphotericin B. (See Amphotericin B, Conventional *on page 74* for suggested management guidelines of side effects.)

Dosage Forms Injection: 100 mg of Abelcet™ in 20 mL of suspension (single use only)

References
De Marie S, "Clinical Use of Liposomal and Lipid-Complexed Amphotericin B," *J Antimicrob Chemother*, 1994, 33(5):907-16.
Kline S, Larsen TA, Fieber L, et al, "Limited Toxicity of Prolonged Therapy With High Doses of Amphotericin B Lipid Complex," *Clin Infect Dis*, 1995, 21(5):1154-8.

Amphotericin B Liposome (am foe TER i sin bee LYE po som)

Brand Names AmBisome®
Synonyms L-AmB
Therapeutic Category Antifungal Agent, Systemic
Use Treatment of aspergillosis, candidiasis, or cryptococcosis in patients who are refractory to or intolerant of conventional amphotericin B therapy (refractory to or intolerant is defined as renal dysfunction with a serum creatinine ≥1.5 mg/dL that develops during therapy, or disease progression after a total dose of conventional amphotericin B of at least 10 mg/kg); empiric therapy for presumed fungal infection in febrile, neutropenic bone marrow transplant patients or febrile, neutropenic acute nonlymphocytic leukemia patients after an unsuccessful trial of antibiotics; treatment of suspected or proven fungal infections in patients with renal impairment

Pregnancy Risk Factor B
Contraindications Hypersensitivity to amphotericin B or any component
Warnings Anaphylaxis has been reported with amphotericin B-containing drugs; facilities for cardiopulmonary resuscitation should be available during administration due to the possibility of anaphylactic reaction
Precautions Due to the nephrotoxic potential of amphotericin B, other nephrotoxic drugs should be avoided
(Continued)

Amphotericin B Liposome *(Continued)*

Adverse Reactions

Cardiovascular: Hypotension, arrhythmias, chest pain, cardiac arrest, vasodilatation

Central nervous system: Headache, transient chills or rigors (18%), fever (17%), anxiety, insomnia, dizziness, hallucinations

Dermatologic: Pruritus, rash, diaphoresis

Endocrine & metabolic: Hypokalemia, bilirubinemia, hypomagnesemia, hyperglycemia, hypocalcemia

Gastrointestinal: Diarrhea, nausea, vomiting

Hematologic: Anemia, thrombocytopenia

Hepatic: Elevated ALT, AST, and alkaline phosphatase

Renal: Renal tubular acidosis, elevated serum creatinine and BUN (19%; occurs to a lesser degree than with conventional amphotericin B), oliguria, hematuria

Respiratory: Dyspnea, respiratory failure, cough

Miscellaneous: Anaphylactoid and other allergic reactions

Drug Interactions Nephrotoxic drugs may cause additive nephrotoxic effects; corticosteroids may increase potassium depletion caused by amphotericin; may predispose patients receiving cardiac glycosides or skeletal muscle relaxants to toxicity secondary to hypokalemia; may result in acute pulmonary toxicity in patients simultaneously receiving leukocyte transfusions; ketoconazole, fluconazole may induce fungal resistance to amphotericin B; may increase toxicity of flucytosine by increasing cellular uptake and/or impairing its renal excretion; may potentiate renal toxicity, bronchospasm and hypotension of antineoplastic agents

Stability Store unopened vials under refrigeration; reconstituted drug is stable for 24 hours under refrigeration. Do not dilute with saline solutions or mix with other drugs or electrolytes since this may cause precipitation of AmBisome®. AmBisome® is stable when further diluted to a concentration of 0.5-2.2 mg/mL in D_5W, $D_{10}W$, and $D_{20}W$ for 72 hours at room temperature or when further diluted in D_5W for 14 days if refrigerated

Pharmacokinetics Exhibits nonlinear kinetics (greater than proportional increase in serum concentration with an increase in dose)

Distribution: V_d: 0.1-0.16 L/kg

Half-life (terminal): 100-153 hours

Usual Dosage Children and Adults: I.V.: 3-5 mg/kg/day given as a once daily infusion; doses as high as 6 mg/kg/day have been used in patients with documented *Aspergillus* infection

Administration Parenteral: I.V.: Do not use in-line filter less than 1 micron to administer AmBisome®. Flush line with D_5W prior to infusion; infusion of diluted AmBisome® should start within 6 hours of preparation; infuse over 2 hours; infusion time may be reduced to 1 hour in patients who tolerate the treatment; AmBisome® may be diluted with D_5W, $D_{10}W$, or $D_{20}W$ to a final concentration of 1-2 mg/mL; lower concentrations (0.2-0.5 mg/mL) may be administered to infants and small children to provide sufficient volume for infusion

Monitoring Parameters BUN, serum creatinine, liver function tests, serum electrolytes, CBC, vital signs, I & O; monitor for signs of hypokalemia (muscle weakness, cramping, drowsiness, EKG changes)

Nursing Implications See Amphotericin B, Conventional *on page 74* for suggested management guidelines of side effects.

Dosage Forms Injection: 50 mg

References

Emminger W, Graninger W, Emminger-Schmidmeir W, et al, "Tolerance of High Dosses of Amphotericin B by Infusion of a Liposomal Formulation in Children With Cancer," *Ann Hematol*, 1994, 68:27-31.

Ringden O, Andstrom E, Remberger M, et al, "Safety of Liposomal Amphotericin B (AmBisome®) In 187 Transplant Recipients Treated With Cyclosporin," *Bone Marrow Transplant*, 1994, 14 Suppl 5:S10-4.

Walsh TJ, Finberg RW, Arndt C, et al, "Liposomal Amphotericin B for Empirical Therapy in Patients With Persistent Fever and Neutropenia," *N Engl J Med*, 1999, 340:764-71.

Ampicillin *(am pi SIL in)*

Related Information

Carbohydrate and Alcohol Content of Liquid Medications for Use in Patients Receiving Ketogenic Diets *on page 1228*

Endocarditis Prophylaxis *on page 1127*

Brand Names Ampicin® [Sodium] (Canada); Apo®-Ampi [Trihydrate] (Canada); Jaa Amp® [Trihydrate] (Canada); Marcillin®; Nu-Ampi® [Trihydrate] (Canada); Omnipen®; Omnipen®-N; Penbritin® (Canada); Polycillin®; Polycillin-N®; Principen®; Pro-Ampi® [Trihydrate] (Canada); Taro-Ampicillin® [Trihydrate] (Canada); Totacillin®; Totacillin®-N

Synonyms Aminobenzylpenicillin
Therapeutic Category Antibiotic, Penicillin
Generic Available Yes
Use Treatment of susceptible bacterial infections caused by streptococci, pneumo-cocci, enterococci, nonpenicillinase-producing staphylococci, *Listeria*, meningo-cocci; some strains of *H. influenzae*, *P. mirabilis*, *Salmonella*, *Shigella*, *E. coli*, *Enterobacter*, and *Klebsiella*; initial empiric treatment of neonates with suspected bacterial sepsis or meningitis used in combination with an aminoglycoside or cefotaxime; endocarditis prophylaxis
Pregnancy Risk Factor B
Contraindications Hypersensitivity to ampicillin (penicillins) or any component
Warnings Epstein-Barr virus infection, acute lymphocytic leukemia or cytomegalo-virus infection increases risk for ampicillin-induced maculopapular rash
Precautions Dosage adjustment may be necessary in patients with renal impair-ment (Cl_{cr} <10-15 mL/minute); use with caution in patients allergic to cephalosporins
Adverse Reactions
Central nervous system: Seizures, headache, dizziness, drug fever
Dermatologic: Rash, urticaria, exfoliative dermatitis, Stevens-Johnson syndrome
Gastrointestinal: Diarrhea (20%), nausea, vomiting, glossitis, pseudomembranous enterocolitis, oral candidiasis
Hematologic: Eosinophilia, hemolytic anemia, thrombocytopenia, neutropenia, prolongation of bleeding time
Renal: Interstitial nephritis
Miscellaneous: Anaphylaxis, hypersensitivity reactions, serum sickness, vasculitis, superinfection
Drug Interactions Estrogen-containing oral contraceptives (decreases contracep-tive effectiveness), aminoglycosides, probenecid (increases ampicillin serum levels), chloroquine (decreases bioavailability of ampicillin), allopurinol (possible increased frequency of ampicillin rash)
Food Interactions Food decreases rate and extent of absorption
Stability Oral suspension is stable for 14 days under refrigeration; reconstituted solutions for I.M. or direct I.V. should be used within 1 hour; solutions for I.V. infusion will be inactivated by dextrose at room temperature; if dextrose-containing solutions are to be used as a diluent, the resultant solution will only be stable for 2 hours vs 8 hours in solutions containing NS
Mechanism of Action Interferes with bacterial cell wall synthesis by binding to one or more penicillin-binding proteins during active multiplication; inhibits the final transpeptidation step of peptidoglycan synthesis causing cell wall death and resultant bactericidal activity against susceptible bacteria
Pharmacokinetics
Absorption: Oral: 50%
Distribution: Into bile; penetration into CSF occurs with inflamed meninges only; low excretion into breast milk
Protein binding:
Neonates: 10%
Adults: 15% to 18%
Half-life:
Neonates:
2-7 days: 4 hours
8-14 days: 2.8 hours
15-30 days: 1.7 hours
Children and Adults: 1-1.8 hours
Anuric patients: 8-20 hours
Time to peak serum concentration: Oral: Within 1-2 hours following administration
Elimination: ~90% of drug excreted unchanged in urine within 24 hours; excreted in bile
~40% is removed by hemodialysis; excreted in bile
Usual Dosage
Children: Oral: 50-100 mg/kg/day divided every 6 hours; maximum dose: 2-3 g/day
Adults: Oral: 250-500 mg every 6 hours
Neonates: I.M., I.V.:
Postnatal age ≤7 days:
≤2000 g: 50 mg/kg/day divided every 12 hours; meningitis: 100 mg/kg/day divided every 12 hours
>2000 g: 75 mg/kg/day divided every 8 hours; meningitis: 150 mg/kg/day divided every 8 hours
Group B streptococcal meningitis: 200 mg/kg/day divided every 8 hours
(Continued)

Ampicillin *(Continued)*

Postnatal age >7 days:

    <1200 g: 50 mg/kg/day divided every 12 hours; meningitis: 100 mg/kg/day divided every 12 hours

    1200-2000 g: 75 mg/kg/day divided every 8 hours; meningitis: 150 mg/kg/day divided every 8 hours

    >2000 g: 100 mg/kg/day divided every 6 hours; meningitis: 200 mg/kg/day divided every 6 hours

Group B streptococcal meningitis: 300 mg/kg/day divided every 6 hours

Infants and Children: I.M., I.V.: 100-200 mg/kg/day divided every 6 hours; meningitis: 200-400 mg/kg/day divided every 6 hours; maximum dose: 12 g/day

Endocarditis prophylaxis:

    50 mg/kg within 30 minutes before procedure (dental, oral, respiratory tract, or esophageal procedures)

    50 mg/kg plus gentamicin 1.5 mg/kg within 30 minutes of starting the procedure; 25 mg/kg 6 hours later (for high-risk patients undergoing genitourinary and GI tract procedures)

Adults: I.M., I.V.: 500 mg to 3 g every 6 hours; maximum dose: 14 g/day

Endocarditis prophylaxis:

    2 g within 30 minutes before procedure (dental, oral, respiratory tract, or esophageal procedures)

    2 g plus gentamicin 1.5 mg/kg (maximum dose: 120 mg) within 30 minutes of starting the procedure; 1 g 6 hours later (for high-risk patients undergoing genitourinary and GI tract procedures)

Dosing interval in renal impairment:

    Cl_{cr} 10-30 mL/minute: Administer every 6-12 hours

    Cl_{cr} <10 mL/minute: Administer every 12 hours

Adults: I.M., I.V.: 500 mg to 3 g every 4-6 hours

Dosing interval in renal impairment: Adults:

    Cl_{cr} 10-30 mL/minute: Administer every 6-12 hours

    Cl_{cr} <10 mL/minute: Administer every 12 hours

Administration

Oral: Administer with water 1-2 hours prior to food on an empty stomach; shake suspension well before using

Parenteral: Ampicillin may be administered IVP over 3-5 minutes at a rate not to exceed 100 mg/minute or I.V. intermittent infusion over 15-30 minutes; final concentration for I.V. administration should not exceed 100 mg/mL (IVP) or 30 mg/mL (I.V. intermittent infusion)

Monitoring Parameters With prolonged therapy monitor renal, hepatic, and hematologic function periodically; observe for change in bowel frequency

Test Interactions False-positive urinary glucose (Benedict's solution, Clinitest®); + Coombs' [direct]

Nursing Implications Ampicillin and gentamicin should not be mixed in the same I.V. tubing or administered concurrently

Additional Information Appearance of a rash should be carefully evaluated to differentiate a nonallergic ampicillin rash from a hypersensitivity reaction. Ampicillin rash occurs in 5% to 10% of children receiving ampicillin and is a generalized dull red, maculopapular rash, generally appearing 3-14 days after the start of therapy. It normally begins on the trunk and spreads over most of the body. It may be most intense at pressure areas, elbows, and knees. Incidence of ampicillin rash is higher in patients with viral infections, infectious mononucleosis, lymphocytic leukemia, or patients with hyperuricemia who are receiving allopurinol.

Sodium content of suspension (250 mg/5 mL, 5 mL): 10 mg (0.4 mEq)

Sodium content of 1 g: 66.7 mg (3 mEq)

Dosage Forms

Capsule, as anhydrous: 250 mg, 500 mg

Capsule, as trihydrate: 250 mg, 500 mg

Powder for injection, as sodium: 125 mg, 250 mg, 500 mg, 1 g, 2 g, 10 g

Powder for oral suspension, as trihydrate: 125 mg/5 mL (5 mL unit dose, 80 mL, 100 mL, 150 mL, 200 mL); 250 mg/5 mL (5 mL unit dose, 80 mL, 100 mL, 150 mL, 200 mL); 500 mg/5 mL (5 mL unit dose, 100 mL)

Powder for oral suspension, drops, as trihydrate: 100 mg/mL (20 mL)

References

Boguniewicz M and Leung DY, "Hypersensitivity Reactions to Antibiotics Commonly Used in Children," *Pediatr Infect Dis J*, 1995, 14(3):221-31.

Brown RD, Campoli-Richards DM, "Antimicrobial Therapy in Neonates, Infants, and Children," *Clin Pharmacokinet*, 1989, 17(Suppl 1):105-15.

Ampicillin and Sulbactam (am pi SIL in & SUL bak tam)

Brand Names Unasyn®

Available Salts Ampicillin Sodium and Sulbactam Sodium

Synonyms Sulbactam and Ampicillin

Therapeutic Category Antibiotic, Beta-lactam and Beta-lactamase Combination; Antibiotic, Penicillin

Generic Available No

Use Treatment of susceptible bacterial infections involved with skin and skin structure, intra-abdominal infections, gynecological infections; spectrum is that of ampicillin plus organisms producing beta-lactamases such as *S. aureus*, *H. influenzae*, *E. coli*, *Klebsiella*, *Acinetobacter*, *Enterobacter*, and anaerobes

Pregnancy Risk Factor B

Contraindications Hypersensitivity to ampicillin, sulbactam, any component, or penicillins

Warnings Epstein-Barr virus infection, acute lymphocytic leukemia or cytomegalovirus infection increases risk for ampicillin-induced maculopapular rash; not FDA approved for children <12 years of age

Precautions Modify dosage in patients with renal impairment; use with caution in patients allergic to cephalosporins

Adverse Reactions

Cardiovascular: Chest pain

Central nervous system: Fatigue, malaise, headache, chills, dizziness

Dermatologic: Rash (2%), itching, urticaria, exfoliative dermatitis, Stevens-Johnson syndrome

Gastrointestinal: Diarrhea (3%), nausea, vomiting, candidiasis, flatulence, pseudomembranous colitis, hairy tongue

Genitourinary: Dysuria, hematuria

Hematologic: Decreased WBC, neutrophils, platelets, hemoglobin, and hematocrit

Hepatic: Increased liver enzymes

Local: Pain at injection site (I.M.: 16%, I.V.: 3%), thrombophlebitis (3%)

Renal: Elevated BUN, elevated serum creatinine

Miscellaneous: Hypersensitivity reactions, anaphylaxis, serum sickness, vasculitis, superinfection

Drug Interactions Probenecid (decreased elimination of ampicillin and sulbactam); allopurinol (possible increased frequency of ampicillin rash); efficacy of oral contraceptives may be reduced

Stability Ampicillin/sulbactam infusion solution is stable for 8 hours in NS at room temperature; incompatible when mixed with aminoglycosides

Mechanism of Action The addition of sulbactam, a beta-lactamase inhibitor, to ampicillin extends the spectrum of ampicillin to include beta-lactamase producing organisms; ampicillin acts by inhibiting bacterial cell wall synthesis during the stage of active multiplication

Pharmacokinetics

Distribution: Into bile, blister and tissue fluids; poor penetration into CSF with uninflamed meninges; higher concentrations attained with inflamed meninges

Protein binding:
Ampicillin: 28%
Sulbactam: 38%

Half-life: Ampicillin and sulbactam are similar: 1-1.8 hours and 1-1.3 hours, respectively in patients with normal renal function

Elimination: ~75% to 85% of both drugs are excreted unchanged in urine within 8 hours following administration

Usual Dosage Unasyn® (ampicillin/sulbactam) is a combination product; each 3 g vial contains 2 g of ampicillin and 1 g of sulbactam. Sulbactam has very little antibacterial activity by itself, but effectively extends the spectrum of ampicillin to include beta-lactamase producing strains that are resistant to ampicillin alone; therefore, dosage recommendations for Unasyn® are based on the **ampicillin** component.

I.M., I.V.:

Infants ≥1 month: 100-150 mg/kg/day divided every 6 hours
Meningitis: 200-300 mg/kg/day divided every 6 hours
Children: 100-200 mg ampicillin/kg/day divided every 6 hours
Meningitis: 200-400 mg/kg/day divided every 6 hours; maximum dose: 8 g ampicillin/day
Adults: 1-2 g ampicillin every 6-8 hours; maximum dose: 12 g ampicillin/day
Dosing interval in renal impairment:
Cl_{cr} 15-29 mL/minute: Administer every 12 hours
(Continued)

Ampicillin and Sulbactam *(Continued)*

Cl_{cr} 5-14 mL/minute: Administer every 24 hours

Administration Parenteral: May be administered by slow I.V. injection over 10-15 minutes at a final concentration for administration not to exceed 45 mg Unasyn® (30 mg ampicillin and 15 mg sulbactam)/mL

Monitoring Parameters With prolonged therapy monitor hematologic, renal, and hepatic function; observe for change in bowel frequency

Test Interactions False-positive urinary glucose levels (Benedict's solution, Clinitest®)

Additional Information Sodium content of 1.5 g (1 g ampicillin plus 0.5 g sulbactam): 5 mEq

Dosage Forms Powder for injection: 1.5 g [ampicillin sodium 1 g and sulbactam sodium 0.5 g]; 3 g [ampicillin sodium 2 g and sulbactam sodium 1 g]

References

Dajani AS, "Sulbactam/Ampicillin in Pediatric Infections," *Drugs*, 1988, 35(Suppl 7):35-8.

Goldfarb J, Aronoff SC, Jaffé A, et al, "Sultamicillin in the Treatment of Superficial Skin and Soft Tissue Infections in Children," *Antimicrob Agents Chemother*, 1987, 31(4):663-4.

Kulhanjian J, Dunphy MG, Hamstra S, et al, "Randomized Comparative Study of Ampicillin/Sulbactam vs Ceftriaxone for Treatment of Soft Tissue and Skeletal Infections in Children," *Pediatr Infect Dis J*, 1989, 8(9):605-10.

Syriopoulou V, Bitsi M, Theodoridis C, et al, "Clinical Efficacy of Sulbactam/Ampicillin in Pediatric Infections Caused by Ampicillin-Resistant or Penicillin-Resistant Organisms," *Rev Infect Dis*, 1986, 8(Suppl 5):S630-3.

♦ **Ampicillin Sodium and Sulbactam Sodium** *see* Ampicillin and Sulbactam *on page 81*

♦ **Ampicin® [Sodium] (Canada)** *see* Ampicillin *on page 78*

Amprenavir *(am PRE na veer)*

Related Information

Adult and Adolescent HIV *on page 1133*
Pediatric HIV *on page 1129*

Brand Names Agenerase®

Therapeutic Category Antiretroviral Agent; HIV Agents (Anti-HIV Agents); Protease Inhibitor

Generic Available No

Use Treatment of HIV infection in combination with other antiretroviral agents (Note: HIV regimens consisting of **three** antiretroviral agents are strongly recommended)

Pregnancy Risk Factor C

Contraindications Hypersensitivity to amprenavir or any component; concurrent therapy with astemizole, bepridil, cisapride, dihydroergotamine, ergotamine, midazolam, or triazolam; due to the high amount of propylene glycol, amprenavir oral **solution** is contraindicated in infants and children <4 years, pregnancy, renal or hepatic failure, and in patients receiving disulfiram or metronidazole

Warnings Amprenavir is a potent CYP3A isoenzyme inhibitor that interacts with numerous drugs. Due to potential serious and/or life-threatening drug interactions, some drugs are contraindicated (see Contraindications and Drug interactions) and the following drugs require concentration monitoring if coadministered with amprenavir: amiodarone, systemic lidocaine, tricyclic antidepressants, and quinidine. Concurrent use with rifampin or certain cholesterol-lowering agents (lovastatin, simvastatin) is not recommended.

Amprenavir oral solution contains a high amount of propylene glycol and should only be used when the capsules or other protease inhibitors are not options; women and certain ethnic groups (Native Americans, Eskimos, Asians) may have a decreased capacity to metabolize propylene glycol and therefore, may be at a higher risk for adverse effects of propylene glycol; when using the oral solution, monitor patients for propylene glycol adverse effects (see Monitoring Parameters); change patient to capsule formulation as soon as patient is able to take capsules.

Severe and life-threatening skin reactions (eg, Stevens-Johnson syndrome) may occur; discontinue amprenavir in patients who develop severe or life-threatening rashes or in patients with moderate rashes and systemic symptoms. Spontaneous bleeding episodes have been reported in patients with hemophilia type A and B receiving protease inhibitors. New onset diabetes mellitus, exacerbations of diabetes, and hyperglycemia have been reported in HIV-infected patients receiving protease inhibitors. Acute hemolytic anemia has been reported.

Precautions Use with caution in patients with diabetes mellitus, sulfonamide allergy, hepatic impairment, or hemophilia. Capsules and oral solution contain high amounts of vitamin E; additional supplements of vitamin E should be avoided.

Adverse Reactions

Central nervous system: Depression or mood disorders (4% to 15%), headache, fatigue

Dermatologic: Rash (28% incidence; usually mild to moderate, maculopapular, some pruritic; median onset: 10 days, range: 7-73 days), Stevens-Johnson syndrome (1% of patients, 4% of patients who develop a rash)

Endocrine & metabolic: Hyperglycemia (37% to 41%), hypertriglyceridemia (36% to 47%), hypercholesterolemia (4% to 9%), new onset diabetes, exacerbation of diabetes mellitus; central redistribution of body fat: central obesity, buffalo hump, facial atrophy, and breast enlargement

Gastrointestinal: Nausea (38% to 73%), vomiting (20% to 29%), diarrhea (33% to 56%), taste disorders (1% to 10%)

Hematologic: Acute hemolytic anemia (rare, one case reported), spontaneous bleeding in hemophiliacs

Neuromuscular & skeletal: Paresthesia (perioral or peripheral)

Drug Interactions Cytochrome P-450 isoenzyme CYP3A4 substrate and inhibitor

Amprenavir may inhibit the metabolism of the following drugs and cause serious or life-threatening adverse effects: Astemizole, bepridil, cisapride, dihydroergotamine, ergotamine, midazolam, and triazolam (concurrent therapy with these drugs and amprenavir is contraindicated); amprenavir may increase the toxic effects of amiodarone, lidocaine, quinidine, warfarin, and tricyclic antidepressants (serum concentration monitoring of these drugs is necessary); amprenavir significantly increases the AUC of rifabutin by 193% (rifabutin dose should be decreased by at least $\frac{1}{2}$ the recommended dose when used in combination with amprenavir); amprenavir may increase the AUC of ketoconazole and zidovudine and decrease the AUC of indinavir and saquinavir; amprenavir may increase serum concentrations or toxicity of diltiazem, nifedipine, alprazolam, clorazepate, diazepam, flurazepam, itraconazole, dapsone, erythromycin, loratadine, sildenafil, carbamazepine, pimozide, and cholesterol-lowering agents (concurrent use of lovastatin or simvastatin is not recommended)

Rifampin significantly reduces amprenavir plasma concentrations (AUC decreased 82%) and should not be used concurrently; the herbal medicine, St John's wort (*Hypericum perforatum*), may significantly decrease concentrations of amprenavir and is not recommended for concurrent use; efavirenz decreases amprenavir concentrations by 39%; saquinavir decreases amprenavir AUC by 32%; phenobarbital, phenytoin, or carbamazepine may decrease amprenavir concentrations; abacavir, clarithromycin, indinavir, ketoconazole, or zidovudine may increase the AUC of amprenavir; nelfinavir may increase the trough concentrations of amprenavir; cimetidine or ritonavir may increase amprenavir concentrations

Amprenavir may decrease the efficacy of hormonal contraceptives (reliable barrier method should be used); antacids or didanosine should be given at least 1 hour before or after amprenavir; vitamin E supplements should be avoided (amprenavir products contain high amounts of vitamin E); alcohol may interact with the high amount of propylene glycol in the oral solution and should be avoided

Food Interactions A high fat meal may decrease mean AUC by 14%

Stability Store at room temperature

Mechanism of Action A protease inhibitor which acts on an enzyme (protease) late in the HIV replication process after the virus has entered into the cell's nucleus; amprenavir binds to the protease activity site and inhibits the activity of the enzyme, thus preventing cleavage of viral polyprotein precursors (gag-pol protein precursors) into individual functional proteins found in infectious HIV; this results in the formation of immature, noninfectious viral particles

Pharmacokinetics

Distribution: V_d (apparent): Adults: 430 L

Protein binding: 90%; high affinity binding protein: alpha$_1$ acid glycoprotein

Metabolism: In the liver via cytochrome P-450 CYP3A4 isoenzyme system; glucuronide conjugation of oxidized metabolites also occurs

Bioavailability: Absolute bioavailability not established; oral solution is 14% less bioavailable than capsules (do not interchange on a mg per mg basis)

Half-life: Adults: 7.1-10.6 hours

Time to peak serum concentrations (single dose): 1-2 hours

Elimination: Minimal excretion of unchanged drug in urine (<3%) and feces; 75% of dose excreted as metabolites via biliary tract into feces and 14% excreted as metabolites in urine

Usual Dosage Oral (use in combination with other antiretroviral agents): Note: Due to differences in bioavailability, capsules and solution are not interchangeable on a mg per mg basis.

(Continued)

Amprenavir *(Continued)*

Neonates, Infants, and Children <4 years:
  Solution: Contraindicated due to potential toxicity from propylene glycol
  Capsules: Not approved for use
Children 4-12 years and Adolescents 13-16 years with a body weight <50 kg:
  Solution: 22.5 mg/kg twice daily or 17 mg/kg 3 times/day; maximum: 2800 mg/day
  Capsules: 20 mg/kg twice daily or 15 mg/kg 3 times/day; maximum: 2400 mg/day
Adolescents 13-16 years with a body weight >50 kg and Adults:
  Capsules: 1200 mg twice daily
Dosing adjustment in hepatic impairment: Adults: Oral: Capsules:
  Child-Pugh score 5-8: 450 mg twice daily
  Child-Pugh score 9-12: 300 mg twice daily

Administration May be administered without regard to meals; avoid administration with high fat meals; do not administer concurrently with antacids

Monitoring Parameters Signs and symptoms of rash or adverse effects; serum glucose, triglycerides, cholesterol, CBC with differential, CD4 cell count, viral load; patients treated with amprenavir oral solution need to be monitored for adverse effects of propylene glycol, such as hyperosmolality, lactic acidosis, seizures, stupor, tachycardia, renal toxicity, and hemolysis

Patient Information Inform your physician if you have a sulfa allergy; amprenavir is not a cure for HIV; notify physician immediately if rash develops; report the use of other medications, nonprescription medications, and herbal or natural products to your physician and pharmacist; take amprenavir everyday as prescribed; do not change dose or discontinue without physician's advice; if a dose is missed, take it as soon as possible, then return to normal dosing schedule; if a dose is skipped, do not double the next dose; avoid alcohol if taking amprenavir oral solution

Additional Information To increase amprenavir solubility, propylene glycol has been added to the oral solution. **Note:** The recommended pediatric dose of the oral solution delivers 1650 mg/kg/day of propylene glycol; the acceptable amount of propylene glycol (when used as an excipient) is not known; treatment of overdose of the oral solution should include monitoring and management of propylene glycol adverse effects including acid-base abnormalities (see Monitoring Parameters); hemodialysis for removal of propylene glycol may be needed .

To increase amprenavir bioavailability, d-alpha tocopherol polyethylene glycol 1000 succinate (a form of vitamin E) has been added in significant concentrations to the product formulations; vitamin E content: 150 mg capsule: 109 international units; oral solution: 46 international units/mL. **Note:** The recommended pediatric dose of the oral solution delivers 138 international units/kg/day of vitamin E; this significantly exceeds the pediatric RDA of 10 international units.

Dosage Forms
Capsules: 50 mg, 150 mg
Solution, oral (grape bubblegum peppermint flavor): 15 mg/mL

References
Adkins JC and Faulds D, "Amprenavir," *Drugs*, 1998, 55(6):837-42.
Panel on Clinical Practices for Treatment of HIV Infection, "Guidelines for the Use of Antiretroviral Agents in HIV-Infected Adults and Adolescents," January 28, 2000, http://www.hivatis.org.
Piscitelli SC, Burstein AH, Chaitt D, et al, "Indinavir Concentrations and St. John's Wort," *Lancet*, 2000, 355(9203):547-8.
Sadler BM, Hanson CD, Chittick GE, et al, "Safety and Pharmacokinetics of Amprenavir (141W94), a Human Immunodeficiency Virus (HIV) Type 1 Protease Inhibitor, Following Oral Administration of Single Doses to HIV-Infected Adults," *Antimicrob Agents Chemother*, 1999, 43(7):1686-92.
Working Group on Antiretroviral Therapy and Medical Management of HIV-Infected Children, "Guidelines for the Use of Antiretroviral Agents in Pediatric HIV Infection," January 7, 2000, http://www.hivatis.org.

♦ **Amrinone** *see* Inamrinone *on page 512*
♦ **Amyl Nitrate Vaporole®** *see* Amyl Nitrite *on page 84*

Amyl Nitrite *(AM il NYE trite)*

Brand Names Amyl Nitrate Vaporole®; Amyl Nitrite Aspirols®
Synonyms Isoamyl Nitrite
Therapeutic Category Antidote, Cyanide; Vasodilator, Coronary
Generic Available Yes
Use Coronary vasodilator in angina pectoris; an adjunct in treatment of cyanide poisoning
Pregnancy Risk Factor X
Contraindications Severe anemia; hypersensitivity to nitrates or any component; recent head trauma or cerebral hemorrhage; hyperthyroidism; recent MI

Precautions Use with caution in patients with increased intracranial pressure, glaucoma, low systolic blood pressure

Adverse Reactions
Cardiovascular: Postural hypotension; cutaneous flushing of head, neck, and clavicular area; tachycardia; palpitations; vasodilation; syncope
Central nervous system: Headache, dizziness, restlessness
Dermatologic: Skin rash (contact dermatitis)
Gastrointestinal: Nausea, vomiting
Hematologic: Hemolytic anemia
Ocular: Increased intraocular pressure

Drug Interactions Alcohol; medications that cause hypotension may increase the postural hypotensive effects of amyl nitrite

Stability Store in cool place, protect from light; flammable, avoid exposure to heat or flame

Mechanism of Action Vasodilator (vascular smooth muscle relaxant) which decreases afterload and improves myocardial blood supply via coronary artery vasodilation; antidote for cyanide poisoning: promotes formation of methemoglobin which combines with cyanide molecule to form cyanmethemoglobin (nontoxic)

Pharmacodynamics
Onset of action: Within 30 seconds
Duration: 3-5 minutes

Pharmacokinetics
Absorption: Inhalation: Readily absorbed through respiratory tract
Metabolism: Hepatic; metabolized by liver to form inorganic nitrates (less potent)
Half-life:
Amyl nitrite: <1 hour
Methemoglobin: 1 hour
Elimination: Renal; ~33%

Usual Dosage Nasal inhalation:
Children and Adults: Cyanide poisoning: Inhale the vapor from a 0.3 mL crushed ampul every minute for 15-30 seconds until I.V. sodium nitrite infusion is available
Adults: Angina: 1-6 inhalations from 1 crushed ampul; may repeat in 3-5 minutes

Administration Give by nasal inhalation; crush ampul in woven covering between finger and hold under patient's nostrils

Monitoring Parameters Blood pressure; with treatment for cyanide poisoning: methemoglobin levels, arterial blood gas

Patient Information Remain seated or lying down during administration because of possible hypotension and dizziness; do not get up suddenly after use; avoid alcohol; if angina pain is not relieved after 2 doses, seek immediate medical attention

Additional Information Amyl nitrite has been used to treat penile erections after urological surgery (eg, circumcisions in adults) and has been used to change the intensity of heart murmurs to aid in their diagnosis

Dosage Forms Inhalant: 0.18 mL, 0.3 mL crushable glass perles (ampuls)

♦ **Anhydrous Glucose** see Dextrose *on page 305*
♦ **Anodynos-DHC®** see Hydrocodone and Acetaminophen *on page 485*
♦ **Ansaid® Oral** see Flurbiprofen *on page 435*
♦ **Ansamycin** see Rifabutin *on page 845*

Antacid Preparations (ant AS id prep a RAE shuns)
Related Information
Calcium Supplements *on page 157*
Carbohydrate and Alcohol Content of Liquid Medications for Use in Patients Receiving Ketogenic Diets *on page 1228*
Magnesium Supplements *on page 588*
Sodium Bicarbonate *on page 870*

Brand Names Amphojel® [OTC]; Basaljel® [OTC]; Gaviscon® [OTC]; Maalox® [OTC]; Maalox® Plus Extra Strength [OTC]; Mylanta® [OTC]; Mylanta®-II [OTC]; Riopan® [OTC]; Tums® [OTC]

Antacid Preparations

Generic/Therapeutic Groupings Brand Names	Al(OH)₃*	Mg(OH)₂*	CaCO₃*	Other Content	Sodium† (mEq)	ANC‡ (mEq)	How Supplied
Aluminum carbonate gel (basic)	400			Simethicone, saccharin, sorbitol	0.13	12	Suspension
Basaljel®	500				0.12	12	Capsule
	500				0.12	13	Tablet
Aluminum hydroxide gel	600			Saccharin, sorbitol	<0.13	16	Suspension
Amphojel®	320			Saccharin, sorbitol	<0.1	10	Suspension
	300				0.08	9	Tablet
	600				0.13	16	Tablet
Aluminum/magnesium hydroxide	225	200		Saccharin, sorbitol	0.06	13.3	Suspension
Maalox®	200	200		Saccharin, sorbitol	0.03	9.7	Tablet/chewable
Maalox® Plus Extra Strength	500	450		Simethicone 40 mg, saccharin, sorbitol (sugar-free)	0.05	29	Suspension
Mylanta®	200	200		Simethicone 20 mg	0.03	12.7	Suspension
	200	200		Simethicone 20 mg	0.03	11.5	Tablet
Mylanta®-II	400	400		Simethicone 40 mg	0.05	25.4	Suspension
	400	400		Simethicone 40 mg	0.06	23	Tablet
Riopan®				Magaldrate 540 mg	0.013	15	Suspension
				Magaldrate 480 mg	≤0.004	13.5	Tablet

Available Salts Aluminum Carbonate; Aluminum Carbonate Gel; Aluminum Hydroxide; Aluminum Hydroxide and Magnesium Carbonate; Aluminum Hydroxide and Magnesium Hydroxide; Aluminum Hydroxide and Magnesium Trisilicate; Aluminum Hydroxide Gel; Aluminum Hydroxide, Magnesium Hydroxide, and Simethicone

Synonyms Magaldrate

Therapeutic Category Antacid; Gastrointestinal Agent, Gastric or Duodenal Ulcer Treatment

Generic Available Yes

Use Adjunct for the relief of peptic ulcer pain and to promote healing of peptic ulcers; relief of stomach upset associated with hyperacidity; prevention of stress ulcer bleeding; treatment of duodenal ulcer and gastroesophageal reflux disease. Aluminum hydroxide is also used to reduce phosphate absorption in hyperphosphatemia; calcium carbonate is used to treat calcium deficiency and to bind phosphate; magnesium oxide is used to treat hypomagnesemia.

Generic/Therapeutic Groupings Brand Names	Al(OH)$_3$*	Mg(OH)$_2$*	CaCO$_3$*	Other Content	Sodium† (mEq)	ANC‡ (mEq)	How Supplied
Aluminum hydroxide/magnesium carbonate							
Gaviscon®	31.7			Magnesium carbonate 119.3 mg, sodium alginate, EDTA, saccharin, sorbitol, parabens	0.57	3-4	Suspension
Aluminum hydroxide/magnesium trisilicate							
Gaviscon®	80			Magnesium trisilicate 20 mg, alginic acid, sodium bicarbonate	0.8	0.5	Tablet/chewable
Calcium carbonate							
Tums®			500		≤0.087	10	Tablet/chewable
Tums E-X® Extra Strength			750		≤0.087		
Calcium carbonate suspension			1250		<0.217		Suspension
			500	Simethicone 20 mg	0.0065	11	Suspension
Titralac Plus®			420	Simethicone 21 mg	≤0.001	7.5	Tablet

*Liquids in mg per 5 mL; capsules and tablets in mg.
†mEq of sodium per tablet, capsule, or 5 mL of liquid (23 mg = 1 mEq sodium)
‡Acid neutralizing capacity per tablet, capsule, or 5 mL of liquid.

(Continued)

Antacid Preparations *(Continued)*

Warnings Use aluminum-containing antacids with caution in patients with decreased bowel motility and dehydration, in patients with gastric outlet obstruction, in patients with renal failure, and in patients who have an upper GI hemorrhage; use magnesium-containing products with caution in patients with renal impairment; use sodium-containing antacids with caution in patients on low-sodium diets, and in patients with CHF, edema, renal failure, or hepatic failure

Adverse Reactions

Aluminum-containing antacids:

Central nervous system: Dementia, encephalopathy, malaise, seizures, confusion, coma

Endocrine & metabolic: Hypophosphatemia, hyperaluminemia, osteoporosis

Gastrointestinal: Constipation, anorexia

Genitourinary: Urinary calculi

Neuromuscular & skeletal: Muscle weakness, osteomalacia

Calcium-containing antacids:

Endocrine & metabolic: Milk-alkali syndrome (hypercalcemia, metabolic alkalosis), hypophosphatemia

Gastrointestinal: Constipation, flatulence

Magnesium-containing antacids:

Endocrine & metabolic: Hypermagnesemia, fluid and electrolyte imbalance

Gastrointestinal: Laxative effects, diarrhea

Sodium-containing antacids:

Cardiovascular: Fluid retention

Endocrine & metabolic: Metabolic alkalosis, sodium overload

Gastrointestinal: Flatulence

Drug Interactions Aluminum-, calcium-, or magnesium-containing antacids (decrease tetracycline and quinolone absorption); antacids decrease absorption of iron, digoxin, phenytoin, indomethacin; increased absorption of buffered or enteric-coated aspirin; aluminum hydroxide (decreased absorption of isoniazid); sucralfate (may impair binding of sucralfate to ulcerated mucosa)

Stability Avoid freezing aluminum hydroxide and magnesium hydroxide

Mechanism of Action Neutralizes gastric acidity increasing gastric pH; inhibits proteolytic activity of pepsin when gastric pH is increased >4

Pharmacodynamics

Duration of action: Dependent on gastric emptying time

Fasting state: 20-60 minutes

1 hour after meals: May be up to 3 hours

Usual Dosage Oral: Aluminum/magnesium hydroxide combination (for extra strength or concentrated suspension, use half the volume of the stated dose):

Peptic ulcer disease:

Infants: 1-2 mL/kg/dose 1-3 hours after meals and at bedtime

Children: 5-15 mL/dose every 3-6 hours or 1-3 hours after meals and at bedtime

Adults: 15-45 mL every 3-6 hours or 1-3 hours after meals and at bedtime

Prophylaxis against GI bleeding:

Neonates: 1 mL/kg every 4 hours as needed

Infants: 2-5 mL/dose every 1-2 hours, titrate to gastric pH >3.5

Children: 5-15 mL/dose every 1-2 hours, titrate to gastric pH >3.5

Adults: 30-60 mL every 1-2 hours, titrate to gastric pH >3.5

Hyperphosphatemia:

Children: Use $Al(OH)_3$ or aluminum carbonate gel product only: 50-150 mg/kg/day (as aluminum hydroxide gel) divided every 4-6 hours; titrate to normal serum phosphorus level

Adults: 30-40 mL of $Al(OH)_3$ 3-4 times/day between meals and at bedtime

Administration Oral: Thoroughly chew tablets before swallowing; shake suspensions well before use

Monitoring Parameters GI complaints, stool frequency; serum phosphate concentrations in patients on hemodialysis receiving chronic aluminum-containing antacid therapy; serum calcium in patients receiving large doses of calcium carbonate; serum electrolytes in patients with renal impairment receiving magnesium-containing antacids

Patient Information Antacids may impair or increase absorption of many drugs, do not take oral medications within 1-2 hours of an antacid dose unless specifically instructed to do so

Dosage Forms See tables on previous pages.

References
Nord KS, "Peptic Ulcer Disease in the Pediatric Population," *Pediatr Clin North Am*, 1988, 35(1):117-140.

♦ **AntibiOtic® Otic** *see* Neomycin, (Bacitracin) Polymyxin B, and Hydrocortisone *on page 679*

♦ **Antidigoxin Fab Fragments** *see* Digoxin Immune Fab *on page 320*

♦ **Antidiuretic Hormone** *see* Vasopressin *on page 971*

♦ **Antiepileptic Drugs** *see page 1176*

Antihemophilic Factor (Human)
(an tee hee moe FIL ik FAK tor HYU man)

Brand Names Alphanate®; Hemofil® M; Humate-P®; Koate®-HP; Koate®-HS; Monoclate-P®; Profilate® HP

Synonyms AHF; AHG; Factor VIII

Therapeutic Category Antihemophilic Agent; Blood Product Derivative

Generic Available Yes

Use Management of hemophilia A in patients whom a deficiency in factor VIII has been demonstrated

Pregnancy Risk Factor C

Contraindications Hypersensitivity to mouse protein (Monoclate-P®; Hemofil® M, Method M, Monoclonal Purified; Antihemophilic Factor (Human), Method M, Monoclonal Purified contain trace amounts of mouse protein)

Precautions Human antihemophilic factor is prepared from pooled plasma and even with heat treated or other viral attenuated processes, the risk of viral transmission (ie, viral hepatitis, HIV) is not totally eradicated. The use of recombinant antihemophilic factor products (such as Bioclate®, Helixate®, Kogenate®, or Recombinate®) substantially decreases the risk of viral transmission because these products are biosynthetically prepared. Progressive anemia and hemolysis may occur in individuals with blood groups A, B, and AB who receive large or frequent doses due to trace amounts of blood group A and B isohemagglutinins.

Adverse Reactions
Cardiovascular: Flushing, tachycardia
Central nervous system: Headache
Gastrointestinal: Nausea, vomiting
Neuromuscular & skeletal: Paresthesia
Miscellaneous: Allergic vasomotor reactions, tightness in neck or chest, development of inhibitor antibodies (3% to 52%); inhibitor antibodies are IgG immunoglobulins that neutralize the activity of factor VIII; an increase of inhibitor antibody concentration is seen at 2-7 days, with peak concentrations at 1-3 weeks after therapy. Children <5 years of age are at greatest risk; higher doses of AHF may be needed if antibody is present; if antibody concentration is >10 Bethesda units/mL, patients may not respond to larger doses and alternative treatment modalities may be needed.

Stability Dried concentrate should be refrigerated, but may be stored at room temperature for up to 6 months depending upon specific product; if refrigerated, the dried concentrate and diluent should be warmed to room temperature before reconstitution; gently agitate or rotate vial after adding diluent, do not shake vigorously; do **not** refrigerate after reconstitution, precipitation may occur; administer within 3 hours after reconstitution; Method M, monoclonal purified products should be administered within 1 hour after reconstitution

Mechanism of Action Factor VIII is a protein in normal plasma which is necessary for clot formation and maintenance of hemostasis; it activates factor X in conjunction with activated factor IX; activated factor X converts prothrombin to thrombin, which converts fibrinogen to fibrin and with factor XIII forms a stable clot

Pharmacodynamics Maximal effect: 1-2 hours

Pharmacokinetics
Distribution: Does not readily cross the placenta
Half-life: 4-24 hours; mean = 12 hours (biphasic)

(Continued)

Antihemophilic Factor (Human) *(Continued)*

Usual Dosage Children and Adults: I.V. (individualize dosage based on coagulation studies performed prior to and during treatment at regular intervals):

Hospitalized patients: 20-50 units/kg/dose; may be higher for special circumstances. Dose can be given every 12-24 hours and more frequently in special circumstances.

Hemophilia A with high titer of inhibitor antibody: 50-75 units/kg/hour has been given

Formula to approximate percentage increase in plasma antihemophilic factor: Units required = body weight (kg) x 0.5 x desired increase factor VIII (% of normal)

Administration Parenteral: I.V. administration only; administer through a separate line, do not mix with drugs or other I.V. fluids; maximum rate of administration is product dependent: Monoclate-P® 2 mL/minute; Humate-P® 4 mL/minute; administration of other AHF products should not exceed 10 mL/minute; use filter needle to draw product into syringe

Monitoring Parameters Heart rate before and during I.V. administration; plasma antihemophilic factor levels prior to and during treatment; inhibitor antibody concentration

Reference Range Plasma antihemophilic factor level: Desired: ~30% of normal for effective hemostasis in patients with hemorrhage; ~5% to 10% of normal for hemarthrosis; ~30% to 50% of normal to prevent hemorrhage for minor surgical procedures; ~80% to 100% of normal for major surgical procedures (give dose 1 hour prior to O.R.); ~30% to 60% of normal may be required for at least 10-14 days postoperatively

Nursing Implications Reduce rate of administration or temporarily discontinue if patient becomes tachycardiac

Additional Information Products using a heat treatment process for viral attenuation include Humate-P®, Koate®-HS, and Monoclate-P®; a solvent/detergent viral inactivation process is used in making Alphanate®

Dosage Forms Injection (approximate factor VIII activity per vial): 200 units, 250 units, 500 units, 750 units, 1000 units, 1250 units, 1500 units; exact potency labeled on each vial

♦ **Antihist-1®** [OTC] *see Clemastine on page 236*

♦ **Antilirium®** Injection *see Physostigmine on page 768*

♦ **Antiminth®** [OTC] *see Pyrantel Pamoate on page 824*

Antipyrine and Benzocaine *(an tee PYE reen & BEN zoe kane)*

Brand Names Allergen® Ear Drops; Auralgan®; Auroto®; Oto®; Otocalm® Ear

Synonyms Benzocaine and Antipyrine

Therapeutic Category Otic Agent, Analgesic; Otic Agent, Cerumenolytic

Generic Available Yes

Use Temporary relief of pain and reduction of inflammation associated with acute congestive and serous otitis media, swimmer's ear, otitis externa; facilitates ear wax removal

Contraindications Hypersensitivity to antipyrine, benzocaine, or any component; perforated tympanic membrane

Warnings Use of otic anesthetics may mask symptoms of a fulminating middle ear infection (acute otitis media); not intended for prolonged use

Adverse Reactions

Hematologic: Methemoglobinemia

Local: Burning, stinging, tenderness, edema

Miscellaneous: Hypersensitivity reactions

Usual Dosage Infants, Children, and Adults: Otic: Fill ear canal; moisten cotton pledget, place in external ear, repeat every 1-2 hours until pain and congestion is relieved; for ear wax removal instill drops 3-4 times/day for 2-3 days

Dosage Forms Solution, otic: Antipyrine 5.4% and benzocaine 1.4% (10 mL, 15 mL)

References

Rodriguez LF, Smolik LM, and Zbehlik AJ, "Benzocaine-Induced Methemoglobinemia: Report of a Severe Reaction and Review of the Literature," *Ann Pharmacother*, 1994, 28(5):643-9.

♦ **Antispas®** Injection *see Dicyclomine on page 314*

♦ **Antithymocyte Globulin (equine)** *see Lymphocyte Immune Globulin on page 586*

♦ **Anti-Tuss®** Expectorant [OTC] *see Guaifenesin on page 464*

Antivenin (*Crotalidae*) Polyvalent
(an tee VEN in (kroe TAL ih die) pol i VAY lent)

Synonyms Crotaline Antivenin, Polyvalent; North and South American Antisnakebite Serum; Snake (Pit Vipers) Antivenin

Therapeutic Category Antivenin

Generic Available No

Use Neutralization of venoms of North and South American crotalids: rattlesnake, copperhead, cottonmouth, tropical moccasins, fer-de-lance, bushmaster

Pregnancy Risk Factor C

Contraindications Not effective against the venoms of coral snakes

Warnings Desensitization may need to be performed on patients with positive skin test reaction or history of sensitivity to equine serum

Precautions Patients with a negative skin test may still react when antivenin is administered; skin test should not be performed unless antivenin is to be used

Adverse Reactions
Cardiovascular: Flushing, cyanosis, shock, edema of the face
Central nervous system: Apprehension
Dermatologic: Urticaria
Gastrointestinal: Vomiting
Neuromuscular & skeletal: Muscle weakness, peripheral neuritis
Respiratory: Dyspnea, cough
Miscellaneous: Anaphylaxis, serum sickness (dose-related; occurs in 83% of patients receiving more than 8 vials)

Stability Avoid storage temperatures >37°C; reconstituted solutions should be used within 48 hours

Usual Dosage The initial dose of antivenin should be administered as soon as possible to be most effective (within 4 hours after the bite). Intradermal sensitivity test should be performed prior to administering antivenin; see Additional Information.

Children and Adults: I.V.:
Minimal envenomation: 20-40 mL
Moderate envenomation: 50-90 mL
Severe envenomation: 100-150 mL
See table.

Dosage Based on Severity of Clinical Picture

Clinical Severity		# of Vials
Minimal	Symptoms confined to bite area; absent of insignificant systemic symptoms	0
Mild	Edema progressing slowly; bite site reveals small amount of ecchymosis; only systemic sign is metallic taste	5
Moderate	Tissue damage beyond immediate bite area; moderate laboratory changes; perioral fasciculation; paresthesias	10
Severe	Tissue damage to entire extremity; major systemic symptoms; significant laboratory abnormalities	>15

Gold BS and Barish RA, "Venomous Snakebites: Current Concepts in Diagnosis, Treatment, and Management," *Emerg Med Clin North Am*, 1992, 10(2):249-67.

Additional doses of antivenin are based on clinical response to the initial dose. If swelling continues to progress, symptoms increase in severity, hypotension occurs, or decrease in hematocrit appears, an additional 10-50 mL should be administered.

Administration Parenteral: Antivenin may be administered I.M. into a large muscle mass for minimal envenomation. I.V. administration of antivenin is preferred for moderate to severe envenomation or in the presence of shock; for I.V. infusion, prepare a 1:1 to 1:10 dilution of reconstituted antivenin in NS or D₅W; infuse the initial 5-10 mL dilution over 3-5 minutes while carefully observing the patient for signs and symptoms of sensitivity reactions. If no reaction occurs, continue infusion at a safe I.V. fluid delivery rate.

Monitoring Parameters Vital signs, hematocrit

Nursing Implications Do not inject into a finger or toe; immediate sensitivity reactions usually occur within 30 minutes after administration; if an immediate reaction occurs, temporarily discontinue antivenin, administer epinephrine and/or
(Continued)

Antivenin *(Crotalidae)* Polyvalent *(Continued)*

an antihistamine; then reinstate infusion at a slower rate after control of the reaction; serum-sickness reaction may occur 5-24 days after a dose

Additional Information Intradermal skin test: 0.02-0.03 mL of a 1:10 dilution of antivenin in NS. If the patient has a history of equine serum sensitivity, administer a 1:100 or greater dilution skin test. Test site is read after 5-30 minutes.

Dosage Forms Injection: Lyophilized serum, diluent (10 mL); one vacuum vial to yield 10 mL of serum

- ◆ **Antivert®** *see* Meclizine *on page 597*
- ◆ **Antizol®** *see* Fomepizole *on page 440*
- ◆ **Antrizine®** *see* Meclizine *on page 597*
- ◆ **Anumed® [OTC]** *see* Hemorrhoidal Preparations *on page 470*
- ◆ **Anusol® [OTC]** *see* Hemorrhoidal Preparations *on page 470*
- ◆ **Anusol® HC-1 Topical [OTC]** *see* Hydrocortisone *on page 486*
- ◆ **Anusol® HC-2.5% Topical [OTC]** *see* Hydrocortisone *on page 486*
- ◆ **Anusol-HC®** **Suppository** *see* Hydrocortisone *on page 486*
- ◆ **Anxanil® Oral** *see* Hydroxyzine *on page 496*
- ◆ **Anzemet®** *see* Dolasetron *on page 337*
- ◆ **Apacet® [OTC]** *see* Acetaminophen *on page 26*
- ◆ **APAP** *see* Acetaminophen *on page 26*
- ◆ **APD** *see* Pamidronate *on page 722*
- ◆ **A.P.L.®** *see* Chorionic Gonadotropin *on page 221*
- ◆ **Apo®-Acetazolamide (Canada)** *see* Acetazolamide *on page 29*
- ◆ **Apo®-Allopurinol (Canada)** *see* Allopurinol *on page 48*
- ◆ **Apo®-Alpraz (Canada)** *see* Alprazolam *on page 50*
- ◆ **Apo®-Amitriptyline (Canada)** *see* Amitriptyline *on page 67*
- ◆ **Apo®-Amoxi (Canada)** *see* Amoxicillin *on page 70*
- ◆ **Apo®-Ampi [Trihydrate] (Canada)** *see* Ampicillin *on page 78*
- ◆ **Apo®-ASA (Canada)** *see* Aspirin *on page 99*
- ◆ **Apo®-Atenol (Canada)** *see* Atenolol *on page 102*
- ◆ **Apo®-Bisacodyl (Canada)** *see* Bisacodyl *on page 133*
- ◆ **Apo®-Capto (Canada)** *see* Captopril *on page 163*
- ◆ **Apo®-Carbamazepine (Canada)** *see* Carbamazepine *on page 165*
- ◆ **Apo®-C (Canada)** *see* Ascorbic Acid *on page 96*
- ◆ **Apo®-Cephalex (Canada)** *see* Cephalexin *on page 196*
- ◆ **Apo®-Chlorpromazine (Canada)** *see* Chlorpromazine *on page 215*
- ◆ **Apo®-Cimetidine (Canada)** *see* Cimetidine *on page 222*
- ◆ **Apo®-Clonidine (Canada)** *see* Clonidine *on page 242*
- ◆ **Apo®-Clorazepate (Canada)** *see* Clorazepate *on page 244*
- ◆ **Apo®-Cloxi (Canada)** *see* Cloxacillin *on page 246*
- ◆ **Apo®-Diazepam (Canada)** *see* Diazepam *on page 307*
- ◆ **Apo®-Diclo (Canada)** *see* Diclofenac *on page 312*
- ◆ **Apo®-Diltiaz (Canada)** *see* Diltiazem *on page 323*
- ◆ **Apo®-Dimenhydrinate (Canada)** *see* Dimenhydrinate *on page 325*
- ◆ **Apo®-Dipyridamole FC (Canada)** *see* Dipyridamole *on page 331*
- ◆ **Apo®-Dipyridamole SC (Canada)** *see* Dipyridamole *on page 331*
- ◆ **Apo®-Doxepin (Canada)** *see* Doxepin *on page 345*
- ◆ **Apo®-Doxy (Canada)** *see* Doxycycline *on page 348*
- ◆ **Apo®-Doxy Tabs (Canada)** *see* Doxycycline *on page 348*
- ◆ **Apo®-Enalapril (Canada)** *see* Enalapril/Enalaprilat *on page 363*
- ◆ **Apo®-Erythro E-C (Canada)** *see* Erythromycin *on page 379*
- ◆ **Apo®-Famotidine (Canada)** *see* Famotidine *on page 401*
- ◆ **Apo®-Ferrous Gluconate (Canada)** *see* Iron Supplements, Oral/Enteral *on page 530*
- ◆ **Apo®-Ferrous Sulfate (Canada)** *see* Iron Supplements, Oral/Enteral *on page 530*
- ◆ **Apo®-Flurazepam (Canada)** *see* Flurazepam *on page 434*
- ◆ **Apo®-Folic (Canada)** *see* Folic Acid *on page 439*
- ◆ **Apo®-Furosemide (Canada)** *see* Furosemide *on page 447*
- ◆ **Apo®-Gain (Canada)** *see* Minoxidil *on page 650*
- ◆ **Apo®-Hydralazine (Canada)** *see* Hydralazine *on page 482*

- **Apo®-Hydro (Canada)** *see* Hydrochlorothiazide *on page 483*
- **Apo®-Hydroxyzine (Canada)** *see* Hydroxyzine *on page 496*
- **Apo®-Ibuprofen (Canada)** *see* Ibuprofen *on page 501*
- **Apo®-Imipramine (Canada)** *see* Imipramine *on page 508*
- **Apo®-Indomethacin (Canada)** *see* Indomethacin *on page 516*
- **Apo®-Lorazepam (Canada)** *see* Lorazepam *on page 583*
- **Apo®-Methyldopa (Canada)** *see* Methyldopa *on page 625*
- **Apo®-Metoclop (Canada)** *see* Metoclopramide *on page 630*
- **Apo®-Metoprolol (Type L) (Canada)** *see* Metoprolol *on page 633*
- **Apo®-Metronidazole (Canada)** *see* Metronidazole *on page 636*
- **Apo®-Nadol (Canada)** *see* Nadolol *on page 665*
- **Apo®-Naproxen (Canada)** *see* Naproxen *on page 672*
- **Apo®-Nifed (Canada)** *see* Nifedipine *on page 687*
- **Apo®-Nitrofurantoin (Canada)** *see* Nitrofurantoin *on page 689*
- **Apo®-Pen VK (Canada)** *see* Penicillin V Potassium *on page 743*
- **Apo®-Piroxicam (Canada)** *see* Piroxicam *on page 777*
- **Apo®-Prazo (Canada)** *see* Prazosin *on page 790*
- **Apo®-Prednisone (Canada)** *see* Prednisone *on page 794*
- **Apo®-Primidone (Canada)** *see* Primidone *on page 796*
- **Apo®-Procainamide (Canada)** *see* Procainamide *on page 799*
- **Apo®-Propranolol (Canada)** *see* Propranolol *on page 816*
- **Apo®-Ranitidine (Canada)** *see* Ranitidine *on page 835*
- **Apo®-Salvent (Canada)** *see* Albuterol *on page 40*
- **Apo®-Sulfamethoxazole (Canada)** *see* Sulfamethoxazole *on page 892*
- **Apo®-Sulfasalazine (Canada)** *see* Sulfasalazine *on page 893*
- **Apo®-Sulfatrim (Canada)** *see* Co-Trimoxazole *on page 258*
- **Apo®-Sulin (Canada)** *see* Sulindac *on page 896*
- **Apo®-Tetra (Canada)** *see* Tetracycline *on page 908*
- **Apo®-Thioridazine (Canada)** *see* Thioridazine *on page 920*
- **Apo®-Timol (Canada)** *see* Timolol *on page 929*
- **Apo®-Timop (Canada)** *see* Timolol *on page 929*
- **Apo®-Triazo (Canada)** *see* Triazolam *on page 950*
- **Apo®-Trihex (Canada)** *see* Trihexyphenidyl *on page 952*
- **Apo®-Verap (Canada)** *see* Verapamil *on page 974*
- **Apo®-Zidovudine (Canada)** *see* Zidovudine *on page 990*
- **APPG** *see* Penicillin G Procaine *on page 742*
- **Apresoline® Injection** *see* Hydralazine *on page 482*
- **Apresoline® Oral** *see* Hydralazine *on page 482*
- **Aprodine® [OTC]** *see* Triprolidine and Pseudoephedrine *on page 957*
- **Apro-Flurbiprofen® (Canada)** *see* Flurbiprofen *on page 435*

Aprotinin (a proe TYE nin)
Brand Names Trasylol®
Therapeutic Category Hemostatic Agent
Use Prophylactic use to reduce perioperative blood loss and the need for blood transfusion in patients undergoing cardiopulmonary bypass in the course of coronary artery bypass graft surgery (CABG); in selected repeat cases of primary CABG surgery where the risk of bleeding is especially high or where transfusion is unavailable or unacceptable
Pregnancy Risk Factor B
Contraindications Hypersensitivity to aprotinin or any component
Warnings Patients with a previous exposure to aprotinin (particularly when re-exposure is within 6 months) are at an increased risk for hypersensitivity reactions including anaphylactic or anaphylactoid reactions; pretreatment with an antihistamine and H_2-blocker before administration of the loading dose is recommended in these patients; delay the addition of aprotinin into the pump prime solution until the loading dose has safely been administered.
Precautions All patients treated with aprotinin should first receive a test dose at least 10 minutes before the loading dose to assess the potential for allergic reactions
(Continued)

Aprotinin *(Continued)*

Adverse Reactions

Cardiovascular: Atrial fibrillation, MI, heart failure, atrial flutter, ventricular tachy-cardia, cerebral embolism, cerebrovascular events, chest pain, hypotension, pericardial effusion, pulmonary hypertension

Central nervous system: Fever, mental confusion, seizures, agitation, dizziness, anxiety

Endocrine & metabolic: Hyperglycemia, hypokalemia, acidosis

Gastrointestinal: Nausea, vomiting, constipation, diarrhea, GI hemorrhage

Hematologic: Hemolysis, anemia, thrombosis

Hepatic: Liver damage, jaundice

Local: Phlebitis

Neuromuscular & skeletal: Arthralgia

Renal: Decreased renal function

Respiratory: Dyspnea, bronchoconstriction, pulmonary edema, apnea, increased cough

Miscellaneous: Anaphylaxis (see Warnings)

Drug Interactions
Decreases effects of fibrinolytic agents such as streptokinase or anistreplase; decreases effects of captopril; prolonged activated clotting time when used with heparin

Stability
Store between 2°C to 25°C (36°F to 77°F); do not freeze; do not mix with other medications; incompatible with corticosteroids, heparin, amino acids, and fat emulsion

Mechanism of Action
Aprotinin, a serine protease inhibitor, modulates the systemic inflammatory response associated with cardiopulmonary bypass surgery; inhibits plasmin, kallikrein, and platelet activation producing antifibrinolytic effects; is a weak inhibitor of plasma pseudocholinesterase; inhibits the contact phase activation of coagulation and preserves adhesive platelet glycoproteins making them resistant to damage from increased circulating plasmin or mechanical injury occurring during bypass

Pharmacokinetics

Metabolism: Aprotinin is slowly degraded by lysosomal enzymes

Half-life, elimination: 150 minutes; terminal elimination: 10 hours

Elimination: <10% excreted unchanged in the urine

Usual Dosage
I.V.: Test dose: All patients should receive a test dose at least 10 minutes prior to the loading dose to assess the potential for allergic reactions

Infants and Children: No conclusive dosage regimen has been established; variable dosage recommendations in the literature. Test dose: (dosage not well documented in studies) 0.1 mg/kg (maximum: 1.4 mg) has been used. Two of the more common recommendations follow (see References for other recommendations):

Body surface area: ≤1.16 m^2:
240 mg/m^2 loading dose
240 mg/m^2 into pump prime volume
56 mg/m^2/hour continuous infusion during surgery

Body surface area: >1.16 m^2:
280 mg/m^2 loading dose
280 mg/m^2 into pump prime volume
70 mg/m^2/hour continuous infusion during surgery

Alternative (based upon body weight only):
30,000 units/kg (4.2 mg/kg) loading dose
30,000 units/kg (4.2 mg/kg) into pump prime volume
30,000 units/kg/hour (4.2 mg/kg/hour) continuous infusion

Adults: Test dose: 1 mL (1.4 mg)

Regimen A (standard dose):
2 million units (280 mg) loading dose
2 million units (280 mg) into pump prime volume
500,000 units/hour (70 mg/hour) continuous infusion during surgery

Regimen B (low dose):
1 million units (140 mg) loading dose
1 million units (140 mg) into pump prime volume
250,000 units/hour (35 mg/hour) continuous infusion during surgery

Administration
Parenteral: For I.V. use only; all I.V. doses should be administered through a central line; infuse test dose over at least 10 minutes; infuse loading dose over 20-30 minutes with patient in the supine position

Monitoring Parameters Bleeding times, prothrombin time, activated clotting time, platelet count, red blood cell counts, hematocrit, hemoglobin, and fibrinogen degradation products

Test Interactions Aprotinin prolongs whole blood clotting time of heparinized blood as determined by the Hemochrom® method or similar surface activation methods; patients may require additional heparin even in the presence of activated clotting time levels that appear to represent adequate anticoagulation

Dosage Forms Injection: 1.4 mg/mL [10,000 units/mL] (100 mL, 200 mL)

References

Boldt J, "Endothelial-Related Coagulation in Pediatric Surgery," *Ann Thorac Surg*, 1998, 65(6 Suppl):S56-9.

Carrel TP, Schwanda M, Vogt P, et al, "Aprotinin in Pediatric Cardiac Operations: A Benefit in Complex Malformations and With High-Dose Regimen Only," *Ann Thorac Surg*, 1998, 66(1):153-8.

Miller BE, Tosone SR, Tam VK, et al, "Hematologic and Economic Impact of Aprotinin in Reoperative Pediatric Cardiac Operations," *Ann Thorac Surg*, 1998, 66(2):535-41.

Penkoske P, Entwistle LM, Marchak BE, et al, "Aprotinin in Children Undergoing Repair of Congenital Heart Defects," *Ann Thorac Surg*, 1995, 60(6 Suppl):S529-32.

Spray TL, "Use of Aprotinin in Pediatric Organ Transplantation," *Ann Thorac Surg*, 1998, 65(6 Suppl):S71-3.

♦ **Aquachloral® Supprettes®** *see* Chloral Hydrate *on page 204*
♦ **Aquacort® (Canada)** *see* Hydrocortisone *on page 486*
♦ **AquaMEPHYTON®** *see* Phytonadione *on page 769*
♦ **Aquaphyllin®** *see* Theophylline *on page 910*
♦ **Aquasol A® [OTC]** *see* Vitamin A *on page 981*
♦ **Aquasol E® Oral [OTC]** *see* Vitamin E *on page 982*
♦ **AquaTar® [OTC]** *see* Coal Tar *on page 247*
♦ **Aqueous Procaine Penicillin G** *see* Penicillin G Procaine *on page 742*
♦ **Aqueous Testosterone** *see* Testosterone *on page 905*
♦ **Ara-A** *see* Vidarabine *on page 977*
♦ **Arabinofuranosyladenine** *see* Vidarabine *on page 977*
♦ **Arabinosylcytosine** *see* Cytarabine *on page 276*
♦ **Ara-C** *see* Cytarabine *on page 276*
♦ **Aralen® Phosphate** *see* Chloroquine *on page 211*
♦ **Aramine®** *see* Metaraminol *on page 612*
♦ **Aredia™** *see* Pamidronate *on page 722*
♦ **Arfonad® Injection** *see* Trimethaphan Camsylate *on page 953*

Arginine (AR ji neen)

Brand Names R-Gene®

Available Salts Arginine Hydrochloride

Therapeutic Category Diagnostic Agent, Growth Hormone Function; Metabolic Alkalosis Agent

Generic Available No

Use Pituitary function test (growth hormone); management of severe, uncompensated, metabolic alkalosis (pH ≥7.55) **after** optimizing therapy with sodium, potassium, or ammonium chloride supplements

Contraindications Hypersensitivity to arginine or any component; renal or hepatic failure

Precautions Arginine hydrochloride is metabolized to nitrogen-containing products for excretion; the temporary effect of a high nitrogen load on the kidneys should be evaluated

Adverse Reactions

Cardiovascular: Flushing (after rapid I.V. administration)

Central nervous system: Headache (after rapid I.V. administration)

Endocrine & metabolic: Hyperglycemia, hyperkalemia, metabolic acidosis secondary to hyperchloremia

Gastrointestinal: Nausea, vomiting, abdominal pain, bloating

Local: Venous irritation

Miscellaneous: Increased serum gastrin concentration

Drug Interactions Estrogen-progesterone combinations, spironolactone (potentially fatal hyperkalemia has been reported in patients with hepatic disease)

Mechanism of Action Stimulates pituitary release of growth hormone and prolactin and pancreatic release of glucagon and insulin; patients with impaired pituitary function have lower or no increase in plasma concentrations of growth hormone after administration of arginine. Arginine hydrochloride has been used for severe metabolic alkalosis due to its high chloride content.

(Continued)

Arginine *(Continued)*

Pharmacokinetics

Absorption: Oral: Well absorbed

Time to peak serum concentration: Within 2 hours

Usual Dosage I.V.:

Growth hormone reserve test:

Children: 500 mg/kg over 30 minutes

Adults: 300 mL over 30 minutes

Inborn errors of urea synthesis: Infants and Children: 0.8 g/kg initially, then 0.2-0.8 g/kg/day as a continuous infusion

Metabolic alkalosis: Infants, Children, and Adults: Arginine hydrochloride dose (g) = weight (kg) x 0.1 x [HCO_3^- - 24] where HCO_3^- = the patient's serum bicarbonate concentration in mEq/L; give $1/2$ to $2/3$ of calculated dose and re-evaluate

Note: Arginine hydrochloride is a fourth-line treatment for uncompensated metabolic alkalosis after sodium chloride, potassium chloride, and ammonium chloride supplementation has been optimized

To correct hypochloremia: Infants, Children, and Adults: Arginine hydrochloride dose (mEq) = 0.2 x weight (kg) x [103 - Cl^-] where Cl^- = the patient's serum chloride concentration in mEq/L; give $1/2$ to $2/3$ of calculated dose and re-evaluate

Note: Arginine hydrochloride should never be used as initial therapy for chloride supplementation but as an alternative in the patient who is unresponsive to sodium chloride or potassium chloride supplementation.

Administration Parenteral: May be infused without further dilution; maximum rate of I.V. infusion: 1 g/kg/hour (4.75 mEq/kg/hour) (maximum dose: 60 g/hour = 285 mEq over 1 hour)

Monitoring Parameters Acid-base status (arterial or capillary blood gases), serum electrolytes, BUN, glucose, plasma growth hormone concentrations (when evaluating growth hormone reserve)

Reference Range If intact pituitary function, human growth hormone levels should rise after arginine administration to 10-30 ng/mL (control range: 0-6 ng/mL)

Nursing Implications I.V. infiltration of arginine hydrochloride may cause necrosis and phlebitis; prolongation of the infusion may diminish the stimulus to the pituitary gland and nullify the test

Dosage Forms Injection, as hydrochloride: 10% [0.475 mEq chloride/mL] (500 mL)

References

Bushinsky DA and Gennari FJ, "Life-Threatening Hyperkalemia Induced by Arginine," *Ann Intern Med*, 1978, 89(5 Pt 1):632-4.

♦ **Arginine Hydrochloride** *see* Arginine *on page 95*

♦ **8-Arginine Vasopressin** *see* Vasopressin *on page 971*

♦ **Aristocort® A Topical** *see* Triamcinolone *on page 946*

♦ **Aristocort® Forte Injection** *see* Triamcinolone *on page 946*

♦ **Aristocort® Intralesional Injection** *see* Triamcinolone *on page 946*

♦ **Aristocort® Oral** *see* Triamcinolone *on page 946*

♦ **Aristocort® Topical** *see* Triamcinolone *on page 946*

♦ **Aristospan® Intra-articular Injection** *see* Triamcinolone *on page 946*

♦ **Aristospan® Intralesional Injection** *see* Triamcinolone *on page 946*

♦ **Arm-a-Med®** *see* Isoetharine *on page 533*

♦ **Arm-a-Med® Isoproterenol** *see* Isoproterenol *on page 536*

♦ **Arm-a-Med® Metaproterenol** *see* Metaproterenol *on page 611*

♦ **Arrestin® Injection** *see* Trimethobenzamide *on page 954*

♦ **Artane®** *see* Trihexyphenidyl *on page 952*

♦ **ASA** *see* Aspirin *on page 99*

♦ **A.S.A. [OTC]** *see* Aspirin *on page 99*

♦ **5-ASA** *see* Mesalamine *on page 608*

♦ **ASA® (Canada)** *see* Aspirin *on page 99*

♦ **Asacol® Oral** *see* Mesalamine *on page 608*

♦ **Asaphen (Canada)** *see* Aspirin *on page 99*

♦ **Asasantine® [with Aspirin also] (Canada)** *see* Dipyridamole *on page 331*

♦ **Ascorbic® 500 (Canada)** *see* Ascorbic Acid *on page 96*

Ascorbic Acid *(a SKOR bik AS id)*

Brand Names Apo®-C (Canada); Ascorbic® 500 (Canada); Ascorbicap® [OTC]; C-Crystals® [OTC]; Cebid®; Cecon® [OTC]; Cetane® [OTC]; Cevalin® [OTC]; Cevi-bid® [OTC]; Ce-Vi-Sol® [OTC]; Dull-C® [OTC]; Duo-CVP® (Canada); Flavorcee®

[OTC]; N'ice®; Redoxon® (Canada); Revitalose C-1000® (Canada); Timecelles® [OTC]; Vita-C® [OTC]; Vitamin C Drops [OTC]

Synonyms Vitamin C

Therapeutic Category   Nutritional Supplement;   Urinary Acidifying Agent; Vitamin, Water Soluble

Generic Available Yes

Use Prevention and treatment of scurvy; urinary acidification; dietary supplementation; prevention and reduction in the severity of colds

Pregnancy Risk Factor A (C if used in doses above RDA recommendation)

Contraindications Large doses during pregnancy

Warnings Some products contain tartrazine or sulfites which may cause allergic reactions in susceptible individuals

Adverse Reactions
Cardiovascular: Flushing
Central nervous system: Faintness, dizziness, headache, fatigue
Gastrointestinal: Nausea, vomiting, heartburn, diarrhea
Renal: Hyperoxaluria

Drug Interactions Aspirin, iron, oral contraceptives (increase estrogen levels), decreased warfarin effect

Stability Injectable form should be stored under refrigeration (2°C to 8°C); protect oral dosage forms from light; ascorbic acid solution is rapidly oxidized

Mechanism of Action Necessary for collagen formation and tissue repair in the body; involved in some oxidation-reduction reactions as well as many other metabolic reactions

Pharmacodynamics Reversal of scurvy symptoms: 2 days to 3 weeks

Pharmacokinetics
Absorption: Oral: Readily absorbed; absorption is an active process and is thought to be dose-dependent
Distribution: Widely distributed
Protein binding: 25%
Metabolism: In the liver by oxidation and sulfation
Elimination: In urine; there is an individual specific renal threshold for ascorbic acid; when blood levels are high, ascorbic acid is excreted in urine, whereas when the levels are subthreshold very little if any ascorbic acid is excreted into urine

Usual Dosage Oral, I.M., I.V., S.C.:
Recommended adequate intake (AI):
0-6 months: 40 mg
6-12 months: 50 mg
Recommended daily allowance (RDA):
1-3 years: 15 mg
4-8 years: 25 mg
9-13 years: 45 mg
14-18 years: Males: 75 mg, females: 65 mg
19 years to Adults: Males: 90 mg, females: 75 mg
Children:
Scurvy: 100-300 mg/day in divided doses
Urinary acidification: 500 mg every 6-8 hours
Dietary supplement (variable): 35-100 mg/day
Adults:
Scurvy: 100-250 mg 1-2 times/day
Urinary acidification: 4-12 g/day in 3-4 divided doses
Dietary supplement (variable): 50-200 mg/day
Prevention and treatment of cold: 1-3 g/day
Children and Adults: Increase iron excretion during deferoxamine administration: 100-200 mg/day during deferoxamine therapy

Administration
Oral: May be administered without regard to meals
Parenteral: Use only in circumstances when the oral route is not possible; I.M. preferred parenteral route due to improved utilization; for I.V. use dilute in equal volume D_5W or NS, and infuse over at least 10 minutes

Reference Range
Normal levels: 10-20 µg/mL
Scurvy: <1-1.5 µg/mL

Test Interactions False-positive urinary glucose with cupric sulfate reagent, false-negative urinary glucose with glucose oxidase method, false-negative amine-dependent stool occult blood test

Additional Information Sodium content of 1 g: ~5 mEq
(Continued)

Ascorbic Acid *(Continued)*

Dosage Forms
Capsule, timed release: 500 mg
Crystals: 4 g/teaspoonful (100 g, 500 g); 5 g/teaspoonful (180 g)
Injection: 250 mg/mL (2 mL, 30 mL); 500 mg/mL (2 mL, 50 mL)
Lozenge: 60 mg
Powder: 4 g/teaspoonful (100 g, 500 g)
Solution, oral: 35 mg/0.6 mL (50 mL); 100 mg/mL (50 mL)
Syrup: 500 mg/5 mL (5 mL, 10 mL, 120 mL, 480 mL)
Tablet: 25 mg, 50 mg, 100 mg, 250 mg, 500 mg, 1000 mg
Tablet:
Chewable: 100 mg, 250 mg, 500 mg, 1000 mg
Timed release: 500 mg, 1000 mg, 1500 mg

References
"Dietary Reference Intakes for Vitamin C, Vitamin E, Selenium, and Carotenoids. A Report of the Panel on Dietary Antioxidants and Related Compounds Food and Nutrition Board, Institute of Medicine," National Academy of Sciences, Washington, DC: National Academy Press, 2000.

♦ **Ascorbicap® [OTC]** *see Ascorbic Acid on page 96*
♦ **Ascriptin® [OTC]** *see Aspirin on page 99*
♦ **Asmalix®** *see Theophylline on page 910*
♦ **ASN-ase** *see Asparaginase on page 98*

Asparaginase *(a SPIR a ji nase)*

Related Information
Emetogenic Potential of Single Chemotherapeutic Agents *on page 1095*

Brand Names Elspar®; Kidrolase® (Canada)
Synonyms A-ase; ASN-ase; Colaspase
Therapeutic Category Antineoplastic Agent, Miscellaneous
Generic Available No
Use In combination therapy for the treatment of acute lymphocytic leukemia, lymphoma
Pregnancy Risk Factor C
Contraindications Pancreatitis; hypersensitivity to *E. coli*, asparaginase, or any component (if a reaction to Elspar® occurs, obtain investigational *Erwinia* preparation from McKesson BioServices at (301) 762-0069 or pegaspargase from Gentiva Health Services at (888) 276-2217 is another alternative - use with caution)
Warnings The FDA currently recommends that procedures for proper handling and disposal of antineoplastic agents be considered; be prepared to treat anaphylaxis at each administration
Precautions Use with caution in patients with impaired renal function; discontinue asparaginase at the first sign of renal failure or pancreatitis

Adverse Reactions
Cardiovascular: Hypotension
Central nervous system: Fever, drowsiness, seizures, chills, malaise, coma, headache, stroke, confusion, dizziness, hallucinations
Dermatologic: Rash, pruritus, urticaria
Endocrine & metabolic: Hyperglycemia, transient diabetes mellitus, hyperammonemia, hyperuricemia, hypoalbuminemia; decreased thyroxine and thyroxine-binding globulin concentration
Gastrointestinal: Vomiting, pancreatitis, nausea, anorexia, abdominal cramps
Hematologic: Leukopenia, coagulation abnormalities (prolonged thrombin, PT, and partial prothrombin times), reduced fibrinogen
Hepatic: Hepatotoxicity (elevated liver enzymes, hyperbilirubinemia)
Renal: Azotemia
Respiratory: Coughing, laryngeal edema, bronchospasm
Miscellaneous: Hypersensitivity reactions (incidence in children is 20% with *E. coli* asparaginase and <5% with *Erwinia* asparaginase); anaphylaxis

Drug Interactions Methotrexate (decreased antineoplastic effect if given prior to methotrexate); vincristine (increases toxicity if given concomitantly); prednisone (increases hyperglycemic effect)
Stability Refrigerate; no loss in potency was noted after storage for 1 week at room temperature, however, the manufacturer recommends that reconstituted solutions should be discarded after 8 hours since there is no preservative; discard immediately if solution becomes cloudy; use of a 0.2 micron filter may result in some loss of potency
Mechanism of Action Inhibits protein synthesis by deaminating asparagine and depriving tumor cells of this essential amino acid

Pharmacokinetics

Absorption: Not absorbed from GI tract, therefore requires parenteral administration

Distribution: Asparaginase not detected in CSF but CSF asparagine is depleted

Half-life:

E. coli L-asparaginase: 24-36 hours

Patients who have had a hypersensitivity reaction to asparaginase have a decreased half-life

Erwinia L-asparaginase: Significantly shorter than for the *E. coli*-derived product; mean half-life *Erwinia* L-asparaginase: 10-15 hours

Elimination: Clearance is unaffected by age, renal function, or hepatic function

Usual Dosage Children and Adults: Refer to individual protocols

Perform intradermal sensitivity testing with 2 units of asparaginase before the initial dose and when a week or more has elapsed between doses:

I.M. (preferred): 6000-10,000 units/m^2/dose 3 times/week for 3 weeks for combination therapy; high-dose I.M. regimen of 25,000 units/m^2/dose once weekly for 9 doses has also been used

I.V.: 1000 units/kg/day for 10 days for combination therapy or 200 units/kg/day for 28 days if combination therapy is inappropriate

Administration

I.M.: Maximum 2 mL volume is recommended for I.M. injections; if the volume to be administered is >2 mL, use multiple injection sites

I.V.: Must be infused over a minimum of 30 minutes

Monitoring Parameters Vital signs during administration, CBC, urinalysis, amylase, liver enzymes, bilirubin, prothrombin time, renal function tests, urine glucose, blood glucose

Patient Information Notify physician if fever, sore throat, painful/burning urination, bruising, bleeding, or shortness of breath occurs

Nursing Implications I.M. route is associated with a more delayed, less severe anaphylactoid reaction compared to the I.V. route; patients should be observed for one hour following an I.M. injection for signs of severe hypersensitivity; appropriate agents for maintenance of an adequate airway and treatment of a hypersensitivity reaction (antihistamine, epinephrine, oxygen, I.V. corticosteroids) should be readily available

Dosage Forms Injection: 10,000 units/vial

References

Asselin BL, Whitin JC, Coppola DJ, et al, "Comparative Pharmacokinetic Studies of Three Asparaginase Preparations," *J Clin Oncol*, 1993, 11(9):1780-6.

Clavell LA, Gelber RD, Cohen HJ, et al, "Four-Agent Induction and Intensive Asparaginase Therapy for Treatment of Childhood Acute Lymphoblastic Leukemia," *N Engl J Med*, 1986, 315(11):657-63.

Nesbit M, Chard R, Evans A, et al, "Evaluation of Intramuscular Versus Intravenous Administration of L-Asparaginase in Childhood Leukemia," *Am J Pediatr Hematol Oncol*, 1979, 1(1):9-13.

Ortega JA, Nesbit ME Jr, and Donaldson MH, "L-Asparaginase, Vincristine, and Prednisone for Induction of First Remission in Acute Lymphocytic Leukemia," *Cancer Res*, 1977, 37(2):535-40.

♦ **A-Spas® S/L** *see* Hyoscyamine *on page 497*

♦ **Aspergum® [OTC]** *see* Aspirin *on page 99*

Aspirin (AS pir in)

Related Information

Drugs and Breast-Feeding *on page 1213*

Overdose and Toxicology *on page 1191*

Brand Names Anacin® [OTC]; Apo®-ASA (Canada); A.S.A. [OTC]; ASA® (Canada); Asaphen (Canada); Ascriptin® [OTC]; Aspergum® [OTC]; Bayer® Aspirin [OTC]; Bufferin® [OTC]; Easprin®; Ecotrin® [OTC]; Empirin® [OTC]; Entrophen® (Canada); Halfprin® [OTC]; Measurin® [OTC]; MSD® Enteric Coated ASA (Canada); Novasen (Canada); ZORprin®

Synonyms Acetylsalicylic Acid; ASA

Therapeutic Category Analgesic, Non-narcotic; Anti-inflammatory Agent; Antiplatelet Agent; Antipyretic; Nonsteroidal Anti-inflammatory Drug (NSAID), Oral; Salicylate

Generic Available Yes

Use Treatment of mild to moderate pain, inflammation and fever; adjunctive treatment of Kawasaki disease; prevention of vascular mortality during suspected acute MI; prevention of recurrent MI; prevention of MI in patients with angina; prevention of recurrent stroke and mortality following TIA or stroke

Pregnancy Risk Factor C (D if full-dose aspirin in 3rd trimester)

Contraindications Bleeding disorders; hypersensitivity to salicylates, any component, or other NSAIDs; hepatic failure

(Continued)

Aspirin *(Continued)*

Warnings Do not use aspirin in children <16 years of age for chickenpox or flu symptoms due to the association with Reye's syndrome

Precautions Use with caution in patients with impaired renal function, erosive gastritis, peptic ulcer, gout, platelet and bleeding disorders

Adverse Reactions

Dermatologic: Rash, urticaria

Gastrointestinal: Nausea, vomiting, GI distress, GI bleeding, ulcers

Hematologic: Inhibition of platelet aggregation

Hepatic: Hepatotoxicity

Respiratory: Bronchospasm

Drug Interactions Aspirin may increase methotrexate serum levels and may displace valproic acid from binding sites which can result in toxicity; aspirin may increase free (unbound) buspirone concentrations; use of warfarin, heparin, low molecular weight heparins, urokinase, streptokinase, and platelet inhibitors (eg, dipyridamole) with aspirin may cause an increase in bleeding; use of NSAIDs with aspirin may cause an increase in GI adverse effects and a possible decrease in serum concentration of NSAIDs; aspirin may antagonize effects of probenecid; aspirin, especially high doses, may decrease the antihypertensive effects of ACE inhibitors; buffered preparations may decrease the oral absorption of tetracycline or ketoconazole, therefore, administer 3-4 hours apart

Food Interactions Aspirin may increase the renal excretion of vitamin C and may decrease serum folate levels; some suggest increasing the dietary intake of foods that are high in vitamin C and folic acid

Stability Keep suppositories in refrigerator, do not freeze; hydrolysis of aspirin occurs upon exposure to water or moist air, resulting in salicylate and acetate; acetate possesses a vinegar-like odor; do not use if a strong odor is present

Mechanism of Action Inhibits prostaglandin synthesis, acts on the hypothalamus heat-regulating center to reduce fever, blocks prostaglandin synthetase action which prevents formation of the platelet-aggregating substance thromboxane A_2

Pharmacokinetics

Absorption: From the stomach and small intestine

Distribution: Readily distributes into most body fluids and tissues; hydrolyzed to salicylate (active) by esterases in the GI mucosa, red blood cells, synovial fluid and blood

Metabolism: Primarily by hepatic microsomal enzymes

Half-life: 15-20 minutes; metabolic pathways are saturable such that salicylate half-life is dose-dependent ranging from 3 hours at lower doses (300-600 mg), 5-6 hours (after 1 g) and 10 hours with higher doses

Time to peak serum concentration: Salicylate: ~1-2 hours; may be delayed with controlled or timed-release preparations

Elimination: Renal as salicylate and conjugated metabolites

Dialyzable: 50% to 100%

Usual Dosage

Children:

Analgesic and antipyretic: Oral, rectal: 10-15 mg/kg/dose every 4-6 hours; maximum dose: 4 g/day

Anti-inflammatory: Oral: Initial: 60-90 mg/kg/day in divided doses; usual maintenance: 80-100 mg/kg/day divided every 6-8 hours; monitor serum concentrations

Antiplatelet effects: Adequate pediatric studies have not been performed; pediatric dosage is derived from adult studies and clinical experience and is not well established; suggested doses have ranged from 3-5 mg/kg/day to 5-10 mg/kg/day given as a single daily dose. Doses are rounded to a convenient amount (eg, 1/2 of 80 mg tablet).

Mechanical prosthetic heart valves: 6-20 mg/kg/day given as a single daily dose (used in combination with an oral anticoagulant in children who have systemic embolism despite adequate oral anticoagulation therapy (INR 2.5-3.5) and used in combination with low-dose anticoagulation (INR 2-3) and dipyridamole when full-dose oral anticoagulation is contraindicated)

Blalock-Taussig shunts: 3-5 mg/kg/day given as a single daily dose

Kawasaki disease: Oral: 80-100 mg/kg/day divided every 6 hours; monitor serum concentrations; after fever resolves: 3-5 mg/kg/day once daily; in patients without coronary artery abnormalities, give lower dose for at least 6-8 weeks or until ESR and platelet count are normal; in patients with coronary artery abnormalities, low-dose aspirin should be continued indefinitely

Adults:
  Analgesic and antipyretic: Oral, rectal: 325-1000 mg every 4-6 hours up to 4 g/day
  Anti-inflammatory: Oral: Initial: 2.4-3.6 g/day in divided doses; usual maintenance: 3.6-5.4 g/day; monitor serum concentrations
  Suspected acute MI: Oral: Initial: 160-162.5 mg as soon as MI is suspected; then 160-162.5 mg once daily for 30 days post MI; then consider further aspirin treatment
  MI prophylaxis: Oral: 75-325 mg once daily (continue indefinitely)
  Prevention of stroke following ischemic stroke or TIA: Oral: 50-325 mg once daily (continue indefinitely)

Administration Oral: Administer with water, food, or milk to decrease GI upset; do not crush controlled release, timed release, or enteric coated tablets; these preparations should be swallowed whole

Monitoring Parameters Serum salicylate concentration with chronic use

Reference Range
  Therapeutic levels:
    Anti-inflammatory effect: 150-300 µg/mL
    Analgesic and antipyretic effect: 30-50 µg/mL
  Timing of serum samples: Peak levels usually occur 2 hours after normal doses but may occur 6-24 hours after acute toxic ingestion.
  Salicylate serum concentrations correlate with the pharmacological actions and adverse effects observed. See table.

Serum Salicylate: Clinical Correlations

Serum Salicylate Concentration (µg/mL)	Desired Effects	Adverse Effects/Intoxication
~100	Antiplatelet Antipyresis Analgesia	GI intolerance and bleeding, hypersensitivity, hemostatic defects
150-300	Anti-inflammatory	Mild salicylism
250-400	Treatment of rheumatic fever	Nausea/vomiting, hyperventilation, salicylism, flushing, sweating, thirst, headache, diarrhea, and tachycardia
>400-500		Respiratory alkalosis, hemorrhage, excitement, confusion, asterixis, pulmonary edema, convulsions, tetany, metabolic acidosis, fever, coma, cardiovascular collapse, renal and respiratory failure

Test Interactions False-negative results for glucose oxidase urinary glucose tests (Clinistix®); false-positives using the cupric sulfate method (Clinitest®); interferes with Gerhardt test, VMA determination; 5-HIAA, xylose tolerance test and T_3 and T_4

Patient Information Watch for bleeding gums or signs of GI bleeding, (bright red blood in emesis or stool, coffee ground-like emesis, black tarry stools); notify physician if ringing in the ears, persistent GI pain, or GI bleeding occurs

Additional Information Bayer® Aspirin has received 5 new FDA indications (see http://www.wonderdrug.com/practitioners3.html)

Dosage Forms
  Suppository, rectal: 60 mg, 120 mg, 125 mg, 130 mg, 195 mg, 200 mg, 300 mg, 325 mg, 600 mg, 650 mg, 1200 mg
  Tablet: 325 mg, 500 mg
  Tablet:
    Buffered:
      325 mg (with aluminum hydroxide and magnesium hydroxide)
      500 mg (with aluminum hydroxide and magnesium hydroxide)
    Chewable: 75 mg, 81 mg
    Chewing gum: 227 mg
    Controlled release: 800 mg
    Enteric coated (delayed release): 80 mg, 165 mg, 325 mg, 500 mg, 650 mg, 975 mg
    Timed release: 650 mg

References
Hathaway WE, "Use of Antiplatelet Agents in Pediatric Hypercoagulable States," Am J Dis Child, 1984, 138(3):301-4.
(Continued)

Aspirin *(Continued)*

Pickering LK, ed, *2000 Red Book, Report of the Committee on Infectious Diseases*, 25th ed, Elk Grove Village IL: American Academy of Pediatrics, 2000, 360-3.

Michelson AD, Bovil E, Monagle P, and Andrew M, "Antithrombotic Therapy in Children," *Chest*, 1998, 114:748S-769S.

♦ **Aspirin and Oxycodone** *see* Oxycodone and Aspirin *on page 717*

♦ **Astelin® Nasal Spray** *see* Azelastine *on page 113*

♦ **Asthma Guidelines** *see page 1178*

♦ **AsthmaHaler® Mist [OTC]** *see* Epinephrine *on page 371*

♦ **AsthmaNefrin® [OTC]** *see* Epinephrine *on page 371*

♦ **Astramorph/PF™ Injection** *see* Morphine Sulfate *on page 657*

♦ **Atarax® Oral** *see* Hydroxyzine *on page 496*

♦ **Atasol® 8, 15, 30 W/ Caffeine (Canada)** *see* Acetaminophen and Codeine *on page 27*

♦ **Atasol® (Canada)** *see* Acetaminophen *on page 26*

Atenolol (a TEN oh lole)

Related Information

Adult ACLS Algorithm, Tachycardia *on page 1010*
Overdose and Toxicology *on page 1191*

Brand Names Apo®-Atenol (Canada); Novo-Atenol® (Canada); Nu-Atenol® (Canada); Taro-Atenol® (Canada); Tenormin®

Therapeutic Category Antianginal Agent; Antihypertensive Agent; Beta-Adrenergic Blocker

Generic Available Yes

Use Treatment of hypertension, alone or in combination with other agents; management of angina pectoris; antiarrhythmic; post-MI patients; acute alcohol withdrawal

Pregnancy Risk Factor D

Contraindications Hypersensitivity to atenolol or any component; Pulmonary edema, cardiogenic shock, bradycardia, heart block, or uncompensated CHF

Warnings Abrupt withdrawal of the drug should be avoided; drug should be discontinued over 1-2 weeks

Precautions Use with caution and modify dosage in patients with renal impairment; use with caution in patients with CHF, bronchospastic disease, diabetes mellitus, and hyperthyroidism. Patients who have a history of anaphylactic hypersensitivity reactions to various substances may be more reactive while receiving beta-blockers; these patients may not be responsive to the normal doses of epinephrine used to treat hypersensitivity reactions.

Adverse Reactions

Cardiovascular: Bradycardia, hypotension, second or third degree A-V block, CHF, chest pain, edema, Raynaud's phenomenon

Central nervous system: Dizziness, fatigue, lethargy, headache, nightmares, insomnia, confusion, mental impairment

Gastrointestinal: Constipation, nausea, diarrhea

Respiratory: Wheezing and dyspnea have occurred with higher doses (eg, >100 mg/day in adults)

Drug Interactions Catecholamine-depleting drugs, such as reserpine, may have additive effects (hypotension, bradycardia); hypotensive agents, diuretics, cardiac glycosides, amiodarone, calcium channel blockers, agents that slow AV conduction, and myocardial depressant general anesthetics may have additive effects with beta-blockers; abrupt withdrawal of clonidine while receiving beta-blockers may result in an exaggerated hypertensive crisis; NSAIDs may decrease the antihypertensive effects of beta-blockers; atenolol (especially at higher doses) may reverse the therapeutic effects of theophylline

Mechanism of Action Competitively blocks response to beta-adrenergic stimulation; selectively blocks beta$_1$-receptors with little or no effect on beta$_2$-receptors except at high doses; does not possess membrane stabilizing or intrinsic sympathomimetic (partial agonist) activities

Pharmacokinetics

Absorption: Incomplete from the GI tract; ~50% absorbed

Distribution: Does not cross the blood-brain barrier; low lipophilicity

Protein binding: Low (6% to 16%)

Half-life, beta:

Neonates: Mean: 16 hours, up to 35 hours

Children 5-16 years of age: Mean: 4.6 hours; range: 3.5-7 hours; children >10 years of age may have longer half-life (>5 hours) compared to children 5-10 years of age (<5 hours)

Adults: 6-7 hours
Prolonged half-life with renal dysfunction
Time to peak serum concentration: Oral: Within 2-4 hours
Elimination: 40% as unchanged drug in urine, 50% in feces
Moderately dialyzable (20% to 50%)

Usual Dosage
Oral:
Children: Initial: 0.8-1 mg/kg/dose given daily; range: 0.8-1.5 mg/kg/day; maximum dose: 2 mg/kg/day
Adults:
Initial: 25-50 mg/dose given daily; usual dose: 50-100 mg/dose given daily
Maximum dose: Hypertension: 100 mg given daily; angina: 200 mg given daily
See table for oral dosing interval in renal impairment.

Creatinine Clearance	Maximum Oral Dose	Frequency of Administration
15-35 mL/min	50 mg or 1 mg/kg/dose	Daily
<15 mL/min	50 mg or 1 mg/kg/dose	Every other day

I.V.: Adults: For early treatment of MI: 5 mg slow I.V. over 5 minutes; may repeat in 10 minutes; if both doses are tolerated, may start oral atenolol 50 mg every 12 hours for 6-9 days post MI

Administration
Oral: May be administered without regard to food
Parenteral: Administer by slow I.V. injection at a rate not to exceed 1 mg/minute; the injection can be administered undiluted or diluted with a compatible I.V. solution

Monitoring Parameters Blood pressure, heart rate, EKG, fluid intake and output, daily weight, respiratory rate

Patient Information Abrupt withdrawal of the drug should be avoided

Additional Information In diabetic patients, atenolol may potentiate hypoglycemia and mask signs and symptoms of hypoglycemia; limited data suggests that atenolol may have a shorter half-life and faster clearance in patients with Marfan syndrome. Higher doses (2 mg/kg/day divided every 12 hours) have been used in patients with Marfan syndrome (6-22 years of age) to decrease aortic root growth rate and prevent aortic dissection or rupture; further studies are needed.

Dosage Forms
Injection: 0.5 mg/mL (10 mL)
Tablet: 25 mg, 50 mg, 100 mg

Extemporaneous Preparations A 2 mg/mL atenolol oral liquid compounded from tablets and a commercially available oral diluent was found to be stable for up to 40 days when stored at 5°C or 25°C
Garner SS, Wiest DB, and Reynolds ER, "Stability of Atenolol in an Extemporaneously Compounded Oral Liquid," *Am J Hosp Pharm*, 1994, 51(4):508-11.

References
Buck ML, Wiest D, Gillette PC, et al, "Pharmacokinetics and Pharmacodynamics of Atenolol in Children," *Clin Pharmacol Ther*, 1989, 46(6):629-33.
Case CL, Trippel DL, and Gillette PC, "New Antiarrhythmic Agents in Pediatrics," *Pediatr Clin North Am*, 1989, 36(5):1293-320.
Trippel DL and Gillette PC, "Atenolol in Children With Supraventricular Tachycardia," *Am J Cardiol*, 1989, 64(3):233-6.
Trippel DL and Gillette PC, "Atenolol in Children With Ventricular Arrhythmias," *Am Heart J*, 1990, 119(6):1312-6.

♦ **ATG** *see* Lymphocyte Immune Globulin *on page 586*
♦ **Atgam®** *see* Lymphocyte Immune Globulin *on page 586*
♦ **Ativan®** *see* Lorazepam *on page 583*
♦ **Atolone® Oral** *see* Triamcinolone *on page 946*

Atovaquone (a TOE va kwone)
Brand Names Mepron®
Synonyms Hydroxy-1,4-naphthoquinone
Therapeutic Category Antiprotozoal
Generic Available No
Use Second-line treatment of mild to moderate *Pneumocystis carinii* pneumonia (PCP) in patients intolerant of trimethoprim/sulfamethoxazole (TMP/SMX); mild to moderate PCP is defined as an alveolar-arterial oxygen diffusion gradient ≤45 mm Hg and PaO$_2$ ≥60 mm Hg on room air; patients intolerant of TMP/SMX are defined as having a significant rash (ie, Stevens-Johnson-like syndrome), neutropenia, or
(Continued)

Atovaquone *(Continued)*

hemolysis; prevention of *Pneumocystis carinii* pneumonia in patients who are intolerant to trimethoprim-sulfamethoxazole; treatment of babesiosis

Pregnancy Risk Factor C

Contraindications Hypersensitivity to atovaquone or any component

Warnings Clinical experience with atovaquone has been limited to patients with mild to moderate PCP; treatment of more severe episodes of PCP has not been systematically studied

Precautions For patients who have difficulty taking atovaquone with food or who have chronic diarrhea, stomach or intestinal problems which may result in drug malabsorption, parenteral therapy with other agents should be considered since a low serum atovaquone concentration could lead to treatment failure

Adverse Reactions

Central nervous system: Fever, headache, insomnia, dizziness, pain

Dermatologic: Maculopapular rash, erythema multiforme, pruritus

Endocrine & metabolic: Hyponatremia

Gastrointestinal: Nausea, vomiting, diarrhea, abdominal pain, constipation, anorexia, elevated amylase

Hematologic: Rare: Neutropenia, anemia

Hepatic: Elevated hepatic enzymes, cholestasis

Respiratory: Cough, sinusitis

Miscellaneous: Diaphoresis

Drug Interactions Rifampin may decrease plasma atovaquone concentration; since atovaquone is highly protein bound, it may compete for protein binding sites with other highly protein-bound agents like warfarin (however, there have been no drug-drug interactions of this type reported to date)

Food Interactions Administration with food enhances absorption

Stability Store at room temperature; do not freeze

Mechanism of Action The mechanism of action against *Pneumocystis carinii* has not been fully elucidated; in *Plasmodium* species, atovaquone selectively inhibits the mitochondrial electron-transport system at the cytochrome bc_1 complex resulting in depletion of dihydroorotate dehydrogenase and ultimately resulting in the inhibition of nucleic acid and adenosine triphosphate synthesis

Pharmacokinetics

Absorption: Oral:

Infants and Children <2 years of age: Decreased absorption

Adults: Oral suspension with food: Absorption is enhanced twofold with food; decreased absorption with single doses exceeding 750 mg

Distribution: V_{dss}: 0.6 L/kg; CSF concentration is <1% of the plasma concentration

Protein binding: >99%

Bioavailability: Suspension (administered with food): 47%

Half-life, elimination:

Children (4 months to 12 years): 60 hours (range: 31-163 hours)

Adults: 2.9 days

Adults with AIDS: 2.2 days

Time to peak serum concentration: Dual peak serum concentrations at 1 to 8 hours and at 24 to 96 hours after dose due to enterohepatic cycling

Elimination: ~94% is recovered as unchanged drug in feces; 0.6% excreted in urine

Usual Dosage Oral:

Children:

Treatment: Dose of 40 mg/kg/day divided twice daily (maximum dose: 1500 mg/day) may be necessary to attain comparable plasma concentrations associated with the successful treatment of PCP as seen in adults.

Prophylaxis of *Pneumocystis carinii* pneumonia:

1-3 months of age and >24 months of age: 30 mg/kg/day once daily (maximum dose: 1500 mg/day)

4-24 months of age: 45 mg/kg/day once daily (maximum dose: 1500 mg/day)

Babesiosis: 40 mg/kg/day divided twice daily (maximum dose: 1500 mg/day) with azithromycin 12 mg/kg/day once daily for 7-10 days

Adolescents 13-16 years and Adults:

Treatment: 750 mg/dose twice daily for 21 days

Prophylaxis of *Pneumocystis carinii* pneumonia: 1500 mg once daily

Babesiosis: 750 mg/dose twice daily for 7-10 days with azithromycin 1000 mg once daily for 3 days then 500 mg once daily for 7 days

Administration Oral: Administer with food or a high-fat meal; shake suspension well before using

Monitoring Parameters CBC with differential, liver enzymes, serum chemistries, serum amylase

Additional Information The suspension contains the inactive ingredients benzyl alcohol and poloxamer 188

Dosage Forms Suspension, oral (citrus flavor): 750 mg/5 mL (210 mL)

References

Centers for Disease Control and Prevention, "1999 USPHS/IDSA Guidelines for the Prevention of Opportunistic Infections in Persons Infected With Human Immunodeficiency Virus," *MMWR Morb Mortal Wkly Rep*, 1999, 48(RR-10):1-59.

Haile LG and Flaherty JF, "Atovaquone: A Review," *Ann Pharmacother*, 1993, 27(12):1488-94.

Hughes W, Leoung G, Kramer F, et al, "Comparison of Atovaquone (566C80) With Trimethoprim-Sulfamethoxazole to Treat *Pneumocystis carinii* Pneumonia in Patients With AIDS," *N Engl J Med*, 1993, 328(21):1521-7.

Pagano G, Kennedy W, Weller S, et al, "The Safety and Pharmacokinetics of Atovaquone in Immunocompromised Children," Abstracts of the IX International Conference on AIDS in Affiliation With the IV STD World Congress: Berlin, 1993, June 6-11; Abs No.PO-B10-1455.

♦ **Atozine® Oral** *see* Hydroxyzine *on page 496*

Atracurium (a tra KYOO ree um)

Brand Names Tracrium®

Available Salts Atracurium Besylate

Therapeutic Category Neuromuscular Blocker Agent, Nondepolarizing; Skeletal Muscle Relaxant, Paralytic

Generic Available No

Use Eases endotracheal intubation as an adjunct to general anesthesia and relaxes skeletal muscle during surgery or mechanical ventilation

Pregnancy Risk Factor C

Contraindications Hypersensitivity to atracurium besylate or any component

Warnings Reduce initial dosage and inject slowly (over 1-2 minutes) in patients in whom substantial histamine release would be potentially hazardous (eg, patients with clinically important cardiovascular disease); maintenance of an adequate airway and respiratory support is critical; avoid use of preservative-containing formulation in neonates; certain clinical conditions may result in potentiation or antagonism of neuromuscular blockade, see table.

Clinical Conditions Affecting Neuromuscular Blockade

Potentiation	Antagonism
Electrolyte abnormalities	Alkalosis
Severe hyponatremia	Hypercalcemia
Severe hypocalcemia	Demyelinating lesions
Severe hypokalemia	Peripheral neuropathies
Hypermagnesemia	Diabetes mellitus
Neuromuscular diseases	
Acidosis	
Acute intermittent porphyria	
Renal failure	
Hepatic failure	

Increased sensitivity in patients with myasthenia gravis, Eaton-Lambert syndrome; resistance to neuromuscular blockade in burn patients (>30% of body) for period of 5-70 days postinjury; resistance in patients with muscle trauma, denervation, immobilization, infection, chronic treatment with atracurium. When used in conjunction with anesthetics, bradycardia may be more common with atracurium than with other neuromuscular blocking agents; it has no clinically significant effects on heart rate to counteract the bradycardia produced by anesthetics.

Precautions Due to potential histamine release, use with caution in patients in whom histamine release may be hazardous (eg, cardiovascular disease, asthma); patients with severe electrolyte disorders; patients with myasthenia gravis

Adverse Reactions

Cardiovascular: Effects are minimal and transient

Dermatologic: Erythema, itching, urticaria

Respiratory: Wheezing, bronchial secretions (increased)

Drug Interactions See table on following page.

Stability Refrigerate; stable at room temperature for 14 days; unstable in alkaline solutions; compatible with D_5W, D_5NS, and NS; do not dilute in LR

(Continued)

Atracurium *(Continued)*

Potential Drug Interactions

Potentiation	Antagonism
Anesthetics	Calcium
Desflurane, sevoflurane, enflurane and	Carbamazepine
isoflurane > halothane > nitrous	Phenytoin
oxide	Steroids (chronic administration)
Antibiotics	Theophylline
Aminoglycosides, polymyxins,	Anticholinesterases*
clindamycin, vancomycin	Neostigmine, pyridostigmine,
Magnesium sulfate	edrophonium, echothiophate
Antiarrhythmics	ophthalmic solution
Quinidine, procainamide, bretylium, and	Caffeine
possibly lidocaine	Azathioprine
Diuretics	
Furosemide, mannitol	
Amphotericin B (secondary to hypokalemia)	
Local anesthetics	
Dantrolene (directly depresses skeletal muscle)	
Beta blockers	
Calcium channel blockers	
Ketamine	
Lithium	
Succinylcholine (when administered prior to nondepolarizing neuromuscular-blocking agent)	
Cyclosporine	

*Can prolong the effects of acetylcholine

Mechanism of Action Blocks neural transmission at the myoneural junction by binding with cholinergic receptor sites

Pharmacodynamics
Onset of action: I.V.: Within 2 minutes
Peak effect: Within 3-5 minutes
Duration: Recovery begins in 20-35 minutes when anesthesia is balanced

Pharmacokinetics
Metabolism: Some metabolites are active; undergoes rapid nonenzymatic degradation (Hofmann elimination) in the bloodstream; additional metabolism occurs via ester hydrolysis
Half-life:
Distributive: 2-3.4 minutes
Terminal: 20 minutes

Usual Dosage I.V.:
Neonates, Infants, and Children ≤2 years: 0.3-0.4 mg/kg initially followed by maintenance doses of 0.3-0.4 mg/kg as needed to maintain neuromuscular blockade
Children >2 years to Adults:
0.4-0.5 mg/kg then 0.08-0.1 mg/kg 20-45 minutes after initial dose to maintain neuromuscular block
or
Continuous infusion: 0.4-0.8 mg/kg/hour or 6.7-13 mcg/kg/minute (range: 2-15 mcg/kg/minute)
Dosage adjustment in hepatic or renal impairment: Not necessary
Dosage adjustment with enflurane or isoflurane: Reduce dosage by 33%
Dosage adjustment with induced hypothermia (cardio-bypass surgery): Reduce dosage by 50%

Administration Parenteral: May be administered without further dilution by rapid I.V. injection; for continuous infusions, dilute to a maximum concentration of 0.5 mg/mL (more concentrated solutions have reduced stability, ie, <24 hours at room temperature); not for I.M. injection due to tissue irritation

Monitoring Parameters Muscle twitch response to peripheral nerve stimulation, heart rate, blood pressure

Additional Information Neuromuscular blockade may be reversed with neostigmine; atropine or glycopyrrolate should be available to treat excessive cholinergic effects from neostigmine

Dosage Forms
Injection, as besylate: 10 mg/mL (5 mL, 10 mL)
Injection, preservative free, as besylate: 10 mg/mL (5 mL)

♦ **Atracurium Besylate** see Atracurium on page 105

♦ **Atropair® Ophthalmic** see Atropine on page 107

Atropine (A troe peen)

Related Information
Adult ACLS Algorithm, Asystole on page 1008
Adult ACLS Algorithm, Bradycardia on page 1012
Adult ACLS Algorithm, Pulseless Electrical Activity on page 1006
Asthma Guidelines on page 1178
Compatibility of Medications Mixed in a Syringe on page 1208
CPR Pediatric Drug Dosages on page 999
Overdose and Toxicology on page 1191
Pediatric ALS Algorithm, Bradycardia on page 1001

Brand Names Atropair® Ophthalmic; Atropine-Care® Ophthalmic; Atropisol® Ophthalmic; Isopto® Atropine Ophthalmic; I-Tropine® Ophthalmic; Ocu-Tropine® Ophthalmic

Available Salts Atropine Sulfate

Therapeutic Category Antiasthmatic; Anticholinergic Agent; Anticholinergic Agent, Ophthalmic; Antidote, Organophosphate Poisoning; Antispasmodic Agent, Gastrointestinal; Bronchodilator; Ophthalmic Agent, Mydriatic

Generic Available Yes

Use Preoperative medication to inhibit salivation and secretions; treatment of sinus bradycardia; management of peptic ulcer; reversal of the muscarinic effects of cholinergic agents such as neostigmine and pyridostigmine; treatment of exercise-induced bronchospasm; antidote for organophosphate pesticide poisoning; used to produce mydriasis and cycloplegia for examination of the retina and optic disk and accurate measurement of refractive errors; treatment of uveitis

Pregnancy Risk Factor C

Contraindications Hypersensitivity to atropine sulfate or any component; narrow-angle glaucoma; tachycardia; thyrotoxicosis; obstructive disease of the GI tract; obstructive uropathy

Precautions Use with caution in children with spastic paralysis or brain damage; children are at increased risk for rapid rise in body temperature due to suppression of sweat gland activity; paradoxical hyperexcitability may occur in children given large doses; infants with Down's syndrome have both increased sensitivity to cardiac effects and mydriasis

Adverse Reactions
Cardiovascular: Tachycardia, palpitations
Central nervous system: Fatigue, delirium, headache, restlessness, ataxia
Dermatologic: Dry hot skin
Gastrointestinal: Impaired GI motility
Neuromuscular & skeletal: Tremor
Ocular: Blurred vision

Drug Interactions Additive effects when administered with other anticholinergic agents; may alter response to beta-adrenergic blockers

Mechanism of Action Blocks the action of acetylcholine at parasympathetic sites in smooth muscle, secretory glands, and the CNS; increases cardiac output, dries secretions, antagonizes histamine and serotonin

Pharmacodynamics
Inhibition of salivation:
Onset:
Oral: 30-60 minutes
I.M.: 30 minutes
Peak effect:
Oral: 2 hours
I.M.: 1-1.6 hours
Duration: Oral, I.M.: Up to 4 hours
Increased heart rate:
Onset:
Oral: 30 minutes to 2 hours
I.M.: 5-40 minutes
(Continued)

Atropine *(Continued)*

Peak effect:
  Oral: 1-2 hours
  I.M.: 20 minutes to 1 hour
  I.V.: 2-4 minutes
Bronchodilation: Oral Inhalation:
  Onset: 15 minutes
  Peak effect: 15 minutes to 1.5 hours

Pharmacokinetics

Absorption: Well absorbed from all dosage forms
Distribution: Widely distributes throughout the body; crosses the placenta; trace amounts appear in breast milk; crosses the blood-brain barrier
Protein binding: 20%
Metabolism: In the liver
Half-life: Adults: 2-3 hours
Elimination: Both metabolites and unchanged drug (30% to 50%) are excreted into urine

Usual Dosage Note: Doses <0.1 mg have been associated with paradoxical bradycardia

Neonates, Infants and Children:
  Preanesthetic: Oral, I.M., I.V., S.C.:
    <5 kg: 0.02 mg/kg/dose 30-60 minutes preop then every 4-6 hours as needed; use of a minimum dosage of 0.1 mg in neonates <5 kg will result in dosages >0.02 mg/kg; there is no documented minimum dosage in this age group
    >5 kg: 0.01-0.02 mg/kg/dose to a maximum 0.4 mg/dose 30-60 minutes preop; minimum dose: 0.1 mg
  Bradycardia: I.V., intratracheal: 0.02 mg/kg, minimum dose 0.1 mg, maximum single dose: 0.5 mg in children and 1 mg in adolescents; may repeat in 5-minute intervals to a maximum total dose of 1 mg in children or 2 mg in adolescents. (**Note:** For intratracheal administration, must be diluted; see Administration.) When treating bradycardia in neonates, reserve use for those patients unresponsive to improved oxygenation and epinephrine.
Children:
  Bronchospasm: Inhalation: 0.03-0.05 mg/kg/dose 3-4 times/day; maximum: 2.5 mg/dose
  Refraction: Ophthalmic:
    Infants <1 year: Instill 1 drop of 0.25% solution 3 times/day for 3 days before the procedure
    Children: 1-5 years: Instill 1 drop of 0.5% solution 3 times/day for 3 days before the procedure
    Children >5 years or Children with dark irides: Instill 1 drop of 1% solution 3 times/day for 3 days before the procedure
  Uveitis: Ophthalmic: Instill 1 drop of 0.5% solution 1-3 times daily
Adults (doses <0.5 mg have been associated with paradoxical bradycardia):
  Asystole: I.V.: 1 mg; may repeat every 3-5 minutes as needed
  Preanesthetic: Oral, I.M., I.V., S.C.: 0.4-0.6 mg 30-60 minutes preop
  Bradycardia: I.V.: 0.5-1 mg every 5 minutes, not to exceed a total of 2 mg or 0.04 mg/kg
  Bronchospasm: Inhalation: 0.025-0.05 mg/kg/dose every 4-6 hours as needed; maximum: 2.5 mg/dose
  Refraction: Ophthalmic: Instill 1-2 drops of 1% solution before the procedure
  Uveitis: Ophthalmic: Instill 1-2 drops of 1% solution up to 4 times/day

Administration

Intratracheal: Dilute with NS to a total volume of 1-2 mL
Parenteral: Administer undiluted by rapid I.V. injection; slow injection may result in paradoxical bradycardia
Ophthalmic: Due to the discontinuance of 0.5% ophthalmic solutions commercially, 0.5% and 0.25% solutions may be prepared by dilution of 1% atropine ophthalmic solution with artificial tears; a 1:1 dilution for 0.5% and a 1:4 dilution for 0.25%; instill solution into conjunctival sac of affected eye(s); avoid contact of bottle tip with eye or skin

Monitoring Parameters Heart rate

Dosage Forms

Injection, as sulfate: 0.1 mg/mL (5 mL, 10 mL); 0.3 mg/mL (1 mL, 30 mL); 0.4 mg/mL (1 mL, 20 mL, 30 mL); 0.5 mg/mL (1 mL, 5 mL, 30 mL); 0.8 mg/mL (0.5 mL, 1 mL); 1 mg/mL (1 mL, 10 mL)
Ointment, ophthalmic, as sulfate: 1% (3.5 g)
Solution, ophthalmic, as sulfate: 1% (1 mL, 2 mL, 5 mL, 15 mL); 2% (1 mL, 2 mL)

Tablet, as sulfate: 0.4 mg
Tablet, soluble, as sulfate: 0.4 mg, 0.6 mg

References

Emergency Cardiac Care Committee and Subcommittees, American Heart Association, "Guidelines for Cardiopulmonary Resuscitation and Emergency Cardiac Care, III: Adult Advanced Cardiac Life Support" and "VI: Pediatric Advanced Life Support," *JAMA*, 1992, 268(16):2199-241 and 2262-75.

♦ **Atropine and Diphenoxylate** *see* Diphenoxylate and Atropine *on page 329*
♦ **Atropine-Care® Ophthalmic** *see* Atropine *on page 107*
♦ **Atropine, Hyoscyamine, Scopolamine, and Phenobarbital** *see* Hyoscyamine, Atropine, Scopolamine, and Phenobarbital *on page 499*
♦ **Atropine Sulfate** *see* Atropine *on page 107*
♦ **Atropisol® Ophthalmic** *see* Atropine *on page 107*
♦ **Atrovent® Aerosol Inhalation** *see* Ipratropium *on page 527*
♦ **Atrovent® Inhalation Solution** *see* Ipratropium *on page 527*
♦ **Atrovent® Nasal Spray** *see* Ipratropium *on page 527*
♦ **A/T/S®** *see* Erythromycin *on page 379*

Attapulgite (at a PULL gite)

Brand Names Children's Kaopectate® [OTC]; Diasorb® [OTC]; Kaopectate® Advanced Formula [OTC]; Kaopectate® Maximum Strength Caplets; Parepectolin®; Rheaban® [OTC]

Therapeutic Category Antidiarrheal

Generic Available Yes

Use Treatment of uncomplicated diarrhea

Pregnancy Risk Factor B

Contraindications Hypersensitivity to attapulgite or any component

Warnings Not to be used for self-medication for diarrhea >48 hours or in the presence of high fever in infants and children <3 years of age; do not use for diarrhea associated with pseudomembranous enterocolitis or in diarrhea caused by toxigenic bacteria

Adverse Reactions
Gastrointestinal: Constipation
Respiratory: Pneumoconiosis (from inhalation of the powder chronically as it contains large amounts of silica)

Drug Interactions May inhibit GI absorption of promazine, digoxin, clindamycin, tetracycline, and penicillamine

Mechanism of Action Controls diarrhea because of its absorbent action

Usual Dosage Adequate controlled clinical studies documenting the efficacy of attapulgite are lacking; its usage and dosage has been primarily empiric; the following are manufacturer's recommended dosages

Oral: Give after each bowel movement
Children:
3-6 years: 300-750 mg/dose; maximum dose: 7 doses/day or 2250 mg/day
6-12 years: 600-1500 mg/dose; maximum dose: 7 doses/day or 4500 mg/day
Children >12 years and Adults: 1200-3000 mg/dose; maximum dose: 8 doses/day or 9000 mg/day

Administration May be administered without regard to meals; shake liquid preparation well before use

Patient Information Do not exceed maximum number of doses per day; drink plenty of fluids; contact your physician if diarrhea persists more than 48 hours or if fever develops in children <3 years of age

Dosage Forms
Liquid: Oral concentrate: 600 mg activated attapulgite/15 mL (180 mL, 240 mL, 360 mL, 480 mL); 750 mg activated attapulgite/15 mL (120 mL)
Tablet: 750 mg
Tablet, chewable: 300 mg, 600 mg

♦ **Augmentin®** *see* Amoxicillin and Clavulanic Acid *on page 71*
♦ **Auralgan®** *see* Antipyrine and Benzocaine *on page 90*

Auranofin (au RANE oh fin)

Brand Names Ridaura®

Therapeutic Category Gold Compound

Generic Available No

Use Management of active stage of classic or definite rheumatoid or psoriatic arthritis in patients who do not respond to or tolerate other agents; adjunctive or alternative therapy for pemphigus

(Continued)

Auranofin (Continued)

Pregnancy Risk Factor C

Contraindications Renal disease; hypersensitivity to auranofin or any component; history of blood dyscrasias; CHF; exfoliative dermatitis; necrotizing enterocolitis; urticaria, eczema, SLE, bone marrow aplasia, pulmonary fibrosis; history of severe toxicity resulting from previous exposure to other heavy metals; patients who have recently received radiation therapy

Warnings Explain the possibility of adverse reactions before initiating therapy; signs of gold toxicity include decrease in hemoglobin, leukocytes, granulocytes and platelets, proteinuria, hematuria, pruritus, stomatitis or persistent diarrhea; advise patients to report any symptoms of toxicity; therapy should be discontinued if platelet count falls to <100,000/mm^3

Adverse Reactions

Central nervous system: Confusion, hallucinations, seizures

Dermatologic: Dermatitis, pruritus, alopecia, chrysiasis, rash, angioedema

Gastrointestinal: Diarrhea, loose stools, stomatitis, abdominal cramping, metallic taste, glossitis, ulcerative enterocolitis, GI hemorrhage, gingivitis, dysphagia

Hematologic: Thrombocytopenia, aplastic anemia, eosinophilia, leukopenia

Hepatic: Elevated liver enzymes, jaundice, hepatitis

Neuromuscular & skeletal: Peripheral neuropathy

Ocular: Conjunctivitis, iritis, corneal ulcers

Renal: Proteinuria, hematuria, nephrotic syndrome

Respiratory: Interstitial pneumonitis, fibrosis, gold bronchitis

Drug Interactions Possible increase of phenytoin serum levels (1 case reported); penicillamine, antimalarials, hydroxychloroquine, cytotoxic drugs, or immunosuppressive agents

Mechanism of Action Unknown, acts principally via immunomodulating effects and by decreasing lysosomal enzyme release; may alter cellular mechanisms by inhibiting sulfhydryl systems

Pharmacodynamics Onset of action: Therapeutic response may not be seen for 3-4 months after start of therapy

Pharmacokinetics

Absorption: Oral: Only about 20% to 25% of gold in a dose is absorbed

Protein binding: 60%

Half-life: 21-31 days (half-life dependent upon single or multiple dosing)

Time to peak blood gold concentrations: Within 2 hours

Elimination: 60% of absorbed gold is eliminated in urine while the remainder is eliminated in feces

Usual Dosage Oral:

Children: Initial: 0.1 mg/kg/day in 1-2 divided doses; usual maintenance: 0.15 mg/kg/day in 1-2 divided doses; maximum dose: 0.2 mg/kg/day in 1-2 divided doses

Adults: 6 mg/day in 1-2 divided doses; after 3 months may be increased to 9 mg/day in 3 divided doses; if still no response after 3 months at 9 mg/day, discontinue drug

Dosing adjustment in renal impairment:

Cl$_{cr}$ 50-80 mL/minute: Reduce dose to 50%

Cl$_{cr}$ <50 mL/minute: Avoid use

Monitoring Parameters CBC with differential, platelet count, urinalysis, baseline renal and liver function tests

Reference Range Gold: Normal: 0-0.1 µg/mL (SI: 0-0.0064 µmol/L); Therapeutic: 1-3 µg/mL (SI: 0.06-0.18 µmol/L); Urine <0.1 µg/24 hours

Test Interactions May enhance the response to a tuberculin skin test

Patient Information Minimize exposure to sunlight; notify your physician of pruritus, sore mouth, indigestion, metallic taste; observe careful oral hygiene

Additional Information Metallic taste may indicate stomatitis

Dosage Forms Capsule: 3 mg [gold 29%]

♦ **Auro® Ear Drops [OTC]** see Carbamide Peroxide on page 167

♦ **Aurolate®** see Gold Sodium Thiomalate on page 460

Aurothioglucose (aur oh thye oh GLOO kose)

Brand Names Solganal®

Therapeutic Category Gold Compound

Generic Available No

Use Management of active stage of classic or definite rheumatoid or psoriatic arthritis in patients that do not respond to or tolerate other agents

Pregnancy Risk Factor C

Contraindications Renal disease; hypersensitivity to aurothioglucose or any component; history of blood dyscrasias; CHF; exfoliative dermatitis; necrotizing enterocolitis; urticaria, eczema, SLE, bone marrow aplasia, pulmonary fibrosis; history of severe toxicity resulting from previous exposure to other heavy metals; patients who have recently received radiation therapy

Warnings Explain the possibility of adverse reactions before initiating therapy; signs of gold toxicity include: decrease in hemoglobin, leukocytes, granulocytes and platelets; proteinuria, hematuria, pruritus, stomatitis, persistent diarrhea, rash, or metallic taste; advise patients to report any symptoms of toxicity; therapy should be discontinued if platelet count <100,000/mm^3, WBC <4000/mm^3, or granulocytes <1500/mm^3

Adverse Reactions

Central nervous system: Confusion, hallucinations, seizures, encephalitis, EEG abnormalities, fever

Dermatologic: Alopecia, urticaria, mild to severe dermatitis, pruritus, chrysiasis, exfoliative dermatitis

Gastrointestinal: Diarrhea, stomatitis, glossitis, metallic taste, gingivitis, ulcerative enterocolitis

Genitourinary: Vaginitis

Hematologic: Eosinophilia, leukopenia, thrombocytopenia, aplastic anemia

Hepatic: Hepatitis, jaundice, elevated liver enzymes

Neuromuscular & skeletal: Peripheral neuropathy

Ocular: Conjunctivitis, corneal ulcers, iritis

Renal: Hematuria, proteinuria, nephrotic syndrome, glomerulitis

Respiratory: Interstitial pneumonitis, fibrosis, gold bronchitis, pharyngitis, pulmonary fibrosis

Miscellaneous: Anaphylactic shock, allergic reaction

Drug Interactions Increased toxicity with penicillamine, antimalarials, hydroxychloroquine, cytotoxic agents, and immunosuppressants

Mechanism of Action Unknown, may decrease prostaglandin synthesis or may alter cellular mechanisms by inhibiting sulfhydryl systems; may decrease lysosomal enzyme release

Pharmacokinetics

Absorption: I.M.: Erratic and slow

Distribution: Crosses the placenta; appears in breast milk

Protein binding: 95% to 99%

Metabolism: Unknown

Half-life: 3-27 days (single dose); 14-40 days (third dose); up to 168 days (11th dose)

Time to peak serum concentration: Within 4-6 hours

Elimination: Majority ultimately excreted in urine (70%) and the remainder in feces (30%)

Usual Dosage I.M. (doses should initially be given at weekly intervals):

Children: Initial: 0.25 mg/kg/dose first week; increment at 0.25 mg/kg/dose increasing with each weekly dose; maintenance: 0.75-1 mg/kg/dose weekly not to exceed 25 mg/dose to a total of 20 doses, then every 2-4 weeks

Adults: 10 mg first week; 25 mg second and third week; then 50 mg/week until 800 mg to 1 g cumulative dose has been given; if improvement occurs without adverse reactions, give 25-50 mg every 2-3 weeks, then every 3-4 weeks

Administration Parenteral: Deep I.M. injection into the upper outer quadrant of the gluteal region; vial should be thoroughly shaken before withdrawing a dose. Do not administer I.V.

Monitoring Parameters CBC with differential, platelet count, urinalysis, baseline renal and liver function tests

Reference Range Gold: Normal: 0-0.1 µg/mL (SI: 0-0.0064 µmol/L); Therapeutic: 1-3 µg/mL (SI: 0.06-0.18 µmol/L); Urine <0.1 µg/24 hours

Patient Information Minimize exposure to sunlight; notify physician of pruritus, sore mouth, indigestion, metallic taste; observe careful oral hygiene

Dosage Forms Injection, suspension: 50 mg/mL [gold 50%] (10 mL)

♦ **Aygestin®** *see* Norethindrone *on page 696*
♦ **Ayr® Nasal [OTC]** *see* Sodium Chloride *on page 871*
♦ **Azactam®** *see* Aztreonam *on page 116*

Azathioprine (ay za THYE oh preen)

Brand Names Imuran®
Available Salts Azathioprine Sodium
Therapeutic Category Antineoplastic Agent, Adjuvant; Immunosuppressant Agent
Generic Available Yes
Use Adjunct with other agents in prevention of transplant rejection; used as an immunosuppressant in a variety of autoimmune diseases such as systemic lupus erythematosus, severe rheumatoid arthritis unresponsive to other agents, and nephrotic syndrome
Pregnancy Risk Factor D
Contraindications Hypersensitivity to azathioprine or any component; pregnancy and lactation
Warnings Chronic immunosuppression increases the risk of neoplasia, particularly lymphoma and skin cancers; mutagenic potential in both men and women; may cause irreversible bone marrow suppression
Precautions Use with caution in patients with liver disease, renal impairment, and those with cadaveric kidneys; modify dosage in patients with renal impairment; reduce dosage to 25% to 33% of usual dosage in patients receiving allopurinol and azathioprine concurrently; discontinue azathioprine therapy in patients with hepatic veno-occlusive disease
Adverse Reactions
Central nervous system: Fever, chills
Dermatologic: Alopecia, erythematous or maculopapular rash
Gastrointestinal: Nausea, vomiting, anorexia, diarrhea, aphthous stomatitis, pancreatitis
Hematologic: Bone marrow depression (leukopenia, thrombocytopenia, anemia)
Hepatic: Hepatotoxicity, jaundice, hepatic veno-occlusive disease
Neuromuscular & skeletal: Arthralgias
Ocular: Retinopathy
Miscellaneous: Rare hypersensitivity reactions which include myalgias, rigors, dyspnea, hypotension, serum sickness, rash
Drug Interactions Allopurinol inhibits the metabolic pathway of azathioprine by inhibiting xanthine oxidase and blocking the conversion of mercaptopurine to inactive products which increases azathioprine's effects; nondepolarizing neuromuscular blockers (decreased blockade); captopril or enalapril in combination with azathioprine has resulted in severe anemia
Stability Reconstituted 10 mg/mL injection is stable for 24 hours at room temperature; stable in neutral or acid solutions, but is hydrolyzed to mercaptopurine in alkaline solutions
Mechanism of Action Antagonizes purine metabolism and may inhibit synthesis of DNA, RNA, and proteins; may also interfere with cellular metabolism and inhibit mitosis
Pharmacokinetics
Distribution: Crosses the placenta
Protein binding: ~30%
Metabolism: Extensive by hepatic xanthine oxidase to 6-mercaptopurine (active)
Bioavailability: ~50%
Half-life:
Parent: 12 minutes
6-mercaptopurine: 0.7-3 hours; with anuria: 50 hours
Elimination: Small amount eliminated as unchanged drug; metabolites eliminated eventually in the urine
Slightly dialyzable (5% to 20%)
Usual Dosage Children and Adults:
Transplantation: Oral, I.V.: Initial: 2-5 mg/kg/dose once daily; maintenance: 1-3 mg/kg/dose once daily
Rheumatoid arthritis: Oral: 1 mg/kg/dose once daily for 6-8 weeks; increase by 0.5 mg/kg every 4 weeks until response or up to 2.5 mg/kg/day
Dosing interval in renal impairment:
Cl$_{cr}$ 10-50 mL/minute: Administer every 36 hours or administer 75% of dose once daily
Cl$_{cr}$ <10 mL/minute: Administer every 48 hours or administer 50% of dose once daily

Administration
Oral: Administer with food to decrease GI upset

Parenteral: Administer IVP over 5 minutes at a concentration not to exceed 10 mg/mL; or may be further diluted with NS or D_5W and administered by intermittent infusion over 15-60 minutes

Monitoring Parameters CBC, platelet counts, creatinine, total bilirubin, alkaline phosphatase, liver function tests

Patient Information Response in rheumatoid arthritis may not occur for up to 2-3 months; inform physician of persistent sore throat, unusual bleeding or bruising, or fatigue

Dosage Forms
Lyophilized powder for injection, as sodium: 100 mg

Tablet: 50 mg

Extemporaneous Preparations A 50 mg/mL suspension compounded from one-hundred twenty of 50 mg tablets comminuted to a fine powder in a mortar with 40 mL of a 1:1 mixture of Ora-Sweet® and Ora-Plus® added and mixed to a fine paste, and then adding the 1:1 mixture of Ora-Sweet® and Ora-Plus® to a total volume of 120 mL, was stable for 60 days at 5°C and 25°C when protected from light. Label "shake well before using" and "protect from light."

Allen LV Jr and Erickson MA, "Stability of Acetazolamide, Allopurinol, Azathioprine, Clonazepam, and Flucytosine in Extemporaneously Compounded Oral Liquids," *Am J Health Syst Pharm*, 1996, 53(16):1944-9.

References
American College of Rheumatology Ad Hoc Committee on Clinical Guidelines, "Guidelines for Monitoring Drug Therapy in Rheumatoid Arthritis," *Arthritis Rheum*, 1996, 39(5):723-31.

Baum D, Bernstein D, Starnes VA, et al, "Pediatric Heart Transplantation at Stanford: Results of a 15-Year Experience," *Pediatrics*, 1991, 88(2):203-14.

Leichter HE, Sheth KJ, Gerlach MJ, et al, "Outcome of Renal Transplantation in Children Aged 1-5 and 6-18 Years," *Child Nephrol Urol*, 1992, 12(1):1-5.

♦ **Azathioprine Sodium** *see Azathioprine on page 112*

Azelastine (a ZEL as teen)
Brand Names Astelin® Nasal Spray; Optivar™

Available Salts Azelastine Hydrochloride

Therapeutic Category Antiallergic, Ophthalmic; Antihistamine, Nasal

Generic Available No

Use
Nasal: Treatment of the symptoms of seasonal allergic rhinitis (SAR) or perennial allergic rhinitis (PAR) such as rhinorrhea, sneezing, and nasal pruritus

Ophthalmic: Treatment of itching of the eye associated with allergic conjunctivitis

Pregnancy Risk Factor C

Contraindications Hypersensitivity to azelastine or any component

Warnings Ophthalmic solution not for use in contact lens-related irritation; preservative in ophthalmic solution may be absorbed by soft contact lenses; wait at least 10 minutes after instillation before inserting soft contact lenses

Precautions Use with caution in asthmatics; patients with hepatic or renal dysfunction may require lower doses

Adverse Reactions
Cardiovascular: Flushing, hypertension, tachycardia

Central nervous system: Drowsiness, headache, somnolence, fatigue, vertigo, depression, nervousness, hypoesthesia

Dermatologic: Contact dermatitis, eczema, hair and follicle infection, furunculosis

Endocrine & metabolic: Weight gain

Gastrointestinal: Nausea, xerostomia, bitter taste, glossitis, ulcerative stomatitis, aphthous stomatitis, constipation, abdominal pain

Genitourinary: Urinary frequency, hematuria

Neuromuscular & skeletal: Myalgia, hyperkinesia

Ocular: Conjunctivitis, watery eyes, eye pain, transient eye burning/stinging (ophthalmic use)

Respiratory: Nasal burning, paroxysmal sneezing, rhinitis, epistaxis, bronchospasm, coughing, throat burning, laryngitis

Drug Interactions May cause additive sedation when concomitantly administered with other CNS depressant medications

Stability Stable 3 months after opening

Mechanism of Action Competes with histamine for H_1-receptor sites on effector cells in the blood vessels and respiratory tract; reduces hyper-reactivity of the airways; increases the motility of bronchial epithelial cilia, improving mucociliary transport

(Continued)

Azelastine *(Continued)*

Pharmacodynamics
Onset of action: 30 minutes to 1 hour
Peak effect: 3 hours
Duration of action: 12 hours

Pharmacokinetics
Protein binding: 88%
Metabolism: Metabolized by cytochrome P-450 enzyme system; active metabolite desmethylazelastine
Bioavailability: After intranasal administration: 40%
Half-life, elimination: 22 hours
Time to peak serum concentration: 2-3 hours

Usual Dosage
Intranasal:
Children 3-12 years: 1 spray each nostril twice daily
Children ≥12 years and Adults: 2 sprays each nostril twice daily
Ophthalmic: Children ≥3 years and Adults: Instill 1 drop into each affected eye twice daily

Administration
Intranasal: Before use, the child-resistant screw cap on the bottle should be replaced with the pump unit and the delivery system should be primed with 4 sprays or until a fine mist appears; when 3 or more days have elapsed since the last use, the pump should be reprimed with 2 sprays or until a fine mist appears
Ophthalmic: Avoid contact of bottle tip with skin or eye

Patient Information
May cause drowsiness and impair ability to perform hazardous activities requiring mental alertness or physical coordination

Dosage Forms
Solution, nasal: 1 mg/mL (137 mcg/spray) (17 mL)
Solution, ophthalmic (Optivar™): 0.05% (6 mL)

References
McNeely W and Wiseman LR, "Intranasal Azelastine. A Review of Its Efficacy in the Management of Allergic Rhinitis," *Drugs*, 1988, 56(1):91-114.

♦ **Azelastine Hydrochloride** *see Azelastine on page 113*
♦ **Azidothymidine** *see Zidovudine on page 990*

Azithromycin *(az ith roe MYE sin)*

Related Information
Carbohydrate and Alcohol Content of Liquid Medications for Use in Patients Receiving Ketogenic Diets *on page 1228*
Endocarditis Prophylaxis *on page 1127*

Brand Names Zithromax™

Therapeutic Category Antibiotic, Macrolide

Generic Available No

Use Treatment of mild to moderate upper and lower respiratory tract infections, infections of the skin and skin structure, acute otitis media, and sexually transmitted diseases due to susceptible strains of *C. trachomatis*, *M. catarrhalis*, *H. influenzae*, *S. aureus*, *S. pneumoniae*, *Mycoplasma pneumoniae*, *M. avium* complex, *C. psittaci*, and *C. pneumoniae*; treatment of babesiosis; endocarditis prophylaxis

Pregnancy Risk Factor B

Contraindications Hypersensitivity to azithromycin, erythromycin, any component, or macrolide antibiotics

Warnings Oral azithromycin should not be used to treat pneumonia that is considered inappropriate for outpatient oral therapy; may mask or delay symptoms of incubating gonorrhea or syphilis so appropriate culture and susceptibility tests should be performed prior to initiating azithromycin; pseudomembranous colitis has been reported with use of macrolide antibiotics; patients who experience allergic reactions to azithromycin may require prolonged periods of observation and symptomatic treatment possibly due to the drug's long tissue half-life

Precautions Use with caution in patients with impaired hepatic function

Adverse Reactions
Cardiovascular: Palpitations, chest pain
Central nervous system: Headache, dizziness, agitation, nervousness, insomnia
Dermatologic: Rash, pruritus, angioedema, photosensitivity, Stevens-Johnson syndrome, toxic epidermal necrolysis
Gastrointestinal: Diarrhea (3.6%), nausea (2.6%), abdominal pain (2.5%), vomiting, anorexia

Genitourinary: Vaginitis
Hepatic: Elevated hepatic enzymes, cholestatic jaundice
Local: Pain at injection site, inflammation
Otic: Ototoxicity
Renal: Nephritis
Miscellaneous: Anaphylaxis

Drug Interactions Aluminum- and magnesium-containing antacids decrease azithromycin peak serum levels by 24%; monitor patients receiving azithromycin and drugs known to interact with erythromycin (ie, theophylline, digoxin, cisapride, anticoagulants, triazolam) since there are still very few studies examining drug-drug interactions with azithromycin

Food Interactions Presence of food decreases bioavailability of the capsule and suspension formulation by up to 50%

Stability After reconstitution, oral suspension may be stored for 10 days at room temperature or in the refrigerator. After reconstituting 500 mg vial for injection at a concentration of 100 mg/mL, solution is stable for 24 hours at room temperature. If solution is further diluted with a compatible diluent to a 1-2 mg/mL concentration, this solution is stable for 24 hours at room temperature or for 7 days if refrigerated.

Mechanism of Action Inhibits bacterial RNA-dependent protein synthesis by binding to the 50S ribosomal subunit which results in the blockage of transpeptidation

Pharmacokinetics
Absorption: Rapid from the GI tract
Distribution: Extensive tissue distribution into skin, lungs, bone, prostate, cervix; CSF concentrations are low
Protein binding: 7% to 50% (concentration-dependent and dependent on alpha$_1$-acid glycoprotein levels)
Metabolism: In the liver to inactive metabolites
Bioavailability: 37%
Half-life, terminal: 68 hours
Time to peak serum concentration: 2-3 hours
Elimination: 50% of dose is excreted unchanged in bile; 6% of dose is excreted unchanged in urine

Usual Dosage
Oral:
Children ≥6 months: Otitis media: 10 mg/kg on day 1 (maximum dose: 500 mg/day) followed by 5 mg/kg/day once daily on days 2-5 (maximum dose: 250 mg/day)
Children ≥2 years: Pharyngitis, tonsillitis: 12 mg/kg/day once daily for 5 days (maximum dose: 500 mg/day)
Children:
Chancroid: Single 20 mg/kg dose (maximum dose: 1 g)
Uncomplicated chlamydial urethritis or cervicitis: Single 10 mg/kg dose (maximum dose: 1 g)
M. avium-infected patients with acquired immunodeficiency syndrome: Not currently FDA approved for use; 5-20 mg/kg/day once daily has been used in clinical trials; prophylaxis for first episode of MAC: 5-12 mg/kg/day once daily (maximum dose: 500 mg/day) or 20 mg/kg (maximum dose: 1200 mg) once weekly
Adolescents ≥16 years and Adults:
Respiratory tract, skin and soft tissue infections: 500 mg on day 1 followed by 250 mg/day on days 2-5 (maximum dose: 500 mg/day)
Chancroid or nongonococcal urethritis and cervicitis due to *C. trachomatis*: Single 1 g dose
Urethritis and cervicitis due to *N. gonorrhoeae*: Single 2 g dose
Prophylaxis of disseminated *M. avium* complex disease in patient with advanced HIV infection: 1200 mg once weekly
I.V.: Adults: 500 mg once daily for 2 days followed by a switch to oral azithromycin therapy

Administration
Oral: Administer capsule or oral suspension on an empty stomach at least 1 hour prior to a meal or 2 hours after a meal; do not administer with food; tablet formulation may be administered with or without food; do not administer with antacids that contain aluminum or magnesium; azithromycin 1 g oral suspension for a single dose regimen should be prepared by mixing contents of 1 packet with approximately 60 mL of water. Have the patient drink the entire contents immediately; add an additional 60 mL of water, mix, and drink (1 g suspension regimen can be taken with or without food).
(Continued)

Azithromycin *(Continued)*

Parenteral: For 1 mg/mL concentration, infuse over 3 hours; for 2 mg/mL concentration, infuse over 1 hour; infuse over a period of not less than 60 minutes

Monitoring Parameters Liver function tests, WBC with differential

Patient Information Report any symptoms of chest pain, heart palpitations, and yellowing of skin or eyes

Dosage Forms

Capsule, as dihydrate: 250 mg

Powder for injection: 500 mg vial

Suspension: 100 mg/5 mL (15 mL); 200 mg/5 mL (15 mL, 22.5 mL, 30 mL); 1 g (single-dose packet)

Tablet, as dihydrate: 250 mg, 600 mg

References

Drew RH and Gallis HA, "Azithromycin-Spectrum of Activity, Pharmacokinetics, and Clinical Applications," *Pharmacotherapy*, 1992, 12(3):161-73.

Foulds G, Shepard RM, and Johnson RB, "The Pharmacokinetics of Azithromycin in Human Serum and Tissues," *J Antimicrob Chemother*, 1990, 25(Suppl A):73-82.

Hammerschlag MR, Golden NH, Oh MK, et al, "Single Dose of Azithromycin for the Treatment of Genital Chlamydial Infections in Adolescents," *J Pediatr*, 1993, 122(6):961-5.

Nahata MC, Koranyi KI, Gadgil SD, et al, "Pharmacokinetics of Azithromycin After Oral Administration of Multiple Doses of Suspension," *Antimicrob Agents Chemother*, 1993, 37(2):314-16.

Starke JR and Correa AG, "Management of Mycobacterial Infection and Disease in Children," *Pediatr Infect Dis J*, 1995, 14(6):455-69.

"1999 USPHS/IDSA Guidelines for the Prevention of Opportunistic Infections in Persons Infected With Human Immunodeficiency Virus. USPHS/IDSA Prevention of Opportunistic Working Group," *MMWR Morb Mortal Wkly Rep*, 1999, 48(RR-10):1-61.

♦ **Azmacort™ Oral Inhaler** see Triamcinolone *on page 946*

♦ **Azo-Standard®** see Phenazopyridine *on page 753*

♦ **AZT** see Zidovudine *on page 990*

♦ **AZT and 3TC** see Lamivudine and Zidovudine *on page 553*

♦ **Azthreonam** see Aztreonam *on page 116*

Aztreonam *(AZ tree oh nam)*

Brand Names Azactam®

Synonyms Azthreonam

Therapeutic Category Antibiotic, Miscellaneous

Generic Available No

Use Treatment of patients with documented multidrug resistant aerobic gram-negative infection in which beta-lactam therapy is contraindicated; used for UTI, lower respiratory tract infections, septicemia, skin/skin structure infections, intra-abdominal infections and gynecological infections caused by susceptible *Enterobacteriaceae, E. coli, K. pneumoniae, P. mirabilis, H. influenzae,* and *P. aeruginosa*

Pregnancy Risk Factor B

Contraindications Hypersensitivity to aztreonam or any component

Warnings Check for hypersensitivity to other beta-lactams (hypersensitivity reactions to aztreonam have occurred rarely in patients with a history of penicillin or cephalosporin hypersensitivity); prolonged use may result in superinfection

Precautions Requires dosage reduction in renal impairment

Adverse Reactions

Cardiovascular: Hypotension, transient EKG changes

Central nervous system: Seizures, confusion

Dermatologic: Rash

Gastrointestinal: Diarrhea, nausea, vomiting, abdominal pain, pseudomembranous colitis

Hematologic: Eosinophilia, leukopenia, neutropenia, thrombocytopenia

Hepatic: Elevated liver enzymes

Local: Pain at injection site, thrombophlebitis, swelling at injection site

Renal: Elevated BUN and serum creatinine

Drug Interactions Avoid antibiotics that induce beta-lactamase production (cefoxitin, imipenem)

Stability Reconstituted solution is stable 48 hours at room temperature and 7 days when refrigerated; incompatible when mixed with nafcillin, metronidazole

Mechanism of Action Binds to penicillin-binding protein 3 which produces filamentation of the bacterium inhibiting bacterial cell wall synthesis and causing cell wall destruction

Pharmacokinetics

Absorption: I.M.: Well absorbed

Distribution: Widely distributed into body tissues, cerebrospinal fluid, bronchial secretions, peritoneal fluid, bone, and breast milk

V_d:
Neonates: 0.26-0.36 L/kg
Children: 0.2-0.29 L/kg
Adults: 0.2 L/kg
Protein binding: 56%
Half-life:
Neonates:
<7 days, ≤2.5 kg: 5.5-9.9 hours
<7 days, >2.5 kg: 2.6 hours
1 week to 1 month: 2.4 hours
Children 2 months to 12 years: 1.7 hours
Children with cystic fibrosis: 1.3 hours
Adults: 1.3-2.2 hours (half-life prolonged in renal failure)
Time to peak serum concentration: Within 60 minutes after an I.M. dose
Elimination: 60% to 70% excreted unchanged in the urine and partially excreted in feces
Moderately dialyzable
Hemodialysis: 27% to 58% in 4 hours
Peritoneal dialysis: 10% with a 6-hour dwell time

Usual Dosage I.M., I.V.:
Neonates:
Postnatal age ≤7 days:
≤2000 g: 60 mg/kg/day divided every 12 hours
>2000 g: 90 mg/kg/day divided every 8 hours
Postnatal age >7 days:
<1200 g: 60 mg/kg/day divided every 12 hours
1200-2000 g: 90 mg/kg/day divided every 8 hours
>2000 g: 120 mg/kg/day divided every 6 hours
Children >1 month: 90-120 mg/kg/day divided every 6-8 hours
Cystic fibrosis: 50 mg/kg/dose every 6-8 hours (ie, up to 200 mg/kg/day); maximum dose: 8 g/day
Adults:
Urinary tract infection: 500 mg to 1 g every 8-12 hours
Moderately severe systemic infections: 1 g I.V. or I.M. or 2 g I.V. every 8-12 hours
Severe systemic or life-threatening infections (especially if caused by *Pseudomonas aeruginosa*): I.V.: 2 g every 6-8 hours; maximum dose: 8 g/day
Dosing adjustment in renal impairment:
Cl_{cr} 10-30 mL/minute: Reduce dose by 50%; give at the usual interval
Cl_{cr} <10 mL/minute: Reduce dose by 75%; give at the usual interval

Administration Parenteral: Administer by IVP over 3-5 minutes at a maximum concentration of 66 mg/mL or by intermittent infusion over 20-60 minutes at a final concentration not to exceed 20 mg/mL
Monitoring Parameters Periodic liver function test
Test Interactions Urine glucose (Clinitest®)
Dosage Forms Powder for injection: 500 mg (15 mL, 100 mL); 1 g (15 mL, 100 mL); 2 g (15 mL, 100 mL)
References
Bosso JA and Black PG, "The Use of Aztreonam in Pediatric Patients: A Review," *Pharmacotherapy,* 1991, 11(1):20-5.
Stutman HR, Chartrand SA, Tolentino T, et al, "Aztreonam Therapy for Serious Gram-Negative Infections in Children," *Am J Dis Child,* 1986, 140(11):1147-51.

♦ **Azulfidine®** *see* Sulfasalazine *on page 893*
♦ **Azulfidine® EN-tabs®** *see* Sulfasalazine *on page 893*
♦ **Babee® Teething [OTC]** *see* Benzocaine *on page 124*
♦ **Bacid® [OTC]** *see* Lactobacillus acidophilus and Lactobacillus bulgaricus *on page 550*
♦ **Baciguent® Topical [OTC]** *see* Bacitracin *on page 117*
♦ **Baci-IM® Injection** *see* Bacitracin *on page 117*
♦ **Bacimyxin (Canada)** *see* Bacitracin and Polymyxin B *on page 119*
♦ **Bacitin (Canada)** *see* Bacitracin *on page 117*

Bacitracin (bas i TRAY sin)
Brand Names AK-Tracin® Ophthalmic; Baciguent® Topical [OTC]; Baci-IM® Injection; Bacitin (Canada)
Therapeutic Category Antibiotic, Ophthalmic; Antibiotic, Topical; Antibiotic, Miscellaneous
Generic Available Yes
(Continued)

Bacitracin *(Continued)*

Use Treatment of pneumonia and empyema caused by susceptible staphylococci; prevention or treatment of superficial skin infections or infections of the eye caused by susceptible organisms; due to its toxicity, use of bacitracin systemically or as an irrigant should be limited to situations where less toxic alternatives would not be effective; treatment of antibiotic-associated colitis

Pregnancy Risk Factor C

Contraindications Hypersensitivity to bacitracin or any component; I.M. use is contraindicated in patients with renal impairment

Warnings I.M. use may cause renal failure due to tubular and glomerular necrosis; do **not** administer intravenously because severe thrombophlebitis occurs; bacitracin may be absorbed from denuded areas and irrigation sites

Precautions Prolonged use may result in overgrowth of nonsusceptible organisms

Adverse Reactions
Cardiovascular: Hypotension, tightness of chest
Central nervous system: Pain
Dermatologic: Rash, itching
Gastrointestinal: Anorexia, nausea, vomiting, diarrhea, rectal itching and burning
Hematologic: Blood dyscrasias
Renal: With I.M. use: Renal tubular and glomerular necrosis, azotemia, renal failure
Miscellaneous: Diaphoresis, edema of lips and face

Drug Interactions Nephrotoxic drugs (increase toxicity), neuromuscular blocking agents and anesthetics (increase neuromuscular blockade)

Stability Sterile powder should be stored in the refrigerator; once reconstituted, bacitracin is stable for 1 week under refrigeration (2°C to 8°C); incompatible with diluents containing parabens

Mechanism of Action Inhibits bacterial cell wall synthesis by preventing transfer of mucopeptides into the growing cell wall

Pharmacokinetics
Absorption: Poor from mucous membranes and intact skin; rapid following I.M. administration
Protein binding: Minimally bound to plasma proteins
Time to peak serum concentration: I.M.: Within 1-2 hours
Elimination: Slow elimination into the urine with 10% to 40% of a dose excreted within 24 hours

Usual Dosage
I.M. (not recommended):
Infants:
≤2.5 kg: 900 units/kg/day in 2-3 divided doses
>2.5 kg: 1000 units/kg/day in 2-3 divided doses
Children: 800-1200 units/kg/day divided every 8 hours
Adults: 10,000-25,000 units/dose every 6 hours; not to exceed 100,000 units/day
Children and Adults:
Topical: Apply 1-5 times/day
Ophthalmic ointment: Instill ¼" to ½" ribbon directly into conjunctival sac(s) every 3-4 hours; reduce frequency of administration as the infection is brought under control to 1-3 times/day
Irrigation, solution: 50-100 units/mL in NS, lactated Ringer's, or sterile water for irrigation; soak sponges in solution for topical compresses 1-5 times/day or as needed during surgical procedures
Antibiotic-associated colitis: Adults: Oral: 25,000 units every 6 hours for 7-10 days

Administration
Ophthalmic: Do not use topical ointment in the eyes; avoid contact of tube tip with skin or eye
Parenteral: For I.M. administration, pH of urine should be kept above 6 by using sodium bicarbonate; bacitracin sterile powder should be dissolved in NS injection containing 2% procaine hydrochloride; administer I.M. injection into the upper outer quadrant of the buttocks; alternate injection sites

Monitoring Parameters I.M.: Urinalysis, renal function tests

Patient Information Ophthalmic ointment may cause blurred vision; topical bacitracin should not be used for longer than 1 week unless directed by a physician

Dosage Forms
Injection: 50,000 units
Ointment:
Ophthalmic: 500 units/g (3.5 g, 3.75 g)
Topical: 500 units/g (1 g, 15 g, 30 g, 120 g, 454 g)

References
Kelly CP, Pothoulakis C, and LaMont JT, "*Clostridium difficile* Colitis," *N Engl J Med*, 1994, 330(4):257-62.

Bacitracin and Polymyxin B (bas i TRAY sin & pol i MIKS in bee)

Brand Names AK-Poly-Bac® Ophthalmic; Bacimyxin (Canada); Betadine® First Aid Antibiotics + Moisturizer [OTC]; Bioderm (Canada); Polysporin® Ophthalmic; Polysporin® Topical; Polytopic® (Canada); Polytracin® (Canada)

Available Salts Bacitracin and Polymyxin B Sulfate

Synonyms Polymyxin B and Bacitracin

Therapeutic Category Antibiotic, Ophthalmic; Antibiotic, Topical

Generic Available Yes

Use Treatment of superficial infections involving the conjunctiva and/or cornea caused by susceptible organisms; prevent infection in minor cuts, scrapes and burns

Pregnancy Risk Factor C

Contraindications Hypersensitivity to polymyxin, bacitracin, or any component

Precautions Prolonged use may result in overgrowth of nonsusceptible organisms

Adverse Reactions
Local: Rash, itching, burning, edema
Ocular: Conjunctival erythema
Miscellaneous: Anaphylactoid reactions

Pharmacokinetics Absorption: Insignificant from intact skin or mucous membrane

Usual Dosage Children and Adults:
Ophthalmic: Instill ¼" to ½" directly into conjunctival sac(s) every 3-4 hours depending on severity of the infection
Topical: Apply a small amount of ointment or dusting of powder to the affected area 1-3 times/day

Administration Ophthalmic: Do not use topical ointment in the eyes; avoid contact of tube tip with skin or eye

Patient Information Do not use longer than 1 week unless directed by physician; ophthalmic ointment may cause blurred vision

Dosage Forms
Ointment:
Ophthalmic: Bacitracin 500 units and polymyxin B sulfate 10,000 units per g (3.5 g)
Topical: Bacitracin 500 units and polymyxin B sulfate 10,000 units per g in white petrolatum (15 g, 30 g)
Powder, topical: Polymyxin B sulfate 10,000 units and bacitracin 500 units per g (10 g)

♦ **Bacitracin and Polymyxin B Sulfate** *see* Bacitracin and Polymyxin B *on page 119*

♦ **Bacitracin. Neomycin, and Polymyxin B** *see* Neomycin, Polymyxin B, and Bacitracin *on page 680*

♦ **Bacitracin, Neomycin, Polymyxin B, and Hydrocortisone** *see* Neomycin, (Bacitracin) Polymyxin B, and Hydrocortisone *on page 679*

Baclofen (BAK loe fen)

Brand Names Alpha-Baclofen® (Canada); Lioresal®; PMS-Baclofen (Canada)

Therapeutic Category Skeletal Muscle Relaxant, Nonparalytic

Generic Available Yes: Tablets only

Use Treatment of cerebral spasticity, reversible spasticity associated with multiple sclerosis or spinal cord lesions; intrathecal use for the management of spasticity in patients who are unresponsive to oral baclofen or experience intolerable CNS side effects; treatment of trigeminal neuralgia; adjunctive treatment of tardive dyskinesia

Pregnancy Risk Factor C

Contraindications Hypersensitivity to baclofen or any component

Warnings Should not be used when spasticity is used to maintain posture or balance; abrupt withdrawal of baclofen has been reported to precipitate hallucinations and/or seizures; due to the life-threatening complications of intrathecal use, physicians must be adequately trained in its use; physostigmine should be available to reverse life-threatening central nervous side effects (eg, respiratory depression); injection for intrathecal use is not recommended or intended for I.V., I.M., S.C. or epidural administration
(Continued)

Baclofen *(Continued)*

Precautions Use with caution in patients with seizure disorder, impaired renal function, peptic ulcer disease, stroke, ovarian cysts, psychotic disorders, autonomic dysreflexia (intrathecal therapy)

Adverse Reactions

Cardiovascular: Hypotension, cardiovascular collapse (with intrathecal therapy), chest pain, palpitations

Central nervous system: Drowsiness, fatigue, vertigo, dizziness, psychiatric disturbances, insomnia, slurred speech, headache, hypotonia, ataxia, life-threatening CNS depression (with intrathecal use)

Dermatologic: Rash, pruritus

Gastrointestinal: Nausea, constipation, anorexia, dysgeusia, diarrhea, abdominal pain, xerostomia

Genitourinary: Impotence, urinary frequency, nocturia

Renal: Hematuria

Respiratory: Respiratory failure (with intrathecal administration), dyspnea

Miscellaneous: Diaphoresis

Drug Interactions Increased CNS depression when administered with other CNS depressants (eg, opiates, alcohol, benzodiazepines, tricyclic antidepressants, MAO inhibitors); baclofen may decrease lithium's effect

Mechanism of Action Inhibits the transmission of both monosynaptic and polysynaptic reflexes at the spinal cord level, possibly by hyperpolarization of primary afferent fiber terminals, with resultant relief of muscle spasticity

Pharmacodynamics

Oral: Muscle relaxation effects require 3-4 days and maximal clinical effects are not seen for 5-10 days

Intrathecal:

Bolus:

Onset of effect: 30 minutes to 1 hour

Peak effect: 4 hours

Duration: 4-8 hours

Continuous intrathecal infusion:

Onset of action: 6-8 hours

Maximum activity: 24-48 hours

Pharmacokinetics

Oral:

Absorption: Rapid; absorption from the GI tract is thought to be dose dependent

Protein binding: 30%

Metabolism: Minimal in the liver (15%)

Half-life: 2.5-4 hours

Time to peak serum concentration: Oral: Within 2-3 hours

Elimination: 85% of dose excreted in urine and feces as unchanged drug

Intrathecal:

Half-life, CSF elimination: 1.5 hours

Clearance, CSF: 30 mL/hour

Usual Dosage

Oral:

Children:

2-7 years: Initial: 10-15 mg/day divided every 8 hours; titrate dose every 3 days in increments of 5-15 mg/day to a maximum of 40 mg/day

≥8 years: Titrate dosage as above to a maximum of 60 mg/day

Adults: 5 mg 3 times/day, may increase 5 mg/dose every 3 days to a maximum of 80 mg/day

Intrathecal: Children and Adults:

Screening dosage: 50 mcg for 1 dose and observe for 4-8 hours; very small children may receive 25 mcg; if ineffective, a repeat dosage increased by 50% (eg, 75 mcg) may be repeated in 24 hours: if still suboptimal, a third dose increased by 33% (eg, 100 mcg) may be repeated in 24 hours; patients who do not respond to 100 mcg intrathecally should not be considered for continuous chronic administration via an implantable pump

Maintenance dose: Continuous infusion: Initial: Depending upon the screening dosage and its duration:

If the screening dose duration >8 hours: Daily dose = effective screening dose

If the screening dose duration <8 hours: Daily dose = **twice** effective screening dose

Continuous infusion dose mcg/hour = daily dose divided by 24 hours

Note: Further adjustments in infusion rate may be done every 24 hours as needed; for spinal cord-related spasticity, increase in 10% to 30% increments/24 hours; for spasticity of cerebral origin, increase in 5% to 10% increments/24 hours

Average daily dose:

Children ≤12 years: 100-300 mcg/day (4.2-12.5 mcg/hour); doses as high as 1000 mcg/day have been used

Children >12 years and Adults: 300-800 mcg/day (12.5-33 mcg/hour); doses as high as 2000 mcg/day have been used

Administration

Oral: Administer with food or milk

Parenteral: Intrathecal: Test dosage: Use dilute concentration (50 mcg/mL) and inject over at least 1 minute; for maintenance infusions, concentrations of 500-2000 mcg/mL may be used

Monitoring Parameters Muscle rigidity, spasticity (decrease in number and severity of spasms), modified Ashworth score

Patient Information Avoid alcohol and other CNS depressants as they may cause drowsiness and impair ability to perform hazardous activities requiring mental alertness or physical coordination

Dosage Forms

Injection, intrathecal, preservative free: 0.05 mg/mL (1 mL); 0.5 mg/mL (20 mL); 2 mg/mL (5 mL)

Tablet: 10 mg, 20 mg

Extemporaneous Preparations Make a 10 mg/mL oral suspension by crushing six 20 mg tablets; gradually add 60 mL Ora-Sweet® or Ora-Plus® and mix until a uniform paste, then add more vehicle to make a total volume of 120 mL; refrigerate; shake well; stable 60 days

Nahata MC and Hipple TF, *Pediatric Drug Formulations*, 3rd ed, Cincinnati, OH: Harvey Whitney Books Co, 1997.

♦ **Bacticort® Otic** *see* Neomycin, (Bacitracin) Polymyxin B, and Hydrocortisone *on page 679*

♦ **Bactine® Hydrocortisone [OTC]** *see* Hydrocortisone *on page 486*

♦ **Bactocill®** *see* Oxacillin *on page 711*

♦ **BactoShield® [OTC]** *see* Chlorhexidine Gluconate *on page 209*

♦ **Bactrim™** *see* Co-Trimoxazole *on page 258*

♦ **Bactrim™ DS** *see* Co-Trimoxazole *on page 258*

♦ **Bactroban®** *see* Mupirocin *on page 660*

♦ **Baking Soda** *see* Sodium Bicarbonate *on page 870*

♦ **BAL in Oil®** *see* Dimercaprol *on page 326*

♦ **Balminil® Decongestant (Canada)** *see* Pseudoephedrine *on page 822*

♦ **Balminil®-DM, -DM Children (Canada)** *see* Dextromethorphan *on page 304*

♦ **Balminil® Expectorant (Canada)** *see* Guaifenesin *on page 464*

♦ **Balnetar® (Canada)** *see* Coal Tar *on page 247*

♦ **Bancap HC®** *see* Hydrocodone and Acetaminophen *on page 485*

♦ **Banophen® Oral [OTC]** *see* Diphenhydramine *on page 327*

♦ **Barbidonna®** *see* Hyoscyamine, Atropine, Scopolamine, and Phenobarbital *on page 499*

♦ **Barbilixir® (Canada)** *see* Phenobarbital *on page 754*

♦ **Barbita®** *see* Phenobarbital *on page 754*

♦ **Baridium®** *see* Phenazopyridine *on page 753*

♦ **Barophen®** *see* Hyoscyamine, Atropine, Scopolamine, and Phenobarbital *on page 499*

♦ **Basaljel® [OTC]** *see* Antacid Preparations *on page 86*

♦ **Bayer® Aspirin [OTC]** *see* Aspirin *on page 99*

♦ **BC® Cold Powder Non-Drowsy Formula (Cold-Sinus) [OTC]** *see* Phenylpropanolamine *on page 761*

♦ **BCNU** *see* Carmustine *on page 172*

♦ **B Complex** *see page 1034*

♦ **B-D Glucose® [OTC]** *see* Dextrose *on page 305*

♦ **Beben® (Canada)** *see* Betamethasone *on page 130*

♦ **Beclodisk® Diskhaler® (Canada)** *see* Beclomethasone *on page 122*

♦ **Becloforte® (Canada)** *see* Beclomethasone *on page 122*

Beclomethasone (be kloe METH a sone)

Related Information

Asthma Guidelines *on page 1178*
Estimated Comparative Daily Dosages for Inhaled Corticosteroids *on page 1185*

Brand Names Beclodisk® Diskhaler® (Canada); Becloforte® (Canada); Beclovent® Oral Inhaler; Beconase AQ® Nasal Inhaler; Beconase® Nasal Inhaler; Propaderm® (Canada); Vancenase® AQ 84 mcg; Vancenase® AQ Inhaler; Vancenase® Nasal Inhaler; Vanceril® 84 mcg Double Strength; Vanceril® Oral Inhaler

Available Salts Beclomethasone Dipropionate

Therapeutic Category Adrenal Corticosteroid; Antiasthmatic; Anti-inflammatory Agent; Corticosteroid, Inhalant (Oral); Corticosteroid, Intranasal; Glucocorticoid

Generic Available No

Use

Oral inhalation: Long-term (chronic) control of persistent bronchial asthma; **NOT** indicated for the relief of acute bronchospasm; 84 mcg/inhalation is also indicated in bronchial asthma patients requiring systemic corticosteroids (84 mcg/inhalation may decrease or eliminate need for systemic steroids)

Intranasal: Management of seasonal or perennial rhinitis and nasal polyposis

Pregnancy Risk Factor C

Contraindications Hypersensitivity to beclomethasone or any component; primary treatment of status asthmaticus

Warnings Fatalities have occurred due to adrenal insufficiency in asthmatic patients during and after switching from systemic corticosteroids to aerosol steroids; several months may be required for full recovery of the adrenal glands; during this period, aerosol steroids do **not** provide the systemic corticosteroid needed to treat patients requiring stress doses (ie, patients with major stress such as trauma, surgery, or infections). When used at high doses hypothalamic - pituitary - adrenal (HPA) suppression may occur; use with inhaled or systemic corticosteroids (even alternate-day dosing) may increase risk of HPA suppression; withdrawal and discontinuation of corticosteroids should be done carefully. Switching from systemic corticosteroids to 84 mcg/inhalation may unmask allergic conditions (such as eczema, conjunctivitis, and rhinitis) that were previously suppressed by systemic steroids. Immunosuppression may occur

Precautions Avoid using higher than recommended dosages; suppression of HPA function, suppression of linear growth, or hypercorticism (Cushing's syndrome) may occur; use with extreme caution in patients with respiratory tuberculosis, untreated systemic infections, or ocular herpes simplex

Adverse Reactions

Central nervous system: Headache

Endocrine & metabolic: Potential adrenal suppression, dysmenorrhea

Gastrointestinal: Xerostomia, sore throat, pharyngitis

Local: Growth of *Candida* in the mouth, throat, or nares

Neuromuscular & skeletal: Growth velocity suppression (reported in asthmatic children receiving oral inhalation 2 puffs 4 times/day)

Respiratory: Cough, sneezing, hoarseness, irritation and burning of the nasal mucosa, nasal ulceration, epistaxis, rhinorrhea, nasal congestion

Drug Interactions Interactions similar to other corticosteroids may potentially occur

Stability Do not store near heat or open flame

Mechanism of Action Controls the rate of protein synthesis, depresses the migration of polymorphonuclear leukocytes and fibroblasts, reverses capillary permeability, and stabilizes lysosomal membranes at the cellular level to prevent or control inflammation

Pharmacodynamics Onset:

Oral inhalation: 1-4 weeks

Nasal inhalation: Within a few days up to 2 weeks

Pharmacokinetics

Absorption: Inhalation: Readily absorbed; quickly hydrolyzed by pulmonary esterases prior to absorption; oral: 90%

Distribution: 10% to 25% of inhaled dose reaches respiratory tract; secreted into breast milk

Protein binding: 87%

Metabolism: Hepatic

Half-life: Biphasic: Initial 3 hours; terminal: 15 hours

Elimination: Primary route of excretion is via feces; 12% to 15% of oral dose excreted in urine as metabolites

Usual Dosage

Aqueous inhalation, nasal:

Vancenase® AQ, Beconase® AQ: Children ≥6 years and Adults: 1-2 inhalations each nostril twice daily

Vancenase® AQ 84 mcg: Children ≥6 years and Adults: 1-2 inhalations in each nostril once daily

Intranasal (Vancenase®, Beconase®):

Children 6-12 years: 1 inhalation in each nostril 3 times/day

Children ≥12 years and Adults: 1 inhalation in each nostril 2-4 times/day or 2 inhalations each nostril twice daily; usual maximum maintenance: 1 inhalation in each nostril 3 times/day

Oral inhalation (doses should be titrated to the lowest effective dose once asthma is controlled):

Beclovent®, Vanceril®:

Children 6-12 years: 1-2 inhalations 3-4 times/day (alternatively: 2-4 inhalations twice daily); maximum dose: 10 inhalations/day

Children ≥12 years and Adults: 2 inhalations 3-4 times/day (alternatively: 4 inhalations twice daily); maximum dose: 20 inhalations/day; patients with severe asthma: Initial: 12-16 inhalations/day (divided 3-4 times/day); dose should be adjusted downward according to patient's response

Vanceril® 84 mcg Double Strength:

Children 6-12 years: 2 inhalations twice daily; maximum dose: 5 inhalations/day

Children ≥12 years and Adults: 2 inhalations twice daily; maximum dose: 10 inhalations/day; patients with severe asthma: Initial: 6-8 inhalations/day (divided twice daily); dose should be adjusted downward according to patient's response

NIH Guidelines (NIH, 1997) [give in divided doses]:

Children:

"Low" dose: 84-336 mcg/day (42 mcg/puff: 2-8 puffs/day or 84 mcg/puff: 1-4 puffs/day)

"Medium" dose: 336-672 mcg/day (42 mcg/puff: 8-16 puffs/day or 84 mcg/puff: 4-8 puffs/day)

"High" dose: >672 mcg/day (42 mcg/puff: >16 puffs/day or 84 mcg/puff >8 puffs/day)

Adults:

"Low" dose: 168-504 mcg/day (42 mcg/puff: 4-12 puffs/day or 84 mcg/puff: 2-6 puffs/day)

"Medium" dose: 504-840 mcg/day (42 mcg/puff: 12-20 puffs/day or 84 mcg/puff: 6-10 puffs/day)

"High" dose: >840 mcg/day (42 mcg/puff: >20 puffs/day or 84 mcg/puff: >10 puffs/day)

Administration

Oral inhalation: Use a spacer device for children <8 years of age

Nasal and oral inhalation: Shake container well before use

Monitoring Parameters Check mucous membranes for signs of fungal infection

Patient Information Notify physician if condition being treated persists or worsens; do not decrease dose or discontinue without physician approval; avoid spraying in eyes; avoid exposure to chicken pox; if exposed, seek medical advice without delay; discard canister when labeled number of metered doses (sprays) have been used

Oral inhalant: Rinse mouth after inhalation to decrease chance of oral candidiasis; report sore mouth or mouth lesions to physician

Additional Information

Oral inhalation: If bronchospasm with wheezing occurs after use, a fast-acting bronchodilator may be used; beclomethasone oral inhalation is also used to help reduce or discontinue oral corticosteroid therapy for asthma

Aqueous beclomethasone nasal spray (2 sprays in each nostril twice daily for 4 weeks, followed by 1 spray in each nostril twice daily) may be useful in reducing adenoidal hypertrophy and nasal airway obstruction in children 5-11 years of age (Demain, 1995)

Dosage Forms

Inhalation, as dipropionate:

Nasal:

Beconase®: 42 mcg/inhalation [80 metered doses] (6.7 g); [200 metered doses] (16.8 g)

Vancenase® Pockethaler: 42 mcg/inhalation [200 metered doses] (7 g)

(Continued)

Beclomethasone *(Continued)*

Oral:

Beclovent®, Vanceril®: 42 mcg/inhalation [80 metered doses] (6.7 g); [200 metered doses] (16.8 g)

Vanceril® 84 mcg Double Strength: 84 mcg/inhalation [40 metered doses] (5.4 g); [120 metered doses] (12.2 g)

Spray, aqueous, nasal, as dipropionate

Beconase AQ®, Vancenase® AQ: 42 mcg/inhalation [200 metered doses] (25 g)

Vancenase® AQ 84 mcg: 84 mcg/inhalation [120 metered doses] (19 g)

References

Demain JG and Goetz DW, "Pediatric Adenoidal Hypertrophy and Nasal Airway Obstruction: Reduction With Aqueous Nasal Beclomethasone," *Pediatrics*, 1995, 95(3):355-64.

Expert Panel Report 2, "Guidelines for the Diagnosis and Management of Asthma," *Clinical Practice Guidelines*, National Institutes of Health, National Heart, Lung, and Blood Institute, NIH Publication No. 94-4051, April, 1997.

Kobayashi RH, Tinkelman DG, Reese ME, et al, "Beclomethasone Dipropionate Aqueous Nasal Spray for Seasonal Allergic Rhinitis in Children," *Ann Allergy*, 1989, 62(3):205-8.

Tinkelman DG, Reed CE, Nelson HS, et al, "Aerosol Beclomethasone Dipropionate Compared With Theophylline as Primary Treatment of Chronic, Mild to Moderately Severe Asthma in Children," *Pediatrics*, 1993, 92(1):64-77.

Wyatt R, Waschek J, Weinberger M, et al, "Effects of Inhaled Beclomethasone Dipropionate and Alternate-Day Prednisone on Pituitary-Adrenal Function in Children With Chronic Asthma," *N Engl J Med*, 1978, 299(25):1387-92.

- ◆ **Beclomethasone Dipropionate** *see Beclomethasone on page 122*
- ◆ **Beclovent® Oral Inhaler** *see Beclomethasone on page 122*
- ◆ **Beconase AQ® Nasal Inhaler** *see Beclomethasone on page 122*
- ◆ **Beconase® Nasal Inhaler** *see Beclomethasone on page 122*
- ◆ **Beepen-VK®** *see Penicillin V Potassium on page 743*
- ◆ **Belix® Oral [OTC]** *see Diphenhydramine on page 327*
- ◆ **Bena-D® Injection** *see Diphenhydramine on page 327*
- ◆ **Benadryl® Injection** *see Diphenhydramine on page 327*
- ◆ **Benadryl® Oral [OTC]** *see Diphenhydramine on page 327*
- ◆ **Benadryl® Topical** *see Diphenhydramine on page 327*
- ◆ **Ben-Allergin-50® Injection** *see Diphenhydramine on page 327*
- ◆ **Ben-Aqua® [OTC]** *see Benzoyl Peroxide on page 126*
- ◆ **Benemid® (Canada)** *see Probenecid on page 798*
- ◆ **Benoxyl®** *see Benzoyl Peroxide on page 126*
- ◆ **Bentyl® Hydrochloride Injection** *see Dicyclomine on page 314*
- ◆ **Bentyl® Hydrochloride Oral** *see Dicyclomine on page 314*
- ◆ **Bentylol® (Canada)** *see Dicyclomine on page 314*
- ◆ **Benuryl™ (Canada)** *see Probenecid on page 798*
- ◆ **Benylin® Cough Syrup [OTC]** *see Diphenhydramine on page 327*
- ◆ **Benylin DM® [OTC]** *see Dextromethorphan on page 304*
- ◆ **Benylin® Expectorant [OTC]** *see Guaifenesin and Dextromethorphan on page 466*
- ◆ **Benylin® Pediatric [OTC]** *see Dextromethorphan on page 304*
- ◆ **Benzac AC® Gel** *see Benzoyl Peroxide on page 126*
- ◆ **Benzac AC® Wash** *see Benzoyl Peroxide on page 126*
- ◆ **Benzac W® Gel** *see Benzoyl Peroxide on page 126*
- ◆ **Benzac W® Wash** *see Benzoyl Peroxide on page 126*
- ◆ **5-Benzagel®** *see Benzoyl Peroxide on page 126*
- ◆ **10-Benzagel®** *see Benzoyl Peroxide on page 126*
- ◆ **Benzagel® Gel (Canada)** *see Benzoyl Peroxide on page 126*
- ◆ **Benzagel® Lotion (Canada)** *see Benzoyl Peroxide on page 126*
- ◆ **Benzagel® Wash (Canada)** *see Benzoyl Peroxide on page 126*
- ◆ **Benzashave® Cream** *see Benzoyl Peroxide on page 126*
- ◆ **Benzathine Benzylpenicillin** *see Penicillin G Benzathine on page 739*
- ◆ **Benzathine Penicillin G** *see Penicillin G Benzathine on page 739*
- ◆ **Benzazoline** *see Tolazoline on page 934*
- ◆ **Benzene Hexachloride** *see Lindane on page 572*
- ◆ **Benzhexol** *see Trihexyphenidyl on page 952*

Benzocaine *(BEN zoe kane)*

Brand Names Americaine® [OTC]; Anbesol® [OTC]; Anbesol® Maximum Strength [OTC]; Babee® Teething [OTC]; Benzocol® [OTC]; Benzodent® [OTC]; Chiggertox®

[OTC]; Cylex® [OTC]; Dermoplast® [OTC]; Foille® [OTC]; Foille® Medicated First Aid [OTC]; Hurricaine®; Lanacane® [OTC]; Mycinettes® [OTC]; Numzitdent® [OTC]; Numzit Teething® [OTC]; Orabase®-B [OTC]; OrabaseGel® [OTC]; Orabase®-O [OTC]; Orajel® Brace-Aid Oral Anesthetic [OTC]; Orajel® Maximum Strength [OTC]; Orajel® Mouth-Aid [OTC]; Orasept® [OTC]; Orasol® [OTC]; Orastect® [OTC]; Rhulicaine® [OTC]; Rid-A-Pain® [OTC]; Slim-Mint® [OTC]; Solarcaine® [OTC]; Spec-T® [OTC]; Vick's Children's Chloraseptic® [OTC]; Vick's Chloraseptic® Sore Throat [OTC]; Zilactin-B® Medicated [OTC]; Topicaine®

Synonyms Ethyl Aminobenzoate

Therapeutic Category Analgesic, Topical; Local Anesthetic, Oral; Local Anesthetic, Topical

Generic Available Yes

Use Temporary relief of pain associated with pruritic dermatosis, pruritus, minor burns, toothache, minor sore throat pain, canker sores, hemorrhoids, rectal fissures; anesthetic lubricant for passage of catheters and endoscopic tubes

Pregnancy Risk Factor C

Contraindications Hypersensitivity to benzocaine, other ester-type local anesthetics, or any component; secondary bacterial infection of area; perforated tympanic membrane (otic formulations only)

Adverse Reactions
Cardiovascular: Edema
Dermatologic: Angioedema, urticaria
Genitourinary: Urethritis
Hematologic: Methemoglobinemia in infants
Local: Contact dermatitis, burning, stinging, tenderness

Mechanism of Action Blocks both the initiation and conduction of nerve impulses from sensory nerves by decreasing the neuronal membrane's permeability to sodium ions, which results in inhibition of depolarization with resultant blockade of conduction

Pharmacokinetics
Absorption: Poor after topical administration to intact skin, but well absorbed from mucous membranes and traumatized skin
Metabolism: Hydrolyzed in plasma and to a lesser extent in the liver by cholinesterase
Elimination: Excretion of the metabolites in urine

Usual Dosage Children and Adults:
Mucous membranes: Dosage varies depending on area to be anesthetized and vascularity of tissues
Oral mouth/throat preparations: Do not administer for >2 days or in children <2 years of age, unless directed by a physician; refer to specific package labeling
Otic: 4-5 drops into ear canal; may repeat every 1-2 hours as needed
Topical: Apply to affected area as needed

Administration
Mucous membranes: Apply to mucous membrane; do not eat for 1 hour after application to oral mucosa
Otic: After instilling into external ear canal, insert cotton pledget into ear canal
Topical: Apply evenly; do not apply to deep or puncture wounds or to serious burns

Patient Information Do not eat for 1 hour after application to oral mucosa; do not chew gum while mouth or throat is anesthetized due to potential biting trauma; do not overuse; do not apply to infected areas or to large areas of broken skin

Dosage Forms
Topical for mucus membranes:
Gel: 6% (7.5 g); 20% (2.5 g, 3.75 g, 7.5 g, 30 g)
Liquid: 20% (3.75 mL, 9 mL, 13.3 mL, 30 mL)
Topical for skin disorders:
Aerosol: 5% (92 mL, 105 mL); 20% (82.5 mL, 90 mL, 92 mL, 150 mL)
Cream: 5% (30 g, 454 g); 6% (28.4 g)
Lotion: 8% (90 mL)
Ointment: 5% (3.5 g, 28 g)
Spray: 5% (97.5 mL); 20% (20 g, 60 g, 120 g, 13.3 mL, 120 mL)
Mouth and throat preparations:
Cream: 5% (10 g)
Gel: 6% (7.5 g); 7.5% (7.2 g, 9.45 g, 14.1 g); 10% (6 g, 9.45 g, 10 g, 15 g); 15% (10.5 g); 20% (9.45 g, 14.1 g)
Liquid: 5% (8.8 mL); 6.3% (9 mL, 22 mL, 14.79 mL); 10% (13 mL); 20% (13.3 mL)
Lotion: 0.2% (15 mL); 2.5% (15 mL)
Lozenges: 5 mg, 6 mg, 10 mg, 15 mg
(Continued)

Benzocaine *(Continued)*

Ointment: 20% (30 g)
Paste: 20% (5 g, 15 g)
Otic preparation: Drops: 20% (15 mL)

♦ **Benzocaine and Antipyrine** *see Antipyrine and Benzocaine on page 90*

♦ **Benzocol® [OTC]** *see Benzocaine on page 124*

♦ **Benzodent® [OTC]** *see Benzocaine on page 124*

Benzoyl Peroxide (BEN zoe il peer OKS ide)

Brand Names Acetoxyl® (Canada); Acnomel® B.P.5 (Canada); Advanced Formula Oxy® Sensitive Gel [OTC]; Ambi 10® [OTC]; Ben-Aqua® [OTC]; Benoxyl®; Benzac AC® Gel; Benzac AC® Wash; Benzac W® Gel; Benzac W® Wash; 5-Benzagel®; 10-Benzagel®; Benzagel® Gel (Canada); Benzagel® Lotion (Canada); Benzagel® Wash (Canada); Benzashave® Cream; BlemErase® Lotion [OTC]; Brevoxyl® Gel; Clear By Design® Gel [OTC]; Clearsil® Maximum Strength [OTC]; Del Aqua-5® Gel; Del Aqua-10® Gel; Desquam-E® Gel; Desquam-X® Gel; Desquam-X® Wash; Dryox® Gel [OTC]; Dryox® Wash [OTC]; Exact® Cream [OTC]; Fostex® 10% BPO Gel [OTC]; Fostex® 10% Wash [OTC]; Fostex® Bar [OTC]; H₂Oxyl® (Canada); Loroxide® [OTC]; Neutrogena® Acne Mask [OTC]; Oxy-5® Advanced Formula for Sensitive Skin [OTC]; Oxy-5® Tinted [OTC]; Oxy-10® Advanced Formula for Sensitive Skin [OTC]; Oxy 10® Wash [OTC]; Oxyderm™ 5%, 10%, 20% (Canada); PanOxyl®-AQ; PanOxyl® Bar [OTC]; Perfectoderm® Gel [OTC]; Peroxin A5®; Peroxin A10®; Persa-Gel®; Solugel® 4, 8 (Canada); Theroxide® Wash [OTC]; Vanoxide® [OTC]

Therapeutic Category Acne Products; Topical Skin Product

Generic Available Yes

Use Adjunctive treatment of mild to moderate acne vulgaris

Pregnancy Risk Factor C

Contraindications Hypersensitivity to benzoyl peroxide, benzoic acid, or any component

Warnings Discontinue if burning, swelling, or undue dryness occurs

Precautions For external use only; may bleach colored fabrics; avoid contact with eyes, eyelids, lips, mucous membranes, and highly inflamed or denuded skin

Adverse Reactions

Dermatologic: Contact dermatitis
Local: Irritation, stinging, dryness, peeling, erythema

Mechanism of Action Releases free-radical oxygen which oxidizes bacterial proteins in the sebaceous follicles decreasing the number of anaerobic bacteria and irritating free fatty acids; exerts a keratolytic activity and a comedolytic effect

Pharmacokinetics

Absorption: ~5% through the skin
Metabolism: Major metabolite is benzoic acid
Elimination: In the urine as benzoate

Usual Dosage Children and Adults: Topical: Apply sparingly 1-3 times/day; initially apply for 15 minutes; length of exposure, strength, and frequency of application are increased as tolerated

Administration Topical: Shake lotion before using; cleanse skin before applying; for external use only; avoid contact with eyes and mucous membranes

Additional Information Granulation may indicate effectiveness; gels are more penetrating than creams and last longer than creams or lotions

Dosage Forms

Bar: 5% (113 g); 10% (106 g, 113 g)
Cream: 5% (18 g, 113.4 g); 10% (18 g, 28 g, 113.4 g)
Gel: 2.5% (30 g, 42.5 g, 45 g, 57 g, 60 g, 90 g, 113 g); 5% (42.5 g, 45 g, 60 g, 80 g, 90 g, 113.4 g); 10% (30 g, 42.5 g, 45 g, 56.7 g, 60 g, 90 g, 113.4 g, 120 g); 20% (30 g, 60 g)
Liquid: 5% (120 mL, 150 mL, 240 mL); 10% (120 mL, 150 mL, 240 mL)
Lotion: 5% (25 mL, 30 mL); 5.5% (25 mL); 10% (12 mL, 29 mL, 30 mL, 60 mL)
Mask: 5% (30 mL, 60 mL, 60 g)

References

Winston MH and Shalita AR, "Acne Vulgaris: Pathogenesis and Treatment," *Pediatr Clin North Am*, 1991, 38(4):889-903.

Benztropine (BENZ troe peen)

Related Information

Overdose and Toxicology *on page 1191*

Brand Names Cogentin®; PMS-Benztropine (Canada)

Available Salts Benztropine Mesylate

Therapeutic Category Anticholinergic Agent; Antidote, Drug-induced Dystonic Reactions; Anti-Parkinson's Agent

Generic Available Yes: Tablet

Use Adjunctive treatment of parkinsonism; also used in treatment of drug-induced extrapyramidal effects (except tardive dyskinesia) and acute dystonic reactions

Pregnancy Risk Factor C

Contraindications Hypersensitivity to benztropine mesylate or any component; children <3 years of age; patients with narrow-angle glaucoma, pyloric or duodenal obstruction, stenosing peptic ulcers; bladder neck obstructions; achalasia; myasthenia gravis

Precautions Use with caution in hot weather or during exercise; may cause anhydrosis and hyperthermia; increased risk of hyperthermia in alcoholics, patients with CNS disease, and with prolonged outdoor exposure

Adverse Reactions

Cardiovascular: Tachycardia, orthostatic hypotension, ventricular fibrillation, palpitations

Central nervous system: Drowsiness, nervousness, hallucinations, coma

Dermatologic: Dry skin, photosensitivity

Endocrine & metabolic: Decreased flow of breast milk

Gastrointestinal: Nausea, vomiting, xerostomia, constipation, dry throat, dysphagia

Neuromuscular & skeletal: Weakness

Ocular: Blurred vision, mydriasis, increased intraocular pain

Respiratory: Dry nose

Miscellaneous: Diaphoresis (decreased)

Drug Interactions As an anticholinergic, benztropine may potentiate the CNS depressant effects of CNS depressants; may inhibit the therapeutic response to neuroleptics; central and/or peripheral anticholinergic syndrome can occur when administered with amantadine, rimantadine, narcotic analgesics, phenothiazides, TCAs, quinidine, and antihistamines

Mechanism of Action Thought to partially block striatal cholinergic receptors to help balance cholinergic and dopaminergic activity

Pharmacodynamics

Onset of action:

Oral: Within 1 hour

Parenteral: Within 15 minutes

Duration of action: 6-48 hours

Usual Dosage

Drug-induced extrapyramidal reaction: Oral, I.M., I.V.:

Children >3 years: 0.02-0.05 mg/kg/dose 1-2 times/day; use in children <3 years should be reserved for life-threatening emergencies

Adults: 1-4 mg/dose 1-2 times/day

Acute dystonia: Adults: I.M., I.V.: 1-2 mg as a single dose

Parkinsonism: Oral: 0.5-6 mg/day in 1-2 divided doses; begin with 0.5 mg/day; increase in 0.5 mg increments at 5- to 6-day intervals to achieve the desired effect

Administration

Oral: Administer with food to decrease GI upset

Parenteral: I.V. route should be reserved for situations when oral or I.M. are not appropriate

Patient Information Causes drowsiness and may impair ability to perform hazardous tasks requiring mental alertness

Dosage Forms

Injection, as mesylate: 1 mg/mL (2 mL)

Tablet, as mesylate: 0.5 mg, 1 mg, 2 mg

♦ **Benztropine Mesylate** see Benztropine on page 126

♦ **Benzylpenicillin Benzathine** see Penicillin G Benzathine on page 739

Benzylpenicilloyl-polylysine (BEN zil pen i SIL oyl pol i LIE seen)

Brand Names Pre-Pen®

Synonyms Penicilloyl-polylysine; PPL

Therapeutic Category Diagnostic Agent, Penicillin Allergy Skin Test

Generic Available No

Use Adjunct in assessing the risk of administering penicillin (penicillin or benzylpenicillin) in patients with a history of clinical penicillin hypersensitivity

Pregnancy Risk Factor C

Contraindications Patients known to be extremely hypersensitive to penicillin

(Continued)

Benzylpenicilloyl-polylysine *(Continued)*

Warnings PPL test alone has a sensitivity rate of 76% and does not identify those patients who react to a minor antigenic determinant; does not appear to reliably predict the occurrence of late reactions and patients at risk for anaphylaxis can be missed

Adverse Reactions

Dermatologic: Erythema, urticaria

Local: Pruritus, wheal, edema

Miscellaneous: Systemic allergic reactions occur rarely

Drug Interactions Antihistamines, tricyclic antidepressants, and sympathomimetic agents may affect skin response

Stability Store in refrigerator; discard if left at room temperature for longer than 1 day

Mechanism of Action Elicits IgE antibodies which produce type I accelerated urticarial reactions to penicillins

Usual Dosage Children and Adults:

Scratch test: Use scratch technique with a 20-gauge needle to make 3-5 mm non-bleeding scratch on epidermis, apply a small drop of solution to scratch, rub in gently with applicator or toothpick. A positive reaction consists of a pale wheal surrounding the scratch site which develops within 10 minutes and ranges from 5-15 mm or more in diameter.

Intradermal test: Use intradermal test with a tuberculin syringe with a 26- to 30-gauge short bevel needle; a dose of 0.01-0.02 mL is injected intradermally. A control of NS should be injected at least $1\frac{1}{2}$" from the PPL test site. Most skin responses to the intradermal test will develop within 5-15 minutes.

Administration Parenteral: PPL is administered by a scratch technique or by intradermal injection. For initial testing, PPL should always be applied via the scratch technique. Do not administer intradermally to patients who have positive reactions to a scratch test.

Nursing Implications Always use scratch test for initial testing

Additional Information Hydroxyzine and diphenhydramine should be discontinued for at least 4 days and astemizole for 6-8 weeks before skin testing

Dosage Forms Solution: 0.25 mL

References

Boguniewicz M and Leung DYM, "Hypersensitivity Reactions to Antibiotics Commonly Used in Children," *Pediatr Infect Dis J*, 1995, 14(3):221-31.

Beractant (ber AKT ant)

Brand Names Survanta®

Synonyms Bovine Lung Surfactant; Natural Lung Surfactant

Therapeutic Category Lung Surfactant

Generic Available No

Use Prevention and treatment of respiratory distress syndrome (RDS) in premature infants

Prophylactic therapy: Infants with body weight <1250 g who are at risk for developing or with evidence of surfactant deficiency

Rescue therapy: Treatment of infants with RDS confirmed by x-ray and requiring mechanical ventilation

Warnings Rapidly affects oxygenation and lung compliance and should be restricted to a highly supervised use in a clinical setting with immediate availability of clinicians experienced with intubation and ventilatory management of premature infants. If transient episodes of bradycardia and decreased oxygen saturation occur, discontinue the dosing procedure and initiate measures to alleviate the condition; produces rapid improvements in lung oxygenation and compliance that may require immediate reductions in ventilator settings and FiO_2.

Precautions Use of beractant in infants <600 g birth weight or >1750 g birth weight has not been evaluated

Adverse Reactions During the dosing procedure:

Cardiovascular: Transient bradycardia, vasoconstriction, hypotension, hypertension, pallor

Respiratory: Oxygen desaturation, endotracheal tube blockage, hypocarbia, hypercarbia, apnea, pulmonary air leaks, pulmonary interstitial emphysema, pulmonary hemorrhage

Miscellaneous: Increased probability of post-treatment nosocomial sepsis

Stability Refrigerate; protect from light; prior to administration warm by standing at room temperature for 20 minutes or hold in hand for 8 minutes; artificial warming methods should **not** be used; unused, unopened vials warmed to room temperature may be returned to the refrigerator within 8 hours of warming only once

Mechanism of Action Replaces deficient or ineffective endogenous lung surfactant in neonates with respiratory distress syndrome (RDS) or in neonates at risk of developing RDS. Surfactant prevents the alveoli from collapsing during expiration by lowering surface tension between air and alveolar surfaces.

Usual Dosage Intratracheal: Neonates:

Prophylactic treatment: Give 4 mL/kg as soon as possible; as many as 4 doses may be administered during the first 48 hours of life, no more frequently than 6 hours apart. The need for additional doses is determined by evidence of continuing respiratory distress or if the infant is still intubated and requiring at least 30% inspired oxygen to maintain a PaO_2 ≤80 torr.

Rescue treatment: Give 4 mL/kg as soon as the diagnosis of RDS is made; may repeat if needed, no more frequently than every 6 hours to a maximum of 4 doses

Administration Intratracheal: For intratracheal administration only. Do not shake; if settling occurs during storage, gently swirl. Suction infant prior to administration; inspect solution to verify complete mixing of the suspension. Administer intratracheally by instillation through a 5-French end-hole catheter inserted into the infant's endotracheal tube. Administer the dose in four 1 mL/kg aliquots. Each quarter-dose is instilled over 2-3 seconds; each quarter-dose is administered with the infant in a different position; slightly downward inclination with head turned to the right, then repeat with head turned to the left; then slightly upward inclination with head turned to the right, then repeat with head turned to the left.

Monitoring Parameters Continuous heart rate and transcutaneous O_2 saturation should be monitored during administration; frequent ABG sampling is necessary to prevent postdosing hyperoxia and hypocarbia.

Dosage Forms Suspension: 100 mg (4 mL); 200 mg (8 mL)

♦ **Berubigen®** see Cyanocobalamin on page 263
♦ **Betachron®** see Propranolol on page 816
♦ **Betacort™ (Canada)** see Betamethasone on page 130
♦ **Betaderm (Canada)** see Betamethasone on page 130
♦ **Betadine® First Aid Antibiotics + Moisturizer [OTC]** see Bacitracin and Polymyxin B on page 119
♦ **9-Beta-D-ribofuranosyladenine** see Adenosine on page 36
♦ **Betagan® Liquifilm® Ophthalmic** see Levobunolol on page 564

Betaine Anhydrous (BAY tayne an HY drus)

Brand Names Cystadane®
Therapeutic Category Homocystinuria, Treatment Agent
Generic Available No
Use Treatment of homocystinuria
Pregnancy Risk Factor C
Contraindications Hypersensitivity to betaine or any component
Adverse Reactions Gastrointestinal: Nausea, vomiting, diarrhea, GI distress
Mechanism of Action Betaine reduces homocysteine blood concentrations by acting as a methyl group donor in the remethylation of homocysteine to methionine
Usual Dosage Oral:

Children <3 years: 100 mg/kg/day divided into 2 doses; increase at weekly intervals in 100 mg/kg/day increments

Children ≥3 years and Adults: 3 g twice daily; doses up to 20 g/day have been needed to control homocysteine plasma concentrations in some patients

Administration Oral: Shake bottle lightly before opening; measure prescribed amount with provided measuring scoop and dissolve in 4-6 ounces of water, juice, milk, or formula; administer immediately; do not use if powder does not completely dissolve or gives a colored solution

Monitoring Parameters Plasma homocysteine concentration (should be low or undetectable)

Additional Information Orphan drug; may only be obtained by contacting Chronimed Inc at 1-800-900-4267; vitamin B_6, vitamin B_{12}, and folate have been helpful in the management of homocystinuria and are often used in conjunction

Dosage Forms Powder: 1 g/scoop (1 scoop = 1.7 mL) (180 g)

♦ **Betalene® Topical** see Betamethasone on page 130
♦ **Betalin®S** see Thiamine on page 916
♦ **Betaloc® (Canada)** see Metoprolol on page 633
♦ **Betaloc® Durules® (Canada)** see Metoprolol on page 633

Betamethasone (bay ta METH a sone)

Related Information
Corticosteroids Comparison, Topical *on page 1033*

Brand Names Alphatrex® Topical; Beben® (Canada); Betacort™ (Canada); Betaderm (Canada); Betalene® Topical; Betatrex® Topical; Beta-Val® Topical; Betnesol® [Disodium Phosphate] (Canada); Betnovate® (Canada); Celestoderm®-V, -EV/2 (Canada); Celestone® Oral; Celestone® Phosphate Injection; Celestone® Soluspan®; Cel-U-Jec® Injection; Diprolene® AF Topical; Diprolene® Glycol [Dipropionate] (Canada); Diprolene® Topical; Diprosone® Topical; Ectosone (Canada); Luxiq™; Maxivate® Topical; Occlucort® (Canada); Psorion® Topical; Rhoprolene® (Canada); Rhoprosone® (Canada); Selestoject® [Sodium Phosphate] (Canada); Selestoject® Injection; Taro-Sone® (Canada); Teladar® Topical; Topilene® (Canada); Topisone® (Canada); Uticort® Topical; Valisone® Topical

Available Salts Betamethasone Benzoate; Betamethasone Dipropionate; Betamethasone Sodium Phosphate; Betamethasone Sodium Phosphate and Acetate; Betamethasone Valerate

Synonyms Flubenisolone

Therapeutic Category Adrenal Corticosteroid; Anti-inflammatory Agent; Corticosteroid, Systemic; Corticosteroid, Topical; Glucocorticoid

Generic Available Yes

Use Anti-inflammatory; immunosuppressant agent; corticosteroid replacement therapy

Topical: Inflammatory dermatoses such as psoriasis, seborrheic or atopic dermatitis, neurodermatitis, inflammatory phase of xerosis, late phase of allergic dermatitis or irritant dermatitis; Foam: Inflammatory and pruritic symptoms of scalp dermatoses responsive to corticosteroids

Pregnancy Risk Factor C

Contraindications Systemic fungal infections; hypersensitivity to betamethasone or any component

Precautions Use with caution in patients with hypothyroidism, cirrhosis, ulcerative colitis; use topical products sparingly in children, systemic effects may be seen

Adverse Reactions
Cardiovascular: Edema, hypertension
Central nervous system: Convulsions, vertigo, confusion, headache
Dermatologic: Thin fragile skin, hyperpigmentation or hypopigmentation, acne, impaired wound healing
Endocrine & metabolic: Cushingoid state, sodium retention, potential pituitary-adrenal axis suppression, potential growth suppression, glucose intolerance, hypokalemia
Gastrointestinal: Peptic ulcer, nausea, vomiting
Local: Burning, itching, stinging, sterile abscess
Neuromuscular & skeletal: Muscle weakness, osteoporosis, fractures
Ocular: Cataracts, glaucoma

Drug Interactions Cytochrome P-450 isoenzyme CYP3A substrate
Barbiturates, phenytoin and rifampin will decrease corticosteroid effects; salicylates; vaccines; NSAIDs; diuretics (potassium depleting); caffeine and alcohol may increase risk for GI ulcer

Food Interactions Systemic use of corticosteroids may require a diet with increased potassium, vitamins A, B_6, C, D, folate, calcium, zinc, and phosphorus and decreased sodium

Stability Foam canister is flammable; store at controlled room temperature; avoid fire, flame, heat; do not store at >120°F (49°C)

Mechanism of Action Controls the rate of protein synthesis, depresses the migration of polymorphonuclear leukocytes and fibroblasts, reverses capillary permeability, and causes lysosomal stabilization at the cellular level to prevent or control inflammation

Pharmacokinetics
Protein binding: 64%
Metabolism: Hepatic
Elimination: <5% of dose excreted renally as unchanged drug; small amounts eliminated via biliary tract

Usual Dosage Base dosage on severity of disease and patient response
Children: Use lowest dose listed as initial dose for adrenocortical insufficiency (physiologic replacement)
I.M.: 0.0175-0.125 mg base/kg/day divided every 6-12 hours **or** 0.5-7.5 mg base/ m^2/day divided every 6-12 hours

Oral: 0.0175-0.25 mg/kg/day divided every 6-8 hours **or** 0.5-7.5 mg/m^2/day divided every 6-8 hours

Adolescents and Adults:

I.M.: 0.6-9 mg/day divided every 12-24 hours

Oral: 2.4-4.8 mg/day in 2-4 doses; range: 0.6-7.2 mg/day

Children and Adults: Topical: Apply thin film 1-3 times/day

Adolescents ≥16 years and Adults: Topical, foam: Apply twice daily (in morning and at night)

Administration

Oral: Administer with food to decrease GI effects

Parenteral: Do not administer injectable suspension I.V.; shake injectable suspension before use

Topical: Apply sparingly, rub in gently until it disappears; do not apply to face or inguinal areas; not for use on broken skin or in areas of infection

Foam: Invert can, dispense small amount of foam onto saucer or other cool surface; foam will melt upon contact with warm skin (do not dispense directly into hands); use fingers to apply small amounts of foam to affected scalp area; rub in gently until it disappears; avoid fire, flame, or smoking during use; contents of can are flammable and under pressure

Test Interactions Skin tests

Patient Information Topical use: Avoid contact with eyes; do not use occlusive dressings unless directed by physician

Additional Information Medium to high potency topical corticosteroid; long-acting corticosteroid with minimal or no sodium-retaining potential

Dosage Forms

Base (Celestone®):
Syrup: 0.6 mg/5 mL
Tablet: 0.6 mg

Benzoate (Uticort®):
Cream, emollient base: 0.025% (60 g)
Gel, topical: 0.025% (15 g, 60 g)
Lotion: 0.025% (60 mL)

Dipropionate (Alphatrex®, Diprosone®, Maxivate®, Teladar®):
Aerosol, topical: 0.1% (85 g)
Cream: 0.05% (15 g, 45 g)
Lotion: 0.05% (20 mL, 30 mL, 60 mL)
Ointment, topical: 0.05% (15 g, 45 g)

Dipropionate (Psorion®):
Cream: 0.05% (15 g, 45 g)

Dipropionate, augmented (Diprolene®, Diprolene® AF):
Cream, emollient base: 0.05% (15 g, 45 g)
Gel, topical: 0.05% (15 g, 45 g)
Lotion: 0.05% (30 mL, 60 mL)
Ointment, topical: 0.05% (15 g, 45 g)

Valerate (Betatrex®, Beta-Val®, Valisone®):
Cream: 0.01% (15 g, 60 g); 0.1% (15 g, 45 g, 110 g, 430 g)
Foam (Luxiq™): 0.12% (100 g)
Lotion: 0.1% (20 mL, 60 mL)
Ointment, topical: 0.1% (15 g, 45 g)
Powder for compounding: 5 g, 10 g

Sodium phosphate (Celestone® Phosphate, Selestoject®):
Injection: Equivalent to 3 mg/mL (5 mL)

Sodium phosphate and acetate (Celestone® Soluspan®):
Injection, suspension: 6 mg/mL [3 mg betamethasone as betamethasone sodium phosphate and 3 mg betamethasone acetate per mL] (5 mL)

♦ **Betamethasone Benzoate** *see* Betamethasone *on page 130*

♦ **Betamethasone Dipropionate** *see* Betamethasone *on page 130*

♦ **Betamethasone Sodium Phosphate** *see* Betamethasone *on page 130*

♦ **Betamethasone Sodium Phosphate and Acetate** *see* Betamethasone *on page 130*

♦ **Betamethasone Valerate** *see* Betamethasone *on page 130*

♦ **Betapen®-VK** *see* Penicillin V Potassium *on page 743*

♦ **Betasept® [OTC]** *see* Chlorhexidine Gluconate *on page 209*

♦ **Beta-Tim® (Canada)** *see* Timolol *on page 929*

♦ **Betatrex® Topical** *see* Betamethasone *on page 130*

♦ **Beta-Val® Topical** *see* Betamethasone *on page 130*

♦ **Betaxin® (Canada)** *see* Thiamine *on page 916*

Bethanechol (be THAN e kole)

Brand Names Duvoid®; Myotonachol™; PMS-Bethanechol Chloride (Canada); Urabeth®; Urecholine®

Available Salts Bethanechol Chloride

Therapeutic Category Cholinergic Agent

Generic Available Yes: Tablet

Use Treatment of nonobstructive urinary retention and retention due to neurogenic bladder; gastroesophageal reflux

Pregnancy Risk Factor C

Contraindications Hypersensitivity to bethanechol chloride or any component; do not use in patients with mechanical obstruction of the GI or GU tract; do not use in patients with hyperthyroidism, peptic ulcer, bronchial asthma, or cardiac disease; contraindicated for I.M. or I.V. use due to severe cholinergic activity

Adverse Reactions
Cardiovascular: Hypotension, cardiac arrest, flushed skin (vasomotor response)
Central nervous system: Headache
Gastrointestinal: Abdominal cramps, diarrhea, nausea, vomiting, salivation
Genitourinary: Urinary frequency
Hepatic: Increased liver enzymes, increased bilirubin
Ocular: Miosis, lacrimation
Respiratory: Bronchial constriction
Miscellaneous: Diaphoresis

Drug Interactions Ganglionic blockers may cause a critical fall in blood pressure; additive effects with other cholinergic agents, epinephrine, and other sympathomimetics; quinidine and procainamide may antagonize cholinergic effects

Mechanism of Action Stimulates cholinergic receptors in the smooth muscle of the urinary bladder and gastrointestinal tract resulting in increased peristalsis, increased GI and pancreatic secretions, bladder muscle contraction, and increased ureteral peristaltic waves

Pharmacodynamics
Onset of action:
Oral 30-90 minutes
S.C.: 5-15 minutes
Duration:
Oral: Up to 6 hours
S.C.: 2 hours

Pharmacokinetics
Absorption: Oral: Variable
Metabolic fate and excretion have not been determined

Usual Dosage
Children:
Oral:
Abdominal distention or urinary retention: 0.6 mg/kg/day divided 3-4 times/day
Gastroesophageal reflux: 0.1-0.2 mg/kg/dose or 3 mg/m^2/dose given 30 minutes to 1 hour before each meal to a maximum of 4 times/day
S.C.: 0.12-0.2 mg/kg/day divided 3-4 times/day
Adults:
Oral: 10-50 mg 2-4 times/day
S.C.: 2.5-5 mg 3-4 times/day, up to 7.5-10 mg every 4 hours for neurogenic bladder

Administration
Oral: Administer on an empty stomach to reduce nausea and vomiting
Parenteral: For S.C. injection only; do not administer I.M. or I.V.

Patient Information Dizziness, lightheadedness, or fainting may occur especially when getting up from a lying position

Dosage Forms
Injection, as chloride: 5 mg/mL (1 mL)
Tablet, as chloride: 5 mg, 10 mg, 25 mg, 50 mg

Extemporaneous Preparations An oral solution of bethanechol 1 mg/mL diluted in sterile water for irrigation is stable for at least 30 days refrigerated.
Schlatter JL and Saulnier J, "Bethanechol Chloride Oral Solutions: Stability and Use in Infants," *Ann Pharmacother*, 31:294-296, 1997.

- ♦ **Bicillin® L-A** *see* Penicillin G Benzathine *on page 739*
- ♦ **Bicitra®** *see* Citrate and Citric Acid *on page 231*
- ♦ **BiCNU®** *see* Carmustine *on page 172*
- ♦ **Biltricide®** *see* Praziquantel *on page 789*
- ♦ **Biocef®** *see* Cephalexin *on page 196*
- ♦ **Bioderm (Canada)** *see* Bacitracin and Polymyxin B *on page 119*
- ♦ **Biomox®** *see* Amoxicillin *on page 70*
- ♦ **Bio-Tab®** *see* Doxycycline *on page 348*

Biotin (BYE oh tin)
Brand Names Biotin® Forte; Biotin® Forte Extra Strength [OTC]; Bio-Tn® [OTC]; d-Biotin
Therapeutic Category Biotinidase Deficiency, Treatment Agent; Nutritional Supplement; Vitamin, Water Soluble
Generic Available Yes
Use Treatment of primary biotinidase deficiency; nutritional biotin deficiency; component of the vitamin B complex
Contraindications Hypersensitivity to biotin or any component
Food Interactions Large amounts of raw egg whites prevent biotin absorption
Mechanism of Action A member of the B-complex group of vitamins; biotin is required for various metabolic functions such as gluconeogenesis, lipogenesis, fatty acid biosynthesis, propionate metabolism, and the catabolism of branched-chain amino acids; there are 9 known biotin-dependent enzymes; the enzyme biotinidase regenerates biotin in the body and is also required for the release of dietary protein-bound biotin.

Biotinidase deficiency is an autosomal recessively inherited metabolic disorder characterized by deficient activity of the enzyme in serum. Children with the disorder usually exhibit seizures, hypotonia, ataxia, skin rash, alopecia, metabolic ketoacidosis, and organic aciduria.
Usual Dosage Oral:
   RDA: Infants, Children, and Adults: There is no official RDA, however 100-200 mcg/day is considered adequate
   Biotinidase deficiency: Neonates, Infants, Children, and Adults: 5-10 mg once daily
   Biotin deficiency: Children and Adults: 5-20 mg once daily
Administration Oral: May be administered without regard to meals
Reference Range Serum biotinidase activity
Dosage Forms Tablet: 300 mcg, 400 mcg, 600 mcg, 800 mcg, 2.5 mg, 3 mg, 5 mg, 10 mg
References
McVoy JR, Levy HL, Lawler M, et al, "Partial Biotinidase Deficiency: Clinical and Biochemical Features," 1990, *J Pediatr*, 116(1):78-83.
Salbert BA, Pellock JM, and Wolf B, "Characterization of Seizures Associated With Biotinidase Deficiency," *Neurology*, 1993, 43(7):1351-5.
Wastell HJ, Bartlett K, Dale G, et al, "Biotinidase Deficiency: A Survey of 10 Cases," *Arch Dis Child*, 1988, 63(10):1244-9.

- ♦ **Biotin® Forte** *see* Biotin *on page 133*
- ♦ **Biotin® Forte Extra Strength [OTC]** *see* Biotin *on page 133*
- ♦ **Bio-Tn® [OTC]** *see* Biotin *on page 133*
- ♦ **Biquin® Durules® (Canada)** *see* Quinidine *on page 830*
- ♦ **Bisac-Evac® [OTC]** *see* Bisacodyl *on page 133*

Bisacodyl (bis a KOE dil)
Brand Names Apo®-Bisacodyl (Canada); Bisac-Evac® [OTC]; Bisacodyl Uniserts®; Bisco-Lax® [OTC]; Carter's Little Pills® [OTC]; Clysodrast®; Dacodyl® [OTC]; Deficol® [OTC]; Dulcolax® [OTC]; Fleet® Laxative [OTC]; PMS-Bisacodyl (Canada)
Therapeutic Category Laxative, Stimulant
Generic Available Yes
Use Treatment of constipation; colonic evacuation prior to procedures or examination
Pregnancy Risk Factor C
Contraindications Hypersensitivity to bisacodyl or any component; do not use in patients with abdominal pain, appendicitis, obstruction, nausea or vomiting; not to be used during pregnancy or lactation
Warnings Safety of bisacodyl tannex usage in children <10 years of age has not been established
Precautions Bisacodyl tannex powder for preparation as a rectal solution should be used with caution in patients with ulceration of the colon
(Continued)

Bisacodyl (Continued)

Adverse Reactions
Endocrine & metabolic: Electrolyte and fluid imbalance (metabolic acidosis or alkalosis, hypocalcemia)

Gastrointestinal: Abdominal cramps, nausea, vomiting, rectal burning

Food Interactions
Administration within 1 hour of ingesting antacids, alkaline material, milk, or dairy products will cause premature dissolution of the enteric coating and resultant gastric irritation

Stability
Store enteric-coated tablets and rectal suppositories at <30°C. Reconstituted bisacodyl tannex solution should be used immediately after preparation.

Mechanism of Action
Stimulates peristalsis by directly irritating the smooth muscle of the intestine, possibly the colonic intramural plexus; alters water and electrolyte secretion producing net intestinal fluid accumulation and laxation

Pharmacodynamics
Onset of action:

Oral: Within 6-10 hours

Rectal: 15-60 minutes

Pharmacokinetics
Absorption: Oral, rectal: <5% absorbed systemically

Metabolism: In the liver

Elimination: Conjugated metabolites excreted in breast milk, bile, and urine

Usual Dosage
Bisacodyl (Dulcolax®) tablet: Oral:

Children 3-12 years: 5-10 mg or 0.3 mg/kg/day as a single dose

Children ≥12 years and Adults: 5-15 mg/day as a single dose

Bisacodyl (Dulcolax®) suppository: Rectal:

Children:

<2 years: 5 mg/day as a single dose

2-11 years: 5-10 mg/day as a single dose

Children ≥12 years and Adults: 10 mg/day as a single dose

Administration
Oral: Administer on an empty stomach with water; patient should swallow tablet whole; do not break or chew enteric-coated tablet; do not administer within 1 hour of ingesting antacids, alkaline material, milk, or dairy products

Patient Information
Should not be used regularly for more than 1 week

Additional Information
In a randomized prospective study of 70 patients, bisacodyl tablets were given orally once daily in the morning for 2 days before colonoscopy to 19 patients (dose for children <5 years: 5 mg; 5-12 years: 10 mg; >12 years: 15 mg) with a Fleet® enema given on the morning of the procedure without any dietary restriction. Results showed that bisacodyl without dietary restriction provided unsatisfactory colon cleansing.

Dosage Forms
Enema: 10 mg/30 mL

Powder: 1.5 mg with tannic acid 2.5 g per packet (25s, 50s)

Suppository, rectal: 5 mg, 10 mg

Tablet, enteric coated: 5 mg

References
Dahshan A, Lin CH, Peters J, et al, "A Randomized, Prospective Study to Evaluate the Efficacy and Acceptance of Three Bowel Preparations for Colonoscopy in Children," Am J Gastroenterol, 1999, 94(12):3497-501.

♦ **Bisacodyl Uniserts®** see Bisacodyl on page 133
♦ **Bisco-Lax® [OTC]** see Bisacodyl on page 133
♦ **Bismatrol® [OTC]** see Bismuth on page 134

Bismuth (BIZ muth)

Brand Names
Bismatrol® [OTC]; Devrom® [OTC]; Pepto-Bismol® [OTC]; Pink Bismuth® [OTC]

Available Salts
Bismuth Subgallate; Bismuth Subsalicylate

Synonyms
BSS

Therapeutic Category
Antidiarrheal; Gastrointestinal Agent, Gastric or Duodenal Ulcer Treatment

Generic Available
Yes

Use
Symptomatic treatment of mild, nonspecific diarrhea including traveler's diarrhea; chronic infantile diarrhea; adjunctive treatment of Helicobacter pylori-associated antral gastritis

Pregnancy Risk Factor
C (D in 3rd trimester)

Contraindications
Do not use subsalicylate in patients with influenza or chickenpox because of risk of Reye's syndrome; do not use in patients with hypersensitivity to salicylates; history of severe GI bleeding or coagulopathy

Warnings Subsalicylate should be used with caution if patient is taking aspirin, due to additive toxicity; use with caution in children <3 years of age and those with viral illness; be aware of salicylate content when prescribing for use in children

Precautions May interfere with radiologic examinations of GI tract as bismuth is radiopaque

Adverse Reactions

Central nervous system: Anxiety, confusion, slurred speech, headache, mental depression

Gastrointestinal: Impaction (infants and debilitated patients), grayish-black stools, darkened tongue

Neuromuscular & skeletal: Muscle spasms, weakness

Otic: Tinnitus, loss of hearing

Drug Interactions Decreases absorption of tetracycline; increased toxicity of aspirin (due to absorption of salicylate), warfarin, hypoglycemics

Mechanism of Action Adsorbs extra water in large intestine, as well as toxins; forms a protective coat on the intestinal mucosa; appears to have antisecretory (salicylate moiety) and antimicrobial effects (bismuth moiety) against bacterial and viral pathogens

Pharmacokinetics

Absorption: Bismuth is minimally absorbed (<1%) across the GI tract while salicylate salt is readily absorbed (80%)

Distribution: Salicylate: V_d: 170 mL/kg

Protein binding, plasma: Bismuth and salicylate: >90%

Metabolism: Bismuth salts undergo chemical dissociation after oral administration; salicylate is extensively metabolized in the liver

Half-life:

Bismuth: Terminal: 21-72 days

Salicylate: Terminal: 2-5 hours

Elimination:

Bismuth: Renal, biliary

Salicylate: Only 10% excreted unchanged in urine

Usual Dosage Oral (bismuth subsalicylate liquid dosages expressed in mL of 262 mg/15 mL concentration):

Nonspecific diarrhea: Bismuth subsalicylate: 100 mg/kg/day divided into 5 equal doses for 5 days (maximum: 4.19 g/day) **or**

Children: Up to 8 doses/24 hours:

3-6 years: 1/3 tablet or 5 mL every 30 minutes to 1 hour as needed

6-9 years: 2/3 tablet or 10 mL every 30 minutes to 1 hour as needed

9-12 years: 1 tablet or 15 mL every 30 minutes to 1 hour as needed

Adults: 2 tablets or 30 mL every 30 minutes to 1 hour as needed up to 8 doses/ 24 hours

Chronic infantile diarrhea: Bismuth subsalicylate:

2-24 months: 2.5 mL every 4 hours

24-48 months: 5 mL every 4 hours

48-70 months: 10 mL every 4 hours

Prevention of traveler's diarrhea: Adults:

Bismuth subgallate: 1-2 tablets 3 times/day with meals

Bismuth subsalicylate: 2.1 g/day or 2 tablets 4 times/day before meals and at bedtime

Helicobacter pylori-associated antral gastritis: Bismuth subsalicylate: Dosage in children is not well established, the following dosages have been used (in conjunction with ampicillin and metronidazole or (in adults) tetracycline and metronidazole):

Children ≤10 years: 15 mL (262 mg) 4 times/day for 6 weeks

Children >10 years and Adults: 30 mL of 262 mg/15 mL solution or two 262 mg tablets 4 times/day for 6 weeks

Dosing adjustment in renal impairment: Avoid use in patients with renal failure

Administration Oral: Shake liquid well before using; chew tablets or allow to dissolve in mouth before swallowing; swallow caplets whole (do not chew)

Test Interactions Bismuth absorbs x-rays and may interfere with diagnostic procedures of GI tract

Patient Information May darken stools; if diarrhea persists for more than 2 days, consult a physician; may tongue black

Additional Information Bismuth subsalicylate: 262 mg = 130 mg nonaspirin salicylate; 525 mg = 236 mg nonaspirin salicylate

Dosage Forms

Caplet, as subsalicylate: 262 mg

(Continued)

Bismuth *(Continued)*

Liquid, as subsalicylate: 262 mg/15 mL (120 mL, 240 mL, 360 mL, 480 mL); 525 mg/15 mL (maximum strength) (120 mL, 240 mL, 360 mL)
Tablet, chewable, as subsalicylate: 262 mg
Tablet, chewable, as subgallate (Devrom®): 200 mg

References

Drumm B, Sherman P, Karmali M, et al, "Treatment of *Campylobacter pylori*-associated Antral Gastritis in Children With Bismuth Subsalicylate and Ampicillin," *J Pediatr*, 1988, 113(5):908-12.

Soriano-Brucher HE, Avendano P, O'Ryan M, et al, "Use of Bismuth Subsalicylate in Acute Diarrhea in Children," *Rev Infect Dis*, 1990, 12(Suppl 1):S51-5.

Walsh JH and Peterson WL, "The Treatment of *Helicobacter pylori* Infection in the Management of Peptic Ulcer Disease," *N Engl J Med*, 1995, 333(15):984-91.

♦ **Bismuth Subgallate** *see* Bismuth *on page 134*

♦ **Bismuth Subsalicylate** *see* Bismuth *on page 134*

♦ **Bistropamide** *see* Tropicamide *on page 959*

Bitolterol *(bye TOLE ter ole)*

Related Information

Asthma Guidelines *on page 1178*

Brand Names Tornalate®

Available Salts Bitolterol Mesylate

Therapeutic Category Adrenergic Agonist Agent; Antiasthmatic; Beta$_2$-Adrenergic Agonist Agent; Bronchodilator; Sympathomimetic

Use Prevention and treatment of bronchial asthma and bronchospasm

Pregnancy Risk Factor C

Contraindications Hypersensitivity to bitolterol or any component

Warnings Excessive use may result in cardiac arrest and death

Precautions Use with caution in patients with unstable vasomotor symptoms, diabetes, hyperthyroidism, prostatic hypertrophy or a history of seizures, cardiovascular disorders such as coronary artery disease, arrhythmias, and hypertension; do not use concurrently with other sympathomimetic bronchodilators

Adverse Reactions

Cardiovascular: Flushing of face, hypertension, pounding heartbeat, chest pain, arrhythmias, tachycardia

Central nervous system: Dizziness, lightheadedness, nervousness, insomnia

Gastrointestinal: Xerostomia, nausea, unpleasant taste, mouth and throat irritation

Neuromuscular & skeletal: Tremors, hyperkinesia, paresthesia

Respiratory: Bronchial irritation, coughing, paradoxical bronchospasm

Drug Interactions Bitolterol decreases the effects of beta-adrenergic blockers (eg, propranolol); inhaled ipratropium may increase duration of bronchodilation; nifedipine may increase FEV-1; increased toxicity with MAO inhibitors, tricyclic antidepressants, sympathomimetic agents, inhaled anesthetics (eg, enflurane)

Stability Solution for nebulization should not be mixed with cromolyn sodium or acetylcysteine; stability when mixed with other nebulized drugs has not been established

Mechanism of Action Bitolterol, a prodrug, undergoes hydrolysis in the lungs to the active agent, colterol. Colterol selectively stimulates beta$_2$-adrenergic receptors in the lungs producing bronchial smooth muscle relaxation. Colterol possesses minor beta$_1$ activity.

Pharmacodynamics

Onset of effect: After oral inhalation: 3-5 minutes

Maximum effect: 0.5-2 hours

Duration of action: 4-8 hours

Pharmacokinetics Since blood levels of colterol (active drug) are too low to be measured by currently available assay methods, the pharmacokinetics of this agent following inhalation are not known.

Usual Dosage Children >12 years and Adults:

Bronchospasm: Oral inhalation: 2 inhalations at an interval of at least 1-3 minutes, followed by a third inhalation if needed

Prevention of bronchospasm: Oral inhalation: 2 inhalations every 8 hours; maximum daily dosage: 3 inhalations every 6 hours or 2 inhalations every 4 hours

Intermittent nebulization: 1 mg (0.5 mL) [range: 0.5-1.5 mg (0.25-0.75 mL)] every 8 hours; treatments may be increased to four times daily, however, the interval between treatments should **not** be less than 4 hours; a dosage of 2 mg (1 mL) may be used in severely obstructed patients; maximum daily dosage: 8 mg (4 mL)

Continuous flow nebulization: 2.5 mg (1.25 mL) 3 times/day [range: 1.5-3.5 mg (0.75-1.75 mL)]; maximum daily dosage 14 mg (7 mL); treatments should be at least 4 hours apart

Administration

Oral inhalation: Shake canister well before use; administer pressurized inhalation during the second half of inspiration, as the airways are open and the aerosol distribution is more extensive. If more than one inhalation per dose is necessary, wait at least 1 full minute between inhalations - second inhalation is best delivered after 10 minutes. Administer every 8 hours rather than 3 times/day, to promote less variation in peak and trough serum levels

Nebulization: Dilute with NS to a total volume of 2-4 mL prior to use; after adding to nebulizer reservoir, swirl contents gently; the patient should breathe deeply until the nebulizer chamber is empty (approximately 5-15 minutes)

Monitoring Parameters Assess lung sounds, heart rate, respiratory rate, peak flow; arterial or capillary blood gases (if patient's condition warrants)

Patient Information Do not exceed recommended dosage, excessive use may lead to adverse effects or loss of effectiveness. May cause nervousness, restlessness, and insomnia; if these effects continue after dosage reduction, notify physician. Also notify physician if palpitations, tachycardia, chest pain, muscle tremors, dizziness, headache, flushing, or if breathing difficulty persists.

Dosage Forms

Aerosol, oral, as mesylate: 0.8% [370 mcg/metered spray, 300 inhalations] (15 mL)
Solution, inhalation, as mesylate: 0.2% (10 mL, 30 mL, 60 mL)

♦ **Bitolterol Mesylate** see Bitolterol on page 136

♦ **Black Draught® [OTC]** see Senna on page 865

♦ **BlemErase® Lotion [OTC]** see Benzoyl Peroxide on page 126

♦ **Blenoxane®** see Bleomycin on page 137

Bleomycin (blee oh MYE sin)

Related Information

Emetogenic Potential of Single Chemotherapeutic Agents on page 1095

Brand Names Blenoxane®

Available Salts Bleomycin Sulfate

Synonyms BLM

Therapeutic Category Antineoplastic Agent, Antibiotic

Generic Available Yes

Use Palliative treatment of squamous cell carcinoma, testicular carcinoma, and germ cell tumors; Hodgkin's lymphoma, non-Hodgkin's lymphoma, renal carcinoma, and soft tissue sarcoma; sclerosing agent to control malignant effusions

Pregnancy Risk Factor D

Contraindications Hypersensitivity to bleomycin sulfate or any component

Warnings The FDA currently recommends that procedures for proper handling and disposal of antineoplastic agents be considered. Occurrence of pulmonary fibrosis is higher in elderly patients and in those receiving a total cumulative dose >400 units; pulmonary toxicity has occurred at a total dosage <200 units or 250 units/m^2 in younger patients; pulmonary irradiation and use of supplemental oxygen increase the chance for developing toxic pulmonary reactions in patients previously treated with bleomycin; a severe idiosyncratic reaction consisting of hypotension, mental confusion, fever, chills, and wheezing is possible.

Precautions Use with caution in patients with renal or pulmonary impairment; dosage modification is recommended in patients with renal impairment; dosage modification may be necessary in patients with a 20% decrease from baseline in FEV_1, FVC, or DL_{co}; administer test dose to lymphoma patients prior to starting therapy

Adverse Reactions

Cardiovascular: Cerebrovascular accident, hypotension, Raynaud's phenomenon

Central nervous system: Fever, chills, malaise

Dermatologic: Hyperpigmentation, hyperkeratosis of hands and nails, rash, alopecia, desquamation

Gastrointestinal: Stomatitis, vomiting, anorexia, mild nausea

Hematologic: Thrombocytopenia, leukopenia

Local: Phlebitis

Respiratory: Interstitial pneumonitis (10%), pulmonary fibrosis (cumulative lifetime dose should not exceed 400 units or 250 units/m^2 in younger patients), dyspnea, tachypnea, nonproductive cough, rales

Miscellaneous: Anaphylactoid reactions

(Continued)

Bleomycin *(Continued)*

Drug Interactions Phenytoin (decreases phenytoin concentrations), cisplatin (decreases bleomycin clearance), bleomycin may decrease digoxin absorption; concurrent use with amphotericin B products may increase nephrotoxicity and risk for hypotension and bronchospasm

Stability Refrigerate; intact vials are stable 28 days at room temperature; reconstituted solution is stable for 24 hours at room temperature; incompatible with amino acid solutions, ascorbic acid, cefazolin, furosemide, diazepam, hydrocortisone, mitomycin, nafcillin, penicillin G, aminophylline, copper; dilution in dextrose solutions may result in a 10% loss of activity within 24 hours

Mechanism of Action Inhibits synthesis of DNA; binds to DNA leading to single- and double-strand breaks by a Fe^{++}-O_2-catalyzed free radical reaction

Pharmacokinetics
Distribution: Into skin, lungs, kidneys, peritoneum, and lymphatics
Protein binding: <10%
Half-life: Dependent upon renal function
Children: 2.1-3.5 hours
Adults, with normal renal function: 2-3 hours
Time to peak serum concentration: I.M.: Within 30-60 minutes
Elimination: 60% to 70% of a dose excreted in the urine as active drug
Not removed by hemodialysis

Usual Dosage Refer to individual protocol
Children and Adults:
I.M., I.V., S.C.:
Test dose for lymphoma patients: 1-2 units of bleomycin for the first 2 doses; monitor vital signs every 15 minutes; wait a minimum of 1 hour before administering remainder of dose
Treatment: 10-20 units/m^2 (0.25-0.5 units/kg) 1-2 times/week in combination regimens or once every 2-4 weeks
Germ cell tumors: 15 units/m^2/dose once weekly for 3 weeks per regimen
Hodgkin's disease: 10 units/m^2/dose on days 1 and 15 of cycle
I.V. continuous infusion: 15-20 units/m^2/day over 24 hours for 3-5 days
Adults: Intracavitary injection for pleural effusion: 15-60 units (dose generally does not exceed 1 unit/kg); drug is diluted with 50-100 mL of NS and is instilled into the pleural cavity via a thoracostomy tube
Dosing adjustment in renal impairment:
Cl_{cr} 25-50 mL/minute: Reduce dose by 25%
Cl_{cr} <25 mL/minute: Reduce dose by 50% to 75%

Administration Parenteral:
I.V.: Administer I.V. slowly over at least 10 minutes (no greater than 1 unit/minute) at a concentration not to exceed 3 units/mL; bleomycin for I.V. continuous infusion can be further diluted in NS (preferred) or D_5W; administration by continuous infusion may produce less severe pulmonary toxicity.
I.M., S.C.: 15 units/mL concentration may be used for I.M., S.C. administration

Monitoring Parameters Pulmonary function tests (total lung volume, forced vital capacity, carbon monoxide diffusion), renal function tests, chest x-ray; vital signs and temperature initially; CBC with differential and platelet count

Patient Information Report any coughing, shortness of breath, or wheezing to physician

Nursing Implications Fever and chills can occur 2-6 hours following parenteral administration; pretreatment with acetaminophen, antihistamine, and hydrocortisone may decrease the severity of fever and chills

Dosage Forms Powder for injection, as sulfate: 15 units (1 unit = 1 mg)

References
Alberts DS, Chen HS, Liu R, et al, "Bleomycin Pharmacokinetics in Man. I. Intravenous Administration," *Cancer Chemother Pharmacol*, 1978, 1(3):177-81.
Berg SL, Grisell DL, Delaney TF, et al, "Principles of Treatment of Pediatric Solid Tumors," *Pediatr Clin North Am*, 1991, 38(2):249-67.

♦ **Botox®** *see* Botulinum Toxin Type A *on page 139*

Botulinum Toxin Type A (BOT yoo lin num TOKS in type aye)
Brand Names Botox®
Synonyms *Clostridium botulinum* Toxin Type A; Oculinum®
Therapeutic Category Muscle Contracture, Treatment; Ophthalmic Agent, Toxin
Generic Available No
Use Treatment of strabismus and blepharospasm associated with dystonia (including benign essential blepharospasm or VII nerve disorders); treatment of dynamic muscle contracture in pediatric cerebral palsy patients (orphan drug)
Pregnancy Risk Factor C
Contraindications Hypersensitivity to botulinum A toxin or any component
Warnings The European formulation of botulinum A toxin (Dysport®) is not equivalent in potency to Botox®; the Dysport®/Botox® equivalency ratio is ~3:1 or 4:1, respectively
Precautions Presence of antibodies to botulinum toxin type A may reduce the effectiveness of therapy; to minimize the development of antibodies, keep the dose of botulinum toxin type A as low as possible; reduced blinking from botulinum toxin type A injection of the orbicularis muscle can lead to corneal exposure, persistent epithelial defect, and corneal ulceration, especially in patients with VII nerve disorders; carefully test corneal sensation in eyes previously operated upon, avoid injection into the lower lid area to avoid ectropion, and vigorously treat any epithelial defect (this may require protective drops, ointment, therapeutic soft contact lenses, or closure of the eye by patching); retrobulbar hemorrhages sufficient to compromise retinal circulation have occurred from needle penetrations into the orbit; have appropriate instruments to decompress the orbit accessible; ocular (globe) penetrations by needles have also occurred (an ophthalmoscope to diagnose this condition should be available)
Adverse Reactions
    Central nervous system: Fever
    Dermatologic: Rash, keratitis
    Local: Pain, bruising at injection site
    Neuromuscular & skeletal: Weakness, temporary loss of function
    Ocular: Dry eyes, lagophthalmos, ptosis, photophobia, vertical deviation, tearing, diplopia, eyelid edema, spatial disorientation, blepharospasm, ectropion, entropion, retrobulbar hemorrhage
Drug Interactions Effects of botulinum toxin may be potentiated by aminoglycoside antibiotics, or any other drug that interferes with neuromuscular transmission
Stability Store lyophilized product in freezer at or below -5°C (23°F); administer within 4 hours after the vial is removed from the freezer and reconstituted; store reconstituted solution in refrigerator (2°C to 8°C/36°F to 46°F)
Mechanism of Action Botulinum A toxin is a neurotoxin produced by *Clostridium botulinum*, a spore-forming anaerobic bacillus; it blocks neuromuscular conduction by binding to receptor sites on motor nerve terminals, entering the nerve terminals and inhibiting the release of acetylcholine. When injected intramuscularly at therapeutic doses, it produces a localized chemical denervation muscle paralysis. When the muscle is chemically denervated, it atrophies and may develop extrajunctional acetylcholine receptors. There is evidence that the nerve can sprout and reinnervate the muscle, with the weakness being reversible. Following several weeks of paralysis, alignment of the eye is measurably changed, despite return of innervation to the injected muscle.
Pharmacodynamics
    Strabismus:
        Onset of action: 1-2 days after injection
        Duration of paralysis: 2-6 weeks
    Blepharospasm:
        Onset of action: 3 days after injection
        Peak effect: 1-2 weeks
        Duration of paralysis: 3 months
    Spasticity associated with cerebral palsy
        Onset of action: Several days
        Duration of paralysis: 3-8 months
Usual Dosage I.M.
    Strabismus:
        Children 2 months to 12 years:
            Horizontal or vertical deviations <20 prism diopters: 1.25 units into any one muscle
(Continued)

Botulinum Toxin Type A *(Continued)*

Horizontal or vertical deviations 20-25 prism diopters: 1-2.5 units into any one muscle

Persistent VI nerve palsy of ≥1 month duration: 1-1.25 units into the medial rectus muscle

Children ≥12 years and Adults:

Horizontal or vertical deviations <20 prism diopters: 1.25-2.5 units into any one muscle

Horizontal or vertical deviations 20-50 prism diopters: 2.5-5 units into any one muscle

Persistent VI nerve palsy of ≥1 month duration: 1.25-2.5 units into the medial rectus muscle

Note: Re-examine patient 7-14 days after each injection to assess effects; dosage may be increased up to twofold of the previously administered dose; do not exceed 25 units as a single injection for any one muscle

Blepharospasm: Adults: Initial: 1.25-2.5 units injected into the medial and lateral pretarsal orbicularis oculi of the upper lid and into the lateral pretarsal orbicularis oculi of the lower lid; dose may be increased up to 2.5-5 units at repeat treatment sessions; do not exceed 5 units per injection or cumulative dose of 200 units in a 30-day period

Spasticity associated with cerebral palsy: Children >18 months to Adolescents: Small muscle: 1-2 units/kg; large muscle: 3-6 units/kg; maximum dose per injection site: 50 units; maximum dose for any one visit: 12 units/kg, up to 400 units; no more than 400 units should be administered during a 3-month period

Administration Parenteral: For I.M. administration only by individuals understanding the relevant neuromuscular and orbital anatomy and any alterations to the anatomy due to prior surgical procedures and standard electromyographic techniques; reconstitute vial with preservative-free NS to obtain an optimal injection volume of 0.1 mL; suggested volumes and concentrations: 1 mL (10 units/0.1 mL); 2 mL (5 units/0.1 mL), 4 mL (2.5 units/0.1 mL) or 8 mL (1.25 units/0.1 mL); gently swirl as botulinum toxin type A is denatured by violent agitation

Patient Information Patients with blepharospasm may have been extremely sedentary for a long time; sedentary patients should be cautioned to resume activity slowly and carefully following injection

Dosage Forms Powder for injection, lyophilized: 100 units

References

Scott AB, Magoon EH, McNeer KW, et al, "Botulinum Treatment of Childhood Strabismus," *Ophthalmology*, 1990, 97(11):1434-8.

Russman BS, Tilton A, and Gormley ME Jr, "Cerebral Palsy: A Rational Approach to a Treatment Protocol, and the Role of Botulinum Toxin in Treatment," *Muscle Nerve Suppl*, 1997, 6:S181-S193.

♦ **Bovine Lung Surfactant** *see* Beractant *on page 128*

♦ **Bovine Lung Surfactant** *see* Calfactant *on page 161*

♦ **Breathe Free® [OTC]** *see* Sodium Chloride *on page 871*

♦ **Breezee® Mist Antifungal [OTC]** *see* Miconazole *on page 641*

♦ **Breonesin® [OTC]** *see* Guaifenesin *on page 464*

♦ **Brethaire®** *see* Terbutaline *on page 903*

♦ **Brethine®** *see* Terbutaline *on page 903*

♦ **Bretylate® (Canada)** *see* Bretylium *on page 140*

Bretylium *(bre TIL ee um)*

Related Information

Adult ACLS Algorithm, Tachycardia *on page 1010*
Adult ACLS Algorithm, V. Fib and Pulseless V. Tach *on page 1004*
CPR Pediatric Drug Dosages *on page 999*
Pediatric ALS Algorithm, Asystole and Pulseless Arrest *on page 1002*

Brand Names Bretylate® (Canada); Bretylol®

Available Salts Bretylium Tosylate

Therapeutic Category Antiarrhythmic Agent, Class III

Generic Available Yes

Use Ventricular tachycardia or ventricular fibrillation; other serious ventricular arrhythmias resistant to lidocaine

Pregnancy Risk Factor C

Contraindications Digitalis intoxication-induced arrhythmias

Precautions Hypotension; patients with fixed cardiac output (severe pulmonary hypertension or aortic stenosis) may experience severe hypotension due to decrease in peripheral resistance without ability to increase cardiac output; reduce dose in renal failure patients

Adverse Reactions
Cardiovascular: Hypotension (incidence 50% to 75%), transient initial hypertension, increase in PVCs, bradycardia, flushing, syncope
Central nervous system: Vertigo, confusion, anxiety, lethargy, hyperthermia
Dermatologic: Rash
Gastrointestinal: Nausea and vomiting with rapid I.V. administration; rarely diarrhea, abdominal pain
Local: Muscle atrophy and necrosis with repeated I.M. injections at same site
Ocular: Conjunctivitis
Renal: Renal impairment
Respiratory: Nasal congestion
Miscellaneous: Hiccups, diaphoresis

Drug Interactions
Other antiarrhythmic agents may potentiate or antagonize cardiac effects, toxic effects may be additive; the pressor effects of catecholamines may be enhanced by bretylium; may potentiate digitalis toxicity; methylphenidate may antagonize effects of bretylium

Mechanism of Action
Class III antiarrhythmic; after an initial release of norepinephrine at the peripheral adrenergic nerve terminals, bretylium inhibits further release by postganglionic nerve endings in response to sympathetic nerve stimulation

Pharmacodynamics
Onset of antiarrhythmic effects:
I.M.: Up to 2 hours
I.V.: Within 6-20 minutes
Maximum effect: Within 6-9 hours

Pharmacokinetics
Protein binding: 1% to 6%
Half-life, adults: 7-11 hours; increases with decreased renal function
Elimination: Unchanged in urine

Usual Dosage
Note: Patients should undergo defibrillation/cardioversion before and after bretylium doses as necessary

Children: (Note: Dose not well established; the following dose has been recommended):
I.M.: 2-5 mg/kg as a single dose
I.V.: 5 mg/kg/dose, may repeat every 10-20 minutes as needed to a total dose of 30 mg/kg
PALS guidelines for treatment of ventricular fibrillation: initial: 5 mg/kg, then attempt electrical defibrillation; repeat with 10 mg/kg and then reattempt electrical defibrillation if ventricular fibrillation persists; may repeat as needed to a total dose of 30 mg/kg
Maintenance dose: I.M., I.V.: 5 mg/kg every 6-8 hours
Adults:
Immediately life-threatening ventricular arrhythmias, ventricular fibrillation, unstable ventricular tachycardia:
Initial dose: I.V.: 5 mg/kg (undiluted) over 1 minute; if arrhythmia persists, give 10 mg/kg (undiluted) over 1 minute and repeat as necessary (usually at 15- to 30-minute intervals) up to a total dose of 30-35 mg/kg
Maintenance dose (for continuous suppression):
I.V. (diluted): 5-10 mg/kg every 6 hours
I.V. continuous infusion (diluted): 1-2 mg/minute (little experience with doses >40 mg/kg/day)
Other ventricular arrhythmias:
Initial dose: I.M., I.V.: 5-10 mg/kg, may repeat every 1-2 hours if arrhythmia persists; give I.V. dose (diluted) over 8-10 minutes
Maintenance dose:
I.M.: 5-10 mg/kg every 6-8 hours
I.V. (diluted): 5-10 mg/kg every 6 hours
I.V. continuous infusion (diluted): 1-2 mg/minute (little experience with doses >40 mg/kg/day)
Dosing interval in renal impairment:
Cl_{cr} 10-50 mL/minute: Administer 25% to 50% of normal dose
Cl_{cr} <10 mL/minute: Administer 25% of normal dose or use alternative agent

Administration
Parenteral:
I.M.: Not recommended for ventricular fibrillation; no more than 5 mL should be injected I.M. per site (adults); rotate injection sites
I.V.:
Life-threatening situations: May administer undiluted I.V. push over <30 seconds
(Continued)

Bretylium *(Continued)*

Nonlife-threatening situations: Dilute to 10 mg/mL and administer slow I.V. push over at least 8 minutes

Monitoring Parameters EKG, heart rate, rhythm, blood pressure

Nursing Implications Avoid extravasation

Additional Information Change patient to oral antiarrhythmic agent as soon as possible (when indicated) for maintenance therapy

Dosage Forms

Injection, as tosylate: 50 mg/mL (10 mL, 20 mL)

Injection, as tosylate, premixed in D$_5$W: 1 mg/mL (500 mL); 2 mg/mL (250 mL); 4 mg/mL (250 mL, 500 mL)

References

Emergency Cardiac Care Committee and Subcommittees, American Heart Association, "Guidelines for Cardiopulmonary Resuscitation and Emergency Cardiac Care, III: Adult Advanced Cardiac Life Support" and "VI: Pediatric Advanced Life Support," *JAMA*, 1992, 268(16):2199-241 and 2262-75.

♦ **Bretylium Tosylate** *see Bretylium on page 140*

♦ **Bretylol®** *see Bretylium on page 140*

♦ **Brevibloc®** *see Esmolol on page 384*

♦ **Brevital® Sodium** *see Methohexital on page 620*

♦ **Brevoxyl® Gel** *see Benzoyl Peroxide on page 126*

♦ **Bricanyl®** *see Terbutaline on page 903*

♦ **Brietal Sodium® (Canada)** *see Methohexital on page 620*

♦ **Bromaline® Elixir [OTC]** *see Brompheniramine and Phenylpropanolamine on page 143*

♦ **Bromanate® Elixir [OTC]** *see Brompheniramine and Phenylpropanolamine on page 143*

♦ **Bromarest® [OTC]** *see Brompheniramine on page 142*

♦ **Bromatapp® [OTC]** *see Brompheniramine and Phenylpropanolamine on page 143*

♦ **Brombay® [OTC]** *see Brompheniramine on page 142*

♦ **Bromphen® Elixir [OTC]** *see Brompheniramine on page 142*

Brompheniramine *(brome fen IR a meen)*

Related Information

OTC Cough & Cold Preparations, Pediatric *on page 1037*

Overdose and Toxicology *on page 1191*

Brand Names Bromarest® [OTC]; Brombay® [OTC]; Bromphen® Elixir [OTC]; Brotane® [OTC]; Chlorphed® [OTC]; Cophene-B®; Diamine T.D.® Oral [OTC]; Dimetane® Extentabs [OTC]; Nasahist B®; ND-Stat®; Oraminic® II; Sinusol-B®; Veltane® Tablet

Available Salts Brompheniramine Maleate

Synonyms Parabromdylamine

Therapeutic Category Antihistamine

Generic Available Yes

Use Perennial and seasonal allergic rhinitis and other allergic symptoms including urticaria

Pregnancy Risk Factor C

Contraindications Hypersensitivity to brompheniramine or any component; narrow-angle glaucoma, bladder neck obstruction, symptomatic prostatic hypertrophy, stenosing peptic ulcer, and pyloroduodenal obstruction

Precautions Use with caution in patients with asthma, heart disease, hypertension, and thyroid disease

Adverse Reactions

Cardiovascular: Palpitations

Central nervous system: Paradoxical excitability, drowsiness, dizziness, headache, fever, nervousness, depression

Dermatologic: Rash, photosensitivity, angioedema

Gastrointestinal: Nausea, anorexia, xerostomia, appetite increase, weight gain, diarrhea, abdominal pain

Hepatic: Hepatitis

Neuromuscular & skeletal: Myalgia, paresthesia

Respiratory: Bronchospasm, epistaxis, thickening of bronchial secretions

Drug Interactions May cause additive sedation with other CNS depressants; may cause additive anticholinergic effects with other anticholinergic agents; MAO inhibitors

Stability Solutions may crystallize if stored below 0°C, crystals will dissolve when warmed

Mechanism of Action Competes with histamine for H_1-receptor sites on effector cells in the gastrointestinal tract, blood vessels, and respiratory tract

Pharmacodynamics
Peak effect: Maximal clinical effects seen within 3-9 hours
Duration: Varies with formulation

Pharmacokinetics
Metabolism: Extensive by the liver
Half-life: 12-34 hours
Time to peak serum concentration: Oral: Within 2-5 hours
Elimination: In urine as inactive metabolites

Usual Dosage
Oral:
Children:
<6 years: 0.125 mg/kg/dose given every 6 hours; maximum dose: 6-8 mg/day
6-12 years: 2-4 mg every 6-8 hours; maximum dose: 12-16 mg/day
Adults: 4-8 mg every 4-6 hours or 8 mg of sustained release form every 8-12 hours or 12 mg of sustained release form every 12 hours; maximum dose: 24 mg/day
I.M., I.V., S.C.:
Children <12 years: 0.5 mg/kg/day or 15 mg/m²/day divided every 6-8 hours
Children ≥12 years and Adults: 10 mg (range: 5-20 mg) every 6-12 hours; maximum dose: 40 mg/day

Administration
Oral: Administer with food or milk; sustained release tablets should be swallowed whole; do not crush or chew
Parenteral: Dilute in 1-10 mL D_5W or NS and infuse over several minutes; the patient should be in a recumbent position during the infusion

Patient Information Causes drowsiness and may impair ability to perform hazardous activities requiring mental alertness or physical coordination

Dosage Forms
Elixir, as maleate: 2 mg/5 mL with 3% alcohol (120 mL, 480 mL, 4000 mL)
Injection, as maleate: 10 mg/mL (10 mL)
Tablet, as maleate: 4 mg, 8 mg, 12 mg
Tablet, sustained release, as maleate: 8 mg, 12 mg

Brompheniramine and Phenylpropanolamine
(brome fen IR a meen & fen il proe pa NOLE a meen)

Related Information
OTC Cough & Cold Preparations, Pediatric *on page 1037*

Brand Names Bromaline® Elixir [OTC]; Bromanate® Elixir [OTC]; Bromatapp® [OTC]; Bromphen® Tablet [OTC]; Cold & Allergy® Elixir [OTC]; DayQuil® Allergy Relief 4 Hour Tablet [OTC]; Dimaphen®; Dimaphen® Elixir [OTC]; Dimetane® Extentabs® [OTC]; Dimetapp® 4 hour Liqui-Gel [OTC]; Dimetapp® Elixir [OTC]; Dimetapp® Tablets [OTC]; Genatap® Elixir [OTC]; Myphetapp® [OTC]; Tamine® [OTC]; Vick's®

Available Salts Brompheniramine Maleate and Phenylpropanolamine Hydrochloride

Synonyms Phenylpropanolamine and Brompheniramine

Therapeutic Category Antihistamine/Decongestant Combination; Decongestant

Generic Available Yes

Use Temporary relief of nasal congestion, running nose, sneezing, and itchy, watery eyes

Pregnancy Risk Factor C

Contraindications Hypersensitivity to brompheniramine, phenylpropanolamine, or any component

Precautions Use with caution in patients with high blood pressure, heart disease, diabetes, thyroid disease, asthma, glaucoma

Adverse Reactions
Cardiovascular: Palpitations
Central nervous system: Excitability, drowsiness, dizziness, headache, fever, depression, fatigue, nervousness
Dermatologic: Rash, photosensitivity, angioedema
Gastrointestinal: Anorexia, nausea, xerostomia, appetite increase, weight gain, diarrhea, abdominal pain
Hematologic: Leukopenia
Hepatic: Hepatitis
Neuromuscular & skeletal: Myalgia, paresthesia, arthralgia
Respiratory: Thickening of bronchial secretions, bronchospasm, epistaxis
(Continued)

Brompheniramine and Phenylpropanolamine *(Continued)*

Drug Interactions May cause additive sedation with other CNS depressants; may cause additive anticholinergic effects with other anticholinergic agents; may inhibit hypotensive effects of propranolol; may cause severe hypertensive reactions in patients receiving MAO inhibitors; hypertension may occur when used with indomethacin or other prostaglandin inhibitor

Usual Dosage Oral:

Children:

1-6 months: 1.25 mL 3-4 times/day

7-24 months: 2.5 mL 3-4 times/day

2-4 years: 3.75 mL 3-4 times/day

4-12 years: 5 mL 3-4 times/day

Adults: 5-10 mL 3-4 times/day or 1 tablet twice daily

Administration Oral: Swallow timed-release tablets whole; do not crush or chew; administer with food

Patient Information Causes drowsiness and may impair ability to perform hazardous activities requiring mental alertness or physical coordination

Dosage Forms

Capsule: Brompheniramine maleate 4 mg and phenylpropanolamine hydrochloride 25 mg

Elixir (grape flavor): Brompheniramine maleate 2 mg and phenylpropanolamine hydrochloride 12.5 mg per 5 mL with alcohol 2.3% (5 mL, 120 mL, 240 mL, 480 mL, 3780 mL)

Tablet: Brompheniramine maleate 4 mg and phenylpropanolamine hydrochloride 25 mg

Tablet, sustained release: Brompheniramine maleate 12 mg and phenylpropanolamine hydrochloride 75 mg

- ♦ **Brompheniramine Maleate** *see* Brompheniramine *on page 142*
- ♦ **Brompheniramine Maleate and Phenylpropanolamine Hydrochloride** *see* Brompheniramine and Phenylpropanolamine *on page 143*
- ♦ **Bromphen® Tablet [OTC]** *see* Brompheniramine and Phenylpropanolamine *on page 143*
- ♦ **Bronalide® (Canada)** *see* Flunisolide *on page 423*
- ♦ **Bronitin® Mist [OTC]** *see* Epinephrine *on page 371*
- ♦ **Bronkaid® Mist [OTC]** *see* Epinephrine *on page 371*
- ♦ **Bronkodyl®** *see* Theophylline *on page 910*
- ♦ **Bronkosol® Inhalation Solution** *see* Isoetharine *on page 533*
- ♦ **Brontex®** *see* Guaifenesin and Codeine *on page 465*
- ♦ **Brotane® [OTC]** *see* Brompheniramine *on page 142*
- ♦ **BSS** *see* Bismuth *on page 134*

Budesonide *(byoo DES oh nide)*

Related Information

Asthma Guidelines *on page 1178*

Estimated Comparative Daily Dosages for Inhaled Corticosteroids *on page 1185*

Brand Names Entocort® (Canada); Pulmicort®, -Nebuamp®, -Turbuhaler® (Canada); Pulmicort® Turbuhaler®; Rhinocort®; Rhinocort® Aqua™; Rhinocort® Turbuhaler® (Canada)

Therapeutic Category Adrenal Corticosteroid; Antiasthmatic; Anti-inflammatory Agent; Corticosteroid, Inhalant (Oral); Corticosteroid, Intranasal; Glucocorticoid

Generic Available No

Use

Oral inhalation: Long-term (chronic) control of persistent bronchial asthma; **NOT** indicated for the relief of acute bronchospasm; also indicated in bronchial asthma patients requiring oral corticosteroids (inhalation may decrease or eliminate need for oral steroids over time)

Intranasal:

Children and Adults: Management of seasonal or perennial allergic rhinitis

Adults: Nonallergic perennial rhinitis

Pregnancy Risk Factor C

Contraindications Hypersensitivity to budesonide or any component; primary treatment of status asthmaticus

Warnings Fatalities have occurred due to adrenal insufficiency in asthmatic patients during and after switching from systemic corticosteroids to aerosol steroids; several months may be required for full recovery of the adrenal glands; during this period, aerosol steroids do **not** provide the systemic corticosteroid needed to treat patients requiring stress doses (ie, patients with major stress such as trauma, surgery, or infections); when used at high doses, hypothalamic-pituitary-adrenal (HPA) suppression may occur; use with inhaled or systemic corticosteroids (even alternate-day dosing) may increase risk of HPA suppression; withdrawal and discontinuation of corticosteroids should be done carefully; immunosuppression may occur

Precautions Avoid using higher than recommended dosages; suppression of HPA function, suppression of linear growth, or hypercorticism (Cushing's syndrome) may occur

Adverse Reactions

Cardiovascular: Facial edema

Central nervous system: Nervousness, migraine, insomnia

Dermatologic: Rash, pruritus, contact dermatitis

Endocrine & metabolic: Potential adrenal suppression

Gastrointestinal: Xerostomia, dysgeusia, GI irritation, nausea, weight gain, abdominal pain, vomiting

Local: Nasal irritation, burning, or ulceration; pharyngitis; growth of *Candida* in the mouth, throat, or nares

Neuromuscular & skeletal: Potential growth suppression, fracture, myalgia, arthralgia

Respiratory: Cough, epistaxis, wheezing, decreased sense of smell, hoarseness, respiratory infection, rhinitis, sinusitis

Drug Interactions Cytochrome P-450 isoenzyme CYP3A substrate

Interactions similar to other corticosteroids may potentially occur

Stability

Intranasal inhaler: Use within 6 months after opening; avoid storage in high humidity; do not store or use by heat or open flame

Oral inhaler: Keep clean and dry; store at controlled room temperature 68°F to 77°F

Mechanism of Action Controls the rate of protein synthesis, depresses the migration of polymorphonuclear leukocytes and fibroblasts, reverses capillary permeability, and stabilizes lysosomal membranes at the cellular level to prevent or control inflammation

Pharmacodynamics Clinical effects are due to direct local effect, rather than systemic absorption

Onset of action: Within 24 hours

Maximum effect:

Intranasal: Inhaler: 3-7 days; spray: 2 weeks

Oral inhalation: 1-2 weeks or more

Duration after discontinuation: Intranasal: Several days

Pharmacokinetics

Absorption:

Intranasal:

Inhaler: 20% of dose delivered reaches systemic circulation

Spray: 34% of dose delivered reaches systemic circulation

Oral inhalation: 39% of the metered dose is systemically available

Distribution: Adults: ~200 L or 2-3 L/kg

Protein binding: 85% to 90%

Metabolism: Extensively metabolized by the liver

Bioavailability: Oral: ~10% (large first pass effect)

Half-life:

Children 10-14 years: 1.5 hours

Adults: 2-3 hours

Elimination: 60% to 66% of dose renally excreted as metabolites; 0% unchanged drug found in urine

Usual Dosage

Intranasal: Children ≥6 years and Adults:

Rhinocort®: Initial: 8 sprays (4 sprays/nostril) per day (256 mcg/day), given as either 2 sprays in each nostril in the morning and evening or as 4 sprays in each nostril in the morning; after symptoms decrease (usually by 3-7 days), reduce dose slowly every 2-4 weeks to the smallest effective dose

Rhinocort® Aqua™ (32 mcg/spray): Initial: 2 sprays (1 spray/nostril) once daily (64 mcg/day); dose may be increased if needed

Maximum dose:

Children <12 years: 4 sprays (2 sprays/nostril) once daily (128 mcg/day)

Children ≥12 years and Adults: 8 sprays (4 sprays/nostril) once daily (256 mcg/day)

(Continued)

Budesonide *(Continued)*

Oral inhalation: **Note:** Doses should be titrated to the lowest effective dose once asthma is controlled; Manufacturer's recommendations:

Children ≥6 years:

Previously treated with bronchodilators alone or with inhaled corticosteroids: Initial 200 mcg (1 puff) twice daily; maximum dose: 400 mcg (2 puffs) twice daily

Treated with oral corticosteroids: 400 mcg (2 puffs) twice daily (maximum dose)

Adults:

Previously treated with bronchodilators alone: Initial: 200-400 mcg (1-2 puffs) twice daily; maximum dose: 400 mcg (2 puffs) twice daily

Treated with inhaled corticosteroids: 200-400 mcg (1-2 puffs) twice daily; maximum dose: 800 mcg (4 puffs) twice daily

Treated with oral corticosteroids: Initial: 400-800 mcg (2-4 puffs) twice daily; maximum dose: 800 mcg (4 puffs) twice daily

NIH Guidelines (NIH, 1997) [give in divided doses twice daily]:

Children:

"Low" dose: 100-200 mcg/day

"Medium" dose: 200-400 mcg/day (1-2 inhalations/day)

"High" dose: >400 mcg/day (>2 inhalation/day)

Adults:

"Low" dose: 200-400 mcg/day (1-2 inhalations/day)

"Medium" dose: 400-600 mcg/day (2-3 inhalations/day)

"High" dose: >600 mcg/day (>3 inhalation/day)

Administration

Intranasal inhaler and intranasal spray: Clear nasal passage by blowing nose prior to use

Intranasal inhaler: Shake well before each use

Intranasal spray: Shake gently before use

Oral inhaler: Do **not** shake inhaler; do not use inhaler with a spacer

Monitoring Parameters Check mucous membranes for signs of fungal infection

Patient Information Notify physician if condition being treated persists or worsens; do not decrease dose or discontinue without physician approval

Oral inhaler: Rinse mouth after inhalation, with water and without swallowing, to decrease chance of oral candidiasis; report sore mouth or mouth lesions to physician; a red mark will appear on the indicator window of the Pulmicort Turbuhaler® when 20 doses are left

Additional Information Budesonide oral inhalation is also used to help reduce or discontinue oral corticosteroid therapy for asthma; if bronchospasm with wheezing occurs after use of oral inhaler, a fast-acting bronchodilator may be used; Pulmicort Turbuhaler® delivers budesonide as a fine powder

Dosage Forms

Oral inhaler (Pulmicort Turbuhaler®): 200 mcg per metered dose [200 doses]

Nasal inhaler (Rhinocort®): 50 mcg released per actuation to deliver ~32 mcg to patient via nasal adapter [200 metered doses] (7 g)

Nasal spray (Rhinocort® Aqua™): 32 mcg per spray [60 metered sprays]

References

Expert Panel Report 2, "Guidelines for the Diagnosis and Management of Asthma," *Clinical Practice Guidelines*, National Institutes of Health, National Heart, Lung, and Blood Institute, NIH Publication No. 94-4051, April, 1997.

♦ **Bufferin® [OTC]** *see* Aspirin *on page 99*

Bumetanide *(byoo MET a nide)*

Brand Names Bumex®; Burinex® (Canada)

Therapeutic Category Antihypertensive Agent; Diuretic, Loop

Generic Available Yes

Use Management of edema secondary to CHF or hepatic or renal disease including nephrotic syndrome; may also be used alone or in combination with antihypertensives in the treatment of hypertension

Pregnancy Risk Factor C (per manufacturer); D (based on expert analysis)

Contraindications Hypersensitivity to bumetanide or any component; in anuria or increasing azotemia

Warnings Loop diuretics are potent diuretics; excess amounts can lead to profound diuresis with fluid and electrolyte loss; close medical supervision and dose evaluation is required; *in vitro* studies using pooled sera from critically ill neonates have shown bumetanide to be a potent displacer of bilirubin; avoid use in neonates at risk for kernicterus; increased risk of ototoxicity with rapid I.V. administration, renal impairment, excessive doses, and concurrent use of other ototoxins

Precautions Use with caution in patients with cirrhosis; allergy to sulfonamides may result in cross hypersensitivity to bumetanide

Adverse Reactions
Cardiovascular: Hypotension, chest pain
Central nervous system: Dizziness, headache, encephalopathy, vertigo
Dermatologic: Rash, pruritus
Endocrine & metabolic: Hyperglycemia, hypokalemia, hypochloremia, hyponatremia
Gastrointestinal: Cramps, nausea, vomiting, diarrhea, abdominal pain
Hepatic: Elevated liver enzymes
Neuromuscular & skeletal: Weakness, muscle cramps, arthritic pain
Otic: Ototoxicity (with rapid I.V. administration)
Renal: Decreased uric acid excretion, elevated serum creatinine

Drug Interactions Decreased blood pressure when used with other antihypertensive agents and ACE inhibitors (may need to decrease dose of one or both agents); indomethacin and probenecid may decrease bumetanide's effect; decreased lithium excretion; ototoxic drugs (aminoglycoside antibiotics, cisplatin); cholestyramine may decrease absorption

Stability Light sensitive, may discolor when exposed to light

Mechanism of Action Inhibits reabsorption of sodium and chloride in the ascending loop of Henle and proximal renal tubule, interfering with the chloride-binding cotransport system, thus causing increased excretion of water, sodium, chloride, magnesium, calcium, and phosphate

Pharmacodynamics
Onset of clinical effects:
Oral, I.M.: Within 30-60 minutes
I.V.: Within a few minutes
Peak effects:
Oral, I.M.: 1-2 hours
I.V.: 15-30 minutes
Duration:
Oral: 4-6 hours
I.V.: 2-3 hours

Pharmacokinetics
Protein binding: 95%
Newborns: 97%
Metabolism: Partial metabolism occurs in the liver
Bioavailability: 72% to 96%
Half-life:
Infants <2 months: 2.5 hours
Infants 2-6 months: 1.5 hours
Adults: 1-1.5 hours
Elimination: Unchanged drug excreted in urine (50%)
Time to peak serum concentration: 0.5-2 hours

Usual Dosage
Oral, I.M., I.V.:
Neonates (see Warnings): 0.01-0.05 mg/kg/dose every 24-48 hours
Infants and Children: 0.015-0.1 mg/kg/dose every 6-24 hours (maximum dose: 10 mg/day)
Adults:
Edema:
Oral: 0.5-2 mg/dose (maximum dose: 10 mg/day) 1-2 times/day
I.M., I.V.: 0.5-1 mg/dose; may repeat in 2-3 hours for up to 2 doses if needed (maximum dose: 10 mg/day)
Continuous I.V. infusion: 0.9-1 mg/hour
Hypertension: Oral: 0.5 mg daily (range: 1-4 mg/day, maximum dose: 5 mg/day); for larger doses, divide into 2-3 doses daily

Administration
Oral: Administer with food to decrease GI irritation
Parenteral: Administer without additional dilution by direct I.V. injection over 1-2 minutes; for continuous infusion, dilute in D_5W, NS, or LR; stability and maximum dilution in I.V. fluid has not been determined

Monitoring Parameters Blood pressure, serum electrolytes, renal function, urine output
(Continued)

Bumetanide *(Continued)*

Additional Information Patients with impaired hepatic function must be monitored carefully, often requiring reduced doses; larger doses may be necessary in patients with impaired renal function to obtain the same therapeutic response

Dosage Forms
Injection: 0.25 mg/mL (2 mL, 4 mL, 10 mL)
Tablet: 0.5 mg, 1 mg, 2 mg

References
Wells TG, "The Pharmacology and Therapeutics of Diuretics in the Pediatric Patient," *Pediatr Clin North Am*, 1990, 37(2):463-504.

♦ **Bumex®** *see* Bumetanide *on page 146*
♦ **Buminate®** *see* Albumin *on page 39*
♦ **Buphenyl®** *see* Sodium Phenylbutyrate *on page 873*

Bupivacaine *(byoo PIV a kane)*

Brand Names Marcaine®; Sensorcaine®; Sensorcaine-MPF®
Available Salts Bupivacaine Hydrochloride
Therapeutic Category Local Anesthetic, Injectable
Generic Available Yes
Use Local anesthetic (injectable) for peripheral nerve block, infiltration, sympathetic block, caudal or epidural block, retrobulbar block
Pregnancy Risk Factor C
Contraindications Hypersensitivity to bupivacaine hydrochloride or any component, PABA or parabens; not recommended for I.V. regional anesthesia (Bier block)
Warnings Convulsions due to systemic toxicity leading to cardiac arrest have been reported, presumably following unintentional intravascular injection; some commercially available formulations contain sodium metabisulfite, which may cause allergic-type reactions; **do not use solutions containing preservatives for caudal or epidural block**
Precautions Use with caution in patients with liver disease
Adverse Reactions
Cardiovascular: Cardiac arrest, hypotension, bradycardia, palpitations
Central nervous system: Headache, restlessness, anxiety, dizziness, seizures
Dermatologic: Pruritus, angioneurotic edema
Gastrointestinal: Nausea, vomiting
Neuromuscular & skeletal: Weakness
Ocular: Blurred vision
Otic: Tinnitus
Respiratory: Apnea, sneezing
Mechanism of Action Blocks both the initiation and conduction of nerve impulses by decreasing the neuronal membrane's permeability to sodium ions, which results in inhibition of depolarization with resultant blockade of conduction
Pharmacodynamics
Onset of anesthetic action: Dependent on route administered, but generally occurs within 4-10 minutes
Duration: 1.5-8.5 hours (depending upon route of administration)
Pharmacokinetics
Protein binding: 84% to 95%
Metabolism: In the liver
Half-life (age-dependent):
Neonates: 8.1 hours
Adults: 1.5-5.5 hours
Elimination: Small amounts (~6%) excreted in urine unchanged
Usual Dosage Dose varies with procedure, depth of anesthesia, vascularity of tissues, duration of anesthesia and condition of patient

Caudal block (with or without epinephrine):
Children: 1-3.7 mg/kg
Adults: 15-30 mL of 0.25% or 0.5%
Epidural block (other than caudal block):
Children: 1.25 mg/kg/dose
Adults: 10-20 mL of 0.25%, 0.5%, or 0.75%
Peripheral nerve block: 5 mL dose of 0.25% or 0.5% (12.5-25 mg); maximum dose: 400 mg/day
Sympathetic nerve block: 20-50 mL of 0.25% (no epinephrine) solution
Administration Solutions containing preservatives should not be used for epidural or caudal blocks

Additional Information Metabisulfites (in epinephrine-containing injection)
Dosage Forms
Injection, as hydrochloride:
Preservative free: 0.25% [2.5 mg/mL]; 0.5% [5 mg/mL]; 0.75% [7.5 mg/mL]
With preservative: 0.25% [2.5 mg/mL]; 0.5% [5 mg/mL]
Injection, as hydrochloride with epinephrine [1:200,000] injection:
Preservative free: 0.25% [2.5 mg/mL]; 0.5% [5 mg/mL]; 0.75% [7.5 mg/mL]
With preservative: 0.25% [2.5 mg/mL]; 0.5% [5 mg/mL]
Injection (spinal), as hydrochloride in dextrose [8.25%]: Preservative free: 0.75%
[7.5 mg/mL]

♦ **Bupivacaine Hydrochloride** *see* Bupivacaine *on page 148*
♦ **Burinex® (Canada)** *see* Bumetanide *on page 146*
♦ **Burow's Solution** *see* Aluminum Acetate *on page 53*
♦ **BuSpar®** *see* Buspirone *on page 149*

Buspirone (byoo SPYE rone)

Related Information
Serotonin Syndrome *on page 1217*
Brand Names BuSpar®
Available Salts Buspirone Hydrochloride
Therapeutic Category Antianxiety Agent
Generic Available No
Use Management of anxiety
Pregnancy Risk Factor B
Contraindications Hypersensitivity to buspirone or any component
Warnings Do not use concurrently with MAO inhibitors or within 10 days of MAO
inhibitors as significant increases in blood pressure may occur
Precautions Use with caution in patients with hepatic or renal dysfunction; use in
severe hepatic or renal impairment is not recommended; buspirone does not
prevent or treat withdrawal from benzodiazepines or sedative/hypnotic drugs
Adverse Reactions
Cardiovascular: Chest pain, tachycardia
Central nervous system: Dizziness, lightheadedness, headache, fatigue, restless-
ness, confusion, insomnia, nightmares, sedation (about $\frac{1}{3}$ of that with benzodi-
azepines), disorientation, excitement, fever, drowsiness (more common with ≥20
mg/day), akathisia; possible psychotic deterioration has been reported (two pedi-
atric cases, see Soni, 1992)
Dermatologic: Rash, urticaria
Gastrointestinal: Nausea, vomiting, diarrhea, flatulence, xerostomia
Hematologic: Rare: Leukopenia, eosinophilia, thrombocytopenia
Neuromuscular & skeletal: Muscle weakness, numbness
Ocular: Blurred vision
Otic: Tinnitus
Drug Interactions Cytochrome P-450 isoenzyme CYP3A4 substrate
Use with MAO inhibitors may cause significant increases in blood pressure; alcohol
or other CNS depressants may increase CNS adverse effects; buspirone may
increase haloperidol levels; buspirone may displace digoxin from serum proteins;
fluoxetine; use with warfarin may increase PT; erythromycin, itraconazole, and
nefazodone increase buspirone plasma concentrations (the dose of buspirone
should be reduced); when used with diazepam, buspirone may increase
nordiazepam serum concentrations; aspirin may increase and flurazepam may
decrease free (unbound) buspirone concentrations
Food Interactions Food may delay oral absorption, decrease the first-pass metabolism effect and increase oral bioavailability
Stability Protect from light; store at room temperature
Mechanism of Action Decreases the spontaneous firing of serotonin-containing
neurons in the CNS by selectively binding to and acting as agonist at presynaptic
CNS serotonin 5-HT$_1$A receptors; possesses partial agonist activity (mixed agonist/
antagonist) at postsynaptic 5-HT$_2$A receptors; does not bind to benzodiazepine-
GABA receptors; binds to dopamine$_2$ receptors; may have other effects on other
neurotransmitter systems; buspirone is "anxiolytic-select" and does not possess
the anticonvulsant, muscle relaxant, or sedative effects of the benzodiazepines;
little potential for abuse, tolerance, or withdrawal reactions
Pharmacodynamics
Onset of effect: Within 2 weeks
Time to maximum effect: 3-4 weeks, up to 4-6 weeks
(Continued)

Buspirone *(Continued)*

Pharmacokinetics

Absorption: Rapid and complete, but bioavailability is limited by extensive first-pass effect; only 1.5% to 13% (mean 4%) of the oral dose reaches the systemic circulation unchanged

Protein binding: 86%

Metabolism: In the liver by oxidation (by cytochrome P-450 isoenzyme CYP3A4) to several metabolites including 1-pyrimidinyl piperazine (about 1/4 as active as buspirone)

Half-life: Adults: Mean: 2-3 hours; increased with renal or liver dysfunction

Elimination: 29% to 63% excreted in urine (primarily as metabolites)

Usual Dosage Oral:

Children and Adolescents: Anxiety disorders: Limited information is available from pediatric case studies and open-labeled trials; dose is not well established; one pilot study of 15 children, 6-14 years of age (mean 10 years), with mixed anxiety disorders, used initial doses of 5 mg daily; doses were individualized with increases in increments of 5 mg/day every week as needed to a maximum dose of 20 mg/day divided into 2 doses; the mean dose required = 18.6 mg/day; some authors (Carrey, 1996 and Kutcher, 1992), based on their clinical experience, recommend higher doses

Adults: Initial: 7.5 mg twice daily; increase in increments of 5 mg/day every 2-3 days as needed to a maximum of 60 mg/day; usual dose: 20-30 mg/day in 2 or 3 divided doses

Dosing adjustment in renal impairment:

Mild to moderate renal dysfunction: Dose reductions not required

Patients with anuria: Reduce dose by 25% to 50%; further studies are needed

Administration Oral: May be administered without regard to food

Monitoring Parameters Mental status, signs and symptoms of anxiety, liver and renal function

Patient Information Avoid alcohol; may cause drowsiness and impair the ability to perform tasks which require mental alertness or physical coordination

Additional Information Not appropriate for "as needed" (prn) use or for brief, situational anxiety; buspirone is equipotent to diazepam on a milligram to milligram basis in the treatment of anxiety; however, unlike diazepam, the onset of buspirone is delayed (see Pharmacodynamics)

Dosage Forms Tablet, as hydrochloride: 5 mg, 10 mg, 15 mg, 30 mg

References

Carrey NJ, Wiggins DM, and Milin RP, "Pharmacological Treatment of Psychiatric Disorders in Children and Adolescents," *Drugs*, 1996, 51(5):750-9.

Hanna GL, Feibusch EL, and Albright KJ, "Buspirone Treatment of Anxiety, Associated With Pharyngeal Dysphagia in a Four-Year Old," *J Child Adolesc Psychopharmacol*, 1997, 7(2):137-43.

Kivisto KT, Lamberg TS, and Kantola T, "Plasma Buspirone Concentrations Are Greatly Increased by Erythromycin and Itraconazole," *Clin Pharmacol Ther*, 1997, 62(3):348-54.

Kutcher SP, Reiter S, Gardner DM, et al, "The Pharmacotherapy of Anxiety Disorders in Children and Adolescents," *Psychiatr Clin North Am*, 1992, 15(1):41-67.

Simeon JG, Knott VJ, DuBois C, et al, "Buspirone Therapy of Mixed Anxiety Disorders in Childhood and Adolescence: A Pilot Study," *J Child Adolesc Psychopharmacol*, 1994, 4(3):159-70.

Soni P and Weintraub AL, "Buspirone-Associated Mental Status Changes," *J Am Acad Child Adolesc Psychiatry*, 1992, 31(6):1098-9.

♦ **Buspirone Hydrochloride** *see* Buspirone *on page 149*

Busulfan *(byoo SUL fan)*

Related Information

Emetogenic Potential of Single Chemotherapeutic Agents *on page 1095*

Brand Names Busulfex®; Myleran®

Therapeutic Category Antineoplastic Agent, Alkylating Agent

Generic Available No

Use Chronic myelogenous leukemia (CML); component of marrow-ablative conditioning regimen prior to bone marrow transplantation (BMT) for refractory leukemias, lymphomas, and pediatric solid tumors

Pregnancy Risk Factor D

Contraindications Hypersensitivity to busulfan or any component; failure to respond to previous courses; should not be used in pregnancy or lactation

Warnings The FDA currently recommends that procedures for proper handling and disposal of antineoplastic agents be considered; discontinue busulfan if lung toxicity develops; busulfan is potentially carcinogenic; malignant tumors and acute leukemias have been reported in patients who received busulfan; busulfan is associated with ovarian failure including failure to achieve puberty in females

Precautions May induce severe bone marrow hypoplasia; reduce dosage in patients with bone marrow suppression; use with extreme caution in patients who have recently received other myelosuppressive drugs or radiation therapy; use with caution in patients with a history of seizure disorder, head trauma, or when receiving other epileptogenic drugs

Adverse Reactions
Central nervous system: Dizziness, seizures
Dermatologic: Hyperpigmentation, alopecia, rash, urticaria
Endocrine & metabolic: Addisonian-like syndrome (hyperpigmentation, wasting, hypotension), hyperuricemia, gynecomastia, testicular atrophy, amenorrhea, sterility
Gastrointestinal: Nausea, vomiting, mucositis, diarrhea
Genitourinary: Hemorrhagic cystitis
Hematologic: Myelosuppression with nadirs of 14-21 days for leukopenia and thrombocytopenia; anemia, aplastic anemia
Hepatic: Hepatic impairment, hepatic veno-occlusive disease, hyperbilirubinemia
Ocular: Blurred vision, subcapsular cataracts, corneal thinning
Respiratory: Pulmonary fibrosis

Drug Interactions Thioguanine (may increase hepatotoxicity); itraconazole (may increase busulfan toxicity); phenytoin lowers busulfan plasma AUC by 15%

Food Interactions No clear or firm data on the effect of food on busulfan bioavailability

Stability Store intact ampuls in the refrigerator; diluted busulfan solution is stable for up to 8 hours at room temperature; infusion must be completed within that 8 hour time frame. If diluted in NS, the solution is stable for 12 hours if refrigerated, but the infusion must be completed within that 12-hour time frame.

Mechanism of Action Interferes with the normal function of DNA by alkylation of intracellular nucleophiles and cross-linking the strands of DNA

Pharmacokinetics
Absorption: Oral: 70% absorbed
Distribution: Crosses into CSF, saliva, placenta, and liver
Protein binding: 32% to 55%
Metabolism: Extensive in the liver
Half-life:
Children: 2.5 hours
Adults: 2.3-2.6 hours
Time to peak plasma concentration: Oral: Within 1-2 hours
Elimination: 10% to 50% excreted in urine as metabolites, 1% excreted unchanged in urine within 24 hours; total plasma clearance rate is 2-4 times higher in children than in adults

Usual Dosage Refer to individual protocols; dose should be based on ideal body weight:
Children: Oral:
Remission induction of CML: 0.06-0.12 mg/kg once daily **or** 1.8-4.6 mg/m^2/day once daily; titrate dose to maintain a leukocyte count >40,000/mm^3; discontinue busulfan if counts fall to ≤20,000/mm^3
BMT marrow-ablative conditioning regimen: 1 mg/kg/dose every 6 hours for 16 doses
Children ≤6 years of age in the hematopoietic stem cell transplant program may receive 40 mg/m^2/dose every 6 hours for 16 doses
Adults:
Oral:
Remission induction of CML: 4-8 mg/day or 0.06 mg/kg/day
Maintenance dose: Controversial; range is from 1-4 mg/day to 2 mg/week; reduce dose in proportion to the decrease in leukocyte count or discontinue busulfan when the leukocyte count falls to ≤20,000/mm^3
I.V.: High-dose BMT conditioning regimen: 0.8 mg/kg/dose every 6 hours for 16 doses ending on day 3 before transplantation

Administration
Oral: May be administered without regard to meals
Parenteral: Dilute busulfan injection with either NS or D$_5$W to a final concentration of ≥0.5 mg/mL (diluent volume should be 10 times the volume of busulfan injection); infuse over 2 hours through a central venous catheter; flush line before and after each infusion with D$_5$W or NS

Monitoring Parameters CBC with differential and platelet count, hemoglobin, liver function tests, bilirubin, alkaline phosphatase

Patient Information Report any difficulty in breathing, cough, fever, sore throat, bleeding or bruising to physician
(Continued)

Busulfan *(Continued)*

Additional Information One method used to prevent seizures during high-dose busulfan (16 mg/kg over 4 days) is to initiate a standard loading dose of phenytoin (15 mg/kg) 1 day prior to starting busulfan therapy followed by a maintenance dose adjusted to maintain a therapeutic phenytoin concentration until 24 hours after the final busulfan dose

Dosage Forms

Injection: 6 mg/mL (10 mL ampul)

Tablet, scored: 2 mg

References

Heard BE and Cooke RA, "Busulphan Lung," *Thorax*, 1968, 23(2):187-93.

Ozkaynak MF, Weinberg K, Kohn D, et al, "Hepatic Veno-Occlusive Disease Post-Bone Marrow Transplantation in Children Conditioned With Busulfan and Cyclophosphamide: Incidence, Risk Factors, and Clinical Outcome," *Bone Marrow Transplant*, 1991, 7(6):467-74.

Regazzi MB, Locatelli F, Buggia I, et al, "Disposition of High Dose Busulfan in Pediatric Patients Undergoing Bone Marrow Transplantation," *Clin Pharmacol Ther*, 1993, 54(1):45-52.

Vassal G, Gouyette A, Hartmann O, et al, "Pharmacokinetics of High-Dose Busulfan in Children," *Cancer Chemother Pharmacol*, 1989, 24(6):386-90.

♦ **Busulfex®** *see* Busulfan *on page 150*

♦ **BW-430C** *see* Lamotrigine *on page 554*

♦ **Byclomine® Injection** *see* Dicyclomine *on page 314*

♦ **Bydramine® Cough Syrup [OTC]** *see* Diphenhydramine *on page 327*

♦ **Cafatine-PB®** *see* Ergotamine *on page 378*

♦ **Cafcit®** *see* Caffeine, Citrated *on page 152*

♦ **Cafergot®** *see* Ergotamine *on page 378*

♦ **Cafetrate®** *see* Ergotamine *on page 378*

Caffeine, Citrated (KAF een, SIT rated)

Related Information

Overdose and Toxicology *on page 1191*

Brand Names Cafcit®

Therapeutic Category Central Nervous System Stimulant, Nonamphetamine; Respiratory Stimulant

Generic Available No

Use Treatment of idiopathic apnea of prematurity

Pregnancy Risk Factor C

Contraindications Hypersensitivity to caffeine or any component

Warnings Do not interchange the caffeine citrate salt formulation with the caffeine sodium benzoate formulation; the sodium benzoate salt has been reported to produce kernicterus (by displacement of bilirubin) and neonatal "gasping syndrome"; its use (sodium benzoate) should be avoided in neonates; during a Cafcit® double-blind, placebo-controlled study, 6 of 85 patients developed necrotizing enterocolitis (NEC); 5 of these 6 patients had received caffeine citrate; although no causal relationship has been established, neonates who receive caffeine citrate should be closely monitored for the development of NEC.

Precautions Use with caution in patients with a history of peptic ulcer, impaired renal or hepatic function, seizure disorders, or cardiovascular disease; avoid in patients with symptomatic cardiac arrhythmias

Adverse Reactions

Cardiovascular: Cardiac arrhythmias, tachycardia, extrasystoles

Central nervous system: Insomnia, restlessness, agitation, irritability, hyperactivity, jitteriness, headache

Endocrine & metabolic: Hypoglycemia, hyperglycemia

Gastrointestinal: Nausea, vomiting, gastric irritation, necrotizing enterocolitis, GI hemorrhage

Genitourinary: Increased urine output

Neuromuscular & skeletal: Muscle tremors or twitches

Drug Interactions Enhances the positive cardiac inotropic and chronotropic effects of beta-adrenergic agonists; cimetidine and phenylpropanolamine may impair caffeine metabolism; decreases hemodynamic effect of adenosine; fluconazole, mexiletine and cimetidine increase caffeine serum levels

Stability Injection and oral solution contain no preservatives; injection is chemically stable for at least 24 hours at room temperature when diluted to 10 mg/mL (as caffeine citrate) with D_5W, $D_{50}W$, Intralipid® 20%, and Aminosyn® 8.5%; also compatible with dopamine (600 mcg/mL), calcium gluconate 10%, heparin (1 unit/mL), and fentanyl (10 mcg/mL) at room temperature for 24 hours

Mechanism of Action Increases levels of 3-5-AMP by inhibiting phosphodiesterase; CNS stimulant which increases medullary respiratory center sensitivity to carbon dioxide, stimulates central inspiratory drive, and improves skeletal muscle contraction (diaphragmatic contractility); prevention of apnea may occur by competitive inhibition of adenosine

Pharmacokinetics

Distribution: V_d:

Neonates: 0.8-0.9 L/kg

Children >9 months to Adults: 0.6 L/kg

Protein binding: 17%

Metabolism: Interconversion between caffeine and theophylline has been reported in preterm neonates (caffeine levels are ~25% of measured theophylline after theophylline administration and ~3% to 8% of caffeine would be expected to be converted to theophylline)

Half-life:

Neonates: 72-96 hours (range: 40-230 hours)

Adults: 5 hours

Time to peak serum concentration: Oral: Within 30 minutes to 2 hours

Elimination:

Neonates ≤1 month: 86% excreted unchanged in urine

Infants >1 month and Adults: Extensively liver metabolized to a series of partially demethylated xanthines and methyluric acids

Clearance:

Neonates: 8.9 mL/hour/kg (range: 2.5-17)

Adults: 94 mL/hour/kg

Usual Dosage Apnea of prematurity: Neonates: Oral, I.V.:

Loading dose: 10-20 mg/kg as caffeine citrate (5-10 mg/kg as caffeine base). If theophylline has been administered to the patient within the previous 3 days, a full or modified loading dose (50% to 75% of a loading dose) may be given (caffeine is a significant metabolite of theophylline in the newborn; see Pharmacokinetics).

Maintenance dose: 5 mg/kg/day as caffeine citrate (2.5 mg/kg/day as caffeine base) once daily starting 24 hours after the loading dose. Maintenance dose is adjusted based on patient's response (efficacy and adverse effects), and serum caffeine concentrations.

Administration

Oral: May be administered without regard to feedings or meals; may administer injectable formulation orally

Parenteral: Infuse loading dose over at least 30 minutes; maintenance dose may be infused over at least 10 minutes; may administer without dilution or diluted with D_5W to 10 mg/mL (caffeine citrate)

Monitoring Parameters Heart rate, number and severity of apnea spells, serum caffeine levels

Reference Range

Therapeutic: Apnea of prematurity: 8-20 µg/mL

Potentially toxic: >20 µg/mL

Toxic: >50 µg/mL

Dosage Forms

Injection: 20 mg/mL as caffeine citrate [equivalent to 10 mg/mL caffeine base] (3 mL)

Solution, oral: 20 mg/mL as caffeine citrate [equivalent to 10 mg/mL caffeine base] (3 mL)

Extemporaneous Preparations An oral solution of 10 mg/mL caffeine citrate, prepared from caffeine citrate powder is stable for 3 months refrigerated.

Nahata MC and Hipple TF, *Pediatric Drug Formulations*, 1st ed, Cincinnati, OH: Harvey Whitney Books Co, 1990.

References

Erenberg A, Leff RD, Haack DG, et al, "Caffeine Citrate for the Treatment of Apnea of Prematurity: A Double-Blind, Placebo-Controlled Study," *Pharmacotherapy*, 2000, 20(6):644-52.

Kriter KE and Blanchard J, "Management of Apnea in Infants," *Clin Pharm*, 1989, 8(8):577-87.

Calamine Lotion (KAL a myne loe shun)

Therapeutic Category Topical Skin Product

Generic Available Yes

Use Employed primarily as an astringent, protectant, and soothing agent for conditions such as poison ivy, poison oak, poison sumac, sunburn, insect bites, or minor skin irritations

Precautions For external use only

(Continued)

Calamine Lotion *(Continued)*

Adverse Reactions
Dermatologic: Rash
Local: Irritation

Usual Dosage Topical: Apply 1-4 times/day as needed; reapply after bathing

Administration Topical: Shake well before using; avoid contact with the eyes; do not use on open wounds or burns

Additional Information Active ingredients: Calamine, zinc oxide

Dosage Forms Lotion:
Topical: Calamine 8%, zinc oxide 8%, glycerin 2% and bentonite magma in calcium hydroxide solution (120 mL, 240 mL, 480 mL)
Topical, phenolated: Calamine 8%, zinc oxide 8%, glycerin 2%, bentonite magma, and phenol 1% in calcium hydroxide solution (120 mL, 240 mL)

♦ **Calan®** *see* Verapamil *on page 974*
♦ **Calan® SR** *see* Verapamil *on page 974*
♦ **Cal Carb-HD® [OTC]** *see* Calcium Supplements *on page 157*
♦ **Calci-Chew™ [OTC]** *see* Calcium Supplements *on page 157*
♦ **Calciday-667® [OTC]** *see* Calcium Supplements *on page 157*
♦ **Calciferol™** *see* Ergocalciferol *on page 377*
♦ **Calcijex™** *see* Calcitriol *on page 155*
♦ **Calcilean® [HepCalium] (Canada)** *see* Heparin *on page 471*
♦ **Calcimar®** *see* Calcitonin *on page 154*
♦ **Calci-Mix™ [OTC]** *see* Calcium Supplements *on page 157*

Calcitonin *(kal si TOE nin)*

Brand Names Calcimar®; Caltine® (Canada); Cibacalcin®; Miacalcin®; Miacalcin® Nasal Spray; Osteocalcin®; Salmonine®

Therapeutic Category Antidote, Hypercalcemia

Generic Available No

Use
Calcitonin (salmon): Treatment of Paget's disease of bone and as adjunctive therapy for hypercalcemia; also used in postmenopausal osteoporosis and osteogenesis imperfecta
Calcitonin (human): Treatment of Paget's disease of bone

Pregnancy Risk Factor C

Contraindications Hypersensitivity to salmon protein or gelatin diluent

Precautions A skin test should be performed prior to initiating therapy with salmon calcitonin only; the skin test is 0.1 mL of 10 unit/mL calcitonin injection in NS (must be prepared) injected intradermally; observe injection site for 15 minutes for wheal or significant erythema

Adverse Reactions
Cardiovascular: Flushing of the face, edema
Central nervous system: Dizziness, headache, chills
Dermatologic: Rash
Gastrointestinal: Nausea, vomiting, diarrhea, anorexia, metallic taste
Local: Inflammatory reactions at the injection site
Neuromuscular & skeletal: Weakness, tingling of palms and soles, back and joint pain
Renal: Diuresis
Respiratory: Shortness of breath, nasal congestion, epistaxis, nasal sores, and sore bridge of nose (nasal spray)

Stability
Salmon calcitonin: Injection: Store under refrigeration; stable for up to 2 weeks at room temperature
Salmon calcitonin: Nasal spray: Store unopened bottle under refrigeration; once the pump has been activated, store at room temperature; stable at room temperature for 30 days
Human calcitonin: Store at room temperature; protect from light

Mechanism of Action Salmon calcitonin is structurally similar to human calcitonin; it directly inhibits osteoclastic bone resorption; promotes the renal excretion of calcium, phosphate, sodium, magnesium and potassium by decreasing tubular reabsorption; increases the jejunal secretion of water, sodium, potassium, and chloride

Pharmacodynamics

Hypercalcemia: Salmon calcitonin:
Onset of action:
I.M., S.C.: 15 minutes
I.V.: Immediate
Peak effect: I.M., S.C.: 4 hours
Duration of effect:
I.M., S.C.: 8-24 hours
I.V.: 30 minutes to 12 hours

Pharmacokinetics

Absorption: Intranasal: Rapidly but highly variable and lower than I.M. administration

Metabolism: Rapidly in the kidneys, blood, and peripheral tissues

Half-life, elimination:
S.C.: Human calcitonin: 1.2 hours
Intranasal: 43 minutes

Time to peak serum concentration: Intranasal: 31-39 minutes

Elimination: As inactive metabolites in urine

Clearance:
Human calcitonin: 8.4 mL/kg/minute
Salmon calcitonin: 3.1 mL/kg/minute

Usual Dosage Dosage for children not established; Adults:

Paget's disease:
Salmon calcitonin (see Precautions):
I.M., S.C.: Initial: 100 units/day; maintenance dose: 50 units/day or 50-100 units every 1-3 days
Intranasal: 200-400 units (1-2 sprays) per day
Human calcitonin: S.C.: Initial: 0.5 mg/day (maximum dose: 0.5 mg twice daily); maintenance: 0.5 mg 2-3 times/week or 0.25 mg/day
Hypercalcemia: Initial: Salmon calcitonin: I.M., S.C.: 4 units/kg every 12 hours; may increase up to 8 units/kg every 12 hours to a maximum of every 6 hours
Osteogenesis imperfecta: Salmon calcitonin: I.M., S.C.: 2 units/kg 3 times/week
Postmenopausal osteoporosis: Salmon calcitonin:
I.M., S.C.: 100 units/day
Intranasal: 200 units (1 spray) per day

Administration

Intranasal: Alternate spray into each nostril daily

Parenteral: Do not exceed 2 mL volume per injection site; human calcitonin should be administered S.C.; salmon calcitonin may be administered S.C. or I.M.

Monitoring Parameters Serum electrolytes and calcium; alkaline phosphatase and 24-hour urine collection for hydroxyproline excretion (Paget's disease); serum calcium

Reference Range Therapeutic: <19 pg/mL (SI: 19 ng/L) basal, depending on the assay

Patient Information Nasal spray: Notify physician if you develop significant nasal irritation; alternate nostrils; in treatment of postmenopausal osteoporosis, maintain adequate vitamin D intake and supplemental calcium

Dosage Forms

Injection:
Human (Cibacalcin®): 0.5 mg/vial
Salmon: 200 units/mL (2 mL)
Spray, nasal: **Salmon** (Miacalcin®): 200 units/activation (0.09 mL/dose) (2 mL glass bottle with pump)

Calcitriol (kal si TRYE ole)

Brand Names Calcijex™; Rocaltrol®

Synonyms 1,25 dihydroxycholecalciferol

Therapeutic Category Rickets, Treatment Agent; Vitamin D Analog; Vitamin, Fat Soluble

Generic Available No

Use Management of hypocalcemia associated with hypoparathyroidism, pseudohypothyroidism, and in patients on chronic renal dialysis; rickets

Pregnancy Risk Factor C

Contraindications Hypercalcemia; vitamin D toxicity; abnormal sensitivity to the effects of vitamin D

Adverse Reactions

Cardiovascular: Increased blood pressure, cardiac arrhythmias
Central nervous system: Somnolence, headache, hyperthermia
(Continued)

Calcitriol *(Continued)*

Dermatologic: Pruritus

Endocrine & metabolic: Hypercholesterolemia, hypercalcemia, polydipsia

Gastrointestinal: Nausea, vomiting, constipation, anorexia, xerostomia, pancreatitis, metallic taste, weight loss

Genitourinary: Nocturia

Hepatic: Increased liver enzymes

Neuromuscular & skeletal: Myalgia, bone pain, weakness

Ocular: Calcific conjunctivitis, photophobia

Renal: Polyuria, uremia, albuminuria

Respiratory: Rhinorrhea

Drug Interactions May antagonize the effects of calcium channel blockers by increasing serum calcium level; may be associated with digoxin toxicity by increasing calcium levels; may result in an additive increase in calcium levels due to decreased calcium excretion by thiazide diuretics; magnesium-containing antacids (potential development of hypermagnesemia); cholestyramine, colestipol, orlistat, and excessive use of mineral oil decrease absorption

Stability Protect from light and heat

Mechanism of Action Promotes absorption of calcium in the intestines and retention via the kidneys thereby increasing calcium levels in the serum; decreases excessive serum phosphatase levels, parathyroid hormone levels, and decreases bone resorption

Pharmacodynamics

Onset of effect: Oral: 2 hours

Peak effect: Oral: 10 hours

Duration: 3-5 days

Pharmacokinetics

Metabolism: Primarily to 1,24,25-trihydroxycholecalciferol and 1,24,25-trihydroxy ergocalciferol

Half-life: 4-6 hours

Elimination: Principally in bile and feces

Usual Dosage Individualize dosage to maintain calcium levels of 9-10 mg/dL

Management of hypocalcemia in patients with chronic renal failure:

Hemodialysis patients:

I.V.:

Children: 0.01-0.05 mcg/kg 3 times/week

Adults: 0.5 mcg (0.01 mcg/kg) 3 times/week; may increase dosage by 0.25-0.5 mcg increments at 2- to 4-week intervals until an optimal response is achieved; range: 0.5-3 mcg (0.01-0.05 mcg/kg)

Oral:

Children: 0.25-2 mcg/day

Adults: 0.25 mcg; may increase in 0.25 mcg increments at 4- to 8-week intervals; range: 0.5-1 mcg/day

Nonhemodialysis patients: Moderate to severe renal failure (Cl_{cr} 15-55 mL/minute; corrected for surface area in children): Oral:

Children <3 years: 0.01-0.015 mcg/kg once daily

Children ≥3 years and Adults: 0.25 mcg/day (maximum dose: 0.5 mcg/day)

Hypoparathyroidism/pseudohypoparathyroidism: Oral (evaluate dosage at 2- to 4-week intervals):

Children:

<1 year: 0.04-0.08 mcg/kg once daily

1-5 years: 0.25-0.75 mcg once daily

Children >6 years and Adults: 0.5-2 mcg once daily

Vitamin D-dependent rickets: Children and Adults: Oral: 1 mcg once daily

Vitamin D-resistant rickets (familial hypophosphatemia): Children and Adults: Oral: Initial: 0.015-0.02 mcg/kg once daily; maintenance: 0.03-0.06 mcg/kg once daily; maximum dose: 2 mcg once daily

Hypocalcemia in premature infants: Oral: 1 mcg once daily for 5 days

Hypocalcemic tetany in premature infants: I.V.: 0.05 mcg/kg once daily for 5-12 days

Administration

Oral: When administering small doses from the liquid-filled capsules, consider the following concentration for Rocaltrol®:

0.25 mcg capsule = 0.25 mcg per 0.17 mL

0.5 mcg capsule = 0.5 mcg per 0.17 mL

Parenteral: May be administered undiluted as a bolus dose I.V. through the catheter at the end of hemodialysis

Monitoring Parameters Serum calcium and phosphorus levels at least twice weekly at the onset of therapy and after each dosage adjustment; weekly for 12 weeks, then monthly after stabilization of dosage; magnesium, 24-hour urinary calcium

Dosage Forms
Capsule: 0.25 mcg, 0.5 mcg
Injection: 1 mcg/mL (1 mL); 2 mcg/mL (1 mL)
Solution, oral: 1 mcg/mL (15 mL)

Calcium Supplements (KAL see um SUP la ments)

Related Information
Antacid Preparations on page 86
Carbohydrate and Alcohol Content of Liquid Medications for Use in Patients Receiving Ketogenic Diets on page 1228
CPR Pediatric Drug Dosages on page 999
Extravasation Treatment on page 1050

Brand Names Alka-Mints® [OTC]; Amitone® [OTC]; Cal Carb-HD® [OTC]; Calci-Chew™ [OTC]; Calciday-667® [OTC]; Calci-Mix™ [OTC]; Calcium Rich [OTC]; Cal-Plus® [OTC]; Caltrate® 600 [OTC]; Caltrate, Jr.® [OTC]; Chooz® [OTC]; Citracal® [OTC]; Dicarbosil® [OTC]; Equilet® [OTC]; Florical® [OTC]; Gencalc® 600 [OTC]; Kalcinate® Cal Plus®; Mallamint® [OTC]; Mylanta® Soothing Antacids [OTC]; Neo-Calglucon® [OTC]; Nephro-Calci® [OTC]; Os-Cal® 500 [OTC]; Oyst-Cal 500 [OTC]; Oystercal® 500; Phos-Ex®; PhosLo®; Posture® [OTC]; Quick Dissolve Maalox® Maximum Strength; Rolaids®; Titralac® [OTC]; Tums® [OTC]; Tums® E-X Extra Strength Tablet [OTC]; Tums® Extra Strength Liquid [OTC]; Tums® Ultra® [OTC]

Available Salts Calcium Acetate; Calcium Carbonate; Calcium Chloride; Calcium Citrate; Calcium Glubionate; Calcium Gluceptate; Calcium Gluconate; Calcium Lactate; Calcium Phosphate, Tribasic

Therapeutic Category Antacid; Antidote, Hydrofluoric Acid; Calcium Salt; Electrolyte Supplement, Oral; Electrolyte Supplement, Parenteral

Generic Available Yes

Use Treatment and prevention of calcium depletion; relief of acid indigestion, heartburn; emergency treatment of hypocalcemic tetany; treatment of hypermagnesemia, cardiac disturbances of hyperkalemia, hypocalcemia, or calcium channel blocking agent toxicity; topical treatment of hydrofluoric acid burns

Pregnancy Risk Factor C

Contraindications Hypercalcemia, renal calculi, ventricular fibrillation

Precautions Use cautiously in patients with sarcoidosis, respiratory failure, acidosis, renal or cardiac disease; avoid too rapid I.V. administration; avoid extravasation; use with caution in digitalized patients; Quick Dissolve Maalox® Maximum Strength tablets contain aspartame, avoid or use with caution in phenylketonuria

Adverse Reactions
Cardiovascular: Vasodilation, hypotension, bradycardia, cardiac arrhythmias, ventricular fibrillation, syncope
Central nervous system: Headache, mental confusion, dizziness, lethargy, coma
Dermatologic: Erythema
Endocrine & metabolic: Hypercalcemia, milk-alkali syndrome, hypophosphatemia, hypercalciuria, hypomagnesemia
Gastrointestinal: Constipation, nausea, vomiting, xerostomia, elevated serum amylase
(Continued)

Calcium Supplements *(Continued)*

Local: Tissue necrosis (I.V. administration)
Neuromuscular & skeletal: Muscle weakness

Drug Interactions May potentiate digoxin toxicity; may antagonize the effects of calcium channel blockers (eg, verapamil); when administered orally, calcium decreases the absorption of tetracycline, atenolol, iron, quinolone antibiotics, alendronate, sodium fluoride, and zinc; high doses of calcium with thiazide diuretics may result in milk-alkali syndrome and hypercalcemia; decreases potassium-binding ability of polystyrene sulfonate

Food Interactions Do not give orally with bran, foods high in oxalates, or whole grain cereals which may decrease calcium absorption

Stability Incompatible with bicarbonates, phosphates, and sulfates

Mechanism of Action Moderates nerve and muscle performance via action potential excitation threshold regulation; neutralizes acidity of stomach (carbonate salt)

Usual Dosage Note: Multiple salt forms of calcium exist; close attention must be paid to the salt form when ordering and administering calcium; incorrect selection or substitution of one salt for another without proper dosage adjustment may result in serious over- or underdosing.

Oral: **Note:** For comparison information of calcium salts, see table.

Elemental Calcium Content of Calcium Salts

Calcium Salt	Elemental Calcium (mg/1 g of salt form)	mEq calcium per gram	Approximate Equivalent Doses (mg of calcium salt)
Calcium acetate	250	12.7	354
Calcium carbonate	400	20	225
Caclium chloride	270	13.5	330
Calcium citrate	211	10.6	425
Calcium glubionate	64	3.2	1400
Calcium gluceptate	82	4.1	1100
Calcium gluconate	90	4.5	1000
Calcium lactate	130	6.5	700
Calcium phosphate, tribasic	390	19.3	233

Recommended daily allowance (RDA): Dosage is in terms of elemental calcium:
<6 months: 400 mg/day
6-12 months: 600 mg/day
1-10 years: 800 mg/day
11-24 years: 1200 mg/day
Adults >24 years: 800 mg/day

Adequate intake (1997 National Academy of Science Recommendations): **Dosage is in terms of elemental calcium:**
0-6 months: 210 mg/day
7-12 months: 270 mg/day
1-3 years: 500 mg/day
4-8 years: 800 mg/day
9-18 years: 1300 mg/day
19-50 years: 1000 mg/day
>50 years: 1200 mg/day

Hypocalcemia (dose depends on clinical condition and serum calcium level): **Oral:**
Dose expressed in mg of **elemental calcium:**
Neonates: 50-150 mg/kg/day in 4-6 divided doses; not to exceed 1 g/day
Children: 45-65 mg/kg/day in 4 divided doses
Adults: 1-2 g or more per day in 3-4 divided doses
Dose expressed in mg of **calcium gluconate:**
Neonates: 500-1500 mg/kg/day in 4-6 divided doses
Infants and Children: 500-725 mg/kg/day in 3-4 divided doses
Adults: 10-20 g daily in 3-4 divided doses
Dose expressed in mg of **calcium glubionate:**
Neonates: 1200 mg/kg/day in 4-6 divided doses

Infants and Children: 600-2000 mg/kg/day in 4 divided up to a maximum of 9 g/day

Adults: 6-18 g/day in divided doses

Dose expressed in mg of **calcium lactate:**

Neonates and Infants: 400-500 mg/kg/day divided every 4-6 hours

Children: 500 mg/kg/day divided every 6-8 hours; maximum daily dose 9 g

Adults: 1.5-3 g divided every 8 hours

Hypocalcemia: I.V.:

Dosage expressed in mg of **calcium chloride:**

Neonates, Infants, and Children: 10-20 mg/kg/dose, repeat every 4-6 hours if needed

Adults: 500 mg to 1 g/dose every 6 hours

Dose expressed in mg of **calcium gluceptate:**

Infants and Children: 200-500 mg/kg/day divided every 6 hours

Adults: 500 mg to 1.1 g/dose as needed

Dose expressed in mg of **calcium gluconate:**

Neonates: 200-800 mg/kg/day as a continuous infusion or in 4 divided doses

Infants and Children: 200-500 mg/kg/day as a continuous infusion or in 4 divided doses

Adults: 2-15 g/day as a continuous infusion or in divided doses

Cardiac arrest in the presence of hyperkalemia or hypocalcemia, magnesium toxicity, or calcium antagonist toxicity: I.V.:

Dosage expressed in mg of **calcium chloride:**

Neonates, Infants, and Children: 20 mg/kg; may repeat in 10 minutes if necessary

Adults: 2-4 mg/kg; may repeat in 10 minutes if necessary

Dose expressed in mg of **calcium gluceptate:**

Infants and Children: 110 mg/kg/dose

Adults: 1.1-1.54 g/dose

Dosage expressed in mg of **calcium gluconate:**

Neonates, Infants, and Children: 100 mg/kg/dose (maximum 3 g/dose)

Adults: 500-800 mg (maximum 3 g/dose)

Hypocalcemia secondary to citrated blood infusion: I.V.: Give 0.45 mEq **elemental** calcium for each 100 mL citrated blood infused

Tetany: I.V.:

Dose expressed in mg of **calcium chloride:**

Neonates, Infants, and Children: 10 mg/kg over 5-10 minutes; may repeat after 6 hours or follow with an infusion with a maximum dose of 200 mg/kg/day

Adults: 1 g over 10-30 minutes; may repeat after 6 hours

Dose expressed in mg of **calcium gluconate:**

Neonates: 100-200 mg/kg/dose; may follow with 500 mg/kg/day in 3-4 divided doses or as a continuous infusion

Infants and Children: 100-200 mg/kg/dose over 5-10 minutes; may repeat after 6 hours or follow with an infusion of 500 mg/kg/day

Adults: 1-3 g may be administered until therapeutic response occurs

Antacid (calcium carbonate): See Antacid Preparations *on page 86*

Hydrofluoric acid (HF) burns (HF concentration <20%): Topical: Various topical calcium preparations have been used anecdotally for treatment of dermal exposure to HF solutions; both calcium gluconate and carbonate at concentrations ranging from 2.5% to 33% have been used: Massage calcium gluconate gel or slurry into exposed area for 15 minutes; topical calcium preparations must be compounded (see Extemporaneous Preparations)

Administration

Oral: Administer with plenty of fluids with or following meals

Parenteral:

I.V.: For direct I.V. injection infuse at a maximum rate of 50-100 mg/minute of calcium salt (gluconate, chloride, or gluceptate)

I.V. infusion: Dilution and infusion rates are dependent upon the salt form; dilute with I.V. fluid to a final concentration not to exceed maximums listed below; infuse over 1 hour without exceeding maximum rates of infusion listed below

Salt form (Maximum dilution; Maximum rate of infusion)

Calcium **chloride:** 20 mg/mL; 45-90 mg/kg over 1 hour; 0.6-1.2 mEq/kg over 1 hour

Calcium **gluceptate:** 55 mg/mL: 150-300 mg/kg over 1 hour; 0.6-1.2 mEq/kg over 1 hour

Calcium **gluconate:** 50 mg/mL; 120-240 mg/kg over 1 hour ; 0.6-1.2 mEq/kg over 1 hour

Do not inject calcium salts I.M. or administer S.C. since severe necrosis and sloughing may occur; extravasation of calcium can result in severe necrosis and (Continued)

Calcium Supplements *(Continued)*

tissue sloughing. Do not use scalp vein or small hand or foot veins for I.V. administration. Not for endotracheal administration.

Monitoring Parameters Serum calcium (ionized calcium preferred if available, see Additional Information), phosphate, magnesium, heart rate, EKG

Reference Range

Calcium: Newborns: 7.0-12.0 mg/dL; 0-2 years: 8.8-11.2 mg/dL; 2 years to adults: 9.0-11.0 mg/dL

Calcium, ionized, whole blood: 4.4-5.4 mg/dL

Additional Information Due to a poor correlation between the serum ionized calcium (free) and total serum calcium, particularly in states of low albumin or acid/base imbalances, direct measurement of ionized calcium is recommended. If ionized calcium is unavailable, in low albumin states, the corrected **total** serum calcium may be estimated by this equation (assuming a normal albumin of 4 g/dL); corrected total calcium = total serum calcium + 0.8 (4 - measured serum albumin)

Dosage Forms Elemental calcium listed in brackets

Calcium acetate:

Capsule: Phos-Ex® 125: 500 mg [125 mg]

Tablet:

Phos-Ex® 62.5: 250 mg [62.5 mg]

Phos-Ex® 167: 668 mg [167 mg]

Phos-Ex® 250: 1000 mg [250 mg]

PhosLo®: 667 mg [169 mg]

Calcium carbonate:

Capsule: 1500 mg [600 mg]

Calci-Mix™: 1250 mg [500 mg]

Florical®: 364 mg [145.6 mg] with sodium fluoride 8.3 mg

Liquid (Tums® Extra Strength): 1000 mg/5 mL [400 mg/5 mL] (360 mL)

Lozenge (Mylanta® Soothing Antacids): 600 mg [240 mg]

Powder (Cal Carb-HD®): 6.5 g/packet [2.6 g]

Suspension, oral: 1250 mg/5 mL [500 mg]

Tablet: 650 mg [260 mg], 1500 mg [600 mg]

Calciday-667®: 667 mg [267 mg]

Os-Cal® 500, Oyst-Cal 500, Oystercal® 500: 1250 mg [500 mg]

Cal-Plus®, Caltrate® 600, Gencalc® 600, Nephro-Calci®: 1500 mg [600 mg]

Tablet, chewable:

Alka-Mints®: 850 mg [340 mg]

Amitone®: 350 mg [140 mg] ®

Caltrate, Jr.®: 750 mg [300 mg]

Calci-Chew™, Os-Cal®: 750 mg [300 mg]

Chooz®, Dicarbosil®, Equilet®, Tums®: 500 mg [200 mg]

Mallamint®: 420 mg [168 mg]

Quick Dissolve Maalox® Maximum Strength: 1000 mg [400 mg]

Rolaids® Calcium Rich: 550 mg [220 mg]

Tums® E-X Extra Strength: 750 mg [300 mg]

Tums® Ultra®: 1000 mg [400 mg]

Florical®: 364 mg [145.6 mg] with sodium fluoride 8.3 mg

Calcium chloride:

Injection: 10% 100 mg/mL [27.2 mg/mL] (10 mL) (1.4 mEq calcium/mL)

Calcium citrate:

Tablet: 950 mg [200 mg]

Tablet, effervescent: 2376 mg [500 mg]

Calcium glubionate: Syrup: 1.8 g/5 mL [115 mg/5mL] (480 mL) (1.2 mEq calcium/mL)

Calcium gluceptate: Injection: 220 mg/mL [18 mg/mL] (5 mL, 50 mL) (0.9 mEq/mL)

Calcium gluconate:

Injection: 10% 100 mg/mL [9 mg/mL] (10 mL, 50 mL, 100 mL, 200 mL) (0.45 mEq/mL)

Tablet: 500 mg [45 mg], 650 mg [58.5 mg], 975 mg [87.75 mg], 1 g [90 mg]

Calcium lactate: Tablet: 325 mg [42.25 mg], 650 mg [84.5 mg]

Calcium phosphate, tribasic: Tablet, sugar free: 1565.2 mg [600 mg]

Extemporaneous Preparations

Calcium gluconate gel: Crush 3.5 g calcium gluconate tablets into a fine powder; add to 5 oz tube of water-soluble surgical lubricant (eg, K-Y® Jelly) or add 3.5 g calcium gluconate injection to 5 oz of water-soluble surgical lubricant (calcium carbonate may be substituted; do not use calcium chloride due to potential for irritation)

Calcium carbonate slurry: 32.5% slurry can be prepared by triturating ten 650 mg tablets into a fine powder and adding 20 mL of water-soluble lubricant gel (eg, K-Y® Jelly)

References

Baker SS, Cochran WJ, Flores CA, et al, "American Academy of Pediatrics. Committee on Nutrition: Calcium Requirements of Infants, Children, and Adolescents, *Pediatrics*, 1999, 104(5):1152-7.

"Dietary Reference Intakes for Calcium, Phosphorus, Magnesium, Vitamin D, and Fluoride. Standing Committee on the Scientific Evaluation of Dietary Reference Intakes, Food and Nutrition Board, Institute of Medicine," National Academy of Sciences, Washington, DC: National Academy Press, 1997.

NIH Consensus Conference, "Optimal Calcium Intake", *JAMA*, 1994, 272(24):1942-8.

♦ **Calcium Undecylenate** *see* Undecylenic Acid and Derivatives *on page 962*

♦ **CaldeCort® Anti-Itch Topical Spray** *see* Hydrocortisone *on page 486*

♦ **CaldeCort® Topical [OTC]** *see* Hydrocortisone *on page 486*

♦ **Caldesene® Topical [OTC]** *see* Undecylenic Acid and Derivatives *on page 962*

Calfactant (cal FAC tant)

Brand Names Infasurf®

Synonyms Bovine Lung Surfactant

Therapeutic Category Lung Surfactant

Generic Available No

Use Prevention and treatment of respiratory distress syndrome (RDS) in premature infants

Prophylactic therapy: Infants <29 weeks at significant risk for RDS

Treatment: Infants ≤72 hours of age with RDS (confirmed by clinical and radiologic findings and requiring endotracheal intubation)

Warnings Rapidly affects oxygenation and lung compliance and should be restricted to a highly supervised use in a clinical setting with immediate availability of clinicians experienced with intubation and ventilatory management of premature infants; if transient episodes of bradycardia and decreased oxygen saturation occur, discontinue the dosing procedure and initiate measures to alleviate the condition; produces rapid improvement in lung oxygenation and compliance that may require immediate reductions in ventilator settings and FiO_2; for intratracheal administration only

Precautions Transient episodes of reflux of calfactant into the endotracheal tube, cyanosis, bradycardia, or airway obstruction have occurred during dosing procedures; such episodes may require stopping administration and taking appropriate measures to alleviate the condition before resuming therapy

Adverse Reactions Most adverse reactions occur during the dosing procedure

Cardiovascular: Bradycardia, cyanosis

Respiratory: Airway obstruction, pneumothorax, pulmonary hemorrhage, apnea

Stability Refrigerate; protect from light; unopened, unused warmed vials of calfactant may be returned to refrigerator within 24 hours for future use; repeated warming to room temperature should be avoided

Mechanism of Action Replaces deficient or ineffective endogenous lung surfactant in neonates with RDS or in neonates at risk of developing RDS; surfactant prevents the alveoli from collapsing during expiration by lowering surface tension between air and alveolar surfaces

Usual Dosage Intratracheal: Neonates: 3 mL/kg every 12 hours up to a total of 3 doses; repeat doses have been administered as early as 6 hours after the previous dose for a total of up to four doses (if the infant was still intubated and required at least 30% inspired oxygen to maintain a PaO_2 ≤80 torr)

Administration Intratracheal: Gently swirl to redisperse suspension; do not shake; administer dosage divided into two aliquots of 1.5 mL/kg each into the endotracheal tube; after each instillation, reposition the infant with either the right or left side dependent; administration is made while ventilation is continued over 20-30 breaths for each aliquot, with small bursts timed only during the inspiratory cycles; a pause followed by evaluation of the respiratory status and repositioning should separate the two aliquots; calfactant dosage has also been divided into four equal aliquots and administered with repositioning in four different positions (prone, supine, right and left lateral)

Monitoring Parameters Continuous heart rate and transcutaneous O_2 saturation should be monitored during administration; frequent ABG sampling is necessary to prevent postdosing hyperoxia and hypocarbia

Dosage Forms Suspension, intratracheal: 6 mL

References

Hudak ML, Martin DJ, Egan EA, et al, "A Multicenter Randomized Masked Comparison Trail of Synthetic Surfactant Versus Calf Lung Surfactant Extract in the Prevention of Neonatal Respiratory Distress Syndrome," *Pediatrics*, 1997, 100(1):39-50.

(Continued)

Calfactant *(Continued)*

Bloom BT, Kattwinkel J, Hall RT, et al, "Comparison of Infasurf® (Calf Lung Surfactant Extract) to Survanta® (Beractant) in the Treatment and Prevention of Respiratory Distress Syndrome," *Pediatrics*, 1997, 100(1):31-8.

♦ **Calmol 4**® *see* Hemorrhoidal Preparations *on page 470*
♦ **Calm-X**® **Oral [OTC]** *see* Dimenhydrinate *on page 325*
♦ **Calmylin Expectorant (Canada)** *see* Guaifenesin *on page 464*
♦ **Cal-Plus**® **[OTC]** *see* Calcium Supplements *on page 157*
♦ **Caltine**® **(Canada)** *see* Calcitonin *on page 154*
♦ **Caltrate**® **600 [OTC]** *see* Calcium Supplements *on page 157*
♦ **Caltrate, Jr.**® **[OTC]** *see* Calcium Supplements *on page 157*
♦ **Camphorated Tincture of Opium** *see* Paregoric *on page 730*
♦ **642**® **(Canada)** *see* Propoxyphene *on page 814*
♦ **Candistatin**® **(Canada)** *see* Nystatin *on page 701*
♦ **Canesten**® **Topical (Canada) Canesten**® **Vaginal (Canada)** *see* Clotrimazole *on page 245*
♦ **Capital**® **and Codeine** *see* Acetaminophen and Codeine *on page 27*
♦ **Capoten**® *see* Captopril *on page 163*

Capsaicin (kap SAY sin)

Brand Names Capsin® [OTC]; Capzasin-P® [OTC]; Dolorac® [OTC]; No Pain-HP® [OTC]; R-Gel® [OTC]; Zostrix® [OTC]; Zostrix®-HP [OTC]
Therapeutic Category Analgesic, Topical; Topical Skin Product
Generic Available No
Use FDA approved for the topical treatment of pain associated with postherpetic neuralgia, rheumatoid arthritis, osteoarthritis, diabetic neuropathy, and postsurgical pain.

Unlabeled uses: Treatment of pain associated with psoriasis, chronic neuralgias unresponsive to other forms of therapy, and intractable pruritus
Contraindications Hypersensitivity to capsaicin or any component
Warnings Avoid contact with eyes, mucous membrane, or with damaged or irritated skin
Precautions Since warm water or excessive sweating may intensify the localized burning sensation after capsaicin application, the affected area should not be tightly bandaged or exposed to direct sunlight or a heat lamp
Adverse Reactions
Dermatologic: Erythema
Local: Itching, burning, or stinging sensation
Respiratory: Cough
Mechanism of Action Induces release of substance P, the principal chemomediator of pain impulses from the periphery to the CNS, from peripheral sensory neurons. After repeated application, capsaicin depletes the neuron of substance P and prevents reaccumulation.
Pharmacodynamics
Onset of action: Pain relief is usually seen within 14-28 days of regular topical application; maximal response may require 4-6 weeks of continuous therapy
Duration: Several hours
Usual Dosage Children ≥2 years and Adults: Topical: Apply to affected area at least 3-4 times/day; application frequency less than 3-4 times/day prevents the total depletion, inhibition of synthesis, and transport of substance P resulting in decreased clinical efficacy and increased local discomfort
Administration Topical: Should not be applied to wounds or damaged skin; avoid eye and mucous membrane exposure
Patient Information For external use only. Avoid washing treated areas for 30 minutes after application
Nursing Implications Wash hands with soap and water after applying to avoid spreading cream to eyes or other sensitive areas of the body
Additional Information In patients with severe and persistent local discomfort, pretreatment with topical lidocaine 5% ointment or concurrent oral analgesics for the first 2 weeks of therapy have been effective in alleviating the initial burning sensation and enabling continuation of topical capsaicin
Dosage Forms
Cream:
Capzasin-P®, Zostrix®: 0.025% (45 g, 90 g)
Dolorac®: 0.25% (28 g)

Zostrix®-HP: 0.075% (30 g, 60 g)
Gel (R-Gel®): 0.025% (15 g, 30 g)
Lotion (Capsin®): 0.025% (59 mL); 0.075% (59 mL)
Roll-on (No Pain-HP®): 0.075% (60 mL)

References

Bernstein JE, Korman NJ, Bickers DR, et al, "Topical Capsaicin Treatment of Chronic Postherpetic Neuralgia," *J Am Acad Dermatol*, 1989, 21(2 Pt 1):265-70.

♦ **Capsin® [OTC]** *see Capsaicin on page 162*

Captopril (KAP toe pril)

Brand Names Apo®-Capto (Canada); Capoten®; Novo-Captopril® (Canada); Nu-Capto® (Canada); Syn-Captopril® (Canada)

Therapeutic Category Angiotensin-Converting Enzyme (ACE) Inhibitor; Antihypertensive Agent

Generic Available Yes

Use Management of hypertension; treatment of CHF; in post-MI patients, improves survival in clinically stable patients with left-ventricular dysfunction

Pregnancy Risk Factor C (1st trimester); D (may cause injury and death to the developing fetus when used during the second and third trimester of pregnancy)

Contraindications Hypersensitivity to captopril, any component, or other ACE inhibitors

Precautions Use with caution and modify dosage in patients with renal impairment (especially those with severe renal artery stenosis); use with caution in patients with collagen vascular disease; risk of neutropenia is increased in patients with collagen vascular disease and renal impairment

Adverse Reactions

Cardiovascular: Hypotension, tachycardia

Central nervous system: Headache, dizziness, fatigue, insomnia, fever

Dermatologic: Rash, angioedema. **Note:** The relative risk of angioedema with ACE inhibitors is higher within the first 30 days of use (compared to >1 year of use), for Black Americans (compared to Whites), for lisinopril or enalapril (compared to captopril), and for patients previously hospitalized within 30 days (Brown, 1996).

Endocrine & metabolic: Hyperkalemia

Gastrointestinal: Ageusia

Hematologic: Neutropenia, agranulocytosis, eosinophilia

Respiratory: Cough, dyspnea

Renal: Elevated BUN and serum creatinine, proteinuria, oliguria

Drug Interactions Captopril plus potassium supplements or potassium-sparing diuretics may cause an additive hyperkalemic effect; captopril plus indomethacin or NSAIDs may result in a reduced antihypertensive response to captopril

Food Interactions Absorption of captopril may be reduced by food; long-term use of captopril may result in a zinc deficiency which can result in a decrease in taste perception; zinc supplements may be used; limit salt substitutes or potassium-rich diet; avoid natural licorice (causes sodium and water retention and increases potassium loss)

Stability Unstable in aqueous solutions

Mechanism of Action Competitive inhibitor of angiotensin-converting enzyme (ACE); prevents conversion of angiotensin I to angiotensin II, a potent vasoconstrictor; results in lower levels of angiotensin II which causes an increase in plasma renin activity and a reduction in aldosterone secretion

Pharmacodynamics

Onset of action: Decrease in blood pressure within 15 minutes

Maximum effect: 60-90 minutes; may require several weeks of therapy before full hypotensive effect is seen

Duration: Dose-related

Pharmacokinetics

Absorption: 60% to 75%

Distribution: 7 L/kg

Protein binding: 25% to 30%

Metabolism: 50% metabolized

Half-life:

Infants with CHF: 3.3 hours; range: 1.2-12.4 hours

Children: 1.5 hours; range: 0.98-2.3 hours

Normal adults (dependent upon renal and cardiac function): 1.9 hours

Adults with CHF: 2.1 hours

Anuria: 20-40 hours

Time to peak serum concentration: Within 1-2 hours

Elimination: 95% excreted in urine in 24 hours

(Continued)

Captopril *(Continued)*

Usual Dosage Note: Dosage must be titrated according to patient's response; use lowest effective dose; lower doses (~½ of those listed) should be used in patients who are sodium and water depleted due to diuretic therapy; Oral:

Newborns and premature Neonates: Initial: 0.01 mg/kg/dose every 8-12 hours; titrate dose

Neonates: Initial: 0.05-0.1 mg/kg/dose every 8-24 hours; titrate dose up to 0.5 mg/kg/dose given every 6-24 hours

Infants: Initial: 0.15-0.3 mg/kg/dose; titrate dose upward to maximum of 6 mg/kg/day in 1-4 divided doses; usual required dose: 2.5-6 mg/kg/day

Children: Initial: 0.3-0.5 mg/kg/dose; titrate upward to maximum of 6 mg/kg/day in 2-4 divided doses

Older Children: Initial: 6.25-12.5 mg/dose every 12-24 hours; titrate upward to maximum of 6 mg/kg/day in 2-4 divided doses

Adolescents and Adults: Initial: 12.5-25 mg/dose given every 8-12 hours; increase by 25 mg/dose to maximum of 450 mg/day

Dosing adjustment in renal impairment:
Cl_{cr} 10-50 mL/minute: Administer 75% of dose
Cl_{cr} <10 mL/minute: Administer 50% of dose

Administration Oral: Administer on an empty stomach 1 hour before meals or 2 hours after meals

Monitoring Parameters Blood pressure, BUN, serum creatinine, renal function, urine dipstick for protein, WBC with differential, serum potassium

Patient Information Limit alcohol; notify physician if swelling of face, lips, tongue, difficulty in breathing, or persistent cough occurs; do not use salt substitute (potassium-containing) without physician advice

Nursing Implications Discontinue if angioedema occurs; monitor blood pressure for hypotension within 1-3 hours after first dose or after a new higher dose

Additional Information Severe hypotension may occur in patients who are sodium and/or volume depleted

Dosage Forms Tablet: 12.5 mg, 25 mg, 50 mg, 100 mg

Extemporaneous Preparations

Captopril has limited stability in aqueous preparations. The addition of an antioxidant (sodium ascorbate) has been shown to increase the stability of captopril in solution; captopril (1 mg/mL) in syrup with methylcellulose is stable for 7 days stored either at 4°C or 22°C. Captopril (1 mg/mL) in distilled water (no additives) is stable for 14 days if stored at 4°C and 7 days if stored at 22°C; captopril (1 mg/mL) with sodium ascorbate (5 mg/mL) in distilled water is stable for 56 days at 4°C and 14 days at 22°C (Nahata, 1994); captopril (1 mg/mL) in an undiluted syrup containing preservatives is stable for 30 days at 5°C in amber glass containers (Lye, 1997).

Captopril (0.75 mg/mL) in cherry syrup is stable for only 2 days in amber clear plastic containers stored at room temperature or under refrigeration; captopril (0.75 mg/mL) in either a 1:1 mixture of Ora-Sweet® and Ora-Plus® or a 1:1 mixture of Ora-Sweet® SF and Ora-Plus® is stable for 10 days or less depending on the storage temperature (see Allen, 1996).

Powder papers can also be made; powder papers are stable for 12 weeks when stored at room temperature (Taketomo, 1990).

Allen LV and Erickson MA, "Stability of Baclofen, Captopril, Diltiazem Hydrochloride, Dipyridamole, and Flecainide Acetate in Extemporaneously Compounded Oral Liquids," *Am J Health Sys Pharm*, 1996, 53(18):2179-84.

Lye MY, Yow KL, Lim LY, et al, "Effects of Ingredients on Stability of Captopril in Extemporaneously Prepared Oral Liquids," *Am J Health Syst Pharm*, 1997, 54(21):2483-7.

Nahata MC, Morosco RS, and Hipple TF, "Stability of Captopril in Three Liquid Dosage Forms," *Am J Hosp Pharm*, 1994, 51(1):95-6.

Taketomo CK, Chu SA, Cheng MH, et al, "Stability of Captopril in Powder Papers Under Three Storage Conditions," *Am J Hosp Pharm*, 1990, 47(8):1799-801.

References

Brown NJ, Ray WA, Snowden M, et al, "Black Americans Have an Increased Rate of Angiotension-Converting Enzyme Inhibitor-Associated Angioedema," *Clin Pharmacol Ther*, 1996, 60(1):8-13.

Friedman WF and George BL, "New Concepts and Drugs in the Treatment of Congestive Heart Failure," *Pediatr Clin North Am*, 1984, 31(6):1197-227.

Levy M, Koren G, Klein J, et al, "Captopril Pharmacokinetics, Blood Pressure Response and Plasma Renin Activity in Normotensive Children With Renal Scarring," *Dev Pharmacol Ther*, 1991, 16(4):185-93.

Mirkin BL and Newman TJ, "Efficacy and Safety of Captopril in the Treatment of Severe Childhood Hypertension: Report of the International Collaborative Study Group," *Pediatrics*, 1985, 75(6):1091-100.

Pereira CM, Tam YK, Collins-Nakai RL, "The Pharmacokinetics of Captopril in Infants With Congestive Heart Failure," *Ther Drug Monit*, 1991, 13(3):209-14.

♦ **Capzasin-P®** [OTC] *see* Capsaicin *on page 162*
♦ **Carafate®** *see* Sucralfate *on page 886*

Carbamazepine (kar ba MAZ e peen)

Related Information
Antiepileptic Drugs *on page 1176*
Blood Level Sampling Time Guidelines *on page 1189*
Carbohydrate and Alcohol Content of Liquid Medications for Use in Patients Receiving Ketogenic Diets *on page 1228*
Overdose and Toxicology *on page 1191*
Serotonin Syndrome *on page 1217*

Brand Names Apo®-Carbamazepine (Canada); Epitol®; Mazepine® (Canada); Novo-Carbamaz® (Canada); Nu-Carbamazepine® (Canada); PMS-Carbamazepine (Canada); Tegretol®; Tegretol®-XR

Synonyms CBZ

Therapeutic Category Anticonvulsant, Miscellaneous

Generic Available Yes: Tablet

Use Prophylaxis of generalized tonic-clonic, partial (especially complex partial), and mixed partial or generalized seizure disorder; to relieve pain in trigeminal neuralgia or diabetic neuropathy; treatment of bipolar disorders

Pregnancy Risk Factor D

Contraindications Patients with a history of bone marrow suppression; hypersensitivity to carbamazepine or any component; cross-sensitivity with tricyclic antidepressants may occur; concomitant therapy with MAO inhibitors

Warnings Potentially fatal blood cell abnormalities have been reported following treatment; early detection of hematologic change is important; advise patients of early signs and symptoms which are: fever, sore throat, mouth ulcers, infections, easy bruising, petechial or purpuric hemorrhage

Substitution of Tegretol® with generic carbamazepine has resulted in decreased carbamazepine levels and increased seizure activity, as well as increased carbamazepine levels and toxicity. Monitoring of carbamazepine serum concentrations is mandatory when patients are switched from any product to another.

Precautions MAO inhibitors should be discontinued for a minimum of 14 days before carbamazepine is begun; administer with caution to patients with history of cardiac disease, hepatic disease, or renal failure; higher peak concentrations occur with the suspension, so treatment is initiated with lower amounts per dose and increased slowly to avoid adverse effects

Adverse Reactions
Cardiovascular: Edema, CHF, syncope, dysrhythmias, heart block
Central nervous system: Sedation, dizziness, drowsiness, fatigue, slurred speech, ataxia, confusion
Dermatologic: Rash, Stevens-Johnson syndrome
Endocrine & metabolic: SIADH, hyponatremia
Gastrointestinal: Nausea, diarrhea, vomiting, abdominal cramps, pancreatitis
Genitourinary: Urinary retention
Hematologic: Neutropenia (can be transient), aplastic anemia, agranulocytosis, thrombocytopenia
Hepatic: Hepatitis
Ocular: Nystagmus, diplopia, blurred vision

Drug Interactions Cytochrome P-450 isoenzyme CYP2C8 and CYP3A3/4 substrate; isoenzyme CYP1A2, CYP2C, and CYP3A3/4 inducer
Clarithromycin, erythromycin, isoniazid, danazol, fluoxetine, ketoconazole, itraconazole, propoxyphene, verapamil, diltiazem, and cimetidine may inhibit hepatic metabolism of carbamazepine with resultant increase of carbamazepine serum concentrations and toxicity; carbamazepine may induce the metabolism of warfarin, cyclosporine, doxycycline, oral contraceptives, phenytoin, theophylline, ritonavir, saquinavir, delavirdine, benzodiazepines, ethosuximide, valproic acid, midazolam, corticosteroids and thyroid hormones; use with lithium may increase neurotic side effects; ritonavir and cefixime may affect the metabolism of carbamazepine; administration of Tegretol® suspension in combination with liquid chlorpromazine or thioridazine results in an orange rubbery precipitate

Stability Store tablets in dry place, protect from moisture

Mechanism of Action May depress activity in the nucleus ventralis of the thalamus or decrease synaptic transmission or decrease summation of temporal stimulation leading to neural discharge, by limiting influx of sodium ions across cell
(Continued)

Carbamazepine *(Continued)*

membrane; other unknown mechanisms; stimulates the release of ADH and potentiates its action in promoting reabsorption of water; chemically related to tricyclic antidepressants; in addition to anticonvulsant effects, carbamazepine has anticholinergic, antineuralgic, antidiuretic, muscle relaxant and antiarrhythmic properties

Pharmacokinetics

Absorption: Slowly from the GI tract

Distribution: V_d:

Neonates: 1.5 L/kg

Children: 1.9 L/kg

Adults: 0.59-2 L/kg

Protein binding: 75% to 90%, bound to alpha$_1$-acid glycoprotein and nonspecific binding sites on albumin; protein binding may be decreased in newborns

Metabolism: Induces liver enzymes to increase metabolism and shorten half-life over time; metabolized in the liver by cytochrome P-450 3A4 to active epoxide metabolite; ratio of serum epoxide to carbamazepine concentrations may be higher in patients receiving polytherapy (vs monotherapy) and in infants (vs older children); boys may have faster carbamazepine clearances and may, therefore, require higher mg/kg/day doses of carbamazepine compared to girls of similar age and weight

Bioavailability, oral: 75% to 85%; relative bioavailability of extended release tablet to suspension: 89%

Half-life:

Initial: 25-65 hours

Multiple dosing:

Children: 8-14 hours

Adults: 12-17 hours

Time to peak serum concentration: Unpredictable, within 4-8 hours

Chronic administration:

Suspension: 1.5 hours

Tablet: 4-5 hours

Extended release tablet: 3-12 hours

Elimination: 1% to 3% excreted unchanged in urine

Usual Dosage Dosage must be adjusted according to patient's response and serum concentrations. Administer tablets (chewable or conventional) in 2-3 divided doses daily and suspension in 4 divided doses daily. (See Additional Information for investigational oral loading dose information.) Oral:

Children:

<6 years: Initial: 10-20 mg/kg/day; increase dose every week until optimal response and therapeutic levels are achieved; maintenance dose: Divide into 3-4 doses daily (tablets or suspension); maximum recommended dose: 35 mg/kg/day

6-12 years: Initial: 100 mg twice daily (tablets or extended release tablets) or 50 mg of suspension 4 times/day (200 mg/day); increase by up to 100 mg/day at weekly intervals using a twice daily regimen of extended release tablets or 3-4 times daily regimen of other formulations until optimal response and therapeutic levels are achieved; usual maintenance: 400-800 mg/day; maximum recommended dose: 1000 mg/day

Children >12 years and Adults: Initial: 200 mg twice daily (tablets or extended release tablets) or 100 mg of suspension 4 times/day (400 mg daily); increase by up to 200 mg/day at weekly intervals using a twice daily regimen of extended release tablets or a 3-4 times/day regimen of other formulations until optimal response and therapeutic levels are achieved; usual dose: 800-1200 mg/day

Maximum recommended doses:

Children 12-15 years: 1000 mg/day

Children >15 years: 1200 mg/day

Adults: 1600 mg/day; however, some patients have required up to 1.6-2.4 g/day

Dosing adjustment in renal impairment: Cl_{cr} <10 mL/minute: Administer 75% of recommended dose; monitor serum levels

Administration

Oral: Administer with food to decrease GI upset; suspension dosage should be administered on a 3-4 times/day schedule vs tablet (conventional or chewable) which can be administered 2-4 times/day; extended release (XR) tablets should be dosed twice daily; do not crush or chew XR tablets

Suspension: Tegretol® should not be administered with diluents or other liquid medicines due to the possibility of a component interaction (see Drug Interactions); shake suspension well before use

Monitoring Parameters CBC with platelet count, liver function tests, serum drug concentration; observe patient for excessive sedation especially when instituting or increasing therapy

Reference Range Therapeutic: 4-12 µg/mL (SI: 17-51 µmol/L). Patients who require higher levels [8-12 µg/mL (SI: 34-51 µmol/L)] should be carefully monitored. Side effects (especially CNS) occur commonly at higher levels. If other anticonvulsants (enzyme inducers) are given, therapeutic range is 4-8 µg/mL (SI: 17-34 µmol/L) due to increase in unmeasured active epoxide metabolite.

Patient Information Avoid alcohol; may cause drowsiness and impair ability to perform activities requiring mental alertness or physical coordination; report fever, sore throat, infection, mouth ulcers, easy bruising, or bleeding to physician; the tablet coating of Tegretol®-XR is not absorbed and may appear in the stool

Additional Information Carbamazepine is not effective in absence, myoclonic, akinetic, or febrile seizures; exacerbation of certain seizure types have been seen after initiation of carbamazepine therapy in children with mixed seizure disorders

Investigationally, loading doses of the suspension (10 mg/kg for children <12 years of age and 8 mg/kg for children >12 years) were given (via NG or ND tubes followed by 5-10 mL of water to flush through tube) to PICU patients with frequent seizures/status; 5 of 6 patients attained mean plasma concentrations of 4.3 mcg/mL and 7.3 mcg/mL at 1 and 2 hours postload; concurrent enteral feeding or ileus may delay absorption of loading dose

Dosage Forms

Suspension, oral (citrus-vanilla flavor): 100 mg/5 mL (450 mL)

Tablet: 200 mg

Tablet, chewable: 100 mg

Tablet, extended release (XR): 100 mg, 200 mg, 400 mg

References

Gilman JT, "Carbamazepine Dosing for Pediatric Seizure Disorders: The Highs and Lows," *DICP*, 1991, 25(10):1109-12.

Korinthenberg R, Haug C, and Hannak D, "The Metabolization of Carbamazepine to CBZ-10,11 Epoxide in Children From the Newborn Age to Adolescence," *Neuropediatrics*, 1994, 25(4):214-6.

Liu H and Delgado MR, "Influence of Sex, Age, Weight, and Carbamazepine Dose on Serum Concentrations, Concentration Ratios, and Level/Dose Ratios of Carbamazepine and Its Metabolites," *Ther Drug Monit*, 1994, 16(5):469-76.

Miles MV, Lawless ST, Tennison MB, et al, "Rapid Loading of Critically Ill Patients With Carbamazepine Suspension," *Pediatrics*, 1990, 86(2):263-6.

Carbamide Peroxide (KAR ba mide per OKS ide)

Brand Names Auro® Ear Drops [OTC]; Clamurid® (Canada); Debrox® Otic [OTC]; E•R•O Ear [OTC]; Gly-Oxide® Oral [OTC]; Mollifene® Ear Wax Removing Formula [OTC]; Murine® Ear Drops [OTC]; Orajel® Perioseptic [OTC]; Proxigel® Oral [OTC]

Synonyms Urea Peroxide

Therapeutic Category Otic Agent, Cerumenolytic

Generic Available Yes

Use

Oral: Relief of minor inflammation of gums, oral mucosal surfaces and lips including canker sores and dental irritation; adjunct in oral hygiene

Otic: Emulsify and disperse ear wax

Pregnancy Risk Factor C

Contraindications Otic preparation should not be used in patients with a perforated tympanic membrane or following otic surgery; ear drainage, ear pain, or rash in the ear; dizziness; oral preparation should not be used for self medication in children <3 years of age; hypersensitivity to carbamide peroxide or any component

Warnings With prolonged use of oral carbamide peroxide, there is a potential for overgrowth of opportunistic organisms, damage to periodontal tissues, delayed wound healing

Adverse Reactions

Central nervous system: Dizziness

Dermatologic: Rash

Local: Irritation, tenderness, pain, redness

Stability Protect from heat and direct light

Mechanism of Action Carbamide peroxide releases hydrogen peroxide which serves as a source of nascent oxygen upon contact with catalase; deodorant action is probably due to inhibition of odor-causing bacteria; softens impacted cerumen due to its foaming action

Pharmacodynamics Onset of effect: Otic: Slight disintegration of hard ear wax in 24 hours

(Continued)

Carbamide Peroxide *(Continued)*

Usual Dosage
Oral: Children and Adults:
Gel: Massage on affected area 4 times/day for up to 7 days
Solution: Apply several drops undiluted to affected area of the mouth 4 times/day and at bedtime for up to 7 days, expectorate after 2-3 minutes; as an adjunct to oral hygiene after brushing, swish 10 drops for 2-3 minutes, then expectorate
Otic: Solution:
Children <12 years: Individualize the dose according to patient size; 3 drops (range: 1-5 drops) twice daily for up to 4 days
Children ≥12 years and Adults: Instill 5-10 drops twice daily for up to 4 days

Administration
Oral: Apply undiluted solution with an applicator or cotton swab to the affected area after meals and at bedtime; or place drops on the tongue, mix with saliva, swish in the mouth for several minutes, then expectorate
Otic: Instill drops into the external ear canal; keep drops in ear for several minutes by keeping head tilted or placing cotton in ear

Patient Information Contact physician if dizziness or otic redness, rash, irritation, tenderness, pain, drainage or discharge develop; do not use in the eye

Nursing Implications Drops foam on contact with ear wax

Dosage Forms
Gel, oral (Proxigel®): 10% (36 g)
Solution:
Oral (Cankaid®, Gly-Oxide®, Orajel® Brace-Aid Rinse): 10% in anhydrous glycerol (15 mL, 22.5 mL, 30 mL, 60 mL)
Otic (Auro® Ear Drops, Debrox®, Murine® Ear Drops): 6.5% in glycerin (15 mL, 30 mL)

Carbenicillin *(kar ben i SIL in)*

Brand Names Geocillin®; Geopen® (Canada)
Available Salts Carbenicillin Indanyl Sodium
Synonyms Carindacillin
Therapeutic Category Antibiotic, Penicillin (Antipseudomonal)
Generic Available No
Use Treatment of urinary tract infections, asymptomatic bacteriuria, or prostatitis caused by susceptible strains of *Pseudomonas aeruginosa*, *E. coli*, indole-positive *Proteus*, and *Enterobacter*
Pregnancy Risk Factor B
Contraindications Hypersensitivity to carbenicillin, any component, or penicillins
Warnings Oral carbenicillin should be limited to treatment of urinary tract infections
Precautions Use with caution in patients with history of cephalosporin hypersensitivity; do not use in patients with severe renal impairment (Cl_{cr} <10 mL/minute) since drug concentration in urine is reduced and inadequate for treatment of UTIs

Adverse Reactions
Dermatologic: Rash, urticaria, pruritus
Gastrointestinal: Nausea, vomiting, diarrhea, abdominal cramps, furry tongue
Genitourinary: Vaginitis
Hematologic: Eosinophilia, hemolytic anemia, neutropenia, leukopenia, thrombocytopenia
Hepatic: Elevated liver enzymes, hepatotoxicity

Drug Interactions Probenecid, lithium
Mechanism of Action Interferes with bacterial cell wall synthesis during active multiplication

Pharmacokinetics
Absorption: Oral: 30% to 40%; in patients with normal renal function, serum concentrations of carbenicillin following oral absorption are inadequate for the treatment of systemic infections
Protein binding: 50%
Half-life:
Neonates:
<7 days, ≤2.5 kg: 4 hours
<7 days, >2.5 kg: 2.7 hours
Children: 0.8-1.8 hours
Adults: 1-1.5 hours; prolonged to 10-20 hours with renal insufficiency
Time to peak serum concentration: Within 30-120 minutes
Elimination: Carbenicillin and its metabolites are excreted in the urine; ~80% to 99% of the dose is excreted unchanged in the urine

Moderately dialyzable (20% to 50%)

Usual Dosage Oral:
Children: 30-50 mg/kg/day divided every 6 hours; maximum dose: 2-3 g/day
Adults:
Urinary tract infections: 1-2 tablets every 6 hours
Prostatitis: 2 tablets every 6 hours

Administration Oral: Administer with water

Monitoring Parameters Renal, hepatic, and hematologic function tests

Test Interactions False-positive urine or serum proteins; false-positive urine glucose (Clinitest®)

Patient Information Tablets have a bitter taste

Additional Information Sodium content of 382 mg tablet: 23 mg (1 mEq)

Dosage Forms Tablet, film coated, as indanyl sodium ester: 382 mg [base]

♦ **Carbenicillin Indanyl Sodium** *see* Carbenicillin *on page 168*

Carbinoxamine and Pseudoephedrine

(kar bi NOKS a meen & soo doe e FED rin)

Brand Names Carbiset® Tablet; Carbiset-TR® Tablet; Carbodec® Syrup; Carbodec® Tablet; Carbodec TR® Tablet; Cardec-S® Syrup; Rondec® Drops; Rondec® Filmtab®; Rondec® Syrup; Rondec-TR®

Available Salts Carbinoxamine Maleate and Pseudoephedrine Hydrochloride

Synonyms Pseudoephedrine and Carbinoxamine

Therapeutic Category Antihistamine/Decongestant Combination

Generic Available Yes

Use Temporary relief of nasal congestion, running nose, sneezing, itching of nose or throat, and itchy, watery eyes due to the common cold, hay fever, or other respiratory allergies

Pregnancy Risk Factor C

Contraindications Hypersensitivity to carbinoxamine, pseudoephedrine, or any component; severe hypertension or coronary artery disease, MAO inhibitor therapy, GI or GU obstruction, narrow-angle glaucoma

Precautions Use with caution in patients with mild to moderate hypertension, heart disease, diabetes, asthma, thyroid disease, or prostatic hypertrophy

Adverse Reactions
Cardiovascular: Hypertension, tachycardia, arrhythmias edema, palpitations
Central nervous system: Sedation, CNS stimulation, headache, seizures, drowsiness, fatigue, nervousness, depression
Dermatologic: Angioedema, photosensitivity, rash
Gastrointestinal: Nausea, vomiting, xerostomia, anorexia, diarrhea, heart burn
Genitourinary: Dysuria
Hepatic: Hepatitis
Neuromuscular & skeletal: Weakness, myalgia, paresthesia
Ocular: Diplopia
Respiratory: Bronchospasm, epistaxis
Renal: Polyuria

Drug Interactions May produce severe hypertensive episodes when used with MAO inhibitors; may inhibit hypotensive effects of beta-adrenergic blocking agents; additive effects with other sympathomimetics, sedatives, alcohol, barbiturates, and other CNS depressants

Mechanism of Action Carbinoxamine competes with histamine for H_1-receptor sites on effector cells in the gastrointestinal tract, blood vessels, and respiratory tract; pseudoephedrine directly stimulates alpha-adrenergic receptors of respiratory mucosa causing vasoconstriction; directly stimulates beta-adrenergic receptors causing bronchial relaxation, increased heart rate and contractility

Usual Dosage Oral:
Children (may dose according to pseudoephedrine component): 4 mg/kg/day **or**
Drops:
1-3 months: 1/4 dropperful (0.25 mL) 4 times/day
3-6 months: 1/2 dropperful (0.5 mL) 4 times/day
6-9 months: 3/4 dropperful (0.75 mL) 4 times/day
9-18 months: 1 dropperful (1 mL) 4 times/day
Syrup or tablet:
18 months to 6 years: 2.5 mL 4 times/day
6 years to Adults: 5 mL or 1 tablet 4 times/day
Extended release tablet: Children >12 years and Adults: 1 tablet 2 times/day

Administration Oral: Do not crush or chew extended release tablets

(Continued)

Carbinoxamine and Pseudoephedrine *(Continued)*

Patient Information May cause drowsiness or impair ability to perform activities requiring mental alertness or physical coordination; may cause blurred vision; may also cause CNS excitation and difficulty sleeping

Dosage Forms

Drops: Carbinoxamine maleate 2 mg and pseudoephedrine hydrochloride 25 mg per mL (30 mL with dropper)

Syrup: Carbinoxamine maleate 4 mg and pseudoephedrine hydrochloride 60 mg per 5 mL (120 mL, 480 mL)

Tablet:

Film-coated: Carbinoxamine maleate 4 mg and pseudoephedrine hydrochloride 60 mg

Sustained release: Carbinoxamine maleate 8 mg and pseudoephedrine hydrochloride 120 mg

♦ **Carbinoxamine Maleate and Pseudoephedrine Hydrochloride** *see Carbinoxamine and Pseudoephedrine on page 169*

♦ **Carbiset® Tablet** *see Carbinoxamine and Pseudoephedrine on page 169*

♦ **Carbiset-TR® Tablet** *see Carbinoxamine and Pseudoephedrine on page 169*

♦ **Carbodec® Syrup** *see Carbinoxamine and Pseudoephedrine on page 169*

♦ **Carbodec® Tablet** *see Carbinoxamine and Pseudoephedrine on page 169*

♦ **Carbodec TR® Tablet** *see Carbinoxamine and Pseudoephedrine on page 169*

♦ **Carbohydrate and Alcohol Content of Liquid Medications for Use in Patients Receiving Ketogenic Diets** *see page 1228*

♦ **Carbolith™ (Canada)** *see Lithium on page 577*

Carboplatin *(KAR boe pla tin)*

Related Information

Emetogenic Potential of Single Chemotherapeutic Agents *on page 1095*

Brand Names Paraplatin®

Synonyms CBDCA

Therapeutic Category Antineoplastic Agent, Alkylating Agent

Generic Available No

Use Treatment of ovarian carcinoma; used in the treatment of small cell lung cancer, squamous cell carcinoma of the esophagus; solid tumors of the bladder, cervix and testes; pediatric brain tumor, neuroblastoma, bony and soft tissue sarcomas, germ cell tumors, and high-dose therapy with stem cell/bone marrow transplants

Pregnancy Risk Factor D

Contraindications Hypersensitivity to carboplatin, cisplatin, any component, other platinum-containing compounds, or mannitol; severe bone marrow suppression or excessive bleeding

Warnings The FDA currently recommends that procedures for proper handling and disposal of antineoplastic agents be considered. When carboplatin is dosed using AUC (area under the concentration versus time curve) as the endpoint, note that the calculated dose is the dose administered, not the dose based on body surface area

Precautions Bone marrow suppression, which may be severe, and vomiting are dose-related; high doses have also resulted in severe abnormalities of liver function; reduce dosage in patients with bone marrow suppression and impaired renal function (creatinine clearance values <60 mL/minute)

Adverse Reactions

Cardiovascular: Hypotension

Central nervous system: Pain

Dermatologic: Urticaria, rash, alopecia, pruritus, erythema

Endocrine & metabolic: Electrolyte abnormalities such as hypocalcemia, hypokalemia, hypomagnesemia

Gastrointestinal: Nausea, vomiting, diarrhea, anorexia, hemorrhagic colitis, mucositis, constipation

Hematologic: Neutropenia, leukopenia, thrombocytopenia (platelet count reaches a nadir between 14-21 days), anemia

Hepatic: Abnormal liver function tests

Neuromuscular & skeletal: Peripheral neuropathy, weakness

Otic: Tinnitus, hearing loss at high tones

Renal: Nephrotoxicity, elevated BUN and serum creatinine, hematuria

Respiratory: Bronchospasm, interstitial pneumonia

Miscellaneous: Anaphylactic-like reactions

Drug Interactions Aminoglycosides (increased ototoxicity and nephrotoxicity); nephrotoxic drugs (increased renal toxicity); decreases phenytoin serum levels

Stability Store unopened vials at room temperature; protect from light; after reconstitution, solutions are stable for 8 hours; 2 mg/mL solutions diluted in D_5W for infusion are stable for 24 hours; 7 mg/mL solutions diluted in NS for infusion are stable for 24 hours; aluminum reacts with carboplatin resulting in a precipitate and loss of potency

Mechanism of Action Platination of DNA results in possible cross-linking and interference with the function of DNA

Pharmacokinetics

Distribution: V_d: 16 L/kg

Protein binding: 0%; however, platinum is 30% protein bound

Half-life: Patients with Cl_{cr} >60 mL/minute: 2.5-5.9 hours

Elimination: ~60% to 80% is excreted renally

Usual Dosage I.V. (refer to individual protocols):

Infants and Children <3 years or ≤12 kg: Various protocols calculate dosage on the basis of body weight rather than body surface area

Children:

Dosing based on target AUC (modified Calvert formula for use in children): Total dose (mg) = [Target AUC (mg/mL/minute)] x [GFR (mL/minute) + (0.36 x body weight in kilograms)]; **Note:** GFR is measured by the plasma clearance of ^{51}Cr-EDTA

Note: The dose of carboplatin calculated is TOTAL mg DOSE not mg/m²; AUC is the area under the concentration versus time curve

Target AUC will vary depending upon: Number of agents in the regimen and treatment status (ie, previously untreated or treated)

Solid tumor: 300-600 mg/m² once every 4 weeks

Brain tumor: 175 mg/m² once weekly for 4 weeks with a 2-week recovery period between courses; dose is then adjusted on platelet count and neutrophil count values; courses should not be repeated until the platelet count is ≥100,000/mm³ and the neutrophil count is ≥2000/mm³

Bone marrow transplant preparative regimen: 500 mg/m²/day for 3 days

Note: Retinoblastoma: Subconjunctival injection of carboplatin for intraocular retinoblastoma has been administered using 1-2 mL of a 10 mg/mL solution per dose to affected eye(s)

Adults:

Single agent: 360 mg/m² once every 4 weeks; dose is then adjusted on platelet count and neutrophil count values; courses should not be repeated until the platelet count is ≥100,000/mm³ and the neutrophil count is ≥2000/mm³

Calvert formula: See table.

Single Agent Carboplatin/No Prior Chemotherapy	Total dose (mg): 6-8 (GFR + 25)
Single Agent Carboplatin/Prior Chemotherapy	Total dose (mg): 4-6 (GFR + 25)
Combination Chemotherapy/No Prior Chemotherapy	Total dose (mg): 4.5-6 (GFR + 25)
Combination Chemotherapy/Prior Chemotherapy	Use a target AUC value <5 for the initial cycle

Dosing adjustment in renal impairment: Adults: Calvert formula:

Total dose (mg) = [Target AUC (mg/mL/minute)] x [GFR (mL/minute) + 25]

Note: The dose of carboplatin calculated is TOTAL mg DOSE not mg/m²; AUC will vary depending upon: Number of agents in the regimen and treatment status (ie, previously untreated or treated)

Administration Parenteral: Administer by I.V. intermittent infusion over 15 minutes to 1 hour, or by continuous infusion (continuous infusion regimens may be less toxic than the bolus route); reconstituted carboplatin 10 mg/mL should be further diluted to a final concentration of 0.5-2 mg/mL with D_5W or NS for administration

Monitoring Parameters CBC with differential and platelet count, serum electrolytes, urinalysis, creatinine clearance, liver function tests

Nursing Implications Needle or intravenous administration sets containing aluminum parts should not be used in the administration or preparation of carboplatin (aluminum can interact with carboplatin resulting in precipitate formation and loss of potency)

Dosage Forms Powder for injection, lyophilized: 50 mg, 150 mg, 450 mg

References

Abramson DH, Frank CM, and Dunkel IJ, "A Phase I/II Study of Subconjunctival Carboplatin for Intraocular Retinoblastoma," *Ophthalmology*, 1999, 106(10):1947-50.

(Continued)

Carboplatin *(Continued)*

Lovett D, Kelsen D, Eisenberger M, et al, "A Phase II Trial of Carboplatin and Vinblastine in the Treatment of Advanced Squamous Cell Carcinoma of the Esophagus," *Cancer*, 1991, 67(2):354-6.

Newell DR, Pearson AD, Balmanno K, et al, "Carboplatin Pharmacokinetics in Children: The Development of a Pediatric Dosing Formula. The United Kingdom Children's Cancer Study Group," *J Clin Oncol*, 1993, 11(12):2314-23.

Oguri S, Sakakibara T, Mase H, et al, "Clinical Pharmacokinetics of Carboplatin," *J Clin Pharmacol*, 1988, 28(3):208-15.

Reece PA, Stafford I, Abbott RI, et al, "Two- Versus 24-Hour Infusion of Cisplatin: Pharmacokinetic Considerations," *J Clin Oncol*, 1989, 7(2):270-5.

Zeltzer PM, Epport K, Nelson MD Jr, et al, "Prolonged Response to Carboplatin in an Infant With Brain Stem Glioma," *Cancer*, 1991, 67(1):43-7.

♦ **Cardec-S® Syrup** *see* Carbinoxamine and Pseudoephedrine *on page 169*

♦ **Cardioquin®** *see* Quinidine *on page 830*

♦ **Cardizem® CD** *see* Diltiazem *on page 323*

♦ **Cardizem® Injectable** *see* Diltiazem *on page 323*

♦ **Cardizem® SR** *see* Diltiazem *on page 323*

♦ **Cardizem® Tablet** *see* Diltiazem *on page 323*

♦ **Carindacillin** *see* Carbenicillin *on page 168*

Carmustine *(kar MUS teen)*

Related Information
Emetogenic Potential of Single Chemotherapeutic Agents *on page 1095*

Brand Names BiCNU®

Synonyms BCNU

Therapeutic Category Antineoplastic Agent, Alkylating Agent (Nitrosourea)

Generic Available No

Use Treatment of brain tumors, multiple myeloma, Hodgkin's disease, and non-Hodgkin's lymphomas; some activity in malignant melanoma, lung and colon cancer

Pregnancy Risk Factor D

Contraindications Hypersensitivity to carmustine or any component

Warnings The FDA currently recommends that procedures for proper handling and disposal of antineoplastic agents be considered. Bone marrow suppression, notably thrombocytopenia and leukopenia, may lead to bleeding and overwhelming infection in an already compromised patient; myelosuppressive effects will last for at least 6 weeks after a dose, do not give courses more frequently than every 6 weeks because the toxicity is cumulative; pulmonary toxicity is more common in patients receiving a cumulative dose >1400 mg/m^2, patients with recent mediastinal irradiation, and in patients with a past history of lung disease; acute leukemia has been reported in patients receiving long-term carmustine.

Precautions Administer with caution to patients with depressed platelet, leukocyte or erythrocyte counts and in patients with renal or hepatic impairment; dosage reduction is recommended in patients with compromised bone marrow function (decreased leukocyte and platelet counts)

Adverse Reactions
Cardiovascular: Flushing; high dose ($\geq$300 mg/m^2) can produce hypotension, tachycardia, and confusion

Central nervous system: Ataxia, dizziness

Dermatologic: Dermatitis, hyperpigmentation, alopecia

Gastrointestinal: Nausea, vomiting, diarrhea, esophagitis, anorexia, mucositis, metallic taste

Hematologic: Myelosuppression (leukopenia, thrombocytopenia) with nadir at 28 days, anemia

Hepatic: Hepatotoxicity, elevated liver enzymes and serum bilirubin, jaundice, veno-occlusive disease with high doses

Local: Pain and thrombophlebitis at injection site, burning sensation

Ocular: Retinitis, optic neuritis

Renal: Renal failure, azotemia

Respiratory: Pulmonary fibrosis, cough, dyspnea, tachypnea

Drug Interactions Cimetidine (potentiates myelosuppressive effects); may potentiate hepatotoxicity with high doses of acetaminophen; may decrease serum digoxin and phenytoin levels; metronidazole (disulfiram reaction)

Stability Store in refrigerator, protect from light and heat; discard vial if oily film is found on the bottom of the vial; reconstituted solution is stable for 8 hours at room temperature, 24 hours when refrigerated, or 48 hours when refrigerated after further dilution in D$_5$W or NS in a glass bottle to a concentration of 0.2 mg/mL;

incompatible with sodium bicarbonate; adsorption of carmustine to plastics and polyvinyl chloride-based infusion containers has been documented

Mechanism of Action Inhibits key enzymatic reactions involved with DNA synthesis; carbamoylation of amine groups on proteins; interferes with the normal function of DNA by alkylation and forms DNA-protein cross-links

Pharmacokinetics

Distribution: Readily crosses the blood-brain barrier since it is highly lipid soluble; CSF:plasma ratio >90%; distributes into breast milk

Protein binding: 75%

Metabolism: Denitrosation through action of microsomal enzymes; some enterohepatic circulation occurs

Half-life, terminal: 20-70 minutes (active metabolites may persist for days)

Elimination: ~60% to 70% excreted as metabolites in the urine and 6% to 10% excreted as CO_2 by the lungs

Usual Dosage I.V. infusion (refer to individual protocols):

Children: 200-250 mg/m^2 every 4-6 weeks as a single dose; next dose is to be determined based on clinical and hematologic response to the previous dose (a repeat course should not be given until platelets are >100,000/mm^3 and leukocytes are >4000/mm^3)

BMT-conditioning agent: 300-600 mg/m^2 over at least 2 hours or may be divided into 2 doses administered 12 hours apart

Adults: 150-200 mg/m^2 every 6 weeks as a single dose or divided into 75-100 mg/m^2/dose on 2 successive days; next dose is to be determined based on clinical and hematologic response to the previous dose (a repeat course should not be given until platelets are >100,000/mm^3 and leukocytes are >4000/mm^3)

Administration Parenteral: Further dilute the 3.3 mg of carmustine per mL solution with NS or D_5W in a glass or polyolefin container to a final concentration of 0.2-1 mg/mL and administer by I.V. infusion over 1-2 hours to prevent vein irritation; carmustine has also been administered over 15-45 minutes diluted in 100-250 mL D_5W with monitoring for vein irritation; burning sensation and pain at I.V. site can be decreased with reduction of infusion rate and further dilution of solution or placing ice pack on I.V. site; flush line before and after carmustine administration to ensure vein patency

Monitoring Parameters CBC with differential and platelet count; pulmonary function, liver function, and renal function tests

Patient Information Report occurrence of fever, sore throat, unusual bleeding or bruising to physician; may discolor skin brown

Nursing Implications Must administer in glass containers; do not mix or administer with solutions containing sodium bicarbonate; accidental skin contact may cause transient burning and brown discoloration of the skin

Additional Information Myelosuppressive effects:

WBC: Moderate (nadir: 5-6 weeks)

Platelets: Severe (nadir: 4-5 weeks)

Dosage Forms Powder for injection: 100 mg/vial packaged with 3 mL of absolute alcohol for use as a sterile diluent

References

Aronin PA, Mahaley MS Jr, Rudnick SA, et al, "Prediction of BCNU Pulmonary Toxicity in Patients With Malignant Gliomas," *N Engl J Med*, 1980, 303(4):183-8.

Colvin M, Hartner J and Summerfield M, "Stability of Carmustine in the Presence of Sodium Bicarbonate," *Am J Hosp Pharm*, 1980, 37(5):677-8.

O'Driscoll BR, Hasleton PS, Taylor PM, et al, "Active Lung Fibrosis Up to 17 Years After Chemotherapy With Carmustine (BCNU) in Childhood," *N Engl J Med*, 1990, 323(6):378-82.

Carnitine (KAR ni teen)

Related Information

Carbohydrate and Alcohol Content of Liquid Medications for Use in Patients Receiving Ketogenic Diets *on page 1228*

Brand Names Carnitor®; Vitacarn®

Synonyms L-carnitine; Levocarnitine

Therapeutic Category Nutritional Supplement

Generic Available Yes

Use Treatment of primary or secondary carnitine deficiency; prevention and treatment of carnitinic deficiency (injection) in patients undergoing dialysis for end stage renal disease (ESRD)

Pregnancy Risk Factor B

Precautions Use with caution in patients with seizure disorders; both new onset seizure activity and increased frequency of seizures have been reported

(Continued)

Carnitine *(Continued)*

Adverse Reactions

Central nervous system: Myasthenia (in uremic patients on D,L-carnitine not L-carnitine), dizziness, fever, depression, seizures

Gastrointestinal: Nausea, vomiting, abdominal cramps, diarrhea, gastritis

Neuromuscular & skeletal: Weakness, paresthesia

Miscellaneous: Body odor (dose-related), allergic reactions

Drug Interactions

Valproic acid, sodium benzoate; D,L-carnitine sold in health food stores as vitamin B_T, competitively inhibits L-carnitine

Stability

Protect from light

Mechanism of Action

Endogenous substance required in energy metabolism; facilitates long chain fatty acid entry into the mitochondria; modulates intracellular coenzyme A homeostasis; carnitine deficiency exists when there is insufficient carnitine to buffer toxic acyl-Co A compounds; secondary carnitine deficiency may be a consequence of inborn errors of metabolism

Pharmacokinetics

Metabolism: Major metabolites: Trimethylamine-N-oxide and acylcarnitine

Half-life, terminal: Adults: 17.4 hours

Bioavailability: 16%

Time to peak serum concentration: Oral: 3.3 hours

Elimination: Renal excretion of free and conjugated metabolites (acylcarnitine)

Usual Dosage

Primary carnitine deficiency:

Oral:

Children: 50-100 mg/kg/day divided 2-3 times/day, maximum 3 g/day; dosage must be individualized based upon patient response; higher dosages have been used

Adults: 330-990 mg/dose 2-3 times/day

I.V.: Children and Adults: 50 mg/kg as a loading dose, followed (in severe cases) by 50 mg/kg/day infusion; maintenance: 50 mg/kg/day divided every 4-6 hours, increase as needed to a maximum of 300 mg/kg/day

ESRD patients on hemodialysis: Adults: I.V.: Predialysis carnitine levels below normal (30-60 μmol): 10-20 mg/kg after each dialysis session; maintenance doses as low as 5 mg/kg may be used after 3-4 weeks of therapy depending upon response (carnitine level)

Supplement to parenteral nutrition: I.V.: Neonates: 10-20 mg/kg/day in parenteral nutrition solution

Administration

Oral: Dilute in beverages or liquid food; administer with meals; consume slowly

Parenteral: May be administered by direct I.V. infusion over 2-3 minutes or as a continuous infusion

Monitoring Parameters

Serum triglycerides, fatty acids, and carnitine levels

Reference Range

Plasma free carnitine level: >20 μmol/L; plasma total carnitine level 30-60 μmol/L; to evaluate for carnitine deficiency determine the plasma acylcarnitine/free carnitine ratio (A/F ratio)

A/F ratio = [plasma total carnitine - free carnitine] divided by free carnitine

Normal plasma A/F ratio = 0.25; in carnitine deficiency A/F ratio >0.4

Additional Information

Routine prophylactic use of carnitine in children receiving valproic acid to avoid carnitine deficiency and hepatotoxicity is probably not indicated

Dosage Forms

Capsule: 250 mg

Injection: 200 mg/mL (2.5 mL, 5 mL)

Liquid (cherry flavor): 100 mg/mL (10 mL)

Tablet: 330 mg

References

Bonner CM, De Brie KL, Hug G, et al, "Effects of Parenteral L-Carnitine Supplementation on Fat Metabolism and Nutrition in Premature Neonates," *J Pediatr*, 1995, 126(2):287-92.

Borum PR, "Carnitine in Neonatal Nutrition," *J Child Neurol*, 1995, 10(Suppl 2):S25-31.

Helms RA, Mauer EC, and Hay WW Jr, "Effect of Intravenous L-Carnitine on Growth Parameters and Fat Metabolism During Parenteral Nutrition in Neonates," *JPEN J Parenter Enteral Nutr*, 1990, 14(5):448-53.

♦ **Carnitor®** *see* Carnitine *on page 173*

♦ **Carter's Little Pills® [OTC]** *see* Bisacodyl *on page 133*

♦ **Casanthranol and Docusate** *see* Docusate and Casanthranol *on page 337*

Cascara Sagrada (kas KAR a sah GRAH dah)

Therapeutic Category Laxative, Stimulant
Generic Available Yes
Use Temporary relief of constipation; sometimes used with milk of magnesia ("black and white" mixture)
Pregnancy Risk Factor C
Contraindications Nausea, vomiting, abdominal pain, fecal impaction, intestinal obstruction, GI bleeding, appendicitis, CHF
Warnings Long-term use may result in laxative dependence
Adverse Reactions
  Cardiovascular: Faintness
  Endocrine & metabolic: Electrolyte and fluid imbalance
  Gastrointestinal: Abdominal cramps, nausea, diarrhea, benign pigmentation of the colonic mucosa (with prolonged use)
  Genitourinary: Discoloration of urine (reddish, pink, or brown)
Stability Protect from light and heat
Mechanism of Action Direct chemical irritation of the intestinal mucosa resulting in an increased rate of colonic motility and change in fluid and electrolyte secretion
Pharmacodynamics Onset of action: 6-10 hours
Pharmacokinetics
  Absorption: Oral: Small amount from small intestine
  Metabolism: In the liver
Usual Dosage Oral (**aromatic fluid extract**):
  Infants: 1.25 mL/day as a single dose (range: 0.5-2 mL) as needed
  Children 2-11 years: 2.5 mL/day as a single dose (range: 1-3 mL) as needed
  Children ≥12 years and Adults: 5 mL/day (range: 2-6 mL) as needed at bedtime
Administration Oral: Administer on an empty stomach; drink plenty of fluids
Patient Information Should not be used regularly for more than 1 week; may discolor urine reddish, pink, or brown
Additional Information Cascara sagrada fluid extract is 5 times more potent than cascara sagrada aromatic fluid extract
Dosage Forms
  Liquid, aromatic fluid extract: 5 mL, 120 mL, 473 mL
  Tablet: 325 mg

Castor Oil (KAS tor oyl)

Brand Names Alphamul® [OTC]; Emulsoil® [OTC]; Fleet® Flavored Castor Oil [OTC]; Neoloid® [OTC]; Purge® [OTC]
Synonyms Oleum Ricini
Therapeutic Category Laxative, Stimulant
Generic Available Yes
Use Preparation for rectal or bowel examination or surgery; rarely used to relieve constipation; also applied to skin as emollient and protectant
Pregnancy Risk Factor X
Contraindications Hypersensitivity to castor oil; nausea, vomiting, abdominal pain, fecal impaction, GI bleeding, appendicitis, CHF, menstruation, dehydration
Warnings Long-term use may result in laxative dependence
Adverse Reactions
  Central nervous system: Dizziness
  Endocrine & metabolic: Electrolyte disturbance, dehydration
  Gastrointestinal: Abdominal cramps, nausea, diarrhea
Stability Protect from heat (emulsion should be protected from freezing)
Mechanism of Action Acts primarily in the small intestine; hydrolyzed to ricinoleic acid which reduces net absorption of fluid and electrolytes and stimulates peristalsis
Pharmacodynamics Onset of action: Oral: Within 2-6 hours
Usual Dosage Oral:
  Castor oil:
    Infants <2 years: 1-5 mL or 15 mL/m^2/dose as a single dose
    Children 2-11 years: 5-15 mL as a single dose
    Children ≥12 years and Adults: 15-60 mL as a single dose
  Emulsified castor oil:
    Infants: 2.5-7.5 mL/dose
    Children:
      <2 years: 5-15 mL/dose
      2-11 years: 7.5-30 mL/dose
    Children ≥12 years and Adults: 30-60 mL/dose
(Continued)

Castor Oil (Continued)

Administration Oral: Do not administer at bedtime because of rapid onset of action; chill or administer with juice or carbonated beverage to improve palatability; administer on an empty stomach

Monitoring Parameters I & O, serum electrolytes, stool frequency

Dosage Forms
Emulsion, oral:
Alphamul®: 60% (90 mL, 3780 mL)
Emulsoil®: 95% (63 mL)
Fleet® Flavored Castor Oil: 67% (45 mL, 90 mL)
Neoloid®: 36.4% (118 mL)
Liquid, oral:
100% (60 mL, 120 mL, 480 mL)
Purge®: 95% (30 mL, 60 mL)

♦ **Cataflam® Oral** see Diclofenac on page 312
♦ **Catapres® Oral** see Clonidine on page 242
♦ **Catapres-TTS® Transdermal** see Clonidine on page 242
♦ **Causes of Neonatal Seizures** see page 1174
♦ **Caverject® Injection** see Alprostadil on page 51
♦ **CBDCA** see Carboplatin on page 170
♦ **CBZ** see Carbamazepine on page 165
♦ **CCNU** see Lomustine on page 578
♦ **C-Crystals® [OTC]** see Ascorbic Acid on page 96
♦ **2-CdA** see Cladribine on page 232
♦ **CDDP** see Cisplatin on page 229
♦ **Cebid®** see Ascorbic Acid on page 96
♦ **Ceclor®** see Cefaclor on page 176
♦ **Ceclor® CD** see Cefaclor on page 176
♦ **Cecon® [OTC]** see Ascorbic Acid on page 96
♦ **CeeNU®** see Lomustine on page 578

Cefaclor (SEF a klor)

Related Information
Carbohydrate and Alcohol Content of Liquid Medications for Use in Patients Receiving Ketogenic Diets on page 1228

Brand Names Ceclor®; Ceclor® CD

Therapeutic Category Antibiotic, Cephalosporin (Second Generation)

Generic Available Yes

Use Infections caused by susceptible organisms including *Staph aureus, S. pneumoniae,* and *H. influenzae*; treatment of otitis media, sinusitis, and infections involving the respiratory tract, skin and skin structure, bone and joint, and urinary tract

Pregnancy Risk Factor B

Contraindications Hypersensitivity to cefaclor, any component, or cephalosporins

Warnings Prolonged use may result in superinfection; do not use in patients with immediate-type hypersensitivity reactions to penicillin

Precautions Use with caution in patients with impaired renal function, history of colitis, or history of penicillin hypersensitivity; modify dosage in patients with severe renal impairment

Adverse Reactions
Dermatologic: Rash, urticaria, pruritus
Gastrointestinal: Nausea, vomiting, diarrhea
Hematologic: Eosinophilia, neutropenia
Hepatic: Elevated liver enzymes, cholestatic jaundice
Miscellaneous: Serum sickness-like reaction (estimated incidence ranges from 0.024% to 0.2% per drug course); majority of reactions have occurred in children <5 years of age with symptoms of rash and arthralgia, often occurring during the second or third exposure

Drug Interactions Probenecid (increased cefaclor concentration); magnesium- or aluminum-containing antacids administered with cefaclor extended-release tablet (decreased cefaclor absorption)

Food Interactions
Capsules and suspension: Food or milk delays and decreases peak concentration
Extended release tablets: Food increases extent of absorption and peak concentrations

Stability Refrigerate suspension after reconstitution; discard after 14 days

Mechanism of Action Inhibits bacterial cell wall synthesis by binding to one or more of the penicillin-binding proteins and interfering with the final transpeptidation step of peptidoglycan synthesis resulting in cell wall death

Pharmacokinetics
Absorption: Oral: Well absorbed; acid stable
Distribution: Distributes into tissues and fluids including bone, pleural and synovial fluid; crosses the placenta; appears in breast milk
Protein binding: 25%
Half-life: 30-60 minutes (prolonged with renal impairment)
Time to peak serum concentration:
Capsule: 60 minutes
Suspension: 45 minutes
Tablet, extended release: 1.5-2.7 hours
Elimination: Most of dose (80%) excreted unchanged in urine
Moderately dialyzable (20% to 50%)

Usual Dosage Oral:
Children >1 month: 20-40 mg/kg/day divided every 8-12 hours; maximum dose: 2 g/day (twice daily option is for treatment of otitis media or pharyngitis)
Adults: 250-500 mg every 8 hours or daily dose can be given in 2 divided doses (twice daily option is for treatment of otitis media or pharyngitis)
Acute bronchitis: 500 mg extended release tablet every 12 hours for 7 days
Pharyngitis and/or tonsillitis: 375 mg extended release tablet every 12 hours for 10 days
Uncomplicated skin and skin structure infection: 375 mg extended release tablet every 12 hours for 7-10 days
Dosing adjustment in renal impairment: Cl_{cr} <10 mL//minute: Administer 50% of dose

Administration Oral:
Capsule, suspension: Administer 1 hour before or 2 hours after a meal; shake suspension well before use
Extended release tablet: Administer with food; do not crush, cut, or chew tablet

Monitoring Parameters With prolonged therapy, monitor CBC and stool frequency periodically

Test Interactions Positive Coombs' [direct], false-positive urine glucose (Clinitest®), false ↑ of serum or urine creatinine

Dosage Forms
Capsule: 250 mg, 500 mg
Powder for oral suspension (strawberry flavor): 125 mg/5 mL (75 mL, 150 mL); 187 mg/5 mL (50 mL, 100 mL); 250 mg/5 mL (75 mL, 150 mL); 375 mg/5 mL (50 mL, 100 mL)
Tablet, extended release: 375 mg, 500 mg

References
Boguniewicz M and Leung DYM, "Hypersensitivity Reactions to Antibiotics Commonly Used in Children," *Pediatr Infect Dis J*, 1995, 14(3):221-31.
Hyslop DL, "Cefaclor Safety Profile: A Ten Year Review," *Clin Ther*, 1988, 11(Suppl A):83-94.
Levine LR, "Quantitative Comparison of Adverse Reactions to Cefaclor vs Amoxicillin in a Surveillance Study," *Pediatr Infect Dis*, 1985, 4(4):358-61.

Cefadroxil Monohydrate (sef a DROKS il mon o HYE drate)

Related Information
Carbohydrate and Alcohol Content of Liquid Medications for Use in Patients Receiving Ketogenic Diets *on page 1228*

Brand Names Duricef®; Ultracef®

Therapeutic Category Antibiotic, Cephalosporin (First Generation)

Generic Available Yes

Use Treatment of susceptible bacterial infections including group A beta-hemolytic streptococcal pharyngitis or tonsillitis; skin and soft tissue infections caused by streptococci or staphylococci; urinary tract infections caused by *Klebsiella*, *E. coli*, and *Proteus mirabilis*

Pregnancy Risk Factor B

Contraindications Hypersensitivity to cefadroxil, any component, or cephalosporins

Warnings Prolonged use may result in superinfection; do not use in patients with immediate-type hypersensitivity reaction to penicillin

Precautions Use with caution in patients who are hypersensitive to penicillin; modify dosage in patients with renal impairment

Adverse Reactions
Dermatologic: Rash
(Continued)

Cefadroxil Monohydrate *(Continued)*

Gastrointestinal: Nausea, vomiting, diarrhea, pseudomembranous colitis
Genitourinary: Vaginitis
Hematologic: Positive Coombs' test, transient neutropenia

Drug Interactions Probenecid may decrease renal tubular secretion and increase cefadroxil serum concentrations

Food Interactions Concomitant administration with food, infant formula, or cow's milk does **not** significantly affect absorption

Stability Refrigerate suspension after reconstitution; discard after 14 days

Mechanism of Action Interferes with bacterial cell wall synthesis during active replication, causing cell wall death and resultant bactericidal activity against susceptible bacteria

Pharmacokinetics
Absorption: Oral: Rapid; well absorbed from GI tract
Distribution: V_d: 0.31 L/kg; crosses the placenta; appears in breast milk
Protein binding: 20%
Half-life: 1-2 hours; 20-24 hours in renal failure
Time to peak serum concentration: Within 70-90 minutes
Elimination: >90% of dose excreted unchanged in urine within 24 hours

Usual Dosage Oral:
Infants and Children: 30 mg/kg/day divided twice daily up to a maximum of 2 g/day
Adolescents and Adults: 1-2 g/day in 1-2 divided doses; maximum dose for adults: 4 g/day

Dosing interval in renal impairment:
Cl_{cr} 10-25 mL/minute: Administer every 24 hours
Cl_{cr} <10 mL/minute: Administer every 36 hours

Administration Oral: May be administered without regard to food; administration with food may decrease nausea or vomiting; shake suspension well before use

Monitoring Parameters Stool frequency, resolution of infection

Test Interactions False-positive with urinary glucose tests using cupric sulfate (Clinitest®, Benedict's solution)

Patient Information Report persistent diarrhea; entire course of medication (eg, 10-14 days) should be taken to ensure eradication of organism

Dosage Forms
Capsule: 500 mg
Powder for oral suspension: 125 mg/5 mL (50 mL, 100 mL); 250 mg/5 mL (50 mL, 100 mL); 500 mg/5 mL (50 mL, 100 mL)
Tablet: 1 g

♦ **Cefadyl®** see Cephapirin *on page 198*
♦ **Cefanex®** see Cephalexin *on page 196*

Cefazolin (sef A zoe lin)

Related Information
Endocarditis Prophylaxis *on page 1127*
Brand Names Ancef®; Kefzol®; Zolicef®
Available Salts Cefazolin Sodium
Therapeutic Category Antibiotic, Cephalosporin (First Generation)
Generic Available Yes

Use Treatment of respiratory tract, skin and skin structure, urinary tract, biliary tract, bone and joint infections and septicemia due to susceptible gram-positive cocci (except enterococcus); some gram-negative bacilli including *E. coli*, *Proteus*, and *Klebsiella* may be susceptible; perioperative prophylaxis; bacterial endocarditis prophylaxis for dental and upper respiratory procedures

Pregnancy Risk Factor B

Contraindications Hypersensitivity to cefazolin sodium, any component, or cephalosporins

Warnings Prolonged use may result in superinfection; do not use in patients with immediate-type hypersensitivity reactions to penicillin

Precautions Use with caution in patients with a history of colitis or in patients with a history of hypersensitivity to penicillins; modify dosage in patients with renal impairment

Adverse Reactions
Central nervous system: Fever, CNS irritation, seizures
Dermatologic: Rash, urticaria
Hematologic: Leukopenia, thrombocytopenia
Hepatic: Transient elevation of liver enzymes

Local: Thrombophlebitis

Drug Interactions Probenecid may decrease renal tubular secretion and increase cefazolin serum concentrations; nephrotoxic agents

Stability Reconstituted solution is stable for 24 hours at room temperature or 96 hours when refrigerated; thawed solutions of the commercially available frozen cefazolin injections are stable for 48 hours at room temperature or 10 days when refrigerated

Mechanism of Action Inhibits bacterial cell wall synthesis by binding to one or more of the penicillin-binding proteins and interfering with the final transpeptidation step of peptidoglycan synthesis resulting in cell wall death

Pharmacokinetics

Distribution: Crosses the placenta; small amounts appear in breast milk; CSF penetration is poor; penetrates bone and synovial fluid well; distributes into bile

Protein binding: 74% to 86%

Metabolism: Hepatic is minimal

Half-life:

Neonates: 3-5 hours

Adults: 90-150 minutes (prolonged with renal impairment)

Time to peak serum concentration:

I.M.: Within 0.5-2 hours

I.V.: Within 5 minutes

Elimination: 80% to 100% excreted unchanged in urine

Moderately dialyzable (20% to 50%)

Usual Dosage I.M., I.V.:

Neonates:

Postnatal age ≤7 days: 40 mg/kg/day divided every 12 hours

Postnatal age >7 days:

≤2000 g: 40 mg/kg/day divided every 12 hours

>2000 g: 60 mg/kg/day divided every 8 hours

Infants and Children: 50-100 mg/kg/day divided every 8 hours; maximum dose: 6 g/day

Bacterial endocarditis prophylaxis for dental and upper respiratory procedures in penicillin allergic patients (see Precautions): 25 mg/kg 30 minutes before procedure; maximum dose: 1 g

Adults: 0.5-2 g every 6-8 hours; maximum dose: 12 g/day

Bacterial endocarditis prophylaxis for dental and upper respiratory procedures in penicillin allergic patients (see Precautions): 1 g 30 minutes before procedure

Perioperative prophylaxis: 1 g 30-60 minutes prior to surgery; 0.5-1 g every 8 hours for 24 hours postoperatively depending on the procedure

Dosing interval in renal impairment:

Cl_{cr} 10-30 mL/minute: Administer every 12 hours

Cl_{cr} <10 mL/minute: Administer every 24 hours

Administration Parenteral: Cefazolin may be administered IVP over 3-5 minutes at a maximum concentration of 100 mg/mL or I.V. intermittent infusion over 10-60 minutes at a final concentration for I.V. administration of 20 mg/mL. In fluid-restricted patients, a concentration of 138 mg/mL has been administered IVP.

Monitoring Parameters Renal function periodically when used in combination with other nephrotoxic drugs, hepatic function tests, and CBC

Test Interactions False-positive urine glucose using Clinitest®, positive Coombs' [direct], false ↑ serum or urine creatinine

Additional Information Sodium content of 1 g: 2 mEq

Dosage Forms

Infusion, premixed, as sodium, in D5W (frozen) (Ancef®): 500 mg (50 mL); 1 g (50 mL)

Injection, as sodium (Kefzol®): 500 mg, 1 g

Powder for injection, as sodium (Ancef®, Zolicef®): 250 mg, 500 mg, 1 g, 5 g, 10 g, 20 g

References

Dajani AS, Taubert KA, Wilson WW, et al, "Prevention of Bacterial Endocarditis. Recommendations by the American Heart Association," *JAMA*, 1997, 277(22):1794-801.

Pickering LK, O'Connor DM, Anderson D, et al, "Clinical and Pharmacologic Evaluation of Cefazolin in Children," *J Infect Dis* 1973, 128(Suppl):S407-1.

Robinson DC, Cookson TL, and Grisafe JA, "Concentration Guidelines for Parenteral Antibiotics in Fluid-Restricted Patients," *Drug Intell Clin Pharm*, 1987, 21(12):985-9.

♦ **Cefazolin Sodium** see Cefazolin *on page 178*

Cefepime (SEF e pim)

Brand Names Maxipime®

Available Salts Cefepime Hydrochloride

(Continued)

Cefepime *(Continued)*

Therapeutic Category Antibiotic, Cephalosporin (Fourth Generation)

Use Treatment of lower respiratory tract infections, cellulitis, other skin and soft tissue infections, and urinary tract infections; empiric monotherapy in febrile neutropenia; considered a fourth generation cephalosporin because it is active against aerobic gram-negative bacteria, including *Pseudomonas aeruginosa*, active against some gram-negative bacteria that are resistant to third-generation cephalosporins, and more active than third-generation cephalosporins against gram-positive bacteria such as *Staphylococcus aureus*

Pregnancy Risk Factor B

Contraindications Hypersensitivity to cefepime, any component, or cephalosporins

Warnings Modify dosage in patients with severe renal impairment; prolonged use may result in superinfection; use with caution in patients with penicillin hypersensitivity; do not use in patients with immediate-type hypersensitivity reactions to penicillin

Adverse Reactions

Central nervous system: Headache, lightheadedness, fever, encephalopathy

Dermatologic: Maculopapular rash, pruritus, urticaria

Gastrointestinal: Dyspepsia, diarrhea, nausea, vomiting, pseudomembranous colitis

Hematologic: Neutropenia after extended therapy, transient leukopenia and thrombocytopenia

Hepatic: Transient elevations in LFTs

Local: Phlebitis

Ocular: Blurred vision

Renal: Elevated BUN, elevated serum creatinine

Miscellaneous: Anaphylaxis

Drug Interactions Probenecid decreases the clearance of cefepime; aminoglycosides increase nephrotoxic potential

Stability Store vial at room temperature and protect from light; incompatible with metronidazole, vancomycin, aminoglycosides, and aminophylline

Mechanism of Action Inhibits bacterial cell wall synthesis by binding to one or more of the penicillin-binding proteins; inhibits the final transpeptidation step of peptidoglycan synthesis in bacterial cell walls

Pharmacokinetics

Distribution: V_d:

Children (2 months to 6 years): 0.32-0.35 L/kg

Adults: 14-20 L; penetrates into inflammatory fluid at concentrations ~80% of serum levels and into bronchial mucosa at levels ~60% of plasma levels; excreted in breast milk at very low concentrations

Protein binding: 16% to 19%

Metabolism: Very little

Half-life:

Children 2 months to 6 years: 1.77-1.96 hours

Adults: 2 hours

Elimination: At least 85% eliminated as unchanged drug in urine

Dialysis: 45% to 68% removed by hemodialysis

Administration Cefepime may be administered by I.V. intermittent infusion over 20-30 minutes; final concentration for I.V. administration should not exceed 40 mg/mL in D_5W, NS, $D_{10}W$, D_5W in 0.9% NaCl, or D_5LR; in clinical trials, cefepime was administered by direct I.V. injection over 3-5 minutes at a final concentration of 100 mg/mL for mild to moderate infections

Usual Dosage I.M., I.V.:

Children 2 months to 16 years, ≤40 kg in weight: 50 mg/kg/dose every 12 hours

Febrile neutropenic patients: 50 mg/kg/dose every 8 hours

Cefepime has been studied in 12 cystic fibrosis patients (ages 4-41 years) with bronchopulmonary infection at a dose of 50 mg/kg/dose every 8 hours (maximum dose: 2 g/dose every 8 hours); cefepime was as effective as cefotaxime in 90 children <15 years of age who were randomized to receive cefepime 50 mg/kg/dose every 8 hours (n=43) or cefotaxime 50 mg/kg/dose every 6 hours (n=47) for the treatment of bacterial meningitis

Adults: 1-2 g every 12 hours; high doses or more frequent administration may be required in pseudomonal infections

UTIs: 500 mg every 12 hours

Empiric monotherapy in febrile neutropenia: 2 g every 8 hours

Dosing Adjustment in Renal Impairment, Adults

Cl$_{cr}$ (mL/min)	Infection		
	Mild to Moderate	Moderate to Severe	Severe
30-60	0.5-1 g I.M./I.V. every 24 hours	1-2 g I.V. every 24 hours	2 g I.V. every 24 hours
11-29	0.5 g I.M./I.V. every 24 hours	0.5-1 g I.V. every 24 hours	1 g I.V. every 24 hours
≤10	0.25 g I.M./I.V. every 24 hours	0.25-0.5 g I.V. every 24 hours	0.5 g I.V. every 24 hours

Monitoring Parameters With prolonged therapy, monitor renal and hepatic function periodically; number and type of stools/day for diarrhea; CBC with differential

Test Interactions Positive Coombs' [direct]; may falsely elevate creatinine values when Jaffé reaction is used; may cause false-positive results in urine glucose tests when using Clinitest®; false-positive urinary proteins and steroids

Patient Information Report side effects such as diarrhea, dyspepsia, headache, blurred vision, and lightheadedness to your physician

Nursing Implications Do not admix with aminoglycosides

Dosage Forms Powder for injection, as hydrochloride: 500 mg, 1 g, 2 g

References

Arguedas AG, Stutman HR, Zaleska M, et al, "Cefepime. Pharmacokinetics and Clinical Response in Patients With Cystic Fibrosis," *Am J Dis Child*, 1992, 146(7):797-802.

Blumer JL, Reed MD, Lemon E, et al, "Pharmacokinetics (PK) of Cefepime in Pediatric Patients Administered Single and Multiple 50 mg/kg Doses Every 8 Hours by the Intravenous (I.V.) or Intramuscular (I.M.) Route," 34th Interscience Conference on Antimicrobial Agents and Chemotherapy, 1994, Orlando, Fl. Abs. A69.

Saez-Llorens X, Castano E, Garcia R, et al, "Prospective Randomized Comparison of Cefepime and Cefotaxime for Treatment of Bacterial Meningitis in Infants and Children", *Antimicrob Agents Chemother*, 1995, 39(4):937-40.

Wynd MA and Paladino JA, "Cefepime: A Fourth-Generation Parenteral Cephalosporin," *Ann Pharmacother*, 1996, 30(12):1414-24.

♦ **Cefepime Hydrochloride** see Cefepime on page 179

Cefixime (sef IKS eem)

Brand Names Suprax®

Therapeutic Category Antibiotic, Cephalosporin (Third Generation)

Generic Available No

Use Treatment of urinary tract infections, otitis media, respiratory infections due to susceptible organisms including *S. pneumoniae* and *pyogenes, H. influenzae, M. catarrhalis*, and many *Enterobacteriaceae*; documented poor compliance with other oral antimicrobials; outpatient therapy of serious soft tissue or skeletal infections due to susceptible organisms; single-dose oral treatment of uncomplicated cervical/urethral gonorrhea due to *N. gonorrhoeae*; treatment of shigellosis in areas with a high rate of resistance to TMP-SMX

Pregnancy Risk Factor B

Contraindications Hypersensitivity to cefixime, any component, or cephalosporins

Warnings Prolonged use may result in superinfection; do not use in patients with immediate-type hypersensitivity reactions to penicillin

Precautions Use with caution in patients hypersensitive to penicillin, patients with impaired renal function, and patients with a history of colitis; modify dosage in patients with renal impairment

Adverse Reactions

Central nervous system: Headache, fever, dizziness, fatigue

Dermatologic: Skin rash, urticaria, pruritus

Gastrointestinal: Nausea, diarrhea (up to 15% of children), abdominal pain, pseudomembranous colitis

Genitourinary: Vaginitis

Hematologic: Eosinophilia, thrombocytopenia, leukopenia

Hepatic: Transient elevation of liver enzymes

Renal: Transient elevation of BUN and serum creatinine

Drug Interactions Probenecid (increases cefixime concentration); cefixime may increase carbamazepine serum concentrations

Food Interactions Presence of food delays the time to reach peak concentrations

Stability After reconstitution, suspension may be stored for 14 days at room temperature

(Continued)

Cefixime (Continued)

Mechanism of Action Inhibits bacterial cell wall synthesis by binding to one or more of the penicillin-binding proteins; inhibits the final transpeptidation step of peptidoglycan synthesis resulting in cell wall death

Pharmacokinetics
Absorption: Oral: 40% to 50%

Distribution: Into bile, sputum, middle ear discharge; crosses the placenta

Protein binding: 65%

Half-life:
Normal renal function: 3-4 hours
Renal failure: Up to 11.5 hours

Time to peak serum concentration: Within 2-6 hours; peak serum concentrations are 15% to 50% higher for the oral suspension versus tablets

Elimination: 50% of absorbed dose excreted as active drug in urine and 10% in bile

Dialysis: 10% removed by hemodialysis

Usual Dosage Oral:
Infants and Children: 8 mg/kg/day divided every 12-24 hours; maximum dose: 400 mg/day

Treatment of acute UTI: 16 mg/kg/day divided every 12 hours on day 1, then 8 mg/kg/day every 24 hours for 13 days

Prophylaxis after sexual victimization: 8 mg/kg in a single dose (maximum dose: 400 mg) **plus** azithromycin 20 mg/kg in a single dose (maximum dose: 1 g); also begin or complete hepatitis B virus immunization and consider prophylaxis for trichomoniasis and bacterial vaginosis

Adolescents and Adults: 400 mg/day divided every 12-24 hours

Uncomplicated cervical/urethral gonorrhea due to *N. gonorrhoeae*: 400 mg as a single dose plus azithromycin 1 g orally in a single dose **or** doxycycline 100 mg orally twice daily for 7 days

Prophylaxis after sexual victimization: 400 mg in a single dose **plus** azithromycin 1 g orally in a single dose **or** doxycycline 100 mg orally twice daily for 7 days **plus** metronidazole 2 g orally in a single dose **plus** hepatitis B virus immunization if not fully immunized plus consider prophylaxis for HIV depending on circumstances

Dosing adjustment in renal impairment:
Cl_{cr} 21-60 mL/minute: Administer 75% of the standard dose

Cl_{cr} <20 mL/minute: Administer 50% of the standard dose

Administration Oral: May be administered with or without food; administer with food to decrease GI distress; shake suspension well before use

Monitoring Parameters With prolonged therapy, monitor renal and hepatic function periodically; number and type of stools/day for diarrhea

Test Interactions False-positive reaction for urine glucose using Clinitest®; false-positive urine ketones using tests with nitroprusside

Patient Information Report problems with diarrhea

Additional Information Otitis media should be treated with the suspension since it results in higher peak blood levels than the tablet

Dosage Forms
Powder for oral suspension (strawberry flavor): 100 mg/5 mL (50 mL, 100 mL)

Tablet, film coated: 200 mg, 400 mg

References
Ashkenazi S, Amir J, Waisman Y, et al, "A Randomized, Double-Blind Study Comparing Cefixime and Trimethoprim-Sulfamethoxazole in the Treatment of Childhood Shigellosis," *J Pediatr*, 1993, 123(5):817-21.

"1998 Guidelines for the Treatment of Sexually Transmitted Diseases. Centers for Disease Control and Prevention," *MMWR Morb Mortal Wkly Rep*, 1998, 47(RR-1):1-111.

Hoberman A, Wald ER, Hickey RW, et al, "Oral Versus Initial Intravenous Therapy for Urinary Tract Infections in Young Febrile Children," *Pediatrics*, 1999, 104(1 Pt 1):79-86.

Johnson CE, Carlin SA, Super DM, et al, "Cefixime Compared With Amoxicillin for Treatment of Acute Otitis Media," *J Pediatr*, 1991, 119(1):117-22.

♦ **Cefizox®** see Ceftizoxime *on page 191*
♦ **Cefobid®** see Cefoperazone *on page 182*

Cefoperazone (sef oh PER a zone)

Brand Names Cefobid®

Available Salts Cefoperazone Sodium

Therapeutic Category Antibiotic, Cephalosporin (Third Generation)

Generic Available No

Use Treatment of susceptible bacterial infections, mainly respiratory tract, skin and skin structure, urinary tract and sepsis; as a third generation cephalosporin, cefoperazone has activity against gram-negative bacilli (eg, *E. coli*, *Klebsiella*, and

Haemophilus) but variable activity against *Streptococcus* and *Staphylococcus* species; it has activity against *Pseudomonas aeruginosa*, but less than ceftazidime

Pregnancy Risk Factor B

Contraindications Hypersensitivity to cefoperazone, any component, or cephalosporins

Warnings Modify dosage in patients who have both severe renal impairment and hepatic dysfunction; prolonged use may result in superinfection; do not use in patients with immediate-type hypersensitivity reactions to penicillin

Precautions Use with caution in patients who are hypersensitive to penicillins

Adverse Reactions
  Dermatologic: Rash
  Gastrointestinal: Nausea, vomiting, diarrhea, pseudomembranous colitis
  Hematologic: Bleeding, bruising, positive Coombs' test
  Local: Pain and induration at I.M. injection site, phlebitis

Drug Interactions Disulfiram-like reaction may occur if taken with alcohol; concomitant use of anticoagulants or other agents that affect blood clotting may increase the risk of severe hemorrhage

Food Interactions Cefoperazone may decrease vitamin K synthesis by suppressing GI flora; vitamin K deficiency may occur and result in an increased risk of hemorrhage; patients at risk include those with malabsorption states (eg, cystic fibrosis) or poor nutritional status; monitor prothrombin time and administer vitamin K as needed

Stability Reconstituted solution and I.V. infusion in NS or D_5W are stable for 24 hours at room temperature, 5 days when refrigerated or 3 weeks when frozen; after freezing, thawed solution is stable for 48 hours at room temperature or 10 days when refrigerated; do not refreeze, do not mix in same bag with aminoglycosides

Mechanism of Action Interferes with bacterial cell wall synthesis during active replication, causing cell wall death and resultant bactericidal activity against susceptible bacteria

Pharmacokinetics
  Half-life:
    Neonates (low birth weight): 6-10 hours
    Adults: 2 hours; half-life increases with hepatic disease or biliary obstruction
  Time to peak serum concentration:
    I.M.: Within 1-2 hours
    I.V.: Within 15-20 minutes (serum levels 2-3 times the serum levels following I.M. administration)
  Elimination: Excreted primarily in the bile (70% to 75%); 20% to 30% recovered unchanged in urine within 12 hours

Usual Dosage I.M., I.V.:
  Neonates: 50 mg/kg/dose every 12 hours
  Infants and Children: 100-150 mg/kg/day divided every 8-12 hours; up to 12 g/day
  Adults: 2-4 g/day in divided doses every 12 hours; maximum dose: 12 g/day divided every 6-12 hours; 16 g/day has been given via continuous infusion to severely immunocompromised patients
    Maximum dose with impaired hepatic function and/or biliary obstruction: 4 g/day
    Maximum dose with combined hepatic and renal dysfunction: 1-2 g/day

Administration Parenteral:
  I.M.: For concentrations >250 mg/mL, may dilute with lidocaine at a final concentration of 0.5%
  Intermittent I.V.: Administer over 15-30 minutes at a maximum concentration of 50 mg/mL
  I.V. continuous infusion: Infuse at a concentration of 2-25 mg/mL

Monitoring Parameters Prothrombin time; number and type of stools/day for diarrhea; resolution of infection

Test Interactions False-positive with urinary glucose tests using cupric sulfate (Clinitest®, Benedict's solution)

Patient Information Avoid alcohol

Nursing Implications Monitor for coagulation abnormalities and diarrhea

Additional Information Sodium content of 1 g cefoperazone sodium: 1.5 mEq (34 mg); chemical structure contains the N-methylthiotetrazole side chain which may be responsible for the increased risk of bleeding and the disulfiram-like reaction with alcohol

Dosage Forms
  Injection, as sodium, premixed (frozen): 1 g (50 mL); 2 g (50 mL)
  Powder for injection, as sodium: 1 g, 2 g

♦ **Cefoperazone Sodium** see Cefoperazone on page 182

CEFOTAXIME

♦ **Cefotan®** see Cefotetan *on page 185*

Cefotaxime (sef oh TAKS eem)
Brand Names Claforan®
Available Salts Cefotaxime Sodium
Therapeutic Category Antibiotic, Cephalosporin (Third Generation)
Generic Available No
Use Treatment of susceptible lower respiratory tract, skin and skin structure, bone and joint, intra-abdominal and genitourinary tract infections; treatment of a documented or suspected meningitis due to susceptible organisms such as *H. influenzae* and *N. meningitidis*; indicated for *Neisseria gonorrhoeae* infections (including uncomplicated cervical and urethral gonorrhea and gonorrhea pelvic inflammatory disease); nonpseudomonal gram-negative rod infection in a patient at risk of developing aminoglycoside-induced nephrotoxicity and/or ototoxicity; infection due to an organism whose susceptibilities clearly favor cefotaxime over cefuroxime or an aminoglycoside
Pregnancy Risk Factor B
Contraindications Hypersensitivity to cefotaxime, any component, or cephalosporins
Warnings Prolonged use may result in superinfection; do not use in patients with immediate-type hypersensitivity reactions to penicillin
Precautions Use with caution in patients with history of penicillin hypersensitivity, impaired renal function, or history of colitis; modify dosage in patients with Cl_{cr} <20 mL/minute
Adverse Reactions
  Central nervous system: Fever, headache
  Dermatologic: Rash, pruritus
  Gastrointestinal: Antibiotic-associated pseudomembranous colitis, diarrhea, nausea, vomiting
  Hematologic: Transient neutropenia, thrombocytopenia, eosinophilia, leukopenia
  Hepatic: Transient elevation of liver enzymes
  Local: Phlebitis, pain at injection site
  Renal: Transient elevation of BUN and serum creatinine
Drug Interactions Probenecid (increases cefotaxime concentration)
Stability Reconstituted solution is stable for 24 hours at room temperature and 10 days when refrigerated
Mechanism of Action Inhibits bacterial cell wall synthesis by binding to one or more of the penicillin-binding proteins; inhibits the final transpeptidation step of peptidoglycan synthesis resulting in cell wall death
Pharmacokinetics
  Distribution: Into bronchial secretions, middle ear effusions, bone, bile; penetration into CSF when meninges are inflamed; crosses the placenta; appears in breast milk
  Protein binding: 31% to 50%
  Metabolism: Partially metabolized in the liver to active metabolite, desacetylcefotaxime
  Half-life:
    Cefotaxime:
      Neonates, premature: <1 week: 5-6 hours
      Neonates, full-term: <1 week: 2-3.4 hours; 1-4 weeks: 2 hours
      Children: 1.5 hours
      Adults: 1-1.5 hours (prolonged with renal and/or hepatic impairment)
      Desacetylcefotaxime: Adults: 1.5-1.9 hours (prolonged with renal impairment)
  Time to peak serum concentration: I.M.: Within 30 minutes
  Elimination: 40% to 60% of a dose excreted as unchanged drug and 24% excreted as desacetylcefotaxime in the urine
  Moderately dialyzable (20% to 50%)
Usual Dosage I.M., I.V.:
  Neonates: 0-4 weeks: <1200 g: 100 mg/kg/day divided every 12 hours
  Postnatal age ≤7 days:
    1200-2000 g: 100 mg/kg/day divided every 12 hours
    >2000 g: 100-150 mg/kg/day divided every 8-12 hours
  Postnatal age >7 days:
    1200-2000 g: 150 mg/kg/day divided every 8 hours
    >2000 g: 150-200 mg/kg/day divided every 6-8 hours
  Infants and Children 1 month to 12 years:
    <50 kg: 100-200 mg/kg/day divided every 6-8 hours

Meningitis: 200 mg/kg/day divided every 6 hours; 225-300 mg/kg/day divided every 6-8 hours has been used to treat invasive pneumococcal meningitis

≥50 kg: Moderate to severe infection: 1-2 g every 6-8 hours; life-threatening infection: 2 g/dose every 4 hours; maximum dose: 12 g/day

Children >12 years and Adults: 1-2 g every 6-8 hours (up to 12 g/day)

Dosing adjustment in renal impairment: Cl_{cr} <20 mL/minute: Reduce dose by 50%

Administration Parenteral: Cefotaxime may be administered IVP over 3-5 minutes at a maximum concentration of 100 mg/mL or I.V. intermittent infusion over 15-30 minutes at a final concentration for I.V. administration of 20-60 mg/mL; in fluid-restricted patients, a concentration of 150 mg/mL may be administered IVP

Monitoring Parameters With prolonged therapy, monitor renal, hepatic, and hematologic function periodically; number and type of stools/day for diarrhea

Test Interactions Positive Coombs' [direct]

Additional Information Sodium content of 1 g: 2.2 mEq

Dosage Forms

Infusion, as sodium, premixed, in D_5W (frozen): 1 g (50 mL); 2 g (50 mL)

Powder for injection, as sodium: 500 mg, 1 g, 2 g, 10 g

References

Spritzer R, Kamp HJ, Dzoljic G, et al, "Five Years of Cefotaxime Use in a Neonatal Intensive Care Unit," Pediatr Infect Dis J, 1990, 9(2):92-6.

♦ **Cefotaxime Sodium** see Cefotaxime on page 184

Cefotetan (SEF oh tee tan)

Brand Names Cefotan®

Available Salts Cefotetan Disodium

Therapeutic Category Antibiotic, Cephalosporin (Second Generation)

Generic Available No

Use Treatment of susceptible lower respiratory tract, skin and skin structure, bone and joint, genitourinary tract, sepsis, gynecologic, and intra-abdominal infections; active against anaerobes including *Bacteroides* species of gastrointestinal tract, gram-negative enteric bacilli including *E. coli*, *Klebsiella*, and *Proteus*; active against many strains of *N. gonorrhoeae*; perioperative prophylaxis

Pregnancy Risk Factor B

Contraindications Hypersensitivity to cefotetan, any component, or cephalosporins

Warnings Prolonged use may result in superinfection; do not use in patients with immediate-type hypersensitivity reactions to penicillin

Precautions Use with caution and modify dosage in patients with renal impairment; use with caution in patients with history of colitis or penicillin hypersensitivity

Adverse Reactions

Central nervous system: Seizures, fever

Dermatologic: Rash, pruritus, urticaria

Gastrointestinal: Diarrhea, nausea, vomiting, pseudomembranous colitis

Hematologic: Neutropenia, leukopenia, thrombocytopenia, hemolytic anemia, bleeding, prolongation of PT

Hepatic: Elevated serum AST, ALT, alkaline phosphatase, LDH

Local: Phlebitis, pain at the injection site, edema

Renal: Elevated BUN, elevated serum creatinine

Drug Interactions Alcohol (disulfiram-like reaction), anticoagulants (may increase the risk of hemorrhage)

Stability Reconstituted solution is stable for 24 hours at room temperature and 96 hours when refrigerated; thawed solutions of the commercially available frozen cefotetan injections are stable for 48 hours at room temperature or 21 days when refrigerated; do not refreeze; incompatible with aminoglycosides, heparin, and tetracycline

Mechanism of Action Inhibits bacterial cell wall synthesis by binding to one or more of the penicillin-binding proteins; inhibits the final transpeptidation step of peptidoglycan synthesis resulting in cell wall death

Pharmacokinetics

Absorption: I.M.: Completely absorbed

Distribution: Distributes into tissues and fluids including gallbladder, kidney, skin, tonsils, uterus, sputum, prostatic and peritoneal fluids; poor penetration into CSF; cross the placenta; small amounts appear in breast milk

Protein binding: 76% to 91%

Half-life: 3.5 hours, prolonged in patients with impaired renal function (up to 10 hours)

Time to peak serum concentration: I.M.: Within 1.5-3 hours

(Continued)

Cefotetan *(Continued)*

Elimination: 49% to 81% excreted as unchanged drug in urine, 20% of dose is excreted in bile
<10% removed by hemodialysis

Usual Dosage I.M., I.V.: Not FDA approved for children
Children: 40-80 mg/kg/day divided every 12 hours; up to 6 g/day
Adolescents and Adults: 2-4 g/day divided every 12 hours; maximum dose: 6 g/day
Urinary tract infections: 1-2 g/day every 12-24 hours
Perioperative prophylaxis: I.V.: 1-2 g 30-60 minutes prior to procedure
Pelvic inflammatory disease: I.V.: 2 g every 12 hours continued for 24-48 hours after significant clinical improvement is demonstrated **plus** doxycycline 100 mg I.V. or orally every 12 hours for 14 days

Dosing interval in renal impairment:
Cl_{cr} 10-30 mL/minute: Administer every 24 hours
Cl_{cr} <10 mL/minute: Administer every 48 hours

Administration Parenteral:
IVP: Administer over 3-5 minutes at a maximum concentration of 100 mg/mL
I.V. intermittent: Infuse over 20-60 minutes at a concentration of 10-40 mg/mL

Monitoring Parameters Prothrombin time, renal function tests; number and type of stools/day for diarrhea

Test Interactions Positive Coombs' [direct], false-positive urine glucose (Clinitest®), falsely elevated serum or urinary creatinine (Jaffé reaction)

Patient Information Avoid alcohol

Additional Information Sodium content of 1 g: 3.5 mEq; chemical structure contains a methyltetrazolethiol side chain which may be responsible for the disulfiram-like reaction with alcohol and increased risk of bleeding

Dosage Forms Powder for injection, as disodium: 1 g (10 mL, 100 mL); 2 g (20 mL, 100 mL); 10 g (100 mL)

References
Martin C, Thomachot L, and Albanese J, "Clinical Pharmacokinetics of Cefotetan," *Clin Pharmacokinet*, 1994, 26(4):248-58.

♦ **Cefotetan Disodium** *see Cefotetan on page 185*

Cefoxitin (se FOKS i tin)

Brand Names Mefoxin®
Available Salts Cefoxitin Sodium
Therapeutic Category Antibiotic, Cephalosporin (Second Generation)
Generic Available No
Use Treatment of susceptible lower respiratory tract, skin and skin structure, bone and joint, genitourinary tract, sepsis, gynecologic, and intra-abdominal infections; active against anaerobes including *Bacteroides* species of the gastrointestinal tract, gram-negative enteric bacilli including *E. coli*, *Klebsiella*, and *Proteus*; active against many strains of *N. gonorrhoeae*; perioperative prophylaxis
Pregnancy Risk Factor B
Contraindications Hypersensitivity to cefoxitin, any component, or cephalosporins
Warnings Prolonged use may result in superinfection; high doses in children have been associated with an increased incidence of eosinophilia and elevation of serum AST; safety and efficacy in infants <3 months have not been established; do not use in patients with immediate-type hypersensitivity reactions to penicillin
Precautions Use with caution and modify dosage in patients with renal impairment; use with caution in patients with history of colitis or penicillin hypersensitivity
Adverse Reactions
Central nervous system: Fever, headache
Dermatologic: Rash, pruritus, exfoliative dermatitis
Gastrointestinal: Pseudomembranous colitis, diarrhea, nausea, vomiting
Hematologic: Transient leukopenia, thrombocytopenia, neutropenia, anemia, eosinophilia
Hepatic: Transient elevation of liver enzymes, AST, ALT, and alkaline phosphatase
Local: Thrombophlebitis, pain at injection site
Renal: Transient elevation of BUN and serum creatinine
Drug Interactions Probenecid (increases serum concentration of cefoxitin)
Stability Reconstituted solution is stable for 24 hours at room temperature and for 1 week under refrigeration; thawed solutions of the commercially available frozen cefoxitin injections are stable for 24 hours at room temperature or 5 days when refrigerated

Mechanism of Action Inhibits bacterial cell wall synthesis by binding to one or more of the penicillin-binding proteins; inhibits the final transpeptidation step of peptidoglycan synthesis resulting in cell wall death

Pharmacokinetics
Distribution: Distributes into tissues and fluids including ascitic, pleural, bile, and synovial fluids; poor penetration into CSF even with inflamed meninges; crosses the placenta; small amounts appear in breast milk
Protein binding: 65% to 79%
Half-life:
Infants (10-53 days of age): 1.4 hours
Adults: 45-60 minutes, increases significantly with renal insufficiency
Time to peak serum concentration: I.M.: Within 20-30 minutes
Elimination: Rapidly excreted as unchanged drug (85%) in the urine
Moderately dialyzable (20% to 50%)

Usual Dosage I.M., I.V.:
Neonates: 90-100 mg/kg/day divided every 8 hours
Infants ≥3 months and Children:
Mild-moderate infection: 80-100 mg/kg/day divided every 6-8 hours
Severe infection: 100-160 mg/kg/day divided every 4-6 hours; maximum dose: 12 g/day
Perioperative prophylaxis: 30-40 mg/kg 30-60 minutes prior to surgery followed by 30-40 mg/kg/dose every 6 hours for no more than 24 hours after surgery depending on the procedure
Adolescents and Adults: 1-2 g every 6-8 hours (I.M. injection is painful); maximum dose: 12 g/day
Pelvic inflammatory disease: I.V.: 2 g every 6 hours continued for 24-48 hours after significant clinical improvement is demonstrated **plus** doxycycline 100 mg I.V. or orally every 12 hours for 14 days
Perioperative prophylaxis: 1-2 g 30-60 minutes prior to surgery followed by 1-2 g every 6-8 hours for no more than 24 hours after surgery depending on the procedure

Dosing interval in renal impairment:
Cl_{cr} 30-50 mL/minute: Administer every 8-12 hours
Cl_{cr} 10-30 mL/minute: Administer every 12-24 hours
Cl_{cr} <10 mL/minute: Administer every 24-48 hours

Administration Parenteral:
IVP: Administer over 3-5 minutes at a maximum concentration of 200 mg/mL
I.V. intermittent infusion: Administer over 10-60 minutes at a final concentration not to exceed 40 mg/mL

Monitoring Parameters Renal function periodically when used in combination with other nephrotoxic drugs; liver function and hematologic function tests; number and type of stools/day for diarrhea

Test Interactions Positive Coombs' [direct]; false-positive urine glucose (Clinitest®), false ↑ in serum or urine creatinine

Additional Information Sodium content of 1 g: 2.3 mEq

Dosage Forms
Infusion, as sodium, premixed, in D_5W (frozen): 1 g (50 mL); 2 g (50 mL)
Powder for injection, as sodium: 1 g, 2 g, 10 g

References
Feldman WE, Moffitt S, and Sprow N, "Clinical and Pharmacokinetic Evaluation of Parenteral Cefoxitin in Infants and Children," *Antimicrob Agents Chemother*, 1980, 17(4):669-74.
Regazzi MB, Chirico G, Cristiani D, et al, "Cefoxitin in Newborn Infants. A Clinical and Pharmacokinetic Study," *Eur J Clin Pharmacol*, 1983, 25(4):507-9.

♦ **Cefoxitin Sodium** *see* Cefoxitin *on page 186*

Cefpodoxime (sef pode OKS eem)
Related Information
Carbohydrate and Alcohol Content of Liquid Medications for Use in Patients Receiving Ketogenic Diets *on page 1228*

Brand Names Vantin®
Available Salts Cefpodoxime Proxetil
Therapeutic Category Antibiotic, Cephalosporin (Third Generation)
Generic Available No
Use Treatment of susceptible acute, community-acquired pneumonia caused by *S. pneumoniae* or nonbeta-lactamase producing *H. influenzae*; alternative regimen for acute uncomplicated gonorrhea caused by *N. gonorrhoeae*; uncomplicated skin and skin structure infections caused by *S. aureus* or *S. pyogenes*; acute otitis media caused by *S. pneumoniae*, *H. influenzae*, or *M. catarrhalis*; pharyngitis or
(Continued)

Cefpodoxime *(Continued)*

tonsillitis; and uncomplicated urinary tract infections caused by *E. coli*, *Klebsiella*, and *Proteus*

Pregnancy Risk Factor B

Contraindications Hypersensitivity to cefpodoxime, any component, or cephalosporins

Warnings Prolonged use may result in superinfection; do not use in patients with immediate-type hypersensitivity reactions to penicillin

Precautions Use with caution in patients with history of penicillin hypersensitivity, impaired renal function, and patients with a history of colitis; modify dosage in patients with renal impairment

Adverse Reactions
Central nervous system: Headache
Dermatologic: Rash
Gastrointestinal: Nausea (3.8%), vomiting, abdominal pain, diarrhea (7.1%), pseudomembranous colitis
Genitourinary: Vaginal fungal infections (3.3%)
Hematologic: Eosinophilia, leukocytosis, thrombocytosis, decrease in hemoglobin or hematocrit, leukopenia, prolonged PT and PTT
Hepatic: Transient elevation in AST, ALT, bilirubin
Renal: Elevated BUN, elevated serum creatinine

Drug Interactions Antacids and H_2-receptor antagonists (reduce absorption and serum concentration of cefpodoxime); probenecid (inhibits renal excretion of cefpodoxime)

Food Interactions Presence of food increases oral bioavailability

Stability After reconstitution, suspension may be stored in refrigerator for 14 days

Mechanism of Action Inhibits bacterial cell wall synthesis by binding to one or more of the penicillin-binding proteins; inhibits the final transpeptidation step of peptidoglycan synthesis resulting in cell wall death

Pharmacokinetics
Absorption: Enhanced in the presence of food or low gastric pH
Distribution: Good tissue penetration, including lung and tonsils; penetrates into pleural fluid
Protein binding: 18% to 23%
Metabolism: Following oral administration, cefpodoxime proxetil is de-esterified in the GI tract to the active metabolite, cefpodoxime
Bioavailability: Oral: 50%
Half-life: 2.2 hours (prolonged with renal impairment)
Time to peak serum concentration: Within 2-3 hours
Elimination: Primarily by the kidney with 80% of absorbed dose excreted unchanged in urine in 24 hours

Usual Dosage Oral:
Children >6 months to 12 years: 10 mg/kg/day divided every 12 hours; maximum dose: 800 mg/day
Children ≥13 years and Adults: 100-400 mg/dose every 12 hours
Uncomplicated gonorrhea: 200 mg as a single dose
Dosing adjustment in renal impairment: Cl_{cr} <30 mL/minute: Administer every 24 hours; patients on hemodialysis, administer dose 3 times/week
Dosing adjustment in hepatic impairment: Not necessary in patient with cirrhosis

Administration Oral:
Tablet: Administer with food
Suspension: May administer with or without food; shake suspension well before use

Monitoring Parameters Observe patient for diarrhea; with prolonged therapy, monitor renal function periodically

Test Interactions Positive Coombs' [direct]

Dosage Forms
Granules for oral suspension, as proxetil (lemon creme flavor): 50 mg/5 mL (100 mL); 100 mg/5 mL (100 mL)
Tablet, film coated, as proxetil: 100 mg, 200 mg

References
Borin MT, "A Review of the Pharmacokinetics of Cefpodoxime Proxetil," *Drugs*, 1991, 42(Suppl 3):13-21.
Fujii R, "Clinical Trials of Cefpodoxime Proxetil Suspension in Pediatrics," *Drugs*, 1991, 42(Suppl 3):57-60.
Mendelman PM, Del-Beccaro MA, McLinn SE, et al, "Cefpodoxime Proxetil Compared With Amoxicillin-Clavulanate for the Treatment of Otitis Media," *J Pediatr*, 1992, 121(3):459-65.

♦ **Cefpodoxime Proxetil** *see* Cefpodoxime *on page 187*

Cefprozil (sef PROE zil)
Related Information
Carbohydrate and Alcohol Content of Liquid Medications for Use in Patients Receiving Ketogenic Diets *on page 1228*
Brand Names Cefzil®
Therapeutic Category Antibiotic, Cephalosporin (Second Generation)
Generic Available No
Use Infections caused by susceptible organisms including *S. pneumoniae, H. influenzae, M. catarrhalis, S. aureus, S. pyogenes*; treatment of infections involving the respiratory tract, skin and skin structure, and otitis media
Pregnancy Risk Factor B
Contraindications Hypersensitivity to cefprozil, any component, or cephalosporins
Warnings Prolonged use may result in superinfection; do not use in patients with immediate-type hypersensitivity reactions to penicillin
Precautions Use with caution in patients with impaired renal function, history of colitis, or in penicillin-sensitive patients; modify dosage in patients with severe renal impairment
Adverse Reactions
Central nervous system: Headache, hyperactivity, insomnia, confusion, dizziness
Dermatologic: Rash, pruritus, diaper rash
Gastrointestinal: Diarrhea, nausea, vomiting, abdominal pain
Genitourinary: Vaginitis
Hematologic: Decrease in leukocyte and platelet count, eosinophilia
Hepatic: Elevated AST, ALT, and alkaline phosphatase; cholestatic jaundice; prolonged PT
Renal: Elevated BUN and serum creatinine
Miscellaneous: Serum sickness-like reactions
Drug Interactions Probenecid increases cefprozil serum levels
Food Interactions Total absorption is not affected by food
Stability Refrigerate suspension after reconstitution; discard after 14 days
Mechanism of Action Inhibits bacterial cell wall synthesis by binding to one or more of the penicillin-binding proteins resulting in disruption of cell wall synthesis and cell lysis
Pharmacokinetics
Absorption: Oral: Well absorbed (95%)
Distribution: Low excretion into breast milk
Protein binding: 35% to 45%
Bioavailability: 94%
Half-life, elimination: 1.3 hours (normal renal function)
Time to peak serum concentration: 1.5 hours (fasting state)
Elimination: 61% excreted unchanged in urine
Hemodialysis: ~55% is removed by hemodialysis
Usual Dosage Oral:
Infants and Children (>6 months to 12 years):
Otitis media: 30 mg/kg/day divided every 12 hours; maximum dose: 1 g/day
Pharyngitis/tonsillitis: 2-12 years: 15 mg/kg/day divided every 12 hours; maximum dose: 1 g/day
Children >12 years and Adults: 250-500 mg every 12 hours or 500 mg every 24 hours
Dosing adjustment in renal impairment: Cl_{cr} <30 mL/minute: Reduce dose by 50%
Administration Oral: May administer with or without food; administer with food if stomach upset occurs; chilling improves flavor of suspension (do not freeze); shake suspension well before use
Monitoring Parameters Evaluate renal function before and during therapy; with prolonged therapy, monitor coagulation tests, CBC, and liver function tests periodically
Test Interactions Positive Coombs' [direct]; may produce false-positive reaction for urine glucose with Clinitest®
Patient Information Report persistent diarrhea to physician
Additional Information Suspension also contains aspartame, FD&C red No. 3, glycine, sodium benzoate, carboxymethylcellulose, sucrose, and phenylalanine
Dosage Forms
Powder for oral suspension, as anhydrous: 125 mg/5 mL (50 mL, 75 mL, 100 mL); 250 mg/5 mL (50 mL, 75 mL, 100 mL)
Tablet, as anhydrous: 250 mg, 500 mg
(Continued)

Cefprozil *(Continued)*

References

Arguedas AG, Zaleska M, Stutman HR, et al, "Comparative Trial of Cefprozil vs Amoxicillin Clavulanate Potassium in the Treatment of Children With Acute Otitis Media With Effusion," *Pediatr Infect Dis J,* 1991, 10(5):375-80.

Barriere SL, "Review of *In Vitro* Activity, Pharmacokinetic Characteristics, Safety, and Clinical Efficacy of Cefprozil, a New Oral Cephalosporin," *Ann Pharmacother,* 1993, 27(9):1082-9.

Lowery N, Kearns GL, Young RA, et al, "Serum Sickness-Like Reactions Associated With Cefprozil Therapy," *J Pediatr,* 1994, 125(2):325-8.

Ceftazidime (SEF tay zi deem)

Brand Names Ceptaz™; Ceptaz™ (Canada); Fortaz®; Pentacef™; Tazicef®; Tazidime®

Available Salts Ceftazidime Sodium

Therapeutic Category Antibiotic, Cephalosporin (Third Generation)

Generic Available No

Use Treatment of infections of the respiratory tract, urinary tract, skin and skin structure, intra-abdominal, osteomyelitis, sepsis, and meningitis caused by susceptible gram-negative aerobic organisms such as Enterobacteriaceae and *Pseudomonas*; pseudomonal infection in patient at risk of developing aminoglycoside-induced nephrotoxicity and/or ototoxicity; empiric therapy for febrile, granulocytopenic patients

Pregnancy Risk Factor B

Contraindications Hypersensitivity to ceftazidime, any component, or cephalosporins

Warnings Prolonged use may result in superinfection; do not use in patients with immediate-type hypersensitivity reactions to penicillin

Precautions Use with caution and modify dosage in patients with impaired renal function; use with caution in patients with history of colitis or patients with penicillin hypersensitivity

Adverse Reactions
Central nervous system: Fever, headache, dizziness
Dermatologic: Rash, pruritus
Gastrointestinal: Pseudomembranous colitis, diarrhea, nausea, vomiting, candidiasis
Hematologic: Transient leukopenia, thrombocytopenia, eosinophilia, thrombocytosis, hemolytic anemia
Hepatic: Transient elevation of liver enzymes
Local: Phlebitis, pain at injection site
Renal: Transient elevation of BUN and serum creatinine

Drug Interactions Probenecid decreases renal clearance of ceftazidime; aminoglycosides may increase risk of nephrotoxicity

Stability Reconstituted solution is stable for 24 hours at room temperature and 10 days when refrigerated; incompatible with sodium bicarbonate; potentially incompatible with aminoglycosides

Mechanism of Action Bactericidal antibiotic with a mechanism similar to that of penicillins by binding to one or more of the penicillin-binding proteins; inhibits mucopeptide synthesis in the bacterial cell wall

Pharmacokinetics
Distribution: Widely distributed throughout the body including bone, bile, skin, CSF (diffuses into CSF at higher concentrations when the meninges are inflamed), endometrium, heart, pleural and lymphatic fluids; distributes into breast milk
Protein binding: 17%
Half-life:
Neonates <23 days: 2.2-4.7 hours
Adults: 1-2 hours (prolonged with renal impairment)
Time to peak serum concentration: I.M.: Within 60 minutes
Elimination: By glomerular filtration with 80% to 90% of the dose excreted as unchanged drug in urine within 24 hours
Dialyzable (50% to 100%)

Usual Dosage I.M., I.V.:
Neonates: 0-4 weeks: <1200 g: 100 mg/kg/day divided every 12 hours
Postnatal age ≤7 days:
1200-2000 g: 100 mg/kg/day divided every 12 hours
>2000 g: 100-150 mg/kg/day divided every 8-12 hours
Postnatal age >7 days: ≥1200 g: 150 mg/kg/day divided every 8 hours
Infants and Children 1 month to 12 years: 100-150 mg/kg/day divided every 8 hours; maximum dose: 6 g/day
Meningitis: 150 mg/kg/day divided every 8 hours; maximum dose: 6 g/day

Adults: 1-2 g every 8-12 hours
Urinary tract infections: 250-500 mg every 12 hours
Dosing interval in renal impairment:
Cl_{cr} 30-50 mL/minute: Administer every 12 hours
Cl_{cr} 10-30 mL/minute: Administer every 24 hours
Cl_{cr} <10 mL/minute: Administer every 24-48 hours

Administration Parenteral: Any carbon dioxide bubbles that may be present in the withdrawn solution should be expelled prior to injection
IVP: Administer over 3-5 minutes at a maximum concentration of 180 mg/mL
I.V. intermittent infusion: Administer over 15-30 minutes at a final concentration ≤40 mg/mL

Monitoring Parameters Renal function periodically when used in combination with aminoglycosides; with prolonged therapy also monitor hepatic and hematologic function periodically; number and type of stools/day for diarrhea

Test Interactions Positive Coombs' [direct], false-positive urine glucose (Clinitest®)

Additional Information Sodium content of 1 g: 2.3 mEq

Dosage Forms
Infusion, premixed (frozen), as sodium (Fortaz®): 1 g (50 mL); 2 g (50 mL)
Powder for injection: 500 mg, 1 g, 2 g, 6 g

References
McCracken GH Jr, Threlkeld N, and Thomas ML, "Pharmacokinetics of Ceftazidime in Newborn Infants," *Antimicrob Agents Chemother*, 1984, 26(4):583-4.
Robinson DG, Cookson TL, and Frisafe JA, "Concentration Guidelines for Parenteral Antibiotics in Fluid-Restricted Patients," *Drug Intell Clin Pharm*, 1987, 21(12):985-9.

♦ **Ceftazidime Sodium** *see Ceftazidime on page 190*

♦ **Ceftin® Oral** *see Cefuroxime on page 194*

Ceftizoxime (sef ti ZOKS eem)

Brand Names Cefizox®
Available Salts Ceftizoxime Sodium
Therapeutic Category Antibiotic, Cephalosporin (Third Generation)
Generic Available No
Use Treatment of susceptible bacterial infections, mainly respiratory tract, skin and skin structure, bone and joint, urinary tract and sepsis; as a third generation cephalosporin, ceftizoxime has activity against gram-negative enteric bacilli (eg, *E. coli*, *Klebsiella*), and cocci (eg, *Neisseria*), and variable activity against gram-positive cocci (*Staphylococcus* and *Streptococcus*); ceftizoxime has some anaerobic coverage but is less active against *B. fragilis* than cefoxitin; also indicated for *Neisseria gonorrhoeae* infections (including uncomplicated cervical and urethral gonorrhea and gonorrhea pelvic inflammatory disease), and *Haemophilus influenzae* meningitis

Pregnancy Risk Factor B

Contraindications Hypersensitivity to ceftizoxime, any component, or cephalosporins

Warnings Prolonged use may result in superinfection; do not use in patients with immediate-type hypersensitivity reaction to penicillin

Precautions Use with caution in patients who are hypersensitive to penicillins; use with caution and modify dosage in patients with renal impairment

Adverse Reactions
Central nervous system: Fever
Dermatologic: Rash, pruritus
Gastrointestinal: Diarrhea, occasionally nausea and vomiting
Genitourinary: Vaginitis (rare)
Hematologic: Positive Coombs' test, eosinophilia, thrombocytosis (transient); rarely: anemia, leukopenia, neutropenia, thrombocytopenia
Hepatic: Elevated bilirubin; transient elevation of AST, ALT, alkaline phosphatase
Local: Pain, burning at injection site
Neuromuscular & skeletal: Numbness
Renal: Transient elevations of BUN and serum creatinine

Drug Interactions Probenecid may decrease renal tubular secretion and increase ceftizoxime serum concentrations

Stability Reconstituted solution is stable for 24 hours at room temperature and 96 hours when refrigerated; for I.V. infusion in NS or D_5W solution is stable for 24 hours at room temperature, 96 hours when refrigerated or 12 weeks when frozen; after freezing, thawed solution is stable for 24 hours at room temperature or 10 days when refrigerated; do not refreeze; do not mix in same bag with aminoglycosides
(Continued)

Ceftizoxime *(Continued)*

Mechanism of Action Interferes with bacterial cell wall synthesis during active replication, causing cell wall death and resultant bactericidal activity against susceptible bacteria

Pharmacokinetics
Distribution: V_d: 0.35-0.5 L/kg; penetrates CSF
Protein binding: 30%
Half-life: 1.6 hours, increases to 25 hours when Cl_{cr} falls to <10 mL/minute
Time to peak serum concentration: I.M.: Within 0.5-1 hour
Elimination: Excreted unchanged in urine
Moderately dialyzable (20% to 50%)

Usual Dosage I.M., I.V.:
Children ≥6 months: 150-200 mg/kg/day divided every 6-8 hours; maximum dose: 12 g/24 hours
Adults: 1-2 g every 8-12 hours
Life-threatening infections: Up to 2 g every 4 hours or 4 g every 8 hours
Uncomplicated gonorrhea: I.M.: 1 g (single dose)
Dosing interval in renal impairment:
Cl_{cr} 50-80 mL/minute: Administer every 8-12 hours
Cl_{cr} 10-50 mL/minute: Administer every 36-48 hours
Cl_{cr} <10 mL/minute: Administer every 48-72 hours

Administration Parenteral:
I.V. intermittent infusion: Administer over 30 minutes; usual dilution: 1 g/50 mL, doses >1 g are usually diluted to 100 mL
I.V. direct (bolus) injection: Administer slowly over 3-5 minutes at a concentration of 95 mg/mL

Test Interactions May falsely elevate creatine values when Jaffé reaction is used; may cause false-positive urinary glucose tests using cupric sulfate (Clinitest®, Benedict's solution)

Additional Information Sodium content of 1 g ceftizoxime: 60 mg (2.6 mEq); ceftizoxime does not cover *Chlamydia trachomatis* infections and must, therefore, be used with appropriate antichlamydial agents when treating pelvic inflammatory disease if *C. trachomatis* is suspected

Dosage Forms
Injection, as sodium, in D_5W (frozen): 1 g (50 mL); 2 g (50 mL)
Powder for injection, as sodium: 500 mg, 1 g, 2 g, 10 g

♦ **Ceftizoxime Sodium** *see* Ceftizoxime *on page 191*

Ceftriaxone (sef trye AKS one)

Brand Names Rocephin®
Available Salts Ceftriaxone Sodium
Therapeutic Category Antibiotic, Cephalosporin (Third Generation)
Generic Available No
Use Treatment of sepsis, meningitis, infections of the lower respiratory tract, skin and skin structure, bone and joint, intra-abdominal and urinary tract due to susceptible organisms; as a third generation cephalosporin, ceftriaxone has activity against gram-negative aerobic bacteria (ie, *H. influenzae*, Enterobacteriaceae, *Neisseria*), and variable activity against gram-positive cocci; documented or suspected infection due to susceptible organisms in home care patients and patients without I.V. line access; treatment of documented or suspected gonococcal infection or chancroid; emergency room management of patients at high risk for bacteremia, periorbital or buccal cellulitis, salmonellosis or shigellosis and pneumonia of unestablished etiology (<5 years of age); treatment of resistant acute otitis media; in children with acute otitis media who are unable to take oral antibiotics

Pregnancy Risk Factor B
Contraindications Hypersensitivity to ceftriaxone sodium, any component, or cephalosporins; do not use in hyperbilirubinemic neonates, particularly those who are premature since ceftriaxone is reported to displace bilirubin from albumin binding sites increasing the risk for kernicterus
Warnings Prolonged use may result in superinfection with yeasts, enterococci, *B. fragilis*, or *P. aeruginosa*; do not use in patients with immediate-type hypersensitivity reactions to penicillin
Precautions Use with caution in patients with gallbladder, biliary tract, liver, or pancreatic disease; or in patients with history of colitis or penicillin hypersensitivity
Adverse Reactions
Central nervous system: Fever, chills, headache, dizziness

Dermatologic: Rash, pruritus

Gastrointestinal: Diarrhea, nausea, vomiting, sludging in the gallbladder, cholelithiasis, pseudomembranous colitis

Genitourinary: Vaginitis, casts in urine

Hematologic: Eosinophilia, leukopenia, anemia, thrombocytopenia, thrombocytosis, bleeding, neutropenia

Hepatic: Transient elevation in liver enzymes, jaundice, elevation in serum bilirubin

Local: Pain at injection site

Renal: Elevated BUN and serum creatinine

Drug Interactions High-dose probenecid (decreases elimination half-life of ceftriaxone); aminoglycosides may increase risk of nephrotoxicity

Stability Reconstituted solution (100 mg/mL) is stable for 3 days at room temperature and 10 days when refrigerated; reconstituted solution (250 mg/mL) is stable for 24 hours at room temperature and 3 days when refrigerated

Mechanism of Action Inhibits bacterial cell wall synthesis by binding to one or more of the penicillin-binding proteins; inhibits the final transpeptidation step of peptidoglycan synthesis resulting in cell wall death

Pharmacokinetics

Distribution: Widely distributed throughout the body including gallbladder, lungs, bone, bile, CSF (diffuses into the CSF at higher concentrations when the meninges are inflamed); crosses the placenta

Protein binding: 85% to 95%

Half-life:

Neonates:

1-4 days: 16 hours

9-30 days: 9 hours

Adults: 5-9 hours (with normal renal and hepatic function)

Time to peak serum concentration: I.M.: Within 1-2 hours

Elimination: Unchanged in the urine (33% to 65%) by glomerular filtration and in feces via bile

Not dialyzable (0% to 5%)

Usual Dosage I.M., I.V.:

Neonates:

Postnatal age ≤7 days: 50 mg/kg/day given every 24 hours

Postnatal age >7 days:

≤2000 g: 50 mg/kg/day given every 24 hours

>2000 g: 50-75 mg/kg/day given every 24 hours

Gonococcal prophylaxis: 25-50 mg/kg as a single dose (dose not to exceed 125 mg)

Gonococcal infection: 25-50 mg/kg/day (maximum dose: 125 mg) given every 24 hours for 7 days, up to 10-14 days if meningitis is documented

Note: Use cefotaxime in place of ceftriaxone in hyperbilirubinemic neonates

Infants and Children: 50-75 mg/kg/day divided every 12-24 hours

Meningitis: 80-100 mg/kg/day divided every 12-24 hours; loading dose of 75 mg/kg may be administered at the start of therapy; maximum dose: 4 g/day

Chemoprophylaxis for high-risk contacts of patients with invasive meningococcal disease:

≤12 years: I.M.: 125 mg in a single dose

>12 years: I.M.: 250 mg in a single dose

Uncomplicated gonococcal infections, sexual assault, and STD prophylaxis: I.M.: 125 mg in a single dose

Complicated gonococcal infections: I.M., I.V.:

<45 kg:

Peritonitis, arthritis, or bacteremia: 50 mg/kg/day once daily for 7 days; maximum dose: 1 g/day

Conjunctivitis: 50 mg/kg (maximum dose: 1 g) in a single dose

Meningitis or endocarditis: 50 mg/kg/day divided every 12 hours for 10-14 days (meningitis), for 28 days (endocarditis); maximum dose: 2 g/day

>45 kg:

Disseminated gonococcal infections: 1 g/day once daily for 7 days

Meningitis: 1-2 g/dose every 12 hours for 10-14 days

Endocarditis: 1-2 g/dose every 12 hours for 28 days

Conjunctivitis: I.M.: 1 g in a single dose

Chancroid: I.M.: 50 mg/kg as a single dose (maximum dose: 250 mg)

Acute epididymitis: I.M.: 250 mg in a single dose

Acute otitis media: 50 mg/kg once daily for 3 days (maximum dose: 1 g/day)

Adults: 1-2 g every 12-24 hours depending on the type and severity of the infection; maximum dose: 4 g/day

(Continued)

Ceftriaxone *(Continued)*

Dosing interval in renal impairment: No change necessary with dose ≤2 g/day

Administration Parenteral:

IVP: Administer over 2-4 minutes at a maximum concentration of 40 mg/mL

I.V. intermittent infusion: Administer over 10-30 minutes; final concentration for I.V. administration should not exceed 40 mg/mL

I.M. injection: May be diluted with sterile water or 1% lidocaine to a final concentration of 250 mg/mL or may be concentrated by using the manufacturer's recommended diluent volume of 1% lidocaine with a resultant concentration of 350 mg/mL; administer I.M. injections deep into a large muscle mass

Monitoring Parameters CBC with differential, PT, renal and hepatic function tests periodically; number and type of stools/day for diarrhea

Test Interactions False-positive urine glucose with Clinitest®

Additional Information Sodium content of 1 g: 3.6 mEq

Dosage Forms

Infusion, as sodium, premixed (frozen): 1 g in $D_{3.8}W$ (50 mL); 2 g in $D_{2.4}W$ (50 mL)

Powder for injection, as sodium: 250 mg, 500 mg, 1 g, 2 g, 10 g

References

Bradley JS, Compogiannis LS, Murray WE, et al, "Pharmacokinetics and Safety of Intramuscular Injection of Concentrated Ceftriaxone in Children," *Clin Pharm*, 1992, 11(11):961-4.

Centers for Disease Control and Prevention, "1998 Guidelines for Treatment of Sexually Transmitted Diseases," *MMWR Morb Mortal Wkly Rep*, 1998, 47(RR-1):1-111.

Committee on Adolescence, American Academy of Pediatrics, "Sexual Assault and the Adolescent," *Pediatrics*, 1994, 94(5):761-5.

Dowell SF, Butler JC, Giebink GS, et al, "Acute Otitis Media: Management and Surveillance in an era of Pneumococcal Resistance--A Report From the Drug-Resistant *Streptococcus pneumoniae* Therapeutic Working Group," *Pediatr Infect Dis J*, 1999, 18(1):1-9.

Richards DM, Heel RC, Brogden RN, et al, "Ceftriaxone: A Review of Its Antibacterial Activity, Pharmacological Properties and Therapeutic Use," *Drugs*, 1984, 27(6):469-527.

♦ **Ceftriaxone Sodium** *see* Ceftriaxone *on page 192*

Cefuroxime *(se fyoor OKS eem)*

Related Information

Carbohydrate and Alcohol Content of Liquid Medications for Use in Patients Receiving Ketogenic Diets *on page 1228*

Brand Names Ceftin® Oral; Kefurox® Injection; Zinacef® Injection

Available Salts Cefuroxime Axetil; Cefuroxime Sodium

Therapeutic Category Antibiotic, Cephalosporin (Second Generation)

Generic Available Yes

Use A second generation cephalosporin useful in infections caused by susceptible staphylococci, group B streptococci, pneumococci, *H. influenzae* (type A and B), *E. coli*, *Enterobacter*, and *Klebsiella*; treatment of susceptible infections of the upper and lower respiratory tract, otitis media, acute bacterial maxillary sinusitis, urinary tract, skin and soft tissue, bone and joint, and sepsis

Pregnancy Risk Factor B

Contraindications Hypersensitivity to cefuroxime, any component, or cephalosporins

Warnings Prolonged use may result in superinfection; safety and efficacy in infants <3 months of age have not been established; do not use in patients with immediate-type hypersensitivity reactions to penicillin

Precautions Use with caution and modify dosage in patients with renal impairment; use with caution in patients with history of colitis or history of penicillin hypersensitivity

Adverse Reactions

Central nervous system: Fever, headache, dizziness, vertigo, seizures

Dermatologic: Rash, pruritus, erythema multiforme, diaper rash

Gastrointestinal: Nausea, vomiting, diarrhea, stomach cramps, GI bleeding, antibiotic-associated colitis, stomatitis

Genitourinary: Vaginitis

Hematologic: Transient neutropenia and leukopenia, decreased hemoglobin and hematocrit, eosinophilia

Hepatic: Transient elevation in liver enzymes

Local: Pain at injection site, thrombophlebitis

Renal: Elevated BUN and serum creatinine

Drug Interactions Probenecid (increases serum cefuroxime concentration); aminoglycosides may increase risk of nephrotoxicity

Food Interactions Presence of food and milk increases bioavailability and peak levels

Stability Reconstituted injectable solution (100 mg/mL) or suspension (200-220 mg/mL) is stable for 24 hours at room temperature or 48 hours when refrigerated; reconstituted oral suspension can be stored in the refrigerator or at room temperature; discard after 10 days

Mechanism of Action Inhibits bacterial cell wall synthesis by binding to one or more of the penicillin-binding proteins; inhibits the final transpeptidation step of peptidoglycan synthesis resulting in cell wall death

Pharmacokinetics

Absorption: Oral: Increased when given with or shortly after food or infant formula

Distribution: Into bronchial secretions, synovial and pericardial fluid, kidneys, heart, liver, bone and bile; penetrates into CSF with inflamed meninges; crosses the placenta; excreted into breast milk

Protein binding: 33% to 50%

Bioavailability: Oral cefuroxime axetil tablets: 37% to 52%; cefuroxime axetil suspension is less bioavailable than the tablet (91% of the AUC for tablets)

Half-life:

Neonates:

≤3 days: 5.1-5.8 hours

6-14 days: 2-4.2 hours

3-4 weeks: 1-1.5 hours

Adults: 1-2 hours (prolonged in renal impairment)

Time to peak serum concentration:

Oral: 2-3 hours

I.M.: Within 15-60 minutes

Elimination: Primarily 66% to 100% as unchanged drug in urine by both glomerular filtration and tubular secretion

Dialyzable

Usual Dosage

I.M., I.V.:

Neonates: 20-100 mg/kg/day divided every 12 hours

Children: 75-150 mg/kg/day divided every 8 hours; maximum dose: 6 g/day

Meningitis: Not recommended (doses of 200-240 mg/kg/day divided every 6-8 hours have been used); maximum dose: 9 g/day

Adults: 750 mg to 1.5 g/dose every 8 hours

Oral: **Cefuroxime axetil film-coated tablets and oral suspension are not bioequivalent and are not substitutable on a mg/mg basis**

Children:

Pharyngitis, tonsillitis:

Suspension: 20 mg/kg/day (maximum dose: 500 mg/day) in 2 divided doses

Tablet: 125 mg every 12 hours

Acute otitis media, acute bacterial maxillary sinusitis, impetigo:

Suspension: 30 mg/kg/day (maximum dose: 1 g/day) in 2 divided doses

Tablet: 250 mg every 12 hours

Adults: 250-500 mg twice daily; uncomplicated urinary tract infection: 125-250 mg every 12 hours

Dosing interval in renal impairment:

Cl_{cr} 10-20 mL/minute: Administer every 12 hours

Cl_{cr} <10 mL/minute: Administer every 24 hours

Administration

Oral: Cefuroxime axetil suspension must be administered with food; shake suspension well before use; tablets may be administered with or without food; administer with food to decrease GI upset; avoid crushing the tablet due to its bitter taste

Parenteral:

IVP: Administer over 3-5 minutes at a maximum concentration of 100 mg/mL

I.V. intermittent infusion: Administer over 15-30 minutes at a final concentration for administration ≤30 mg/mL; in fluid restricted patients, a concentration of 137 mg/mL may be administered

I.M.: I.M. injection is less painful when administered as an injectable suspension rather than a solution, and is less painful when administered into the buttock rather than the thigh

Monitoring Parameters With prolonged therapy, monitor renal, hepatic, and hematologic function periodically; number and type of stools/day for diarrhea

Test Interactions Positive Coombs' [direct]; false-positive urine glucose with Clinitest®

Additional Information Sodium content of 1 g: 2.4 mEq

Dosage Forms

Infusion, premixed (frozen), as sodium (Zinacef®): 750 mg (50 mL); 1.5 g (50 mL)

(Continued)

Cefuroxime *(Continued)*

Powder for injection, as sodium (Kefurox®, Zinacef®): 750 mg, 1.5 g, 7.5 g
Suspension, as axetil (Ceftin®): 125 mg/5 mL (50 mL, 100 mL, 200 mL)
Tablet, as axetil (Ceftin®): 125 mg, 250 mg, 500 mg

References

de Louvois J, Mulhall A, and Hurley R, "Cefuroxime in the Treatment of Neonates," *Arch Dis Child*, 1982, 57(1):59-62.

Gooch WM 3rd, Blair E, Puopolo A, et al, "Effectiveness of Five Days of Therapy With Cefuroxime Axetil Suspension for Treatment of Acute Otitis Media," *Pediatr Infect Dis J*, 1996, 15(2):157-64.

Nelson JD, "Cefuroxime: A Cephalosporin With Unique Applicability to Pediatric Practice," *Pediatr Infect Dis*, 1983, 2(5):394-6.

Thoene DE and Johnson CE, "Pharmacotherapy of Otitis Media," *Pharmacotherapy*, 1991, 11(3):212-21.

+ **Cefuroxime Axetil** *see Cefuroxime on page 194*
+ **Cefuroxime Sodium** *see Cefuroxime on page 194*
+ **Cefzil®** *see Cefprozil on page 189*
+ **Celestoderm®-V, -EV/2 (Canada)** *see Betamethasone on page 130*
+ **Celestone® Oral** *see Betamethasone on page 130*
+ **Celestone® Phosphate Injection** *see Betamethasone on page 130*
+ **Celestone® Soluspan®** *see Betamethasone on page 130*
+ **CellCept®** *see Mycophenolate on page 663*
+ **Celontin®** *see Methsuximide on page 624*
+ **Celontin® (Canada)** *see Methsuximide on page 624*
+ **Cel-U-Jec® Injection** *see Betamethasone on page 130*
+ **Cenafed® [OTC]** *see Pseudoephedrine on page 822*
+ **Cenafed® Plus [OTC]** *see Triprolidine and Pseudoephedrine on page 957*
+ **Cena-K®** *see Potassium Supplements on page 786*

Cephalexin *(sef a LEKS in)*

Related Information

Carbohydrate and Alcohol Content of Liquid Medications for Use in Patients Receiving Ketogenic Diets *on page 1228*
Endocarditis Prophylaxis *on page 1127*

Brand Names Apo®-Cephalex (Canada); Biocef®; Cefanex®; Keflex®; Keftab®; Novo-Lexin® (Canada); Nu-Cephalex® (Canada); Zartan®

Available Salts Cephalexin Hydrochloride

Therapeutic Category Antibiotic, Cephalosporin (First Generation)

Generic Available Yes

Use Treatment of susceptible bacterial infections, including those caused by group A beta-hemolytic *Streptococcus*, *Staphylococcus*, *Klebsiella pneumoniae*, *E. coli*, and *Proteus mirabilis*; not active against enterococci; used to treat susceptible infections of the respiratory tract, skin and skin structure, bone, genitourinary tract, and otitis media

Pregnancy Risk Factor B

Contraindications Hypersensitivity to cephalexin, any component, or cephalosporins

Warnings Prolonged use may result in gastrointestinal or genitourinary superinfection; do not use in patients with immediate-type hypersensitivity reactions to penicillin

Precautions Use with caution and modify dosage in patients with renal impairment; use with caution in patients with history of colitis or history of penicillin hypersensitivity

Adverse Reactions

Central nervous system: Dizziness, headache, fatigue, fever
Dermatologic: Rash
Gastrointestinal: Nausea, vomiting, pseudomembranous colitis, diarrhea, cramps
Hematologic: Transient neutropenia, anemia, eosinophilia
Hepatic: Transient elevation in liver enzymes

Drug Interactions Probenecid increases serum concentration of cephalexin

Food Interactions Presence of food may delay absorption

Stability Refrigerate suspension after reconstitution; discard after 14 days

Mechanism of Action Inhibits bacterial cell wall synthesis by binding to one or more of the penicillin-binding proteins; inhibits the final transpeptidation step of peptidoglycan synthesis resulting in cell wall death

Pharmacokinetics

Absorption: Delayed in young children and may be decreased up to 50% in neonates

Distribution: Into tissues and fluids including bone, pleural and synovial fluid; crosses the placenta; appears in breast milk

Protein binding: 6% to 15%

Half-life:
Neonates: 5 hours
Children 3-12 months: 2.5 hours
Adults: 0.5-1.2 hours (prolonged with renal impairment)

Time to peak serum concentration: Oral: Within 60 minutes

Elimination: 80% to 100% of dose excreted as unchanged drug in urine within 8 hours

Moderately dialyzable (20% to 50%)

Usual Dosage Oral:

Children: 25-100 mg/kg/day divided every 6-8 hours; maximum dose: 4 g/day
Adults: 250-500 mg every 6 hours; maximum dose: 4 g/day

Dosing interval in renal impairment:
Cl_{cr} 10-40 mL/minute: Administer every 8-12 hours
Cl_{cr} <10 mL/minute: Administer every 12-24 hours

Administration Oral: Administer on an empty stomach (ie, 1 hour prior to, or 2 hours after meals); administer with food if GI upset occurs; shake suspension well before use

Monitoring Parameters With prolonged therapy, monitor renal, hepatic, and hematologic function periodically; number and type of stools/day for diarrhea

Test Interactions False-positive urine glucose with Clinitest®; positive Coombs' [direct]; false $\uparrow$ serum or urine creatinine

Dosage Forms

Capsule, as monohydrate: 250 mg, 500 mg
Powder for oral suspension, as monohydrate: 125 mg/5 mL (5 mL unit dose, 60 mL, 100 mL, 200 mL); 250 mg/5 mL (5 mL unit dose, 100 mL, 200 mL)
Suspension, oral, as monohydrate, pediatric: 100 mg/mL [5 mg/drop] (10 mL)
Tablet, as monohydrate: 500 mg, 1 g
Tablet, as hydrochloride: 500 mg

♦ **Cephalexin Hydrochloride** see Cephalexin on page 196

Cephalothin (sef A loe thin)

Brand Names Ceporacin® (Canada); Keflin® Injection

Available Salts Cephalothin Sodium

Therapeutic Category Antibiotic, Cephalosporin (First Generation)

Generic Available Yes

Use Treatment of respiratory tract, skin and skin structure, urinary tract, bone and joint infections, endocarditis, and septicemia due to susceptible gram-positive cocci (except enterococcus); some gram-negative bacilli including *E. coli*, *Proteus*, and *Klebsiella* may be susceptible; perioperative prophylaxis

Pregnancy Risk Factor B

Contraindications Hypersensitivity to cephalothin, any component, or cephalosporins

Warnings Prolonged use may result in superinfection; do not use in patients with immediate-type hypersensitivity reactions to penicillin

Precautions Use with caution in patients with a history of colitis or in patients with a history of hypersensitivity to penicillins; modify dosage in patients with renal impairment

Adverse Reactions

Central nervous system: Dizziness, headache, fever
Dermatologic: Rash, urticaria, pruritus
Gastrointestinal: Nausea, vomiting, diarrhea, dyspepsia, pseudomembranous colitis
Hematological: Hemolytic anemia, granulocytopenia, eosinophilia, thrombocytopenia, prolonged PT, bleeding
Hepatic: Transient elevation in AST and alkaline phosphatase
Local: Severe phlebitis (especially with doses >6 g/day for longer than 3 days), thrombophlebitis, pain and induration at injection site
Renal: Elevated BUN and serum creatinine, nephrotoxicity

Drug Interactions Probenecid decreases renal clearance of cephalothin; aminoglycosides may increase risk of nephrotoxicity

Stability Reconstituted solution is stable for 12-24 hours at room temperature and 96 hours when refrigerated; thawed solution of the commercially available frozen (Continued)

Cephalothin *(Continued)*

cephalothin injection is stable for 12 hours at room temperature or 7 days when refrigerated

Mechanism of Action Inhibits bacterial cell wall synthesis by binding to one or more of the penicillin-binding proteins and interfering with the final transpeptidation step of peptidoglycan synthesis

Pharmacokinetics

Distribution: Widely distributed throughout the body but with poor penetration into CSF and bile; crosses the placenta

Protein binding: 65% to 80%

Metabolism: 10% to 40% metabolized in the liver and kidneys to desacetylcephalothin (active metabolite)

Half-life:

Neonates <7 days: 90-120 minutes

Adults with normal renal function: 30-60 minutes (cephalothin) and 12 minutes (desacetylcephalothin)

Time to peak serum concentration: I.M.: Within 30 minutes

Elimination: 50% to 75% of a dose is excreted in the urine as unchanged drug

Usual Dosage

Neonates: I.V.:

Postnatal age ≤7 days:

≤2000 g: 40 mg/kg/day divided every 12 hours

>2000 g: 60 mg/kg/day divided every 8 hours

Postnatal age >7 days:

<1200 g: 40 mg/kg/day divided every 12 hours

1200-2000 g: 60 mg/kg/day divided every 8 hours

>2000 g: 80 mg/kg/day divided every 6 hours

Children: I.M., I.V.: 80-150 mg/kg/day divided every 4-6 hours; maximum dose: 12 g/day

Perioperative prophylaxis: I.V.: 20-30 mg/kg 30-60 minutes prior to surgery and 20-30 mg/kg every 6 hours for no more than 24 hours after surgery depending on the procedure

Adults: I.M., I.V.: 500 mg to 2 g every 4-6 hours; maximum dose: 12 g/day

Perioperative prophylaxis: I.V.: 1-2 g 30-60 minutes prior to surgery and 1-2 g every 6 hours for no more than 24 hours after surgery depending on the procedure

Dosing interval in renal impairment:

Cl_{cr} 10-50 mL/minute: Administer every 6-8 hours

Cl_{cr} <10 mL/minute: Administer every 12 hours

Administration Parenteral:

IVP: Administer over 3-5 minutes at a maximum concentration of 100 mg/mL

I.V. intermittent infusion: Administer over 30-60 minutes at a final concentration for I.V. administration ≤100 mg/mL

Monitoring Parameters Periodic renal function tests when used in combination with other nephrotoxic drugs, hepatic function tests, and CBC; number and type of stools/day for diarrhea

Test Interactions False-positive urine glucose, using Clinitest®, positive Coombs' [direct], false ↑ serum or urine creatinine

Nursing Implications Monitor patient for vein irritation

Additional Information Sodium content of 1 g: 2.8 mEq

Dosage Forms

Infusion, as sodium, in $D_{1.1}W$ (frozen): 2 g (50 mL)

Infusion, as sodium, in $D_{3.5}W$ (frozen): 1 g (50 mL)

Powder for injection, as sodium: 1 g, 2 g

References

Pickering LK, O'Connor DM, Anderson D, et al, "Comparative Evaluation of Cefazolin and Cephalothin in Children," *J Pediatr*, 1974, 85(6):842-7.

♦ **Cephalothin Sodium** *see* Cephalothin *on page 197*

Cephapirin *(sef a PYE rin)*

Brand Names Cefadyl®

Available Salts Cephapirin Sodium

Therapeutic Category Antibiotic, Cephalosporin (First Generation)

Generic Available No

Use Treatment of respiratory tract, skin and skin structure, urinary tract, bone and joint infections, endocarditis and septicemia due to susceptible gram-positive cocci (except enterococcus); some gram-negative bacilli including *E. coli*, *Proteus*, and *Klebsiella*, may be susceptible; perioperative prophylaxis

Pregnancy Risk Factor B

Contraindications Hypersensitivity to cephapirin sodium, any component, or cephalosporins

Warnings Prolonged use may result in superinfection; safety and efficacy in infants <3 months of age have not been established; do not use in patients with immediate-type hypersensitivity reactions to penicillin

Precautions Use with caution in patients with a history of colitis or in patients with a history of hypersensitivity to penicillins; modify dosage in patients with renal impairment

Adverse Reactions

Central nervous system: Fever

Dermatologic: Rash, urticaria

Gastrointestinal: Diarrhea, pseudomembranous colitis

Hematologic: Neutropenia, eosinophilia, leukopenia, thrombocytopenia

Hepatic: Elevated AST, ALT, alkaline phosphatase, and bilirubin; jaundice

Local: Thrombophlebitis, pain on injection

Renal: Nephrotoxicity, acute interstitial nephritis, elevated BUN, elevated serum creatinine

Drug Interactions Probenecid decreases renal clearance of cephapirin; aminoglycosides may increase risk of nephrotoxicity

Stability Reconstituted solution is stable for 12 hours at room temperature and 10 days when refrigerated; after freezing, thawed solution is stable for 12 hours at room temperature or 10 days when refrigerated

Mechanism of Action Inhibits bacterial cell wall synthesis by binding to one or more of the penicillin-binding proteins and interfering with the final transpeptidation step of peptidoglycan synthesis

Pharmacokinetics

Distribution: Widely distributed to tissues and fluids including heart, bone, pericardial, pleural and synovial fluid; crosses the placenta; only small amounts distribute into CSF and breast milk

Protein binding: 44% to 50%

Metabolism: Partially metabolized in the liver, kidneys, and plasma to desacetylcephapirin (active metabolites)

Half-life: 21-48 minutes (adults with normal renal function) and 26 minutes (desacetylcephapirin)

Time to peak serum concentration: I.M.: Within 30 minutes

Elimination: 30% to 70% excreted as unchanged drug in urine

Hemodialysis: 23% of a dose is removed by hemodialysis

Usual Dosage I.M., I.V.:

Infants >3 months of age and Children: 40-80 mg/kg/day divided every 6 hours; maximum dose: 12 g/day

Adults: 500 mg to 1 g every 6 hours up to 12 g/day

Perioperative prophylaxis: 1-2 g 30-60 minutes prior to surgery and 1-2 g every 6 hours for no more than 24 hours after surgery depending on the procedure

Dosing interval in renal impairment:

Cl$_{cr}$ 10-50 mL/minute: Administer every 6-8 hours

Cl$_{cr}$ <10 mL/minute: Administer every 12 hours

Administration Parenteral:

IVP: Administer over 3-5 minutes at a maximum concentration of 100 mg/mL

I.V. intermittent infusion: Administer over 30 minutes; maximum cephapirin concentration that can be administered to fluid-restricted patients is 200 mg/mL

Monitoring Parameters Periodic renal function tests, CBC; number and type of stools/day for diarrhea

Test Interactions False-positive urine glucose using Clinitest®; positive Coombs' [direct]; false ↑ serum or urine creatinine

Nursing Implications Monitor patient for vein irritation

Additional Information Sodium content of 1 g: 2.4 mEq

Dosage Forms Powder for injection, as sodium: 500 mg, 1 g, 2 g, 4 g, 20 g

References

Khan AJ and Pryles CV, "Clinical and Pharmacological Evaluation of Cephapirin Sodium (BL-P-1322) in Infants and Children (Cephapirin in Pediatric Patients)," *Curr Ther Res Clin Exp*, 1973, 15(4):198-204.

♦ **Cephapirin Sodium** *see* Cephapirin *on page 198*

Cephradine (SEF ra deen)

Related Information
  Carbohydrate and Alcohol Content of Liquid Medications for Use in Patients Receiving Ketogenic Diets *on page 1228*

Brand Names Velosef®

Therapeutic Category Antibiotic, Cephalosporin (First Generation)

Generic Available Yes

Use Treatment of susceptible bacterial infections, including skin and skin structure infections caused by *Streptococcus* or *Staphylococcus*; urinary tract infections caused by *Klebsiella, E. coli,* and *Proteus mirabilis*; respiratory tract infections caused by group A beta-hemolytic streptococci and *Streptococcus pneumoniae*; otitis media caused by group A beta-hemolytic streptococci, *Streptococcus pneumoniae,* or *H. influenzae*

Pregnancy Risk Factor B

Contraindications Hypersensitivity to cephradine, any component, or cephalosporins

Warnings Prolonged use may result in superinfection; do not use in patients with immediate-type hypersensitivity reaction to penicillin

Precautions Use with caution in patients with a history of penicillin hypersensitivity; reduce dose in patients with renal impairment

Adverse Reactions
  Dermatologic: Rash
  Gastrointestinal: Diarrhea, nausea, vomiting, pseudomembranous colitis
  Genitourinary: Vaginitis
  Hematologic: Positive Coombs' test, transient neutropenia
  Hepatic: Increased hepatic enzymes, increased bilirubin
  Neuromuscular & skeletal: Arthralgia
  Renal: Elevated BUN, elevated serum creatinine

Drug Interactions Probenecid may decrease renal tubular secretion and increase cephradine serum concentrations

Food Interactions Food will decrease the rate, but not the extent of oral absorption

Stability Oral suspension: Stable for 7 days at room temperature, or 14 days at 2°C to 8°C after reconstitution

Mechanism of Action Interferes with bacterial cell wall synthesis during active replication, causing cell wall death and resultant bactericidal activity against susceptible bacteria

Pharmacokinetics
  Absorption: Well absorbed from GI tract
  Distribution: V_d: 0.25 L/kg; crosses the placenta; appears in breast milk
  Protein binding: 6% to 20%
  Half-life: Adults: 0.7-2 hours; Children: 1 hour; half-life increases with renal dysfunction
  Time to peak serum concentration: Oral: Within 1-2 hours
  Elimination: Excreted unchanged in the urine (80% to 90%) via glomerular filtration and tubular secretion

Usual Dosage Oral:
  Infants ≥9 months and children:
    Usual: 25-50 mg/kg/day in divided doses every 6-12 hours
    Otitis media: 75-100 mg/kg/day in divided doses every 6-12 hours
    Maximum dose: 4 g/day
  Adults:
    Oral: 250-500 mg every 6-12 hours
  Dosing adjustment in renal impairment:
    Cl_{cr} 10-50 mL/minute: Administer 50% of dose given at normal interval
    Cl_{cr} <10 mL/minute: Administer 25% of dose given at normal interval
    or
    Cl_{cr} 25-50 mL/minute: Administer normal dose every 12 hours
    Cl_{cr} 10-25 mL/minute: Administer normal dose every 24 hours
    Cl_{cr} <10 mL/minute: Administer normal dose every 36 hours

Administration Oral: May be administered without regard to food; shake suspension well before use

Test Interactions False-positive Coombs' test; may falsely elevate creatinine values when Jaffé reaction is used; may cause false-positive results in urine glucose tests using cupric sulfate (Benedict's solution, Clinitest®)

Patient Information Report persistent diarrhea; entire course of medication (eg, 10-14 days) should be taken to ensure eradication of organism

Additional Information Efficacy not established for twice daily dosing in infants <9 months of age; parenteral product no longer available in the United States

Dosage Forms
Capsule: 250 mg, 500 mg
Powder for oral suspension: 125 mg/5 mL (5 mL, 100 mL, 200 mL); 250 mg/5 mL (5 mL, 100 mL, 200 mL)

References
Donowitz GR and Mandell GL, "Drug Therapy. Beta-Lactam Antibiotics (1)," *N Engl J Med*, 1988, 318(7):419-26.
Donowitz GR and Mandell GL, "Drug Therapy. Beta-Lactam Antibiotics (2)," *N Engl J Med*, 1988, 318(8):490-500.
Gustaferro CA and Steckelberg JM, "Cephalosporin Antimicrobial Agents and Related Compounds," *Mayo Clin Proc*, 1991, 66(10):1064-73.
Smith GH, "Oral Cephalosporins in Perspective," *DICP*, 1990, 24(1):45-51.

- ◆ **Cephulac®** *see* Lactulose *on page 550*
- ◆ **Ceporacin® (Canada)** *see* Cephalothin *on page 197*
- ◆ **Ceptaz™** *see* Ceftazidime *on page 190*
- ◆ **Ceptaz™ (Canada)** *see* Ceftazidime *on page 190*
- ◆ **Cerebyx®** *see* Fosphenytoin *on page 443*
- ◆ **Ceredase® Injection** *see* Alglucerase *on page 47*
- ◆ **Cerezyme®** *see* Imiglucerase *on page 506*
- ◆ **Cerubidine®** *see* Daunorubicin *on page 285*
- ◆ **Cerumenex® Otic** *see* Triethanolamine Polypeptide Oleate-Condensate *on page 951*
- ◆ **C.E.S.** *see* Estrogens, Conjugated *on page 387*
- ◆ **C.E.S.™ (Canada)** *see* Estrogens, Conjugated *on page 387*
- ◆ **Cetacort® Topical** *see* Hydrocortisone *on page 486*
- ◆ **Cetamide®** *see* Sulfacetamide *on page 888*
- ◆ **Cetane® [OTC]** *see* Ascorbic Acid *on page 96*

Cetirizine (se TI ra zeen)

Brand Names Reactine™ (Canada); Zyrtec®
Available Salts Cetirizine Hydrochloride
Synonyms P-071; UCB-P071
Therapeutic Category Antihistamine
Generic Available No
Use Perennial and seasonal allergic rhinitis; chronic idiopathic urticaria
Pregnancy Risk Factor B
Contraindications Hypersensitivity to cetirizine, hydroxyzine, or any component
Warnings Doses >10 mg/day may cause significant drowsiness
Precautions Use with caution in patients with hepatic or renal dysfunction
Adverse Reactions
Central nervous system: Headache, drowsiness, somnolence, fatigue, dizziness, depression, confusion, vertigo, ataxia
Gastrointestinal: Diarrhea, flatulence, constipation, xerostomia, dyspepsia, abdominal pain, pharyngitis
Neuromuscular & skeletal: Paresthesias, hyperkinesia, hypertonia, tremor, leg cramps
Respiratory: Cough, epistaxis, bronchospasm
Drug Interactions Increased cetirizine toxicity: CNS depressants, anticholinergics; theophylline may decrease cetirizine clearance with potential increased toxicity
Stability Store at room temperature; protect syrup from light
Mechanism of Action Cetirizine, a metabolite of hydroxyzine, competes with histamine for H_1-receptor sites on effector cells in the gastrointestinal tract, blood vessels, and respiratory tract
Pharmacodynamics
Onset of effect: 20-60 minutes
Duration of effect: 24 hours
Pharmacokinetics
Absorption: Well absorbed from the GI tract
Distribution: V_d:
Children: 0.7 L/kg
Adults: 0.5-0.8 L/kg
Protein binding: 93%
Metabolism: Exact fate is unknown, limited hepatic metabolism
Half-life:
Children: 6.2 hours
(Continued)

Cetirizine *(Continued)*

Adults: 7.4-9 hours

Adults with mild-moderate renal failure: 19-21 hours

Time to peak serum concentration: 1 hour

Elimination: 60% to 70% excreted unchanged in urine

Usual Dosage Oral:

Children <2 years: Limited data: 0.25 mg/kg/day as a single dose

Children 2-5 years: 2.5 mg/day; may be increased to a maximum of 5 mg/day given either as a single dose or divided into 2 doses

Children ≥6 years to Adults: 5-10 mg/day as a single dose or divided into 2 doses

Dosing interval in renal or hepatic impairment: Adults with Cl$_{cr}$ ≤31 mL/minute, dialysis patients with Cl$_{cr}$ <7 mL/minute, or hepatic impairment: Administer 5 mg/day

Administration Oral: Administer with or without food

Patient Information Causes drowsiness and may impair ability to perform hazardous tasks requiring mental alertness

Dosage Forms

Syrup, as hydrochloride: 5 mg/5mL

Tablet, film-coated, as hydrochloride: 5 mg, 10 mg

♦ **Cetirizine Hydrochloride** *see Cetirizine on page 201*

♦ **Cevalin® [OTC]** *see Ascorbic Acid on page 96*

♦ **Cevi-bid® [OTC]** *see Ascorbic Acid on page 96*

♦ **Ce-Vi-Sol® [OTC]** *see Ascorbic Acid on page 96*

♦ **CG** *see Chorionic Gonadotropin on page 221*

♦ **CharcoAid® [OTC]** *see Charcoal on page 202*

♦ **CharcoAid® 2000 [OTC]** *see Charcoal on page 202*

Charcoal *(CHAR kole)*

Brand Names Actidose-Aqua® [OTC]; Actidose® With Sorbitol [OTC]; CharcoAid® [OTC]; CharcoAid® 2000 [OTC]; Charcocaps® [OTC]; Insta-Char® [OTC]; Liqui-Char® [OTC]

Synonyms Activated Carbon; Activated Charcoal; Adsorbent Charcoal; Liquid Antidote; Medicinal Carbon; Medicinal Charcoal

Therapeutic Category Antidiarrheal; Antidote, Adsorbent; Antiflatulent

Generic Available Yes

Use Emergency treatment in poisoning by drugs and chemicals; repetitive doses for gastrointestinal dialysis in drug overdose to enhance the elimination of certain drugs (eg, theophylline, phenobarbital, carbamazepine, dapsone, quinine) and in uremia to adsorb various waste products

Pregnancy Risk Factor C

Contraindications Patients with an unprotected airway (eg, depressed CNS state without endotracheal intubation); patients at increased risk and severity of aspiration (eg, ingestion of hydrocarbon with a high potential for aspiration); patients at risk of GI perforation or hemorrhage due to medical conditions, recent surgery, or other pathology; **Note:** Ingestion of a corrosive (caustic) substance is **not** a contraindication if charcoal is used for co-ingested systemic toxin. Charcoal is not effective for cyanide, mineral acids, caustic alkalis, organic solvents, iron, ethanol, methanol or lithium poisonings; do not use charcoal with sorbitol in patients with fructose intolerance; charcoal with sorbitol is not recommended in children <1 year of age

Warnings If charcoal in sorbitol is administered, doses should be limited to prevent excessive fluid and electrolyte losses

Precautions When using ipecac with charcoal, induce vomiting with ipecac before administering activated charcoal since charcoal adsorbs ipecac syrup; charcoal may cause vomiting which is hazardous in petroleum distillate and caustic ingestions; charcoal (especially in multiple doses) may adsorb maintenance medications and place the patient at risk for exacerbation of concomitant disorders

Adverse Reactions

Gastrointestinal: Vomiting (**Note:** Use of charcoal with sorbitol may increase rate of emesis), constipation, intestinal obstruction, black stools; diarrhea if product contains sorbitol

Ocular: Corneal abrasions if spilled into eyes

Miscellaneous: Aspiration may cause tracheal obstruction in infants, but usually not a major problem in adults; aspiration pneumonitis, bronchiolitis obliterans, and ARDS have been reported following aspiration of charcoal; however, these problems may be due to the aspiration of gastric contents and not charcoal per se

Food Interactions Milk, ice cream, sherbet, or marmalade may reduce charcoal's effectiveness; chocolate or fruit syrup do not appear to reduce efficacy

Stability Adsorbs gases from air; store in closed container

Mechanism of Action Adsorbs toxic substances or irritants, thus inhibiting GI absorption; for select drugs, increases drug clearance by interfering with enterohepatic recycling or dialysis across intestine; adsorbs intestinal gas; the addition of sorbitol results in hyperosmotic laxative action causing catharsis

Pharmacodynamics In studies using adult human volunteers: Mean **reduction** in drug absorption following a single dose of activated charcoal:

All size doses of activated charcoal:
  Given within 30 minutes after ingestion: 69.1% reduction
  Given at 60 minutes after ingestion: 34.4% reduction
50 g activated charcoal:
  Given within 30 minutes after ingestion: 88.6% reduction
  Given at 60 minutes after ingestion: 37.3% reduction

Pharmacokinetics
  Absorption: Not absorbed from the GI tract
  Metabolism: Not metabolized
  Elimination: Excreted as charcoal in feces

Usual Dosage Oral:
  Acute poisoning:
    Single dose: Charcoal with sorbitol (**Note:** The use of repeated oral charcoal with sorbitol doses is not recommended):
      Infants <1 year: Not recommended
      Children 1-12 years: 1-2 g/kg or 25-50 g or approximately 5-10 times the weight of the ingested poison on a gram-to-gram basis; 1 g adsorbs 100-1000 mg of poison; in young children sorbitol should be repeated **no more** than 1-2 times/day
      Adolescents and Adults: 30-100 g
    Single dose: Charcoal in water (a cathartic such as sorbitol should be added in appropriate doses):
      Infants <1 year: 1 g/kg
      Children 1-12 years: 1-2 g/kg or 25-50 g
      Adolescents and Adults: 30-100 g or 1-2 g/kg
    Multiple dose: Charcoal in water (doses are repeated until clinical observations of toxicity subside and serum drug concentrations have returned to a subtherapeutic range or until the development of absent bowel sounds or ileus; use only one dose of cathartic daily):
      Infants <1 year: 1 g/kg every 4-6 hours
      Children 1-12 years: 1-2 g/kg or 15-30 g every 2-6 hours
      Adolescents and Adults: 25-60 g or 1-2 g/kg every 2-6 hours
  Gastric dialysis: Adults: 20-50 g every 6 hours for 1-2 days

Administration Oral: Administer as soon as possible after ingestion, preferably within 1 hour for greatest effect; shake well before use; do not mix with milk, ice cream, sherbet, or marmalade; may be mixed with chocolate or fruit syrup to increase palatability; instruct patient to drink slowly, rapid administration may increase frequency of vomiting; if patient has persistent vomiting, multiple doses may be administered as a continuous enteral infusion

Monitoring Parameters Fluid status, sorbitol intake, number of stools, electrolytes if increase in stools or diarrhea occurs

Patient Information Charcoal causes the stools to turn black

Nursing Implications Charcoal slurries that are too concentrated may clog airways, if aspirated

Additional Information 5-6 tablespoonfuls is approximately equal to 30 g of activated charcoal; minimum dilution of 240 mL water per 20-30 g activated charcoal should be mixed as an aqueous slurry; multiple dose activated charcoal has been shown to be effective in increasing the elimination of certain drugs (carbamazepine, theophylline, phenobarbital) even after these drugs have been absorbed

The Position Statement of The American Academy of Clinical Toxicology and The European Association of Poisons Centres and Clinical Toxicologists does not advocate routine use of single dose activated charcoal in the treatment of poisoned patients; scientific literature supports the use of activated charcoal within 1 hour of toxin ingestion, when it will be more likely to produce benefit. Therefore, this publication states that activated charcoal may be considered up to 1 hour following ingestion of a potentially toxic amount of poison; the use of activated charcoal may be considered greater than 1 hour following ingestion, but there are no studies to support or exclude its use; furthermore, based on current literature, the routine administration of a cathartic with activated charcoal is not recommended; when (Continued)

Charcoal *(Continued)*

cathartics are used, only a single dose should be administered so as to decrease adverse effects.

Dosage Forms

Capsule (Charcocaps®): 260 mg

Granules, activated: CharcoAid® 2000: 15 g (120 mL)

Liquid, activated:

Actidose-Aqua®: 12.5 g (60 mL); 25 g (120 mL)

CharcoAid® 2000: 15 g (120 mL); 50 g (240 mL)

Liqui-Char®: 12.5 g (60 mL); 15 g (75 mL); 25 g (120 mL); 30 g (120 mL); 50 g (240 mL)

Liquid, activated, with propylene glycol: 12.5 g (60 mL); 25 g (120 mL)

Liquid, activated, with sorbitol:

Actidose® With Sorbitol: 25 g (120 mL); 50 g (240 mL)

Charcoaid®: 15 g (120 mL); 30 g (150 mL)

CharcoAid® 2000: 15 g (120 mL); 50 g (240 mL)

Powder for suspension, activated: 15 g, 30 g, 40 g, 120 g, 240 g

References

Burns MM, "Activated Charcoal as the Sole Intervention for Treatment After Childhood Poisoning," *Curr Opin Pediatr*, 2000, 12(2):166-71.

Farley TA, "Severe Hypernatremic Dehydration After Use of an Activated Charcoal-Sorbitol Suspension," *J Pediatr*, 1986, 109(4):719-22.

"Position Statement: Cathartics. American Academy of Clinical Toxicology; European Association of Poisons Centres and Clinical Toxicologists," *J Toxicol Clin Toxicol*, 1997, 35(7):743-52.

"Position Statement: Single-Dose Activated Charcoal. American Academy of Clinical Toxicology; European Association of Poisons Centres and Clinical Toxicologists," *J Toxicol Clin Toxicol*, 1997, 35(7):721-41.

Shannon M, "Ingestion of Toxic Substances by Children," *N Engl J Med*, 2000, 342(3):186-91.

♦ **Charcocaps® [OTC]** *see* Charcoal *on page 202*

♦ **Chealamide®** *see* Edetate Disodium *on page 358*

♦ **Chemet®** *see* Succimer *on page 883*

♦ **Cheracol®** *see* Guaifenesin and Codeine *on page 465*

♦ **Cheracol D® [OTC]** *see* Guaifenesin and Dextromethorphan *on page 466*

♦ **Chiggertox® [OTC]** *see* Benzocaine *on page 124*

♦ **Children's Advil® Suspension** *see* Ibuprofen *on page 501*

♦ **Children's Hold® [OTC]** *see* Dextromethorphan *on page 304*

♦ **Children's Kaopectate® [OTC]** *see* Attapulgite *on page 109*

♦ **Children's Motrin® Suspension [OTC]** *see* Ibuprofen *on page 501*

♦ **Children's Silfedrine® [OTC]** *see* Pseudoephedrine *on page 822*

♦ **Chlo-Amine® Oral [OTC]** *see* Chlorpheniramine *on page 214*

♦ **Chloral** *see* Chloral Hydrate *on page 204*

Chloral Hydrate *(KLOR al HYE drate)*

Related Information

Carbohydrate and Alcohol Content of Liquid Medications for Use in Patients Receiving Ketogenic Diets *on page 1228*

Preprocedure Sedatives in Children *on page 1169*

Brand Names Aquachloral® Supprettes®; Novo-Chlorhydrate® (Canada); PMS-Chloral Hydrate (Canada)

Synonyms Chloral; Hydrated Chloral; Trichloroacetaldehyde Monohydrate

Therapeutic Category Hypnotic; Sedative

Generic Available Yes

Use Short-term sedative and hypnotic (<2 weeks), sedative/hypnotic prior to nonpainful therapeutic or diagnostic procedures (eg, EEG, CT scan, MRI, ophthalmic exam, dental procedure)

Restrictions C-IV

Pregnancy Risk Factor C

Contraindications Hypersensitivity to chloral hydrate or any component; hepatic or renal impairment; gastritis or ulcers; severe cardiac disease

Warnings Trichloroethanol (TCE), an active metabolite of chloral hydrate, is a carcinogen in mice; there is no data in humans

Precautions Use with caution in neonates, drug and metabolites may accumulate with repeated use; prolonged use in neonates is associated with direct hyperbilirubinemia (active metabolite [TCE] competes with bilirubin for glucuronide conjugation in the liver); use with caution in patients with porphyria. Tolerance to hypnotic effect develops, therefore, not recommended for use >2 weeks; taper dosage to avoid withdrawal with prolonged use. Avoid use in patients with moderate to severe renal failure (Cl_{cr} <50 mL/minute).

Adverse Reactions
Central nervous system: Disorientation, sedation, excitement (paradoxical), dizziness, fever, headache, ataxia

Dermatologic: Rash, urticaria

Gastrointestinal: Gastric irritation, nausea, vomiting, diarrhea, flatulence

Hematologic: Leukopenia, eosinophilia

Respiratory: Respiratory depression when combined with other sedatives or narcotics

Miscellaneous: Physical and psychological dependence with prolonged use

Drug Interactions
May potentiate effects of warfarin, central nervous system depressants, alcohol; vasodilation reaction (flushing, tachycardia, etc) may occur with concurrent use of alcohol; concomitant use of furosemide (I.V.) may result in flushing, sweating, and blood pressure changes; chloral hydrate may increase the conversion of cyclophosphamide and ifosfamide to active metabolites and may increase toxicity

Stability
Sensitive to light; exposure to air causes volatilization; store in light-resistant, airtight container

Mechanism of Action
Central nervous system depressant effects are primarily due to its active metabolite trichloroethanol, mechanism unknown; in neonates, chloral hydrate itself may play a role in the immediate sedative effects

Pharmacodynamics
Onset of action: 10-20 minutes

Peak effects: Within 30-60 minutes

Duration: 4-8 hours

Pharmacokinetics
Absorption: Oral, rectal: Well absorbed

Distribution: Crosses the placenta; negligible amounts appear in breast milk

Protein binding: Trichloroethanol: 35% to 40%; trichloroacetic acid: ~94% (may compete with bilirubin for albumin binding sites)

Metabolism: Rapidly metabolized by alcohol dehydrogenase to trichloroethanol (active metabolite); trichloroethanol undergoes glucuronidation in the liver; variable amounts of chloral hydrate and trichloroethanol are metabolized in liver and kidney to trichloroacetic acid (inactive)

Half-life:
Chloral hydrate: Infants: 1 hour

Trichloroethanol (active metabolite):
Neonates: Range: 8.5-66 hours

Half-life decreases with increasing postconceptional age (PCA):
Preterm infants (PCA 31-37 weeks): Mean half-life: 40 hours

Term infants (PCA 38-42 weeks): Mean half-life: 28 hours

Older children (PCA 57-708 weeks): Mean half-life: 10 hours

Adults: 8-11 hours

Trichloroacetic acid: Adults: 67.2 hours

Elimination: Metabolites excreted in urine; small amounts excreted in feces via bile

Dialyzable (50% to 100%)

Usual Dosage
Oral, rectal:

Neonates: 25 mg/kg/dose for sedation prior to a procedure; **Note:** Repeat doses should be used with great caution, as drug and metabolites accumulate with repeated use; toxicity has been reported after 3 days in a preterm neonate and after 7 days in a term neonate receiving chloral hydrate 40-50 mg/kg every 6 hours

Infants and Children:
Sedation, anxiety: 25-50 mg/kg/day divided every 6-8 hours, maximum dose: 500 mg/dose

Prior to EEG: 25-50 mg/kg/dose 30-60 minutes prior to EEG; may repeat in 30 minutes to a total maximum of 100 mg/kg or 1 g total for infants and 2 g total for children

Hypnotic: 50 mg/kg; maximum dose: 2 g/dose/day

Sedation, nonpainful procedure: 50-75 mg/kg/dose 30-60 minutes prior to procedure; may repeat 30 minutes after initial dose if needed, to a total maximum dose of 120 mg/kg or 1 g total for infants and 2 g total for children

Adults:
Sedation, anxiety: 250 mg 3 times/day

Hypnotic: 500-1000 mg at bedtime or 30 minutes prior to procedure, not to exceed 2 g/24 hours

Dosing adjustment in renal impairment:
Cl_{cr} ≥50 mL/minute: No dosage adjustment needed

(Continued)

Chloral Hydrate *(Continued)*

Cl$_{cr}$ <50 mL/minute: Avoid use

Administration Oral: Minimize unpleasant taste and gastric irritation by administering with water, infant formula, fruit juice, or ginger ale; do not crush capsule, contains drug in liquid form with unpleasant taste

Monitoring Parameters Level of sedation; vital signs and O$_2$ saturation with doses used for sedation prior to procedure

Test Interactions False-positive urine glucose using Clinitest® method; may interfere with fluorometric urine catecholamine and urinary 17-hydroxycorticosteroid tests

Patient Information May cause drowsiness and impair ability to perform hazardous duties requiring mental alertness; avoid alcohol and other CNS depressants

Nursing Implications May cause irritation of skin and mucous membranes

Additional Information Not an analgesic; osmolality of 500 mg/5 mL syrup is approximately 3500 mOsm/kg

Dosage Forms

Capsule: 500 mg

Suppository, rectal: 324 mg, 500 mg, 648 mg

Syrup: 250 mg/5 mL (10 mL); 500 mg/5 mL (5 mL, 10 mL, 480 mL)

References

American Academy of Pediatrics, Committee on Drugs and Committee on Environmental Health, "Use of Chloral Hydrate for Sedation in Children," *Pediatrics*, 1993, 92(3):471-3.

Buck ML, "Chloral Hydrate Use During Infancy," *Neonatal Pharmacology Quarterly*, 1992, 1(1):31-7.

Mayers DJ, Hindmarsh KW, Gorecki DK, et al, "Sedative/Hypnotic Effects of Chloral Hydrate in the Neonate: Trichloroethanol or Parent Drug?" *Dev Pharmacol Ther*, 1992, 19(2-3):141-6.

Mayers DJ, Hindmarsh KW, Sankaran K, et al, "Chloral Hydrate Disposition Following Single-Dose Administration to Critically Ill Neonates and Children," *Dev Pharmacol Ther*, 1991, 16(2):71-7.

Steinberg AD, "Should Chloral Hydrate be Banned?" *Pediatrics*, 1993, 92(3)442-6.

Chlorambucil *(klor AM byoo sil)*

Related Information

Emetogenic Potential of Single Chemotherapeutic Agents *on page 1095*

Brand Names Leukeran®

Therapeutic Category Antineoplastic Agent, Alkylating Agent (Nitrogen Mustard)

Generic Available No

Use Treatment of chronic lymphocytic leukemia (CLL), Hodgkin's and non-Hodgkin's lymphoma; breast and ovarian carcinoma, testicular carcinoma, choriocarcinoma; Waldenström's macroglobulinemia, and nephrotic syndrome unresponsive to conventional therapy

Pregnancy Risk Factor D

Contraindications Hypersensitivity to chlorambucil or any component, or previous resistance

Warnings The FDA currently recommends that procedures for proper handling and disposal of antineoplastic agents be considered. Chlorambucil can severely suppress bone marrow function; affects human fertility; carcinogenic in humans and probably mutagenic and teratogenic as well; chromosomal damage has been documented; secondary AML may be associated with chronic therapy.

Precautions Use with caution in patients with seizure disorder and bone marrow suppression; reduce initial dosage if patient has received radiation therapy, myelosuppressive drugs or has a depressed baseline leukocyte or platelet count within the previous 4 weeks

Adverse Reactions

Central nervous system: Seizures, fever, agitation, irritability, hyperactivity, confusion, ataxia

Dermatologic: Rash, pruritus, erythema multiforme, toxic epidermal necrolysis

Endocrine & metabolic: Hyperuricemia, menstrual cramps, amenorrhea

Gastrointestinal: Nausea, vomiting, abdominal pain, stomatitis, diarrhea

Genitourinary: Oligospermia

Hematologic: Leukopenia, thrombocytopenia, anemia, lymphocytopenia, neutropenia

Hepatic: Hepatotoxicity, jaundice

Neuromuscular & skeletal: Tremor, muscular twitching, weakness

Respiratory: Pulmonary fibrosis

Drug Interactions Phenobarbital (possible increased chlorambucil toxicity)

Food Interactions Avoid acidic foods, hot foods, and spices; increased bioavailability when administered with food

Mechanism of Action Interferes with DNA replication and RNA transcription by alkylation and cross-linking the strands of DNA; immunosuppressive activity due to suppression of lymphocytes

Pharmacokinetics

Absorption: Oral: 70% to 80% from GI tract

Distribution: To liver, ascitic fluid, fat; extensively bound to plasma and tissue proteins; crosses the placenta

Protein binding: ~99%

Metabolism: In the liver to an active metabolite, phenylacetic acid mustard

Bioavailability: 56% to 100% (increased when taken with food)

Half-life: Chlorambucil: 1.5 hours; phenylacetic acid mustard: 2.5 hours

Elimination: 60% excreted in urine within 24 hours principally as metabolites; <1% excreted as unchanged drug in urine

Probably not dialyzable

Usual Dosage Oral (refer to individual protocols):

Children:

General short courses: 0.1-0.2 mg/kg/day or 4.5 mg/m^2/day once daily for 3-6 weeks for remission induction (usual: 4-10 mg/day); maintenance therapy: 0.03-0.1 mg/kg/day (usual: 2-4 mg/day)

Nephrotic syndrome: 0.1-0.2 mg/kg/day every day for 5-12 weeks with low dose prednisone

CLL:

Biweekly regimen: Initial: 0.4 mg/kg/dose every 2 weeks; increase dose by 0.1 mg/kg every 2 weeks until a response occurs and/or myelosuppression occurs

Monthly regimen: Initial: 0.4 mg/kg every 4 weeks, increase dose by 0.2 mg/kg every 4 weeks until a response occurs and/or myelosuppression occurs

Malignant lymphomas:

Non-Hodgkin's lymphoma: 0.1 mg/kg/day

Hodgkin's: 0.2 mg/kg/day

Adults: 0.1-0.2 mg/kg/day or 3-6 mg/m^2/day once daily for 3-6 weeks, then adjust dose on basis of blood counts

Administration Oral: Administer with food

Monitoring Parameters Liver function tests, CBC, leukocyte and platelet counts, serum uric acid

Patient Information Notify physician if fever, sore throat, or bleeding occurs

Additional Information Myelosuppressive effects:

WBC: Moderate

Platelets: Moderate

Onset (days): 7

Nadir (days): 14-21

Dosage Forms Tablet, sugar coated: 2 mg

Extemporaneous Preparations A 2 mg/mL suspension was stable for 7 days when refrigerated and compounded as follows: Pulverize sixty 2 mg tablets; levigate with a small amount of glycerin; add 20 mL Cologel® and levigate until a uniform mixture is obtained; add a 2:1 simple syrup/cherry syrup mixture to make a total volume of 60 mL; label "refrigerate" and "shake well before use"

Handbook on Extemporaneous Formulations, 3rd ed, Bethesda, MD: American Society of Hospital Pharmacists, 1997.

References

Baluarte HJ, Hiner L, and Gruskin AB, "Chlorambucil Dosage in Frequently Relapsing Nephrotic Syndrome: A Controlled Clinical Trial," *J Pediatr*, 1978, 92(2):295-8.

Chloramphenicol (klor am FEN i kole)

Related Information

Blood Level Sampling Time Guidelines *on page 1189*

Drugs and Breast-Feeding *on page 1213*

Brand Names AK-Chlor® Ophthalmic; Chloromycetin®; Chloroptic® Ophthalmic; Diochloram (Canada); Ophthochlor® Ophthalmic; Ortho-Chloram® (Canada); Pentamycetin® (Canada); Sopamycetin® (Canada)

Available Salts Chloramphenicol Sodium Succinate

Therapeutic Category Antibacterial, Otic; Antibiotic, Ophthalmic; Antibiotic, Otic; Antibiotic, Miscellaneous

Generic Available Yes

Use Treatment of serious infections due to organisms resistant to other less toxic antibiotics or when its penetrability into the site of infection is clinically superior to other antibiotics to which the organism is sensitive; useful in infections caused by (Continued)

Chloramphenicol *(Continued)*

Bacteroides, H. influenzae, Neisseria meningitidis, S. pneumoniae, Salmonella, and *Rickettsia*

Pregnancy Risk Factor C

Contraindications Hypersensitivity to chloramphenicol or any component

Warnings Serious and fatal blood dyscrasias have occurred after both short-term and prolonged therapy; should not be used when less potentially toxic agents are effective; prolonged use may result in superinfection; breast-feeding is not recommended

Precautions Use with caution in patients with G-6-PD deficiency, impaired renal or hepatic function and in neonates; monitor serum concentrations and CBC in all patients; reduce dose in patients with hepatic and renal impairment

Adverse Reactions

Cardiovascular: Cardiotoxicity (left ventricular dysfunction), gray baby syndrome (see Additional Information)

Central nervous system: Nightmares, headache

Dermatologic: Rash

Gastrointestinal: Diarrhea, stomatitis, enterocolitis, vomiting

Hematologic: Bone marrow suppression, aplastic anemia, neutropenia, thrombocytopenia, hemolysis in patients with G-6-PD deficiency, anemia (see additional information)

Hepatic: Hepatitis-pancytopenia syndrome

Neuromuscular & skeletal: Peripheral neuropathy

Ocular: Optic neuritis

Miscellaneous: Anaphylaxis

Drug Interactions Chloramphenicol inhibits the metabolism of chlorpropamide, phenytoin, oral anticoagulants; phenobarbital and rifampin may decrease concentration of chloramphenicol; phenytoin may increase chloramphenicol concentration

Food Interactions May decrease intestinal absorption of vitamin B_{12}; may have increased dietary need for riboflavin, pyridoxine, and vitamin B_{12}

Stability Store ophthalmic solution in the refrigerator; reconstituted parenteral solution (100 mg/mL) is stable for 30 days at room temperature

Mechanism of Action Reversibly binds to 50S ribosomal subunits of susceptible organisms preventing amino acids from being transferred to growing peptide chains thus inhibiting protein synthesis

Pharmacokinetics

Distribution: Readily crosses the placenta; appears in breast milk; distributes to most tissues and body fluids; good CSF and brain penetration

CSF concentration with uninflamed meninges: 21% to 50% of plasma concentration

CSF concentration with inflamed meninges: 45% to 89% of plasma concentration

Protein binding: 60%

Metabolism: Extensive in the liver (90%) to inactive metabolites, principally by glucuronidation; chloramphenicol sodium succinate must be hydrolyzed by esterases to active base.

Half-life:

Neonates:

1-2 days: 24 hours

10-16 days: 10 hours

Adults: 1.6-3.3 hours (prolonged with hepatic insufficiency)

Elimination: 5% to 15% excreted as unchanged drug in urine and 4% excreted in bile; in neonates, 6% to 80% of the dose may be excreted unchanged in urine

Slightly dialyzable (5% to 20%)

Usual Dosage

Neonates: Initial loading dose: I.V. (I.M. administration is not recommended): 20 mg/kg (the first maintenance dose should be given 12 hours after the loading dose)

Maintenance dose: Postnatal age:

≤7 days: 25 mg/kg/day once every 24 hours

>7 days, ≤2000 g: 25 mg/kg/day once every 24 hours

>7 days, >2000 g: 50 mg/kg/day divided every 12 hours

Meningitis: I.V.: Infants and Children: Maintenance dose: 75-100 mg/kg/day divided every 6 hours

Other infections: I.V.:

Infants and Children: 50-75 mg/kg/day divided every 6 hours; maximum daily dose: 4 g/day

Adults: 50 mg/kg/day in divided doses every 6 hours; maximum daily dose: 4 g/day

Dosing adjustment in renal and/or hepatic impairment: Dose reduction should be based upon serum chloramphenicol concentrations

Children and Adults:
Ophthalmic: Apply 1-2 drops or small amount of ointment every 3-6 hours; increase interval between applications after 48 hours
Otic: Place 2-3 drops into the affected ear 3 times/day
Topical: Gently rub into the affected area 3-4 times/day

Administration
Ophthalmic: Solution: Reconstitute powder with sterile water to make a final concentration of 0.5%, 0.25%, or 0.16% chloramphenicol; avoid contact of tube or bottle tip with skin or eye
Otic: Apply topically to external ear
Parenteral:
IVP: Administer over 5 minutes at a maximum concentration of 100 mg/mL
I.V. intermittent infusion: Administer over 15-30 minutes at a final concentration for administration ≤20 mg/mL

Monitoring Parameters CBC with reticulocyte and platelet counts, serum iron level, iron-binding capacity, periodic liver and renal function tests, serum drug concentration

Reference Range
Meningitis:
Peak: 15-25 µg/mL
Trough: 5-15 µg/mL
Other infections:
Peak: 10-20 µg/mL
Trough: 5-10 µg/mL

Nursing Implications Draw peak levels 90 minutes after the end of a 30-minute infusion; trough levels should be drawn just prior to the next dose

Additional Information Sodium content of 1 g injection: 2.25 mEq
Three (3) major toxicities associated with chloramphenicol include:
Aplastic anemia, an idiosyncratic reaction which can occur with any route of administration; usually occurs 3 weeks to 12 months after initial exposure to chloramphenicol; incidence: 1 in 40,000 cases
Bone marrow suppression is thought to be dose-related with serum concentrations >25 mcg/mL and reversible once chloramphenicol is discontinued; anemia and neutropenia may occur during the first week of therapy
Gray baby syndrome is characterized by circulatory collapse, hypothermia, cyanosis, acidosis, abdominal distention, myocardial depression, coma, and death; reaction appears to be associated with serum levels ≥50 mcg/mL; may result from drug accumulation in patients with impaired hepatic or renal function; may occur after 3-4 days of therapy or within hours of initiating therapy

Dosage Forms
Cream (Chloromycetin®): 1% (30 g)
Ointment, ophthalmic (AK-Chlor®, Chloromycetin®, Chloroptic®): 1% [10 mg/g] (3.5 g)
Powder for injection, as sodium succinate: 1 g
Powder for ophthalmic solution (Chloromycetin®): 25 mg/vial
Solution:
Ophthalmic (AK-Chlor®, Chloroptic®, Ophthochlor®): 0.5% [5 mg/mL] (2.5 mL, 7.5 mL, 15 mL)
Otic (Chloromycetin®): 0.5% (15 mL)

References
Nahata MC and Powell DA, "Bioavailability and Clearance of Chloramphenicol After Intravenous Chloramphenicol Succinate," *Clin Pharmacol Ther*, 1981, 30(3):368-72.

♦ **Chloramphenicol Sodium Succinate** *see* Chloramphenicol *on page 207*
♦ **Chlorate® Oral [OTC]** *see* Chlorpheniramine *on page 214*

Chlorhexidine Gluconate (klor HEKS i deen GLOO koe nate)

Brand Names BactoShield® [OTC]; Betasept® [OTC]; Dyna-Hex® [OTC]; Exidine® Scrub [OTC]; Hibiclens® [OTC]; Hibidil® 1:2000 (Canada); Hibistat® [OTC]; Hibitane® Skin Cleanser (Canada); Oro-Clense (Canada); Peridex®; Periochip®; PerioGard®

Therapeutic Category Antibacterial, Topical; Antibiotic, Oral Rinse

Generic Available Yes

Use Skin cleanser for surgical scrub; cleanser for skin wounds; germicidal hand rinse; antibacterial dental rinse to reduce plaque formation and control gingivitis; (Continued)

Chlorhexidine Gluconate *(Continued)*

prophylactic dental rinse to prevent oral infections in immunocompromised patients, particularly bone marrow transplant patients receiving cytotoxic therapy; and short-term substitute for toothbrushing in situations where the patient is unable to tolerate mechanical stimulation of the gums; chip, for periodontal pocket insertion (indicated as an adjunct to scaling and root planing procedures)

Pregnancy Risk Factor B

Contraindications Hypersensitivity to chlorhexidine gluconate or any component; do not use as a preoperative skin preparation of the face or head (except Hibiclens® liquid) as serious, permanent eye injury has occurred when chlorhexidine gluconate enters and remains in the eye during surgery.

Warnings For topical use only; there have been several case reports of anaphylaxis following disinfection with chlorhexidine; a case of bradycardic episodes after breast-feeding in a 2 day old infant whose mother used chlorhexidine gluconate topically on her breasts to prevent mastitis has been reported; use of periodontal chip has not been studied in patients with an acutely abscessed periodontal pocket and is not recommended

Precautions Staining of oral surfaces, teeth, restorations, and dorsum of tongue may occur and may be visible as soon as 1 week after therapy begins; staining is more pronounced when there is a heavy accumulation of unremoved plaque and when teeth fillings have rough surfaces; stain does not have clinically adverse effect, but because removal may not be possible, patients with frontal restoration should be advised of the potential permanency of the stain; avoid contact with meninges; corneal injury has been associated with direct eye contact (see Contraindications); deafness has been associated with direct instillation into the middle ear through a perforated eardrum

Adverse Reactions

Dermatologic: Skin irritation, photosensitivity (rare)

Gastrointestinal: Tongue irritation, minor irritation and superficial desquamation of oral mucosa (particularly among children), increased tartar on teeth, staining of oral surfaces (mucosa, teeth, and dorsum of tongue; see Warnings), dysgeusia, transient parotiditis; toothache (chip)

Ophthalmic: Corneal damage (see Precautions)

Otic: Deafness (see Precautions)

Respiratory: Nasal congestion, shortness of breath

Miscellaneous: Edema of face, anaphylactoid reactions

Drug Interactions When combined with nystatin, *in vitro*, the minimum inhibitory concentrations (MIC) of susceptible organisms, were increased to both agents.

Stability Store away from heat and direct light; do not freeze

Mechanism of Action The bactericidal effect of chlorhexidine is a result of the binding of this cationic molecule to negatively charged bacterial cell walls and extramicrobial complexes. At low concentrations, this causes an alteration of bacterial cell osmotic equilibrium and leakage of potassium and phosphorous resulting in a bacteriostatic effect. At high concentrations of chlorhexidine, the cytoplasmic contents of the bacterial cell precipitate and result in cell death. Chlorhexidine is active against gram-positive and gram-negative organisms, facultative anaerobes, anaerobes, and yeast.

Pharmacokinetics

Absorption: ~30% of chlorhexidine is retained in the oral cavity following rinsing and is slowly released into the oral fluids; chlorhexidine is poorly absorbed from the GI tract and is not absorbed topically through intact skin

Serum concentrations: Detectable levels are not present in the plasma 12 hours after administration

Elimination: Primarily through the feces (~90%); <1% excreted in the urine

Usual Dosage

Chip: Adults: 1-8 chips per procedure; repeat every 3 months

Oral rinse (Peridex® or PerioGard®) (see Administration: Oral):

Children and Adults: 15 mL twice daily

Immunocompromised patient: 10-15 mL, 2-3 times/day

Cleanser: Children and Adults: Apply 5 mL per scrub or hand wash; apply 25 mL per body wash or hair wash

Administration

Chip: Pocket should be isolated and surrounding area dried prior to chip insertion; chip should be grasped using forceps with the rounded edges away from the forceps; chip should be inserted into the periodontal pocket to its maximum depth; it may be maneuvered into position using the tips of the forceps or a flat instrument; the chip biodegrades completely and does not need to be removed

Oral rinse: Precede use of solution by flossing and brushing teeth, completely rinse toothpaste from mouth; swish undiluted oral rinse around in mouth for 30 seconds, then expectorate; caution patient not to swallow the medicine; avoid eating for 2-3 hours after treatment.

Topical:

Surgical scrub: Scrub 3 minutes and rinse thoroughly, wash for an additional 3 minutes

Hand wash: Wash for 15 seconds and rinse

Hand rinse: Rub vigorously for 15 seconds

Body wash: Wet body and/or hair, apply, rinse thoroughly, repeat.

Monitoring Parameters Improvement in gingival inflammation and bleeding; development of teeth or denture discoloration; dental prophylaxis to remove stains at regular intervals of no greater than 6 months.

Test Interactions If chlorhexidine is used as a disinfectant before midstream urine collection, a false-positive urine protein may result (when using dipstick method based upon a pH indicator color change).

Patient Information

Chip: Mild to moderate sensitivity may be noted in the first week following insertion; avoid using dental floss at site of insertion for 10 days after insertion; notify dentist if pain or swelling occurs.

Oral rinse: Use after tooth brushing; do not swallow, do not rinse after use; may cause reduced taste perception which is reversible; may cause discoloration of teeth which may be removed with professional dental cleaning; notify dentist or physician if difficulty breathing or flushing or swelling of face occurs

Topical administration is for external use only; if accidentally enters eyes or ears, rinse out promptly and thoroughly with water

Dosage Forms

Chip for periodontal pocket insertion (Periochip®): 2.5 mg

Foam, topical, with isopropyl alcohol 4% (BactoShield®): 4% (180 mL)

Liquid, topical, with isopropyl alcohol 4%:

Skin cleanser:

DynaHex®, Exidine®, Hibiclens®: 2% (120 mL, 240 mL, 480 mL, 960 mL)

BactoShield® 2.2% (960 mL); 4% (15 mL, 120 mL, 240 mL, 480 mL, 4000 mL);

Sponge/brush (Hibiclens®): 4% (22 mL)

Rinse:

Oral (Peridex®, PerioGard®): 0.12% with alcohol 11.6% (480 mL)

Topical (Hibistat® Hand Rinse): 0.5% with isopropyl alcohol 70% (120 mL, 240 mL)

Wipes, topical (Hibistat®): 0.5% with 70% isopropanol

References

Quinn MW and Bini RM, "Bradycardia Associated With Chlorhexidine Spray," *Arch Dis Child*, 1989, 64(6):892-3.

Yong D, Parker FC, and Foran SM, "Severe Allergic Reactions and Intra-Urethral Chlorhexidine Gluconate," *Med J Aust*, 1995, 162(5):257-8.

◆ **2-Chlorodeoxyadenosine** *see* Cladribine *on page 232*

◆ **Chloromycetin®** *see* Chloramphenicol *on page 207*

◆ **Chloroptic® Ophthalmic** *see* Chloramphenicol *on page 207*

Chloroquine (KLOR oh kwin)

Brand Names Aralen® Phosphate

Available Salts Chloroquine Phosphate

Therapeutic Category Amebicide; Antimalarial Agent

Generic Available Yes

Use Suppression or chemoprophylaxis of malaria in chloroquine-sensitive areas; treatment of uncomplicated or mild-moderate malaria due to susceptible *Plasmodium* species, except chloroquine-resistant *Plasmodium falciparum*; extraintestinal amebiasis; rheumatoid arthritis; discoid lupus erythematosus, scleroderma, pemphigus

Pregnancy Risk Factor C

Contraindications Retinal or visual field changes; patients with psoriasis; hypersensitivity to chloroquine or any component

Precautions Use with caution in patients with liver disease, G-6-PD deficiency, or in conjunction with hepatotoxic drugs

Adverse Reactions

Cardiovascular: Hypotension, EKG changes

Central nervous system: Fatigue, personality changes, headache, confusion, agitation, psychotic episodes, seizures

Dermatologic: Pruritus, hair bleaching, skin eruptions, exfoliative dermatitis

(Continued)

Chloroquine *(Continued)*

Gastrointestinal: Anorexia, nausea, vomiting, diarrhea, stomatitis, weight loss

Hematologic: Blood dyscrasias (neutropenia, aplastic anemia, thrombocytopenia)

Neuromuscular & skeletal: Peripheral neuropathy, neuromyopathy, myalgia

Ocular: Retinopathy, blurred vision, corneal opacity, photophobia

Otic: Tinnitus, deafness

Drug Interactions Intradermally administered rabies vaccine; cimetidine increases levels of chloroquine; urinary acidifiers increase the elimination of chloroquine

Stability Protect from light

Mechanism of Action Binds to and inhibits DNA and RNA polymerase; interferes with metabolism and hemoglobin utilization by parasites; inhibits prostaglandin effects

Pharmacokinetics

Absorption: Oral: Rapid

Distribution: Widely distributed in body tissues including eyes, heart, kidneys, liver, and lungs where retention is prolonged; crosses the placenta; appears in breast milk

Protein binding: 50% to 65%

Metabolism: Partial hepatic

Half-life: 3-5 days

Time to peak serum concentration: Oral: Within 1-2 hours

Elimination: ~70% of dose excreted unchanged in urine; acidification of the urine increases elimination of drug; small amounts of drug may be present in urine months following discontinuation of therapy

Minimally removed by hemodialysis

Usual Dosage (Dosage expressed in terms of base):

Oral:

Suppression or prophylaxis of malaria:

Children: Administer 5 mg base/kg/week on the same day each week (not to exceed 300 mg base/dose); begin 1-2 weeks prior to exposure; continue for 4 weeks after leaving endemic area; if suppressive therapy is not begun prior to exposure, double the initial loading dose to 10 mg base/kg and give in 2 divided doses 6 hours apart, followed by the usual dosage regimen

Adults: 300 mg/week (base) on the same day each week; begin 1-2 weeks prior to exposure; continue for 4 weeks after leaving endemic area; if suppressive therapy is not begun prior to exposure, double the initial loading dose to 600 mg base and give in 2 divided doses 6 hours apart, followed by the usual dosage regimen

Acute attack:

Children: 10 mg base/kg (maximum dose: 600 mg) stat, then 5 mg base/kg (maximum dose: 300 mg base) 6 hours later and then 5 mg base/kg/day (maximum daily dose: 300 mg base) once daily for 2 days

Adults: 600 mg base/dose one time, then 300 mg base/dose 6 hours later, and then 300 mg base/dose once daily for 2 days

Extraintestinal amebiasis:

Children: 10 mg base/kg once daily for 2-3 weeks (up to 300 mg base/day)

Adults: 600 mg base/day for 2 days followed by 300 mg base/day for at least 2-3 weeks

Rheumatoid arthritis: Adults: 150 mg base once daily

I.M.:

Severe malaria when oral therapy is not feasible:

Children: 5 mg base/kg (maximum dose: 200 mg base); dose may be repeated in 6 hours; maximum dose: 10 mg base/kg in a 24-hour period

Adults: 200 mg base every 6 hours

Administration

Oral: Administer with meals to decrease GI upset; chloroquine phosphate tablets have also been mixed with chocolate syrup or enclosed in gelatin capsules to mask the bitter taste

Parenteral: Cautious administration of frequent small doses by I.M. or S.C. injection in children may reduce risk of severe adverse effects (eg, 2.5 mg base/kg every 4 hours not to exceed 10 mg base/kg in a 24-hour period)

Monitoring Parameters Periodic CBC, examination for muscular weakness and ophthalmologic examination in patients receiving prolonged therapy

Patient Information Report any visual disturbances, muscular weakness, or difficulty in hearing or ringing in the ears; tablets are bitter tasting

Dosage Forms

Injection, as phosphate: 40 mg [base] per mL (5 mL)

Tablet, as phosphate: 250 mg [150 mg base]; 500 mg [300 mg base]

Extemporaneous Preparations A 15 mg chloroquine base/mL suspension is made by pulverizing three Aralen® 500 mg phosphate = 300 mg base/tablet, levigating with 15 mL of a 1:1 vehicle of Ora-Sweet® and Ora-Plus®, and adding vehicle by geometric proportion, levigating until a uniform mixture is obtained; qsad to 100 mL with vehicle, stable for up to 60 days when stored at 5°C or 25°C and protected from light. Label "shake well before using" and "protect from light."

Allen LV Jr and Erickson MA, "Stability of Alprazolam, Chloroquine Phosphate, Cisapride, Enalapril Maleate, and Hydralazine Hydrochloride in Extemporaneously Compounded Oral Liquids," *Am J Health Syst Pharm*, 1998, 55(18):1915-20.

References
Wyler DJ, "Malaria Chemoprophylaxis for the Traveler," *N Engl J Med*, 1993, 329(1):31-7.

♦ **Chloroquine Phosphate** *see* Chloroquine *on page 211*

Chlorothiazide (klor oh THYE a zide)

Related Information
Carbohydrate and Alcohol Content of Liquid Medications for Use in Patients Receiving Ketogenic Diets *on page 1228*

Brand Names Diurigen®; Diuril®

Available Salts Chlorothiazide Sodium

Therapeutic Category Antihypertensive Agent; Diuretic, Thiazide

Generic Available Yes: Tablet

Use Management of mild to moderate hypertension; edema associated with CHF, pregnancy, or nephrotic syndrome

Pregnancy Risk Factor D

Contraindications Hypersensitivity to chlorothiazide or any component; cross-sensitivity with other thiazides or sulfonamides; do not use in anuric patients

Warnings The injection must not be administered subcutaneously or I.M.

Precautions Use with caution in patients with severe renal disease, impaired hepatic function, moderate-high cholesterol concentrations, and in patients with high triglycerides

Adverse Reactions
Cardiovascular: Hypotension, arrhythmia, weak pulse
Central nervous system: Dizziness, vertigo, headache, fever
Dermatologic: Rash, photosensitivity
Endocrine & metabolic: Hypokalemia, hypochloremic alkalosis, hyperglycemia, hyperlipidemia, hyperuricemia
Gastrointestinal: Anorexia, nausea, vomiting, cramping, diarrhea, pancreatitis, constipation
Hematologic: Rarely blood dyscrasias
Hepatic: Intrahepatic cholestasis
Neuromuscular & skeletal: Muscle weakness, paresthesia
Ophthalmic: Blurred vision
Renal: Prerenal azotemia, hematuria

Drug Interactions NSAIDs with chlorothiazide may result in decreased antihypertensive effect; additive potassium losses with steroids, loop diuretics and amphotericin B; decreases lithium clearance; increases hypersensitivity reactions to allopurinol; increases hyperglycemia with diazoxide; decreases absorption of chlorothiazide when administered with cholestyramine; milk-alkali syndrome with high calcium dosages

Food Interactions Avoid natural licorice (causes sodium and water retention and increases potassium loss); may need to decrease sodium and calcium, may need to increase potassium, zinc, magnesium, and riboflavin in diet

Stability Reconstituted injection is stable for 24 hours at room temperature

Mechanism of Action Inhibits sodium reabsorption in the distal tubules causing increased excretion of sodium, chloride, potassium, bicarbonate, magnesium, phosphate, calcium (transiently) and water

Pharmacodynamics
Diuresis: Onset of effect: Oral: Within 2 hours
Duration:
  Oral: ~6-12 hours
  I.V.: 2 hours

Pharmacokinetics
Absorption: Oral: Poor (~10% to 20%); dose dependent
Distribution: Breast milk to plasma ratio: 0.05
Half-life: Adults: 45-120 minutes
Time to peak serum concentration: Within 4 hours
Elimination: Excreted unchanged in urine
(Continued)

Chlorothiazide *(Continued)*

Usual Dosage I.V. dosage in infants and children has not been well established. The following I.V. dosages in infants and children have been extrapolated from oral absorption data (~10% to 20%) and have been used successfully. Equivalent I.V./ oral doses have been used safely in adult patients.

Neonates and Infants <6 months:
Oral: 20-40 mg/kg/day in 2 divided doses; maximum: 375 mg/day
I.V.: 2-8 mg/kg/day in 2 divided doses
Infants >6 months and Children:
Oral: 20 mg/kg/day in 2 divided doses; maximum: 1 g/day
I.V.: 4 mg/kg/day divided in 1-2 doses
Adults:
Oral: 500 mg to 2 g/day divided in 1-2 doses
I.V.:100-500 mg/day divided in 1-2 doses

Administration

Oral: Administer with food; shake suspension well before use
Parenteral: Dilute 500 mg vial with 18 mL sterile water (resulting in 27.8 mg/mL concentration); administer by direct I.V. infusion over 3-5 minutes or infusion over 30 minutes in dextrose or NS; avoid extravasation of parenteral solution since it is extremely irritating to tissues

Monitoring Parameters Serum electrolytes (sodium, potassium, chloride, and bicarbonate), glucose, uric acid, triglycerides

Dosage Forms

Powder for injection, lyophilized, as sodium: 500 mg
Suspension, oral: 250 mg/5 mL (237 mL)
Tablet: 250 mg, 500 mg

♦ **Chlorothiazide Sodium** *see* Chlorothiazide *on page 213*
♦ **Chlorphed® [OTC]** *see* Brompheniramine *on page 142*
♦ **Chlorphed®-LA Nasal Solution [OTC]** *see* Oxymetazoline *on page 718*

Chlorpheniramine (klor fen IR a meen)

Related Information

OTC Cough & Cold Preparations, Pediatric *on page 1037*
Overdose and Toxicology *on page 1191*

Brand Names Aller-Chlor® Oral [OTC]; AL-Rr® Oral [OTC]; Chlo-Amine® Oral [OTC]; Chlorate® Oral [OTC]; Chlor-Pro® Injection; Chlor-Trimeton® Injection; Chlor-Trimeton® Oral [OTC]; Chlor-Tripolon® (Canada); Klorominr® Oral [OTC]; Phenetron® Oral; Polaramine®; Telachlor® Oral; Teldrin® Oral [OTC]

Available Salts Chlorpheniramine Maleate; Chlorpheniramine Tannate; Dexchlorpheniramine Maleate

Therapeutic Category Antihistamine

Generic Available Yes

Use Perennial and seasonal allergic rhinitis and other allergic symptoms including urticaria

Pregnancy Risk Factor B

Contraindications Hypersensitivity to chlorpheniramine maleate or any component; narrow-angle glaucoma, bladder neck obstruction, symptomatic prostatic hypertrophy, stenosing peptic ulcer, pyloroduodenal obstruction

Precautions Use with caution in patients with asthma; young children may be more susceptible to side effects and CNS stimulation

Adverse Reactions

Cardiovascular: Palpitations
Central nervous system: Drowsiness, vertigo, headache, excitability (children may be at increased risk for developing central nervous system stimulation), nervousness, fatigue, dizziness, depression
Dermatologic: Dermatitis, photosensitivity, angioedema
Gastrointestinal: Nausea, xerostomia, diarrhea, abdominal pain, appetite increase, weight gain
Genitourinary: Urinary retention
Neuromuscular & skeletal: Weakness, arthralgia, paresthesia
Ocular: Diplopia, blurred vision
Renal: Polyuria
Respiratory: Thickening of bronchial secretions, pharyngitis, epistaxis

Drug Interactions May cause additive sedation when concomitantly administered with other CNS depressant medications

Mechanism of Action Competes with histamine for H_1-receptor sites on effector cells in the gastrointestinal tract, blood vessels, and respiratory tract

Pharmacodynamics

Onset: Oral: 6 hours

Duration: Oral: 24 hours

Pharmacokinetics (Data from chlorpheniramine maleate)

Distribution: V_d:

Children: 3.8 L/kg

Adults: 2.5-3.2 L/kg

Protein binding: 69% to 72%

Metabolism: Substantial metabolism in GI mucosa and on first pass through liver

Bioavailability: Chlorpheniramine:

Solution: 35% to 60%

Tablet: 25% to 45%

Half-life:

Children: Average: 9.6-13.1 hours (range: 5.2-23.1 hours)

Adults: 12-43 hours

Time to peak serum concentration: Oral (solution and conventional tablets): 2-6 hours

Elimination: 35% excreted in 48 hours

Usual Dosage

Chlorpheniramine maleate: Oral:

Children <12 years: Oral: 0.35 mg/kg/day in divided doses every 4-6 hours or as an alternative

2-5 years: 1 mg every 4-6 hours

6-11 years: 2 mg every 4-6 hours, not to exceed 12 mg/day or timed release 8 mg every 12 hours

Children ≥12 years and Adults: 4 mg every 4-6 hours, not to exceed 24 mg/day or timed release 8-12 mg every 12 hours

Chlorpheniramine maleate: I.M., I.V., S.C.:

Children <12 years: 0.0875 mg/kg or 2.5 mg/m^2 4 times/day

Children ≥12 years and Adults: 5-20 mg as a single dose; not to exceed 40 mg/day

Dexchlorpheniramine maleate: Oral:

Children 2-5 years: 0.5 mg every 4-6 hours, not to exceed 3 mg/day

Children 6-11 years: 1 mg every 4-6 hours, not to exceed 6 mg/day **or** as timed release tablets: 4 mg once daily at bedtime

Children ≥12 years and Adults: 2 mg every 4-6 hours **or** as timed release tablets: 4-6 mg at bedtime or every 8-10 hours; not to exceed 12 mg/day

Administration

Oral: Administer with food to decrease GI distress; do not crush or chew timed release tablets

Parenteral: May be given I.M., I.V., or S.C.; do not administer intradermally

Patient Information Causes drowsiness and may impair ability to perform hazardous activities requiring mental alertness or physical coordination

Dosage Forms

Capsule, as chlorpheniramine maleate: 12 mg

Capsule, timed release, as chlorpheniramine maleate: 8 mg, 12 mg

Injection: as chlorpheniramine maleate: 10 mg/mL

Solution, as dexchlorpheniramine maleate (Polaramine®): 2 mg/5 mL

Syrup, as chlorpheniramine maleate: 2 mg/5 mL (120 mL, 473 mL)

Tablet, as chlorpheniramine maleate: 4 mg, 8 mg, 12 mg

Tablet, chewable, as chlorpheniramine maleate: 2 mg

Tablet, as dexchlorpheniramine maleate (Polaramine®): 2 mg

Tablet, timed release, as chlorpheniramine maleate: 8 mg, 12 mg

Tablet, timed release, as dexchlorpheniramine maleate (Polaramine®): 4 mg

♦ **Chlorpheniramine Maleate** see Chlorpheniramine on page 214

♦ **Chlorpheniramine Tannate** see Chlorpheniramine on page 214

♦ **Chlor-Pro® Injection** see Chlorpheniramine on page 214

♦ **Chlorpromanyl® (Canada)** see Chlorpromazine on page 215

Chlorpromazine (klor PROE ma zeen)

Related Information

Carbohydrate and Alcohol Content of Liquid Medications for Use in Patients Receiving Ketogenic Diets on page 1228

Compatibility of Medications Mixed in a Syringe on page 1208

Drugs and Breast-Feeding on page 1213

Overdose and Toxicology on page 1191

(Continued)

Chlorpromazine *(Continued)*

Prochlorperazine *on page 803*

Brand Names Apo®-Chlorpromazine (Canada); Chlorpromanyl® (Canada); Chlorprom® (Canada); Largactil® (Canada); Novo-Chlorpromazine® (Canada); Ormazine®; Thorazine®

Available Salts Chlorpromazine Hydrochloride

Therapeutic Category Antiemetic; Antipsychotic Agent; Phenothiazine Derivative

Generic Available Yes

Use Treatment of nausea and vomiting, psychoses, Tourette's syndrome, mania, intractable hiccups (adults), behavioral problems (children)

Pregnancy Risk Factor C

Contraindications Hypersensitivity to chlorpromazine hydrochloride or any component; cross-sensitivity with other phenothiazines may exist; avoid use in patients with narrow-angle glaucoma, bone marrow suppression, severe liver or cardiac disease

Warnings Significant hypotension may occur, especially when the drug is administered parenterally; extended release capsules and injection contain benzyl alcohol; injection also contains sulfites which may cause allergic reaction

Precautions Use with caution in patients with cardiovascular disease, seizures, significant medical disorders or children with acute illnesses

Adverse Reactions

Cardiovascular: Hypotension (especially with I.V. use), orthostatic hypotension, tachycardia, arrhythmias

Central nervous system: Sedation, drowsiness, restlessness, anxiety, extrapyramidal reactions, pseudoparkinsonian signs and symptoms, tardive dyskinesia, neuroleptic malignant syndrome, seizures, altered central temperature regulation

Dermatologic: Hyperpigmentation, pruritus, rash, photosensitivity; oral solution or injection may cause contact dermatitis (avoid contact with skin)

Endocrine & metabolic: Amenorrhea, galactorrhea, gynecomastia

Gastrointestinal: Xerostomia, constipation, GI upset, weight gain

Genitourinary: Impotence, urinary retention

Hematologic: Agranulocytosis, leukopenia (usually in patients with large doses for prolonged periods), thrombocytopenia, hemolytic anemia, eosinophilia

Hepatic: Cholestatic jaundice (rare)

Local: Thrombophlebitis

Ocular: Retinal pigmentation, blurred vision

Miscellaneous: Anaphylactoid reactions

Drug Interactions Cytochrome P-450 isoenzyme CYP1A2, CYP2D6, and CYP3A/4 substrate; isoenzyme CYP2D6 inhibitor

Additive effects with other CNS depressants; epinephrine may cause hypotension in patients receiving chlorpromazine due to phenothiazine-induced alpha-adrenergic blockade and unopposed epinephrine beta$_2$ action; chlorpromazine may increase valproic acid serum concentrations; absorption may be decreased if administered concomitantly with aluminum- or magnesium-containing antacids; liquid preparations of chlorpromazine will form an orange rubbery precipitate if mixed with or administered simultaneously with carbamazepine suspension; may interact with metyrapone and reduce test effectiveness; may interact with tranexamic acid

Food Interactions Interferes with riboflavin metabolism and may induce depletion; some may recommend increasing riboflavin in diet; may also decrease absorption of vitamin B$_{12}$; undiluted oral concentrate may precipitate tube feeding

Stability Protect oral dosage forms from light; discard solution if markedly discolored; diluted injection (1 mg/mL) with NS stored in 5 mL vials remains stable for 30 days; brown precipitate may occur when chlorpromazine is mixed with caffeine-containing liquids

Mechanism of Action Blocks postsynaptic mesolimbic dopaminergic receptors in the brain; exhibits a strong alpha-adrenergic blocking effect and depresses the release of hypothalamic and hypophyseal hormones

Pharmacodynamics

Onset of action:

Oral tablet: 30-60 minutes

Rectal suppository: >60 minutes

Antipsychotic effects: Gradual, may take up to several weeks

Time to peak antipsychotic effects: 6 weeks to 6 months

Duration of action:

Oral tablets: 4-6 hours

Rectal suppository: 3-4 hours

Pharmacokinetics

Absorption: Oral: Rapid and virtually complete; large first-pass effect due to metabolism during absorption in the GI mucosa

Distribution: Widely distributed into most body tissues and fluids; crosses blood-brain barrier and placenta; appears in breast milk; V_d: 8-160 L/kg (adults)

Protein binding: 90% to 99%

Metabolism: Extensively in the liver by demethylation (followed by glucuronide conjugation) and amine oxidation

Bioavailability: Oral: ~32%

Half-life, biphasic:
Initial: 2 hours
Terminal: 30 hours

Elimination: <1% excreted in urine as unchanged drug within 24 hours

Not dialyzable (0% to 5%)

Usual Dosage

Neonates: Neonatal abstinence syndrome (withdrawal from maternal narcotic use): I.M. and Oral: Initial: I.M.: 0.5-0.7 mg/kg/dose given every 6 hours; change to oral after ~4 days, decrease dose gradually over 2-3 weeks. **Note:** Chlorpromazine is rarely used for neonatal abstinence syndrome due to adverse effects such as hypothermia and eosinophilia. Other agents (eg, phenobarbital or a 25-fold dilution of tincture of opium) are preferred.

Children >6 months:

Psychosis:
Oral: 0.5-1 mg/kg/dose every 4-6 hours; older children may require 200 mg/day or higher
I.M., I.V.: 0.5-1 mg/kg/dose every 6-8 hours; maximum I.M./I.V. dose for <5 years (<22.7 kg) = 40 mg/day; maximum I.M./I.V. for 5-12 years (22.7-45.5 kg) = 75 mg/day

Nausea and vomiting:
Oral: 0.5-1 mg/kg/dose every 4-6 hours as needed
I.M., I.V.: 0.5-1 mg/kg/dose every 6-8 hours; maximum dose: Same as psychosis
Rectal: 1 mg/kg/dose every 6-8 hours as needed

Adults:

Psychosis:
Oral: Range: 30-800 mg/day in 1-4 divided doses, initiate at lower doses and titrate as needed; usual dose is 200 mg/day; some patients may require 1-2 g/day
I.M., I.V.: 25 mg initially, may repeat (25-50 mg) in 1-4 hours, gradually increase to a maximum of 400 mg/dose every 4-6 hours until patient controlled; usual dose 300-800 mg/day

Nausea and vomiting:
Oral: 10-25 mg every 4-6 hours
I.M., I.V.: 25-50 mg every 4-6 hours
Rectal: 50-100 mg every 6-8 hours

Administration

Oral: Administer with water, food, or milk to decrease GI upset; sustained release capsule should be swallowed whole; dilute oral concentrate solution in juice before administration; do not administer chlorpromazine liquid preparations simultaneously with carbamazepine suspension (see Drug Interactions)

Parenteral: Do not administer S.C. (tissue damage and irritation may occur); for direct I.V. injection: Dilute with NS to a maximum concentration of 1 mg/mL, administer slow I.V. at a rate not to exceed 1 mg/minute in adults and 0.5 mg/minute in children

Monitoring Parameters Periodic eye exam with prolonged therapy; blood pressure with parenteral administration; CBC with differential

Reference Range Relationship of plasma concentration to clinical response is not well established
Therapeutic: 50-300 ng/mL (SI: 157-942 nmol/L)
Toxic: >750 ng/mL (SI: >2355 nmol/L)

Test Interactions False-positives for phenylketonuria, amylase, uroporphyrins, urobilinogen; possible false-negative pregnancy urinary test

Patient Information May cause drowsiness and impair ability to perform activities requiring mental alertness or physical coordination; may cause dry mouth, photosensitivity; avoid excessive sunlight; use sunscreen

Nursing Implications Avoid contact of oral solution or injection with skin (may cause contact dermatitis)

(Continued)

Chlorpromazine *(Continued)*

Additional Information Although chlorpromazine has been used in combination with meperidine and promethazine as a premedication ("lytic cocktail"), this combination may have a higher rate of adverse effects compared to alternative sedatives/analgesics; see References. Use decreased doses in elderly or debilitated patients; dystonic reactions may be more common in patients with hypocalcemia; extrapyramidal reactions may be more common in pediatric patients, especially those with dehydration or acute illnesses (viral or CNS infections); avoid rectal administration in immunocompromised patients.

Dosage Forms
Capsule, as hydrochloride, sustained action: 30 mg, 75 mg, 150 mg, 200 mg, 300 mg
Concentrate, oral, as hydrochloride: 30 mg/mL (120 mL); 100 mg/mL (60 mL, 240 mL)
Injection, as hydrochloride: 25 mg/mL (1 mL, 2 mL, 10 mL)
Suppository, rectal, as base: 25 mg, 100 mg
Syrup, as hydrochloride: 10 mg/5 mL (120 mL)
Tablet, as hydrochloride: 10 mg, 25 mg, 50 mg, 100 mg, 200 mg

References
American Academy of Pediatrics Committee on Drugs, "Reappraisal of Lytic Cocktail/Demerol®, Phenergan®, and Thorazine® (DPT) for the Sedation of Children," *Pediatrics*, 1995, 95(4):598-602.

♦ **Chlorpromazine Hydrochloride** *see* Chlorpromazine *on page 215*
♦ **Chlorprom® (Canada)** *see* Chlorpromazine *on page 215*
♦ **Chlor-Trimeton® Injection** *see* Chlorpheniramine *on page 214*
♦ **Chlor-Trimeton® Oral [OTC]** *see* Chlorpheniramine *on page 214*
♦ **Chlor-Tripolon® (Canada)** *see* Chlorpheniramine *on page 214*

Chlorzoxazone (klor ZOKS a zone)

Brand Names Flexaphen®; Paraflex®; Parafon Forte™ DSC
Therapeutic Category Skeletal Muscle Relaxant, Nonparalytic
Generic Available Yes
Use Symptomatic treatment of muscle spasm and pain associated with acute musculoskeletal conditions
Pregnancy Risk Factor C
Contraindications Hypersensitivity to chlorzoxazone or any component; impaired liver function
Warnings Serious (including fatal) hepatocellular toxicity has been reported rarely
Adverse Reactions
Cardiovascular: Tachycardia, tightness in chest, flushing of face, syncope
Central nervous system: Drowsiness, dizziness, lightheadedness, headache, paradoxical stimulation, ataxia
Dermatologic: Rash, urticaria, petechiae, angioneurotic edema, erythema multiforme
Gastrointestinal: Nausea, vomiting, diarrhea, GI bleeding (rare), stomach cramps
Genitourinary: Discoloration of urine (orange or purple-red)
Hematologic: Anemia, granulocytopenia, eosinophilia
Hepatic: Hepatitis
Neuromuscular & skeletal: Paresthesia, trembling
Ocular: Burning of eyes
Respiratory: Shortness of breath
Miscellaneous: Hiccups
Drug Interactions May cause additive sedation when concomitantly administered with other CNS depressant medications
Food Interactions Watercress may decrease chlorzoxazone clearance
Mechanism of Action Acts on the spinal cord and subcortical levels by depressing polysynaptic reflexes
Pharmacodynamics
Onset of effects: Within 60 minutes
Duration: 3-4 hours
Pharmacokinetics
Absorption: Oral: Readily
Metabolism: Extensive in the liver by glucuronidation
Half-life: ~60 minutes
Elimination: In urine as conjugates
Usual Dosage Oral:
Children: 20 mg/kg/day or 600 mg/m²/day in 3-4 divided doses
Adults: 250-750 mg 3-4 times/day

Administration Oral: Administer with food

Monitoring Parameters Periodic liver function tests

Patient Information May color urine orange or purple-red; causes drowsiness and may impair ability to perform hazardous activities requiring mental alertness; notify physician if experiencing fever, rash, anorexia, right upper quadrant pain, dark urine, or jaundice

Dosage Forms
Caplet (Parafon Forte™ DSC): 500 mg
Capsule (Flexaphen®): 250 mg with acetaminophen 300 mg
Tablet: 250 mg

♦ **Cholac®** see Lactulose on page 550

Cholestyramine Resin (koe LES tir a meen REZ in)

Brand Names LoCHOLEST®; LoCHOLEST® Light; PMS-Cholestyramine (Canada); Prevalite®; Questran®; Questran® Light

Therapeutic Category Antilipemic Agent

Generic Available Yes

Use Adjunct in the management of primary hypercholesterolemia; pruritus associated with elevated levels of bile acids; diarrhea associated with excess fecal bile acids; pseudomembraneous colitis

Pregnancy Risk Factor C

Contraindications Hypersensitivity to cholestyramine or any component; avoid using in complete biliary obstruction or biliary atresia

Precautions Use with caution in patients with constipation; Prevalite® and Questran® Light contain aspartame, caution in patients with phenylketonuria

Adverse Reactions
Dermatologic: Rash
Endocrine & metabolic: Hyperchloremic acidosis
Gastrointestinal: Constipation, nausea, vomiting, abdominal distention and pain, malabsorption of fat-soluble vitamins
Genitourinary: Increased urinary calcium excretion
Local: Irritation of perianal area, skin, or tongue

Drug Interactions May decrease oral absorption of digitalis glycosides, warfarin, thyroid hormones, thiazide diuretics, propranolol, phenobarbital, amiodarone, methotrexate, NSAIDs, and other drugs by binding to the drug in the intestine

Food Interactions Cholestyramine (especially high doses or long-term therapy) may decrease the absorption of fat-soluble vitamins (vitamins A, D, E, and K), folic acid, calcium, and iron; deficiencies may occur including hypoprothrombinemia and increased bleeding from vitamin K deficiency; supplementation of vitamins A, D, E, and K, folic acid, and iron may be required with high-dose, long-term therapy

Mechanism of Action Forms a nonabsorbable complex with bile acids in the intestine, releasing chloride ions in the process; inhibits enterohepatic reuptake of intestinal bile salts and thereby increases the fecal loss of bile salt-bound low density lipoprotein cholesterol

Pharmacodynamics
Peak effect on serum cholesterol levels: Within 4 weeks

Pharmacokinetics
Absorption: Not absorbed from the GI tract
Elimination: Forms an insoluble complex with bile acids which is excreted in feces

Usual Dosage Oral (dosages are expressed in terms of anhydrous resin):
Children: 240 mg/kg/day in 3 divided doses; need to titrate dose depending on indication
Adults: 3-4 g 3-4 times/day to a maximum of 16-32 g/day in 2-4 divided doses

Administration Oral: Administer before meals; do not administer the powder in its dry form; just prior to administration, mix with water, noncarbonated liquid, or applesauce; to minimize binding of concomitant medications, administer other drugs including vitamins or mineral supplements at least 1 hour before or at least 4-6 hours after cholestyramine

Monitoring Parameters Serum cholesterol, serum triglycerides; with prolonged use, prothrombin time, liver enzymes, CBC, electrolytes; number of stools/day

Nursing Implications Maintain adequate oral fluid intake to avoid constipation; with high-dose, long-term therapy, use of daily multivitamin with iron and folic acid is recommended

Additional Information Overdose may result in GI obstruction

Dosage Forms
Powder: 4 g of resin/9 g of powder (9 g, 378 g)
(Continued)

Cholestyramine Resin *(Continued)*

Powder, for oral suspension, with aspartame:
Prevalite®: 4 g of resin/5.5 g of powder (5.5 g)
Questran® Light: 4 g of resin/5 g of powder (5 g, 210 g)

Choline Magnesium Trisalicylate

(KOE leen mag NEE zhum trye sa LIS i late)

Related Information
Overdose and Toxicology *on page 1191*

Brand Names Tricosal®; Trilisate®

Therapeutic Category Analgesic, Non-narcotic; Anti-inflammatory Agent;
Nonsteroidal Anti-inflammatory Drug (NSAID), Oral; Salicylate

Generic Available Yes

Use Management of osteoarthritis, rheumatoid arthritis, and other arthritides

Pregnancy Risk Factor C (D in 3rd trimester)

Contraindications Hypersensitivity to salicylates, any component, or other
nonacetylated salicylates

Warnings Avoid use in patients with suspected varicella or influenza (salicylates
have been associated with Reye's syndrome in children <16 years of age when
used to treat symptoms of chickenpox or the flu)

Precautions Use with extreme caution in patients with impaired renal function,
erosive gastritis or peptic ulcer

Adverse Reactions
Dermatologic: Rash, pruritus, urticaria
Gastrointestinal: Nausea, vomiting, GI distress, ulceration
Hepatic: Hepatotoxicity
Otic: Tinnitus
Respiratory: Pulmonary edema

Drug Interactions Antacids may decrease salicylate concentration; salicylates may
increase hypoprothrombinemic effect of warfarin

Mechanism of Action Inhibits prostaglandin synthesis; acts on the hypothalamus
heat-regulating center to reduce fever; blocks the generation of pain impulses

Pharmacokinetics
Absorption: From stomach and small intestine
Distribution: Readily distributes into most body fluids and tissues; crosses the
placenta; appears in breast milk
Protein binding: 90% to 95%
Metabolism: Hepatic microsomal enzyme system
Half-life: Dose-dependent, ranging from 2-3 hours at low doses to 30 hours at high
doses
Time to peak serum concentration:
Solution: 20-35 minutes
Tablet: Within ~2 hours
Elimination: 10% excreted as unchanged drug

Usual Dosage Oral (based on **total salicylate content**):
Children: 30-60 mg/kg/day given in 3-4 divided doses
Adults: 500 mg to 1.5 g 1-3 times/day

Administration Oral: Administer with food or milk to decrease GI upset; liquid may
be mixed with fruit juice just before drinking; do not administer with antacids

Monitoring Parameters Serum salicylate levels; serum magnesium with high
doses or in patients with decreased renal function

Reference Range
Salicylate blood levels for anti-inflammatory effect: 150-300 µg/mL
Analgesia and antipyretic effect: 30-50 µg/mL

Test Interactions False-negative results for Clinistix® urine test; false-positive
results with Clinitest®

Choline Magnesium Trisalicylate

Brand Name	Dosage Form	Total Salicylate	Choline Salicylate	Magnesium Salicylate
Trilisate®	Liquid	500 mg/5 mL	293 mg/5 mL	362 mg/5 mL
Trilisate 500®	Tablet	500 mg	293 mg	362 mg
Trilisate 750®	Tablet	750 mg	440 mg	544 mg
Trilisate 1000®	Tablet	1000 mg	587 mg	725 mg

Patient Information Avoid alcohol; notify physician if ringing in ears or persistent GI pain occurs

Additional Information Salicylate salts do not inhibit platelet aggregation and, therefore, should not be substituted for aspirin in the prophylaxis of thrombosis (ie, for aspirin's antiplatelet effects)

Dosage Forms See table on previous page.

References

Berde C, Ablin A, Glazer J, et al, "American Academy of Pediatrics Report of the Subcommittee on Disease-Related Pain in Childhood Cancer," *Pediatrics*, 1990, 86(5 Pt 2):818-25.

♦ **Chooz® [OTC]** *see* Calcium Supplements *on page 157*
♦ **Chorex®** *see* Chorionic Gonadotropin *on page 221*

Chorionic Gonadotropin (kor ee ON ik goe NAD oh troe pin)

Brand Names A.P.L.®; Chorex®; Choron®; Corgonject®; Follutein®; Glukor®; Gonic®; Pregnyl®; Profasi® HP

Synonyms CG; hCG

Therapeutic Category Gonadotropin; Ovulation Stimulator

Generic Available Yes

Use Treatment of hypogonadotropic hypogonadism, prepubertal cryptorchidism; induce ovulation

Pregnancy Risk Factor X

Contraindications Hypersensitivity to chorionic gonadotropin or any component; precocious puberty, prostatic carcinoma or similar neoplasms

Warnings hCG is **not** effective in the treatment of obesity; Pregnyl® contains benzyl alcohol; avoid use in neonates

Precautions Use with caution in patients with asthma, seizure disorders, migraine, cardiac or renal disease; may induce precocious puberty

Adverse Reactions
Cardiovascular: Edema
Central nervous system: Irritability, restlessness, depression, fatigue, headache, aggressive behavior
Endocrine & metabolic: Gynecomastia, precocious puberty
Local: Pain at the injection site
Neuromuscular & skeletal: Premature closure of epiphyses

Stability Following reconstitution with provided diluent, stable for 30-90 days (depending upon preparation) when stored at 2°C to 15°C

Mechanism of Action Stimulates production of gonadal steroid hormones by causing production of androgen by the testis; as a substitute for luteinizing hormone (LH) to stimulate ovulation

Pharmacokinetics
Half-life, biphasic:
Initial: 11 hours
Terminal: 23 hours
Elimination: Excreted unchanged in urine within 3-4 days

Usual Dosage Children: I.M. (many regimens have been described):
Prepubertal cryptorchidism:
1000-2000 units/m^2/dose 3 times/week for 3 weeks or 4000 units 3 times/week for 3 weeks
or
5000 units every second day for 4 injections
or
500 units 3 times/week for 4-6 weeks
Hypogonadotropic hypogonadism:
500-1000 units 3 times/week for 3 weeks, followed by the same dose twice weekly for 3 weeks
or
1000-2000 units 3 times/week
or
4000 units 3 times/week for 6-9 months; reduce dosage to 2000 units 3 times/week for additional 3 months
Induction of ovulation: 5000-10,000 units the day following the last dose of menotropins

Administration Parenteral: Administer I.M. only

Reference Range Depends on application and methodology; <3 milli international units/mL (SI: <3 units/L) usually normal (nonpregnant)

Dosage Forms Powder for injection: 200 units/mL (10 mL, 25 mL); 500 units/mL (10 mL); 1000 units/mL (10 mL); 2000 units/mL (10 mL)

♦ **Choron**® *see* Chorionic Gonadotropin *on page 221*
♦ **Chroma-Pak**® *see* Trace Metals *on page 940*
♦ **Chromium Chloride** *see* Trace Metals *on page 940*
♦ **Chronulac**® *see* Lactulose *on page 550*
♦ **Cibacalcin**® *see* Calcitonin *on page 154*
♦ **Cidomycin**® **(Canada)** *see* Gentamicin *on page 452*
♦ **Cilastatin and Imipenem** *see* Imipenem and Cilastatin *on page 506*
♦ **Cilastatin Sodium** *see* Imipenem and Cilastatin *on page 506*
♦ **Ciloxan**™ **Ophthalmic** *see* Ciprofloxacin *on page 224*

Cimetidine (sye MET i deen)

Related Information
Carbohydrate and Alcohol Content of Liquid Medications for Use in Patients Receiving Ketogenic Diets *on page 1228*

Brand Names Apo®-Cimetidine (Canada); Novo-Cimetidine® (Canada); Nu-Cimet® (Canada); Peptol® (Canada); Tagamet®; Tagamet-HB® [OTC]

Available Salts Cimetidine Hydrochloride

Therapeutic Category Gastrointestinal Agent, Gastric or Duodenal Ulcer Treatment; Histamine H_2 Antagonist

Generic Available Yes

Use Short-term treatment of active duodenal ulcers and benign gastric ulcers; long-term prophylaxis of duodenal ulcer; gastric hypersecretory states; gastroesophageal reflux (GERD); prevention of upper GI bleeding in critically ill patients; over-the-counter (OTC) formulation for relief of acid indigestion, heartburn, or sour stomach

Pregnancy Risk Factor B

Contraindications Hypersensitivity to cimetidine or any component

Warnings Rapid I.V. administration may cause hypotension or cardiac arrhythmias

Precautions Modify dosage in patients with renal and/or hepatic impairment; multiple drug interactions exist requiring dose modifications of other medications or cimetidine (see Drug Interactions)

Adverse Reactions
Cardiovascular: Bradycardia, hypotension, cardiac arrhythmias (after rapid I.V. administration), tachycardia
Central nervous system: Dizziness, mental confusion, agitation, headache, psychosis, drowsiness, fever
Dermatologic: Rash
Endocrine & metabolic: Gynecomastia
Gastrointestinal: Mild diarrhea, nausea, vomiting
Hematologic: Neutropenia, agranulocytosis, thrombocytopenia
Hepatic: Elevated AST and ALT
Neuromuscular & skeletal: Myalgia
Renal: Elevated serum creatinine

Drug Interactions Cimetidine reduces the hepatic metabolism of drugs metabolized by the cytochrome P-450 pathway which may result in decreased elimination of lidocaine, diazepam, theophylline, phenytoin, gabapentin, metronidazole, triamterene, procainamide, quinidine, propranolol, carbamazepine, chloroquine, lomustine, warfarin, flecainide, and tricyclic antidepressants; antacids, metoclopramide, and anticholinergics may reduce the absorption of cimetidine; cimetidine may decrease the absorption of iron, melphalan, indomethacin, ketoconazole, tetracyclines, delavirdine, and possibly fluconazole; cimetidine may decrease digoxin serum levels; may increase diltiazem, flecainide, praziquantel, tacrolimus, cyclosporin, nevirapine, mexiletine, and pentoxifylline serum levels; cimetidine decreases the renal clearance of zalcitabine and zidovudine; potentiates myelosuppressive effects of carmustine; may increase didanosine absorption

Food Interactions Limit xanthine-containing foods and beverages

Stability Protect from light; store at room temperature; do not refrigerate the injection since precipitation may occur (can be redissolved by warming without degradation); stable in parenteral nutrition solutions for up to 7 days when protected from light

Mechanism of Action Competitive inhibition of histamine at H_2-receptors of the gastric parietal cells resulting in reduced gastric acid secretion

Pharmacokinetics
Distribution: Crosses the placenta; breast milk to plasma ratio: 4.6-11.76
Protein binding: 13% to 25%
Bioavailability: 60% to 70%

Half-life:
Neonates: 3.6 hours
Children: 1.4 hours
Adults with normal renal function: 2 hours
Time to peak serum concentration: Oral: Within 1-2 hours
Elimination: Principally as unchanged drug by the kidney; some excretion in bile and feces

Usual Dosage

Neonates: Oral, I.M., I.V.: 5-10 mg/kg/day in divided doses every 8-12 hours
Infants: Oral, I.M., I.V.: 10-20 mg/kg/day divided every 6-12 hours
Children: Oral, I.M., I.V.: 20-40 mg/kg/day in divided doses every 6 hours
Adults:
Short-term treatment of active ulcers:
Oral: 300 mg 4 times/day or 800 mg at bedtime or 400 mg twice daily for up to 8 weeks
I.M., I.V.: 300 mg every 6 hours or 150 mg single dose followed by 37.5 mg/hour by continuous infusion; adjust dosage to maintain an intragastric pH ≥5 or acid secretory rate of <10 mEq/hour; (average dose 160 mg/hour; range: 40-600 mg/hour)
Duodenal ulcer prophylaxis: Oral: 400-800 mg at bedtime
Gastric hypersecretory conditions: Oral, I.M., I.V.: 300-600 mg every 6 hours; dosage not to exceed 2.4 g/day
GERD: Oral: 800 mg twice daily or 400 mg 4 times/day for 12 weeks
Acid indigestion, heartburn, sour stomach relief (OTC use): Oral: 100 mg right before or up to 30 minutes before a meal; no more than 2 tablets per day
Prevention of upper GI bleeding: Continuous I.V. infusion of 50 mg/hour

Dosing interval in renal impairment using 5-10 mg/kg/dose in children or 300 mg in adults (titrate dose to gastric pH and Cl_{cr}):
Cl_{cr} >40 mL/minute: Administer every 6 hours
Cl_{cr} 20-40 mL/minute: Administer every 8 hours or reduce dose by 25%
Cl_{cr} <20 mL/minute: Administer every 12 hours or reduce dose by 50%
Hemodialysis: Administer after dialysis and every 12 hours during the interdialysis period

Dosing adjustment in hepatic impairment: Reduce dosage in severe liver disease

Administration

Oral: Administer with food; do not administer with antacids
Parenteral: Can be administered as a slow I.V. push over 15 minutes (minimum 5 minutes; rapid administration has been associated with hypotension and cardiac arrhythmias) at a concentration not to exceed 15 mg/mL; or preferably as an I.V. intermittent or I.V. continuous infusion. Intermittent infusions are administered over 15-30 minutes at a final concentration not to exceed 6 mg/mL; for patients with an active bleed, preferred method of administration is continuous infusion; may be administered intramuscularly

Monitoring Parameters Blood pressure and heart rate with I.V. push administration; CBC; gastric pH

Patient Information Avoid excessive amount of coffee and aspirin; when self medicating, if symptoms of heartburn, acid indigestion, or sour stomach persist after 2 weeks of continuous use of the drug, consult a clinician; notify your physician if taking other medications (multiple drug interactions exist)

Dosage Forms

Infusion, as hydrochloride, in NS: 300 mg (50 mL); 900 mg (150 mL); 1200 mg (200 mL)
Injection, as hydrochloride: 150 mg/mL (2 mL, 8 mL)
Liquid, oral, as hydrochloride (mint-peach flavor): 300 mg/5 mL with alcohol 2.8% (5 mL, 240 mL)
Tablet: 100 mg, 200 mg, 300 mg, 400 mg, 800 mg

References

Lambert J, Mobassaleh M, and Grand RJ, "Efficacy of Cimetidine for Gastric Acid Suppression in Pediatric Patients," *J Pediatr*, 1992, 120(3):474-8.
Lloyd CW, Martin WJ, Taylor BD, et al, "Pharmacokinetics and Pharmacodynamics of Cimetidine and Metabolites in Critically Ill Children," *J Pediatr*, 1985, 107(2):295-300.
Lloyd CW, Martin WJ, and Taylor BD, "The Pharmacokinetics of Cimetidine and Metabolites in a Neonate," *Drug Intell Clin Pharm*, 1985, 19(3):203-5.
Somogyi A and Gugler R, "Clinical Pharmacokinetics of Cimetidine," *Clin Pharmacokinet*, 1983, 8(6):463-95.

♦ **Cimetidine Hydrochloride** *see* Cimetidine *on page 222*

Ciprofloxacin (sip roe FLOKS a sin)

Brand Names Ciloxan™ Ophthalmic; Cipro® HC Otic; Cipro™ Injection; Cipro™ Oral
Available Salts Ciprofloxacin Hydrochloride
Therapeutic Category Antibiotic, Ophthalmic; Antibiotic, Quinolone
Generic Available No

Use Treatment of documented or suspected pseudomonal infection of the respiratory or urinary tract, skin and soft tissue, bone and joint, eye and ear; documented multidrug-resistant, aerobic gram-negative bacilli, some gram-positive staphylococci, and *Mycobacterium tuberculosis*; documented infectious diarrhea due to *Campylobacter jejuni*, *Shigella*, or *Salmonella*; osteomyelitis caused by susceptible organisms in which parenteral therapy is not feasible; pulmonary exacerbation of cystic fibrosis; used ophthalmically for treatment of corneal ulcers and conjunctivitis due to susceptible organisms; otic suspension is used for treatment of acute bacterial otitis externa due to susceptible strains of *S. aureus*, *P. aeruginosa*, or *Proteus mirabilis*

Pregnancy Risk Factor C

Contraindications Hypersensitivity to ciprofloxacin, any component, or other quinolones; not recommended for use in pregnant women or during breast-feeding

Warnings Not recommended in children <18 years of age; ciprofloxacin has caused arthropathy with erosions of the cartilage in weight bearing joints of immature animals; green discoloration of teeth in newborns has been reported; Achilles tendonitis and tendon rupture have been reported with fluoroquinolones; prolonged use may result in superinfection; CNS stimulation may occur resulting in tremors, restlessness, confusion, and very rarely hallucinations or convulsive seizures

Precautions Use with caution in patients with seizure disorders or renal impairment; modify dosage in patients with renal impairment

Adverse Reactions
Central nervous system: Headache, restlessness, dizziness, confusion, seizures, insomnia, hallucinations
Dermatologic: Rash, photosensitivity, pruritus, urticaria
Gastrointestinal: Nausea, diarrhea, vomiting, GI bleeding, abdominal pain, pseudomembranous colitis
Genitourinary: Crystalluria
Hematologic: Anemia, eosinophilia, neutropenia
Hepatic: Elevated liver enzymes
Local: With I.V.: Phlebitis, burning, pain, erythema, and swelling (occurs more frequently with infusion time <30 minutes)
Neuromuscular & skeletal: Arthralgia, joint and back pain, tremor, joint stiffness, arthritis, tendonitis
Renal: Elevated BUN and serum creatinine, acute renal failure, interstitial nephritis
Miscellaneous: Anaphylaxis

Drug Interactions Magnesium-, aluminum- or calcium-containing antacids and sucralfate decrease ciprofloxacin absorption by up to 90% if given at the same time; antacids in didanosine formulation chelate ciprofloxacin and decrease its absorption (administer ciprofloxacin 2 hours before or 6 hours after didanosine); probenecid decreases renal clearance of ciprofloxacin and can increase ciprofloxacin concentrations; ciprofloxacin decreases theophylline, warfarin, and cyclosporine clearance; NSAID (increase CNS stimulation)

Food Interactions Dairy foods (milk, yogurt) and mineral supplements decrease ciprofloxacin concentrations; ciprofloxacin increases caffeine concentrations; use caution with xanthine-containing foods and beverages

Stability Premixed bags: Out of overwrap stability: 14 days at room temperature; reconstituted oral suspension: Stable for 14 days when stored at room temperature or refrigerated; store tablets at room temperature; protect from intense light

Mechanism of Action Inhibits DNA-gyrase in susceptible organisms; inhibits relaxation of supercoiled DNA and promotes breakage of double-stranded DNA

Pharmacokinetics
Absorption: Oral: Well absorbed
Distribution: Widely distributed into body tissues and fluids with high concentration in bile, urine, sputum, stool, lungs, liver, skin, muscle, and bone; low concentration in CSF; crosses the placenta; appears in breast milk
Protein binding: 16% to 43%
Metabolism: Partially in the liver to active metabolites
Bioavailability: Oral: 50% to 85%; younger CF patients have a lower bioavailability of 68% versus CF patients >13 years of age with bioavailability of 95%
Half-life:
Infants: 2.73 hours

Children:
  1-5 years: 1.28 hours
  6-12 years: 2.5-2.6 hours
Adults with normal renal function: 3-5 hours
Time to peak serum concentration: Oral: Within 0.5-2 hours
Elimination: 30% to 50% excreted as unchanged drug in urine; 20% to 40% excreted in feces primarily from biliary excretion
Clearance: After I.V.:
  CF child: 0.84 L/hour/kg
  Adult: 0.5-0.6 L/hour/kg
Only small amounts of ciprofloxacin are removed by dialysis (<10%)

Usual Dosage

Neonates: I.V. ciprofloxacin has been used in 23 neonates at doses ranging from 7-40 mg/kg/day divided every 12 hours (Schaad, 1995)
Children:
  Oral: 20-30 mg/kg/day in 2 divided doses; maximum dose: 1.5 g/day
  I.V.: 20-30 mg/kg/day divided every 12 hours; maximum dose: 800 mg/day
  Cystic fibrosis:
    Oral: 40 mg/kg/day divided every 12 hours; maximum dose: 2 g/day
    I.V.: 30 mg/kg/day divided every 8-12 hours; maximum dose: 1.2 g/day
Adults:
  Oral: 250-750 mg every 12 hours, depending on severity of infection and susceptibility
    Chemoprophylaxis regimen for high-risk contacts of invasive meningococcal disease: 500 mg as a single dose
    Uncomplicated gonorrhea: 500 mg as a single dose
    Chancroid: 500 mg twice daily for 3 days
  I.V.: 200-400 mg every 12 hours depending on severity of infection
  Ophthalmic: Instill 1-2 drops into the affected eye(s) every 2 hours while awake for 2 days, then 1-2 drops every 4 hours while awake for the next 5 days **or** instill 1/2" ointment ribbon 3 times/day for 2 days, then twice daily for the next 5 days
    Treatment of corneal ulcers: Instill 2 drops every 15 minutes for the first 6 hours, then 2 drops every 30 minutes for the remainder of the first day; on the second day, 2 drops every hour; then 2 drops every 4 hours thereafter
Children ≥1 year and Adults: Otic: Instill 3 drops into the affected ear(s) twice daily for 7 days
Dosing interval in renal impairment: Cl$_{cr}$ <30 mL/minute: Administer every 18-24 hours

Administration

Oral: Administer tablets 2 hours after a meal; may administer with food to minimize GI upset; oral suspension may be administered with or without food; to prepare oral suspension, pour the microcapsules (small bottle) completely into the large bottle of diluent - DO NOT ADD WATER TO THE SUSPENSION. Shake suspension vigorously before use. Avoid antacid use. Drink plenty of fluids to maintain proper hydration and urine output
Parenteral: Administer by slow I.V. infusion over 60 minutes to reduce the risk of venous irritation (burning, pain, erythema, and swelling); final concentration for administration should not exceed 2 mg/mL
Ophthalmic: Ointment: Instill ointment in the lower conjunctival sac
Otic: Warm suspension by holding bottle in hand prior to instillation; shake well before use; patient should lie with affected ear upward and maintain position for 30-60 seconds after suspension is instilled into the ear canal

Monitoring Parameters Patients receiving concurrent ciprofloxacin and theophylline should have serum levels of theophylline monitored; monitor INR in patients receiving warfarin; patients receiving concurrent ciprofloxacin and cyclosporine should have cyclosporine levels monitored; monitor renal, hepatic, and hematopoietic function periodically; number and type of stools/day for diarrhea

Reference Range Avoid peak serum concentrations >5 µg/mL

Patient Information Do not chew microcapsules of the oral suspension; avoid caffeine; may cause dizziness or lightheadedness and impair ability to perform activities which require mental alertness; avoid excessive exposure to sunlight; notify physician if tendon pain or swelling occurs; remove contact lenses prior to administration of ophthalmic solution and ointment

Nursing Implications Do not administer antacids with or within 4 hours of a ciprofloxacin dose; ensure adequate patient hydration

Dosage Forms

Infusion, as lactate, in D$_5$W: 400 mg (200 mL)
Infusion, as lactate, in NS or D$_5$W: 200 mg (100 mL)
(Continued)

Ciprofloxacin *(Continued)*

Injection, as lactate: 200 mg (20 mL); 400 mg (40 mL)
Ointment, ophthalmic, as hydrochloride: 0.3% (3.5 g)
Solution, ophthalmic, as hydrochloride: 3.5 mg/mL (2.5 mL, 5 mL)
Suspension, oral: 5% (50 mg/mL); 10% (100 mg/mL)
Suspension, otic, as hydrochloride: 0.2% with hydrocortisone 1% (10 mL)
Tablet, as hydrochloride: 100 mg, 250 mg, 500 mg, 750 mg

References

Campoli-Richards DM, Monk JP, Price A, et al, "Ciprofloxacin: A Review of Its Antibacterial Activity, Pharmacokinetic Properties and Therapeutic Use," *Drugs*, 1988, 35(4):373-447.

Rodriguez WJ, and Wiedermann BL, "The Role of Newer Oral Cephalosporins, Fluoroquinolones, and Macrolides in the Treatment of Pediatric Infections," *Adv Pediatr Infect Dis*, 1994, 9:125-59.

Rubio TT, Miles MV, Lettieri JT, et al, "Pharmacokinetic Disposition of Sequential Intravenous/Oral Ciprofloxacin in Pediatric Cystic Fibrosis Patients with Acute Pulmonary Exacerbation," *Pediatr Infect Dis J*, 1997, 16:112-7

Schaad UB, abdus Salam M, Aujard Y, et al, "Use of Fluoroquinolones in Pediatrics: Consensus Report of an International Society of Chemotherapy Commission," *Pediatr Infect Dis J*, 1995, 14(1):1-9.

♦ **Ciprofloxacin Hydrochloride** *see* Ciprofloxacin *on page 224*
♦ **Cipro® HC Otic** *see* Ciprofloxacin *on page 224*
♦ **Cipro™ Injection** *see* Ciprofloxacin *on page 224*
♦ **Cipro™ Oral** *see* Ciprofloxacin *on page 224*

Cisapride *U.S. - Available Via Limited-Access Protocol Only* (SIS a pride)

Related Information

Carbohydrate and Alcohol Content of Liquid Medications for Use in Patients Receiving Ketogenic Diets *on page 1228*

Brand Names Prepulsid® (Canada); Propulsid®

Therapeutic Category Gastrointestinal Agent, Prokinetic

Generic Available No

Use Treatment of nocturnal symptoms of gastroesophageal reflux disease (GERD), also demonstrated effectiveness for gastroparesis, refractory constipation, and nonulcer dyspepsia in patients failing other therapies (see Warnings)

Pregnancy Risk Factor C

Contraindications Hypersensitivity to cisapride or any component; GI hemorrhage, mechanical obstruction, GI perforation, or other situations when GI motility stimulation is dangerous; patients with CHF, renal failure, multisystem organ failure, and COPD; patients at risk for developing or who have hypokalemia, hypocalcemia, or hypomagnesemia (eg, severe dehydration, vomiting, diarrhea, malnutrition, or receiving chronic diuretic therapy); patients with a known family history of congenital long-QT syndrome; prolonged Q-T intervals (QT$_c$ >450), ventricular arrhythmias, ischemic heart disease, sinus node dysfunction, clinically significant bradycardia, and second or third degree AV block; patients receiving medications known to prolong the Q-T interval such as quinidine, procainamide, sotalol, amitriptyline (and other tricyclic antidepressants), maprotiline, phenothiazines, sertindole, astemizole, bepridil, or sparfloxacin, (see Warnings and Drug Interactions); serious cardiac arrhythmias including ventricular tachycardia, ventricular fibrillation, torsades de pointes, and Q-T prolongations have been reported in patients taking medications which inhibit cytochrome P-450 3A4; some of these events have been fatal; do not coadminister with ketoconazole, itraconazole, fluconazole, miconazole, erythromycin, clarithromycin, nefazodone, delavirdine, indinavir, nelfinavir, ritonavir, saquinavir, or troleandomycin; do not coadminister with grapefruit juice

Warnings Serious cardiac arrhythmias including ventricular tachycardia, ventricular fibrillation, torsades de pointes, and QT prolongation have been reported in patients receiving cisapride; more than 270 cases have been reported including 70 fatalities; 85% of these cases occurred in patients with known risk factors (see Contraindications); for this reason, cisapride is available only for use in patients with severely debilitating conditions who meet specific criteria for a limited-access program directly through Janssen Pharmaceutical Company; for more information contact Janssen at 1-800-Janssen

Precautions Use with caution in neonates, particularly if premature due to a potential increased risk of serious cardiac arrhythmias; decreased cisapride clearance found in neonates may result in increased serum levels; a 12-lead EKG (measuring Q-T intervals) should be done in all patients before beginning therapy

Adverse Reactions

Cardiovascular: Sinus tachycardia, Q-T interval prolongation, serious cardiac arrhythmias (see Warnings and Contraindications)

Central nervous system: Headache, insomnia, anxiety, nervousness, confusion

Dermatologic: Rash, pruritus, photosensitivity

Endocrine & metabolic: Hypoglycemia with acidosis, hyperglycemia

Gastrointestinal: Diarrhea, abdominal pain, nausea, flatulence, dyspepsia, constipation, xerostomia

Genitourinary: Vaginitis (rare), urinary frequency

Hematologic: Thrombocytopenia, leukopenia, aplastic anemia, pancytopenia, hemolytic anemia, methemoglobinemia

Hepatic: Hepatitis, elevated liver enzymes

Neuromuscular & skeletal: Arthralgia, tremor

Respiratory: Rhinitis, sinusitis, cough, apnea

Miscellaneous: Positive ANA

Drug Interactions Cytochrome P-450 isoenzyme CYP3A3/4 substrate

Decreased absorption of digoxin; decreased effect with atropine

Increased effect/toxicity of warfarin, diazepam (increased levels); increased bioavailability of cisapride with cimetidine and ranitidine use

Concomitant administration with ketoconazole has resulted in markedly elevated cisapride plasma concentrations and prolonged Q-T intervals on the EKG. These prolonged intervals have rarely been associated with serious ventricular arrhythmias and torsade de pointes; some of these adverse reactions have been fatal. Since the interaction is due to a decrease in cytochrome P-450 metabolism induced by ketoconazole, it is expected that similar reactions would occur with itraconazole, miconazole, fluconazole, troleandomycin, delavirdine, indinavir, erythromycin, clarithromycin, nefazodone, nelfinavir, amprenavir, ritonavir, and saquinavir; see Contraindications and Food Interactions

Food Interactions Do not use with grapefruit juice which increases cisapride bioavailability

Mechanism of Action A GI prokinetic agent which enhances the release of acetylcholine at the myenteric plexus. *In vitro* studies have shown cisapride to have serotonin-4 receptor agonistic properties; it has no dopamine receptor blocking activity and, therefore, no extrapyramidal side effects or central antiemetic activity. It increases lower esophageal sphincter pressure, increases the amplitude of peristalsis, accelerates gastric emptying, improves antroduodenal coordination, increases colonic motility, and enhances cecal and ascending colonic emptying.

Pharmacodynamics Onset of effect: 0.5-1 hour

Pharmacokinetics

Distribution: Breast milk to plasma ratio: 0.045

Protein binding: 98%

Metabolism: Extensive in liver via cytochrome P-450 isoenzyme CYP 3A3/4 to norcisapride, which is eliminated in urine and feces

Bioavailability: 40% to 50%

Half-life: 7-10 hours

Elimination: <10% of dose excreted into feces and urine

Usual Dosage Oral:

Neonates: 0.15-0.2 mg/kg/dose 3-4 times/day; maximum dose: 0.8 mg/kg/day

Infants and Children: 0.15-0.3 mg/kg/dose 3-4 times/day; maximum dose: 10 mg/dose

Adults: Initial: 10 mg 4 times/day at least 15 minutes before meals and at bedtime; in some patients the dosage will need to be increased to 20 mg to obtain a satisfactory result

Dosage adjustment in liver dysfunction: Reduce daily dosage by 50%

Administration Oral: Administer 15 minutes before meals or feeding

Monitoring Parameters EKG (prior to beginning therapy), serum electrolytes in patients on diuretic therapy (prior to beginning therapy and periodically thereafter); see Contraindications

Dosage Forms

Suspension, cherry cream flavor: 1 mg/mL (450 mL)

Tablet: 10 mg, 20 mg

References

Cucchiara S, Staiano A, Boccieri A, et al, "Effects of Cisapride on Parameters of Oesophageal Motility and on the Prolonged Intraoesophageal pH Test in Infants With Gastro-Oesophageal Reflux Disease," *Gut*, 1990, 31(1):21-5.

Hill SL, Evangelista KJ, Pizzi AM, et al, "Proarrhythmia Associated With Cisapride in Children," *Pediatrics*, 1998, 101(6):1053-6.

Khongphatthanayothin A, Lane J, Thomas D, et al, "Effects of Cisapride on QT Interval in Children," *J Pediatr*, 1998, 133(1):51-6.

Lander A, "The Risks and Benefits of Cisapride in Premature Neonates, Infants and Children," *Arch Dis Child*, 1998, 79:469-71.

Lewin MB, Bryant RM, Fenrich AL, et al, "Cisapride-Induced QT Interval," *J Pediatr*, 1996, 128(2):279-81.

(Continued)

Cisapride *U.S. - Available Via Limited-Access Protocol Only* (Continued)

Tolia V, "Long-Term Use of Cisapride in Premature Neonates of <34 Weeks Gestational Age," *J Pediatr Gastroenterol Nutr*, 1990, 11:420-2.

Van Eygen M and Van Ravensteyn H, "Effect of Cisapride on Excessive Regurgitation in Infants," *Clin Ther*, 1989, 11(5):669-77.

Cisatracurium (sis a tra KYOO ree um)
Brand Names Nimbex®
Available Salts Cisatracurium Besylate
Therapeutic Category Neuromuscular Blocker Agent, Nondepolarizing; Skeletal Muscle Relaxant, Paralytic
Generic Available No
Use Eases endotracheal intubation as an adjunct to general anesthesia and relaxes skeletal muscle during surgery or mechanical ventilation
Pregnancy Risk Factor B
Contraindications Hypersensitivity to cisatracurium or any component
Warnings Maintenance of an adequate airway and respiratory support is critical; 10 mL multiple use vials contain benzyl alcohol as a preservative; avoid use in neonates; due to its intermediate onset of action, it is not recommended for rapid sequence intubation; certain clinical conditions may result in potentiation or antagonism of neuromuscular blockade, see table.

Increased sensitivity in patients with myasthenia gravis, Eaton-Lambert syndrome, resistance to neuromuscular blockade in burn patients (>30% of body) for period of 5-70 days postinjury; resistance to neuromuscular blockade in patients with muscle trauma, denervation, immobilization, infection

Precautions Certain clinical conditions may result in potentiation or antagonism of neuromuscular blockade, see table.

Clinical Conditions Affecting Neuromuscular Blockade

Potentiation	Antagonism
Electrolyte abnormalities	Alkalosis
Severe hyponatremia	Hypercalcemia
Severe hypocalcemia	Demyelinating lesions
Severe hypokalemia	Peripheral neuropathies
Hypermagnesemia	Diabetes mellitus
Neuromuscular diseases	
Acidosis	
Acute intermittent porphyria	
Renal failure	
Hepatic failure	

Adverse Reactions
Cardiovascular: Rarely mild histamine release, cardiovascular effects are minimal and transient
Dermatologic: Rash
Respiratory: Bronchospasm
Miscellaneous: Hypersensitivity reactions including anaphylaxis
Drug Interactions See table on following page.
Stability Protect from light; refrigerate; once removed from refrigerator, stable 21 days even if re-refrigerated; unstable in alkaline solutions; **compatible** with D_5W, D_5NS, and NS; do not dilute in LR; **incompatible** for Y-site administration with propofol or ketorolac; **compatible** for Y-site administration with sufentanil, alfentanil, fentanyl, midazolam, and droperidol.
Mechanism of Action Blocks neural transmission at the myoneural junction by binding with cholinergic receptor sites
Pharmacodynamics
Onset of action: I.V.: Within 2-3 minutes
Peak effect: Within 3-5 minutes
Clinical duration: Dose dependent, 35-45 minutes after a single 0.1 mg/kg dose; recovery begins in 20-35 minutes when anesthesia is balanced; recovery is attained in 90% of patients in 25-93 minutes
Pharmacokinetics
Metabolism: Some metabolites are active; 80% of drug clearance is via a rapid

nonenzymatic degradation (Hofmann elimination) in the bloodstream; additional metabolism occurs via ester hydrolysis

Half-life: 22-31 minutes

Elimination: <10% of dose excreted as unchanged drug in urine

Potential Drug Interactions

Potentiation	Antagonism
Anesthetics	Calcium
Desflurane, sevoflurane, enflurane and	Carbamazepine
isoflurane > halothane > nitrous	Phenytoin
oxide	Steroids (chronic administration)
Antibiotics	Theophylline
Aminoglycosides, polymyxins,	Anticholinesterases*
clindamycin, vancomycin	Neostigmine, pyridostigmine,
Magnesium sulfate	edrophonium, echothiophate
Antiarrhythmics	ophthalmic solution
Quinidine, procainamide, bretylium, and	Caffeine
possibly lidocaine	Azathioprine
Diuretics	
Furosemide, mannitol	
Amphotericin B (secondary to hypokalemia)	
Local anesthetics	
Dantrolene (directly depresses skeletal muscle)	
Beta blockers	
Calcium channel blockers	
Ketamine	
Lithium	
Succinylcholine (when administered prior to nondepolarizing neuromuscular-blocking agent)	
Cyclosporine	

*Can prolong the effects of acetylcholine

Usual Dosage I.V.:

  Children 2-12 years: Initial: 0.1 mg/kg followed by maintenance dose of 0.03 mg/kg as needed to maintain neuromuscular blockade

  Children >12 years to Adults: Initial: 0.15-0.2 mg/kg followed by maintenance dose of 0.03 mg/kg 40-65 minutes later or as needed to maintain neuromuscular blockade

  Continuous infusion: Children ≥2 years to Adults: 1-3 mcg/kg/minute (range 0.5-10 mcg/kg/minute) or 0.06-0.18 mg/kg/hour

Administration Parenteral: May be administered without further dilution by rapid I.V. injection over 5-10 seconds; for continuous infusions, dilute to a concentration of 0.1-0.4 mg/mL in D_5W or NS; not for I.M. injection due to tissue irritation

Monitoring Parameters Muscle twitch response to peripheral nerve stimulation, heart rate, blood pressure

Additional Information Neuromuscular blocking potency is 3 times that of atracurium; maximum block is up to 2 minutes longer than for equipotent doses of atracurium; laudanosine, a metabolite without neuromuscular blocking activity has been associated with hypotension and seizure activity in animal studies.

Dosage Forms Injection, as besylate: 2 mg/mL (5 mL, 10 mL); 10 mg/mL (20 mL)

♦ **Cisatracurium Besylate** *see* Cisatracurium *on page 228*

Cisplatin (SIS pla tin)

Related Information

  Emetogenic Potential of Single Chemotherapeutic Agents *on page 1095*

  Extravasation Treatment *on page 1050*

Brand Names Platinol®; Platinol®-AQ

Synonyms CDDP

Therapeutic Category Antineoplastic Agent, Alkylating Agent

Generic Available No

(Continued)

Cisplatin *(Continued)*

Use Treatment of testicular, ovarian, and breast cancer; advanced bladder cancer, osteosarcoma, Hodgkin's and non-Hodgkin's lymphoma, head or neck cancer, cervical cancer, lung cancer, brain tumors, neuroblastoma; used alone or in combination with other agents

Pregnancy Risk Factor D

Contraindications Hypersensitivity to cisplatin, platinum-containing agents, or any component; pre-existing renal impairment, hearing impairment, and myelosuppression; pregnancy

Warnings The FDA currently recommends that procedures for proper handling and disposal of antineoplastic agents be considered. Cumulative renal toxicity may be severe; dose-related toxicities include myelosuppression, nausea and vomiting; ototoxicity, especially pronounced in children, is manifested by tinnitus or loss of high frequency hearing and occasionally, deafness

Precautions All patients should receive adequate hydration prior to and for 24 hours after cisplatin administration with a sodium chloride-containing intravenous solution to promote chloruresis, with or without mannitol and/or furosemide, to ensure good urine output and decrease the chance of nephrotoxicity; reduce dosage in renal impairment and in infants <6 months of age due to their decreased renal function and renal tubular secretion; serum magnesium, as well as electrolytes, should be monitored before and within 48 hours after cisplatin therapy. Patients who are magnesium-depleted should receive replacement therapy before the start of cisplatin.

Adverse Reactions

Cardiovascular: Bradycardia, arrhythmias, Raynaud's phenomenon

Central nervous system: Seizures, encephalopathy

Dermatologic: Mild alopecia

Endocrine & metabolic: Hypomagnesemia, hypocalcemia, hypokalemia, hypophosphatemia, hyperuricemia

Gastrointestinal: Nausea and vomiting occur in 76% to 100% of patients and is dose-related

Hematologic: Myelosuppression

Hepatic: Elevated liver enzymes

Local: Phlebitis

Neuromuscular & skeletal: Peripheral neuropathy (related to cumulative doses >200 mg/m^2)

Ocular: Papilledema, optic neuritis

Otic: Ototoxicity (especially pronounced in children; hearing loss in the high-frequency range is related to a cumulative dose of cisplatin >400 mg/m^2)

Renal: Nephrotoxicity (damage to the proximal tubules), azotemia, elevated BUN and serum creatinine

Miscellaneous: Anaphylactoid reactions

Drug Interactions Aminoglycosides, amphotericin B, and other nephrotoxic drugs (increase risk of nephrotoxicity); loop diuretics, aminoglycosides (potentiate ototoxicity); synergistic antineoplastic activity with cytarabine, 5-fluorouracil, etoposide; reduces renal elimination of methotrexate

Stability Reconstituted powder for injection is stable for 20 hours at room temperature; do not refrigerate reconstituted solution since precipitation may occur; protect from light; incompatible with sodium bicarbonate; do not infuse in solutions containing <0.2% sodium chloride; stable when combined with mannitol (12.5-50 g mannitol/L)

Mechanism of Action Platination of DNA leads to reactive intermediates that bind to DNA and form intrastrand and interstrand DNA cross-links

Pharmacokinetics

Distribution: I.V.: Rapid tissue distribution; CSF unbound platinum concentration: 40% of the plasma concentration

Protein binding: >90%; only the free (unbound) platinum and parent drug are cytotoxic

Metabolism: Undergoes nonenzymatic metabolism

Half-life, terminal: Children:

Free drug: 1.3 hours

Total platinum: 44 hours

Elimination: ~50% of dose excreted in urine within 5 days in an inactive form

Minimally removed by hemodialysis

Usual Dosage Children and Adults: I.V. (refer to individual protocols): **TO PREVENT POSSIBLE OVERDOSE, VERIFY ANY CISPLATIN DOSE EXCEEDING 120 mg/m^2 PER COURSE.**

Intermittent dosing schedule: 37-75 mg/m² once every 2-3 weeks or 50-100 mg/m² over 4-6 hours, once every 21-28 days

Daily dosing schedule: 15-20 mg/m²/day for 5 days every 3-4 weeks

Osteogenic sarcoma or neuroblastoma: 60-100 mg/m² on day 1 every 3-4 weeks

Recurrent brain tumors: 60 mg/m² once daily for 2 consecutive days every 3-4 weeks

Bone marrow/blood cell transplantation: Continuous infusion: High dose: 55 mg/m²/day for 72 hours; total dose = 165 mg/m²

Dosing adjustment in renal impairment:
Cl_{cr} 10-50 mL/minute: Administer 75% of dose
Cl_{cr} <10 mL/minute: Administer 50% of dose

Administration Parenteral: I.V.: Administer according to protocol; rate of administration has varied from a 15- to 20-minute infusion, 1 mg/minute infusion, 6- to 8-hour infusion or 24-hour infusion; rapid I.V. injection may be associated with increased nephrotoxicity or ototoxicity compared to a slower I.V. infusion

Monitoring Parameters Renal function tests (serum creatinine, BUN, Cl_{cr}), electrolytes (particularly magnesium, calcium, potassium), hearing test, neurologic exam (with high dose), liver function tests periodically, CBC with differential and platelet count, urine output, urinalysis

Nursing Implications Needles, syringes, catheters, or I.V. administration sets that contain aluminum parts should not be used for administration of drug; methods to prevent nephrotoxicity include prehydration, diuresis with mannitol, and administration of hypertonic sodium chloride solutions to promote chloruresis. Adequate hydration and urinary output should be maintained for 24 hours after administration.

Additional Information Myelosuppressive effects:
WBC: Mild
Platelets: Mild
Onset (days): 10
Nadir (days): 18-23
Recovery (days): 21-40

Dosage Forms
Injection, aqueous: 1 mg/mL (50 mL, 100 mL)
Powder for injection: 10 mg, 50 mg

References
Costello MA, Dominick C, and Clerico A, "A Pilot Study of 5-Day Continuous Infusion of High-Dose Cisplatin and Pulsed Etoposide in Childhood Solid Tumors," Am J Pediatr Hematol Oncol, 1988, 10:103-8.

Reece PA, Stafford I, Abbott RL, et al, "Two-Versus 24-Hour Infusion of Cisplatin: Pharmacokinetic Considerations," J Clin Oncol, 1989, 7(2):270-5.

♦ **13-*cis*-Retinoic Acid** *see* Isotretinoin *on page 537*
♦ **Citracal® [OTC]** *see* Calcium Supplements *on page 157*

Citrate and Citric Acid (SIT rate & SIT rik AS id)

Related Information
Carbohydrate and Alcohol Content of Liquid Medications for Use in Patients Receiving Ketogenic Diets *on page 1228*

Brand Names Bicitra®; Oracit®; Polycitra®; Polycitra K®; Polycitra-LC®; Urocit®-K; PMS-Dicitrate™ (Can)

Available Salts Potassium Citrate; Sodium Citrate and Citric Acid

Synonyms Citrate/Citric Acid; Citric Acid and Citrate; Shohl's Solution, Modified

Therapeutic Category Alkalinizing Agent, Oral

Generic Available No

Use Treatment of metabolic acidosis; alkalinizing agent in conditions where long-term maintenance of an alkaline urine is desirable

Potassium citrate: Prevention of uric acid nephrolithiasis, prevention of calcium renal stones in patients with hypocitraturia; urinary alkalizer when sodium citrate is contraindicated

Pregnancy Risk Factor C

Contraindications Patients receiving sodium-restricted diet (sodium salts); severe renal impairment with oliguria, azotemia, or anuria; untreated Addison's disease, acute dehydration, heat cramps, severe myocardial damage, hyperkalemia (potassium salts)

Warnings Conversion to bicarbonate may be impaired in patients with hepatic failure, in shock, or who are severely ill

Precautions Use sodium salts with caution in patients with CHF, hypertension, pulmonary edema; may predispose patient to urolithiasis
(Continued)

Citrate and Citric Acid *(Continued)*

Adverse Reactions
Central nervous system: Tetany

Endocrine & metabolic: Metabolic alkalosis, hypernatremia (if sodium salt used), hypocalcemia, hyperkalemia (if potassium salt used)

Gastrointestinal: Diarrhea, nausea, vomiting

Drug Interactions
Decreased effect/levels of chlorpropamide, lithium, methenamine, methotrexate, salicylates, and tetracycline due to urinary alkalinization

Increased toxicity/levels of amphetamines, flecainide, ephedrine, pseudoephedrine, quinidine, and quinine due to urinary alkalinization

Potassium-sparing diuretics, salt substitutes, captopril, and enalapril may result in increased serum potassium (potassium-containing salt forms only)

Mechanism of Action
Citrate salts are oxidized in the body to form bicarbonate

Usual Dosage
Oral (dilute in water or juice):

Infants and Children: 2-3 mEq/kg/day in divided doses 3-4 times/day or 5-15 mL with water after meals and at bedtime

Adults: Solution: 15-30 mL with water after meals and at bedtime

Administration
Oral: Dilute with water or juice and administer after meals

Monitoring Parameters
Serum sodium, bicarbonate, potassium, urine pH

Dosage Forms
Solution, oral:

Bicitra® (alcohol free) : Sodium citrate 500 mg and citric acid 334 mg per 5 mL **(1 mEq sodium and 1 mEq bicarbonate equivalent per mL)** (15 mL unit dose, 480 mL)

Oracit®: Sodium citrate 490 mg and citric acid 640 mg per 5 mL **(1 mEq sodium and 1 mEq bicarbonate equivalent per mL)**

Polycitra® (alcohol free): Sodium citrate 500 mg and citric acid 334 mg with potassium citrate 550 mg per 5 mL **(1 mEq potassium, 1 mEq sodium, 2 mEq bicarbonate equivalent per mL)**

Polycitra-LC® (alcohol free and sugar free): Potassium citrate monohydrate 550 mg, sodium citrate dihydrate 500 mg, citric acid monohydrate 334 mg per 5 mL **(1 mEq potassium, 1 mEq sodium, 2 mEq bicarbonate equivalent per mL)**

Polycitra K® (alcohol free): Crystals and solution: Potassium citrate monohydrate 1100 mg, citric acid monohydrate 334 mg per 5 mL **(2 mEq potassium and 2 mEq bicarbonate equivalent per mL)**

- ♦ **Citrate/Citric Acid** *see* Citrate and Citric Acid *on page 231*
- ♦ **Citrate of Magnesia (Magnesium Citrate)** *see* Magnesium Supplements *on page 588*
- ♦ **Citric Acid and Citrate** *see* Citrate and Citric Acid *on page 231*
- ♦ **Citrovorum Factor** *see* Leucovorin *on page 559*
- ♦ **CL-65336** *see* Tranexamic Acid *on page 943*

Cladribine *(KLA dri been)*

Brand Names
Leustatin™

Synonyms
2-CdA; 2-Chlorodeoxyadenosine

Therapeutic Category
Antineoplastic Agent, Antimetabolite (Purine)

Use
Treatment of hairy cell leukemia, chronic myeloid leukemia, and chronic lymphocytic leukemia; cladribine has activity in the treatment of Langerhans cell histiocytosis (LCH), non-Hodgkin's lymphomas, T-cell lymphomas, relapsed acute lymphocytic leukemia and relapsed acute myeloid leukemia

Pregnancy Risk Factor
D

Contraindications
Hypersensitivity to cladribine or any component

Warnings
The FDA currently recommends that procedures for proper handling and disposal of antineoplastic agents be considered. Serious neurological toxicity has been reported in patients who received cladribine by continuous infusion at high doses (0.4-0.8 mg/kg/day or >16 mg/m²/day); neurologic toxicity appears to be dose-related. Severe neurologic toxicity has been reported rarely with standard dosing regimens. Acute nephrotoxicity has been observed with cladribine doses of 0.4-0.8 mg/kg/day, especially in patients concurrently receiving other nephrotoxic agents.

Precautions
Dose-limiting toxicity is myelosuppression; use with caution in patients with pre-existing hematologic or immunologic abnormalities; prophylactic administration of allopurinol should be considered in patients receiving cladribine due to the potential for hyperuricemia secondary to tumor lysis; appropriate antibiotic therapy should be administered promptly in patients exhibiting signs and symptoms of neutropenia and infection.

Adverse Reactions

Cardiovascular: Edema, tachycardia

Central nervous system: Fever (69%), fatigue (45%), headache, dizziness, insomnia, malaise, irreversible neurologic toxicity (paraparesis/quadriparesis) at high doses (0.4-0.8 mg/kg/day or >16 mg/m^2/day)

Dermatologic: Pruritus, erythema, rash

Gastrointestinal: Constipation, abdominal pain, nausea, vomiting, decreased appetite, diarrhea

Hematologic: Myelosuppression (prolonged pancytopenia), aplastic anemia, hemolytic anemia

Hepatic: Reversible, mild elevations of bilirubin and transaminase levels

Local: Injection site reactions, pain

Neuromuscular & skeletal: Myalgia, trunk pain

Renal: Acute nephrotoxicity reported at high doses (rare)

Respiratory: Abnormal breath sounds, cough, shortness of breath

Stability Refrigerate unopened vials (2°C to 8°C/36°F to 46°F); protect from light. Solutions should be administered immediately after the initial dilution or stored in the refrigerator (2°C to 8°C) for ≤8 hours. **The use of D$_5$W as a diluent is not recommended due to increased degradation of cladribine;** should not be mixed with other intravenous drugs or additives or infused simultaneously via a common intravenous line. Diluted solution of cladribine in NS is stable for 24 hours at room temperature under normal room light in polyvinyl chloride infusion containers.

Mechanism of Action A purine nucleoside analogue; prodrug which enters the cells through a transport system and is activated via phosphorylation by deoxycytidine kinase to a 5'-triphosphate derivative. This active form incorporates into DNA resulting in inhibition of DNA synthesis and early chain termination. The induction of strand breaks results in a drop in the cofactor nicotinamide adenine dinucleotide and disruption of cell metabolism. ATP is depleted to deprive cells of an important source of energy. Cladribine kills both resting as well as dividing cells.

Pharmacokinetics

Distribution: V$_d$:

Children: 305 L/m^2

Adults: 0.5-9 L/kg (53-160 L/m^2)

CSF: Plasma concentration ratio: 18.2%

Protein binding: 20%

Bioavailability: S.C.: 100%

Half-life: 19.7 hours ± 3.4 hours; (range: 14.3-25.8 hours)

Elimination: 21% to 44% renally excreted

Usual Dosage I.V. (refer to individual protocols):

Children:

Hairy cell leukemia: 0.09 mg/kg/day continuous infusion for 7 days

AML:

<3 years: 0.3 mg/kg/day over 2 hours daily for 5 days

≥3 years: 9 mg/m^2/day over 2 hours daily for 5 days

Langerhans cell histiocytosis: 5-10 mg/m^2/day over 2 hours daily for 5 days; do not administer if platelet count <100,000

Adults: 0.09-0.1 mg/kg/day continuous infusion for 7 consecutive days

Administration Parenteral: I.V.: **Single daily infusion:** May administer diluted in NS as an intermittent infusion or continuous infusion; administer through a 0.22 micron in-line filter

Monitoring Parameters CBC with differential and platelet count; creatinine clearance before initial dose; periodic renal and hepatic function tests

Nursing Implications Cladribine I.V. solution for administration should be inspected visually for particulates. A precipitate may occur at low temperatures and may be resolubilized at room temperature or by shaking the solution vigorously.

Dosage Forms Injection, preservative free: 1 mg/mL (10 mL)

References

Kearns CM, Blakley RL, Santane VM, et al, "Pharmacokinetics of Cladribine (2-Chlorodioxyadenosine) in Children with Acute Leukemia," *Cancer Research,* 1994, 54:1235-39.

Larson RA, et al, "Dose Escalation Trial of Cladribine Using 5 Daily I.V. Infusions in Patients with Advanced Hematologic Malignancies," *J Clin Oncol,* 1996, 14(1):188-95.

Liliemark J, "The Clinical Pharmacokinetics of Cladribine," *Clin Pharmacokinet,* 1997, 32:120-131.

Stine KC, Saylors RL, Williams LL, et al, "2-Chlorodeoxyadenosine (2-CDA) for the Treatment of Refractory or Recurrent Langerhans Cell Histiocytosis (LCH) in Pediatric Patients," *Med Pediatr Oncol,* 1997, 29:288-92.

♦ **Claforan®** see Cefotaxime *on page 184*

♦ **Clamurid® (Canada)** see Carbamide Peroxide *on page 167*

Clarithromycin (kla RITH roe mye sin)
Related Information
Carbohydrate and Alcohol Content of Liquid Medications for Use in Patients Receiving Ketogenic Diets *on page 1228*
Endocarditis Prophylaxis *on page 1127*
Brand Names Biaxin™
Therapeutic Category Antibiotic, Macrolide
Generic Available No
Use Treatment of upper and lower respiratory tract infections, acute otitis media, and infections of the skin and skin structure due to susceptible strains of *S. aureus*, *S. pyogenes*, *S. pneumoniae*, *H. influenzae*, *M. catarrhalis*, *Mycoplasma pneumoniae*, *C. trachomatis*, and *Legionella* sp; prophylaxis and treatment of *Mycobacterium avium* complex (MAC) disease in patients with advanced HIV infection; treatment of *Helicobacter pylori* infection; prophylaxis of bacterial endocarditis in penicillin-allergic patients
Pregnancy Risk Factor C
Contraindications Hypersensitivity to clarithromycin, any component, erythromycin, or any macrolide antibiotics; concomitant administration of terfenadine, astemizole, or cisapride with clarithromycin may result in Q-T interval prolongation, ventricular tachycardia, ventricular fibrillation, hypotension, palpitations, cardiac arrest, and death
Warnings Safety and efficacy of clarithromycin have not been established in children <6 months of age; pseudomembranous colitis has been reported with use of clarithromycin
Precautions Use with caution in patients with hepatic or renal impairment; reduce dosage or prolong dosing interval in patients with severe renal impairment with or without coexisting hepatic impairment
Adverse Reactions
Central nervous system: Headache, hallucinations
Dermatologic: Pruritus, rash, Stevens-Johnson syndrome
Gastrointestinal: Diarrhea, nausea, vomiting, abdominal pain, dysgeusia, stomatitis; incidence of adverse GI effects (diarrhea, nausea, vomiting, dyspepsia, abdominal pain) is lower (13%) compared to erythromycin treated patients (32%)
Hematologic: Increased prothrombin time, decreased WBC
Hepatic: Elevated liver enzymes, hyperbilirubinemia
Otic: Hearing loss
Renal: Elevated BUN and serum creatinine
Drug Interactions Cytochrome P-450 isoenzyme CYP3A3/4 substrate; CYP1A2 and CYP3A3/4 isoenzyme inhibitor
Clarithromycin has been shown to increase serum **theophylline** levels by as much as 20%; **carbamazepine** levels have been shown to increase after a single dose of clarithromycin; hepatic metabolism of terfenadine, astemizole, and cisapride are reduced by clarithromycin (see Contraindications); increases serum level of digoxin, cyclosporine, tacrolimus, ergot alkaloids, omeprazole, lovastatin, simvastatin, and triazolam; potentiates the effects of warfarin; fluconazole and ritonavir increase serum level of clarithromycin; efavirenz decreases clarithromycin levels while increasing the levels of its metabolite
Food Interactions Food may delay the rate but not the extent of oral absorption
Stability Reconstituted oral suspension should **not** be refrigerated because it might gel; microencapsulated particles of clarithromycin in suspension is stable for 14 days when stored at room temperature
Mechanism of Action Inhibits bacterial RNA-dependent protein synthesis by binding to the 50S ribosomal subunit; the 14-hydroxy metabolite of clarithromycin is twice as active as the parent compound
Pharmacokinetics
Absorption: Rapid from the GI tract; food delays onset of absorption and formation of active metabolite, but does not affect the extent of tablet absorption; in pediatric patients, coadministration of the suspension with food did not significantly alter the extent of clarithromycin absorption or formation of the 14-OH metabolite
Distribution: Widely distributed throughout the body with tissue concentrations higher than serum concentrations
Protein binding: 65% to 70%
Metabolism: In the liver to active and inactive metabolites; undergoes extensive first-pass metabolism
Bioavailability: 50% to 68%
Half-life: Dose-dependent, prolonged with renal dysfunction
Clarithromycin:
250 mg dose: 3-4 hours

500 mg dose: 5-7 hours
14-hydroxy metabolite:
250 mg dose: 5-6 hours
500 mg dose: 7 hours
Time to peak serum concentration (tablet and suspension): 1-4 hours
Elimination: After a 250 mg dose, 20% is excreted unchanged in urine, 10% to 15% is excreted as active metabolite 14-OH clarithromycin, and 4% is excreted in feces

Usual Dosage Oral:

Infants and Children:
Acute otitis media: 15 mg/kg/day divided every 12 hours for 10 days
Respiratory, skin and skin structure infections: 15 mg/kg/day divided every 12 hours for 7-14 days
Prophylaxis for bacterial endocarditis: 15 mg/kg 1 hour before procedure
Prophylaxis for first episode of MAC with the following CD4$^+$ T-lymphocyte counts (see below): 15 mg/kg/day divided every 12 hours; maximum dose: 1 g/day
Children <12 months: <750 cells/µL
1-2 years: <500 cells/µL
2-6 years: <75 cells/µL
≥6 years: <50 cells/µL
Prophylaxis for recurrence of MAC: 15 mg/kg/day divided every 12 hours; maximum dose: 1 g/day (use in combination with ethambutol and with or without rifabutin)

Adolescents and Adults: 250 mg every 12 hours for 7-14 days for all indications except sinusitis and chronic bronchitis due to *H. influenzae*; for these indications, 500 mg every 12 hours for 7-14 days
Prophylaxis for bacterial endocarditis: 500 mg 1 hour before procedure
Prophylaxis for first episode of MAC in patients with CD4$^+$ T-lymphocyte count <50 cells/µL: 500 mg twice daily
Prophylaxis for recurrence of MAC: 500 mg twice daily in combination with ethambutol and with or without rifabutin
Helicobacter pylori (combination therapy with omeprazole or with bismuth subsalicylate, tetracycline, and an H$_2$ receptor antagonist): 250 mg twice daily up to 500 mg 3 times/day

Dosing adjustment in renal impairment: Cl$_{cr}$ <30 mL/minute: Decrease dose by 50% and administer once or twice daily

Administration Oral: May administer with or without meals; may administer with milk; shake suspension well before use

Monitoring Parameters Monitor serum concentration of other drugs in patients receiving clarithromycin and drugs known to interact with erythromycin (ie, theophylline, digoxin, anticoagulants, triazolam) since there are still very few studies examining drug-drug interactions with clarithromycin; liver function tests; hearing (in patients receiving long-term treatment with clarithromycin); observe for changes in bowel frequency

Dosage Forms
Suspension, oral: 125 mg/5 mL (50 mL, 100 mL); 250 mg/5 mL (50 mL, 100 mL)
Tablet, film coated: 250 mg, 500 mg

References

Aspin MM, Hoberman A, McCarty J, et al, "Comparative Study of the Safety and Efficacy of Clarithromycin and Amoxicillin-Clavulanate in the Treatment of Acute Otitis Media in Children," *J Pediatr*, 1994, 125(1):136-41.

Guay DR and Craft JC, "Overview of the Pharmacology of Clarithromycin Suspension in Children and a Comparison With That in Adults," *Pediatr Infect Dis J*, 1993, 12(12 Suppl 3):S106-11.

Husson RN, Ross LA, Sandelli S, et al, "Orally Administered Clarithromycin for the Treatment of Systemic *Mycobacterium avium* Complex Infection in Children With Acquired Immunodeficiency Syndrome," *J Pediatr*, 1994, 124(5 Pt 1):807-14.

Neu HC, "The Development of Macrolides: Clarithromycin in Perspective," *J Antimicrob Chemother*, 1991, 27(Suppl A):1-9.

"1999 USPHS/IDSA Guidelines for the Prevention of Opportunistic Infections in Persons Infected With Human Immunodeficiency Virus. USPHS/IDSA Prevention of Opportunistic Infections Working Group," *MMWR Morb Mortal Wkly Rep*, 1999, 48(RR-10):1-66.

♦ **Claritin®** *see* Loratadine *on page 582*

♦ **Claritin® RediTab®** *see* Loratadine *on page 582*

♦ **Clavulanate Potassium and Ticarcillin** *see* Ticarcillin and Clavulanate Potassium *on page 928*

♦ **Clavulanic Acid and Amoxicillin** *see* Amoxicillin and Clavulanic Acid *on page 71*

♦ **Clavulin® (Canada)** *see* Amoxicillin and Clavulanic Acid *on page 71*

♦ **Clear Away® Disc [OTC]** *see* Salicylic Acid *on page 854*

♦ **Clear By Design® Gel [OTC]** *see Benzoyl Peroxide on page 126*
♦ **Clear Eyes® [OTC]** *see Naphazoline on page 671*
♦ **Clearsil® Maximum Strength [OTC]** *see Benzoyl Peroxide on page 126*
♦ **Clear Tussin® 30** *see Guaifenesin and Dextromethorphan on page 466*

Clemastine (KLEM as teen)

Related Information
Carbohydrate and Alcohol Content of Liquid Medications for Use in Patients Receiving Ketogenic Diets *on page 1228*
Drugs and Breast-Feeding *on page 1213*

Brand Names Antihist-1® [OTC]; Tavist®; Tavist®-1 [OTC]

Available Salts Clemastine Fumarate

Synonyms Meclastine; Mecloprodin

Therapeutic Category Antihistamine

Generic Available Yes

Use Perennial and seasonal allergic rhinitis and other allergic symptoms including urticaria

Pregnancy Risk Factor C

Contraindications Narrow-angle glaucoma; hypersensitivity to clemastine or any component; patients receiving MAO inhibitors

Precautions Use with caution in patients with stenosing peptic ulcer, GI or GU obstruction, asthma, or prostatic hypertrophy

Adverse Reactions
Cardiovascular: Bradycardia, edema, palpitations
Central nervous system: Drowsiness, fatigue, headache, dizziness, vertigo, ataxia, CNS stimulation (more common in children)
Dermatologic: Rash, angioedema, photosensitivity
Gastrointestinal: Nausea, vomiting, xerostomia, gastritis, appetite increase, weight gain, diarrhea, abdominal pain
Hepatic: Hepatitis
Neuromuscular & skeletal: Arthralgia, myalgia, paresthesia
Respiratory: Shortness of breath, pharyngitis, bronchospasm, epistaxis

Drug Interactions Increased toxicity (CNS depression or excessive anticholinergic activity): CNS depressants, MAO inhibitors, tricyclic antidepressants, phenothiazines

Mechanism of Action Competes with histamine for H_1-receptor sites on effector cells in the gastrointestinal tract, blood vessels, and respiratory tract

Pharmacodynamics
Onset of effect: 2 hours after administration
Peak effect: 5-7 hours
Duration of action: 10-12 hours

Pharmacokinetics
Absorption: Oral: Well absorbed
Distribution: Breast milk to plasma ratio: 0.25-0.5
Metabolism: In the liver
Time to peak serum concentration: 2-4 hours
Elimination: Majority of an oral dose eliminated in the urine

Usual Dosage Oral:
Infants and Children <6 years: 0.05 mg/kg/day as **clemastine base** or 0.335-0.67 mg/day clemastine fumarate (0.25-0.5 mg base/day) divided into two or three doses; maximum daily dosage: 1.34 mg (1 mg base)
Children 6-12 years: 0.67-1.34 mg clemastine fumarate (0.5-1 mg base) twice daily; do not exceed 4.02 mg/day (3 mg/day base)
Children ≥12 years and Adults: 1.34 mg clemastine fumarate (1 mg base) twice daily to 2.68 mg (2 mg base) 3 times/day; do not exceed 8.04 mg/day (6 mg base)

Administration Oral: Administer with food

Monitoring Parameters Look for a reduction of rhinitis, urticaria, eczema, pruritus, or other allergic symptoms

Patient Information Avoid alcohol; may cause drowsiness and impair ability to perform hazardous activities requiring mental alertness or physical coordination

Dosage Forms
Syrup, as fumarate (citrus flavor): 0.67 mg/5 mL (0.5 mg base/5 mL) with alcohol 5.5% (120 mL)
Tablet, as fumarate: 1.34 mg (1 mg base), 2.68 mg (2 mg base)

♦ **Clemastine Fumarate** *see Clemastine on page 236*
♦ **Cleocin HCl® Oral** *see Clindamycin on page 237*

♦ **Cleocin Pediatric® Oral** *see* Clindamycin *on page 237*
♦ **Cleocin Phosphate® Injection** *see* Clindamycin *on page 237*
♦ **Cleocin T® Topical** *see* Clindamycin *on page 237*
♦ **Cleocin® Vaginal** *see* Clindamycin *on page 237*
♦ **Climara® Transdermal** *see* Estradiol *on page 386*
♦ **Clinda-Derm® Topical** *see* Clindamycin *on page 237*

Clindamycin (klin da MYE sin)

Related Information
Carbohydrate and Alcohol Content of Liquid Medications for Use in Patients Receiving Ketogenic Diets *on page 1228*
Endocarditis Prophylaxis *on page 1127*

Brand Names Cleocin HCl® Oral; Cleocin Pediatric® Oral; Cleocin Phosphate® Injection; Cleocin T® Topical; Cleocin® Vaginal; Clinda-Derm® Topical; Dalacin® C [Hydrochloride] Topical (Canada); Dalacin® C [Hydrochloride] Vaginal Cream (Canada)

Available Salts Clindamycin Hydrochloride; Clindamycin Palmitate; Clindamycin Phosphate

Therapeutic Category Acne Products; Antibiotic, Anaerobic; Antibiotic, Miscellaneous

Generic Available Yes

Use Useful agent against most aerobic gram-positive staphylococci and streptococci (except enterococci); useful against *Fusobacterium*, *Bacteroides* sp and *Actinomyces* for treatment of respiratory tract infections, skin and soft tissue infections, sepsis, intra-abdominal infections, and infections of the female pelvis and genital tract; bacterial endocarditis prophylaxis for dental and upper respiratory procedures in penicillin-allergic patients; treatment of babesiosis; used topically in treatment of severe acne; used intravaginally for treatment of bacterial vaginosis

Pregnancy Risk Factor B

Contraindications Hypersensitivity to clindamycin or any component; previous pseudomembranous colitis, hepatic impairment

Warnings Can cause severe and possibly fatal colitis characterized by severe persistent diarrhea, severe abdominal cramps and possibly, the passage of blood and mucus; discontinue drug if significant diarrhea occurs

Precautions Use with caution and modify dosage in patients with severe renal and/or hepatic impairment

Adverse Reactions
Cardiovascular: Hypotension, cardiac arrest (with rapid I.V. administration); arrhythmia due to Q-T$_c$ prolongation
Dermatologic: Urticaria, rash, Stevens-Johnson syndrome
Gastrointestinal: Diarrhea, nausea, vomiting, pseudomembranous colitis, esophagitis
Hematologic: Eosinophilia, granulocytopenia, thrombocytopenia
Hepatic: Elevated liver enzymes
Local: Sterile abscess at I.M. injection site; thrombophlebitis, erythema, pain, swelling
Renal: Rare: Renal dysfunction

Drug Interactions Clindamycin may increase the neuromuscular blocking action of tubocurarine, pancuronium

Stability Do **not** refrigerate the reconstituted oral solution because it will thicken; oral solution stable for 2 weeks at room temperature following reconstitution; I.V. clindamycin is incompatible with aminophylline, tobramycin

Mechanism of Action Reversibly binds to 50S ribosomal subunits preventing peptide bond formation thus inhibiting bacterial protein synthesis; bacteriostatic or bactericidal depending on drug concentration, infection site, and organism

Pharmacokinetics
Absorption:
Oral: 90% of clindamycin hydrochloride is rapidly absorbed; clindamycin palmitate must be hydrolyzed in the GI tract before it is active
Topical: ~10% absorbed systemically
Distribution: No significant levels are seen in CSF, even with inflamed meninges; crosses the placenta; distributes into breast milk, saliva, ascites fluid, pleural fluid, bone, and bile
Protein binding: 94%
Bioavailability: Oral: ~90%
(Continued)

Clindamycin *(Continued)*

Half-life:
Neonates:
Premature: 8.7 hours
Full-term: 3.6 hours
Infants 1 month to 1 year: 3 hours
Children and Adults with normal renal function: 2-3 hours
Time to peak serum concentration:
Oral: Within 60 minutes
I.M.: Within 1-3 hours
Elimination: Most of the drug is eliminated by hepatic metabolism; 10% of an oral dose excreted in urine and 3.6% excreted in feces as active drug and metabolites
Not dialyzable (0% to 5%)

Usual Dosage

Neonates: I.M., I.V.:
Postnatal age ≤7 days:
≤2000 g: 10 mg/kg/day divided every 12 hours
>2000 g: 15 mg/kg/day divided every 8 hours
Postnatal age >7 days:
<1200 g: 10 mg/kg/day divided every 12 hours
1200-2000 g: 15 mg/kg/day divided every 8 hours
>2000 g: 20-30 mg/kg/day divided every 6-8 hours
Infants and Children:
Oral: 10-30 mg/kg/day divided every 6-8 hours; maximum dose: 1.8 g/day
I.M., I.V.: 25-40 mg/kg/day divided every 6-8 hours; maximum dose: 4.8 g/day
Bacterial endocarditis prophylaxis for dental and upper respiratory procedures in penicillin allergic patients:
Oral: 20 mg/kg 1 hour before procedure **or** I.V.: 20 mg/kg 30 minutes before procedure; maximum dose: 600 mg
Babesiosis: Oral: 20-40 mg/kg/day divided every 8 hours for 7 days plus quinine
Children and Adults: Topical: Apply twice daily
Adolescents and Adults:
Oral: 150-450 mg/dose every 6-8 hours; maximum dose: 1.8 g/day
I.M., I.V.: 1.2-1.8 g/day in 2-4 divided doses; maximum dose: 4.8 g/day
Vaginal: One full applicator (100 mg) inserted intravaginally once daily before bedtime for seven consecutive days
Bacterial endocarditis prophylaxis for dental and upper respiratory procedures in penicillin allergic patients:
Oral: 600 mg 1 hour before procedure **or** I.V.: 600 mg 30 minutes before procedure
Pelvic inflammatory disease: 900 mg I.V. every 8 hours for 24-48 hours after significant clinical improvement, followed by 600 mg orally 3 times/day to complete a 14-day course
Babesiosis:
I.V.: 1.2 g twice daily plus quinine
or
Oral: 600 mg 3 times/day for 7 days plus quinine
Dosing interval in renal/hepatic impairment: Reduce dosage in patients with severe renal or hepatic impairment

Administration

Intravaginal: Do not use for topical therapy, instillation in the eye, or oral administration
Oral: Adults: Capsule should be taken with a full glass of water to avoid esophageal irritation; shake oral solution well before use; may administer with or without meals
Parenteral: Administer by I.V. intermittent infusion over at least 10-60 minutes, at a rate **not** to exceed 30 mg/minute; hypotension and cardiopulmonary arrest have been reported following rapid I.V. administration; final concentration for administration should not exceed 18 mg/mL
Topical: Do not use intravaginally, instill in the eye, or administer orally

Monitoring Parameters Observe for changes in bowel frequency; during prolonged therapy monitor CBC, liver and renal function tests periodically

Patient Information Report any severe diarrhea immediately; clindamycin vaginal cream (oil-based) may weaken latex condoms for up to 72 hours after completing therapy

Dosage Forms

Capsule, as hydrochloride: 75 mg, 150 mg, 300 mg

Cream, vaginal, as phosphate: 2% (40 g)
Gel, topical, as phosphate: 1% (7.5 g, 30 g)
Granules for oral solution, as palmitate: 75 mg/5 mL (100 mL)
Infusion, as phosphate, in D_5W: 300 mg (50 mL); 600 mg (50 mL)
Injection, as phosphate: 150 mg/mL (2 mL, 4 mL, 6 mL, 50 mL, 60 mL)
Lotion, as phosphate: 1% (60 mL)
Solution, topical, as phosphate: 1% (30 mL, 60 mL, 480 mL)

References
Dajani AS, Taubert KA, Wilson W, et al, "Prevention of Bacterial Endocarditis. Recommendations by the American Heart Association," *JAMA*, 1997, 277(22):1794-801.

♦ **Clindamycin Hydrochloride** *see* Clindamycin *on page 237*
♦ **Clindamycin Palmitate** *see* Clindamycin *on page 237*
♦ **Clindamycin Phosphate** *see* Clindamycin *on page 237*
♦ **Clinoril®** *see* Sulindac *on page 896*

Clioquinol (klye oh KWIN ole)

Brand Names Clioquinol® (Canada); Vioform® [OTC]
Synonyms Iodochlorhydroxyquin
Therapeutic Category Antifungal Agent, Topical
Generic Available Yes: Cream
Use Used topically in the treatment of tinea pedis, tinea cruris, and skin infections caused by dermatophytic fungi (ringworm)
Contraindications Not effective in the treatment of scalp or nail fungal infections; children <2 years of age; hypersensitivity to clioquinol, hydroxyquinoline, quinoline derivatives, iodides, or any component
Warnings Topical application poses a potential risk of toxicity to infants and children; known to cause serious and irreversible optic atrophy and peripheral neuropathy with muscular weakness, sensory loss, and blindness
Precautions Routine use is not recommended; may irritate sensitized skin; use with caution in patients with iodine intolerance
Adverse Reactions
Dermatologic: Skin irritation, rash, discoloration of skin
Neuromuscular & skeletal: Peripheral neuropathy
Ocular: Optic atrophy
Stability Store in tight, light-resistant container; avoid freezing
Mechanism of Action Chelates bacterial surface and trace metals needed for bacterial growth
Pharmacokinetics
Absorption: With an occlusive dressing up to 40% of a dose can be absorbed systemically during a 12-hour period; drug absorption is enhanced when applied under diapers
Half-life: 11-14 hours
Elimination: Conjugated and excreted in urine
Usual Dosage Children ≥2 years and Adults: Topical: Apply 2-4 times/day; do not use for >7 days
Administration Topical: Do not apply to the eyes; apply after cleansing the affected area with soap and water and drying thoroughly
Test Interactions Thyroid function tests (decreases ^{131}I uptake); false-positive ferric chloride test for phenylketonuria
Patient Information Can stain skin and fabrics; for external use only; avoid contact with eyes and mucous membranes
Dosage Forms
Cream: 3% (30 g)
Ointment, topical: 3% (30 g)
References
American Academy of Pediatrics Committee on Drugs, "Clioquinol (Iodochlorhydroxyquin, Vioform®) and Iodoquinol (Diiodohydroxyquin): Blindness and Neuropathy," *Pediatrics*, 1990, 86(5):797-8.

♦ **Clioquinol® (Canada)** *see* Clioquinol *on page 239*
♦ **Clocort® Maximum Strength [OTC]** *see* Hydrocortisone *on page 486*

Clofazimine (kloe FA zi meen)

Brand Names Lamprene®
Therapeutic Category Antibiotic, Miscellaneous; Leprostatic Agent
Generic Available No
Use Treatment of dapsone-resistant lepromatous leprosy (*Mycobacterium leprae*); multibacillary dapsone-sensitive leprosy; erythema nodosum leprosum; **Note:** (Continued)

Clofazimine *(Continued)*

Clofazimine has been associated with an adverse outcome in the treatment of MAC disease and should not be used

Pregnancy Risk Factor C

Contraindications Hypersensitivity to clofazimine or any component

Precautions Well tolerated when administered in dosages ≤100 mg/day; dosages >100 mg/day should be used for as short a duration as possible; use with caution in patients with GI problems; patients with abdominal pain, colic, nausea, vomiting, or diarrhea during clofazimine therapy may require a dosage adjustment or discontinuation of therapy

Adverse Reactions

Central nervous system: Dizziness, drowsiness, fatigue, headache, fever

Dermatologic: Discoloration of the skin and conjunctiva (pink to brownish-black), dry skin, rash, pruritus, acneiform eruptions, erythema multiforme, phototoxicity

Endocrine & metabolic: Hyperglycemia

Gastrointestinal: Constipation, abdominal pain, diarrhea, nausea, anorexia, vomiting, bowel obstruction, GI bleeding, dysgeusia

Hepatic: Hepatitis, jaundice

Ocular: Irritation of the eyes

Neuromuscular & skeletal: Peripheral neuropathy

Drug Interactions Isoniazid increases clofazimine plasma and urinary concentration and decreases clofazimine skin concentration

Food Interactions Presence of food increases the extent of absorption

Stability Protect from moisture

Mechanism of Action Binds preferentially to mycobacterial DNA at the guanine base to inhibit mycobacterial growth; also has some anti-inflammatory activity through an unknown mechanism

Pharmacokinetics

Absorption: Oral: 45% to 70% slowly absorbed

Distribution: Clofazimine remains in tissues for prolonged periods and distributes into fatty tissues of the reticuloendothelial system, mesenteric lymph nodes, adrenal glands, liver, bile, spleen, small intestine, lungs, muscles, bone, skin, breast milk; does not appear to penetrate into the CSF

Metabolism: In the liver to three metabolites

Half-life:

Terminal: 8 days

Tissue: 70 days

Elimination: Principally in feces; only negligible amounts excreted unchanged in the urine; small amounts excreted in sputum, saliva, and sweat

Usual Dosage Oral:

Children: Leprosy: 1 mg/kg/day every 24 hours in combination with dapsone and rifampin

Adults:

Dapsone-resistant leprosy: 50-100 mg once daily in combination with one or more antileprosy drugs for 2 years; then alone 50-100 mg/day

Dapsone-sensitive multibacillary leprosy: 50-100 mg once daily in combination with two or more antileprosy drugs for at least 2 years and continue until negative skin smears are obtained, then institute single-drug therapy with appropriate agent

Erythema nodosum leprosum: 100-200 mg/day for up to 3 months or longer then taper dose to 100 mg/day when possible

Administration Oral: Administer with meals or milk to maximize absorption

Monitoring Parameters GI complaints, periodic liver function tests

Patient Information May discolor skin, conjunctiva, tears, sweat, urine, feces, and nasal secretions to a pink to brownish-black color; skin discoloration reversal may take several months after discontinuation of clofazimine

Nursing Implications Clofazimine-induced dry skin may be relieved by applying petrolatum or an emollient lotion containing 25% urea to the affected areas

Dosage Forms Capsule: 50 mg, 100 mg

References

Chesney PJ, "New Concepts for Antimicrobial Use in Opportunistic Infections," *Semin Pediatr Infect Dis*, 1991, 2(1):67-73.

Garrelts JC, "Clofazimine: A Review of Its Use in Leprosy and *Mycobacterium avium* Complex Infection," *DICP*, 1991, 25(5):525-31.

"1999 USPHS/IDSA Guidelines for the Prevention of Opportunistic Infections in Persons Infected With Human Immunodeficiency Virus. USPHS/IDSA Prevention of Opportunistic Infections Working Group," *MMWR Morb Mortal Wkly Rep*, 1999, 48(RR-10):1-66.

Clonazepam (kloe NA ze pam)

Related Information
Antiepileptic Drugs *on page 1176*
Overdose and Toxicology *on page 1191*

Brand Names Klonopin™; PMS-Clonazepam (Canada); Rivotril® (Canada)

Therapeutic Category Anticonvulsant, Benzodiazepine; Benzodiazepine

Generic Available Yes

Use Treatment of absence (petit mal), petit mal variant (Lennox-Gastaut), infantile spasms, akinetic, and myoclonic seizures

Restrictions C-IV

Pregnancy Risk Factor C

Contraindications Hypersensitivity to clonazepam, any component, or other benzodiazepines; severe liver disease, acute narrow-angle glaucoma

Precautions Use with caution in patients with chronic respiratory disease or impaired renal function; abrupt discontinuance may precipitate withdrawal symptoms, status epilepticus or seizures

Adverse Reactions
Cardiovascular: Hypotension
Central nervous system: Drowsiness, changes in behavior or personality, vertigo, confusion, memory impairment, decreased concentration, headache, ataxia, choreiform movements, hypotonia
Dermatologic: Rash
Gastrointestinal: Nausea, xerostomia, vomiting, diarrhea, constipation, anorexia, hypersalivation
Hematologic: Thrombocytopenia, anemia, leukopenia, eosinophilia
Neuromuscular & skeletal: Tremor
Ocular: Nystagmus, blurred vision
Respiratory: Bronchial hypersecretion, respiratory depression
Miscellaneous: Physical and psychological dependence

Drug Interactions Cytochrome P-450 isoenzyme CYP3A3/4 substrate
CNS depressants or alcohol increase sedation; phenytoin, carbamazepine, rifampin, or barbiturates increase clonazepam clearance; drugs that inhibit cytochrome P-450 isoenzyme CYP3A3/4 may increase levels and effects of clonazepam; monitor for altered benzodiazepine response

Mechanism of Action Suppresses the spike-and-wave discharge in absence seizures by depressing nerve transmission in the motor cortex; depresses all levels of the CNS, including the limbic and reticular formation, by binding to the benzodiazepine site on the gamma-aminobutyric acid (GABA) receptor complex and modulating GABA, which is a major inhibitory neurotransmitter in the brain

Pharmacodynamics
Onset of effect: 20-60 minutes
Duration:
Infants and young children: Up to 6-8 hours
Adults: Up to 12 hours

Pharmacokinetics
Absorption: Oral: Well absorbed
Distribution: V_d: Adults: 1.5-4.4 L/kg
Protein binding: 85%
Metabolism: Extensively metabolized; glucuronide and sulfate conjugation
Half-life:
Children: 22-33 hours
Adults: 19-50 hours
Elimination: Metabolites excreted as glucuronide or sulfate conjugates; less than 2% excreted unchanged in urine

Usual Dosage Oral:
Infants and Children <10 years or 30 kg:
Initial daily dose: 0.01-0.03 mg/kg/day (maximum dose: 0.05 mg/kg/day) given in 2-3 divided doses; increase by no more than 0.5 mg every third day until seizures are controlled or adverse effects seen
Maintenance dose: 0.1-0.2 mg/kg/day divided 3 times/day; not to exceed 0.2 mg/kg/day
Children ≥10 years (>30 kg) and Adults:
Initial daily dose not to exceed 1.5 mg given in 3 divided doses; may increase by 0.5-1 mg every third day until seizures are controlled or adverse effects seen
Maintenance dose: 0.05-0.2 mg/kg; do not exceed 20 mg/day

Administration Oral: May administer with food or water to decrease GI distress
(Continued)

241

Clonazepam *(Continued)*

Reference Range Relationship between serum concentration and seizure control is not well established; measurement at random times postdose may contribute to this problem; predose concentrations are recommended
Proposed therapeutic levels: 20-80 ng/mL
Potentially toxic concentration: >80 ng/mL

Patient Information Avoid alcohol; may cause drowsiness and impair ability to perform hazardous activities requiring mental alertness or physical coordination

Additional Information Ethosuximide or valproic acid may be preferred for treatment of absence (petit mal) seizures; clonazepam-induced behavioral disturbances may be more frequent in mentally handicapped patients; when discontinuing therapy in children, the clonazepam dose may be safely reduced by ≤0.04 mg/kg/week and discontinued when the daily dose is ≤0.04 mg/kg/day

Dosage Forms Tablet: 0.5 mg, 1 mg, 2 mg

Extemporaneous Preparations A 0.1 mg/mL oral liquid can be made using 3 different vehicles (cherry syrup; a 1:1 mixture of Ora-Sweet® and Ora-Plus®; or a 1:1 mixture of Ora-Sweet® SF and Ora-Plus®); crush six 2 mg tablets into a fine powder in a mortar; add 10 mL of the vehicle and mix to make a uniform paste; mix while adding the vehicle in geometric portions to **almost** 120 mL; transfer to a calibrated bottle and qsad with vehicle to 120 mL; preparation is stable for 60 days when stored in amber prescription bottles in the dark at room temperature (25°C) or under refrigeration (5°C); label "shake well" and "protect from light"

Allen LV and Erickson MA, "Stability of Acetazolamide, Allopurinol, Azathioprine, Clonazepam, and Flucytosine in Extemporaneously Compounded Oral Liquids," *Am J Health Syst Pharm*, 1996, 53(16):1944-9.

References

Sugai K, "Seizures With Clonazepam: Discontinuation and Suggestions for Safe Discontinuation Rates in Children," *Epilepsia*, 1993, 34(6):1089-97.

Clonidine (KLOE ni deen)

Brand Names Apo®-Clonidine (Canada); Catapres® Oral; Catapres-TTS® Transdermal; Dixarit® (Canada); Duraclon™ Injection; Novo-Clonidine® (Canada); Nu-Clonidine® (Canada)

Available Salts Clonidine Hydrochloride

Therapeutic Category Adrenergic Agonist Agent; Alpha-Adrenergic Agonist; Analgesic, Non-narcotic (Epidural); Antihypertensive Agent

Generic Available Yes: Tablet

Use Management of hypertension; aid in the diagnosis of pheochromocytoma and growth hormone deficiency; used for heroin withdrawal and smoking cessation therapy in adults; alternate agent for the treatment of attention-deficit/hyperactivity disorder (ADHD); epidural form is used in combination with opiates for relief of severe pain in cancer patients whose pain was not relieved by opiates alone

Pregnancy Risk Factor C

Contraindications Hypersensitivity to clonidine hydrochloride or any component; epidural injection is contraindicated in patients receiving anticoagulation therapy, patients with a bleeding diathesis, or an infection at the injection site. Administration of epidural clonidine above the C_4 dermatome is contraindicated.

Warnings Do not abruptly discontinue as rapid increase in blood pressure and symptoms of sympathetic overactivity (such as increased heart rate, tremors, agitation, anxiety, insomnia, sweating, palpitations) may occur; if need to discontinue, taper dose gradually over more than 1 week. EKG abnormalities and 4 cases of sudden cardiac death have been reported in children receiving clonidine with methylphenidate; reduce dose of methylphenidate by 40% when used concurrently with clonidine; consider EKG monitoring. Epidural clonidine is not recommended for perioperative, obstetrical, or postpartum pain [due to the risk of hemodynamic instability (hypotension, bradycardia)], in patients with severe cardiovascular disease, or those who are hemodynamically unstable.

Precautions Dosage modification is required in patients with renal impairment; use with caution in cerebrovascular disease, coronary insufficiency, renal impairment, sinus node dysfunction; monitor patients for signs of depression (especially those with a history of affective disorders)

Adverse Reactions
Cardiovascular: Raynaud's phenomenon, hypotension, bradycardia, palpitations, tachycardia, CHF, rebound hypertension if discontinued abruptly
Central nervous system: Drowsiness, sedation, headache, dizziness, fatigue, insomnia, anxiety, depression
Dermatologic: Rash, local skin reactions with patch
Endocrine & metabolic: Sodium and water retention, parotid pain

Gastrointestinal: Constipation, anorexia, xerostomia

Respiratory: Respiratory depression and ventilatory abnormalities with high epidural doses

Drug Interactions Use with methylphenidate may potentially increase EKG effects (see Warnings); tricyclic antidepressants antagonize hypotensive effects of clonidine; beta-blockers may potentiate bradycardia in patients receiving clonidine and may increase the rebound hypertension seen with clonidine withdrawal; discontinue beta-blocker several days before clonidine is tapered off; CNS depressants and alcohol may increase sedative effects; use with opiates may increase hypotension; epidural clonidine may prolong the effects of epidural local anesthetics

Food Interactions Hypertensive patients may need to decrease sodium and calories in diet

Stability Epidural injection: Discard unused portion of vial (preservative free)

Mechanism of Action Stimulates alpha$_2$-adrenoreceptors in the brain stem, thus activating an inhibitory neuron, resulting in reduced sympathetic outflow, producing a decrease in vasomotor tone and heart rate

Epidural use: Prevents pain signal transmission to the brain and produces analgesia at presynaptic and postjunctional alpha$_2$-adrenoreceptors in the spinal cord

Pharmacodynamics Oral:

Onset of effects: 30-60 minutes

Peak effects: Within 2-4 hours

Duration: 6-10 hours

Pharmacokinetics

Distribution: V_d: Adults: 2.1 L/kg

Protein binding: 20% to 40%

Metabolism: Hepatic to inactive metabolites

Bioavailability, oral: 75% to 95%

Half-life, serum:

Neonates: 44-72 hours

Adults:

Normal renal function: 6-20 hours

Renal impairment: 18-41 hours

Half-life, CSF: Adults: 1.3 ± 0.5 hours

Elimination: 65% excreted in urine (32% unchanged) and 22% excreted in feces via enterohepatic recirculation

Not dialyzable (0% to 5%)

Usual Dosage

Children:

Hypertension: Oral: Initial: 5-10 mcg/kg/day in divided doses every 8-12 hours; increase gradually, if needed, to 5-25 mcg/kg/day in divided doses every 6 hours; maximum dose: 0.9 mg/day

ADHD: Oral: Initial: 0.05 mg/day, increase every 3-7 days by 0.05 mg/day to 3-5 mcg/kg/day given in divided doses 3-4 times/day; maximum dose: 0.3-0.4 mg/day

Clonidine tolerance test (test of growth hormone release from the pituitary): Oral: 0.15 mg/m^2 or 4 mcg/kg as a single dose

Analgesia: Epidural (continuous infusion): Reserved for cancer patients with severe intractable pain, unresponsive to other analgesics or epidural or spinal opiates: Initial: 0.5 mcg/kg/hour; adjust with caution, based on clinical effect

Adults:

Hypertension:

Oral: Initial dose: 0.1 mg twice daily, usual maintenance dose: 0.2-1.2 mg/day in 2-4 divided doses; maximum recommended dose: 2.4 mg/day

Transdermal: Applied once weekly as transdermal delivery system; initial therapy with 0.1 mg/24 hours applied once every 7 days; adjust dosage based on response; hypotensive action may not begin until 2-3 days after initial application

Analgesia: Epidural (continuous infusion): Initial: 30 mcg/hour; titrate to clinical effect; usual maximum dose: 40 mcg/hour

Administration

Oral: May be administered without regard to meals

Transdermal: Patches should be applied at bedtime to a clean, hairless area of the upper arm or chest; rotate patch sites weekly in adults; in children, the patch may need to be changed more frequently (eg, every 3-5 days); **Note:** Transdermal patch is a membrane-controlled system; do **not** cut the patch to deliver partial doses; rate of drug delivery, reservoir contents, and adhesion may be affected if cut; if partial dose is needed, surface area of patch can be blocked proportionally using adhesive bandage (see Lee, 1997)

(Continued)

Clonidine *(Continued)*

Monitoring Parameters Blood pressure, heart rate; consider EKG monitoring in patients with history of heart disease or concurrent use of medications affecting conduction

Patient Information Avoid alcohol; may cause drowsiness and impair ability to perform hazardous duties requiring mental alertness; do not stop drug abruptly

Nursing Implications Counsel patient/parent about compliance and danger of withdrawal reaction if doses are missed or drug is discontinued

Additional Information Epidural clonidine may be more effective in the treatment of neuropathic pain compared to somatic or visceral pain; clonidine-induced symptomatic bradycardia may be treated with atropine

Dosage Forms

Injection, epidural, preservative free, as hydrochloride: 100 mcg/mL (10 mL); 500 mcg/mL (10 mL)

Patch, transdermal, as hydrochloride: 1, 2, and 3 (0.1 mg, 0.2 mg, 0.3 mg/day to 7-day duration)

Tablet, as hydrochloride: 0.1 mg, 0.2 mg, 0.3 mg

Extemporaneous Preparations A 0.1 mg/mL oral suspension compounded from tablets is stable for 28 days when stored in amber glass bottles and refrigerated (4°C); thirty 0.2 mg tablets are crushed in a glass mortar and ground to a fine powder; 2 mL Purified Water USP is slowly added, and triturated to make a fine paste; Simple Syrup, NF is slowly added in 15 mL increments and triturated; qsad 60 mL; shake well before use

Levinson ML and Johnson CE, "Stability of an Extemporaneously Compounded Clonidine Hydrochloride Oral Liquid," *Am J Hosp Pharm*, 1992, 49(1):122-5.

References

Hart-Santora D and Hart LL, "Clonidine in Attention Deficit Hyperactivity Disorder," *Ann Pharmacother*, 1992, 26(1):37-9.

Hunt RD, Minderaa RB, and Cohen DJ, "The Therapeutic Effect of Clonidine in Attention Deficit Disorder With Hyperactivity: A Comparison With Placebo and Methylphenidate," *Psychopharmacol Bull*, 1986, 22(1):229-35.

Lee NA and Anderson PO, "Giving Partial Doses of Transdermal Patches," *Am J Health Syst Pharm*, 1997, 54(15):1759-60.

Rocchini AP, "Childhood Hypertension: Etiology, Diagnosis, and Treatment," *Pediatr Clin North Am*, 1984, 31(6):1259-73.

Sinaiko AR, "Pharmacologic Management of Childhood Hypertension," *Pediatr Clin North Am*, 1993, 40(1):195-212.

♦ **Clonidine Hydrochloride** *see* Clonidine *on page 242*

♦ **Clopra®** *see* Metoclopramide *on page 630*

Clorazepate *(klor AZ e pate)*

Related Information

Antiepileptic Drugs *on page 1176*

Overdose and Toxicology *on page 1191*

Brand Names Apo®-Clorazepate (Canada); Gen-XENE®; Novo-Clopate® (Canada); Tranxene®

Available Salts Clorazepate Dipotassium

Therapeutic Category Anticonvulsant, Benzodiazepine; Benzodiazepine; Sedative

Generic Available Yes

Use Treatment of generalized anxiety and panic disorders; management of alcohol withdrawal; adjunct anticonvulsant in management of partial seizures

Restrictions C-IV

Pregnancy Risk Factor D

Contraindications Hypersensitivity to clorazepate dipotassium or any component; cross-sensitivity with other benzodiazepines may exist; avoid using in patients with pre-existing CNS depression, severe uncontrolled pain, or narrow-angle glaucoma

Warnings Abrupt discontinuation may cause withdrawal symptoms or seizures

Precautions Use with caution in patients with hepatic or renal disease

Adverse Reactions

Cardiovascular: Hypotension

Central nervous system: Drowsiness, dizziness, confusion, amnesia, headache, depression, ataxia

Dermatologic: Rash

Gastrointestinal: Nausea, xerostomia

Hematologic: Reduced hematocrit (with long-term use)

Ocular: Blurred vision

Miscellaneous: Physical and psychological dependence with long-term use; long-term use may also be associated with renal or hepatic injury

Drug Interactions Cimetidine or other hepatic enzyme inhibitors may decrease hepatic clearance, monitor for altered benzodiazepine response; concurrent use of clorazepate with ritonavir is not recommended

Stability Unstable in water

Mechanism of Action Depresses all levels of the CNS, including the limbic and reticular formation, by binding to the benzodiazepine site on the gamma-aminobutyric acid (GABA) receptor complex and modulating GABA, which is a major inhibitory neurotransmitter in the brain

Pharmacokinetics
Absorption: Rapidly decarboxylated to desmethyldiazepam (active) in acidic stomach prior to absorption
Distribution: Crosses the placenta
Metabolism: In the liver to oxazepam (active)
Half-life, adults:
Desmethyldiazepam: 48-96 hours
Oxazepam: 6-8 hours
Time to peak serum concentration: Oral: Within 1 hour
Elimination: Primarily in urine

Usual Dosage Oral:
Anticonvulsant:
Children 9-12 years: Initial: 3.75-7.5 mg/dose twice daily; increase dose by 3.75 mg at weekly intervals, not to exceed 60 mg/day in 2-3 divided doses
Children >12 years and Adults: Initial: Up to 7.5 mg/dose 2-3 times/day; increase dose by 7.5 mg at weekly intervals; usual dose: 0.5-1 mg/kg/day; not to exceed 90 mg/day (up to 3 mg/kg/day has been used)
Anxiety: Adults: 7.5-15 mg 2-4 times/day, or given as single dose of 15-22.5 mg at bedtime
Alcohol withdrawal: Adults: Initial: 30 mg, then 15 mg 2-4 times/day on first day; maximum daily dose: 90 mg; gradually decrease dose over subsequent days

Administration Oral: May administer with food or water to decrease GI upset

Monitoring Parameters Excessive CNS depression, respiratory rate, and cardiovascular stress

Reference Range Therapeutic: 0.12-1 µg/mL (SI: 0.36-3.01 µmol/L)

Patient Information Avoid alcohol; may cause drowsiness and impair ability to perform hazardous duties requiring mental alertness

Dosage Forms
Capsule, as dipotassium: 3.75 mg, 7.5 mg, 15 mg
Tablet, as dipotassium: 3.75 mg, 7.5 mg, 15 mg
Tablet, as dipotassium, single dose: 11.25 mg, 22.5 mg

♦ **Clorazepate Dipotassium** see Clorazepate on page 244
♦ **Clostridium botulinum Toxin Type A** see Botulinum Toxin Type A on page 139
♦ **Clotrimaderm (Canada)** see Clotrimazole on page 245

Clotrimazole (kloe TRIM a zole)

Brand Names Canesten® Topical (Canada) Canesten® Vaginal (Canada); Clotrimaderm (Canada); Gyne-Lotrimin® Vaginal [OTC]; Lotrimin AF® Topical [OTC]; Lotrimin® Topical; Mycelex®-G Topical; Mycelex®-G Vaginal [OTC]; Mycelex® Troche; Myclo-Derm® (Canada); Myclo-Gyne® (Canada)

Therapeutic Category Antifungal Agent, Oral Nonabsorbed; Antifungal Agent, Topical; Antifungal Agent, Vaginal

Generic Available Yes

Use Treatment of susceptible fungal infections, including oropharyngeal candidiasis, dermatophytoses, superficial mycoses, cutaneous candidiasis, as well as vulvovaginal candidiasis; limited data suggests that the use of clotrimazole troches may be effective for prophylaxis against oropharyngeal candidiasis in neutropenic patients

Pregnancy Risk Factor B (topical); C (troches)

Contraindications Hypersensitivity to clotrimazole or any component

Warnings Clotrimazole troches should not be used for treatment of systemic fungal infection

Precautions Safety and effectiveness of clotrimazole lozenges (troches) in children <3 years of age have not been established

Adverse Reactions
Dermatologic: Erythema, pruritus, urticaria, skin fissures, blistering
Gastrointestinal: Nausea and vomiting may occur in patients on clotrimazole troches; lower abdominal cramps may occur in patients receiving clotrimazole vaginal tablets
(Continued)

Clotrimazole *(Continued)*

Hepatic: Abnormal liver function tests (causal relationship between troches and elevated LFTs not clearly established)

Local: Mild burning, irritation, stinging of skin or vaginal area

Mechanism of Action Binds to phospholipids in the fungal cell membrane altering cell wall permeability resulting in loss of essential intracellular elements

Pharmacokinetics

Absorption: Negligible through intact skin when administered topically; 3% to 10% of an intravaginal dose is absorbed

Distribution: Following oral/topical administration, clotrimazole is present in saliva for up to 3 hours following 30 minutes of dissolution time in the mouth

Usual Dosage

Children >3 years and Adults:

Topical/Oral: 10 mg troche dissolved slowly 5 times/day

Topical: Apply twice daily

Children >12 years and Adults: Vaginal: 100 mg/day at bedtime for 7 days or 200 mg/day at bedtime for 3 days or 500 mg single dose; or 5 g (= 1 applicatorful) of 1% vaginal cream daily at bedtime for 7-14 days

Administration

Oral: Dissolve lozenge (troche) in mouth over 15-30 minutes

Topical: Apply sparingly and rub gently into the cleansed, affected area and surrounding skin; do not apply to the eye

Monitoring Parameters Periodic liver function tests during oral therapy with clotrimazole lozenges

Patient Information Vaginal cream and tablet are oil-based and may weaken latex condoms and diaphragms

Dosage Forms

Cream:

Topical (Lotrimin®, Lotrimin® AF, Mycelex®, Mycelex® OTC): 1% (15 g, 30 g, 45 g, 90 g)

Vaginal (Gyne-Lotrimin®, Mycelex®-G): 1% (45 g, 90 g)

Lotion (Lotrimin®): 1% (30 mL)

Solution, topical (Lotrimin®, Lotrimin® AF, Mycelex®, Mycelex® OTC): 1% (10 mL, 30 mL)

Tablet, vaginal (Gyne-Lotrimin®, Mycelex®-G): 100 mg (7s); 500 mg (1s)

Troche (Mycelex®): 10 mg

Twin pack (Mycelex®): Tablet 500 mg (1's) and vaginal cream 1% (7 g)

Cloxacillin *(kloks a SIL in)*

Related Information

Carbohydrate and Alcohol Content of Liquid Medications for Use in Patients Receiving Ketogenic Diets *on page 1228*

Brand Names Apo®-Cloxi (Canada); Cloxapen®; Novo-Cloxin® (Canada); Nu-Cloxi® (Canada); Orbenin® (Canada); Taro-Cloxacillin® (Canada); Tegopen®

Available Salts Cloxacillin Sodium

Therapeutic Category Antibiotic, Penicillin (Antistaphylococcal)

Generic Available Yes

Use Treatment of susceptible bacterial infections of the respiratory tract, skin and skin structure, bone and joint caused by penicillinase-producing staphylococci

Pregnancy Risk Factor B

Contraindications Hypersensitivity to cloxacillin, any component, or penicillins

Precautions Use with caution in patients with a history of cephalosporin hypersensitivity

Adverse Reactions

Central nervous system: Fever

Dermatologic: Rash

Gastrointestinal: Nausea, vomiting, diarrhea

Hematologic: Eosinophilia, leukopenia, neutropenia, thrombocytopenia, agranulocytosis

Hepatic: Hepatotoxicity

Renal: Hematuria, elevated BUN, elevated serum creatinine

Miscellaneous: Serum sickness-like reactions

Drug Interactions Probenecid (increases serum cloxacillin concentration)

Food Interactions Presence of food decreases extent of absorption

Stability Refrigerate oral solution after reconstitution; discard after 14 days; stable for 3 days at room temperature

Mechanism of Action Inhibits bacterial cell wall synthesis by binding to one or more of the penicillin-binding proteins; inhibits the final transpeptidation step of peptidoglycan synthesis resulting in cell wall death

Pharmacokinetics
Absorption: Oral: ~50%
Distribution: Into pleural and synovial fluid, bone, liver, and kidneys; poor penetration into CSF; crosses the placenta; appears in breast milk
Protein binding: 90% to 98%
Metabolism: Significant in the liver to active and inactive metabolites
Half-life: 30-90 minutes (prolonged with renal impairment and in neonates)
Time to peak serum concentration: Oral: Within 0.5-2 hours
Elimination: In the urine and through the bile
Not dialyzable (0% to 5%)

Usual Dosage Oral:
Children >1 month: 50-100 mg/kg/day in divided doses every 6 hours; up to a maximum of 4 g/day
Adults: 250-500 mg every 6 hours

Administration Oral: Administer 1 hour before or 2 hours after meals; shake suspension well before use

Monitoring Parameters CBC with differential, urinalysis, BUN, serum creatinine, and liver enzymes

Test Interactions False-positive urine and serum proteins

Additional Information
Sodium content of 250 mg capsule: 0.6 mEq
Sodium content of 5 mL of 125 mg/5 mL solution, oral: 0.48 mEq

Dosage Forms
Capsule, as sodium: 250 mg, 500 mg
Powder for oral suspension, as sodium: 125 mg/5 mL (100 mL, 200 mL)

♦ **Cloxacillin Sodium** see Cloxacillin on page 246
♦ **Cloxapen®** see Cloxacillin on page 246
♦ **Clysodrast®** see Bisacodyl on page 133

Coal Tar (KOLE tar)

Brand Names AquaTar® [OTC]; Balnetar® (Canada); Denorex® [OTC]; DHS® Tar [OTC]; Duplex® T [OTC]; Estar® [OTC]; Fototar® [OTC]; Ionil-T® Plus (Canada); Neutrogena® T/Derm; Pentrax® [OTC]; Polytar® [OTC]; psoriGel® [OTC]; T/Gel® [OTC]; Zetar® [OTC]

Synonyms LCD

Therapeutic Category Antipsoriatic Agent, Topical; Antiseborrheic Agent, Topical

Generic Available Yes

Use Topically for controlling dandruff, seborrheic dermatitis, or psoriasis

Contraindications Hypersensitivity to coal tar or any ingredient in the formulation

Warnings Due to a potential carcinogenic risk, do not use around the rectum or in the genital area or groin

Precautions Do not apply to acutely inflamed skin; avoid exposure to sunlight for at least 24 hours

Adverse Reactions Dermatologic: Dermatitis, folliculitis, irritation, acneiform eruption, photosensitization

Drug Interactions Tetracyclines, phenothiazines, tretinoin, and sulfonamides also have phototoxic potential

Mechanism of Action Reduces the number and size of epidermal cells produced

Usual Dosage Children and Adults: Topical:
Bath: 60-90 mL of a 5% to 20% solution or 15-25 mL of 30% lotion is added to bath water; soak 5-20 minutes, then pat dry; use once daily to once every 3 days
Shampoo: Apply twice weekly for the first 2 weeks then once weekly or more often if needed
Skin: Apply to the affected area 1-4 times/day; decrease frequency to 2-3 times/week once condition has been controlled
Atopic dermatitis: 2% to 5% coal tar cream may be applied once daily or every other day to reduce inflammation
Scalp psoriasis: Tar oil bath or coal tar solution may be painted sparingly to the lesions 3-12 hours before each shampoo
Psoriasis of the body, arms, legs: Apply at bedtime; if thick scales are present, use product with salicylic acid and apply several times during the day
(Continued)

Coal Tar *(Continued)*

Administration Topical:
  Bath: Add appropriate amount of coal tar to lukewarm bath water and mix thoroughly
  Shampoo: Rub shampoo onto wet hair and scalp, rinse thoroughly; repeat; leave on 5 minutes; rinse thoroughly

Patient Information Avoid contact with eyes, genital, or rectal area; coal tar preparations frequently stain the skin and hair; avoid exposure to direct sunlight; shake suspension well before use

Dosage Forms
  Cream: 1% to 5%
  Gel: Coal tar 5%
  Lotion: 2.5% to 30%
  Lotion: Coal tar 2% to 5%
  Shampoo: Coal tar extract 2% with salicylic acid 2% (60 mL)
  Shampoo, topical: Coal tar: 0.5% to 5%
  Solution:
    Coal tar: 2.5%, 5%, 20%
    Coal tar extract: 5%
  Suspension, coal tar: 30% to 33.3%

References
  Greaves MW, Weinstein GD, "Treatment of Psoriasis," *N Engl J Med*, 1995, 332(9):581-8.
  Hanifin JM, "Atopic Dermatitis in Infants and Children," *Pediatr Clin North Am*, 1991, 38(4):763-89.

♦ Cobex® *see* Cyanocobalamin *on page 263*

Cocaine (koe KANE)

Related Information
  Drugs and Breast-Feeding *on page 1213*
  Laboratory Detection of Drugs in Urine *on page 1204*

Available Salts Cocaine Hydrochloride

Therapeutic Category Analgesic, Topical; Local Anesthetic, Topical

Generic Available Yes

Use Topical anesthesia for mucous membranes

Restrictions C-II

Pregnancy Risk Factor C (X if nonmedical use)

Contraindications Systemic use; hypersensitivity to cocaine or any component

Precautions Use with caution in patients with hypertension, severe cardiovascular disease, thyrotoxicosis, and in infants; use with caution in patients with severely traumatized mucosa in the region of intended application

Adverse Reactions
  Cardiovascular: Hypertension, tachycardia, cardiac arrhythmias
  Central nervous system: Restlessness, nervousness, euphoria, excitement, hallucinations, seizures
  Gastrointestinal: Vomiting
  Neuromuscular & skeletal: Tremor
  Ocular: Topical: Sloughing of the corneal epithelium, ulceration of the cornea
  Respiratory: Tachypnea

Drug Interactions Cytochrome P-450 isoenzyme CYP3A3/4 substrate
  MAO inhibitors, inhalational anesthetics, levodopa, methyldopa, sympathomimetics and ethanol may increase risk of cardiac arrhythmias; CNS stimulants; beta-adrenergic blocking agents; cholinesterase inhibitors

Stability Store in well closed, light-resistant containers

Mechanism of Action Blocks both the initiation and conduction of nerve impulses by decreasing the neuronal membrane's permeability to sodium ions. This results in inhibition of depolarization with resultant blockade of conduction; interferes with the uptake of norepinephrine by adrenergic nerve terminals producing vasoconstriction.

Pharmacodynamics Following topical administration to mucosa:
  Onset of action: Within 1 minute
  Peak action: Within 5 minutes
  Duration: ≥30 minutes, depending upon route and dosage administered

Pharmacokinetics
  Absorption: Well absorbed through mucous membranes; absorption is limited by drug-induced vasoconstriction and enhanced by inflammation
  Distribution: V_d: ~2 L/kg; appears in breast milk (see Additional Information)
  Metabolism: In the liver; major metabolites are ecgonine methyl ester and benzoyl ecgonine

Half-life: 75 minutes

Elimination: Primarily in urine as metabolites and unchanged drug (<10%); cocaine metabolites may appear in the urine of neonates for up to 5 days after birth due to maternal cocaine use shortly before birth

Usual Dosage Topical application (ear, nose, throat, bronchoscopy): Concentrations of 1% to 4% are used; use lowest effective dose; do not exceed 1 mg/kg; patient tolerance, anesthetic technique, vascularity of tissue, and area to be anesthetized will determine dose needed. Solutions >4% are not recommended due to increased risk and severity of systemic toxicities.

Administration Topical: Use only on mucous membranes of the oral, laryngeal, and nasal cavities; do not use on extensive areas of broken skin; do not apply commercially available products to the eye (an extemporaneously prepared ophthalmic product must be made)

Monitoring Parameters Heart rate, blood pressure, respiratory rate, temperature

Additional Information Repeated ophthalmic applications to the eye may cause cornea to become clouded or pitted, therefore, NS should be used to irrigate and protect cornea during surgery; not for injection; cocaine intoxication of infants who are receiving breast milk from their mothers abusing cocaine has been reported

Dosage Forms

Powder, as hydrochloride: 5 g, 25 g

Solution, topical, as hydrochloride: 4% [40 mg/mL] (2 mL, 4 mL, 10 mL); 10% [100 mg/mL] (4 mL, 10 mL)

Solution, topical, viscous, as hydrochloride: 4% [40 mg/mL] (4 mL, 10 mL); 10% [100 mg/mL] (4 mL, 10 mL)

Tablet, soluble, for topical solution, as hydrochloride: 135 mg

References

Chasnoff IJ, Lewis DE, and Squires L, "Cocaine Intoxication in Breast-Fed Infants," *Pediatrics*, 1987, 80(6):836-8.

Greenglass EJ, "The Adverse Effects of Cocaine on the Developing Human," Yaffe SJ and Arana JV, eds, *Pediatric Pharmacology: Therapeutic Principles in Practice*, 2nd ed, Philadelphia, PA: WB Saunders Co, 1992, 598-604.

♦ **Cocaine Hydrochloride** *see* Cocaine *on page 248*

Codeine (KOE deen)

Related Information

Compatibility of Medications Mixed in a Syringe *on page 1208*
Laboratory Detection of Drugs in Urine *on page 1204*
Narcotic Analgesics Comparison *on page 1035*
Overdose and Toxicology *on page 1191*

Brand Names Codeine Conhn® (Canada); Linctus Codeine Blac (Canada); Linctus With Codeine Phosphate (Canada); Paveral Stanley Syrup With Codeine Phosphate (Canada)

Available Salts Codeine Phosphate; Codeine Sulfate

Synonyms Methylmorphine

Therapeutic Category Analgesic, Narcotic; Antitussive; Cough Preparation

Generic Available Yes

Use Treatment of mild to moderate pain; antitussive in lower doses

Restrictions C-II

Pregnancy Risk Factor C (D if used for prolonged periods or in high doses at term)

Contraindications Hypersensitivity to codeine or any component

Warnings Some preparations contain sulfites which may cause allergic reactions

Precautions Use with caution in patients with hypersensitivity reactions to other phenanthrene derivative opioid agonists (morphine, hydrocodone, hydromorphone, levorphanol, oxycodone, oxymorphone); respiratory diseases including: asthma, emphysema, COPD or severe liver or renal insufficiency

Adverse Reactions

Cardiovascular: Palpitations, bradycardia, peripheral vasodilation, hypotension due to vasodilation from histamine release

Central nervous system: CNS depression, increased intracranial pressure, dizziness, drowsiness, sedation

Dermatologic: Pruritus from histamine release

Endocrine & metabolic: Antidiuretic hormone release

Gastrointestinal: Nausea, vomiting, constipation, biliary tract spasm

Genitourinary: Urinary tract spasm

Ocular: Miosis

Respiratory: Respiratory depression

Miscellaneous: Physical and psychological dependence, histamine release

(Continued)

Codeine *(Continued)*

Drug Interactions Cytochrome P-450 isoenzyme CYP2D6 and CYP3A3/4 substrate; isoenzyme CYP2D6 inhibitor

CNS depressants, phenothiazines, tricyclic antidepressants may potentiate the adverse effects of codeine

Mechanism of Action Binds to opiate receptors in the CNS, causing inhibition of ascending pain pathways, altering the perception of and response to pain; causes cough suppression by direct central action in the medulla; produces generalized CNS depression

Pharmacodynamics

Onset:
Oral: 30-60 minutes
I.M.: 10-30 minutes
Peak action:
Oral: 60-90 minutes
I.M.: 30-60 minutes
Duration: 4-6 hours

Pharmacokinetics

Absorption: Oral: Adequate
Distribution: Crosses the placenta; appears in breast milk
Protein binding: 7%
Metabolism: Hepatic to morphine (active); undergoes hydroxylation and O-demethylation via cytochrome P-450 isoenzyme CYP2D6 and demethylation via CYP3A3/4
Half-life: 2.5-3.5 hours
Elimination: 3% to 16% in urine as unchanged drug, norcodeine, and free and conjugated morphine

Usual Dosage Doses should be titrated to appropriate analgesic effect; when changing routes of administration, note that oral dose is $^2/_3$ as effective as parenteral dose

Analgesic: Oral, I.M., S.C.:
Children: 0.5-1 mg/kg/dose every 4-6 hours as needed; maximum dose: 60 mg/dose
Adults: Usual: 30 mg/dose; range: 15-60 mg every 4-6 hours as needed
Antitussive: Oral (for nonproductive cough):
Infants and Children <2 years: Not recommended
Children ≥2 years: 1-1.5 mg/kg/day in divided doses every 4-6 hours as needed:
Alternatively dose according to age:
2-5 years: 2.5-5 mg every 4-6 hours as needed; maximum dose: 30 mg/day
6-12 years: 5-10 mg every 4-6 hours as needed; maximum dose: 60 mg/day
Children >12 years and Adults: 10-20 mg/dose every 4-6 hours as needed; maximum dose: 120 mg/day

Dosing adjustment in renal impairment:
Cl_{cr} 10-50 mL/minute: Administer 75% of dose
Cl_{cr} <10 mL/minute: Administer 50% of dose

Administration

Oral: Administer with food or water to decrease nausea and GI upset
Parenteral: I.M., S.C.: Not intended for I.V. use due to large histamine release and cardiovascular effects

Monitoring Parameters Respiratory rate, heart rate, blood pressure, pain relief

Patient Information Increase fluid and fiber intake to avoid constipation; avoid alcohol; may cause drowsiness and impair ability to perform hazardous duties requiring mental alertness

Nursing Implications Observe patient for excessive sedation and respiratory depression; implement safety measures; may need to assist with ambulation

Additional Information Not recommended for use for cough control in patients with a productive cough; equianalgesic doses: 120 mg codeine phosphate I.M. approximately equals morphine 10 mg I.M.

Dosage Forms

Injection, as phosphate: 30 mg (1 mL, 2 mL); 60 mg (1 mL, 2 mL)
Solution, oral: 15 mg/5 mL
Tablet, as sulfate: 15 mg, 30 mg, 60 mg
Tablet, as phosphate, soluble: 30 mg, 60 mg
Tablet, as sulfate, soluble: 15 mg, 30 mg, 60 mg

♦ **Codeine and Acetaminophen** *see* Acetaminophen and Codeine *on page 27*
♦ **Codeine and Glycerol Guaiacolate** *see* Guaifenesin and Codeine *on page 465*
♦ **Codeine and Guaifenesin** *see* Guaifenesin and Codeine *on page 465*

Colchicine (KOL chi seen)

Therapeutic Category Antigout Agent; Anti-inflammatory Agent

Generic Available Yes

Use Treatment of acute gouty arthritis attacks and prevention of recurrences of such attacks; management of familial Mediterranean fever

Pregnancy Risk Factor D

Contraindications Hypersensitivity to colchicine or any component; severe renal, GI disease, or cardiac disorders

Warnings Patients who become pregnant while receiving colchicine therapy may be at greater risk of producing trisomic offspring

Precautions Modify dosage in patients with renal impairment

Adverse Reactions
Dermatologic: Rash, alopecia
Endocrine & metabolic: Azoospermia, hypothyroidism
Gastrointestinal: Nausea, vomiting, diarrhea, abdominal pain, steatorrhea, paralytic ileus
Hematologic: Agranulocytosis, aplastic anemia
Hepatic: Elevated liver enzymes
Local: Irritation if extravasation occurs
Neuromuscular & skeletal: Myopathy, peripheral neuropathy
Renal: Hematuria, renal damage

Drug Interactions Colchicine may decrease absorption of Vitamin B_{12}

Food Interactions May need low purine diet during acute gouty attack

Stability I.V. colchicine is incompatible with dextrose or I.V. solutions with preservatives; protect from light

Mechanism of Action Decreases leukocyte motility, phagocytosis in joints and lactic acid production, thereby reducing the deposition of urate crystals that perpetuates the inflammatory response; inhibits secretion of serum amyloid A protein

Pharmacodynamics Onset of effect:
Oral: Relief of pain and inflammation occurs after 24-48 hours
I.V.: 6-12 hours

Pharmacokinetics
Distribution: Concentrates in leukocytes, kidney, spleen, and liver; does not distribute in heart, skeletal muscle, and brain
Metabolism: Partially deacetylated in the liver
Half-life, terminal: 9.3-10.6 hours
Time to peak serum concentration: Oral: Within 30-120 minutes then declines for 2 hours before increasing again due to enterohepatic recycling
Elimination: Primarily in the feces via bile; 10% to 20% excreted in urine
Not dialyzable (0% to 5%)

Usual Dosage
Prophylaxis of familial Mediterranean fever: Oral:
Children:
≤5 years: 0.5 mg/day
>5 years: 1-1.5 mg/day in 2-3 divided doses
Adults: 1-2 mg/day in 2-3 divided doses
Gouty arthritis: Acute attacks: Adults:
Oral: Initial: 0.5-1.2 mg, then 0.5-0.6 mg every 1-2 hours or 1-1.2 mg every 2 hours until relief or GI side effects occur to a maximum total dose of 8 mg
I.V.: Initial: 1-3 mg, then 0.5 mg every 6 hours until response, not to exceed 4 mg/day; if pain recurs, it may be necessary to administer a daily dose of 1-2 mg for several days, however, do not give more colchicine by any route for at

(Continued)

Colchicine *(Continued)*

least 7 days after a full course of I.V. therapy (4 mg); transfer to oral colchicine in a dose similar to that being given I.V.

Prophylaxis of recurrent attacks: Oral: 0.5-0.6 mg every day or every other day

Dosing adjustment in renal impairment: Cl_{cr} <10 mL/minute: Decrease dose by 50%

Administration

Oral: Administer with water and maintain adequate fluid intake

Parenteral: Administer I.V. over 2-5 minutes into tubing of free-flowing I.V. with compatible fluid

Monitoring Parameters CBC and renal function test

Test Interactions May cause false-positive results in urine tests for erythrocytes or hemoglobin

Patient Information If taking for acute gouty attacks, discontinue if pain is relieved or if nausea, vomiting or diarrhea occur; avoid alcohol

Nursing Implications Severe local irritation can occur if inadvertently administered S.C. or I.M.; extravasation can cause tissue irritation

Dosage Forms

Injection: 0.5 mg/mL (2 mL)

Tablet: 0.5 mg, 0.6 mg

References

Levy M, Spino M, and Read SE, "Colchicine: A State-of-the-Art Review," *Pharmacotherapy*, 1991, 11(3):196-211.

Majeed HA, Carroll JE, Khuffash FA, et al, "Long-term Colchicine Prophylaxis in Children With Familial Mediterranean Fever (Recurrent Hereditary Polyserositis)," *J Pediatr*, 1990, 116(6):997-9.

♦ **Cold & Allergy® Elixir [OTC]** *see* Brompheniramine and Phenylpropanolamine *on page 143*

♦ **Coldloc®** *see* Guaifenesin, Phenylpropanolamine, and Phenylephrine *on page 467*

Colfosceril *(kole FOS er il)*

Brand Names Exosurf® Neonatal

Available Salts Colfosceril Palmitate

Synonyms Dipalmitoylphosphatidylcholine; DPPC; Synthetic Lung Surfactant

Therapeutic Category Lung Surfactant

Generic Available No

Use Neonatal respiratory distress syndrome (RDS):

Prophylactic therapy: Infants at risk for developing RDS with body weight <1350 g; infants with evidence of pulmonary immaturity with body weight >1350 g

Rescue therapy: Treatment of infants with RDS based on respiratory distress not attributable to any other causes and chest radiographic findings consistent with RDS

Warnings This drug may rapidly affect oxygenation and lung compliance. If chest expansion improves substantially the ventilator peak inspiratory pressure setting should be reduced immediately. Hyperoxia and hypocarbia (hypocarbia can decrease blood flow to the brain) may occur requiring appropriate ventilator adjustments.

Adverse Reactions Respiratory: Pulmonary hemorrhage, apnea, mucous plugging, decrease in transcutaneous O_2 >20%

Stability Reconstituted suspension is stable 12 hours after reconstitution; **do not refrigerate**

Mechanism of Action Replaces deficient or ineffective endogenous lung surfactant in neonates with RDS or in neonates at risk of developing RDS; reduces surface tension and stabilizes the alveoli from collapsing

Pharmacokinetics Absorption: Following intratracheal administration, colfosceril is absorbed from the alveolus; catabolized and reutilized for further synthesis and secretion in lung tissue

Usual Dosage Intratracheal: Neonates:

Prophylactic treatment: Give 5 mL/kg as soon as possible; the second and third doses should be administered at 12 and 24 hours later to those infants remaining on ventilators

Rescue treatment: Give 5 mL/kg as soon as the diagnosis of RDS is made. The second 5 mL/kg dose should be administered 12 hours later

Administration Reconstitute with 8 mL preservative free sterile water for injection; each mL contains 13.5 mg colfosceril; if the suspension appears to separate, gently swirl vial to resuspend contents; do not use if persistent large flakes or particulates appear

Intratracheal: For intratracheal administration only. Suction infant prior to administration; inspect solution to verify complete mixing of the suspension. Administer via sideport on the special endotracheal tube adapter without interrupting mechanical ventilation. Administer the dose in two 2.5 mL/kg aliquots. Each half-dose is instilled slowly over 1-2 minutes in small bursts with each inspiration. After the first 2.5 mL/kg dose turn the infants head and torso 45° right for 30 seconds, then return to the midline position and administer the second dose as above. Following the second dose, turn the infant's head and torso 45° to the left for 30 seconds and return the infant to the midline position.

Monitoring Parameters Continuous EKG and transcutaneous O_2 saturation should be monitored during administration; frequent ABG sampling is necessary to prevent postdosing hyperoxia and hypocarbia.

Dosage Forms Suspension, intratracheal, as palmitate: 108 mg (10 mL)

- **Colfosceril Palmitate** see Colfosceril on page 252
- **Colocort™ Rectal** see Hydrocortisone on page 486
- **Colonic Lavage Solution** see Polyethylene Glycol-Electrolyte Solution on page 782
- **Colovage®** see Polyethylene Glycol-Electrolyte Solution on page 782
- **CoLyte®** see Polyethylene Glycol-Electrolyte Solution on page 782
- **CoLyte®-Flavored** see Polyethylene Glycol-Electrolyte Solution on page 782
- **Comalose-R (Canada)** see Lactulose on page 550
- **Combantrin® (Canada)** see Protirelin on page 821
- **Combivir®** see Lamivudine and Zidovudine on page 553
- **Comfort® Ophthalmic [OTC]** see Naphazoline on page 671
- **Comparison of Adverse Effects of Antidepressants** see page 1030
- **Comparison of Usual Adult Dosage and Mechanism of Action of Antidepressants** see page 1029
- **Compatibility of Medications Mixed in a Syringe** see page 1208
- **Compazine®** see Prochlorperazine on page 803
- **Compound F** see Hydrocortisone on page 486
- **Compound S** see Zidovudine on page 990
- **Compoz® Gel Caps [OTC]** see Diphenhydramine on page 327
- **Compoz® Nighttime Sleep Aid [OTC]** see Diphenhydramine on page 327
- **Congest (Canada)** see Estrogens, Conjugated on page 387
- **Conjugated Estrogens** see Estrogens, Conjugated on page 387
- **Constilac®** see Lactulose on page 550
- **Constulose®** see Lactulose on page 550
- **Contac® Cough Formula Liquid [OTC]** see Guaifenesin and Dextromethorphan on page 466
- **Control® [OTC]** see Phenylpropanolamine on page 761
- **Contuss®** see Guaifenesin, Phenylpropanolamine, and Phenylephrine on page 467
- **Cophene-B®** see Brompheniramine on page 142
- **Copper Sulfate** see Trace Metals on page 940
- **Coptin® (Canada)** see Sulfadiazine on page 889
- **Cordarone®** see Amiodarone on page 63
- **Corgard®** see Nadolol on page 665
- **Corgonject®** see Chorionic Gonadotropin on page 221
- **CortaGel® Topical [OTC]** see Hydrocortisone on page 486
- **Cortaid® Maximum Strength Topical [OTC]** see Hydrocortisone on page 486
- **Cortaid® with Aloe Topical [OTC]** see Hydrocortisone on page 486
- **Cortamed® (Canada)** see Hydrocortisone on page 486
- **Cortate® (Canada)** see Hydrocortisone on page 486
- **Cortatrigen® Otic** see Neomycin, (Bacitracin) Polymyxin B, and Hydrocortisone on page 679
- **Cort-Dome® High Potency Suppository** see Hydrocortisone on page 486
- **Cort-Dome® Topical** see Hydrocortisone on page 486
- **Cortef® Feminine Itch Topical** see Hydrocortisone on page 486
- **Cortef® Oral** see Hydrocortisone on page 486
- **Cortenema® Rectal** see Hydrocortisone on page 486
- **Corticosteroids Comparison, Systemic** see page 1032
- **Corticosteroids Comparison, Topical** see page 1033

Corticotropin (kor ti koe TROE pin)

Related Information
Antiepileptic Drugs *on page 1176*

Brand Names H.P. Acthar® Gel

Synonyms ACTH; Adrenocorticotropic Hormone; Corticotropin, Repository

Therapeutic Category Adrenal Corticosteroid; Diagnostic Agent, Adrenocortical Insufficiency; Infantile Spasms, Treatment

Generic Available Yes

Use Infantile spasms; diagnostic aid in adrenocortical insufficiency; acute exacerbations of multiple sclerosis; severe muscle weakness in myasthenia gravis

Pregnancy Risk Factor C

Contraindications Scleroderma, osteoporosis, systemic fungal infections, ocular herpes simplex, peptic ulcer, hypertension, CHF; hypersensitivity to corticotropin, porcine proteins, or any component

Warnings May mask signs of infection; do not administer live vaccines; long-term therapy in children may retard bone growth; acute adrenal insufficiency may occur with abrupt withdrawal after chronic use or with stress

Precautions Use with caution in patients with hypothyroidism, cirrhosis, thromboembolic disorders, seizure disorders or renal insufficiency

Adverse Reactions
Cardiovascular: Hypertension
Central nervous system: Seizures, mood swings, headache, pseudotumor cerebri
Dermatologic: Skin atrophy, bruising, hyperpigmentation, acne, hirsutism
Endocrine & metabolic: Amenorrhea, sodium and water retention, Cushing's syndrome, hyperglycemia, bone growth suppression, hypokalemia
Gastrointestinal: Abdominal distention, ulcerative esophagitis, pancreatitis
Neuromuscular & skeletal: Muscle wasting
Miscellaneous: Hypersensitivity reactions, including anaphylaxis

Drug Interactions NSAIDs (increase risk of ulcers, increase clearance of NSAIDs), loop diuretics, thiazide diuretics, amphotericin B (increases potassium wasting), antidiabetic agents (may require increased doses due to hyperglycemic activity of adrenal glucocorticoids), live virus vaccines (increase risk of viral infection), vaccines may have decreased effect

Food Interactions May increase renal loss of potassium, calcium, zinc, and vitamin C; may need to increase dietary intake or give supplements

Stability Store repository injection (gel) in the refrigerator; warm gel before administration

Mechanism of Action Stimulates the adrenal cortex to secrete adrenal steroids (including hydrocortisone, cortisone), androgenic substances, and a small amount of aldosterone. Exact mechanism of action for treatment of infantile spasms is unknown, but may be an independent antiepileptic effect (unrelated to stimulation of release of adrenocorticosteroids). One theory is that ACTH suppresses corticotropin-releasing hormone (CRH). CRH is an excitatory neuropeptide that has a greater potency in infants. Infants with infantile spasms may have increased CRH activity. ACTH may decrease CRH release and, therefore, decrease infantile spasms.

Pharmacodynamics
Peak effect on cortisol levels: I.M., S.C. (gel): 3-12 hours
Duration: Repository (gel): 10-25 hours, up to 3 days

Pharmacokinetics
Absorption: I.M. (repository): Over 8-16 hours
Half-life: 15 minutes
Elimination: In urine

Usual Dosage
Children: I.M.: Gel (repository) formulation:
Anti-inflammatory/immunosuppressant: 0.8 units/kg/day or 25 units/m^2/day divided every 12-24 hours
Infantile spasms: Various regimens have been used. Some neurologists recommend low-dose ACTH (5-40 units/day) for short periods (1-6 weeks), while others recommend larger doses of ACTH (40-160 units/day) for long periods of treatment (3-12 months)
A prospective, single-blind study (Hrachovy, 1994) found no major difference in effectiveness between high-dose long-duration versus low-dose short-duration ACTH therapy. Hypertension, however, occurred more frequently in

the high-dose group. Further studies comparing long-term outcomes are needed. Low-dose regimen used in this study:

Initial: 20 units/day for 2 weeks, if patient responds, taper and discontinue over a 1-week period; if patient does not respond, increase dose to 30 units/day for 4 weeks then taper and discontinue over a 1-week period

Usual dose: 20-40 units/day or 5-8 units/kg/day in 1-2 divided doses; range: 5-160 units/day

Adults: I.M.: Gel (repository) formulation:

Acute exacerbation of multiple sclerosis: 80-120 units/day in divided doses for 2-3 weeks

Diagnostic purposes: 25 units

Anti-inflammatory/immunosuppressant: 40-80 units every 24-72 hours

Administration Parenteral: Gel should be administered I.M. only

Monitoring Parameters Electrolytes, glucose, blood pressure, height, and weight; for infantile spasms, monitor seizure frequency, type, and duration

Test Interactions Skin tests

Patient Information Do not abruptly discontinue the medication; tell your physician you are using this drug if you are going to have skin tests, immunizations, surgery, emergency treatment, or if you have a serious infection or injury

Additional Information Cosyntropin is preferred over corticotropin for diagnostic test of adrenocortical insufficiency (cosyntropin is less allergenic and test is shorter in duration); oral prednisone (2 mg/kg/day) was as effective as I.M. ACTH gel (20 units/day) in controlling infantile spasms; corticotropin zinc hydroxide (Cortrophin® Zinc) and corticotropin aqueous (Acthar®) have been discontinued by the manufacturer

Dosage Forms Injection, repository (H.P. Acthar® Gel): 40 units/mL (1 mL, 5 mL); 80 units/mL (1 mL, 5 mL)

References

Haines ST and Casto DT, "Treatment of Infantile Spasms," Ann Pharmacother, 1994, 28(6):779-91.
Hrachovy RA and Frost JD Jr, "Infantile Spasms," Pediatr Clin North Am, 1989, 36(2):311-29.
Hrachovy RA, Frost JD Jr, and Glaze DG, "High-Dose, Long-Duration Versus Low-Dose, Short-Duration Corticotropin Therapy for Infantile Spasms," J Pediatr, 1994, 124(5 Pt 1):803-6.
Hrachovy RA, Frost JD Jr, Kellaway P, et al, "Double-Blind Study of ACTH vs Prednisone Therapy in Infantile Spasms," J Pediatr, 1983, 103(4):641-5.

♦ **Corticotropin, Repository** see Corticotropin on page 254
♦ **Corticreme® (Canada)** see Hydrocortisone on page 486
♦ **Cortifoam® Rectal** see Hydrocortisone on page 486
♦ **Cortiment® (Canada)** see Hydrocortisone on page 486
♦ **Cortisol** see Hydrocortisone on page 486

Cortisone (KOR ti sone)

Related Information

Corticosteroids Comparison, Systemic on page 1032

Brand Names Cortone® Acetate

Available Salts Cortisone Acetate

Therapeutic Category Adrenal Corticosteroid; Anti-inflammatory Agent; Corticosteroid, Systemic; Glucocorticoid

Generic Available Yes

Use Management of adrenocortical insufficiency

Pregnancy Risk Factor D

Contraindications Serious infections, except septic shock or tuberculous meningitis; hypersensitivity to corticosteroids; systemic fungal or viral infections

Warnings May retard bone growth; acute adrenal insufficiency may occur with abrupt withdrawal after long-term therapy or with stress

Precautions Use with caution in patients with hypothyroidism, cirrhosis, hypertension, CHF, ulcerative colitis, thromboembolic disorders, osteoporosis, peptic ulcer, diabetes mellitus, seizure disorders

Adverse Reactions

Cardiovascular: Edema, hypertension

Central nervous system: Vertigo, seizures, headache, psychoses, pseudotumor cerebri

Dermatologic: Acne, skin atrophy

Endocrine & metabolic: Cushing's syndrome, pituitary-adrenal axis suppression, growth suppression, glucose intolerance, hypokalemia, alkalosis

Gastrointestinal: Peptic ulcer, nausea, vomiting

Neuromuscular & skeletal: Muscle weakness, osteoporosis, fractures

Ocular: Cataracts, glaucoma

Drug Interactions Cytochrome P-450 isoenzyme CYP3A3/4 substrate

(Continued)

Cortisone *(Continued)*

Barbiturates, phenytoin, rifampin, salicylates, estrogens, NSAID, diuretics (potassium depleting), anticholinesterase agents, warfarin; caffeine and alcohol may increase risk for GI ulcer; live virus vaccines (increase risk of viral infection); vaccines may have decreased effects

Food Interactions Systemic use of corticosteroids may require a diet with increased potassium, vitamins A, B_6, C, D, folate, calcium, zinc, phosphorus, and decreased sodium

Mechanism of Action Controls the rate of protein synthesis, depresses the migration of polymorphonuclear leukocytes and fibroblasts, reverses capillary permeability, and stabilizes lysosomal membranes at the cellular level to prevent or control inflammation

Pharmacodynamics
Peak effect:
Oral: Within 2 hours
I.M.: Within 20-48 hours
Duration: 30-36 hours

Pharmacokinetics
Absorption: I.M.: Slow rate of absorption, over 24-48 hours
Distribution: Crosses the placenta; appears in breast milk; distributes to muscles, liver, skin, intestines, and kidneys
Metabolism: In the liver to inactive metabolites
Half-life: 30 minutes
Elimination: In bile and urine

Usual Dosage Depends upon the condition being treated and the response of the patient. Supplemental doses may be warranted during times of stress in the course of withdrawing therapy.

Children:
Anti-inflammatory or immunosuppressive:
Oral: 2.5-10 mg/kg/day or 20-300 mg/m²/day in divided doses every 6-8 hours
I.M.: 1-5 mg/kg/day or 14-375 mg/m²/day in divided doses every 12-24 hours
Physiologic replacement:
Oral: 0.5-0.75 mg/kg/day or 20-25 mg/m²/day in divided doses every 8 hours
I.M.: 0.25-0.35 mg/kg/day or 12.5 mg/m²/day once daily
Stress coverage for surgery: I.M.: 1 and 2 days before preanesthesia, and 1-3 days after surgery: 50-62.5 mg/m²/day; 4 days after surgery: 31-50 mg/m²/day; 5 days after surgery, resume presurgical corticosteroid dose
Adults: Oral, I.M.: 20-300 mg/day divided every 12-24 hours

Administration
Oral: Administer with meals, food, or milk to decrease GI effects
Parenteral: Injection is for I.M. use only; do not administer I.V.; administer I.M. daily dose before 9 AM to minimize adrenocortical suppression; shake vial before withdrawing I.M. dose

Monitoring Parameters Long-term use: Electrolytes, glucose, blood pressure, height, weight

Test Interactions Skin tests

Patient Information Do not discontinue or reduce dose without physician's approval; limit caffeine; avoid alcohol

Nursing Implications Taper dose gradually with long-term use

Additional Information Insoluble in water

Dosage Forms
Injection, as acetate: 50 mg/mL (10 mL)
Tablet, as acetate: 5 mg, 10 mg, 25 mg

♦ **Cortisone Acetate** *see* Cortisone *on page 255*
♦ **Cortisporin® Ophthalmic Suspension** *see* Neomycin, (Bacitracin) Polymyxin B, and Hydrocortisone *on page 679*
♦ **Cortisporin® Otic** *see* Neomycin, (Bacitracin) Polymyxin B, and Hydrocortisone *on page 679*
♦ **Cortisporin® Topical Cream** *see* Neomycin, (Bacitracin) Polymyxin B, and Hydrocortisone *on page 679*
♦ **Cortizone®-5 Topical [OTC]** *see* Hydrocortisone *on page 486*
♦ **Cortizone®-10 Topical [OTC]** *see* Hydrocortisone *on page 486*
♦ **Cortoderm (Canada)** *see* Hydrocortisone *on page 486*
♦ **Cortone® Acetate** *see* Cortisone *on page 255*
♦ **Cortrosyn®** *see* Cosyntropin *on page 257*
♦ **Cosmegen®** *see* Dactinomycin *on page 281*

Cosyntropin (koe sin TROE pin)

Brand Names Cortrosyn®; Synacthen® Depot (Canada)

Synonyms Synacthen; Tetracosactide

Therapeutic Category Adrenal Corticosteroid; Diagnostic Agent, Adrenocortical Insufficiency

Generic Available No

Use Diagnostic test to differentiate primary adrenal from secondary (pituitary) adrenocortical insufficiency

Pregnancy Risk Factor C

Contraindications Hypersensitivity to cosyntropin or any component

Precautions Use with caution in patients with pre-existing allergic disease or a history of allergic reactions to corticotropin

Adverse Reactions

Dermatologic: Pruritus, flushing

Endocrine & metabolic: Decreased carbohydrate tolerance; increased requirements for insulin or oral hypoglycemic agents in diabetics; activation of latent diabetes mellitus

Miscellaneous: Hypersensitivity reactions, including anaphylaxis

Drug Interactions Cortisone, hydrocortisone, estrogens, spironolactone

Stability Reconstituted solution is stable for 24 hours at room temperature and 21 days when refrigerated; for I.V. infusion in NS or D_5W, solution is stable for 12 hours at room temperature

Mechanism of Action Stimulates the adrenal cortex to secrete adrenal steroids (including hydrocortisone, cortisone), androgenic substances, and a small amount of aldosterone

Pharmacodynamics I.M., I.V.:

Onset of action: Plasma cortisol levels rise in healthy individuals in 5 minutes

Peak levels: Within 45-60 minutes

Pharmacokinetics Metabolism: Unknown

Usual Dosage Diagnostic test doses:

Adrenocortical insufficiency: I.M., I.V.:

Preterm neonates: Dose not well defined (see Additional Information)

Neonates: 0.015 mg/kg/dose

Children <2 years: 0.125 mg

Children >2 years and Adults: 0.25 mg

When greater cortisol stimulation is needed, an I.V. infusion may be used:

Children >2 years and Adults: 0.25 mg administered over 4-8 hours (usually 6 hours)

Congenital adrenal hyperplasia evaluation: 1 mg/m²/dose up to a maximum of 1 mg

Administration Parenteral: Administer I.V. push doses over 2 minutes; for I.V. infusion, may dilute with D_5W or NS

Reference Range Plasma cortisol concentrations should be measured immediately before and exactly 30 minutes after the dose; dose should be given in the early morning; normal morning baseline cortisol >5 µg/dL (SI: >138 nmol/L); normal response 30 minutes after cosyntropin injection: an increase in serum cortisol concentration of ≥7 µg/dL (SI: ≥193 nmol/L) or peak response >18 µg/dL (SI: >497 nmol/L).

Nursing Implications Patient should not receive corticosteroids or spironolactone the day prior to and the day of the test

Additional Information Each 0.25 mg of cosyntropin is equivalent to 25 units of corticotropin; Korte 1996 used physiologic doses of cosyntropin (0.1 mcg/kg) to test adrenal function in VLBW infants [mean weight 900 g; mean gestational age 27 weeks (range: 23-32 weeks)]; only 36% of infants responded; increasing the dose to 0.2 mcg/kg resulted in 67% of the infants responding, but sensitivity of the test was decreased. Cole 1999 used cosyntropin doses of 3.5 mcg/kg to test adrenal function in 44 preterm infants [mean birthweight 823 g; mean gestational age 26.2 weeks; mean postmenstrual age 30.1 weeks] during inhaled beclomethasone therapy.

Dosage Forms Powder for injection: 0.25 mg

References

Cole CH, Shah B, Abbasi S, et al, "Adrenal Function in Premature Infants During Inhaled Beclomethasone Therapy," *J Pediatr*, 1999, 135(1):65-70.

Korte C, Styne D, Merritt TA, et al, "Adrenocortical Function in the Very Low Birth Weight Infant: Improved Testing Sensitivity and Association With Neonatal Outcome," *J Pediatr*, 1996, 128(2):257-63.

♦ **Cotazym®** *see* Pancrelipase *on page 724*

♦ **Cotazym-S®** *see* Pancrelipase *on page 724*

♦ **Cotrim®** see Co-Trimoxazole on page 258
♦ **Cotrim® DS** see Co-Trimoxazole on page 258

Co-Trimoxazole (koe trye MOKS a zole)

Related Information

Carbohydrate and Alcohol Content of Liquid Medications for Use in Patients Receiving Ketogenic Diets on page 1228

Brand Names Apo®-Sulfatrim (Canada); Bactrim™; Bactrim™ DS; Cotrim®; Cotrim® DS; Novo-Trimel® (Canada); Nu-Cotrimox® (Canada); Pro-Trin® (Canada); Roubac® (Canada); Septra®; Septra® DS; Sulfamethoprim®; Sulfatrim®; Sulfatrim® DS; Trisulfa® (Canada); Trisulfa-S® (Canada); Uroplus® DS; Uroplus® SS

Synonyms SMX-TMP; Sulfamethoxazole and Trimethoprim; TMP-SMX; Trimethoprim and Sulfamethoxazole

Therapeutic Category Antibiotic, Sulfonamide Derivative

Generic Available Yes

Use Treatment of urinary tract infections caused by susceptible E. coli, Klebsiella, Enterobacter, Proteus mirabilis, Proteus (indole positive); acute otitis media due to amoxicillin-resistant H. influenzae, S. pneumoniae, and M. catarrhalis; acute exacerbations of chronic bronchitis; prophylaxis and treatment of Pneumocystis carinii pneumonitis (PCP); treatment of susceptible shigellosis, typhoid fever, Nocardia asteroides infection, and Xanthomonas maltophilia infection; the I.V. preparation is used for treatment of Pneumocystis carinii pneumonitis, Shigella, and severe urinary tract infections

Pregnancy Risk Factor C

Contraindications Hypersensitivity to any sulfa drug or any component; porphyria; megaloblastic anemia due to folate deficiency; infants <2 months of age (for exception, see Additional Information)

Warnings Fatalities associated with sulfonamides, although rare, have occurred due to severe reactions including Stevens-Johnson syndrome, toxic epidermal necrolysis, hepatic necrosis, agranulocytosis, aplastic anemia, and other blood dyscrasias; discontinue use at first sign of rash or any sign of adverse reaction; injectable formulation contains benzyl alcohol, propylene glycol, and sodium metabisulfite; metabisulfites may cause allergic type reactions in susceptible patients

Precautions Use with caution in patients with G-6-PD deficiency, impaired renal or hepatic function; adjust dosage in patients with renal impairment

Adverse Reactions

Central nervous system: Confusion, depression, hallucinations, seizures, fever, ataxia, kernicterus in neonates, aseptic meningitis

Dermatologic: Rash (more common in patients taking large dosages or in patients with AIDS), erythema multiforme, epidermal necrolysis, Stevens-Johnson syndrome

Endocrine & metabolic: Hyperkalemia

Gastrointestinal: Nausea, vomiting, glossitis, stomatitis, diarrhea, pseudomembranous colitis, pancreatitis, splenomegaly

Hematologic: Thrombocytopenia, megaloblastic anemia, granulocytopenia, aplastic anemia, hemolysis (with G-6-PD deficiency)

Hepatic: Hepatitis, cholestatic jaundice

Local: Local irritation, pain, phlebitis

Renal: Interstitial nephritis, renal tubular acidosis

Miscellaneous: Serum sickness

Drug Interactions Co-trimoxazole decreases the clearance of warfarin; methotrexate (displaced from protein binding sites); increases the effect of sulfonylureas, phenytoin, and thiopental; decreases serum cyclosporine concentrations

Stability Do not refrigerate concentrate for injection; for I.V. administration, a 1:25 dilution is stable for 48 hours in D_5W or NS; 1:20 dilution is stable for 24 hours in D_5W or 14 hours in NS; 1:15 dilution is stable for 4 hours in D_5W or 2 hours in NS; 1:10 dilution is stable for 1 hour in D_5W or NS; do not mix with other drugs or solutions

Mechanism of Action Sulfamethoxazole interferes with bacterial folic acid synthesis and growth via inhibition of dihydrofolic acid formation from para-aminobenzoic acid; trimethoprim inhibits dihydrofolic acid reduction to tetrahydrofolate resulting in sequential inhibition of enzymes of the folic acid pathway

Pharmacokinetics

Absorption: Oral: Almost completely (90% to 100%)

Distribution: Crosses the placenta; distributes into breast milk, joint fluid, sputum, middle ear fluid, bile, and CSF

Protein binding:
TMP: 45%

SMX: 68%
Metabolism:
TMP: Metabolized to oxide and hydroxylated metabolites
SMX: N-acetylated and glucuronidated
Half-life:
TMP: 6-11 hours, prolonged in renal failure
SMX: 9-12 hours, prolonged in renal failure
Time to peak serum concentration: Oral: Within 1-4 hours
Elimination: Both excreted in urine as metabolites and unchanged drug

Usual Dosage Oral, I.V. **(dosage recommendations are based on the trimethoprim (TMP) component):**

Children >2 months and Adults:
Mild-moderate infections: 6-12 mg TMP/kg/day in divided doses every 12 hours
Serious infection/*Pneumocystis*: 15-20 mg TMP/kg/day in divided doses every 6-8 hours
Prophylaxis of *Pneumocystis* (see Note in Additional Information): 150 mg TMP/m^2/day in divided doses every 12 hours 3 days/week on consecutive days; acceptable alternative dosage schedules include 150 mg TMP/m^2/day as a single daily dose 3 times/week on consecutive days or 150 mg TMP/m^2/day in divided doses every 12 hours administered 7 days/week, or 150 mg TMP/m^2/day in divided doses every 12 hours administered 3 times/week on alternate days; dose should not exceed 320 mg trimethoprim and 1600 mg sulfamethoxazole/day
Urinary tract infection prophylaxis: 2 mg TMP/kg/dose daily or 5 mg TMP/kg/dose twice weekly

Adults:
Urinary tract infection/chronic bronchitis: 1 double strength tablet every 12 hours for 10-14 days
Prophylaxis of *Pneumocystis*: One double-strength tablet daily or an acceptable alternative is 1 single-strength tablet daily

Dosing adjustment in renal impairment (frequency may need to be adjusted):
Cl_{cr} 15-30 mL/minute: Reduce dose by 50%
Cl_{cr} <15 mL/minute: Not recommended

Administration
Oral: May administer with water on an empty stomach; shake suspension well before use
Parenteral: Infuse I.V. co-trimoxazole over 60-90 minutes; must be further diluted 1:25 (5 mL drug to 125 mL diluent, ie, D_5W); in patients who require fluid restriction, a 1:15 dilution (5 mL drug to 75 mL diluent, ie, D_5W) or a 1:10 dilution (5 mL drug to 50 mL diluent, ie, D_5W) may be administered; see Stability

Monitoring Parameters CBC, renal function test, liver function test, urinalysis; observe for change in bowel frequency

Patient Information Maintain adequate fluid intake

Additional Information Note: Guidelines for prophylaxis of *Pneumocystis carinii* pneumonia: Initiate PCP prophylaxis in the following patients: Children born to HIV-infected mothers should be given prophylaxis with TMP/SMZ beginning at 4-6 weeks of age and continue through the first year of life or until HIV infection has been reasonably excluded; children 1-5 years of age with CD4+ count <500 or CD4+ percentage <15%; children 6-12 years of age with CD4+ count <200 or CD4+ percentage <15%; adolescents and adults with CD4+ count <200 or oropharyngeal candidiasis. Folinic acid should be given if bone marrow suppression occurs.

Dosage Forms The 5:1 ratio (SMX to TMP) remains constant in all dosage forms:
Injection: Sulfamethoxazole 80 mg and trimethoprim 16 mg per mL (5 mL, 10 mL, 20 mL, 30 mL, 50 mL)
Suspension, oral: Sulfamethoxazole 200 mg and trimethoprim 40 mg per 5 mL (20 mL, 100 mL, 150 mL, 200 mL, 480 mL)
Tablet: Sulfamethoxazole 400 mg and trimethoprim 80 mg
Tablet, double strength: Sulfamethoxazole 800 mg and trimethoprim 160 mg

References
Jarosinki PF, Kennedy PE, and Gallelli JF, "Stability of Concentrated Trimethoprim-Sulfamethoxazole Admixtures," *AJHP*, 1989, 46(4):732-7.
Hughes WT, "*Pneumocystis carinii* Pneumonia: New Approaches to Diagnosis, Treatment, and Prevention," *Pediatr Infect Dis J*, 1991, 10(5):391-9.
"1999 USPHS/IDSA Guidelines for the Prevention of Opportunistic Infections in Persons Infected With Human Immunodeficiency Virus. USPHS/IDSA Prevention of Opportunistic Infections Working Group," *MMWR Morb Mortal Wkly Rep*, 1999, 48(RR-10):1-66.

♦ **Coumadin®** *see* Warfarin *on page 984*
♦ **Covera-HS®** *see* Verapamil *on page 974*

♦ **CPI® [OTC]** *see* Hemorrhoidal Preparations *on page 470*
♦ **CPM** *see* Cyclophosphamide *on page 268*
♦ **CPR Pediatric Drug Dosages** *see page 999*
♦ **Creon®** *see* Pancreatin *on page 723*
♦ **Creon® 10** *see* Pancrelipase *on page 724*
♦ **Creon® 20** *see* Pancrelipase *on page 724*
♦ **Creo-Terpin® [OTC]** *see* Dextromethorphan *on page 304*
♦ **Crixivan®** *see* Indinavir *on page 514*
♦ **Crolom®** *see* Cromolyn *on page 260*
♦ **Cromoglycic Acid** *see* Cromolyn *on page 260*

Cromolyn (KROE moe lin)

Related Information
Asthma Guidelines *on page 1178*

Brand Names Crolom®; Gastrocrom®; Intal®; Nasalcrom® [OTC]; Novo-Cromolyn® (Canada); Opticrom®; Opticrom® (Canada); PMS-Sodium Cromoglycate (Canada); Rynacrom® (Canada)

Available Salts Cromolyn Sodium

Synonyms Cromoglycic Acid; Disodium Cromoglycate; DSCG

Therapeutic Category Antiasthmatic; Inhalation, Miscellaneous

Generic Available Yes

Use
Oral inhalation and nebulization: Prophylactic agent used for long-term (chronic) control of persistent asthma; NOT indicated for the relief of acute bronchospasm; also used for the prevention of allergen- or exercise-induced bronchospasm

Intranasal: Management of seasonal or perennial allergic rhinitis

Ophthalmologic: Vernal conjunctivitis, vernal keratoconjunctivitis, and vernal keratitis

Systemic: Mastocytosis, food allergy, and treatment of inflammatory bowel disease

Pregnancy Risk Factor B

Contraindications Hypersensitivity to cromolyn or any component; primary treatment of status asthmaticus

Warnings Cromolyn is a prophylactic drug with no benefit for acute situations; rare but severe anaphylactic reactions can occur; discontinue if eosinophilic pneumonia occurs

Precautions Use with caution and decrease dose in patients with renal and hepatic impairment; use inhalation aerosol with caution in patients with coronary artery disease or history of cardiac arrhythmias (due to propellants); use with caution when tapering the dose or withdrawing the drug since symptoms may reoccur; patients should not wear contact lenses during treatment with ophthalmic solution

Adverse Reactions
Central nervous system: Dizziness, headache

Dermatologic: Rash, urticaria, angioedema

Gastrointestinal: Nausea, vomiting, diarrhea, xerostomia, unpleasant taste (inhalation aerosol)

Local: Nasal burning

Neuromuscular & skeletal: Arthralgia

Ocular (topical): Ocular stinging, lacrimation

Respiratory: Coughing, wheezing, sneezing, nasal congestion, throat irritation, eosinophilic pneumonia, pulmonary infiltrates, hoarseness

Stability Protect from direct light and heat; nebulization solution is compatible with beta agonists, anticholinergic solutions, acetylcysteine and NS; incompatible with alkaline solutions, calcium and magnesium salts; store oral concentrate ampuls in foil pouch until ready for use

Mechanism of Action Prevents the mast cell release of histamine, leukotrienes and slow-reacting substance of anaphylaxis by inhibiting degranulation after contact with antigens

Pharmacodynamics Not effective for immediate relief of symptoms in acute asthmatic attacks; must be used at regular intervals for 2-4 weeks to be effective

Pharmacokinetics
Absorption:
Oral: 0.5% to 2%
Inhalation: ~8% of dose reaches the lungs upon inhalation of the powder and is well absorbed

Half-life: 80-90 minutes

Time to peak serum concentration: Within 15 minutes after inhalation

Elimination: Equally excreted unchanged in urine and feces (via bile); small amounts after inhalation are exhaled

Usual Dosage

Inhalation:

For chronic control of asthma, taper frequency to the lowest effective dose (ie, 4 times/day to 3 times/day to twice daily):

Nebulization solution: Children >2 years and Adults: Initial: 20 mg 4 times/day; usual dose: 20 mg 3-4 times/day

Metered spray:

Children 5-12 years: Initial: 2 inhalations 4 times/day; usual dose: 1-2 inhalations 3-4 times/day

Children ≥12 years and Adults: Initial: 2 inhalations 4 times/day; usual dose: 2-4 inhalations 3-4 times/day

Prevention of allergen- or exercise-induced bronchospasm: Administer 10-15 minutes prior to exercise or allergen exposure but no longer than 1 hour before:

Nebulization solution: Children >2 years and Adults: Single dose of 20 mg

Metered spray: Children >5 years and Adults: Single dose of 2 inhalations

Intranasal: Children ≥6 years and Adults: 1 spray in each nostril 3-6 times/day

Ophthalmic: Children >4 years and Adults: Instill 1-2 drops 4-6 times/day

Oral:

Systemic mastocytosis:

Neonates and Preterm Infants: Not recommended

Infants and Children <2 years: 20 mg/kg/day in 4 divided doses; may increase in patients 6 months to 2 years of age if benefits not seen after 2-3 weeks; do not exceed 30 mg/kg/day

Children 2-12 years: 100 mg 4 times/day; not to exceed 40 mg/kg/day

Children >12 years and Adults: 200 mg 4 times/day

Food allergy and inflammatory bowel disease:

Children <2 years: Not recommended

Children 2-12 years: Initial dose: 100 mg 4 times/day; may double the dose if effect is not satisfactory within 2-3 weeks; not to exceed 40 mg/kg/day

Children >12 years and Adults: Initial dose: 200 mg 4 times/day; may double the dose if effect is not satisfactory within 2-3 weeks; up to 400 mg 4 times/day

Once desired effect is achieved, dose may be tapered to lowest effective dose

Administration

Oral concentrate: Open ampul and squeeze contents into glass of water; stir well; administer at least 30 minutes before meals and at bedtime; do not mix with juice, milk, or food

Oral inhalation: Shake canister gently before use; do not immerse canister in water

Nasal inhalation: Clear nasal passages by blowing nose prior to use

Monitoring Parameters Asthma: Periodic pulmonary function tests; signs and symptoms of disease state when tapering dose

Additional Information Reserve systemic use in children <2 years of age for severe disease; avoid systemic use in premature infants; inhalation aerosol contains fluorocarbon propellants

Dosage Forms

Inhalation, as sodium, oral (Intal®): 800 mcg/spray [112 metered inhalations (56 doses)[(8.1 g); [200 metered inhalation (100 doses)] (14.2 g)

Oral concentrate, as sodium, (Gastrocrom®): 100 mg/5 mL ampul

Solution, as sodium, for nebulization (Intal®): 10 mg/mL (2 mL)

Solution, as sodium, nasal (Nasalcrom® [OTC]): 40 mg/mL (13 mL)

Solution, as sodium, ophthalmic:

Crolom®: 4% (2.5 mL, 10 mL)

Opticrom®: 4% (10 mL)

References

Expert Panel Report 2, "Guidelines for the Diagnosis and Management of Asthma," *Clinical Practice Guidelines*, National Institutes of Health, National Heart, Lung, and Blood Institute, NIH Publication No. 94-4051, April, 1997.

♦ **Cromolyn Sodium** *see* Cromolyn *on page 260*

♦ **Crotaline Antivenin, Polyvalent** *see* Antivenin (*Crotalidae*) Polyvalent *on page 91*

Crotamiton (kroe TAM i tonn)

Brand Names Eurax®

Therapeutic Category Scabicidal Agent

Generic Available No

Use Treatment of scabies (*Sarcoptes scabiei*) in infants and children

(Continued)

Crotamiton *(Continued)*

Pregnancy Risk Factor C

Contraindications Hypersensitivity to crotamiton or any component; patients who manifest a primary irritation response to topical medications

Precautions Avoid contact with face, eyes, mucous membranes, and urethral meatus; do not apply to acutely inflamed or raw skin

Adverse Reactions
Dermatologic: Pruritus, contact dermatitis
Local: Irritation

Mechanism of Action Mechanism for scabicidal activity is unknown

Usual Dosage Scabicide: Topical: Infants, Children, and Adults: Apply over entire body below the head; apply once daily for 2 days followed by a cleansing bath 48 hours after the last application; treatment may be repeated after 7-10 days if mites appear

Administration Topical: Wash thoroughly and scrub away loose scales, then towel dry; apply a thin layer and gently massage drug onto skin of the entire body from the neck to the toes (with special attention to skin folds, creases, and interdigital spaces); since scabies can affect the head, scalp, and neck in infants and young children, apply to head, neck, and body of this age group; do not apply to the face, eyes, mouth, mucous membranes, or urethral meatus; shake lotion well before use

Patient Information For topical use only; all contaminated clothing and bed linen should be washed to avoid reinfestation

Additional Information Treatment may be repeated after 7-10 days if live mites are still present

Dosage Forms
Cream: 10% (60 g)
Lotion: 10% (60 mL, 480 mL)

References
Eichenfield LF, Honig PJ, "Blistering Disorders in Childhood," *Pediatr Clin North Am*, 1991, 38(4):959-76.

Hogan DJ, Schachner L, Tanglertsampan C, "Diagnosis and Treatment of Childhood Scabies and Pediculosis," *Pediatr Clin North Am*, 1991, 38(4):941-57.

♦ **Cruex® Topical [OTC]** *see* Undecylenic Acid and Derivatives *on page 962*
♦ **Crystalline Penicillin** *see* Penicillin G, Parenteral, Aqueous *on page 741*
♦ **Crystal Violet** *see* Gentian Violet *on page 455*
♦ **Crystamine®** *see* Cyanocobalamin *on page 263*
♦ **Crysticillin® A.S.** *see* Penicillin G Procaine *on page 742*
♦ **CsA** *see* Cyclosporine *on page 270*
♦ **C-Solve-2®** *see* Erythromycin *on page 379*
♦ **CTX** *see* Cyclophosphamide *on page 268*
♦ **Cupric Chloride** *see* Trace Metals *on page 940*
♦ **Cuprimine®** *see* Penicillamine *on page 738*
♦ **Curosurf®** *see* Poractant Alfa *on page 784*
♦ **Curretab® Oral** *see* Medroxyprogesterone *on page 599*
♦ **Cutivate®** *see* Fluticasone *on page 436*
♦ **CyA** *see* Cyclosporine *on page 270*

Cyanide Antidote Kit *(SYE a nide AN tee dote kit)*

Available Salts Sodium Thiosulfate, Sodium Nitrite, and Amyl Nitrite

Therapeutic Category Antidote, Cyanide

Generic Available Yes

Use Treatment agents for cyanide poisoning

Pregnancy Risk Factor Sodium thiosulfate and sodium nitrite: C; amyl nitrite: X

Contraindications Hypersensitivity to amyl nitrite, sodium nitrite, sodium thiosulfate, or any component

Warnings Excessive methemoglobin results when sodium nitrite dosage is exceeded; use only enough sodium nitrite to achieve a satisfactory clinical response; avoid methemoglobin levels >30%; patients with malignancy and G6PD deficiency have increased sensitivity to the methemoglobin-generating activities of sodium nitrite

Precautions When cyanide poisoning is related to smoke inhalation, if possible, the patient should be at pressure in a hyperbaric chamber before the kit is administered; the methemoglobin initially produced by sodium nitrite injection may otherwise exacerbate concomitant carbon monoxide poisoning that has already severely diminished oxygen-carrying capacity in red cells

Adverse Reactions Reactions listed are those of sodium nitrite; see individual monographs for Amyl Nitrite *on page 84* and Sodium Thiosulfate *on page 875*:
Cardiovascular: Tachycardia, syncope, cyanosis, hypotension (associated with rapid infusion), flushing
Central nervous system: Dizziness, headache
Gastrointestinal: Nausea, vomiting
Miscellaneous: Methemoglobin formation

Drug Interactions Sodium nitrite antagonizes acetylcholine, epinephrine, and histamine effects; sodium nitrite potentiates hypotensive effects and/or anticholinergic effects of tricyclic antidepressants, antihistamines, and meperidine and related CNS depressants; also see Amyl Nitrite *on page 84*

Stability Sodium nitrite is stable at room temperature; do not mix with other medications; see individual monographs Amyl Nitrite *on page 84* and Sodium Thiosulfate *on page 875*

Mechanism of Action Amyl nitrite and sodium nitrite promote the formation of methemoglobin which binds with cyanide to form cyanomethemoglobin (nontoxic); sodium thiosulfate, by providing an extra sulfur group to the enzyme rhodanese, increases the rate of detoxification of cyanide

Usual Dosage Administer in sequential order:
Amyl nitrite: Infants, Children, and Adults: Inhale vapors from 1 ampul continuously for 15-30 seconds, followed by a rest for 15 seconds (this interrupted schedule is important because continuous use of amyl nitrite may prevent adequate oxygenation); reapply until sodium nitrite can be administered
Sodium nitrite: I.V.:
Infants and Children: 6-8 mL/m^2 (~0.2 mL/kg); maximum: 10 mL; follow immediately with sodium thiosulfate
or as an alternative:
<25 kg: 4.5-10 mg/kg
>25 kg: 300 mg
Follow immediately with sodium thiosulfate
Adolescents and Adults: 300 mg; follow immediately with sodium thiosulfate
Sodium thiosulfate: I.V.:
Infants and Children: 7 mg/m^2; maximum: 12.5 g
or as an alternative:
<25 kg: 50 mg/kg
>25 kg: 12.5 g
Adolescents and Adults: 12.5 g
Patients should be watched for at least 24-48 hours; if signs of poisoning reappear, injection of both sodium nitrite and sodium thiosulfate should be repeated, but each in $^1/_2$ of the original dose; even if the patient is asymptomatic, repeat $^1/_2$ doses of both sodium nitrite and sodium thiosulfate may be given for prophylactic purposes 2 hours after the first injection

Administration
Inhalation: **Amyl nitrite:** Crush ampul in cloth and hold under patient's nares for 15-30 seconds; remove for 15 seconds; repeat
Parenteral: I.V.:
Sodium nitrite: Administer undiluted at a rate of 2.5-5 mL/minute
Sodium thiosulfate: Administer undiluted over at least 10 minutes; rapid administration may cause hypotension

Monitoring Parameters Blood cyanide levels, methemoglobin levels, arterial blood gases, oxygen saturation, vital signs

Reference Range Symptoms associated with blood cyanide levels:
Flushing and tachycardia: 0.5-1 µg/mL
Obtundation: 1-2.5 µg/mL
Coma and respiratory depression: >2.5 µg/mL
Death: >3 µg/mL

Dosage Forms Kit:
Injection: Sodium nitrite 300 mg/10 mL (2 ampuls); sodium thiosulfate 12.5 g/50 mL (2 ampuls)
Inhalant: Amyl nitrite 0.3 mL (12 crushable ampuls)

Cyanocobalamin (sye an oh koe BAL a min)

Brand Names Berubigen®; Cobex®; Crystamine®; Cyanoject®; Cyomin®; Ener-B® [OTC]; Kaybovite-1000®; Redisol®; Rubramin® (Canada); Rubramin-PC®; Sytobex®
Synonyms Vitamin B$_{12}$
Therapeutic Category Nutritional Supplement; Vitamin, Water Soluble
Generic Available Yes
(Continued)

Cyanocobalamin *(Continued)*

Use Pernicious anemia; vitamin B$_{12}$ deficiency; increased B$_{12}$ requirements due to pregnancy, thyrotoxicosis, hemorrhage, malignancy, liver or kidney disease; nutritional supplement

Pregnancy Risk Factor A *(C if dose exceeds RDA recommendation)*

Contraindications Hypersensitivity to cyanocobalamin, any component, or cobalt; patients with hereditary optic nerve atrophy

Warnings Vitamin B$_{12}$ deficiency for >3 months results in irreversible degenerative CNS lesions; vegetarian diets may result in vitamin B$_{12}$ deficiency

Precautions Serum potassium concentrations should be monitored early as severe hypokalemia has occurred after the conversion of megaloblastic anemia to normal erythropoiesis

Adverse Reactions
Cardiovascular: Peripheral vascular thrombosis
Dermatologic: Itching, urticaria, exanthema
Endocrine & metabolic: Hypokalemia
Gastrointestinal: Diarrhea
Miscellaneous: Allergic reactions

Drug Interactions Decreased absorption of cyanocobalamin from GI tract; aminoglycoside antibiotics, colchicine, extended release potassium products, aminosalicylic acid, phenytoin, and phenobarbital; antagonism of hematopoietic response to cyanocobalamin: chloramphenicol; chemical degradation of cyanocobalamin; large doses of ascorbic acid

Stability Clear pink to red solutions are stable at room temperature; protect from light; **incompatible** with chlorpromazine, phytonadione, prochlorperazine, warfarin, ascorbic acid, dextrose, heavy metals, oxidizing or reducing agents

Mechanism of Action Coenzyme for various metabolic functions, including fat and carbohydrate metabolism and protein synthesis, used in cell replication and hematopoiesis

Pharmacodynamics
Onset:
Megaloblastic anemia: I.M.:
Conversion of megaloblastic to normoblastic erythroid hyperplasia within bone marrow: 8 hours
Increased reticulocytes: 2-5 days
Complicated vitamin B$_{12}$ deficiency: I.M., S.C.: Resolution of:
Psychiatric sequelae: 24 hours
Thrombocytopenia: 10 days
Granulocytopenia: 2 weeks

Pharmacokinetics
Absorption: Oral: Drug is absorbed from the terminal ileum in the presence of calcium; for absorption to occur, gastric "intrinsic factor" must be present to transfer the compound across the intestinal mucosa
Distribution: Principally stored in the liver, also stored in the kidneys and adrenals
Protein binding: Bound to transcobalamin II
Metabolism: Converted in the tissues to active coenzymes methylcobalamin and deoxyadenosylcobalamin
Bioavailability: Oral: Pernicious anemia: 1.2%
Time to peak serum concentration:
I.M., S.C.: 30 minutes to 2 hours
Intranasal: 1.6 hours
Elimination: 50% to 98% unchanged in the urine

Usual Dosage
I.M. or deep S.C. (oral use is recommended only as a nutritional supplement or as maintenance of vitamin B$_{12}$ deficiency):
Recommended daily allowance (RDA):
Children: 0.3-2 mcg
Adults: 2 mcg
Adults, pregnancy: 2.2 mcg
Adults, lactation: 2.6 mcg
Adults, vegetarians: 6 mcg
Pernicious anemia, congenital (if evidence of neurologic involvement): 1000 mcg/day for at least 2 weeks; maintenance: 50 mcg/month
Children: 30-50 mcg/day for 2 or more weeks (to a total dose of 1000 mcg), then follow with 100 mcg monthly as maintenance dosage
Adults: 100 mcg/day for 6-7 days; if improvement, give same dose on alternate days for 7 doses; then every 3-4 days for 2-3 weeks; once hematologic values have returned to normal, maintenance dosage: 100 mcg/month

Vitamin B$_{12}$ deficiency:

Children: I.M., S.C.: 100 mcg/day for 10-15 days (total dose of 1-1.5 mg), then once or twice weekly for several months; may taper to 60 mcg every month

Adults:

Uncomplicated: Initial: (I.M. or deep S.C. are the preferred routes)

Oral: 25-1000 mcg/day until remission is complete

I.M. or deep S.C.: 100 mcg/day for 5-10 days, followed by 100-200 mcg monthly until remission is complete **or** as an alternative: 100 mcg/ day for 7 days, followed by 100 mcg every other day for 2 weeks, followed by 100 mcg every 3-4 days until remission is complete

Complicated (severe anemia, CHF, thrombocytopenia with bleeding, severe neurologic damage or granulocytopenia with infection): Initial: I.M. or deep S.C.: 1000 mcg with I.M. or I.V. folic acid 15 mg as single doses, followed by 1000 mcg/day plus oral folic acid 5 mg/day for 1 week; **Note:** Oral therapy is **not** indicated for treatment of complicated deficiency

Maintenance: Oral, I.M., deep S.C.: 100-200 mcg monthly

Dosage adjustment in renal impairment: Increased dosage may be required in vitamin B$_{12}$-deficient patients

Administration

Oral: Not generally recommended for treatment of severe vitamin B$_{12}$ deficiency due to poor oral absorption (lack of intrinsic factor); oral administration may be used in less severe deficiencies and maintenance therapy; may be administered without regard to food

Parenteral: I.M. or deep S.C.: Avoid I.V. administration due to a more rapid system elimination with resulting decreased utilization

Monitoring Parameters Serum potassium, erythrocyte and reticulocyte count, hemoglobin, hematocrit

Reference Range Serum vitamin B$_{12}$ levels: Normal: 200-900 pg/mL; vitamin B$_{12}$ deficiency: <200 pg/mL; megaloblastic anemia: <100 pg/mL

Dosage Forms

Gel, nasal (Ener-B®) [OTC]: 400 mcg/0.1 mL

Injection: 30 mcg/mL (30 mL); 100 mcg/mL (1 mL, 10 mL, 30 mL); 1000 mcg/mL (1 mL, 10 mL, 30 mL)

Tablet [OTC]: 25 mcg, 50 mcg, 100 mcg, 250 mcg, 500 mcg, 1000 mcg

♦ **Cyanoject®** see Cyanocobalamin on page 263

Cyclobenzaprine (sye kloe BEN za preen)

Brand Names Flexeril®; Novo-Cycloprine® (Canada)

Available Salts Cyclobenzaprine Hydrochloride

Therapeutic Category Skeletal Muscle Relaxant, Nonparalytic

Generic Available Yes

Use Treatment of muscle spasm associated with acute painful musculoskeletal conditions; supportive therapy in tetanus

Pregnancy Risk Factor B

Contraindications Hypersensitivity to cyclobenzaprine or any component; hyperthyroidism, CHF, arrhythmias, heart block; do not use concomitantly or within 14 days of MAO inhibitors

Warnings Abrupt withdrawal after prolonged administration may result in nausea, headache, and malaise; not effective in the treatment of spasticity due to cerebral or spinal cord disease

Precautions Use with caution in patients with urinary retention, angle-closure glaucoma

Adverse Reactions

Cardiovascular: Tachycardia, hypotension, arrhythmias, edema of face/lips, syncope

Central nervous system: Drowsiness, headache, dizziness, fatigue, nervousness, confusion

Dermatologic: Rash

Gastrointestinal: Dyspepsia, nausea, constipation, xerostomia, vomiting, diarrhea, paralytic ileus, dysgeusia, stomach cramps

Genitourinary: Urinary frequency or retention

Hepatic: Hepatitis, cholestasis, jaundice

Neuromuscular & skeletal: Weakness, muscle twitching

Ocular: Blurred vision

Otic: Tinnitus

Drug Interactions MAO inhibitors; additive effects with sedatives, alcohol, anticholinergic agents, and other CNS depressants

(Continued)

Cyclobenzaprine *(Continued)*

Mechanism of Action Centrally-acting skeletal muscle relaxant pharmacologically related to tricyclic antidepressants; reduces tonic somatic motor activity influencing both alpha and gamma motor neurons

Pharmacodynamics

Onset of action: Within 1 hour

Duration: 12-24 hours

Pharmacokinetics

Absorption: Oral: Complete

Metabolism: Hepatic

Half-life: 1-3 days

Time to peak serum concentration: Within 3-8 hours

Elimination: Primarily renal as inactive metabolites and in the feces (via bile) as unchanged drug; may undergo enterohepatic recycling

Usual Dosage Oral:

Children: Dosage has not been established

Adults: 10 mg 3 times/day (range: 20-40 mg/day in 2-4 divided doses); maximum dose: 60 mg/day; usage for more than 2-3 weeks is not recommended

Administration Oral: May be administered without regard to meals

Patient Information Avoid alcohol; causes drowsiness and may impair ability to perform hazardous tasks involving mental alertness or physical coordination

Dosage Forms Tablet, as hydrochloride: 10 mg

♦ **Cyclobenzaprine Hydrochloride** *see* Cyclobenzaprine *on page 265*

♦ **Cyclogyl®** *see* Cyclopentolate *on page 266*

♦ **Cyclomydril® Ophthalmic** *see* Cyclopentolate and Phenylephrine *on page 267*

Cyclopentolate *(sye kloe PEN toe late)*

Brand Names AK-Pentolate®; Cyclogyl®; I-Pentolate®; Ocu-Pentolate®

Available Salts Cyclopentolate Hydrochloride

Therapeutic Category Anticholinergic Agent, Ophthalmic; Ophthalmic Agent, Mydriatic

Generic Available Yes

Use Diagnostic procedures requiring mydriasis and cycloplegia

Pregnancy Risk Factor C

Contraindications Narrow-angle glaucoma; hypersensitivity to cyclopentolate or any component

Warnings Use of cyclopentolate has been associated with psychotic reactions and behavioral disturbances in pediatric patients; increased susceptibility to these effects has been reported in young infants, young children, and in children with spastic paralysis or brain damage, particularly with concentrations >1%; observe neonates and infants closely for at least 30 minutes after administration; may cause transient elevation of intraocular pressure

Adverse Reactions Central nervous system and cardiovascular reactions most commonly seen in children after receiving 2% solution:

Cardiovascular: Tachycardia, hypertension

Central nervous system: Psychotic and behavioral disturbances manifested by ataxia, restlessness, hallucinations, psychosis, hyperactivity, seizures, incoherent speech

Local: Burning sensation

Ocular: Increase in intraocular pressure, loss of visual accommodation

Miscellaneous: Allergic reactions

Mechanism of Action Prevents the muscle of the ciliary body and the sphincter muscle of the iris from responding to cholinergic stimulation, causing mydriasis and cycloplegia

Pharmacodynamics

Peak effects:

Cycloplegia: 15-60 minutes

Mydriasis: Within 15-60 minutes, with recovery taking up to 24 hours

Usual Dosage Ophthalmic:

Neonates and Infants: See Cyclopentolate and Phenylephrine *on page 267* (preferred agent for use in neonates and infants due to lower cyclopentolate concentration and reduced risk for systemic reactions)

Children: 1 drop of 0.5% or 1% in eye followed by 1 drop of 0.5% or 1% in 5 minutes, if necessary, approximately 40-50 minutes before procedure

Adults: 1 drop of 1% followed by another drop in 5 minutes; approximately 40-50 minutes prior to the procedure, may use 2% solution in heavily pigmented iris

Administration Ophthalmic: Instill drops into conjunctival sac of affected eye(s); avoid contact of bottle tip with skin or eye; to avoid excessive systemic absorption, finger pressure should be applied on the lacrimal sac during and for 1-2 minutes following application

Patient Information May cause blurred vision and increased sensitivity to light

Additional Information Pilocarpine ophthalmic drops applied after the examination may reduce recovery time to 3-6 hours

Dosage Forms Solution, ophthalmic, as hydrochloride: 0.5% (2 mL, 5 mL, 15 mL); 1% (2 mL, 5 mL, 15 mL); 2% (2 mL, 5 mL, 15 mL)

Cyclopentolate and Phenylephrine

(sye kloe PEN toe late & fen il EF rin)

Brand Names Cyclomydril® Ophthalmic

Available Salts Cyclopentolate Hydrochloride and Phenylephrine Hydrochloride

Synonyms Phenylephrine and Cyclopentolate

Therapeutic Category Adrenergic Agonist Agent, Ophthalmic; Anticholinergic Agent, Ophthalmic; Ophthalmic Agent, Mydriatic

Generic Available No

Use Diagnostic procedures requiring mydriasis and cycloplegia; preferred agent for use in neonates and infants

Pregnancy Risk Factor C

Contraindications Narrow-angle glaucoma or untreated anatomically narrow angles; hypersensitivity to cyclopentolate, phenylephrine, or any component

Warnings Use of cyclopentolate has been associated with psychotic reactions and behavioral disturbances in pediatric patients; increased susceptibility to these effects has been reported in young infants, young children, and in children with spastic paralysis or brain damage, particularly with concentrations >1%; observe neonates and infants closely for at least 30 minutes after administration; may cause transient elevation of intraocular pressure

Precautions Use with caution in patient's with Down's syndrome, cardiovascular disease, hypertension, and hyperthyroidism; feeding intolerance may follow ophthalmic use of this product in neonates and infants; withhold feedings for 4 hours after examination

Adverse Reactions

Cardiovascular: Tachycardia, hypertension

Central nervous system: Psychotic and behavioral disturbances manifested by ataxia, restlessness, hallucinations, psychosis, hyperactivity, seizures, incoherent speech, hyperpyrexia

Gastrointestinal: Feeding intolerance, decreased gastric motility

Genitourinary: Urinary retention

Local: Burning sensation

Ocular: Increased intraocular pressure, loss of visual accommodation, transient stinging, browache, photophobia, lacrimation, superficial punctate keratitis

Miscellaneous: Allergic reactions

Drug Interactions May interfere with the ocular antihypertensive action of carbachol, pilocarpine, or ophthalmic cholinesterase inhibitors

Stability Store at room temperature

Mechanism of Action See individual monographs for Cyclopentolate *on page 266* and Phenylephrine *on page 758*

Pharmacodynamics Onset of action and duration of effect are partially dependent upon eye pigment; dark eyes have a prolonged onset of action and shorter duration than blue eyes

Onset: 15-60 minutes

Duration: 4-12 hours

Usual Dosage Ophthalmic:

Neonates, Infants, Children, and Adults: Instill 1 drop into the eye every 5-10 minutes, for up to 3 doses, approximately 40-50 minutes before the examination

Administration Ophthalmic: Instill drops into conjunctival sac of affected eye(s); avoid contact of bottle tip with skin or eye; to avoid excessive systemic absorption, finger pressure should be applied on the lacrimal sac during and for 1-2 minutes following application

Patient Information May cause blurred vision and increased sensitivity to light

Nursing Implications Do not repeat dosage within at least 4 hours, but preferably 24 hours, after initial treatment to prevent drug accumulation and potential systemic toxicity; see Warnings

(Continued)

Cyclopentolate and Phenylephrine *(Continued)*

Additional Information Cyclomydril® is the preferred agent for use in neonates and infants because lower concentrations of both cyclopentolate and phenylephrine provide optimal dilation while minimizing the systemic side effects noted with a higher concentration of each agent used alone

Dosage Forms Solution, ophthalmic, as hydrochloride: Cyclopentolate hydrochloride 0.2% and phenylephrine hydrochloride 1% (2 mL, 5 mL)

♦ **Cyclopentolate Hydrochloride** *see Cyclopentolate on page 266*
♦ **Cyclopentolate Hydrochloride and Phenylephrine Hydrochloride** *see Cyclopentolate and Phenylephrine on page 267*

Cyclophosphamide *(sye kloe FOS fa mide)*

Related Information
Drugs and Breast-Feeding *on page 1213*
Emetogenic Potential of Single Chemotherapeutic Agents *on page 1095*

Brand Names Cytoxan®; Neosar®; Procytox® (Canada)
Synonyms CPM; CTX; CYT
Therapeutic Category Antineoplastic Agent, Alkylating Agent (Nitrogen Mustard)
Generic Available No

Use Treatment of Hodgkin's disease, malignant lymphomas, multiple myeloma, leukemias, sarcomas, mycosis fungoides, neuroblastoma, ovarian carcinoma, breast carcinoma, a variety of other tumors; conditioning regimen for bone marrow transplantation; nephrotic syndrome, lupus erythematosus, severe rheumatoid arthritis, and rheumatoid vasculitis

Pregnancy Risk Factor D
Contraindications Hypersensitivity to cyclophosphamide or any component
Warnings The FDA currently recommends that procedures for proper handling and disposal of antineoplastic agents be considered; cyclophosphamide is potentially carcinogenic and mutagenic; it may impair fertility or cause sterility and birth defects

Precautions Use with caution in patients with bone marrow suppression and impaired renal or hepatic function; modify dosage in patients with renal impairment or compromised bone marrow function. Patients with compromised bone marrow function may require a 33% to 50% reduction in initial dose.

Adverse Reactions
Cardiovascular: Cardiotoxicity with high-dose therapy, pericardial effusion, CHF
Dermatologic: Alopecia, rash
Endocrine & metabolic: Hypokalemia, amenorrhea, SIADH, hyperuricemia, hyperkalemia, hyponatremia
Gastrointestinal: Nausea, vomiting, dysgeusia, anorexia, diarrhea, mucositis
Genitourinary: Oligospermia, hemorrhagic cystitis (5% to 10%)
Hematologic: Leukopenia nadir at 8-15 days, hemolytic anemia, thrombocytopenia, hypothrombinemia
Hepatic: Dose-related hepatotoxicity, jaundice
Renal: Nephrotoxicity
Respiratory: Interstitial pulmonary fibrosis, nasal stuffiness

Drug Interactions Allopurinol (increases myelotoxicity of cyclophosphamide); phenobarbital, phenytoin, and chloral hydrate may increase conversion of cyclophosphamide to active metabolites; chloramphenicol, phenothiazines, imipramine may inhibit the metabolism of cyclophosphamide (increased bone marrow suppression); cyclophosphamide may prolong the neuromuscular blocking activity of succinylcholine

Stability Reconstituted I.V. solution is stable for 24 hours at room temperature or 6 days if refrigerated

Mechanism of Action Interferes with the normal function of DNA by alkylation and cross-linking the strands of DNA, and by possible protein modification

Pharmacokinetics
Absorption: 75% to 95% with low doses
Distribution: Crosses the placenta; appears in breast milk; distributes throughout the body including the brain and CSF
Protein binding: 20%; metabolite: 60%
Metabolism: Inactive prodrug must undergo hydroxylation to form active alkylating mustards; further oxidation leads to formation of inactive metabolites
Half-life: Range 3-12 hours
  Children: 4 hours
  Adults: 6-8 hours
Time to peak serum concentration: Oral: Within 1 hour

Elimination: In urine as unchanged drug (<20%) and as metabolites (85% to 90%)
Moderately dialyzable (20% to 50%)

Usual Dosage Refer to individual protocols

Children and Adults with no hematologic problems:

Induction:

Oral, I.V.: Children: 2-8 mg/kg or 60-250 mg/m^2/day

I.V.: 40-50 mg/kg (1.5-1.8 g/m^2) in divided doses over 2-5 days

Maintenance:

Oral: Children: 2-5 mg/kg or 50-150 mg/m^2 twice weekly

Oral: Adults: 1-5 mg/kg/day

I.V.: 10-15 mg/kg (350-550 mg/m^2) every 7-10 days or 3-5 mg/kg (110-185 mg/m^2) twice weekly

Children:

SLE: I.V.: 500-750 mg/m^2 every month; maximum dose: 1 g/m^2

JRA/vasculitis: I.V.: 10 mg/kg every 2 weeks

BMT conditioning regimen: I.V.: 50 mg/kg/day once daily for 3-4 days

Nephrotic syndrome: Oral: 2-3 mg/kg/day every day for up to 12 weeks when corticosteroids are unsuccessful

Dosing adjustment in renal impairment:

Cl_{cr} >10 mL/minute: Administer 100% of normal dose

Cl_{cr} ≤10 mL/minute: Administer 75% of normal dose

Administration

Oral: Administer with food only if GI distress occurs

Parenteral: May administer IVP, I.V. intermittent, or continuous infusion at a final maximum concentration for administration of 20-25 mg/mL; usually administered as a single bolus dose or in fractionated doses over 2-3 days. Most protocols use a 30-60 minute infusion time; doses >1800 mg/m^2 need to be infused over a longer period (ie, 4- or 6-hour infusions)

Monitoring Parameters CBC with differential and platelet count, ESR, BUN, urinalysis, serum electrolytes, serum creatinine, urine specific gravity, urine output

Test Interactions Positive Coombs' [direct]

Patient Information Maintain high fluid intake and urine output

Nursing Implications Encourage adequate hydration and frequent voiding to help prevent hemorrhagic cystitis; before initiating cyclophosphamide therapy, verify that urine specific gravity is <1.010 and that urine output is >100 mL/m^2/hour (or 3 mL/kg/hour)

Additional Information Aggressive hydration using fluid containing at least 0.45% sodium chloride at 125 mL/m^2/hour, frequent emptying of the bladder, and concurrent administration of mesna are used to reduce the potential of hemorrhagic cystitis (use mesna with cyclophosphamide doses >1 g/m^2/day; doses ≤1 g/m^2/day may not require use of mesna)

Myelosuppressive effects:

WBC: Moderate

Platelets: Moderate

Onset (days): 7

Nadir (days): 8-14

Recovery (days): 21

Dosage Forms

Powder for injection: 100 mg, 200 mg, 500 mg, 1 g, 2 g

Tablet: 25 mg, 50 mg

Extemporaneous Preparations To make a 2 mg/mL oral elixir, reconstitute a 200 mg vial with aromatic elixir, withdraw the solution, and add sufficient aromatic elixir to make a final volume of 100 mL in a graduate; store in amber glass; stable for 14 days in the refrigerator

Nahata MC and Hipple TF, *Pediatric Drug Formulations*, 3rd ed, Cincinnati, OH: Harvey Whitney Books Co, 1997.

References

Bostrom BC, Weisdorf DJ, Kim TH, et al, "Bone Marrow Transplantation for Advanced Acute Leukemia: A Pilot Study of High-Energy Total Body Irradiation, Cyclophosphamide and Continuous Infusion Etoposide," *Bone Marrow Transplant*, 1990, 5(2):83-9.

McCune WJ, Golbus J, Zeldes W, et al, "Clinical and Immunologic Effects of Monthly Administration of Intravenous Cyclophosphamide in Severe Systemic Lupus Erythematosus," *N Engl J Med*, 1988, 318(22):1423-31.

Cycloserine (sye kloe SER een)

Brand Names Seromycin® Pulvules®

Therapeutic Category Antibiotic, Miscellaneous; Antitubercular Agent

Generic Available No

(Continued)

Cycloserine *(Continued)*

Use Adjunctive treatment in pulmonary or extrapulmonary tuberculosis; treatment of acute urinary tract infections caused by *E. coli* or *Enterobacter* sp when less toxic conventional therapy has failed or is contraindicated

Pregnancy Risk Factor C

Contraindications Hypersensitivity to cycloserine or any component; epilepsy, depression, severe anxiety or psychosis, severe renal insufficiency, chronic alcoholism

Precautions Dosage must be adjusted in patients with renal impairment

Adverse Reactions

Cardiovascular: Cardiac arrhythmias, CHF

Central nervous system: Drowsiness, headache, dizziness, vertigo, seizures, confusion, psychosis, paresis, coma, anxiety, nervousness, depression, personality changes

Dermatologic: Rash, photosensitivity

Endocrine & metabolic: Vitamin B_{12} deficiency, folate deficiency

Hepatic: Elevated liver enzymes

Neuromuscular & skeletal: Tremor, dysarthria

Drug Interactions Cycloserine inhibits metabolism of phenytoin; alcohol may increase risk of seizures; ethionamide, isoniazid (additive neurotoxicity with cycloserine)

Food Interactions May increase vitamin B_{12} and folic acid dietary requirements

Mechanism of Action Inhibits bacterial cell wall synthesis by competing with amino acid (D-alanine) for incorporation into the bacterial cell wall

Pharmacokinetics

Absorption: ~70% to 90% from the GI tract

Distribution: Crosses the placenta; appears in breast milk, bile, sputum, synovial fluid and CSF

Protein binding: Not plasma protein bound

Half-life: Patients with normal renal function: 10 hours

Time to peak serum concentration: Within 3-4 hours

Elimination: 60% to 70% of an oral dose excreted unchanged in urine by glomerular filtration within 72 hours, small amounts excreted in feces, remainder is metabolized

Usual Dosage Oral:

Tuberculosis:

Children: 10-20 mg/kg/day divided every 12 hours up to 1000 mg/day

Adults: Initial: 250 mg every 12 hours for 14 days, then give 500 mg to 1 g/day in 2 divided doses

Urinary tract infection: Adults: 250 mg every 12 hours for 14 days

Dosing adjustment in renal impairment:

Cl_{cr} 10-50 mL/minute: Administer every 24 hours

Cl_{cr} <10 mL/minute: Administer every 36-48 hours

Administration Oral: May administer without regard to meals

Monitoring Parameters Periodic renal, hepatic, hematological tests, and plasma cycloserine concentrations

Reference Range Adjust dosage to maintain blood cycloserine concentrations <30 µg/mL

Patient Information May cause drowsiness and impair ability to perform tasks requiring mental alertness or physical coordination; avoid alcohol

Nursing Implications Some of the neurotoxic effects may be relieved or prevented by the concomitant administration of pyridoxine; sedatives may be effective in reducing anxiety or tremor

Dosage Forms Capsule: 250 mg

Cyclosporine *(SYE kloe spor een)*

Related Information

Blood Level Sampling Time Guidelines *on page 1189*

Carbohydrate and Alcohol Content of Liquid Medications for Use in Patients Receiving Ketogenic Diets *on page 1228*

Drugs and Breast-Feeding *on page 1213*

Brand Names Neoral®; Sandimmune®; SangCya™

Synonyms CsA; CyA; Cyclosporine A

Therapeutic Category Immunosuppressant Agent

Generic Available No

Use Immunosuppressant used with corticosteroids to prevent graft vs host disease in patients with kidney, liver, lung, heart, and bone marrow transplants; treatment of nephrotic syndrome in patients with documented focal glomerulosclerosis when corticosteroids and cyclophosphamide are unsuccessful; severe psoriasis; severe autoimmune disease that is resistant to corticosteroids and other therapy

Pregnancy Risk Factor C

Contraindications Hypersensitivity to cyclosporine or any component (ie, polyoxyl 35 castor oil is an ingredient of the parenteral formulation and polyoxyl 40 hydrogenated castor oil is an ingredient of the cyclosporine capsules and solution for microemulsion)

Warnings Immunosuppression with cyclosporine may result in an increased susceptibility to infection and an increased risk of malignancy (lymphomas, lymphoproliferative disorders and squamous cell carcinoma); closely monitor and be prepared to treat anaphylaxis in patients receiving I.V. cyclosporine; serious nephrotoxicity, hypertension, and/or seizures may occur in children receiving cyclosporine; **adjust dosage to avoid toxicity or possible organ rejection via cyclosporine blood or plasma concentration monitoring.**

Precautions Close monitoring and dosage adjustment is required in patients with renal and hepatic impairment

Adverse Reactions

Cardiovascular: Hypertension, flushing, edema

Central nervous system: Seizures, headache, confusion, fever

Dermatologic: Hirsutism, gingival hyperplasia, acne

Endocrine & metabolic: Hyperkalemia, hypomagnesemia, hyperuricemia, hyperchloremic metabolic acidosis, gynecomastia, hyperlipidemia (in patients receiving I.V. cyclosporine)

Gastrointestinal: Abdominal discomfort, diarrhea, nausea, vomiting, anorexia, pancreatitis

Hepatic: Hepatotoxicity (elevated liver enzymes, hyperbilirubinemia)

Neuromuscular & skeletal: Myositis, tremor, paresthesia, leg cramps

Renal: Nephrotoxicity (elevated BUN and serum creatinine)

Respiratory: Sinusitis

Miscellaneous: Lymphoproliferative disorder, increased susceptibility to infection, sensitivity to temperature extremes, anaphylaxis in patients receiving I.V. cyclosporine (reaction includes flushing of the face, respiratory distress with dyspnea and wheezing, hypotension, tachycardia)

Drug Interactions Cytochrome isoenzyme P-450 CYP3A3/4 substrate

Ketoconazole, itraconazole, clarithromycin, fluconazole, azithromycin, erythromycin, tacrolimus, diltiazem, verapamil, and methylprednisolone increase cyclosporine concentration by inhibiting hepatic metabolism; acyclovir, amphotericin B, aminoglycosides, diclofenac, co-trimoxazole, melphalan, and vancomycin may increase nephrotoxicity of cyclosporine; erythromycin and metoclopramide increase cyclosporine absorption; phenytoin and octreotide decrease cyclosporine bioavailability; phenytoin, phenobarbital, carbamazepine, primidone, ticlopidine, rifabutin, rifampin, trimethoprim, and nafcillin decrease cyclosporine concentration by increasing hepatic metabolism of cyclosporine; potassium-sparing diuretics increase risk of hyperkalemia; cimetidine may increase cyclosporine concentration

Food Interactions High-fat meal increases volume of distribution of cyclosporine; grapefruit and grapefruit juice may affect cyclosporine metabolism resulting in increased cyclosporine concentrations; St John's wort significantly reduces cyclosporine levels

Stability Do **not** store oral solution or oral solution for emulsion in the refrigerator; store oral solutions in original container only and use contents within 2 months after opening; I.V. cyclosporine prepared in NS is stable 6 hours in a polyvinyl chloride container or 12 hours in a glass container; I.V. cyclosporine diluted in D_5W to a final concentration of 2 mg/mL is stable for 24 hours in glass or polyvinyl chloride containers; I.V. cyclosporine may bind to the plastic tubing in I.V. administration sets and to polyvinyl chloride bags. Polyoxyethylated castor oil (Cremophor EI®) surfactant in cyclosporine injection may leach phthalate from PVC containers such as bags and tubing.

Mechanism of Action Inhibition of production and release of interleukin II and inhibits interleukin II-induced activation of resting T lymphocytes

Pharmacokinetics

Absorption: Oral:

Solution or soft gelatin capsule (Sandimmune®): Erratically and incompletely absorbed; dependent on the presence of food, bile acids, and GI motility; larger oral doses of cyclosporine are needed in pediatric patients vs adults due to a shorter bowel length resulting in limited intestinal absorption

(Continued)

Cyclosporine *(Continued)*

Solution in a microemulsion or soft gelatin capsule in a microemulsion are bioequivalent (Neoral®): Erratically and incompletely absorbed; increased absorption, up to 30% when compared to Sandimmune®; absorption is less dependent on food intake, bile, or GI motility when compared to Sandimmune®

Distribution: Widely distributed in tissues and body fluids including the liver, pancreas, and lungs; crosses the placenta; excreted into breast milk

V_{dss}: 4-6 L/kg in renal, liver, and marrow transplant recipients (slightly lower values in cardiac transplant patients; children <10 years of age have higher values)

Protein binding: 90% to 98% of dose binds to blood lipoproteins

Metabolism: Undergoes extensive first-pass metabolism following oral administration; extensively metabolized by the cytochrome P-450 system in the liver

Bioavailability:

Solution or soft gelatin capsule (Sandimmune®): Dependent on patient population and transplant type (<10% in adult liver transplant patients and as high as 89% in renal patients)

Children: 28% (range: 17% to 42%); with gut dysfunction commonly seen in BMT recipients, oral bioavailability is further reduced

Solution or soft gelatin capsule in a microemulsion (Neoral®):

Children: 43% (range: 30% to 68%)

Adults: 23% greater than with Sandimmune® in renal transplant patients, 50% greater in liver transplant patients

Half-life:

Solution or soft gelatin capsule (Sandimmune®): Biphasic

Alpha phase: 1.4 hours

Terminal phase: 6-24 hours, prolonged in patients with hepatic dysfunction

Solution or soft gelatin capsule in a microemulsion (Neoral®): 8.4 hours; lower in pediatric patients vs adults due to a higher metabolism rate

Time to peak serum concentration:

Oral solution or capsule (Sandimmune®): 2-6 hours; some patients have a second peak at 5-6 hours

Oral solution or capsule in a microemulsion (Neoral®): 1.5-2 hours (in renal transplant patients)

Elimination: Primarily biliary with 6% of the dose excreted in urine as unchanged drug (0.1%) and metabolites; clearance is more rapid in pediatric patients than in adults

Usual Dosage Children and Adults (oral dosage is ~3 times the I.V. dosage):

I.V.:

Initial: 5-6 mg/kg/dose administered 4-12 hours prior to organ transplantation

Maintenance: 2-10 mg/kg/day in divided doses every 8-24 hours; patients should be switched to oral cyclosporine as soon as possible; cyclosporine doses should be adjusted to maintain whole blood HPLC trough concentrations in the reference range

Oral: Solution or soft gelatin capsule:

Initial: 14-18 mg/kg/dose administered 4-12 hours prior to organ transplantation

Maintenance, postoperative: 5-15 mg/kg/day divided every 12-24 hours; maintenance dose is usually tapered to 3-10 mg/kg/day

Focal segmental glomerulosclerosis: Initial: 3 mg/kg/day divided every 12 hours

Oral: Solution or soft gelatin capsule in a microemulsion (Neoral®): Based on the organ transplant population:

Initial: Same as the initial dose for solution or soft gelatin capsule

or

Renal: 9 mg/kg/day (range: 6-12 mg/kg/day)

Liver: 8 mg/kg/day (range: 4-12 mg/kg/day)

Heart: 7 mg/kg/day (range: 4-10 mg/kg/day)

Note: A 1:1 ratio conversion from Sandimmune® to Neoral® has been recommended initially; however, lower doses of Neoral® may be required after conversion to prevent overdose. Total daily doses should be adjusted based on the cyclosporine trough blood concentration and clinical assessment of organ rejection. Cyclosporine blood trough levels should be determined prior to conversion. After conversion to Neoral®, cyclosporine trough levels should be monitored every 4-7 days. **Neoral®, SangCya™, and Sandimmune® are not bioequivalent and cannot be used interchangeably.** (SangCya™ oral solution was **voluntarily withdrawn form the market.**)

Conditions for dosage adjustments, see table on following page.

Cyclosporine

Condition	Cyclosporine Dosing Adjustment
Switch from I.V. to oral therapy	Threefold increase in dose
T-tube clamping	Decrease dose; increase availability of bile facilitates absorption of cyclosporine
Pediatric patients	May require higher weight-based dose compared to adults
Hepatic dysfunction	Decrease I.V. dose; increase oral dose
Renal dysfunction	Monitor drug levels; may need to decrease dose
Dialysis	Not removed
Inhibitors of hepatic metabolism	Decrease dose
Inducers of hepatic metabolism	Monitor drug level; may need to increase dose

Administration
Oral: Administer consistently at the same time twice daily; use oral syringe, glass dropper, or glass container (not plastic or styrofoam cup); to improve palatability, oral solution may be mixed with milk, chocolate milk, orange juice, or apple juice that is at room temperature; dilution of Neoral® with milk can be unpalatable; stir well and drink at once; do not allow to stand before drinking; rinse with more diluent to ensure that the total dose is taken; after use, dry outside of glass dropper, do not rinse with water or other cleaning agents

Parenteral: May administer by I.V. intermittent infusion or continuous infusion; for intermittent infusion, administer over 2-6 hours at a final concentration not to exceed 2.5 mg/mL

Monitoring Parameters Blood/serum drug concentration (trough), renal and hepatic function tests, serum electrolytes, blood pressure, heart rate

Reference Range Reference ranges are method dependent and specimen dependent; use the same analytical method consistently; trough levels should be obtained immediately prior to next dose

Therapeutic: Not well defined, dependent on organ transplanted, time after transplant, organ function, and cyclosporine toxicity. Empiric therapeutic concentration ranges for trough cyclosporine concentrations:
Kidney: 100-200 ng/mL (serum, RIA)
BMT: 100-250 ng/mL (serum, RIA)
Heart: 100-200 ng/mL (serum, RIA)
Liver: 100-400 ng/mL (blood, HPLC)
Method dependent (optimum cyclosporine trough concentrations):
Serum, RIA: 150-300 ng/mL; 50-150 ng/mL (late post-transplant period)
Whole blood, RIA: 250-800 ng/mL; 150-450 ng/mL (late post-transplant period)
Whole blood, HPLC: 100-500 ng/mL

Test Interactions Cyclosporine adsorbs to silicone; specific whole blood assay for cyclosporine may be falsely elevated if sample is drawn from the same central venous line through which dose was administered (even if flush has been administered and/or dose was given hours before); cyclosporine metabolites cross-react with radioimmunoassay and fluorescence polarization immunoassay

Patient Information Take dose at the same time each day; do not allow diluted oral solution to stand before drinking; do not change brands of cyclosporine unless directed by your physician

Nursing Implications Adequate airway, supportive measures, and agents for treating anaphylaxis should be present when I.V. cyclosporine is administered

Additional Information Diltiazem has been used to prevent cyclosporine nephrotoxicity, reduce the frequency of delayed graft function when administered before and after surgery, and used to treat the mild hypertension that occurs in most patients after transplantation; diltiazem increases cyclosporine blood concentration by delaying its clearance resulting in decreased dosage requirements for cyclosporine

Dosage Forms
Capsule (in a microemulsion): Neoral®: 25 mg, 100 mg
Capsule, soft gelatin: Sandimmune®: 25 mg, 50 mg, 100 mg
Injection: 50 mg/mL (5 mL)
Solution (in a microemulsion): Neoral®: 100 mg/mL

References
Burckart GJ, Canafax DM, and Yee GC, "Cyclosporine Monitoring," *Drug Intell Clin Pharm*, 1986, 20(9):649-52.
(Continued)

Cyclosporine (Continued)

Holt DW, Mueller EA, Kovarik JM, et al, "Sandimmune® Neoral® Pharmacokinetics: Impact of the New Oral Formulation," *Transplant Proc*, 1995, 27(1):1434-7.

Lin CY and Lee SF, "Comparison of Pharmacokinetics Between CsA Capsules and Sandimmune® Neoral® in Pediatric Patients," *Transplant Proc*, 1994, 26(5):2973-4.

Niese D, "A Double-Blind Randomized Study of Sandimmune® Neoral® vs Sandimmune® in New Renal Transplant Recipients: Results After 12 Months," *Transplant Proc*, 1995, 27(2):1849-56.

Taesch S, Niese D, and Mueller EA, "Sandimmune® Neoral®, A New Oral Formulation of Cyclosporine With Improved Pharmacokinetic Characteristics: Safety and Tolerability in Renal Transplant Patients," *Transplant Proc*, 1994, 26(6):3147-9.

Wandstrat TL, Schroeder TJ, and Myre SA, "Cyclosporine Pharmacokinetics in Pediatric Transplant Recipients," *Ther Drug Monit*, 1989, 11(5):493-6.

Yee GC, "Recent Advances in Cyclosporine Pharmacokinetics," *Pharmacotherapy*, 1991, 11(5):130S-134S.

♦ **Cyclosporine A** see Cyclosporine on page 270
♦ **Cycrin® Oral** see Medroxyprogesterone on page 599
♦ **Cyklokapron®** see Tranexamic Acid on page 943
♦ **Cylert®** see Pemoline on page 736
♦ **Cylex® [OTC]** see Benzocaine on page 124
♦ **Cyomin®** see Cyanocobalamin on page 263

Cyproheptadine (si proe HEP ta deen)

Related Information
Overdose and Toxicology on page 1191
Brand Names Periactin®; PMS-Cyproheptadine (Canada)
Available Salts Cyproheptadine Hydrochloride
Therapeutic Category Antihistamine
Generic Available Yes
Use Perennial and seasonal allergic rhinitis and other allergic symptoms including urticaria; appetite stimulant (useful in the management of anorexia nervosa); prophylactic treatment of cluster and migraine headaches; spasticity associated with spinal cord damage associated with spasticity
Pregnancy Risk Factor B
Contraindications Hypersensitivity to cyproheptadine or any component; narrow-angle glaucoma, bladder neck obstruction, acute asthmatic attack, stenosing peptic ulcer, GI tract obstruction, those on MAO inhibitors
Adverse Reactions
Cardiovascular: Tachycardia, palpitations, edema
Central nervous system: Sedation, CNS stimulation, seizures, fatigue, headache, nervousness, depression
Dermatologic: Photosensitivity, rash, angioedema
Gastrointestinal: Appetite stimulation, xerostomia, nausea, diarrhea, abdominal pain
Hematologic: Hemolytic anemia, leukopenia, thrombocytopenia
Hepatic: Hepatitis
Neuromuscular & skeletal: Myalgia, paresthesia, arthralgia
Respiratory: Bronchospasm, epistaxis, pharyngitis
Miscellaneous: Allergic reactions
Drug Interactions MAO inhibitors; enhances sedative effects of other CNS depressants; enhances anticholinergic effects of other anticholinergic agents
Mechanism of Action A potent antihistamine and serotonin antagonist, competes with histamine for H_1-receptor sites on effector cells in the gastrointestinal tract, blood vessels, and respiratory tract
Pharmacokinetics
Absorption: Well absorbed
Metabolism: Extensively by conjugation
Elimination: >50% excreted in urine (primarily as metabolites); approximately 25% excreted in feces
Usual Dosage Oral:
Allergic conditions:
Children: 0.25 mg/kg/day or 8 mg/m²/day in 2-3 divided doses or
2-6 years: 2 mg every 8-12 hours (not to exceed 12 mg/day)
7-14 years: 4 mg every 8-12 hours (not to exceed 16 mg/day)
Adults: 4-20 mg/day divided every 8 hours (not to exceed 0.5 mg/kg/day)
Appetite stimulation (anorexia nervosa): Children >13 years and Adults: 2 mg 4 times/day; may be increased gradually over a 3-week period to 8 mg 4 times/day
Cluster headaches: Adults: 4 mg 4 times/day
Migraine headaches:
Children: 4 mg 2-3 times/day

Adults: 4-8 mg 3 times/day

Spasticity associated with spinal cord damage: Children ≥12 years and Adults: 4 mg at bedtime; increase by a 4 mg dose every 3-4 days; average daily dose: 16 mg in divided doses; not to exceed 36 mg/day

Dosage adjustment in hepatic impairment: Reduce dosage in patients with significant hepatic dysfunction

Administration Oral: Administer with food or milk

Test Interactions Diagnostic antigen skin tests; ↑ amylase (S); ↓ fasting glucose (S)

Patient Information Causes drowsiness and may impair ability to perform hazardous duties requiring mental alertness or physical coordination

Dosage Forms

Syrup, as hydrochloride: 2 mg/5 mL with alcohol 5% (473 mL)

Tablet, as hydrochloride: 4 mg

References

Gracies JM, Nance P, Elovic E, et al, "Traditional Pharmacological Treatments for Spasticity. Part II: General and Regional Treatments," *Muscle Nerve Suppl*, 1997, 6:S92-120.

♦ **Cyproheptadine Hydrochloride** *see* Cyproheptadine *on page 274*

♦ **Cystadane®** *see* Betaine Anhydrous *on page 129*

♦ **Cystagon®** *see* Cysteamine *on page 275*

Cysteamine (sis TEE a meen)

Brand Names Cystagon®

Available Salts Cysteamine Bitartrate

Therapeutic Category Cystinosis, Treatment Agent

Use Management of nephropathic cystinosis

Pregnancy Risk Factor C

Contraindications Hypersensitivity to cysteamine, penicillamine, or any component

Warnings Leukocyte cystine levels should be monitored during oral cysteamine therapy; cysteamine should be given in the lowest doses possible to achieve adequate leukocyte cystine depletion; toxicity can be reduced by initiating therapy with a slowly increasing dose schedule (See Usual Dosage)

Precautions Use with caution in patients with a history of blood dyscrasias, gastric or duodenal ulcer, or neurologic disorder

Adverse Reactions

Cardiovascular: Hypertension

Central nervous system: Somnolence, encephalopathy, headache, seizures, ataxia, confusion, dizziness, jitteriness, nervousness, impaired cognition, emotional changes, hallucinations, nightmares, fever, lethargy

Dermatologic: Urticaria, rash

Endocrine & metabolic: Dehydration

Gastrointestinal: Bad breath, abdominal pain, dyspepsia, constipation, gastroenteritis, duodenitis, duodenal ulceration, vomiting, anorexia, diarrhea

Hematologic: Anemia, leukopenia

Hepatic: Abnormal liver enzymes

Neuromuscular & skeletal: Tremor, hyperkinesia

Otic: Decreased hearing

Mechanism of Action Reacts with cystine in the lysosome to convert it to cysteine and to a cysteine-cysteamine mixed disulfide, both of which can then exit the lysosome in patients with cystinosis, an inherited defect of lysosomal transport

Pharmacokinetics

Absorption: Rapid

Protein binding: 10% to 18%

Half-life: 1 hour

Usual Dosage Oral:

Children <12 years: Initial: 10 mg/kg/day divided into 4 doses; increase by 10 mg/kg/day every 3 weeks to a maximum of 90 mg/kg/day (average effective dose: 50-60 mg/kg/day) **or** 0.16-0.32 g/m²/day divided into 4 doses; increasing every 3 weeks to a maximum of 1.3 g/m²/day

Children ≥12 years and Adults (>110 lb): 2 g/day in 4 divided doses; dosage may be increased gradually to 1.95 g/m²/day

Administration Oral: Contents of capsule may be sprinkled over food

Monitoring Parameters Blood counts and liver enzymes during therapy; monitor leukocyte cystine measurements to determine adequate dosage and compliance (measure 5-6 hours after administration)

Reference Range Leukocyte cystine: <1 nmol of half-cystine/mg protein

(Continued)

Cysteamine *(Continued)*

Patient Information May cause drowsiness or impair ability to perform activities which require mental alertness or physical coordination

Dosage Forms Capsule, as bitartrate: 50 mg, 150 mg

♦ **Cysteamine Bitartrate** *see Cysteamine on page 275*

Cysteine *(SIS teen)*

Available Salts Cysteine Hydrochloride

Therapeutic Category Nutritional Supplement

Generic Available Yes

Use Supplement to crystalline amino acid solutions, in particular the specialized pediatric formulas (eg, Aminosyn® PF, TrophAmine®) to meet the intravenous amino acid nutritional requirements of infants receiving parenteral nutrition (PN)

Contraindications Hypersensitivity to cysteine or any component; patients with hepatic coma or metabolic disorders involving impaired nitrogen utilization

Warnings Metabolic acidosis has occurred in infants related to the "hydrochloride" component of cysteine; each 1 mmol cysteine (175 mg) delivers 1 mEq chloride and 1 mEq hydrogen ion; to balance the extra hydrochloride ions and prevent acidosis addition to the PN solution of a 1 mEq acetate electrolyte salt for each mmole (175 mg) of cysteine may be needed; each 40 mg cysteine (equal to every 1 g amino acid when used in the recommended ratio) adds 0.228 mEq chloride and hydrogen

Precautions Use with caution in patients with renal dysfunction and hepatic insufficiency

Adverse Reactions

Central nervous system: Fever

Endocrine & metabolic: Metabolic acidosis (see Warnings)

Gastrointestinal: Nausea

Renal: Elevated BUN, azotemia

Stability Avoid excessive heat, do not freeze; when combined with parenteral amino acid solutions, cysteine is relatively unstable; it is intended to be added immediately prior to administration to the patient; infusion of the admixture should begin within 1 hour of mixing or refrigerated until use; stable 24 hours in PN solution; opened vials must be used within 4 hours of entry

Mechanism of Action Cysteine is a sulfur-containing amino acid synthesized from methionine via the transsulfuration pathway. It is a precursor of the tripeptide glutathione and also of taurine. Newborn infants have a relative deficiency of the enzyme necessary to affect this conversion. Cysteine may be considered an essential amino acid in infants.

Usual Dosage I.V.: Neonates and Infants: Added as a fixed ratio to crystalline amino acid solution: 40 mg cysteine per g of amino acids; dosage will vary with the daily amino acid dosage (eg, 0.5-2.5 g/kg/day amino acids would result in 20-100 mg/kg/day cysteine); individual doses of cysteine of 0.8-1 mmol/kg/day have also been added directly to the daily PN solution; the duration of treatment relates to the need for PN; patients on chronic PN therapy have received cysteine until 6 months of age and in some cases until 2 years of age

Administration Parenteral: Use only after dilution into PN solution; dilute with amino acid solution in a ratio of 40 mg cysteine to 1 g amino acid: eg, 500 mg cysteine is added to 12.5 g (250 mL) of 5% amino acid solution

Monitoring Parameters BUN, ammonia, electrolytes, pH, acid-base balance, serum creatinine, liver function tests, growth curve

Additional Information Addition of cysteine to PN solutions enhances the solubility of calcium and phosphate by lowering the overall pH of the solution

Dosage Forms Injection, as hydrochloride: 50 mg/mL [~0.285 mmol/mL] (10 mL)

♦ **Cysteine Hydrochloride** *see Cysteine on page 276*

♦ **Cystospaz®** *see Hyoscyamine on page 497*

♦ **Cystospaz-M®** *see Hyoscyamine on page 497*

♦ **CYT** *see Cyclophosphamide on page 268*

Cytarabine *(sye TARE a been)*

Related Information

Emetogenic Potential of Single Chemotherapeutic Agents *on page 1095*

Brand Names Cytosar-U®; Tarabine® PFS

Available Salts Cytarabine Hydrochloride

Synonyms Arabinosylcytosine; Ara-C; Cytosine Arabinosine

Therapeutic Category Antineoplastic Agent, Antimetabolite

Generic Available Yes

Use Used in combination regimens for the treatment of leukemias, meningeal leukemia, Hodgkin's lymphoma, and non-Hodgkin's lymphoma

Pregnancy Risk Factor D

Contraindications Hypersensitivity to cytarabine or any component

Warnings The FDA currently recommends that procedures for proper handling and disposal of antineoplastic agents be considered. Must monitor for drug toxicity; drug toxicity includes bone marrow suppression with leukopenia, thrombocytopenia, and anemia along with nausea, vomiting, diarrhea, abdominal pain, oral ulceration, and hepatic dysfunction; irreversible cerebellar toxicity may occur with a cumulative dose ≥ 30 g/m^2; cytarabine is potentially mutagenic and carcinogenic.

Precautions Marked bone marrow suppression necessitates dosage reduction or a reduction in the number of days of administration; with severe hepatic dysfunction, dosage may need to be reduced

Adverse Reactions

Cardiovascular: Cardiomegaly, chest pain, pericarditis

Central nervous system: Headache, malaise, confusion, seizures, fever, irritability, cerebral and cerebellar dysfunction (somnolence, personality changes, coma, ataxia)

Dermatologic: Alopecia, rash

Endocrine & metabolic: Hyperuricemia

Gastrointestinal: Nausea, vomiting, oral and anal inflammation with ulceration, anorexia, diarrhea, GI hemorrhage, mucositis

Hematologic: Myelosuppression (leukopenia, thrombocytopenia, anemia)

Hepatic: Hepatic dysfunction, jaundice, elevated serum bilirubin and liver enzymes

Local: Thrombophlebitis

Neuromuscular & skeletal: Myalgia, bone pain, peripheral neuropathy, weakness, gait disturbances

Ocular: Conjunctivitis, hemorrhagic conjunctivitis, corneal toxicity, photophobia, blurred vision

Respiratory: Syndrome of sudden respiratory distress progressing to pulmonary edema and diffuse interstitial pneumonitis have been reported with high-dose regimens

Miscellaneous: Ara-C syndrome (fever, myalgia, bone pain, rash, conjunctivitis, malaise occurring 6-12 hours after administration); headache and vomiting with I.T. administration; anaphylactoid reaction

Drug Interactions Decreases digoxin oral tablet absorption

Stability Reconstituted solutions containing 20-100 mg/mL cytarabine are stable for 48 hours at room temperature; I.T. Ara-C is compatible with methotrexate and hydrocortisone mixed in the same syringe; physically incompatible with fluorouracil, heparin

Mechanism of Action Converted intracellularly to the active metabolite cytarabine triphosphate; inhibits DNA polymerase by competing with deoxycytidine triphosphate resulting in inhibition of DNA synthesis; incorporated into DNA chain resulting in termination of chain elongation; cell cycle-specific for the S-phase of cell division

Pharmacokinetics

Distribution: Penetrates the CSF in limited amounts, crosses the placenta

Protein binding: 13%

Metabolism: Deactivated by cytidine deaminase primarily in the liver, but also in kidneys, GI mucosa, and granulocytes

Half-life, terminal: 1-3 hours

Elimination: ~80% of dose excreted in urine as metabolites within 24 hours; 10% excreted in urine as unchanged drug

Usual Dosage Children and Adults (refer to individual protocols):

Induction remission:

I.V.: 200 mg/m^2/day for 5 days at 2-week intervals as a single agent; in combination chemotherapy, 100-200 mg/m^2/day for 5- to 10-day therapy course every 2-4 weeks, or every day until remission, given as an I.V. continuous drip or in 2 divided doses/day

I.T.: 5-75 mg/m^2 every 2-7 days until CNS findings normalize

Maintenance remission:

I.V.: 70-200 mg/m^2/day for 2-5 days at monthly intervals

I.M., S.C.: 1-1.5 mg/kg single dose for maintenance at 1- to 4-week intervals

I.T.: 5-75 mg/m^2 every 2-7 days until CNS findings normalize **or**

<1 year: 20 mg

1-2 years: 30 mg

2-3 years: 50 mg

(Continued)

Cytarabine *(Continued)*

>3 years: 70 mg

High-dose regimen: Refractory leukemias or refractory non-Hodgkin's lymphoma: I.V. infusion: 3 g/m^2/dose every 12 hours for up to 12 doses

Administration Parenteral: May administer S.C., I.M., IVP, I.V. infusion, or I.T. at a concentration not to exceed 100 mg/mL

High-dose regimens or for use in neonates: Diluents containing benzyl alcohol should not be used to reconstitute the drug; high-dose regimens (dose >1 g/m^2) are usually administered by I.V. infusion over 2 hours or longer, or as an I.V. continuous infusion

IVP: May administer over 15 minutes; rapid administration is associated with greater neurotoxicity

I.T. administration: Reconstitute with preservative free NS, Elliotts B solution, or preservative free LR solution; use preservative free injection formulation for I.T. use; filter through a 0.22 micron filter; the volume to be given I.T. is in the range of 3-10 mL and should correspond to an equivalent volume of CSF removed; antiemetic therapy should be administered prior to intrathecal doses of cytarabine

S.C. administration: Rotate injection sites to thigh, abdomen, and flank regions; avoid repeated administration to a single site

Monitoring Parameters Liver function tests, CBC with differential and platelet count, serum creatinine, BUN, serum uric acid; signs of neurotoxicity

Patient Information Notify physician of any fever, sore throat, bleeding, or bruising

Nursing Implications Administer corticosteroid eye drops for prophylaxis of conjunctivitis around-the-clock prior to, during, and for 2-7 days after high-dose Ara-C; pyridoxine has been administered on days of high-dose Ara-C therapy for prophylaxis of CNS toxicity.

Additional Information Myelosuppressive effects:

WBC: Severe

Platelets: Severe

Onset (days): 4-7

Nadir (days): 14-18

Recovery (days): 21-28

Dosage Forms

Injection, preservative free, as hydrochloride (Tarabine® PFS): 20 mg/mL (5 mL, 50 mL)

Powder for injection, as hydrochloride (Cytosar-U®): 100 mg, 500 mg, 1 g, 2 g

References

Grossman L, Baker MA, Sutton DM, et al, "Central Nervous System Toxicity of High-Dose Cytosine Arabinoside," *Med Pediatr Oncol*, 1983, 11(4):246-50.

Dacarbazine *(da KAR ba zeen)*

Related Information

Emetogenic Potential of Single Chemotherapeutic Agents *on page 1095*

Brand Names DTIC-Dome®

Synonyms DIC; Imidazole Carboxamide

Therapeutic Category Antineoplastic Agent, Miscellaneous

Generic Available Yes

Use Treatment of malignant melanoma, Hodgkin's disease, soft-tissue sarcomas (fibrosarcomas, rhabdomyosarcoma), islet cell carcinoma, medullary carcinoma of the thyroid, and neuroblastoma

Pregnancy Risk Factor C

Contraindications Hypersensitivity to dacarbazine or any component

Warnings The FDA currently recommends that procedures for proper handling and disposal of antineoplastic agents be considered. Hematopoietic depression is common; hepatic necrosis is also possible; dacarbazine has been reported to cause sterility and is mutagenic and teratogenic in rats

Precautions Use with caution in patients with bone marrow suppression, renal and/or hepatic impairment; dosage reduction may be necessary in patients with renal or hepatic insufficiency; avoid extravasation of the drug

Adverse Reactions

Cardiovascular: Facial flushing, hypotension

Central nervous system: Malaise, headache, fever, seizure

Dermatologic: Alopecia, rash, photosensitivity

Gastrointestinal: Anorexia, nausea, vomiting, metallic taste

Hematologic: Myelosuppression (nadir: 2-4 weeks): Leukopenia, thrombocytopenia

Hepatic: Hepatotoxicity, hepatic vein thrombosis, hepatocellular necrosis

Local: Pain and burning at infusion site, thrombophlebitis

Neuromuscular & skeletal: Myalgia, paresthesia

Ocular: Blurred vision

Respiratory: Sinus congestion

Miscellaneous: Flu-like syndrome, anaphylactic reactions

Drug Interactions Phenytoin, phenobarbital may induce dacarbazine metabolism

Stability Store in refrigerator; intact vials are stable for 4 weeks at room temperature; protect dacarbazine solutions from light; reconstituted dacarbazine solution 10 mg/mL is stable for 72 hours when refrigerated or 8 hours at room temperature; drug decomposition has occurred if the solution turns pink; dacarbazine is incompatible with hydrocortisone sodium succinate

Mechanism of Action Alkylating agent which forms methyldiazonium ions that attack nucleophilic groups in DNA; inhibits DNA, RNA, and protein synthesis by cross-linking DNA strands

Pharmacokinetics

Distribution: Distributes to the liver; very little distribution into CSF

V_{dss}: 17 L/m^2

Protein binding: Minimal, 5%

Metabolism: N-demethylated in the liver by microsomal enzymes; metabolites may also have an antineoplastic effect

Half-life, biphasic: Initial: 20-40 minutes; terminal: 5 hours (in patients with normal renal/hepatic function)

Elimination: ~30% to 50% of dose excreted in urine by tubular secretion, 15% to 25% is excreted in urine as unchanged drug

Usual Dosage I.V. (refer to individual protocols):

Children:

Pediatric solid tumors: 200-470 mg/m^2/day over 5 days every 21-28 days

Pediatric neuroblastoma: 800-900 mg/m^2 as a single dose on day 1 of therapy every 3-4 weeks in combination therapy

Hodgkin's disease: 375 mg/m^2 on days 1 and 15 of treatment course, repeat every 28 days

Adults:

Malignant melanoma: 2-4.5 mg/kg/day for 10 days, repeat in 4 weeks or may use 250 mg/m^2/day for 5 days, repeat in 3 weeks

Hodgkin's disease: 150 mg/m^2/day for 5 days, repeat every 4 weeks **or** 375 mg/m^2 on day 1, repeat in 15 days of each 28-day cycle in combination with other agents

Administration Parenteral: Reconstitute vial for IVP doses with at least 2 mL of D$_5$W or NS; administer dose diluted in 5-10 mL D$_5$W or NS by slow IVP over 2-3 minutes or by I.V. infusion over 15-120 minutes at a concentration not to exceed 10 mg/mL

Monitoring Parameters CBC with differential, erythrocytes and platelet count; liver function tests

Patient Information Avoid exposure to sunlight; restrict intake of food for 4-6 hours prior to dacarbazine dose to decrease vomiting; flu-like symptoms (ie, malaise, fever, myalgia) may occur 1 week after infusion

(Continued)

279

Dacarbazine *(Continued)*

Nursing Implications Avoid extravasation; use a D_5W or NS flush before and after a dacarbazine infusion; local pain, burning sensation, and irritation at the injection site may be relieved by local application of hot packs, slowing the I.V. rate and further dilution in I.V. fluid

Dosage Forms Injection: 100 mg (10 mL, 20 mL); 200 mg (20 mL, 30 mL); 500 mg (50 mL)

References

Berg SL, Grisell DL, DeLaney TF, et al, "Principles of Treatment of Pediatric Solid Tumors," *Pediatr Clin North Am*, 1991, 38(2):249-67.

Finklestein JZ, Albo V, Ertel I, et al, "5-(3,3-Dimethyl-l-triazeno) imidazole-4-carboxamide (NSC-45388) in the Treatment of Solid Tumors in Children," *Cancer Chemother Rep*, 1975, 59(2 Pt 1):351-7.

Mutz ID and Urban CE, "Dimethyl-triazeno-imidazole-carboxamide (DTIC) in Combination Chemotherapy for Childhood Neuroblastoma," *Wien Klin Wochenschr*, 1978, 90(24):867-70.

Daclizumab *(da CLI zoo mab)*

Brand Names Zenapax®

Synonyms HAT Antibody; Humanized Anti-CD25 mo Ab; Humanized Anti-interleukin-2 Receptor mo Ab; Humanized Anti-Tac mo Ab

Therapeutic Category Immunosuppressant Agent

Use In combination with an immunosuppressive regimen, including cyclosporine and corticosteroids, for prophylaxis of acute organ rejection in patients receiving renal transplants; daclizumab has also been studied in pediatric bone marrow patients; steroid-refractory graft-versus-host disease

Pregnancy Risk Factor C

Contraindications Hypersensitivity to daclizumab or any component

Warnings Should only be used by physicians experienced in immunosuppressive therapy or management of transplant patients; adequate laboratory and supportive medical resources must be readily available in the facility for patient management; may result in an increased susceptibility to infection or an increased risk for developing lymphoproliferative disorders

Adverse Reactions

Cardiovascular: Edema, hypertension (48% in pediatric patients), hypotension, tachycardia, thrombosis

Central nervous system: Headache, dizziness, insomnia, depression, anxiety, fever, chills

Dermatologic: Impaired wound healing, acne, pruritus, rash, hirsutism

Endocrine & metabolic: Dehydration (frequency may be higher for pediatric patients than for adults), diabetes mellitus

Genitourinary: Oliguria, dysuria

Gastrointestinal: Constipation, nausea, diarrhea (36%), vomiting (32%), abdominal pain, abdominal distention

Neuromuscular & skeletal: Tremors, back pain, arthralgia, myalgia

Ocular: Blurred vision

Renal: Renal tubular necrosis, hematuria

Respiratory: Atelectasis, congestion, hypoxia, pharyngitis, pleural effusion

Miscellaneous: Diaphoresis

Stability Refrigerate; do not shake or freeze; protect from direct light; diluted daclizumab solution is stable for 24 hours if refrigerated or for 4 hours at room temperature; discard solution if colored or if particulate matter is present

Mechanism of Action A humanized IgG1 monoclonal antibody produced by recombinant DNA technology that binds specifically to the alpha subunit (p55 alpha, CD25, or Tac subunit) of the human high affinity interleukin-2 receptor (IL-2R) on the surface of activated lymphocytes inhibiting IL-2 binding; inhibits IL-2 mediated activation of lymphocytes which is involved in allograft rejection

Pharmacokinetics Daclizumab serum levels appeared to be somewhat lower in pediatric renal transplant patients than in adult transplant patients administered the same 1 mg/kg dosing regimen

Distribution: V_d: Adults: ~6 L

Half-life: 20 days

Usual Dosage I.V. (refer to individual protocols): Children and Adults:

Initial dose: 1 mg/kg given no more than 24 hours before transplantation, followed by 1 mg/kg/dose administered every 14 days for a total of 5 doses; maximum dose: 100 mg

Steroid-refractory graft-versus-host disease: 0.5-1.5 g/kg as a single dose administered for transient response (repeat doses have been given 11-48 days following the initial dose)

Dosing interval in renal impairment: No dosage adjustment necessary

Administration Parenteral: Daclizumab dose should be diluted in 50 mL NS solution. In fluid-restricted patients, a final concentration of 1 mg/mL can be administered over 15 minutes. When mixing the solution, gently invert the bag to avoid foaming; do not shake. Daclizumab solution should be administered within 4 hours of preparation if stored at room temperature; infuse over a 15-minute period via a peripheral or central vein

Monitoring Parameters CBC with differential, vital signs, immunologic monitoring of T cells

Reference Range Serum trough levels: 5-10 µg/mL

Dosage Forms Injection: 5 mg/mL (5 mL)

References
Vincenti F, Kirkman R, Light S, et al, "Interleukin-2-Receptor Blockade With Daclizumab to Prevent Acute Rejection in Renal Transplantation. Daclizumab Triple Therapy Study Group," *N Engl J Med*, 1998, 338(3):161-5.

♦ **Dacodyl® [OTC]** *see* Bisacodyl *on page 133*

Dactinomycin (dak ti noe MYE sin)

Related Information
Emetogenic Potential of Single Chemotherapeutic Agents *on page 1095*

Brand Names Cosmegen®

Synonyms ACT; Act-D; Actinomycin D

Therapeutic Category Antineoplastic Agent, Antibiotic

Generic Available No

Use Management (either alone or in combination with other treatment modalities) of Wilms' tumor, rhabdomyosarcoma, neuroblastoma, retinoblastoma, Ewing's sarcoma, trophoblastic neoplasms, testicular tumors and uterine sarcomas

Pregnancy Risk Factor C

Contraindications Hypersensitivity to dactinomycin or any component; patients with chickenpox or herpes zoster; avoid in infants <6 months of age since the incidence of adverse effects is increased in infants

Warnings The FDA currently recommends that procedures for proper handling and disposal of antineoplastic agents be considered. Dactinomycin is extremely irritating to tissues. If extravasation occurs during I.V. use, severe damage to soft tissue may occur leading to pain, swelling, ulceration, and necrosis.

Precautions Use with caution in patients with hepatobiliary dysfunction or in patients who have received radiation therapy; reduce dosage in patients receiving concurrent radiation therapy and in patients with hepatobiliary dysfunction; avoid administering live virus vaccinations after dactinomycin

Adverse Reactions
Central nervous system: Fatigue, fever
Dermatologic: Alopecia, erythema, hyperpigmentation of skin, desquamation, acne, maculopapular rash
Endocrine & metabolic: Hypocalcemia, hyperuricemia
Gastrointestinal: Anorexia, vomiting, diarrhea, stomatitis, proctitis, nausea
Hematologic: Myelosuppression (nadir: 2-3 weeks), leukopenia, thrombocytopenia, anemia
Hepatic: Hepatitis, hepatic veno-occlusive disease, elevated liver enzymes
Local: Soft tissue damage with extravasation
Miscellaneous: Anaphylactoid reaction, immunosuppression

Drug Interactions Dactinomycin potentiates the effects of radiation therapy; enflurane, halothane (increased hepatotoxicity); decreased effectiveness of vaccines given following dactinomycin

Stability Binds to cellulose filters, therefore, avoid in-line filtration; adsorbs to glass and plastic so dactinomycin should not be given by continuous or intermittent infusion; use of a diluent containing preservatives for reconstitution may result in a precipitate; any unused portion of the reconstituted 0.5 mg/mL solution should be discarded after 24 hours

Mechanism of Action Binds to the guanine portion of DNA intercalating between guanine and cytosine base pairs blocking replication and transcription of the DNA template; causes topoisomerase-mediated single-strand breaks in DNA

Pharmacokinetics
Distribution: Concentrates in nucleated cells and bone marrow; crosses the placenta; poor penetration into CSF (CSF:plasma ratio is <10%); distributes into submaxillary gland, liver, and kidney
Half-life: 3.5 hours (using radioimmunoassay)
Time to peak serum concentration: I.V.: Within 2-5 minutes
Elimination: ~10% of dose excreted as unchanged drug in urine; 15% recovered in feces; 50% appears in bile
(Continued)

Dactinomycin *(Continued)*

Usual Dosage Dosage should be based on body surface area in obese or edematous patients

Children >6 months and Adults: I.V. (refer to individual protocols): 15 mcg/kg/day or 400-600 mcg/m²/day (maximum dose: 500 mcg/day) for 5 days, may repeat every 3-6 weeks; or 2.5 mg/m² given in divided doses over 1 week; or 0.75-2 mg/m² as a single dose given at intervals of 3-6 weeks has been used

Administration Parenteral: I.V.: For I.V. administration only; since drug is extremely irritating to tissues, **do not give I.M. or S.C.;** avoid extravasation; use a D₅W or NS flush before and after a dactinomycin dose to ensure venous patency; administer by slow IVP over a few minutes at a concentration not to exceed 500 mcg/mL into the side-port of a freely flowing I.V. infusion; if extravasation occurs, apply cold compresses to the site

Monitoring Parameters CBC with differential and platelet count, liver function tests and renal function tests

Patient Information Notify physician if fever, sore throat, bleeding, or bruising occurs

Dosage Forms Powder for injection, lyophilized: 0.5 mg

References

Berg SL, Grisell DL, DeLaney TF, et al, "Principles of Treatment of Pediatric Solid Tumors," *Pediatr Clin North Am*, 1991, 38(2):249-67.

Berkowitz RS and Goldstein DP, "Gestational Trophoblastic Disease," *Cancer*, 1995, 76(10 Suppl):2079-85.

Carli M, Pastore G, Perilongo G, et al, "Tumor Response and Toxicity After Single High-Dose Versus Standard Five-Day Divided Dose Dactinomycin in Childhood Rhabdomyosarcoma," *J Clin Oncol*, 1988, 6(4):654-8.

♦ **Dalacin® C [Hydrochloride] Topical (Canada)** *see* Clindamycin *on page 237*

♦ **Dalacin® C [Hydrochloride] Vaginal Cream (Canada)** *see* Clindamycin *on page 237*

♦ **Dalalone D.P.® Injection** *see* Dexamethasone *on page 294*

♦ **Dalalone® Injection** *see* Dexamethasone *on page 294*

♦ **Dalalone L.A.® Injection** *see* Dexamethasone *on page 294*

♦ **Dalmane®** *see* Flurazepam *on page 434*

♦ **d-Alpha Tocopherol** *see* Vitamin E *on page 982*

♦ **Dantrium®** *see* Dantrolene *on page 282*

Dantrolene *(DAN troe leen)*

Brand Names Dantrium®

Available Salts Dantrolene Sodium

Therapeutic Category Antidote, Malignant Hyperthermia; Hyperthermia, Treatment; Skeletal Muscle Relaxant, Nonparalytic

Generic Available No

Use Treatment of spasticity associated with upper motor neuron disorders such as spinal cord injury, stroke, cerebral palsy, or multiple sclerosis; also used as treatment of malignant hyperthermia

Pregnancy Risk Factor C

Contraindications Active hepatic disease; should not be administered where spasticity is used to maintain posture or balance

Warnings May cause hepatotoxicity; overt hepatitis has been most frequently observed between the third and twelfth month of therapy; hepatic injury appears to be greater in females and in patients >35 years of age

Precautions Use with caution in patients with impaired cardiac or pulmonary function or history of previous liver disease

Adverse Reactions

Cardiovascular/respiratory: Pleural effusion with pericarditis, tachycardia

Central nervous system: Seizures, drowsiness, dizziness, lightheadedness, confusion, headache, fatigue, speech disturbances, mental depression, chills, fever

Dermatologic: Rash, photosensitization, acne-like rash, pruritus, urticaria, abnormal hair growth

Gastrointestinal: Diarrhea, nausea, vomiting, severe constipation, GI bleeding, abdominal cramps, dysphagia

Genitourinary: Urinary retention or frequency, urinary incontinence

Hepatic: Hepatitis

Local: Phlebitis

Neuromuscular & skeletal: Muscle weakness, myalgia, backache

Ocular: Visual disturbances, excessive tearing

Renal: Hematuria

Drug Interactions Use with verapamil may result in hyperkalemia and myocardial depression; estrogen increases incidence of hepatotoxicity when used concomitantly; additive CNS depressive effects with other CNS depressants; increased toxicity with MAO inhibitors, phenothiazines, clindamycin, warfarin, clofibrate, and tolbutamide

Stability Protect from light; use reconstituted injection within 6 hours; incompatible with dextrose, NS, or bacteriostatic water for injection; precipitates when placed in glass containers for infusion

Mechanism of Action Acts directly on skeletal muscle by interfering with release of calcium ion from the sarcoplasmic reticulum; prevents or reduces the increase in myoplasmic calcium ion concentration that activates the acute catabolic processes associated with malignant hyperthermia

Pharmacokinetics
Absorption: Oral: 35%
Metabolism: Extensive
Half-life:
Children: 7.3 hours
Adults: 8.7 hours
Elimination: 25% excreted in urine as metabolites and unchanged drug; 45% to 50% excreted in feces via bile

Usual Dosage
Spasticity: Oral:
Children: Initial: 0.5 mg/kg/dose twice daily, increase frequency to 3-4 times/day at 4- to 7-day intervals, then increase dose by 0.5 mg/kg to a maximum of 3 mg/kg/dose 2-4 times/day up to 400 mg/day
Adults: 25 mg/day to start, increase frequency to 2-4 times/day, then increase dose by 25 mg every 4-7 days to a maximum of 100 mg 2-4 times/day or 400 mg/day
Hyperthermia: Children and Adults:
Preoperative prophylaxis:
Oral: 4-8 mg/kg/day in 4 divided doses given 1-2 days prior to surgery for those patients at risk; to prevent recurrence, administer last dosage 3-4 hours before scheduled surgery
I.V.: 2.5 mg/kg 1¼ hours before surgery and infused over 1 hour; additional doses may be needed during surgery especially for prolonged surgery
Crisis: I.V.: 1 mg/kg; may repeat as needed to a maximum cumulative dose of 10 mg/kg; if physiologic and metabolic abnormalities reappear, repeat regimen
Postcrisis follow-up: Oral: 4-8 mg/kg/day in 4 divided doses for 1-3 days; I.V. dantrolene may be used when oral therapy is not practical; individualize dosage beginning with 1 mg/kg or more as the clinical situation dictates

Administration
Oral: Contents of capsule may be mixed with juice or liquid
Parenteral: Reconstitute by adding 60 mL sterile water (**not bacteriostatic water for injection**), resultant concentration 0.333 mg/mL; administer by rapid I.V. injection; for infusion, do **not** further dilute with NS or dextrose; place solution in plastic container for continuous infusion

Monitoring Parameters Baseline and periodic liver function tests; temperature (hyperthermia use)

Patient Information Avoid unnecessary exposure to sunlight; avoid alcohol; causes drowsiness and may impair ability to perform hazardous functions requiring mental alertness or physical coordination

Nursing Implications Avoid extravasation since dantrolene is a tissue irritant

Dosage Forms
Capsule, as sodium: 25 mg, 50 mg, 100 mg
Powder for injection, as sodium: 20 mg

Extemporaneous Preparations A 5 mg/mL suspension may be made by adding five 100 mg capsules to a citric acid solution (150 mg citric acid powder in 10 mL water) and then adding syrup to a total volume of 100 mL; shake well; stable 2 days in refrigerator
Nahata MC and Hipple TF, *Pediatric Drug Formulations*, 3rd ed, Cincinnati, OH: Harvey Whitney Books Co, 1997.

♦ **Dantrolene Sodium** see Dantrolene on page 282
♦ **Dapa® [OTC]** see Acetaminophen on page 26
♦ **Dapacin® [OTC]** see Acetaminophen on page 26

Dapsone (DAP sone)
Brand Names Avlosulfon®
Synonyms Diaminodiphenylsulfone
(Continued)

Dapsone *(Continued)*

Therapeutic Category Antibiotic, Sulfone; Leprostatic Agent

Generic Available Yes

Use Treatment of leprosy due to susceptible strains of *M. leprae*; treatment of dermatitis herpetiformis; prophylaxis against *Pneumocystis carinii* pneumonia (PCP) in patients who cannot tolerate sulfamethoxazole/trimethoprim or aerosolized pentamidine; prophylaxis against toxoplasmic encephalitis in patients who cannot tolerate sulfamethoxazole/trimethoprim

Pregnancy Risk Factor C

Contraindications Hypersensitivity to dapsone or any component; patients with severe anemia

Precautions Use with caution in patients with G-6-PD deficiency, methemoglobin reductase deficiency or hemoglobin M; in patients receiving drugs capable of inducing hemolysis; hypersensitivity to other sulfonamides

Adverse Reactions

Cardiovascular: Tachycardia

Central nervous system: Psychotic episodes, hallucinations, insomnia, vertigo, irritability, headache, fever, uncoordinated speech

Dermatologic: Exfoliative dermatitis, erythema multiforme, toxic epidermal necrolysis, urticaria, morbilliform reactions, erythema nodosum, photosensitivity

Endocrine & metabolic: Hyperkalemia, hypoalbuminemia

Gastrointestinal: Nausea, vomiting, abdominal pain, anorexia

Hematologic: Hemolytic anemia, methemoglobinemia, leukopenia, agranulocytosis, aplastic anemia, neutropenia

Hepatic: Hepatitis, cholestatic jaundice; elevated alkaline phosphatase, AST, bilirubin, and LDH

Neuromuscular & skeletal: Muscle weakness, peripheral neuropathy

Ocular: Blurred vision

Otic: Tinnitus

Renal: Acute tubular necrosis, nephrotic syndrome, albuminuria

Miscellaneous: Lupus erythematosus, mononucleosis-like syndrome

Drug Interactions Didanosine (decreases dapsone absorption); rifampin (decreases dapsone concentrations); trimethoprim (increases dapsone concentration); pyrimethamine, nitrofurantoin, primaquine (increase risk of hematologic side effects)

Food Interactions Do not administer with antacids, alkaline foods, or alkaline drugs (may decrease dapsone absorption)

Stability Protect from light

Mechanism of Action Dapsone is a sulfone antimicrobial. The mechanism of action of the sulfones is similar to that of the sulfonamides. Sulfonamides are competitive antagonists of para-aminobenzoic acid (PABA) and inhibit folic acid synthesis in susceptible organisms.

Pharmacokinetics

Absorption: Oral: 86% to 100%

Distribution: Distributes into skin, muscle, kidneys, liver, sweat, sputum, tears, and bile; distributes into breast milk

Protein binding: 50% to 90%

Metabolism: Acetylated and hydroxylated in the liver

Half-life:

Children: 15.1 hours

Adults: 13-83 hours (mean: 20-30 hours)

Time to peak serum concentration: Within 2-8 hours

Elimination: 5% to 20% of dose excreted in urine as unchanged drug; 70% to 85% excreted in urine as metabolites; small amount excreted in feces

Usual Dosage Oral:

Children ≥1 month of age:

Prophylaxis for first episode of opportunistic disease due to *Toxoplasma gondii*: 2 mg/kg or 15 mg/m^2 (maximum dose: 25 mg) once daily in combination with pyrimethamine 1 mg/kg once daily and leucovorin 5 mg every 3 days

Primary and secondary PCP prophylaxis (see "Note" in Additional Information): 2 mg/kg/day once daily (maximum dose: 100 mg/day), or 4 mg/kg/dose once weekly (maximum dose: 200 mg)

Children:

Leprosy: 1-2 mg/kg/day given once daily in combination therapy; maximum dose: 100 mg/day

Adults:

Leprosy: 50-100 mg once daily; combination therapy with one or more antileprosy drugs is recommended to avoid dapsone resistance

Dermatitis herpetiformis: Initial: 50 mg once daily; maintenance dosage range: 25-400 mg/day

PCP treatment: 100 mg once daily in combination with trimethoprim

Primary and secondary PCP prophylaxis: 50 mg twice daily; or dapsone 50 mg once daily plus pyrimethamine 50 mg orally every week plus leucovorin 25 mg orally every week; or dapsone 200 mg orally plus pyrimethamine 75 mg orally plus leucovorin 25 mg orally every week

Toxoplasma gondii prophylaxis: 50 mg once daily plus pyrimethamine 50 mg orally every week, plus leucovorin 25 mg orally every week

Administration Oral: Administer with water

Monitoring Parameters CBC with differential, platelet count, hemoglobin, hematocrit, liver function tests, and urinalysis

Patient Information May cause photosensitivity; notify physician if fever, sore throat, pallor, fatigue, rash, purpura, or jaundice occurs

Additional Information Note: Guidelines for prophylaxis of *Pneumocystis carinii* pneumonia: Initiate PCP prophylaxis in the following patients: In all HIV-exposed children at 4-6 weeks of age and continue through the first year of life or until HIV infection has been reasonably excluded; children 1-5 years of age with CD4+ count <500 or CD4+ percentage <15%; children 6-12 years of age with CD4+ count <200 or CD4+ percentage <15%. Folinic acid (leucovorin) should be given if bone marrow suppression occurs.

Dosage Forms Tablet: 25 mg, 100 mg

Extemporaneous Preparations One report indicated that dapsone may not be well absorbed when administered to children as suspensions made from pulverized tablets

Mirochnick M, Clarke D, Brenn A, et al, "Low Serum Dapsone Concentrations in Children Receiving an Extemporaneously Prepared Oral Formulation," [Abstract Th B 365], APS-SPR, Baltimore, MD: 1992.

Jacobus Pharmaceutical Company (609) 921-7447 makes a 2 mg/mL proprietary liquid formulation available under an IND for the prophylaxis of *Pneumocystis carinii* pneumonia

References

1999 USPHS/IDSA Guidelines for the Prevention of Opportunistic Infections in Persons Infected With Human Immunodeficiency Virus. USPHS/IDSA Prevention of Opportunistic Infections Working Group," *MMWR Morb Mortal Wkly Rep*, 1999, 48(RR-10): 1-66.

Barnett ED, Pelton SI, Mirochnick M, et al, "Dapsone for Prevention of *Pneumocystis* Pneumonia in Children With Acquired Immunodeficiency Syndrome," *Pediatr Infect Dis J*, 1994, 13(1):72-4.

Mirochnick M, Michaels M, Clarke D, et al, "Pharmacokinetics of Dapsone in Children," *J Pediatr*, 1993, 122(5 Pt 1):806-9.

Stavola JJ and Noel GJ, "Efficacy and Safety of Dapsone Prophylaxis Against *Pneumocystis carinii* Pneumonia in Human Immunodeficiency Virus-Infected Children," *Pediatr Infect Dis J*, 1993, 12(8):644-7.

♦ **Daraprim®** *see* Pyrimethamine *on page 828*

♦ **Darvocet-N®** *see* Propoxyphene and Acetaminophen *on page 815*

♦ **Darvocet-N® 100** *see* Propoxyphene and Acetaminophen *on page 815*

♦ **Darvon®** *see* Propoxyphene *on page 814*

♦ **Darvon-N®** *see* Propoxyphene *on page 814*

♦ **Daunomycin** *see* Daunorubicin *on page 285*

Daunorubicin (daw noe ROO bi sin)

Related Information

Extravasation Treatment *on page 1050*

Brand Names Cerubidine®

Available Salts Daunorubicin Hydrochloride

Synonyms Daunomycin; DNR; Rubidomycin

Therapeutic Category Antineoplastic Agent, Anthracycline; Antineoplastic Agent, Antibiotic

Generic Available No

Use In combination with other agents in the treatment of leukemias (ALL, AML)

Pregnancy Risk Factor D

Contraindications Hypersensitivity to daunorubicin or any component; CHF, left ventricular ejection fraction <30% to 40%, or arrhythmias; pre-existing bone marrow suppression

Warnings The FDA currently recommends that procedures for proper handling and disposal of antineoplastic agents be considered; I.V. use only; severe local tissue necrosis will result if extravasation occurs; irreversible myocardial toxicity may occur as total dosage approaches 550 mg/m^2 in adults, 400 mg/m^2 in patients receiving chest radiation, 300 mg/m^2 in children ≥2 years of age, or 10 mg/kg in children <2 years; this may occur during therapy or several months after therapy; (Continued)

Daunorubicin *(Continued)*

total cumulative dose should take into account previous or concomitant treatment with cardiotoxic agents or irradiation of chest; infants and children may be more susceptible to anthracycline-induced cardiotoxicity than adults; severe myelosuppression is possible when used in therapeutic doses

Precautions Reduce dosage in patients with hepatic, biliary, or renal impairment

Adverse Reactions

Cardiovascular: Cardiotoxicity, CHF (dose-related, may occur 7-8 years after treatment), arrhythmias, EKG abnormalities

Central nervous system: Fever, chills

Dermatologic: Alopecia, hyperpigmentation of skin and nail beds, urticaria, pruritus

Endocrine & metabolic: Hyperuricemia, infertility, sterility

Gastrointestinal: Stomatitis, esophagitis, nausea, vomiting, diarrhea

Genitourinary: Discoloration of urine (red-orange)

Hematologic: Myelosuppression (thrombocytopenia, leukopenia)

Hepatic: Elevated serum bilirubin, AST, and alkaline phosphatase

Local: Severe tissue necrosis with extravasation

Stability Protect from light; reconstituted solution is stable for 48 hours when refrigerated and 24 hours at room temperature; a color change from red to blue/purple indicates decomposition of the drug; unstable in solutions with a pH >8; incompatible with heparin, sodium bicarbonate, 5-FU, and dexamethasone

Mechanism of Action Inhibition of DNA and RNA synthesis by intercalating between DNA base pairs, uncoiling of the helix, and by steric obstruction; not cell cycle-specific for the S-phase of cell division; may cause free radical damage to DNA

Pharmacokinetics

Distribution: Widely distributed in tissues such as spleen, heart, kidneys, liver, and lungs; does not cross the blood-brain barrier; crosses the placenta

Metabolism: To daunorubicinol (active)

Half-life, terminal: 14-18.5 hours

Daunorubicinol, active metabolite: 26.7 hours

Elimination: 40% of dose excreted in bile; ~14% to 23% excreted in urine as metabolite and unchanged drug

Usual Dosage I.V. (refer to individual protocols):

Children <2 years or <0.5 m^2: Dosage should be calculated on the basis of body weight rather than body surface area: 1 mg/kg or per protocol with frequency dependent on regimen employed

Children:

ALL combination therapy: Remission induction: 25-45 mg/m^2 on days 1 and 8 of cycle, or 30-45 mg/m^2/day for 3 days every 3-4 weeks, or 25 mg/m^2 every week for 4 weeks

AML combination therapy: Induction: I.V. continuous infusion: 30-60 mg/m^2/day on days 1-3 of cycle, or 20 mg/m^2/day for 4 days every 14 days

Adults: 30-60 mg/m^2/day for 3-5 days, repeat dose in 3-4 weeks; total cumulative dose should not exceed 400-600 mg/m^2

AML: Single agent induction: 60 mg/m^2/day for 3 days; repeat every 3-4 weeks

AML: Combination therapy induction: 45 mg/m^2/day for 3 days of the first course of induction therapy; subsequent courses: Every day for 2 days

ALL: Combination therapy: Remission induction: 45 mg/m^2 on days 1, 2, and 3 of induction course

Dosing adjustment in hepatic or renal impairment: Reduce dose by 25% in patients with serum bilirubin of 1.2-3 mg/dL; reduce dose by 50% in patients with serum bilirubin and/or creatinine >3 mg/dL

Administration Parenteral: Drug is very irritating, do not inject I.M. or S.C.; administer IVP diluting the reconstituted dose in 10-15 mL NS and administering over 2-3 minutes into the tubing of a rapidly infusing I.V. solution of D$_5$W or NS; daunorubicin has also been diluted in 100 mL of D$_5$W or NS and infused over 30-45 minutes or as a continuous 24-hour infusion

Monitoring Parameters CBC with differential and platelet count, liver function test, EKG, ventricular ejection fraction, renal function test; patency of I.V. line

Patient Information Transient red-orange discoloration of urine can occur for up to 48 hours after a dose; notify physician if fever, sore throat, bleeding, or bruising occurs

Nursing Implications Leukemic patients should receive prophylactic allopurinol to prevent acute urate nephropathy; avoid extravasation; if extravasation occurs, apply a cold compress immediately for 30-60 minutes, then alternate off/on every 15 minutes for 1 day; apply 1.5 mL of dimethylsulfoxide 99% (w/v) solution to the site every 6 hours for 14 days; allow to air-dry; do not cover

Additional Information Myelosuppressive effects:
  WBC: Severe
  Platelets: Severe
  Onset (days): 7
  Nadir (days): 10-14
  Recovery (days): 21-28
Dosage Forms
  Injection, as hydrochloride: 5 mg/mL (4 mL)
  Powder for injection, lyophilized, as hydrochloride: 20 mg
References
  Crom WR, Glynn-Barnhart AM, Rodman JH, et al, "Pharmacokinetics of Anticancer Drugs in Children," *Clin Pharmacokinet*, 1987, 12(3):168-213.

Deferoxamine (de fer OKS a meen)

Brand Names Desferal® Mesylate
Available Salts Deferoxamine Mesylate
Therapeutic Category Antidote, Aluminum Toxicity; Antidote, Iron Toxicity; Chelating Agent, Parenteral
Generic Available No
Use Acute iron intoxication; chronic iron overload secondary to multiple transfusions; diagnostic test for iron overload; used investigationally in the treatment of aluminum accumulation in renal failure
Pregnancy Risk Factor C
Contraindications Patients with severe renal disease, anuria, or primary hemochromatosis
Warnings Cataracts, decreased visual acuity, impaired peripheral and color vision, impaired night vision, and retinal pigmentary abnormalities have been reported after usage for prolonged periods at high dosages or in patients with low ferritin levels; periodic eye exams are recommended while on chronic therapy; neurotoxicity-related auditory abnormalities have been reported including high frequency sensorineural hearing loss; periodic auditory exams are recommended
Precautions Use with caution in patients with pyelonephritis; may increase susceptibility to *Yersinia enterocolitica* infections; flushing of the skin, urticaria, hypotension, and shock have been reported after rapid I.V. administration
Adverse Reactions
  Cardiovascular: Flushing, hypotension with rapid I.V. injection, tachycardia, shock, edema
  Central nervous system: Fever
  Dermatologic: Erythema, urticaria, pruritus, rash, cutaneous wheal formation
  Endocrine & Metabolic: Growth impairment
  Gastrointestinal: Abdominal discomfort, diarrhea
  Genitourinary: Discoloration of urine (reddish color)
  Local: Pain, induration at injection site
  Neuromuscular & skeletal: Leg cramps
  (Continued)

Deferoxamine *(Continued)*

Ocular: Blurred vision; cataracts; impaired peripheral, color, and night vision; retinal pigmentary abnormalities

Otic: Hearing loss, tinnitus

Miscellaneous: Anaphylaxis, possible increased risk of infections particularly with *Y. enterocolitica*

Stability Protect from light; reconstituted solutions are stable for 7 days at room temperature

Mechanism of Action Complexes with trivalent ions (ferric ions) to form ferrioxamine, which is removed by the kidneys

Pharmacokinetics

Absorption: Oral: <15%

Metabolism: By plasma enzymes to ferrioxamine

Half-life:

Deferoxamine: 6.1 hours

Ferrioxamine: 5.8 hours

Elimination: Renal excretion of the metabolite iron chelate and unchanged drug

Usual Dosage

Children:

Acute iron intoxication:

I.M.: 50 mg/kg/dose every 6 hours; maximum dose: 6 g/day

I.V.: 15 mg/kg/hour; maximum dose: 6 g/day

Alternative dosing I.M. or I.V.: 20 mg/kg or 600 mg/m^2 initially followed by 10 mg/kg or 300 mg/m^2 at 4-hour intervals for 2 doses; subsequent doses of 10 mg/kg or 300 mg/m^2 every 4-12 hours may be repeated depending upon the clinical response; maximum dose: 6 g/day

Chronic iron overload:

I.V.: 15 mg/kg/hour; maximum dose: 12 g/day

S.C. infusion via a portable, controlled infusion device: 20-50 mg/kg/day over 8-12 hours; maximum dose: 2 g/day

Adults:

Acute iron intoxication:

I.M.: 1 g stat, then 0.5 g every 4 hours for two doses, additional doses of 0.5 g every 4-12 hours up to 6 g/day may be needed depending upon the clinical response

I.V.: 15 mg/kg/hour; maximum dose: 6 g/day

Chronic iron overload:

I.M.: 0.5-1 g/day

I.V.: 15 mg/kg/hour; maximum dose: 12 g/day

S.C. infusion via a portable, controlled infusion device: 1-2 g/day over 8-24 hours

Aluminum-induced bone disease: 20-40 mg/kg every hemodialysis treatment, frequency dependent on clinical status of the patient

Administration Parenteral: Add 2 mL sterile water to 500 mg vial; for I.M. or S.C. administration, no further dilution is required; for I.V. infusion, dilute in dextrose, NS, LR: 10 mg/mL (maximum concentration: 250 mg/mL); maximum rate of infusion: 15 mg/kg/hour; local reactions at the site of subcutaneous infusion may be minimized by diluting the deferoxamine in 5-10 mL sterile water and adding 1 mg hydrocortisone to each mL of deferoxamine solution

Monitoring Parameters Serum ferritin, iron, total iron binding capacity; ophthalmologic exam and audiometry with chronic use

Reference Range Effective plasma concentration: 3-15 mcg/mL

Patient Information Report any hearing loss, night blindness, decreased visual acuity, impaired peripheral vision, or loss of color vision; may cause the urine to turn a reddish color

Nursing Implications Local injection site reactions may be minimized by daily rotation of subcutaneous injection sites and by applying topical corticosteroids; painful lumps formed under the skin may indicate that the rate of S.C. administration exceeds the rate of absorption from the injection site or the needle is inserted too close to the dermis

Additional Information Has been used investigationally as a single 40 mg/kg I.V. dose over 2 hours, to promote mobilization of aluminum from tissue stores as an aid in the diagnosis of aluminum-associated osteodystrophy

Dosage Forms Powder for injection, as mesylate: 500 mg

References

Bentur Y, McGuigan M, and Koren G, "Deferoxamine (Desferrioxamine): New Toxicities for an Old Drug," *Drug Saf*, 1991, 6(1):37-46.

Cohen AR, Mizanin J, and Schwartz E, "Rapid Removal of Excessive Iron With Daily, High-Dose Intravenous Chelation Therapy," *J Pediatr*, 1989, 115(1):151-5.

Freedman MH, Olivieri N, Benson L, et al, "Clinical Studies on Iron Chelation in Patients With Thalassemia Major," *Haematologica*, 1990, 75(Suppl 5):74-83.

Giardina PJ, Grady RW, Ehlers KH, et al, "Current Therapy of Cooley's Anemia: A Decade of Experience With Subcutaneous Desferrioxamine," *Ann N Y Acad Sci*, 1990, 612:275-85.

Kirking MH, "Treatment of Chronic Iron Overload," *Clin Pharm*, 1991, 10(10):775-83.

Pippard MJ, "Iron Metabolism and Iron Chelation in the Thalassemia Disorders," *Haematologica*, 1990, 75(Suppl 5):66-71.

♦ **Deferoxamine Mesylate** *see Deferoxamine on page 287*
♦ **Deficol® [OTC]** *see Bisacodyl on page 133*
♦ **Degas® [OTC]** *see Simethicone on page 868*
♦ **Degest® 2 Ophthalmic [OTC]** *see Naphazoline on page 671*
♦ **Dehydral™ (Canada)** *see Methenamine on page 615*
♦ **Dehydrated Alcohol Injection** *see Ethyl Alcohol on page 394*
♦ **Dekasol® Injection** *see Dexamethasone on page 294*
♦ **Dekasol-L.A.® Injection** *see Dexamethasone on page 294*
♦ **Del Aqua-5® Gel** *see Benzoyl Peroxide on page 126*
♦ **Del Aqua-10® Gel** *see Benzoyl Peroxide on page 126*
♦ **Delatest® Injection** *see Testosterone on page 905*
♦ **Delatestryl® Injection** *see Testosterone on page 905*
♦ **Delaxin®** *see Methocarbamol on page 619*
♦ **Delcort® Topical** *see Hydrocortisone on page 486*
♦ **Delestrogen®** *see Estradiol on page 386*
♦ **Delsym® [OTC]** *see Dextromethorphan on page 304*
♦ **Delta-Cortef® Oral** *see Prednisolone on page 791*
♦ **Deltacortisone** *see Prednisone on page 794*
♦ **Deltadehydrocortisone** *see Prednisone on page 794*
♦ **Deltahydrocortisone** *see Prednisolone on page 791*
♦ **Deltasone®** *see Prednisone on page 794*
♦ **Delta-Tritex® Topical** *see Triamcinolone on page 946*
♦ **Del-Vi-A®** *see Vitamin A on page 981*
♦ **Demadex® Injection** *see Torsemide on page 939*
♦ **Demadex® Oral** *see Torsemide on page 939*

Demeclocycline (dem e kloe SYE kleen)

Brand Names Declomycin®
Available Salts Demeclocycline Hydrochloride
Synonyms Demethylchlortetracycline
Therapeutic Category Antibiotic, Tetracycline Derivative
Generic Available No
Use Treatment of susceptible bacterial infections (acne, gonorrhea, pertussis, chronic bronchitis, and urinary tract infections) caused by both gram-negative and gram-positive organisms; treatment of chronic syndrome of inappropriate antidiuretic hormone (SIADH) secretion
Pregnancy Risk Factor D
Contraindications Hypersensitivity to demeclocycline, tetracyclines, or any component
Warnings Photosensitivity reactions occur frequently with this drug, avoid prolonged exposure to sunlight; do not use tanning equipment. Do not administer to children ≤8 years of age; use of tetracyclines during tooth development may cause permanent discoloration of the teeth and enamel hypoplasia; do not administer to pregnant women; use of tetracyclines in pregnant women may result in retardation of bone growth and skeletal development of the fetus; prolonged use may result in superinfection. Use of outdated tetracyclines have caused a Fanconi-like syndrome.
Precautions Modify dosage in patients with impaired renal function
Adverse Reactions
Central nervous system: Increased intracranial pressure, bulging fontanels in infants
Dermatologic: Rash, pruritus, photosensitivity, exfoliative dermatitis, discoloration of nails, Stevens-Johnson syndrome
Endocrine & metabolic: Diabetes insipidus syndrome
Gastrointestinal: Nausea, vomiting, diarrhea, anorexia, pancreatitis
Hematologic: Leukopenia, neutropenia, thrombocytopenia
Hepatic: Hepatotoxicity
(Continued)

Demeclocycline *(Continued)*

Neuromuscular & skeletal: Paresthesia
Renal: Azotemia
Miscellaneous: Superinfections

Drug Interactions Antacids, calcium, magnesium, zinc, and iron preparations may decrease absorption of demeclocycline

Food Interactions Food, milk, milk formulas, and dairy products decrease absorption of demeclocycline

Mechanism of Action Inhibits protein synthesis by binding with the 30S ribosomal subunits and preventing the binding of transfer RNA to those ribosomes of susceptible bacteria; may also cause alterations in the cytoplasmic membrane

Pharmacodynamics Onset of action for diuresis in SIADH: Within 5 days

Pharmacokinetics

Absorption: ~60% to 80% of dose absorbed from the GI tract; food and dairy products reduce absorption by 50% or more
Distribution: Excreted into breast milk
Protein binding: 90% to 95%
Metabolism: Small amounts metabolized in the liver to inactive metabolites; enterohepatically recycled
Half-life: 10-17 hours (prolonged with reduced renal function)
Time to peak serum concentration: Oral: Within 3-6 hours
Elimination: Excreted as unchanged drug (42% to 50%) in urine

Usual Dosage Oral:

Children >8 years: 8-12 mg/kg/day divided every 6-12 hours
Adults: 150 mg 4 times/day or 300 mg twice daily
Uncomplicated gonorrhea: 600 mg stat, 300 mg every 12 hours for 4 days (3 g total)
SIADH: 900-1200 mg/day or 13-15 mg/kg/day divided every 6-8 hours initially, then decrease to 600-900 mg/day

Dosing adjustment in renal impairment: Not recommended

Administration Oral: Administer 1 hour before or 2 hours after food or milk with plenty of fluids; do not administer with food, milk, dairy products, antacids, zinc, or iron supplements

Monitoring Parameters CBC, renal and hepatic function tests

Test Interactions May interfere with tests for urinary glucose (false-negative urine glucose using Clinistix®, Tes-Tape®)

Patient Information Avoid prolonged exposure to sunlight or sunlamps; sunscreens provide only limited protection against photosensitivity reactions; may discolor fingernails; avoid taking dosages at bedtime

Dosage Forms

Capsule, as hydrochloride: 150 mg
Tablet, as hydrochloride: 150 mg, 300 mg

References

Abdi EA and Bishop S, "The Syndrome of Inappropriate Antidiuretic Hormone Secretion With Carcinoma of the Tongue," Med Pediatr Oncol, 1988, 16(3):210-5.
Troyer AD, "Demeclocycline. Treatment for Syndrome of Inappropriate Antidiuretic Hormone Secretion," JAMA, 1977, 237(25):2723-6.

♦ **Deponit® Patch** *see* Nitroglycerin *on page 690*

♦ **Depopred® Injection** *see* Methylprednisolone *on page 629*

♦ **Depo-Provera® Injection** *see* Medroxyprogesterone *on page 599*

♦ **Depotest® Injection** *see* Testosterone *on page 905*

♦ **Depo®-Testosterone Injection** *see* Testosterone *on page 905*

♦ **Dermacort® Topical** *see* Hydrocortisone *on page 486*

♦ **Dermarest Dricort® Topical** *see* Hydrocortisone *on page 486*

♦ **Derma-Smoothe/FS® Topical** *see* Fluocinolone *on page 425*

♦ **Dermazin™ (Canada)** *see* Silver Sulfadiazine *on page 867*

♦ **Dermolate® Topical [OTC]** *see* Hydrocortisone *on page 486*

♦ **Dermoplast® [OTC]** *see* Benzocaine *on page 124*

♦ **Dermtex® HC with Aloe Topical [OTC]** *see* Hydrocortisone *on page 486*

♦ **Desenex® [OTC]** *see* Tolnaftate *on page 936*

♦ **Desenex® (Canada)** *see* Undecylenic Acid and Derivatives *on page 962*

♦ **Desferal® Mesylate** *see* Deferoxamine *on page 287*

Desipramine (des IP ra meen)

Related Information
Comparison of Adverse Effects of Antidepressants *on page 1030*
Comparison of Usual Adult Dosage and Mechanism of Action of Antidepressants
on page 1029
Drugs and Breast-Feeding *on page 1213*
Overdose and Toxicology *on page 1191*

Brand Names Norpramin®; PMS-Desipramine (Canada)

Available Salts Desipramine Hydrochloride

Therapeutic Category Antidepressant, Tricyclic

Generic Available Yes: Tablet

Use Treatment of various forms of depression, often in conjunction with psycho-therapy; analgesic in chronic pain, peripheral neuropathies

Pregnancy Risk Factor C

Contraindications Hypersensitivity to desipramine (cross-sensitivity with other tricyclic antidepressants may occur) or any component; patients receiving MAO inhibitors within past 14 days; narrow-angle glaucoma

Warnings Do not discontinue abruptly in patients receiving long-term high-dose therapy; some formulations contain tartrazine which may cause allergic reaction

Precautions Use with caution in patients with cardiovascular disease, conduction disturbances, urinary retention, seizure disorders, hyperthyroidism or those receiving thyroid replacement

Adverse Reactions Less sedation and anticholinergic adverse effects than amitriptyline or imipramine

Cardiovascular: Arrhythmias, hypotension; asymptomatic EKG changes and minor increases in diastolic blood pressure and heart rate have been noted in children receiving >3.5 mg/kg/day; **Note:** 4 cases of sudden death have been reported in children 5-14 years of age; an association between desipramine and sudden death was not shown to be significant in one retrospective study; further studies are needed

Central nervous system: Sedation, confusion, dizziness

Dermatologic: Photosensitivity

Endocrine & metabolic: SIADH

Gastrointestinal: Constipation, nausea, vomiting, xerostomia, weight gain

Genitourinary: Urinary retention, discoloration of urine (blue-green)

Hematologic: Blood dyscrasias

Hepatic: Hepatitis

Ocular: Blurred vision, increases intraocular pressure

Otic: Tinnitus

Miscellaneous: Hypersensitivity reactions

Drug Interactions Cytochrome P-450 isoenzyme CYP1A2 and CYP2D6 substrate; isoenzyme CYP2D6 inhibitor

May decrease effects of guanethidine and clonidine; may increase effects of CNS depressants, alcohol, adrenergic agents, anticholinergic agents; with MAO inhibitors, fever, tachycardia, hypertension, seizures, and death may occur; cimetidine may decrease desipramine clearance and increase plasma concentrations; interactions similar to other tricyclics may occur

Food Interactions May increase riboflavin dietary requirements
(Continued)

Desipramine *(Continued)*

Mechanism of Action Increases the synaptic concentration of serotonin and/or norepinephrine in the central nervous system by inhibition of their reuptake by the presynaptic neuronal membrane

Pharmacodynamics
Onset of antidepressant effects: Occasionally seen in 2-5 days
Maximum antidepressant effects: After more than 2 weeks

Pharmacokinetics
Absorption: Well absorbed from the GI tract
Distribution: V_d: Adults: 21 L/kg; distributes into breast milk (concentrations approximately equal to maternal plasma)
Protein binding: 90%
Metabolism: In the liver
Half-life, adults: 12-57 hours
Elimination: 70% in urine

Usual Dosage Oral:
Children 6-12 years: 1-3 mg/kg/day in divided doses; monitor carefully with doses >3 mg/kg/day; maximum dose: 5 mg/kg/day
Adolescents: Initial: 25-50 mg/day; gradually increase to 100 mg/day in single or divided doses; maximum dose: 150 mg/day
Adults: Initial: 75 mg/day in divided doses; increase gradually to 150-200 mg/day in divided or single dose; maximum dose: 300 mg/day

Administration Oral: Administer with food to decrease GI upset

Monitoring Parameters Blood pressure, heart rate, EKG, mental status, weight
Long-term use: CBC with differential, liver enzymes, serum concentrations

Reference Range
Therapeutic: 150-300 ng/mL (SI: 560-1125 nmol/L)
Possible toxicity: >300 ng/mL (SI: >1070 nmol/L)
Toxic: >1000 ng/mL (SI: >3750 nmol/L)

Patient Information May cause drowsiness and impair ability to perform activities requiring mental alertness or physical coordination; may cause dry mouth; avoid alcohol; limit caffeine; may discolor urine to blue-green color; do not discontinue medication abruptly; may increase appetite; avoid unnecessary exposure to sunlight

Additional Information Place in therapy (treatment of depression): Desipramine is considered by some clinicians to be the first or second drug of choice for depressed children with excessive daytime sleepiness

Dosage Forms Tablet, as hydrochloride (Norpramin®): 10 mg, 25 mg (with tartrazine), 50 mg (with tartrazine), 75 mg (with tartrazine), 100 mg (with tartrazine), 150 mg

References
Biederman J, Thisted RA, Greenhill LL, et al, "Estimation of the Association Between Desipramine and the Risk for Sudden Death in 5-14 Year-Old Children," *J Clin Psychiatry*, 1995, 56(3):87-93.
Levy HB, Harper CR, and Weinberg WA, "A Practical Approach to Children Failing in School," *Pediatr Clin North Am*, 1992, 39(4):895-928.

♦ **Desipramine Hydrochloride** *see* Desipramine *on page 291*

Desmopressin *(des moe PRES in)*

Brand Names DDAVP®; Octostim® (Canada); Stimate®
Available Salts Desmopressin Acetate
Synonyms 1-Deamino-8-D-Arginine Vasopressin
Therapeutic Category Antihemophilic Agent; Hemostatic Agent; Vasopressin Analog, Synthetic
Generic Available No
Use Treatment of diabetes insipidus, control of bleeding in hemophilia A (with factor VIII levels >5%), mild to moderate type I von Willebrand disease, and thrombocytopenia; primary nocturnal enuresis
Pregnancy Risk Factor B
Contraindications Hypersensitivity to desmopressin or any component; avoid using in patients with severe type I, type IIB or platelet-type (pseudo) von Willebrand disease, hemophilia A with factor VIII levels ≤5% or hemophilia B
Warnings Avoid intranasal use in patients with nasal mucosa changes (scarring, edema, discharge, obstruction, or severe atopic rhinitis)
Precautions Use with caution in patients with predisposition to thrombus formation, conditions associated with fluid and electrolyte imbalance (eg, cystic fibrosis), and in patients with coronary artery disease and/or hypertensive cardiovascular disease

Adverse Reactions

Cardiovascular: Facial flushing, increase in blood pressure, chest pain, palpitations, tachycardia

Central nervous system: Headache, somnolence, dizziness, insomnia, agitation

Endocrine & metabolic: Hyponatremia, water intoxication

Gastrointestinal: Nausea, abdominal cramps, dyspepsia, vomiting

Genitourinary: Vulval pain, balanitis

Local: Pain at the injection site

Ocular: Itchy or light-sensitive eyes

Respiratory: Rhinitis, upper respiratory infections, epistaxis, nasal congestion

Drug Interactions Decreased antidiuretic response with lithium, large doses of epinephrine, demeclocycline, and heparin; increased antidiuretic response with carbamazepine, chlorpropamide, fludrocortisone, and clofibrate

Stability Refrigerate injection, nasal solution and Stimate® nasal spray; nasal solution and Stimate® nasal spray are stable for 3 weeks when stored at room temperature if unopened; injection stable for 2 weeks at room temperature; DDAVP® nasal spray is stable at room temperature

Mechanism of Action Enhances reabsorption of water in the kidneys by increasing cellular permeability of the collecting ducts; possibly causes smooth muscle constriction with resultant vasoconstriction; dose-dependent increase in plasma factor VIII and plasminogen activator

Pharmacodynamics

Oral administration:

Onset of ADH effects: 1 hour

Peak effect: 2-7 hours

Duration: 6-8 hours

Intranasal administration:

Onset of ADH effects: Within 1 hour

Peak effect: Within 1.5 hours

Duration: 5-21 hours

I.V. infusion:

Onset of increased factor VIII activity: Within 15-30 minutes

Peak effect: 90 minutes to 3 hours

Pharmacokinetics

Absorption:

Oral tablets: 5% to 15%

Nasal solution: 10% to 20%

Nasal spray (1.5 mg/mL concentration): 3.3% to 4.1%

Metabolism: Unknown

Half-life:

Oral: 1.5-2.5 hours

I.V.:

Mean initial: 7.8 minutes

Terminal: 75.5 minutes (range: 0.4-4 hours)

Intranasal: 3.3-3.5 hours

Usual Dosage

Diabetes insipidus:

Oral:

Children ≤12 years: Initial: 0.05 mg 2 times daily; titrate to desired response (range: 0.1-0.8 mg daily)

Children >12 years and Adults: 0.05 mg 2 times daily; titrate to desired response (range: 0.1-1.2 mg divided 2-3 times/day)

Intranasal:

Children 3 months to ≤12 years: Initial (using 100 mcg/mL nasal solution): 5 mcg/day (0.05 mL/day) divided 1-2 times/day; range: 5-30 mcg/day (0.05-0.3 mL/day); adjust morning and evening doses separately for an adequate diurnal rhythm of water turnover

Children >12 years and Adults: Initial (using 100 mcg/mL nasal solution): 5-40 mcg (0.05-0.4 mL) divided 1-3 times/day; adjust morning and evening doses separately for an adequate diurnal rhythm of water turnover. **Note:** The nasal spray pump can only deliver doses of 10 mcg (0.1 mL) or multiples of 10 mcg (0.1 mL), if doses other than this are needed, the rhinal tube delivery system is preferred

I.V., S.C.: Children >12 years and Adults: 2-4 mcg/day in 2 divided doses or ¹/₁₀ of the maintenance intranasal dose

Hemophilia:

I.V.: Children ≥3 months and Adults: 0.3 mcg/kg beginning 30 minutes before procedure; may repeat dose if needed

(Continued)

Desmopressin *(Continued)*

Intranasal: Children >12 years and Adults: Using high concentration Stimate® nasal spray:

≤50 kg: 150 mcg (1 spray)

>50 kg: 300 mcg (1 spray each nostril)

Repeat use is determined by the patients clinical condition and laboratory work; if using preoperatively, administer 2 hours before surgery

Nocturnal enuresis:

Intranasal: Children ≥6 years: (Using 100 mcg/mL nasal solution): Initial: 20 mcg (0.2 mL) at bedtime; range: 10-40 mcg; it is recommended that ½ of the dose be given in each nostril

Oral: Children >12 years: 0.2-0.4 mg once before bedtime

Administration

Intranasal: Using rhinal tube delivery system, draw solution into flexible, calibrated rhinal; insert one end into nostril; blow on the other end to deposit the solution deep into the nasal cavity. The Stimate® spray pump must be primed prior to first use; to prime pump, press down 4 times. Avoid spray use in children <6 years of age due to difficulty in titrating dosage; discard any solution remaining after 25 or 50 doses (2.5 or 5 mL vials, respectively) because the amount delivered may be substantially less than prescribed

Parenteral: I.V.: Dilute to a maximum concentration of 0.5 mcg/mL in NS and infuse over 15-30 minutes; if desmopressin I.V. is given preoperatively, administer 30 minutes prior to surgery

Monitoring Parameters I.V. infusion: Blood pressure and pulse should be monitored

Diabetes insipidus: Fluid intake, urine volume, specific gravity, plasma and urine osmolality, serum electrolytes

Hemophilia: Factor VIII antigen levels, APTT, Factor VIII activity level

Patient Information Avoid overhydration; blow nose before using nasal solution or spray; notify physician if headache, shortness of breath, heartburn, nausea, abdominal cramps, or vulval pain occur

Dosage Forms

Injection, as acetate (DDAVP®): 4 mcg/mL (1 mL); 15 mcg/mL (1mL, 2 mL)

Solution, nasal, as acetate, (DDAVP®): 100 mcg/mL (2.5 mL, 5 mL)

Spray, nasal, as acetate:

DDAVP®: 10 mcg/spray (5 mL)

Stimate® (DDAVP® high concentration): 1.5 mg/mL (2.5 mL)

Tablet, as acetate: 0.1 mg, 0.2 mg

References

Stenberg A and Läckgren G, "Desmopressin Tablets in the Treatment of Severe Nocturnal Enuresis in Adolescents," *Pediatrics*, 1994, 94(6 Pt 1):841-46.

♦ **Desmopressin Acetate** *see* Desmopressin *on page 292*

♦ **Despec®** *see* Guaifenesin, Phenylpropanolamine, and Phenylephrine *on page 467*

♦ **Desquam-E® Gel** *see* Benzoyl Peroxide *on page 126*

♦ **Desquam-X® Gel** *see* Benzoyl Peroxide *on page 126*

♦ **Desquam-X® Wash** *see* Benzoyl Peroxide *on page 126*

♦ **Desyrel®** *see* Trazodone *on page 944*

♦ **Detensol® (Canada)** *see* Propranolol *on page 816*

♦ **Devrom® [OTC]** *see* Bismuth *on page 134*

♦ **Dex4 Glucose [OTC]** *see* Dextrose *on page 305*

♦ **Dexacidin® Ophthalmic** *see* Dexamethasone, Neomycin, and Polymyxin B *on page 297*

♦ **Dexacort™ Phosphate Respihaler® Oral Inhaler** *see* Dexamethasone *on page 294*

♦ **Dexacort™ Phosphate Turbinaire® Intranasal Aerosol** *see* Dexamethasone *on page 294*

♦ **Dex-A-Diet® [OTC]** *see* Phenylpropanolamine *on page 761*

Dexamethasone *(deks a METH a sone)*

Related Information

Carbohydrate and Alcohol Content of Liquid Medications for Use in Patients Receiving Ketogenic Diets *on page 1228*

Corticosteroids Comparison, Systemic *on page 1032*

Brand Names Aeroseb-Dex® Topical Aerosol; AK-Dex® Ophthalmic; Dalalone D.P.® Injection; Dalalone® Injection; Dalalone L.A.® Injection; Decadron®-LA Injection; Decadron® Oral; Decadron® Phosphate Cream; Decadron® Phosphate Injection; Decadron® Phosphate Nasal Turbinaire®; Decadron® Phosphate Ophthalmic;

Decaject® Injection; Decaject-LA® Injection; Decaspray® Topical Aerosol; Dekasol® Injection; Dekasol-L.A.® Injection; Dexacort™ Phosphate Respihaler® Oral Inhaler; Dexacort™ Phosphate Turbinaire® Intranasal Aerosol; Dexameth® Oral; Dexasone® Injection; Dexasone® L.A. Injection; Dexone® Injection; Dexone® LA Injection; Dexone® Tablet; Hexadrol® Phosphate Injection; Hexadrol® Tablet; Maxidex® Ophthalmic; Solurex® Injection; Solurex L.A.® Injection

Available Salts Dexamethasone Acetate; Dexamethasone Sodium Phosphate

Therapeutic Category Adrenal Corticosteroid; Antiasthmatic; Antiemetic; Anti-inflammatory Agent; Anti-inflammatory Agent, Ophthalmic; Corticosteroid, Inhalant (Oral); Corticosteroid, Intranasal; Corticosteroid, Ophthalmic; Corticosteroid, Systemic; Corticosteroid, Topical; Glucocorticoid

Generic Available Yes

Use

Intranasal: Management of allergic or inflammatory nasal conditions and nasal polyps

Oral inhalation: Long-term (chronic) control of persistent bronchial asthma; **NOT** indicated for the relief of acute bronchospasm

Systemically and locally for chronic inflammation, allergic, hematologic, neoplastic, and autoimmune diseases; may be used in management of cerebral edema, septic shock, and as a diagnostic agent

Pregnancy Risk Factor C

Contraindications Active untreated infections; viral, fungal, or tuberculous diseases of the eye; hypersensitivity to dexamethasone or any component; primary treatment of status asthmaticus

Warnings Fatalities have occurred due to adrenal insufficiency in asthmatic patients during and after switching from systemic corticosteroids to aerosol steroids; several months may be required for full recovery of the adrenal glands; during this period, aerosol steroids do **not** provide the systemic corticosteroid needed to treat patients requiring stress doses (ie, patients with major stress such as trauma, surgery, or infections); when used at high doses hypothalamic - pituitary - adrenal (HPA) suppression may occur; use with inhaled or systemic corticosteroids (even alternate-day dosing) may increase risk of HPA suppression; withdrawal and discontinuation of corticosteroids should be done carefully; immunosuppression may occur

Precautions Avoid using higher than recommended doses; suppression of HPA function, suppression of linear growth, or hypercorticism (Cushing's syndrome) may occur; use with extreme caution in patients with respiratory tuberculosis, untreated systemic infections, or ocular herpes simplex

Adverse Reactions

Cardiovascular: Edema, hypertension

Central nervous system: Headache, vertigo, seizures, psychosis, pseudotumor cerebri

Dermatologic: Acne, skin atrophy

Endocrine & metabolic: Pituitary-adrenal axis suppression, growth suppression, glucose intolerance, hypokalemia, alkalosis, Cushing's syndrome

Gastrointestinal: Peptic ulcer, nausea, vomiting

Neuromuscular & skeletal: Muscle weakness, osteoporosis, fractures

Ocular: Cataracts, glaucoma

Drug Interactions Cytochrome P-450 isoenzyme CYP3A3/4 substrate; isoenzyme CYP3A3/4 inducer; isoenzyme CYP3A3/4 inhibitor

Barbiturates, phenytoin, rifampin, ritonavir, saquinavir, salicylates, NSAIDs, toxoids; alcohol and caffeine may increase adverse GI effects; live virus vaccines (increase risk of viral infection); vaccines may have decreased effects

Food Interactions Systemic use of corticosteroids may require a diet with increased potassium, vitamins A, B_6, C, D, folate, calcium, zinc, and phosphorus and decreased sodium

Stability Dilution of dexamethasone sodium phosphate injection with D_5W or NS is stable for at least 24 hours

Mechanism of Action Decreases inflammation by suppression of migration of polymorphonuclear leukocytes and reversal of increased capillary permeability; suppresses normal immune response

Pharmacodynamics Duration: Metabolic effects can last for 72 hours

Pharmacokinetics

Metabolism: In the liver

Half-life: Terminal:

Extremely low birth weight infants with BPD: 9.3 hours

Children 3 months to 16 years: 4.3 hours

Healthy adults: 3 hours

(Continued)

Dexamethasone *(Continued)*

Time to peak serum concentration:
Oral: Within 1-2 hours
I.M.: Within 8 hours
Elimination: In urine and bile

Usual Dosage
Neonates:
Airway edema or extubation: I.V.: Usual: 0.25 mg/kg/dose given ~4 hours prior to scheduled extubation and then every 8 hours for 3 doses total; range: 0.25-1 mg/kg/dose for 1-3 doses; maximum dose: 1 mg/kg/day. **Note:** A longer duration of therapy may be needed with more severe cases.
Bronchopulmonary dysplasia (to facilitate ventilator weaning): Oral, I.V.: Numerous dosing schedules have been proposed; range: 0.5-0.6 mg/kg/day given in divided doses every 12 hours for 3-7 days, then taper over 1-6 weeks
Children:
Airway edema or extubation: Oral, I.M., I.V.: 0.5-2 mg/kg/day in divided doses every 6 hours; begin 24 hours prior to extubation and continue for 4-6 doses after extubation
Antiemetic (chemotherapy induced): I.V.: Initial: 10 mg/m^2/dose (maximum dose: 20 mg) then 5 mg/m^2/dose every 6 hours
Anti-inflammatory: Oral, I.M., I.V.: 0.08-0.3 mg/kg/day or 2.5-10 mg/m^2/day in divided doses every 6-12 hours
Bacterial meningitis: Infants and Children >2 months: I.V.: 0.6 mg/kg/day divided every 6 hours for the first 4 days of antibiotic treatment; start dexamethasone at the time of the first dose of antibiotic
Cerebral edema: Oral, I.M., I.V.: Loading dose: 1-2 mg/kg/dose as a single dose; maintenance: 1-1.5 mg/kg/day (maximum dose: 16 mg/day) in divided doses every 4-6 hours
Inhalation: Oral: 2 inhalations 3-4 times/day to a maximum of 8 inhalations/day; doses should be titrated to lowest effective dose once asthma is controlled
Intranasal: Children: 6-12 years: 1-2 sprays into each nostril twice daily to a maximum of 8 sprays/day; decrease dose according to patient response
Physiologic replacement: Oral, I.M., I.V.: 0.03-0.15 mg/kg/day or 0.6-0.75 mg/m^2/day in divided doses every 6-12 hours
Children and Adults: Ophthalmic:
Ointment: Apply thin coating to conjunctival sac 3-4 times/day, gradually taper dose to discontinue
Suspension: Instill 2 drops every hour during the day and every other hour during the night; gradually reduce dose to every 3-4 hours, then to 3-4 times/day
Children and Adults: Topical: Apply 1-4 times/day
Adults:
Acute nonlymphoblastic leukemia (ANLL) protocol: I.V.: 2 mg/m^2/dose every 8 hours for 12 doses
Anti-inflammatory: Oral, I.M., I.V.: 0.75-9 mg/day in divided doses every 6-12 hours
Cerebral edema: I.V.: Initial: 10 mg then 4 mg I.M./I.V. every 6 hours
Diagnosis for Cushing's syndrome: Oral: 1 mg at 11 PM, draw blood at 8 AM
Inhalation: Oral: 3 inhalations 3-4 times/day to a maximum of 12 inhalations/day; doses should be titrated to lowest effective dose once asthma is controlled
Intranasal: 2 sprays into each nostril 2-3 times/day to a maximum of 12 sprays/day; decrease dose according to patient response

Administration
Oral: May administer with food or milk to decrease GI adverse effects
Oral inhalation: Shake aerosol container well prior to use
Parenteral: **Acetate injection is not for I.V. use**; I.V. (as sodium phosphate): Administer undiluted solution (4 mg/mL) I.V. push over 1-4 minutes if dose is <10 mg; high-dose therapy must be diluted in D$_5$W or NS and administered by I.V. intermittent infusion over 15-30 minutes
Topical: Use sparingly, do not apply to open wounds

Monitoring Parameters Hemoglobin, occult blood loss, blood pressure, serum potassium and glucose

Reference Range Dexamethasone suppression test: 8 AM cortisol less than 6 µg/100 mL in adults given dexamethasone 1 mg at 11 PM the previous night

Test Interactions Skin tests

Patient Information Avoid alcohol; limit caffeine; do not decrease dose or discontinue drug without physician's approval; inform physician you are taking corticosteroid prior to any surgery or with any injury

Additional Information Due to long duration of effect, not suitable for every other day dosing

Dosage Forms

Dexamethasone **acetate**:
  Injection: 8 mg/mL (5 mL); 16 mg/mL (1 mL, 5 mL)

Dexamethasone **base**:
  Aerosol, topical:
    Aeroseb-Dex®: 0.01% (58 g)
    Decaspray®: 0.04% (25 g)
  Elixir: 0.5 mg/5 mL (5 mL, 20 mL, 100 mL, 120 mL, 237 mL, 240 mL, 500 mL)
  Solution, oral: 0.5 mg/5 mL (5 mL, 20 mL, 500 mL)
  Solution, oral concentrate: 0.5 mg/0.5 mL (30 mL)
  Suspension, ophthalmic: 0.1% (5 mL, 15 mL)
  Tablet: 0.25 mg, 0.5 mg, 0.75 mg, 1 mg, 1.5 mg, 2 mg, 4 mg, 6 mg
  Therapeutic pack (Hexadrol®): Six 1.5 mg tablets and eight 0.75 mg tablets

Dexamethasone **sodium phosphate**:
  Aerosol, nasal (Dexacort™ Phosphate Turbinaire®, Decadron® Phosphate Turbinaire®): 84 mcg/activation [170 metered doses] (12.6 g)
  Aerosol, oral (Dexacort™ Phosphate Respihaler®): 84 mcg/activation [170 metered doses] (12.6 g)
  Cream (Decadron® Phosphate): 0.1% (15 g, 30 g)
  Injection: 4 mg/mL (1 mL, 2 mL, 2.5 mL, 5 mL, 10 mL, 30 mL); 10 mg/mL (1 mL, 10 mL); 20 mg/mL (5 mL); 24 mg/mL (5 mL, 10 mL)
  Ointment, ophthalmic: 0.05% (3.5 g)
  Solution, ophthalmic: 0.1% (5 mL)

References

American Academy of Pediatrics Committee on Infectious Diseases, "Dexamethasone Therapy for Bacterial Meningitis in Infants and Children," *Pediatrics*, 1990, 86(1):130-3.

Bahal N and Nahata MC, "The Role of Corticosteroids in Infants and Children With Bacterial Meningitis," *DICP*, 1991, 25(5):542-5.

Couser RJ, Ferrara TB, Falde B, et al, "Effectiveness of Dexamethasone in Preventing Extubation Failure in Preterm Infants at Increased Risk for Airway Edema," *J Pediatr*, 1992, 121(4):591-6.

Durand M, Sardesai S, and McEvoy C, "Effects of Early Dexamethasone Therapy on Pulmonary Mechanics and Chronic Lung Disease in Very Low Birth Weight Infants: A Randomized, Controlled Trial," *Pediatrics*, 1995, 95(4):584-90.

Ng PC, "The Effectiveness and Side Effects of Dexamethasone in Preterm Infants With Bronchopulmonary Dysplasia," *Arch Dis Child*, 1993, 68(3 Spec No):330-6.

♦ **Dexamethasone Acetate** *see* Dexamethasone *on page 294*

Dexamethasone, Neomycin, and Polymyxin B

(deks a METH a sone, nee oh MYE sin, & pol i MIKS in bee)

Brand Names AK-Trol® Ophthalmic; Dexacidin® Ophthalmic; Dexasporin® Ophthalmic; Infectrol® Ophthalmic; Maxitrol® Ophthalmic; Ocu-Trol® Ophthalmic

Available Salts Dexamethasone, Neomycin Sulfate, and Polymyxin B Sulfate

Synonyms Neomycin, Dexamethasone, and Polymyxin B Polymyxin B, Dexamethasone, and Neomycin

Therapeutic Category Antibiotic, Ophthalmic; Corticosteroid, Ophthalmic

Generic Available Yes

Use Steroid-responsive inflammatory ocular conditions in which a corticosteroid is indicated and where bacterial infection or a risk of bacterial infection exists

Pregnancy Risk Factor C

Contraindications Hypersensitivity to dexamethasone, polymyxin, neomycin, or any component; viral diseases of the cornea and conjunctiva; mycobacterial infection of the eye; fungal disease of ocular structures; dendritic keratitis; use after uncomplicated removal of a corneal foreign body

Warnings Prolonged use may result in glaucoma, defects in visual acuity, posterior subcapsular cataract formation, and secondary ocular infections

Adverse Reactions

Dermatologic: Contact dermatitis, cutaneous sensitization (sensitivity to topical neomycin has been reported to occur in 5% to 15% of patients)

Local: Pain, stinging

Ocular: Development of glaucoma, cataract, increased intraocular pressure, optic nerve damage, visual defects, blurred vision

Miscellaneous: Delayed wound healing, secondary infections

Usual Dosage Children and Adults: Ophthalmic:

Ointment: Apply a small amount (~½") in the affected eye 3-4 times/day or apply at bedtime as an adjunct with drops

Suspension: Instill 1-2 drops into affected eye(s) every 4-6 hours; in severe disease, drops may be used hourly and tapered to discontinuation

(Continued)

297

Dexamethasone, Neomycin, and Polymyxin B
(Continued)

Administration Ophthalmic: Shake suspension well before using; instill drop into affected eye; avoid contacting bottle tip with skin or eye

Monitoring Parameters Intraocular pressure with use >10 days

Patient Information May cause temporary blurring of vision or stinging following administration

Dosage Forms

Ointment, ophthalmic: Dexamethasone 0.1%, neomycin sulfate 3.5 mg, and polymyxin B sulfate 10,000 units per g (3.5 g)

Suspension, ophthalmic: Dexamethasone 0.1%, neomycin sulfate 3.5 mg, and polymyxin B sulfate 10,000 units per mL (5 mL)

- ♦ **Dexamethasone, Neomycin Sulfate, and Polymyxin B Sulfate** *see* Dexamethasone, Neomycin, and Polymyxin B *on page 297*
- ♦ **Dexamethasone Sodium Phosphate** *see* Dexamethasone *on page 294*
- ♦ **Dexameth®️ Oral** *see* Dexamethasone *on page 294*
- ♦ **Dexasone®️ Injection** *see* Dexamethasone *on page 294*
- ♦ **Dexasone®️ L.A. Injection** *see* Dexamethasone *on page 294*
- ♦ **Dexasporin®️ Ophthalmic** *see* Dexamethasone, Neomycin, and Polymyxin B *on page 297*
- ♦ **Dexatrim®️ [OTC]** *see* Phenylpropanolamine *on page 761*
- ♦ **Dexchlorpheniramine Maleate** *see* Chlorpheniramine *on page 214*
- ♦ **Dexedrine®️** *see* Dextroamphetamine *on page 300*
- ♦ **Dexferrum®️** *see* Iron Dextran Complex *on page 528*
- ♦ **Dexone®️ Injection** *see* Dexamethasone *on page 294*
- ♦ **Dexone®️ LA Injection** *see* Dexamethasone *on page 294*
- ♦ **Dexone®️ Tablet** *see* Dexamethasone *on page 294*

Dexrazoxane (deks ray ZOKS ane)

Brand Names Zinecard®️

Therapeutic Category Antineoplastic Agent; Chelating Agent; Chemoprotectant Agent

Use Reduction of anthracycline-induced (doxorubicin, daunorubicin) cardiotoxicity. Not generally recommended for use with the initiation of anthracycline therapy. Most dexrazoxane studies have been done in women with metastatic breast cancer who had received a cumulative doxorubicin dose of 300 mg/m^2.

Pregnancy Risk Factor C

Contraindications Hypersensitivity to dexrazoxane or any component; should only be used with chemotherapy regimens containing an anthracycline

Warnings Due to limited experience, the possibility of dexrazoxane interference with antineoplastic efficacy may exist; dose-limiting toxicity is myelosuppression; dexrazoxane may add to the myelosuppression caused by chemotherapeutic agents; dexrazoxane should be handled, prepared, and disposed as an antineoplastic agent

Precautions Do not give doxorubicin prior to dexrazoxane administration. Doxorubicin should be given within 30 minutes from the beginning of a dexrazoxane infusion.

Adverse Reactions

Central nervous system: Low grade fever

Dermatologic: Alopecia (possibly dose-related)

Endocrine/metabolic: Elevated serum iron and serum triglyceride levels, decreased serum zinc and calcium levels

Gastrointestinal: Mild nausea and vomiting, diarrhea, elevated serum amylase levels

Hepatic: Transient elevation of serum transaminase level

Hematologic: **Dose-limiting, additive myelosuppression** (leukopenia and thrombocytopenia at high doses >1000 mg/m^2)

Local: Pain at injection site (13%)

Drug Interactions Dexrazoxane can have either a synergistic or inhibitory activity with different anthracyclines

Stability Reconstituted solution is stable for 6 hours at room temperature or under refrigeration. Dexrazoxane degrades rapidly at pH >7.

Mechanism of Action Dexrazoxane is a piperazine EDTA derivative that rapidly penetrates the myocardial cell membrane. It binds intracellular iron and prevents generation of oxygen free radicals by anthracyclines. Dexrazoxane is hydrolyzed intracellularly to an open-ring chelating agent which is responsible for chelating heavy metals and preventing formation of superhydroxide free radicals believed to be responsible for anthracycline-induced cardiomyopathy. Dexrazoxane may also have antitumor activity and have synergistic activity with certain cytotoxic agents.

Pharmacokinetics Minimal data in the pediatric population
Distribution: V_d:
  Children: 0.67 L/kg
  Adults: 1.3 L/kg
Protein binding: Insignificant
Half-life: Biphasic
  Distribution half-life: 8-21 minutes
  Terminal half-life: 2-3 hours
Elimination: 40% to 60% of dose excreted renally within 24 hours; removed by peritoneal or hemodialysis

Usual Dosage I.V. (refer to individual protocols):
Children: 10:1 dose ratio with doxorubicin (example: 250 mg/m^2 dexrazoxane: 25 mg/m^2 doxorubicin) is currently recommended; 20:1 ratio with doxorubicin has been studied, but due to higher incidence of adverse reactions is no longer recommended
Adults: 10:1 ratio with doxorubicin (example: 500 mg/m^2 dexrazoxane: 50 mg/m^2 doxorubicin); administer 30 minutes before doxorubicin

Administration Parenteral: Reconstitute with 0.167 Molar sodium lactate injection to a concentration of 10 mg/mL. Administer slow I.V. push or further dilute in NS or D$_5$W to a final concentration of 1.3-5 mg/mL and give as a rapid I.V. infusion over 15-30 minutes

Monitoring Parameters Complete blood count; cardiac function tests; serum iron, calcium, and zinc levels; liver function tests

Nursing Implications To ensure optimal chemoprotectant effect, do not allow chemotherapy to be delayed following completion of dexrazoxane

Dosage Forms Injection: 250 mg

References
Sehested M, et al, "Dexrazoxane for Protection Against Cardiotoxic Effects of Anthracyclines," *J Clin Oncol*, 1996, 14:2884.
Swain SM, et al, "Cardioprotection With Dexrazoxane for Doxorubicin-Containing Therapy in Advanced Breast Cancer," *J Clin Oncol*, 1997, 15:1318-32.
Swain SM, et al, "Delayed Administration of Dexrazoxane Provides Cardioprotection for Patients With Advanced Breast Cancer Treated With Doxorubicin-Containing Therapy," *J Clin Oncol*, 1997, 15:1333-40.
Wexler LH, et al, "Randomized Trial of the Cardioprotective Agent ICRF-187 in Pediatric Sarcoma Patients Treated With Doxorubicin," *J Clin Oncol*, 1996, 14:362-72.

Dextran (DEKS tran)

Brand Names Gentran®; Hyskon® (Canada); LMD®; Macrodex®; Rheomacrodex®
Synonyms Dextran 40; Dextran 70; Dextran, High Molecular Weight; Dextran, Low Molecular Weight
Therapeutic Category Plasma Volume Expander
Generic Available Yes
Use Fluid replacement and blood volume expander used in the treatment of hypovolemia, shock, or near shock states
Pregnancy Risk Factor C
Contraindications Hypersensitivity to dextrans or any component; renal failure, severe thrombocytopenia
Warnings Use with caution in patients with CHF, pulmonary edema, renal insufficiency, thrombocytopenia, or active hemorrhage; watch for anaphylactoid reactions, have epinephrine and diphenhydramine at bedside
Precautions Use with caution in patients with extreme dehydration, renal failure may occur
Adverse Reactions
Cardiovascular: Mild hypotension
Central nervous system: Fever
Dermatologic: Urticaria
Gastrointestinal: Nausea, vomiting
Hematologic: Prolongation of bleeding time with higher doses (may interfere with platelet function)
Neuromuscular & skeletal: Arthralgia
Respiratory: Wheezing, pulmonary edema with high doses, tightness of chest, nasal congestion
Miscellaneous: Anaphylaxis
Stability Store at room temperature; discard partially used containers
(Continued)

Dextran *(Continued)*

Mechanism of Action Produces plasma volume expansion due to high colloidal osmotic effect (similar to albumin); draws interstitial fluid into the intravascular space; dextran 40 may also increase blood flow in microcirculation

Pharmacodynamics

Maximum effect on plasma volume:

Dextran 40: Within several minutes

Dextran 70 and dextran 75: ~1 hour

Pharmacokinetics

Metabolism: Molecules with molecular weight ≥50,000 are metabolized to glucose

Elimination:

Molecules with molecular weight ≤15,000: Rapidly eliminated in the kidney

Dextran 40: ~70% excreted in urine (unchanged) within 24 hours

Dextran 70 & 75: ~50% excreted in urine within 24 hours

Usual Dosage I.V. (dose and infusion rate are dependent upon the patient's fluid status and must be individualized):

Children: Total dose should not be >20 mL/kg during first 24 hours and not >10 mL/kg/day thereafter; do not treat for >5 days

Adults: 500-1000 mL at rate of 20-40 mL/minute

Maximum daily dose: First 24 hours: 20 mL/kg and 10 mL/kg/day thereafter; therapy should not continue beyond 5 days

Administration Parenteral: I.V. infusion only; usual maximum infusion rate (adults): 4 mL/minute; maximum infusion rate in emergency situations (adults): 20-40 mL/minute

Monitoring Parameters Vital signs, signs of allergic/anaphylactoid reaction especially when starting infusions; signs of circulatory overload (ie, heart rate, blood pressure, central venous pressure, hematocrit); urine output; urine specific gravity

Nursing Implications Be prepared to treat anaphylaxis with epinephrine, antihistamines, supportive therapy, and alternative agents to dextran to maintain circulation; do not administer if cloudy or if solution contains dextran flakes; discontinue dextran if urine specific gravity is low, if oliguria or anuria occur, or if there is a rapid acute rise in central venous pressure or other signs of circulatory overload

Additional Information Dextran in sodium chloride 0.9% contains sodium chloride 154 mEq/L

Dosage Forms Injection:

High molecular weight:

6% dextran 75 in dextrose 5% (500 mL)

Gentran®: 6% dextran 75 in sodium chloride 0.9% (500 mL)

Gentran®, Macrodex®: 6% dextran 70 in sodium chloride 0.9% (500 mL)

Macrodex®: 6% dextran 70 in dextrose 5% (500 mL)

Low molecular weight: Gentran®, LMD®, Rheomacrodex®:

10% dextran 40 in dextrose 5% (500 mL)

10% dextran 40 in sodium chloride 0.9% (500 mL)

- ◆ **Dextran 40** *see Dextran on page 299*
- ◆ **Dextran 70** *see Dextran on page 299*
- ◆ **Dextran, High Molecular Weight** *see Dextran on page 299*
- ◆ **Dextran, Low Molecular Weight** *see Dextran on page 299*

Dextroamphetamine (deks troe am FET a meen)

Related Information

Drugs and Breast-Feeding *on page 1213*

Laboratory Detection of Drugs in Urine *on page 1204*

Brand Names Dexedrine®

Available Salts Dextroamphetamine Sulfate

Therapeutic Category Amphetamine; Anorexiant; Central Nervous System Stimulant, Amphetamine

Generic Available Yes

Use Adjunct in treatment of attention-deficit/hyperactivity disorder (ADHD) in children, narcolepsy, exogenous obesity

Restrictions C-II

Pregnancy Risk Factor C

Contraindications Hypersensitivity to dextroamphetamine or any component; advanced arteriosclerosis, hypertension, hyperthyroidism, glaucoma; concurrent use or use within 14 days of MAO inhibitors (hypertensive crisis may occur)

Warnings High potential for abuse; use in weight reduction programs only when alternative therapy has been ineffective; prolonged administration may lead to drug dependence; use in psychotic children may exacerbate symptoms of thought disorder and behavior disturbance; may potentially be associated with growth inhibition (monitor growth); 5 mg tablets and 5 mg, 10 mg, and 15 mg Dexedrine® Spansule® capsules contain tartrazine

Precautions Use with caution in patients with psychopathic personalities

Adverse Reactions

Cardiovascular: Hypertension, tachycardia, palpitations, cardiac arrhythmias

Central nervous system: Insomnia, headache, nervousness, dizziness, irritability, depression

Endocrine & metabolic: Growth suppression, weight loss

Gastrointestinal: Anorexia, nausea, vomiting, diarrhea, abdominal cramps, metallic taste, xerostomia

Neuromuscular & skeletal: Movement disorders, tremor

Ocular: Mydriasis

Miscellaneous: Physical and psychologic dependence with long-term use

Drug Interactions Amphetamines may decrease hypotensive effects of antihypertensives and sedative effect of antihistamines; may increase effects of tricyclic antidepressants or sympathomimetics; may precipitate hypertensive crisis in patients receiving MAO inhibitors (avoid use within 14 days) and arrhythmias in patients receiving general anesthetics; may delay oral absorption of ethosuximide, phenobarbital, and phenytoin. With propoxyphene overdose, CNS stimulation from amphetamines is potentiated (fatal convulsions may occur); tricyclic antidepressants may enhance the effects of amphetamines (avoid use or monitor for cardiovascular effects); chlorpromazine and haloperidol may inhibit the CNS stimulant effects of amphetamines. Antacids may increase the oral absorption of amphetamines; urinary alkalinizers or large doses of antacids may decrease urinary excretion of amphetamines and increase their half-life and duration of action (dosage decrease may be needed). Acids or acidifiers may decrease the oral absorption of amphetamines; urinary acidifiers may increase urinary excretion of amphetamines and decrease their half-life and duration of action (dosage adjustment may be needed).

Food Interactions Acidic foods, juices, or vitamin C may decrease GI absorption

Mechanism of Action Blocks reuptake of dopamine and norepinephrine from the synapse, thus increases the amounts of circulating dopamine and norepinephrine in cerebral cortex to reticular activating system; inhibits the action of monoamine oxidase and causes catecholamines to be released; peripherally increases blood pressure and acts as a respiratory stimulant and weak bronchodilator

Pharmacodynamics Onset of action: Oral: 60-90 minutes

Pharmacokinetics

Metabolism: In the liver

Half-life, adults: 34 hours (pH dependent)

Time to peak serum concentration: Oral: Within 3 hours

Elimination: In urine as unchanged drug and inactive metabolites; urinary excretion is pH dependent and is increased with acid urine (low pH)

Usual Dosage Oral: **Note:** Use lowest effective individualized dose; administer first dose as soon as awake

ADHD: Children:

<3 years: Not recommended

3-5 years: Initial: 2.5 mg/day given every morning; increase by 2.5 mg/day at weekly intervals until optimal response is obtained, usual range is 0.1-0.5 mg/kg/dose every morning with maximum of 40 mg/day given in 1-3 divided doses per day

≥6 years: 5 mg once or twice daily; increase in increments of 5 mg/day at weekly intervals until optimal response is reached, usual range is 0.1-0.5 mg/kg/dose every morning (5-20 mg/day) with maximum of 40 mg/day given in 1-3 divided doses per day

Narcolepsy:

Children 6-12 years: Initial: 5 mg/day, may increase at 5 mg increments at weekly intervals until optimal response is obtained; maximum dose: 60 mg/day

Children >12 and Adults: Initial: 10 mg/day, may increase at 10 mg increments at weekly intervals until optimal response is obtained; maximum dose: 60 mg/day

Exogenous obesity: Children >12 years and Adults: 5-30 mg/day in divided doses of 5-10 mg given 30-60 minutes before meals

Administration Oral: Sustained release preparations should be used for once daily dosing; do not crush or chew sustained release preparations; to avoid insomnia, last daily dose should be administered no less than 6 hours before retiring

Monitoring Parameters CNS activity, blood pressure, height, weight

Patient Information Do not discontinue abruptly

(Continued)

Dextroamphetamine *(Continued)*

Additional Information Treatment for ADHD should include "drug holiday" or periodic discontinuation in order to assess the patient's requirements, decrease tolerance, and limit suppression of linear growth and weight

Dosage Forms

Capsule, sustained release, as sulfate (Dexedrine® Spansule® capsules contain tartrazine): 5 mg, 10 mg, 15 mg

Tablet, as sulfate: 5 mg (with tartrazine), 10 mg

Dextroamphetamine and Amphetamine

(deks troe am FET a meen & am FET a meen)

Related Information

Dextroamphetamine *on page 300*

Drugs and Breast-Feeding *on page 1213*

Laboratory Detection of Drugs in Urine *on page 1204*

Brand Names Adderall®

Available Salts Amphetamine Aspartate, Amphetamine Sulfate, Dextroamphetamine Saccharate, and Dextroamphetamine Sulfate

Synonyms Amphetamine and Dextroamphetamine

Therapeutic Category Amphetamine; Anorexiant; Central Nervous System Stimulant, Amphetamine

Generic Available No

Use Attention-deficit/hyperactivity disorder (ADHD); narcolepsy

Restrictions C-II

Pregnancy Risk Factor C

Contraindications Hypersensitivity or idiosyncrasy to dextroamphetamine, amphetamine, sympathomimetic amines, or any component; advanced arteriosclerosis, moderate to severe hypertension, symptomatic cardiovascular disease, hyperthyroidism, glaucoma, agitated states, history of drug abuse; concurrent use or use within 14 days of MAO inhibitors (hypertensive crisis may occur)

Warnings High potential for abuse; prolonged administration may lead to drug dependence; use in psychotic children may exacerbate symptoms of thought disorder and behavior disturbance; may potentially be associated with growth inhibition (monitor growth)

Precautions Use with caution in patients with mild hypertension; prescribe or dispense least amount feasible to minimize chance of overdose

Adverse Reactions

Cardiovascular system: Hypertension: tachycardia, palpitations; cardiomyopathy (chronic use)

Central nervous system: Insomnia, headache, nervousness, overstimulation, dizziness, euphoria, dysphoria, dyskinesia, exacerbation of phonic and motor tics; psychotic episodes (rare at recommended doses)

Dermatologic: Rash, urticaria

Endocrine and metabolic: Growth suppression, weight loss

Gastrointestinal: Anorexia, diarrhea, constipation, xerostomia, unpleasant taste

Neuromuscular and skeletal: Tremor

Miscellaneous: Physical and psychological dependence with long-term use

Drug Interactions Amphetamines may decrease hypotensive effects of antihypertensives and sedative effect of antihistamines; may increase effects of tricyclic antidepressants or sympathomimetics; may precipitate hypertensive crisis in patients receiving MAO inhibitors (avoid use within 14 days) and arrhythmias in patients receiving general anesthetics; may delay oral absorption of ethosuximide, phenobarbital, and phenytoin. With propoxyphene overdose, CNS stimulation from amphetamines is potentiated (fatal convulsions may occur); tricyclic antidepressants may enhance the effects of amphetamines (avoid use or monitor for cardiovascular effects); chlorpromazine and haloperidol may inhibit the CNS stimulant effects of amphetamines. Antacids may increase the oral absorption of amphetamines; urinary alkalinizers or large doses of antacids may decrease urinary excretion of amphetamines and increase their half-life and duration of action (dosage decrease may be needed). Acids or acidifiers may decrease the oral absorption of amphetamines; urinary acidifiers may increase urinary excretion of amphetamines and decrease their half-life and duration of action (dosage adjustment may be needed).

Food Interactions Acidic foods, juices, or vitamin C may decrease oral absorption

Stability Store tablets at controlled room temperature; dispense in tight, light-resistant container

Mechanism of Action Blocks reuptake of dopamine and norepinephrine from the synapse, thus increases the amounts of circulating dopamine and norepinephrine in cerebral cortex to reticular activating system; inhibits the action of monoamine oxidase and causes catecholamines to be released; peripherally increases blood pressure and acts as a respiratory stimulant and weak bronchodilator

Pharmacodynamics Oral:
Onset: 30-60 minutes
Duration: 4-6 hours

Pharmacokinetics
Absorption: Oral: Well-absorbed
Distribution: V_d: Adults: 3.5-4.6 L/kg; concentrates in breast milk (avoid breast-feeding); distributes into CNS, mean CSF concentrations are 80% of plasma
Metabolism: In the liver by cytochrome P-450 monoxygenase and glucuronidation
Elimination: 70% of a single dose is eliminated within 24 hours; excreted as unchanged amphetamine (30%), benzoic acid, hydroxy-amphetamine, hippuric acid, norephedrine and p-hydroxynorephedrine

Usual Dosage Oral: **Note:** Use lowest effective individualized dose; administer first dose as soon as awake; use intervals of 4-6 hours between additional doses
ADHD:
  Children: <3 years: Not recommended
  Children: 3-5 years: Initial 2.5 mg/day given every morning; increase daily dose by 2.5 mg at weekly intervals until optimal response is obtained; maximum dose: 40 mg/day given in 1-3 divided doses per day
  Children: ≥6 years: Initial: 5 mg once or twice daily; increase daily dose by 5 mg at weekly intervals until optimal response is obtained; usual maximum dose: 40 mg/day given in 1-3 divided doses per day
Narcolepsy:
  Children:
    Children: 6-12 years: Initial: 5 mg/day; increase daily dose by 5 mg at weekly intervals until optimal response is obtained; maximum dose: 60 mg/day given in 1-3 divided doses per day
    Children >12 years and Adults: Initial: 10 mg/day; increase daily dose by 10 mg at weekly intervals until optimal response is obtained; maximum dose: 60 mg/day given in 1-3 divided doses per day

Administration Oral: To avoid insomnia, last daily dose should be administered no less than 6 hours before retiring

Monitoring Parameters CNS activity, blood pressure, height, weight

Patient Information May impair ability to perform potentially hazardous activities; do not discontinue abruptly; limit caffeine; avoid alcohol

Additional Information Treatment of ADHD should include "drug holidays" or periodic discontinuation of medication in order to assess the patient's requirments, decrease tolerance, and limit suppression of linear growth and weight; the combination of equal parts of *d, l*-amphetamine aspartate, *d, l*-amphetamine sulfate, dextroamphetamine saccharate and dextroamphetamine sulfate results in a 75:25 ratio of the dextro- and levo isomers of amphetamine.

The duration of action of Adderall® is longer than methylphenidate; behavioral effects of a single morning dose of Adderall® may last throughout the school day; a single morning dose of Adderall® has been shown in several studies to be as effective as twice daily dosing of methylphenidate for the treatment of ADHD (see Pelham et al, *Pediatrics*, 1999, 104(6):1300-11; Manos 1999, Pliszka 2000).

Dosage Forms Tablet:
5 mg (amphetamine aspartate 1.25 mg, amphetamine sulfate 1.25 mg, dextroamphetamine saccharate 1.25 mg, dextroamphetamine sulfate 1.25 mg) [total amphetamine base equivalence: 3.13 mg]
10 mg (amphetamine aspartate 2.5 mg, amphetamine sulfate 2.5 mg, dextroamphetamine saccharate 2.5 mg, dextroamphetamine sulfate 2.5 mg) [total amphetamine base equivalence: 6.3 mg]
20 mg (amphetamine aspartate 5 mg, amphetamine sulfate 5 mg, dextroamphetamine saccharate 5 mg, dextroamphetamine sulfate 5 mg) [total amphetamine base equivalence: 12.6 mg]
30 mg (amphetamine aspartate 7.5 mg, amphetamine sulfate 7.5 mg, dextroamphetamine saccharate 7.5 mg, dextroamphetamine sulfate 7.5 mg) [total amphetamine base equivalence: 18.8 mg]

References
Manos MJ, Short EJ, and Findling RL, "Differential Effectiveness of Methylphenidate and Adderall® in School-Age Youths With Attention-Deficit/Hyperactivity Disorder," *J Am Acad Child Adolesc Psychiatry*, 1999, 38(7):813-9.
Pelham WE, Aronoff HR, Midlam JK, et al, "A Comparison of Ritalin® and Adderall®: Efficacy and Time-Course in Children With Attention-Deficit/Hyperactivity Disorder," *Pediatrics*, 1999, 103(4):e43. URL: http://www.pediatrics.org/cgi/content/full/103/4/e43

(Continued)

Dextroamphetamine and Amphetamine *(Continued)*

Pelham WE, Gnagy EM, Chronis AM, et al, "A Comparison of Morning-Only and Morning/Late After-noon Adderall® to Morning-Only, Twice-Daily, and Three Times-Daily Methylphenidate in Children With Attention-Deficit/Hyperactivity Disorder," *Pediatrics*, 1999, 104(6):1300-11.

Pliszka SR, Browne RG, Olvera RL, et al, "A Double-Blind, Placebo-Controlled Study of Adderall® and Methylphenidate in the Treatment of Attention-Deficit/Hyperactivity Disorder," *J Am Acad Child Adolesc Psychiatry*, 2000, 39(5):619-26.

Swanson JM, Wigal S, Greenhill LL, et al, "Analog Classroom Assessment of Adderall® in Children With ADHD," *J Am Acad Child Adolesc Psychiatry*, 1998, 37(5):519-26.

♦ **Dextroamphetamine Sulfate** *see* Dextroamphetamine *on page 300*

Dextromethorphan (deks troe meth OR fan)

Brand Names Balminil®-DM, -DM Children (Canada); Benylin DM® [OTC]; Benylin® Pediatric [OTC]; Children's Hold® [OTC]; Creo-Terpin® [OTC]; Delsym® [OTC]; Drixoral® Cough Liquid Caps [OTC]; Hold® DM [OTC]; Koffex® DM, -DM Children (Canada); Pertussin® CS [OTC]; Pertussin® ES [OTC]; Robitussin® Cough Calmers [OTC]; Robitussin® Pediatric [OTC]; Scot-Tussin DM® Cough Chasers [OTC]; Silphen DM® [OTC]; St. Joseph® Cough Suppressant [OTC]; Sucrets® Cough Calmers [OTC]; Suppress® [OTC]; Triaminic DM (Canada); Trocal® [OTC]; Vicks Formula 44® [OTC]; Vicks Formula 44® Pediatric Formula [OTC]

Available Salts Dextromethorphan Hydrobromide; Dextromethorphan Hydrochloride

Synonyms DM

Therapeutic Category Antitussive; Cough Preparation

Generic Available Yes

Use Symptomatic relief of coughs caused by minor viral upper respiratory tract infections or inhaled irritants

Pregnancy Risk Factor C

Contraindications Hypersensitivity to dextromethorphan or any component; concomitant use or use within 14 days of MAO inhibitors

Warnings Do not use for persistent or chronic cough, or for cough accompanied by excessive secretions

Precautions Anecdotal reports of abuse of dextromethorphan-containing cough/cold products have increased, especially among teenagers

Adverse Reactions

Central nervous system: Drowsiness, dizziness

Gastrointestinal: Nausea

Drug Interactions MAO inhibitors (increased risk of serotonin syndrome); haloperidol and fluoxetine decrease dextromethorphan metabolism; dextromethorphan decreases fluoxetine metabolism

Mechanism of Action Non-narcotic chemical relative of morphine; controls cough by depressing the medullary cough center

Pharmacodynamics

Onset of antitussive action: Within 15-30 minutes

Duration: Up to 6 hours

Pharmacokinetics

Metabolism: In the liver

Half-Life: 1.4-3.9 hours

Time to peak serum concentration: 2-2.5 hours

Elimination: Principally in urine

Usual Dosage Dosage in children <2 years of age is not well established; the following dosage recommendations in children <2 years are consistent with the dosages received when using combination products containing dextromethorphan.

Oral:

Children:

1-3 months: 0.5-1 mg every 6-8 hours

3-6 months: 1-2 mg every 6-8 hours

7 months to 1 year: 2-4 mg every 6-8 hours

≥2-6 years : 2.5-7.5 mg every 4-8 hours; extended release formulation: 15 mg twice daily (maximum: 30 mg/24 hours)

7-12 years: 5-10 mg every 4 hours or 15 mg every 6-8 hours; extended release formulation: 30 mg twice daily (maximum: 60 mg/24 hours)

Children >12 years and Adults: 10-30 mg every 4-8 hours or extended release formulation: 60 mg twice daily (maximum: 120 mg/24 hours)

Administration Oral: May administer without regard to meals

Monitoring Parameters Cough, mental status

Test Interactions Can give a false-positive on phencyclidine qualitative immunoassay screen

Patient Information If cough lasts more than 1 week or is accompanied by fever or headache, notify physician

Additional Information Dextromethorphan 15-30 mg equals 8-15 mg codeine as an antitussive

Dosage Forms

Capsule, as hydrobromide (Drixoral® Cough Liquid Caps): 30 mg

Liquid: (Creo-Terpin®): 10 mg/15 mL (120 mL)

Liquid, as hydrobromide:

Pertussin® CS: 3.5 mg/5 mL (120 mL)

Robitussin® Pediatric, St. Joseph® Cough Suppressant: 7.5 mg/5 mL (60 mL, 120 mL, 240 mL)

Pertussin® ES, Vicks Formula 44®: 15 mg/5 mL (120 mL, 240 mL)

Liquid, sustained release, as polistirex, as hydrobromide (Delsym®): 30 mg/5 mL (89 mL)

Lozenges, as hydrobromide:

Scot-Tussin DM® Cough Chasers: 2.5 mg

Children's Hold®, Hold® DM, Robitussin® Cough Calmers, Sucrets® Cough Calmers: 5 mg

Suppress®, Trocal®: 7.5 mg

Syrup, as hydrobromide:

Benylin® Pediatric: 7.5 mg/mL (118 mL)

Benylin DM®, Silphen DM®: 10 mg/5 mL (120 mL, 3780 mL)

Vicks Formula 44® Pediatric Formula: 15 mg/15 mL (120 mL)

♦ **Dextromethorphan and Glycerol Guaiacolate** *see* Guaifenesin and Dextromethorphan *on page 466*

♦ **Dextromethorphan and Guaifenesin** *see* Guaifenesin and Dextromethorphan *on page 466*

♦ **Dextromethorphan Hydrobromide** *see* Dextromethorphan *on page 304*

♦ **Dextromethorphan Hydrochloride** *see* Dextromethorphan *on page 304*

♦ **Dextropropoxyphene** *see* Propoxyphene *on page 814*

Dextrose (DEKS trose)

Related Information

Fluid and Electrolyte Requirements in Children *on page 1068*

Parenteral Nutrition (PN) *on page 1072*

Brand Names B-D Glucose® [OTC]; Dex4 Glucose [OTC]; Glutose® [OTC]; Insta-Glucose® [OTC]; Insulin Reaction [OTC]

Synonyms Anhydrous Glucose; D_5W; $D_{10}W$; $D_{25}W$; $D_{30}W$; $D_{40}W$; $D_{50}W$; $D_{60}W$; $D_{70}W$; Dextrose Monohydrate; Glucose; Glucose Monohydrate; Glycosum

Therapeutic Category Antidote, Insulin; Antidote, Oral Hypoglycemic; Fluid Replacement, Enteral; Fluid Replacement, Parenteral; Hyperglycemic Agent; Hyperkalemia, Adjunctive Treatment Agent; Intravenous Nutritional Therapy

Generic Available Yes

Use

5% and 10% solutions: Peripheral infusion to provide calories and fluid replacement

10% solution: Treatment of hypoglycemia in premature neonates

25% (hypertonic) solution: Treatment of acute symptomatic episodes of hypoglycemia in infants and children to restore depressed blood glucose levels; adjunctive treatment of hyperkalemia when combined with insulin

50% (hypertonic) solution: Treatment of insulin-induced hypoglycemia (hyperinsulinemia or insulin shock) and adjunctive treatment of hyperkalemia in adolescents and adults

≥10% solutions: Infusion after admixture with amino acids for nutritional support

Pregnancy Risk Factor C

Contraindications Diabetic coma with hyperglycemia; hypertonic solutions in patients with intracranial or intraspinal hemorrhage; patients with delirium tremens and dehydration; patients with anuria, hepatic coma, or glucose-galactose malabsorption syndrome

Warnings Hypertonic solutions (>10%) may cause thrombosis if infused via peripheral veins; administer hypertonic solutions via a central venous catheter; rapid administration of hypertonic solutions may produce significant hyperglycemia, glycosuria, and shifts in electrolytes; this may result in dehydration, hyperosmolar syndrome, coma, and death especially in patients with chronic uremia or carbohydrate intolerance; hyperglycemia and glycosuria may be functions of the rate of administration of dextrose; to minimize these effects, reduce the rate of infusion; addition of insulin may be necessary; administration of potassium free I.V. dextrose solutions may result in significant hypokalemia, particularly if highly concentrated (Continued)

Dextrose *(Continued)*

solutions are used; add potassium to dextrose solutions for patients with adequate renal function; abrupt withdrawal of dextrose solution may be associated with rebound hypoglycemia; an unexpected rise in blood glucose level in an otherwise stable patient may be an early symptom of infection; glucose is not absorbed from the buccal cavity; it must be swallowed to be effective; do not use oral forms in unconscious patients

Precautions Use with caution in premature infants, especially very low birth weight infants, as rapid changes is osmolality may produce profound effects on the brain, including intraventricular hemorrhage; small incremental changes in infusion rates are necessary in these patients; use with caution also in patients with diabetes mellitus

Adverse Reactions Note: Most adverse effects are associated with excessive dosage or rate of infusion

Cardiovascular: Venous thrombosis, phlebitis, hypovolemia, hypervolemia, dehydration, edema

Central nervous system: Fever, mental confusion, unconsciousness, hyperosmolar syndrome

Endocrine & metabolic: Hyperglycemia, hypokalemia, acidosis, hypophosphatemia, hypomagnesemia

Local: Pain, vein irritation, tissue necrosis

Genitourinary: Polyuria, glycosuria, ketonuria

Gastrointestinal: Polydipsia, nausea

Respiratory: Tachypnea, pulmonary edema

Drug Interactions Corticosteroids

Stability Stable at room temperature; protect from freezing and extreme heat; store oral dextrose in airtight containers

Mechanism of Action Dextrose, a monosaccharide, is a source of calories and fluids in patients unable to obtain adequate oral intake; may decrease body protein and nitrogen losses; promotes glycogen deposition in the liver; for the treatment of hyperkalemia, when combined with insulin, dextrose stimulates the uptake of potassium by cells, especially in muscle tissue

Pharmacodynamics

Onset: Treatment of hypoglycemia: Oral: 10 minutes

Peak effect: Treatment of hyperkalemia: I.V.: 30 minutes

Pharmacokinetics

Absorption: Rapidly from the small intestine by an active mechanism

Metabolism: Metabolized to carbon dioxide and water

Time to peak concentration: Oral: 40 minutes

Usual Dosage

Hypoglycemia: Doses may be repeated in severe cases

I.V.:

Premature neonates: 0.1-0.2 g/kg/dose (1-2 mL/kg/dose of 10% solution); followed by continuous infusion at a rate of 4-6 mg/kg/minute

Infants ≤6 months: 0.25-0.5 g/kg/dose (1-2 mL/kg/dose of 25% solution); maximum: 25 g/dose

Infants >6 months and Children: 0.5-1 g/kg/dose (2-4 mL/kg/dose of 25% solution); maximum: 25 g/dose

Adolescents and Adults: 10-25 g (40-100 mL of 25% solution or 20-50 mL of 50% solution)

Oral:

Children >2 years and Adults: 10-20 g as single dose; repeat in 10 minutes if necessary

Treatment of Hyperkalemia: I.V. (in combination with insulin):

Infants and Children: 0.5-1 g/kg (using 25% or 50% solution) combined with regular insulin 1 unit for every 4-5 g dextrose given; infuse over 2 hours (infusions as short as 30 minutes have been recommended); repeat as needed

Adolescents and Adults: 0.1 mL/kg (using 50% solution) with regular insulin 1 unit for every 4-5 g dextrose given (repeat as needed) **or** as an alternative 10 units regular insulin added to 250 mL $D_{10}W$ and infuse over 30-60 minutes

Fluid therapy: See Fluid and Electrolyte Requirements in Children *on page 1068*
Nutrition: See Parenteral Nutrition (PN) *on page 1072*

Administration

Oral: Must be swallowed to be absorbed (see Warnings)

Parenteral: Not for S.C. or I.M. administration; dilute concentrated dextrose solutions for peripheral venous administration to a maximum concentration of 12.5%; in emergency situations, 25% dextrose has been used peripherally; for direct I.V.

infusion, infuse at a maximum rate of 200 mg/kg over 1 minute; continuous infusion rates very with tolerance (see Parenteral Nutrition (PN) *on page 1072*) and range from 4.5-15 mg/kg/minute; hyperinsulinemic neonates may require up to 15-25 mg/kg/minute infusion rates

Monitoring Parameters Blood and urine sugar, serum electrolytes, I & O, caloric intake

Reference Range Normal blood sugar:
Neonates: 110-270 mg/dL
0-2 years: 60-105 mg/dL
Children >2 years and Adults: 70-110 mg/dL

Additional Information Each g of I.V. dextrose contains 3.4 kcal; glucose monohydrate 1 g is equal to 1 g anhydrous dextrose

Dosage Forms
Gel, as 40% dextrose: (Glutose®, Insta-Glucose®, Insulin Reaction): 25 g, 30.8 g, 80 g
Infusion, as 5% dextrose: 10 mL, 25 mL, 50 mL, 150 mL, 250 mL, 500 mL, 1000 mL
Infusion, as 10% dextrose: 3 mL, 250 mL, 500 mL, 1000 mL
Infusion, as 20% dextrose: 500 mL, 1000 mL
Infusion, as 25% dextrose: 10 mL
Infusion, as 30% dextrose: 500 mL, 1000 mL
Infusion, as 40% dextrose: 500 mL, 1000 mL
Infusion, as 50% dextrose: 50 mL, 500 mL, 1000 mL, 2000 mL
Infusion, as 60% dextrose: 500 mL, 1000 mL
Infusion, as 70% dextrose: 70 mL, 500 mL, 1000 mL, 2000 mL
Tablet, chewable (B-D Glucose®): 5 g

♦ **Dextrose Monohydrate** *see* Dextrose *on page 305*
♦ **Dey-Dose® Isoproterenol** *see* Isoproterenol *on page 536*
♦ **Dey-Dose® Metaproterenol** *see* Metaproterenol *on page 611*
♦ **Dey-Drop® Ophthalmic Solution** *see* Silver Nitrate *on page 866*
♦ **Dey-Lute® Isoetharine** *see* Isoetharine *on page 533*
♦ **DHAD** *see* Mitoxantrone *on page 653*
♦ **DHPG** *see* Ganciclovir *on page 450*
♦ **DHS® Tar [OTC]** *see* Coal Tar *on page 247*
♦ **DHT™** *see* Dihydrotachysterol *on page 321*
♦ **Diabetic Tussin DM® [OTC]** *see* Guaifenesin and Dextromethorphan *on page 466*
♦ **Diabetic Tussin EX® [OTC]** *see* Guaifenesin *on page 464*
♦ **Dialose® [OTC]** *see* Docusate *on page 336*
♦ **Dialose® Plus Capsule [OTC]** *see* Docusate and Casanthranol *on page 337*
♦ **Diamine T.D.® Oral [OTC]** *see* Brompheniramine *on page 142*
♦ **Diaminodiphenylsulfone** *see* Dapsone *on page 283*
♦ **Diamox®** *see* Acetazolamide *on page 29*
♦ **Diamox Sequels®** *see* Acetazolamide *on page 29*
♦ **Diar-aid® [OTC]** *see* Loperamide *on page 580*
♦ **Diasorb® [OTC]** *see* Attapulgite *on page 109*
♦ **Diastat® Rectal Delivery System** *see* Diazepam *on page 307*
♦ **Diazemuls® (Canada)** *see* Diazepam *on page 307*
♦ **Diazemuls® Injection** *see* Diazepam *on page 307*

Diazepam (dye AZ e pam)
Related Information
Adult ACLS Algorithm, Electrical Conversion *on page 1014*
Carbohydrate and Alcohol Content of Liquid Medications for Use in Patients Receiving Ketogenic Diets *on page 1228*
Drugs and Breast-Feeding *on page 1213*
Laboratory Detection of Drugs in Urine *on page 1204*
Overdose and Toxicology *on page 1191*
Preprocedure Sedatives in Children *on page 1169*

Brand Names Apo®-Diazepam (Canada); Diastat® Rectal Delivery System; Diazemuls® (Canada); Diazemuls® Injection; Diazepam Intensol®; Dizac® Injectable Emulsion; E Pam® (Canada); Meval® (Canada); Novo-Dipam® (Canada); PMS-Diazepam (Canada); Valium® Injection; Valium® Oral; Vivol® (Canada)

Therapeutic Category Antianxiety Agent; Anticonvulsant, Benzodiazepine; Benzodiazepine; Hypnotic; Sedative
(Continued)

Diazepam *(Continued)*

Generic Available
Yes: Injection, tablets, solution
No: Extended release capsules, emulsified injection, rectal gel

Use Management of general anxiety disorders, panic disorders; to provide preoperative sedation, light anesthesia, and amnesia; treatment of status epilepticus, alcohol withdrawal symptoms; used as a skeletal muscle relaxant; rectal gel is indicated for intermittent episodes of markedly increased seizure activity in epilepsy patients on stable regimens of anticonvulsants

Restrictions C-IV

Pregnancy Risk Factor D

Contraindications Hypersensitivity to diazepam or any component (emulsified diazepam injection contains soybean oil, egg yolk phospholipids); there may be a cross-sensitivity with other benzodiazepines; do not use in a comatose patient, in those with pre-existing CNS depression, respiratory depression, narrow-angle glaucoma, or severe uncontrolled pain

Warnings Rapid I.V. push may cause sudden respiratory depression, apnea, or hypotension

Precautions Use with caution in patients receiving other CNS depressants, patients with low albumin, renal or hepatic dysfunction, and in the elderly and young infants; use with extreme caution in neonates; injection and rectal gel contain sodium benzoate and benzoic acid which may displace bilirubin from protein binding sites and at larger doses can cause the gasping syndrome; neonates have decreased metabolism of diazepam and desmethyldiazepam (active metabolite), both can accumulate with repeated use and cause increased toxicity

Adverse Reactions
Cardiovascular: Cardiac arrest, hypotension, bradycardia, cardiovascular collapse
Central nervous system: Drowsiness, somnolence, confusion, dizziness, fatigue, amnesia, slurred speech, ataxia, impaired coordination, paradoxical excitement or rage (rare)
Dermatologic: Rash, dermatitis
Local: Phlebitis, pain with injection (less with emulsified injection)
Ocular: Blurred vision, diplopia
Respiratory: Decrease in respiratory rate, apnea, laryngospasm
Miscellaneous: Physical and psychological dependence with prolonged use

Drug Interactions Cytochrome P-450 isoenzyme CYP1A2, CYP2C8, CYP2C19 (minor), and CYP3A3/4 (minor) substrate; desmethyldiazepam is a CYP2C19 isoenzyme substrate

CNS depressants (alcohol, barbiturates, opioids) may enhance sedation and respiratory depression of diazepam; enzyme inducers may increase the hepatic metabolism of diazepam; cimetidine and erythromycin may decrease the metabolism of diazepam; valproic acid may displace diazepam from binding sites which may result in an increase in sedative effects; concurrent use of diazepam with ritonavir is not recommended

Stability Do not mix either I.V. product with other medications; protect I.V. products from light; diazepam injectable emulsion does not contain preservative, discard unused portion; diazepam injectable emulsion is incompatible with morphine and glycopyrrolate

Mechanism of Action Depresses all levels of the CNS, including the limbic and reticular formation by binding to the benzodiazepine site on the gamma-aminobutyric acid (GABA) receptor complex and modulating GABA, which is a major inhibitory neurotransmitter in the brain

Pharmacodynamics Status epilepticus:
Onset of action:
I.V.: 1-3 minutes
Rectal: 2-10 minutes
Duration: 15-30 minutes

Pharmacokinetics Note: No significant differences exist in pharmacokinetics between conventional and emulsified diazepam formulations

Absorption:
Oral: 85% to 100%
I.M.: Poor
Rectal (gel): Well absorbed
Distribution: Widely distributed; crosses blood-brain barrier and placenta; distributes into breast milk
Protein binding:
Neonates: 84% to 86%

Adults: 98%

Metabolism: In the liver to desmethyldiazepam (active metabolite) and N-methyloxazepam (active metabolite); these are metabolized to oxazepam (active) which undergoes glucuronide conjugation before being excreted

Bioavailability:
Emulsified diazepam: I.V.: 93%
Rectal (gel): 90%

Half-life:
Diazepam:
Infants 1 month to 2 years: 40-50 hours
Children 2-12 years: 15-21 hours
Children 12-16 years: 18-20 hours
Adults: 20-50 hours; emulsified diazepam: 30-60 hours
Increased half-life in neonates (50-95 hours), elderly, and those with severe hepatic disorders
Desmethyldiazepam (active metabolite): 50-100 hours and can be prolonged in neonates

Time to peak serum concentration: Rectal (gel): 1.5 hours

Elimination: In urine, primarily as conjugated oxazepam (75%), desmethyldiazepam, and N-methyloxazepam

Usual Dosage
Children:
Conscious sedation for procedures: Oral: 0.2-0.3 mg/kg (maximum dose: 10 mg) 45-60 minutes prior to procedure
Febrile seizure prophylaxis: Oral: 1 mg/kg/day divided every 8 hours; initiate therapy at first sign of fever and continue for 24 hours after fever is gone
Sedation or muscle relaxation or anxiety:
Oral: 0.12-0.8 mg/kg/day in divided doses every 6-8 hours
I.M., I.V.: 0.04-0.3 mg/kg/dose every 2-4 hours to a maximum of 0.6 mg/kg within an 8-hour period if needed
Status epilepticus: I.V.:
Neonates: (Not recommended as a first-line agent; conventional injection contains sodium benzoate and benzoic acid; see Precautions) 0.1-0.3 mg/kg/dose given over 3-5 minutes, every 15-30 minutes to a maximum total dose of 2 mg
Infants >30 days and Children <5 years: 0.05-0.3 mg/kg/dose given over 3-5 minutes, every 15-30 minutes to a maximum total dose of 5 mg or 0.2-0.5 mg/dose every 2-5 minutes to a maximum total dose of 5 mg; repeat in 2-4 hours as needed
Children ≥5 years: 0.05-0.3 mg/kg/dose given over 3-5 minutes, every 15-30 minutes to a maximum total dose of 10 mg or 1 mg/dose every 2-5 minutes to a maximum of 10 mg; repeat in 2-4 hours as needed
Muscle spasm associated with tetanus: I.V., I.M.:
Infants >30 days: 1-2 mg/dose every 3-4 hours as needed
Children ≥5 years: 5-10 mg/dose every 3-4 hours as needed
Anticonvulsant: Acute treatment:
Rectal gel formulation:
Infants <6 months: Not recommended
Children <2 years: Safety and efficacy have not been studied
Children 2-5 years: 0.5 mg/kg
Children 6-11 years: 0.3 mg/kg
Children ≥12 years and Adults: 0.2 mg/kg
Note: Round dose to 2.5, 5, 10, 15, and 20 mg/dose; dose may be repeated in 4-12 hours if needed; do not use more than 5 times per month or more than once every 5 days
Rectal: Undiluted 5 mg/mL conventional parenteral formulation (filter if using ampul): 0.5 mg/kg/dose then 0.25 mg/kg/dose in 10 minutes if needed
Adolescents: Conscious sedation for procedures:
Oral: 10 mg
I.V.: 5 mg; may repeat with 2.5 mg if needed
Adults:
Anxiety:
Oral: 2-10 mg 2-4 times/day
I.M., I.V.: 2-10 mg, may repeat in 3-4 hours if needed
Skeletal muscle relaxation:
Oral: 2-10 mg 2-4 times/day
I.M., I.V.: 5-10 mg, may repeat in 2-4 hours
Status epilepticus: I.V.: 5-10 mg every 10-15 minutes up to 30 mg in an 8-hour period; may repeat in 2-4 hours
(Continued)

Diazepam *(Continued)*

Preoperative medication: I.M.: 10 mg before surgery

Administration

Oral: Administer with food or water; oral concentrate solution (5 mg/mL) should be diluted or mixed with water, juice, soda, applesauce, or pudding before use

Parenteral: I.V.: Infants and children: Do not exceed 1-2 mg/minute I.V. push; adult maximum infusion rate: 5 mg/minute; rapid injection may cause respiratory depression or hypotension; emulsified diazepam injection is for I.V. use only; do not add emulsified diazepam injection to infusion sets containing polyvinyl chloride

Monitoring Parameters Heart rate, respiratory rate, blood pressure

Reference Range Effective therapeutic range not well established

Proposed therapeutic:

Diazepam: 0.2-1.5 µg/mL (SI: 0.7-5.3 µmol/L)

N-desmethyldiazepam (nordiazepam): 0.1-0.5 µg/mL (SI: 0.35-1.8 µmol/L)

Test Interactions False-negative urinary glucose determinations with Clinistix® or Diastix®

Patient Information Avoid alcohol; limit caffeine; may cause drowsiness and impair ability to perform activities that require mental alertness or physical coordination; avoid abrupt discontinuation after prolonged use

Nursing Implications Avoid extravasation; infuse I.V. into secure line using larger veins

Additional Information Diazepam does not have any analgesic effects; diarrhea in a 9 month old infant receiving high-dose oral diazepam was attributed to the diazepam oral solution that contained polyethylene glycol and propylene glycol (both are osmotically active); diarrhea resolved when crushed tablets were substituted for the oral solution (see Marshall, 1995); emulsified diazepam injection is an oil-in-water emulsion; rectal gel contains sodium benzoate, benzyl alcohol (1.5%) and benzoic acid

Dosage Forms

Gel, rectal delivery system (Diastat®):

Pediatric rectal tip (4.4 cm): 5 mg/mL (2.5 mg, 5 mg, 10 mg) [twin packs]

Adult rectal tip (6 cm): 5 mg/mL (10 mg, 15 mg, 20 mg) [twin packs]

Injection: 5 mg/mL (1 mL, 2 mL, 5 mL, 10 mL)

Injection, emulsified:

Dizac®: 5 mg/mL (3 mL)

Diazemuls®: 5 mg/mL (2 mL)

Solution, oral (wintergreen-spice flavor): 5 mg/5 mL (5 mL, 10 mL, 500 mL)

Solution, oral concentrate (Diazepam Intensol®): 5 mg/mL (30 mL)

Tablet: 2 mg, 5 mg, 10 mg

References

Marshall JD, Farrar HC, and Kearns GL, "Diarrhea Associated With Enteral Benzodiazepine Solutions," *J Pediatr*, 1995, 126(4):657-9.

Rosman NP, Colton T, Labazzo J, et al, "A Controlled Trial of Diazepam Administered During Febrile Illnesses to Prevent Recurrence of Febrile Seizures," *N Engl J Med*, 1993, 329(2):79-84.

Zeltzer LK, Altman A, Cohen D, et al, "Report of the Subcommittee on the Management of Pain Associated With Procedures in Children With Cancer," *Pediatrics*, 1990, 86(5 Pt 2):826-31.

♦ Diazepam Intensol® *see* Diazepam *on page 307*

Diazoxide *(dye az OKS ide)*

Brand Names Hyperstat® I.V.; Proglycem® Oral

Therapeutic Category Antihypertensive Agent; Antihypoglycemic Agent; Vasodilator

Generic Available Yes: Injection

Use

I.V.: Emergency lowering of blood pressure

Oral: Hypoglycemia related to hyperinsulinism secondary to islet cell adenoma, carcinoma, or hyperplasia; adenomatosis; nesidioblastosis (persistent hyperinsulinemic hypoglycemia of infancy); leucine sensitivity, or extrapancreatic malignancy

Pregnancy Risk Factor C

Contraindications Hypersensitivity to diazoxide, any component, thiazides, or other sulfonamide derivatives; aortic coarctation, arteriovenous shunts, dissecting aortic aneurysm

Precautions Diabetes mellitus, renal or liver disease, coronary artery disease, or cerebral vascular insufficiency; use care when switching oral dosage forms, oral suspension may result in higher blood concentrations than capsule in some patients

Adverse Reactions
Cardiovascular: Hypotension, tachycardia, flushing
Central nervous system: Dizziness, seizure, headache
Dermatologic: Rash, hirsutism
Endocrine & metabolic: Hyperglycemia, ketoacidosis, hyperuricemia, sodium and water retention, edema (more common in young infants and adults)
Gastrointestinal: Nausea, vomiting, anorexia, constipation
Hematologic: Leukopenia, thrombocytopenia
Local: Pain, burning, cellulitis/phlebitis upon extravasation
Neuromuscular & skeletal: Weakness
Miscellaneous: Extrapyramidal symptoms and development of abnormal facies with chronic oral use

Drug Interactions Diuretics and hypotensive agents may potentiate diazoxide adverse effects; diazoxide may increase phenytoin metabolism or free fraction; diazoxide may decrease warfarin protein binding

Stability Protect from light, heat, and freezing; avoid using darkened solutions

Mechanism of Action Inhibits insulin release from the pancreas; produces direct smooth muscle relaxation of the peripheral arterioles which results in decrease in blood pressure and reflex increase in heart rate and cardiac output

Pharmacodynamics
Hyperglycemic effects (oral):
Onset of action: Within 1 hour
Duration (normal renal function): 8 hours
Hypotensive effects (I.V.):
Peak: Within 5 minutes
Duration: Usually 3-12 hours

Pharmacokinetics
Protein binding: 90%
Half-life:
Children: 9-24 hours
Adults: 20-36 hours
Elimination: 50% excreted unchanged in urine

Usual Dosage
Hyperinsulinemic hypoglycemia: Oral (**Note:** Use lower dose listed as initial dose):
Newborns and Infants: 8-15 mg/kg/day in divided doses every 8-12 hours
Children and Adults: 3-8 mg/kg/day in divided doses every 8-12 hours
Hypertension: I.V.: Children and Adults: 1-3 mg/kg (maximum dose: 150 mg in a single injection); repeat dose in 5-15 minutes until blood pressure adequately reduced; repeat administration every 4-24 hours; monitor blood pressure closely

Administration
Oral: Administer on an empty stomach 1 hour before or 1 hour after meals; shake suspension well before use
Parenteral: Do not administer I.M. or S.C.; administer I.V. (undiluted) by rapid I.V. injection over a period of 30 seconds or less

Monitoring Parameters Blood pressure, blood glucose

Additional Information Patients may require a diuretic with repeated doses

Dosage Forms
Capsule (Proglycem®): 50 mg
Injection (Hyperstat®): 15 mg/mL (1 mL, 20 mL)
Suspension, oral (chocolate-mint flavor) (Proglycem®): 50 mg/mL (30 mL)

♦ **Dibent® Injection** see Dicyclomine on page 314
♦ **Dibenzyline®** see Phenoxybenzamine on page 756

Dibucaine (DYE byoo kane)
Brand Names Nupercainal® [OTC]
Therapeutic Category Analgesic, Topical; Local Anesthetic, Topical
Generic Available Yes
Use Fast, temporary relief of pain and itching due to hemorrhoids, minor burns, other minor skin conditions
Pregnancy Risk Factor C
Contraindications Hypersensitivity to amide-type anesthetics
Warnings Products may contain sulfites; avoid use in sensitive individuals
Adverse Reactions
Cardiovascular: Edema
Dermatologic: Urticaria, cutaneous lesions, contact dermatitis
Local: Burning, tenderness, irritation, inflammation
(Continued)

Dibucaine *(Continued)*

Mechanism of Action Blocks both the initiation and conduction of nerve impulses by decreasing the neuronal membrane's permeability to sodium ions, which results in inhibition of depolarization with resultant blockade of conduction

Pharmacodynamics
Onset of action: Within 15 minutes
Duration: 2-4 hours

Pharmacokinetics Absorption: Poor through intact skin, but well absorbed through mucous membranes and excoriated skin

Usual Dosage Children and Adults:
Rectal: Hemorrhoids: Administer each morning, evening, and after each bowel movement
Topical: Apply gently to the affected areas; no more than 30 g for adults or 7.5 g for children should be used in any 24-hour period

Administration
Rectal: Insert ointment into rectum using a rectal applicator
Topical: Apply gently to affected areas; do not use near the eyes or over denuded surfaces or blistered areas

Dosage Forms
Cream: 0.5% (45 g)
Ointment, topical: 1% (30 g, 60 g)

♦ **DIC** *see* Dacarbazine *on page 278*
♦ **Dicarbosil® [OTC]** *see* Calcium Supplements *on page 157*
♦ **Dichysterol** *see* Dihydrotachysterol *on page 321*

Diclofenac *(dye KLOE fen ak)*

Brand Names Apo®-Diclo (Canada); Cataflam® Oral; Novo-Difenac® (Canada); Novo-Difenac-SR® (Canada); Nu-Diclo® (Canada); Voltaren® Ophthalmic; Voltaren® Oral; Voltaren®-XR Oral

Available Salts Diclofenac Potassium; Diclofenac Sodium

Therapeutic Category Analgesic, Non-narcotic; Anti-inflammatory Agent; Nonsteroidal Anti-inflammatory Drug (NSAID), Ophthalmic; Nonsteroidal Anti-inflammatory Drug (NSAID), Oral

Generic Available Yes

Use
Oral: Acute treatment of mild to moderate pain; acute and chronic treatment of rheumatoid arthritis, ankylosing spondylitis, and osteoarthritis; used for juvenile rheumatoid arthritis, gout, dysmenorrhea
Ophthalmic solution: Postoperative inflammation after cataract extraction; temporary relief of pain and photophobia in patients undergoing corneal refractive surgery

Pregnancy Risk Factor B

Contraindications Hypersensitivity to diclofenac, any component, aspirin, or NSAIDs; porphyria

Precautions Use with caution in patients with CHF, hypertension, decreased renal or hepatic function, history of GI disease, or those receiving anticoagulants; patients should not wear soft contact lenses while using ophthalmic solution

Adverse Reactions
Central nervous system: Dizziness, headache
Dermatologic: Rash, pruritus
Endocrine & metabolic: Fluid retention
Gastrointestinal: Abdominal pain, indigestion, peptic ulcer, GI bleeding, GI perforation, constipation, diarrhea
Hematologic: Agranulocytosis, aplastic anemia (rare), inhibition of platelet aggregation
Hepatic: Elevated ALT or AST, possible hepatitis
Ocular: With ophthalmic use, itching, tearing (allergic reaction); irritation, redness, burning; ocular irritation with use of hydrogel soft contact lenses
Otic: Tinnitus
Renal: Renal impairment, nephrotic-like syndrome

Drug Interactions Cytochrome P-450 isoenzyme CYP2C8 and CYP2C9 substrate; CYP2C9 isoenzyme inhibitor
Diclofenac may increase serum concentrations of digoxin, methotrexate and lithium; may increase nephrotoxicity of cyclosporin; may decrease diuretic and antihypertensive effects of thiazides and furosemide; diclofenac plus potassium-sparing diuretics may increase serum potassium; concomitant insulin or oral hypoglycemic agents may increase or decrease serum glucose; aspirin may

decrease serum concentration of diclofenac (combination not recommended); gastric irritants (eg, aspirin, other NSAIDs, potassium supplements) may increase risk of GI irritation

Food Interactions Delayed oral absorption has been reported with food for single doses but not with chronic multiple-dose administration

Stability Ophthalmic solution: Store at room temperature; protect from light

Mechanism of Action Inhibits prostaglandin synthesis by decreasing the activity of the enzyme, cyclo-oxygenase, which results in decreased formation of prostaglandin precursors

Usual Dosage
Oral:
Children: 2-3 mg/kg/day divided 2-4 times/day
Adults:
Rheumatoid arthritis:
Cataflam® or Voltaren®: 100-200 mg/day in 2-4 divided doses; maximum dose: 225 mg/day
Voltaren®-XR: 100 mg/day; dose may be increased to 100 mg twice daily; maximum dose: 225 mg/day
Osteoarthritis:
Cataflam® or Voltaren®: 100-150 mg/day in 2-3 divided doses
Voltaren®-XR: 100 mg/day
Ankylosing spondylitis: Voltaren®: 100-125 mg/day in 4-5 divided doses
Analgesia and primary dysmenorrhea: Cataflam®: 50 mg given 3 times/day; some patients may have better relief with an initial dose of 100 mg
Ophthalmic:
Cataract surgery: Instill 1 drop into affected eye 4 times/day beginning 24 hours after cataract surgery and continuing for 2 weeks
Corneal refractive surgery: Instill 1-2 drops into operative eye within the hour prior to surgery, within 15 minutes after surgery, and continuing 4 times/day for up to 3 days

Administration Oral: Administer with milk or food to decrease GI upset; do not chew or crush tablets, swallow whole

Monitoring Parameters CBC, liver enzymes; monitor urine output, BUN, serum creatinine in patients receiving diuretics

Patient Information Avoid alcohol; report any signs of blood in stool; do not use hydrogel soft contact lenses during ophthalmic diclofenac therapy

Additional Information Vomiting, drowsiness, and acute renal failure have been reported with overdoses; Cataflam® tablets are immediate release and is the formulation which should be used when prompt onset of pain relief is desired; Voltaren®-XR should not be used for acute pain relief due to its extended release

Dosage Forms
Solution, ophthalmic, as sodium (Voltaren®): 0.1% (2.5 mL, 5 mL)
Tablet, delayed release, as sodium (Voltaren®): 25 mg, 50 mg, 75 mg
Tablet, extended release, as sodium (Voltaren®-XR): 100 mg
Tablet, as potassium (Cataflam®): 50 mg

References
Brogden RN, Heel RC, Pakes GE, et al, "Diclofenac Sodium: A Review of Its Pharmacological Properties and Therapeutic Use in Rheumatic Diseases and Pain of Varying Origin," *Drugs*, 1980, 20(1):24-48.
Haapasaari J, Wuolijoki E, and Ylijoki H, "Treatment of Juvenile Rheumatoid Arthritis With Diclofenac Sodium" *Scand J Rheumatol*, 1983, 12(4):325-30.

♦ **Diclofenac Potassium** *see Diclofenac on page 312*
♦ **Diclofenac Sodium** *see Diclofenac on page 312*

Dicloxacillin (dye kloks a SIL in)

Brand Names Dycill®; Dynapen®; Pathocil®
Available Salts Dicloxacillin Sodium
Therapeutic Category Antibiotic, Penicillin (Antistaphylococcal)
Generic Available Yes
Use Treatment of skin and soft tissue infections, pneumonia and follow-up therapy of osteomyelitis caused by susceptible penicillinase-producing staphylococci
Pregnancy Risk Factor B
Contraindications Hypersensitivity to dicloxacillin, penicillin, or any component
Warnings Elimination is prolonged in neonates
Adverse Reactions
Central nervous system: Fever
Dermatologic: Rash
Gastrointestinal: Nausea, vomiting, diarrhea, *C. difficile* colitis
(Continued)

Dicloxacillin (Continued)

Hematologic: Eosinophilia, neutropenia, leukopenia, thrombocytopenia
Hepatic: Elevation in liver enzymes
Miscellaneous: Serum sickness-like reaction

Drug Interactions Oral contraceptives (decreased effectiveness), probenecid (increase serum concentration of dicloxacillin)

Food Interactions Presence of food decreases the rate and extent of absorption

Stability Reconstituted dicloxacillin suspension is stable for 7 days at room temperature or 14 days if refrigerated

Mechanism of Action Inhibits bacterial cell wall synthesis by binding to one or more of the penicillin-binding proteins and interfering with the final transpeptidation step of peptidoglycan synthesis

Pharmacokinetics
Absorption: 35% to 76% absorbed from the GI tract
Distribution: Into bone, bile, pleural fluid, synovial fluid, and amniotic fluid; appears in breast milk
Protein binding: 96% to 98%
Half-life: Adults: 0.6-0.8 hours; slightly prolonged in patients with renal impairment
Time to peak serum concentration: Within 0.5-2 hours
Elimination: Partially eliminated by the liver and excreted in bile; 31% to 65% eliminated in urine as unchanged drug and active metabolite
Neonates: Prolonged
CF patients: More rapid elimination than healthy patients
Not dialyzable (0% to 5%)

Usual Dosage Oral:
Children <40 kg: 25-50 mg/kg/day divided every 6 hours; doses of 50-100 mg/kg/day in divided doses every 6 hours have been used for follow-up therapy of osteomyelitis; maximum dose: 2 g/day
Children >40 kg and Adults: 125-500 mg every 6 hours; maximum dose: 2 g/day

Administration Oral: Administer with water 1 hour before or 2 hours after meals on an empty stomach

Monitoring Parameters Periodic monitoring of CBC, BUN, serum creatinine, urinalysis, and liver enzymes during prolonged therapy

Additional Information
Sodium content of 250 mg capsule: 0.6 mEq
Sodium content of 5 mL suspension: 2.9 mEq

Dosage Forms
Capsule, as sodium: 125 mg, 250 mg, 500 mg
Powder for oral suspension, as sodium: 62.5 mg/5 mL (80 mL, 100 mL, 200 mL)

♦ **Dicloxacillin Sodium** see Dicloxacillin on page 313

Dicyclomine (dye SYE kloe meen)

Related Information
Carbohydrate and Alcohol Content of Liquid Medications for Use in Patients Receiving Ketogenic Diets on page 1228
Overdose and Toxicology on page 1191

Brand Names Antispas® Injection; Bentyl® Hydrochloride Injection; Bentyl® Hydrochloride Oral; Bentylol® (Canada); Byclomine® Injection; Dibent® Injection; Dilomine® Injection; Di-Spaz® Injection; Di-Spaz® Oral; Or-Tyl® Injection; Spasmoject® Injection

Available Salts Dicyclomine Hydrochloride

Synonyms Dicycloverine

Therapeutic Category Anticholinergic Agent; Antispasmodic Agent, Gastrointestinal

Generic Available Yes

Use Treatment of functional disturbances of GI motility such as irritable bowel syndrome

Pregnancy Risk Factor B

Contraindications Hypersensitivity to any anticholinergic drug; narrow-angle glaucoma, tachycardia, GI obstruction, obstruction of the urinary tract, myasthenia gravis; should not be used in infants <6 months of age due to reports of respiratory distress, seizures, syncope, asphyxia, pulse rate fluctuations, muscular hypotonia, and coma

Precautions Use with caution in patients with hepatic or renal disease, ulcerative colitis, hyperthyroidism, cardiovascular disease, hypertension, hiatal hernia, autonomic neuropathy

Adverse Reactions Children with Down's syndrome, spastic paralysis, or brain damage are more sensitive to toxic effects than adults

Cardiovascular: Tachycardia, palpitations, orthostatic hypotension

Central nervous system: Seizures, coma, nervousness, excitement, confusion, insomnia, headache

Dermatologic: Urticaria, pruritus, dry skin, photosensitivity

Gastrointestinal: Nausea, vomiting, constipation, xerostomia, dry throat, dysphagia

Genitourinary: Urinary retention

Local: Injection site reactions

Neuromuscular & skeletal: Muscular hypotonia, weakness

Ocular: Blurred vision, photophobia

Respiratory: Respiratory distress, asphyxia, dry nose

Miscellaneous: Decreased diaphoresis

Drug Interactions Additive adverse effects when given with medications with anticholinergic activity; may alter GI absorption of various drugs due to prolonged GI transit time; antacids; antagonizes effects of antiglaucoma agents

Stability Protect from light

Mechanism of Action Blocks the action of acetylcholine at parasympathetic sites in smooth muscle, secretory glands and the CNS

Pharmacodynamics

Onset of effects: 1-2 hours

Duration: Up to 4 hours

Pharmacokinetics

Absorption: Oral: Well absorbed

Distribution: V_d: 3.65 L/kg

Bioavailability: 67%

Half-life:

Initial phase: 1.8 hours

Terminal phase: 9-10 hours

Time to peak serum concentration: Oral: 1-1.5 hours

Elimination: 80% in urine; 10% in feces

Usual Dosage

Infants >6 months: Oral: 5 mg/dose 3-4 times/day

Children: Oral: 10 mg/dose 3-4 times/day

Adults:

Oral: Initial: 20 mg 4 times/day, then increase up to 40 mg 4 times/day

I.M.: 20 mg/dose 4 times/day; oral therapy should replace I.M. therapy as soon as possible

Administration

Oral: Administer 30 minutes before eating

Parenteral: I.M. only; not for I.V. use

Patient Information Limit alcohol

Dosage Forms

Capsule, as hydrochloride: 10 mg, 20 mg

Injection, as hydrochloride: 10 mg/mL (2 mL, 10 mL)

Syrup, as hydrochloride: 10 mg/5 mL (118 mL, 473 mL, 946 mL)

Tablet, as hydrochloride: 20 mg

♦ **Dicyclomine Hydrochloride** *see* Dicyclomine *on page 314*

♦ **Dicycloverine** *see* Dicyclomine *on page 314*

Didanosine (dye DAN oh seen)

Related Information

Adult and Adolescent HIV *on page 1133*

Brand Names Videx® Oral

Synonyms DDI; Dideoxyinosine

Therapeutic Category Antiretroviral Agent; HIV Agents (Anti-HIV Agents); Nucleoside Reverse Transcriptase Inhibitor (NRTI)

Generic Available No

Use Treatment of HIV infection in combination with other antiretroviral agents; (Note: HIV regimens consisting of **three** antiretroviral agents are strongly recommended)

Pregnancy Risk Factor B

Contraindications Hypersensitivity to didanosine or any component

Warnings Major clinical toxicities of didanosine include pancreatitis and peripheral neuropathy; fatal and nonfatal pancreatitis has been reported during therapy; risk factors for developing pancreatitis include a previous history of the condition, didanosine dosage >10 mg/kg/day, concurrent cytomegalovirus or *Mycobacterium* (Continued)

Didanosine (Continued)

avium-intracellulare infection, and concomitant use of stavudine with or without hydroxyurea, pentamidine, or co-trimoxazole. Dose-related (treatment-limiting) peripheral neuropathy occurs most often after 2-6 months of continuous didanosine administration; may cause retinal depigmentation in children receiving doses >300 mg/m²/day. Fatal cases of lactic acidosis and severe hepatomegaly with steatosis have been reported with use of didanosine and other NRTIs; obesity and prolonged nucleoside exposure may be risk factors

Precautions Use with caution in patients with phenylketonuria, patients on sodium-restricted diets, patients with history of pancreatitis, and patients with renal or hepatic impairment; adjust dosage in patients with renal impairment or peripheral neuropathy; discontinue didanosine if clinical signs of pancreatitis occur; only after pancreatitis has been ruled out should dosing be resumed

Adverse Reactions
Central nervous system: Headache (32% to 36%), insomnia, malaise, CNS depression, fever

Dermatologic: Rash, pruritus, alopecia

Endocrine & metabolic: Hypokalemia, hyperuricemia, increased triglycerides, hyperglycemia

Gastrointestinal: Diarrhea (18%), nausea, vomiting, anorexia, stomatitis, pancreatitis (9%, dose-related, less common in children than adults), abdominal pain

Hepatic: Elevated liver enzymes, hepatic failure, elevated amylase

Neuromuscular & skeletal: Peripheral neuropathy (dose-related), myalgia, arthritis, weakness

Ocular: Retinal depigmentation, optic neuritis

Respiratory: Cough, dyspnea

Drug Interactions Antacids, omeprazole, ganciclovir, cimetidine, and ranitidine may increase absorption of didanosine; decreases absorption of ketoconazole, itraconazole, indinavir, ganciclovir, dapsone, ciprofloxacin, tetracyclines (administer at least 2 hours before or 2 hours after didanosine); drugs associated with peripheral neuropathy (cisplatin, isoniazid, metronidazole, phenytoin, vincristine, stavudine, zalcitabine, dapsone, ethambutol ethionamide, hydralazine, and nitrofurantoin) may increase the risk for didanosine peripheral neuropathy; drugs associated with pancreatitis (alcohol, I.V. pentamidine) may increase the risk of pancreatitis; concomitant administration of didanosine and delavirdine may decrease absorption of both drugs (separate dosing by at least 2 hours); concomitant administration of didanosine and ritonavir may decrease AUC of didanosine

Food Interactions Presence of food decreases oral bioavailability by as much as 50%; do not mix with fruit juice or other acid-containing liquid since didanosine is unstable in acidic solutions

Stability Undergoes rapid degradation when exposed to an acidic environment; tablets dispersed in water are stable for 1 hour at room temperature; reconstituted buffered solution is stable for 4 hours at room temperature; reconstituted unbuffered solution is stable for 30 days if refrigerated; unbuffered powder for oral solution must be reconstituted with water and mixed with an equal volume of double strength antacid at time of preparation; when unbuffered powder for oral solution is reconstituted and admixed with a double-strength antacid to make a 20 mg/mL solution for adult once-daily dosing, the admixture is stable for 24 hours at room temperature and for 30 days if refrigerated

Mechanism of Action A purine dideoxynucleoside analog converted within the cell to an active metabolite, dideoxyadenosine triphosphate which serves as a substrate and inhibitor of viral RNA-directed DNA polymerase resulting in premature termination of viral DNA synthesis

Pharmacokinetics
Distribution: Extensive intracellular distribution; low penetration into CNS; crosses the placenta
V_d:
Children: 35.6 L/m²; range: 18.4-61 L/m²
Adults: 18.4-60.7 L/m²

Protein binding: <5%

Metabolism: Converted intracellularly to active triphosphate form

Bioavailability: Variable and affected by the presence of food in the GI tract, gastric pH, and the dosage form administered
Children and Adolescents: 32% to 42% (ranges from 13% to 78%)
Adults:
Tablet: 40%
Powder: 30%

Half-life:
  Plasma:
    Children and Adolescents: 0.8 hour
    Adults: 1.3-1.6 hours
  Intracellular: Adults: 25-40 hours
  Elimination: Excreted in urine
    Children: 6% to 30%
    Adults: 20% to 55%

Usual Dosage Oral: (Use in combination with other antiretroviral agents):
  Neonates <90 days: Based on clinical study data from PACTG 239: 50 mg/m²/dose every 12 hours
  Children <13 years: Dosing is based on body surface area (m²): 180-300 mg/m²/day divided every 12 hours. (**Note:** Use lower dosage range for patients on combination therapy with other antiretrovirals; may need higher dose in patients with central nervous system disease.)
  Children ≥13 years and Adults:
    <60 kg: 125 mg every 12 hours using 2 tablets/dose **or** 250 mg once daily using 2 tablets/dose
      Buffered oral solution: 167 mg every 12 hours
    ≥60 kg: 200 mg every 12 hours using 2 tablets/dose **or** 400 mg once daily using 2 tablets/dose or a special Videx® solution in double-strength antacid which provides 400 mg/20 mL for once-daily dosing
      Buffered oral solution: 250 mg every 12 hours

Administration Oral: Administer on an empty stomach 1 hour before or at least 2 hours after a meal; tablets should be chewed, crushed, or dispersed in water for oral administration; tablets dispersed in water must be administered within 1 hour; unbuffered pediatric powder should be reconstituted with water and admixed in equal parts with a double-strength antacid to provide a final concentration of 10 mg/mL; unbuffered pediatric powder has also been reconstituted and admixed with a double-strength antacid to provide a final concentration of 20 mg/mL to be used for once-daily dosing in adults; shake oral solution well before use; administer at least 1 hour apart from indinavir or 2 hours apart from ritonavir; when administering chewable tablets, at least 2 tablets should be taken per dose to ensure adequate buffering capacity

Monitoring Parameters Serum potassium, uric acid, creatinine; hemoglobin, CBC with neutrophil and platelet count, CD4 cells; HIV RNA plasma level; liver function tests, serum amylase and triglyceride levels; weight gain; perform dilated retinal exam every 6 months; signs and symptoms of peripheral neuropathy

Patient Information The buffered oral vehicle may contribute to the development of diarrhea; inform physician if numbness, tingling, persistent severe abdominal pain, nausea, or vomiting occurs; shake oral solution well before use and keep refrigerated; discard solution after 30 days and obtain new supply

Additional Information
  Contents of each tablet: 11.5 mEq of sodium, 15.7 mEq of magnesium, along with phenylalanine; tablets are buffered with dihydroxyaluminum sodium carbonate, magnesium hydroxide, and sodium citrate
  Sodium content of each packet of buffered powder for oral solution: 60 mEq

Dosage Forms
  Powder for oral solution:
    Buffered (single dose packet): 100 mg, 167 mg, 250 mg
    Pediatric (for 10 mg/mL solution): 2 g, 4 g
  Tablet, buffered, chewable (mint flavor): 25 mg, 50 mg, 100 mg, 150 mg, 200 mg

References
Balis FM, Pizzo PA, Butler KM, et al, "Clinical Pharmacology of 2', 3'-Dideoxyinosine in Human Immunodeficiency Virus-Infected Children," *J Infect Dis*, 1992, 165(1):99-104.

Butler KM, Husson RN, Balis FM, et al, "Dideoxyinosine in Children With Symptomatic Human Immunodeficiency Virus Infection," *N Engl J Med*, 1991, 324(3):137-44.

Panel on Clinical Practices for Treatment of HIV Infection, "Guidelines for the Use of Antiretroviral Agents in HIV-Infected Adults and Adolescents," January 28, 2000, http://www.hivatis.org.

Working Group on Antiretroviral Therapy and Medical Management of HIV-Infected Children, "Guidelines for the Use of Antiretroviral Agents in Pediatric HIV Infection," January 15, 2000, http://www.hivatis.org.

Digoxin (di JOKS in)

Related Information

Adult ACLS Algorithm, Hypotension, Shock *on page 1016*
Adult ACLS Algorithm, Tachycardia *on page 1010*
Blood Level Sampling Time Guidelines *on page 1189*
Carbohydrate and Alcohol Content of Liquid Medications for Use in Patients Receiving Ketogenic Diets *on page 1228*
Overdose and Toxicology *on page 1191*

Brand Names Lanoxicaps®; Lanoxin®; Novo-Digoxin® (Canada)

Therapeutic Category Antiarrhythmic Agent, Miscellaneous; Cardiac Glycoside

Generic Available Yes: Tablet

Use Treatment of CHF; slows the ventricular rate in tachyarrhythmias such as atrial fibrillation, atrial flutter, supraventricular tachycardia

Pregnancy Risk Factor C

Contraindications Hypersensitivity to digoxin, other digitalis preparations, or any component; ventricular fibrillation, A-V block, idiopathic hypertrophic subaortic stenosis, or constrictive pericarditis

Warnings Use with extreme caution in patients with hypoxia, hypothyroidism, acute myocarditis, electrolyte disorders, acute MI

Precautions Use with caution and reduce dosage in patients with renal impairment

Adverse Reactions

Cardiovascular: Sinus bradycardia, A-V block, S-A block, atrial or nodal ectopic beats, ventricular arrhythmias, bigeminy, trigeminy, atrial tachycardia with A-V block

Central nervous system: Drowsiness, fatigue, headache, lethargy, vertigo, disorientation

Endocrine & metabolic: Hyperkalemia with acute toxicity

Gastrointestinal: Vomiting, nausea, feeding intolerance, abdominal pain, diarrhea

Neuromuscular & skeletal: Neuralgia

Ocular: Blurred vision, halos, yellow or green vision, diplopia, photophobia, flashing lights

Drug Interactions Antacids, kaolin-pectin, cholestyramine, cisapride, colestipol, sucralfate, and metoclopramide may decrease absorption of digoxin; quinidine, nifedipine, itraconazole, indomethacin, verapamil, amiodarone, erythromycin, propafenone, tetracycline, and spironolactone may increase digoxin serum concentration; penicillamine may decrease digoxin's pharmacologic effects; calcium (especially rapid I.V. use) may cause severe arrhythmias; paroxetine may decrease the AUC of digoxin by 15%; ritonavir may increase or decrease digoxin levels, close monitoring of digoxin levels is recommended; suspected interaction with nevirapine, careful monitoring is recommended

Food Interactions Meals containing increased fiber (bran) or foods high in pectin, may decrease oral absorption of digoxin; avoid natural licorice (causes sodium and water retention and increases potassium loss); maintain adequate amounts of potassium in diet to decrease risk of hypokalemia (hypokalemia may increase risk of digoxin toxicity)

Stability I.V. solution compatibility: D_5W, $D_{10}W$, NS, sterile water for injection (when diluted fourfold or greater); do not mix with other drugs; store at room temperature; protect from light

Mechanism of Action Increases the influx of calcium ions, from extracellular to intracellular cytoplasm by inhibition of sodium and potassium ion movement across the myocardial membranes; this increase in calcium ions results in a potentiation of the activity of the contractile heart muscle fibers and an increase in the force of myocardial contraction (positive inotropic effect); inhibits adenosine triphosphatase (ATPase); decreases conduction through the S-A and A-V nodes

Pharmacodynamics

Onset of effects:
Oral: 0.5-2 hours
I.V.: 5-30 minutes

Maximum effect:
Oral: 2-8 hours
I.V.: 1-4 hours

Duration (adults): 3-4 days

Pharmacokinetics

Distribution: Distribution phase: 6-8 hours
V_d:
Neonates, full-term: 7.5-10 L/kg
Children: 16 L/kg
Adults: 7 L/kg

Renal disease: Decreased V_d
Protein binding: 20% to 25%
Bioavailability (dependent upon formulation):
  Capsules: 90% to 100%
  Elixir: 70% to 85%
  Tablets: 60% to 80%
Half-life, elimination (dependent upon age, renal and cardiac function):
  Premature: 61-170 hours
  Neonates, full-term: 35-45 hours
  Infants: 18-25 hours
  Children: 35 hours
  Adults: 38-48 hours
  Anephric adults: >4.5 days
  Anuric adults: 3.5-5 days
Elimination: 50% to 70% excreted unchanged in urine
Nondialyzable (0% to 5%)
Usual Dosage Dosage must be individualized due to substantial individual variation; table lists dose based on average patient response.

Dosage Recommendations for Digoxin*

Age	Total Digitalizing Dose† (mcg/kg)		Daily Maintenance Dose‡ (mcg/kg)	
	P.O.	I.V. or I.M.	P.O.	I.V. or I.M.
Neonates				
Preterm	20-30	15-25	5-7.5	4-6
Full-term	25-35	20-30	6-10	5-8
Infants and Children				
1 mo - 2 y	35-60	30-50	10-15	7.5-12
2-5 y	30-40	25-35	7.5-10	6-9
5-10 y	20-35	15-30	5-10	4-8
>10 y	10-15	8-12	2.5-5	2-3
Adults	0.75-1.5 mg	0.5-1 mg	0.125-0.5 mg	0.1-0.4 mg

*Based on lean body weight and normal renal function for age. Decrease maintenance dose in patients with decreased renal function and decrease total digitalizing dose by 50% in end-stage renal disease.

†Give one-half of the total digitalizing dose (TDD) in the initial dose, then give one-quarter of the TDD in each of two subsequent doses at 6- to 12-hour intervals. Obtain EKG 6 hours after each dose to assess potential toxicity.

‡Divided every 12 hours in infants and children <10 years of age. Given once daily to children >10 years of age and adults.

Dosing adjustment in renal impairment: (Monitor patient closely):
  Total digitalizing dose: Reduce by 50% in end stage renal disease
  Maintenance dose:
    Cl_{cr} 10-50 mL/minute: Administer 25% to 75% of normal daily dose (divided and given at normal intervals) or administer normal dose every 36 hours
    Cl_{cr} <10 mL/minute: Administer 10% to 25% of normal daily dose (divided and given at normal intervals) or give normal dose every 48 hours
Administration
  Oral: Administer consistently with relationship to meals; avoid concurrent administration (ie, administer digoxin 1 hour before or 2 hours after) with meals high in fiber or pectin and with drugs that decrease oral absorption of digoxin
  Parenteral: Administer I.V. doses (undiluted or diluted at least fourfold) slowly over 5-10 minutes; I.M. route not usually recommended due to local irritation, pain, and tissue damage
Monitoring Parameters Heart rate and rhythm, periodic EKG; follow serum potassium, magnesium, and calcium closely (especially in patients receiving diuretics or amphotericin); decreased serum potassium and magnesium, or increased serum magnesium and calcium may increase digoxin toxicity; assess renal function (serum BUN, S_{cr}) in order to adjust dose; obtain serum drug concentrations at least 8-12 hours after a dose, preferably prior to next scheduled dose
Reference Range Therapeutic: 0.8-2 ng/mL (SI: 1.0-2.6 nmol/L); Adults: <0.5 ng/mL (SI: <0.6 nmol/L) probably indicates underdigitalization unless there are special circumstances. Toxicity usually associated with levels >2 ng/mL (SI: >2.6 nmol/L).
Note: Serum concentration must be used in conjunction with clinical symptoms and EKG to confirm diagnosis of digoxin intoxication.
(Continued)

Digoxin *(Continued)*

Test Interactions Spironolactone may interfere with radioimmunoassay

Patient Information Notify physician if decreased appetite, nausea, vomiting, diarrhea, or visual changes occur

Additional Information Digoxin-like immunoreactive substance (DLIS) may cross-react with digoxin immunoassay and falsely increase serum concentrations; DLIS has been found in patients with renal dysfunction, liver disease, CHF, neonates, and pregnant women (third trimester)

Dosage Forms

Capsule: 50 mcg, 100 mcg, 200 mcg

Elixir, pediatric (lime flavor): 50 mcg/mL with alcohol 10% (60 mL)

Injection: 250 mcg/mL (1 mL, 2 mL)

Injection, pediatric: 100 mcg/mL (1 mL)

Tablet: 125 mcg, 250 mcg, 500 mcg

References

Bakir M and Bilgic A, "Single Daily Dose of Digoxin for Maintenance Therapy of Infants and Children With Cardiac Disease: Is It Reliable?" *Pediatr Cardiol*, 1994, 15(5):229-32.

Bendayan R and McKenzie MW, "Digoxin Pharmacokinetics and Dosage Requirements in Pediatric Patients," *Clin Pharm*, 1983, 2(3):224-35.

Park MK, "Use of Digoxin in Infants and Children With Specific Emphasis on Dosage," *J Pediatr*, 1986, 108(6):871-7.

Digoxin Immune Fab *(di JOKS in i MYUN fab)*

Brand Names Digibind®

Synonyms Antidigoxin Fab Fragments

Therapeutic Category Antidote, Digoxin

Generic Available No

Use Treatment of potentially life-threatening digoxin or digitoxin intoxication in carefully selected patients; use in life-threatening ventricular arrhythmias secondary to digoxin, acute digoxin ingestion (ie, >10 mg in adults or >4 mg in children), hyperkalemia (serum potassium >5 mEq/L) in the setting of digoxin toxicity

Pregnancy Risk Factor C

Contraindications Hypersensitivity to ovine (sheep) proteins; renal or cardiac failure

Warnings Hypokalemia has been reported to occur following reversal of digitalis intoxication; monitor serum potassium levels closely; Fab fragments may be eliminated more slowly in patients with renal failure; heart failure may be exacerbated as digoxin level is reduced; total serum digoxin concentration may rise precipitously following administration of Digibind®, but this will be almost entirely bound to the Fab fragment and not able to react with receptors in the body; Digibind® will interfere with digitalis immunoassay measurements - this will result in clinically misleading serum digoxin concentrations until the Fab fragment is eliminated from the body (several days to >1 week after Digibind® administration); serum digoxin levels drawn prior to therapy may be difficult to evaluate if 6-8 hours have not elapsed after the last dose of digoxin (time to equilibration between serum and tissue); redigitalization should not be initiated until Fab fragments have been eliminated from the body, which may occur over several days or greater than a week in patients with impaired renal function

Precautions Use with caution in renal or cardiac failure; allergic reactions possible; epinephrine should be immediately available; patients may deteriorate due to withdrawal of digoxin and may require I.V. inotropic support (eg, dobutamine) or vasodilators

Adverse Reactions

Cardiovascular: Worsening of low cardiac output or CHF, rapid ventricular response in patients with atrial fibrillation as digoxin is withdrawn

Dermatologic: Urticarial rash

Endocrine & metabolic: Hypokalemia

Miscellaneous: Facial edema and redness, allergic reactions

Stability Reconstituted solutions are stable 4 hours at 2°C to 8°C

Mechanism of Action Binds with molecules of free (unbound) digoxin or digitoxin and then is removed from the body by renal excretion

Pharmacodynamics Onset of action: Improvement in signs and symptoms occurs within 2-30 minutes following I.V. infusion

Pharmacokinetics

Half-life: 15-20 hours, prolonged in patients with renal impairment

Elimination: Renal with levels declining to undetectable amounts within 5-7 days

Usual Dosage To determine the dose of digoxin immune Fab, first determine the total body load of digoxin (TBL) or digitoxin (depending upon which product was ingested) as follows (using either an approximation of the amount ingested or a postdistribution serum digoxin/digitoxin concentration (C)):

TBL of **digoxin** (in mg) = C (in ng/mL) x 5.6 x body weight (in kg)/1000
or
TBL = mg of **digoxin** ingested (as tablets or elixir) x 0.8

TBL of **digitoxin** (mg) = C (in ng/mL) x 0.56 x body weight (in kg)/1000
or
TBL of **digitoxin** (in mg) = mg digitoxin ingested
Dose of digoxin immune Fab **(in mg)** I.V. = TBL x 76
Dose of digoxin immune Fab **(# vials)** I.V. = TBL/0.5
See tables.

Infants and Children Dose Estimates of Digibind® (in mg) From Serum Digoxin Concentration

Patient Weight (kg)	Serum Digoxin Concentration (ng/mL)						
	1	2	4	8	12	16	20
1	0.4 mg*	1 mg*	1.5 mg*	3 mg	5 mg	6 mg	8 mg
3	1 mg*	2 mg*	5 mg	9 mg	14 mg	18 mg	23 mg
5	2 mg*	4 mg	8 mg	15 mg	23 mg	30 mg	38 mg
10	4 mg	8 mg	15 mg	30 mg	46 mg	61 mg	76 mg
20	8 mg	15 mg	30 mg	61 mg	91 mg	122 mg	152 mg

*Dilution of reconstituted vial to 1 mg/mL may be desirable.

Adult Dose Estimate of Digibind® (in # of Vials) From Serum Digoxin Concentration

Patient Weight (kg)	Serum Digoxin Concentration (ng/mL)						
	1	2	4	8	12	16	20
40	0.5 v*	1 v	2 v	3 v	5 v	7 v	8 v
60	0.5 v	1 v	3 v	5 v	7 v	10 v	12 v
70	1 v	2 v	3 v	6 v	9 v	11 v	14 v
80	1 v	2 v	3 v	7 v	10 v	13 v	16 v
100	1 v	2 v	4 v	8 v	12 v	16 v	20 v

* v = vials

Administration Parenteral: I.V.: Digoxin immune Fab is reconstituted by adding 4 mL sterile water, resulting in a 9.5 mg/mL concentration for I.V. infusion; the reconstituted solution may be further diluted with NS to a convenient volume (eg, 1 mg/mL); infuse over 15-30 minutes; to remove protein aggregates, 0.22 micron in-line filter is needed

Monitoring Parameters Serum potassium; serum digoxin/digitoxin level prior to first dose of digoxin immune Fab; (digoxin levels will greatly increase with Digibind® use and are not an accurate determination of body stores); continuous EKG monitoring

Additional Information Each 38 mg vial will bind approximately 0.5 mg digoxin or digitoxin; for individuals at increased risk of sensitivity (see Contraindications) an intradermal or scratch technique skin test using a 1:100 dilution of reconstituted digoxin immune Fab diluted in NS has been used. Skin test volume is 0.1 mL of 1:100 dilution; evaluate after 20 minutes.

Dosage Forms Powder for injection, lyophilized: 38 mg

References

Hickey AR, Wenger TL, Carpenter VP, et al, "Digoxin Immune Fab Therapy in the Management of Digitalis Intoxication: Safety and Efficacy Results of an Observational Surveillance Study," *J Am Coll Cardiol*, 1991, 17(3):590-8.

Dihydrotachysterol (dye hye droe tak IS ter ole)

Brand Names DHT™; Hytakerol®

Synonyms Dichysterol

Therapeutic Category Nutritional Supplement; Vitamin D Analog; Vitamin, Fat Soluble

Generic Available Yes

(Continued)

Dihydrotachysterol *(Continued)*

Use Treatment of hypocalcemia associated with hypoparathyroidism; prophylaxis of hypocalcemic tetany following thyroid surgery; suppression of hyperparathyroidism and treatment of renal osteodystrophy in patients with chronic renal failure

Pregnancy Risk Factor C

Contraindications Hypercalcemia; hypersensitivity to dihydrotachysterol or any component

Warnings Use cautiously in patients with renal stones, renal failure, and heart disease; calcium phosphate may precipitate if the product of serum calcium multiplied by phosphate (Ca x P) >70; adequate dietary calcium is necessary for a clinical response to therapy

Adverse Reactions Related to accompanying hypercalcemia
Central nervous system: Convulsions
Endocrine & metabolic: Hypercalcemia, metastatic calcification, polydipsia
Gastrointestinal: Nausea, vomiting, anorexia, weight loss
Hematologic: Anemia
Neuromuscular & skeletal: Weakness
Renal: Renal damage, polyuria

Drug Interactions Cholestyramine may reduce absorption; clofibrate, thiazides, phenobarbital, and phenytoin decrease the half-life of dihydrotachysterol; potential dihydrotachysterol-induced hypercalcemia may precipitate arrhythmias with cardiac glycosides

Mechanism of Action A synthetic reduction product of tachysterol, a close isomer of vitamin D; stimulates calcium and phosphate absorption from the small intestine, promotes secretion of calcium from bone to blood

Pharmacodynamics
Maximum hypercalcemic effects: Within 2 weeks
Duration: As long as 9 weeks

Pharmacokinetics
Absorption: Well absorbed from the GI tract
Metabolism: Hydroxylated in liver to 25-hydroxy-dihydrotachysterol

Usual Dosage Oral:
Hypoparathyroidism:
Neonates: 0.05-0.1 mg/day
Infants and young Children: Initial: 1-5 mg/day for 4 days, then 0.5-1.5 mg/day
Older Children and Adults: Initial: 0.75-2.5 mg/day for 4 days, then 0.2-1 mg/day; maximum dose: 1.5 mg/day
Nutritional rickets: 0.5 mg as a single dose or 13-50 mcg/day until healing occurs
Renal osteodystrophy:
Children and Adolescents: 0.1-0.5 mg/day
Adults: 0.1-0.6 mg/day

Administration Oral: May administer without regard to meals

Monitoring Parameters Serum calcium and phosphate, renal function, alkaline phosphatase, 24-hour urinary calcium

Additional Information 1 mg is approximately equivalent to 120,000 international units vitamin D_2

Dosage Forms
Capsule (Hytakerol®): 0.125 mg
Solution:
Oral Concentrate (DHT™): 0.2 mg/mL (30 mL)
Oral, in oil (Hytakerol®): 0.25 mg/mL (15 mL)
Tablet (DHT™): 0.125 mg, 0.2 mg, 0.4 mg

♦ **1,25 dihydroxycholecalciferol** *see* Calcitriol *on page 155*
♦ **Dihyrex® Injection** *see* Diphenhydramine *on page 327*
♦ **Diiodohydroxyquin** *see* Iodoquinol *on page 526*
♦ **Dilacor XR®** *see* Diltiazem *on page 323*
♦ **Dilantin®** *see* Phenytoin *on page 762*
♦ **Dilaudid® Cough Syrup** *see* Hydromorphone *on page 491*
♦ **Dilaudid-HP® Injection** *see* Hydromorphone *on page 491*
♦ **Dilaudid® Injection** *see* Hydromorphone *on page 491*
♦ **Dilaudid® Oral** *see* Hydromorphone *on page 491*
♦ **Dilaudid® Suppository** *see* Hydromorphone *on page 491*
♦ **Dilocaine® Injection** *see* Lidocaine *on page 568*
♦ **Dilomine® Injection** *see* Dicyclomine *on page 314*

Diltiazem (dil TYE a zem)

Related Information

Adult ACLS Algorithm, Tachycardia *on page 1010*

Brand Names Apo®-Diltiaz (Canada); Cardizem® CD; Cardizem® Injectable; Cardizem® SR; Cardizem® Tablet; Dilacor XR®; Novo-Diltiazem® (Canada); Nu-Diltiaz® (Canada); Syn-Diltiazem® (Canada); Tiamate®; Tiazac®

Available Salts Diltiazem Hydrochloride

Therapeutic Category Antianginal Agent; Antihypertensive Agent; Calcium Channel Blocker

Generic Available Yes

Use

Oral: Hypertension; chronic stable angina or angina from coronary artery spasm

Injection: Atrial fibrillation or atrial flutter; paroxysmal supraventricular tachycardias (PSVT)

Pregnancy Risk Factor C

Contraindications Hypersensitivity to diltiazem or any component; severe hypotension; second or third degree heart block; sick-sinus syndrome; acute MI with pulmonary congestion

Warnings May cause bradycardia, second or third degree heart block, hypotension, hepatic injury; may worsen CHF; use with certain medications may result in additive effects on cardiac condition (see Drug Interactions)

Precautions Use with caution in patients with CHF or impaired renal or hepatic function

Adverse Reactions

Cardiovascular: Arrhythmia, bradycardia, hypotension, A-V block, tachycardia (rare), flushing, peripheral edema, CHF

Central nervous system: Headache, dizziness, insomnia, nervousness

Dermatologic: Urticaria, rash; erythema multiforme, exfoliative dermatitis (rare)

Gastrointestinal: Nausea, vomiting, constipation, dyspepsia, dysgeusia

Hematologic: Leukopenia (rare), thrombocytopenia (rare)

Hepatic: Mild to marked elevations in liver enzyme tests (rare)

Neuromuscular & skeletal: Gait abnormality, tremor, paresthesia, weakness

Drug Interactions Cytochrome P-450 isoenzyme CYP3A3/4 substrate; isoenzyme CYP1A2, CYP2D6, and CYP3A3/4 inhibitor

Cimetidine may increase diltiazem serum concentration; digoxin, beta-adrenergic blocking agents may increase risk of bradycardia or heart block; diltiazem may decrease metabolism and increase concentrations of cyclosporine, carbamazepine, digoxin, midazolam; diltiazem may increase the effect/toxicity of digitalis glycosides, encainide, fentanyl; rifampin may decrease diltiazem serum concentrations

Food Interactions Food may increase absorption of diltiazem from sustained-release preparation; high fat meal does not effect extent of absorption of Cardizem® CD or Tiazac®

Stability Injection: May dilute with NS, D_5W or $D_5\frac{1}{2}NS$ for continuous infusion; refrigerate; may store at room temperature for up to 1 month; not compatible with furosemide

Mechanism of Action Inhibits calcium ion from entering the "slow channels" or select voltage-sensitive areas of vascular smooth muscle and myocardium during depolarization; produces a relaxation of coronary vascular smooth muscle and coronary vasodilation; increases myocardial oxygen delivery in patients with vasospastic angina

Pharmacodynamics

Onset:

Oral:

Tablet: 30-60 minutes

Sustained release: 2-3 hours

Parenteral: I.V. (bolus): Within 3 minutes

Maximum effect:

Antiarrhythmic (I.V. bolus): 2-7 minutes

Antihypertensive (Oral): Within 2 weeks

Pharmacokinetics

Absorption: 80%

Distribution: V_d: 1.7 L/kg; appears in breast milk

Protein binding: 70% to 80%

Metabolism: Extensive first-pass effect; metabolized in the liver; desacetyldiltiazem is an active metabolite (25% to 50% as potent as diltiazem based on coronary (Continued)

Diltiazem *(Continued)*

vasodilation effects); desacetyldiltiazem may accumulate with plasma concentrations 10% to 20% of diltiazem levels

Bioavailability: ~40%

Half-life: 3-4.5 hours, up to 8 hours with chronic high dosing

Time to peak serum concentration:

Tablet: 2-3 hours

Cardizem® CD: 10-14 hours

Cardizem® SR: 6-11 hours

Elimination: In urine and bile mostly as metabolites; 2% to 4% excreted as unchanged drug in urine

Not dialyzable

Usual Dosage

Children: Minimal information available; some centers use the following:

Hypertension: Oral: Initial: 1.5-2 mg/kg/day in 3-4 divided doses; maximum dose: 3.5 mg/kg/day

Note: Doses up to 8 mg/kg/day given in 4 divided doses have been used for investigational therapy of Duchenne muscular dystrophy

Adolescents and Adults:

Oral: Hypertension:

Capsule, sustained release:

Cardizem® CD: 180-300 mg once daily; maximum: 480 mg once daily

Cardizem® SR: 60-120 mg twice daily

Dilacor™ XR: 180-240 mg once daily

Tiazac®: 120-240 mg once daily; maximum: 540 mg once daily

Tablet: 30-120 mg 3-4 times/day; dosage should be increased gradually, at 1- to 2-day intervals until optimum response is obtained; usual maintenance dose: 180-360 mg/day

I.V. (antiarrhythmic): Initial: 0.25 mg/kg as a bolus over 2 minutes, if response is inadequate a second bolus dose (0.35 mg/kg) may be administered after 15 minutes; further bolus doses should be individualized

I.V. continuous infusion (start after I.V. bolus doses): 5-15 mg/hour for up to 24 hours

Conversion from I.V. diltiazem to oral diltiazem: Start first oral dose approximately 3 hours after bolus dose

Oral dose (mg/day) is approximately equal to [rate (mg/hour) x 3 + 3] x 10;

Note: Dose per day may need to be divided depending on formulation used (see Usual Dosage above)

3 mg/hour = 120 mg/day

5 mg/hour = 180 mg/day

7 mg/hour = 240 mg/day

11 mg/hour = 360 mg/day (maximum recommended dose)

Administration

Oral: May be administered with or without food, but should be administered consistently with relation to meals; administer with a full glass of water; swallow sustained release preparation (CD, SR, XR, Tiazac®) whole, do not chew or crush

Tiazac® capsules (extended release) may be opened and sprinkled on applesauce; swallow applesauce immediately, do not chew; follow with some cool water (adults: 1 glass) to ensure complete swallowing; do not divide capsule contents (ie, do not administer partial doses); do not store mixture of applesauce and capsule contents, use immediately

Parenteral:

I.V. bolus: Adults: Infuse over 2 minutes

I.V. continuous: Maximum final concentration: 1 mg/mL

Monitoring Parameters Blood pressure, renal function, liver enzymes

Patient Information Do not discontinue abruptly; report any dizziness, shortness of breath, palpitations, or edema; avoid alcohol

Nursing Implications Do not crush sustained release capsules (CD, SR, XR, Tiazac®)

Dosage Forms

Capsule, sustained release, as hydrochloride:

Cardizem® CD: 120 mg, 180 mg, 240 mg, 300 mg, 360 mg

Cardizem® SR: 60 mg, 90 mg, 120 mg

Dilacor™ XR: 120 mg, 180 mg, 240 mg

Tiazac®: 120 mg, 180 mg, 240 mg, 300 mg, 360 mg, 420 mg

Injection, as hydrochloride: 5 mg/mL (5 mL, 10 mL)

Cardizem®: 5 mg/mL (5 mL, 10 mL)

Tablet, as hydrochloride (Cardizem®): 30 mg, 60 mg, 90 mg, 120 mg

Tablet, extended release, as hydrochloride (Tiamate®): 120 mg, 180 mg, 240 mg

Extemporaneous Preparations A 12 mg/mL oral liquid preparation made from tablets (regular, not sustained release) and 3 different vehicles (cherry syrup, a 1:1 mixture of Ora-Sweet® and Ora-Plus®, or a 1:1 mixture of Ora-Sweet® SF and Ora-Plus®) was stable for 60 days when stored in amber plastic prescription bottles in the dark at room temperature (25°C) or under refrigeration (5°C); grind sixteen 90 mg tablets in a mortar into a fine powder; add 10 mL of the vehicle and mix well to form a uniform paste; mix while adding the vehicle in geometric proportions to almost 120 mL; transfer to a calibrated bottle and qsad with vehicle to 120 mL; label "shake well" and "protect from light"

Allen LV and Erickson MA, "Stability of Baclofen, Captopril, Diltiazem Hydrochloride, Dipyridamole, and Flecainide Acetate in Extemporaneously Compounded Oral Liquids," *Am J Health Sys Pharm*, 1996, 53(18):2179-84.

References
Bertorini TE, Palmieri GMA, Griffin JW, et al, "Effect of Chronic Treatment With the Calcium Antagonist Diltiazem in Duchenne Muscular Dystrophy," *Neurology*, 1988, 38(4):609-13.

♦ **Diltiazem Hydrochloride** *see* Diltiazem *on page 323*

♦ **Dimaphen®** *see* Brompheniramine and Phenylpropanolamine *on page 143*

♦ **Dimaphen® Elixir [OTC]** *see* Brompheniramine and Phenylpropanolamine *on page 143*

Dimenhydrinate (dye men HYE dri nate)

Related Information

Overdose and Toxicology *on page 1191*

Brand Names Apo®-Dimenhydrinate (Canada); Calm-X® Oral [OTC]; Dimetabs® Oral; Dinate® Injection; Dramamine® Oral [OTC]; Dramilin® Injection; Dramoject® Injection; Dymenate® Injection; Gravol® (Canada); Hydrate® Injection; Marmine® Injection; Marmine® Oral [OTC]; PMS-Dimenhydrinate (Canada); Tega-Vert® Oral; Travel Aid® (Canada); Travel Tabs (Canada); TripTone® Caplets® [OTC]

Therapeutic Category Antiemetic; Antihistamine

Generic Available Yes

Use Treatment and prevention of nausea, vertigo, and vomiting associated with motion sickness

Pregnancy Risk Factor B

Contraindications Hypersensitivity to dimenhydrinate or any component

Warnings Parenteral product contains benzyl alcohol which has been associated with a fatal "gasping syndrome" in premature infants; chewable tablets contain the dye tartrazine which may cause allergic reactions in sensitive individuals (particularly if sensitive to aspirin)

Precautions Use with caution in patients with a history of seizure disorder; may produce excitation in the young child; use with caution in any condition which may be aggravated by anticholinergic symptoms such as prostatic hypertrophy, asthma, bladder neck obstruction, narrow-angle glaucoma, etc

Adverse Reactions

Cardiovascular: Hypotension, palpitations, tachycardia

Central nervous system: Drowsiness, headache, paradoxical CNS stimulation, dizziness

Dermatologic: Photosensitivity, urticaria, rash

Gastrointestinal: Anorexia, xerostomia, dry mucous membranes, constipation

Genitourinary: Urinary frequency, dysuria

Hematologic: Hemolytic anemia

Local: Pain at the injection site

Ocular: Blurred vision, diplopia

Otic: Tinnitus

Respiratory: Chest tightness, wheezing, thickened secretions

Drug Interactions Enhances sedative effects of other CNS depressants, may potentiate anticholinergic effects; may mask early signs and symptoms of ototoxicity in patients on aminoglycosides, furosemide, etc

Mechanism of Action Competes with histamine for H_1-receptor sites on effector cells in the gastrointestinal tract, blood vessels, and respiratory tract; diminishes vestibular stimulation and depresses labyrinthine function through its central anticholinergic activity; consists of equimolar proportions of diphenhydramine and chlorotheophylline

Pharmacodynamics

Onset of action:

Oral: Within 15-30 minutes

I.M.: 20-30 minutes

(Continued)

325

Dimenhydrinate *(Continued)*

I.V.: Immediate

Duration: ~3-6 hours

Pharmacokinetics

Absorption: Well absorbed from the GI tract

Metabolism: Extensive in the liver

Usual Dosage Oral, I.M., I.V.:

Children:

2-5 years: 12.5-25 mg every 6-8 hours, maximum dose: 75 mg/day

6-12 years: 25-50 mg every 6-8 hours, maximum dose: 150 mg/day

or

Alternately: 5 mg/kg/day or 150 mg/m^2/day in 4 divided doses, not to exceed 300 mg/day

Children ≥12 years and Adults: 50-100 mg every 4-6 hours, not to exceed 400 mg/day

Administration

Oral: Administer with food or water

Parenteral: Dilute to a maximum concentration of 5 mg/mL in NS and infuse over 2 minutes; may be administered I.M.

Patient Information Causes drowsiness and may impair ability to perform hazardous tasks requiring mental alertness

Dosage Forms

Capsule: 50 mg

Injection: 50 mg/mL (1 mL, 5 mL, 10 mL)

Liquid: 12.5 mg/4 mL; 16.62 mg/5 mL

Tablet: 50 mg

Tablet, chewable: 50 mg

Dimercaprol (dye mer KAP role)

Brand Names BAL in Oil®

Therapeutic Category Antidote, Arsenic Toxicity; Antidote, Gold Toxicity; Antidote, Lead Toxicity; Antidote, Mercury Toxicity; Chelating Agent, Parenteral

Generic Available No

Use Antidote to gold, arsenic, and mercury poisoning; adjunct to edetate calcium disodium in lead poisoning

Pregnancy Risk Factor C

Contraindications Hepatic insufficiency; patients with hypersensitivity reactions to peanuts (injection in peanut oil); do not use in iron, cadmium, or selenium poisoning; do not use iron supplements during therapy

Precautions Use with caution in patients with renal impairment or hypertension; produces hemolysis in persons with G-6-PD deficiency, especially in the presence of infection or other stressful situations; due to increased frequency of histamine-release related side effects, pretreatment with antihistamines is recommended; urine should be kept alkaline to prevent dissociation of chelate

Adverse Reactions

Cardiovascular: Hypertension, tachycardia

Central nervous system: Nervousness, seizures, fever (30% of children), headache, anxiety

Gastrointestinal: Vomiting, nausea, salivation

Hematologic: Transient neutropenia

Local: Pain at the injection site, sterile abscesses

Neuromuscular & skeletal: Paresthesia of hands

Ocular: Blepharospasm, conjunctivitis, lacrimation, burning eyes

Renal: Nephrotoxicity

Respiratory: Rhinorrhea

Miscellaneous: Burning sensation of the lips, mouth, throat, and penis

Drug Interactions Iron (chelation product toxic to kidneys)

Stability Do not mix in the same syringe with edetate calcium disodium

Mechanism of Action Sulfhydryl group combines with ions of various heavy metals (arsenic, gold, mercury, lead) to form relatively stable, nontoxic, soluble chelates which are excreted in the urine

Pharmacokinetics

Distribution: To all tissues including the brain

Metabolism: Rapid to inactive products

Time to peak serum concentration: 30-60 minutes

Elimination: In urine and feces via bile

Usual Dosage Children and Adults: I.M.:

Mild arsenic and gold poisoning: 2.5 mg/kg/dose every 6 hours for 2 days, then every 12 hours on the third day, and once daily thereafter for 10 days

Severe arsenic and gold poisoning: 3 mg/kg/dose every 4 hours for 2 days then every 6 hours on the third day, then every 12 hours thereafter for 10 days

Mercury poisoning: 5 mg/kg initially followed by 2.5 mg/kg/dose 1-2 times/day for 10 days

Lead poisoning: (use with edetate calcium disodium):

Mild: 4 mg/kg/dose for one dose then 3 mg/kg/dose every 4 hours for 2-7 days

Severe and acute encephalopathy: (**blood levels >70 mcg/dL**): 4 mg/kg/dose every 4 hours in combination with edetate calcium disodium for at least 72 hours; may use for up to 5 days; if additional days of therapy (>5 days) are indicated, a minimum of 2 days without treatment should elapse before considering another treatment course

Administration Parenteral: Administer undiluted, deep I.M.

Monitoring Parameters Specific heavy metal levels, urine pH

Dosage Forms Injection: 100 mg/mL (3 mL)

References

"Treatment Guidelines for Lead Exposure in Children. American Academy of Pediatrics Committee on Drugs," *Pediatrics,* 1995, 96(1 Pt 1):155-60.

♦ **Dimetabs® Oral** *see* Dimenhydrinate *on page 325*

♦ **Dimetane® Extentabs [OTC]** *see* Brompheniramine *on page 142*

♦ **Dimetane® Extentabs® [OTC]** *see* Brompheniramine and Phenylpropanolamine *on page 143*

♦ **Dimetapp® 4 hour Liqui-Gel [OTC]** *see* Brompheniramine and Phenylpropanolamine *on page 143*

♦ **Dimetapp® Elixir [OTC]** *see* Brompheniramine and Phenylpropanolamine *on page 143*

♦ **Dimetapp® Tablets [OTC]** *see* Brompheniramine and Phenylpropanolamine *on page 143*

♦ **Dimethoxyphenyl Penicillin** *see* Methicillin *on page 616*

♦ **β,β-Dimethylcysteine** *see* Penicillamine *on page 738*

♦ **Dinate® Injection** *see* Dimenhydrinate *on page 325*

♦ **Diocaine(Canada)** *see* Proparacaine *on page 811*

♦ **Diocarpine (Canada)** *see* Pilocarpine *on page 770*

♦ **Diochloram (Canada)** *see* Chloramphenicol *on page 207*

♦ **Diocto® [OTC]** *see* Docusate *on page 336*

♦ **Diocto C® [OTC]** *see* Docusate and Casanthranol *on page 337*

♦ **Diocto-K® [OTC]** *see* Docusate *on page 336*

♦ **Diocto-K Plus® [OTC]** *see* Docusate and Casanthranol *on page 337*

♦ **Dioctolose Plus® [OTC]** *see* Docusate and Casanthranol *on page 337*

♦ **Dioctyl Calcium Sulfosuccinate** *see* Docusate *on page 336*

♦ **Dioctyl Potassium Sulfosuccinate** *see* Docusate *on page 336*

♦ **Dioctyl Sodium Sulfosuccinate** *see* Docusate *on page 336*

♦ **Diodoquin® (Canada)** *see* Iodoquinol *on page 526*

♦ **Dioeze® [OTC]** *see* Docusate *on page 336*

♦ **Diomycin (Canada)** *see* Erythromycin *on page 379*

♦ **Dionephrine (Canada)** *see* Phenylephrine *on page 758*

♦ **Diotrope (Canada)** *see* Tropicamide *on page 959*

♦ **Dioval®** *see* Estradiol *on page 386*

♦ **Dipalmitoylphosphatidylcholine** *see* Colfosceril *on page 252*

♦ **Dipentum®** *see* Olsalazine *on page 705*

♦ **Diphenacen-50® Injection [OTC]** *see* Diphenhydramine *on page 327*

♦ **Diphen® Cough [OTC]** *see* Diphenhydramine *on page 327*

♦ **Diphenhist [OTC]** *see* Diphenhydramine *on page 327*

Diphenhydramine (dye fen HYE dra meen)

Related Information

Carbohydrate and Alcohol Content of Liquid Medications for Use in Patients Receiving Ketogenic Diets *on page 1228*

Compatibility of Medications Mixed in a Syringe *on page 1208*

OTC Cough & Cold Preparations, Pediatric *on page 1037*

Overdose and Toxicology *on page 1191*

Brand Names Allerdryl® (Canada); AllerMax® Oral [OTC]; Allernix® (Canada); Banophen® Oral [OTC]; Belix® Oral [OTC]; Bena-D® Injection; Benadryl® Injection; Benadryl® Oral [OTC]; Benadryl® Topical; Ben-Allergin-50® Injection; Benylin® (Continued)

Diphenhydramine *(Continued)*

Cough Syrup [OTC]; Bydramine® Cough Syrup [OTC]; Compoz® Gel Caps [OTC]; Compoz® Nighttime Sleep Aid [OTC]; Dihyrex® Injection; Diphenacen-50® Injection [OTC]; Diphen® Cough [OTC]; Diphenhist [OTC]; Dormarex® 2 Oral [OTC]; Dormin® Oral [OTC]; Genahist® Oral; Hydramyn® Syrup [OTC]; Hyrexin-50® Injection; Maximum Strength Nytol® [OTC]; Miles Nervine® Caplets [OTC]; Nordryl® Injection; Nordryl® Oral; Nytol® Oral [OTC]; Phendry® Oral [OTC]; Siladryl® Oral [OTC]; Silphen® Cough [OTC]; Sleep-eze 3® Oral [OTC]; Sleepinal® [OTC]; Sleep-well 2-nite® [OTC]; Sominex® Oral [OTC]; Tusstat® Syrup; Twilite® Oral [OTC]; Uni-Bent® Cough Syrup; Winks® [OTC]

Available Salts Diphenhydramine Hydrochloride

Therapeutic Category Antidote, Drug-induced Dystonic Reactions; Antidote, Hypersensitivity Reactions; Antihistamine; Sedative

Generic Available Yes

Use Symptomatic relief of allergic symptoms caused by histamine release which include nasal allergies and allergic dermatosis; mild nighttime sedation, prevention of motion sickness, as an antitussive; treatment of phenothiazine-induced dystonic reactions

Pregnancy Risk Factor B

Contraindications Hypersensitivity to diphenhydramine or any component; should not be used in acute attacks of asthma

Warnings Topical diphenhydramine should not be used to treat chickenpox, poison ivy, or sunburn, on large areas of the body, or on blistered or oozing skin, due to potential for causing toxic psychosis, particularly in children

Precautions Use with caution in patients with angle-closure glaucoma, peptic ulcer, urinary tract obstruction, hyperthyroidism; may cause paradoxical excitation in young children

Adverse Reactions

Cardiovascular: Hypotension, palpitations, tachycardia

Central nervous system: Sedation, dizziness, paradoxical excitement, fatigue, insomnia

Dermatologic: Photosensitivity, rash, urticaria

Gastrointestinal: Nausea, vomiting, xerostomia, dry mucous membranes, anorexia, constipation, epigastric distress

Genitourinary: Urinary retention, dysuria

Hematologic: Rare: Hemolytic anemia, aplastic anemia, thrombocytopenia

Neuromuscular & skeletal: Paresthesia of hands, tremor

Ocular: Blurred vision

Respiratory: Chest tightness, thickened bronchial secretions, wheezing

Drug Interactions Additive sedation when given with drugs which depress the central nervous system; may impair absorption of aminosalicylic acid

Stability Compatible when mixed in the same syringe: atropine, chlorpromazine, cimetidine, droperidol, fentanyl, glycopyrrolate, hydromorphone, meperidine, metoclopramide, midazolam, morphine, promethazine, and ranitidine

Mechanism of Action Competes with histamine for H_1-receptor sites on effector cells in the gastrointestinal tract, blood vessels, and respiratory tract

Pharmacodynamics

Maximum sedative effect: 1-3 hours after administration

Duration of action: 4-7 hours

Pharmacokinetics

Absorption: Oral: Well absorbed but 40% to 60% of an oral dose reaches the systemic circulation due to first-pass metabolism

Protein-binding: 78%

Metabolism: Extensive in the liver

Half-life: 2-8 hours

Time to peak serum concentration: 2-4 hours

Usual Dosage

Oral, I.M., I.V.:

Treatment of phenothiazine dystonic reactions and moderate to severe allergic reactions:

Children: 5 mg/kg/day or 150 mg/m^2/day in divided doses every 6-8 hours, not to exceed 300 mg/day

Adults: 25-50 mg every 4 hours, not to exceed 400 mg/day

Minor allergic rhinitis or motion sickness:

Children 2 to <6 years: 6.25 mg every 4-6 hours; maximum: 37.5 mg/day

Children 6 to <12 years: 12.5-25 mg every 4-6 hours; maximum: 150 mg/day

Children ≥12 years and Adults: 25-50 mg every 4-6 hours; maximum: 300 mg/day

Antitussive: Oral:
Children 2 to <6 years: 6.25 mg every 4 hours; maximum 37.5 mg/day
Children 6 to <12 years: 12.5 mg every 4 hours; maximum 75 mg/day
Children ≥12 years and Adults: 25 mg every 4 hours; maximum 150 mg/day

Night-time sleep aid: 30 minutes before bedtime:
Children 2 to <12 years: 1 mg/kg/dose; maximum: 50 mg/dose
Children ≥12 years and Adults: 50 mg

Administration
Oral: Administer with food to avoid GI distress
Parenteral: I.V.: Dilute with compatible I.V. fluid to a maximum concentration of 25 mg/mL and infuse over 10-15 minutes (maximum rate of infusion: 25 mg/minute)

Test Interactions May suppress the wheal and flare reactions to skin test antigens; discontinue 4 days prior to skin testing procedures

Patient Information May cause drowsiness and impair ability to perform hazardous activities which require mental alertness or physical coordination

Dosage Forms
Capsule, as hydrochloride: 25 mg, 50 mg
Cream, as hydrochloride: 1%, 2%
Elixir, as hydrochloride: 12.5 mg/5 mL (5 mL, 10 mL, 20 mL, 120 mL, 480 mL, 3780 mL)
Injection, as hydrochloride: 10 mg/mL (10 mL, 30 mL); 50 mg/mL (1 mL, 10 mL)
Lotion, as hydrochloride: 1% (75 mL)
Solution, topical spray, as hydrochloride: 1% (60 mL)
Syrup, as hydrochloride: 12.5 mg/5 mL (5 mL, 120 mL, 240 mL, 480 mL, 3780 mL)
Tablet, as hydrochloride: 25 mg, 50 mg

♦ **Diphenhydramine Hydrochloride** *see* Diphenhydramine *on page 327*

Diphenoxylate and Atropine (dye fen OKS i late & A troe peen)

Brand Names Lofene®; Logen®; Lomanate®; Lomodix®; Lomotil®; Lonox®; Low-Quel®

Available Salts Diphenoxylate Hydrochloride and Atropine Sulfate

Synonyms Atropine and Diphenoxylate

Therapeutic Category Antidiarrheal

Generic Available Yes

Use Treatment of diarrhea

Restrictions C-V

Pregnancy Risk Factor C

Contraindications Hypersensitivity to diphenoxylate, atropine, or any component; severe liver disease, jaundice, dehydration, and narrow-angle glaucoma; do not use in children <2 years of age

Warnings Reduction of intestinal motility may be deleterious in diarrhea resulting from *Shigella, Salmonella*, toxigenic strains of *E. coli* and from pseudomembranous enterocolitis associated with broad spectrum antibiotics; children (especially those with Down syndrome) may develop signs of atropinism (dry skin and mucous membranes, thirst, hyperthermia, tachycardia, urinary retention, flushing) even at the recommended dosages

Precautions Use with extreme caution in patients with dehydration, cirrhosis, hepatorenal disease, renal dysfunction, and acute ulcerative colitis

Adverse Reactions
Cardiovascular: Tachycardia
Central nervous system: Sedation, dizziness, euphoria, headache, hyperthermia
Dermatologic: Pruritus, urticaria
Gastrointestinal: Nausea, vomiting, abdominal discomfort, paralytic ileus, pancreatitis, xerostomia
Genitourinary: Urinary retention
Neuromuscular & skeletal: Weakness
Ocular: Blurred vision
Respiratory: Respiratory depression (young children may be at greater risk)
Miscellaneous: Physical and psychological dependence with prolonged use

Drug Interactions MAO inhibitors (hypertensive crisis), CNS depressants, alcohol, anticholinergic agents, naltrexone

Stability Protect from light

Mechanism of Action Diphenoxylate inhibits excessive GI motility and GI propulsion; commercial preparations contain a subtherapeutic amount of atropine to discourage abuse

(Continued)

Diphenoxylate and Atropine *(Continued)*

Pharmacodynamics
Onset of action: Within 45-60 minutes
Peak effect: Within 2 hours
Duration: 3-4 hours
Tolerance to antidiarrheal effects may occur with prolonged use

Pharmacokinetics
Absorption: Oral: Well absorbed
Metabolism: Extensive in the liver to diphenoxylic acid (active)
Half-life:
Diphenoxylate: 2.5 hours
Diphenoxylic acid: 12-24 hours
Time to peak serum concentration: ~2 hours
Elimination: Primarily in feces (via bile); ~14% is excreted in urine as metabolites; <1% excreted unchanged in urine

Usual Dosage Oral (as diphenoxylate):
Children: Liquid: 0.3-0.4 mg/kg/day in 2-4 divided doses **or**
<2 years: Not recommended
2-5 years: 2 mg 3 times/day
5-8 years: 2 mg 4 times/day
8-12 years: 2 mg 5 times/day
Note: Do not exceed recommended doses; reduce dose as soon as symptoms are initially controlled; maintenance doses may be as low as 25% of initial dose; if no improvement within 48 hours of therapy, diphenoxylate is not likely to be effective.
Adults: 15-20 mg/day in 3-4 divided doses; maintenance: 5-15 mg/day in 2-3 divided doses

Administration Oral: May be administered with food to decrease GI upset

Monitoring Parameters Bowel frequency, signs and symptoms of atropinism, fluid and electrolytes

Patient Information Avoid alcohol; may cause drowsiness or dizziness and impair ability to perform activities requiring mental alertness or physical coordination; may cause dry mouth

Additional Information Naloxone reverses toxicity due to diphenoxylate; Lomotil® solution also contains sorbitol, cherry flavoring, and yellow dye 6

Dosage Forms
Solution, oral: Diphenoxylate hydrochloride 2.5 mg and atropine sulfate 0.025 mg per 5 mL (4 mL, 10 mL, 60 mL)
Tablet: Diphenoxylate hydrochloride 2.5 mg and atropine sulfate 0.025 mg

- **Diphenoxylate Hydrochloride and Atropine Sulfate** *see* Diphenoxylate and Atropine *on page 329*
- **Diphenylan Sodium®** *see* Phenytoin *on page 762*
- **Diphenylhydantoin** *see* Phenytoin *on page 762*
- **Diphtheria and Tetanus Toxoids** *see page 1138*
- **Diphtheria, Tetanus, and Accellular Pertussis Vaccine** *see page 1138*
- **Diphtheria, Tetanus Toxoids, and Whole-Cell Pertussis Vaccine** *see page 1138*
- **Dipivalyl Epinephrine** *see* Dipivefrin *on page 330*

Dipivefrin *(dye PI ve frin)*

Brand Names DPE™ (Canada); Optho-Dipivefrin™ (Canada); Propine®
Available Salts Dipivefrin Hydrochloride
Synonyms Dipivalyl Epinephrine; DPE
Therapeutic Category Adrenergic Agonist Agent, Ophthalmic; Ophthalmic Agent, Vasoconstrictor
Generic Available Yes
Use Reduces elevated intraocular pressure in chronic open-angle glaucoma; treatment of ocular hypertension
Pregnancy Risk Factor B
Contraindications Hypersensitivity to dipivefrin, any component, sulfites (commercial preparation contains sodium metabisulfite), or epinephrine; contraindicated in patients with angle-closure glaucoma
Precautions Use with caution in patients with vascular hypertension or cardiac disorders and in aphakic patients (dipivefrin may cause cystoid macular edema in aphakic patients)

Adverse Reactions
Central nervous system: Headache
Local: Burning, stinging
Ocular: Ocular congestion, photophobia, mydriasis, blurred vision, ocular pain, bulbar conjunctival follicles, blepharoconjunctivitis, cystoid macular edema

Drug Interactions Effects of lowering IOP may be additive when used with topical miotics, timolol, betaxolol, or carbonic anhydrase inhibitors

Stability Protect from light and avoid exposure to air; discolored or darkened solutions indicate loss of potency

Mechanism of Action Dipivefrin is a prodrug of epinephrine which is the active agent that stimulates alpha- and/or beta-adrenergic receptors increasing aqueous humor outflow

Pharmacodynamics
Onset of action:
Ocular pressure effects: Within 30 minutes
Mydriasis: Within 30 minutes
Duration:
Ocular pressure effects: 12 hours or longer
Mydriasis: Several hours

Pharmacokinetics Absorption: Rapid into the aqueous humor; converted to epinephrine

Usual Dosage Children and Adults: Ophthalmic: Initial: Instill 1 drop every 12 hours

Administration Ophthalmic: Instill drop into eye; avoid contacting bottle tip with skin or eye

Monitoring Parameters Intraocular pressure

Patient Information Discolored solutions should be discarded; may cause burning or stinging, blurred vision, and sensitivity to light

Additional Information Contains sodium metabisulfite

Dosage Forms Solution, ophthalmic, as hydrochloride: 0.1% (5 mL, 10 mL, 15 mL)

♦ **Dipivefrin Hydrochloride** see Dipivefrin on page 330
♦ **Diprivan® Injection** see Propofol on page 812
♦ **Diprolene® AF Topical** see Betamethasone on page 130
♦ **Diprolene® Glycol [Dipropionate] (Canada)** see Betamethasone on page 130
♦ **Diprolene® Topical** see Betamethasone on page 130
♦ **Dipropylacetic Acid** see Valproic Acid and Derivatives on page 966
♦ **Diprosone® Topical** see Betamethasone on page 130

Dipyridamole (dye peer ID a mole)

Brand Names Apo®-Dipyridamole FC (Canada); Apo®-Dipyridamole SC (Canada); Asasantine® [with Aspirin also] (Canada); Novo-Dipiradol® (Canada); Persantine®

Therapeutic Category Antiplatelet Agent; Vasodilator, Coronary

Generic Available Yes

Use Maintain patency after surgical grafting procedures including coronary artery bypass; with warfarin to decrease thrombosis in patients after artificial heart valve replacement; for chronic management of angina pectoris; with aspirin to prevent coronary artery thrombosis; in combination with aspirin or warfarin to prevent other thromboembolic disorders; dipyridamole may also be given 2 days prior to open heart surgery to prevent platelet activation by extracorporeal bypass pump; diagnostic agent I.V. (dipyridamole stress test) for coronary artery disease

Pregnancy Risk Factor C

Contraindications Hypersensitivity to dipyridamole or any component

Precautions May further decrease blood pressure in patients with hypotension due to peripheral vasodilation

Adverse Reactions
Cardiovascular: Vasodilatation, flushing, syncope
Central nervous system: Dizziness, headache (dose-related)
Dermatologic: Rash, pruritus
Gastrointestinal: Abdominal distress, nausea, vomiting, diarrhea
Neuromuscular & skeletal: Weakness

Drug Interactions Heparin, warfarin, streptokinase, urokinase, aspirin, NSAIDs, cefamandole, cefoperazone, cefotetan, and valproic acid may increase risk of bleeding; decreased coronary artery vasodilation from I.V. dipyridamole may occur in patients receiving theophylline or caffeine

Stability Do not freeze; protect I.V. preparation from light

Mechanism of Action Inhibits the activity of adenosine deaminase and phosphodiesterase, which causes an accumulation of adenosine, adenine nucleotides, and
(Continued)

Dipyridamole *(Continued)*

cyclic AMP; these mediators then inhibit platelet aggregation and may cause vasodilation; may also stimulate release of prostacyclin or PGD_2; causes coronary vasodilation

Pharmacokinetics Oral:

Absorption: Slow and variable

Distribution: V_d: Adults: 2-3 L/kg

Protein binding: 91% to 99%

Metabolism: In the liver to glucuronide conjugate

Bioavailability: Ranges from 27% to 66%

Half-life, terminal: 10-12 hours

Time to peak serum concentration: Within 2-2.5 hours

Elimination: In feces via bile as glucuronide conjugates and unchanged drug

Usual Dosage

Children:

Oral: 3-6 mg/kg/day in 3 divided doses

Doses of 4-10 mg/kg/day have been used investigationally to treat proteinuria in pediatric renal disease

Mechanical prosthetic heart valves: 2-5 mg/kg/day (used in combination with an oral anticoagulant in children who have systemic embolism despite adequate oral anticoagulant therapy (INR 2.5-3.5), and used in combination with low-dose oral anticoagulation (INR 2-3) plus aspirin in children in whom full-dose oral anticoagulation is contraindicated)

Adults:

Oral: 75-400 mg/day in 3-4 divided doses

Dipyridamole stress test (for evaluation of myocardial perfusion): I.V.: 0.142 mg/kg/minute for a total of 4 minutes (0.57 mg/kg total); maximum dose: 60 mg; inject thallium 201 within 5 minutes after end of injection of dipyridamole

Platelet aggregation inhibitor: I.V. infusion: 250 mg/day at a rate of 10 mg/hour; maximum dose: 400 mg/day (use lower doses with aspirin)

Administration

Oral: Administer with water before meals

Parenteral: I.V.: Dilute in at least a 1:2 ratio with NS, ½NS, or D_5W; infusion of undiluted dipyridamole may cause local irritation; see Usual Dosage for infusion rates

Monitoring Parameters Blood pressure, heart rate

Test Interactions Patients on theophylline may show false-negative thallium scan result

Patient Information Notify physician or pharmacist if taking other medications that affect bleeding, such as warfarin or NSAIDs

Dosage Forms

Injection: 5 mg/mL (2 mL, 10 mL)

Tablet: 25 mg, 50 mg, 75 mg

Extemporaneous Preparations A 10 mg/mL oral liquid preparation made from tablets and 3 different vehicles (cherry syrup, a 1:1 mixture of Ora-Sweet® and Ora-Plus®, or a 1:1 mixture of Ora-Sweet® SF and Ora-Plus®) was stable for 60 days when stored in amber plastic prescription bottles in the dark, at room temperature (25°C) or under refrigeration (5°C); grind twenty-four 50 mg tablets in a mortar into a fine powder; add 20 mL of the vehicle and mix well to form a uniform paste; mix while adding the vehicle in geometric proportions to **almost** 120 mL; transfer to a calibrated bottle and qsad with vehicle to 120 mL; label "shake well" and "protect from light"

Allen LV and Erickson MA, "Stability of Baclofen, Captopril, Diltiazem Hydrochloride, Dipyridamole, and Flecainide Acetate in Extemporaneously Compounded Oral Liquids," *Am J Health Sys Pharm*, 1996, 53(18):2179-84.

References

Michelson AD, Bovill E, Monagle P, et al, "Antithrombotic Therapy in Children," *Chest*, 1998, 114(5 Suppl):748S-69S.

Rao PS, Solymar L, Mardini MK, et al, "Anticoagulant Therapy in Children With Prosthetic Valves," *Ann Thorac Surg*, 1989, 47(4):589-92.

Ueda N, Kawaguchi S, Niinomi Y, et al, "Effect of Dipyridamole Treatment on Proteinuria in Pediatric Renal Disease," *Nephron*, 1986, 44(3):174-9.

♦ **Disanthrol®** [OTC] *see* Docusate and Casanthranol *on page 337*

♦ **Disodium Cromoglycate** *see* Cromolyn *on page 260*

♦ **Disodium Thiosulfate Pentahydrate** *see* Sodium Thiosulfate *on page 875*

♦ **d-Isoephedrine** *see* Pseudoephedrine *on page 822*

♦ **Disonate®** [OTC] *see* Docusate *on page 336*

Disopyramide (dye soe PEER a mide)

Brand Names Norpace®; Norpace® CR; Rythmodan®, -LA (Canada)

Available Salts Disopyramide Phosphate

Therapeutic Category Antiarrhythmic Agent, Class I-A

Generic Available Yes

Use Suppression and prevention of unifocal and multifocal ventricular premature complexes, coupled ventricular premature complexes, and/or paroxysmal ventricular tachycardia; also effective in the conversion and prevention of recurrence of atrial fibrillation, atrial flutter, and paroxysmal atrial tachycardia

Pregnancy Risk Factor C

Contraindications Pre-existing second or third degree A-V block; cardiogenic shock or hypersensitivity to disopyramide or any component

Precautions Pre-existing urinary retention, family history or existing angle-closure glaucoma, myasthenia gravis, hypotension during initiation of therapy, CHF unless caused by an arrhythmia, widening of QRS complex during therapy or lengthening of Q-T interval (>25% to 50% of baseline QRS complex or Q-T interval), sick sinus syndrome, Wolf Parkinson White syndrome (WPW) or bundle-branch block; may increase ventricular rate in patients with atrial flutter who have not received digoxin; use with caution and decrease dose in patients with renal or hepatic impairment; not recommended for use 48 hours before or 24 hours after verapamil; do not administer with clarithromycin or erythromycin (see Drug Interactions)

Adverse Reactions

Cardiovascular: CHF, edema, chest pain, syncope and hypotension, conduction disturbances including A-V block, widening QRS complex and lengthening of Q-T interval

Central nervous system: Fatigue, headache, malaise, nervousness, acute psychosis, depression, dizziness

Dermatologic: Generalized rashes

Endocrine & metabolic: Hypoglycemia, increased cholesterol and triglycerides; may initiate contractions of pregnant uterus; hyperkalemia may enhance toxicities

Gastrointestinal: Xerostomia, constipation, nausea, vomiting, diarrhea, pain, gas, anorexia, weight gain

Genitourinary: Urinary retention/hesitancy

Hepatic: Elevated liver enzymes, hepatic cholestasis

Neuromuscular & skeletal: Weakness

Ocular: Blurred vision

Respiratory: Dyspnea (<1%)

Miscellaneous: Dry nose, eyes, and throat

Drug Interactions Cytochrome P-450 isoenzyme CYP3A4 substrate

Hepatic microsomal enzyme inducing agents (ie, phenytoin, phenobarbital, rifampin) may increase metabolism of disopyramide and lower serum concentrations; clarithromycin and erythromycin may increase disopyramide serum concentrations which can be life-threatening; other antiarrhythmic agents (quinidine, procainamide, lidocaine, propranolol) may increase adverse conduction effects (widening QRS complex, lengthening Q-T interval)

Mechanism of Action Class IA antiarrhythmic: Decreases myocardial excitability and conduction velocity; reduces disparity in refractory period between normal and infarcted myocardium; possesses anticholinergic, peripheral vasoconstrictive and negative inotropic effects

Pharmacodynamics

Capsules, regular:
Onset of action: 30-210 minutes
Duration: 1.5-8.5 hours

Pharmacokinetics

Protein binding: Concentration dependent, stereoselective, and ranges from 20% to 60%

Distribution: V_d: Children: 1 L/kg

Metabolism: In the liver; major metabolite has anticholinergic and antiarrhythmic effects

Bioavailability: 60% to 83%

Half-life:
Children: 3.15 hours
Adults: 4-10 hours (mean: 6.7 hours), increased half-life with hepatic or renal disease

Elimination: 40% to 60% excreted unchanged in urine and 10% to 15% in feces

Clearance is greater and half-life shorter in children vs adults; clearance (children): 3.76 mL/minute/kg

(Continued)

Disopyramide *(Continued)*

Usual Dosage Oral:

Children (start with lower dose listed):

<1 year: 10-30 mg/kg/day in 4 divided doses

1-4 years: 10-20 mg/kg/day in 4 divided doses

4-12 years: 10-15 mg/kg/day in 4 divided doses

12-18 years: 6-15 mg/kg/day in 4 divided doses

Adults: **Note:** Some patients may require initial loading dose; see product information for details

<50 kg: 100 mg every 6 hours **or** 200 mg every 12 hours (controlled release)

>50 kg: 150 mg every 6 hours **or** 300 mg every 12 hours (controlled release); if no response, may increase to 200 mg every 6 hours; maximum dose required for patients with severe refractory ventricular tachycardia is 400 mg every 6 hours. **Note:** Use lower doses (100 mg of nonsustained release every 6-8 hours) in adults with cardiomyopathy or cardiac decompensation.

Adult dosing adjustment in renal impairment: 100 mg (nonsustained release) given at the following intervals: See table

Creatinine Clearance (mL/min)	Dosage Interval
30-40	Every 8 hours
15-30	Every 12 hours
<15	Every 24 hours

Administration Oral: Administer on an empty stomach; do not crush, break, or chew controlled release capsules, swallow whole

Monitoring Parameters Blood pressure, EKG, drug level; serum potassium, glucose, cholesterol, triglycerides, and liver enzymes; especially important to monitor EKG in patients with hepatic or renal disease, heart disease, or others with increased risk of adverse effects

Reference Range Therapeutic:

Atrial arrhythmias: 2.8-3.2 µg/mL (SI: 8.3-9.4 µmol/L)

Ventricular arrhythmias: 3.3-7.5 µg/mL (SI: 9.7-22 µmol/L)

Toxic: >7 µg/mL (SI: >20.7 µmol/L)

Patient Information Avoid alcohol; notify physician if urinary retention or worsening of CHF occurs

Dosage Forms

Capsule, as phosphate (Norpace®): 100 mg, 150 mg

Capsule, sustained action, as phosphate (Norpace® CR): 100 mg, 150 mg

Extemporaneous Preparations Extemporaneous suspensions in cherry syrup (1 mg/mL and 10 mg/mL) are stable for 4 weeks in amber glass bottles stored at 5°C, 30°C, or at room temperature; shake well before use; do not use extended release capsules for this suspension

Mathur LK, Lai PK, and Shively CD, "Stability of Disopyramide Phosphate in Cherry Syrup," *J Hosp Pharm,* 1982, 39(2):309-10.

References

Chiba K, Koike K, Nakamoto M, et al, "Steady-State Pharmacokinetics and Bioavailability of Total and Unbound Disopyramide in Children With Cardiac Arrhythmias," *Ther Drug Monit,* 1992, 14(2):112-8.

Echizen H, Takahashi H, Nakamura H, et al, "Stereoselective Disposition and Metabolism of Disopyramide in Pediatric Patients," *J Pharmacol Exp Ther,* 1991, 259(3):953-60.

- ♦ **DM** *see* Dextromethorphan *on page 304*
- ♦ **D-Mannitol** *see* Mannitol *on page 593*
- ♦ **4-DMDR** *see* Idarubicin *on page 503*
- ♦ **D-Med® Injection** *see* Methylprednisolone *on page 629*
- ♦ **DMSA** *see* Succimer *on page 883*
- ♦ **DNase** *see* Dornase Alfa *on page 341*
- ♦ **DNR** *see* Daunorubicin *on page 285*

Dobutamine (doe BYOO ta meen)

Related Information
Adult ACLS Algorithm, Hypotension, Shock *on page 1016*
Emergency Pediatric Drip Calculations *on page 1000*
Extravasation Treatment *on page 1050*

Brand Names Dobutrex®

Available Salts Dobutamine Hydrochloride

Therapeutic Category Adrenergic Agonist Agent; Sympathomimetic

Generic Available Yes

Use Short-term management of patients with cardiac decompensation

Pregnancy Risk Factor B

Contraindications Hypersensitivity to sulfites (commercial preparation contains sodium bisulfite); patients with idiopathic hypertrophic subaortic stenosis (IHSS)

Warnings Potent drug; must be diluted prior to use. Patient's hemodynamic status should be monitored.

Precautions Hypovolemia should be corrected prior to use; infiltration causes local inflammatory changes, extravasation may cause dermal necrosis

Adverse Reactions
Cardiovascular: Ectopic heartbeats, increased heart rate, chest pain, angina, palpitations, elevation in blood pressure; in higher doses ventricular tachycardia or arrhythmias may be seen; patients with atrial fibrillation or flutter are at risk of developing a rapid ventricular response
Central nervous system: Headache
Gastrointestinal: Nausea, vomiting
Local: Phlebitis
Neuromuscular & skeletal: Mild leg cramps, paresthesia
Respiratory: Dyspnea

Drug Interactions Beta-adrenergic blocking agents, general anesthetics

Stability Stable in various parenteral solutions for 24 hours; incompatible with alkaline solutions, do not give through same I.V. line as heparin, sodium bicarbonate, ethacrynic acid, cefazolin, or penicillin; compatible when coadministered with dopamine, nitroprusside, potassium chloride, protamine sulfate, tobramycin, epinephrine, atracurium, vecuronium, isoproterenol, and lidocaine; pink discoloration of dobutamine hydrochloride indicates slight oxidation, but no significant loss of potency if administered within the recommended time period

Mechanism of Action Stimulates beta$_1$-adrenergic receptors, causing increased contractility and heart rate, with little effect on beta$_2$- or alpha-receptors

Pharmacodynamics
Onset of action: I.V.: 1-10 minutes
Peak effect: Within 10-20 minutes

Pharmacokinetics
Metabolism: In tissues and the liver to inactive metabolites
Half-life: 2 minutes

Usual Dosage I.V. continuous infusion:
Neonates: 2-15 mcg/kg/minute, titrate to desired response
Children and Adults: 2.5-15 mcg/kg/minute, titrate to desired response; maximum dose: 40 mcg/kg/minute

Administration Parenteral: Dilute in dextrose or NS; maximum recommended concentration: 5000 mcg/mL (5 mg/mL); rate of infusion (mL/hour) = dose (mcg/kg/minute) x weight (kg) x 60 minutes/hour divided by the concentration (mcg/mL); administer into large vein; use infusion device to control rate of flow

Monitoring Parameters EKG, heart rate, CVP, MAP, urine output; if pulmonary artery catheter is in place, monitor CI, PCWP, RAP, and SVR. Dobutamine lowers central venous pressure and wedge pressure but has little effect on pulmonary vascular resistance.

Dosage Forms Injection, as hydrochloride: 12.5 mg/mL (20 mL, 100 mL)

- ♦ **Dobutamine Hydrochloride** *see* Dobutamine *on page 335*
- ♦ **Dobutrex®** *see* Dobutamine *on page 335*

Docusate (DOK yoo sate)

Brand Names Albert® Docusate (Canada); Colace® [OTC]; Colax-C® (Canada); DC 240® Softgel® [OTC]; Dialose® [OTC]; Diocto® [OTC]; Diocto-K® [OTC]; Dioeze® [OTC]; Disonate® [OTC]; DOK® [OTC]; DOS® Softgel® [OTC]; D-S-S® [OTC]; Kasof® [OTC]; Modane® Soft [OTC]; PMS-Docusate Calcium (Canada); Pro-Cal-Sof® [OTC]; Regulax SS® [OTC]; Regulex® (Canada); Regutol® [OTC]; Selax® (Canada); Soflax™ (Canada); Sulfalax® [OTC]; Surfak® [OTC]

Available Salts Dioctyl Calcium Sulfosuccinate; Dioctyl Potassium Sulfosuccinate; Dioctyl Sodium Sulfosuccinate; Docusate Calcium; Docusate Potassium; Docusate Sodium

Synonyms DOSS; DSS

Therapeutic Category Laxative, Surfactant; Stool Softener

Generic Available Yes

Use Stool softener in patients who should avoid straining during defecation; constipation associated with hard, dry stools; ceruminolytic

Pregnancy Risk Factor C

Contraindications Concomitant use of mineral oil; intestinal obstruction, acute abdominal pain, nausea, vomiting; hypersensitivity to docusate or any component

Adverse Reactions
Dermatologic: Rash
Gastrointestinal: Intestinal obstruction, diarrhea, abdominal cramping
Local: Throat irritation

Drug Interactions Docusate may increase absorption of mineral oil and the rate of phenolphthalein absorption; docusate may increase the GI toxicity of aspirin

Mechanism of Action Reduces surface tension of the oil-water interface of the stool resulting in enhanced incorporation of water and fat allowing for stool softening

Pharmacodynamics Onset of action: 12-72 hours

Usual Dosage
Infants and Children: Oral: 5 mg/kg/day in 1-4 divided doses or dose by age:
   <3 years: 10-40 mg/day in 1-4 divided doses
   3-6 years: 20-60 mg/day in 1-4 divided doses
   6-12 years: 40-150 mg/day in 1-4 divided doses
Adolescents and Adults: Oral: 50-400 mg/day in 1-4 divided doses
Older Children and Adults: Rectal: Add 50-100 mg of docusate liquid (not syrup) to enema fluid (saline or water)

Administration
Oral: Administer docusate liquid (not syrup) with milk, fruit juice, or infant formula to mask the bitter taste; ensure adequate fluid intake
Rectal: Administer as a retention or flushing enema

Additional Information Docusate sodium 5-10 mg/mL liquid instilled in the ear as a ceruminolytic produces substantial ear wax disintegration within 15 minutes and complete disintegration after 24 hours

Dosage Forms
Capsule, as calcium: 240 mg
   DC 240® Softgel®, Pro-Cal-Sof®, Sulfalax®: 240 mg
   Surfak®: 50 mg, 240 mg
Capsule, as potassium:
   Diocto-K®: 100 mg
   Kasof®: 240 mg
Capsule, as sodium: 50 mg, 100 mg, 250 mg
   Colace®: 50 mg, 100 mg
   Dioeze®: 250 mg
   Disonate®: 100 mg, 240 mg
   DOK®: 100 mg, 250 mg
   DOS® Softgel®: 100 mg, 250 mg
   Doxinate®: 250 mg
   D-S-S®: 100 mg
   Modane® Soft: 100 mg
   Pro-Sof®: 100 mg, 250 mg
   Regulax SS®: 100 mg, 250 mg
Liquid, as sodium (Diocto®, Colace®, Disonate®, DOK®): 150 mg/15 mL (30 mL, 60 mL, 480 mL)
Solution, oral, as sodium (Doxinate®): 50 mg/mL with alcohol 5% (60 mL, 3780 mL)
Syrup, as sodium: 50 mg/15 mL (15 mL, 30 mL); 60 mg/15 mL (480 mL, 3780 mL)
   Colace®, Diocto®, Disonate®, DOK®, Pro-Sof®: 60 mg/15 mL (240 mL, 480 mL, 3780 mL)
Tablet, as sodium (Dialose®, Regutol®): 100 mg

References
Chen DA and Caparosa RJ, "A Nonprescription Cerumenolytic," *Am J Otol*, 1991, 12(6):475-6.

Docusate and Casanthranol (DOK yoo sate & ka SAN thra nole)

Brand Names Dialose® Plus Capsule [OTC]; Diocto C® [OTC]; Diocto-K Plus® [OTC]; Dioctolose Plus® [OTC]; Disanthrol® [OTC]; DSMC Plus® [OTC]; D-S-S Plus® [OTC]; Genasoft® Plus [OTC]; Peri-Colace® [OTC]; Pro-Sof® Plus [OTC]; Regulace® [OTC]

Available Salts Docusate Potassium and Casanthranol; Docusate Sodium and Casanthranol

Synonyms Casanthranol and Docusate; DSS With Casanthranol

Therapeutic Category Laxative, Stimulant; Laxative, Surfactant; Stool Softener

Generic Available Yes

Use Treatment of constipation generally associated with dry, hard stools and decreased intestinal motility

Pregnancy Risk Factor C

Contraindications Concomitant use of mineral oil; intestinal obstruction; acute abdominal pain; nausea, vomiting; hypersensitivity to docusate, casanthranol, or any component

Warnings Do not use when abdominal pain, nausea, or vomiting are present

Precautions Casanthranol is habit-forming; may result in laxative dependence and loss of normal bowel function with prolonged use

Adverse Reactions
Dermatologic: Rash
Gastrointestinal: Intestinal obstruction, diarrhea, abdominal cramping
Local: Throat irritation

Drug Interactions Docusate may increase absorption of mineral oil and the rate of phenolphthalein absorption; docusate may increase the GI toxicity of aspirin

Mechanism of Action Combination stool softener (docusate) which lowers surface tension of the stool allowing water and lipids to penetrate and a stimulant laxative (casanthranol) which produces a net intestinal fluid accumulation and laxation

Pharmacodynamics Onset of action: 8-12 hours after administration but may require up to 24 hours

Usual Dosage Oral:
Children: 5-15 mL of syrup at bedtime or 1 capsule at bedtime
Adults: 1-2 capsules or 15-30 mL syrup at bedtime, may be increased to 2 capsules or 30 mL twice daily or 3 capsules at bedtime

Administration Oral: Administer with plenty of fluids

Monitoring Parameters Bowel frequency

Dosage Forms
Capsule (Dialose® Plus, Diocto-K Plus®, Dioctolose Plus®, DSMC Plus®): Docusate potassium 100 mg and casanthranol 30 mg
Capsule (Disanthrol®, D-S-S Plus®, Genasoft® Plus, Peri-Colace®, Pro-Sof® Plus, Regulace®): Docusate sodium 100 mg and casanthranol 30 mg
Syrup (Diocto C®, Peri-Colace®): Docusate sodium 60 mg and casanthranol 30 mg per 15 mL (240 mL, 480 mL, 4000 mL)

♦ **Docusate Calcium** *see Docusate on page 336*
♦ **Docusate Potassium** *see Docusate on page 336*
♦ **Docusate Potassium and Casanthranol** *see Docusate and Casanthranol on page 337*
♦ **Docusate Sodium** *see Docusate on page 336*
♦ **Docusate Sodium and Casanthranol** *see Docusate and Casanthranol on page 337*
♦ **DOK® [OTC]** *see Docusate on page 336*
♦ **Doktors® Nasal Solution [OTC]** *see Phenylephrine on page 758*
♦ **Dolacet®** *see Hydrocodone and Acetaminophen on page 485*

Dolasetron (dol A se tron)

Brand Names Anzemet®
Available Salts Dolasetron Mesylate
Synonyms Hydrodolasetron
Therapeutic Category Antiemetic
Generic Available No
Use Prevention of chemotherapy-induced nausea and vomiting; prevention and treatment of postoperative nausea and vomiting
Pregnancy Risk Factor B
(Continued)

Dolasetron *(Continued)*

Contraindications Hypersensitivity to dolasetron or any component

Warnings Dolasetron may cause EKG interval changes (PR, QT_c, JT prolongation and QRS widening) related in magnitude and frequency to blood levels of the active metabolite, hydrodolasetron; interval prolongation could lead to cardiovascular consequences such as heart block or cardiac arrhythmias

Precautions Use with caution in patients with, or who may develop, prolongation of cardiac conduction intervals, particularly QT_c; conditions include hypokalemia, hypomagnesemia, or congenital QT syndrome; use with caution in patients receiving antiarrhythmic or other medications known to prolong the QT interval (eg, class I or III antiarrhythmic agents) or medications known to reduce potassium or magnesium levels (eg, diuretics)

Adverse Reactions

Cardiovascular: Prolonged QT interval and other EKG changes (see Warnings), hypertension, hypotension, edema, increased sweating

Central nervous system: Headache, fatigue, dizziness, fever, chills, shivering, agitation, sleep disorder, confusion, anxiety, abnormal dreams

Dermatologic: Rash, urticaria

Gastrointestinal: Diarrhea, abdominal pain, constipation, dyspepsia, anorexia, pancreatitis (rarely), taste perversion

Genitourinary: Urinary retention, acute renal failure (rarely), polyuria (rarely), dysuria (rarely)

Hepatic: Transient increases in liver enzymes

Neuromuscular & skeletal: Myalgia, arthralgia

Ocular: Photophobia (rarely), abnormal vision

Otic: Tinnitus (rarely)

Miscellaneous: Hypersensitivity reactions

Drug Interactions Increased hydrodolasetron (active metabolite) serum levels with cimetidine; decreased hydrodolasetron serum levels with rifampin; decreased clearance of hydrodolasetron with atenolol; (see Warnings and Precautions)

Stability Injection is stable after dilution in NS, D_5W, $D_5\frac{1}{2}NS$, D_5LR, LR, and 10% mannitol injection for 24 hours at room temperature and 48 hours under refrigeration

Mechanism of Action Dolasetron and its major metabolite, hydrodolasetron, are selective $5\text{-}HT_3$ receptor antagonists, blocking serotonin, both peripherally on vagal nerve terminals and centrally in the chemoreceptor trigger zone

Pharmacokinetics Due to the rapid metabolism of dolasetron to hydrodolasetron (primary active metabolite), the majority of the following pharmacokinetic parameters relate to hydrodolasetron:

Distribution:
Children: 5.9-7.4 L/kg
Adults: 4.15-5.5 L/kg

Metabolism: Rapidly converted by carbonyl reductase to active major metabolite, hydrodolasetron; hydrodolasetron is metabolized by the cytochrome P-450 CYP2D6 and CYP3A enzyme systems and flavin mono-oxygenase

Bioavailability: Oral: Children: 59% (formulation not specified), adults: 70% to 80%

Half-life, elimination:
Dolasetron: <10 minutes
Hydrodolasetron:
Oral: Children: 5.7 hours, adults: 8.1 hours (range: 5-10 hours)
I.V.: Children: 4.8 hours, adults: 7.3 hours (range: 4-8 hours)

Time to peak concentration:
Oral: 1-1.5 hours
I.V.: 0.6 hours

Elimination: Dolasetron: <1% excreted unchanged in urine; hydrodolasetron: 53% to 61% excreted unchanged in urine within 36 hours

Usual Dosage

Prevention of chemotherapy-induced nausea and vomiting: **Oral:** Administered within 1 hour before chemotherapy; or **I.V.:** Administered 30 minutes before chemotherapy:

Children ≥2 years to 16 years:
Oral, I.V.: 1.8 mg/kg as a single dose (maximum: 100 mg)

Adults:
Oral: 100 mg as a single dose
I.V.: 1.8 mg/kg or alternatively 100 mg as a single dose

Prevention or treatment of postoperative nausea and vomiting: **Oral:** Administered 2 hours before surgery and; **I.V.:** Administered 15 minutes prior to cessation of anaesthesia or as soon as symptoms present

Children ≥2 years to 16 years:
    Oral: 1.2 mg/kg as a single dose (maximum: 100 mg)
    I.V.: 0.35 mg/kg as a single dose (maximum: 12.5 mg)
Adults:
    Oral: 100 mg as a single dose
    I.V.: 12.5 mg as a single dose

Dosage adjustment in hepatic or renal impairment: No dosage adjustment needed

Administration
Oral: May be administered with or without food; injection may be used orally, dilute injection in apple or apple-grape juice; stable for 2 hours at room temperature
Parenteral: I.V.: Infuse undiluted over 30 seconds or dilute in 50 mL compatible I.V. fluid and infuse over ≤15 minutes; do not mix with other medications

Monitoring Parameters Baseline EKG in high-risk patients (see Warnings and Precautions), emesis episodes

Dosage Forms
Injection, as mesylate: 20 mg/mL (0.625 mL, 5 mL)
Tablet: 50 mg, 100 mg

References
Coppes MJ, Lau R, Ingram LC, et al, "Open-Label Comparison of the Antiemetic Efficacy of Single Intravenous Doses of Dolasetron Mesylate in Pediatric Cancer Patients Receiving Moderately to Highly Emetogenic Chemotherapy," *Med Pediatr Oncol*, 1999, 33(2):99-105.

♦ **Dolasetron Mesylate** *see Dolasetron on page 337*

♦ **Dolene®** *see Propoxyphene on page 814*

♦ **Dolophine®** *see Methadone on page 613*

♦ **Dolorac® [OTC]** *see Capsaicin on page 162*

♦ **Domeboro® [OTC]** *see Aluminum Acetate on page 53*

♦ **Donnagel®-MB (Canada)** *see Kaolin and Pectin on page 540*

♦ **Donnamar®** *see Hyoscyamine on page 497*

♦ **Donnamor®** *see Hyoscyamine, Atropine, Scopolamine, and Phenobarbital on page 499*

♦ **Donnapine®** *see Hyoscyamine, Atropine, Scopolamine, and Phenobarbital on page 499*

♦ **Donna-Sed®** *see Hyoscyamine, Atropine, Scopolamine, and Phenobarbital on page 499*

♦ **Donnatal®** *see Hyoscyamine, Atropine, Scopolamine, and Phenobarbital on page 499*

♦ **Donnazyme®** *see Pancreatin on page 723*

♦ **Donphen®** *see Hyoscyamine, Atropine, Scopolamine, and Phenobarbital on page 499*

♦ **Dopamet® (Canada)** *see Methyldopa on page 625*

Dopamine (DOE pa meen)

Related Information
Adult ACLS Algorithm, Bradycardia *on page 1012*
Adult ACLS Algorithm, Hypotension, Shock *on page 1016*
Emergency Pediatric Drip Calculations *on page 1000*
Extravasation Treatment *on page 1050*

Brand Names Intropin®

Available Salts Dopamine Hydrochloride

Therapeutic Category Adrenergic Agonist Agent; Sympathomimetic

Generic Available Yes

Use Increase cardiac output, blood pressure, and urine flow as an adjunct in the treatment of shock or hypotension which persists after adequate fluid volume replacement; in low dosage to increase renal perfusion

Pregnancy Risk Factor C

Contraindications Hypersensitivity to sulfites (commercial preparation contains sodium bisulfite); pheochromocytoma, or ventricular fibrillation

Warnings Potent drug; must be diluted prior to use. Patient's hemodynamic status should be monitored.

Precautions Blood volume depletion should be corrected, if possible, before starting dopamine therapy. Dopamine must not be used as sole therapy in hypovolemic patients. Extravasation may cause tissue necrosis (treat extravasation with phentolamine; see Extravasation Treatment *on page 1050*); due to potential gangrene of extremities, use with caution in patients with occlusive vascular disease.
(Continued)

Dopamine *(Continued)*

Adverse Reactions

Cardiovascular: Ectopic heartbeats, tachycardia, vasoconstriction, cardiac conduction abnormalities, widened QRS complex, hypertension, ventricular arrhythmias, gangrene of the extremities (with high doses for prolonged periods or even with low doses in patients with occlusive vascular disease), anginal pain, palpitations

Central nervous system: Anxiety, headache

Gastrointestinal: Nausea, vomiting

Genitourinary: Decreased urine output

Neuromuscular & skeletal: Piloerection

Ocular: Dilated pupils

Renal: Azotemia

Respiratory: Dyspnea

Drug Interactions Dopamine's cardiac and pressor response are prolonged and intensified by MAO inhibitors, alpha- and beta-adrenergic agonists, and oxytocic drugs; tricyclic antidepressants may decrease effects; use with phenytoin has resulted in seizures, severe hypotension, and bradycardia; use with halogenated hydrocarbon anesthetics may lead to serious arrhythmias; dopamine's cardiac effects are antagonized by beta-adrenergic blocking agents; vasoconstrictive effects are antagonized by alpha-adrenergic blocking agents

Stability Protect from light; solutions that are darker than slightly yellow should not be used; incompatible with alkaline solutions or iron salts; compatible when coadministered with dobutamine, epinephrine, isoproterenol, lidocaine, atracurium, vecuronium

Mechanism of Action Stimulates both adrenergic and dopaminergic receptors; low doses are mainly dopaminergic which stimulate and produce renal and mesenteric vasodilation; intermediate doses stimulate both dopaminergic and $beta_1$-adrenergic receptors and produce cardiac stimulation (increased heart rate and cardiac index) and increased renal blood flow; high doses stimulate alpha-adrenergic receptors primarily (vasoconstriction and increased blood pressure)

Pharmacodynamics

Onset of action: Adults: 5 minutes

Duration: Due to its short duration of action (<10 minutes) a continuous infusion must be used

Pharmacokinetics

Metabolism: In plasma, kidneys, and liver; 75% to inactive metabolites by monoamine oxidase and catechol-o-methyltransferase and 25% to norepinephrine (active)

Half-life: 2 minutes

Clearance: Neonatal clearance varies and appears to be age related. Clearance is more prolonged with combined hepatic and renal dysfunction. Dopamine has exhibited nonlinear kinetics in children; dose changes in children may not achieve steady-state for approximately 1 hour rather than 20 minutes seen in adults.

Usual Dosage I.V. infusion:

The hemodynamic effects of dopamine are dose-dependent:

Low dosage: 1-5 mcg/kg/minute, increased renal blood flow and urine output

Intermediate dosage: 5-15 mcg/kg/minute, increased renal blood flow, heart rate, cardiac contractility, cardiac output, and blood pressure

High dosage: >15 mcg/kg/minute, alpha-adrenergic effects begin to predominate, vasoconstriction, increased blood pressure

Neonates: 1-20 mcg/kg/minute continuous infusion, titrate to desired response

Children: 1-20 mcg/kg/minute, maximum dose: 50 mcg/kg/minute continuous infusion, titrate to desired response

Adults: 1 mcg/kg/minute up to 50 mcg/kg/minute, titrate to desired response

If dosages >20-30 mcg/kg/minute are needed, a more direct-acting pressor may be beneficial (ie, epinephrine, norepinephrine)

Administration Parenteral: Must be diluted prior to administration; maximum concentration: 3200 mcg/mL (3.2 mg/mL); (concentrations as high as 6000 mcg/mL have been infused into large veins, safely and with efficacy, in cases of extreme fluid restriction); rate of infusion (mL/hour) = dose (mcg/kg/minute) x weight (kg) x 60 minutes/hour divided by concentration (mcg/mL); administer into large vein to prevent the possibility of extravasation; use infusion device to control rate of flow; administration into an umbilical arterial catheter is **not** recommended

Monitoring Parameters EKG, heart rate, CVP, MAP, urine output; if pulmonary artery catheter is in place, monitor CI, PWCP, SVR, RAP, and PVR

Dosage Forms
Infusion, as hydrochloride, in D$_5$W: 0.8 mg/mL (250 mL, 500 mL); 1.6 mg/mL (250 mL, 500 mL); 3.2 mg/mL (250 mL, 500 mL)

Injection, as hydrochloride: 40 mg/mL (5 mL, 10 mL, 20 mL); 80 mg/mL (5 mL, 20 mL); 160 mg/mL (5 mL)

References
Banner W, Jr, Vernon DD, Dean JM, et al, "Nonlinear Dopamine Pharmacokinetics in Pediatric Patients," *J Pharmacol Exp Ther*, 1989, 249(1):131-3.

♦ **Dopamine Hydrochloride** *see* Dopamine *on page 339*

♦ **Dopar®** *see* Levodopa *on page 565*

♦ **Dopram®** *see* Doxapram *on page 343*

♦ **Dorcol® [OTC]** *see* Acetaminophen *on page 26*

♦ **Dormarex® 2 Oral [OTC]** *see* Diphenhydramine *on page 327*

♦ **Dormin® Oral [OTC]** *see* Diphenhydramine *on page 327*

Dornase Alfa (DOOR nase AL fa)
Brand Names Pulmozyme®

Synonyms DNase; Recombinant Human Deoxyribonuclease

Therapeutic Category Enzyme, Inhalant; Mucolytic Agent

Generic Available No

Use Management of cystic fibrosis patients to reduce the frequency of respiratory infections and to improve pulmonary function

Pregnancy Risk Factor B

Contraindications Hypersensitivity to dornase alfa, Chinese hamster ovary cell products (eg, epoetin alfa), or any component

Warnings Safety and efficacy has not been established in children <5 years of age or in patients with forced vital capacity <40% of normal; no data exists regarding safety during lactation

Adverse Reactions
Cardiovascular: Chest pain
Dermatologic: Skin rash
Gastrointestinal: Sore throat
Hepatic: Liver disease
Ocular: Conjunctivitis
Respiratory: Increased cough, dyspnea, hemoptysis, wheezing, laryngitis, rhinitis, pharyngitis
Miscellaneous: Voice alteration, hoarseness

Drug Interactions None known at this time

Stability Must be stored in the refrigerator at 2°C to 8°C (36°F to 46°F) and protected from strong light; unopened vials left at room temperature for a total time of 24 hours should be discarded; discard solution if cloudy or discolored

Mechanism of Action Dornase alfa is a deoxyribonuclease (DNA) enzyme produced by recombinant gene technology. Dornase selectively cleaves DNA, thus reducing mucous viscosity seen in the pulmonary secretions of cystic fibrosis patients. As a result, airflow in the lung is improved and the risk of bacterial infection may be decreased.

Pharmacodynamics Onset of improved pulmonary function tests (PFTs): 3-8 days; PFTs will return to baseline 2-3 weeks after discontinuation of therapy

Pharmacokinetics Following nebulization, enzyme levels are measurable in the sputum within 15 minutes and decline rapidly thereafter

Usual Dosage
Infants and Children ≤5 years: Not approved for use, however studies using this therapy in small numbers of children as young as 3 months of age have reported efficacy and similar side effects. See References.
Children >5 years and Adults: Inhalation: 2.5 mg/day through selected nebulizers in conjunction with a Pulmo-Aide® or a Pari-Proneb® compressor; some patients, especially older than 21 years of age or with forced vital capacity (FVC) >85%, may benefit from twice daily administration

Administration Nebulization: Should not be diluted or mixed with any other drugs in the nebulizer, this may inactivate the drug

Dosage Forms Solution, inhalation: 1 mg/mL (2.5 mL)

References
Fuchs HJ, Borowitz DS, Christiansen DH, et al, "Effect of Aerosolized Recombinant Human DNase on Exacerbations of Respiratory Symptoms and on Pulmonary Function in Patients With Cystic Fibrosis," *N Engl J Med*, 1994, 331(10):637-42.

Mueller GA, Rubins G, Wessel D, et al, "Effects of Dornase Alfa on Pulmonary Function Tests in Infants with Cystic Fibrosis," *Am J Respir Crit Care Med*, 1996, 153:A70.

(Continued)

Dornase Alfa *(Continued)*

Rock M, Kirchner K, McCubbin M, et al, "Aerosol Delivery and Safety of rhDNASE in Young Children With Cystic Fibrosis: A Bronchoscopic Study," *Pediatr Pulmonol*, 1996, 13(Suppl):A268.

♦ **Doryx®** *see Doxycycline on page 348*
♦ **DOSS** *see Docusate on page 336*
♦ **DOS® Softgel® [OTC]** *see Docusate on page 336*

Doxacurium (doks a KYOO ri um)

Brand Names Nuromax® Injection
Available Salts Doxacurium Chloride
Therapeutic Category Neuromuscular Blocker Agent, Nondepolarizing; Skeletal Muscle Relaxant, Paralytic
Generic Available No
Use Doxacurium is indicated for use as an adjunct to general anesthesia. It provides skeletal muscle relaxation during surgery or endotracheal intubation; increases pulmonary compliance during mechanical ventilation
Pregnancy Risk Factor C
Contraindications Hypersensitivity to doxacurium or any component
Warnings Ventilation must be supported during neuromuscular blockade
Precautions Contains benzyl alcohol; avoid use in neonates; use with caution in patients with neuromuscular disease such as myasthenia gravis, cardiovascular disease; use with caution and reduce dosage in patients with renal or hepatic impairment; certain clinical conditions may result in potentiation or antagonism of neuromuscular blockade, see table.

Clinical Conditions Affecting Neuromuscular Blockade

Potentiation	Antagonism
Electrolyte abnormalities	Alkalosis
Severe hyponatremia	Hypercalcemia
Severe hypocalcemia	Demyelinating lesions
Severe hypokalemia	Peripheral neuropathies
Hypermagnesemia	Diabetes mellitus
Neuromuscular diseases	
Acidosis	
Acute intermittent porphyria	
Renal failure	
Hepatic failure	

Adverse Reactions The most frequent adverse reactions appear as an extension of the agent's neuromuscular blocking actions

Cardiovascular: Hypotension (rare), bradycardia (rare)
Central nervous system: Fever
Dermatologic: Cutaneous flushing, urticaria
Neuromuscular & skeletal: Muscle weakness
Ocular: Diplopia
Respiratory: Respiratory insufficiency and apnea, bronchospasm, wheezing

Drug Interactions See table on following page.
Stability Stable for 24 hours at room temperature when diluted in concentrations up to 0.1 mg/mL in D_5W or NS; compatible with sufentanil, alfentanil, and fentanyl; incompatible with alkaline solutions
Mechanism of Action Doxacurium is a long-acting nondepolarizing skeletal muscle relaxant. The drug is a bis-quaternary benzylisoquinolinium diester, with a chemical structure similar to that of atracurium. Similar to other nondepolarizing neuromuscular blocking agents, doxacurium produces muscle relaxation by competing with acetylcholine for cholinergic receptor sites on the postjunctional membrane; significant presynaptic depressant activity is also observed.
Pharmacodynamics
Onset of effects: 5-11 minutes
Duration: 30 minutes (range: 12-54 minutes)
Pharmacokinetics
Protein binding: 30%
Half-life:
Normal: 1.5 hours

Renal dysfunction: 3.7 hours
Liver dysfunction: 1.9 hours
Elimination: Primarily as unchanged drug via the kidneys and biliary tract

Potential Drug Interactions

Potentiation	Antagonism
Anesthetics	Calcium
Desflurane, sevoflurane, enflurane and	Carbamazepine
isoflurane > halothane > nitrous	Phenytoin
oxide	Steroids (chronic administration)
Antibiotics	Theophylline
Aminoglycosides, polymyxins,	Anticholinesterases*
clindamycin, vancomycin	Neostigmine, pyridostigmine,
Magnesium sulfate	edrophonium, echothiophate
Antiarrhythmics	ophthalmic solution
Quinidine, procainamide, bretylium, and	Caffeine
possibly lidocaine	Azathioprine
Diuretics	
Furosemide, mannitol	
Amphotericin B (secondary to hypokalemia)	
Local anesthetics	
Dantrolene (directly depresses skeletal muscle)	
Beta blockers	
Calcium channel blockers	
Ketamine	
Lithium	
Succinylcholine (when administered prior to nondepolarizing neuromuscular-blocking agent)	
Cyclosporine	

*Can prolong the effects of acetylcholine

Usual Dosage I.V. (in obese patients, use ideal body weight):
Children 2-12 years: Initial: 0.03-0.05 mg/kg/dose (30-50 mcg/kg/dose); maintenance: 0.005-0.01 mg/kg (5-10 mcg/kg/dose) every 30-45 minutes, or as needed depending upon individual patient response
Children >12 years and Adults: Initial: 0.025-0.05 mg/kg/dose (25-50 mcg/kg/dose); maintenance: 0.005-0.01 mg/kg/dose (5-10 mcg/kg/dose) every 60-100 minutes
Dosing adjustment in renal or hepatic impairment: Reduce initial dose and titrate carefully as duration may be prolonged
Administration Parenteral: I.V.: May be administered by rapid I.V. injection undiluted
Monitoring Parameters Peripheral nerve stimulation testing (measures twitch response), heart rate, blood pressure, assisted ventilation status
Additional Information Doxacurium is a long-acting nondepolarizing neuromuscular blocker with virtually no cardiovascular side effects. The characteristics of this agent make it especially useful in procedures requiring careful maintenance of hemodynamic stability for prolonged periods
Dosage Forms Injection, as chloride: 1 mg/mL (5 mL)

♦ **Doxacurium Chloride** see Doxacurium on page 342

Doxapram (DOKS a pram)
Brand Names Dopram®
Available Salts Doxapram Hydrochloride
Therapeutic Category Central Nervous System Stimulant, Nonamphetamine; Respiratory Stimulant
Generic Available No
Use Respiratory and CNS stimulant; idiopathic apnea of prematurity refractory to xanthines
Pregnancy Risk Factor B
(Continued)

Doxapram *(Continued)*

Contraindications Hypersensitivity to doxapram or any component; epilepsy, cerebral edema, head injury, asthma or restrictive pulmonary disease, pheochromocytoma, cardiovascular or coronary artery disease, hypertension, hyperthyroidism, cardiac arrhythmias

Warnings Should be used with caution in newborns as the U.S. product contains benzyl alcohol (0.9%); recommended doses of doxapram for neonates will deliver 5.4-27 mg/kg/day of benzyl alcohol; large amounts of benzyl alcohol (>100 mg/kg/day) have been associated with fatal toxicity (gasping syndrome); the use of doxapram in newborns should be reserved for neonates who are unresponsive to the treatment of apnea with therapeutic serum concentrations of theophylline or caffeine; not an antagonist to muscle relaxant drugs nor a specific narcotic antagonist; doxapram alone may not stimulate adequate spontaneous breathing or provide sufficient arousal in patients who are severely depressed; use as an adjunct to establish supportive measures

Adverse Reactions

Cardiovascular: Hypertension (dose-related), tachycardia, arrhythmias, hypotension, flushing

Central nervous system: CNS stimulation, restlessness, lightheadedness, jitters, hallucinations, irritability, seizures, headache, fever, hypothermia

Hematologic: Hemolysis

Gastrointestinal: Abdominal distension, nausea, vomiting, retching, increased gastric residuals

Local: Phlebitis

Metabolic: Hyperglycemia

Neuromuscular & skeletal: Tremor, hyper-reflexia

Ocular: Lacrimation, mydriasis

Renal: Glucosuria

Respiratory: Coughing, laryngospasm, dyspnea

Miscellaneous: Diaphoresis

Drug Interactions Sympathomimetic drugs and MAO inhibitors may cause significant increase in blood pressure; general anesthetics

Stability Stable at room temperature; incompatible with aminophylline, sodium bicarbonate, thiopental sodium, and other alkaline solutions

Mechanism of Action Stimulates respiration through action on respiratory center in medulla or through reflex stimulation of carotid, aortic, or other peripheral chemoreceptors; antagonizes opiate-induced respiratory depression, but does not affect analgesia

Pharmacodynamics Following I.V. injection:

Onset of respiratory stimulation: Within 20-40 seconds

Peak effect: Within 1-2 minutes

Duration: 5-12 minutes

Pharmacokinetics

Metabolism: Extensive in the liver

Distribution: V_d: Neonates: 4-7.3 L/kg

Half-life:

Neonates, premature: 6.6-8.2 hours; clearance: 0.44-0.7 L/hour/kg

Adults: Mean: 3.4 hours (range: 2.4-4.1 hours)

Usual Dosage I.V.:

Neonatal apnea (apnea of prematurity): Initial loading dose: 2.5-3 mg/kg followed by a continuous infusion of 1 mg/kg/hour titrated to the lowest rate at which apnea is controlled (maximum dose: 2.5 mg/kg/hour)

Adults: Respiratory depression following anesthesia:

Initial: 0.5-1 mg/kg; may repeat at 5-minute intervals; maximum total dose: 2 mg/kg

I.V. infusion: Initial: 5 mg/minute until adequate response or adverse effects seen; decrease to 1-3 mg/minute; usual total dose: 0.5-4 mg/kg or 300 mg

Administration Parenteral: I.V. use only: Dilute loading dose to a maximum concentration of 2 mg/mL and infuse over 15-30 minutes; for infusion, dilute in NS or dextrose to 1 mg/mL (maximum concentration: 2 mg/mL); irritating to tissues; avoid extravasation

Monitoring Parameters Blood pressure, heart rate, deep tendon reflexes; for apnea: number, duration, and severity of apneic episodes

Reference Range Initial studies suggest a therapeutic serum level of at least 1.5 mg/L; toxicity becomes frequent at serum levels >5 mg/L

Dosage Forms Injection, as hydrochloride: 20 mg/mL (20 mL)

References
Barrington KJ, Finer NN, Torok-Both G, et al, "Dose-Response Relationship of Doxapram in the Therapy for Refractory Idiopathic Apnea of Prematurity," *Pediatrics*, 1987, 80(1):22-7.

♦ **Doxapram Hydrochloride** *see* Doxapram *on page 343*

Doxepin (DOKS e pin)

Related Information
Comparison of Adverse Effects of Antidepressants *on page 1030*
Comparison of Usual Adult Dosage and Mechanism of Action of Antidepressants *on page 1029*
Drugs and Breast-Feeding *on page 1213*
Overdose and Toxicology *on page 1191*

Brand Names Adapin® Oral; Apo®-Doxepin (Canada); Novo-Doxepin® (Canada); Sinequan® Oral; Triadapin® (Canada); Zonalon® Topical Cream

Available Salts Doxepin Hydrochloride

Therapeutic Category Antianxiety Agent; Antidepressant, Tricyclic

Generic Available Yes

Use
Oral: Treatment of various forms of depression, usually in conjunction with psychotherapy; treatment of anxiety disorders; analgesic for certain chronic and neuropathic pain

Topical: Adults: Short-term (<8 days) therapy of moderate pruritus due to atopic dermatitis or lichen simplex chronicus

Pregnancy Risk Factor C

Contraindications Hypersensitivity to doxepin or any component (cross-sensitivity with other tricyclic antidepressants may occur); narrow-angle glaucoma

Warnings Do not discontinue abruptly in patients receiving chronic high dose therapy

Precautions Use with caution in patients with cardiovascular disease, conduction disturbances, seizure disorders, urinary retention, hyperthyroidism or those receiving thyroid replacement; avoid use during lactation; use with caution in pregnancy

Adverse Reactions Pronounced sedation and anticholinergic adverse effects may occur
Cardiovascular: Hypotension, arrhythmias
Central nervous system: Sedation, confusion, dizziness
Dermatologic: Photosensitivity
Endocrine & metabolic: SIADH (rare)
Gastrointestinal: Constipation, nausea, vomiting, xerostomia, increased appetite, weight gain
Genitourinary: Urinary retention
Hematologic: Blood dyscrasias (rare)
Hepatic: Hepatitis
Neuromuscular & skeletal: Fine tremor
Ocular: Blurred vision
Otic: Tinnitus
Miscellaneous: Hypersensitivity reactions

Drug Interactions Cytochrome P-450 isoenzyme CYP2D6 substrate
CNS depressants, alcohol, MAO inhibitors, guanethidine, clonidine, antithyroid agents, cimetidine, carbamazepine

Food Interactions Oral solution is physically incompatible with carbonated beverages and grape juice

Stability Protect from light

Mechanism of Action Increases the synaptic concentration of serotonin and/or norepinephrine in the central nervous system by inhibition of their reuptake by the presynaptic neuronal membrane

Pharmacodynamics Maximum antidepressant effects: Usually occur after >2 weeks; anxiolytic effects may occur sooner

Pharmacokinetics
Distribution: Crosses the placenta; appears in breast milk
Protein binding: 80% to 85%
Metabolism: Hepatic to metabolites, including desmethyldoxepin (active)
Half-life, adults: 6-8 hours
Elimination: Renal

Usual Dosage
Oral:
Children: 1-3 mg/kg/day in single or divided doses
(Continued)

Doxepin *(Continued)*

Adolescents: Initial: 25-50 mg/day in single or divided doses; gradually increase to 100 mg/day

Adults: Initial: 30-150 mg/day at bedtime or in 2-3 divided doses; may increase up to 300 mg/day; single dose should not exceed 150 mg; select patients may respond to 25-50 mg/day

Topical: Adults: Apply to affected area 4 times/day

Administration Oral: Administer with food to decrease GI upset; oral concentrate should be diluted in water, milk, or juice (but not grape juice) prior to administration (use 120 mL for adults); do not mix with carbonated beverages

Monitoring Parameters Blood pressure, heart rate, mental status, weight, liver enzymes, CBC with differential

Reference Range Utility of serum level monitoring controversial

Therapeutic concentration: Doxepin plus desmethyldoxepin: 110-250 ng/mL (SI: 4-9 nmol/L)

Toxic concentration: >300 ng/mL (SI: >11 nmol/L)

Patient Information May cause drowsiness and impair ability to perform activities requiring mental alertness or physical coordination; may cause dry mouth; avoid alcohol; limit caffeine; may increase appetite; do not discontinue abruptly; avoid unnecessary exposure to sunlight

Nursing Implications Do not use occlusive dressings with cream (increases dermal absorption)

Additional Information Place in therapy (treatment of depression): Considered by some to be the drug of choice in nonobese, depressed children with prominent anxiety, phobias, and somatic symptoms and a third drug of choice for nonobese, depressed children without excessive daytime sleepiness

Dosage Forms

Capsule, as hydrochloride: 10 mg, 25 mg, 50 mg, 75 mg, 100 mg, 150 mg

Concentrate, oral, as hydrochloride: 10 mg/mL (120 mL)

Cream: 5% (30 g)

References

Levy HB, Harper CR, and Weinberg WA, " A Practical Approach to Children Failing in School," *Pediatr Clin North Am*, 1992, 39(4):895-928.

♦ **Doxepin Hydrochloride** *see Doxepin on page 345*

Doxorubicin (doks oh ROO bi sin)

Related Information

Drugs and Breast-Feeding *on page 1213*

Emetogenic Potential of Single Chemotherapeutic Agents *on page 1095*

Extravasation Treatment *on page 1050*

Brand Names Adriamycin PFS™; Adriamycin RDF™; Rubex®

Available Salts Doxorubicin Hydrochloride

Synonyms ADR; Hydroxydaunomycin

Therapeutic Category Antineoplastic Agent, Anthracycline; Antineoplastic Agent, Antibiotic

Generic Available Yes

Use Treatment of various solid tumors including ovarian, breast, and bladder tumors; various lymphomas and leukemias (AML, ALL), soft tissue sarcomas, neuroblastoma, osteosarcoma

Pregnancy Risk Factor D

Contraindications Hypersensitivity to doxorubicin or any component; severe CHF, cardiomyopathy, pre-existing myelosuppression; patients who have received a total dose of 550 mg/m^2 of doxorubicin or 400 mg/m^2 in patients with previous or concomitant treatment with daunorubicin, idarubicin, mitoxantrone, cyclophosphamide, or irradiation of the cardiac region

Warnings The FDA currently recommends that procedures for proper handling and disposal of antineoplastic agents be considered. **I.V. use only,** severe local tissue necrosis will result if extravasation occurs; irreversible myocardial toxicity may occur if the total cumulative dose approaches 450 mg/m^2 in adults with normal cardiac function or 300 mg/m^2 in adults with prior mediastinal irradiation, concurrent cyclophosphamide therapy, or pre-existing heart disease; severe myelosuppression is also possible. Pediatric patients are at increased risk for developing delayed cardiac toxicity and CHF during early adulthood due to an increasing census of long-term survivors; periodic long-term monitoring of cardiac function is recommended. Pediatric patients are at risk of developing secondary acute myeloid leukemia.

Precautions Modify dosage in patients with impaired hepatic function

Adverse Reactions

Cardiovascular: CHF, cardiomyopathy, cardiotoxicity (transient type with abnormal EKG and arrhythmias, or a chronic, cumulative, dose-dependent type which progresses to CHF), cardiorespiratory decompensation, facial flushing

Dermatologic: Alopecia, hyperpigmentation of nail beds, urticaria

Endocrine & metabolic: Hyperuricemia, infertility

Gastrointestinal: Stomatitis, esophagitis, nausea, vomiting, mucositis, diarrhea

Genitourinary: Discoloration of urine (red/orange), cystitis

Hematologic: Leukopenia (nadir: 10-14 days), thrombocytopenia, anemia

Hepatic: Transient elevation of liver function tests

Local: Tissue necrosis upon extravasation, erythematous streaking along the vein if administered too rapidly, phlebitis

Ocular: Lacrimation

Drug Interactions May potentiate the toxicity of cyclophosphamide, mercaptopurine; ritonavir and cyclosporine decrease doxorubicin metabolism; doxorubicin decreases carbamazepine, digoxin, and phenytoin levels

Stability Protect from light; store vials containing powder at room temperature, refrigerate vials containing liquid; reconstituted vials stable for 24 hours at room temperature and 48 hours if refrigerated. Discard unused portion of preservative free injection vial. Incompatible with hydrocortisone, fluorouracil, furosemide, sodium bicarbonate, aminophylline, heparin, cephalothin, dexamethasone; unstable in solutions with a pH <3 or >7. Color change from red to purple indicates decomposition of drug.

Mechanism of Action Inhibits DNA and RNA synthesis by intercalating between DNA base pairs and by steric obstruction; produces oxygen-free radicals which cause DNA denaturation; inhibits DNA topoisomerase I resulting in DNA strand breaks

Pharmacokinetics

Distribution: Into breast milk; does not penetrate into CSF; distributes into cells rapidly with high concentrations in lung, kidney, muscle, spleen, and liver

Protein binding: 75%

Metabolism: In both the liver and in plasma to both active and inactive metabolites

Half-life:

Primary: 30 minutes

Secondary: 3-3.5 hours for its metabolites

Terminal: 17-30 hours for doxorubicin and its metabolites

Elimination: Undergoes triphasic elimination; 40% to 60% eventually excreted in bile and feces; <5% excreted in urine, primarily as unchanged drug and metabolites

Clearance:

Infants <2 years: 813 mL/minute/m^2

Children >2 years: 1540 mL/minute/m^2

Usual Dosage Patient's ideal weight should be used to calculate body surface area. Lower dose regimens should be given to patients with decreased bone marrow reserve, prior radiation therapy, or marrow infiltration with malignant cells.

I.V. (refer to individual protocols):

Children: 35-75 mg/m^2 as a single dose, repeat every 21 days; or 20-30 mg/m^2 once weekly; or 60-90 mg/m^2 given as a continuous infusion over 96 hours every 3-4 weeks

Adults: 60-75 mg/m^2 as a single dose, repeat every 21 days; or 20-30 mg/m^2/day for 2-3 days, repeat in 4 weeks or 20 mg/m^2 once weekly

Dosing adjustment in hepatic impairment:

Bilirubin 1.2-3 mg/dL: Reduce dose by 50%

Bilirubin >3 mg/dL: Reduce dose by 75%

Administration Parenteral: I.V. use only; reconstitute IVP doses with D_5W or NS to ensure isotonicity of the final solution; administer slow IVP at a rate no faster than over 3-5 minutes or by I.V. infusion over 1-4 hours at a concentration not to exceed 2 mg/mL, or by I.V. continuous infusion

Monitoring Parameters CBC with differential, erythrocyte and platelet count; echocardiogram, liver function tests including AST, ALT, alkaline phosphatase, and bilirubin; observe I.V. injection site for infiltration and vein irritation

Patient Information Transient red-orange discoloration of urine can occur for up to 48 hours after a dose; avoid unnecessary exposure to sunlight; notify physician if fever, sore throat, bleeding, or bruising occurs; report any stinging sensation at the injection site during infusion

Nursing Implications Local erythematous streaking along the vein and/or facial flushing may indicate too rapid a rate of administration; drug is very irritating; avoid extravasation; if extravasation occurs, apply cold packs immediately for 30-60 (Continued)

Doxorubicin *(Continued)*

minutes, then alternate off/on every 15 minutes for 1 day; apply 1.5 mL of dimethyl-sulfoxide 99% (w/v) solution to the site every 6 hours for 14 days; allow to air-dry; do not cover. Take precautions to prevent contact with the patient's urine and other body fluids for at least 5 days after each treatment.

Additional Information Myelosuppressive effects:
WBC: Moderate
Platelets: Moderate
Onset (days): 7
Nadir (days): 10-14
Recovery (days): 21-28

Dosage Forms
Injection, as hydrochloride:
Aqueous, with NS: 2 mg/mL (5 mL, 10 mL, 25 mL)
Preservative free (Adriamycin PFS™): 2 mg/mL (5 mL, 10 mL, 25 mL, 100 mL)
Powder for injection, as hydrochloride, lyophilized: 10 mg, 20 mg, 50 mg
Rubex®: 10 mg, 50 mg, 100 mg
Powder for injection, as hydrochloride, lyophilized, rapid dissolution formula (Adriamycin RDF™): 10 mg, 20 mg, 50 mg, 150 mg

References
Berg SL, Grisell DL, DeLaney TF, et al, "Principles of Treatment of Pediatric Solid Tumors," *Pediatr Clin North Am*, 1991, 38(2):249-67.
Ishii E, Hara T, Ohkubo K, et al, "Treatment of Childhood Acute Lymphoblastic Leukemia With Intermediate Dose Cytosine Arabinoside and Adriamycin," *Med Pediatr Oncol*, 1986, 14(2):73-7.
Legha SS, Benjamin RS, Mackay B, et al, "Reduction of Doxorubicin Cardiotoxicity by Prolonged Continuous Intravenous Infusion," *Ann Intern Med*, 1982, 96(2):133-9.

♦ **Doxorubicin Hydrochloride** *see Doxorubicin on page 346*

♦ **Doxy-200®** *see Doxycycline on page 348*

♦ **Doxy-Caps®** *see Doxycycline on page 348*

♦ **Doxychel®** *see Doxycycline on page 348*

♦ **Doxycin (Canada)** *see Doxycycline on page 348*

Doxycycline *(doks i SYE kleen)*

Brand Names Apo®-Doxy (Canada); Apo®-Doxy Tabs (Canada); Bio-Tab®; Doryx®; Doxy-200®; Doxy-Caps®; Doxychel®; Doxycin (Canada); Doxy-Tabs®; Doxytec (Canada); Dynacin®; Monodox®; Novo-Doxylin® (Canada); Nu-Doxycycline® (Canada); Vibramycin®; Vibra-Tabs®

Available Salts Doxycycline Calcium; Doxycycline Hyclate

Therapeutic Category Antibiotic, Tetracycline Derivative

Generic Available Yes

Use
Children, Adolescents, Adults: Treatment of Rocky Mountain spotted fever caused by susceptible *Rickettsia*; treatment of ehrlichiosis
Older Children, Adolescents, Adults: Treatment of Lyme disease, *Mycoplasma* infection, or *Legionella*; management of malignant pleural effusions when intrapleural therapy is indicated
Adolescents and Adults: Treatment of nongonococcal pelvic inflammatory disease and urethritis due to *Chlamydia*; treatment for victims of sexual assault

Pregnancy Risk Factor D

Contraindications Hypersensitivity to doxycycline, tetracycline, or any component; children <8 years; severe hepatic dysfunction

Warnings Photosensitivity reaction may occur with this drug; avoid prolonged exposure to sunlight or tanning equipment. Do not administer to children <8 years of age due to associated retardation in skeletal development; use of tetracyclines during tooth development may cause permanent discoloration of the teeth and enamel hypoplasia; staining of teeth is dose-related so that duration of therapy should be minimized; doxycycline may be less likely to stain developing teeth than tetracycline since it binds less strongly to calcium; prolonged use may result in superinfection.

Adverse Reactions
Central nervous system: Increased intracranial pressure, bulging fontanels in infants
Dermatologic: Rash, photosensitivity, discoloration of nails
Gastrointestinal: Nausea, diarrhea, esophagitis and esophageal ulceration with the hyclate salt formulation; anorexia, pseudomembranous colitis, oral candidiasis
Hematologic: Neutropenia, eosinophilia
Hepatic: Hepatotoxicity
Local: Phlebitis, pain at the injection site

Neuromuscular & skeletal: Retardation of skeletal development in infants

Miscellaneous: May cause discoloration of teeth in children <8 years of age

Drug Interactions Antacids containing aluminum, calcium, or magnesium; zinc, kaolin, pectin, iron, and bismuth subsalicylate may decrease doxycycline bioavailability; rifampin, barbiturates, phenytoin, and carbamazepine decrease doxycycline's half-life; doxycycline enhances the hypoprothrombinemic effect of warfarin

Food Interactions Administration with iron, calcium, milk or dairy products may decrease doxycycline absorption; may decrease absorption of calcium, iron, magnesium, zinc and amino acids

Stability Reconstituted oral doxycycline suspension is stable for 2 weeks at room temperature; I.V. doxycycline solutions must be protected from direct sunlight

Mechanism of Action Inhibits protein synthesis by binding to the 30S and possibly the 50S ribosomal subunit(s) of susceptible bacteria preventing additions of amino acids to the growing peptide chain; may also cause alterations in the cytoplasmic membrane

Pharmacokinetics

Absorption: Almost completely from the GI tract; absorption can be reduced by food or milk by 20%

Distribution: Widely distributed into body tissues and fluids including synovial and pleural fluid, bile, bronchial secretions; poor penetration into the CSF; appears in breast milk

Protein binding: 80% to 85%

Metabolism: Not metabolized in the liver; partially inactivated in the GI tract by chelate formation

Bioavailability: 90% to 100%

Half-life: 12-15 hours (usually increases to 22-24 hours with multiple dosing)

Time to peak serum concentration: Oral: Within 1.5-4 hours

Elimination: In the urine (23%) and feces (30%)

Not dialyzable (0% to 5%)

Usual Dosage

Children ≥8 years: Oral, I.V.: 2-4 mg/kg/day divided every 12-24 hours, not to exceed 200 mg/day

Lyme disease: Oral: 100 mg/dose twice daily for 14-21 days

Chlamydial infections: Oral: 100 mg/dose twice daily for 7-10 days

Adolescents and Adults: Oral, I.V.: 100-200 mg/day in 1-2 divided doses

Lyme disease: Oral: 100 mg/dose twice daily for 14-21 days

Pelvic inflammatory disease:

Hospitalized regimen: Oral, I.V.: 100 mg every 12 hours for 14 days administered with cefoxitin or cefotetan

Outpatient regimen: Oral: 100 mg every 12 hours for 14 days plus single dose ceftriaxone

Sclerosing agent for pleural effusion: 500 mg in 25-30 mL of NS instilled into the pleural space to control pleural effusions associated with metastatic tumors; or for recurrent malignant pleural effusions: 500 mg in 250 mL NS

Administration

Oral: Administer capsules or tablets with adequate amounts of fluid; avoid antacids, infant formula, milk, dairy products, and iron for 1 hour before or 2 hours after administration of doxycycline; may be administered with food to decrease GI upset; shake suspension well before use

Parenteral: For I.V. use only; administer by slow I.V. intermittent infusion over a minimum of 1-2 hours at a concentration not to exceed 1 mg/mL (may be infused over 1-4 hours); concentrations <0.1 mg/mL are not recommended

Sclerosing agent:

To control pleural effusions associated with metastatic tumors: Instill into the pleural space through a thoracostomy tube following drainage of the accumulated pleural fluid; clamp the tube then remove the fluid

For recurrent malignant pleural effusions: Administer via chest tube lavage, clamp tube for 24 hours then drain

Monitoring Parameters Periodic monitoring of renal, hematologic, and hepatic function tests; observe for changes in bowel frequency

Test Interactions False-negative urine glucose using Clinistix®, Tes-Tape®

Patient Information Avoid unnecessary exposure to sunlight; may discolor teeth if <8 years of age; may discolor fingernails

Nursing Implications Check for signs of phlebitis; I.V. doxycycline should not be given I.M. or S.C.; avoid extravasation

Dosage Forms

Capsule, as hyclate: 50 mg, 100 mg

Doxychel®, Monodox®, Vibramycin®: 50 mg

(Continued)

Doxycycline *(Continued)*

Doxy®, Doxychel®, Monodox®, Vibramycin®: 100 mg
Capsule, coated pellets, as hyclate (Doryx®): 100 mg
Powder for injection, as hyclate: 100 mg, 200 mg
Doxy®, Doxychel®, Vibramycin® IV: 100 mg, 200 mg
Powder for oral suspension, as monohydrate (raspberry flavor) (Vibramycin®): 25 mg/5 mL (60 mL)
Syrup, as calcium (raspberry-apple flavor) (Vibramycin®): 50 mg/5 mL (30 mL, 473 mL)
Tablet, as hyclate
Doxychel®: 50 mg
Bio-Tab®, Doxychel®, Vibra-Tabs®: 100 mg

References

Centers for Disease Control and Prevention, "1998 Guidelines for Treatment of Sexually Transmitted Diseases, *MMWR Morb Mortal Wkly Rep*, 1998, 47(RR-1):1-111.

- ◆ **Doxycycline Calcium** *see Doxycycline on page 348*
- ◆ **Doxycycline Hyclate** *see Doxycycline on page 348*
- ◆ **Doxy-Tabs®** *see Doxycycline on page 348*
- ◆ **Doxytec (Canada)** *see Doxycycline on page 348*
- ◆ **DPA** *see Valproic Acid and Derivatives on page 966*
- ◆ **DPE** *see Dipivefrin on page 330*
- ◆ **DPE™ (Canada)** *see Dipivefrin on page 330*
- ◆ **D-Penicillamine** *see Penicillamine on page 738*
- ◆ **DPH** *see Phenytoin on page 762*
- ◆ **DPPC** *see Colfosceril on page 252*
- ◆ **Dramamine® II [OTC]** *see Meclizine on page 597*
- ◆ **Dramamine® Oral [OTC]** *see Dimenhydrinate on page 325*
- ◆ **Dramilin® Injection** *see Dimenhydrinate on page 325*
- ◆ **Dramoject® Injection** *see Dimenhydrinate on page 325*
- ◆ **Drisdol®** *see Ergocalciferol on page 377*
- ◆ **Dristan® Long Lasting Nasal Solution [OTC]** *see Oxymetazoline on page 718*
- ◆ **Dristan® Saline Spray [OTC]** *see Sodium Chloride on page 871*
- ◆ **Drixoral® Cough Liquid Caps [OTC]** *see Dextromethorphan on page 304*
- ◆ **Drixoral® Nasal (Canada)** *see Oxymetazoline on page 718*
- ◆ **Drixoral® Non-Drowsy [OTC]** *see Pseudoephedrine on page 822*

Dronabinol *(droe NAB i nol)*

Brand Names Marinol®
Synonyms Tetrahydrocannabinol; THC
Therapeutic Category Antiemetic
Generic Available Yes
Use Treatment of nausea and vomiting secondary to cancer chemotherapy in patients who have not responded to conventional antiemetics; treatment of anorexia associated with weight loss in AIDS patients
Restrictions C-III
Pregnancy Risk Factor B
Contraindications Should not be used in patients with a history of schizophrenia; hypersensitivity to dronabinol, any component, marijuana, or sesame oil
Warnings Dronabinol has a high potential for abuse; limit antiemetic therapy availability to current cycle of chemotherapy
Precautions Use with caution in patients with heart disease, hepatic disease, or seizure disorders; reduce dosage in patients with severe hepatic impairment
Adverse Reactions
Cardiovascular: Orthostatic hypotension, tachycardia, palpitations, vasodilation, hypotension
Central nervous system: Drowsiness, dizziness, vertigo, difficulty in concentrating, mood change, euphoria, detachment, depression, anxiety, paranoia, hallucinations, nervousness, ataxia, headache, memory lapse
Gastrointestinal: Xerostomia, diarrhea
Hepatic: Increased liver enzymes
Neuromuscular & skeletal: Myalgia, tremor, paresthesia, weakness
Ocular: Vision difficulties
Respiratory: Sinusitis, cough, rhinitis
Miscellaneous: Diaphoresis

Drug Interactions Additive tachycardia, hypertension with amphetamines, cocaine, sympathomimetics, tricyclic antidepressants; additive CNS effects with sedatives, antihistamines, hypnotics, psychomimetics, tricyclic antidepressants, alcohol; hypomanic state with disulfiram, fluoxetine; increases theophylline metabolism; decreases barbiturate clearance

Stability Store in a cool place

Mechanism of Action Dronabinol is the principal psychoactive substance found in *Cannabis sativa* (marijuana); its mechanism of action as an antiemetic is not well defined, it probably inhibits the vomiting center in the medulla oblongata

Pharmacodynamics
Onset of action: 30 minutes to 1 hour
Peak effect: 2-4 hours
Duration: 4-6 hours

Pharmacokinetics
Absorption: Oral: 90% to 95%; first-pass metabolism results in low systemic bioavailability
Distribution: V_d: ~10L/kg
Protein binding: 97% to 99%
Metabolism: Extensive first-pass; metabolized in the liver to several metabolites some of which are active
Bioavailability: 10% to 20%
Half-life:
Biphasic: Alpha: 4 hours
Terminal: 25-36 hours
Time to peak serum concentration: Within 2-3 hours
Elimination: Biliary excretion is the major route of elimination

Usual Dosage Oral:
Antiemetic: Children and Adults: 5 mg/m² 1-3 hours before chemotherapy, then give 5 mg/m²/dose every 2-4 hours after chemotherapy for a total of 4-6 doses/day; dose may be increased up to a maximum of 15 mg/m² per dose if needed (dosage may be increased in 2.5 mg/m² increments)
Appetite stimulant: Adults: 2.5 mg twice daily before lunch and dinner; if intolerant, a dosage of 2.5 mg once daily at night may be tried; maximum dosage (escalating): 5 mg 4 times/day (20 mg/day)

Administration May be administered without regard to meals; take before meals if used to stimulate appetite

Monitoring Parameters Heart rate, blood pressure

Patient Information Causes drowsiness and may impair ability to perform hazardous tasks requiring mental alertness or physical coordination

Dosage Forms Capsule, gelatin: 2.5 mg, 5 mg, 10 mg

References
Lane M, Smith FE, Sullivan RA, et al, "Dronabinol and Prochlorperazine Alone and in Combination as Antiemetic Agents for Cancer Chemotherapy," *Am J Clin Oncol*, 1990, 13(6):480-4.

Droperidol (droe PER i dole)

Related Information
Compatibility of Medications Mixed in a Syringe on page 1208

Brand Names Inapsine®

Therapeutic Category Antiemetic; Antipsychotic Agent

Generic Available Yes

Use Tranquilizer and antiemetic in surgical and diagnostic procedures; antiemetic for cancer chemotherapy; preoperative medication

Pregnancy Risk Factor C

Contraindications Hypersensitivity to droperidol or any component

Precautions Use with caution in patients with impaired hepatic or renal function

Adverse Reactions
Cardiovascular: Hypotension (especially in hypovolemic patients), tachycardia
Central nervous system: Extrapyramidal reactions such as dystonic reactions, akathisia, and oculogyric crisis; anxiety, hyperactivity, drowsiness, dizziness, hallucinations, chills
Respiratory: Laryngospasm, bronchospasm

Drug Interactions Use with other CNS depressants may have additive effects (CNS, respiratory depression, etc); droperidol plus fentanyl or other analgesics may increase blood pressure; conduction anesthesia may increase hypotension; droperidol plus epinephrine may decrease blood pressure due to alpha-adrenergic blockade effects of droperidol; droperidol plus atropine may cause tachycardia

Stability Physically compatible and chemically stable with D_5W, LR, NS at a concentration of 20 mg/L
(Continued)

Droperidol *(Continued)*

Mechanism of Action Alters the action of dopamine in the CNS, at subcortical levels, to produce sedation and a dissociative state; also possesses alpha-adrenergic blockade effects

Pharmacodynamics
Onset of action: 3-10 minutes
Peak effects: Within 30 minutes
Duration: 2-4 hours (up to 12 hours)

Pharmacokinetics
Metabolism: In the liver
Half-life, adults: 2.3 hours
Elimination: In urine (75%) and feces (22%)

Usual Dosage Titrate carefully to desired effect
Children 2-12 years:
Premedication: I.M.: 0.088-0.165 mg/kg
Adjunct to general anesthesia: I.V. induction: 0.088-0.165 mg/kg
Nausea and vomiting: I.M., I.V.: 0.05-0.06 mg/kg/dose every 4-6 hours as needed
Postop antiemetic: I.V.: 0.01-0.03 mg/kg/dose every 6-8 hours as needed
Adults:
Premedication: I.M.: 2.5-10 mg 30-60 minutes preoperatively
Adjunct to general anesthesia: I.V. induction: 0.22-0.275 mg/kg; maintenance: 1.25-2.5 mg/dose
Alone in diagnostic procedures: I.M.: Initial: 2.5-10 mg 30-60 minutes before, then 1.25-2.5 mg if needed
Nausea and vomiting: I.M., I.V.: 2.5-5 mg/dose every 3-4 hours as needed

Administration Parenteral: Administer by slow I.V. injection over 2-5 minutes

Monitoring Parameters Blood pressure, heart rate, respiratory rate

Additional Information Does not possess analgesic effects; has little or no amnesic properties

Dosage Forms Injection: 2.5 mg/mL (1 mL, 2 mL, 5 mL, 10 mL)

References
Yaster M, Sola JE, Pegoli W Jr, et al, "The Night After Surgery: Postoperative Management of the Pediatric Outpatient - Surgical and Anesthetic Aspects," *Pediatr Clin North Am*, 1994, 41(1):199-220.

Droperidol and Fentanyl (droe PER i dole & FEN ta nil)

Related Information
Overdose and Toxicology *on page 1191*

Brand Names Innovar®

Available Salts Droperidol and Fentanyl Citrate

Synonyms Fentanyl and Droperidol

Therapeutic Category Analgesic, Narcotic

Generic Available Yes

Use To produce and maintain analgesia and sedation during diagnostic or surgical procedures (neuroleptanalgesia and neuroleptanesthesia); adjunct to general anesthesia

Restrictions C-II

Pregnancy Risk Factor C

Contraindications Hypersensitivity to droperidol, any component, or fentanyl; patients who have taken MAO inhibitors within 14 days

Warnings Rapid I.V. injection can cause muscle rigidity, particularly involving the muscles of respiration

Precautions Use with caution in patients with impaired hepatic, renal, or respiratory function and those with pre-existing cardiac bradyarrhythmias

Adverse Reactions
Cardiovascular: Hypotension, hypertension, bradycardia
Central nervous system: Postoperative drowsiness, dysphoria, disorientation, restlessness, delirium, extrapyramidal symptoms, hypothermia
Endocrine & metabolic: Hyperglycemia
Gastrointestinal: Nausea, vomiting
Neuromuscular & skeletal: Muscular rigidity
Ocular: Miosis
Respiratory: Respiratory depression, apnea, laryngospasm, bronchospasm
Miscellaneous: Shivering

Drug Interactions Fentanyl is a cytochrome P-450 isoenzyme CYP3A3/4 substrate

CNS depressant drugs may have additive effects; MAO inhibitors may cause hypertensive crisis

Mechanism of Action See individual monographs for Droperidol *on page 351* and Fentanyl *on page 406*

Usual Dosage

Children:

Premedication: I.M.: 0.03 mL/kg (maximum dose: 2 mL) 30-60 minutes prior to procedure

Adjunct to general anesthesia: I.V.: Total dose: 0.05 mL/kg as slow infusion (1 mL/1-2 minutes) until sleep occurs

Adults:

Premedication: I.M.: 0.5-2 mL 30-60 minutes prior to surgery

Adjunct to general anesthesia: I.V.: 0.09-0.11 mL/kg as slow infusion (1 mL/1-2 minutes) until sleep occurs

Administration Parenteral: I.V.: Infuse slowly at a rate of 1 mL per 1-2 minutes

Monitoring Parameters Vital signs, oxygen saturation, blood pressure

Nursing Implications An opioid antagonist, resuscitative and intubation equipment, and oxygen should be available

Dosage Forms Injection: Droperidol 2.5 mg and fentanyl 50 mcg per mL (2 mL, 5 mL)

d-Xylose (dee ZYE lose)

Brand Names Xylo-Pfan® [OTC]

Synonyms Wood Sugar; Xylose

Therapeutic Category Diagnostic Agent, Intestinal Absorption

Generic Available No

Use Diagnostic agent used in the determination of intestinal disorders due to disease or injury, which result in carbohydrate malabsorption, such as celiac disease, malabsorptive enteropathy, giardiasis, and food- or protein-induced enterocolitis

Pregnancy Risk Factor Unknown

Contraindications Hypersensitivity to d-xylose or any component

Warnings False-positive results may occur in patients with renal impairment, dehydration, edema, massive ascites, iron deficiency, inadequate circulating blood volume, anemia, pernicious anemia, severe diarrhea, vomiting, gastric stasis, thyroid dysfunction, and massive overgrowth of intestinal bacteria due to abnormally low excretion of d-xylose

Adverse Reactions Gastrointestinal: Nausea, intestinal bloating, vomiting, cramping, abdominal discomfort, diarrhea

Drug Interactions Indomethacin and neomycin inhibit the intestinal absorption of d-xylose; aspirin inhibits the urinary excretion of d-xylose

Stability Store powder at room temperature in an airtight container

Mechanism of Action D-xylose is a 5 carbon monosaccharide which is absorbed from the small intestine; its mechanism of absorption is not completely understood, however, a small portion is absorbed via an active transport system as seen with glucose; it does not depend upon bile or pancreatic juices for absorption; measurement of d-xylose blood or urinary concentrations evaluates the extent of carbohydrate absorption

Pharmacokinetics

Absorption: Oral: 35% in the small intestine; absorption is dose-dependent (eg, 5 g doses are absorbed more readily than 25 g doses)

Distribution: 0.21-0.32 L/kg

Metabolism: Via Krebs cycle and phosphoglucuronic pathways to carbon dioxide, water, and unidentified metabolites

Elimination: 25% of 25 g dose or 35% of 5 g dose is excreted unchanged in urine within 5 hours; decreased rate of elimination and renal clearance may be observed in geriatric patients

Usual Dosage Oral: Give after fasting at least 4 hours in infants and overnight in children and adults (see Administration):

Infants and Children: 500 mg/kg or 14.5 g/m^2 or 5 g as a single dose; maximum dose: 25 g

Adults: 5 g or 25 g as a single dose

Administration Oral:

Infants and Children: Dissolve powder in sufficient water to result in 5% to 10% solution (50-100 mg/mL; eg, 25 g in 250-500 mL water)

Adults: Dissolve 5 g or 25 g in 200-300 mL water, then after the dose is taken, administer 200-400 mL water

Monitoring Parameters Blood and urinary d-xylose concentrations

Reference Range The following peak blood d-xylose concentration and urinary excretion values indicate **NORMAL** absorption of d-xylose: See tables.

Blood d-Xylose Concentration (mg/dL)

Time After Dose (minutes)	Infants/Children	Adults (after 5 g or 25 g dose)
30	≥15	–
60	≥20	≥30
120	≥20	≥30

ALTERNATIVE METHOD: If using 5 g dosage instead of dosage per weight: Measure blood d-xylose concentration (mg/dL) prior to administration (baseline) and 60 minutes after administration. Calculate corrected d-xylose blood value as follows:

Corrected d-xylose blood value $= \dfrac{\text{(value at 60 min - baseline value)} \times \text{actual surface area}}{1.73}$

NORMAL CORRECTED BLOOD VALUE = 9.8-20 mg/dL

Urinary Excretion

Mean 5-hour excretion expressed as a percentage of ingested d-xylose*		
Infants/Children		Adults (after 25 g dose)
<6 mo	11% to 30%	
6-12 mo	20% to 32%	
1-3 y	20% to 42%	4.5 g total urinary excretion
3-10 y	25% to 45%	
>10 y	25% to 50%	
or % excretion > (0.2 x age/months) + 12		

*The lower the d-xylose blood or urine concentration findings, the greater the chance of intestinal disease or abnormal condition.

Patient Information Do not eat for at least 5 hours after the test; fluids may be consumed after the test; contact your physician if abdominal pain or discomfort is severe or continues for >5 hours

Dosage Forms Powder for oral solution: 25 g

References
Buts JP, Morin CL, Roy CC, et al, "One-Hour Blood Xylose Test: A Reliable Index of Small Bowel Function," *J Pediatr*, 1978, 92(5):729-33.

♦ **Dycill®** *see* Dicloxacillin *on page 313*
♦ **Dyclone®** *see* Dyclonine *on page 355*

Dyclonine (DYE kloe neen)

Brand Names Dyclone®; Sucrets® [OTC]

Available Salts Dyclonine Hydrochloride

Therapeutic Category Local Anesthetic, Oral

Generic Available No

Use As a local anesthetic prior to laryngoscopy, bronchoscopy, or endotracheal intubation; used topically for temporary relief of pain associated with oral mucosa, skin, episiotomy, or anogenital lesions; the 0.5% topical solution may be used to block the gag reflex, and to relieve the pain of oral ulcers or stomatitis; the lozenge is used for temporary relief of sore throat pain and gum irritation

Pregnancy Risk Factor C

Contraindications Contraindicated in patients allergic to chlorobutanol (preservative used in dyclonine), dyclonine, or any component

Warnings Resuscitative equipment, oxygen and resuscitative drugs should be immediately available when dyclonine topical solution is administered to mucous membranes; may impair swallowing and enhance the danger of aspiration

Precautions Use with caution in patients with sepsis or traumatized mucosa in the area of application to avoid rapid systemic absorption; use with caution in patients with shock or heart block

Adverse Reactions Excessive dosage and rapid absorption may result in adverse CNS and cardiovascular effects

Cardiovascular: Hypotension, bradycardia, cardiac arrest, edema
Central nervous system: Excitation, drowsiness, nervousness, dizziness, seizures
Dermatologic: Rash, urticaria
Local: Slight irritation and stinging may occur when applied
Ocular: Blurred vision
Respiratory: Respiratory arrest
Miscellaneous: Allergic reactions

Stability Store in tight, light-resistant container; avoid freezing

Mechanism of Action Blocks impulses at peripheral nerve endings in skin and mucous membranes by altering cell membrane permeability to ionic transfer

Pharmacodynamics
Onset of local anesthesia: 2-10 minutes
Duration: 30-60 minutes

Usual Dosage
Children and Adults:
Topical solution: Mouth sores: 5-10 mL of 0.5% or 1% to oral mucosa (swab or swish and then spit) 3-4 times/day as needed; maximum single dose: 200 mg (40 mL of 0.5% solution or 20 mL of 1% solution); solution may be diluted 1:1 with water

(Continued)

Dyclonine *(Continued)*

Bronchoscopy: Use 2 mL of the 1% solution or 4 mL of the 0.5% solution sprayed onto the larynx and trachea every 5 minutes for 2-3 applications until the reflex has been abolished

Children >3 years: Topical: Slowly dissolve 1 lozenge (1.2 mg) in mouth every 2 hours, if necessary

Children >12 years and Adults: Topical: Slowly dissolve 1 lozenge (3 mg) in mouth every 2 hours, if necessary

Administration Topical: Apply to mucous membranes of the mouth or throat area: food should not be ingested for 60 minutes following application in the mouth or throat area

Patient Information Do not chew lozenge; numbness of the tongue and buccal mucosa may result in increased risk of biting trauma; may impair swallowing

Nursing Implications Use the lowest dose needed to provide effective anesthesia; not for injection; do not apply nasally or to the eye

Dosage Forms

Lozenges, as hydrochloride: 1.2 mg, 3 mg

Solution, topical, as hydrochloride: 0.5% (30 mL); 1% (30 mL)

References

Carnel SB, Blakeslee DB, Oswald SG, et al, "Treatment of Radiation- and Chemotherapy-Induced Stomatitis," *Otolaryngol Head Neck Surg*, 1990, 102(4):326-30.

♦ **Dyclonine Hydrochloride** *see* Dyclonine *on page 355*

♦ **Dymenate® Injection** *see* Dimenhydrinate *on page 325*

♦ **Dynacin®** *see* Doxycycline *on page 348*

♦ **Dyna-Hex® [OTC]** *see* Chlorhexidine Gluconate *on page 209*

♦ **Dynapen®** *see* Dicloxacillin *on page 313*

♦ **Dyrenium®** *see* Triamterene *on page 949*

♦ **Easprin®** *see* Aspirin *on page 99*

♦ **EC-Naprosyn®** *see* Naproxen *on page 672*

♦ **E-Complex-600® [OTC]** *see* Vitamin E *on page 982*

Econazole *(e KONE a zole)*

Brand Names Ecostatin® (Canada); Spectazole™

Available Salts Econazole Nitrate

Therapeutic Category Antifungal Agent, Topical

Generic Available No

Use Topical treatment of tinea pedis, tinea cruris, tinea corporis, tinea versicolor, and cutaneous candidiasis

Pregnancy Risk Factor C

Contraindications Hypersensitivity to econazole or any component

Warnings Not for ophthalmic or intravaginal use

Precautions Discontinue the drug if sensitivity or chemical irritation occurs; cross-sensitization may occur with other imidazole derivatives (ie, clotrimazole, miconazole)

Adverse Reactions

Dermatologic: Pruritus, erythema

Local: Burning, stinging

Mechanism of Action Alters fungal cell wall membrane permeability; may interfere with RNA and protein synthesis, and lipid metabolism

Pharmacokinetics

Absorption: Following topical administration, <10% is percutaneously absorbed

Metabolism: In the liver to >20 metabolites

Elimination: <1% of an applied dose recovered in urine or feces

Usual Dosage Children and Adults: Topical:

Tinea cruris, corporis, pedis, and tinea versicolor: Apply once daily

Cutaneous candidiasis: Apply twice daily

Administration Topical: Apply a sufficient amount of cream to cover affected areas; do not apply to the eye or intravaginally

Patient Information For external use only

Additional Information Candidal infections and tinea cruris, versicolor, and corporis should be treated for 2 weeks and tinea pedis for 1 month; occasionally, longer treatment periods may be required

Dosage Forms Cream, as nitrate: 1% (15 g, 30 g, 85 g)

♦ **Econazole Nitrate** *see* Econazole *on page 356*

♦ **Econopred® Ophthalmic** *see* Prednisolone *on page 791*

- ◆ **Econopred® Plus Ophthalmic** *see* Prednisolone *on page 791*
- ◆ **Ecostatin® (Canada)** *see* Econazole *on page 356*
- ◆ **Ecotrin® [OTC]** *see* Aspirin *on page 99*
- ◆ **Ectosone (Canada)** *see* Betamethasone *on page 130*
- ◆ **Edathamil Disodium** *see* Edetate Disodium *on page 358*
- ◆ **Edecrin® Oral** *see* Ethacrynic Acid *on page 390*
- ◆ **Edecrin® Sodium Injection** *see* Ethacrynic Acid *on page 390*

Edetate Calcium Disodium (ED e tate KAL see um dye SOW dee um)

Brand Names Calcium Disodium Versenate®

Synonyms Calcium Disodium Edathamil; Calcium Disodium Edetate; Calcium Edetate; Calcium EDTA

Therapeutic Category Antidote, Lead Toxicity; Chelating Agent, Parenteral

Generic Available No

Use Treatment of acute and chronic lead poisoning; also used as an aid in the diagnosis of lead poisoning

Pregnancy Risk Factor B

Contraindications Severe renal disease, anuria

Warnings Do not exceed recommended daily dose; avoid rapid I.V. infusion in the management of lead encephalopathy, intracranial pressure may be increased to lethal levels; intramuscular administration is the preferred route in these patients; if anuria, increasing proteinuria, or hematuria occurs during therapy, discontinue calcium EDTA

Precautions Renal tubular necrosis and fatal nephrosis may occur, especially with high doses; establish urine flow prior to administration

Adverse Reactions
Cardiovascular: Hypotension, arrhythmias, EKG changes
Central nervous system: Fever, headache, chills
Dermatologic: Skin lesions, cheilosis
Endocrine & metabolic: Hypercalcemia, zinc deficiency
Gastrointestinal: GI upset, anorexia, nausea, vomiting
Hematologic: Transient marrow suppression, anemia
Hepatic: Mild increase in liver function tests
Local: Pain at injection site following I.M. injection, thrombophlebitis following I.V. infusion (when concentration >5 mg/mL)
Neuromuscular & skeletal: Arthralgia, tremor, numbness, paresthesia
Ocular: Lacrimation
Renal: Renal tubular necrosis, proteinuria, microscopic hematuria
Respiratory: Sneezing, nasal congestion

Drug Interactions Do not use simultaneously with zinc insulin preparations

Stability Dilute with NS or D_5W; physically incompatible with $D_{10}W$, LR; do not mix in the same syringe with dimercaprol

Mechanism of Action Calcium is displaced by divalent and trivalent heavy metals, forming a nonionizing soluble complex that is excreted in the urine

Pharmacodynamics
Onset of chelation with I.V. administration: 1 hour
Peak excretion of chelated lead with I.V. administration: 24-48 hours

Pharmacokinetics
Absorption: I.M., S.C.: Well absorbed
Distribution: Into extracellular fluid; minimal CSF penetration
Half-life, plasma:
 I.M.: 1.5 hours
 I.V.: 20 minutes
Elimination: Rapid in urine as metal chelates or unchanged drug

Usual Dosage Several regimens have been recommended:
Diagnosis of lead poisoning: Mobilization test (not recommended by AAP guidelines): I.M., I.V.:
 Children: 500 mg/m²/dose, (maximum dose: 1 g) as a single dose or divided into 2 doses
 Adults: 500 mg/m²/dose
 Note: Urine is collected for 24 hours after first EDTA dose and analyzed for lead content; if the ratio of mcg of lead in urine to mg calcium EDTA given is >1, then test is considered positive; for convenience, an 8-hour urine collection may be done after a single 50 mg/kg I.M. (maximum dose: 1 g) or 500 mg/m² I.V. dose; a positive test occurs if the ratio of lead excretion to mg calcium EDTA >0.5-0.6.

(Continued)

357

Edetate Calcium Disodium *(Continued)*

Treatment of lead poisoning: Children and Adults (each regimen is specific for route):

Symptoms of lead encephalopathy and/or blood lead level >70 mcg/dL: Treat 5 days; give in conjunction with dimercaprol; wait a minimum of 2 days with no treatment before considering a repeat course:

I.M.: 250 mg/m²/dose every 4 hours

I.V.: 50 mg/kg/day as 24-hour continuous I.V. infusion **or** 1-1.5 g/m² I.V. as either an 8- to 24-hour infusion or divided into 2 doses every 12 hours

Symptomatic lead poisoning **without** encephalopathy **or** asymptomatic with blood lead level >70 mcg/dL: Treat 3-5 days; treatment with dimercaprol is recommended until the blood lead level concentration <50 mcg/dL:

I.M.: 167 mg/m² every 4 hours

I.V.: 1 g/m² as an 8- to 24-hour infusion or divided every 12 hours

Asymptomatic **children** with blood lead level 45-69 mcg/dL: I.V.: 25 mg/kg/day for 5 days as an 8- to 24-hour infusion or divided into 2 doses every 12 hours

Depending upon the blood lead level, additional courses may be necessary; repeat at least 2-4 days and preferably 2-4 weeks apart

Adults with lead nephropathy: An alternative dosing regimen reflecting the reduction in renal clearance is based upon the serum creatinine (see table):

Alternative Dosing Regimen for Adults With Lead Nephropathy

Serum Creatinine (mg/dL)	Ca EDTA dosage
≤2	1 g/m²/day for 5 days
>2-3	500 mg/m²/day for 5 days
>3-4	500 mg/m²/dose every 48 hours for 3 doses
>4	500 mg/m²/week

Repeat these regimens monthly until lead excretion is reduced toward normal.

Administration Parenteral:

Intermittent I.V. infusion: Administer the dose I.V. over at least 1 hour in asymptomatic patients, 2 hours in symptomatic patients

Single daily I.V. continuous infusion: Dilute to 2-4 mg/mL in D_5W or NS and infuse over at least 8 hours, usually over 12-24 hours

I.M. injection: To minimize pain at the injection site, 1.67 mL of 2% procaine may be added to 5 mL calcium EDTA, resulting in 150 mg/mL concentration with 0.5% procaine (stable 3 months; see Nahata, 1997)

Monitoring Parameters BUN, serum creatinine, urinalysis, fluid balance, EKG, blood and urine lead concentrations

Test Interactions If calcium EDTA is given as a continuous I.V. infusion, stop the infusion for at least 1 hour before blood is drawn for lead concentration to avoid a falsely elevated value

Dosage Forms Injection: 200 mg/mL (5 mL)

References
American Academy of Pediatrics Committee on Drugs, "Treatment Guidelines for Lead Exposure in Children," *Pediatrics*, 1995, 96(1 Pt 1):155-60.

Nahata MC and Hipple TF, *Pediatric Drug Formulations*, 3rd ed, Cincinnati, OH: Harvey Whitney Books Co, 1997.

Edetate Disodium *(ED e tate dye SOW dee um)*

Brand Names Chealamide®; Disotate®; Endrate®

Synonyms Edathamil Disodium; EDTA; Sodium Edetate

Therapeutic Category Antidote, Hypercalcemia; Chelating Agent, Parenteral

Generic Available Yes

Use Emergency treatment of hypercalcemia; control digitalis-induced cardiac dysrhythmias (ventricular arrhythmias)

Pregnancy Risk Factor C

Contraindications Severe renal failure or anuria, hypocalcemia, patients with active tuberculosis or healed calcified tubercular lesions

Warnings Use of this drug is recommended only when the severity of the clinical condition justifies the aggressive measures associated with this type of therapy. Use with caution in patients with intracranial lesions, seizure disorders, coronary or peripheral vascular disease; cardiac function should be evaluated prior to therapy

Precautions Sudden, precipitous decreases of serum calcium may occur, a source of I.V. calcium replacement should be readily available; blood sugar and insulin requirements may be lower when used in insulin-dependent diabetics

Adverse Reactions
Cardiovascular: Arrhythmias, hypotension
Central nervous system: Seizures, headache, chills, fever
Dermatologic: Skin eruptions
Endocrine/metabolic: Hypomagnesemia, hypokalemia, hypocalcemia, hyperuricemia
Gastrointestinal: Vomiting, diarrhea, abdominal cramps
Genitourinary: Urinary urgency, dysuria
Hematologic: Anemia
Local: Thrombophlebitis, pain at injection site
Neuromuscular & skeletal: Back pain, muscle cramps, paresthesia, tetany
Renal: Nephrotoxicity, acute tubular necrosis, polyuria, oliguria, glucosuria
Respiratory: Respiratory arrest

Drug Interactions May reduce insulin requirements in diabetic patients treated with insulin

Stability Physically compatible with dextrose and saline I.V. solutions

Mechanism of Action Chelates with divalent or trivalent metals to form a soluble complex that is then eliminated in urine

Pharmacokinetics
Metabolism: Not metabolized
Half-life: 20-60 minutes
Elimination: Following chelation, 95% excreted in urine as chelates within 24-48 hours

Usual Dosage I.V.:
Hypercalcemia:
Children: 40-70 mg/kg/day slow infusion over 3-4 hours or more to a maximum of 3 g/24 hours; administer for 5 days and allow 5 days between courses of therapy **or** 50 mg/kg **or** 1.5 g/m^2 as a single dose
Adults: 50 mg/kg/day over 3 or more hours to a maximum of 3 g/24 hours; a suggested regimen of 5 days followed by 2 days without drug and repeated courses up to 15 total doses
Digitalis-induced arrhythmias: Children and Adults: 15 mg/kg/hour (maximum dose: 60 mg/kg/day) as continuous infusion

Administration Parenteral: I.V.: Must be diluted before I.V. use in D$_5$W or NS to a maximum concentration of 30 mg/mL (3%) and infused over at least 3 hours; avoid extravasation; not for I.M. use

Monitoring Parameters Serum and urine electrolytes (including calcium and magnesium), blood pressure (during infusion), renal function (before and during therapy), liver function, EKG

Test Interactions Colorimetric, oxalate, or other precipitation methods for measuring serum calcium

Nursing Implications Patient should remain supine for a short period after infusion

Additional Information Sodium content of 1 g: 5.4 mEq

Dosage Forms Injection: 150 mg/mL (20 mL)

♦ **Edex® Injection** see Alprostadil on page 51

Edrophonium (ed roe FOE nee um)
Related Information
Overdose and Toxicology on page 1191
Brand Names Enlon®; Reversol®; Tensilon®
Available Salts Edrophonium Chloride
Therapeutic Category Antidote, Neuromuscular Blocking Agent; Cholinergic Agent; Diagnostic Agent, Myasthenia Gravis
Generic Available No
Use Diagnosis of myasthenia gravis; differentiation of cholinergic crises from myasthenia crises; reversal of nondepolarizing neuromuscular blockers; treatment of paroxysmal atrial tachycardia
Pregnancy Risk Factor C
Contraindications Hypersensitivity to edrophonium or any component (injection contains sodium sulfite and phenol); GI or GU mechanical obstruction
Warnings Overdosage can cause cholinergic crisis which may be fatal; I.V. atropine should be readily available for treatment of cholinergic reactions; contains sodium sulfite; avoid use in sensitive individuals
(Continued)

Edrophonium *(Continued)*

Precautions Use with caution in asthmatic patients and those receiving a cardiac glycoside

Adverse Reactions

Cardiovascular: Arrhythmias (especially bradycardia), hypotension, A-V block

Central nervous system: Seizures, drowsiness, headache, dysphoria

Gastrointestinal: Nausea, vomiting, diarrhea, excessive salivation, stomach cramps

Genitourinary: Urinary frequency

Local: Thrombophlebitis

Neuromuscular & skeletal: Weakness, muscle cramps, muscle spasms

Ocular: Diplopia, miosis, lacrimation

Respiratory: Laryngospasm, bronchospasm, respiratory paralysis, increased bronchial secretions

Miscellaneous: Diaphoresis, hypersensitivity reactions

Drug Interactions Digoxin may enhance bradycardia potential of edrophonium; succinylcholine and decamethonium effects are prolonged by edrophonium; quinidine may antagonize effects of edrophonium; antagonizes effects of nondepolarizing muscle relaxants (eg, pancuronium, vecuronium)

Mechanism of Action Inhibits destruction of acetylcholine by acetylcholinesterase. This facilitates transmission of impulses across myoneural junction and results in increased cholinergic responses such as miosis, increased tonus of intestinal and skeletal muscles, bronchial and ureteral constriction, bradycardia, and increased salivary and sweat gland secretions

Pharmacodynamics

Onset:

I.M.: 2-10 minutes

I.V.: 30-60 seconds

Duration:

I.M.: 5-30 minutes

I.V.: 5-10 minutes

Usual Dosage Usually administered I.V., however, if not possible, I.M. or S.C. may be used

Infants: Diagnosis of myasthenia gravis: Initial:

I.M.: 0.5-1 mg

I.V.: Initial: 0.1 mg, followed by 0.4 mg (if no response); total dose = 0.5 mg

Children:

Diagnosis of myasthenia gravis: Initial:

I.M.: ≤34 kg: 2 mg; >34 kg: 5 mg

I.V.: 0.04 mg/kg given over 1 minute followed by 0.16 mg/kg given within 45 seconds (if no response) (maximum dose: 10 mg total)

Titration of oral anticholinesterase therapy: I.V.: 0.04 mg/kg once given 1 hour after oral intake of the drug being used in treatment; if strength improves, an increase in neostigmine or pyridostigmine dose is indicated

Adults:

Diagnosis of myasthenia gravis: Initial:

I.M.: Initial: 10 mg; if no cholinergic reaction occurs, administer 2 mg 30 minutes later to rule out false-negative reaction

I.V.: 2 mg test dose administered over 15-30 seconds; 8 mg given 45 seconds later (if no response is seen); test dose may be repeated after 30 minutes.

Titration of oral anticholinesterase therapy: I.V.: 1-2 mg given 1 hour after oral dose of anticholinesterase; if strength improves, an increase in neostigmine or pyridostigmine dose is indicated

Differentiation of cholinergic from myasthenic crisis: I.V.: 1 mg, may repeat after 1 minute **(Note:** Intubation and controlled ventilation may be required if patient has cholinergic crises.)

Reversal of nondepolarizing neuromuscular blocking agents (neostigmine with atropine usually preferred): I.V.: 10 mg over 30-45 seconds, may repeat every 5-10 minutes up to 40 mg total dose

Termination of paroxysmal atrial tachycardia: I.V.: 5-10 mg

Dosing adjustment in renal impairment: Dose may need to be reduced in patients with chronic renal failure

Administration Parenteral: Edrophonium is administered by direct I.V. or I.M. injection; see Usual Dosage

Monitoring Parameters Pre- and postinjection strength (cranial musculature is most useful); heart rate, respiratory rate, blood pressure, changes in fasciculations

Dosage Forms Injection, as chloride: 10 mg/mL (1 mL, 10 mL, 15 mL)

◆ **Edrophonium Chloride** *see* Edrophonium *on page 359*

◆ **ED-SPAZ®** *see* Hyoscyamine *on page 497*

◆ **EDTA** *see* Edetate Disodium *on page 358*

◆ **E.E.S.®** *see* Erythromycin *on page 379*

◆ **E.E.S. 400®** *see* Erythromycin *on page 379*

◆ **E.E.S.® Chewable** *see* Erythromycin *on page 379*

◆ **E.E.S.® Granules** *see* Erythromycin *on page 379*

Efavirenz (eh FAH vih rehnz)

Related Information
Adult and Adolescent HIV *on page 1133*
Pediatric HIV *on page 1129*

Brand Names Sustiva™

Therapeutic Category Antiretroviral Agent; HIV Agents (Anti-HIV Agents); Non-nucleoside Reverse Transcriptase Inhibitor (NNRTI)

Generic Available No

Use Treatment of HIV-1 infection in combination with other antiretroviral agents. (**Note:** HIV regimens consisting of **three** antiretroviral agents are strongly recommended)

Pregnancy Risk Factor C

Contraindications Hypersensitivity to efavirenz or any component; concurrent therapy with astemizole, cisapride, midazolam, triazolam, or ergot derivatives

Warnings Efavirenz is a mixed inducer/inhibitor of CYP450 enzymes and numerous drug interactions occur. Due to potential serious and/or life-threatening drug interactions, certain drugs are contraindicated (see Contraindications and Drug Interactions). Resistance emerges rapidly if administered as monotherapy; always use efavirenz in combination with at least two other antiretroviral agents; do not add efavirenz as a single agent to antiretroviral regimens that are failing; initiate in combination with at least one other antiretroviral agent to which the patient is naive.

Precautions Use with caution in patients with a history of mental illness or substance abuse (delusions, inappropriate behavior, and severe acute depression may occur); serious CNS and psychiatric symptoms may occur (see Adverse Effects); discontinue if severe rash (involving blistering, desquamation, mucosal involvement, or fever) occurs; rash is more common and more severe in children versus adults, **consider prophylaxis with antihistamines in children**; use with caution in patients with known or suspected hepatitis B or C, those receiving other hepatotoxic medications, and those with hepatic impairment; weigh risk versus benefit in patients with persistent elevations of serum transaminases (ie, >5 times normal); cross resistance with other non-nucleoside reverse transcriptase inhibitors may occur

Adverse Reactions
Central nervous system: (Note: Overall incidence of CNS adverse effects was 53% versus 25% in controls; CNS effects in children have been reported in one study to be 9%) somnolence, dizziness, drowsiness, abnormal dreams, insomnia, confusion, headache, hypoesthesia, impaired concentration, abnormal thinking, agitation, amnesia, depersonalization, euphoria, hallucinations, delusions, inappropriate behavior; fever (children 26%); anxiety, nervousness; serious psychiatric adverse effects (patients with history of psychiatric disorders may be at greater risk): Suicidal ideation/attempts, severe acute depression, aggressive behavior, paranoid reactions, manic reactions

Dermatologic: Rash, usually pruritic maculopapular skin eruptions (incidence: children 40%, adults 26%; median onset, adults: 11 days, children: 9 days [range 6-205 days], **Note:** Most rashes in children appeared within 14 days after starting therapy; median duration, adults: 16 days, children: 6 days [range 2-37 days], **Note:** Median duration of rash in children who continued therapy was 9 days; rash may be treated with antihistamines and corticosteroids and usually resolves within one month while continuing therapy; **Note:** Blistering, desquamation, fever, mucosal involvement, or ulceration may occur and requires discontinuation of drug, see Precautions); pruritus, increased sweating

Endocrine & metabolic: Hypercholesterolemia, hypertriglyceridemia

Gastrointestinal: Nausea or vomiting (children 16%), diarrhea/loose stools (children 39%), abdominal pain, asymptomatic elevations in serum amylase, pancreatitis (several cases)

Hepatic: Elevated liver enzymes (patients with hepatitis B or C may be at greater risk)

Respiratory: Cough (children 25%)

Miscellaneous: Alcohol intolerance

(Continued)

Efavirenz *(Continued)*

Drug Interactions Cytochrome P-450 isoenzyme CYP3A4 and CYP2B6 substrate; mixed inducer/inhibitor of CYP450 enzymes: Induces CYP3A4 and inhibits isoenzymes CYP2C9, 2C19, and 3A4

Concurrent use of efavirenz with astemizole, cisapride, midazolam, triazolam, or ergot derivatives is contraindicated (efavirenz may inhibit the metabolism of these drugs and result in serious or life-threatening effects); efavirenz decreases serum concentrations of indinavir (indinavir dosage increase is recommended), saquinavir (use of saquinavir as sole protease inhibitor with efavirenz is not recommended), amprenavir, and clarithromycin; efavirenz increases serum concentrations of nelfinavir, ritonavir, ethinyl estradiol, and 14-hydroxy metabolite of clarithromycin; efavirenz may increase or decrease the effects of warfarin

Saquinavir, rifampin, rifabutin, phenobarbital and other enzyme inducing agents may decrease efavirenz serum concentrations; the herbal medicine, St John's wort (*Hypericum perforatum*) may significantly decrease concentrations of efavirenz and is not recommended for concurrent use; ritonavir may increase efavirenz AUC by 20%; alcohol or other CNS depressants may increase adverse effects; rash may be more common when efavirenz is used with clarithromycin (consider azithromycin use); interaction with oral contraceptives is not fully characterized (use reliable barrier method)

Food Interactions Food does not usually effect bioavailability; high fat meals increase bioavailability by 50%

Stability Store at room temperature

Mechanism of Action A non-nucleoside reverse transcriptase inhibitor which specifically binds to HIV-1 reverse transcriptase and blocks RNA-dependent and DNA-dependent DNA polymerase activity including HIV-1 replication; does not require intracellular phosphorylation for antiviral activity

Pharmacokinetics Note: Pharmacokinetics in children ≥3 years of age are thought to be similar to adults

Distribution: CSF concentrations are 0.69% of plasma (range 0.26% to 1.2%); however, CSF: Plasma concentration ratio is 3 times higher than free fraction in plasma

Protein binding: 99.5% to 99.8%, primarily to albumin

Metabolism: In the liver, primarily by cytochrome P-450 enzymes (mainly isoenzymes CYP3A4 and CYP2B6) to hydroxylated metabolites which then undergo glucuronidation; induces P-450 enzymes and it's own metabolism

Bioavailability: 42% (increased with fatty meal)

Half-life, adults:
Single dose: 52-76 hours
Multiple dose: 40-55 hours

Time to peak concentration: 3-5 hours

Elimination: <1% excreted unchanged in the urine; 14% to 34% excreted as metabolites in the urine and 16% to 61% in feces (primarily as unchanged drug)

Usual Dosage Oral: (use in combination with other antiretroviral agents)
Neonates, Infants, and Children <3 years: Not approved for use (no information available)
Children ≥3 years: Dose according to body weight:
10 kg to <15 kg: 200 mg once daily
15 kg to <20 kg: 250 mg once daily
20 kg to <25 kg: 300 mg once daily
25 kg to <32.5 kg: 350 mg once daily
32.5 kg to <40 kg: 400 mg once daily
≥40 kg: 600 mg once daily
Adults: 600 mg once daily

Administration Administer dose at bedtime to decrease CNS adverse effects (especially during the first 2-4 weeks of therapy); may be administered without regard to food; avoid administration with high fat meals; capsules may be opened and added to food or liquids, but efavirenz tastes peppery (grape jelly may be used to improve taste)

Monitoring Parameters Signs and symptoms of rash; viral load; CD4 counts; serum amylase; liver enzymes in patients with known or suspected hepatitis B or C, those receiving concomitant ritonavir, and those receiving other hepatotoxic medications; serum cholesterol, triglycerides

Test Interactions False positive test for cannabinoids using the CEDIA DAU Multilevel THC assay

Patient Information May cause drowsiness and impair ability to perform activities requiring mental alertness or physical coordination; avoid alcohol; efavirenz is not a cure for HIV; notify physician immediately if rash develops; report the use of other medications, nonprescription medications and herbal or natural products to your physician and pharmacist; take efavirenz everyday as prescribed; do not change dose or discontinue without physician's advice; if a dose is missed, take it as soon as possible, then return to normal dosing schedule; if a dose is skipped, do **not** double the next dose

Additional Information An oral liquid formulation of efavirenz (strawberry/mint-flavored solution) is available on an investigational basis from DuPont Pharmaceuticals Company as part of an expanded access program for HIV-infected children and adolescents 3-16 years of age.

Dosage Forms Capsule: 50 mg, 100 mg, 200 mg

References

Adkins JC and Noble S, "Efavirenz," *Drugs*, 1998, 56(6):1055-64.

Panel on Clinical Practices for Treatment of HIV Infection, "Guidelines for the Use of Antiretroviral Agents in HIV-Infected Adults and Adolescents," January 28, 2000, http://www.hivatis.org.

Piscitelli SC, Burstein AH, Chaitt D, et al, "Indinavir Concentrations and St John's Wort," *Lancet*, 2000, 355(9203):547-8.

Starr SE, Fletcher CV, Spector SA, et al, "Combination Therapy With Efavirenz, Nelfinavir, and Nucleoside Reverse-transcriptase Inhibitors in Children Infected with Human Immunodeficiency Virus Type 1. Pediatric AIDS Clinical Trials Group 382 Team," *N Engl J Med* 1999, 341(25):1874-81.

Working Group on Antiretroviral Therapy and Medical Management of HIV-Infected Children, "Guidelines for the Use of Antiretroviral Agents in Pediatric HIV Infection," January 7, 2000, http://www.hivatis.org.

♦ **Effer-Syllium® [OTC]** *see* Psyllium *on page 823*

♦ **Efidac/24® [OTC]** *see* Pseudoephedrine *on page 822*

♦ **Efudex® Topical** *see* Fluorouracil *on page 430*

♦ **EHDP** *see* Etidronate Disodium *on page 396*

♦ **Elavil®** *see* Amitriptyline *on page 67*

♦ **Eldecort® Topical** *see* Hydrocortisone *on page 486*

♦ **Electrolyte Lavage Solution** *see* Polyethylene Glycol-Electrolyte Solution *on page 782*

♦ **Elimite™ Cream** *see* Permethrin *on page 752*

♦ **Elixomin®** *see* Theophylline *on page 910*

♦ **Elixophyllin®** *see* Theophylline *on page 910*

♦ **Elspar®** *see* Asparaginase *on page 98*

♦ **Eltor® (Canada)** *see* Pseudoephedrine *on page 822*

♦ **Eltroxin®** *see* Levothyroxine *on page 566*

♦ **Eltroxin® (Canada)** *see* Levothyroxine *on page 566*

♦ **Emergency Pediatric Drip Calculations** *see page 1000*

♦ **Emetogenic Potential of Single Chemotherapeutic Agents** *see page 1095*

♦ **Emgel®** *see* Erythromycin *on page 379*

♦ **EMLA®** *see* Lidocaine and Prilocaine *on page 570*

♦ **Emo-Cort™ (Canada)** *see* Hydrocortisone *on page 486*

♦ **Empirin® [OTC]** *see* Aspirin *on page 99*

♦ **Empracet®-30, -60 (Canada)** *see* Acetaminophen and Codeine *on page 27*

♦ **Emtec-30® (Canada)** *see* Acetaminophen and Codeine *on page 27*

♦ **Emulsoil® [OTC]** *see* Castor Oil *on page 175*

♦ **E-Mycin®** *see* Erythromycin *on page 379*

♦ **E-Mycin-E®** *see* Erythromycin *on page 379*

Enalapril/Enalaprilat (e NAL a pril/e NAL a pril at)

Brand Names Apo®-Enalapril (Canada); Vasotec® I.V.; Vasotec® Oral

Available Salts Enalapril Maleate

Therapeutic Category Angiotensin-Converting Enzyme (ACE) Inhibitor; Antihypertensive Agent

Generic Available No

Use Management of mild to severe hypertension, CHF, and asymptomatic left ventricular dysfunction

Pregnancy Risk Factor C (1st trimester); D (may cause injury and death to the developing fetus when used during the 2nd and 3rd trimesters of pregnancy)

Contraindications Hypersensitivity to enalapril, enalaprilat, any component, or other ACE inhibitors; patients with idiopathic or hereditary angioedema or a history of angioedema with ACE inhibitors

Precautions Use with caution and modify dosage in patients with renal impairment (especially renal artery stenosis), hyponatremia, hypovolemia, severe CHF, left ventricular outflow tract obstruction, or with coadministered diuretic therapy; experience in children is limited; severe hypotension may occur in patients who are
(Continued)

Enalapril/Enalaprilat *(Continued)*

sodium and/or volume depleted, initiate lower doses and monitor closely when starting therapy in these patients; use with caution in neonates; injectable product contains benzyl alcohol 9 mg/mL (benzyl alcohol is converted to benzoic acid which may displace bilirubin from protein binding sites and at larger doses can cause the gasping syndrome in neonates)

Adverse Reactions
Cardiovascular: Hypotension, syncope
Central nervous system: Fatigue, vertigo, insomnia, dizziness, headache
Dermatologic: Rash, angioedema. **Note:** The relative risk of angioedema with ACE inhibitors is higher within the first 30 days of use (compared to >1 year of use), for Black Americans (compared to Whites), for lisinopril or enalapril (compared to captopril), and for patients previously hospitalized within 30 days (Brown, 1996).
Endocrine & metabolic: Hypoglycemia, hyperkalemia
Gastrointestinal: Nausea, diarrhea, ageusia
Genitourinary: Impotence
Hematologic: Agranulocytosis, neutropenia, anemia
Neuromuscular & skeletal: Muscle cramps
Renal: Deterioration in renal function
Respiratory: Cough, dyspnea, eosinophilic pneumonitis

Drug Interactions Cytochrome P-450 isoenzyme CYP3A3/4 substrate
Use with potassium-sparing diuretics may result in an additive hyperkalemic effect; diuretics or other antihypertensive agents may increase hypotensive effect; indomethacin may decrease hypotensive effect; enalapril may increase lithium levels; use with NSAIDs in patients with compromised renal function may increase renal dysfunction (usually reversible)

Food Interactions Food does not affect absorption; limit salt substitutes or potassium-rich diet; avoid natural licorice (causes sodium and water retention and increases potassium loss)

Stability To deliver small I.V. doses, a dilution with NS to a final concentration of 25 mcg/mL can be made; solutions for I.V. infusion mixed in NS or D_5W are stable for 24 hours at room temperature

Mechanism of Action Competitive inhibitor of angiotensin-converting enzyme (ACE); prevents conversion of angiotensin I to angiotensin II, a potent vasoconstrictor; results in lower levels of angiotensin II which causes an increase in plasma renin activity and a reduction in aldosterone secretion

Pharmacodynamics
Onset of action:
Oral: Within 1 hour
I.V.: Within 15 minutes
Maximum effect:
Oral: Within 4-8 hours
I.V.: Within 1 hour
Duration:
Oral: 12-24 hours
I.V.: Dose dependent, usually 4-6 hours

Pharmacokinetics
Absorption: Oral: 55% to 75% (enalapril)
Protein binding: 50% to 60%
Metabolism: Enalapril is a prodrug (inactive) and undergoes biotransformation to enalaprilat (active) in the liver
Half-life:
Enalapril:
CHF neonates 10-19 days of age (n=3): 10.3 hours (range: 4.2-13.4 hours)
CHF infants >27 days and children ≤6.5 years of age (n=11): 2.7 hours (range: 1.3-6.3 hours)
Healthy adults: 2 hours
CHF adults: 3.4-5.8 hours
Enalaprilat:
CHF neonates 10-19 days of age (n=3): 11.9 hours (range 5.9-15.6 hours)
CHF infants >27 days and children ≤6.5 years of age (n=11): 11.1 hours (range: 5.1-20.8 hours)
Infants 6 weeks to 8 months: 6-10 hours
Adults: 35-38 hours
Time to peak serum concentration: Oral:
Enalapril: Within 0.5-1.5 hours
Enalaprilat (active): Within 3-4.5 hours
Elimination: Principally in urine (60% to 80%) with some fecal excretion

Usual Dosage Use lower listed initial dose in patients with hyponatremia, hypovolemia, severe CHF, decreased renal function, or in those receiving diuretics

Neonates:

Oral: **Enalapril**: Initial: 0.1 mg/kg/day given every 24 hours; increase dose and interval as required every few days (see Additional Information)

I.V.: **Enalaprilat**: 5-10 mcg/kg/dose administered every 8-24 hours (as determined by blood pressure readings) has been used for the treatment of neonatal hypertension; monitor patients carefully; select patients may require higher doses

Infants and Children:

Oral: **Enalapril**: Initial: 0.1 mg/kg/day in 1-2 divided doses; increase as required over 2 weeks to maximum of 0.5 mg/kg/day; mean dose required for CHF improvement in 39 children (9 days to 17 years of age) was 0.36 mg/kg/day; investigationally, select individuals have been treated with doses up to 0.94 mg/kg/day (Leversha, 1994)

I.V.: **Enalaprilat**: 5-10 mcg/kg/dose administered every 8-24 hours (as determined by blood pressure readings); monitor patients carefully; select patients may require higher doses

Adolescents and Adults:

Oral: **Enalapril**: Initial: 2.5-5 mg/day then increase as required; usual dose for hypertension: 10-40 mg/day in 1-2 divided doses; usual dose for CHF: 5-20 mg/day in 2 divided doses; maximum dose: 40 mg/day

Asymptomatic left ventricular dysfunction: Initial: 2.5 mg twice daily; increase as tolerated; usual dose: 20 mg/day in 2 divided doses

I.V.: **Enalaprilat**: 0.625-1.25 mg/dose every 6 hours; doses as high as 5 mg/dose every 6 hours have been tolerated for up to 36 hours; little experience with doses >20 mg/day

Dosing adjustment in renal impairment:

Cl_{cr} 10-50 mL/minute: Administer 75% to 100% of dose

Cl_{cr} <10 mL/minute: Administer 50% of dose

Administration

Oral: May administer without regard to food

Parenteral: I.V.: Administer as I.V. infusion (undiluted solution or further diluted) over 5 minutes

Monitoring Parameters Blood pressure, renal function, WBC, serum potassium

Patient Information Limit alcohol; notify physician if vomiting, diarrhea, excessive perspiration, or dehydration occurs, or if swelling of face, lips, tongue, or difficulty in breathing occurs; do not use a salt substitute (potassium-containing) without physician advice

Nursing Implications Discontinue if angioedema occurs; observe closely for hypotension within 1-3 hours of first dose or with new higher dose

Additional Information Severe hypotension was reported in a **preterm** neonate (birth weight 835 g, gestational age 26 weeks, postnatal age 9 days) who was treated with enalapril 0.1 mg/kg orally; hypotension responded to I.V. plasma and dopamine; the authors suggest starting enalapril in preterm infants at 0.01 mg/kg and increasing upwards in a stepwise fashion with very close monitoring of blood pressure and urine output. However, in this case report, oral enalapril at doses of 0.01 mg/kg to 0.04 mg/kg did not adequately control blood pressure. Further studies are needed. (Schilder, 1995)

Dosage Forms

Injection, as enalaprilat: 1.25 mg/mL (1 mL, 2 mL)

Tablet, as maleate: 2.5 mg, 5 mg, 10 mg, 20 mg

Extemporaneous Preparations

A 1 mg/mL oral liquid preparation made from tablets and 3 different vehicles (cherry syrup, a 1:1 mixture of Ora-Sweet® and Ora-Plus®, or a 1:1 mixture of Ora-Sweet® SF and Ora-Plus®) was stable for 60 days when stored in amber plastic prescription bottles in the dark at room temperature (25°C) or under refrigeration (5°C); grind six 20 mg tablets in a mortar into a fine powder; add 15 mL of the vehicle and mix well to form a uniform paste; mix while adding the vehicle in geometric proportions to **almost** 120 mL; transfer to a calibrated bottle and qsad with vehicle to 120 mL; label "shake well" and "protect from light" (Allen, 1998).

A 1 mg/mL oral liquid preparation made from tablets and 3 different vehicles (deionized water, citrate buffer solution at pH 5.0, or a 1:1 mixture of Ora-Sweet® and Ora-Plus®) was stable for 91 days when stored in plastic prescription bottles in the dark under refrigeration (4°C). When stored at room temperature (25°C), the preparations made in citrate buffer solution at pH 5.0 and the 1:1 mixture of Ora-Sweet® and Ora-Plus® were also stable for 91 days, but the preparation

(Continued)

Enalapril/Enalaprilat *(Continued)*

made in deionized water was stable for only 56 days. Grind twenty 10 mg tablets in a mortar; add a small amount of vehicle and mix well to form a smooth paste; mix while adding increasing amounts of the vehicle to make the mixture pourable; transfer to a graduated cylinder and qsad to 200 mL; **Note:** To prepare the isotonic citrate buffer solution (pH 5.0), see reference; label "shake well" and "protect from light" (Nahata, 1998).

Allen LV and Erickson MA, "Stability of Alprazolam, Chloroquine Phosphate, Cisapride, Enalapril Maleate, and Hydralazine Hydrochloride in Extemporaneously Compounded Oral Liquids," *Am J Health Syst Pharm*, 1998, 55(18):1915-20.

Nahata MC, Morosco RS, and Hipple TF, "Stability of Enalapril Maleate in Three Extemporaneously Prepared Oral Liquids," *Am J Health Syst Pharm*, 1998, 55(11):1155-7.

References

Brown NJ, Ray WA, Snowden M, et al, "Black Americans Have an Increased Rate of Angiotension-Converting Enzyme Inhibitor-Associated Angioedema," *Clin Pharmacol Ther*, 1996, 60(1):8-13.

Bult Y and van den Anker J, "Hypertension in a Preterm Infant Treated With Enalapril," *J Pediatr Pharm Pract*, 1997, 2(4):229-31.

Frenneaux M, Stewart RA, Newman CM, et al, "Enalapril for Severe Heart Failure in Infancy," *Arch Dis Child*, 1989, 64(2):219-23.

Leversha AM, Wilson NJ, Clarkson PM, et al, "Efficacy and Dosage of Enalapril in Congenital and Acquired Heart Disease," *Arch Dis Child*, 1994, 70(1):35-9.

Lloyd TR, Mahoney LT, Knoedel D, et al, "Orally Administered Enalapril for Infants With Congestive Heart Failure: A Dose Finding Study," *J Pediatr*, 1989, 114(4 Pt 1):650-4.

Marcadis ML, Kraus DM, Hatzopoulos FK, et al, "Use of Enalaprilat for Neonatal Hypertension," *J Pediatr*, 1991, 119(3):505-6.

Nakamura H, Ishii M, Sugimura T, et al, "The Kinetic Profiles of Enalapril and Enalaprilat and Their Possible Developmental Changes in Pediatric Patients With Congestive Heart Failure," *Clin Pharmacol Ther*, 1994, 56(2):160-8.

Schilder JL and Van den Anker JN, "Use of Enalapril in Neonatal Hypertension," *Acta Paediatr*, 1995, 84(12):1426-8.

Wells TG, Bunchman TE, Kearns GL, "Treatment of Neonatal Hypertension With Enalaprilat," *J Pediatr*, 1990, 117(4):664-7.

♦ **Enalapril Maleate** *see* Enalapril/Enalaprilat *on page 363*

♦ **Enbrel®** *see* Etanercept *on page 388*

♦ **Endantadine™ (Canada)** *see* Amantadine *on page 53*

♦ **Endocarditis Prophylaxis** *see page 1127*

♦ **Endocet® (Canada)** *see* Oxycodone and Acetaminophen *on page 716*

♦ **Endodan® (Canada)** *see* Oxycodone and Aspirin *on page 717*

♦ **Endrate®** *see* Edetate Disodium *on page 358*

♦ **Ener-B® [OTC]** *see* Cyanocobalamin *on page 263*

♦ **Enlon®** *see* Edrophonium *on page 359*

♦ **Enomine®** *see* Guaifenesin, Phenylpropanolamine, and Phenylephrine *on page 467*

♦ **Enovil®** *see* Amitriptyline *on page 67*

Enoxaparin *(e noks ah PAIR in)*

Brand Names Lovenox®

Available Salts Enoxaparin Sodium

Therapeutic Category Anticoagulant; Low Molecular Weight Heparin

Generic Available No

Use Prophylaxis and treatment of thromboembolic disorders, specifically: (in adults) prevention of DVT following hip or knee replacement surgery, and abdominal surgery in patients at thromboembolic risk (ie, >40 years of age, obese, general anesthesia >30 minutes, malignancy, history of DVT or pulmonary embolism); administered with warfarin for inpatient treatment of acute DVT (with or without pulmonary embolism) and outpatient treatment of acute DVT (without pulmonary embolism); administered with aspirin for prevention of ischemic complications of non-Q-wave MI and unstable angina

Pregnancy Risk Factor B

Contraindications Active major bleeding; hypersensitivity to enoxaparin, heparin, any component, or pork products (enoxaparin is derived from porcine intestinal mucosa); acute heparin-induced (or low molecular weight heparin-induced) thrombocytopenia

Warnings Bleeding or thrombocytopenia may occur. Use with extreme caution in patients with an increased risk of hemorrhage (eg, active GI ulceration or bleeding, angiodysplastic GI disease, bacterial endocarditis, bleeding disorders, hemorrhagic stroke); recent brain, spinal, or ophthalmological surgery; concomitant platelet inhibitor therapy (see Drug Interactions); or a history of heparin-induced thrombocytopenia. Do not use unit-for-unit in place of heparin or other low molecular weight heparins.

Epidural or spinal hematoma resulting in long-term or permanent paralysis may occur in patients receiving low molecular weight heparins or heparinoids during epidural/spinal anesthesia or spinal puncture; these patients must be monitored frequently for neurological impairment and treated immediately if compromised; the use of indwelling spinal catheters for analgesia, concomitant use of platelet inhibitors, NSAIDs, or other anticoagulants, and repeated or traumatic epidural/spinal puncture increase the risk for epidural/spinal hematoma; potential benefits must be weighed against the risks.

Precautions Use with caution in patients with uncontrolled arterial hypertension, bleeding diathesis, history of recent GI ulceration, diabetic retinopathy, and hemorrhage; use with caution and consider dosage decrease in patients with severe renal dysfunction (Cl_{cr} <30 mL/minute); institute appropriate therapy if thromboembolism occurs despite enoxaparin prophylaxis

Adverse Reactions
Cardiovascular: Edema

Central nervous system: Fever

Endocrine & metabolic: Hyperlipidemia (very rare)

Gastrointestinal: Nausea

Hematologic: Hemorrhage, thrombocytopenia (incidence of heparin-induced thrombocytopenia is less than with heparin therapy)

Hepatic: Elevated SGOT and SGPT (asymptomatic, fully reversible, rarely associated with elevated bilirubin levels)

Local: Irritation, pain, hematoma, ecchymosis, erythema at S.C. injection site

Drug Interactions Anticoagulants, platelet inhibitors (aspirin, salicylates, NSAIDs including ketorolac, dipyridamole, and sulfinpyrazone) may increase the risk of bleeding

Stability Store at room temperature; does not contain preservatives, discard unused portions; do not mix with other injections or infusions

Mechanism of Action Potentiates the action of antithrombin III and inactivates coagulation factor Xa; also inactivates factor IIa (thrombin), but to a much lesser degree; ratio of antifactor Xa to antifactor IIa activity is ~4:1 (ratio for unfractionated heparin is 1:1)

Pharmacodynamics Antifactor Xa and antithrombin (antifactor IIa) activities:
Maximum effect: S.C.: 3-5 hours

Duration: ~12 hours following a 40 mg daily dose given S.C.

Pharmacokinetics Based on antifactor Xa activity
Distribution: Does not cross the placental barrier

Mean V_d: Adults: 6 L

Protein binding: Does not bind to most heparin binding proteins

Bioavailability: S.C.: 92%

Half-life: S.C.: Adults: 4.5 hours (range 2.2-6 hours)

Elimination: 40% of I.V. dose is excreted in urine as active and inactive fragments; 8% to 20% of antifactor Xa activity is recovered within 24 hours in the urine

Clearance: Decreased by 30% in patients with Cl_{cr} <30 mL/minute

Usual Dosage S.C.:

Neonates, Infants, and Children: Few studies have been conducted; the Fifth American College of Chest Physicians Consensus Conference on Antithrombotic Therapy (Michelson, 1998) recommends low molecular weight heparin as an alternative to heparin therapy in children ≥2 months with DVT or pulmonary embolism and in newborns with DVT, pulmonary embolism, or arterial thrombosis; the following initial doses and titration schedule, based on therapeutic antifactor Xa levels of 0.5-1 unit/mL, are recommended

Note: For treatment of DVT or pulmonary embolism in children ≥2 months of age, enoxaparin should be continued for 5-10 days and oral anticoagulation should be overlapped for 4-5 days (see Michelson, 1998)

Infants <2 months:
Prophylaxis: Initial: 0.75 mg/kg every 12 hours
Treatment: Initial: 1.5 mg/kg every 12 hours

Infants >2 months and Children ≤18 years:
Prophylaxis: Initial: 0.5 mg/kg every 12 hours
Treatment: Initial: 1 mg/kg every 12 hours

See **Dosage Titration** table on the following page.

Adults: **Note:** Consider lower doses for patients <45 kg
(Continued)

Enoxaparin *(Continued)*

Enoxaparin Dosage Titration

Antifactor Xa	Dose Titration	Time to Repeat Antifactor Xa Level
<0.35 units/mL	Increase dose by 25%	4 h after next dose
0.35-0.49 units/mL	Increase dose by 10%	4 h after next dose
0.5-1 unit/mL	Keep same dosage	Next day, then 1 wk later (4 h after dose)
1.1-1.5 units/mL	Decrease dose by 20%	Before next dose
1.6-2 units/mL	Hold dose for 3 h and decrease dose by 30%	Before next dose, then 4 h after next dose
>2 units/mL	Hold all doses until antifactor Xa is 0.5 units/mL, then decrease dose by 40%	Before next dose and every 12 h until antifactor Xa <0.5 units/mL

Prevention of DVT:
    Knee replacement surgery: 30 mg every 12 hours; give first dose 12-24 hours after surgery (provided hemostasis has been established); average duration 7-10 days, up to 14 days

    Hip replacement surgery: Initial phase: 30 mg every 12 hours with first dose 12-24 hours after surgery (provided hemostasis has been established) or consider 40 mg once daily with first dose given 12 ± 3 hours prior to surgery; average duration of initial phase: 7-10 days, up to 14 days; after initial phase, give 40 mg once daily for 3 weeks

    Abdominal surgery in patients at risk: 40 mg once daily; give first dose 2 hours prior to surgery; average duration: 7-10 days, up to 12 days

Treatment of acute DVT and pulmonary embolism: Note: Initiate warfarin therapy when appropriate (usually within 72 hours of starting enoxaparin), continue enoxaparin for a minimum of 5 days (average 7 days) until INR is therapeutic

    Inpatient treatment of acute DVT with or without pulmonary embolism: 1 mg/kg every 12 hours or 1.5 mg/kg once daily

    Outpatient treatment of acute DVT without pulmonary embolism: 1 mg/kg every 12 hours

Dosage adjustment in renal impairment: No specific guidelines are available, but clearance is decreased when Cl_{cr} <30 mL/minute; monitor antifactor Xa activity to adjust dosage

Administration Parenteral: For S.C. use only; do not administer I.M. or I.V.; administer by deep S.C. injection; do not rub injection site after S.C. administration as bruising may occur

Monitoring Parameters CBC with platelets, stool occult blood tests, antifactor Xa activity in select patients (eg, neonates, infants, and children, and patients with significant renal impairment, active bleeding, or abnormal coagulation parameters); **Note:** Routine monitoring of PT and APTT is not warranted since PT and APTT are relatively insensitive measures of low molecular weight heparin activity; consider monitoring bone density in infants and children with long-term use

Reference Range Antifactor Xa level of 0.5-1 unit/mL measured 4-6 hours after S.C. administration

Additional Information Discontinue therapy if platelets fall <100,000/mm^3; each 10 mg of enoxaparin sodium equals ~1000 international units of antifactor Xa activity; enoxaparin should be withheld (at least 2 doses) and antifactor Xa activity should be determined (if possible), prior to lumbar or epidural procedures.

Enoxaparin contains fragments of unfractionated heparin produced by alkaline degradation (depolymerization) of heparin benzyl ester; enoxaparin has mean molecular weights of 3500-5600 daltons, which are much lower than mean molecular weights of unfractionated heparin (12,000-15,000 daltons). Low molecular weight heparins (LMWH) have several advantages over unfractionated heparin: better S.C. bioavailability, more convenient administration (S.C. versus I.V.), longer half-life (longer dosing interval), more predictable pharmacokinetics and pharmacodynamic (anticoagulant) effect, less intensive laboratory monitoring, reduced risk of heparin-induced thrombocytopenia, potential for outpatient use, and probable reduced risk of osteoporosis (further studies are needed).

Accidental overdosage may be treated with protamine sulfate; 1 mg protamine sulfate neutralizes 1 mg enoxaparin; first dose of protamine sulfate should equal the dose of enoxaparin injected, a second dose of 0.5 mg protamine sulfate per 1 mg enoxaparin may be given if APTT remains prolonged 2-4 hours after first dose (see Protamine *on page 820*)

Dosage Forms Injection, as sodium, preservative free:
Prefilled syringe: 30 mg/0.3 mL; 40 mg/0.4 mL
Graduated prefilled syringe: 60 mg/0.6 mL, 80 mg/0.8 mL, 100 mg/1 mL
Ampul: 30 mg/0.3 mL

References

deVeber G, Chan A, Monagle P, et al, "Anticoagulation Therapy in Pediatric Patients With Sinovenous Thrombosis: A Cohort Study," *Arch Neurol*, 1998, 55(12):1533-7.

Hirsh J, Warkentin TE, Raschke R, et al, "Heparin and Low-Molecular-Weight Heparin: Mechanisms of Action, Pharmacokinetics, Dosing Considerations, Monitoring, Efficacy, and Safety," *Chest*, 1998, 114(5 Suppl):489S-510S.

Martineau P and Tawil N, "Low-Molecular-Weight Heparins in the Treatment of Deep-Vein Thrombosis," *Ann Pharmacother*, 1998, 32(5):588-98, 601.

Massicotte P, Adams M, Marzinotto V, et al, "Low-Molecular-Weight Heparin in Pediatric Patients With Thrombotic Disease: A Dose Finding Study," *J Pediatr*, 1996, 128(3):313-8.

Michelson AD, Bovill E, Monagle P, et al, "Antithrombotic Therapy in Children," *Chest*, 1998, 114(5 Suppl):748S-69S.

♦ **Enoxaparin Sodium** *see* Enoxaparin *on page 366*

♦ **Entex**® *see* Guaifenesin, Phenylpropanolamine, and Phenylephrine *on page 467*

♦ **Entocort**® **(Canada)** *see* Budesonide *on page 144*

♦ **Entozyme**® *see* Pancreatin *on page 723*

♦ **Entrophen**® **(Canada)** *see* Aspirin *on page 99*

♦ **Enulose**® *see* Lactulose *on page 550*

♦ **E Pam**® **(Canada)** *see* Diazepam *on page 307*

♦ **Ephedra** *see* Ephedrine *on page 369*

Ephedrine (e FED rin)

Available Salts Ephedrine Sulfate

Synonyms Ephedra; Ephedrinum; Ma Huang

Therapeutic Category Adrenergic Agonist Agent; Antiasthmatic; Bronchodilator; Sympathomimetic

Generic Available Yes

Use Treatment of mild asthma, nasal congestion, acute bronchospasm, idiopathic orthostatic hypotension; adjunctive agent for treatment of shock

Pregnancy Risk Factor C

Contraindications Hypersensitivity to ephedrine or any component; patients with hypertension, cardiac arrhythmias, angle-closure glaucoma, and psychoneurosis; use during halothane or cyclopropane anesthesia (see Drug Interactions)

Warnings Use of ephedrine as a pressor is not a substitute for replacement of blood, plasma, fluids, and electrolytes; blood volume should be corrected as fully as possible before ephedrine therapy; must not be used as sole therapy in hypovolemic patients; hypoxia, hypercapnia, and acidosis may reduce the effectiveness and increase the incidence of side effects of ephedrine; may cause hypertension which may result in intracranial hemorrhage; long-term use may cause anxiety and symptoms of paranoid schizophrenia; the FDA has issued warnings concerning ephedrine-containing nonprescription products with claims of producing such effects as euphoria, increased sexual sensation, increased energy, and weight loss; healthcare professionals are urged to be aware of these products and counsel patients, when appropriate, about the potential adverse effects of ephedrine such as headache, dizziness, heart irregularities, seizures, and possibly death

Precautions Use with caution in patients with hyperthyroidism, diabetes mellitus, prostatic hypertrophy, coronary insufficiency, and angina

Adverse Reactions

Cardiovascular: Hypertension, precordial pain, edema, palpitations, tachycardia, arrhythmias

Central nervous system: Nervousness, anxiety, apprehension, fear, tension, agitation, excitation, restlessness, irritability, insomnia, dizziness, vertigo, confusion, delirium, hallucinations, euphoria, paranoid psychosis, headache

Dermatologic: Rash

Gastrointestinal: Nausea, vomiting, xerostomia, mild epigastric distress, anorexia

Genitourinary: Urinary retention

Neuromuscular & skeletal: Tremors, hyperactive reflexes, weakness

Drug Interactions Increased effects with other sympathomimetic agents; reduced pressor response to ephedrine with alpha-adrenergic blocking agents and methyldopa; increased cardiac irritability and arrhythmias with halothane and cyclopropane anesthesia; increased pressor effects with MAO inhibitors; cardiac glycosides may increase cardiac stimulation; medications which alkalinize or acidify the urine

(Continued)

369

Ephedrine *(Continued)*

may result in increased or decreased ephedrine effects (see Pharmacokinetics); increased CNS and GI effects when used with theophylline

Stability Protect from light

Mechanism of Action Stimulates both alpha- and beta-adrenergic receptors and also stimulates the release of norepinephrine from storage sites resulting in bronchodilation, cardiac stimulation, and increased systolic and diastolic blood pressure; tachyphylaxis may occur

Pharmacodynamics

Bronchodilation:
Onset of effect: Oral: 15-60 minutes
Duration: Oral: 2-4 hours
Pressor/cardiac effects: Duration:
Oral: 4 hours
I.M., S.C.: 1 hour

Pharmacokinetics

Absorption: Oral: Complete
Metabolism: Liver by oxidative deamination, demethylation, aromatic hydroxylation, and conjugation
Bioavailability: Oral: 85%
Half-life: 4.9-6.5 hours
Elimination: Dependent upon urinary pH with greatest excretion in acid pH; urine pH 5: 74% to 99% excreted unchanged; urine pH 8: 22% to 25% excreted unchanged

Usual Dosage

Bronchodilation and nasal decongestion: Oral:
Children >2-6 years: 2-3 mg/kg/day or 100 mg/m^2/day in 4-6 divided doses
Children 7-11 years: 6.25-12.5 mg every 4 hours; not to exceed 75 mg/day
Children ≥12 years and Adults: 12.5-50 mg every 3-4 hours; not to exceed 150 mg/day

Orthostatic hypotension: Oral: Adults: 25 mg 1-4 times/day

Adjunctive agent in the treatment of shock: Use the smallest effective dose for the shortest time:
Children <12 years: I.M., I.V., S.C.: 3 mg/kg/day in 4-6 divided doses
Children ≥12 years and Adults:
I.M., S.C.: 25-50 mg (range: 10-50 mg); may repeat with a second dose of 50 mg; not to exceed 150 mg/24 hours
I.V.: 10-25 mg; may repeat with a second dose in 5-10 minutes of 25 mg; not to exceed 150 mg/24 hours

Administration

Parenteral:
I.M., S.C.: May be administered undiluted
I.V.: May be administered by slow I.V. push
Oral: May be administered without regard to food

Monitoring Parameters Vital signs, pulmonary function tests, respiratory rate (when applicable)

Test Interactions May cause a false-positive test for amphetamine (by EMIT assay)

Patient Information Use for self-medication for asthma only under physician's direction; contact your physician if nervousness, tremor, insomnia, nausea, or loss of appetite occur; see Warnings

Additional Information Because ephedrine has been used to synthesize methamphetamine, restrictions are in place to reduce the potential for misuse (diversion) and abuse; 24 g of ephedrine (in terms of base) is the limit for a single transaction for drug products containing ephedrine regardless of the form in which these drugs are packaged

Dosage Forms

Capsule, as sulfate: 25 mg
Injection, as sulfate: 50 mg/mL (1 mL)

♦ **Ephedrine Sulfate** *see Ephedrine on page 369*
♦ **Ephedrinum** *see Ephedrine on page 369*
♦ **Epidermal Thymocyte Activating Factor** *see Aldesleukin on page 42*
♦ **Epi E-Z Pen™, -Jr (Canada)** *see Epinephrine on page 371*
♦ **Epifrin®** *see Epinephrine on page 371*
♦ **Epimorph® (Canada)** *see Morphine Sulfate on page 657*

Epinephrine (ep i NEF rin)

Related Information

Adult ACLS Algorithm, Asystole *on page 1008*
Adult ACLS Algorithm, Bradycardia *on page 1012*
Adult ACLS Algorithm, Pulseless Electrical Activity *on page 1006*
Adult ACLS Algorithm, V. Fib and Pulseless V. Tach *on page 1004*
Asthma Guidelines *on page 1178*
CPR Pediatric Drug Dosages *on page 999*
Emergency Pediatric Drip Calculations *on page 1000*
Extravasation Treatment *on page 1050*
Pediatric ALS Algorithm, Asystole and Pulseless Arrest *on page 1002*
Pediatric ALS Algorithm, Bradycardia *on page 1001*

Brand Names Adrenalin® Chloride; AsthmaHaler® Mist [OTC]; AsthmaNefrin® [OTC]; Bronitin® Mist [OTC]; Bronkaid® Mist [OTC]; Epi E-Z Pen™, -Jr (Canada); Epifrin®; EpiPen®; EpiPen® Jr; Glaucon®; Medihaler-Epi® [OTC]; microNefrin® [OTC]; Primatene® Mist [OTC]; Sus-Phrine®; Vaponefrin® [OTC]

Available Salts Epinephrine Bitartrate; Epinephrine Hydrochloride

Synonyms Adrenaline; Racemic Epinephrine

Therapeutic Category Adrenergic Agonist Agent; Antiasthmatic; Antidote, Hypersensitivity Reactions; Bronchodilator; Decongestant, Nasal; Sympathomimetic

Generic Available Yes

Use Treatment of bronchospasm, anaphylactic reactions, cardiac arrest, and management of open-angle (chronic simple) glaucoma; nasal decongestant (topical nasal formulation)

Pregnancy Risk Factor C

Contraindications Hypersensitivity to epinephrine or any component; cardiac arrhythmias, angle-closure glaucoma

Precautions Patients with diabetes mellitus, cardiovascular disease (angina, tachycardia, myocardial infarction), thyroid disease, or cerebral arteriosclerosis; rebound nasal congestion may occur after frequent nasal use

Adverse Reactions

Cardiovascular: Pallor, tachycardia, hypertension, increased myocardial oxygen consumption, cardiac arrhythmias, sudden death

Central nervous system: Anxiety, headache

Gastrointestinal: Nausea

Genitourinary: Acute urinary retention in patients with bladder outflow obstruction

Neuromuscular & skeletal: Weakness, tremor

Ocular: Precipitation of or exacerbation of narrow-angle glaucoma

Renal: Decreased renal and splanchnic blood flow

Drug Interactions Increased cardiac irritability if administered concurrently with halogenated inhalational anesthetics; beta-blocking agents (ie, propranolol); alpha-blocking agents (eg, phentolamine); alpha- and beta-blocking agents (labetalol); phenothiazines with alpha-blocking activity; tricyclic antidepressants enhance pressor response to epinephrine

Stability Protect from light; incompatible with alkaline solutions (sodium bicarbonate); compatible when coadministered with dopamine, dobutamine, inamrinone (amrinone), atracurium, pancuronium, and vecuronium

Mechanism of Action Stimulates alpha-, beta$_1$- and beta$_2$-adrenergic receptors resulting in relaxation of smooth muscle of the bronchial tree, cardiac stimulation, and dilation of skeletal muscle vasculature; small doses can cause vasodilation via beta$_2$-vascular receptors; large doses may produce constriction of skeletal and vascular smooth muscle; decreases production of aqueous humor and increases aqueous outflow; dilates the pupil by contracting the dilator muscle

Pharmacodynamics

Local vasoconstriction (topical):
Onset: 5 minutes
Duration: <1 hour
Onset of bronchodilation:
Inhalation: Within 1 minute
S.C.: Within 5-10 minutes
Peak ocular effect: Following conjunctival instillation intraocular pressures fall within 1 hour with a maximal response occurring within 4-8 hours
Duration: Ocular effects persist for 12-24 hours

Pharmacokinetics

Absorption: Orally ingested doses are rapidly metabolized in GI tract and liver; pharmacologically active concentrations are **not** achieved
Distribution: Crosses placenta but not blood-brain barrier
(Continued)

Epinephrine *(Continued)*

Metabolism: Extensive in the liver and other tissues by the enzymes catechol-o-methyltransferase and monoamine oxidase

Usual Dosage

Neonates: I.V., Intratracheal: 0.01-0.03 mg/kg (0.1-0.3 mL/kg of **1:10,000** solution) every 3-5 minutes as needed; dilute intratracheal doses to 1-2 mL with NS

Infants and Children:

I.M.: EpiPen® and EpiPen® Jr: 0.01 mg/kg

or as alternative

<30 kg: 0.15 mg; >30 kg: 0.3 mg

S.C.: 0.01 mg/kg (0.01 mL/kg/dose of **1:1000** solution) not to exceed 0.5 mg **or**
Suspension: 0.005 mL/kg/dose (1:200); not to exceed 0.15 mL every 8-12 hours

Bradycardia:

I.V.: 0.01 mg/kg (0.1 mL/kg) of **1:10,000** solution (maximum dose: 1 mg or 10 mL)

Intratracheal: 0.1 mg/kg (0.1 mL/kg) of **1:1000** solution; doses as high as 0.2 mg/kg may be effective

Asystole or pulseless arrest:

I.V. or intraosseous: **First dose:** 0.01 mg/kg (0.1 mL/kg) of **1:10,000** solution; **Subsequent doses:** 0.1 mg/kg (0.1 mL/kg of **1:1000** solution; doses as high as 0.2 mg/kg may be effective); repeat every 3-5 minutes as needed

Intratracheal: 0.1 mg/kg (0.1 mL/kg) of **1:1000** solution (doses as high as 0.2 mg/kg may be effective)

Continuous I.V. infusion rate: 0.1-1 mcg/kg/minute; titrate dosage to desired effect

Nebulization: 0.25-0.5 mL of 2.25% **racemic epinephrine** solution diluted in 3 mL NS, or L-epinephrine at an equivalent dose; racemic epinephrine 10 mg = 5 mg L-epinephrine; use lower end of dosing range for younger infants

Ophthalmic: Instill 1-2 drops in eye(s) once or twice daily

Nasal: Children ≥6 years and Adults: Apply drops locally as needed; do not exceed 1 mL every 15 minutes

Adults:

Asystole: I.V.: 1 mg every 3-5 minutes; if this approach fails, alternative regimens include:

Intermediate: 2-5 mg every 3-5 minutes

Escalating: 1 mg, 3 mg, 5 mg at 3-minute intervals

High: 0.1 mg/kg every 3-5 minutes

Intratracheal: 1 mg (although the optimal dose is unknown, doses of 2-2.5 times the I.V. dose may be needed)

I.M., S.C.: 0.1-0.5 mg every 10-15 minutes

Continuous I.V. infusion rate: Initial: 1 mcg/minute (range: 1-10 mcg/minute); titrate dosage to desired effect

Ophthalmic: Instill 1-2 drops in eye(s) once or twice daily; when treating open-angle glaucoma, the concentration and dosage must be adjusted to the response of the patient

Administration

Inhalation: Nebulization: Dilute in 3 mL NS

Nasal: Apply as drops or with sterile swab

Ophthalmic: Instill drops into affected eye(s); avoid contacting bottle tip with skin or eye

Oral inhalation: Shake well before use; use spacer in children <8 years of age

Parenteral:

Direct I.V. administration: Dilute to a maximum concentration of 100 mcg/mL (if using 1:10,000 concentration, no dilution is necessary)

Continuous I.V. infusion: Rate of infusion (mL/hour) = dose (mcg/kg/minute) x weight (kg) x 60 minutes/hour divided by the concentration (mcg/mL); maximum concentration: 64 mcg/mL

I.M. (EpiPen® and EpiPen® Jr): Intramuscularly into anterolateral aspect of thigh

S.C.: Use only 1:1000 solution or 1:200 suspension

Monitoring Parameters
Heart rate, blood pressure, site of infusion for excessive blanching/extravasation

Nursing Implications
Tissue irritant; extravasation may be treated by local small injections of a diluted phentolamine solution (mix 5 mg with 9 mL NS)

Dosage Forms

Aerosol, oral:

Bitartrate (AsthmaHaler® Mist, Bronitin® Mist, Medihaler-Epi®, Primatene® Mist Suspension): 0.3 mg/spray [epinephrine base 0.16 mg/spray] (10 mL, 15 mL, 22.5 mL)

Bronkaid® Mist: 0.5% (10 mL, 15 mL, 22.5 mL)

Primatene® Mist: 0.2 mg/spray (15 mL, 22.5 mL)

Emergency kit, auto-injector:

EpiPen®: Delivers 0.3 mg I.M. of epinephrine 1:1000 (2 mL)

EpiPen® Jr.: Delivers 0.15 mg I.M. of epinephrine 1:2000 (2 mL)

Solution:

Inhalation:

Adrenalin®: 1% [10 mg/mL - 1:100] (7.5 mL)

AsthmaNefrin®, microNefrin®, Nephron®: Racepinephrine 2% [epinephrine base 1.125%] (7.5 mL, 15 mL, 30 mL)

Vaponefrin®: Racepinephrine 2% [epinephrine base 1%] (15 mL, 30 mL)

Injection: 0.01 mg/mL [1:100,000] (5 mL); 0.1 mg/mL [1:10,000] (3 mL, 10 mL); 1 mg/mL [1:1000] (1 mL, 2 mL, 30 mL)

Adrenalin®: 1 mg/mL [1:1000] (1 mL, 30 mL)

Nasal (Adrenalin®): 0.1% [1 mg/mL - 1:1000] (30 mL)

Ophthalmic, as hydrochloride: 0.1% (1 mL)

Epifrin®, Glaucon®: 0.1% (1 mL, 30 mL); 0.5% (15 mL); 1% (1mL, 10 mL, 15 mL); 2% (10 mL, 15mL)

Topical (Adrenalin®): 0.1% [1 mg/mL, 1:1000] (10 mL, 30 mL)

Suspension for injection (Sus-Phrine®): 5 mg/mL [1:200] (0.3 mL, 5 mL)

References

American College of Cardiology, American Heart Association Task Force, "Adult Advanced Cardiac Life Support" and "Pediatric Advanced Life Support Guidelines," *JAMA*, 1992, 268(16):2199-241 and 2262-75.

Waisman Y, Klein BL, Boenning DA, et al, "Prospective Randomized Double-Blind Study Comparing L-Epinephrine and Racemic Epinephrine Aerosols in the Treatment of Laryngotracheitis (Croup)," *Pediatrics*, 1992, 89(2):302-6.

- ♦ **Epinephrine and Lidocaine** *see Lidocaine and Epinephrine on page 570*
- ♦ **Epinephrine Bitartrate** *see Epinephrine on page 371*
- ♦ **Epinephrine Hydrochloride** *see Epinephrine on page 371*
- ♦ **EpiPen®** *see Epinephrine on page 371*
- ♦ **EpiPen® Jr** *see Epinephrine on page 371*
- ♦ **Epitol®** *see Carbamazepine on page 165*
- ♦ **Epivir®** *see Lamivudine on page 552*
- ♦ **Epivir-HBV®** *see Lamivudine on page 552*
- ♦ **EPO** *see Epoetin Alfa on page 373*

Epoetin Alfa (e POE e tin AL fa)

Brand Names Epogen®; Eprex® (Canada); Procrit®

Synonyms EPO; Erythropoietin; rHuEPO; rHuEPO-α

Therapeutic Category Colony-Stimulating Factor; Recombinant Human Erythropoietin

Generic Available No

Use Anemia associated with end-stage renal disease; anemia in cancer patients with nonmyeloid malignancies on chemotherapy; anemia related to AIDS and therapy with zidovudine-treated, HIV-infected patients; endogenous serum erythropoietin (EPO) levels which are inappropriately low for hemoglobin level (eg, anemia of neoplasia); anemia of prematurity; patients undergoing autologous blood donation prior to surgery (EPO may accelerate recovery of hemoglobin level and, in some cases, permit more units of blood to be donated)

Pregnancy Risk Factor C

Contraindications Hypersensitivity to albumin (human) or mammalian cell-derived products; uncontrolled hypertension; neutropenia in newborns

Warnings The multidose formulation contains benzyl alcohol; avoid use in neonates. Pooled use of unused portions of preservative-free EPO has resulted in microbial contamination, bacteremia, and pyrogenic reactions. Preservative-free formulations are intended for single use only.

Precautions Use with caution in patients with porphyria or a history of seizures. Decrease the EPO dose if an increase in hematocrit exceeds 4 points in any 2-week period. EPO is not intended for patients who require acute corrections of anemia and is not a substitute for emergency blood transfusion.

Assessment of iron stores and therapeutic iron supplementation is essential to optimal EPO therapy. Iron supplementation is necessary to provide for increased (Continued)

Epoetin Alfa *(Continued)*

requirements during expansion of the red cell mass secondary to marrow stimulation by EPO, unless iron stores are already in excess.

Factors Limiting Response to Epoetin Alfa

Factor	Mechanism
Iron deficiency	Limits hemoglobin synthesis
Blood loss/hemolysis	Counteracts epoetin alfa-stimulated erythropoiesis
Infection/inflammation	Inhibits iron transfer from storage to bone marrow
	Suppresses erythropoiesis through activated macrophages
Aluminum overload	Inhibits iron incorporation into heme protein
Bone marrow replacement Hyperparathyroidsm Metastatic, neoplastic	Limits bone marrow volume
Folic acid/vitamin B$_{12}$ deficiency	Limits hemoglobin synthesis
Patient compliance	Self-administered epoetin alfa or iron therapy

Adverse Reactions

Cardiovascular: Hypertension, edema, chest pain, myocardial infarction, CVA/TIA
Central nervous system: Fatigue, dizziness, headache, seizure, fever
Dermatologic: Rash, urticaria
Local: Pain, irritation at injection site (S.C. injection)
Gastrointestinal: Nausea, diarrhea, vomiting
Hematologic: Neutropenia
Neuromuscular & skeletal: Arthralgias, weakness
Respiratory: Cough
Miscellaneous: Hypersensitivity reactions

Stability Refrigerate; single-dose vials contain no preservatives; discard after entry (see Warnings). Multiple-dose vials contain benzyl alcohol preservative and are stable 2 weeks at room temperature and when refrigerated, may be used up to 21 days after initial entry. EPO is stable for 24 hours when diluted in dextrose I.V. fluid which contains at least 0.05% human albumin or parenteral nutrition solutions containing at least 0.5% amino acids. EPO may be diluted with NS or bacteriostatic NS in a 1:1 ratio at the time of S.C. administration.

Mechanism of Action Epoetin alfa, a glycoprotein manufactured by recombinant DNA technology, has the same effects as endogenous erythropoietin. EPO induces erythropoiesis by stimulating the division and differentiation of committed erythroid progenitor cells. It induces the release of reticulocytes from the bone marrow into the bloodstream, where they mature to erythrocytes (dose response relationship) resulting in an increase in reticulocyte counts followed by a rise in hematocrit and hemoglobin levels. There is normally an inverse correlation between the plasma EPO level and the hemoglobin concentration (only when the hemoglobin concentration is <10.5 g/dL).

Pharmacodynamics

Onset of action: Several days
Peak effect: 2-6 weeks

Pharmacokinetics

Absorption: S.C.: 31.9%
Distribution: Adults: V$_d$: 9 L; rapid in the plasma compartment; majority of drug is taken up by the liver, kidneys, and bone marrow
Bioavailability: S.C.: ~21% to 31%
Half-life:
Neonates: S.C.: 17.6 hours on day 3 of therapy, 11.2 hours on day 10 of therapy
Adults: 4-13 hours in patients with chronic renal failure (CRF); half-life is 20% shorter in patients with normal renal function
Time to peak serum concentration: S.C.: 5-24 hours
Elimination: Some metabolic degradation does occur with small amounts recovered in the urine
Clearance: Neonates: S.C. or continuous I.V. infusion: 26-35 mL/hour/kg on day 3 of therapy and 65-87 mL/hour/kg on day 10 of therapy
Note: While a much higher peak plasma concentration is achieved after I.V. bolus administration, it declines at a more rapid rate (over 2-3 days) than after subcutaneous administration (plasma concentrations greater than endogenous are maintained for at least 4 days). Subcutaneous administration is associated with a 30% to 50% lower EPO dose requirement.

Usual Dosage Dosing schedules need to be individualized and careful monitoring of patients receiving the drug is recommended. EPO may be ineffective if other factors such as iron or B_{12}/folate deficiency limit marrow response. Dosage based upon S.C. administration; use of I.V. administration may result in the need to increase doses by as much as 30% to 50% to achieve the same outcome: I.V., S.C.:

Neonates: Anemia of prematurity: Variable regimens: 25-100 units/kg/dose 3 times/week **or** 100 units/kg/dose 5 times/week **or** 200 units/kg/dose every other day for 10 doses

Children and Adults:

Anemia in cancer patients: 150 units/kg/dose 3 times/week; maximum 1200 units/kg/week

Anemia in chronic renal failure: 50-150 units/kg/dose 3 times/week

Note: Once weekly dosage has been studied in chronic renal failure patients. When transitioning from multiple doses/week to once weekly, begin with a weekly dosage equal to the current total dose per week. Allow at least 4 weeks to determine full effects of the new regimen.

Epoetin Alfa Dosage Adjustments

Target hematocrit range	30% to 33% (maximum 36%)
Reduce dose when	Target range is reached **or** hematocrit increases >4 points in any 2-week period
Increase dose when	Hematocrit does not increase by 5-6 points after 8 weeks of therapy **and** hematocrit is below target range
Stop therapy when	Hematocrit ≥40%; reinstate therapy at a lower dose after the hematocrit decreases to 36%
Maintenance dose (chronic renal failure)	Individualize: General dosage range: 25 units/kg 3 times/week

Zidovudine-treated, HIV-infected patients: Initial: 100 units/kg/dose 3 times/week for 8 weeks; after 8 weeks of therapy the dose may be adjusted by 50-100 units/kg increments 3 times/week to a maximum dose of 300 units/kg 3 times/week

Presurgery, autologous blood donation: Adults: 300 units/kg/day for 10 days before surgery, the day of surgery, and 4 days after **or as an alternative**, 600 units/kg/week at 21-, 14-, and 7 days before surgery and on the day of surgery

Administration Parenteral:

S.C. is the preferred route of administration; 1:1 dilution with bacteriostatic NS (containing benzyl alcohol) acts as a local anesthetic to reduce pain at the injection site. Multiple-dose vials already contain benzyl alcohol.

I.V.: Dilute with an equal volume of NS and infuse over 1-3 minutes; it may be administered into the venous line at the end of the dialysis procedure

Monitoring Parameters

Careful monitoring of blood pressure is indicated; problems with hypertension have been noted especially in renal failure patients treated with rHuEPO. Other patients are less likely to develop this complication. See table.

Test	Initial Phase Frequency	Maintenance Phase Frequency
Hematocrit/hemoglobin	2 times/week	2-4 times/month
Blood pressure	3 times/week	3 times/week
Serum ferritin	Monthly	Quarterly
Transferrin saturation	Monthly	Quarterly
Serum chemistries including CBC with differential, creatinine, blood urea nitrogen, potassium, phosphorous	Regularly per routine	Regularly per routine
Reticulocyte count	Baseline prior to starting therapy	After 10 days of therapy

Hematocrit should be determined twice weekly until stabilization within the target range (30% to 36%), and twice weekly for at least 2-6 weeks after a dose increase.

Reference Range The decision to initiate EPO therapy may be made by utilizing an endogenous erythropoietin serum level measurement. Endogenous erythropoietin (Continued)

Epoetin Alfa *(Continued)*

levels are inversely related to the hemoglobin (and hematocrit) level in anemias that are not attributed to impaired erythropoietin production (eg, iron deficiency anemia). A normal erythropoietin level, for subjects with normal hemoglobin and hematocrit, is 4.1-22.2 mIU/mL. Baseline erythropoietin levels in anemic patients may increase up to 100-1000 fold in untreated patients with a normal release of erythropoietin. The following table illustrates the "normal" response to anemia. EPO is indicated in patients who do not exhibit a normal response to anemia (eg, the measurement of endogenous erythropoietin is low relative to a normal response). If the patient has exhibited a normal response, addition of exogenous EPO may not be beneficial. Clinical studies involving the following disease states have established criteria for assessment of endogenous erythropoietin levels prior to initiating EPO therapy:

Zidovudine-treated HIV patients: Available evidence indicates patients with endogenous serum erythropoietin levels >500 mIU/mL are unlikely to respond

Cancer chemotherapy patients: Treatment of patients with endogenous serum erythropoietin levels >200 mIU/mL is not recommended.

Inverse Relationship of Endogenous Erythropoietin to Hemoglobin

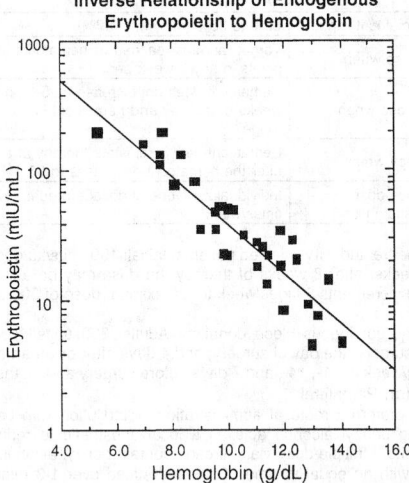

Patient Information Frequent blood tests are needed to determine the correct dose; notify physician if any severe headache develops; due to increased risk of seizure activity in CRF patients during the first 90 days of therapy, avoid potentially hazardous activities (eg, driving during this period)

Additional Information Do not shake as this may denature the glycoprotein rendering the drug biologically inactive; optimal response is achieved when iron stores are maintained with supplemental iron if necessary; evaluate iron stores prior to and during therapy

Reimbursement Hotline (Epogen®): 1-800-272-9376
Professional Services [Amgen]: 1-800-77-AMGEN
Reimbursement Hotline (Procrit®): 1-800-553-3851
Professional Services [Ortho Biotech]: 1-800-325-7504

Dosage Forms

Injection, preservative free: 2000 units (1 mL); 3000 units (1 mL); 4000 units (1 mL); 10,000 units (1 mL)

Injection, with preservative: 10,000 units/mL (2 mL); 20,000 units/mL (1 mL); 40,000 units/mL (1 mL)

References

Blanche S, Caniglia M, Fischer A, et al, "Zidovudine Therapy in Children With Acquired Immunodeficiency Syndrome," *Am J Med*, 1988, 85(2A):203-7.

Halperin DS, Wacker P, Lacourt G, et al, "Effects of Recombinant Human Erythropoietin in Infants With the Anemia of Prematurity: A Pilot Study," *J Pediatr*, 1990, 116(5):779-86.

Ohls RK and Christensen, RD, "Stability of Human Recombinant Epoetin Alfa in Commonly Used Neonatal Intravenous Solutions," *Ann Pharmacother*, 1996, 30(5):466-468.

Ohls RK, Veerman MW, and Christensen RD, "Pharmacokinetics and Effectiveness of Recombinant Erythropoietin Administered to Preterm Infants by Continuous Infusion in Total Parenteral Nutrition Solution," *J Pediatr*, 1996, 128(4):518-23.

Rhondeau SM, Christensen RD, Ross MP, et al, "Responsiveness to Recombinant Human Erythropoietin of Marrow Erythroid Progenitors From Infants With the Anemia of Prematurity," *J Pediatr*, 1988, 112(6):935-40.

Shannon KM, Keith JF 3rd, Mentzer WC, et al, "Recombinant Human Erythropoietin Stimulates Erythropoiesis and Reduces Erythrocyte Transfusions in Very Low Birth Weight Preterm Infants," *Pediatrics*, 1995, 95(1):1-8.

Sinai-Trieman L, Salusky IB, and Fine RN, "Use of Subcutaneous Recombinant Human Erythropoietin in Children Undergoing Continuous Cycling Peritoneal Dialysis," *J Pediatr*, 1989, 114(4 Pt 1):550-4.

◆ **Epogen®** see Epoetin Alfa *on page 373*

◆ **Eprex® (Canada)** see Epoetin Alfa *on page 373*

◆ **Epsom Salts (Magnesium Sulfate)** see Magnesium Supplements *on page 588*

◆ **Equilet® [OTC]** see Calcium Supplements *on page 157*

◆ **Ercaf®** see Ergotamine *on page 378*

Ergocalciferol (er goe kal SIF e role)

Brand Names Calciferol™; Drisdol®; Ostoforte®(Canada); Radiostol® (Canada)

Synonyms Activated Ergosterol; Viosterol; Vitamin D_2

Therapeutic Category Nutritional Supplement; Vitamin D Analog; Vitamin, Fat Soluble

Generic Available Yes

Use Refractory rickets; hypophosphatemia; hypoparathyroidism

Pregnancy Risk Factor A (C if dose exceeds RDA recommendation)

Contraindications Hypercalcemia; hypersensitivity to ergocalciferol or any component; malabsorption syndrome; evidence of vitamin D toxicity

Precautions Use with caution in patients with coronary artery disease, renal stones, and impaired renal function; adequate calcium intake is necessary for clinical response to ergocalciferol therapy; maintain adequate fluid intake; avoid hypercalcemia

Adverse Reactions
Cardiovascular: Hypertension, arrhythmias, hypotension
Central nervous system: Drowsiness, irritability, headache, psychosis
Dermatologic: Pruritus
Endocrine & metabolic: Mild acidosis, hypercholesterolemia, polydipsia
Gastrointestinal: Nausea, vomiting, anorexia, constipation, metallic taste, xerostomia, pancreatitis, weight loss
Genitourinary: Albuminuria, nocturia, polyuria
Neuromuscular & skeletal: Weakness, myalgia, bone pain
Ocular: Photophobia
Renal: Polyuria, nephrocalcinosis

Drug Interactions May antagonize the effects of calcium channel blockers by increasing serum calcium level; may be associated with digoxin toxicity by increasing calcium levels; may result in an additive increase in calcium levels due to decreased calcium excretion by thiazide diuretics; magnesium-containing antacids (potential development of hypermagnesemia); cholestyramine, colestipol, orlistat, and excessive use of mineral oil decrease absorption

Stability Protect from light

Mechanism of Action Vitamin D stimulates calcium and phosphate absorption from the small intestine; promotes secretion of calcium from bone to blood; promotes renal tubule phosphate resorption; acts directly on bone cells (osteoblasts) to stimulate skeletal growth and on the parathyroid glands to suppress PTH synthesis and secretion

Pharmacodynamics Peak effect occurs in ~1 month following daily doses

Pharmacokinetics
Absorption: Readily absorbed from GI tract; absorption requires intestinal presence of bile
Metabolism: Inactive until hydroxylated in the liver and the kidney to calcifediol and then to calcitriol (most active form)

Usual Dosage Oral dosing is preferred; use I.M. only in patients with GI, liver, or biliary disease associated with malabsorption of vitamin D:
Adequate Intake (AI) (1997 National Academy of Science Recommendations):
Neonates, Children and Adults: 200 international units/day

Dietary supplementation (each mcg = 40 USP units):
Premature infants: 10-20 mcg/day (400-800 units), up to 750 mcg/day (30,000 units)
Infants and healthy Children: 10 mcg/day (400 units)
Adults: 10 mcg/day (400 units)
(Continued)

Ergocalciferol *(Continued)*

Renal failure:
Children: 100-1000 mcg/day (4000-40,000 units)
Adults: 500 mcg/day (20,000 units)
Hypoparathyroidism:
Children: 1.25-5 mg/day (50,000-200,000 units) with calcium supplements
Adults: 625 mcg to 5 mg/day (25,000-200,000 units) with calcium supplements
Vitamin D-dependent rickets:
Children: 75-125 mcg/day (3000-5000 units); maximum dose: 1500 mcg/day
Adults: 250 mcg to 1.5 mg/day (10,000-60,000 units)
Nutritional rickets and osteomalacia:
Children and Adults (with normal absorption): 25-125 mcg/day (1000-5000 units)
for 6-12 weeks
Children with malabsorption: 250-625 mcg/day (10,000-25,000 units)
Adults with malabsorption: 250-7500 mcg/day (10,000-300,000 units)
Vitamin D-resistant rickets:
Children: Initial: 1000-2000 mcg/day (40,000-80,000 units) with phosphate
supplements; daily dosage is increased at 3- to 4-month intervals in 250-500
mcg (10,000-20,000 units) increments
Adults: 250-1500 mcg/day (10,000-60,000 units) with phosphate supplements

Administration
Oral: May be administered without regard to meals; for oral liquid, use accompanying dropper for dosage measurements
Parenteral: Injection for I.M. use only

Monitoring Parameters Serum calcium and phosphorus levels; alkaline phosphatase, BUN; bone x-ray (hypophosphatemia or hypoparathyroidism)

Reference Range Serum calcium times serum phosphorus should not exceed 70 mg/dL to avoid ectopic calcification; ergocalciferol levels: 10-60 ng/mL

Additional Information 1.25 mg ergocalciferol provides 50,000 units of vitamin D activity; 1 drop of 8000 units/mL = 200 units (40 drops = 1 mL)

Dosage Forms
Capsule (Drisdol®): 50,000 units [1.25 mg]
Injection (Calciferol™): 500,000 units/mL [12.5 mg/mL] (1 mL)
Liquid (Calciferol™, Drisdol®): 8000 units/mL [200 mcg/mL] (60 mL)
Tablet (Calciferol™): 50,000 units [1.25 mg]

References
"Dietary Reference Intakes for Calcium, Phosphorus, Magnesium, Vitamin D, and Fluoride. Standing Committee on the Scientific Evaluation of Dietary Reference Intakes, Food and Nutrition Board, Institute of Medicine," National Academy of Sciences, Washington, DC: National Academy Press, 1997.

♦ **Ergomar®** *see Ergotamine on page 378*
♦ **Ergomar® (Canada)** *see Ergotamine on page 378*

Ergotamine *(er GOT a meen)*

Related Information
Drugs and Breast-Feeding *on page 1213*
Overdose and Toxicology *on page 1191*

Brand Names Cafatine-PB®; Cafergot®; Cafetrate®; Ercaf®; Ergomar®; Ergomar® (Canada); Ergotamine Tartrate and Caffeine Cafatine®; Gynergen® (Canada); Phenerbel-S®; Wigraine®

Available Salts Ergotamine Tartrate; Ergotamine Tartrate and Caffeine

Synonyms Ergotamine and Caffeine

Therapeutic Category Alpha-Adrenergic Blocking Agent, Oral; Antimigraine Agent; Ergot Alkaloid and Derivative

Generic Available Yes

Use Prevent or abort vascular headaches, such as migraine or cluster

Pregnancy Risk Factor X

Contraindications Hypersensitivity to ergotamine, caffeine, or any component; peripheral vascular disease, hepatic or renal disease, hypertension, peptic ulcer disease, sepsis, coronary heart disease

Warnings Avoid during pregnancy; patients who take ergotamine for extended periods of time may become dependent on it; may be harmful due to reduction in cerebral blood flow; may precipitate angina, MI, or aggravate intermittent claudication

Precautions Avoid prolonged administration or excessive dosage because of the danger of ergotism and gangrene

Adverse Reactions

Cardiovascular: Angina-like precordial pain, transient tachycardia or bradycardia, vasospasm, vasoconstriction, claudication

Central nervous system: Rebound headaches (with abrupt withdrawal), drowsiness, dizziness

Dermatologic: Pruritus

Gastrointestinal: Nausea, vomiting, diarrhea, xerostomia

Local: Edema

Neuromuscular & skeletal: Leg cramps, myalgia, weakness, paresthesia of the extremities

Drug Interactions Increased peripheral ischemia with macrolides, enhanced vasoconstriction with beta-blocking agents; increased vasoconstrictor effects with methysergide

Food Interactions Caffeine may increase GI absorption of ergotamine

Mechanism of Action Ergot alkaloid alpha-adrenergic blocker directly stimulates vascular smooth muscle to vasoconstrict peripheral and cerebral vessels; may also have antagonist effects on serotonin

Pharmacokinetics

Absorption: Oral, rectal: Erratic; absorption is enhanced by caffeine coadministration

Metabolism: Extensive in the liver

Bioavailability: Poor overall (<5%)

Time to peak serum concentration: Oral: Within 0.5-3 hours

Elimination: In bile as metabolites (90%)

Usual Dosage

Older Children and Adolescents: Oral, S.L.: 1 mg at onset of attack; then 1 mg every 30 minutes as needed, up to a maximum of 3 mg per attack

Adults:

Oral:

Cafergot®: 2 mg at onset of attack; then 1-2 mg every 30 minutes as needed; maximum dose: 6 mg per attack; do not exceed 10 mg/week

Ergomar®: 1 tablet under tongue at first sign, then 1 tablet every 30 minutes; maximum: 3 tablets/24 hours, 5 tablets/week

Rectal, suppositories (Cafergot®, Wigraine®, Cafatine®): 1 suppository at first sign of an attack; follow with second dose after 1 hour, if needed; maximum dose: 2 per attack; do not exceed 5/week

Administration Place sublingual tablets under tongue; oral tablets may be taken without regard to meals

Patient Information Any symptoms such as nausea, vomiting, numbness or tingling, and chest, muscle, or abdominal pain should be reported to the physician at the first sign of an attack; do **not** exceed recommended dosage; avoid coffee, tea, and cola

Dosage Forms

Suppository, rectal (Cafatine®, Cafergot®, Cafetrate®, Wigraine®): Ergotamine tartrate 2 mg and caffeine 100 mg (12s)

Tablet (Ercaf®, Wigraine®): Ergotamine tartrate 1 mg and caffeine 100 mg

Tablet, sublingual (Ergomar®): Ergotamine tartrate 2 mg

Erythromycin (er ith roe MYE sin)

Related Information

Carbohydrate and Alcohol Content of Liquid Medications for Use in Patients Receiving Ketogenic Diets on page 1228

(Continued)

Erythromycin *(Continued)*

Brand Names AK-Mycin®; Akne-Mycin®; Apo®-Erythro E-C (Canada); A/T/S®; C-Solve-2®; Diomycin (Canada); E.E.S.®; E.E.S. 400®; E.E.S.® Chewable; E.E.S.® Granules; Emgel®; E-Mycin®; E-Mycin-E®; Erybid™ (Canada); Eryc®; Erycette®; EryDerm®; Erygel®; Erymax®; Ery-Tab®; Erythro-Base® (Canada); Erythrocin®; E-Solve-2®; ETS-2%®; Ilosone®; Ilosone® Pulvules®; Ilotycin®; Ilotycin® (Canada); Novo-Rythro Encap (Canada); PCE®; PMS-Erythromycin (Canada); Staticin®; T-Stat®; Wyamycin® S

Available Salts Erythromycin Estolate; Erythromycin Ethylsuccinate; Erythromycin Glucepate; Erythromycin Lactobionate; Erythromycin Stearate

Synonyms Erythromycin Base

Therapeutic Category Antibiotic, Macrolide; Antibiotic, Ophthalmic

Generic Available Yes

Use Treatment of mild to moderately severe infections of the upper and lower respiratory tract, pharyngitis and skin infections due to susceptible streptococci and staphylococci; other susceptible bacterial infections including *Mycoplasma pneumoniae*, *Legionella* pneumonia, Lyme disease, diphtheria, pertussis, chancroid, *Chlamydia*, and *Campylobacter* gastroenteritis; used in conjunction with neomycin for decontaminating the bowel for surgery; ophthalmic ointment used to prevent gonococcal ophthalmia neonatorum

Pregnancy Risk Factor B

Contraindications Hepatic impairment; concomitant administration with astemizole, terfenadine, or cisapride; hypersensitivity to erythromycin or any component

Warnings Hepatic impairment with or without jaundice has occurred primarily in older children and adults; it may be accompanied by malaise, nausea, vomiting, abdominal colic, and fever; discontinue use if these occur; avoid using erythromycin lactobionate in neonates since formulation may contain benzyl alcohol which is associated with a fatal gasping syndrome in neonates; risk of serious cardiac arrhythmias exist in patients receiving erythromycin and astemizole, terfenadine, or cisapride (do not use concurrently with erythromycin)

Adverse Reactions

Cardiovascular: Ventricular arrhythmias, prolongation of the Q-T interval; bradycardia, hypotension with I.V. administration

Central nervous system: Fever, dizziness

Dermatologic: Skin rash, pruritus

Gastrointestinal: Abdominal pain, cramping, nausea, vomiting, diarrhea, stomatitis

Hematologic: Eosinophilia

Hepatic: Cholestatic hepatitis, jaundice; (incidence of erythromycin-associated hepatotoxicity is ~0.1% in children and 0.25% in adults)

Local: Thrombophlebitis (I.V. form)

Otic: Ototoxicity (after I.V. use)

Miscellaneous: Allergic reactions, anaphylaxis

Drug Interactions Erythromycin decreases clearance of astemizole, terfenadine, carbamazepine, cisapride, cyclosporine, midazolam, phenytoin, and triazolam; erythromycin may decrease theophylline clearance, increase theophylline's half-life by up to 60%, and result in theophylline toxicity (patients on high dose theophylline and erythromycin or who have received erythromycin for >5 days may be at higher risk); may potentiate anticoagulant effect of warfarin; may increase toxicity of ergotamine; may increase serum levels of digoxin, disopyramide, and quinidine

Stability Erythromycin lactobionate should be reconstituted with sterile water for injection without preservatives to avoid gel formation; the reconstituted solution is stable for 2 weeks when refrigerated or 24 hours at room temperature. Erythromycin I.V. infusion solution is stable at pH 6-8.

Mechanism of Action Inhibits bacterial RNA-dependent protein synthesis at the chain elongation step; binds to the 50S ribosomal subunit resulting in blockage of transpeptidation

Pharmacokinetics

Absorption: Variable but better with salt forms like the estolate than with base form; 18% to 45% absorbed orally; ethylsuccinate may be better absorbed with food

Distribution: Crosses the placenta; distributes into body tissues, fluids, and breast milk with poor penetration into the CSF

V_d: 0.64 L/kg

Protein binding: 75% to 90%

Metabolism: In the liver by demethylation

Half-life:

Neonates (≤15 days of age): 2.1 hours

Adults: 1.5-2 hours

Time to peak serum concentration: Oral:
  Base: 4 hours
  Stearate: 3 hours
  Ethylsuccinate: 0.5-2.5 hours
  Estolate: 2-4 hours (time to peak is delayed in the presence of food except when using estolate)
Elimination: 2% to 5% unchanged drug excreted in urine, major excretion in feces (via bile); not removed by peritoneal dialysis or hemodialysis

Usual Dosage

Neonates:
  Oral: Ethylsuccinate: Postnatal age:
    ≤7 days: 20 mg/kg/day in divided doses every 12 hours
    >7 days, <1200 g: 20 mg/kg/day in divided doses every 12 hours
    >7 days, 1200-2000 g: 30 mg/kg/day in divided doses every 8 hours
    >7 days, >2000 g: 30-40 mg/kg/day in divided doses every 6-8 hours
  Ophthalmic: Prophylaxis of neonatal gonococcal ophthalmia: 0.5-1 cm ribbon of ointment should be instilled into each conjunctival sac once
  I.V.: One study (n=14, ≤15 days of age, birth weight ≤1500 g) used erythromycin lactobionate in doses of 25 or 40 mg/kg/day divided every 6 hours for treatment of *Ureaplasma urealyticum* infection
  Chlamydial conjunctivitis and pneumonia: Oral: Ethylsuccinate: 50 mg/kg/day divided every 6 hours for 14 days
Infants and Children:
  Oral:
    Base and ethylsuccinate: 30-50 mg/kg/day divided every 6-8 hours; do not exceed 2 g/day (as base) or 3.2 g/day (as ethylsuccinate); **(Note:** Due to differences in absorption, 200 mg erythromycin ethylsuccinate produces the same serum levels as 125 mg erythromycin base or estolate)
    Estolate: 30-50 mg/kg/day divided every 6-12 hours; do not exceed 2 g/day
    Stearate: 30-50 mg/kg/day divided every 6 hours; do not exceed 2 g/day
  Chlamydia trachomatis: Oral: 50 mg/kg/day divided every 6 hours for 10-14 days
  Pertussis: Oral: 40-50 mg/kg/day divided every 6 hours for 14 days (some experts recommend using the estolate salt)
  Preop bowel preparation: Oral: 20 mg/kg erythromycin base at 1, 2, and 11 PM on the day before surgery combined with mechanical cleansing of the large intestine and oral neomycin
  I.V.:
    Lactobionate: 15-50 mg/kg/day divided every 6 hours, not to exceed 4 g/day
    Gluceptate: 15-50 mg/kg/day divided every 6 hours, not to exceed 4 g/day
Children and Adults:
  Ophthalmic: Instill ointment one or more times daily depending on the severity of the infection
  Topical: Apply 2% solution over the affected area twice daily after the skin has been thoroughly washed and patted dry
Adults:
  Oral:
    Base, delayed release: 333 mg every 8 hours
    Estolate, stearate or base: 250-500 mg every 6-12 hours
    Ethylsuccinate: 400-800 mg every 6-12 hours
  Chancroid: Oral: Base: 500 mg 4 times/day for 7 days
  Chlamydia trachomatis: Oral:
    Base: 500 mg 4 times/day for 7 days **or**
    Ethylsuccinate: 800 mg 4 times/day for 7 days
  Preop bowel preparation: Oral: 1 g erythromycin base at 1, 2, and 11 PM on the day before surgery combined with mechanical cleansing of the large intestine and oral neomycin
  I.V.: Lactobionate or gluceptate: 15-20 mg/kg/day divided every 6 hours or given as a continuous infusion over 24 hours, not to exceed 4 g/day
Prokinetic agent (to improve gastric emptying time and intestinal motility):
  Children: Lactobionate or gluceptate: Initial: 3 mg/kg I.V. infused over 60 minutes followed by 20 mg/kg/day orally in 3-4 divided doses before meals, or before meals and at bedtime
  Adults: Lactobionate or gluceptate: Initial: 200 mg I.V. followed by 250 mg orally 3 times/day 30 minutes before meals

Administration

Ophthalmic ointment for prevention of neonatal ophthalmia: Wipe each eyelid gently with sterile cotton; instill 0.5-1 cm ribbon of ointment in each lower conjunctival sac; massage eyelids gently to spread the ointment; after 1 minute, excess ointment can be wiped away with sterile cotton
(Continued)

Erythromycin *(Continued)*

Oral: Avoid milk and acidic beverages 1 hour before or after a dose; administer after food to decrease GI discomfort; ethylsuccinate chewable tablets should not be swallowed whole; do not chew delayed release capsule or enteric coated tablets, swallow whole

Parenteral: Administer by I.V. intermittent or continuous infusion diluted in either dextrose or saline solutions to a concentration of 1-2.5 mg/mL; maximum concentration: 5 mg/mL; I.V. intermittent infusions may be administered over 20-60 minutes; to decrease vein irritation, administer as a continuous infusion at a concentration ≤1 mg/mL; prolonging the infusion duration over 60 minutes or longer has been recommended to decrease the cardiotoxic effects of erythromycin

Monitoring Parameters Liver function tests

Test Interactions False-positive urinary catecholamines, 17-hydroxycorticosteroids and 17-ketosteroids

Nursing Implications Do not crush enteric coated or delayed release drug products

Additional Information Treatment of erythromycin-associated cardiac toxicity with prolongation of the Q-T interval and ventricular tachydysrhythmias includes discontinuing erythromycin and administering magnesium.

Dosage Forms

Capsule, as estolate: 125 mg, 250 mg

Capsule, delayed release: 250 mg

Injection, gluceptate: 1 g (30 mL)

Injection, lactobionate: 500 mg, 1 g

Gel, topical: 2% (30 g)

Ointment, ophthalmic: 5 mg/g (3.5 g)

Ointment, topical: 2% (25 g)

Solution, topical: 1.5% (60 mL); 2% (60 mL)

Suspension:

Oral, as estolate: 125 mg/5 mL (480 mL); 250 mg/5 mL (480 mL)

Oral, as ethylsuccinate: 200 mg/5 mL (480 mL); 400 mg/5 mL (480 mL)

Oral drops, as estolate: 100 mg/mL (10 mL)

Oral drops, as ethylsuccinate: 100 mg/2.5 mL (30 mL)

Swab: 2% (60s)

Tablet:

Chewable, as estolate: 125 mg, 250 mg

Chewable, as ethylsuccinate: 200 mg

Delayed release, as base: 250 mg, 333 mg, 500 mg

Film coated: 250 mg, 500 mg

Film coated, as ethylsuccinate: 400 mg

Film coated, as stearate: 250 mg, 500 mg

Polymer coated particles, as base: 333 mg

Polymer coated particles, as estolate: 500 mg

References

Di Lorenzo C, Lachman R, and Hyman PE, "Intravenous Erythromycin for Postpyloric Intubation," *J Pediatr Gastroenterol Nutr*, 1990, 11(1):45-7.

Janssens J, Peeters TL, Vantrappen G, et al, "Improvement of Gastric Emptying in Diabetic Gastroparesis by Erythromycin," *N Engl J Med*, 1990, 322(15):1028-31.

Reid B, DiLorenzo C, Travis L, et al, "Diabetic Gastroparesis Due to Postprandial Antral Hypomotility in Childhood," *Pediatrics*, 1992, 90(1 Pt 1):43-6.

Thoene DE and Johnson CE, "Pharmacotherapy of Otitis Media," *Pharmacotherapy*, 1991, 11(3):212-21.

Waites KB, Sims PJ, Crouse DT, et al, "Serum Concentrations of Erythromycin After Intravenous Infusion in Preterm Neonates Treated for *Ureaplasma urealyticum* Infection," *Pediatr Infect Dis J*, 1994, 13(4):287-93.

Erythromycin and Sulfisoxazole

(er ith roe MYE sin & sul fi SOKS a zole)

Related Information

Carbohydrate and Alcohol Content of Liquid Medications for Use in Patients Receiving Ketogenic Diets *on page 1228*

Brand Names Eryzole®; Pediazole®; Sulfimycin®

Available Salts Erythromycin Ethylsuccinate and Sulfisoxazole Acetyl

Synonyms Sulfisoxazole and Erythromycin

Therapeutic Category Antibiotic, Macrolide; Antibiotic, Sulfonamide Derivative

Generic Available Yes

Use Treatment of susceptible bacterial infections of the upper and lower respiratory tract; otitis media in children caused by susceptible strains of *Haemophilus influenzae*; other infections in patients allergic to penicillin

Pregnancy Risk Factor C

Contraindications Hepatic dysfunction; hypersensitivity to erythromycin, any component, or sulfonamides; infants <2 months of age (sulfas compete with bilirubin for binding sites which may result in kernicterus in newborns); patients with porphyria; pregnant women at term; mothers nursing infants <2 months of age; concomitant administration of astemizole, terfenadine, or cisapride

Warnings Risk of serious cardiac arrhythmias exist in patients receiving erythromycin, astemizole, terfenadine, or cisapride (do not use concurrently); fatalities due to Stevens-Johnson syndrome, toxic epidermal necrolysis, fulminant hepatic necrosis, agranulocytosis, and aplastic anemia have occurred with the administration of sulfonamides; prolonged use may result in superinfection or pseudomembranous colitis

Precautions Use with caution in patients with impaired renal or hepatic function, G-6-PD deficiency (hemolysis may occur)

Adverse Reactions
Cardiovascular: Tachycardia, palpitations, syncope
Central nervous system: Headache, disorientation, fever, dizziness
Dermatologic: Rash, photosensitivity, Stevens-Johnson syndrome, toxic epidermal necrolysis, pruritus, urticaria
Gastrointestinal: Abdominal cramping, nausea, vomiting, diarrhea, pseudomembranous colitis, anorexia, stomatitis, pancreatitis
Genitourinary: Crystalluria, hematuria
Hematologic: Agranulocytosis, aplastic anemia, leukopenia, eosinophilia, thrombocytopenia
Hepatic: Hepatic necrosis, jaundice
Renal: Toxic nephrosis, elevated BUN and serum creatinine, acute renal failure
Respiratory: Cough, shortness of breath, pulmonary infiltrates
Miscellaneous: Anaphylaxis

Drug Interactions Erythromycin may decrease theophylline clearance, increase theophylline's half-life by up to 60%, and result in theophylline toxicity (patients on high doses of theophylline and erythromycin or on >5 days of erythromycin may be at higher risk); erythromycin inhibits carbamazepine metabolism; erythromycin decreases clearance of cyclosporine, triazolam, midazolam, phenytoin, digoxin, alfentanil, disopyramide, quinidine, cisapride, astemizole, and terfenadine; may potentiate anticoagulant effects of warfarin; may increase toxicity of ergotamine; sulfisoxazole may decrease the amount of thiopental needed for anesthesia; sulfisoxazole may displace methotrexate from plasma protein-binding sites increasing free methotrexate concentrations

Stability Reconstituted suspension is stable for 14 days when refrigerated

Mechanism of Action Erythromycin inhibits bacterial protein synthesis by binding to the 50S ribosomal subunit; sulfisoxazole competitively inhibits bacterial synthesis of folic acid from para-aminobenzoic acid

Pharmacokinetics
Erythromycin ethylsuccinate:
Absorption: Well absorbed from the GI tract
Distribution: Widely distributed into most body tissues and fluids; poor penetration into CSF; crosses the placenta; excreted in breast milk
Protein binding: 75% to 90%
Metabolism: In the liver by demethylation
Half-life: 1-1.5 hours
Elimination: Unchanged drug is excreted and concentrated in bile; <5% of dose eliminated in urine; not removed by peritoneal dialysis or hemodialysis
Sulfisoxazole acetyl:
Absorption: Hydrolyzed in the GI tract to sulfisoxazole which is rapidly and completely absorbed; the small intestine is the major site of absorption
Distribution: Into extracellular space; CSF concentration ranges from 8% to 57% of blood concentration in patients with normal meninges; crosses the placenta, excreted in breast milk
Protein binding: 85%
Metabolism: Undergoes N-acetylation and N-glucuronide conjugation in the liver
Half-life: 4.6-7.8 hours, prolonged in renal impairment
Elimination: 50% in urine as unchanged drug

Usual Dosage Oral (dosage recommendation is based on the product's erythromycin content):

Children ≥2 months: 40-50 mg/kg/day in divided doses every 6-8 hours; not to

(Continued)

Erythromycin and Sulfisoxazole *(Continued)*

exceed 2 g erythromycin or 6 g sulfisoxazole/day

Adults: 400 mg erythromycin and 1200 mg sulfisoxazole every 6 hours

Administration Oral: Administer with or without food; maintain adequate fluid intake to prevent crystalluria and kidney stone formation

Monitoring Parameters CBC, urinalysis; periodic liver function and renal function tests; observe patient for diarrhea

Test Interactions False-positive urinary protein; false-positive urinary catecholamines, 17-hydroxycorticosteroids and 17-ketosteroids

Patient Information Avoid prolonged exposure to sunlight

Dosage Forms Suspension, oral: Erythromycin ethylsuccinate 200 mg and sulfisoxazole acetyl 600 mg per 5 mL (100 mL, 150 mL, 200 mL, 250 mL)

References

Rodriguez WJ, Schwartz RH, Sait T, et al, "Erythromycin-Sulfisoxazole vs Amoxicillin in the Treatment of Acute Otitis Media in Children," *Am J Dis Child*, 1985, 139(8):766-70.

◆ **Erythromycin Base** *see* Erythromycin *on page 379*

◆ **Erythromycin Estolate** *see* Erythromycin *on page 379*

◆ **Erythromycin Ethylsuccinate** *see* Erythromycin *on page 379*

◆ **Erythromycin Ethylsuccinate and Sulfisoxazole Acetyl** *see* Erythromycin and Sulfisoxazole *on page 382*

◆ **Erythromycin Gluceptate** *see* Erythromycin *on page 379*

◆ **Erythromycin Lactobionate** *see* Erythromycin *on page 379*

◆ **Erythromycin Stearate** *see* Erythromycin *on page 379*

◆ **Erythropoietin** *see* Epoetin Alfa *on page 373*

◆ **Eryzole®** *see* Erythromycin and Sulfisoxazole *on page 382*

◆ **Eserine** *see* Physostigmine *on page 768*

◆ **Esidrix®** *see* Hydrochlorothiazide *on page 483*

◆ **Eskalith®** *see* Lithium *on page 577*

Esmolol *(ES moe lol)*

Related Information

Adult ACLS Algorithm, Tachycardia *on page 1010*

Overdose and Toxicology *on page 1191*

Brand Names Brevibloc®

Available Salts Esmolol Hydrochloride

Therapeutic Category Antiarrhythmic Agent, Class II; Antihypertensive Agent; Beta-Adrenergic Blocker

Generic Available No

Use Supraventricular tachycardia (primarily to control ventricular rate) and hypertension (especially perioperatively)

Pregnancy Risk Factor C

Contraindications Sinus bradycardia or heart block, uncompensated CHF, cardiogenic shock; hypersensitivity to esmolol, any component, or other beta-blockers

Warnings Caution should be exercised when discontinuing esmolol infusions to avoid withdrawal effects

Precautions Use with extreme caution in patients with hyper-reactive airway disease; use lowest dose possible and discontinue infusion if bronchospasm occurs; use with caution in diabetes mellitus, hypoglycemia, renal failure; avoid extravasation

Adverse Reactions

Cardiovascular: Hypotension (especially with doses >200 mcg/kg/minute), bradycardia, Raynaud's phenomena

Central nervous system: Dizziness, somnolence, confusion, lethargy, depression, headache

Gastrointestinal: Nausea, vomiting

Local: Phlebitis, skin necrosis after extravasation

Respiratory: Bronchoconstriction (less than propranolol, but more likely with higher doses)

Miscellaneous: Diaphoresis, adverse reactions similar to other beta-blockers may occur

Drug Interactions Esmolol may increase digoxin or theophylline serum concentrations; morphine may increase esmolol blood concentrations; xanthines (eg, theophylline, caffeine) may decrease effects of esmolol

Food Interactions Avoid xanthine-containing foods or beverages

Mechanism of Action Class II antiarrhythmic: Competitively blocks response to beta$_1$-adrenergic stimulation with little or no effect on beta$_2$-receptors except at high doses (ie, cardioselective at lower doses); no intrinsic sympathomimetic activity; no membrane-stabilizing activity; ultrashort-acting

Pharmacodynamics
Onset of action: I.V.: Beta blockade occurs within 2-10 minutes (onset of effects is quickest when loading doses are administered)
Duration: Short (10-30 minutes)

Pharmacokinetics
Protein binding: 55%
Distribution: V$_d$:
Children: 2 L/kg
Adults: 3.5 L/kg (range: 2-5 L/kg)
Metabolism: In blood by esterases
Half-life, elimination:
Children:
18 months to 14 years (n=12): 2.88 ± 2.67 minutes
2.5-16 years (n=20): 4.5 ± 2.1 minutes
Adults: 9 minutes
Elimination: ~69% of dose excreted in urine as metabolites and 2% as unchanged drug

Usual Dosage Must be adjusted to individual response and tolerance
Children: I.V.: Limited information available
Supraventricular tachycardia (SVT): Some centers have utilized initial doses of 100-500 mcg/kg given over 1 minute followed by a continuous infusion for control of SVT. One electrophysiologic study assessing esmolol-induced beta-blockade (n=20, 2-16 years of age) used an initial dose of 600 mcg/kg over 2 minutes followed by an infusion of 200 mcg/kg/minute; the infusion was titrated upward by 50-100 mcg/kg/minute every 5-10 minutes until a reduction >10% in heart rate or mean blood pressure occurred. Mean dose required: 550 mcg/kg/minute with a range of 300-1000 mcg/kg/minute.
Postoperative hypertension: Loading doses of 500 mcg/kg/minute over 1 minute with doses of 125-250 mcg/kg/minute (mean 173) have been used in addition to nitroprusside in a small number of patients (7 patients, 7-19 years of age, median age 13 years) after coarctation of aorta repair.
Adults: I.V.: Loading dose: 500 mcg/kg over 1 minute; follow with a 50 mcg/kg/minute infusion for 4 minutes; if response is inadequate, rebolus with another 500 mcg/kg loading dose over 1 minute, and increase the maintenance infusion to 100 mcg/kg/minute. Repeat this process until a therapeutic effect has been achieved or to a maximum recommended maintenance dose of 200 mcg/kg/minute. Usual dosage range: 50-200 mcg/kg/minute with average dose = 100 mcg/kg/minute.

Administration Parenteral: I.V.: The 250 mg/mL ampul is **not** for direct I.V. injection, but must first be diluted to a final concentration not to exceed 10 mg/mL (ie, 2.5 g in 250 mL or 5 g in 500 mL); infuse I.V. loading dose over 1-2 minutes

Monitoring Parameters Blood pressure, EKG, heart rate, respiratory rate, I.V. site

Nursing Implications Decrease infusion rate or discontinue if hypotension, CHF, etc occur

Dosage Forms Injection, as hydrochloride: 10 mg/mL (10 mL); 250 mg/mL (10 mL)

References
Cuneo BF, Zales VR, Blahunka PC, et al, "Pharmacodynamics and Pharmacokinetics of Esmolol, A Short-Acting Beta-Blocking Agent in Children," *Pediatr Cardiol*, 1994, 15(6):296-301.
Trippel DL, Wiest DB, and Gillette PC, "Cardiovascular and Antiarrhythmic Effects of Esmolol in Children," *J Pediatr*, 1991, 119(1):142-7.
Vincent RN, Click LA, Williams HM, et al, "Esmolol As an Adjunct in the Treatment of Systemic Hypertension After Operative Repair of Coarctation of the Aorta," *Am J Cardiol*, 1990, 65(13):941-3.
Wiest DB, Trippel DL, Gillette PC, et al, "Pharmacokinetics of Esmolol in Children," *Clin Pharmacol Ther*, 1991, 49(6):618-23.

◆ **Esmolol Hydrochloride** see Esmolol on page 384
◆ **E-Solve-2®** see Erythromycin on page 379
◆ **Estar® [OTC]** see Coal Tar on page 247
◆ **Estimated Comparative Daily Dosages for Inhaled Corticosteroids** see page 1185
◆ **Estivin® II Ophthalmic [OTC]** see Naphazoline on page 671
◆ **Estrace®** see Estradiol on page 386
◆ **Estraderm®** see Estradiol on page 386

Estradiol (es tra DYE ole)

Brand Names Climara® Transdermal; Delestrogen®; depGynogen®; Depo®-Estradiol; Depogen®; Dioval®; Dura-Estrin®; Estrace®; Estraderm®; Estro-Cyp®; Estroject-L.A.®; Estronol-LA®; Gynogen L.A.® 20; Vagifem®; Valergen®; Vivelle® Transdermal

Available Salts Estradiol Cypionate; Estradiol Valerate

Therapeutic Category Estrogen Derivative; Estrogen Derivative, Vaginal

Generic Available Yes

Use Atrophic vaginitis, atrophic dystrophy of vulva, menopausal symptoms, female hypogonadism; prevention of postmenopausal osteoporosis

Pregnancy Risk Factor X

Contraindications Thromboembolic disorders, active arterial thrombosis, thyroid dysfunction, blood dyscrasias; hypersensitivity to estradiol or any component; known or suspected pregnancy

Warnings Estrogens have been reported to increase the risk of endometrial carcinoma; do not use estrogens during pregnancy

Precautions Use with caution in patients with renal or hepatic insufficiency, or diseases that may be exacerbated by fluid retention; estrogens may cause premature closure of the epiphyses in young individuals

Adverse Reactions

Cardiovascular: Hypertension, edema, thromboembolic disorders

Central nervous system: Depression, headache

Dermatologic: Chloasma, melasma

Endocrine & metabolic: Hypercalcemia, folate deficiency, change in menstrual flow; increased risk for endometrial hyperplasia

Gastrointestinal: Nausea, vomiting

Hepatic: Cholestatic jaundice

Local: Pain at injection site; topical may cause burning or irritation

Neuromuscular & skeletal: Premature closure of epiphyses in young patients (large and repeated doses over an extended period of time)

Drug Interactions Cytochrome P-450 isoenzyme CYP1A2 and CYP3A3/4 substrate

Rifampin (decreased effect of estrogens); anticoagulants, bromocriptine, dantrolene (increased risk of hepatotoxicity); estrogens may decrease the clearance and increase serum concentrations and toxic effects of corticosteroids and cyclosporine

Food Interactions Larger doses of vitamin C (eg, 1 g/day in adults) may increase the serum concentrations and adverse effects of estradiol; vitamin C supplements are not recommended, but this effect may be decreased if vitamin C supplement is given 2-3 hours after estrogen; dietary intake of folate and pyridoxine may need to be increased

Mechanism of Action Increases the synthesis of DNA, RNA, and various proteins in target tissues; reduces the release of gonadotropin-releasing hormone from the hypothalamus; reduces FSH and LH release from the pituitary

Usual Dosage Adolescents and Adults: All dosage needs to be adjusted based upon the patient's response

Female hypogonadism:
I.M.:
Cypionate: 1.5-2 mg given once each month
Valerate: 10-20 mg given once each month
Oral: 0.5-2 mg/day in a cyclic regimen (3 weeks on drug, 1 week off)
Transdermal: Initial: 0.05 mg patch (titrate dosage to response) applied twice weekly in a cyclic regimen

Vaginal and vulval atrophy: Intravaginal: Initial: 200-400 mcg of estradiol once daily for 1-2 weeks; taper dose gradually to 100-200 mcg of estradiol once daily for 1-2 weeks; maintenance, cyclic regimen (after vaginal mucosa restored): 100 mcg of estradiol 1-3 times/week for 3 weeks, then no drug for the 4th week per cycle

Administration

Oral: Administer with food or after a meal to reduce GI upset

Parenteral: Injection for I.M. use only

Monitoring Parameters Blood pressure, serum calcium, glucose, liver enzymes; bone maturation and epiphyseal effects in young patients in whom bone growth is not complete

Test Interactions Thyroid function tests: Estrogens may increase thyroid binding globulin and circulating total thyroid hormone (when measured by T_4 RIA, T_4 by column, or by PBI); decreases free T_3 resin uptake; concentration of free T_4 is not altered

Patient Information Limit alcohol; limit caffeine; notify physician if sudden severe headache or vomiting, disturbance of vision or speech, numbness or weakness of extremity, sharp or crushing chest pain, calf pain, shortness of breath, severe abdominal pain or mass, mental depression, or unusual bleeding occurs

Nursing Implications Do not apply transdermal system to breasts; do not apply transdermal system to waistline (may loosen patch)

Dosage Forms

Cream, vaginal (Estrace®): 0.1 mg/g (42.5 g)

Injection, as **cypionate** (depGynogen®, Depo®-Estradiol, Depogen®, Dura-Estrin®, Estra-D®, Estro-Cyp®, Estroject-L.A.®): 5 mg/mL (5 mL, 10 mL)

Injection, as **valerate**:

Delestrogen®, Valergen®: 10 mg/mL (5 mL, 10 mL); 20 mg/mL (1 mL, 5 mL, 10 mL); 40 mg/mL (5 mL, 10 mL)

Dioval®, Estra-L®, Gynogen L.A.®: 20 mg/mL (10 mL); 40 mg/mL (10 mL)

Tablet, micronized (Estrace®): 0.5 mg, 1 mg, 2 mg

Tablet, vaginal (Vagifem®): 25 mcg

Transdermal system:

Climara®:

0.025 mg/24 hours [6.5 cm^2]

0.05 mg/24 hours [12.5 cm^2]

0.075 mg/24 hours [18.75 cm^2]

0.1 mg/24 hours [25 cm^2]

Estraderm®:

0.05 mg/24 hours [10 cm^2]

0.1 mg/24 hours [20 cm^2]

Vivelle®:

0.0375 mg/24 hours [11 cm^2]

0.05 mg/24 hours [14.5 cm^2]

0.075 mg/24 hours [22 cm^2]

0.1 mg/24 hours [29 cm^2]

- ◆ **Estradiol Cypionate** *see Estradiol on page 386*
- ◆ **Estradiol Valerate** *see Estradiol on page 386*
- ◆ **Estro-Cyp®** *see Estradiol on page 386*
- ◆ **Estrogenic Substances, Conjugated** *see Estrogens, Conjugated on page 387*

Estrogens, Conjugated (ES troe jenz KON joo gate ed)

Brand Names C.E.S.™ (Canada); Congest (Canada); Premarin®

Synonyms C.E.S.; Conjugated Estrogens; Estrogenic Substances, Conjugated

Therapeutic Category Estrogen Derivative; Estrogen Derivative, Vaginal

Generic Available No

Use Dysfunctional uterine bleeding, hypogonadism, atrophic vaginitis, vasomotor symptoms of menopause; postmenopausal hormonal replacement therapy

Pregnancy Risk Factor X

Contraindications Undiagnosed vaginal bleeding; hypersensitivity to estrogens or any component; thrombophlebitis or thromboembolic disorders; pregnancy; known or suspected breast cancer (except in select patients being treated for metastatic disease); estrogen-dependent neoplasia

Warnings Estrogens have been reported to increase the risk of endometrial carcinoma; do not use estrogens during pregnancy

Precautions Use with caution in patients with asthma, epilepsy, migraine, diabetes, hypercalcemia, cardiac, liver, or renal dysfunction; estrogens may cause premature closure of the epiphyses in young individuals; may greatly increase triglycerides and lead to pancreatitis and other problems in patients with familial defects of lipoprotein

Adverse Reactions

Cardiovascular: Hypertension, edema, thromboembolic disorder

Central nervous system: Depression, headache

Dermatologic: Chloasma, melasma

Endocrine & metabolic: Breast tenderness, change in menstrual flow, hypercalcemia, folate deficiency; increased risk of endometrial hyperplasia

Gastrointestinal: Nausea, vomiting

Hepatic: Cholestatic jaundice

Local: Pain at injection site

Neuromuscular & skeletal: Premature closure of epiphyses in young patients

Drug Interactions Rifampin (decreased effect of estrogens), anticoagulants, bromocriptine, dantrolene (increased risk of hepatotoxicity); estrogens may (Continued)

Estrogens, Conjugated *(Continued)*

decrease the clearance and increase the serum concentrations and toxic effects of corticosteroids and cyclosporine

Food Interactions Larger doses of vitamin C (eg, 1 g/day in adults) may increase the serum concentrations and adverse effects of estrogens; vitamin C supplements are not recommended, but this effect may be decreased if vitamin C supplement is given 2-3 hours after estrogen; dietary intake of folate and pyridoxine may need to be increased

Stability Injection: Store in the refrigerator; compatible with NS, dextrose, and invert sugar solutions; not compatible with ascorbic acid, protein hydrolysate, or acidic pH

Mechanism of Action Increases the synthesis of DNA, RNA, and various proteins in target tissues; reduces the release of gonadotropin-releasing hormone from the hypothalamus; reduces FSH and LH release from the pituitary

Usual Dosage Adolescents and Adults:

Hypogonadism: Oral: 2.5-7.5 mg/day in divided doses for 20 days, off 10 days and repeat until menses occur

Dysfunctional uterine bleeding:

Stable hematocrit: Oral: 1.25 mg twice daily for 21 days; if bleeding persists after 48 hours, increase to 2.5 mg twice daily; if bleeding persists after 48 more hours, increase to 2.5 mg 4 times/day; some recommend starting at 2.5 mg 4 times/day (**Note:** Medroxyprogesterone acetate 10 mg/day is also given on days 17-21; see References)

Alternatively: Oral: 2.5-5 mg/day for 7-10 days; then decrease to 1.25 mg/day for 2 weeks

Unstable hematocrit: Oral, I.V.: 5 mg 2-4 times/day; if bleeding is profuse, 20-40 mg every 4 hours up to 24 hours may be used; a progestational-weighted contraception pill should also be given (eg, Ovral® 2 tablets stat and 1 tablet 4 times/day or medroxyprogesterone acetate 5-10 mg 4 times/day; see References)

Alternatively: I.M., I.V.: 25 mg every 6-12 hours until bleeding stops

Vaginal and vulval atrophy: Intravaginal or topical: Cyclic regimen: 1.25-2.5 mg/day of conjugated estrogens for 3 weeks, then no drug for the 4th week per cycle; repeat as clinically needed

Administration

Oral: Administer with food or after eating to reduce GI upset; administration of dose at bedtime may decrease adverse effects

Parenteral: Add sterile diluent provided by manufacturer and shake gently; I.V.: Administer slow I.V. to avoid vascular flushing; I.M.: may be administered I.M. for dysfunctional uterine bleeding, but I.V. use is preferred (more rapid response)

Monitoring Parameters Blood pressure, serum calcium, glucose, liver enzymes; dysfunctional uterine bleeding: Hematocrit, hemoglobin, PT; bone maturation and epiphyseal effects in young patients in whom bone growth is not complete

Test Interactions Thyroid function tests: Estrogens may increase thyroid binding globulin and circulating total thyroid hormone (when measured by T_4 RIA, T_4 by column, or by PBI); decreases free T_3 resin uptake; concentration of free T_4 is not altered

Patient Information Limit caffeine; notify physician if sudden severe headache, vomiting, disturbance of vision or speech, numbness or weakness of extremity, sharp or crushing chest pain, calf pain, shortness of breath, severe abdominal pain or mass, mental depression, or unusual bleeding occurs

Dosage Forms

Cream, vaginal: 0.625 mg/g (42.5 g)

Injection: 25 mg (5 mL)

Tablet: 0.3 mg, 0.625 mg, 0.9 mg, 1.25 mg, 2.5 mg

References

Neinstein LS, *Adolescent Health Care - A Practical Guide*, 2nd ed, Baltimore: Urban & Schwarzenberg, 1991, 661-6.

♦ **Estroject-L.A.**® *see* Estradiol *on page 386*

♦ **Estronol-LA**® *see* Estradiol *on page 386*

♦ **ETAF** *see* Aldesleukin *on page 42*

Etanercept *(et a NER cept)*

Brand Names Enbrel®

Therapeutic Category Antirheumatic, Disease Modifying

Generic Available No

Use Treatment of polyarticular-course juvenile rheumatoid arthritis in patients who have had an inadequate response to one or more disease-modifying antirheumatic drugs; treatment of signs and symptoms of moderately to severely active rheumatoid arthritis in patients who have had an inadequate response to one or more disease-modifying antirheumatic drugs or in combination with methotrexate in patients who do not respond adequately to methotrexate alone

Pregnancy Risk Factor B

Contraindications Hypersensitivity to etanercept or any component (ie, mannitol, sucrose, tromethamine, and benzyl alcohol); patients with any serious active infection or sepsis

Warnings Some patients have developed serious infections and several have died from their infections while taking etanercept; patients who develop a new infection while being treated with etanercept should be monitored closely

Precautions Use with caution in patients with a history of recurrent infections or illnesses such as poorly controlled diabetes which predisposes the patient to infection; discontinue etanercept in a child who develops varicella infection or who has a significant exposure to varicella virus and consider prophylactic treatment with varicella-zoster immune globulin; patients with latex allergy should not handle the needle cover of the diluent syringe since it contains latex; anti-TNF therapies such as etanercept may affect host defenses against infections and malignancies

Adverse Reactions

Central nervous system: Headache (19%), depression, personality disorder, dizziness

Dermatologic: Rash

Gastrointestinal: Nausea (9%), abdominal pain (19%), vomiting (13%), esophagitis/gastritis

Local: Injection site reactions (erythema, discomfort, itching, swelling)

Respiratory: Respiratory tract infection, rhinitis

Miscellaneous: Allergic reaction (hives, difficulty breathing), positive antinuclear antibodies, positive antidouble-stranded DNA antibodies

Drug Interactions Live vaccines (unknown whether secondary transmission of infection in live vaccines can occur)

Stability Store vial in the refrigerator; do not freeze; etanercept solution should be used within 6 hours of reconstitution; do not shake or agitate vigorously; do not use if discolored or cloudy; do not filter reconstituted solution; do not add or mix with other medications

Mechanism of Action Binds to tumor necrosis factor and blocks its interaction with cell surface TNF receptors rendering TNF biologically inactive; modulates biological responses that are induced or regulated by TNF

Pharmacodynamics

Onset of action: One week of treatment

Peak effect: Full effect is usually seen within 3 months

Pharmacokinetics

Absorption: Absorbed slowly after subcutaneous injection

Distribution: V_d: 1.78-3.39 L/m^2

Bioavailability: S.C.: 60%

Half-life: Adults: 115 hours (range: 98-300 hours)

Time to peak serum concentration: S.C.: 72 hours (range: 48-96 hours)

Elimination: Clearance:

Children 4-17 years: 46 mL/hour/m^2

Adults: 52 mL/hour/m^2

Usual Dosage S.C.:

Children 4-17 years: 0.4 mg/kg/dose twice weekly given 72-96 hours apart; maximum dose: 25 mg

Adult: 25 mg twice weekly given 72-96 hours apart

Administration Parenteral: Administer by S.C. injection into thigh, abdomen, or upper arm; injection sites should be rotated with subsequent doses given at least 1 inch from an old site; do not inject into areas where the skin is tender, bruised, red, or hard

Monitoring Parameters Assess for joint swelling, pain, and tenderness; ESR or C-reactive protein level

Dosage Forms Powder for injection: 25 mg vial

References

Lovell DJ, Giannini EH, Whitmore JB, et al, "Safety and Efficacy of Tumor Necrosis Factor Receptor P75Fc Fusion Protein (TNFR:Fc, ENBREL) in Polyarticular Course Juvenile Rheumatoid Arthritis," Presented at American College of Rheumatology National Meeting, San Diego, CA, 1998.

Moreland LW, Baumgartner SW, Schiff MH, et al, "Treatment of Rheumatoid Arthritis With a Recombinant Human Tumor Necrosis Factor Receptor (p75)-Fc Fusion Protein," N Engl J Med, 1997, 337(3):141-7.

♦ **Ethacrynate Sodium** *see Ethacrynic Acid on page 390*

Ethacrynic Acid (eth a KRIN ik AS id)

Brand Names Edecrin® Oral; Edecrin® Sodium Injection
Available Salts Ethacrynate Sodium
Therapeutic Category Antihypertensive Agent; Diuretic, Loop
Generic Available No
Use Management of edema secondary to CHF; hepatic or renal disease, hypertension
Pregnancy Risk Factor B
Contraindications Hypersensitivity to ethacrynic acid or any component; hypotension, hyponatremic dehydration, metabolic alkalosis with hypokalemia, or anuria
Warnings Loop diuretics are potent diuretics; excess amounts can lead to profound diuresis with fluid and electrolyte loss; close medical supervision and dose evaluation is required; may increase risk of gastric hemorrhage associated with corticosteroid treatment
Precautions Avoid use in patients with severe renal dysfunction (Cl_{cr} <10 mL/minute)
Adverse Reactions
  Cardiovascular: Hypotension
  Central nervous system: Headache, fatigue, mental confusion, vertigo
  Dermatologic: Rash, photosensitivity
  Endocrine & metabolic: Hyperglycemia, fluid and electrolyte imbalances (fluid depletion, hypokalemia, hyponatremia, hypomagnesemia, hypocalcemia), hyperuricemia
  Gastrointestinal: GI irritation, diarrhea, anorexia, abdominal pain, dysphagia, GI bleed
  Hematologic: Thrombocytopenia, neutropenia, agranulocytosis
  Hepatic: Abnormal liver function tests, jaundice, hepatocellular damage
  Local: Local irritation, pain at injection site
  Otic: Ototoxicity, tinnitus
  Renal: Renal injury, hematuria
Drug Interactions Additive potassium depletion with drugs which cause potassium depletion: amphotericin, steroids, corticotropin; decreased renal clearance of lithium; decreased hypoglycemic effect of insulin or oral antidiabetic agents; decreased excretion of ethacrynic acid by probenecid; increased risk of ototoxicity with aminoglycosides; increased warfarin activity due to displacement from protein-binding sites
Food Interactions Need diet rich in potassium and magnesium
Stability When reconstituted with 50 mL D_5W or NS, resultant solution (1 mg/mL) is stable for 24 hours at room temperature
Mechanism of Action Inhibits reabsorption of sodium and chloride in the ascending loop of Henle and distal renal tubule, interfering with the chloride-binding cotransport system, thus causing increased excretion of water, sodium, chloride, magnesium, and calcium
Pharmacodynamics
  Onset of action:
    Oral: Within 30 minutes
    I.V.: 5 minutes
  Peak effect:
    Oral: 2 hours
    I.V.: 15-30 minutes
  Duration:
    Oral: 6-8 hours
    I.V.: 2 hours
Pharmacokinetics
  Absorption: Oral: Rapid
  Protein binding: >90%
  Metabolism: In the liver to active cysteine conjugate (35% to 40%)
  Elimination: In bile, 30% to 60% excreted unchanged in urine
Usual Dosage
  Children:
    Oral: 1 mg/kg/dose once daily, increase at intervals of 2-3 days to a maximum of 3 mg/kg/day
    I.V.: 1 mg/kg/dose; repeat doses are not routinely recommended, however if indicated, repeat doses every 8-12 hours
  Adults:
    Oral: 25-400 mg/day in 1-2 divided doses

I.V.: 0.5-1 mg/kg/dose (maximum dose: 100 mg/dose); repeat doses not routinely recommended, however if indicated, repeat every 8-12 hours

Administration
Oral: Administer with food or milk
Parenteral: Dilute injection with 50 mL D$_5$W or NS (1 mg/mL concentration resulting); maximum concentration 2 mg/mL; may be injected without further dilution over a period of several minutes or infused over 20-30 minutes; tissue irritant; not to be administered I.M. or S.C.

Monitoring Parameters Serum electrolytes, blood pressure, renal function, hearing

Additional Information Injection contains thimerosal

Dosage Forms
Powder for injection, as ethacrynate sodium: 50 mg (50 mL)
Tablet: 25 mg, 50 mg

Extemporaneous Preparations To make a 1 mg/mL suspension: Dissolve 120 mg ethacrynic acid powder in a small amount of 10% alcohol. Add a small amount of 50% sorbitol solution and stir. Adjust pH to 7 with 0.1N sodium hydroxide solution. Add sufficient 50% sorbitol solution to make a final volume of 120 mL. (Methylparaben 6 mg and propylparaben 2.4 mg are added as preservatives.) Stable 220 days at room temperature. Shake well before use.
Handbook on Extemporaneous Formulations, 3rd ed, Bethesda, MD: American Society of Hospital Pharmacists, 1997.

Ethambutol (e THAM byoo tole)
Brand Names Etibi® (Canada); Myambutol®
Available Salts Ethambutol Hydrochloride
Therapeutic Category Antitubercular Agent
Generic Available No
Use Treatment of tuberculosis and other mycobacterial diseases in conjunction with other antimycobacterial agents
Pregnancy Risk Factor B
Contraindications Hypersensitivity to ethambutol or any component; optic neuritis
Warnings Use only in children whose visual acuity can accurately be determined and monitored; not recommended for use in children <13 years of age unless benefit outweighs risk of therapy
Precautions Use with caution in patients with ocular defects or impaired renal function; modify dose in patients with renal impairment
Adverse Reactions
Central nervous system: Malaise, mental confusion, fever, headache, dizziness
Dermatologic: Rash, pruritus
Endocrine & metabolic: Elevated uric acid levels
Gastrointestinal: Nausea, vomiting, anorexia, abdominal pain
Hepatic: Abnormal liver function tests
Neuromuscular & skeletal: Peripheral neuropathy, arthralgia
Ocular: Optic neuritis, decreased visual acuity, decreased red-green color discrimination
Miscellaneous: Anaphylaxis
Mechanism of Action Suppresses mycobacterial multiplication by interfering with RNA synthesis
Pharmacokinetics
Absorption: Oral: ~80%
Distribution: Well distributed throughout the body with high concentrations in kidneys, lungs, saliva, CSF, and red blood cells; crosses the placenta; excreted into breast milk
Protein binding: 20% to 30%
Metabolism: 20% by the liver to inactive metabolite
Half-life: 2.5-3.6 hours (up to 7 hours or longer with renal impairment)
Time to peak serum concentration: Within 2-4 hours
Elimination: ~50% in urine and 20% excreted in feces as unchanged drug
Slightly dialyzable (5% to 20%)
Usual Dosage Oral:
Tuberculosis: Infants, Children, Adolescents, and Adults: 15-25 mg/kg/day once daily **or** 50 mg/kg/dose twice weekly, not to exceed 2.5 g/dose
Nontuberculous mycobacterial infection: Children, Adolescents, and Adults: 15 mg/kg/day, not to exceed 1 g/day
Dosing interval in renal impairment:
Cl$_{cr}$ 10-50 mL/minute: Administer every 24-36 hours
Cl$_{cr}$ <10 mL/minute: Administer every 48 hours and/or reduce usual dose
(Continued)

Ethambutol *(Continued)*

Administration Oral: Administer with or without food; if GI upset occurs, administer with food

Monitoring Parameters Monthly examination of visual acuity and color discrimination in patients receiving >15 mg/kg/day; periodic renal, hepatic, and hematologic function tests

Patient Information Report to physician any visual changes, numbness or tingling in hands or feet, rash, fever, and chills

Dosage Forms Tablet, as hydrochloride: 100 mg, 400 mg

References
American Academy of Pediatrics, Committee on Infectious Diseases, "Chemotherapy for Tuberculosis in Infants and Children," *Pediatrics*, 1992, 89(1):161-5.

Starke JR and Correa AG, "Management of Mycobacterial Infection and Disease in Children," *Pediatr Infect Dis J*, 1995, 14:455-70.

♦ **Ethambutol Hydrochloride** see Ethambutol *on page 391*

♦ **Ethanol** see Ethyl Alcohol *on page 394*

Ethionamide (e thye on AM ide)

Brand Names Trecator®-SC

Therapeutic Category Antitubercular Agent

Generic Available No

Use In conjunction with other antituberculosis agents in the treatment of tuberculosis and other mycobacterial diseases

Pregnancy Risk Factor C

Contraindications Severe hepatic impairment; hypersensitivity to ethionamide or any component

Precautions Use with caution in patients receiving cycloserine or isoniazid or in diabetic patients

Adverse Reactions
Cardiovascular: Postural hypotension
Central nervous system: Drowsiness, dizziness, seizures, headache, encephalopathy, depression
Dermatologic: Rash
Endocrine & metabolic: Hypoglycemia, goiter, gynecomastia
Gastrointestinal: Nausea, vomiting, abdominal pain, diarrhea, anorexia, stomatitis, metallic taste, weight loss
Hematologic: Thrombocytopenia
Hepatic: Hepatitis; jaundice; elevated AST, ALT, and serum bilirubin
Neuromuscular & skeletal: Peripheral neuropathy, tremor
Ocular: Optic neuritis
Miscellaneous: Excessive salivation

Food Interactions Increase dietary intake of pyridoxine to prevent neurotoxic effects of ethionamide

Mechanism of Action Inhibits peptide synthesis in susceptible organisms

Pharmacokinetics
Absorption: ~80% is rapidly absorbed from the GI tract
Distribution: Crosses the placenta; widely distributed into body tissues and fluids including liver, kidneys, and CSF
Protein binding: 10%
Metabolism: In the liver to active and inactive metabolites
Bioavailability: 80%
Half-life: 2-3 hours
Time to peak serum concentration: Oral: Occur within 3 hours
Elimination: As metabolites (active and inactive) and parent drug in the urine

Usual Dosage Oral:
Children: 15-20 mg/kg/day in 2-3 divided doses, not to exceed 1 g/day
Adults: 500-1000 mg/day in 1-3 divided doses

Administration Oral: Administer with meals to decrease GI distress

Monitoring Parameters Initial and periodic serum AST and ALT, blood glucose

Nursing Implications Neurotoxic effects may be relieved by the administration of pyridoxine

Dosage Forms Tablet: 250 mg

References
Donald PR and Seifart HI,"Cerebrospinal Fluid Concentrations of Ethionamide in Children With Tuberculous Meningitis," *J Pediatr*, 1989, 115(3):483-6.

Starke JR and Correa AG, "Management of Mycobacterial Infection and Disease in Children," *Pediatr Infect Dis J*, 1995, 14(6):455-69.

Ethosuximide (eth oh SUKS i mide)

Related Information

Antiepileptic Drugs *on page 1176*

Blood Level Sampling Time Guidelines *on page 1189*

Carbohydrate and Alcohol Content of Liquid Medications for Use in Patients Receiving Ketogenic Diets *on page 1228*

Brand Names Zarontin®

Therapeutic Category Anticonvulsant, Succinimide

Generic Available Yes

Use Management of absence (petit mal) seizures, myoclonic seizures, and akinetic epilepsy

Pregnancy Risk Factor C

Contraindications Hypersensitivity to ethosuximide or any component

Warnings Ethosuximide may increase tonic-clonic seizures in patients with mixed seizure disorders; ethosuximide must be used in combination with other anticonvulsants in patients with both absence and tonic-clonic seizures

Precautions Use with caution in patients with hepatic or renal disease; abrupt withdrawal of the drug may precipitate absence status

Adverse Reactions

Central nervous system: Sedation, dizziness, lethargy, euphoria, hallucinations, insomnia, agitation, behavioral changes, headache

Dermatologic: Rashes, urticaria

Gastrointestinal: Nausea, vomiting, anorexia, abdominal pain

Hematologic: Rare: Leukopenia, aplastic anemia, thrombocytopenia

Miscellaneous: Hiccups, rarely systemic lupus erythematosus

Drug Interactions Cytochrome P-450 isoenzyme CYP3A3/4 substrate

Phenytoin, carbamazepine, primidone, phenobarbital may increase the hepatic metabolism of ethosuximide; isoniazid may inhibit hepatic metabolism with a resultant increase in ethosuximide serum concentrations; CNS depressants, alcohol may increase adverse effects; haloperidol may change the frequency or pattern of seizure activity; valproic acid (increases or decreases ethosuximide serum concentrations)

Food Interactions Folate requirements may be increased

Mechanism of Action Increases the seizure threshold and suppresses paroxysmal spike-and-wave pattern in absence seizures; depresses nerve transmission in the motor cortex

Pharmacokinetics

Distribution: V_d: Adults: 0.62-0.72 L/kg

Protein binding: <10%

Metabolism: ~80% metabolized in the liver to three inactive metabolites

Half-life:

Children: 30 hours

Adults: 50-60 hours

Time to peak serum concentration:

Capsule: Within 2-4 hours

Syrup: <2-4 hours

Elimination: Slow in urine as metabolites (50%) and as unchanged drug (10% to 20%); small amounts excreted in feces

Dialysis: Removed by hemodialysis and peritoneal dialysis

Usual Dosage Oral:

Children <6 years: Initial: 15 mg/kg/day in 2 divided doses (maximum dose: 250 mg/dose); increase every 4-7 days; usual maintenance dose: 15-40 mg/kg/day in 2 divided doses; maximum dose: 1.5 g/day

Children >6 years and Adults: Initial: 250 mg twice daily; increase by 250 mg/day as needed every 4-7 days up to 1.5 g/day in 2 divided doses; usual maintenance dose: 20-40 mg/kg/day in 2 divided doses

Administration Oral: Administer with food or milk to decrease GI upset

Monitoring Parameters Seizure frequency, trough serum concentrations; CBC with differential, platelets, liver enzymes, urinalysis

Reference Range

Therapeutic: 40-100 µg/mL (SI: 280-710 µmol/L)

Toxic: >150 µg/mL (SI: >1062 µmol/L)

Patient Information Avoid alcohol; causes drowsiness and may impair ability to perform hazardous activities requiring mental alertness and coordination; do not discontinue abruptly

Additional Information Considered to be drug of choice for simple absence seizures

(Continued)

Ethosuximide *(Continued)*

Dosage Forms
    Capsule: 250 mg
    Syrup (raspberry flavor): 250 mg/5 mL (473 mL)

References
    Marquardt ED, Ishisaka DY, Batra KK, et al, "Removal of Ethosuximide and Phenobarbital by Peritoneal Dialysis in a Child," *Clin Pharm*, 1992, 11(12):1030-1.

♦ **Ethoxynaphthamido Penicillin** *see* Nafcillin *on page 666*

Ethyl Alcohol (ETH il AL koe hol)

Brand Names AHD 2000®; Lavacol® [OTC]

Synonyms Alcohol; Dehydrated Alcohol Injection; Ethanol; EtOH

Therapeutic Category Antidote, Ethylene Glycol Toxicity; Antidote, Methanol Toxicity; Anti-infective Agent, Topical; Fat Occlusion (Central Venous Catheter), Treatment Agent; Neurolytic

Generic Available Yes

Use Antidote for the treatment of methanol and ethylene glycol intoxication; neurolysis of nerves or ganglia for the relief of intractable, chronic pain in such conditions as inoperable cancer and trigeminal neuralgia (dehydrated alcohol injection); topical anti-infective; treatment of occluded central venous catheters due to lipid deposition from fat emulsion infusion (particularly 3-in-1 admixture)

Pregnancy Risk Factor D (X if used for prolonged periods or in high doses at term)

Contraindications Hypersensitivity to ethyl alcohol; seizure disorder and diabetic coma; subarachnoid injection of dehydrated alcohol in patients receiving anticoagulants

Warnings Ethanol is a flammable liquid and should be kept cool and away from any heat source; proper positioning of the patient for neurolytic administration is essential to control localization of the injection of dehydrated alcohol (which is hypobaric) into the subarachnoid space; avoid extravasation; not for S.C. administration; do not administer simultaneously with blood due to the possibility of pseudoagglutination or hemolysis; may potentiate severe hypoprothrombic bleeding; clinical evaluation and periodic lab determinations, including serum ethanol levels, are necessary to monitor effectiveness, changes in electrolyte concentrations, and acid-base balance (when used as an antidote)

Precautions Use with caution in diabetics (alcohol decreases blood sugar), patients with gout, shock, following cranial surgery, and in anticipated postpartum hemorrhage; monitor blood glucose closely, particularly in children as treatment of ingestions is associated with hypoglycemia; avoid extravasation during I.V. administration; ethanol passes freely into breast milk at a level approximately equivalent to maternal serum level; affects on the infant are insignificant until maternal blood level reaches 300 mg/dL; minimize dermal exposure of ethanol in infants as significant systemic absorption and toxicity can occur

Adverse Reactions
    Cardiovascular: Tachycardia, hypertension, hypotension, arrhythmias, cardiomegaly, angina, chest pain, CHF, vasodilation, flushing, hypothermia
    Central nervous system: Ataxia, dementia, Wernicke-Korsakoff syndrome, amnesia, paranoia, hyperthermia, vertigo, lethargy, sedation, coma, seizures, hallucinations
    Endocrine & metabolic: Hypoglycemia, acidosis, hypokalemia, hypomagnesemia, increased serum osmolality
    Dermatologic: Dry skin, irritation
    Gastrointestinal: Nausea, diarrhea, abdominal pain, dyspepsia, vomiting, gastrointestinal hemorrhage, anorexia, pancreatitis, hiccups
    Hematologic: Porphyria, megaloblastic anemia
    Hepatic: Hepatic cirrhosis, fatty degeneration of liver, hepatic steatosis
    Local: Phlebitis
    Neuromuscular & skeletal: Hypotonia, dysarthria, myopathy, neuropathy (peripheral); post-injection neuritis with persistent pain, hyperesthesia, and paresthesia (after neurolytic use)
    Ophthalmic: Eye stinging (from vapors)
    Respiratory: Respiratory depression, tachypnea, bronchial irritation

Drug Interactions Increased CNS depressant effects with sedative hypnotic agents, antihistamines, antidepressants, narcotic analgesics, dronabinol, phenothiazines, benzodiazepines, and metoclopramide; disulfiram-like reaction with cephalosporins, chlorpropamide, disulfiram, furazolidone, metronidazole, and procarbazine; increased GI blood loss and bleeding time with aspirin and salicylates; altered glucose metabolism resulting in either hypoglycemic or hyperglycemic effects with insulin, phenformin, and sulfonylureas; increases phenytoin serum levels; increased oral bioavailability of ethyl alcohol with aspirin, ranitidine, cimetidine, and nizatidine; increases theophylline levels

Stability Store at room temperature (see Warnings); do not use unless solution is clear and container is intact

Mechanism of Action Competitively inhibits the oxidation of methanol and ethylene oxide by alcohol dehydrogenase to their more toxic metabolites; as a neurolytic, ethyl alcohol produces injury to tissue cells by producing dehydration and precipitation of protoplasm; when injected in close proximity to nerve cells, it produces neuritis and nerve degeneration

Pharmacokinetics

Distribution: V_d: 0.6 L/kg

Metabolism: Hepatic to acetaldehyde or acetate by alcohol dehydrogenase

Clearance: 10-20 mL/hour

Hemodialysis clearance: 300-400 mL/minute with an ethanol removal rate of 280 mg/minute

Usual Dosage

Absolute ethanol/ethyl alcohol (EtOH):

Treatment of methanol or ethylene glycol ingestion: Children, Adolescents, and Adults:

Loading dose:

Oral: 0.8-1 mL/kg of 95% EtOH or 2 mL/kg of 40% EtOH

I.V.: 8-10 mL/kg of 10% EtOH solution (see Administration), not to exceed 200 mL

Modified loading dose (if ingestion of both EtOH **and** methanol or ethylene glycol):

Oral:

$$95\% \text{ EtOH (mL)} = \frac{[(100 \text{ mg/dL} - [\text{Blood EtOH level (mg/dL})] \times 0.6 \text{ mL/kg} \times \text{Wt (kg)}}{(754 \text{ mg/mL}) \times 0.95}$$

I.V.:

$$10\% \text{ EtOH (mL)} = \frac{[(100 \text{ mg/dL} - [\text{Blood EtOH level (mg/dL})] \times 0.6 \text{ mL/kg} \times \text{Wt (kg)}}{(790 \text{ mg/mL}) \times 0.1}$$

Note: The modified loading dose is reduced related to the measured EtOH blood level.

Maintenance dose:	Non-Drinker	Average Drinker	Chronic Drinker
EtOH dosage (by wt)	66 mg/kg/h	110 mg/kg/h	154 mg/kg/h
Oral: 40% EtOH	0.2 mL/kg/h	0.3 mL/kg/h	0.4 mL/kg/h
Oral: 95% EtOH	0.1 mL/kg/h	0.15 mL/kg/h	0.2 mL/kg/h
I.V.: 10% EtOH	0.8 mL/kg/h	1.4 mL/kg/h	2 mL/kg/h

Note: Continue therapy until methanol or ethylene glycol blood level <10 mg/dL

Dosage adjustment for hemodialysis: Increase maintenance dosage by 150 mg/kg/h during hemodialysis

Treatment of fat occlusion of central venous catheters: Children and Adults:

I.V. (see institutional-based protocol for catheter clearance assessment, the following assessment is a general methodology): Up to 3 mL of 70% ethanol (maximum 0.55 mL/kg); the volume to instill is equal to the internal volume of the catheter; may repeat if patency not restored after 30 minute dwell time; if dose repeated, reassess after 4-hour dwell time

Dehydrated alcohol injection: Therapeutic neurolysis (nerve or ganglion block): Adults: Intraneural: Dosage variable depending upon the site of injection, eg, trigeminal neuralgia: 0.05-0.5 mL as a single injection per interspace vs subarachnoid injection: 0.5-1 mL as a single injection per interspace; single doses >1.5 mL are seldom required

Liquid denatured alcohol: Topical: Children and Adults: Apply as needed

Administration

Oral: Dilute ethanol in 6 ounces orange juice and give over 30 minutes

Parenteral: Not for S.C. administration; I.V.: Dilute absolute alcohol for I.V. administration to a final concentration of 5% to 10% v/v in D_5W or $D_{10}W$ (I.V. ethanol is also available commercially in both 5% and 10% solutions; see Dosage Forms); infuse loading dose plus 1 hour of maintenance dosage over 60 minutes; for treatment of occluded central venous catheter, a 70% dilution of ethanol may be made by adding 0.8 mL sterile water to 2 mL 98% ethanol; instill with a volume equal to the internal volume of the catheter; assess patency at 30 minutes (or per institutional protocol); may repeat (see Usual Dosage)

(Continued)

395

Ethyl Alcohol *(Continued)*

Intraneural: Separate needles should be used for each of multiple injections or sites to prevent residual alcohol deposition at sites not intended for tissue destruction; inject slowly after determining proper placement of needle; since dehydrated alcohol is hypobaric when compared with spinal fluid, proper positioning of the patient is essential to control localization of injections into the subarachnoid space

Monitoring Parameters Antidotal therapy: Blood ethanol levels (at the end of the loading dose, every hour until stabilized, and then every 8-12 hours thereafter); blood glucose, electrolytes, arterial pH, blood gases, methanol or ethylene glycol blood levels

Reference Range

Symptoms associated with serum ethanol levels:

Nausea and vomiting: Serum level >100 mg/dL

Coma: Serum level >300 mg/dL

Antidote for methanol/ethylene glycol: Goal range: Blood ethanol level: 100-130 mg/dL (22-28 mmol/liter)

Patient Information May cause drowsiness and impair ability to perform hazardous activities which require mental alertness or physical coordination

Additional Information Eighty-proof spirits contain 40% ethanol

Dosage Forms

Infusion, in D_5W: 5% alcohol (1000 mL)

Infusion, in D_5W: 10% alcohol (1000 mL)

Injection, absolute: 98% (2 mL)

Injection, dehydrated: 98% (1 mL, 5 mL)

Liquid, topical, denatured: 70% (473 mL)

References

Chernow B, ed, "Poisoning", *Essentials of Critical Care Pharmacology*, 2nd ed, Baltimore: Williams & Wilkins, 1994, 501-29.

Pennington CR and Pithie AD, "Ethanol Lock in the Management of Catheter Occlusion", *JPEN J Parenter Enteral Nutr*, 1987, 11(5):507-8.

Werlin SL, Lausten T, Jessens, et al, "Treatment of Central Venous Catheter Occlusions With Ethanol and Hydrochloric Acid", *JPEN J Parenter Enteral Nutr*, 1995, 19(5):416-8.

♦ **Ethyl Aminobenzoate** *see* Benzocaine *on page 124*

♦ **Ethyol®** *see* Amifostine *on page 55*

♦ **Etibi® (Canada)** *see* Ethambutol *on page 391*

Etidronate Disodium (e ti DROE nate dye SOW dee um)

Brand Names Didronel®

Synonyms EHDP; Sodium Etidronate

Therapeutic Category Antidote, Hypercalcemia; Bisphosphonate Derivative

Generic Available No

Use Symptomatic treatment of Paget's disease and heterotopic ossification due to spinal cord injury; hypercalcemia associated with malignancy

Pregnancy Risk Factor B (oral), C (parenteral)

Contraindications Patients with serum creatinine >5 mg/dL; clinically overt osteomalacia; hypersensitivity to biphosphonates or any component

Precautions Use with caution in patients with restricted calcium and vitamin D intake; I.V. form may be nephrotoxic and should be used with caution, if at all, in patients with impaired renal function; dosage modification required in renal impairment

Adverse Reactions Generally dose-related and most significant when taking oral doses >5 mg/kg/day

Central nervous system: Fever, convulsions, pain

Dermatologic: Angioedema, rash

Endocrine & metabolic: Hyperphosphatemia, hypocalcemia, hypomagnesemia, fluid overload

Gastrointestinal: Diarrhea, nausea, vomiting, occult blood in stools, dysgeusia

Neuromuscular & skeletal: Bone pain, increased risk of fractures, rachitic syndrome (found in children taking dosage >10 mg/kg/day over 1 year or longer)

Renal: Nephrotoxicity

Miscellaneous: Hypersensitivity reactions

Stability When diluted in 250 mL NS, solutions are stable 48 hours at room temperature

Mechanism of Action Decreases bone resorption by inhibiting osteocystic osteolysis; decreases mineral release and matrix or collagen breakdown in bone

Pharmacodynamics
Onset of therapeutic effects: Within 1-3 months of therapy
Duration: Persists for 12 months without continuous therapy

Pharmacokinetics
Absorption: Dependent upon dose administered
Half-life: 8.7 hours (range: 6.9-10 hours)
Elimination: Primarily as unchanged drug in urine with unabsorbed drug eliminated in feces

Usual Dosage
Children and Adults: Heterotopic ossification with spinal cord injury: Oral: 20 mg/kg once daily (or in divided doses if GI discomfort occurs) for 2 weeks, then 10 mg/kg/day for 10 weeks (**Note:** This dosage has been used in children, however, treatment >1 year has been associated with a rachitic syndrome)

Adults:
Paget's disease: Oral: 5-10 mg/kg once daily for no more than 6 months; may give 11-20 mg/kg/day for up to 3 months. Daily dose may be divided if adverse GI effects occur; courses of therapy should be separated by drug-free periods of at least 3 months.

Hypercalcemia associated with malignancy:
I.V.: 7.5 mg/kg once daily for 3 days, may be continued up to 7 days if necessary; courses of therapy should be separated by at least 7 drug-free days
Oral: Start 20 mg/kg once daily (or in divided doses if GI discomfort occurs) on the last day of infusion and continue for 30-90 days

Dosing adjustment in renal impairment:
S_{cr} 2.5-4.9 mg/dL: Use with caution
S_{cr} ≥5 mg/dL: **Not recommended**

Administration
Oral: Administer on an empty stomach, 2 hours before meals; avoid giving foods/supplements with calcium, iron, or magnesium within 2 hours of drug
Parenteral: I.V.: Dilute in a minimum volume of 250 mL NS; infuse over at least 2 hours

Monitoring Parameters Serum calcium, phosphate, creatinine, BUN

Patient Information Maintain adequate intake of calcium and vitamin D

Dosage Forms
Injection: 50 mg/mL (6 mL)
Tablet: 200 mg, 400 mg

♦ **EtOH** *see* Ethyl Alcohol *on page 394*

Etoposide (e toe POE side)

Related Information
Emetogenic Potential of Single Chemotherapeutic Agents *on page 1095*

Brand Names VePesid®

Synonyms VP-16; VP-16-213

Therapeutic Category Antineoplastic Agent, Mitotic Inhibitor

Generic Available Yes

Use Treatment of testicular and lung carcinomas, malignant lymphoma, Hodgkin's disease, leukemias (ALL, ANLL, AML), neuroblastoma; treatment of Ewing's sarcoma, rhabdomyosarcoma, osteosarcoma, Wilms' tumor, brain tumors; conditioning regimen with hematopoietic stem cell support

Pregnancy Risk Factor D

Contraindications Hypersensitivity to etoposide or any component

Warnings The FDA currently recommends that procedures for proper handling and disposal of antineoplastic agents be considered. Severe myelosuppression with resulting infection or bleeding may occur; injectable etoposide contains polysorbate 80 (polysorbate 80 has caused thrombocytopenia, ascites, and renal, pulmonary, and hepatic failure in premature infants who received an injectable vitamin E product containing polysorbate 80). Higher rates of anaphylactoid reactions have been reported in children who received I.V. infusions of etoposide at higher than recommended concentrations; injection contains benzyl alcohol as a preservative; use with caution in neonates

Precautions Use with caution and consider dosage reduction in patients with hepatic impairment, bone marrow suppression, and renal impairment

Adverse Reactions
Cardiovascular: Hypotension, tachycardia, facial flushing
Central nervous system: Somnolence, fatigue, fever, headache, chills
Dermatologic: Alopecia, rash, urticaria, angioedema
(Continued)

Etoposide *(Continued)*

Gastrointestinal: Nausea, vomiting, diarrhea, mucositis, anorexia, constipation

Hematologic: Myelosuppression, anemia (granulocyte nadir: ~7-14 days, platelet nadir: ~9-16 days)

Hepatic: Hepatotoxicity

Local: Thrombophlebitis

Neuromuscular & skeletal: Peripheral neuropathy, weakness

Respiratory: Bronchospasm

Miscellaneous: Anaphylactoid reactions

Food Interactions Administration of food does not affect GI absorption with doses ≤200 mg

Stability Stability of diluted injection is concentration dependent (ie, 0.2 mg/mL: 96 hours; 0.4 mg/mL: 48 hours; 1 mg/mL: 2 hours; 2 mg/mL: 1 hour); at a concentration of 1 mg/mL in NS or D_5W, crystallization has occurred within 30 minutes; **incidence of precipitation increases when final infusion concentration is >0.4 mg/mL;** intact vials remain stable for 2 years at room temperature; refrigerate capsules

Mechanism of Action Inhibits mitotic activity; inhibits DNA type II topoisomerase producing single- and double-strand DNA breaks

Pharmacokinetics

Absorption: Oral: Large variability

Distribution: CSF concentration is <5% of plasma concentration

Children V_{dss}: 10 L/m^2

Adults V_{dss}: 7-17 L/m^2

Protein binding: 94% to 97%

Metabolism: In the liver (with a biphasic decay)

Bioavailability: Averages 50% (range: 10% to 80%, dose-dependent)

Half-life, terminal:

Children: 6-8 hours

Adults: 4-15 hours with normal renal and hepatic function

Time to peak serum concentration: Oral: Within 1-1.5 hours

Elimination: Both unchanged drug and metabolites are excreted in urine and a small amount (2% to 16%) in feces; up to 55% of an I.V. dose is excreted unchanged in urine in children

Usual Dosage Refer to individual protocols

Children: I.V.: 60-150 mg/m^2/day for 2-5 days every 3-6 weeks

AML:

Remission induction: 150 mg/m^2/day for 2-3 days for 2-3 cycles

Intensification or consolidation: 250 mg/m^2/day for 3 days, on courses 2-5

Brain tumor: 150 mg/m^2/day on days 2 and 3 of treatment course

Neuroblastoma: 100 mg/m^2/day over 1 hour on days 1-5 of cycle; repeat cycle every 4 weeks

High-dose conditioning regimen for allogeneic BMT: 60 mg/kg/dose as a single dose

BMT conditioning regimen used in patients with rhabdomyosarcoma or neuroblastoma: I.V. continuous infusion: 160 mg/m^2/day for 4 days

Adults:

Testicular cancer: I.V.: 50-100 mg/m^2/day on days 1-5 or 100 mg/m^2/day on days 1, 3 and 5 every 3-4 weeks for 3-4 courses

Small cell lung cancer:

Oral: Twice the I.V. dose rounded to the nearest 50 mg given once daily if total dose ≤400 mg/day or in divided doses if >400 mg/day

I.V.: 35 mg/m^2/day for 4 days or 50 mg/m^2/day for 5 days every 3-4 weeks

Dosing adjustment in renal impairment:

Cl_{cr} 10-50 mL/minute: Administer 75% of normal dose

Cl_{cr} <10 mL minute: Administer 50% of normal dose

Dosing adjustment in patients with elevated serum bilirubin: Reduce dose by 50% for bilirubin 1.5-3 mg/dL; reduce dose by 75% for bilirubin >3 mg/dL

Administration

Oral: If necessary, the injection may be used for oral administration. Mix with orange juice, apple juice, or lemonade at a final concentration not to exceed 0.4 mg/mL to prevent precipitation. Etoposide has been found to be stable with no loss of potency over 3 hours when administered in apple juice or lemonade at concentrations of 1 mg/mL.

Parenteral: I.V.: Do not administer by rapid I.V. injection or by intrathecal, intraperitoneal, or intrapleural routes due to possible severe toxicity. Administer I.V. infusion via an in-line 0.22 micron filter over at least 60 minutes at a rate not to exceed 100 mg/m^2/hour (or 3.3 mg/kg/hour) to minimize the risk of hypotensive reactions at a final concentration for administration of 0.2-0.4 mg/mL in NS or D_5W. More concentrated I.V. solutions (0.6-1 mg/mL) can be infused but have shorter stability times (see Stability). For high-dose etoposide infusions, undiluted etoposide (20 mg/mL) has been infused as a single dose from a glass syringe via syringe pump through a central venous catheter over 1-4 hours. Problems associated with higher than recommended concentrations of etoposide infusions include cracking of hard plastic in chemo venting pins and infusion lines; inspect infusion solution for particulate matter and plastic devices for cracks and leaks.

Monitoring Parameters CBC with differential and platelet count, hemoglobin, vital signs (blood pressure), bilirubin, and renal function tests; inspect solution and tubing for precipitation before and during infusion

Patient Information Notify physician if fever, sore throat, painful/burning urination, bruising, bleeding or shortness of breath occurs

Nursing Implications Adequate airway and other supportive measures and agents for treating hypotension or anaphylactoid reactions should be present when I.V. etoposide is given

Dosage Forms
Capsule: 50 mg
Injection: 20 mg/mL (5 mL, 25 mL)

References
Berg SL, Grisell DL, DeLaney TF, et al, "Principles of Treatment of Pediatric Solid Tumors," *Pediatr Clin North Am*, 1991, 38(2):249-67.

Boos J, Krümpelmann S, Schulze-Westhoff P, et al, "Steady-State Levels and Bone Marrow Toxicity of Etoposide in Children and Infants: Does Etoposide Require Age-Dependent Dose Calculation?" *J Clin Oncol*, 1995, 13(12):2954-60.

Clark PL and Slevin ML, "The Clinical Pharmacology of Etoposide and Teniposide," *Clin Pharmacokinet*, 1987, 12(4):223-52.

Lazarus HM, Creger RJ, and Diaz D, "Simple Method for the Administration of High-Dose Etoposide During Autologous Bone Marrow Transplantation," *Cancer Treat Rep*, 1985, 70(6):819-20.

Nishikawa A, Nakamura Y, Nobori U, et al, "Acute Monocytic Leukemia in Children. Response to VP-16-213 as a Single Agent," *Cancer*, 1987, 60(9):2146-9.

O'Dwyer PJ, Leyland-Jones B, Alonso MT, et al, "Etoposide (VP-16-213): Current Status of an Active Anticancer Drug," *N Engl J Med*, 1985, 312(11):692-700.

Factor IX Complex (Human) (FAK ter nyne KOM pleks HYU man)

Brand Names Konӱne® 80; Profilnine® Heat-Treated; Proplex® SX-T; Proplex® T

Therapeutic Category Antihemophilic Agent; Blood Product Derivative

Generic Available No

Use To control bleeding in patients with factor IX deficiency (hemophilia B or Christmas disease); prevention/control of bleeding in hemophilia A patients with inhibitors to factor VIII; Proplex® T is indicated to prevent or control bleeding due to factor VII deficiency

Pregnancy Risk Factor C

Contraindications Liver disease, intravascular coagulation or fibrinolysis

Precautions Use with caution in patients with liver dysfunction; risk of viral transmission is not totally eradicated, prepared from pooled human plasma

Adverse Reactions
Cardiovascular: Flushing
Central nervous system: Somnolence, fever, headache, chills
(Continued)

Factor IX Complex (Human) *(Continued)*

Dermatologic: Urticaria
Gastrointestinal: Nausea, vomiting
Hematologic: Disseminated intravascular coagulation, thrombosis following high dosages in hemophilia B patients
Neuromuscular & skeletal: Paresthesia
Miscellaneous: Tightness in chest and neck

Drug Interactions Increased risk of thrombosis with aminocaproic acid (some recommend to delay the administration of aminocaproic acid 8 hours after factor IX complex administration)

Stability Administer within 3 hours after reconstitution; store unopened vials in refrigerator

Mechanism of Action Replaces deficient clotting factors including factors II, VII, IX, and X

Pharmacokinetics Cleared rapidly from the serum in two phases
Half-life:
First phase: 4-6 hours
Terminal: 22.5 hours

Usual Dosage Dose is expressed in terms of factor IX units; dose must be individualized; **Note:** 1 unit/kg raises factor IX levels 1%

Children and Adults: I.V.:
Factor IX deficiency: Hospitalized patients: 20-50 units/kg/dose; may be higher in special cases; may be given every 24 hours or more often in special cases
Factor VIII inhibitor patients: 75-100 units/kg/dose; may be given every 6-12 hours

Administration Parenteral: I.V. administration only; rate of administration should be individualized for patient's comfort; maximum rates of administration: Konÿne® 80: 100 international units/minute; Profilnine® heat treated: 10 mL/minute; Proplex® T: 2-3 mL/minute; use filter needle to draw product into syringe

Monitoring Parameters Levels of factors II, IX, and X; signs/symptoms of bleeding; hemoglobin, hematocrit

Reference Range Patients with severe hemophilia will have factor IX levels <1%, often undetectable. Moderate forms of the disease have levels of 1% to 10% while some mild cases may have 11% to 49% of normal factor IX. Plasma concentration is about 4 mg/L.

Additional Information AlphaNine® and Mononine® contain only factor IX and should not be confused with factor IX **complex**

Dosage Forms Injection: **(Note:** Exact potency labeled on each vial)
Konÿne® 80: 10 mL, 20 mL
Profilnine® Heat-Treated: Single dose vial
Proplex® SX-T: Vial
Proplex® T: Vial

References
Lusher JM, "Thrombogenicity Associated With Factor IX Complex Concentrates," *Semin Hematol*, 1991, 28(3 Suppl 6):3-5.

♦ **Factor VIII** *see* Antihemophilic Factor (Human) *on page 89*
♦ **Factrel®** *see* Gonadorelin *on page 461*

Famciclovir *(fam SYE kloe veer)*

Brand Names Famvir®
Therapeutic Category Antiviral Agent, Oral
Generic Available No
Use Management of acute herpes zoster (shingles); treatment or suppression of recurrent genital herpes in the immunocompetent; treatment of recurrent mucocutaneous herpes simplex infections in HIV patients
Pregnancy Risk Factor B
Contraindications Hypersensitivity to famciclovir, penciclovir, or any component
Precautions Use with caution and decrease dose in patients with renal dysfunction; dosage adjustment may be needed in patients with poorly compensated hepatic impairment

Adverse Reactions
Central nervous system: Headache, fatigue, dizziness, fever, somnolence
Dermatologic: Pruritus, rash
Gastrointestinal: Nausea, diarrhea, vomiting, constipation, anorexia, abdominal pain
Neuromuscular & skeletal: Rigors, paresthesia

Drug Interactions Potentially probenecid

Food Interactions Rate of absorption and/or conversion to penciclovir and peak concentration are reduced with food, but bioavailability is not affected

Mechanism of Action Synthetic guanine derivative, prodrug for penciclovir; penciclovir has inhibitory activity against varicella zoster virus (VZV) and herpes simplex virus type 1 and 2 (HSV 1 and HSV 2); penciclovir is converted to penciclovir monophosphate (by viral thymidine kinase in VZV-, HSV 1-, and HSV 2-infected cells), then to penciclovir triphosphate which competes with deoxyguanosine triphosphate for viral DNA polymerase and incorporation into viral DNA; therefore, inhibits DNA synthesis and viral replication

Pharmacokinetics Penciclovir:

Absorption: Rapid

Distribution: V_{dss}: Healthy adults: 73-85 L

Protein binding: <20%

Metabolism: Famciclovir is a prodrug which is metabolized via deacetylation and oxidation in the intestinal wall and liver to penciclovir (active) during extensive first-pass metabolism

Bioavailability: 72% to 83%

Half-life:

Serum: 2-3 hours; increased with renal dysfunction

Mean half-life, terminal:

Cl_{cr} >80 mL/minute: 2.15 hours

Cl_{cr} 60-80 mL/minute: 2.47 hours

Cl_{cr} 30-59 mL/minute: 3.87 hours

Cl_{cr} <29 mL/minute: 9.85 hours

Intracellular penciclovir triphosphate: HSV 1: 10 hours; HSV 2: 20 hours; VZV: 7 hours

Time to peak serum concentration: ~1 hour

Elimination: Primary route is the kidney with 73% excreted in urine (predominantly as penciclovir) and 27% in feces; penciclovir undergoes tubular secretion; requires dosage adjustment with renal impairment

Usual Dosage Adult: Oral:

Herpes zoster: 500 mg every 8 hours for 7 days; initiate as soon as diagnosed; initiation of therapy within 48 hours of rash onset may be more beneficial; no efficacy data available for treatment initiated >72 hours after onset of rash

Recurrent genital herpes: 125 mg twice daily for 5 days; initiate at first sign or symptom

Suppression of recurrent genital herpes: 250 mg twice daily for up to 1 year

HIV patients with recurrent orolabial or genital herpes: 500 mg twice daily for 7 days

Dosing interval in renal impairment: Adults:

Cl_{cr} 40-59 mL/minute: Administer 500 mg every 12 hours

Cl_{cr} 20-39 mL/minute: Administer 500 mg every 24 hours

Administration Oral: May be administered without regard to meals; may be administered with food to decrease GI upset

Monitoring Parameters Resolution of rash

Patient Information Famciclovir is not a cure for genital herpes

Dosage Forms Tablet: 125 mg, 250 mg, 500 mg

References

Boike SC, Pue MA, and Freed MI, "Pharmacokinetics of Famciclovir in Subjects With Varying Degrees of Renal Impairment," *Clin Pharmacol Ther*, 1994, 55(4):418-26.

Famotidine (fa MOE ti deen)

Related Information

Carbohydrate and Alcohol Content of Liquid Medications for Use in Patients Receiving Ketogenic Diets *on page 1228*

Brand Names Apo®-Famotidine (Canada); Novo-Famotidine® (Canada); Nu-Famotidine® (Canada); Pepcid®; Pepcid® AC Acid Controller [OTC]; Pepcid RPD®

Therapeutic Category Gastrointestinal Agent, Gastric or Duodenal Ulcer Treatment; Histamine H_2 Antagonist

Generic Available No

Use Short-term therapy and treatment of duodenal ulcer, gastric ulcer, control gastric pH in critically ill patients, symptomatic relief in gastritis, gastroesophageal reflux disease (GERD), active benign ulcer, and pathological hypersecretory conditions; over-the-counter (OTC) formulation for use in the relief of heartburn, acid indigestion, and sour stomach

Pregnancy Risk Factor B

(Continued)

Famotidine *(Continued)*

Contraindications Hypersensitivity to famotidine, any component, or other H$_2$ antagonists

Warnings Use with caution and modify dose in patients with renal impairment

Precautions Pepcid RPD® tablets contain phenylalanine; avoid use in phenylketonurics

Adverse Reactions

Cardiovascular: Bradycardia, tachycardia, palpitations, hypertension

Central nervous system: Headache, vertigo, anxiety, dizziness, seizures, depression, insomnia, drowsiness, confusion, fever

Dermatologic: Acne, pruritus, urticaria, dry skin, alopecia

Gastrointestinal: Constipation, nausea, vomiting, diarrhea, abdominal discomfort, flatulence, belching, dysgeusia, dry mouth, anorexia

Genitourinary: Impotence

Hematologic: Thrombocytopenia, pancytopenia, leukopenia (rare)

Hepatic: Increased liver enzymes, hepatomegaly, cholestatic jaundice

Neuromuscular & skeletal: Weakness, arthralgias, paresthesia, muscle cramps

Ocular: Orbital edema

Otic: Ototoxicity, tinnitus

Renal: Elevated BUN, elevated serum creatinine, proteinuria

Respiratory: Bronchospasm

Drug Interactions Decreased absorption of ketoconazole, triamterene, delavirdine, itraconazole, cefpodoxime, cyanocobalamin, indomethacin, melphalan; decreased effect of tolazoline

Food Interactions Limit xanthine-containing foods and beverages

Stability Concentrate for injection must be refrigerated but is stable for 48 hours at room temperature; if concentrated injection is diluted in D$_5$W or NS it is stable 48 hours at room temperature; commercially available diluted solution in NS is stable at room temperature for 15 months; injection is also compatible with D$_{10}$W, LR injection, 5% bicarbonate injection, and standard parenteral nutrition solutions with electrolytes, multivitamins, and trace minerals; reconstituted oral solution is stable for 30 days at room temperature

Mechanism of Action Competitive inhibition of histamine at H$_2$-receptors of the gastric parietal cells, which results in inhibition of gastric acid secretion

Pharmacodynamics

Onset of GI effect: Oral, I.V.: Within 1 hour

Peak effect:

Oral: 1-4 hours

I.V.: 30 minutes to 3 hours

Duration: 10-12 hours

Pharmacokinetics

Distribution: V$_d$:

Children: 2 ±1.5 L/kg

Adults: 0.94-1.33 L/kg

Protein binding: 15% to 20%

Metabolism: 30% to 35% liver metabolism

Bioavailability: Oral: 40% to 45%

Half-life:

Children: 3.3 ±2.5 hours

Adults: 2.5-3.5 hours; increases with renal impairment; if Cl$_{cr}$ <10 mL/minute, half-life ≥12 hours

Anuria: 24 hours

Elimination: 65% to 70% unchanged drug in urine

Usual Dosage

Infants and Children <16 years: Oral, I.V.:

Peptic ulcer: 0.5 mg/kg/day at bedtime or divided twice daily (maximum: 40 mg/day)

GERD: 1 mg/kg/day divided twice daily (maximum: 80 mg/day)

Adults:

Oral:

Duodenal ulcer, gastric ulcer: 40 mg/day at bedtime for 4-8 weeks (a regimen of 20 mg twice daily is also effective); maintenance therapy: 20 mg at bedtime

Hypersecretory conditions: Initial: 20 mg every 6 hours, may increase up to 160 mg every 6 hours

Esophagitis: 20-40 mg twice daily for up to 12 weeks

GERD: 20 mg twice daily for 6 weeks

Acid indigestion, heartburn, or sour stomach (OTC use): 10 mg 15-60 minutes before eating; not more than 2 tablets per day
I.V.: 20 mg every 12 hours

Dosing adjustment in renal impairment:
Cl_{cr} 30-60 mL/minute: Administer normal dose every 24 hours or 50% of dose at normal dosing interval
Cl_{cr} <30 mL/minute: Administer normal dose every 36-48 hours or 25% of dose at normal dosing interval

Administration

Oral: May administer with food and antacids; shake suspension vigorously for 10-15 seconds prior to each use; Pepcid RPD® tablets should be placed on the tongue to disintegrate and be swallowed with saliva

Parenteral: I.V.: Dilute to a maximum concentration of 4 mg/mL; may be administered I.V. push at 10 mg/minute over 2 minutes or as an infusion over 15-30 minutes

Patient Information Avoid excessive amounts of coffee and aspirin; when self medicating, if the symptoms of heartburn, acid indigestion, or sour stomach persist after 2 weeks of continuous use of the drug, consult a clinician.

Dosage Forms

Capsule, gelatin: 10 mg
Infusion, premixed in NS: 20 mg (50 mL)
Injection: 10 mg/mL (2 mL, 4 mL)
Powder for oral suspension (cherry-banana-mint flavor): 40 mg/5 mL (50 mL)
Tablet, chewable: 10 mg
Tablet, film coated: 20 mg, 40 mg
Pepcid® AC Acid Controller: 10 mg
Tablet, orally disintegrating (Pepcid RPD®): 20 mg, 40 mg

References
James LP and Kearns GL, "Pharmacokinetics and Pharmacodynamics of Famotidine in Paediatric Patients," *Clin Pharmacokinet*, 1996, 31(2):103-10.
Treem WR, Davis PM, and Hyams JS, "Suppression of Gastric Acid Secretion by Intravenous Administration of Famotidine in Children," *J Pediatr*, 1991, 118(5):812-6.

♦ **FAMP** *see* Fludarabine *on page 419*
♦ **Famvir**® *see* Famciclovir *on page 400*
♦ **Fansidar**® *see* Sulfadoxine and Pyrimethamine *on page 890*
♦ **F-ara-AMP** *see* Fludarabine *on page 419*

Fat Emulsion (fat e MUL shun)

Related Information
Parenteral Nutrition (PN) *on page 1072*

Brand Names Intralipid®; Liposyn®; Nutrilipid®; Soyacal®

Synonyms Intravenous Fat Emulsion; Lipid Emulsion

Therapeutic Category Caloric Agent; Intravenous Nutritional Therapy

Generic Available Yes

Use Source of calories and essential fatty acids for patients requiring parenteral nutrition of extended duration

Pregnancy Risk Factor B/C

Contraindications Pathologic hyperlipidemia; lipoid nephrosis; hypersensitivity to fat emulsion and severe egg or legume (soybean) allergies; pancreatitis with hyperlipemia

Precautions Use with caution in patients with severe liver damage, pulmonary disease, anemia, or blood coagulation disorder, and in jaundiced or premature infants

Adverse Reactions
Cardiovascular: Cyanosis, flushing, chest pain
Hepatic: Hyperlipemia, hepatomegaly
Local: Thrombophlebitis
Respiratory: Dyspnea
Miscellaneous: Sepsis

Stability May be stored at room temperature; do not use if emulsion appears to be layering out; exposure to light, particularly phototherapy light, used in treatment or prevention of hyperbilirubinemia has been associated with increased lipid oxidation; the clinical significance remains to be established

Mechanism of Action Essential for normal structure and function of cell membranes

Usual Dosage I.V. infusion: Fat emulsion should not exceed 60% of the total daily calories
(Continued)

Fat Emulsion *(Continued)*

Note: At the onset of therapy, the patient should be observed for any immediate allergic reactions such as dyspnea, cyanosis, and fever. Slower initial rates of infusion may be used for the first 10-15 minutes of the infusion (eg, 0.1 mL/minute of 10% or 0.05 mL/minute of 20% solution).

Premature infants: Initial dose: 0.25-0.5 g/kg/day, increase by 0.25-0.5 g/kg/day to a maximum of 3-4 g/kg/day; maximum rate of infusion: 0.15 g/kg/hour (0.75 mL/kg/hour of 20% solution)

Infants and Children: Initial dose: 0.5-1 g/kg/day, increase by 0.5 g/kg/day to a maximum of 3-4 g/kg/day; maximum rate of infusion: 0.25 g/kg/hour (1.25 mL/kg/hour of 20% solution)

Adolescents and Adults: Initial dose: 1 g/kg/day, increase by 0.5-1 g/kg/day to a maximum of 2.5 g/kg/day; maximum rate of infusion: 0.25 g/kg/hour (1.25 mL/kg/hour of 20% solution); do not exceed 50 mL/hour (20%) or 100 mL/hour (10%)

Children and Adults: Fatty acid deficiency: 8% to 10% of total caloric intake; infuse once or twice weekly

Administration Parenteral: May be simultaneously infused with amino acid, dextrose mixtures by means of Y-connector located near infusion site into either central or peripheral line

Monitoring Parameters Serum triglycerides, free fatty acids

Additional Information 10% = 1.1 Kcal/mL, 20% = 2 Kcal/mL; both solutions are isotonic and may be administered peripherally; avoid use of 10% fat emulsion in preterm infants; a greater accumulation of plasma lipids occurs due to the greater phospholipid load of the 10% fat emulsion

Dosage Forms Injection: 10% [100 mg/mL] (100 mL, 250 mL, 500 mL); 20% [200 mg/mL] (100 mL, 250 mL, 500 mL)

References
Haumont D, Richelle M, Deckelbaum RJ, et al, "Effect of Liposomal Content of Lipid Emulsions of Plasma Lipid Concentrations in Low Birth Weight Infants Receiving Parenteral Nutrition," *J Pediatr,* 1992, 121(5 Pt 1):759-63.

Neuzil J, Darlow BA, Inder TE, et al, "Oxidation of Parenteral Lipid Emulsion by Ambient and Photo-therapy Lights: Potential Toxicity of Routine Parenteral Feeding," *J Pediatr,* 1995, 126(5 Pt 1):785-90.

♦ **5-FC** *see* Flucytosine *on page 418*

Felbamate *(FEL ba mate)*
Related Information
Antiepileptic Drugs *on page 1176*
Carbohydrate and Alcohol Content of Liquid Medications for Use in Patients Receiving Ketogenic Diets *on page 1228*
Brand Names Felbatol®
Therapeutic Category Anticonvulsant, Miscellaneous
Generic Available No
Use Not a first-line agent, see Warnings; reserved for patients who do not adequately respond to alternative agents and whose epilepsy is so severe that benefit outweighs risk of liver failure or aplastic anemia; used as monotherapy and adjunctive therapy in patients ≥14 years of age with partial seizures with and without secondary generalization; adjunctive therapy in children ≥2 years of age who have partial and generalized seizures associated with Lennox-Gastaut syndrome
Pregnancy Risk Factor C
Contraindications History of or current blood dyscrasia or hepatic dysfunction; hypersensitivity to felbamate, any component, or other carbamates (eg, meprobamate)
Warnings Thirty-three cases of aplastic anemia (with 8 deaths) and 14 cases of hepatic failure (with 8 deaths) have been reported in patients who received felbamate. The manufacturer (Carter Wallace) and the FDA recommend the use of this agent be suspended unless withdrawal of the product would place a patient at greater risk.

Aplastic anemia: Of the 27 cases analyzed by the manufacturer, 26 occurred in adult patients (mean age: 42 years) exposed to felbamate for a mean of 170 days at a mean dose of 3168 mg/day. One case occurred in a 13-year old exposed to felbamate for 276 days at a dose of ~69 mg/kg/day. Twenty-three of 27 patients received other antiepileptic drugs (AEDs) and 9 received drugs associated with blood dyscrasias. The 8 deaths occurred in adults (mean age: 47 years). Six of the 8 patients had a history of blood dyscrasias and 6 had allergies to medications (3 to AEDs). The onset of aplastic anemia ranged from 5-30 weeks.

Hepatic failure: Of the 14 cases, 6 cases occurred in children 3-12 years of age (mean: 6 years) exposed to felbamate for 30-218 days (mean: 115 days) at a mean dose of 1520 mg/day

All patients receiving felbamate **must** be monitored closely; in addition, a CBC with differential and platelet count should be taken before, during, and for a significant time after discontinuing felbamate therapy; liver enzyme tests and bilirubin should be obtained before initiation and every 1-2 weeks during therapy. Felbamate should be immediately withdrawn if abnormal liver function tests or bone marrow suppression occur.

The FDA and the manufacturer strongly recommend that physicians discuss the risks of felbamate with each patient and a written informed consent be obtained from the patient prior to starting therapy or before continuing therapy. A patient information consent form is included as part of the package insert and is available from the local Wallace representative or by calling 609-655-6147.

Precautions Use with caution in patients concurrently receiving other antiepileptic drugs due to the potential for drug interactions; decrease dosage of phenytoin, carbamazepine, or valproic acid by 20% to 30% when felbamate is added to the regimen and when felbamate doses are titrated upwards; monitor serum levels of concomitant antiepileptic drug therapy

Adverse Reactions

Central nervous system: Headache, insomnia, somnolence, fatigue, dizziness, anxiety, drowsiness, depression, behavior changes, ataxia

Dermatologic: Acne, rash, pruritus

Gastrointestinal: Anorexia, vomiting, nausea, diarrhea, constipation, dyspepsia, gum bleeding or hyperplasia, weight loss

Hematologic: Thrombocytopenia, granulocytopenia, agranulocytosis, purpura, leukopenia, aplastic anemia (100-fold increase in risk; see Warnings)

Hepatic: Increased liver enzymes, hepatitis, acute liver failure, can be associated with death (see Warnings)

Drug Interactions Cytochrome P-450 isoenzyme CYP2C19 inhibitor

Phenytoin, carbamazepine may increase and valproic acid may decrease the clearance of felbamate; felbamate increases the concentrations of phenytoin and valproic acid; felbamate decreases carbamazepine concentrations but increases the concentration of carbamazepine epoxide (active metabolite)

Food Interactions Food does **not** affect absorption

Stability Store in tightly closed container at room temperature away from excessive heat, moisture, or direct sunlight

Mechanism of Action Mechanism of action is unknown but may be similar to other anticonvulsants; has weak inhibitory effects on GABA and benzodiazepine receptor binding; does not have activity at the MK-801 receptor binding site of the NMDA receptor-ionophore complex.

Pharmacokinetics

Absorption: Oral: Rapid and almost complete

Distribution: V_d: Adults: Mean: 0.75 L/kg; range: 0.7-1.1 L/kg

Protein binding: 20% to 25%, primarily to albumin

Metabolism: In the liver via hydroxylation and conjugation

Bioavailability: >90%

Half-life: Adults: Mean: 20-30 hours, shorter (ie, 14 hours) with concomitant enzyme-inducing drugs

Time to peak serum concentration: 1-4 hours

Elimination: 40% to 50% excreted as unchanged drug and 40% as inactive metabolites in urine

Usual Dosage See Precautions regarding concomitant antiepileptic drugs

Children 2-14 years with Lennox-Gastaut: Adjunctive therapy: Initial: 15 mg/kg/day in 3-4 divided doses; increase dose by 15 mg/kg/day increments at weekly intervals; maximum dose: 45 mg/kg/day or 3600 mg/day (whichever is less)

Children ≥14 years and Adults:

Adjunctive therapy: Initial: 1200 mg/day in 3-4 divided doses; increase daily dose by 1200 mg increments every week to a maximum dose of 3600 mg/day

Conversion to monotherapy: Initial: 1200 mg/day in 3 or 4 divided doses; at week 2, increase daily dose by 1200 mg increments every week up to a maximum dose of 3600 mg/day. Decrease dose of other anticonvulsants by 1/3 their original dose at initiation of felbamate, and when felbamate dose is increased at week 2; continue to reduce other anticonvulsants as clinically needed.

Monotherapy: Initial: 1200 mg/day in 3 or 4 divided doses; titrate dosage upward according to clinical response and monitor patients closely; increase daily dose in 600 mg increments every 2 weeks to 2400 mg/day; maximum dose: 3600 mg/day

(Continued)

Felbamate *(Continued)*

Administration Oral: May be administered without regard to meals; shake suspension well before use

Monitoring Parameters Serum concentrations of concomitant anticonvulsant therapy; liver enzymes, bilirubin, CBC with differential, platelet count prior to therapy and every 1-2 weeks

Reference Range Not necessary to routinely monitor serum drug levels; dose should be titrated to clinical response; therapeutic range not fully determined; proposed 30-100 µg/mL

Patient Information Do not abruptly discontinue, an increase in seizure activity may result; report any unusual symptoms, such as a rash, bruises, bleeding, sore throat, fever, and/or dark urine to physician immediately

Additional Information Monotherapy has not been associated with gingival hyperplasia, impaired concentration, weight gain, or abnormal thinking

Dosage Forms

Suspension, oral: 600 mg/5 mL (240 mL, 960 mL)

Tablet: 400 mg, 600 mg

References

Dodson WE, "Felbamate in the Treatment of Lennox-Gastaut Syndrome: Results of a 12-Month Open-Label Study Following a Randomized Clinical Trial," *Epilepsia*, 1993, 34(Suppl 7):S18-24.

Graves NM, "Felbamate," *Ann Pharmacother*, 1993, 27(9):1073-81.

Leppik IE, "Felbamate," *Epilepsia*, 1995, 36(Suppl 2):S66-72.

The Felbamate Study Group in Lennox-Gastaut Syndrome, "Efficacy of Felbamate in Childhood Epileptic Encephalopathy (Lennox-Gastaut Syndrome)," *N Engl J Med*, 1993, 328(1):29-33.

Written Communication, Elisabeth Neumann, Director Medical Services, Wallace Laboratories, June 13, 1995.

♦ **Felbatol®** *see* Felbamate *on page 404*

♦ **Feldene®** *see* Piroxicam *on page 777*

♦ **Femiron® [OTC]** *see* Iron Supplements, Oral/Enteral *on page 530*

♦ **Fenesin™ [OTC]** *see* Guaifenesin *on page 464*

♦ **Fenesin DM®** *see* Guaifenesin and Dextromethorphan *on page 466*

Fentanyl *(FEN ta nil)*

Related Information

Adult ACLS Algorithm, Electrical Conversion *on page 1014*

Compatibility of Medications Mixed in a Syringe *on page 1208*

Narcotic Analgesics Comparison *on page 1035*

Overdose and Toxicology *on page 1191*

Preprocedure Sedatives in Children *on page 1169*

Serotonin Syndrome *on page 1217*

Brand Names Actiq®; Duragesic® Transdermal; Fentanyl Oralet®; Sublimaze® Injection

Available Salts Fentanyl Citrate

Therapeutic Category Analgesic, Narcotic; General Anesthetic

Generic Available Injection: Yes

Use Sedation; relief of pain; preoperative medication; adjunct to general or regional anesthesia; management of chronic pain (transdermal product)

Oral transmucosal:

Fentanyl Oralet®: Hospital setting use only, as preoperative anesthetic agent or to induce conscious sedation before procedures

Actiq®: Breakthrough cancer pain in adult patients tolerant to opioid therapy and who are currently receiving opiates for persistent cancer pain. Patients are considered opioid tolerant if they are receiving at least 60 mg/day of morphine, 50 mcg/hour of transdermal fentanyl, or an equivalent dose of another opioid for 1 week or longer.

Restrictions C-II

Pregnancy Risk Factor C (D if used for prolonged periods or in high doses at term)

Contraindications Hypersensitivity or intolerance to fentanyl or any component; transdermal system is contraindicated in patients with hypersensitivity to contact adhesives; increased intracranial pressure; severe respiratory depression; severe liver or renal insufficiency; Fentanyl Oralet® is contraindicated in children <15 kg, for use at home or any setting other than a hospital, and for the treatment of acute or chronic pain; Actiq® is contraindicated in patients who are not opioid tolerant and in the treatment of acute or postoperative pain.

Warnings Physical and psychological dependence may occur with prolonged use.

I.V. use: Rapid I.V. infusion may result in skeletal muscle and chest wall rigidity → impaired ventilation → respiratory distress → apnea, bronchoconstriction, laryngospasm; inject slowly over 3-5 minutes; nondepolarizing skeletal muscle relaxant may be required

Fentanyl Oralet®: Due to risk of hypoventilation, use only in a closely monitored setting that has immediate access to advanced life support equipment and medications; directly observe and monitor patients carefully (eg, a patient-dedicated observer and pulse oximetry); should be administered by qualified health care professionals trained in anesthetic drug use and advanced cardiac life support (eg, anesthesiologists); doses should be titrated, use lowest effective dose

Actiq®: Use only for the care of cancer patients; should be used only by specialists who are knowledgeable in treating cancer pain; keep out of the reach of children and discard any open units properly; contains an amount of medication that can be fatal to children

Precautions Use with caution in patients with bradycardia, hepatic, renal, or respiratory disease or those with increased ICP, head injuries, or impaired consciousness; patients must be monitored until fully recovered; decrease dose in patients with hepatic and/or renal disease; not recommended if patient received MAO inhibitors within 14 days; use of transdermal system is not recommended in children <12 years or those <18 years and <50 kg

Adverse Reactions

Cardiovascular: Hypotension, bradycardia, flushing

Central nervous system: CNS depression, drowsiness, dizziness, sedation, euphoria

Dermatologic: Erythema, pruritus, facial pruritus with oral transmucosal product

Endocrine & metabolic: ADH release

Gastrointestinal: Nausea, vomiting, constipation, biliary tract spasm

Genitourinary: Urinary tract spasm

Local: Transdermal system: Edema, erythema, pruritus

Neuromuscular & skeletal: Skeletal and thoracic muscle rigidity especially following rapid I.V. administration

Ocular: Miosis

Respiratory: Respiratory depression, apnea

Miscellaneous: Physical and psychological dependence with prolonged use. **Note:** Neonates who receive a total fentanyl dose >1.6 mg/kg or continuous infusion duration >5 days are more likely to develop narcotic withdrawal symptoms; children 1 week to 22 months who receive a total dose of 1.5 mg/kg or duration >5 days have a 50% chance of developing narcotic withdrawal and those receiving a total dose >2.5 mg/kg or duration of infusion >9 days have a 100% chance of developing withdrawal. Doses should be tapered to prevent withdrawal symptoms.

Drug Interactions Cytochrome P-450 isoenzyme CYP3A3/4 substrate

CNS depressants, alcohol, phenothiazines, MAO inhibitors, tricyclic antidepressants may potentiate fentanyl's adverse effects

Stability Protect from light

Mechanism of Action Binds with stereospecific opioid mu receptors at many sites within the CNS, increases pain threshold, alters pain reception, inhibits ascending pain pathways

Pharmacodynamics Respiratory depressant effect may last longer than analgesic effect

Onset of analgesia:

I.M.: 7-15 minutes

I.V.: Almost immediate

Transdermal: 6-8 hours

Transmucosal: 5-15 minutes

Maximum effect:

Transdermal: 24 hours

Transmucosal: 20-30 minutes

Duration:

I.M.: 1-2 hours

I.V.: 30-60 minutes

Transdermal: 72 hours

Transmucosal: 1-2 hours

Pharmacokinetics

Absorption: Transmucosal: Rapid; ~25% absorbed from buccal mucosa; 75% swallowed with saliva and slowly absorbed from GI tract

Distribution: Highly lipophilic, redistributes into muscle and fat

V_d: Adults: 4 L/kg

(Continued)

Fentanyl *(Continued)*

V_{dss}: Children: 0.05-14 years of age (after long-term continuous infusion): ~15 L/kg (range: 5-30 L/kg)

Protein binding: 80% to 85%, primarily to alpha-1-acid glycoprotein

Metabolism: >90% metabolized in the liver via N-dealkylation and hydroxylation to inactive metabolites

Bioavailability: Transmucosal: ~50% (range: 36% to 71%)

Half-life:

Children 5 months to 4.5 years: Mean: 2.4 hours

Children 0.5-14 years (after long-term continuous infusion): ~21 hours (range: 11-36 hours)

Adults: I.V.: 2-4 hours

Transdermal: 17 hours (range: 13-22); apparent half-life increased with transdermal due to continued absorption

Transmucosal: 6.6 hours (range: 5-15 hours)

Elimination: In urine primarily as metabolites and <10% as unchanged drug

Usual Dosage Doses should be titrated to appropriate effects; wide range of doses, dependent upon desired degree of analgesia/anesthesia, clinical environment, and patient's status

Neonates and younger Infants:

Sedation/analgesia: Slow I.V. push: 1-4 mcg/kg/dose; may repeat every 2-4 hours

Continuous sedation/analgesia: Initial I.V. bolus: 1-2 mcg/kg, then 0.5-1 mcg/kg/hour; titrate upward

Mean required dose: Neonates with gestational age <34 weeks: 0.64 mcg/kg/hour; neonates with gestational age ≥34 weeks: 0.75 mcg/kg/hour

Continuous sedation/analgesia during ECMO: Initial I.V. bolus: 5-10 mcg/kg slow I.V. push over 10 minutes, then 1-5 mcg/kg/hour; titrate upward; tolerance may develop; higher doses (up to 20 mcg/kg/hour) may be needed by day 6 of ECMO

Older Infants and Children 1-12 years:

Sedation for minor procedures/analgesia: I.M., I.V.: 1-2 mcg/kg/dose; may repeat at 30- to 60-minute intervals. **Note:** Children 18-36 months of age may require 2-3 mcg/kg/dose.

Continuous sedation/analgesia: Initial I.V. bolus: 1-2 mcg/kg then 1 mcg/kg/hour; titrate upward; usual: 1-3 mcg/kg/hour; some require 5 mcg/kg/hour

Transdermal: Not recommended

Children >12 years and Adults:

Sedation for minor procedures/analgesia: I.V.: 0.5-1 mcg/kg/dose; may repeat after 30-60 minutes; **or** 25-50 mcg, repeat full dose in 5 minutes if needed, may repeat 4-5 times with 25 mcg at 5-minute intervals if needed. **Note:** Higher doses are used for major procedures.

Preoperative sedation, adjunct to regional anesthesia, postoperative pain: I.M., I.V.: 50-100 mcg/dose

Adjunct to general anesthesia: I.M., I.V.: 2-50 mcg/kg

General anesthesia without additional anesthetic agents: I.V. 50-100 mcg/kg with O_2 and skeletal muscle relaxant

Transdermal: Initial: 25 mcg/hour system; use short-acting analgesics for first 24 hours with supplemental PRN doses thereafter; dose may be increased after 3 days; if currently receiving opiates, convert to fentanyl equivalent and administer equianalgesic dosage; (see package insert for further information); transdermal patch is usually administered every 72 hours but select patients may require every 48-hour administration; dosage increase should be tried before 48-hour schedule is used

Fentanyl Oralet®: Conscious sedation/preoperative anesthetic transmucosal:

Children <15 kg: Contraindicated

Children ≥2 years of age who are ≥15 kg to <40 kg: 5-15 mcg/kg; maximum dose: 15 mcg/kg or 400 mcg (whichever is less)

Children who are **not** apprehensive at onset may only require 5 mcg/kg/dose; children who are apprehensive at onset and younger children may require 5-15 mcg/kg/dose

Children ≥40 kg and Adults: 5 mcg/kg; maximum dose: 5 mcg/kg or 400 mcg/dose (whichever is less)

Note: Use 1/4 to 1/3 the starting dose of other narcotics if given within 6-12 hours of Fentanyl Oralet®

Actiq®: Breakthrough cancer pain: Transmucosal: Adults: Titrate dose to provide adequate analgesia: Initial: 200 mcg; may redose 15 minutes after completion of first dose if needed; no more than 2 units are recommended for each break-through cancer pain episode; titrate dose up to next higher strength if treatment of several consecutive breakthrough episodes requires >1 Actiq® per episode; evaluate each new dose over several breakthrough cancer pain episodes (generally 1-2 days) to determine proper dose of analgesia with acceptable side effects. Once dose has been determined, consumption should be limited to ≤4 units per day. Re-evaluate long-acting opioid dose if patient requires >4 units/day. If signs of excessive opioid effects occur before a dose is complete, the unit should be removed from the mouth immediately, and subsequent doses decreased.

Dosing adjustment in renal impairment:
  Cl_{cr} 10-50 mL/minute: Administer 75% of dose
  Cl_{cr} <10 mL/minute: Administer 50% of dose

Administration

Transdermal: Apply to nonhairy, dry, nonirritated flat area of front or back of upper torso; do **not** shave area; do not apply new patch to same place as old patch; **Note:** Transdermal patch is a membrane-controlled system; do **not** cut the patch to deliver partial doses; rate of drug delivery, reservoir contents, and adhesion may be affected if cut; if partial dose is needed, surface area of patch can be blocked proportionally using adhesive bandage (see Lee, 1997)

Transmucosal: Foil overwrap should be removed just prior to administration; once removed, patient should place the unit in mouth and suck (not chew) it

  Fentanyl Oralet®: Begin 20-40 minutes prior to the anticipated start of surgery, diagnostic, or therapeutic procedure; unit should be removed after it is consumed or if patient has achieved an adequate sedation and anxiolytic level, and/or shows signs of respiratory depression

  Actiq®: Place in mouth between cheek and lower gum; occasionally move unit from one side of the mouth to the other; consume unit over 15 minutes; remove unit from mouth if signs of excessive opioid effects appear before unit is totally consumed

Parenteral: I.V.: Administer by slow I.V. push over 3-5 minutes or by continuous infusion; larger bolus doses (>5 mcg/kg) should be given slow I.V. push over 5-10 minutes

Monitoring Parameters
Respiratory rate, blood pressure, heart rate, oxygen saturation, bowel sounds, abdominal distention

Patient Information
Avoid alcohol; may cause drowsiness and impair ability to perform activities requiring mental alertness or physical coordination; an Actiq® Welcome Kit, containing educational materials and safe storage containers (to keep medication away from children), as well as a patient safety video, is available from the manufacturer; these can be obtained by healthcare professionals who call 1-888-818-4113; dispose of transmucosal and transdermal products properly; keep all products (even if used) out of the reach of children; see Actiq® Patient Leaflet for details on proper storage, administration, and disposal of Actiq®, as well as, instructions about overdose management.

Nursing Implications
Patients with elevated temperature may have increased fentanyl absorption transdermally, observe for adverse effects, dosage adjustment may be needed; pharmacologic and adverse effects can be seen after discontinuation of transdermal system, observe patients for at least 12 hours after transdermal product removed; destroy unused portion of fentanyl Oralet® and Actiq® according to hospital policy on controlled substances; partial unused doses of Actiq® can be dissolved under hot running tap water; dispose of handle properly; keep out of the reach of children

Additional Information
An opioid antagonist, resuscitative and intubation equipment, and oxygen should be available; fentanyl is 50-100 times as potent as morphine; morphine 10 mg I.M. = fentanyl 0.1-0.2 mg I.M.; fentanyl has less hypotensive effects than morphine or meperidine due to minimal or no histamine release; keep transmucosal and transdermal products (both used and unused) out of the reach of children; special child-resistant containers are available to temporarily store partially-consumed units that cannot be disposed of immediately; do **not** use soap, alcohol, or other solvents to remove transdermal gel if it accidentally touches skin as they may increase transdermal absorption, use copious amounts of water; Fentanyl Oralet® 5 mcg/kg = fentanyl 0.75-1.25 mcg/kg I.M.

Dosage Forms
Injection, preservative free, as citrate: 0.05 mg/mL (2 mL, 5 mL, 10 mL, 20 mL, 30 mL, 50 mL)

Lozenge, oral transmucosal, as citrate (raspberry flavored) mounted on a plastic radiopaque handle:
  Actiq®: 200 mcg, 400 mcg, 600 mcg, 800 mcg, 1200 mcg, 1600 mcg
  Fentanyl Oralet®: 100 mcg, 200 mcg, 300 mcg, 400 mcg
(Continued)

Fentanyl *(Continued)*

Transdermal system: 25 mcg/hour [10 cm^2]; 50 mcg/hour [20 cm^2]; 75 mcg/hour [30 cm^2]; 100 mcg/hour [40 cm^2] (all available in 5s)

References

Billmire DA, Neale HW, and Gregory RO, "Use of I.V. Fentanyl in the Outpatient Treatment of Pediatric Facial Trauma," *J Trauma*, 1985, 25(11):1079-80.

Katz R, Kelly HW, and Hsi A, "Prospective Study on the Occurrence of Withdrawal in Critically Ill Children Who Receive Fentanyl by Continuous Infusion," *Crit Care Med*, 1994, 22(5):763-7.

Lee NA and Anderson PO, "Giving Partial Doses of Transdermal Patches," *Am J Health Syst Pharm*, 1997, 54(15):1759-60.

Leuschen MP, Willett LD, Hoie EB, et al, "Plasma Fentanyl Levels in Infants Undergoing Extracorporeal Membrane Oxygenation," *J Thorac Cardiovasc Surg*, 1993, 105(5):885-91.

Roth B, Schlunder C, Houben F, et al, "Analgesia and Sedation in Neonatal Intensive Care Using Fentanyl by Continuous Infusion," *Dev Pharmacol Ther*, 1991, 17(3-4):121-7.

Schechter NL, Weisman SJ, Rosenblum M, et al, "The Use of Oral Transmucosal Fentanyl Citrate for Painful Procedures in Children," *Pediatrics*, 1995, 95(3):335-9.

Zeltzer LK, Altman A, Cohen D, et al, "Report of the Subcommittee on the Management of Pain Associated With Procedures in Children With Cancer," *Pediatrics*, 1990, 86(5 Pt 2):826-31.

♦ **Fentanyl and Droperidol** *see* Droperidol and Fentanyl *on page 352*

♦ **Fentanyl Citrate** *see* Fentanyl *on page 406*

♦ **Fentanyl Oralet®** *see* Fentanyl *on page 406*

♦ **Feosol® [OTC]** *see* Iron Supplements, Oral/Enteral *on page 530*

♦ **Feostat® [OTC]** *see* Iron Supplements, Oral/Enteral *on page 530*

♦ **Feratab® [OTC]** *see* Iron Supplements, Oral/Enteral *on page 530*

♦ **Fergon® [OTC]** *see* Iron Supplements, Oral/Enteral *on page 530*

♦ **Fer-In-Sol® [OTC]** *see* Iron Supplements, Oral/Enteral *on page 530*

♦ **Fer-Iron® [OTC]** *see* Iron Supplements, Oral/Enteral *on page 530*

♦ **Fermalac® (Canada)** *see* Lactobacillus acidophilus and Lactobacillus bulgaricus *on page 550*

♦ **Fero-Gradumet® [OTC]** *see* Iron Supplements, Oral/Enteral *on page 530*

♦ **Ferospace® [OTC]** *see* Iron Supplements, Oral/Enteral *on page 530*

♦ **Ferralet® [OTC]** *see* Iron Supplements, Oral/Enteral *on page 530*

♦ **Ferralyn® Lanacaps® [OTC]** *see* Iron Supplements, Oral/Enteral *on page 530*

♦ **Ferra-TD® [OTC]** *see* Iron Supplements, Oral/Enteral *on page 530*

Ferric Gluconate (FER ik GLOO koe nate)

Brand Names Ferrlecit®

Available Salts Sodium Ferric Gluconate

Synonyms Sodium Ferric Gluconate Complex in Sucrose Injection

Therapeutic Category Iron Salt, Parenteral; Mineral, Parenteral

Generic Available No

Use Treatment of microcytic, hypochromic anemia resulting from iron deficiency in patients who are undergoing hemodialysis in conjunction with erythropoietin therapy, when oral iron administration is not feasible or ineffective

Pregnancy Risk Factor B

Contraindications Hypersensitivity to ferric gluconate or any component; use in any anemia not associated with iron deficiency; hemochromatosis, hemolytic anemia

Warnings Potentially serious hypersensitivity reactions may occur; fatal immediate hypersensitivity reactions have occurred with other iron carbohydrate complexes; treatment agents for anaphylactic reactions (eg, epinephrine, steroids, diphenhydramine) should be immediately available; a test dose is recommended prior to initial therapy; rapid administration is associated with flushing and hypotension; contains benzyl alcohol, avoid use in neonates

Precautions Use with caution in patients with histories of significant allergies; safety and efficacy have not been established in children

Adverse Reactions

Note: Anaphylactoid reactions: Respiratory difficulties and cardiovascular collapse have been reported with other iron carbohydrate complexes and occur most frequently within the first several minutes of administration

Cardiovascular: Hypotension, chest pain, hypertension, syncope, tachycardia, angina, MI, hypovolemia

Central nervous system: Headache, fatigue, fever, malaise, dizziness, insomnia, agitation, somnolence

Dermatologic: Pruritus, rash

Endocrine & metabolic: Hyperkalemia, hypoglycemia, hypokalemia

Gastrointestinal: Abdominal pain, nausea, vomiting, diarrhea, dyspepsia, flatulence, melena, eructation

Genitourinary: Urinary tract infection
Hematologic: Abnormal erythrocytes, lymphadenopathy
Local: Injection site reactions, pain
Neuromuscular & skeletal: Weakness, back pain, leg cramps, myalgia, arthralgia, paresthesia
Ocular: Blurred vision, conjunctivitis
Respiratory: Dyspnea, cough, rhinitis, upper respiratory infection, pulmonary edema, pneumonia
Miscellaneous: Anaphylactoid reactions, infection, rigors, chills, flu-like syndrome, sepsis, carcinoma, diaphoresis

Stability Use immediately after dilution in NS; do not mix with other medications or add to parenteral nutrition solutions

Mechanism of Action Replaces iron found in hemoglobin, myoglobin, and specific enzymes; allows transportation of oxygen via hemoglobin

Pharmacokinetics Not dialyzable

Usual Dosage I.V.: Test dose is required before repletion dose: Dosage expressed in mg **elemental** iron:
Adults:
Test dose: 25 mg (2 mL)
Repletion dose: 125 mg (10 mL) during hemodialysis; most patients will require a cumulative dose of 1 g over ~8 sequential dialysis treatments to achieve a favorable response

Administration Parenteral: Dilute test dose in 50 mL NS and infuse over 1 hour; dilute repletion dose (125 mg) in 100 mL NS and infuse over at least 1 hour; do not exceed 2.1 mg/minute

Monitoring Parameters Frequent vital signs during infusion; hemoglobin, hematocrit, serum iron, serum ferritin, iron saturation, reticulocyte count

Additional Information Iron storage may lag behind the appearance of normal red blood cell morphology; use periodic hematologic determination to assess therapy

Dosage Forms Injection: 12.5 mg/mL (5 mL) [expressed in mg of **elemental** iron]

♦ **Ferrlecit®** see Ferric Gluconate on page 410
♦ **Ferro-Sequels® [OTC]** see Iron Supplements, Oral/Enteral on page 530
♦ **Ferrous Fumarate** see Iron Supplements, Oral/Enteral on page 530
♦ **Ferrous Gluconate** see Iron Supplements, Oral/Enteral on page 530
♦ **Ferrous Sulfate** see Iron Supplements, Oral/Enteral on page 530
♦ **FeSO₄ (Ferrous Sulfate)** see Iron Supplements, Oral/Enteral on page 530
♦ **Feverall™ [OTC]** see Acetaminophen on page 26
♦ **Fiberall® Powder [OTC]** see Psyllium on page 823
♦ **Fiberall® Wafer [OTC]** see Psyllium on page 823
♦ **Fibrepur® (Canada)** see Psyllium on page 823

Filgrastim (fil GRA stim)

Brand Names Neupogen®
Synonyms G-CSF; Granulocyte Colony Stimulating Factor
Therapeutic Category Colony Stimulating Factor
Generic Available No

Use Reduction of the duration of neutropenia and the associated risk of infection in patients with malignancies receiving myelosuppressive chemotherapeutic regimens associated with a significant incidence of severe neutropenia with fever; cancer patients receiving bone marrow transplant; severe chronic neutropenia which includes patients with congenital neutropenia, cyclic neutropenia, or idiopathic neutropenia; mobilization of peripheral blood progenitor cells into the peripheral blood for collection by leukapheresis; AIDS patients on zidovudine and in neonatal neutropenia

Pregnancy Risk Factor C

Contraindications Hypersensitivity to E. coli-derived proteins, G-CSF, or any component; use in patients receiving concomitant chemotherapy and radiation therapy

Warnings Leukocytosis (white blood cell counts ≥100,000/mm³) has been observed in approximately 2% of patients receiving G-CSF at doses >5 mcg/kg/day

Precautions Do not administer 24 hours prior to or within 24 hours following the administration of chemotherapy; use with caution in any malignancy with myeloid characteristics due to G-CSF's potential to act as a growth factor; use with caution in patients with gout, psoriasis; monitor patients with pre-existing cardiac conditions as cardiac events (MIs, arrhythmias) have been reported in premarketing clinical studies. Be alert to the possibility of ARDS in septic patients.

Premature discontinuation of G-CSF therapy prior to the time of recovery from the expected neutrophil nadir is generally not recommended. A transient increase in neutrophil counts is typically seen 1-2 days after initiation of therapy. For a (Continued)

Filgrastim *(Continued)*

sustained therapeutic response, G-CSF should be continued until the post nadir absolute neutrophil count (ANC) reaches:

10,000/mm^3 in chemotherapy treated patients, or

>1000/mm^3 for 3 consecutive days in bone marrow transplant patients

Most patients experience a 30% to 50% decrease in circulating leukocytes within 1-2 days following discontinuation of G-CSF

Adverse Reactions

Cardiovascular: Transient decrease in blood pressure, vasculitis, chest pain

Central nervous system: Fever, headache

Dermatologic: Exacerbation of pre-existing skin disorders, alopecia

Endocrine & metabolic: Reversible increase in uric acid, lactate dehydrogenase

Gastrointestinal: Splenomegaly, nausea, vomiting, diarrhea, mucositis

Hematologic: Thrombocytopenia, leukocytosis

Hepatic: Elevated alkaline phosphatase

Neuromuscular & skeletal: Medullary bone pain (24% incidence) is generally dose-related, localized to the lower back, posterior iliac crests, and sternum; osteoporosis

Renal: Hematuria, proteinuria

Stability Store in refrigerator; do not freeze; stable for 24 hours at room temperature; solutions with concentration ≥15 mcg/mL in D$_5$W are stable for 24 hours; incompatible with salt solutions

Mechanism of Action Stimulates the production, maturation, and activation of neutrophils; G-CSF activates neutrophils to increase both their migration and cytotoxicity

Pharmacodynamics

Onset of action: Immediate transient leukopenia with the nadir occurring 5-15 minutes after an I.V. dose or 30-60 minutes after a S.C. dose followed by a sustained elevation in neutrophil levels within the first 24 hours reaching a plateau in 3-5 days

Duration: Upon discontinuation of G-CSF, ANC decreases by 50% within 2 days and returns to pretreatment levels within 1 week; white counts return to the normal range in 4-7 days

Pharmacokinetics

Distribution: V$_d$: 150 mL/kg

Bioavailability: Not bioavailable after oral administration

Half-life: 1.8-3.5 hours; Neonates: 4.4 hours

Time to peak serum concentration: S.C.: Within 2-6 hours

Elimination: No evidence of drug accumulation over a 11- to 20-day period

Usual Dosage I.V., S.C. (refer to individual protocols):

Neonates: 5-10 mcg/kg/day once daily for 3-5 days has been administered to neutropenic neonates with sepsis. There was a rapid and significant increase in peripheral neutrophil counts and the neutrophil storage pool.

Children and Adults: 5-10 mcg/kg/day (~150-300 mcg/m^2/day) once daily for up to 14 days until ANC = 10,000/mm^3; dose escalations at 5 mcg/kg/day may be required in some individuals when response at 5 mcg/kg/day is not adequate; in phase 3 trials, efficacy was observed at dosages of 4-8 mcg/kg/day with myelosuppressive chemotherapy

Peripheral blood progenitor cell (PBPC) mobilization: S.C.: 10 mcg/kg/day given for 4 days before the first leukapheresis procedure and continued until the last leukapheresis

Patients with congenital neutropenia: S.C.: Initial: 6 mcg/kg/dose twice daily; dosages of 2-60 mcg/kg/day individualized according to neutrophil count have been administered to children and adults

Patients with idiopathic or cyclic neutropenia: S.C.: 5 mcg/kg/day once daily

Cancer patients receiving bone marrow transplant: I.V. infusion, S.C.: 5-10 mcg/kg/day administered ≥24 hours after cytotoxic chemotherapy and ≥24 hours after bone marrow infusion

Dosage adjustment during neutrophil recovery period: see table

Filgrastim Dose Based on Neutrophil Response

Absolute Neutrophil Count	Filgrastim Dose Adjustment
When ANC >1000/mm^3 for 3 consecutive days	Reduce to 5 mcg/kg/day
If ANC remains >1000/mm^3 for 3 more consecutive days	Discontinue filgrastim
If ANC decreases to <1000/mm^3	Resume at 5 mcg/kg/day

If ANC decreases <1000/mm^3 during the 5 mcg/kg/day dose, increase filgrastim to 10 mcg/kg/day and follow the above steps in the table.

Administration Parenteral:

S.C.: Administer undiluted solution

S.C. continuous infusion: Dilute dose in 10 mL D₅W and infuse at a rate of 10 mL/ 24 hours

I.V. continuous infusion; Administer over 15-60 minutes or as a continuous I.V. infusion at a final concentration of at least 15 mcg/mL in D₅W. If the final concentration of G-CSF in D₅W is <15 mcg/mL, then add 2 mg albumin/mL to I.V. fluid; the solution is stable for 24 hours; albumin acts as a carrier molecule to prevent drug adsorption to the I.V. tubing. Albumin should be added to the D₅W prior to addition of G-CSF; final concentration of G-CSF for administration <5 mcg/mL is not recommended; do not shake solution to avoid foaming.

Monitoring Parameters CBC with differential and platelet count, hematocrit, uric acid, urinalysis, liver function tests

Reference Range Blood samples for monitoring the hematologic effects of G-CSF should be drawn just before the next dose at least twice weekly

Patient Information Possible bone pain

Nursing Implications Bone pain management is usually successful with non-narcotic analgesic therapy

Dosage Forms Injection, preservative free: 300 mcg/mL (1 mL, 1.6 mL), produced by recombinant DNA technology using an *E. coli* expression system

References

"Update of Recommendations for the Use of Hematopoietic Colony-Stimulating Factors: Evidence-based Clinical Practice Guidelines. American Society of Clinical Oncology," *J Clin Oncol*, 1996, 14(6):1957-60.

Bonilla MA, Gillio AP, Ruggeiro M, et al, "Effects of Recombinant Human Granulocyte Colony-Stimulating Factor on Neutropenia in Patients With Congenital Agranulocytosis," *N Engl J Med*, 1989, 320(24):1574-80.

Gilmore MM, Stroncek DF, and Korones DN, "Treatment of Alloimmune Neonatal Neutropenia With Granulocyte Colony-Stimulating Factor," *J Pediatr*, 1994, 125(6 Pt 1):948-51

Hollingshead LM, Goa KL, "Recombinant Granulocyte Colony-Stimulating Factor (rG-CSF). A Review of Its Pharmacological Properties and Prospective Role in Neutropenic Conditions," *Drugs*, 1991, 42(2):300-30.

Morstyn G, Campbell L, Lieschke G, et al, "Treatment of Chemotherapy-Induced Neutropenia by Subcutaneously Administered Granulocyte Colony-Stimulating Factor With Optimization of Dose and Duration of Therapy," *J Clin Oncol*, 1989, 7(10):1554-62.

Wolach B, "Neonatal Sepsis: Pathogenesis and Supportive Therapy," *Semin Perinatol*, 1997, 21(1):28-38.

♦ **Fisalamine** *see* Mesalamine *on page 608*

♦ **FK506** *see* Tacrolimus *on page 901*

♦ **Flagyl® Oral** *see* Metronidazole *on page 636*

♦ **Flamazine® (Canada)** *see* Silver Sulfadiazine *on page 867*

♦ **Flarex®** *see* Fluorometholone *on page 429*

♦ **Flatulex® [OTC]** *see* Simethicone *on page 868*

♦ **Flavorcee® [OTC]** *see* Ascorbic Acid *on page 96*

Flecainide (fle KAY nide)

Brand Names Tambocor®

Available Salts Flecainide Acetate

Therapeutic Category Antiarrhythmic Agent, Class I-C

Generic Available No

Use Prevention and suppression of documented life-threatening ventricular arrhythmias (ie, sustained ventricular tachycardia); prevention of symptomatic, disabling supraventricular tachycardias in patients without structural heart disease

Pregnancy Risk Factor C

Contraindications Pre-existing second or third degree A-V block; right bundle-branch block associated with left hemiblock (bifascicular block) or trifascicular block; cardiogenic shock, myocardial depression; hypersensitivity to flecainide or any component

Warnings The manufacturer and FDA recommend that this drug be reserved for life-threatening ventricular arrhythmias unresponsive to conventional therapy. Its use for symptomatic nonsustained ventricular tachycardia, frequent premature ventricular complexes (PVCs), uniform and multiform PVCs and/or coupled PVCs is no longer recommended. Flecainide can worsen or cause arrhythmias with an associated risk of death. Proarrhythmic effects range from an increased number of PVCs to more severe ventricular tachycardias (ie, tachycardias that are more sustained or more resistant to conversion to sinus rhythm).

Precautions Worsening arrhythmias, pre-existing sinus node dysfunction, sick sinus syndrome, history of CHF or myocardial dysfunction; increases in P-R interval ≥300 MS, QRS ≥180 MS, Q-T$_c$ interval increases and/or new bundle-branch block; patients with pacemakers, renal impairment and/or hepatic impairment; use decreased doses and cautiously titrate dose according to serum concentrations and effects in patients with CHF, or myocardial, liver or renal dysfunction

(Continued)

Flecainide *(Continued)*

Adverse Reactions
Cardiovascular: Bradycardia, heart block, worsening ventricular arrhythmias, CHF, palpitations, chest pain, edema; increased P-R, QRS duration

Central nervous system: Dizziness, fatigue, nervousness, hypoesthesia, headache

Dermatologic: Rash

Gastrointestinal: Nausea

Hematologic: Blood dyscrasias

Hepatic: Possible hepatic dysfunction

Neuromuscular & skeletal: Paresthesia, tremor

Ocular: Blurred vision

Respiratory: Dyspnea

Drug Interactions Cytochrome P-450 isoenzyme CYP2D6 substrate

Other antiarrhythmic agents may increase adverse cardiac effects; flecainide may increase plasma digoxin concentrations; use with beta-blockers, disopyramide, or verapamil may result in possible additive negative inotropic effects; alkalinizing agents (high-dose antacids, carbonic anhydrase inhibitors or sodium bicarbonate) may decrease flecainide's clearance; urinary acidifiers may increase flecainide's clearance; amiodarone and cimetidine increase flecainide serum concentrations; concurrent use of flecainide with ritonavir is not recommended

Food Interactions Dairy products (milk, infant formula, yogurt) may interfere with the absorption of flecainide in infants; there is one case report of a neonate (GA 34 weeks PNA >6 days) who required extremely large doses of oral flecainide when administered every 8 hours with feedings ("milk feeds"); changing the feedings from "milk feeds" to 5% glucose feeds alone resulted in a doubling of the flecainide serum concentration and toxicity (see Russell, et al); clearance of flecainide may be decreased in patients with strict vegetarian diets due to urinary pH ≥8

Mechanism of Action Class IC antiarrhythmic; slows conduction in cardiac tissue by altering transport of ions across cell membranes; causes slight prolongation of refractory periods; decreases the rate of rise of the action potential without affecting its duration; increases electrical stimulation threshold of ventricle, HIS-Purkinje system; possesses local anesthetic and moderate negative inotropic effects

Pharmacokinetics
Absorption: Oral: Rapid and nearly complete

Distribution: V_d: Adults: 5-13.4 L/kg

Protein binding: 40% to 50% (alpha$_1$ glycoprotein)

Metabolism: In the liver

Bioavailability: 85% to 90%

Half-life, elimination: Increased half-life with CHF or renal dysfunction

Newborns: ~29 hours

Infants: 11-12 hours

Children: 8 hours

Adults: ~20 hours (range: 12-27 hours)

Time to peak serum concentration: ~3 hours (range 1-6 hours)

Elimination: In urine as unchanged drug (10% to 50%) and metabolites

Usual Dosage Oral:
Children: Initial: 1-3 mg/kg/day or 50-100 mg/m^2/day in 3 divided doses; usual: 3-6 mg/kg/day or 100-150 mg/m^2/day in 3 divided doses; up to 8 mg/kg/day or 200 mg/m^2/day for uncontrolled patients with subtherapeutic levels; higher doses have been reported, however they may be associated with an increased risk of proarrhythmias; a review of world literature reports the average effective dose to be 4 mg/kg/day or 140 mg/m^2/day

Adults: Life-threatening ventricular arrhythmias: Initial: 100 mg every 12 hours, increase by 100 mg/day (given in 2 doses/day) every 4 days to maximum of 400 mg/day; for patients receiving 400 mg/day who are not controlled and have trough concentrations <0.6 mcg/mL, dosage may be increased to 600 mg/day

Prevention of paroxysmal supraventricular arrhythmias in patients with disabling symptoms but no structural heart disease: Initial: 50 mg every 12 hours; maximum dose: 300 mg/day

Dosing adjustment in renal failure: Children and Adults: Decrease the usual dose by 25% to 50%

Administration Oral: May be administered in children and adults without regard to food; in infants receiving milk based formulas, avoid concurrent administration with feedings; monitor serum concentrations and decrease the dose when the diet changes to a decreased consumption of milk

Monitoring Parameters EKG, serum concentrations; **Note:** Obtain serum trough concentrations at steady state (after at least 3 days when doses are started or changed) or when dietary changes due to maturation or concurrent illness occur

Reference Range Therapeutic: 0.2-1 µg/mL (SI: 0.4-2 µmol/L). **Note:** Pediatric patients may respond at the lower end of the recommended therapeutic range.

Patient Information May cause dizziness; notify physician if chest pain, faintness, palpitations, dizziness or visual disturbances occur

Additional Information Single oral dose flecainide for termination of PSVT in children and young adults (n=25) and combination therapy of flecainide with amiodarone for refractory tachyarrhythmias in infancy (n=9) have been reported (See References)

Dosage Forms Tablet, as acetate: 50 mg, 100 mg, 150 mg

Extemporaneous Preparations

A 5 mg/mL suspension compounded from tablets and an oral flavored commercially available diluent (Roxane®) was stable for up to 45 days when stored at 5°C or 25°C in amber glass bottles (Wiest, 1992)

A 20 mg/mL oral liquid preparation made from tablets and 3 different vehicles (cherry syrup, a 1:1 mixture of Ora-Sweet® and Ora-Plus®, or a 1:1 mixture of Ora-Sweet® SF and Ora-Plus®) was stable for 60 days when stored in amber plastic prescription bottles in the dark at room temperature (25°C) or under refrigeration (5°C); grind twenty-four 100 mg tablets in a mortar into a fine powder; add 20 mL of the vehicle and mix well to form a uniform paste; mix while adding the vehicle in geometric proportions to **almost** 120 mL; transfer to a calibrated bottle and qsad with vehicle to 120 mL; label "shake well" and "protect from light" (Allen, 1996).

Allen LV and Erickson MA, "Stability of Baclofen, Captopril, Diltiazem Hydrochloride, Dipyridamole, and Flecainide Acetate in Extemporaneously Compounded Oral Liquids," *Am J Health Syst Pharm*, 1996, 53(18):2179-84.

Wiest DB, Garner SS, and Pagacz LR, "Stability of Flecainide Acetate in an Extemporaneously Compounded Oral Suspension," *Am J Hosp Pharm*, 1992, 49(6):1467-70.

References

Fenrich AL Jr, Perry JC, and Friedman RA, "Flecainide and Amiodarone: Combined Therapy for Refractory Tachyarrhythmias in Infants," *J Am Coll Cardiol*, 1995, 25(5):1195-8.

Musto B, Cavallaro C, Musto A, et al, "Flecainide Single Oral Dose for Management of Paroxysmal Supraventricular Tachycardia in Children and Young Adults," *Am Heart J*, 1992, 124(1):110-5.

Perry JC and Garson A Jr, "Flecainide Acetate for Treatment of Tachyarrhythmias in Children: Review of World Literature on Efficacy, Safety, and Dosing," *Am Heart J*, 1992, 124(6):1614-21.

Perry JC, McQuinn RL, Smith RT Jr, et al, "Flecainide Acetate for Resistant Arrhythmias in the Young: Efficacy and Pharmacokinetics," *J Am Coll Cardiol*, 1989, 14(1):185-91.

Priestley KA, Ladusans EJ, Rosenthal E, et al, "Experience With Flecainide for the Treatment of Cardiac Arrhythmias in Children," *Eur Heart J*, 1988, 9(12):1284-90.

Russell GA and Martin RP, "Flecainide Toxicity," *Arch Dis Child*, 1989, 64(6):860-2.

Zeigler V, Gillette PC, Ross BA, et al, "Flecainide for Supraventricular and Ventricular Arrhythmias in Children and Young Adults," *Am J Cardiol*, 1988, 62(10 Pt 1):818-20.

♦ **Flecainide Acetate** *see Flecainide on page 413*
♦ **Fleet® Babylax® Rectal [OTC]** *see Glycerin on page 457*
♦ **Fleet® Enema [OTC]** *see Phosphate Supplements on page 765*
♦ **Fleet® Flavored Castor Oil [OTC]** *see Castor Oil on page 175*
♦ **Fleet® Laxative [OTC]** *see Bisacodyl on page 133*
♦ **Fleet® Mineral Oil Enema [OTC]** *see Mineral Oil on page 649*
♦ **Fleet® Phospho®-Soda [OTC]** *see Phosphate Supplements on page 765*
♦ **Fleet® Relief®** *see Hemorrhoidal Preparations on page 470*
♦ **Flexaphen®** *see Chlorzoxazone on page 218*
♦ **Flexeril®** *see Cyclobenzaprine on page 265*
♦ **Flodine® (Canada)** *see Folic Acid on page 439*
♦ **Flonase®** *see Fluticasone on page 436*
♦ **Flo-Pack®** *see Succinylcholine on page 884*
♦ **Florical® [OTC]** *see Calcium Supplements on page 157*
♦ **Florinef® Acetate** *see Fludrocortisone on page 420*
♦ **Flovent®** *see Fluticasone on page 436*
♦ **Flovent® Rotadisk®** *see Fluticasone on page 436*
♦ **Flubenisolone** *see Betamethasone on page 130*

Fluconazole (floo KOE na zole)

Related Information

Carbohydrate and Alcohol Content of Liquid Medications for Use in Patients Receiving Ketogenic Diets *on page 1228*

(Continued)

Fluconazole *(Continued)*

Brand Names Diflucan®

Therapeutic Category Antifungal Agent, Systemic

Generic Available No

Use Treatment of susceptible fungal infections including oropharyngeal, esophageal, and vaginal candidiasis; treatment of systemic candidal infections including urinary tract infection, peritonitis, cystitis, and pneumonia; strains of *Candida* with decreased *in vitro* susceptibility to fluconazole are being isolated with increasing frequency; fluconazole is more active against *C. albicans* than other candidal strains like *C. parapsilosis*, *C. glabrata*, and *C. tropicalis*; treatment and suppression of cryptococcal meningitis; prophylaxis of candidiasis in patients undergoing bone marrow transplantation; alternative to amphotericin B in patients with pre-existing renal impairment or when requiring concomitant therapy with other potentially nephrotoxic drugs

Pregnancy Risk Factor C

Contraindications Hypersensitivity to fluconazole, other azoles, or any component; concurrent use of astemizole, cisapride, and terfenadine

Warnings Patients who develop abnormal liver function tests during fluconazole therapy should be monitored closely for the development of more severe hepatic injury; if clinical signs and symptoms consistent with liver disease develop that may be attributable to fluconazole, fluconazole should be discontinued

Precautions Use with caution and modify dosage in patients with impaired renal function

Adverse Reactions

Cardiovascular: Pallor

Central nervous system: Dizziness, headache (1.9%), seizures

Dermatologic: Skin rash (1.8%), exfoliative skin disorders, Stevens-Johnson syndrome

Endocrine & metabolic: Hypokalemia, hypercholesterolemia, hypertriglyceridemia

Gastrointestinal: Nausea (2%), abdominal pain (3%), vomiting (5%), diarrhea (2%)

Hematologic: Eosinophilia, leukopenia, thrombocytopenia

Hepatic: Elevated AST, ALT, or alkaline phosphatase; hepatitis; cholestasis

Miscellaneous: Anaphylaxis

Drug Interactions Cytochrome P-450 isoenzyme CYP2CP substrate; CYP2C19 and CYP3A3/4 (weak) isoenzyme inhibitor

Oral antidiabetic agents (fluconazole reduces the metabolism and increases the concentration of tolbutamide, glyburide, and glipizide); hydrochlorothiazide (increases fluconazole AUC); warfarin (increased prothrombin time); fluconazole increases plasma cyclosporine, zidovudine, cisapride, (fatal arrhythmias including ventricular tachycardia, ventricular fibrillation, torsades de pointes, and QT prolongation have been reported in patients taking cisapride concurrently with fluconazole), astemizole, terfenadine, rifabutin, and phenytoin concentrations; rifampin increases fluconazole metabolism; antagonism may occur if amphotericin B and fluconazole are used concomitantly

Food Interactions Food decreases the rate but not the extent of absorption

Stability Incompatible with ampicillin, calcium gluconate, ceftazidime, cefotaxime, cefuroxime, ceftriaxone, clindamycin, furosemide, imipenem, ticarcillin, and piperacillin; reconstituted oral suspension is stable for 14 days at room temperature or if refrigerated

Mechanism of Action Interferes with fungal cytochrome P-450 sterol C-14 alpha-demethylation activity, decreasing ergosterol synthesis (principal sterol in fungal cell membrane) and inhibiting cell membrane formation

Pharmacokinetics

Absorption: Oral: Well absorbed; food does not affect extent of absorption

Distribution: Distributes widely into body tissues and fluids including the CSF, saliva, sputum, vaginal fluid, skin, eye; excreted in breast milk

Protein binding: 11% to 12%

Bioavailability: Oral: >90%

Half-life:

Premature newborns: 73.6 hours; 6 days PNA: 53.2 hours; 12 days PNA: 46.6 hours

Children:

9 months to 13 years: 19.5-25 hours (with oral dose)

5-15 years: 15.2-17.6 hours (with multiple I.V. dosing)

Adults: 25-30 hours with normal renal function

Time to peak serum concentration: Oral: Within 2-4 hours (1-2 hours in fasted patients)

Elimination: 80% of dose excreted unchanged in urine; 11% of dose excreted in urine as metabolites

Hemodialysis: 3-hour session decreases plasma concentration 50%

Usual Dosage Daily dose of fluconazole is the same for oral and I.V. administration:

Oral, I.V.:

Premature neonates:

≤29 weeks gestation:

Postnatal age 0-14 days: 5-6 mg/kg/dose every 72 hours

Postnatal age >14 days: 5-6 mg/kg/dose every 48 hours

30-36 weeks gestation: Postnatal age 0-14 days: 3-6 mg/kg/dose every 48 hours

Neonates >14 days, Infants, Children: Once daily: See table

Safety profile of fluconazole has been studied in 577 children ages 1 day to 17 years. Doses as high as 12 mg/kg/day once daily (equivalent to adult doses of 400 mg/day) have been used to treat candidiasis in immunocompromised children; 10-12 mg/kg/day doses once daily have been used prophylactically against fungal infections in pediatric bone marrow transplantation patients. Do not exceed 600 mg/day.

Adults: Oral, I.V.: Once daily: See table

Indication	Day 1	Daily Therapy	Minimum Duration of Therapy
Neonates 0-14 days: Same dosage as older children but administered every 24-72 h			
Neonates >14 days, infants, and children			
Oropharyngeal candidiasis	6 mg/kg	3 mg/kg	14 d
Esophageal candidiasis	6 mg/kg	3 mg/kg up to 12 mg/kg/d	21 d
Systemic candidiasis	6-12 mg/kg/d		28 d
Cryptococcal meningitis			
acute	12 mg/kg	6 mg/kg up to 12 mg/kg/d	10-12 wk after CSF culture becomes negative
relapse	6 mg/kg		
Adults			
Oropharyngeal candidiasis	200 mg	100 mg	14 d
Esophageal candidiasis	200 mg	100-400 mg	21 d
Systemic candidiasis	400 mg	200-800 mg	28 d
Cryptococcal meningitis			
acute	400 mg	200-800 mg	10-12 wk after CSF culture becomes negative
relapse	200 mg	200 mg	

Vaginal candidiasis: Oral: 150 mg single dose

Prophylaxis against fungal infections in bone marrow transplantation patients: Oral, I.V.: 400 mg/day once daily

Dosing adjustment in renal impairment:

Cl$_{cr}$ 21-50 mL/minute: Administer 50% of recommended dose

Cl$_{cr}$ <20 mL/minute: Administer 25% of recommended dose

Patients receiving hemodialysis: One recommended dose after each dialysis

Administration

Oral: Administer with or without food; shake suspension well before use

Parenteral: Fluconazole must be administered by I.V. infusion over approximately 1-2 hours at a rate not to exceed 200 mg/hour and a final concentration for administration of 2 mg/mL; for pediatric patients receiving doses ≥6 mg/kg/day, administer I.V. infusion over 2 hours

Monitoring Parameters Periodic liver function and renal function tests

Patient Information Notify physician of unusual bleeding or bruising, yellowing of skin and eyes, or severe skin rash

Additional Information Oral suspension contains sucrose and sodium benzoate as inactive ingredients

Dosage Forms

Injection: 2 mg/mL (100 mL, 200 mL)

Suspension, oral: 10 mg/mL (35 mL), 40 mg/mL (35 mL)

Tablet: 50 mg, 100 mg, 150 mg, 200 mg

References

Como JA and Dismukes WE, "Oral Azole Drugs as Systemic Antifungal Therapy," *N Engl J Med*, 1993, 330(4):263-72.

(Continued)

Fluconazole *(Continued)*

Goodman JL, Winston DJ, Greenfield RA, et al, "A Controlled Trial of Fluconazole to Prevent Fungal Infections in Patients Undergoing Bone Marrow Transplantation," *N Engl J Med,* 1992, 326(13):845-51.

Lee JW, Seibel NL, Amantea M, et al, "Safety and Pharmacokinetics of Fluconazole in Children With Neoplastic Diseases," *J Pediatr,* 1992, 120(6):987-93.

Moncino MD and Gutman LT, "Severe Systemic Cryptococcal Disease in a Child: Review of Prognostic Indicators Predicting Treatment Failure and an Approach to Maintenance Therapy With Oral Fluconazole," *Pediatr Infect Dis J,* 1990, 9(5):363-8.

Viscoli C, Castagnola E, Fioredda F, et al, "Fluconazole in the Treatment of Candidiasis in Immunocompromised Children," *Antimicrob Agents Chemother,* 1991, 35(2):365-7.

Flucytosine *(floo SYE toe seen)*

Related Information
Blood Level Sampling Time Guidelines *on page 1189*

Brand Names Ancobon®; Ancotil® (Canada)

Synonyms 5-FC; 5-Flurocytosine

Therapeutic Category Antifungal Agent, Systemic

Generic Available No

Use In combination with amphotericin B in the treatment of serious *Candida, Aspergillus, Cryptococcus,* and *Torulopsis* infections (resistance emerges if flucytosine is used as a single agent)

Pregnancy Risk Factor C

Contraindications Hypersensitivity to flucytosine or any component

Precautions Use with extreme caution in patients with renal impairment, bone marrow suppression, patients with AIDS; dosage modification required in patients with impaired renal function; monitor serum concentration

Adverse Reactions
Central nervous system: Confusion, headache, sedation, hallucinations, vertigo, ataxia

Dermatologic: Rash

Endocrine & metabolic: Temporary growth failure

Gastrointestinal: Nausea, vomiting, diarrhea, enterocolitis

Hematologic: Bone marrow suppression (often observed after 10-26 days of therapy and occurs more frequently with sustained concentrations >100 mcg/mL), anemia, leukopenia, thrombocytopenia

Hepatic: Elevated liver enzymes, hepatitis

Neuromuscular & skeletal: Neuropathy

Renal: Elevated BUN and serum creatinine

Miscellaneous: Anaphylaxis

Drug Interactions Increased efficacy as well as toxicity (enterocolitis, myelosuppression) with concurrent amphotericin administration; antacids and aluminum or magnesium salts delay the rate of absorption

Food Interactions Food decreases the rate, but not the extent of absorption

Mechanism of Action Penetrates fungal cells and is converted to fluorouracil which competes with uracil interfering with fungal RNA and protein synthesis

Pharmacokinetics
Absorption: Oral: 75% to 90%; bioavailability decreased in neonates; rate of absorption is delayed in patients with renal impairment

Distribution: Widely distributed into body tissues and fluids including CSF, aqueous humor, peritoneal fluid, bronchial secretions, liver, kidney, heart, and joints

Protein binding: 2% to 4%

Metabolism: Minimal

Half-life:
Neonates: 4-34 hours
Adults: 3-8 hours (prolonged as high as 200 hours in anuria)

Time to peak serum concentration: Oral: Within 2-6 hours

Elimination: 75% to 90% excreted unchanged in urine by glomerular filtration

Dialyzable (50% to 100%)

Usual Dosage Oral:
Neonates: Initial: 50-100 mg/kg/day in divided doses every 12-24 hours

Infants, Children, Adults: 100-150 mg/kg/day in divided doses every 6 hours

Dosing adjustment in renal impairment:
Cl_{cr} 10-50 mL/minute: Administer every 12 hours
Cl_{cr} <10 mL/minute: Administer every 24 hours

Administration Oral: Administer with food over a 15-minute period to decrease nausea and vomiting

Monitoring Parameters Serum creatinine, BUN, alkaline phosphatase, AST, ALT, CBC, platelet count; serum flucytosine concentrations

Reference Range Therapeutic levels: 25-100 µg/mL; with invasive candidiasis, maintain peak plasma concentration between 40-60 mcg/mL; increased bone marrow suppression with sustained serum flucytosine concentration >100 µg/mL; obtain flucytosine concentration 60 minutes after an oral dose; obtain trough level immediately before the next dose

Test Interactions Flucytosine causes markedly false elevations in serum creatinine values when the Ektachem® analyzer is used

Additional Information Resistance develops rapidly if used alone; more rapid emergence of fungal resistance may occur when lower doses are used; maintain trough ≥25 mcg/mL to prevent emergence of resistant strains

Dosage Forms Capsule: 250 mg, 500 mg

Extemporaneous Preparations Flucytosine oral liquid has been prepared by using the contents of ten 500 mg capsules triturated in a mortar and pestle with a small amount of distilled water; the mixture was transferred to a 500 mL volumetric flask; the mortar was rinsed several times with a small amount of distilled water and the fluid added to the flask; sufficient distilled water was added to make a total volume of 500 mL of a 10 mg/mL liquid; oral liquid was stable for 70 days when stored in glass or plastic prescription bottles at 4°C or for up to 14 days at room temperature.

Wintermeyer SM and Nahata MC, "Stability of Flucytosine in an Extemporaneously Compounded Oral Liquid," *Am J Health-Syst Pharm*, 1996, 53:407-9.

References
Baley JE, Meyers C, Kliegman RM, et al, "Pharmacokinetics, Outcome of Treatment, and Toxic Effects of Amphotericin B and 5-Fluorocytosine in Neonates," *J Pediatr*, 1990, 116(5):791-7.

Fludarabine (floo DARE a been)

Related Information
Emetogenic Potential of Single Chemotherapeutic Agents *on page 1095*

Brand Names Fludara®

Available Salts Fludarabine Phosphate

Synonyms FAMP; F-ara-AMP

Therapeutic Category Antineoplastic Agent, Antimetabolite

Generic Available No

Use Treatment of B-cell chronic lymphocytic leukemia unresponsive to previous therapy with an alkylating agent containing regimen; non-Hodgkin's lymphoma. Fludarabine has been tested in patients with refractory acute lymphocytic leukemia and acute nonlymphocytic leukemia, but required a highly toxic dose to achieve response.

Pregnancy Risk Factor D

Contraindications Hypersensitivity to fludarabine phosphate or any component

Warnings The FDA currently recommends that procedures for proper handling and disposal of antineoplastic agents be considered; doses ≥77 mg/m²/day for 5-7 days were associated with severe neurotoxicity. Neurotoxicity can occur 21-60 days after completing a course of fludarabine and appears to be dose related. Severe bone marrow suppression has been observed at therapeutic doses. Hematologic function must be frequently monitored. Concomitant therapy with pentostatin may be associated with severe pulmonary toxicity.

Precautions Use with caution in patients with pre-existing neurologic problems and in patients with renal insufficiency; dosage adjustment may be needed in patients with impaired renal function or bone marrow suppression

Adverse Reactions
Cardiovascular: Edema
Central nervous system: Neurotoxicity (primarily progressive demyelinating encephalopathy with mental status deterioration), somnolence, seizures, fever, agitation, confusion, depression, chills, fatigue, headache
Dermatologic: Pruritus, rash, alopecia
Endocrine & metabolic: Metabolic acidosis, tumor lysis syndrome, (hyperuricemia, hyperphosphatemia, hypocalcemia, hyperkalemia), hyperglycemia
Gastrointestinal: Nausea, vomiting, diarrhea, stomatitis, metallic taste, gastrointestinal bleeding, anorexia
Hematologic: Leukopenia, neutropenia, thrombocytopenia, lymphocytopenia, autoimmune hemolytic anemia, anemia
Hepatic: Elevated transaminase levels
Neuromuscular & skeletal: Myalgia, peripheral neuropathy, weakness, blurred vision, photophobia
Ocular: Blindness, blurred vision, photophobia
Renal: Hematuria, renal failure
Respiratory: Interstitial pneumonitis

Drug Interactions Cytarabine when administered with or prior to a fludarabine dose competes for deoxycytidine kinase decreasing the phosphorylation of fludarabine to the active F-ara-ATP (inhibits the antineoplastic effect of (Continued)

Fludarabine *(Continued)*

fludarabine); however, administering fludarabine prior to cytarabine may stimulate activation of cytarabine; pentostatin (increased pulmonary toxicity)

Stability Store vial in refrigerator; reconstituted 25 mg/mL fludarabine solution should be used within 8 hours after preparation since it contains no preservatives. When fludarabine is diluted in D_5W or NS to a final concentration of 1 mg/mL, the solution is stable for 24 hours at room temperature. Discard solution if a slight haze develops.

Mechanism of Action F-ara-AMP is dephosphorylated to 2-fluoro-ara-A which enters the cell by a carrier mediated transport process; it is phosphorylated intracellularly to the active metabolite F-ara-ATP. F-ara-ATP competes with deoxy-adenosine triphosphate for incorporation into the A-sites of the DNA strand inhibiting DNA synthesis in the S-phase via inhibition of DNA polymerases and RNA reductase.

Pharmacokinetics
Distribution: Widely distributed with extensive tissue binding
Half-life: Terminal:
Children: 12.4-19 hours
Adults: 7-20 hours
Elimination: Fludarabine clearance appears to be inversely correlated with serum creatinine; at a dose of 25 mg/m²/day for 5 days, 24% of dose excreted in urine; at higher doses, 41% to 60% of dose renally excreted

Usual Dosage Not currently FDA approved for use in children (refer to individual protocols): I.V.:

Children:
Acute leukemia: 10 mg/m² bolus over 15 minutes followed by a continuous infusion of 30.5 mg/m²/day over 5 days; or 10.5 mg/m² bolus over 15 minutes followed by a continuous infusion of 30.5 mg/m²/day over 48 hours followed by cytarabine has been used in clinical trials
Solid tumors: 9 mg/m² bolus followed by 27 mg/m²/day continuous infusion over 5 days
Adults: Chronic lymphocytic leukemia: 20-25 mg/m²/day over 30 minutes for 5 days; doses up to 30 mg/m²/day as single daily doses for 5 days have also been used; courses are usually repeated every 28 days

Dosing adjustment in renal impairment: Cl_{cr} <50 mL/minute: Dose reduction is indicated in patients with renal failure; no specific guidelines are available; monitor closely for toxicity

Administration Parenteral: Fludarabine phosphate has been administered by intermittent I.V. infusion over 15-30 minutes and by continuous infusion; in clinical trials the loading dose has been diluted in 20 mL D_5W and administered over 15 minutes and the continuous infusion diluted to 240 mL in D_5W and administered at a constant rate of 10 mL/hour; in other clinical studies fludarabine has been diluted to a concentration of 0.25-1 mg/mL in D_5W or NS

Monitoring Parameters CBC with differential, platelet count, AST, ALT, creatinine, serum albumin, uric acid, and examination for visual changes

Patient Information Notify physician if fever, sore throat, bleeding, bruising, tachypnea, respiratory distress, or neurologic changes occur

Nursing Implications Prophylactic allopurinol, adequate hydration, and urinary alkalinization should be considered for patients with large initial tumor burdens

Additional Information Myelosuppressive effects:
Granulocyte nadir: 13 days (3-25)
Platelet nadir: 16 days (2-32)
Recovery: 5-7 weeks

Dosage Forms Powder for injection, as phosphate, lyophilized: 50 mg

References
Avramis VI, Champagne J, Sato J, et al, "Pharmacology of Fludarabine Phosphate After a Phase I/II Trial by a Loading Bolus and Continuous Infusion in Pediatric Patients," *Cancer Res*, 1990, 50(22):7226-31.
Von Hoff DD, "Phase I Clinical Trials With Fludarabine Phosphate," *Semin Oncol*, 1990, 17(5 Suppl 8):33-8.

♦ **Fludarabine Phosphate** *see* Fludarabine *on page 419*

Fludrocortisone *(floo droe KOR ti sone)*

Related Information
Corticosteroids Comparison, Systemic *on page 1032*
Brand Names Florinef® Acetate
Available Salts Fludrocortisone Acetate

Synonyms Fluohydrisone; Fluohydrocortisone; 9α-Fluorohydrocortisone

Therapeutic Category Adrenal Corticosteroid; Corticosteroid, Systemic; Glucocorticoid; Mineralocorticoid

Generic Available No

Use Addison's disease; partial replacement therapy for adrenal insufficiency; treatment of salt-losing forms of congenital adrenogenital syndrome; has been used with increased sodium intake for the treatment of idiopathic orthostatic hypotension

Pregnancy Risk Factor C

Contraindications Hypersensitivity to fludrocortisone or any component; CHF, systemic fungal infections

Precautions Dosage should be tapered gradually if therapy is discontinued; use with caution in patients with hypertension, edema, or renal dysfunction

Adverse Reactions
Cardiovascular: Hypertension, edema, CHF
Central nervous system: Convulsions, headache
Dermatologic: Acne, rash, bruising
Endocrine & metabolic: Hypokalemic alkalosis, suppression of growth, hyperglycemia, hypothalamic-pituitary-adrenal suppression
Gastrointestinal: Peptic ulcer
Neuromuscular & skeletal: Muscle weakness
Ocular: Cataracts

Drug Interactions Digoxin (fludrocortisone-induced hypokalemia may increase digoxin toxicity); phenytoin and rifampin may increase metabolism of fludrocortisone; hypokalemia-causing medications may increase risk of hypokalemia

Food Interactions Systemic use of mineralocorticoids/corticosteroids may require a diet with increased potassium, vitamins A, B_6, C, D, folate, calcium, zinc, and phosphorus, and decreased sodium; with fludrocortisone a decrease in dietary sodium is often not required as the increased retention of sodium is usually the desired therapeutic effect

Mechanism of Action Potent mineralocorticoid with glucocorticoid activity; promotes increased reabsorption of sodium and loss of potassium from distal tubules

Pharmacodynamics Duration: 1-2 days

Pharmacokinetics
Absorption: Rapid and complete from GI tract
Protein binding: 42%
Metabolism: In the liver
Half-life:
Plasma: ~3.5 hours
Biological: 18-36 hours

Usual Dosage Oral:
Infants and Children: 0.05-0.1 mg/day
Adults: 0.05-0.2 mg/day

Administration Oral: May administer with food to decrease GI upset

Monitoring Parameters Serum electrolytes, blood pressure, serum renin

Patient Information Notify physician if dizziness, severe or continuing headache, swelling of feet or lower legs, or unusual weight gain occurs

Additional Information In patients with salt-losing forms of congenital adrenogenital syndrome, use along with cortisone or hydrocortisone; fludrocortisone 0.1 mg has sodium retention activity equal to DOCA® 1 mg

Dosage Forms Tablet, as acetate: 0.1 mg

♦ **Fludrocortisone Acetate** see Fludrocortisone on page 420

♦ **Fluid and Electrolyte Requirements in Children** see page 1068

♦ **Flumadine® Oral** see Rimantadine on page 848

Flumazenil (FLO may ze nil)

Brand Names Anexate® (Canada); Romazicon® Injection

Therapeutic Category Antidote, Benzodiazepine

Generic Available No

Use Benzodiazepine antagonist; reverses sedative effects of benzodiazepines used in general anesthesia or conscious sedation; management of benzodiazepine overdose; **not indicated** for ethanol, barbiturate, general anesthetic or narcotic overdose

Pregnancy Risk Factor C

Contraindications Hypersensitivity to flumazenil, any component, or benzodiazepines; patients given benzodiazepines for control of potentially life-threatening (Continued)

Flumazenil *(Continued)*

conditions (eg, control of intracranial pressure or status epilepticus); patients with signs of serious cyclic-antidepressant overdosage

Warnings Seizures may occur in patients physically dependent on benzodiazepines, in patients treated with benzodiazepines for seizure disorders or other reasons, in overdose patients with seizure activity prior to flumazenil, or in patients with serious cyclic antidepressant overdoses; higher than normal doses of benzodiazepines may be required to treat these seizures; mixed drug overdose patients who have ingested drugs that increase the likelihood of seizures (eg, cocaine, lithium, cyclosporine, cyclic antidepressants, bupropion, methylxanthines, MAO inhibitors, isoniazid, or propoxyphene) are at extremely high risk for seizures (flumazenil may be contraindicated in these patients)

Precautions Resedation may occur with flumazenil use (due to its short half-life in comparison to some benzodiazepines); pediatric patients (especially 1-5 years of age) may experience resedation; these patients may require repeat bolus doses or continuous infusion; monitor patients for return of sedation and respiratory depression. Flumazenil should be used with caution in the intensive care unit because of increased risk of unrecognized benzodiazepine dependence in such settings. Flumazenil may provoke panic attacks in patients with panic disorder. Do not use flumazenil until effects of neuromuscular blockers have been fully reversed.

Adverse Reactions

Cardiovascular: Arrhythmias, bradycardia, tachycardia, chest pain, hypertension, hypotension

Central nervous system: Seizures (more common in patients physically dependent on benzodiazepines or with cyclic antidepressant overdoses, see Warnings), fatigue, dizziness, headache, agitation, emotional lability, anxiety, euphoria, depression, abnormal crying

Endocrine & metabolic: Hot flashes

Gastrointestinal: Nausea, vomiting, xerostomia

Local: Pain at injection site

Ocular: Blurred vision

Miscellaneous: Increased diaphoresis, shivering, hiccups, sensation of coldness; can precipitate acute withdrawal symptoms in patients physically dependent on benzodiazepines

Drug Interactions Use with caution in mixed drug overdose; toxic effects of other drugs (especially with cyclic antidepressants) may occur with reversal of benzodiazepine effects

Stability Compatible with D_5W, LR, or NS for 24 hours; discard any unused solution after 24 hours

Mechanism of Action Antagonizes the effect of benzodiazepines on the GABA/benzodiazepine receptor complex. Flumazenil is benzodiazepine specific and does not antagonize other nonbenzodiazepine GABA agonists (including ethanol, barbiturates, general anesthetics); does not reverse the effects of opiates.

Pharmacodynamics

Onset of benzodiazepine reversal: Within 1-3 minutes

Peak effect: 6-10 minutes

Duration: Usually <1 hour; duration is related to dose given and benzodiazepine plasma concentrations; reversal effects of flumazenil may wear off before effects of benzodiazepine and resedation may occur

Pharmacokinetics Follows a two compartment open model; **Note:** Clearance and V_d per kg are similar for children and adults, but children display more variability

Distribution: Adults:

Initial V_d: 0.5 L/kg

V_{dss} 0.77-1.6 L/kg

Protein binding: ~50%

Metabolism: In the liver to the de-ethylated free acid and its glucuronide conjugate

Half-life

Children: Terminal: 20-75 minutes (mean: 40 minutes)

Adults:

Alpha: 7-15 minutes

Terminal: 41-79 minutes

Elimination: Clearance dependent upon hepatic blood flow, hepatically eliminated; <1% excreted unchanged in urine

Usual Dosage I.V.:

Children:

Reversal of benzodiazepine when used in conscious sedation or general anesthesia: Initial dose: 0.01 mg/kg (maximum dose: 0.2 mg) given over 15 seconds; may repeat 0.01 mg/kg (maximum dose: 0.2 mg) after 45 seconds, and then every minute to a maximum total cumulative dose of 0.05 mg/kg or 1 mg, whichever is lower; usual total dose: 0.08-1 mg (mean: 0.65 mg)

Management of benzodiazepine overdose: Minimal information available; initial dose: 0.01 mg/kg (maximum dose: 0.2 mg) with repeat doses of 0.01 mg/kg (maximum dose: 0.2 mg) given every minute to a maximum total cumulative dose of 1 mg; as an alternative to repeat bolus doses, follow up continuous infusions of 0.005-0.01 mg/kg/hour have been used; further studies are needed

Adults:

Reversal of benzodiazepine when used in conscious sedation or general anesthesia: 0.2 mg given over 15 seconds; may repeat 0.2 mg after 45 seconds and then every 60 seconds up to a total of 1 mg, usual total dose: 0.6-1 mg. In event of resedation, may repeat doses at 20-minute intervals with maximum of 1 mg/dose (given at 0.2 mg/minute); maximum dose: 3 mg in 1 hour.

Management of benzodiazepine overdose: 0.2 mg over 30 seconds; may give 0.3 mg dose after 30 seconds if desired level of consciousness is not obtained; additional doses of 0.5 mg can be given over 30 seconds at 1-minute intervals up to a cumulative dose of 3 mg; usual cumulative dose: 1-3 mg; rarely, patients with partial response at 3 mg may require additional titration up to total dose of 5 mg; if patient has not responded 5 minutes after cumulative dose of 5 mg, the major cause of sedation is not likely due to benzodiazepines. In the event of resedation, may repeat doses at 20-minute intervals with maximum of 1 mg/dose (given at 0.5 mg/minute); maximum dose: 3 mg in 1 hour.

Dosing adjustment in hepatic impairment: Initial dose: Use normal dose; repeat doses should be decreased in size or frequency

Administration Parenteral: For I.V. use only; administer by rapid I.V. injection over 15-30 seconds via a freely running I.V. infusion into larger vein (to decrease chance of pain, phlebitis). Children: Do not exceed 0. 2 mg/minute. Adults: Repeat doses: Do not exceed 0.2 mg/minute for reversal of general anesthesia and do not exceed 0.5 mg/minute for reversal of benzodiazepine overdose.

Monitoring Parameters Level of consciousness and resedation, blood pressure, heart rate, respiratory rate, continuous pulse oximetry; monitor for resedation for 1-2 hours after reversal of sedation in patients who receive benzodiazepine sedation

Patient Information Flumazenil does not consistently reverse amnesia; do not engage in activities requiring alertness for 18-24 hours after discharge; resedation may occur in patients on long-acting benzodiazepines (such as diazepam); avoid alcohol or OTC medications for 18-24 hours after flumazenil is used or if benzodiazepine effects persist

Nursing Implications Flumazenil does not effectively reverse hypoventilation, even in alert patients

Additional Information In one study of conscious sedation reversal in 107 pediatric patients (1-17 years of age), resedation occurred between 19-50 minutes after the start of flumazenil. Flumazenil has been used to successfully treat paradoxical reactions in children associated with midazolam use (eg, agitation, restlessness, combativeness) (see Massanari, 1997).

Dosage Forms Injection: 0.1 mg/mL (5 mL, 10 mL)

References

Baktai G, Szekely E, Marialigeti T, et al, "Use of Midazolam (Dormicum) and Flumazenil (Anexate) in Paediatric Bronchology," *Curr Med Res Opin*, 1992, 12(9):552-9.

Clark RF, Sage TA, Tunget C, et al, "Delayed Onset Lorazepam Poisoning Successfully Reversed By Flumazenil in a Child: Case Report and Review of the Literature," *Pediatr Emerg Care*, 1995, 11(1):32-4.

Jones RD, Lawson AD, Andrew LJ, et al, "Antagonism of the Hypnotic Effect of Midazolam in Children: A Randomized, Double Blind Study of Placebo and Flumazenil Administered After Midazolam-Induced Anaesthesia," *Br J Anaesth*, 1991, 66(6):660-6.

Massanari M, Novitsky J, and Reinstein LJ, "Paradoxical Reactions in Children Associated With Midazolam Use During Endoscopy," *Clin Pediatr*, 1997, 36(12):681-4.

Richard P, Autret E, Bardol J, et al, "The Use of Flumazenil in a Neonate," *J Toxicol Clin Toxicol*, 1991, 29(1):137-40.

Roald OK and Dahl V, "Flunitrazepam Intoxication in a Child Successfully Treated With the Benzodiazepine Antagonist Flumazenil," *Crit Care Med*, 1989, 17(12):1355-6.

Shannon M, Albers G, Burkhart K, et al, "Safety and Efficacy of Flumazenil in the Reversal of Benzodiazepine-Induced Conscious Sedation. The Flumazenil Pediatric Study Group," *J Pediatr*, 1997, 131(4):582-6.

Sugarman JM and Paul RI, "Flumazenil: A Review," *Pediatr Emerg Care*, 1994, 10(1):37-43.

Flunisolide (floo NIS oh lide)

Related Information

Asthma Guidelines *on page 1178*
Estimated Comparative Daily Dosages for Inhaled Corticosteroids *on page 1185*
(Continued)

Flunisolide (Continued)

Brand Names AeroBid®-M Oral Aerosol Inhaler; AeroBid® Oral Aerosol Inhaler; Bronalide® (Canada); Nasalide® Nasal Spray; Nasarel® Nasal Spray; Rhinalar® (Canada); Rhinaris-F® (Canada); Syn-Flunisolide® (Canada)

Therapeutic Category Adrenal Corticosteroid; Antiasthmatic; Anti-inflammatory Agent; Corticosteroid, Inhalant (Oral); Corticosteroid, Intranasal; Glucocorticoid

Generic Available No

Use

Oral inhalation: Long-term (chronic) control of persistent bronchial asthma; **NOT** indicated for the relief of acute bronchospasm

Intranasal: Management of seasonal or perennial rhinitis

Pregnancy Risk Factor C

Contraindications Hypersensitivity to flunisolide or any component; primary treatment of status asthmaticus; untreated nasal mucosa infection

Warnings Fatalities have occurred due to adrenal insufficiency in asthmatic patients during and after switching from systemic corticosteroids to aerosol steroids; several months may be required for full recovery of the adrenal glands; during this period, aerosol steroids do **not** provide the systemic corticosteroid needed to treat patients requiring stress doses (ie, patients with major stress such as trauma, surgery, or infections); when used at high doses, hypothalamic-pituitary-adrenal (HPA) suppression may occur; use with inhaled or systemic corticosteroids (even alternate-day dosing) may increase risk of HPA suppression; withdrawal and discontinuation of corticosteroids should be done carefully; immunosuppression may occur

Precautions Avoid using higher than recommended doses; suppression of HPA function, suppression of linear growth, or hypercorticism (Cushing's syndrome) may occur; use with extreme caution in patients with respiratory tuberculosis, untreated systemic infections, or ocular herpes simplex

Adverse Reactions

Cardiovascular: Palpitations (oral inhalation), hypertension (oral inhalation)

Central nervous system: Dizziness, headache, nervousness

Dermatologic: Rash, itching, eczema

Endocrine & metabolic: Adrenal suppression, potential growth suppression

Gastrointestinal: Nausea, vomiting, diarrhea, upset stomach, sore throat, bitter taste, aftertaste

Genitourinary: Menstrual disturbances (oral inhalation)

Local: Nasal burning

Respiratory: Sneezing, nasal congestion, nasal dryness, pharyngitis, epistaxis, Candida infections of the nose or pharynx, atrophic rhinitis, upper respiratory infections

Drug Interactions Expected interactions similar to other corticosteroids

Stability Store intranasal solutions at 59°F to 86°F

Mechanism of Action Controls the rate of protein synthesis, depresses the migration of polymorphonuclear leukocytes and fibroblasts, reverses capillary permeability, and stabilizes lysosomal membranes at the cellular level to prevent or control inflammation

Pharmacodynamics Clinical effects are due to a direct local effect rather than systemic absorption

Onset of action: Intranasal: Within a few days

Maximum effects: Intranasal: 1-2 weeks

Pharmacokinetics

Absorption: Nasal inhalation: ~50%; oral inhalation: ~40%

Metabolism: Rapid in the liver to a less active metabolite, followed by glucuronide and sulfate conjugation

Half-life: 1.8 hours

Elimination: Excreted in urine and feces

Usual Dosage Manufacturer recommendation:

Intranasal:

Children 6-14 years: Initial: 1 spray to each nostril 3 times/day or 2 sprays to each nostril 2 times/day; maximum dose: 4 sprays to each nostril per day; after symptoms are controlled, dose should be reduced to lowest effective amount; maintenance: 1 spray each nostril once daily

Adults: Initial: 2 sprays to each nostril twice daily; may increase in 4-7 days if needed to 2 sprays to each nostril 3 times/day; maximum dose: 8 sprays to each nostril per day; after symptoms are controlled, dose should be reduced to lowest effective amount; maintenance: 1 spray to each nostril once daily

Oral inhalation: Doses should be titrated to the lowest dose once asthma is controlled:

Children: 6-15 years: 2 inhalations twice daily

Adults: 2 inhalations twice daily; maximum dose: 8 inhalations/day

NIH Guidelines (NIH, 1997) [give in divided doses twice daily]

Children:

"Low" dose: 500-750 mcg/day (2-3 puffs/day)

"Medium" dose: 1000-1250 mcg/day (4-5 puffs/day)

"High" dose: >1250 mcg/day (>5 puffs/day)

Adults:

"Low" dose: 500-1000 mcg/day (2-4 puffs/day)

"Medium" dose: 1000-2000 mcg/day (4-8 puffs/day)

"High" dose: >2000 mcg/day (>8 puffs/day)

Administration Do not spray in eyes

Oral inhalant: Use a spacer for children <8 years of age; shake well before use; rinse mouth after inhalation to decrease chance of oral candidiasis

Intranasal: Clear nasal passages by blowing nose prior to use; shake well before use

Monitoring Parameters Check mucus membranes for signs of fungal infection

Patient Information Notify physician if condition being treated persists or worsens; do not decrease dose or discontinue without physician approval

Oral inhalant: Report sore mouth or mouth lesions to physician

Additional Information Nasalide® and Nasarel™ do not contain fluorocarbons. AeroBid® and AeroBid-M® contain fluorocarbon propellants. The efficacy of Nasalide® and Nasarel™ are similar; however, more nasal burning and stinging were reported with Nasalide®, and more taste problems (eg, aftertaste) were reported with Nasarel™. These differences are due to the different vehicles of the two products. If bronchospasm with wheezing occurs after use of oral inhalation, a fast-acting bronchodilator may be used. Flunisolide oral inhalation is also used to help reduce or discontinue oral corticosteroid therapy for asthma.

Dosage Forms Inhalant:

Oral:

AeroBid®: 250 mcg/actuation [100 metered doses] (7 g)

AeroBid-M® (menthol flavor): 250 mcg/actuation [100 metered doses] (7 g)

Nasal (Nasalide®, Nasarel®): 25 mcg/actuation [200 sprays] (25 mL)

References

Expert Panel Report 2, "Guidelines for the Diagnosis and Management of Asthma," *Clinical Practice Guidelines*, National Institutes of Health, National Heart, Lung, and Blood Institute, NIH Publication No. 94-4051, April, 1997.

Fluocinolone (floo oh SIN oh lone)

Related Information

Corticosteroids Comparison, Topical *on page 1033*

Brand Names Derma-Smoothe/FS® Topical; Fluonid® Topical; Flurosyn® Topical; FS Shampoo® Topical; Lidemol® (Canada); Synalar-HP® Topical; Synalar® Topical; Synemol® Topical

Available Salts Fluocinolone Acetonide

Therapeutic Category Adrenal Corticosteroid; Anti-inflammatory Agent; Corticosteroid, Topical; Glucocorticoid

Generic Available Yes

Use Relief of susceptible inflammatory dermatosis

Derma-Smoothe/FS®: Children ≥6 years: Moderate to severe atopic dermatitis (for use ≤4 weeks); Adults: Atopic dermatitis or psoriasis of the scalp

Pregnancy Risk Factor C

Contraindications Fungal infection, hypersensitivity to fluocinolone or any component, TB of skin, herpes (including varicella)

Warnings Infants and small children may be more susceptible to adrenal axis suppression from topical corticosteroid therapy; systemic effects may occur when used on large areas of the body, denuded areas, for prolonged periods of time, or with an occlusive dressing; Derma-Smoothe/FS® contains peanut oil, use with caution in patients with peanut hypersensitivity

Adverse Reactions

Dermatologic: Acne, hypopigmentation, allergic dermatitis, maceration of the skin, skin atrophy, folliculitis, hypertrichosis

Endocrine & metabolic: Hypothalamic-pituitary-adrenal suppression, Cushing's syndrome, growth retardation

Local: Burning, itching, irritation, dryness

Miscellaneous: Secondary infection

(Continued)

Nursing Implications Do not use tight fitting diapers or plastic pants on a child being treated in the diaper area

Additional Information Considered to be a high potency steroid

Dosage Forms
Cream:
Anhydrous, emollient (Lidex®): 0.05% (15 g, 30 g, 60 g, 120 g)
Aqueous, emollient (Lidex-E®): 0.05% (15 g, 30 g, 60 g, 120 g)
Gel, topical (Lidex®): 0.05% (15 g, 30 g, 60 g, 120 g)
Ointment, topical (Lidex®): 0.05% (15 g, 30 g, 60 g, 120 g)
Solution, topical (Lidex®): 0.05% (20 mL, 60 mL)

♦ **Fluoderm (Canada)** see Fluocinonide on page 426
♦ **Fluohydrisone** see Fludrocortisone on page 420
♦ **Fluohydrocortisone** see Fludrocortisone on page 420
♦ **Fluonid® Topical** see Fluocinolone on page 425
♦ **Fluor-A-Day® (Canada)** see Fluoride on page 427
♦ **FluorCare® Neutral** see Fluoride on page 427

Fluoride (FLOR ide)

Brand Names ACT® [OTC]; Fluor-A-Day® (Canada); FluorCare® Neutral; Fluorigard® [OTC]; Fluorinse®; Fluoritab®; Fluotic® (Canada); Flura®; Flura-Drops®; Flura-Loz®; Gel-Kam®; Gel-Tin® [OTC]; Karidium®; Karigel®; Karigel®-N; Listermint® with Fluoride [OTC]; Lozi-Tab®; Luride®; Luride®-SF; Minute-Gel®; Pediaflor®; Pedi-Dent™ (Canada); Pharmaflur®; Phos-Flur®; Point-Two®; Prevident®; Stop® [OTC]; Thera-Flur®; Thera-Flur-N®

Available Salts Acidulated Phosphate Fluoride; Sodium Fluoride; Stannous Fluoride

Therapeutic Category Mineral, Oral; Mineral, Oral Topical

Generic Available Yes

Use Prevention of dental caries

Pregnancy Risk Factor C

Contraindications Hypersensitivity to fluoride, tartrazine, or any component; when fluoride content of drinking water exceeds 0.7 ppm; low sodium or sodium-free diets; do not use 1 mg tablets in children <3 years of age or when drinking water fluoride content is ≥0.3 ppm; do not use 1 mg/5 mL rinse (as supplement) in children <6 years of age

Precautions Prolonged ingestion with excessive doses may result in dental fluorosis and osseous changes; dosage should be adjusted in proportion to the amount of fluoride in the drinking water; do **not** exceed recommended dosage

Adverse Reactions
Central nervous system: Headache
Dermatologic: Rash, eczema, atopic dermatitis, urticaria
Gastrointestinal: GI upset, nausea, vomiting
Miscellaneous: Products containing stannous fluoride may stain the teeth

Drug Interactions Magnesium-, aluminum-, and calcium-containing products may decrease absorption of fluoride

Food Interactions Do not administer with milk

Stability Sodium fluoride solutions decompose in glass containers; store only in tightly closed plastic containers; aqueous solutions of stannous fluoride decompose within hours of preparation; prepare solutions immediately before use

Mechanism of Action Promotes remineralization of decalcified enamel; inhibits the cariogenic microbial process in dental plaque; increases tooth resistance to acid dissolution

Pharmacokinetics
Absorption: Via GI tract, lungs, and skin
Distribution: 50% of fluoride is deposited in teeth and bone after ingestion; crosses placenta; appears in breast milk; topical application works superficially on enamel and plaque
Elimination: In urine and feces

Usual Dosage Oral:
Adequate Intake (AI) (1997 National Academy of Science Recommendations):
Children:
0-6 months: 0.01 mg/day
7-12 months: 0.5 mg/day
1-3 years: 0.7 mg/day
4-8 years: 1 mg/day
9-13 years: 2 mg/day
14-18 years: 3 mg/day
(Continued)

427

Fluoride *(Continued)*

Children >19 and Adults:
Males: 4 mg/day
Females: 3 mg/day

The recommended daily fluoride intake is adjusted in proportion to the fluoride content of available drinking water; see **Recommended Daily Fluoride Dose** table

Recommended Daily Fluoride Dose

Fluoride Content of Drinking Water	Daily Dose, Oral Fluoride (mg)
<0.3 ppm	
Birth - 6 mo	0
6 mo to 3 y	0.25
3-6 y	0.5
6-16 y	1
0.3-06 ppm	
Birth - 3 y	0
3-6 y	0.25
6-16 y	0.5
>0.6 ppm	
All ages	0

Adapted from *AAP News*, 1995, 11(2):18.

Dental rinse: See **Sodium Fluoride Dental Rinse Dosing** table
Sodium fluoride (dosage based upon concentration of solution):
Note: 2% concentrations are administered by dental personnel only

Sodium Fluoride Dental Rinse Dosing

Age	% Solution	Dosage
6 y	0.05%	10 mL daily
6-12 y	0.02%	10 mL twice daily
	0.2%	5 mL once weekly
>12 y	0.02%	10 mL twice daily
	0.2%	10 mL once weekly

Acidulated phosphate fluoride rinse: Children 6 years and Adults: 5-10 mL of 0.02% daily at bedtime

Gel:
Acidulated phosphate fluoride: Adults: 4-8 drops of 0.5% gel daily or for desensitizing exposed root surfaces, use a few drops of 0.5% to 1.2% gel applied and brushed onto affected area each night
Stannous fluoride: Children >6 years and Adults: Apply 0.4% gel to teeth once daily

Administration Oral:
Dental gel: Do **not** swallow; gel drops are placed in trough of applicator; applicator is applied over upper and lower teeth at same time; bite down for 6 minutes
Dental rinse: Swish or rinse in mouth then expectorate; do not swallow
Tablet: Dissolve in mouth, chew, swallow whole, or add to drinking water or fruit juice; administer with food (but not milk) to eliminate GI upset

Reference Range Total plasma fluoride: 0.14-0.19 µg/mL

Dosage Forms Fluoride ion content listed in brackets
Gel, topical:
Acidulated phosphate fluoride (Minute-Gel®): 1.23% (480 mL)
Sodium fluoride (Karigel®, Karigel®-N, PreviDent®): 1.1% [0.5%] (24 g, 30 g, 60 g, 120 g, 130 g, 250 g)
Stannous fluoride (Gel Kam®, Gel-Tin®, Stop®): 0.4% [0.1%] (60 g, 65 g, 105 g, 120 g)
Lozenge, as sodium (Flura-Loz®) (sugar free) (raspberry flavor): 2.2 mg [1 mg]
Rinse, topical, as sodium:
ACT®, Fluorigard®: 0.05% [0.02%] (90 mL, 180 mL, 300 mL, 360 mL, 480 mL)
Fluorinse® (alcohol free) , Point-Two®: 0.2% [0.09%] (240 mL, 480 mL, 3780 mL)

Listermint® with Fluoride: 0.02% [0.01%] (180 mL, 300 mL, 360 mL, 480 mL, 540 mL, 720 mL, 960 mL, 1740 mL)

Solution, oral, as sodium:

Phos-Flur® Daily Oral Rinse, Liqui-Flur®, Acidulated Phosphate Fluoride Oral Rinse®: 0.044% [0.02% mg/mL]

Flura-Drops®: 0.55 mg/drop [0.25 mg/drop] (22.8 mL, 24 mL)

Karidium®, Luride® (sugar free): 0.275 mg/drop [0.125 mg/drop] (30 mL, 60 mL)

Luride®, Pediaflor® (sugar free): 1.1 mg/mL [0.5 mg/mL] (50 mL)

Fluoritab® Liquid: 11 mg/mL [5 mg/mL]

Tablet, as sodium:

Chewable:

Fluoritab®, Flura-Loz®, Luride® 0.25 mg F Lozi-Tabs® Quarter-Strength: 0.55 mg [0.25 mg]

Fluoritab® (sugar free), Luride® 0.5 mg F Lozi-Tab® Half-Strength (sugar free), Pharmaflur® (sugar free): 1.1 mg [0.5 mg]

Karidium®, Luride® 1.0 mg F Lozi-Tab® Full-Strength (sugar free), Luride®-SF Lozi-Tab® (sugar free), Pharmaflur® (sugar free): 2.2 mg [1 mg]

Fluoritab® (sugar free), Flura® Tab® (sugar free), Karidium®: 2.2 mg [1 mg]

Topical, foam (FluoroCare® Neutral Foam, Neutra-Foam®): Sodium fluoride 2% [0.9% fluoride ion]

Topical, gel:

Acidulated phosphate fluoride: Phos-Flur® Gel: 1.1% [0.5%]

Sodium fluoride: FluoroCare® Neutral: 2%

References

"Dietary Reference Intakes for Calcium, Phosphorus, Magnesium, Vitamin D, and Fluoride. Standing Committee on the Scientific Evaluation of Dietary Reference Intakes, Food and Nutrition Board, Institute of Medicine," National Academy of Sciences, Washington, DC: National Academy Press, 1997.

♦ **Fluorigard® [OTC]** see Fluoride on page 427

♦ **Fluorinse®** see Fluoride on page 427

♦ **Fluoritab®** see Fluoride on page 427

♦ **9α-Fluorohydrocortisone** see Fludrocortisone on page 420

Fluorometholone (flure oh METH oh lone)

Brand Names Flarex®; Fluor-Op®; FML®; FML® Forte

Therapeutic Category Adrenal Corticosteroid; Anti-inflammatory Agent, Ophthalmic; Corticosteroid, Ophthalmic; Glucocorticoid

Generic Available No

Use Inflammatory conditions of the eye, including keratitis, iritis, cyclitis, and conjunctivitis

Pregnancy Risk Factor C

Contraindications Herpes simplex, fungal diseases, most viral diseases

Warnings Not recommended for children <2 years of age; some products contain sulfites

Precautions Prolonged use may result in glaucoma, increased intraocular pressure, or other ocular damage

Adverse Reactions

Local: Stinging, burning

Ocular: Increased intraocular pressure, open-angle glaucoma, defect in visual acuity and field of vision, cataracts, photosensitivity

Mechanism of Action Decreases inflammation by suppression of migration of polymorphonuclear leukocytes and reversal of increased capillary permeability

Pharmacokinetics Absorption: Into aqueous humor with slight systemic absorption

Usual Dosage Children >2 years and Adults: Ophthalmic:

Ointment: May be applied every 4 hours in severe cases or 1-3 times/day in mild to moderate cases.

Drops: Instill 1-2 drops into conjunctival sac every hour during day, every 2 hours at night until favorable response is obtained, then use 1 drop every 4 hours; in mild or moderate inflammation: 1-2 drops into conjunctival sac 2-4 times/day.

Administration Ophthalmic: Avoid contact of medication tube or bottle tip with skin or eye; shake suspension well before use

Patient Information May cause blurring of vision and photosensitivity; do not discontinue without consulting physician; notify physician if improvement does not occur after 7-8 days

Dosage Forms Ophthalmic:

Ointment (FML®): 0.1% (3.5 g)

Suspension:

Flarex®, Fluor-Op®, FML®: 0.1% (5 mL, 10 mL, 15 mL)

(Continued)

Fluorometholone *(Continued)*

FML® Forte: 0.25% (2 mL, 5 mL, 10 mL, 15 mL)

- ♦ **Fluor-Op®** *see Fluorometholone on page 429*
- ♦ **Fluoroplex® Topical** *see Fluorouracil on page 430*

Fluorouracil (flure oh YOOR a sil)

Related Information
Emetogenic Potential of Single Chemotherapeutic Agents *on page 1095*
Brand Names Adrucil® Injection; Efudex® Topical; Fluoroplex® Topical
Synonyms 5-Fluorouracil; 5-FU
Therapeutic Category Antineoplastic Agent, Antimetabolite
Generic Available Yes: Injection
Use Treatment of carcinoma of stomach, colon, rectum, breast, and pancreas; topically for management of multiple actinic keratoses and superficial basal cell carcinomas
Pregnancy Risk Factor D
Contraindications Hypersensitivity to fluorouracil or any component; patients with poor nutritional status, bone marrow suppression, thrombocytopenia; pregnancy
Warnings The FDA currently recommends that procedures for proper handling and disposal of antineoplastic agents be considered; if intractable vomiting, diarrhea, or hemorrhage occurs, discontinue fluorouracil immediately
Precautions Use with caution and modify dosage in patients with renal or hepatic impairment
Adverse Reactions
Cardiovascular: Cardiac arrhythmias, heart failure, hypotension
Central nervous system: Headache, cerebellar ataxia (gait and speech abnormalities), somnolence, dizziness
Dermatologic: Alopecia, skin pigmentation, pruritic maculopapular rash, partial loss of nails or hyperpigmentation of nail bed, photosensitivity
Gastrointestinal: Nausea, vomiting, diarrhea, anorexia, GI hemorrhage, stomatitis, esophagitis
Hematologic: Myelosuppression, granulocytopenia, thrombocytopenia
Hepatic: Hepatotoxicity
Ocular: Visual disturbances, nystagmus, conjunctivitis
Miscellaneous: Palmar-plantar erythrodysethesias (erythematous, desquamative rash involving hands and feet accompanied by pain, tingling, and swollen palms; this adverse effect may be treated with oral pyridoxine)
Drug Interactions Cimetidine (increases 5-FU concentration); leucovorin may potentiate the antitumor activity of 5-FU
Food Interactions Use of acidic solutions such as orange juice or other fruit juices to dilute 5-FU for oral administration may result in precipitation of the drug and decreased absorption; increase dietary intake of thiamine
Stability Store at room temperature; protect from light; slight discoloration of injection during storage does not affect potency; if precipitate forms, redissolve drug by heating to 140°F, shake well; allow to cool to body temperature before administration; incompatible with cytarabine, diazepam, doxorubicin, methotrexate
Mechanism of Action A pyrimidine antimetabolite that inhibits thymidylate synthase leading to depletion of the DNA precursor thymidine; incorporated into RNA, DNA
Pharmacokinetics
Absorption: Oral: Erratic
Distribution: Into tumors, intestinal mucosa, liver, bone marrow, and CSF
Protein binding: <10%
Metabolism: Inactive metabolites are formed following metabolism in the liver
Bioavailability: 50% to 80%; variable due to saturable first-pass elimination process
Half-life, biphasic:
Primary: 10-20 minutes
Terminal: 15-19 hours
Elimination: Biphasic elimination with <10% of dose excreted unchanged in the urine
Usual Dosage Children and Adults (refer to individual protocols with dose based on lean body weight):
I.V.:
Initial: 400-500 mg/m^2/day (12 mg/kg/day; maximum dose: 800 mg/day) for 4-5 days
Maintenance: 200-250 mg/m^2/dose (6 mg/kg) every other day for 4 doses; repeat in 4 weeks

Single weekly bolus dose of 15 mg/kg or 500 mg/m^2 can be administered depending on the patient's reaction to the previous course of treatment; maintenance dose of 5-15 mg/kg/week as a single dose not to exceed 1 g/week

I.V. infusion: 15 mg/kg/day or 500 mg/m^2/day (maximum daily dose: 1 g) has been given by I.V. infusion over 4 hours for 5 days; or 800-1200 mg/m^2 for continuous infusion over 24-120 hours

Oral: 15-20 mg/kg/day for 5-8 days has been used for colorectal carcinoma; 15 mg/kg/week for hepatoma

Dosing adjustment in hepatic impairment: Bilirubin >5 mg/dL: Not recommended for use

Topical: Cream or solution: Apply twice daily

Administration

Oral: Administer in early morning on an empty stomach; do not eat for 2 hours before and after dosage administration; dilute injectable fluorouracil solution dose in 4 oz of water or a diluted bicarbonate buffer solution to increase absorption

Parenteral: Administer by direct I.V. injection (50 mg/mL solution needs no further dilution) over several minutes or by I.V. intermittent or continuous infusion diluted in saline or dextrose solutions; toxicity (eg, myelosuppression) may be reduced by giving the drug as a continuous infusion. Doses >750-800 mg/m^2 should be administered as a continuous infusion, **not** by bolus injection; dose-limiting toxicity with continuous infusion is mucous membrane toxicity (ie, stomatitis, diarrhea)

Topical: Apply with a nonmetallic applicator or gloved fingers in a sufficient amount to cover affected area

1% or 2%: Apply to lesions on the head and neck for the treatment of multiple actinic keratoses

5%: Use on lesions in areas other than the head and neck for multiple actinic keratoses; only 5% preparations are used for the treatment of superficial basal cell carcinoma

Monitoring Parameters CBC with differential and platelet count, renal function tests, liver function tests

Patient Information Avoid unnecessary exposure to sunlight

Nursing Implications Wash hands immediately after topical application of the cream or solution

Additional Information Myelosuppressive effects:

WBC: Mild

Platelets: Mild

Onset (days): 7-10

Nadir (days): 9-14

Recovery (days): 21

Dosage Forms

Cream, topical:

Efudex®: 5% (25 g)

Fluoroplex®: 1% (30 g)

Injection (Adrucil®): 50 mg/mL (10 mL, 20 mL, 50 mL, 100 mL)

Solution, topical:

Efudex®: 2% (10 mL); 5% (10 mL)

Fluoroplex®: 1% (30 mL)

References

Balis FM, Holcenberg JS and Bleyer WA, "Clinical Pharmacokinetics of Commonly Used Anticancer Drugs," *Clin Pharmacokinet*, 1983, 8(3):202-32.

♦ **5-Fluorouracil** see Fluorouracil on page 430

♦ **Fluotic® (Canada)** see Fluoride on page 427

Fluoxetine (floo OKS e teen)

Related Information

Carbohydrate and Alcohol Content of Liquid Medications for Use in Patients Receiving Ketogenic Diets on page 1228

Comparison of Adverse Effects of Antidepressants on page 1030

Comparison of Usual Adult Dosage and Mechanism of Action of Antidepressants on page 1029

Drugs and Breast-Feeding on page 1213

Serotonin Syndrome on page 1217

Brand Names Prozac®; Sarafem™

Available Salts Fluoxetine Hydrochloride

Therapeutic Category Antidepressant, Serotonin Reuptake Inhibitor

Generic Available No

Use Treatment of depression, obsessive-compulsive disorder, bulimia nervosa; **Note:** in July, 2000, the FDA approved fluoxetine (under the trade name Sarafem™) for the treatment of premenstrual dysphoric disorder (PMDD)

(Continued)

Fluoxetine *(Continued)*

Pregnancy Risk Factor C

Contraindications Hypersensitivity to fluoxetine or any component; patients receiving MAO inhibitors currently or in past 2 weeks

Warnings Rash or urticaria may occur along with leukocytosis, fever, edema, arthralgia, lymphadenopathy, respiratory distress, and other symptoms; rare cases of vasculitis have been reported; discontinue use if rash or other allergic reaction occurs

Precautions Due to limited experience, use with caution in patients with renal or hepatic impairment, seizure disorders, cardiac dysfunction, diabetes mellitus; decrease dose in liver dysfunction; use with caution in patients at high risk for suicide; discontinue MAO inhibitors at least 14 days before initiating fluoxetine; add or initiate other antidepressants with caution for up to 5 weeks after stopping fluoxetine

Adverse Reactions Predominant adverse effects are CNS and GI:

Central nervous system: Headache, nervousness, insomnia, drowsiness, anxiety, dizziness, fatigue, sedation, mania, suicidal ideation, extrapyramidal reactions (rare)

Dermatologic: Rash, urticaria (7%), pruritus

Endocrine & metabolic: Hypoglycemia, hyponatremia (elderly or volume-depleted patients)

Gastrointestinal: Nausea, diarrhea, xerostomia, anorexia, dyspepsia, constipation, weight loss

Neuromuscular & skeletal: Tremor

Ocular: Visual disturbances

Miscellaneous: Anaphylactoid reactions, allergies, diaphoresis

Drug Interactions Cytochrome P-450 isoenzyme CYP2D6 substrate (minor pathway), CYP3A3/4 substrate; CYP2C9 isoenzyme inducer; CYP1A2 (at higher doses), CYP2C9, CYP2C19, CYP2D6, CYP3A3/4 isoenzyme inhibitor (extent of CYP3A4 inhibition may not be clinically significant; however, the metabolite norfluoxetine is a more potent CYP3A inhibitor)

With MAO inhibitors, fever, tremors, seizures, delirium, coma may occur; tryptophan may increase CNS and GI toxic effects; fluoxetine may inhibit metabolism and increase effects of tricyclic antidepressants, trazodone, and possibly diazepam; may antagonize buspirone effects; may displace highly protein bound drugs

Food Interactions Tryptophan supplements may increase CNS and GI adverse effects (eg, restlessness, agitation, GI problems); food does not affect bioavailability

Mechanism of Action Inhibits CNS neuron serotonin uptake; minimal or no effect on reuptake of norepinephrine or dopamine; does not significantly bind to alpha-adrenergic, histamine or cholinergic receptors; may therefore be useful in patients at risk from sedation, hypotension and anticholinergic effects of tricyclic antidepressants

Pharmacodynamics Peak effect: Maximum antidepressant effects usually occur after more than 4 weeks; due to long half-life, resolution of adverse reactions after discontinuation may be slow

Pharmacokinetics

Absorption: Oral: Well absorbed

Distribution: Adults: V_d: 20-45 L/kg; widely distributed

Protein binding: ~95% (albumin and alpha$_1$-glycoprotein)

Metabolism: In the liver to norfluoxetine (active) and other metabolites

Half-life: Adults:

Fluoxetine: Acute dosing: 1-3 days; chronic dosing: 4-6 days

Norfluoxetine: Acute and chronic dosing: 4-16 days

Time to peak serum concentration: Within 4-8 hours

Elimination: In urine as fluoxetine (2.5% to 5%) and norfluoxetine (10%)

Usual Dosage Oral:

Children <5 years: No dosing information available

Children 5-18 years: Dose and safety not established; initial doses of 5-10 mg/day (or even 10 mg given 3 times a week) may result in less adverse effects; dose is titrated upwards as needed; usual maximum dose: 20 mg/day; **Note:** A study in children 8-15 years of age with obsessive compulsive disorder (n=14) used a fixed dose of 20 mg/day (Riddle, 1992); a study of children 10-18 years of age with obsessive compulsive symptoms and Tourette's syndrome (n=5) used 20-40 mg/day (Kurlan, 1993); 6 children 6-12 years of age with elective mutism were treated with initial doses of 0.2 mg/kg/day for 1 week, then 0.4 mg/kg/day for 1 week, then 0.6 mg/kg/day for 10 weeks (Black,1994); further studies are needed

Adults:

Depression or obsessive-compulsive disorder: Initial dose: 20 mg/day administered in the morning; may increase after several weeks by 20 mg/day increments; maximum dose: 80 mg/day; doses >20 mg/day can be given either once daily (in the morning) or divided into morning or noon doses

Bulimia nervosa: 60 mg/day administered in the morning; may need to titrate up to this dose over several days in some patients

Dosage adjustment in renal impairment: Adjustment not routinely needed

Dosage adjustment in hepatic impairment: Lower doses or less frequent administration are recommended

Administration Oral: May be administered without regard to food

Reference Range

Therapeutic: Fluoxetine 100-800 ng/mL (SI: 289-2314 nmol/L); norfluoxetine 100-600 ng/mL (SI: 289-1735 nmol/L)

Toxic: (Fluoxetine plus norfluoxetine): >2000 ng/mL (SI: >5784 nmol/L)

Patient Information Avoid alcohol and tryptophan; may cause dizziness or drowsiness and impair ability to perform activities requiring mental alertness or physical coordination; may cause dry mouth

Nursing Implications Last dose of the day should be given before 4 PM (to avoid insomnia)

Additional Information Oral solution contains benzoic acid

Dosage Forms

Capsule, as hydrochloride: 10 mg, 20 mg, 40 mg

Solution, oral, as hydrochloride (mint flavor): 20 mg/5 mL (120 mL)

Tablet, as hydrochloride: 10 mg

References

Black B and Uhde TW, "Treatment of Elective Mutism With Fluoxetine: A Double Blind, Placebo-Controlled Study," *J Am Acad Child Adolesc Psychiatry*, 1994, 33(7):1000-6.

Como PG and Kurlan R, "An Open-Label Trial of Fluoxetine for Obsessive-Compulsive Disorder in Gilles de la Tourette's Syndrome," *Neurology*, 1991, 41(6):872-4.

Kurlan R, Como PG, Deeley C, et al, "A Pilot Controlled Study of Fluoxetine for Obsessive-Compulsive Symptoms in Children With Tourette's Syndrome," *Clin Neuropharmacol*, 1993, 16(2):167-72.

Riddle MA, Hardin MT, King R, et al, "Fluoxetine Treatment of Children and Adolescents With Tourette's and Obsessive-Compulsive Disorders: Preliminary Clinical Experience," *J Am Acad Child Adolesc Psychiatry*, 1990, 29(1):45-8.

Riddle MA, Scahill L, King RA, et al, "Double-Blind, Crossover Trial of Fluoxetine and Placebo in Children and Adolescents With Obsessive-Compulsive Disorder," *J Am Acad Child Adolesc Psychiatry*, 1992, 31(6):1062-9.

♦ **Fluoxetine Hydrochloride** *see* Fluoxetine *on page 431*

Fluoxymesterone (floo oks i MES te rone)

Brand Names Halotestin®

Therapeutic Category Androgen

Generic Available Yes

Use Replacement of endogenous testicular hormone; in female used as palliative treatment of breast cancer, postpartum breast engorgement

Restrictions C-III

Pregnancy Risk Factor X

Contraindications Serious cardiac disease, liver or kidney disease; hypersensitivity to fluoxymesterone or any component

Precautions May accelerate bone maturation without producing compensatory gain in linear growth; in prepubertal children perform radiographic examination of the hand and wrist every 6 months to determine the rate of bone maturation and to assess the effect of treatment on the epiphyseal centers

Adverse Reactions

Cardiovascular: Edema

Central nervous system: Anxiety, mental depression, headache

Dermatologic: Acne, hirsutism

Endocrine & metabolic: Gynecomastia, amenorrhea, hypercalcemia, female virilization

Gastrointestinal: Nausea

Genitourinary: Priapism

Hematologic: Polycythemia, suppression of clotting factors II, VII, IX, X

Hepatic: Cholestatic hepatitis

Neuromuscular & skeletal: Paresthesia

Miscellaneous: Hypersensitivity reactions

Drug Interactions May potentiate the action of oral anticoagulants; may decrease blood glucose concentrations and insulin requirements in patients with diabetes; may elevate cyclosporin levels; may increase extrapyramidal side effects and other (Continued)

Fluoxymesterone *(Continued)*

CNS effects when coadministered with lithium; may potentiate respiratory depressant effects of narcotics

Mechanism of Action Synthetic androgenic anabolic steroid hormone responsible for the normal growth and development of male sex organs and maintenance of secondary sex characteristics; synthetic testosterone derivative with significant androgen activity; stimulates RNA polymerase activity resulting in an increase in protein production; increases bone development

Pharmacokinetics

Absorption: Oral: Rapid

Protein binding: 98%

Metabolism: In the liver

Half-life: 10-100 minutes

Elimination: Enterohepatic circulation and urinary excretion (90%)

Halogenated derivative of testosterone with up to 5 times the activity of methyltestosterone

Usual Dosage Adults: Oral:

Male:

Hypogonadism: 5-20 mg/day

Delayed puberty: 2.5-20 mg/day for 4-6 months

Female:

Inoperable breast carcinoma: 10-40 mg/day in divided doses for 1-3 months

Breast engorgement: 2.5 mg after delivery, 5-10 mg/day in divided doses for 4-5 days

Monitoring Parameters Periodic radiographic exams of hand and wrist (when used in children); hemoglobin hematocrit (if receiving high dosages or long-term therapy)

Dosage Forms Tablet: 2 mg, 5 mg, 10 mg

♦ **Flura®** *see Fluoride on page 427*

♦ **Flura-Drops®** *see Fluoride on page 427*

♦ **Flura-Loz®** *see Fluoride on page 427*

Flurazepam *(flure AZ e pam)*

Related Information

Overdose and Toxicology *on page 1191*

Brand Names Apo®-Flurazepam (Canada); Dalmane®; Novo-Flupam® (Canada); PMS-Flupam (Canada); Somnol® (Canada); Som Pam® (Canada)

Available Salts Flurazepam Hydrochloride

Therapeutic Category Benzodiazepine; Hypnotic; Sedative

Generic Available Yes

Use Short-term treatment of insomnia

Restrictions C-IV

Pregnancy Risk Factor X

Contraindications Hypersensitivity to flurazepam or any component (there may be cross-sensitivity with other benzodiazepines), pregnancy, pre-existing CNS depression, respiratory depression, narrow-angle glaucoma

Precautions Use with caution in patients receiving other CNS depressants, patients with low albumin, hepatic dysfunction and in the elderly

Adverse Reactions

Central nervous system: Drowsiness, dizziness, confusion; residual daytime sedation; paradoxical reactions, hyperactivity, and excitement (rare), ataxia

Miscellaneous: Physical and psychological dependence with prolonged use

Drug Interactions Additive CNS depression with other CNS depressants, alcohol; cimetidine may decrease and enzyme inducers may increase metabolism of flurazepam; concurrent use of flurazepam with ritonavir is not recommended

Mechanism of Action Depresses all levels of the CNS, including the limbic and reticular formation, by binding to the benzodiazepine site on the gamma-aminobutyric acid (GABA) receptor complex and modulating GABA, which is a major inhibitory neurotransmitter in the brain

Pharmacodynamics Hypnotic effects:

Onset of action: 15-20 minutes

Peak: 3-6 hours

Duration: 7-8 hours

Pharmacokinetics

Metabolism: In the liver to N-desalkylflurazepam (active)

Half-life, metabolite (adults): 40-114 hours

Usual Dosage Oral:
  Children:
    <15 years: Dose not established
    >15 years: 15 mg at bedtime
  Adults: 15-30 mg at bedtime
Patient Information Avoid alcohol and other CNS depressants; may be habit-forming; avoid abrupt discontinuation after prolonged use
Dosage Forms Capsule, as hydrochloride: 15 mg, 30 mg

♦ **Flurazepam Hydrochloride** *see* Flurazepam *on page 434*

Flurbiprofen (flure BI proe fen)

Brand Names Ansaid® Oral; Apro-Flurbiprofen® (Canada); Froben® (Canada); Froben-SR® (Canada); Novo-Flurprofen® (Canada); Nu-Flurprofen® (Canada); Ocufen® Ophthalmic
Available Salts Flurbiprofen Sodium
Therapeutic Category Analgesic, Non-narcotic; Anti-inflammatory Agent; Anti-inflammatory Agent, Ophthalmic; Nonsteroidal Anti-inflammatory Drug (NSAID), Ophthalmic; Nonsteroidal Anti-inflammatory Drug (NSAID), Oral
Generic Available Tablet: Yes
Use
  Ophthalmic: For inhibition of intraoperative trauma-induced miosis; the value of flurbiprofen for the prevention and management of postoperative ocular inflammation and postoperative cystoid macular edema remains to be determined
  Systemic: Management of inflammatory disease and rheumatoid disorders; dysmenorrhea; pain
Pregnancy Risk Factor B (D in 3rd trimester)
Contraindications Dendritic keratitis; hypersensitivity to flurbiprofen, any component, aspirin, or other NSAIDs
Warnings Use with caution in patients with history of herpes simplex, keratitis, and patients who might be affected by inhibition of platelet aggregation; use with caution in patients in whom asthma, rhinitis, or urticaria is precipitated by aspirin or other NSAIDs
Precautions Use oral form with caution in renal or hepatic impairment, GI disease, cardiac disease, and patients receiving anticoagulants
Adverse Reactions
  Cardiovascular: Edema
  Central nervous system: Headache, fatigue, drowsiness, vertigo
  Dermatologic: Pruritus, rash
  Gastrointestinal: Abdominal discomfort, nausea, heartburn, constipation, vomiting, GI bleeding, ulcers, perforation
  Hematologic: Thrombocytopenia, inhibits platelet aggregation; prolongs bleeding time; agranulocytosis
  Hepatic: Hepatitis
  Ocular: Slowing of corneal wound healing, mild ocular stinging, itching, burning, ocular irritation
  Otic: Tinnitus
  Renal: Renal dysfunction
Drug Interactions Cytochrome P-450 isoenzyme CYP2C9 substrate and inhibitor
  Oral: Drug interactions similar to other NSAIDs may occur
  Ophthalmic: Carbachol and acetylcholine chloride may not be effective when used concurrently with flurbiprofen
Food Interactions Food may decrease the rate but not the extent of absorption
Mechanism of Action Inhibits prostaglandin synthesis by decreasing the activity of the enzyme, cyclo-oxygenase, which results in decreased formation of prostaglandin precursors
Pharmacokinetics Oral:
  Time to peak serum concentration: Within 1.5-2 hours
  Elimination: 95% in urine
Usual Dosage
  Children and Adults: Ophthalmic: Instill 1 drop every 30 minutes starting 2 hours prior to surgery (total of 4 drops to each affected eye)
  Adults: Oral:
    Arthritis: 200-300 mg/day in 2-4 divided doses; maximum dose: 100 mg/dose; maximum: 300 mg/day
    Dysmenorrhea: 50 mg 4 times/day
Administration
  Oral: Administer with food, milk, or antacid to decrease GI effects
(Continued)

Flurbiprofen (Continued)

Ophthalmic: Instill drops into affected eye(s); avoid contact of container tip with skin or eye

Monitoring Parameters Systemic use: CBC, BUN, serum creatinine, liver enzymes, occult blood loss, periodic eye exams

Patient Information Ophthalmic solution may cause mild burning or stinging, notify physician if this becomes severe or is persistent

Dosage Forms
Solution, ophthalmic, as sodium (Ocufen®): 0.03% (2.5 mL, 5 mL, 10 mL)
Tablet, as sodium (Ansaid®): 50 mg, 100 mg

- **Flurbiprofen Sodium** see Flurbiprofen on page 435
- **5-Flurocytosine** see Flucytosine on page 418
- **Flurosyn® Topical** see Fluocinolone on page 425
- **Flutex® Topical** see Triamcinolone on page 946

Fluticasone (floo TIK a sone)

Related Information
Asthma Guidelines on page 1178
Estimated Comparative Daily Dosages for Inhaled Corticosteroids on page 1185

Brand Names Cutivate®; Flonase®; Flovent®; Flovent® Rotadisk®

Available Salts Fluticasone Propionate

Therapeutic Category Adrenal Corticosteroid; Antiasthmatic; Anti-inflammatory Agent; Corticosteroid, Inhalant (Oral); Corticosteroid, Intranasal; Corticosteroid, Topical; Glucocorticoid

Generic Available No

Use
Oral inhalation: Long-term (chronic) control of persistent bronchial asthma; NOT indicated for the relief of acute bronchospasm
Intranasal: Management of seasonal and perennial allergic and nonallergic rhinitis
Topical: Relief of inflammation and pruritus associated with corticosteroid-responsive dermatoses [medium potency topical corticosteroid]

Pregnancy Risk Factor C

Contraindications Hypersensitivity to fluticasone or any component; primary treatment of status asthmaticus

Warnings Fatalities have occurred due to adrenal insufficiency in asthmatic patients during and after switching from systemic corticosteroids to aerosol steroids (see Additional Information); several months may be required for full recovery of the adrenal glands; during this period, aerosol steroids do **not** provide the systemic corticosteroid needed to treat patients requiring stress doses (ie, patients with major stress such as trauma, surgery, or infections); when used at high doses, hypothalamic-pituitary-adrenal (HPA) suppression may occur; use with inhaled or systemic corticosteroids (even alternate-day dosing) may increase risk of HPA suppression; withdrawal and discontinuation of corticosteroids should be done carefully; immunosuppression may occur

Topical use: Adverse systemic effects may occur when used on large areas of the body, denuded areas, for prolonged periods of time, with an occlusive dressing, and/or in infants or small children; use with caution in pediatric patients

Precautions Avoid using higher than recommended doses; suppression of HPA function, suppression of linear growth, or hypercorticism (Cushing's syndrome) may occur; these adverse effects (as well as intracranial hypertension) may occur with topical use and have been reported in pediatric patients (see also Additional Information); use with extreme caution in patients with respiratory tuberculosis, untreated systemic infections, or ocular herpes simplex. Eosinophilic conditions (eosinophilia, vasculitic rash, cardiac complications, worsening pulmonary symptoms, and/or neuropathy) may occur and are usually associated with withdrawal or decrease of oral corticosteroids after the initiation of fluticasone (oral inhalation); a causal relationship by fluticasone has not been established

Adverse Reactions
Central nervous system: Headache, dizziness, malaise, fatigue, insomnia
Dermatologic:
Inhalational use: Dermatitis, rash
Topical use: Pruritus, dry skin, numbness of fingers, acne, hypopigmentation, allergic dermatitis, maceration of the skin, skin atrophy, folliculitis, hypertrichosis, itching
Endocrine & metabolic: HPA suppression, Cushing's syndrome, growth suppression

Gastrointestinal: Oral candidiasis, nausea, vomiting, diarrhea, dyspepsia

Local: Burning, irritation

Neuromuscular & skeletal: Muscular soreness

Ocular: Eye pain

Respiratory: Respiratory infection, pharyngitis, nasal congestion, sinusitis, nasal discharge, rhinitis, epistaxis (intranasal), dysphonia (oral inhalation),

Miscellaneous: Secondary infection, eosinophilic conditions (see Precautions)

Drug Interactions Ketoconazole and other P-450 3A4 isoenzyme inhibitors may increase fluticasone serum concentrations

Stability

Oral inhalation: Store canister between 36°F to 86°F with nozzle end down; do not store at >120°F; protect from freezing and direct sunlight; store Rotadisk® at controlled room temperature; keep dry; discard Rotadisk® blisters 2 months after opening moisture-proof foil overwrap (or before expiration date)

Intranasal: Store nasal spray between 39°F to 86°F

Mechanism of Action Controls the rate of protein synthesis, depresses the migration of polymorphonuclear leukocytes and fibroblasts, reverses capillary permeability, and stabilizes lysosomal membranes at the cellular level to prevent or control inflammation

Pharmacodynamics

Oral inhalation: Clinical effects are due to direct local effect rather than systemic absorption

Onset of action: Within 24 hours

Maximum effect: 1-2 weeks or more

Duration after discontinuation: Several days or more

Pharmacokinetics

Distribution: V_d: Adults: 4.2 L/kg

Protein binding: 91%

Metabolism: Via cytochrome P-450 3A4 pathway

Bioavailability: Oral inhalation: 30% of dose delivered from activator

Half-life: 7.8 hours

Usual Dosage

Intranasal:

Children <4 years: Not recommended

Children ≥4 years and Adolescents: Initial: 1 spray (50 mcg/spray) to each nostril daily (100 mcg/day); if response is inadequate, give 2 sprays to each nostril daily (200 mcg/day); once symptoms are controlled, reduce dose to 100 mcg/day (1 spray to each nostril daily); maximum dose: 200 mcg/day (4 sprays/day)

Adults: Initial: 200 mcg/day given as 2 sprays (50 mcg/spray) to each nostril daily or 1 spray to each nostril twice daily; dosage may be reduced to 100 mcg/day (1 spray to each nostril daily) after the first few days if symptoms are controlled; maximum dose: 200 mcg/day (4 sprays/day)

Oral inhalation: If adequate response is not seen after 2 weeks of initial dosage, increase dosage; doses should be titrated to the lowest effective dose once asthma is controlled; Manufacturer recommendations:

Inhalation aerosol (Flovent®): Children ≥12 years and Adults:

Patients previously treated with bronchodilators only: Initial: 88 mcg twice daily; maximum dose: 440 mcg twice daily

Patients treated with an inhaled corticosteroid: Initial: 88-220 mcg twice daily; maximum dose: 440 mcg twice daily; may start doses above 88 mcg twice daily in poorly controlled patients or in those who previously required higher doses of inhaled corticosteroids

Patients previously treated with oral corticosteroids: Initial: 880 mcg twice daily; maximum dose: 880 mcg twice daily

NIH Guidelines (NIH, 1997) [give in divided doses twice daily]:

Children:

"Low" dose: 88-176 mcg/day (44 mcg/puff: 2-4 puffs/day)

"Medium" dose: 176-440 mcg/day (44 mcg/puff: 4-10 puffs/day or 110 mcg/puff: 2-4 puffs/day)

"High" dose: >440 mcg/day (110 mcg/puff: >4 puffs/day or 220 mcg/puff: >2 puffs/day)

Adults:

"Low" dose: 88-264 mcg/day (44 mcg/puff: 2-6 puffs/day or 110 mcg/puff: 2 puffs/day)

"Medium" dose: 264-660 mcg/day (110 mcg/puff: 2-6 puffs/day)

"High" dose: >660 mcg/day (110 mcg/puff: >6 puffs/day or 220 mcg/puff: >3 puffs/day)

(Continued)

Fluticasone *(Continued)*

Inhalation powder (Flovent® Rotadisk®):
  Children 4-11 years: Patients previously treated with bronchodilators alone or inhaled corticosteroids: Initial: 50 mcg twice daily; maximum dose: 100 mcg twice daily; may start higher initial dose in poorly controlled patients or in those who previously required higher doses of inhaled corticosteroids
  Adolescents and Adults:
    Patients previously treated with bronchodilators alone: Initial: 100 mcg twice daily; maximum dose: 500 mcg twice daily
    Patients previously treated with inhaled corticosteroids: Initial: 100-250 mcg twice daily; maximum dose: 500 mcg twice daily; may start doses above 100 mcg twice daily in poorly controlled patients or in those who previously required higher doses of inhaled corticosteroids
    Patients previously treated with oral corticosteroids: Initial: 1000 mcg twice daily; maximum dose: 1000 mcg twice daily
Topical:
  Cream:
    Infants <3 months: Not approved for use
    Infants ≥3 months, Children, and Adults: **Note:** Safety and efficacy of use >4 weeks in pediatric patients have not been established:
      Atopic dermatitis: Apply a thin film to affected area once or twice daily
      Other dermatoses: Apply a thin film to affected area twice daily
  Ointment: Adolescents and Adults: Apply sparingly in a thin film twice daily

Administration
Intranasal spray: Shake bottle gently before use; clear nasal passages by blowing nose prior to use; nasal spray pump must be primed (6 actuations) before first use or after ≥1 week of non-use; discard unit after 120 metered sprays are used
Oral inhalant: Shake aerosol canister well before use; use a spacer device for children <8 years of age; rinse mouth after inhalation to decrease chance of oral candidiasis; do not puncture Rotadisk® blister until taking dose with Diskhaler®
Topical: Apply sparingly to affected area, gently rub in until disappears; do not use on open skin; avoid application on face, underarms, or groin area unless directed by physician; avoid contact with eyes; do not occlude area unless directed; do not apply to diaper area

Monitoring Parameters
Oral inhalation: Check mucus membranes for signs of fungal infection

Patient Information
Notify physician if condition being treated persists or worsens; do not decrease dose or discontinue without physician approval
Oral inhalant: Report sore mouth or mouth lesions to physician

Additional Information
Fluticasone oral inhalation is also used to help reduce or discontinue oral corticosteroid therapy for asthma; do not decrease prednisone faster than 2.5 mg/day on a weekly basis, beginning after at least 1 week of fluticasone inhalation therapy; monitor patients for signs of asthma instability and adrenal insufficiency (see Warnings); decrease fluticasone to lowest effective dose **after** prednisone reduction is complete. If bronchospasm with wheezing occurs after oral inhalation use, a fast-acting bronchodilator may be used.
Topical: HPA axis suppression occurred in 2 children (2 and 5 years old) of 43 pediatric patients treated topically for 4 weeks; application covered at least 35% of body surface area

Dosage Forms
Powder, oral inhalation, as propionate (Flovent® Rotadisk®; 4 blisters of the drug per Rotadisk®, 15 Rotadisks® per pack) : 50 mcg (delivers 44 mcg/inhalation); 100 mcg (delivers 88 mcg/inhalation); 250 mcg (delivers 220 mcg/inhalation)
Spray, aerosol, oral inhalation, as propionate (Flovent®): 44 mcg/actuation (7.9 g = 60 actuations or 13 g = 120 actuations); 110 mcg/actuation (7.9 g = 60 actuations or 13 g = 120 actuations); 220 mcg/actuation (7.9 g = 60 actuations or 13 g = 120 actuations)
Spray, intranasal, as propionate (Flonase®): 50 mcg/actuation (16 g = 120 actuations)
Topical, as propionate (Cutivate®):
  Cream: 0.05% (15 g, 30 g, 60 g)
  Ointment: 0.005% (15 g, 30 g, 60 g)

References
Expert Panel Report 2, "Guidelines for the Diagnosis and Management of Asthma," *Clinical Practice Guidelines*, National Institutes of Health, National Heart, Lung, and Blood Institute, NIH Publication No. 94-4051, April, 1997.

♦ **Fluticasone Propionate** *see* Fluticasone *on page 436*
♦ **FML®** *see* Fluorometholone *on page 429*

♦ **FML® Forte** *see* Fluorometholone *on page 429*
♦ **Foille® [OTC]** *see* Benzocaine *on page 124*
♦ **Foille® Medicated First Aid [OTC]** *see* Benzocaine *on page 124*
♦ **Folacin** *see* Folic Acid *on page 439*
♦ **Folate** *see* Folic Acid *on page 439*

Folic Acid (FOE lik AS id)

Brand Names Apo®-Folic (Canada); Flodine® (Canada); Folvite®; Novo-Folacid® (Canada)

Synonyms Folacin; Folate; Pteroylglutamic Acid

Therapeutic Category Nutritional Supplement; Vitamin, Water Soluble

Generic Available Yes

Use Treatment of megaloblastic and macrocytic anemias due to folate deficiency; dietary supplement to prevent neural tube defects

Pregnancy Risk Factor A (C if dose exceeds RDA recommendation)

Contraindications Pernicious, aplastic, or normocytic anemias

Warnings Large doses may mask the hematologic effects of B_{12} deficiency, thus obscuring the diagnosis of pernicious anemia while allowing the neurologic complications due to B_{12} deficiency to progress; injection contains benzyl alcohol (1.5%) as preservative, therefore, avoid use in premature infants

Adverse Reactions
Cardiovascular: Slight flushing
Central nervous system: Irritability, difficulty sleeping, confusion, malaise
Dermatologic: Pruritus, rash
Gastrointestinal: GI upset
Miscellaneous: Hypersensitivity reactions

Drug Interactions May decrease phenytoin serum concentration; hematologic response antagonized by chloramphenicol; folic acid antagonists (ie, methotrexate, pyrimethamine, trimethoprim) prevent the formation of tetrahydrofolic acid (active metabolite), therefore, folic acid is not effective for the treatment of overdosage of these drugs (leucovorin must be used); decreased folic acid absorption with sulfa-salazine and aminosalicylic acid; decreased folic acid concentration with phenytoin, primidone, para-aminosalicylic acid

Mechanism of Action Folic acid is necessary for formation of a number of coenzymes in many metabolic systems, particularly for purine and pyrimidine synthesis; required for nucleoprotein synthesis and maintenance in erythropoiesis; stimulates WBC and platelet production in folate deficiency anemia

Pharmacodynamics Peak effect: Within 30-60 minutes following oral administration

Pharmacokinetics
Absorption: In the proximal part of the small intestine
Time to peak serum concentration: Oral: 1 hour
Elimination: Primarily via liver metabolism

Usual Dosage
Recommended daily allowance (RDA): Oral:
Premature neonates: 50 mcg (~15 mcg/kg/day)
Neonates to 6 months: 25-35 mcg
Children:
6 months to 3 years: 50 mcg
4-6 years: 75 mcg
7-10 years: 100 mcg
11-14 years: 150 mcg
Children >15 years and Adults: 200 mcg
Pregnant women: 400 mcg
Folic acid deficiency: Oral, I.M., I.V., S.C.:
Infants: 15 mcg/kg/dose daily or 50 mcg/day
Children: 1 mg/day initial dosage; maintenance dose: 1-10 years: 0.1-0.4 mg/day
Children >11 years and Adults: 1 mg/day initial dosage; maintenance dose: 0.5 mg/day

Administration
Oral: May be administered without regard to meals
Parenteral: I.V.: Dilute with sterile water, dextrose or saline solution to 0.1 mg/mL; if I.M. route used, administer deep I.M.; may also administer S.C.

Monitoring Parameters CBC with differential

Reference Range Total folate: Normal: 5-15 ng/mL; folate deficiency: <5 ng/mL; megaloblastic anemia: <2 ng/mL
(Continued)

439

Folic Acid *(Continued)*

Additional Information Oral liquid vitamin drops (eg, Vi-Daylin®) do not contain folic acid due to the instability of folic acid in the pH of these formulations.

Dosage Forms
Injection, as sodium folate: 5 mg/mL (10 mL); 10 mg/mL (10 mL)
Tablet: 0.1 mg, 0.4 mg, 0.8 mg, 1 mg

Extemporaneous Preparations A 50 mcg/mL solution may be made by mixing 1 mL (5 mg) folic acid injection in 90 mL purified water; adjust pH to 9 with sodium hydroxide 0.1 N (approximately 2.8 mL), then add purified water to make a total volume of 100 mL; stable 30 days at room temperature
    Nahata MC and Hipple TF, *Pediatric Drug Formulations*, 3rd ed, Cincinnati, OH: Harvey Whitney Books Company, 1997.

♦ **Folinic Acid** *see Leucovorin on page 559*

♦ **Follutein®** *see Chorionic Gonadotropin on page 221*

♦ **Folvite®** *see Folic Acid on page 439*

Fomepizole *(foe ME pi zole)*

Brand Names Antizol®
Synonyms 4-Methylpyrazole; 4-MP
Therapeutic Category Antidote, Ethylene Glycol Toxicity; Antidote, Methanol Toxicity
Generic Available No
Use Ethylene glycol (antifreeze) and methanol toxicity; may be useful in propylene glycol toxicity
Pregnancy Risk Factor C
Contraindications Hypersensitivity to fomepizole, other pyrazoles, or any component
Warnings By inhibiting the action of alcohol dehydrogenase, fomepizole reduces the elimination of alcohol; this must be considered when using fomepizole, as alcohol is often ingested concomitantly by patients with ethylene glycol intoxication; likewise, alcohol may reduce the elimination of fomepizole by the same mechanism; safety and efficacy in pediatric patients has not been established
Precautions Management of ethylene glycol ingestion may require treatment of metabolic acidosis, acute renal failure, adult respiratory distress syndrome, and hypocalcemia; dialysis should be considered, in addition to fomepizole therapy, in patients with acute renal failure, severe metabolic acidosis, or a serum ethylene glycol concentration >50 mg/dL; adjust dosage for renal dysfunction (see Usual Dosage)
Adverse Reactions
Cardiovascular: Bradycardia, tachycardia, hypotension
Central nervous system: Headache, dizziness, seizure, slurred speech, fever, somnolence
Dermatologic: Rash
Gastrointestinal: Nausea, vomiting, diarrhea, anorexia, heartburn, metallic taste, abdominal pain
Hematologic: Eosinophilia, anemia
Hepatic: Transient elevations in transaminase levels
Local: Phlebosclerosis, vein irritation
Ocular: Nystagmus, blurred vision
Respiratory: Pharyngitis, hiccups
Miscellaneous: Hypersensitivity reactions
Drug Interactions Alcohol (see Warnings)
Stability Store at room temperature; fomepizole solidifies at temperatures <25°C (77°F); if solidification occurs, liquefy by running the vial under warm water or by holding in the hand; solidification does not affect the efficacy, safety, or stability of fomepizole; stabile diluted in NS or D_5W for 48 hours; does not contain a preservative; use within 24 hours of dilution
Mechanism of Action A competitive alcohol dehydrogenase inhibitor, fomepizole complexes and inactivates alcohol dehydrogenase thus preventing formation of the toxic metabolites of the alcohols
Pharmacokinetics
Distribution: V_d: 0.6-2.03 L/kg; rapidly distributes into total body water
Protein binding: Negligible
Metabolism: Liver; primarily to 4-carboxypyrazole; after single doses, exhibits saturable, Michaelis-Menton kinetics; with multiple dosing, fomepizole induces its own metabolism via the cytochrome P-450 system; after enzyme induction elimination follows first order kinetics

Elimination: 1% to 3.5% excreted unchanged in the urine
Dializable

Usual Dosage I.V.:

Children: Has not been studied

Adults **not requiring** hemodialysis: Initial: 15 mg/kg loading dose; followed by 10 mg/kg every 12 hours for 4 doses; then 15 mg/kg every 12 hours until ethylene glycol levels have been reduced to <20 mg/dL

Adults **requiring** hemodialysis: Since fomezipole is dialyzable, follow the above dose recommendations at intervals related to institution of hemodialysis and its duration:

Dose at the beginning of hemodialysis:

If <6 hours since last fomezipole dose: Do **not** administer dose

If ≥6 hours since last fomezipole dose: Administer next scheduled dose

Dose during hemodialysis: Administer every 4 hours

Dose at the time hemodialysis is completed (dependent upon the time between the last dose and the end of hemodialysis):

<1 hour: Do **not** administer at the end of hemodialysis

1-3 hours: Administer ½ of the next scheduled dose

>3 hours: Administer the next scheduled dose

Maintenance dose off hemodialysis: Give next scheduled dose 12 hours from last dose administered

Dosage adjustment in renal impairment: Fomepizole is substantially excreted by the kidney and the risk of toxic reactions to this drug may be increased in patients with impaired renal function; no dosage recommendations for patients with impaired renal function have been established

Administration Parenteral: I.V. Dilute in at least 100 mL NS or D_5W (<25 mg/mL); infuse over 30 minutes; rapid infusion of concentrations ≥25 mg/mL has been associated with vein irritation and phlebosclerosis

Monitoring Parameters Vital signs, arterial blood gases, acid-base status, plasma and urinary ethylene glycol, urinary oxalate, anion and osmolar gaps, ethylene glycol level, clinical signs and symptoms of toxicity (arrhythmias, seizures, coma)

Reference Range Ethylene glycol: Goal: <20 mg/dL

Additional Information If ethylene glycol poisoning is left untreated, the natural progression of the poisoning leads to accumulation of toxic metabolites, including glycolic and oxalic acids; these metabolites can induce metabolic acidosis, seizures, stupor, coma, calcium oxaluria, acute tubular necrosis and death; as ethylene glycol levels diminish in the blood when metabolized to glycolate, the diagnosis of this poisoning may be difficult

Dosage Forms Injection, concentrate: 1 g/mL (1.5 mL)

- ♦ **5-Formyl Tetrahydrofolate** *see Leucovorin on page 559*
- ♦ **Fortaz®** *see Ceftazidime on page 190*
- ♦ **Fortovase®** *see Saquinavir on page 857*

Foscarnet (fos KAR net)

Brand Names Foscavir®

Synonyms PFA; Phosphonoformate

Therapeutic Category Antiviral Agent, Parenteral

Generic Available No

Use Alternative to ganciclovir for treatment of CMV infections and is possibly the preferred initial agent for the treatment of CMV retinitis except for those patients with decreased renal function; treatment of acyclovir-resistant mucocutaneous herpes simplex virus infections in immunocompromised patients and acyclovir-resistant herpes zoster infections

Pregnancy Risk Factor C

Contraindications Hypersensitivity to foscarnet or any component; Cl_{cr} <0.4 mL/minute/kg

Warnings Renal impairment occurs to some degree in the majority of patients treated with foscarnet; renal impairment may occur at any time and is usually reversible within 1 week following dose adjustment or discontinuation of therapy; however, several patients have died with renal failure within 4 weeks of stopping foscarnet; foscarnet is deposited in teeth and bone of young, growing animals; it has adversely affected tooth enamel development in rats; safety and effectiveness in children has not been studied

Patients with a low ionized calcium may experience perioral tingling, numbness, parasthesia, tetany, and seizures. Risk factor for seizures include a low baseline ANC, impaired renal function, and low total serum calcium.

(Continued)

Foscarnet *(Continued)*

Precautions Use with caution in patients with renal impairment, patients with altered electrolyte levels, and patients with neurologic or cardiac abnormalities; adjust dose for patients with impaired renal function; discontinue treatment in adults if serum creatinine ≥2.9 mg/dL; therapy can be restarted if serum creatinine ≤2 mg/dL

Adverse Reactions

Cardiovascular: Hypertension, palpitations, chest pain, EKG abnormalities

Central nervous system: Fatigue, fever, headache, seizures, hallucinations, dizziness, agitation, amnesia

Endocrine & metabolic: Hypocalcemia, hypomagnesemia, hypokalemia, hypo- or hyperphosphatemia

Gastrointestinal: Nausea, diarrhea, vomiting, weight loss, pancreatitis

Genitourinary: Vulvovaginal ulceration, penile epithelium ulceration, dysuria, urethral disorder

Hematologic: Decreases in hemoglobin and hematocrit

Hepatic: Elevated liver enzymes, cholecystitis, hepatitis

Local: Thrombophlebitis

Neuromuscular & skeletal: Peripheral neuropathy, paresthesia, tremor

Renal: Elevated BUN and serum creatinine, polyuria, oliguria, renal failure, proteinuria

Respiratory: Coughing, dyspnea, bronchospasm

Drug Interactions Pentamidine (additive hypocalcemia); aminoglycosides, amphotericin B (additive nephrotoxicity)

Stability Store at room temperature; refrigeration may result in crystallization of the drug; incompatible with dextrose ≥30%, I.V. solutions containing calcium, magnesium, vancomycin, TPN

Mechanism of Action Pyrophosphate analog which inhibits DNA synthesis by interfering with viral DNA polymerase and reverse transcriptase

Pharmacokinetics

Distribution: V_d: Adults: 0.74 L/kg; minimal penetration of the drug across the blood-brain barrier

Protein binding: 14% to 17%

Half-life, plasma: Adults with normal renal function: 3-4.5 hours

Terminal: 18-42 hours

Elimination: 80% to 90% excreted unchanged in urine

Usual Dosage Adolescents and Adults: I.V.:

CMV retinitis: Induction treatment: 180 mg/kg/day divided every 8 hours for 14-21 days

Maintenance therapy: 90-120 mg/kg/day as a single infusion once daily

Acyclovir-resistant herpes simplex virus infection: 40 mg/kg/dose every 8 hours or 40-60 mg/kg/dose every 12 hours for up to 3 weeks or until lesions heal; repeat treatment may lead to the development of resistance

Dosing interval in renal impairment: See tables.

Induction Treatment

Cl_{cr} (mL/min/kg)	mg/kg/8h
≥1.6	60
1.5	56.5
1.4	53
1.3	49.4
1.2	45.9
1.1	42.4
1	38.9
0.9	35.3
0.8	31.8
0.7	28.3
0.6	24.8
0.5	21.2
0.4	17.7

Maintenance Therapy

Cl_cr (mL/min/kg)	mg/kg/day
≥1.4	90-120
1.2-1.4	78-104
1-1.2	75-100
0.8-1	71-94
0.6-0.8	63-84
0.4-0.6	57-76

Administration Parenteral: 24 mg/mL solution may be administered without further dilution when using a central venous catheter for infusion; for peripheral vein administration, the solution **must** be diluted to a final concentration **not to exceed** 12 mg/mL with either NS or D$_5$W; administer by I.V. infusion at a rate **not to exceed** 60 mg/kg/dose over 1 hour or 120 mg/kg/dose over 2 hours

Monitoring Parameters Serum creatinine, calcium, phosphorus, potassium, magnesium; hemoglobin, ophthalmologic exams

Reference Range Therapeutic for CMV: 150 µg/mL

Patient Information Report any numbness in the extremities, paresthesias, or perioral tingling

Nursing Implications Provide adequate hydration with I.V. NS or D$_5$W prior to and during treatment to minimize nephrotoxicity

Dosage Forms Injection: 24 mg/mL (250 mL, 500 mL)

References

Butler KM, DeSmet MD, Husson RN, et al, "Treatment of Aggressive Cytomegalovirus Retinitis With Ganciclovir in Combination With Foscarnet in a Child Infected With Human Immunodeficiency Virus," *J Pediatr,* 1992, 120(3):483-6.

Polis MA, "Foscarnet and Ganciclovir in the Treatment of Cytomegalovirus Retinitis," *J Acquir Immune Defic Syndr,* 1992, 5(Suppl 1):S3-10.

Fosphenytoin (FOS fen i toyn)

Related Information
Blood Level Sampling Time Guidelines *on page 1189*

Brand Names Cerebyx®

Available Salts Fosphenytoin Sodium

Synonyms 3-Phosphoryloxymethyl Phenytoin Disodium

Therapeutic Category Anticonvulsant, Hydantoin

Generic Available No

Use Management of generalized convulsive status epilepticus; used for short-term parenteral administration of phenytoin; prevention and management of seizures responsive to phenytoin

Pregnancy Risk Factor D

Contraindications Hypersensitivity to fosphenytoin, phenytoin, or any other component; heart block, sinus bradycardia

Warnings Abrupt withdrawal may precipitate status epilepticus; monitor blood pressure and EKG with I.V. loading doses; use with caution in patients with severe myocardial insufficiency and hypotension; discontinue if skin rash develops, do not resume drug if rash is exfoliative, purpuric, bullous, or if SLE, Stevens-Johnson syndrome, or toxic epidermal necrolysis is suspected; discontinue if acute hepatotoxicity occurs

Precautions Use with caution in patients with porphyria; consider the amount of phosphate delivered by fosphenytoin in patients who require phosphate restriction; use with caution and modify dosage in patients with hepatic or renal dysfunction

Adverse Reactions
Cardiovascular: Hypotension (with rapid I.V. administration), vasodilation, tachycardia, bradycardia
Central nervous system: Slurred speech, dizziness, drowsiness, headache, somnolence, ataxia, fever
Dermatologic: Rash, exfoliative dermatitis, facial edema
Endocrine & metabolic: Folic acid depletion, hyperglycemia
Gastrointestinal: Nausea, vomiting, taste perversion
Genitourinary: Pelvic pain
Hematologic: Neutropenia, thrombocytopenia, anemia (megaloblastic)
Local: Pain on injection; since fosphenytoin is water soluble and has a lower pH (8.8) than phenytoin (12), irritation at injection site or phlebitis is reduced; I.M.: Local itching
Neuromuscular & skeletal: Osteomalacia
(Continued)

Fosphenytoin *(Continued)*

Ocular: Nystagmus, blurred vision, diplopia

Otic: Tinnitus

Miscellaneous: Lymphadenopathy; sensory disturbances (burning, pruritus, tingling, paresthesia) occur predominately in the groin area, but may occur in the lower back, abdomen, head or neck (these effects may be related to the phosphate load); paresthesia and pruritus are more common with I.V. vs I.M. administration and are dose and infusion rate related

Drug Interactions No drugs are known to interfere with the conversion of fosphenytoin to phenytoin; see Phenytoin *on page 762* for phenytoin interactions

Stability Store unopened vials in the refrigerator; fosphenytoin at concentrations of 1, 8, and 20 mg phenytoin sodium equivalents **(PE)**/mL in D_5W or NS is stable for 30 days when stored at 25°C or 4°C in glass bottles or polyvinyl chloride infusion bags, and when frozen at -20°C in polyvinyl chloride infusion bags. After removal from the freezer, these solutions are stable for 7 days at 25°C or 4°C.

Undiluted fosphenytoin injection (50 mg **PE**/mL) is stable in polypropylene syringes for 30 days at 25°C, 4°C, or frozen at -20°C.

Fosphenytoin at concentrations of 1, 8, and 20 mg **PE**/mL prepared in D_5/$\frac{1}{2}$NS, D_5/$\frac{1}{2}$NS with KCl 20 mEq/L, D_5/$\frac{1}{2}$NS with 40 mEq/L, LR, D_5/LR, D_{10}W, amino acid 10%, mannitol 20%, hetastarch 6% in NS or Plasma-Lyte A® injection is stable in polyvinyl chloride bags for 7 days when stored at 25°C (room temperature).

Mechanism of Action Diphosphate ester salt of phenytoin which acts as a water soluble prodrug of phenytoin; after administration, plasma and tissue esterases convert fosphenytoin to phosphate, formaldehyde and phenytoin (as the active moiety); phenytoin works by stabilizing neuronal membranes and decreasing seizure activity by increasing efflux or decreasing influx of sodium ions across cell membranes in the motor cortex during generation of nerve impulses

Pharmacokinetics The pharmacokinetics of fosphenytoin-derived phenytoin are the same as those for phenytoin (see Phenytoin *on page 762*). Parameters listed below are for fosphenytoin (the prodrug) unless otherwise noted. **Note:** The pharmacokinetics of fosphenytoin have been studied in a limited number of children 5-18 years of age and have been found to be similar to the pharmacokinetics observed in young adults (see Pellock, 1996).

Bioavailability: I.M., I.V.: 100%

Distribution: Adults: V_d: 4.3-10.8 L; V_d of fosphenytoin increases with dose and rate of administration

Protein binding: 95% to 99% primarily to albumin; binding of fosphenytoin to protein is saturable (the percent bound decreases as total concentration increases); fosphenytoin displaces phenytoin from protein binding sites; during the time fosphenytoin is being converted to phenytoin, fosphenytoin may temporarily increase the free fraction of phenytoin up to 30% unbound

Metabolism: Each millimole of fosphenytoin is metabolized to 1 millimole of phenytoin, phosphate, and formaldehyde; formaldehyde is converted to formate, which is then metabolized by a folate-dependent mechanism; conversion of fosphenytoin to phenytoin increases with increasing dose and infusion rate, most likely due to a decrease in fosphenytoin protein binding

Conversion of fosphenytoin to phenytoin: Half-life: 15 minutes

Time for complete conversion to phenytoin:

    I.M.: 4 hours after injection

    I.V.: 2 hours after the end of infusion

Elimination: 0% fosphenytoin excreted in urine

Usual Dosage

The dose, concentration in solutions, and infusion rates for fosphenytoin are expressed as PHENYTOIN SODIUM EQUIVALENTS (PE)

Fosphenytoin should ALWAYS be prescribed and dispensed in mg of PE; otherwise significant medication errors may occur

Children 5-18 years: I.V.: A limited number of children have been studied. Seven children received a single I.V. loading dose of fosphenytoin 10-20 mg **PE**/kg for the treatment of acute generalized convulsive status epilepticus (Pellock, 1996). Some centers are using the phenytoin dosing guidelines in children and dosing fosphenytoin using **PE** doses equal to the phenytoin doses (ie, phenytoin 1 mg = fosphenytoin 1 mg **PE**). Further pediatric studies are needed.

Adults:

    Loading dose:

        Status epilepticus: I.V.: 15-20 mg **PE**/kg

        Nonemergent loading: I.M., I.V.: 10-20 mg **PE**/kg

Initial daily maintenance dose: I.M., I.V.: 4-6 mg **PE**/kg; I.M. dose may be administered as a single daily dose using 1 or 2 injection sites; some patients may require more frequent dosing

I.M. or I.V. substitution for oral phenytoin: Initial: Use the same total daily dose in **PE** of fosphenytoin (ie, phenytoin 1 mg = fosphenytoin 1 mg **PE**); plasma concentrations may increase slightly with this method because oral phenytoin sodium is 90% bioavailable and phenytoin derived from I.M. or I.V. fosphenytoin is 100% bioavailable. Monitor clinical response and phenytoin concentrations to further guide dosage adjustments after 3-4 days

Dosing adjustments in renal/hepatic impairment:

Cirrhosis: Phenytoin clearance may be substantially reduced and monitoring of plasma concentrations with dosage adjustments is advisable

Renal or hepatic disease and patients with hypoalbuminemia: Fosphenytoin conversion to phenytoin may be increased (due to lower protein binding) without a similar increase in phenytoin clearance, leading to a potential increase in the frequency and severity of adverse effects

Administration Dilute with D$_5$W or NS to 1.5-25 mg **PE**/mL

Children 5-18 years: An administration rate of 3 mg **PE**/kg/minute with a maximum of 150 mg **PE**/minute was used in 7 patients (see Pellock, 1996)

Adults: Administer at a rate of 100-150 mg **PE**/minute with a maximum infusion rate of 150 mg **PE**/minute

Monitoring Parameters Serum phenytoin concentrations, CBC with differential, liver enzymes; blood pressure, vital signs (with I.V. use); free (unbound) and total serum phenytoin concentrations in patients with hyperbilirubinemia, hypoalbuminemia, renal dysfunction, uremia, or hepatic disease

Reference Range Monitor **phenytoin** serum concentrations; obtain phenytoin concentrations 2 hours after the end of an I.V. infusion or 4 hours after an I.M. injection of fosphenytoin; see Phenytoin *on page 762* for phenytoin reference range

Additional Information Dosing equivalency: Fosphenytoin sodium 1.5 mg is equivalent to phenytoin sodium 1 mg which is equivalent to fosphenytoin 1 mg **PE**

Phosphate load: Each mg **PE** of fosphenytoin delivers 0.0037 mmol of phosphate

Formaldehyde production from fosphenytoin is not expected to be clinically significant in adults with short-term use (eg, 1 week); potentially harmful amounts of phosphate and formaldehyde could occur with an overdose of fosphenytoin; fosphenytoin is more water soluble than phenytoin and, therefore, the injection does not contain propylene glycol; antiarrhythmic effects should be similar to phenytoin

Dosage Forms Injection, as sodium: 150 mg [equivalent to phenytoin sodium 100 mg (ie, 100 mg **PE**)] in 2 mL vials; 750 mg [equivalent to phenytoin sodium 500 mg (ie, 500 mg **PE**)] in 10 mL vials

References

Boucher BA, Feler CA, Dean JC, et al, "The Safety, Tolerability, and Pharmacokinetics of Fosphenytoin After Intramuscular and Intravenous Administration in Neurosurgery Patients," *Pharmacotherapy*, 1996, 16(4):638-45.

Boucher BA, "Fosphenytoin: A Novel Phenytoin Prodrug," *Pharmacotherapy*, 1996, 16(5):777-91.

Fischer JH, Cwik MS, Luer MS, et al, "Stability of Fosphenytoin Sodium With Intravenous Solutions in Glass Bottles, Polyvinyl Chloride Bags, and Polypropylene Syringes," *Ann Pharmacother*, 1997, 31(5):553-9.

Pellock JM, "Fosphenytoin Use in Children," *Neurology*, 1996, 46(6 Suppl 1):S14-6.

Wilder BJ, Campbell K, Ramsay RE, et al, "Safety and Tolerance of Multiple Doses of Intramuscular Fosphenytoin Substituted for Oral Phenytoin in Epilepsy or Neurosurgery," *Arch Neurol*, 1996, 53(8):764-8.

♦ **Fosphenytoin Sodium** *see* Fosphenytoin *on page 443*
♦ **Fostex® [OTC]** *see* Sulfur and Salicylic Acid *on page 896*
♦ **Fostex® 10% BPO Gel [OTC]** *see* Benzoyl Peroxide *on page 126*
♦ **Fostex® 10% Wash [OTC]** *see* Benzoyl Peroxide *on page 126*
♦ **Fostex® Bar [OTC]** *see* Benzoyl Peroxide *on page 126*
♦ **Fototar® [OTC]** *see* Coal Tar *on page 247*
♦ **Freezone® Solution [OTC]** *see* Salicylic Acid *on page 854*
♦ **Froben® (Canada)** *see* Flurbiprofen *on page 435*
♦ **Froben-SR® (Canada)** *see* Flurbiprofen *on page 435*
♦ **FS Shampoo® Topical** *see* Fluocinolone *on page 425*
♦ **5-FU** *see* Fluorouracil *on page 430*
♦ **Fulvicin® P/G** *see* Griseofulvin *on page 463*
♦ **Fulvicin-U/F®** *see* Griseofulvin *on page 463*
♦ **Fumasorb® [OTC]** *see* Iron Supplements, Oral/Enteral *on page 530*

- ♦ **Fumerin® [OTC]** *see* Iron Supplements, Oral/Enteral *on page 530*
- ♦ **Fungizone®** *see* Amphotericin B, Conventional *on page 74*
- ♦ **Fungoid® Creme** *see* Miconazole *on page 641*
- ♦ **Fungoid® Tincture** *see* Miconazole *on page 641*
- ♦ **Fungoid® Topical Solution** *see* Undecylenic Acid and Derivatives *on page 962*
- ♦ **Furadantin®** *see* Nitrofurantoin *on page 689*
- ♦ **Furalan®** *see* Nitrofurantoin *on page 689*
- ♦ **Furan®** *see* Nitrofurantoin *on page 689*
- ♦ **Furanite®** *see* Nitrofurantoin *on page 689*

Furazolidone (fyoor a ZOE li done)

Brand Names Furoxone®

Therapeutic Category Antibiotic, Miscellaneous; Antiprotozoal

Generic Available No

Use Treatment of bacterial or protozoal diarrhea and enteritis caused by susceptible organisms: *Giardia lamblia* and *Vibrio cholerae*

Pregnancy Risk Factor C

Contraindications Hypersensitivity to furazolidone or any component; concurrent use of alcohol; infants <1 month of age because of the possibility of producing hemolytic anemia; MAO inhibitors, tyramine-containing foods

Precautions Use with caution in patients with G-6-PD deficiency

Adverse Reactions
Cardiovascular: Hypotension
Central nervous system: Dizziness, drowsiness, malaise, fever, headache, polyneuritis
Dermatologic: Rash
Endocrine & metabolic: Hypoglycemia, disulfiram-like reaction after alcohol ingestion
Gastrointestinal: Nausea, vomiting, diarrhea
Genitourinary: Discoloration of urine (brown)
Hematologic: Agranulocytosis, hemolysis in patients with G-6-PD deficiency and neonates, leukopenia
Respiratory: Pulmonary infiltration
Miscellaneous: Hypersensitivity reactions including angioedema, hypotension, fever, urticaria, arthralgia

Drug Interactions Adrenergic agents, tricyclic antidepressants, MAO inhibitors (may increase hypertensive effect); alcohol (may cause disulfiram-like reactions)

Food Interactions Avoid tyramine-containing foods (cheese, broad beans, dry or aged sausage, nonfresh meat, liver, salami, mortadella, concentrated yeast extracts, liquid and powdered protein supplements, fermented bean curd and soya bean, meat extract and hydrolyzed protein extracts, raspberries, Chianti wine, Kimchee, or sauerkraut)

Stability Protect from light

Mechanism of Action Inhibits several vital enzymatic reactions causing antibacterial and antiprotozoal action; acts as a monoamine oxidase inhibitor and may prevent acetylation of coenzyme A

Pharmacokinetics
Absorption: Oral: Poor
Metabolism: Inactivated in the intestine
Elimination: 5% of oral dose excreted in urine as active drug and metabolites

Usual Dosage Oral:
Children >1 month: 5-8.8 mg/kg/day divided every 6 hours, not to exceed 400 mg/day
Adults: 100 mg 4 times/day

Administration Oral: May be administered without regard to food

Monitoring Parameters CBC

Test Interactions False-positive results for urine glucose with Clinitest®

Patient Information May discolor urine to a brown tint; avoid alcohol during treatment and for 4 days after discontinuing furazolidone

Dosage Forms
Suspension: 50 mg/15 mL (60 mL, 473 mL)
Tablet: 100 mg

References
Murphy TV and Nelson JD, "Five vs Ten Days' Therapy With Furazolidone for Giardiasis," *Am J Dis Child,* 1983, 137(3):267-70.
Turner JA, "Giardiasis and Infections With Dientamoeba Fragilis," *Pediatr Clin North Am,* 1985, 32(4):865-80.

♦ **Furazosin** *see Prazosin on page 790*

Furosemide (fyoor OH se mide)
Related Information
Adult ACLS Algorithm, Hypotension, Shock *on page 1016*
Carbohydrate and Alcohol Content of Liquid Medications for Use in Patients Receiving Ketogenic Diets *on page 1228*
Brand Names Apo®-Furosemide (Canada); Furoside® (Canada); Lasix® Injection; Lasix® Oral; Lasix® Special (Canada); Novo-Semide® (Canada); Uritol® (Canada)
Therapeutic Category Antihypertensive Agent; Diuretic, Loop
Generic Available Yes
Use Management of edema associated with CHF and hepatic or renal disease; used alone or in combination with antihypertensives in treatment of hypertension
Pregnancy Risk Factor C
Contraindications Hypersensitivity to furosemide or any component; anuria
Warnings Loop diuretics are potent diuretics; excess amounts can lead to profound diuresis with fluid and electrolyte loss
Precautions Hepatic cirrhosis (rapid alterations in fluid/electrolytes may precipitate coma)
Adverse Reactions
Cardiovascular: Orthostatic hypotension
Central nervous system: Dizziness, vertigo, headache
Dermatologic: Urticaria, photosensitivity
Endocrine & metabolic: Hypokalemia, hyponatremia, hypomagnesemia, hypocalcemia, hyperglycemia, hypochloremia, alkalosis, dehydration, hyperuricemia
Gastrointestinal: Pancreatitis, nausea; oral solutions may cause diarrhea due to sorbitol content; anorexia, vomiting, constipation, abdominal cramping
Hematologic: Agranulocytosis, anemia, thrombocytopenia
Hepatic: Ischemic hepatitis, jaundice
Otic: Potential ototoxicity
Renal: Nephrocalcinosis, prerenal azotemia, interstitial nephritis, hypercalciuria
Drug Interactions Indomethacin decreases the effect of furosemide; decreased lithium excretion; decreased glucose tolerance with antidiabetic agents; increased ototoxicity with aminoglycosides and ethacrynic acid; drugs affected by potassium depletion (ie, digoxin); increased anticoagulant activity of warfarin; increased salicylate toxicity due to decreased excretion; decreased furosemide effects when administered at the same time as sucralfate
Food Interactions Do not mix with acidic solutions; limit intake of natural licorice (causes sodium and water retention and increases potassium loss)
Stability Furosemide injection should be stored at controlled room temperature and protected from light; exposure to light may cause discoloration; do not use furosemide solutions if they have a yellow color; refrigeration may result in precipitation or crystallization, however, resolubilization at room temperature or warming may be performed without affecting the drugs stability; furosemide solutions are unstable in acidic media but very stable in basic media; I.V. infusion solution mixed in NS or D_5W solution is stable for 24 hours at room temperature
Mechanism of Action Inhibits reabsorption of sodium and chloride in the ascending loop of Henle and distal renal tubule, interfering with the chloride-binding cotransport system, thus causing increased excretion of water, potassium, sodium, chloride, magnesium, and calcium
Pharmacodynamics
Onset of action:
Oral: Within 30-60 minutes
I.M.: 30 minutes
I.V.: 5 minutes
Peak effect: Oral: Within 1-2 hours
Duration:
Oral: 6-8 hours
I.V.: 2 hours
Pharmacokinetics
Absorption: 65% in patients with normal renal function, decreases to 45% in patients with renal failure
Protein binding: 98%
Half-life: Adults:
Normal renal function: 30 minutes
Renal failure: 9 hours
(Continued)

Furosemide *(Continued)*

Elimination: 50% of oral dose and 80% of I.V. dose excreted in urine within 24 hours; the remainder is eliminated by other nonrenal pathways including liver metabolism and excretion of unchanged drug in feces

Usual Dosage

Neonates, premature: (see Additional Information)

Oral: Bioavailability is poor by this route; doses of 1-4 mg/kg/dose 1-2 times/day have been used

I.M., I.V.: 1-2 mg/kg/dose given every 12-24 hours

Infants and Children:

Oral: 1-6 mg/kg/day divided every 6-12 hours

I.M., I.V.: 1-2 mg/kg/dose every 6-12 hours

Continuous infusion: 0.05 mg/kg/hour; titrate dosage to clinical effect

Adults:

Oral: Initial: 20-80 mg/dose; increase in increments of 20-40 mg/dose at intervals of 6-8 hours; usual maintenance dose interval is twice daily or every day; may be titrated up to 600 mg/day with severe edematous states

I.M., I.V.: 20-40 mg/dose; repeat in 1-2 hours as needed and increase by 20 mg/dose until the desired effect has been obtained; usual dosing interval: 6-12 hours; for acute pulmonary edema, the usual dose is 40 mg I.V.; if not adequate, may increase dose to 80 mg

Continuous I.V. infusion: Initial I.V. bolus dose of 0.1 mg/kg followed by continuous I.V. infusion doses of 0.1 mg/kg/hour doubled every 2 hours to a maximum of 0.4 mg/kg/hour

Dosing adjustment in renal impairment: Acute renal failure: High doses (up to 1-3 g/day - oral/I.V.) have been used to initiate desired response; avoid use in oliguric states

Dialysis: Not removed by hemo- or peritoneal dialysis; supplemental dose is not necessary

Dosing adjustment in hepatic disease: Diminished natriuretic effect with increased sensitivity to hypokalemia and volume depletion in cirrhosis; monitor effects, particularly with high doses

Administration

Oral: May administer with food or milk to decrease GI distress

Parenteral: I.V.: May be administered undiluted direct I.V. at a maximum rate of 0.5 mg/kg/minute for doses <120 mg and 4 mg/minute for doses >120 mg; may also be diluted for infusion 1-2 mg/mL (maximum concentration: 10 mg/mL) over 10-15 minutes (following maximum rate as above)

Monitoring Parameters Serum electrolytes, renal function, blood pressure, hearing (if high dosages used)

Additional Information Nebulized furosemide at 1 mg/kg/dose (diluted to a final volume of 2 mL with NS) has been shown to be effective in improving pulmonary function in eight preterm infants with bronchopulmonary dysplasia undergoing mechanical ventilation; no diuresis or systemic side effects were noted

Dosage Forms

Injection: 10 mg/mL (2 mL, 4 mL, 5 mL, 6 mL, 8 mL, 10 mL, 12 mL)

Solution, oral: 10 mg/mL (60 mL, 120 mL); 40 mg/5 mL (5 mL, 10 mL, 500 mL)

Tablet: 20 mg, 40 mg, 80 mg

References

Copeland JG, Campbell DW, Plachetka JR, et al, "Diuresis With Continuous Infusion of Furosemide After Cardiac Surgery," *Am J Surg*, 1983, 146(6):796-9.

Rastogi A, Luayon M, Ajayi OA, et al, "Nebulized Furosemide in Infants With Bronchopulmonary Dysplasia," *J Pediatr*, 1994, 125(6 Pt 1):976-9.

Rudy DW, Voelker JR, Greene PK, et al, "Loop Diuretics for Chronic Renal Insufficiency: A Continuous Infusion Is More Efficacious Than Bolus Therapy," *Ann Intern Med*, 1991, 115(5):360-6.

♦ **Furoside®** (Canada) *see* Furosemide *on page 447*

♦ **Furoxone®** *see* Furazolidone *on page 446*

Gabapentin *(GA ba pen tin)*

Related Information

Antiepileptic Drugs *on page 1176*

Brand Names Neurontin®

Therapeutic Category Anticonvulsant, Miscellaneous

Generic Available No

Use Adjunct for treatment of partial and secondarily generalized seizures

Pregnancy Risk Factor C

Contraindications Hypersensitivity to gabapentin or any component

Warnings Abrupt withdrawal may precipitate status epilepticus or increase in seizures; decrease dose gradually over at least 1 week

Precautions Use with caution and decrease the dose in patients with renal dysfunction; in male (but not female) rats receiving gabapentin, a high incidence of pancreatic acinar adenocarcinoma was noted, the clinical significance in humans is unknown

Adverse Reactions

Central nervous system: Somnolence, dizziness, ataxia, fatigue, depression, nervousness; behavioral changes such as hyperactivity, aggression, oppositional behavior, conduct disorders; children with mental retardation and attention deficit disorders may be at increased risk for behavioral side effects

Dermatologic: Pruritus

Gastrointestinal: Dyspepsia, constipation, nausea, vomiting, weight gain

Genitourinary: Impotence

Hematologic: Leukopenia

Neuromuscular & skeletal: Back pain, dysarthria, tremor, myalgia

Ocular: Nystagmus, diplopia

Drug Interactions Antacids reduce the bioavailability of gabapentin by 20% (separate administration times by at least 2 hours); cimetidine may decrease the clearance of gabapentin (minor effect); gabapentin may increase levels of norethindrone (minor effect); gabapentin does not alter the pharmacokinetics of other antiepileptic drugs

Food Interactions Food does not affect rate or extent of absorption

Mechanism of Action Not fully elucidated, most likely binds to an undefined neuroreceptor in the brain that is possibly linked with, or identical to a site resembling the L-system amino acid carrier protein; although structurally similar to the inhibitory neurotransmitter, gamma-aminobutyric acid (GABA), gabapentin does not significantly affect the GABA system; it does **not** bind to GABA receptors, affect GABA neuronal uptake nor mimic GABA effects

Pharmacokinetics

Absorption: Very rapid; via an active (ie, facilitated transport) saturable process; dose-dependent

Distribution: V_d: Adults: 50-60 L or 0.65-1.04 L/kg; CSF concentrations are ~20% of plasma concentrations

Protein binding: <3% (not clinically significant)

Metabolism: Not metabolized

Bioavailability: ~60% (300 mg dose); bioavailability decreases with increasing doses

Time to peak serum concentration: Adults: 2-3 hours

Half-life, elimination (adults, normal): 5.3 hours (range: 5-9); increased half-life with decreased renal function; anuric patients: 132 hours; patients on hemodialysis: 51 hours

Elimination: Excreted unchanged in the urine (75% to 80%) and feces (10% to 20%)

Usual Dosage Oral:

Children 2-12 years: Minimal information exists; one abstract (Leiderman, 1993) described doses of 8-35 mg/kg/day divided every 8 hours to be well tolerated in 21 children 4-12 years of age. An open-label clinical study (Khurana, 1996) in 32 children with refractory partial seizures (age range: 2-16 years; mean age: 7 years) used initial doses of 5 mg/kg daily rounded to the nearest 100 mg; doses were increased, if tolerated, over a period of 3-4 days to 20 mg/kg/day; doses were increased further, if clinically indicated and tolerated with a maximum dose of 50 mg/kg/day; further studies are needed.

Children >12 years and Adults: Initial: 300 mg 3 times/day; titrate dose upward if needed; usual dose: 900-1800 mg/day; doses up to 2400 mg/day divided into 3 doses/day are well tolerated long-term; maximum dose: 3600 mg/day; do not exceed 12 hours between doses with 3 times/day dosing

Dosing adjustment in renal impairment: Children >12 years and Adults:

Cl_{cr} >60 mL/minute: Administer 400 mg 3 times daily

Cl_{cr} 30-60 mL/minute: 300 mg twice daily

Cl_{cr} 15-30 mL/minute: 300 mg/day

Cl_{cr} <15 mL/minute: 150 mg/day or 300 mg every other day

Hemodialysis patients >12 years of age: Initial: Loading dose of 300-400 mg; give 200-300 mg after each 4-hour dialysis

Administration Oral: May be administered without regard to meals; administration with meals may decrease adverse GI effects; do not administer within 2 hours of magnesium- or aluminum-containing antacids.

(Continued)

Gabapentin *(Continued)*

One pediatric study (Khurana, 1996) mixed the contents of the capsule in drinks (eg, orange juice) or food (eg, applesauce) for patients who could not swallow the capsule

Reference Range Minimum effective serum concentration may be 2 µg/mL; **routine monitoring of drug levels is not required**

Test Interactions False positive urinary protein with N-Multistix SG® test

Patient Information Take only as prescribed; may cause dizziness and impair the ability to perform activities requiring mental alertness or physical coordination; may cause somnolence, and other symptoms and signs of CNS depression; do not operate machinery or drive a car until you have experience with the drug

Nursing Implications Doses should be titrated based on clinical response; content of capsule is bitter tasting

Additional Information Gabapentin is not effective for absence seizures; gabapentin does not induce liver enzymes

Dosage Forms

Capsule: 100 mg, 300 mg, 400 mg

Solution, oral: 250 mg/5 mL (Approved by FDA March, 2000; projected availability October, 2000)

Tablet, film-coated: 600 mg, 800 mg

References

Andrews CO and Fischer JH, "Gabapentin: A New Agent for the Management of Epilepsy," *Ann Pharmacother*, 1994, 28(10):1188-96.

Bourgeois BF, "Antiepileptic Drugs in Pediatric Practice," *Epilepsia*, 1995, 36(Suppl 2):S34-45.

Khurana DS, Riviello J, Helmers S, et al, "Efficacy of Gabapentin Therapy in Children With Refractory Partial Seizures," *J Pediatr*, 1996, 128(6):829-33.

Lee DO, Steingard RJ, Cesena M, et al, "Behavioral Side Effects of Gabapentin in Children," *Epilepsia*, 1996, 37(1):87-90.

Leiderman D, Garofalo E, and LaMoreaux L, "Gabapentin Patients With Absence Seizures: Two Double-Blind, Placebo Controlled Studies," *Epilepsia*, 1993, 34(Suppl 6):45 (abstract).

♦ **Gabitril®** *see* Tiagabine *on page 924*

♦ **Gamimune® N** *see* Immune Globulin, Intravenous *on page 510*

♦ **Gamma Benzene Hexachloride** *see* Lindane *on page 572*

♦ **Gammagard S/D®** *see* Immune Globulin, Intravenous *on page 510*

♦ **Gammar®-IV** *see* Immune Globulin, Intravenous *on page 510*

Ganciclovir *(gan SYE kloe veer)*

Brand Names Cytovene®

Available Salts Ganciclovir Sodium

Synonyms DHPG; GCV; Nordeoxyguanosine

Therapeutic Category Antiviral Agent, Parenteral

Generic Available No

Use Treatment of cytomegalovirus (CMV) retinitis in immunocompromised patients, as well as CMV GI infections and pneumonitis; prevention of CMV disease in transplant patients who have been diagnosed with latent or active CMV; ganciclovir also has antiviral activity against herpes simplex virus types 1 and 2

Pregnancy Risk Factor C

Contraindications Absolute neutrophil count <500/mm^3; platelet count <25,000/mm^3; hypersensitivity to ganciclovir, acyclovir, or any component

Warnings Ganciclovir may adversely affect spermatogenesis and fertility; due to its mutagenic potential, contraceptive precautions for female and male patients need to be followed during and for at least 90 days after therapy with the drug; ganciclovir is potentially carcinogenic

Precautions Dosage adjustment or interruption of ganciclovir therapy may be necessary in patients with neutropenia and/or thrombocytopenia and patients with impaired renal function; use with extreme caution in children since long-term safety has not been determined and due to ganciclovir's potential for long-term carcinogenic and adverse reproductive effects

Adverse Reactions

Cardiovascular: Edema, arrhythmias, hypertension

Central nervous system: Headaches, seizure, confusion, nervousness, dizziness, hallucinations, coma, fever, encephalopathy, malaise

Dermatologic: Rash, pruritus, urticaria, acne

Gastrointestinal: Nausea, vomiting, diarrhea, pancreatitis

Hematologic: Neutropenia, thrombocytopenia, leukopenia, anemia, eosinophilia

Hepatic: Elevated liver function tests

Local: Phlebitis

Ocular: Retinal detachment, photophobia, abnormal vision, loss of vision

Renal: Hematuria, elevated BUN, elevated serum creatinine

Respiratory: Dyspnea

Drug Interactions Zidovudine (pancytopenia), imipenem/cilastatin (seizures), immunosuppressive agents increase suppression of bone marrow; amphotericin B, tacrolimus, cyclosporine increase nephrotoxicity; probenecid decreases renal clearance of ganciclovir; increases didanosine AUC (increases risk of peripheral neuropathy, pancreatitis)

Food Interactions High fat meal may increase AUC by 22%

Stability Reconstituted solution is stable for 12 hours at room temperature; **do not refrigerate**; reconstitute with sterile water **not** bacteriostatic water because parabens may cause precipitation; diluted I.V. ganciclovir solutions in D_5W or NS with a concentration <10 mg/mL are stable for 24 hours

Mechanism of Action Ganciclovir is phosphorylated to a substrate which competitively inhibits the binding of deoxyguanosine triphosphate to DNA polymerase; ganciclovir triphosphate competes with deoxyguanosine triphosphate for incorporation into viral DNA and interferes with viral DNA chain elongation resulting in inhibition of viral replication

Pharmacokinetics

Absorption: Oral: Poor

Distribution: Distributes to most body fluids, tissues, and organs including the brain

Protein binding: 1% to 2%

Bioavailability: Fasting: 5%; following food: 6% to 9%

Half-life (prolonged with impaired renal function):

Neonates 2-49 days of age: 2.4 hours

Adults: 2.5-3.6 hours (range: 1.7-5.8 hours)

Elimination: Majority (80% to 99%) excreted as unchanged drug in the urine

40% to 50% removed by a 4-hour hemodialysis

Usual Dosage

Slow I.V. infusion:

Retinitis: Children >3 months and Adults:

Induction therapy: 10 mg/kg/day divided every 12 hours as a 1- to 2-hour infusion for 14-21 days

Maintenance therapy: 5 mg/kg/day as a single daily dose for 7 days/week or 6 mg/kg/day for 5 days/week

Prevention of CMV disease in transplant recipients: Children and Adults:

Initial: 10 mg/kg/day divided every 12 hours for 7-14 days, followed by 5 mg/kg/day once daily 7 days/week or 6 mg/kg/day once daily 5 days/week

Lung/heart-lung transplant patients (CMV + donor with CMV + recipient): 6 mg/kg/day once daily for 28 days

Other CMV infections: Children and Adults: Initial: 10 mg/kg/day divided every 12 hours for 14-21 days or 7.5 mg/kg/day divided every 8 hours; maintenance therapy: 5 mg/kg/day as a single daily dose for 7 days/week or 6 mg/kg/day for 5 days/week

Note: Preliminary data indicates that a higher initial dose of 15 mg/kg/day divided every 12 hours and more prolonged treatment may be more effective in infants with symptomatic congenital CMV infection

Oral: Adults (following induction treatment with I.V. ganciclovir): Maintenance: 1000 mg 3 times/day **or** 500 mg 6 times/day every 3 hours during waking hours

Sustained release intravitreal implant: CMV retinitis: Adults: One implant every 6-9 months; following depletion of ganciclovir, as evidenced by progression of retinitis, implant may be removed and replaced

Dosing interval in renal impairment:

Oral:

Cl_{cr} 50-69 mL/minute: Administer 1500 mg/day or 500 mg 3 times/day

Cl_{cr} 25-49 mL/minute: Administer 1000 mg/day or 500 mg twice daily

Cl_{cr} 10-24 mL/minute: Administer 500 mg/day

Cl_{cr} <10 mL/minute: Administer 500 mg 3 times/week following hemodialysis

I.V. induction:

Cl_{cr} 50-69 mL/minute: Administer 2.5 mg/kg every 12 hours

Cl_{cr} 25-49 mL/minute: Administer 2.5 mg/kg every 24 hours

Cl_{cr} 10-24 mL/minute: Administer 1.25 mg/kg every 24 hours

Cl_{cr} <10 mL/minute: Administer 1.25 mg/kg/dose 3 times/week following hemodialysis

Administration

Oral: Do not open or crush ganciclovir capsules; administer with food

Parenteral: Do not administer I.M. or S.C. since the reconstituted ganciclovir injection may cause severe tissue irritation due to its high pH; administer by slow I.V. infusion over at least 1 hour at a final concentration for administration not to exceed 10 mg/mL

(Continued)

Ganciclovir *(Continued)*

Monitoring Parameters CBC with differential and platelet count, urine output, serum creatinine, ophthalmologic exams

Nursing Implications Handle and dispose according to guidelines issued for cytotoxic drugs; avoid direct contact of skin or mucous membranes with the powder contained in capsules or the I.V. solution; to minimize the risk of phlebitis, infuse through a large vein with adequate blood flow; maintain adequate patient hydration

Additional Information Sodium content of 1 g: 4 mEq

Dosage Forms

Capsule: 250 mg

Implant, intravitreal: 4.5 mg released gradually over 5-8 months

Powder for injection, lyophilized, as sodium: 500 mg

References

Fletcher C, Sawchuk R, Chinnock B, et al, "Human Pharmacokinetics of the Antiviral Drug DHPG," *Clin Pharmacol Ther*, 1986, 40(3):281-6.

Goodrich JM, Bowden RA, Fisher L, et al, "Ganciclovir Prophylaxis to Prevent Cytomegalovirus Disease After Allogeneic Marrow Transplant," *Ann Intern Med*, 1993, 118(3):173-8.

Gudnason T, Belani KK, and Balfour HH Jr, "Ganciclovir Treatment of Cytomegalovirus Disease in Immunocompromised Children," *Pediatr Infect Dis J*, 1989, 8(7):436-40.

Merigan TC, Renlund DG, Keay S, et al, "A Controlled Trial of Ganciclovir to Prevent Cytomegalovirus Disease After Heart Transplantation," *N Engl J Med*, 1992, 326(18):1182-6.

- **Ganciclovir Sodium** *see Ganciclovir on page 450*
- **Gantanol®** *see Sulfamethoxazole on page 892*
- **Gantrisin®** *see Sulfisoxazole on page 894*
- **Garamycin®** *see Gentamicin on page 452*
- **Garatec (Canada)** *see Gentamicin on page 452*
- **Gastrocrom®** *see Cromolyn on page 260*
- **Gastrosed™** *see Hyoscyamine on page 497*
- **Gas-X® [OTC]** *see Simethicone on page 868*
- **Gaviscon® [OTC]** *see Antacid Preparations on page 86*
- **G-CSF** *see Filgrastim on page 411*
- **GCV** *see Ganciclovir on page 450*
- **Gee Gee® [OTC]** *see Guaifenesin on page 464*
- **Gel-Kam®** *see Fluoride on page 427*
- **Gel-Tin® [OTC]** *see Fluoride on page 427*
- **Genabid®** *see Papaverine on page 728*
- **Genac® [OTC]** *see Triprolidine and Pseudoephedrine on page 957*
- **Genagesic®** *see Propoxyphene and Acetaminophen on page 815*
- **Genahist® Oral** *see Diphenhydramine on page 327*
- **Genapap® [OTC]** *see Acetaminophen on page 26*
- **Genasoft® Plus [OTC]** *see Docusate and Casanthranol on page 337*
- **Genaspor® [OTC]** *see Tolnaftate on page 936*
- **Genatap® Elixir [OTC]** *see Brompheniramine and Phenylpropanolamine on page 143*
- **Genatuss® [OTC]** *see Guaifenesin on page 464*
- **Genatuss DM® [OTC]** *see Guaifenesin and Dextromethorphan on page 466*
- **Gencalc® 600 [OTC]** *see Calcium Supplements on page 157*
- **Genebs® [OTC]** *see Acetaminophen on page 26*
- **Genex® [OTC]** *see Phenylpropanolamine on page 761*
- **Gen-K®** *see Potassium Supplements on page 786*
- **Gen-Lac (Canada)** *see Lactulose on page 550*
- **Gen-Minoxidil (Canada)** *see Minoxidil on page 650*
- **Gen-Nifedipine (Canada)** *see Nifedipine on page 687*
- **Genoptic®** *see Gentamicin on page 452*
- **Genotropin® Injection** *see Human Growth Hormone on page 478*
- **Genpril® [OTC]** *see Ibuprofen on page 501*
- **Gentacidin®** *see Gentamicin on page 452*
- **Gent-AK®** *see Gentamicin on page 452*

Gentamicin *(jen ta MYE sin)*

Related Information

Blood Level Sampling Time Guidelines *on page 1189*

Endocarditis Prophylaxis *on page 1127*

Overdose and Toxicology *on page 1191*

Brand Names Cidomycin® (Canada); Garamycin®; Garatec (Canada); Genoptic®; Gentacidin®; Gent-AK®; Gentrasul®; G-myticin®; Jenamicin®; Lomicin® Ophthalmic (Canada); Ocugram® (Canada)

Available Salts Gentamicin Sulfate

Therapeutic Category Antibiotic, Aminoglycoside; Antibiotic, Ophthalmic; Antibiotic, Topical

Generic Available Yes

Use Treatment of susceptible bacterial infections, normally gram-negative organisms including *Pseudomonas*, *Proteus*, *Serratia*, and gram-positive *Staphylococcus*; treatment of bone infections, CNS infections, respiratory tract infections, skin and soft tissue infections, as well as abdominal and urinary tract infections, endocarditis, and septicemia; used in combination with ampicillin as empiric therapy for sepsis in newborns; used topically to treat superficial infections of the skin or ophthalmic infections caused by susceptible bacteria

Pregnancy Risk Factor D

Contraindications Hypersensitivity to gentamicin, any component, or other aminoglycosides

Warnings Parenteral aminoglycosides are associated with significant nephrotoxicity or ototoxicity; the ototoxicity is directly proportional to the amount of drug given and the duration of treatment; tinnitus or vertigo are indications of vestibular injury and impending irreversible bilateral deafness; renal damage is usually reversible; some formulations contain sulfites which may cause allergic reactions. Aminoglycosides can cause fetal harm when administered to a pregnant woman; aminoglycosides have been associated with several reports of total irreversible bilateral congenital deafness in pediatric patients exposed *in utero*.

Precautions Use with caution in neonates due to renal immaturity that results in a prolonged gentamicin half-life and in patients with pre-existing renal impairment, auditory or vestibular impairment, hypocalcemia, myasthenia gravis, and in conditions which depress neuromuscular transmission; modify dosage in patients with renal impairment and in neonates on extracorporeal membrane oxygenation (ECMO)

Adverse Reactions
Central nervous system: Vertigo, ataxia, gait instability, dizziness, headache, fever
Dermatologic: Rash, pruritus, erythema
Endocrine & metabolic: Hypomagnesemia
Gastrointestinal: Nausea, vomiting, anorexia
Genitourinary: Decrease in urine specific gravity, casts in urine, possible electrolyte wasting
Hematologic: Granulocytopenia, thrombocytopenia, eosinophilia
Hepatic: Elevated AST and ALT
Local: Thrombophlebitis
Neuromuscular & skeletal: Neuromuscular blockade, muscle cramps, tremor, weakness
Ocular: Optic neuritis; ophthalmic use: burning, stinging, redness, lacrimation
Otic: Ototoxicity (may be associated with high serum aminoglycoside concentrations persisting for prolonged periods) with tinnitus, hearing loss; early toxicity usually affects high-pitched sound
Renal: Nephrotoxicity (high trough levels) with proteinuria, reduction in glomerular filtration rate, elevated serum creatinine

Drug Interactions Increased toxicity: Concurrent use of amphotericin B, cephalosporins, penicillins, loop diuretics, vancomycin, cisplatin, indomethacin; potentiates effect of neuromuscular blocking agents and botulinum toxin

Stability Incompatible with penicillins, cephalosporins, heparin

Mechanism of Action Inhibits cellular initiation of bacterial protein synthesis by binding to 30S and 50S ribosomal subunits resulting in a defective bacterial cell membrane

Pharmacokinetics
Absorption: Oral: Poorly absorbed (<2%)
Distribution: Crosses the placenta; distributes primarily in the extracellular fluid volume and in most tissues; poor penetration into CSF; drug accumulates in the renal cortex; small amounts distribute into bile, sputum, saliva, tears, and breast milk
V_d: Increased in neonates and with fever, edema, ascites, fluid overload; V_d is decreased in patients with dehydration
Neonates: 0.45 ± 0.1 L/kg
Infants: 0.4 ± 0.1 L/kg
Children: 0.35 ± 0.15 L/kg
Adolescents: 0.3 ± 0.1 L/kg
(Continued)

Gentamicin *(Continued)*

Adults: 0.2-0.3 L/kg
Protein binding: <30%
Half-life:
Neonates:
<1 week: 3-11.5 hours
1 week to 1 month: 3-6 hours
Infants: 4 ± 1 hour
Children: 2 ± 1 hour
Adolescents: 1.5 ± 1 hour
Adults with normal renal function: 1.5-3 hours
Anuria: 36-70 hours
Time to peak serum concentration:
I.M.: Within 30-90 minutes
I.V.: 30 minutes after 30-minute infusion
Elimination: Clearance is directly related to renal function; eliminated almost completely by glomerular filtration of unchanged drug with excretion into urine
Clearance:
Neonates: 0.045 ± 0.01 L/hour/kg
Infants: 0.1 ± 0.05 L/hour/kg
Children: 0.1 ± 0.03 L/hour/kg
Adolescents: 0.09 ± 0.03 L/hour/kg
Dialyzable (50% to 100%)

Usual Dosage Dosage should be based on an estimate of ideal body weight, except in neonates (neonatal dosage should be based on actual weight unless the patient has hydrocephalus or hydrops fetalis):
Neonates: I.M., I.V.:
Premature neonate, <1000 g: 3.5 mg/kg/dose every 24 hours
0-4 weeks, <1200 g: 2.5 mg/kg/dose every 18-24 hours
Postnatal age ≤7 days: 2.5 mg/kg/dose every 12 hours
Postnatal age >7 days:
1200-2000 g: 2.5 mg/kg/dose every 8-12 hours
>2000 g: 2.5 mg/kg/dose every 8 hours
Initial dose for term neonates receiving ECMO: I.V.: 2.5 mg/kg/dose every 18 hours; subsequent doses should be individualized by monitoring serum drug concentrations; when ECMO is discontinued, dosage may require readjustment due to large shifts in body water
Infants and Children <5 years: I.M., I.V.: 2.5 mg/kg/dose every 8 hours*
Pulmonary infection in cystic fibrosis: 2.5-3.3 mg/kg/dose every 6-8 hours
Patients on hemodialysis: 1.25-1.75 mg/kg/dose postdialysis
Children ≥5 years: I.M., I.V.: 2-2.5 mg/kg/dose every 8 hours*
Pulmonary infection in cystic fibrosis: 2.5-3.3 mg/kg/dose every 6-8 hours
Patients on hemodialysis: 1.25-1.75 mg/kg/dose postdialysis
*Some patients may require larger or more frequent doses (eg, every 6 hours) if serum levels document the need (ie, cystic fibrosis, patients with major burns, or febrile granulocytopenic patients); modify dose based on individual patient requirements as determined by renal function, serum drug concentrations, and patient-specific clinical parameters
Intraventricular/intrathecal **(use a preservative free preparation):**
Newborns: 1 mg/day
Infants >3 months and Children: 1-2 mg/day
Adults: 4-8 mg/day
Infants, Children, and Adults:
Topical: Apply 3-4 times/day
Ophthalmic:
Ointment: Apply 2-3 times/day
Solution: Instill 1-2 drops every 2-4 hours, up to 2 drops every hour for severe infections
Adults: I.M., I.V.: 3-6 mg/kg/day in divided doses every 8 hours; studies of once daily dosing have used I.V. doses of 4-6.6 mg/kg once daily
Patients on hemodialysis: 0.5-0.7 mg/kg/dose postdialysis
Dosing adjustment in renal impairment: I.M., I.V.: 2.5 mg/kg** (Cl$_{cr}$ <60 mL/minute/1.73 m^2)
**2-3 serum level measurements should be obtained after the initial dose to measure the patient's pharmacokinetic parameters (eg, half-life, V$_d$) in order to determine the frequency and amount of subsequent doses
Administration Parenteral: Administer by I.M., I.V. slow intermittent infusion over 30-60 minutes or by direct injection over 15 minutes; final concentration for I.V.

administration should not exceed 10 mg/mL; administer other antibiotics, such as penicillins and cephalosporins, at least 1 hour before or after gentamicin

Monitoring Parameters Urinalysis, urine output, BUN, serum creatinine, peak and trough serum gentamicin concentrations, hearing test

Not all infants and children who receive aminoglycosides require monitoring serum aminoglycoside concentrations. Indications for use of aminoglycoside serum concentration monitoring include:

Treatment course >5 days

Patients with decreased or changing renal function

Patients with poor therapeutic response

Infants <3 months of age

Atypical body constituency (obesity, expanded extracellular fluid volume)

Clinical need for higher doses or shorter intervals (eg, cystic fibrosis, burns, endocarditis, meningitis, critically ill patients, relatively resistant organism)

Patients on hemodialysis or chronic ambulatory peritoneal dialysis

Signs of nephrotoxicity or ototoxicity

Concomitant use of other nephrotoxic agents

Reference Range

Peak: 4-12 µg/mL; peak values are 2-3 times greater with once daily dosing regimens

Trough: 0.5-2 µg/mL

Test Interactions Aminoglycoside levels measured in blood taken from Silastic® central line catheters can sometimes give falsely high readings

Patient Information Report any dizziness or sensations of ringing or fullness in ears to the physician

Nursing Implications Obtain drug levels after the third or fourth dose except in neonates and patients with rapidly changing renal function in whom levels need to be measured sooner; peak gentamicin serum concentrations are drawn 30 minutes after the end of a 30-minute I.V. infusion, immediately on completion of a 1-hour I.V. infusion, or 1 hour after an intramuscular injection; trough levels are drawn within 30 minutes before the next dose; provide adequate patient hydration and perfusion

Dosage Forms

Cream, topical, as sulfate: 0.1% (15 g)

Infusion, in D_5W, as sulfate: 60 mg, 80 mg, 100 mg

Infusion, in NS, as sulfate: 40 mg, 60 mg, 80 mg, 90 mg, 100 mg, 120 mg

Injection, as sulfate: 40 mg/mL (1 mL, 1.5 mL, 2 mL)

Pediatric, as sulfate: 10 mg/mL (2 mL)

Ointment:

Ophthalmic, as sulfate: 0.3% (3.5 g)

Topical, as sulfate: 0.1% (15 g)

Solution, ophthalmic, as sulfate: 0.3% (1 mL, 5 mL, 15 mL)

References

Bhatt-Mehta V, Johnson CE and Schumacher RE, "Gentamicin Pharmacokinetics in Term Neonates Receiving Extracorporeal Membrane Oxygenation," *Pharmacotherapy*, 1992, 12(1):28-32.

Gilbert DN, "Once-Daily Aminoglycoside Therapy," *Antimicrob Agents Chemother*, 1991, 35(3):399-405.

Reimche LD, Rooney, ME, Hindmarsh KW, et al, "An Evaluation of Gentamicin Dosing According to Renal Function in Neonates With Suspected Sepsis," *Am J Perinatol*, 1987, 4(3):262-5.

Shevchuk YM and Taylor DM, "Aminoglycoside Volume of Distribution in Pediatric Patients," *DICP*, 1990, 24(3):273-6.

♦ **Gentamicin and Prednisolone** *see* Prednisolone and Gentamicin *on page 793*

♦ **Gentamicin Sulfate** *see* Gentamicin *on page 452*

Gentian Violet (JEN shun VYE oh let)

Synonyms Crystal Violet; Methylrosaniline Chloride

Therapeutic Category Antibacterial, Topical; Antifungal Agent, Topical

Generic Available Yes

Use Treatment of cutaneous or mucocutaneous infections caused by *Candida albicans* and other superficial skin infections refractory to topical nystatin, clotrimazole, miconazole, or econazole

Pregnancy Risk Factor C

Contraindications Hypersensitivity to gentian violet; ulcerated areas; patients with porphyria

Warnings May result in tattooing of the skin when applied to granulation tissue

Adverse Reactions

Dermatological: Staining of skin (purple)

Gastrointestinal: Esophagitis

(Continued)

Gentian Violet *(Continued)*

Local: Burning, irritation, vesicle formation, sensitivity reactions, ulceration of mucous membranes

Respiratory: Laryngitis, tracheitis may result from swallowing gentian violet solution, laryngeal obstruction following frequent or prolonged use

Mechanism of Action Topical antiseptic/germicide effective against some vegetative gram-positive bacteria, particularly *Staphylococcus* species, and some yeast; it is much less effective against gram-negative bacteria and is ineffective against acid-fast bacteria

Usual Dosage Topical:

Infants: Apply 3-4 drops of a 0.5% solution under the tongue or on lesion after feedings

Children and Adults: Apply 0.5% to 2% solution to lesion 2-3 times/day for 3 days, do not swallow

Administration Topical: Apply to lesions with cotton; do not apply to ulcerative lesions on the face

Patient Information Drug stains skin and clothing purple; proper hygiene and skin care need to be used to prevent spread of infection and reinfection

Nursing Implications Keep affected area dry and exposed to air

Additional Information 0.25% or 0.5% solution is less irritating than a 1% to 2% solution and is reported to be as effective

Dosage Forms Solution, topical: 1% (30 mL); 2% (30 mL)

♦ **Gen-Timolol® (Canada)** *see* Timolol *on page 929*
♦ **Gentran®** *see* Dextran *on page 299*
♦ **Gentrasul®** *see* Gentamicin *on page 452*
♦ **Gen-Triazolam® (Canada)** *see* Triazolam *on page 950*
♦ **Gen-XENE®** *see* Clorazepate *on page 244*
♦ **Geocillin®** *see* Carbenicillin *on page 168*
♦ **Geopen® (Canada)** *see* Carbenicillin *on page 168*
♦ **Geridium®** *see* Phenazopyridine *on page 753*
♦ **GG** *see* Guaifenesin *on page 464*
♦ **GG-Cen® [OTC]** *see* Guaifenesin *on page 464*
♦ **Glaucon®** *see* Epinephrine *on page 371*
♦ **GlucaGen®** *see* Glucagon (rDNA Origin) *on page 456*
♦ **Glucagon Diagnostic Kit** *see* Glucagon (rDNA Origin) *on page 456*
♦ **Glucagon Emergency Kit** *see* Glucagon (rDNA Origin) *on page 456*
♦ **Glucagon Hydrochloride** *see* Glucagon (rDNA Origin) *on page 456*

Glucagon (rDNA Origin) (GLOO ka gon)

Brand Names GlucaGen®; Glucagon Diagnostic Kit; Glucagon Emergency Kit

Available Salts Glucagon Hydrochloride

Therapeutic Category Antihypoglycemic Agent

Generic Available No

Use Management of hypoglycemia; diagnostic aid in the radiologic examination of GI tract when a hypotonic state is needed; used with some success as a cardiac stimulant in management of severe cases of beta-adrenergic blocking agent overdosage

Pregnancy Risk Factor B

Contraindications Hypersensitivity to glucagon or any component

Warnings Use with caution in patients with a history of insulinoma and/or pheochromocytoma; because glucagon depletes glycogen stores, the patient should be given supplemental carbohydrates as soon as physically possible

Adverse Reactions

Cardiovascular: Hypotension

Dermatologic: Urticaria

Gastrointestinal: Nausea, vomiting

Respiratory: Respiratory distress

Miscellaneous: Hypersensitivity reactions

Drug Interactions Enhances anticoagulant effect of warfarin; phenytoin inhibits the stimulant effect of glucagon on insulin release by the islet cells; propranolol partially inhibits the hyperglycemic effect of glucagon

Stability Glucagon (rDNA origin) for injection (Lilly) should be stored at controlled room temperature; glucagon (rDNA origin) for injection (GlucaGen®) should be refrigerated; both injections should be used immediately after reconstitution

Mechanism of Action Glucagon (rDNA origin) is genetically engineered and identical to human glucagon. It stimulates adenylate cyclase to produce increased cyclic AMP. It promotes hepatic glycogenolysis and gluconeogenesis, causing an increase in blood glucose levels; produces both positive inotropic and chronotropic effects.

Pharmacodynamics

Blood glucose effects (after 1 mg dosage):
Onset of action: I.M.: 8-10 minutes; I.V.: 1 minute
Duration: I.M.: 12-27 minutes; I.V.: 9-17 minutes

GI tract effects:
Onset of action: Within 1-10 minutes
Duration: 12-30 minutes

Pharmacokinetics

Distribution: V_d: 0.25 L/kg
Metabolism: Extensively degraded in liver and kidneys
Half-life, plasma: 8-18 minutes
Clearance: 13.5 mL/minute/kg

Usual Dosage

Hypoglycemia or insulin shock therapy: I.M., I.V., S.C. (may repeat in 20 minutes as needed):
Neonates, Infants and Children ≤20 kg: 0.5 mg or 0.02-0.03 mg/kg
Children >20 kg and Adults: 1 mg
Diagnostic aid: Adults:
I.M.: 1-2 mg 10 minutes prior to procedure
I.V.: 0.25-2 mg 10 minutes prior to procedure

Administration Parenteral: Dilute with manufacturer provided diluent resulting in 1 mg/mL; if doses exceeding 2 mg are used, dilute with sterile water instead of diluent; administer by direct I.V. injection, I.M., or S.C.

Monitoring Parameters Blood glucose, blood pressure

Additional Information 1 unit = 1 mg

Dosage Forms

Powder for injection, lyophilized (Glucagon Diagnostic Kit, Glucagon Emergency Kit): 1 mg [1 unit] (diluent available in disposable syringe)
Powder for injection, lyophilized, as hydrochloride (GlucaGen®): 1 mg [1 unit]

♦ **Glucocerebrosidase** see Alglucerase on page 47

♦ **Glucose** see Dextrose on page 305

♦ **Glucose Monohydrate** see Dextrose on page 305

♦ **Glukor®** see Chorionic Gonadotropin on page 221

♦ **Glutose® [OTC]** see Dextrose on page 305

♦ **Glyate® [OTC]** see Guaifenesin on page 464

Glycerin (GLIS er in)

Brand Names Fleet® Babylax® Rectal [OTC]; Ophthalgan® Ophthalmic; Osmoglyn® Ophthalmic; Sani-Supp® Suppository [OTC]

Synonyms Glycerol

Therapeutic Category Laxative, Osmotic

Generic Available Yes

Use Constipation; reduction of intraocular pressure; reduction of corneal edema; glycerin has been administered orally to reduce intracranial pressure

Pregnancy Risk Factor C

Contraindications Hypersensitivity to glycerin or any component; severe dehydration, anuria

Precautions Use oral glycerin with caution in patients with cardiac, renal or hepatic disease and in diabetics

Adverse Reactions

Central nervous system: Dizziness, headache, confusion, disorientation
Endocrine & metabolic: Hyperglycemia, dehydration
Gastrointestinal: Diarrhea, nausea, tenesmus, thirst, cramping pain, vomiting, rectal irritation
Local: Pain/irritation with ophthalmic solution (may need to apply a topical ophthalmic anesthetic before glycerin administration)

Stability Protect from heat; freezing should be avoided

Mechanism of Action Osmotic dehydrating agent which increases osmotic pressure; draws fluid into colon and thus stimulates evacuation; glycerin ophthalmic solution's osmotic action reduces edema and causes clearing of corneal haze; when given orally, glycerin increases osmotic pressure of the plasma drawing

(Continued)

Glycerin *(Continued)*

water from the extravascular spaces into the blood producing a decrease in intra-ocular pressure

Pharmacodynamics

Onset of action for glycerin suppository or enema: 15-30 minutes
Onset of action in decreasing intraocular pressure: Within 10-30 minutes
Duration: 4-8 hours
Increased intracranial pressure decreases within 10-60 minutes following an oral dose
Duration: ~2-3 hours

Pharmacokinetics

Absorption:
Oral: Well absorbed
Rectal: Poorly absorbed
Metabolism: Primarily in the liver with 20% metabolized in the kidney
Half-life: 30-45 minutes
Time to peak serum concentration: Oral: Within 60-90 minutes
Elimination: Only a small percentage of drug is excreted unchanged in urine

Usual Dosage

Constipation: Rectal: Administered in single doses only at infrequent intervals
Neonates: 0.5 mL/kg/dose of rectal solution as an enema
Children <6 years: 1 infant suppository as needed or 2-5 mL of rectal solution as an enema
Children ≥6 years and Adults: 1 adult suppository as needed or 5-15 mL of rectal solution as an enema
Children and Adults:
Reduction of intraocular pressure: Oral: 1-1.8 g/kg 1-1½ hours preoperatively; additional doses may be administered at 5-hour intervals
Reduction of intracranial pressure: Oral: 1.5 g/kg/day divided every 4 hours; 1 g/kg/dose every 6 hours has also been used
Reduction of corneal edema: Ophthalmic: Instill 1-2 drops in eye(s) every 3-4 hours

Administration

Oral: Orange or lemon juice may be added to unflavored 50% oral solution; pour solution over crushed ice and drink through a straw to improve palatability
Rectal: Insert suppository high in the rectum and retain 15 minutes

Monitoring Parameters Blood glucose, intraocular pressure

Patient Information Do not use if experiencing abdominal pain, nausea, or vomiting

Nursing Implications Use caution during insertion of suppository to avoid intestinal perforation, especially in neonates; instruct patient to lie down after oral glycerin administration to prevent or relieve headaches

Dosage Forms

Solution:
Ophthalmic, sterile (Ophthalgan®): Glycerin with chlorobutanol 0.55% (7.5 mL)
Oral (lime flavor)(Osmoglyn®): 50% (220 mL)
Rectal (Fleet® Babylax®): 4 mL/applicator (6s)
Suppository, rectal (Sani-Supp®): Glycerin with sodium stearate (infant and adult sizes)

References

Heinemeyer G, "Clinical Pharmacokinetic Considerations in the Treatment of Increased Intracranial Pressure," *Clin Pharmacokinet,* 1987, 13(1):1-25.
Rottenberg DA, Hurwitz BJ, and Posner JB, "The Effect of Oral Glycerol on Intraventricular Pressure in Man," *Neurology,* 1977, 27(7):600-8.

♦ **Glycerol** *see Glycerin on page 457*
♦ **Glycerol Guaiacolate** *see Guaifenesin on page 464*
♦ **Glycerol Guaiacolate, Phenylpropanolamine, and Phenylephrine** *see Guaifenesin, Phenylpropanolamine, and Phenylephrine on page 467*
♦ **Glyceryl Trinitrate** *see Nitroglycerin on page 690*

Glycopyrrolate *(glye koe PYE roe late)*

Related Information

Compatibility of Medications Mixed in a Syringe *on page 1208*
Overdose and Toxicology *on page 1191*

Brand Names Robinul®; Robinul® Forte

Available Salts Glycopyrrolate Bromide

Synonyms Glycopyrronium

Therapeutic Category Anticholinergic Agent; Antispasmodic Agent, Gastrointestinal

Generic Available Yes

Use Adjunct in treatment of peptic ulcer disease; inhibition of salivation and excessive secretions of the respiratory tract; reversal of the muscarinic effects of cholinergic agents such as neostigmine and pyridostigmine during reversal of neuromuscular blockade

Pregnancy Risk Factor B

Contraindications Narrow-angle glaucoma; acute hemorrhage; tachycardia; hypersensitivity to glycopyrrolate or any component; ulcerative colitis; obstructive uropathy; paralytic ileus; myasthenia gravis

Warnings Infants, patients with Down syndrome, and children with spastic paralysis or brain damage may be hypersensitive to antimuscarinic effects

Precautions Use with caution in patients with fever, hyperthyroidism, hepatic or renal disease, hypertension, CHF, GI infections, diarrhea, reflux esophagitis

Adverse Reactions
　　Cardiovascular: Tachycardia, orthostatic hypotension, ventricular fibrillation, palpitations
　　Central nervous system: Drowsiness, nervousness, headache, insomnia, confusion, loss of memory, fatigue, ataxia
　　Dermatologic: Rash, dry skin
　　Gastrointestinal: Xerostomia, constipation, nausea, vomiting, dry throat, dysphagia
　　Genitourinary: Urinary retention, dysuria
　　Local: Irritation at injection site
　　Neuromuscular & skeletal: Weakness
　　Ocular: Blurred vision
　　Respiratory: Dry nose
　　Miscellaneous: Decreased diaphoresis

Drug Interactions Phenothiazines, meperidine, amantadine, tricyclic antidepressants, and quinidine (additive anticholinergic effect); wax-matrix potassium chloride (increased severity of potassium-induced GI mucosal lesions); antacids (decreased absorption); decreased effect of levodopa

Stability Unstable at pH >6; compatible in the same syringe with atropine, benzquinamide, chlorpromazine, codeine, diphenhydramine, droperidol, fentanyl, hydromorphone, hydroxyzine, lidocaine, meperidine, promethazine, morphine, neostigmine, oxymorphone, procaine, prochlorperazine, promazine, pyridostigmine, scopolamine, triflupromazine, and trimethobenzamide

Mechanism of Action Inhibits the muscarinic action of acetylcholine at postganglionic parasympathetic neuroeffector sites in smooth muscle, secretory glands, and CNS

Pharmacodynamics
　　Onset of action:
　　　　Oral: Within 1 hour
　　　　I.M., S.C.: 15-30 minutes
　　　　I.V.: 1-10 minutes
　　Peak effect: I.M., S.C.: 30-45 minutes
　　Duration of effect (anticholinergic effects):
　　　　Oral: 8-12 hours
　　　　Parenteral: 7 hours

Pharmacokinetics
　　Absorption: Oral: Poor and erratic; 10% absorption
　　Distribution: Does not adequately penetrate into CNS
　　Elimination: Primarily unchanged via biliary elimination (70% to 90%)

Usual Dosage
　　Children:
　　　　Control of secretions:
　　　　　　Oral: 40-100 mcg/kg/dose 3-4 times/day
　　　　　　I.M., I.V.: 4-10 mcg/kg/dose every 3-4 hours
　　　　Preoperative: I.M.:
　　　　　　<2 years: 4.4-8.8 mcg/kg 30-60 minutes before procedure
　　　　　　>2 years: 4.4 mcg/kg 30-60 minutes before procedure
　　Children and Adults: Reversal of muscarinic effects of cholinergic agents: I.V.: 0.2 mg for each 1 mg of neostigmine or 5 mg of pyridostigmine administered
　　Adults:
　　　　Peptic ulcer:
　　　　　　Oral: 1-2 mg 2-3 times/day
　　　　　　I.M., I.V.: 0.1-0.2 mg 3-4 times/day
　　　　Preoperative: I.M.: 4.4 mcg/kg 30-60 minutes before procedure
(Continued)

Glycopyrrolate *(Continued)*

Administration
Oral: May be administered without regard to meals

Parenteral: Dilute to a concentration of 2 mcg/mL (maximum concentration: 200 mcg/mL); infuse over 15-20 minutes; may be administered direct I.V. at a maximum rate of 20 mcg/minute; may be administered I.M.

Monitoring Parameters Heart rate

Dosage Forms
Injection, as bromide: 0.2 mg/mL (1 mL, 2 mL, 5 mL, 20 mL)
Robinul®: 0.2 mg/mL (1 mL, 2 mL, 5 mL, 20 mL)
Tablet, as bromide:
Robinul®: 1 mg
Robinul® Forte: 2 mg

♦ **Glycopyrrolate Bromide** *see Glycopyrrolate on page 458*

♦ **Glycopyrronium** *see Glycopyrrolate on page 458*

♦ **Glycosum** *see Dextrose on page 305*

♦ **Glycotuss® [OTC]** *see Guaifenesin on page 464*

♦ **Glycotuss-dM® [OTC]** *see Guaifenesin and Dextromethorphan on page 466*

♦ **Gly-Oxide® Oral [OTC]** *see Carbamide Peroxide on page 167*

♦ **Glysennid® (Canada)** *see Senna on page 865*

♦ **Glytuss® [OTC]** *see Guaifenesin on page 464*

♦ **GM-CSF** *see Sargramostim on page 858*

♦ **G-myticin®** *see Gentamicin on page 452*

♦ **Go-Evac®** *see Polyethylene Glycol-Electrolyte Solution on page 782*

Gold Sodium Thiomalate (gold SOW dee um thye oh MAL ate)

Brand Names Aurolate®; Myochrysine®

Therapeutic Category Gold Compound

Generic Available Yes

Use Treatment of progressive rheumatoid arthritis

Pregnancy Risk Factor C

Contraindications Severe hepatic or renal dysfunction; hypersensitivity to gold compounds or other heavy metals; systemic lupus erythematosus; history of blood dyscrasias; CHF, exfoliative dermatitis, or colitis; avoid concomitant use of antimalarials, immunosuppressive agents, penicillamine, or phenylbutazone

Warnings Explain the possibility of adverse reactions before initiating therapy; signs of gold toxicity include: decrease in hemoglobin, leukocytes, granulocytes and platelets, proteinuria, hematuria, pigmentation, pruritus, stomatitis or persistent diarrhea, rash, metallic taste; advise patient to report any symptoms of toxicity

Precautions Frequent monitoring of patients for signs and symptoms of toxicity will prevent serious adverse reactions; NSAIDs and corticosteroids may be discontinued after initiating gold therapy; must not be injected I.V.

Adverse Reactions
Cardiovascular: Flushing

Central nervous system: Seizures, headache

Dermatologic: Exfoliative urticaria, dermatitis, erythema nodosum, alopecia, shedding of nails, pruritus, gray-to-blue pigmentation of skin and mucous membranes

Gastrointestinal: Stomatitis, nausea, diarrhea, abdominal cramps, metallic taste, gingivitis, glossitis, ulcerative enterocolitis, GI hemorrhage, dysphagia

Genitourinary: Vaginitis

Hematologic: Eosinophilia, leukopenia, agranulocytosis, thrombocytopenia

Hepatic: Hepatitis

Neuromuscular & skeletal: Arthralgias, peripheral neuropathy

Ocular: Blurred vision, conjunctivitis, corneal ulcers, iritis

Renal: Hematuria, proteinuria, nephrotic syndrome

Respiratory: Interstitial pneumonitis and fibrosis

Miscellaneous: Hypersensitivity reactions including anaphylaxis (rare)

Drug Interactions Decreased effect with penicillamine, acetylcysteine

Mechanism of Action Unknown, may decrease prostaglandin synthesis or may alter cellular mechanisms by inhibiting sulfhydryl systems

Pharmacokinetics
Distribution: Breast milk to plasma ratio: 0.02-0.3

Half-life: 3-27 days (may lengthen with multiple doses)

Time to peak serum concentration: I.M.: Within 3-6 hours

Elimination: Majority (50% to 90%) excreted in urine with smaller amounts (10% to 50%) excreted in feces (via bile)

Usual Dosage I.M.:

Children: Initial: Test dose of 10 mg I.M. is recommended, followed by 1 mg/kg I.M. weekly for 20 weeks (maximum dose: 50 mg); maintenance: 1 mg/kg/dose at 2- to 4-week intervals thereafter for as long as therapy is clinically beneficial and toxicity does not develop. Administration for 2-4 months is usually required before clinical improvement is observed.

Adults: 10 mg first week; 25 mg second week; then 25-50 mg/week until clinical improvement or a 1 g cumulative dose has been given. If improvement occurs without adverse reactions, give 25-50 mg every 2 weeks for 2-20 weeks; if continues stable, give 25-50 mg every 3-4 weeks indefinitely.

Dosage adjustment in renal impairment:
Cl_{cr} 50-80 mL/minute: Administer 50% of dose
Cl_{cr} <50 mL/minute: Avoid use

Administration Parenteral: Administer I.M. only, preferably intragluteally; addition of 0.1 mL of 1% lidocaine to each injection may reduce the discomfort associated with I.M. administration; patients should be recumbent during injection and for 10 minutes afterwards; observe closely for 15 minutes after injection

Monitoring Parameters CBC, platelets, hemoglobin, urinalysis, renal and liver function tests

Reference Range Gold: Normal: 0-0.1 µg/mL (SI: 0-0.0064 µmol/L); Therapeutic: 1-3 µg/mL (SI: 0.06-0.18 µmol/L); Urine <0.1 µg/24 hours

Dosage Forms Injection: 50 mg/mL (1 mL, 2 mL, 10 mL)

♦ **GoLYTELY®** see Polyethylene Glycol-Electrolyte Solution on page 782

Gonadorelin (goe nad oh REL in)

Brand Names Factrel®; Lutrepulse®
Available Salts Gonadorelin Acetate; Gonadorelin Hydrochloride
Synonyms LH-RH; LRH
Therapeutic Category Diagnostic Agent, Gonadotrophic Hormone; Gonadotropin
Generic Available No
Use Evaluation of hypothalamic-pituitary gonadotropic function; used to evaluate abnormal gonadotropin regulation as in precocious puberty and delayed puberty; treatment of primary hypothalamic amenorrhea
Pregnancy Risk Factor B
Contraindications Hypersensitivity to gonadorelin or any component
Adverse Reactions
Cardiovascular: Flushing
Central nervous system: Lightheadedness, headache
Dermatologic: Skin rash
Gastrointestinal: Nausea, abdominal discomfort
Local: Pain, pruritus, edema
Miscellaneous: Hypersensitivity reactions
Drug Interactions Androgens, estrogens, progestins, glucocorticoids affect pituitary secretion of gonadotropins; spironolactone, levodopa may increase gonadotropin levels; oral contraceptives, digoxin may suppress gonadotropin levels; phenothiazines, dopamine antagonists may blunt response to gonadorelin
Stability Prepare immediately prior to use; after reconstitution, store at room temperature and use within 1 day; discard unused portion
Mechanism of Action Stimulates the release of luteinizing hormone (LH) from the anterior pituitary gland
Pharmacodynamics
Onset of action: Following administration maximal LH release occurs within 20 minutes
Duration: 3-5 hours
Pharmacokinetics Half-life: 4 minutes
Usual Dosage
Children: I.V. **(as hydrochloride salt)**: 100 mcg to evaluate abnormal gonadotropin regulation
Children >12 years and Adults: I.V., S.C. **(as hydrochloride salt)**: 100 mcg; administer to women during early phase of menstrual cycle (day 1-7)
Adults: I.V. (as acetate salt): 5 mcg (range: 1-20 mcg) every 90 minutes via the Lutrepulse® pump; recommended treatment interval: 21 days
Administration Parenteral: Dilute (hydrochloride salt) in 3 mL of NS; administer I.V. push over 30 seconds
Monitoring Parameters Plasma LH and FSH
(Continued)

Gonadorelin *(Continued)*

Hypothalamic/pituitary function evaluation: Draw blood samples for LH 15 minutes before and immediately before gonadorelin dose, then at 15, 30, 45, 60, and 120 minutes after dose

Dosage Forms

Injection, as acetate (Lutrepulse®): 0.8 mg, 3.2 mg

Injection, as hydrochloride (Factrel®): 100 mcg, 500 mcg

References

Pescovitz OH, Comite F, Hench K, et al, "The NIH Experience With Precocious Puberty: Diagnostic Subgroups and Response to Short-Term Luteinizing Hormone-Releasing Hormone Analogue Therapy," *J Pediatr,* 1986, 108(1):47-54.

♦ **Gonadorelin Acetate** *see* Gonadorelin *on page 461*

♦ **Gonadorelin Hydrochloride** *see* Gonadorelin *on page 461*

♦ **Gonic®** *see* Chorionic Gonadotropin *on page 221*

♦ **Gordofilm® Liquid** *see* Salicylic Acid *on page 854*

Granisetron *(gra NI se tron)*

Brand Names Kytril™ Injection

Therapeutic Category Antiemetic

Generic Available No

Use Prophylaxis and treatment of chemotherapy and radiation-related nausea and emesis

Pregnancy Risk Factor B

Contraindications Hypersensitivity to granisetron or any component

Warnings Use with caution in patients with liver disease or in pregnant patients

Adverse Reactions

Cardiovascular: Hypertension, hypotension, arrhythmias such as bradycardia, atrial fibrillation, A-V block

Central nervous system: Agitation, anxiety, CNS stimulation, headache, insomnia, somnolence, fever

Dermatologic: Skin rashes

Gastrointestinal: Constipation, diarrhea, dysgeusia, abdominal pain

Hepatic: Increased liver enzymes

Drug Interactions Because granisetron is metabolized by hepatic cytochrome P-450 drug metabolizing enzymes, inducers or inhibitors of this system may change the clearance and half-life

Stability Stable when mixed in NS, D_5W for at least 24 hours

Mechanism of Action Selective 5-HT$_3$ receptor antagonist, blocking serotonin, both peripherally on vagal nerve terminals and centrally in the chemoreceptor trigger zone

Pharmacodynamics

Onset of action: I.V.: 1-3 minutes

Duration: I.V.: ≤24 hours

Pharmacokinetics

Distribution: V_d: 2-3 L/kg; widely distributed throughout the body

Half-life:

Cancer patients: 10-12 hours

Healthy volunteers: 3-4 hours

Elimination: Primarily nonrenal, 8% to 15% of dose excreted unchanged in urine

Usual Dosage

Children ≥2 years and Adults: I.V.:

10-20 mcg/kg given just prior to chemotherapy (15-60 minutes before).

As intervention therapy for breakthrough nausea and vomiting, during the first 24 hours following chemotherapy, 2 or 3 repeat infusions (same dose) have been administered

Single doses of 40 mcg/kg have been used safely and effectively

Adults: Oral: 2 mg once daily or 1 mg twice daily (1 hour before chemotherapy and 12 hours later)

Administration

Oral: Given at least 1 hour prior to chemotherapy and then 12 hours later; shake oral suspension well before use

Parenteral: I.V.: Infuse over 30 seconds undiluted **or** dilute in small volume NS or D_5W and administer over 5 minutes **or** dilute in 20-50 mL of NS or D_5W and infuse over 30 minutes to 1 hour

Dosage Forms

Injection, preservative free: 1 mg/mL (1 mL)

Injection, with benzyl alcohol: 1 mg/mL (4 mL)

Tablet: 1 mg

Extemporaneous Preparations

A 0.2 mg/mL suspension may be made by crushing twelve 1 mg tablets. Add 30 mL distilled water, mix well, and transfer to a bottle. Rinse the mortar with 10 mL cherry syrup and add to bottle. Add enough cherry syrup to make a final volume of 60 mL. Label "shake well"; stable 14 days at room temperature or refrigerated (Quercia, 1997).

A 50 mcg/mL suspension may be made by crushing one 1 mg tablet. Add 1% methylcellulose and syrup NF to a total volume of 20 mL (may also use Ora-Sweet® or Ora-Plus® instead of methylcellulose and syrup); shake well; stable 91 days refrigerated.

Nahata MC and Hipple TF, *Pedatric Drug Formulations*, 3rd ed, Cincinnati, OH: Harvey Whitney Books Company, 1997.

Quercia RA, Zhang J, Fan C, et al, "Stability of Granisetron Hydrochloride in an Extemporaneously Prepared Oral Liquid," *Am J Health-Syst Pharm*, 1997, 54(12):1404-6.

References

Hahlen K, Quintana E, Pinkerton CR, et al, "A Randomized Comparison of Intravenously Administered Granisetron Versus Chlorpromazine Plus Dexamethasone in the Prevention of Ifosfamide-Induced Emesis in Children," *J Pediatr*, 1995, 126(2):309-13.

Lemerle J, Amaral D, Southall DP, et al, "Efficacy and Safety of Granisetron in the Prevention of Chemotherapy-Induced Emesis in Paediatric Patients," *Eur J Cancer*, 1991, 27(9):1081-3.

♦ **Granulocyte Colony Stimulating Factor** *see* Filgrastim *on page 411*

♦ **Granulocyte Macrophage Colony Stimulating Factor** *see* Sargramostim *on page 858*

♦ **Gravol® (Canada)** *see* Dimenhydrinate *on page 325*

♦ **Grifulvin® V** *see* Griseofulvin *on page 463*

♦ **Grisactin®** *see* Griseofulvin *on page 463*

♦ **Grisactin® Ultra** *see* Griseofulvin *on page 463*

Griseofulvin (gri see oh FUL vin)

Related Information

Carbohydrate and Alcohol Content of Liquid Medications for Use in Patients Receiving Ketogenic Diets *on page 1228*

Brand Names Fulvicin® P/G; Fulvicin-U/F®; Grifulvin® V; Grisactin®; Grisactin® Ultra; Grisovin®-FP (Canada); Gris-PEG®

Synonyms Griseofulvin Microsize; Griseofulvin Ultramicrosize

Therapeutic Category Antifungal Agent, Systemic

Generic Available Yes

Use Treatment of tinea infections of the skin, hair, and nails caused by susceptible species of *Microsporum*, *Epidermophyton*, or *Trichophyton*

Pregnancy Risk Factor C

Contraindications Hypersensitivity to griseofulvin or any component; severe liver disease, porphyria (interferes with porphyrin metabolism); pregnant women

Precautions Avoid exposure to intense sunlight to prevent photosensitivity reactions; use with caution in patients with penicillin hypersensitivity

Adverse Reactions

Central nervous system: Fatigue, confusion, impaired judgment, insomnia, headache, incoordination, dizziness

Dermatologic: Rash, urticaria, photosensitivity reaction

Endocrine & metabolic: Estrogen-like effects in children

Gastrointestinal: Nausea, vomiting, diarrhea, oral thrush

Hematologic: Leukopenia, granulocytopenia

Hepatic: Hepatotoxicity

Neuromuscular & skeletal: Paresthesia

Renal: Proteinuria

Miscellaneous: Lupus-like syndrome

Drug Interactions Phenobarbital decreases griseofulvin concentrations; griseofulvin decreases warfarin effectiveness; griseofulvin decreases oral contraceptive efficacy; griseofulvin potentiates the effects of alcohol and causes flushing and tachycardia

Food Interactions Fatty meal will increase griseofulvin absorption

Mechanism of Action Inhibits fungal cell mitosis at metaphase by disrupting the cell's mitotic spindle structure; binds to human keratin making it resistant to fungal invasion

(Continued)

Griseofulvin *(Continued)*

Pharmacokinetics

Absorption: Ultramicrosize griseofulvin absorption is almost complete; absorption of microsize griseofulvin is variable (25% to 70% of an oral dose); absorbed from the duodenum

Distribution: Deposited in the keratin layer of skin, hair, and nails; concentrates in liver, fat, and skeletal muscles; crosses the placenta

Metabolism: Extensive in the liver

Half-life: 9-22 hours

Elimination: <1% excreted unchanged in urine; also excreted in feces and perspiration

Usual Dosage Oral:

Children:

Microsize: 10-20 mg/kg/day in single or 2 divided doses

Ultramicrosize: >2 years: 5-10 mg/kg/day in single or 2 divided doses

Adults:

Microsize: 500-1000 mg/day in single or divided doses

Ultramicrosize: 330-375 mg/day in single or divided doses; doses up to 750 mg/day have been used for infections more difficult to eradicate such as tinea unguium

Duration of therapy depends on the site of infection:

Tinea corporis: 2-4 weeks

Tinea capitis: 4-6 weeks or longer

Tinea pedis: 4-8 weeks

Tinea unguium: 3-6 months or longer

Administration Oral: Administer with a fatty meal (peanuts or ice cream to increase absorption), or with food or milk to avoid GI upset

Monitoring Parameters Periodic renal, hepatic, and hematopoietic function tests

Test Interactions False-positive urinary VMA levels

Patient Information Avoid exposure to sunlight; avoid alcohol

Dosage Forms

Microsize:

Capsule (Grisactin®): 125 mg, 250 mg

Suspension, oral (Grifulvin V): 125 mg/5 mL with alcohol 0.2% (120 mL)

Tablet:

Fulvicin-U/F®, Grifulvin® V: 250 mg

Fulvicin-U/F®, Grifulvin® V, Grisactin-500®: 500 mg

Ultramicrosize:

Tablet:

Fulvicin® P/G: 165 mg, 330 mg

Fulvicin® P/G, Grisactin® Ultra, Gris-PEG®: 125 mg, 250 mg

Grisactin® Ultra: 330 mg

References

Ginsburg CM, McCracken GH Jr, Petruska M, et al, "Effect of Feeding on Bioavailability of Griseofulvin in Children," *J Pediatr*, 1983, 102(2):309-11.

- ♦ **Griseofulvin Microsize** *see* Griseofulvin *on page 463*
- ♦ **Griseofulvin Ultramicrosize** *see* Griseofulvin *on page 463*
- ♦ **Grisovin®-FP (Canada)** *see* Griseofulvin *on page 463*
- ♦ **Gris-PEG®** *see* Griseofulvin *on page 463*
- ♦ **Growth Hormone** *see* Human Growth Hormone *on page 478*

Guaifenesin *(gwye FEN e sin)*

Related Information

OTC Cough & Cold Preparations, Pediatric *on page 1037*

Brand Names Anti-Tuss® Expectorant [OTC]; Balminil® Expectorant (Canada); Breonesin® [OTC]; Calmylin Expectorant (Canada); Diabetic Tussin EX® [OTC]; Duratuss-G®; Fenesin™ [OTC]; Gee Gee® [OTC]; Genatuss® [OTC]; GG-Cen® [OTC]; Glyate® [OTC]; Glycotuss® [OTC]; Glytuss® [OTC]; Guaifenex LA®; GuaiCough® Expectorant [OTC]; Guiatuss® [OTC]; Halotussin® [OTC]; Humibid® L.A. [OTC]; Humibid® Sprinkle [OTC]; Hytuss® [OTC]; Hytuss-2X® [OTC]; Liquibid® Malotuss® [OTC]; Medi-Tuss® [OTC]; Monafed®; Muco-Fen-LA®; Mytussin® [OTC]; Naldecon® Senior EX [OTC]; Organidin NR®; Pneumomist®; Respa-GF; Robitussin® [OTC]; Scot-Tussin® [OTC]; Siltussin® [OTC]; Sinumist®-SR Capsulets® [OTC]; Touro Ex®; Tusibron® [OTC]; Uni-tussin® [OTC]

Synonyms GG; Glycerol Guaiacolate

Therapeutic Category Expectorant

Generic Available Yes

Use Temporary control of cough due to minor throat and bronchial irritation

Pregnancy Risk Factor C

Contraindications Hypersensitivity to guaifenesin or any component

Adverse Reactions
Central nervous system: Drowsiness, headache
Dermatologic: Rash
Gastrointestinal: Nausea, vomiting

Mechanism of Action Thought to act as an expectorant by irritating the gastric mucosa and stimulating respiratory tract secretions, thereby increasing respiratory fluid volumes and decreasing phlegm viscosity

Usual Dosage Oral:
Children:
<2 years: 12 mg/kg/day in 6 divided doses
2-5 years: 50-100 mg every 4 hours, not to exceed 600 mg/day
6-11 years: 100-200 mg every 4 hours, not to exceed 1.2 g/day
Children >12 years and Adults: 200-400 mg every 4 hours to a maximum of 2.4 g/day

Administration Oral: Administer with a large quantity of fluid to ensure proper action

Test Interactions May cause a colorimetric interference with certain laboratory determinations of 5-hydroxyindoleacetic acid (5-HIAA) and vanillylmandelic acid (VMA)

Dosage Forms
Caplet, sustained release (Touro Ex®): 600 mg
Capsule (Breonesin®, GG-Cen®, Hytuss-2X®): 200 mg
Capsule, sustained release (Humibid® Sprinkle): 300 mg
Liquid:
Diabetic Tussin EX®, Organidin® NR, Tusibron®: 100 mg/5 mL (118 mL)
Naldecon® Senior EX: 200 mg/5 mL (118 mL, 480 mL)
Syrup (Anti-Tuss® Expectorant, Genatuss®, Glyate®, GuiaCough® Expectorant, Guiatuss®, Halotussin®, Malotuss®, Medi-Tuss®, Mytussin®, Robitussin®, Scot-Tussin®, Siltussin®, Tusibron®, Uni-Tussin®): 100 mg/5 mL with alcohol 3.5% (30 mL, 120 mL, 240 mL, 473 mL, 946 mL)
Tablet (Duratuss-G®): 1200 mg
Gee Gee®, Glytuss®, Organidin®:200 mg
Glycotuss®, Hytuss®: 100 mg
Sustained release (Fenesin™, Guaifenex LA®, Humibid® L.A., Liquibid®, Monafed®, Muco-Fen-LA®, Pneumomist®, Respa-GF®, Sinumist®-SR Capsulets®): 600 mg

Guaifenesin and Codeine (gwye FEN e sin & KOE deen)

Related Information
OTC Cough & Cold Preparations, Pediatric on page 1037

Brand Names ACRobafen® AC; Brontex®; Cheracol®; Guaituss AC®; Guiatussin® With Codeine; Mytussin®; Robitussin® A-C; Tussi-Organidin® NR

Available Salts Guaifenesin and Codeine Phosphate

Synonyms Codeine and Glycerol Guaiacolate; Codeine and Guaifenesin

Therapeutic Category Antitussive; Cough Preparation; Expectorant

Generic Available Yes

Use Temporary control of cough due to minor throat and bronchial irritation

Restrictions C-V

Pregnancy Risk Factor C

Contraindications Hypersensitivity to guaifenesin, codeine, or any component

Adverse Reactions
Codeine:
Cardiovascular: Palpitations, bradycardia, peripheral vasodilation
Central nervous system: CNS depression, dizziness, drowsiness, sedation, increased intracranial pressure
Dermatologic: Pruritus from histamine release
Endocrine & metabolic: Antidiuretic hormone release
Gastrointestinal: Nausea, vomiting, constipation, biliary tract spasm
Genitourinary: Urinary tract spasm
Ocular: Miosis
Respiratory: Respiratory depression
Miscellaneous: Histamine release, physical and psychological dependence with prolonged use
Guaifenesin:
Central nervous system: Drowsiness, headache
(Continued)

Guaifenesin and Codeine *(Continued)*

Dermatologic: Rash

Gastrointestinal: Nausea, vomiting

Drug Interactions CNS depressant medications produce additive sedative properties

Mechanism of Action See individual monographs for Guaifenesin *on page 464* and Codeine *on page 249*

Usual Dosage Oral:

Children:

2-6 years: 1-1.5 mg/kg codeine/day divided into 4 doses administered every 4-6 hours (maximum dose: 30 mg/24 hours)

6-12 years: 5 mL every 4 hours, not to exceed 30 mL/24 hours

>12 years: 10 mL every 4 hours, up to 60 mL/24 hours

Adults: 5-10 mL or 1 tablet every 4-6 hours; not to exceed 120 mg (60 mL) codeine/day or 6 tablets/day

Administration Oral: Administer with a large quantity of fluid to ensure proper action

Test Interactions May cause a colorimetric interference with certain laboratory determinations of 5-hydroxy indoleacetic acid (5-HIAA) and vanillylmandelic acid (VMA)

Dosage Forms

Syrup: Guaifenesin 100 mg and codeine phosphate 10 mg per 5 mL (60 mL, 120 mL, 480 mL)

Tablet: Guaifenesin 300 mg and codeine phosphate 10 mg

♦ **Guaifenesin and Codeine Phosphate** *see* Guaifenesin and Codeine *on page 465*

Guaifenesin and Dextromethorphan

(gwye FEN e sin & deks troe meth OR fan)

Related Information

OTC Cough & Cold Preparations, Pediatric *on page 1037*

Brand Names Benylin® Expectorant [OTC]; Cheracol D® [OTC]; Clear Tussin® 30; Contac® Cough Formula Liquid [OTC]; Diabetic Tussin DM® [OTC]; Extra Action Cough Syrup [OTC]; Fenesin DM®; Genatuss DM® [OTC]; Glycotuss-dM® [OTC]; Guaifenex DM®; GuiaCough® [OTC]; Guiatuss DM® [OTC]; Halotussin® DM [OTC]; Humibid® DM [OTC]; Iobid DM®; Kolephrin® GG/DM [OTC]; Muco-Fen-DM®; Mytussin® DM [OTC]; Naldecon® Senior DX [OTC]; Phanatuss® [OTC]; Phenadex® Senior [OTC]; Respa-DM®; Rhinosyn-DMX® [OTC]; Robafen DM® [OTC]; Robitussin®-DM [OTC]; Safe Tussin® 30 [OTC]; Scot-Tussin® Senior Clear [OTC]; Siltussin DM® [OTC]; Syracol-CF® [OTC]; Tolu-Sed® DM [OTC]; Tusibron-DM® [OTC]; Tuss-DM® [OTC]; Tussi-Organidin® DM NR; Uni-tussin® DM [OTC]; Vicks® 44E [OTC]; Vicks® Pediatric Formula 44E [OTC]

Available Salts Guaifenesin and Dextromethorphan Hydrobromide

Synonyms Dextromethorphan and Glycerol Guaiacolate; Dextromethorphan and Guaifenesin

Therapeutic Category Antitussive; Cough Preparation; Expectorant

Generic Available Yes

Use Temporary control of cough due to minor throat and bronchial irritation

Pregnancy Risk Factor C

Contraindications Hypersensitivity to guaifenesin, dextromethorphan, or any component

Adverse Reactions

Central nervous system: Drowsiness, dizziness, headache

Dermatologic: Rash

Gastrointestinal: Nausea

Mechanism of Action See individual monographs for Guaifenesin *on page 464* and Dextromethorphan *on page 304*

Pharmacodynamics Onset of action: Antitussive effect: Oral: 15-30 minutes

Pharmacokinetics Absorption: Dextromethorphan is rapidly absorbed from the GI tract

Usual Dosage Oral (dose expressed in mg of dextromethorphan):

Children: 1-2 mg/kg/day every 6-8 hours

Adults: 60-120 mg/day divided every 6-8 hours

Administration Oral: Administer with a large quantity of fluid to ensure proper effect

Test Interactions May cause a colorimetric interference with certain laboratory determinations of 5-hydroxy indoleacetic acid (5-HIAA) and vanillylmandelic acid (VMA)

Dosage Forms

Syrup:

Benylin® Expectorant: Guaifenesin 100 mg and dextromethorphan hydrobromide 5 mg per 5 mL (118 mL, 236 mL)

Cheracol D®, Clear Tussin®, Genatuss DM®, Mytussin® DM, Robitussin®-DM, Siltussin DM®, Tolu-Sed® DM, Tussi-Organidin® DM NR: Guaifenesin 100 mg and dextromethorphan hydrobromide 10 mg per 5 mL (5 mL, 10 mL, 120 mL, 240 mL, 360 mL, 480 mL, 3780 mL)

Contac® Cough Formula Liquid: Guaifenesin 67 mg and dextromethorphan hydrobromide 10 mg per 5 mL (120 mL)

Extra Action Cough Syrup, GuiaCough®, Guiatuss DM®, Halotussin® DM, Rhinosyn-DMX®, Tusibron-DM®, Uni-Tussin® DM: Guaifenesin 100 mg and dextromethorphan hydrobromide 15 mg per 5 mL (120 mL, 240 mL, 480 mL)

Kolephrin® GG/DM: Guaifenesin 150 mg and dextromethorphan hydrobromide 10 mg per 5 mL (120 mL)

Naldecon® Senior DX: Guaifenesin 200 mg and dextromethorphan hydrobromide 15 mg per 5 mL (118 mL, 480 mL)

Phanatuss®: Guaifenesin 85 mg and dextromethorphan hydrobromide 10 mg per 5 mL

Vicks® 44E: Guaifenesin 66.7 mg and dextromethorphan hydrobromide 6.7 mg per 5 mL

Tablet, extended release:

Guaifenex DM®, Iobid DM®, Fenesin DM®, Humibid® DM, Monafed® DM, Respa-DM®: Guaifenesin 600 mg and dextromethorphan hydrobromide 30 mg

Glycotuss-dM®: Guaifenesin 100 mg and dextromethorphan hydrobromide 10 mg

Queltuss®: Guaifenesin 100 mg and dextromethorphan hydrobromide 15 mg

Syracol-CF®: Guaifenesin 200 mg and dextromethorphan hydrobromide 15 mg

Tuss-DM®: Guaifenesin 200 mg and dextromethorphan hydrobromide 10 mg

♦ **Guaifenesin and Dextromethorphan Hydrobromide** see Guaifenesin and Dextromethorphan on page 466

Guaifenesin, Phenylpropanolamine, and Phenylephrine

(gwye FEN e sin, fen il proe pa NOLE a meen, & fen il EF rin)

Brand Names Coldloc®; Contuss®; Despec®; Dura-Gest®; Enomine®; Entex®; Guaifenex®; Guiatex®; Respinol-G®; ULR®

Available Salts Guaifenesin, Phenylpropanolamine Hydrochloride, and Phenylephrine Hydrochloride

Synonyms Glycerol Guaiacolate, Phenylpropanolamine, and Phenylephrine; Phenylephrine, Guaifenesin, and Phenylpropanolamine; Phenylpropanolamine, Guaifenesin, and Phenylephrine

Therapeutic Category Decongestant; Expectorant

Generic Available Yes

Use Temporary relief of nasal congestion, running nose, sneezing, itching of nose and throat, and itchy, watery eyes due to common cold, hay fever, or other upper respiratory allergies

Pregnancy Risk Factor C

Contraindications Hypersensitivity to guaifenesin, phenylephrine, phenylpropanolamine, or any component; severe hypertension or coronary artery disease; MAO inhibitor therapy; GI or GU obstruction, narrow-angle glaucoma, peripheral vascular disease

Adverse Reactions

Cardiovascular: Hypertension, tachycardia, arrhythmias

Central nervous system: Sedation, nervousness, insomnia, restlessness, headache

Dermatologic: Rash

Gastrointestinal: Nausea, gastric irritation, vomiting, anorexia

Genitourinary: Urinary retention

Neuromuscular & skeletal: Tremor

Drug Interactions MAO inhibitors, alpha- and beta-adrenergic blocking agents, sympathomimetics, aspirin, NSAIDs

Mechanism of Action Phenylephrine and phenylpropanolamine are alpha-adrenergic receptor agonists which produce vasoconstriction resulting in shrinking of swollen nasal mucous membranes and reduction of tissue hyperemia and edema; for guaifenesin, see Guaifenesin on page 464

(Continued)

Guaifenesin, Phenylpropanolamine, and Phenylephrine
(Continued)

Usual Dosage Oral (safety and efficacy in children <2 years of age have not been established):

Children:
   2-4 years: 2.5 mL every 6 hours
   4-6 years: 5 mL every 6 hours
   6 to ≤12 years: 7.5 mL every 6 hours **or** ½ extended release tablet every 12 hours
   Children >12 years and Adults: 10 mL every 6 hours **or** 1 capsule every 6 hours **or** 1 extended release tablet every 12 hours

Administration Oral: Administer with a large quantity of fluid to ensure proper effect; extended release tablets may be cut in half and still maintain effective release properties, do not crush or chew them

Test Interactions May cause a colorimetric interference with certain laboratory determinations of 5-hydroxy indoleacetic acid (5-HIAA) and vanillylmandelic acid (VMA)

Patient Information Causes drowsiness and may impair ability to perform hazardous activities requiring mental alertness or physical coordination

Dosage Forms

Capsule (Contuss®, Dura-Gest®, Enomine®, Entex®, Guiatex®, ULR®): Guaifenesin 200 mg, phenylpropanolamine hydrochloride 45 mg, and phenylephrine hydrochloride 5 mg

Liquid (Coldloc®, Contuss®, Despec®, Entex®, Guaifenex®): Guaifenesin 100 mg, phenylpropanolamine hydrochloride 20 mg, and phenylephrine hydrochloride 5 mg per 5 mL (118 mL, 480 mL)

Tablet (Respinol-G®): Guaifenesin 200 mg, phenylpropanolamine hydrochloride 45 mg, and phenylephrine hydrochloride 5 mg

♦ **Guaifenesin, Phenylpropanolamine Hydrochloride, and Phenylephrine Hydrochloride** *see* Guaifenesin, Phenylpropanolamine, and Phenylephrine *on page 467*

♦ **Guaifenex®** *see* Guaifenesin, Phenylpropanolamine, and Phenylephrine *on page 467*

♦ **Guaifenex DM®** *see* Guaifenesin and Dextromethorphan *on page 466*

♦ **Guaifenex LA®** *see* Guaifenesin *on page 464*

♦ **Guaituss AC®** *see* Guaifenesin and Codeine *on page 465*

♦ **GuiaCough® [OTC]** *see* Guaifenesin and Dextromethorphan *on page 466*

♦ **GuiaCough® Expectorant [OTC]** *see* Guaifenesin *on page 464*

♦ **Guiatex®** *see* Guaifenesin, Phenylpropanolamine, and Phenylephrine *on page 467*

♦ **Guiatuss® [OTC]** *see* Guaifenesin *on page 464*

♦ **Guiatuss DM® [OTC]** *see* Guaifenesin and Dextromethorphan *on page 466*

♦ **Guiatussin® With Codeine** *see* Guaifenesin and Codeine *on page 465*

♦ **G-well®** *see* Lindane *on page 572*

♦ **Gynecort® Topical [OTC]** *see* Hydrocortisone *on page 486*

♦ **Gyne-Lotrimin® Vaginal [OTC]** *see* Clotrimazole *on page 245*

♦ **Gynergen® (Canada)** *see* Ergotamine *on page 378*

♦ **Gynogen L.A.® 20** *see* Estradiol *on page 386*

♦ **H₂O₂** *see* Hydrogen Peroxide *on page 490*

♦ **H₂Oxyl® (Canada)** *see* Benzoyl Peroxide *on page 126*

♦ *Haemophilus* **b Oligosaccharide Conjugate Vaccine** *see page 1138*

♦ **Halcion®** *see* Triazolam *on page 950*

♦ **Haldol®** *see* Haloperidol *on page 468*

♦ **Haldol® Decanoate** *see* Haloperidol *on page 468*

♦ **Haley's M-O®** *see* Magnesium Supplements *on page 588*

♦ **Halfprin® [OTC]** *see* Aspirin *on page 99*

Haloperidol (ha loe PER i dole)

Related Information

Carbohydrate and Alcohol Content of Liquid Medications for Use in Patients Receiving Ketogenic Diets *on page 1228*
Drugs and Breast-Feeding *on page 1213*

Brand Names Haldol®; Haldol® Decanoate; Peridol (Canada)

Available Salts Haloperidol Decanoate; Haloperidol Lactate

Therapeutic Category Antipsychotic Agent; Phenothiazine Derivative

Generic Available Yes

Use Treatment of psychoses, Tourette's disorder, and severe behavioral problems in children

Pregnancy Risk Factor C

Contraindications Hypersensitivity to haloperidol or any component; narrow-angle glaucoma, bone marrow suppression, CNS depression, severe liver or cardiac disease, parkinsonism

Warnings Safety and efficacy have not been established in children <3 years of age; 1 mg, 5 mg, and 10 mg tablets contain tartrazine which may cause allergic reactions

Precautions Use with caution in patients with renal or hepatic dysfunction, thyrotoxicosis, cardiovascular disease, or history of seizures

Adverse Reactions

Cardiovascular: Tachycardia, hypotension

Central nervous system: Extrapyramidal reactions, neuroleptic malignant syndrome, tardive dyskinesia, drowsiness

Dermatologic: Rash, contact dermatitis

Endocrine & metabolic: Galactorrhea, gynecomastia, decreased serum magnesium levels

Gastrointestinal: Xerostomia, constipation

Genitourinary: Urinary retention

Hematologic: Leukopenia, leukocytosis, anemia

Hepatic: Hepatotoxicity (rare)

Ocular: Blurred vision

Drug Interactions Cytochrome P-450 isoenzyme CYP1A2, CYP2D6 (minor), and CYP3A3/4 substrate; CYP2D6 and CYP3A3/4 isoenzyme inhibitor

CNS depressants may increase adverse effects; epinephrine may cause hypotension; carbamazepine and phenobarbital may increase metabolism and decrease effectiveness of haloperidol; use of haloperidol with anticholinergic agents may increase intraocular pressure; concurrent use with lithium has occasionally caused acute encephalopathy-like syndrome

Food Interactions Drug may precipitate if oral concentrate is mixed with coffee or tea

Mechanism of Action Competitive blockade of postsynaptic dopamine receptors in the mesolimbic dopaminergic system; depresses cerebral cortex and hypothalamus; exhibits a strong alpha-adrenergic and anticholinergic blocking activity

Pharmacokinetics

Absorption: Oral: Well absorbed, undergoes first-pass metabolism in the liver

Distribution: Crosses the placenta; appears in breast milk

Protein binding: 92%

Metabolism: In the liver, hydroxy-metabolite is active

Bioavailability: Oral: 60%

Half-life: Adults: 20 hours; range: 13-35 hours

Elimination: Excreted in urine and feces as drug and metabolites

Usual Dosage

Children: (see also Additional Information)

3-12 years (15-40 kg): Oral: Initial: 0.25-0.5 mg/day given in 2-3 divided doses; increase by 0.25-0.5 mg every 5-7 days; maximum dose: 0.15 mg/kg/day; usual maintenance:

Agitation or hyperkinesia: 0.01-0.03 mg/kg/day once daily

Tourette's disorder: 0.05-0.075 mg/kg/day in 2-3 divided doses

Psychotic disorders: 0.05-0.15 mg/kg/day in 2-3 divided doses

6-12 years: I.M. **(as lactate)**: 1-3 mg/dose every 4-8 hours to a maximum of 0.15 mg/kg/day; switch to oral therapy as soon as able

Adults:

Oral: 0.5-5 mg 2-3 times/day; usual maximum dose: 30 mg/day; some patients may require 100 mg/day

I.M.:

As **lactate**: 2-5 mg every 4-8 hours as needed

As **decanoate**: Initial: 10-15 times the individual patients' stabilized oral dose, given at 3- to 4-week intervals

Administration

Oral: Administer with food or milk to decrease GI distress; do not mix oral concentrate with coffee or tea

Parenteral: Decanoate product is for I.M. use only, do not give I.V.; although not FDA-approved, haloperidol **lactate** has been administered I.V.

Monitoring Parameters Blood pressure, CBC with differential

Patient Information Avoid alcohol; may cause drowsiness and impair ability to perform activities requiring mental alertness or physical coordination

(Continued)

469

Haloperidol *(Continued)*

Nursing Implications Observe for extrapyramidal effects

Additional Information Preliminary findings of a double-blind, placebo controlled study reported the mean optimal dose in 12 schizophrenic children 5-12 years to be ~2 mg/day (range: 0.5-3.5 mg/day or 0.02-0.12 mg/kg/day) given in 3 divided doses

Dosage Forms

Concentrate, oral, as lactate: 2 mg/mL (5 mL, 10 mL, 15 mL, 120 mL, 240 mL)

Injection, as decanoate: 50 mg/mL (1 mL, 5 mL); 100 mg/mL (1 mL, 5 mL)

Injection, as lactate: 5 mg/mL (1 mL, 2 mL, 2.5 mL, 10 mL)

Tablet: 0.5 mg, 1 mg, 2 mg, 5 mg, 10 mg, 20 mg

References

Serrano AC, "Haloperidol - Its Use in Children," *J Clin Psychiatry*, 1981, 42(4):154-6.

Spencer EK, Kafantaris V, Padron-Gayol MV, et al, "Haloperidol in Schizophrenic Children: Early Findings From a Study in Progress," *Psychopharmacol Bull*, 1992, 28(2):183-6.

♦ **Haloperidol Decanoate** *see Haloperidol on page 468*
♦ **Haloperidol Lactate** *see Haloperidol on page 468*

Haloprogin *(ha loe PROE jin)*

Brand Names Halotex®

Therapeutic Category Antifungal Agent, Topical

Generic Available No

Use Topical treatment of tinea pedis, tinea cruris, tinea corporis, tinea manuum caused by *Trichophyton rubrum*, *Trichophyton tonsurans*, *Trichophyton mentagrophytes*, *Microsporum canis*, or *Epidermophyton floccosum*

Pregnancy Risk Factor C

Contraindications Hypersensitivity to haloprogin or any component

Warnings Safety and efficacy have not been established in children

Adverse Reactions

Dermatologic: Pruritus, folliculitis, vesicle formation, erythema, scaling

Local: Irritation, burning sensation

Mechanism of Action Inhibits yeast cell respiration and disrupts its cell membrane

Pharmacokinetics Absorption: Poor through the skin (~11%)

Usual Dosage Children and Adults: Topical: Twice daily for 2-3 weeks; intertriginous areas may require up to 4 weeks of treatment

Administration Topical: A small amount of cream or 2-3 drops of the solution should be rubbed gently into the affected area

Patient Information Avoid contact with eyes, for topical use only; contact physician if increased irritation occurs

Dosage Forms

Cream: 1% (15 g, 30 g)

Solution, topical: 1% with alcohol 75% (10 mL, 30 mL)

♦ **Halotestin®** *see Fluoxymesterone on page 433*
♦ **Halotex®** *see Haloprogin on page 470*
♦ **Halotussin® [OTC]** *see Guaifenesin on page 464*
♦ **Halotussin® DM [OTC]** *see Guaifenesin and Dextromethorphan on page 466*
♦ **Haltran® [OTC]** *see Ibuprofen on page 501*
♦ **HAT Antibody** *see Daclizumab on page 280*
♦ **hCG** *see Chorionic Gonadotropin on page 221*
♦ **HCTZ** *see Hydrochlorothiazide on page 483*
♦ **Heavy Mineral Oil** *see Mineral Oil on page 649*
♦ **Hemet® Rectal [OTC]** *see Hemorrhoidal Preparations on page 470*
♦ **Hemocaine® [OTC]** *see Hemorrhoidal Preparations on page 470*
♦ **Hemocyte® [OTC]** *see Iron Supplements, Oral/Enteral on page 530*
♦ **Hemofil® M** *see Antihemophilic Factor (Human) on page 89*

Hemorrhoidal Preparations *(HEM or oyd al prep a RAY shuns)*

Brand Names A-Caine® Rectal [OTC]; Anumed® [OTC]; Anusol® [OTC]; Calmol 4®; CPI® [OTC]; Fleet® Relief®; Hemet® Rectal [OTC]; Hemocaine® [OTC]; Hem-Prep® [OTC]; Nupercainal®; Pazo® Hemorrhoid [OTC]; Perifoam® [OTC]; Posterisan® [OTC]; Preparation H® [OTC]; Proctofoam® [OTC]; Rectal Medicone® [OTC]; Tronolane®

Therapeutic Category Topical Skin Product

Generic Available Yes

Use Symptomatic relief of pain and discomfort in external and internal hemorrhoids, proctitis, papillitis, cryptitis, anal fissures, incomplete fistulas and relief of local pain following anorectal surgery

Contraindications Hypersensitivity to any component

Warnings Some preparations contain a sulfite which may cause allergic-type reactions

Adverse Reactions
Dermatologic: Rash
Local: Irritation, burning, itching

Mechanism of Action
Dibucaine, benzocaine, pramoxine: Temporarily relieves pain, itching, and irritation by blocking nerve impulses at the sensory nerve endings in the skin and mucous membranes
Emollient/protectant (glycerin, lanolin, mineral oil, petrolatum, zinc oxide, cocoa butter, shark liver oil): Form a physical barrier and lubricate tissues preventing irritation of the anorectal area and water loss

Pharmacodynamics
Onset of effect: Topical:
Pramoxine: 3-5 minutes
Dibucaine: <15 minutes
Benzocaine: 1 minute

Usual Dosage
Children and Adults: Topical: Apply ointment as a thin layer to the perianal area and the anal canal 3-6 times/day
Benzocaine-containing preparations: Apply up to 6 times/day
Dibucaine-containing preparations: Apply ointment into the rectum each morning and evening and after each bowel movement; ointment may be applied topically to anal tissues; apply up to 3-4 times/day
Children: No more than 7.5 g in a 24-hour period
Adults: No more than 30 g in a 24-hour period
Pramoxine-containing preparations: Apply up to 5 times/day (2-3 times/day and after bowel movements)
Adults: Rectal: Insert 1 suppository in the morning and at bedtime and after each bowel movement

Administration
Rectal: Foam, ointment, and cream for rectal use are instilled using a rectal applicator. The aerosol should not be inserted into the anus.
Topical: Apply cream or ointment to affected areas and rub in gently. A small amount of foam may be applied to the affected area using a cleansing tissue or pad.

Patient Information If anorectal symptoms do not improve in 7 days, or if bleeding, protrusion or seepage occurs, consult physician; avoid contact of topical preparations to the eyes

Dosage Forms
Dibucaine: 1%: Nupercainal® hemorrhoidal and anesthetic ointment
Pramoxine:
Cream: 1%: Tronolane®
Foam: 1%: Proctofoam®: 15 g, 45 g
Ointment: 1%: Fleet Relief®; Anusol®
Rectal suppository: 1%: Tronolane®
Benzocaine: 20%: Americaine® hemorrhoidal ointment
Emollient/protectants (glycerin, lanolin, mineral oil, petrolatum, zinc oxide, cocoa butter, shark liver oil):
Cream: Preparation H®
Ointment: Preparation H®
Suppository: Preparation H®, Calmol 4®; Wyanoids® Relief Factor; Nupercainal®

♦ **Hem-Prep® [OTC]** *see* Hemorrhoidal Preparations *on page 470*

♦ **Hepalean®, -LOK, -LCO (Canada)** *see* Heparin *on page 471*

Heparin (HEP a rin)

Related Information
Adult ACLS Algorithm, Tachycardia *on page 1010*
Overdose and Toxicology *on page 1191*

Brand Names Calcilean® [HepCalium] (Canada); Hepalean®, -LOK, -LCO (Canada); Hep-Lock®; Liquaemin®

Available Salts Heparin Sodium

Synonyms Heparin Lock Flush

Therapeutic Category Anticoagulant
(Continued)

Heparin *(Continued)*

Generic Available Yes

Use Prophylaxis and treatment of thromboembolic disorders

Pregnancy Risk Factor C

Contraindications Hypersensitivity to heparin or any component; severe thrombocytopenia, subacute bacterial endocarditis, suspected intracranial hemorrhage, shock, severe hypotension, uncontrollable bleeding (unless secondary to disseminated intravascular coagulation)

Warnings Some preparations contain benzyl alcohol as a preservative. In neonates, large amounts of benzyl alcohol (>100 mg/kg/day) have been associated with fatal toxicity (gasping syndrome); the use of preservative free heparin is, therefore, recommended in neonates. Some preparations contain sulfites which may cause allergic reactions.

Precautions Use with caution as hemorrhage may occur; risk factors for hemorrhage include: I.M. injections; peptic ulcer disease; intermittent I.V. injections (vs continuous I.V. infusion); increased capillary permeability; menstruation; recent surgery or invasive procedures; severe renal, hepatic, or biliary disease; and indwelling catheters

Heparin does not possess fibrinolytic activity and, therefore, cannot lyse established thrombi; discontinue heparin if hemorrhage occurs; severe hemorrhage or overdosage may require protamine

Adverse Reactions

Central nervous system: Fever, headache, chills

Dermatologic: Urticaria, alopecia

Gastrointestinal: Nausea, vomiting

Hematologic: Hemorrhage, thrombocytopenia (may be more common with beef lung heparin vs porcine mucosa heparin; however, if a patient receiving beef lung heparin experiences severe thrombocytopenia it is **not** recommended to switch to porcine mucosa heparin because a similar reaction may occur)

Hepatic: Elevated liver enzymes

Local: Irritation, ulceration, cutaneous necrosis has been rarely reported with deep S.C. injections

Neuromuscular & skeletal: Osteoporosis (with long-term use)

Drug Interactions Thrombolytic agents (urokinase, streptokinase) and drugs which affect platelet function (eg, aspirin, NSAIDs, dipyridamole) may potentiate the risk of hemorrhage; digoxin, tetracycline, nicotine, antihistamines, and I.V. nitroglycerin may decrease heparin's anticoagulant effect.

Mechanism of Action Potentiates the action of antithrombin III and thereby inactivates thrombin (as well as activated coagulation factors IX, X, XI, XII, and plasmin) and prevents the conversion of fibrinogen to fibrin; heparin also stimulates release of lipoprotein lipase (lipoprotein lipase hydrolyzes triglycerides to glycerol and free fatty acids)

Pharmacodynamics Onset of anticoagulation effect:

S.C.: 20-60 minutes

I.V.: Immediate

Pharmacokinetics

Absorption: S.C., I.M.: Erratic

Distribution: Does not cross the placenta; does not appear in breast milk

Metabolism: Believed to be partially metabolized in the reticuloendothelial system

Half-life: Mean: 90 minutes (range: 1-2 hours); affected by obesity, renal function, hepatic function, malignancy, presence of pulmonary embolism, and infections

Elimination: Renal; small amount excreted unchanged in urine

Usual Dosage

Line flushing: When using daily flushes of heparin to maintain patency of single and double lumen central catheters, 10 units/mL is commonly used for younger infants (eg, <10 kg) while 100 units/mL is used for older infants, children, and adults. Capped polyvinyl chloride catheters and peripheral heparin locks require flushing more frequently (eg, every 6-8 hours). Volume of heparin flush is usually similar to volume of catheter (or slightly greater) or may be standardized according to specific hospital's policy (eg, 2-5 mL/flush). Dose of heparin flush used should not approach therapeutic unit per kg dose. Additional flushes should be given when stagnant blood is observed in catheter, after catheter is used for drug or blood administration, and after blood withdrawal from catheter.

TPN: Heparin 1 unit/mL (final concentration) may be added to TPN solutions, both central and peripheral. (Addition of heparin to peripheral TPN has been shown to increase duration of line patency.) The final concentration of heparin used for TPN solutions may need to be decreased to 0.5 units/mL in small infants receiving larger TPN volumes in order to avoid approaching therapeutic amounts.

Arterial lines: Heparinize with a usual final concentration of 1 unit/mL; range: 0.5-2 units/mL; in order to avoid large total doses and systemic effects, use 0.5 unit/mL in low birth weight/premature newborns and in other patients receiving multiple lines containing heparin

Prophylaxis for cardiac catheterization via an artery: Newborns and Children: I.V.: Bolus: 100-150 units/kg (see Michelson, 1998)

Neonates and Infants <1 year: I.V. infusion: Initial loading dose: 75 units/kg given over 10 minutes; then initial maintenance dose: 28 units/kg/hour; adjust dose to maintain APTT of 60-85 seconds (assuming this reflects an antifactor Xa level of 0.3-0.7); see table.

Children >1 year:

Intermittent I.V.: Initial: 50-100 units/kg, then 50-100 units/kg every 4 hours

I.V. infusion: Initial loading dose: 75 units/kg given over 10 minutes, then initial maintenance dose: 20 units/kg/hour; adjust dose to maintain APTT of 60-85 seconds (assuming this reflects an anti-factor Xa level of 0.3-0.7); see table.

PEDIATRIC PROTOCOL FOR SYSTEMIC HEPARIN ADJUSTMENT

To be used after initial loading dose and maintenance dose (see Usual Dosage) to maintain APTT of 60-85 seconds (assuming this reflects antifactor Xa level of 0.3-0.7)

Obtain blood for APTT 4 hours after heparin loading dose and 4 hours after every infusion rate change

Obtain daily CBC and APTT after APTT is therapeutic

APTT (seconds)	Dosage Adjustment	Time to Repeat APTT
<50	Give 50 units/kg bolus and increase infusion rate by 10%	4 h after rate change
50-59	Increase infusion rate by 10%	4 h after rate change
60-85	Keep rate the same	Next day
86-95	Decrease infusion rate by 10%	4 h after rate change
96-120	Hold infusion for 30 minutes and decrease infusion rate by 10%	4 h after rate change
>120	Hold infusion for 60 minutes and decrease infusion rate by 15%	4 h after rate change

Modified from Michelson AD, Bovill E, Monagle P, et al, "Antithrombotic Therapy in Children," *Chest*, 1998, 114(5 Suppl):748S-69S.

Adults:

Prophylaxis (low dose heparin): S.C.: 5000 units every 8-12 hours

Intermittent I.V.: Initial: 10,000 units, then 50-70 units/kg (5000-10,000 units) every 4-6 hours

I.V. infusion: Initial loading dose: 80 units/kg; initial maintenance dose: 18 units/kg/hour with dose adjusted according to APTT; usual range: 10-30 units/kg/hour

Administration Parenteral: Continuous I.V. infusion is preferred vs I.V. intermittent injections

Monitoring Parameters Platelet counts, signs of bleeding, hemoglobin, hematocrit, APTT; for full-dose heparin (ie, non-low dose), the dose should be titrated according to APTT (see table). For intermittent I.V. injections, APTT is measured 3.5-4 hours after I.V. injection.

Reference Range Treatment of venous thrombotic disease: Recommended APTT should reflect a heparin level by protamine titration of 0.2-0.4 units/mL or an anti-factor Xa level of 0.3-0.7 units/mL; this usually reflects an APTT of 60-85 seconds

Test Interactions ↑ thyroxine (S) (competitive protein binding methods)

Patient Information Limit alcohol

Nursing Implications Do not administer I.M. due to pain, irritation, and hematoma formation

Additional Information To reverse the effects of heparin, use protamine (see Protamine *on page 820* for specifics); heparin is available from beef lung and from porcine intestinal mucosa sources

Duration of heparin therapy (pediatric):

DVT: At least 5 days

Extensive DVT or pulmonary embolism (PE): 7-10 days

(Continued)

Heparin *(Continued)*

Note: Oral anticoagulation can be started on day 1 of heparin, except for extensive DVT or PE, when it should be delayed; oral anticoagulation should be overlapped with heparin for 4-5 days

Dosage Forms

Heparin sodium:

Lock flush injection:

Beef lung source: 10 units/mL (1 mL, 2 mL, 2.5 mL, 3 mL, 5 mL, 10 mL, 30 mL); 100 units/mL (1 mL, 2 mL, 2.5 mL, 3 mL, 5 mL, 10 mL, 30 mL)

Porcine intestinal mucosa source: 10 units/mL (1 mL, 2 mL, 10 mL, 30 mL); 100 units/mL (1 mL, 2 mL, 10 mL, 30 mL)

Porcine intestinal mucosa source, preservative free: 10 units/mL (1 mL); 100 units/mL (1 mL)

Multiple-dose vial injection:

Beef lung source, with preservative: 1000 units/mL (5 mL, 10 mL, 30 mL); 5000 units/mL (10 mL); 10,000 units/mL (4 mL, 5 mL, 10 mL); 20,000 units/mL (2 mL, 5 mL, 10 mL); 40,000 units/mL (5 mL)

Porcine intestinal mucosa source, with preservative: 1000 units/mL (10 mL, 30 mL); 5000 units/mL (10 mL); 10,000 units/mL (4 mL); 20,000 units/mL (2 mL, 5 mL)

Single-dose vial injection:

Beef lung source: 1000 units/mL (1 mL); 5000 units/mL (1 mL); 10,000 units/mL (1 mL); 20,000 units/mL (1 mL); 40,000 units/mL (1 mL)

Porcine intestinal mucosa: 1000 units/mL (1 mL); 5000 units/mL (1 mL); 10,000 units/mL (1 mL); 20,000 units/mL (1 mL); 40,000 units/mL (1 mL)

Unit dose injection:

Porcine intestinal mucosa source, with preservative: 1000 units/dose (1 mL, 2 mL); 2500 units/dose (1 mL); 5000 units/dose (0.5 mL, 1 mL); 7500 units/dose (1 mL); 10,000 units/dose (1 mL); 15,000 units/dose (1 mL); 20,000 units/dose (1 mL)

Heparin sodium infusion, porcine intestinal mucosa source:

D_5W: 40 units/mL (500 mL); 50 units/mL (250 mL, 500 mL); 100 units/mL (100 mL, 250 mL)

NaCl 0.45%: 2 units/mL (500 mL, 1000 mL); 50 units/mL (250 mL); 100 units/mL (250 mL)

NaCl 0.9%: 2 units/mL (500 mL, 1000 mL); 5 units/mL (1000 mL); 50 units/mL (250 mL, 500 mL, 1000 mL)

References

Andrew M, Marzinotto V, Massicotte P, et al, "Heparin Therapy in Pediatric Patients: A Prospective Cohort Study," *Pediatr Res*, 1994, 35(1):78-83.

Hirsh J, Warkentin TE, Raschke R, et al, "Heparin and Low-Molecular Weight-Heparin: Mechanisms of Action, Pharmacokinetics, Dosing Considerations, Monitoring, Efficacy and Safety," *Chest*, 1998, 114(5 Suppl):489S-510S.

Michelson AD, Bovill E, Monagle P, et al, "Antithrombotic Therapy in Children," *Chest*, 1998, 114(5 Suppl):748S-69S.

- ♦ **Heparin Lock Flush** *see Heparin on page 471*
- ♦ **Heparin Sodium** *see Heparin on page 471*
- ♦ **Hepatitis A Vaccine** *see page 1138*
- ♦ **Hepatitis B Immune Globulin** *see page 1138*
- ♦ **Hepatitis B Vaccine** *see page 1138*
- ♦ **Hep-Lock®** *see Heparin on page 471*
- ♦ **Heptalac®** *see Lactulose on page 550*
- ♦ **HES** *see Hetastarch on page 474*
- ♦ **Hespan®** *see Hetastarch on page 474*

Hetastarch *(HET a starch)*

Brand Names Hespan®

Synonyms HES; Hydroxyethyl Starch

Therapeutic Category Plasma Volume Expander

Generic Available No

Use Blood volume expander used in treatment of shock or impending shock when blood or blood products are not available; does not have oxygen-carrying capacity and is not a substitute for blood or plasma

Pregnancy Risk Factor C

Contraindications Severe bleeding disorders, renal failure with oliguria or anuria, or severe CHF; management of cerebral vasospasm associated with subarachnoid hemorrhage or for conditions other than leukapheresis which necessitate repeated use of the drug over several days

Warnings Anaphylactoid reactions have occurred; use with caution in patients with thrombocytopenia (may interfere with platelet function); large volume may cause drops in hemoglobin concentrations; use with caution in patients at risk from overexpansion of blood volume, including the very young or aged patients, those with CHF or pulmonary edema; large volumes may interfere with platelet function and prolong PT and PTT times; use with caution in patients with a history of liver disease

Adverse Reactions
Cardiovascular: Heart failure, circulatory overload, peripheral edema
Central nervous system: Headache, fever, chills
Dermatologic: Urticaria, pruritus
Endocrine & metabolic: Parotid gland enlargement, hyperchloremic metabolic acidosis, hypernatremia
Gastrointestinal: Vomiting, increased amylase levels
Hematologic: Thrombocytopenia, transient prolongation of PT, PTT, clotting time, and bleeding time
Hepatic: Increased indirect bilirubin
Neuromuscular & skeletal: Myalgia
Ocular: Periorbital edema
Respiratory: Wheezing
Miscellaneous: Anaphylactoid reactions

Stability Do not use if crystalline precipitate forms or is turbid deep brown

Mechanism of Action Hetastarch. a synthetic polymer, produces plasma volume expansion by virtue of its highly colloidal starch structure

Pharmacodynamics
Onset of volume expansion: I.V.: Within 30 minutes
Duration: 24-36 hours

Pharmacokinetics
Metabolism: Molecules >50,000 daltons require enzymatic degradation by the reticuloendothelial system or amylases in the blood prior to urinary and fecal excretion
Elimination: Smaller molecular weight molecules are readily excreted in urine; approximately 40% of dose excreted in first 24 hours in patients with normal renal function

Usual Dosage I.V. infusion:
Children: 10 mL/kg/dose; the total daily dose should not exceed 20 mL/kg
Adults: 500-1000 mL (30-60 g) per dose; the total daily dose should not exceed 1.2 g/kg or 90 g (1500 mL)
Dosing adjustment in renal impairment: Cl_{cr} <10 mL/minute: Initial dose is the same but subsequent doses should be reduced by 20% to 50% of normal

Administration Parenteral: I.V.: Maximum rate of infusion: 1.2 g/kg/hour (20 mL/ kg/hour)

Monitoring Parameters Volume expansion: capillary refill time, CVP, RAP, MAP, urine output, heart rate, if pulmonary artery catheter in place, monitor PWCP, SVR, and PVR; hemoglobin, hematocrit; for leukapheresis, monitor CBC, total leukocyte and platelet counts, leukocyte differential count, hemoglobin, hematocrit, prothrombin time, and partial thromboplastin time

Additional Information Each 500 mL provides 77 mEq sodium chloride; currently available product in the United States is high molecular weight (HMW); low molecular weight (LMW) products available in Europe may have an improved adverse reaction profile

Dosage Forms Infusion, in sodium chloride 0.9%: 6% (250 mL, 500 mL)

References
Brutocao D, Bratton SL, Thomas JR, et al, "Comparison of Hetastarch With Albumin for Postoperative Volume Expansion in Children After Cardiopulmonary Bypass," *J Cardiothoracic Vasc Anesth,* 1996, 10(3):348-51.

♦ **Hexachlorocyclohexane** *see* Lindane *on page 572*

Hexachlorophene (heks a KLOR oh feen)
Brand Names pHisoHex®; Septisol®
Therapeutic Category Antibacterial, Topical; Soap
Generic Available Yes
Use Surgical scrub and as a bacteriostatic skin cleanser; to control an outbreak of gram-positive staphylococcal infection when other infection control procedures have been unsuccessful
Pregnancy Risk Factor C
(Continued)

Hexachlorophene *(Continued)*

Contraindications Hypersensitivity to halogenated phenol derivatives or hexachlorophene; use in premature infants; use on burned or denuded skin; use with an occlusive dressing; application to mucous membranes

Warnings Do not use for bathing infants; do not apply to mucous membranes; premature and low birth weight infants are particularly susceptible to hexachlorophene topical absorption; irritability, generalized clonic muscular contractions, decerebrate rigidity, and brain lesions in the white matter have occurred in infants following topical use of 6% hexachlorophene; exposure of preterm infants or patients with extensive burns has been associated with apnea, convulsions, agitation, and coma

Adverse Reactions

Central nervous system: CNS injury, seizures, irritability

Dermatologic: Dermatitis, erythema, dry skin, photosensitivity

Drug Interactions Polysorbate 80, nonionic detergents with concentration >8% may decrease antibacterial activity of hexachlorophene

Stability Store in nonmetallic container (incompatible with many metals); protect from light

Mechanism of Action Bacteriostatic polychlorinated biphenol which inhibits membrane-bound enzymes and disrupts the cell membrane

Pharmacokinetics

Absorption: Percutaneously through inflamed, excoriated and intact skin

Distribution: Crosses the placenta

Half-life, infants: 6.1-44.2 hours

Usual Dosage Children and Adults: Topical: Apply 5 mL cleanser and water to area to be cleansed; lather and rinse thoroughly under running water; for use as a surgical scrub, a second application of 5 mL cleanser should be made and the hands and forearms scrubbed for an additional 3 minutes, rinsed thoroughly with running water and dried

Administration Topical: For external use only; rinse thoroughly after each use

Patient Information Avoid prolonged contact with skin

Dosage Forms

Foam (Septisol®): 0.23% with alcohol 56% (180 mL, 600 mL)

Liquid, topical (pHisoHex®): 3% (8 mL, 150 mL, 500 mL, 3840 mL)

References

Lester RS, "Topical Formulary for the Pediatrician," *Pediatr Clin North Am*, 1983, 30(4):749-65.

♦ **Hexadrol® Phosphate Injection** *see* Dexamethasone *on page 294*

♦ **Hexadrol® Tablet** *see* Dexamethasone *on page 294*

♦ **Hexamethylenetetramine** *see* Methenamine *on page 615*

♦ **Hexit® (Canada)** *see* Lindane *on page 572*

♦ **Hibiclens® [OTC]** *see* Chlorhexidine Gluconate *on page 209*

♦ **Hibidil® 1:2000 (Canada)** *see* Chlorhexidine Gluconate *on page 209*

♦ **Hibistat® [OTC]** *see* Chlorhexidine Gluconate *on page 209*

♦ **Hibitane® Skin Cleanser (Canada)** *see* Chlorhexidine Gluconate *on page 209*

♦ **Hi-Cor-1.0® Topical** *see* Hydrocortisone *on page 486*

♦ **Hi-Cor-2.5® Topical** *see* Hydrocortisone *on page 486*

♦ **Hiprex®** *see* Methenamine *on page 615*

♦ **Histantil (Canada)** *see* Promethazine *on page 805*

♦ **Histerone® Injection** *see* Testosterone *on page 905*

Histrelin *(his TREL in)*

Brand Names Supprelin™

Synonyms ORF17070; RWJ17070

Therapeutic Category Gonadotropin Releasing Hormone Analog

Generic Available No

Use Central idiopathic precocious puberty; also used to treat estrogen-associated gynecological disorders [ie, endometriosis, intermittent porphyria, possibly premenstrual syndrome, leiomyomata uteri (uterine fibroids)]

Pregnancy Risk Factor X

Contraindications Hypersensitivity to histrelin or any component; pregnancy or expected pregnancy, breast-feeding

Precautions Inadequate control of pubertal process may occur with noncompliance or changes in the dosing schedule

Adverse Reactions

Central nervous system: Anxiety, depression, irritability, insomnia, headaches, rarely increase in seizure frequency

Endocrine & metabolic: Prevention of ovulation and menses, inhibition of spermatogenesis, breast tenderness, amenorrhea, transient testicular enlargement

Gastrointestinal: Nausea, vomiting

Genitourinary: Vaginal dryness, dyspareunia, increase in urinary calcium excretion

Local: Irritation at injection site

Neuromuscular & skeletal: Joint stiffness, possible osteoporosis

Miscellaneous: Severe hypersensitivity reactions (ie, angioedema, urticaria, hypotension, etc)

Stability Protect from light, store in refrigerator, discard unused portion

Mechanism of Action Central idiopathic precocious puberty: Histrelin is a synthetic long-acting gonadotropin-releasing hormone analog; with daily administration, it desensitizes the pituitary to endogenous gonadotropin-releasing hormone (ie, suppresses gonadotropin release by causing down regulation of the pituitary); this results in a decrease in gonadal sex steroid production which stops the secondary sexual development

Pharmacodynamics Precocious puberty: Onset of hormonal response: Physical evidence of reduction in secretion of sex steroids within 3 months

Usual Dosage S.C.:

Children ≥2 years: Central idiopathic precocious puberty: 10 mcg/kg/day; give as a single daily injection

Adult female:

Acute intermittent porphyria: 5 mcg/day

Endometriosis: 100 mcg/day

Leiomyomata uteri: 20-50 mcg/day or 4 mcg/day

Administration Parenteral: S.C.: Vary the injection site daily; administer dose at the same time each day; allow vial to warm to room temperature before giving dose

Monitoring Parameters Precocious puberty: Prior to initiating therapy: Height and weight, hand and wrist x-rays, total sex steroid levels, beta-hCG level, adrenal steroid level, gonadotropin-releasing hormone stimulation test, pelvic/adrenal/testicular ultrasound/head CT; during therapy monitor 3 months after initiation and then every 6-12 months; serial levels of sex steroids and gonadotropin-releasing hormone testing; physical exam; secondary sexual development

Additional Information Noncompliance or changing the dosage schedule may result in inadequate control; histrelin may be discontinued when the patient reaches the appropriate age for puberty

Dosage Forms Injection: 7-day kits of single use: 120 mcg/0.6 mL; 300 mcg/0.6 mL; 600 mcg/0.6 mL

♦ **Hi-Vegi-Lip®** see Pancreatin on page 723

♦ **Hivid®** see Zalcitabine on page 988

♦ **HMS Liquifilm®** see Medrysone on page 600

♦ **HN₂** see Mechlorethamine on page 595

♦ **Hold® DM [OTC]** see Dextromethorphan on page 304

Homatropine (hoe MA troe peen)

Brand Names AK-Homatropine®; Isopto® Homatropine

Available Salts Homatropine Hydrobromide

Therapeutic Category Anticholinergic Agent, Ophthalmic; Ophthalmic Agent, Mydriatic

Generic Available Yes

Use Producing cycloplegia and mydriasis for refraction; treatment of acute inflammatory conditions of the uveal tract

Pregnancy Risk Factor C

Contraindications Hypersensitivity to homatropine or any component; narrow-angle glaucoma, acute hemorrhage

Precautions Use with caution in patients with hypertension, cardiac disease, increased intraocular pressure, obstructive uropathy, paralytic ileus, or ulcerative colitis

Adverse Reactions

Cardiovascular: Vascular congestion, edema

Central nervous system: Drowsiness

Dermatologic: Eczematoid dermatitis

Ocular: Follicular conjunctivitis, blurred vision, increased intraocular pressure, stinging, exudate

(Continued)

Homatropine *(Continued)*

Mechanism of Action Blocks response of iris sphincter muscle and the accommodative muscle of the ciliary body to cholinergic stimulation resulting in dilation and loss of accommodation

Pharmacodynamics Ophthalmic:
Onset of accommodation and pupil effect:
Maximum mydriatic effect: Within 10-30 minutes
Maximum cycloplegic effect: Within 30-90 minutes
Duration:
Mydriasis: Persists for 6 hours to 4 days
Cycloplegia: 10-48 hours

Usual Dosage Ophthalmic:
Children:
Mydriasis and cycloplegia for refraction: Instill 1 drop of 2% solution immediately before the procedure; repeat at 10-minute intervals as needed
Uveitis: Instill 1 drop of 2% solution 2-3 times/day
Adults:
Mydriasis and cycloplegia for refraction: Instill 1-2 drops of 2% solution or 1 drop of 5% solution before the procedure; repeat at 5- to 10-minute intervals as needed
Uveitis: Instill 1-2 drops of either 2% or 5% solution 2-3 times/day up to every 3-4 hours as needed

Administration Ophthalmic: Finger pressure should be applied to lacrimal sac for 1-2 minutes after instillation to decrease risk of absorption and systemic reactions

Dosage Forms Solution, ophthalmic, as hydrobromide:
2% (1 mL, 5 mL); 5% (1 mL, 2 mL, 5 mL)
AK-Homatropine®: 5% (15 mL)
Isopto® Homatropine 2% (5 mL, 15 mL); 5% (5 mL, 15 mL)

♦ **Homatropine Hydrobromide** *see* Homatropine *on page 477*

♦ **Horse Antihuman Thymocyte Gamma Globulin** *see* Lymphocyte Immune Globulin *on page 586*

♦ **H.P. Acthar® Gel** *see* Corticotropin *on page 254*

♦ **Humalog®** *see* Insulin Preparations *on page 518*

♦ **Humalog® Mix 50/50™** *see* Insulin Preparations *on page 518*

♦ **Humalog® Mix 75/25™** *see* Insulin Preparations *on page 518*

Human Growth Hormone (HYU man grothe HOR mone)

Brand Names Genotropin® Injection; Humatrope® Injection; Norditropin® Injection; Nutropin® AQ Injection; Nutropin® Depot™; Nutropin® Injection; Protropin® Injection; Saizen® Injection; Serostim® Injection

Synonyms Growth Hormone; Somatrem; Somatropin

Therapeutic Category Growth Hormone

Generic Available No

Use Long-term treatment of growth failure from lack of or inadequate endogenous growth hormone secretion; Nutropin®: Treatment of children who have growth failure associated with chronic renal insufficiency up until the time of renal transplantation; short stature associated with Turner syndrome in patients whose epiphyses are not closed; adults with growth hormone deficiency as a result of pituitary disease, hypothalamic disease, surgery, radiation, or trauma; Serostim®: AIDS-related wasting or cachexia

Pregnancy Risk Factor C; Serostim® (only): B

Contraindications Do not use for growth promotion in pediatric patients with closed epiphyses; hypersensitivity to human growth hormone, benzyl alcohol (sometrem), M-cresol, or glycerin (somatropin) or any component; evidence of active malignancy; progression of any underlying intracranial lesion or actively growing intracranial tumor; patients with acute critical illness due to complications following open heart or abdominal surgery, multiple accidental trauma, or acute respiratory failure

Precautions Use with caution in patients with diabetes or family history of diabetes; somatrem contains benzyl alcohol, use with caution in neonates; insulin dosage may require adjustment when growth hormone therapy is instituted; patients with hypopituitarism may develop hypothyroidism during growth hormone therapy; children may develop slipped capital epiphyses during therapy

Adverse Reactions
Cardiovascular: Mild transient edema
Central nervous system: Headache, intracranial hypertension

Dermatologic: Increased growth of pre-existing nevi; local lipoatrophy or lipodystrophy (S.C. administration)

Endocrine & metabolic: Reversible hypothyroidism (reported in pituitary-derived growth hormone), mild hyperglycemia; gynecomastia (rare)

Gastrointestinal: pancreatitis (rare)

Hematologic: Small risk for developing leukemia

Local: Pain at injection site

Neuromuscular & skeletal: Carpal tunnel syndrome (rare), pain in hip/knee

Renal: Glucosuria

Drug Interactions Corticosteroids may inhibit growth hormone activity

Stability Refrigerate once reconstituted (all products except Nutropin® Depot™); stable for 14 days after reconstitution when refrigerated; Nutropin® AQ (aqueous form) is stable for 28 days after initial entry; Nutropin® Depot™ must be used immediately after reconstitution

Mechanism of Action Somatropin and somatrem are purified polypeptide hormones of recombinant DNA origin; somatropin contains the identical sequence of amino acids found in human growth hormone while somatrem's amino acid sequence is identical plus an additional amino acid, methionine; human growth hormone stimulates growth of linear bone, skeletal muscle, and organs; stimulates erythropoietin which increases red blood cell mass; exerts both insulin-like and diabetogenic effects

Pharmacokinetics Somatrem and somatropin have equivalent pharmacokinetic profiles

Absorption: I.M.: Well absorbed

Distribution: V_d: 50 mL/kg

Metabolism: ~90% of dose metabolized in the liver and kidney cells

Bioavailability: S.C.: 81 ± 20%

Half-life: S.C.: 2.3 ± 0.42 hours

Elimination: 0.1% of dose excreted in urine unchanged

Usual Dosage

Children: I.M., S.C.:

Growth hormone inadequacy:

Somatrem: 0.3 mg/kg (0.9 international units/kg) **weekly** divided into daily doses

Somatropin:

Humatrope®: 0.18 mg/kg (0.54 international units/kg) **weekly** divided into equal doses given either on alternate days or 6 times per week; maximum **weekly** dosage: 0.3 mg/kg (0.9 international units/kg)

Norditropin®: 0.024-0.034 mg/kg/dose (0.07-0.1 international units/kg/dose) 6-7 times per week

Nutropin®: 0.3 mg/kg (0.9 international units/kg) **weekly** divided into daily doses; in pubertal patients, dosage may be increased to 0.7 mg/kg (2.1 international units/kg) **weekly** divided into daily doses

Saizen®: 0.06 mg/kg (0.18 international units/kg) 3 times per week

Nutropin® Depot™: S.C. only:

Once-monthly injection: 1.5 mg/kg body weight administered on the same day of each month; patients >15 kg will require more than one injection per dose

Twice-monthly injection: 0.75 mg/kg body weight administered twice each month on the same days of each month (eg, days 1 and 15 of each month); patients >30 kg will require more than one injection per dose; twice monthly dosing is recommended in patients >45 kg

Note: Human growth hormone therapy should be discontinued when the patient has reached satisfactory adult height, when epiphyses have fused, or when the patient ceases to respond. Growth of ≥5 cm/year is expected, if growth rate does not exceed 2.5 cm in a 6-month period, double the dose for the next 6 months, if there is still no satisfactory response, discontinue therapy

Chronic renal insufficiency: Nutropin®: Weekly dosage of 0.35 mg/kg (approximately 1.05 international units/kg); may be continued until time of transplantation

Turner syndrome: Weekly dosage ≤0.375 mg/kg (1.125 international units/kg) divided into equal doses daily or on 3 alternate days

Adults: Growth hormone deficiency: 0.006 mg/kg/day (0.018 international units/kg/day) once daily; may be increased to a maximum of 0.025 mg/kg/day (0.075 international units/kg) in patients <35 years of age and to a maximum of 0.0125 mg/kg/day (0.0375 international units/kg/day) in patients >35 years of age

AIDS-related wasting or cachexia: Serostim®:

Children (limited information): 0.04-0.07 mg/kg/day for 4 weeks

Adults: Administered once daily at bedtime:

<35 kg: 0.1 mg/kg

(Continued)

Human Growth Hormone *(Continued)*

35-44 kg: 4 mg
45-55 kg: 5 mg
>55 kg: 6 mg

Administration Parenteral: Administer S.C. or I.M.; do not shake; rotate injection site

Somatrem: Reconstitute each 5 mg vial with 1-5 mL bacteriostatic water for injection, USP (benzyl alcohol preserved) only; when using in newborns, reconstitute with preservative free sterile water

Somatropin: Reconstitute each 5 mg vial with 1.5-5 mL diluent; when using in newborns, reconstitute with preservative free sterile water

Nutropin® Depot™: Reconstitute vials with provided diluent only, resulting in 19 mg/mL concentration; swirl vigorously for 2 minutes until all the powder is fully dispersed; withdraw measured dose, change to a new needle, and administer immediately to avoid settling of the suspension in the syringe; inject S.C. at a continuous rate over no more than 5 seconds

Note: When treating chronic renal insufficiency patients, growth hormone should be administered as follows: in hemodialysis patients, administer injection at night just prior to sleeping and at least 3-4 hours after dialysis; in chronic cycling peritoneal dialysis patients, administer injection in the morning after dialysis; in chronic ambulatory peritoneal dialysis patients administer injection in the evening at the time of the overnight exchange.

Monitoring Parameters Growth curve, periodic thyroid function tests, bone age (annually), periodical urine testing for glucose, somatomedin C levels

Patient Information Report the development of a severe headache, acute visual changes, a limp or complaints of hip or knee pain to your physician

Additional Information S.C. administration can cause local lipoatrophy or lipodystrophy and may enhance the development of neutralizing antibodies

Dosage Forms Powder for injection (lyophilized):

Somatropin:

Genotropin®: 1.5 mg [1.3 mg/mL (4 international units/mL)]; 5.8 mg [5 mg/mL (15 international units/mL)]; 13.8 mg [12 mg/mL (36 international units/mL)]

Humatrope®: 5 mg ~15 international units

Norditropin®: 4 mg ~12 international units; 8 mg ~24 international units

Nutropin® (rDNA origin): 5 mg ~15 international units (10 mL); 10 mg ~30 international units (10 mL)

Nutropin® AQ (rDNA origin): 10 mg ~30 international units (2 mL)

Nutropin® Depot™ (rDNA origin): 13.5 mg (3 mL); 18 mg (3 mL); 22.5 mg (3 mL)

Saizen® (rDNA origin): 5 mg ~15 international units

Serostim®: 4 mg (12 international units); 5 mg (15 international units); 10 mg (30 international units)

Somatrem, Protropin®: 5 mg ~15 international units (10 mL); 10 mg ~30 international units (10 mL)

References

Howrie DL, "Growth Hormone for the Treatment of Growth Failure in Children," *Clin Pharm*, 1987, 6(4):283-91.

Hyaluronidase (hye al yoor ON i dase)

Related Information
Extravasation Treatment *on page 1050*

Brand Names Wydase®

Therapeutic Category Antidote, Extravasation

Generic Available No

Use Increase the dispersion and absorption of other drugs; increase rate of absorption of parenteral fluids given by hypodermoclysis; management of I.V. extravasations

Pregnancy Risk Factor C

Contraindications Hypersensitivity to hyaluronidase or any component; do not inject in or around infected, inflamed, or cancerous areas

Warnings Drug infiltrates in which hyaluronidase is **not** the extravasation management of choice include dopamine and alpha agonists

Precautions Hypersensitivity reactions may occur; a preliminary intradermal skin test should be performed utilizing 0.02 mL of a 150 units/mL solution

Adverse Reactions
Cardiovascular: Tachycardia, hypotension
Central nervous system: Dizziness, chills
Dermatologic: Urticaria, erythema
Gastrointestinal: Nausea, vomiting

Drug Interactions Salicylates, cortisone, ACTH, estrogens, antihistamines (decrease effectiveness of hyaluronidase)

Stability Reconstituted hyaluronidase solution prepared from a 150 unit vial of lyophilized powder for injection is stable for 24 hours; refrigerate the stabilized hyaluronidase solution for injection

Mechanism of Action Modifies the permeability of connective tissue through hydrolysis of hyaluronic acid, one of the chief ingredients of tissue cement which offers resistance to diffusion of liquids through tissues; hyaluronidase increases both the distribution and absorption of locally injected substances

Pharmacodynamics
Onset by the S.C. or intradermal routes for the treatment of extravasation: Immediate
Duration: 24-48 hours

Usual Dosage
Infants and Children: Management of I.V. extravasation: S.C., intradermal: Reconstitute the 150 unit vial of lyophilized powder with 1 mL NS; take 0.1 mL of this solution and dilute with 0.9 mL NS to yield 15 units/mL; using a 25- or 26-gauge needle, five 0.2 mL injections are made subcutaneously or intradermally into the extravasation site at the leading edge, changing the needle after each injection; **Note:** Some sites utilize a 150 units/mL hyaluronidase solution and, without further dilution, administer 0.2 mL injections subcutaneously or intradermally into the extravasation site at the leading edge

Adults: Absorption and dispersion of drugs: I.M., S.C.: 150 units is added to the vehicle containing the drug

Hypodermoclysis: S.C.: 15 units is added to each 100 mL of I.V. fluid to be administered

Premature Infants and Neonates: Volume of a single clysis should not exceed 25 mL/kg and the rate of administration should not exceed 2 mL/minute

Children <3 years: Volume of a single clysis should not exceed 200 mL

Children ≥3 years and Adults: Rate and volume of administration should not exceed those used for I.V. infusion

Administration Management of intravenous extravasations: Do not administer I.V.; stop the infusion and remove needle; elevate extremity; administer hyaluronidase within the first few minutes to 1 hour after the extravasation is recognized

Monitoring Parameters Observe appearance of lesion for induration, swelling, discoloration, blanching, and blister formation every 15 minutes for ~2 hours

Dosage Forms
Injection, stabilized solution: 150 units/mL (1 mL, 10 mL)
Powder for injection, lyophilized: 150 units, 1500 units

References
Raszka WV, Keuser TK, Smith FR, et al, "The Use of Hyaluronidase in the Treatment of Intravenous Extravasation Injuries," *J Perinatol*, 1990, 10(2):146-9.

Zenk KE, "Hyaluronidase: An Antidote for Intravenous Extravasations," *CSHP Voice*, 1981, 66-8.

Zenk KE, Dungy CI, and Greene GR, "Nafcillin Extravasation Injury: Use of Hyaluronidase as an Antidote," *Am J Dis Child*, 1981, 135(12):1113-4.

♦ **Hycort® Topical** *see* Hydrocortisone *on page 486*

♦ **Hyderm (Canada)** *see* Hydrocortisone *on page 486*

Hydralazine (hye DRAL a zeen)

Brand Names Apo®-Hydralazine (Canada); Apresoline® Injection; Apresoline® Oral; Novo-Hylazin® (Canada); Nu-Hydral® (Canada)

Available Salts Hydralazine Hydrochloride

Therapeutic Category Antihypertensive Agent; Vasodilator

Generic Available Yes

Use Management of moderate to severe hypertension, CHF, hypertension secondary to pre-eclampsia/eclampsia, primary pulmonary hypertension

Pregnancy Risk Factor C

Contraindications Hypersensitivity to hydralazine or any component; dissecting aortic aneurysm, mitral valve rheumatic heart disease, coronary artery disease

Warnings Monitor blood pressure closely with I.V. use; modify dosage in patients with severe renal impairment; some formulations may contain tartrazines or sulfites

Precautions Discontinue hydralazine in patients who develop SLE-like syndrome or positive ANA; use with caution in patients with severe renal disease or cerebral vascular accidents

Adverse Reactions

Cardiovascular: Palpitations, flushing, tachycardia, edema, orthostatic hypotension (rare)

Central nervous system: Malaise, fever, headache, dizziness

Dermatologic: Rash

Gastrointestinal: Anorexia, nausea, vomiting, diarrhea

Neuromuscular & skeletal: Arthralgias, weakness, pyridoxine deficiency-induced peripheral neuropathy (paresthesia, numbness)

Miscellaneous: Positive ANA, positive LE cells, SLE-like syndrome

Drug Interactions MAO inhibitors may cause a significant decrease in blood pressure; indomethacin may decrease hypotensive effects

Food Interactions Avoid natural licorice (causes sodium and water retention and increases potassium loss); long-term use of hydralazine may cause pyridoxine deficiency resulting in numbness, tingling, and paresthesias; if symptoms develop, pyridoxine supplements may be needed

Stability Changes color after contact with a metal filter; do not store intact ampuls in refrigerator

Mechanism of Action Direct vasodilation of arterioles (with little effect on veins) which results in decreased systemic resistance

Pharmacodynamics

Onset of action:

Oral: 20-30 minutes

I.V.: 5-20 minutes

Duration:

Oral: 2-4 hours

I.V.: 2-6 hours

Pharmacokinetics

Distribution: Crosses placenta; appears in breast milk

Protein-binding: 85% to 90%

Metabolism: Acetylated in the liver

Bioavailability: 30% to 50%; large first-pass effect orally

Half-life, adults: 2-8 hours; half-life varies with genetically determined acetylation rates

Elimination: 14% excreted unchanged in urine

Usual Dosage

Infants and Children:

Oral: Initial: 0.75-1 mg/kg/day in 2-4 divided doses, not to exceed 25 mg/dose; increase over 3-4 weeks to maximum of 5 mg/kg/day in infants and 7.5 mg/kg/day in children, given in 2-4 divided doses; maximum daily dose: 200 mg/day

I.M., I.V.: Initial: 0.1-0.2 mg/kg/dose (not to exceed 20 mg) every 4-6 hours as needed; up to 1.7-3.5 mg/kg/day divided in 4-6 doses

Adults:

Oral: Initial: 10 mg 4 times/day, increase by 10-25 mg/dose every 2-5 days to maximum of 300 mg/day

I.M., I.V.: Hypertension: Initial: 10-20 mg/dose every 4-6 hours as needed, may increase to 40 mg/dose

I.M., I.V.: Pre-eclampsia/eclampsia: 5 mg/dose then 5-10 mg every 20-30 minutes as needed

Dosing interval in renal impairment:

Cl_{cr} 10-50 mL/minute: Administer every 8 hours

Cl$_{cr}$ <10 mL/minute: Administer every 8-16 hours in fast acetylators and every 12-24 hours in slow acetylators

Administration
Oral: Administer with food
Parenteral: I.V.: Do not exceed rate of 0.2 mg/kg/minute; maximum concentration for I.V. use: 20 mg/mL

Monitoring Parameters Heart rate, blood pressure, ANA titer

Patient Information Limit alcohol; notify physician if flu-like symptoms occur

Nursing Implications I.V. use: Monitor blood pressure closely

Additional Information Slow acetylators, patients with decreased renal function and patients receiving >200 mg/day (chronically) are at higher risk for SLE. Titrate dosage to patient's response. Usually administered with diuretic and a beta-blocker to counteract hydralazine's side effects of sodium and water retention and reflex tachycardia.

Dosage Forms
Injection, as hydrochloride: 20 mg/mL (1 mL)
Tablet, as hydrochloride: 10 mg, 25 mg, 50 mg, 100 mg

Extemporaneous Preparations
An oral solution (20 mg/5 mL) has been made from 20 mL of the hydralazine injection (20 mg/mL), 8 mL of propylene glycol and purified water USP qsad 100 mL; expected stability: 30 days if refrigerated (Nahata, 1997)

A flavored syrup (1.25 mg/mL) has been made using seventy-five hydralazine hydrochloride 50 mg tablets, dissolved in 250 mL of distilled water with 2250 g of Lycasin® (75% w/w maltitol syrup vehicle); edetate disodium 3 g and sodium saccharin 3 g dissolved in 50 mL distilled water was added; solution was preserved with 30 mL of a solution containing methylparaben 10% (w/v) and propylparaben 2% (w/v) in propylene glycol; flavored with 3 mL orange flavoring; qsad to 3 L with distilled water and then pH adjusted to pH of 3.7 using glacial acetic acid; measured stability was 5 days at room temperature (25°C); less than 2% loss of hydralazine occurred at 2 weeks when syrup was stored at 5°C (Alexander, 1993)

A 4 mg/mL oral liquid preparation made from tablets was **not** stable for very long; preparation made in cherry syrup was not even stable for 1 day; preparation made in a 1:1 mixture of Ora-Sweet® and Ora-Plus® was stable for only 1 day under refrigeration (5°C) and not even 1 day at room temperature (25°C); preparation made in a 1:1 mixture of Ora-Sweet® SF and Ora-Plus® was stable for only 2 days under refrigeration (5°C), but not even 1 day at room temperature (25°C) (Allen, 1998).

Alexander KS, Pudipeddi M, and Parker GA, "Stability of Hydralazine Hydrochloride Syrup Compounded From Tablets," *Am J Hosp Pharm*, 1993, 50(4):683-6.

Allen LV and Erickson MA, "Stability of Alprazolam, Chloroquine Phosphate, Cisapride, Enalapril Maleate, and Hydralazine Hydrochloride in Extemporaneously Compounded Oral Liquids," *Am J Health Syst Pharm*, 1998, 55(18):1915-20.

Nahata MC and Hipple TF, *Pediatric Drug Formulations*, 3rd ed, Cincinnati, OH: Harvey Whitney Books Co, 1997.

♦ **Hydralazine Hydrochloride** see Hydralazine on page 482
♦ **Hydramyn® Syrup [OTC]** see Diphenhydramine on page 327
♦ **Hydrated Chloral** see Chloral Hydrate on page 204
♦ **Hydrate® Injection** see Dimenhydrinate on page 325
♦ **Hydrea®** see Hydroxyurea on page 494
♦ **Hydrocet®** see Hydrocodone and Acetaminophen on page 485

Hydrochlorothiazide (hye droe klor oh THYE a zide)

Related Information
Carbohydrate and Alcohol Content of Liquid Medications for Use in Patients Receiving Ketogenic Diets on page 1228

Brand Names Apo®-Hydro (Canada); Diuchlor® (Canada); Esidrix®; Ezide®; Hydro-DIURIL®; Hydro-Par®; Microzide®; Neo-Codema® (Canada); Novo-Hydrazide® (Canada); Oretic®; Urozide® (Canada)

Synonyms HCTZ

Therapeutic Category Antihypertensive Agent; Diuretic, Thiazide

Generic Available Yes: Tablet

Use Management of mild to moderate hypertension; treatment of edema in CHF and nephrotic syndrome

Pregnancy Risk Factor B (per manufacturer), D (based upon expert analysis)

(Continued)

Hydrochlorothiazide *(Continued)*

Contraindications Hypersensitivity to hydrochlorothiazide or any component; cross-sensitivity with other thiazides or sulfonamides; anuria

Precautions Use with caution in patients with severe renal disease (Cl_{cr} <10 mL/minute), impaired hepatic function, hepatic disease, gout, lupus erythematosus, diabetes mellitus; some products may contain tartrazine

Adverse Reactions

Cardiovascular: Hypotension

Central nervous system: Drowsiness, vertigo, headache

Dermatologic: Photosensitivity

Endocrine & metabolic: Hypokalemia, hyperglycemia, hypochloremic metabolic alkalosis, hyperlipidemia, hyperuricemia

Gastrointestinal: Nausea, vomiting, anorexia, diarrhea, cramping, pancreatitis

Hematologic: Aplastic anemia, hemolytic anemia, leukopenia, agranulocytosis, thrombocytopenia

Hepatic: Hepatitis, intrahepatic cholestasis

Neuromuscular & skeletal: Muscle weakness, paresthesia

Renal: Polyuria, prerenal azotemia

Drug Interactions NSAIDs decrease antihypertensive effect; steroids, amphotericin B increase potassium losses; hydrochlorothiazide increases hypersensitivity reactions to allopurinol; decreased clearance of lithium; increased hyperglycemia with diazoxide; hydrochlorothiazide decreases effectiveness of antidiabetic agents in blood sugar control; cholestyramine decreases hydrochlorothiazide absorption

Food Interactions Avoid natural licorice (causes sodium and water retention and increases potassium loss); may need to decrease sodium and calcium and increase potassium, zinc, magnesium, and riboflavin in diet

Mechanism of Action Inhibits sodium reabsorption in the distal tubules causing increased excretion of sodium and water as well as potassium, hydrogen, magnesium, phosphate, calcium, and bicarbonate ions

Pharmacodynamics

Onset of diuretic action: Oral: Within 2 hours

Peak effects: Within 3-6 hours

Duration: 6-12 hours

Pharmacokinetics

Absorption: Oral: ~60% to 80%

Distribution: Breast milk to plasma ratio: 0.25

Half-life: 5.6-14.8 hours

Elimination: Unchanged in urine

Usual Dosage Oral: (daily dosages should be decreased if used with other antihypertensives):

Neonates and Infants <6 months: 2-4 mg/kg/day in 2 divided doses; maximum daily dosage: 37.5 mg

Infants >6 months and Children: 2 mg/kg/day in 2 divided doses; maximum daily dosage: 200 mg

Adults: 25-100 mg/day in 1-2 doses; maximum dose: 200 mg/day

Dosage adjustment in renal impairment: Cl_{cr} <25-50 mL/minute: May not be effective

Administration Oral: Administer with food or milk

Monitoring Parameters Serum electrolytes, BUN, creatinine, blood pressure, fluid balance, body weight

Dosage Forms

Capsule: 12.5 mg

Solution, oral (mint flavor): 50 mg/5 mL (50 mL)

Tablet: 25 mg, 50 mg, 100 mg

Hydrochlorothiazide and Spironolactone

(hye droe klor oh THYE a zide & speer on oh LAK tone)

Brand Names Alazide®; Aldactazide®; Spironazide®; Spirozide®

Synonyms Spironolactone and Hydrochlorothiazide

Therapeutic Category Antihypertensive Agent, Combination; Diuretic, Combination

Generic Available Yes

Use Management of mild to moderate hypertension; treatment of edema in CHF and nephrotic syndrome

Pregnancy Risk Factor C

Contraindications Anuria, hyperkalemia, renal or hepatic failure; hypersensitivity to hydrochlorothiazide, spironolactone, or any component; cross-sensitivity with other thiazides or sulfonamides; patients receiving triamterene or amiloride

Warnings This fixed combination is not indicated for initial therapy of hypertension; therapy requires titration to the individual patient; if dosage so determined represents this fixed combination, its use may be more convenient

Adverse Reactions See individual components, Hydrochlorothiazide *on page 483* and Spironolactone *on page 877*, for full adverse drug reaction information

Drug Interactions Drugs that increase serum potassium (amiloride, triamterene, indomethacin, ACE inhibitors); digoxin decreases renal clearance; see individual components, Hydrochlorothiazide *on page 483* and Spironolactone *on page 877*, for full adverse drug reaction information

Food Interactions Avoid food with high potassium content, natural licorice (causes sodium and water retention and increases potassium loss), and salt substitutes

Usual Dosage Oral: As the product is in a fixed combination of equal mg doses, the following dosages represent mg of either spironolactone **or** hydrochlorothiazide

Children: 1.5-3 mg/kg/day in 2-4 divided doses; maximum daily dosage: 200 mg
Adults: 25-200 mg in 1-2 divided doses

Administration Oral: Administer in the morning; administer the last dose of multiple doses before 6 PM unless instructed otherwise; administer with food or milk

Monitoring Parameters Blood pressure, serum electrolytes, renal function

Test Interactions Spironolactone may interfere with plasma and urinary cortisol levels and the radioimmunoassay for digoxin

Dosage Forms Tablet:
25/25: Hydrochlorothiazide 25 mg and spironolactone 25 mg
50/50: Hydrochlorothiazide 50 mg and spironolactone 50 mg

Extemporaneous Preparations A 5 mg/mL oral suspension may be compounded by crushing twenty-four 25 mg (spironolactone/HCTZ) Aldactazide® tablets; add geometric amounts of a 1:1 mixture of Ora-Sweet® and Ora-Plus®, or Ora-Sweet® SF and Ora-Plus®, or cherry syrup alone to a final volume of 120 mL; shake well, refrigerate; stable 60 days

Allen LV and Erickson MA, "Stability of Labetalol Hydrochloride, Metoprolol Tartrate, Verapamil Hydrochloride, and Spironolactone With Hydrochlorothiazide in Extemporaneously Compounded Oral Liquids," *Am J Health Syst Pharm*, 1996, 53(19):2304-9.

♦ **Hydrocil® [OTC]** *see* Psyllium *on page 823*
♦ **Hydro-Cobex®** *see* Hydroxocobalamin *on page 492*

Hydrocodone and Acetaminophen
(hye droe KOE done & a seet a MIN oh fen)

Related Information
Narcotic Analgesics Comparison *on page 1035*
Overdose and Toxicology *on page 1191*

Brand Names Anexsia®; Anodynos-DHC®; Bancap HC®; Co-Gesic®; Dolacet®; DuoCet™; Duradyne DHC®; Hydrocet®; Hydrogesic®; Hy-Phen®; Lorcet®; Lorcet® 10/650; Lorcet®-HD; Lorcet® Plus; Lortab®; Margesic® H; Norcet®; Stagesic®; T-Gesic®; Vapocet®; Vicodin®; Vicodin® ES; Zydone®

Available Salts Hydrocodone Bitartrate and Acetaminophen

Synonyms Acetaminophen and Hydrocodone

Therapeutic Category Analgesic, Narcotic; Antitussive; Cough Preparation

Generic Available Yes

Use Relief of moderate to severe pain; antitussive (hydrocodone)

Restrictions C-III

Pregnancy Risk Factor C

Contraindications CNS depression; hypersensitivity to hydrocodone, acetaminophen, or any component; severe respiratory depression

Warnings Some tablets contain sulfites which may cause allergic reactions

Precautions Use with caution in patients with hypersensitivity reactions to other phenanthrene derivative opioid agonists (morphine, codeine, hydromorphone, oxycodone, oxymorphone, levorphanol)

Adverse Reactions
Cardiovascular: Hypotension, bradycardia, peripheral vasodilation
Central nervous system: CNS depression, drowsiness, dizziness, sedation, increased intracranial pressure
Endocrine & metabolic: Antidiuretic hormone release
Gastrointestinal: Nausea, vomiting, constipation, biliary tract spasm
(Continued)

Hydrocodone and Acetaminophen *(Continued)*

Genitourinary: Urinary tract spasm
Ocular: Miosis
Respiratory: Respiratory depression
Miscellaneous: Histamine release, physical and psychological dependence with prolonged use

Drug Interactions CNS depressants, alcohol, phenothiazines, tricyclic antidepressants may potentiate the adverse effects of hydrocodone

Food Interactions Rate of absorption of acetaminophen may be decreased when given with food high in carbohydrates

Mechanism of Action Inhibits the synthesis of prostaglandins in the central nervous system and peripherally blocks pain impulse generation; produces antipyresis from inhibition of hypothalamic heat-regulating center

Pharmacodynamics Narcotic analgesia: Oral:
Onset of action: Within 10-20 minutes
Duration: 3-6 hours

Usual Dosage Oral:
Antitussive (doses based on hydrocodone):
Children: 0.6 mg/kg/day or 20 mg/m²/day divided in 3-4 doses/day
<2 years: Do not exceed 1.25 mg/single dose
2-12 years: Do not exceed 5 mg/single dose
>12 years: Do not exceed 10 mg/single dose
Analgesic: Doses should be titrated to appropriate analgesic effect
Children: Dose has not been established
Adults: 1-2 tablets or capsules every 4-6 hours as needed

Administration Oral: May administer with food or milk to decrease GI distress

Monitoring Parameters Pain relief, respiratory rate, blood pressure

Patient Information Avoid alcohol; may cause drowsiness and impair ability to perform hazardous activities requiring mental alertness; may be habit-forming

Dosage Forms
Capsule:
Bancap HC®, Dolacet®, Hydrocet®, Hydrogesic®, Lorcet®-HD, Margesic® H, Norcet®, Stagesic®, T-Gesic®, Zydone®: Hydrocodone bitartrate 5 mg and acetaminophen 500 mg
Elixir, oral (tropical fruit punch flavor) (Lortab®): Hydrocodone bitartrate 2.5 mg and acetaminophen 167 mg per 5 mL with alcohol 7% (480 mL)
Tablet: Hydrocodone bitartrate 5 mg and acetaminophen 400 mg; hydrocodone bitartrate 7.5 mg and acetaminophen 400 mg; hydrocodone bitartrate 10 mg and acetaminophen 400 mg; hydrocodone bitartrate 5 mg and acetaminophen 500 mg; hydrocodone bitartrate 7.5 mg and acetaminophen 500 mg; hydrocodone bitartrate 7.5 mg and acetaminophen 650 mg; hydrocodone bitartrate 7.5 mg and acetaminophen 750 mg; hydrocodone bitartrate 10 mg and acetaminophen 650 mg
Lortab® 2.5/500: Hydrocodone bitartrate 2.5 mg and acetaminophen 500 mg
Anexsia® 5/500, Anodynos-DHC®, Co-Gesic®, DuoCet™, Duradyne DHC®, Hy-Phen®, Lorcet®, Lortab®® 5/500, Vicodin®: Hydrocodone bitartrate 5 mg and acetaminophen 500 mg
Lortab® 7.5/500: Hydrocodone bitartrate 7.5 mg and acetaminophen 500 mg
Anexsia® 7.5/650, Lorcet® Plus: Hydrocodone bitartrate 7.5 mg and acetaminophen 650 mg
Vicodin® ES: Hydrocodone bitartrate 7.5 mg and acetaminophen 750 mg
Lortab® 10/500: Hydrocodone bitartrate 10 mg and acetaminophen 500 mg
Lortab® 10/650: Hydrocodone bitartrate 10 mg and acetaminophen 650 mg
Lorcet® 10/650: Hydrocodone bitartrate 10 mg and acetaminophen 650 mg
Zydone®: Hydrocodone bitartrate 5 mg and acetaminophen 400 mg; hydrocodone bitartrate 7.5 mg and acetaminophen 400 mg; Hydrocodone bitartrate 10 mg and acetaminophen 400 mg

♦ **Hydrocodone Bitartrate and Acetaminophen** *see* Hydrocodone and Acetaminophen *on page 485*

Hydrocortisone *(hye droe KOR ti sone)*
Related Information
Carbohydrate and Alcohol Content of Liquid Medications for Use in Patients Receiving Ketogenic Diets *on page 1228*
Corticosteroids Comparison, Systemic *on page 1032*
Corticosteroids Comparison, Topical *on page 1033*

Brand Names Acticort® Topical; Aeroseb-HC® Topical; A-hydroCort® Injection; Ala-Cort® Topical; Ala-Scalp® Topical; Anusol® HC-1 Topical [OTC]; Anusol® HC-2.5% Topical [OTC]; Anusol-HC® Suppository; Aquacort® (Canada); Bactine® Hydrocortisone [OTC]; CaldeCort® Anti-Itch Topical Spray; CaldeCort® Topical [OTC]; Cetacort® Topical; Clocort® Maximum Strength [OTC]; Colocort™ Rectal; CortaGel® Topical [OTC]; Cortaid® Maximum Strength Topical [OTC]; Cortaid® with Aloe Topical [OTC]; Cortamed® (Canada); Cortate® (Canada); Cort-Dome® High Potency Suppository; Cort-Dome® Topical; Cortef® Feminine Itch Topical; Cortef® Oral; Cortenema® Rectal; Corticreme® (Canada); Cortifoam® Rectal; Cortiment® (Canada); Cortizone®-5 Topical [OTC]; Cortizone®-10 Topical [OTC]; Cortoderm (Canada); Delcort® Topical; Dermacort® Topical; Dermarest Dricort® Topical; Dermolate® Topical [OTC]; Dermtex® HC with Aloe Topical [OTC]; Eldecort® Topical; Emo-Cort™ (Canada); Gynecort® Topical [OTC]; Hi-Cor-1.0® Topical; Hi-Cor-2.5® Topical; Hycort® Topical; Hyderm (Canada); Hydrocortone® Acetate Injection; Hydrocortone® Oral; Hydrocortone® Phosphate Injection; Hydrocort® Topical; Hydro-Tex® Topical [OTC]; Hytone® Topical; LactiCare-HC® Topical; Lanacort® Topical [OTC]; Locoid® Topical; Nutracort® Topical; Orabase® HCA Topical; Penecort® Topical; Prevex™ HC (Canada); Proctocort™ Rectal; Rectocort (Canada); Scalpicin® Topical; Solu-Cortef® Injection; S-T Cort® Topical; Synacort® Topical; Tegrin®-HC Topical [OTC]; Texacort® Topical; U-Cort™ Topical; Westcort® Topical

Available Salts Hydrocortisone Acetate; Hydrocortisone Butyrate; Hydrocortisone Cypionate; Hydrocortisone Sodium Phosphate; Hydrocortisone Sodium Succinate; Hydrocortisone Valerate

Synonyms Compound F; Cortisol

Therapeutic Category Adrenal Corticosteroid; Antiasthmatic; Anti-inflammatory Agent; Anti-inflammatory Agent, Rectal; Corticosteroid, Rectal; Corticosteroid, Systemic; Corticosteroid, Topical; Glucocorticoid

Generic Available Yes

Use Management of adrenocortical insufficiency; relief of inflammation of corticosteroid-responsive dermatoses; adjunctive treatment of ulcerative colitis

Pregnancy Risk Factor C

Contraindications Serious infections, except septic shock or tuberculous meningitis; hypersensitivity to hydrocortisone or any component; viral, fungal, or tubercular skin lesions

Warnings Acute adrenal insufficiency may occur with abrupt withdrawal after long-term therapy or with stress; infants and small children may be more susceptible to hypothalamic-pituitary-adrenal (HPA) suppression from topical therapy; some preparations and manufacturer supplied diluents contain benzyl alcohol (eg, Act-o-vial®, A-hydroCort®)

Precautions Use with caution in patients with hyperthyroidism, cirrhosis, nonspecific ulcerative colitis, hypertension, osteoporosis, thromboembolic tendencies, CHF, convulsive disorders, myasthenia gravis, thrombophlebitis, peptic ulcer, diabetes; suppression of HPA function, suppression of linear growth, or hypercorticism (Cushing's syndrome) may occur

Adverse Reactions

Cardiovascular: Hypertension, edema

Central nervous system: Euphoria, insomnia, headache

Dermatologic: Acne, dermatitis, skin atrophy

Endocrine & metabolic: Hypokalemia, hyperglycemia, Cushing's syndrome, growth suppression; suppression of HPA function

Gastrointestinal: Peptic ulcer

Ocular: Cataracts

Miscellaneous: Immunosuppression

Drug Interactions Cytochrome P-450 isoenzyme CYP2D6 and CYP3A3/4 substrate

Barbiturates, phenytoin, rifampin, salicylates, NSAIDs, diuretics (potassium depleting), warfarin; caffeine and alcohol may increase risk for GI ulcer; live virus vaccines (increase risk of viral infection); vaccines may have decreased effects

Food Interactions Systemic use of corticosteroids may require a diet with increased potassium, vitamins A, B_6, C, D, folate, calcium, zinc, phosphorus, and decreased sodium

Mechanism of Action Decreases inflammation by suppression of migration of polymorphonuclear leukocytes and reversal of increased capillary permeability

Pharmacodynamics Anti-inflammatory effects:

Peak effect:

Oral: 12-24 hours

I.V.: 4-6 hours

(Continued)

Hydrocortisone *(Continued)*

Duration: 8-12 hours

Pharmacokinetics

Absorption: Rapid by all routes, except rectally

Metabolism: In the liver

Half-life, biologic: 8-12 hours

Elimination: Renally, mainly as 17-hydroxysteroids and 17-ketosteroids

Usual Dosage Dose should be based on severity of disease and patient response

Acute adrenal insufficiency: I.M., I.V.:

Infants and young Children: 1-2 mg/kg/dose I.V. bolus, then 25-150 mg/day in divided doses every 6-8 hours

Older Children: 1-2 mg/kg I.V. bolus, then 150-250 mg/day in divided doses every 6-8 hours

Adults: 100 mg I.V. bolus, then 300 mg/day in divided doses every 8 hours or as a continuous infusion for 48 hours; once patient is stable change to oral, 50 mg every 8 hours for 6 doses, then taper to 30-50 mg/day in divided doses

Anti-inflammatory or immunosuppressive:

Infants and Children:

Oral: 2.5-10 mg/kg/day or 75-300 mg/m^2/day divided every 6-8 hours

I.M., I.V.: 1-5 mg/kg/day or 30-150 mg/m^2/day divided every 12-24 hours

Adolescents and Adults: Oral, I.M., I.V., S.C.: 15-240 mg every 12 hours

Congenital adrenal hyperplasia: Oral: Initial: 30-36 mg/m^2/day with $^1/_3$ of dose every morning and $^2/_3$ every evening or $^1/_4$ every morning and midday and $^1/_2$ every evening; maintenance: 20-25 mg/m^2/day in divided doses

Physiologic replacement: Children:

Oral: 0.5-0.75 mg/kg/day or 20-25 mg/m^2/day divided every 8 hours

I.M.: 0.25-0.35 mg/kg/day or 12-15 mg/m^2/day once daily

Shock: I.V.: **Sodium succinate:**

Children: Initial: 50 mg/kg then repeated in 4 hours and/or every 24 hours if needed

Adolescents and Adults: 500 mg to 2 g every 2-6 hours

Status asthmaticus:

Children: I.V.: Optional loading dose: 4-8 mg/kg; maximum: 250 mg; then maintenance: 2 mg/kg/dose every 6 hours

Adults: 100-500 mg every 6 hours

Adolescents and Adults: Rectal: Apply 1 application 1-2 times/day for 2-3 weeks

Ulcerative colitis: One enema nightly for 21 days, or until remission occurs; clinical symptoms should subside within 3-5 days; discontinue use if no improvement within 2-3 weeks; some patients may require 2-3 months of therapy; if therapy lasts >21 days, discontinue slowly by decreasing use to every other night for 2-3 weeks

Children and Adults: Topical: Apply 3-4 times/day

Administration

Oral: Administer with food or milk to decrease GI upset

Parenteral:

I.V. bolus: Dilute to 50 mg/mL and administer over 3-5 minutes

I.V. intermittent infusion: Dilute to 1 mg/mL and administer over 20-30 minutes; maximum concentration: 5 mg/mL

Rectal: Patient should lie on left side during administration and for 30 minutes after; retain enema for at least 1 hour, preferably all night

Topical: Apply a thin film to clean, dry skin and rub in gently

Monitoring Parameters Blood pressure, weight, serum glucose, electrolytes

Reference Range Hydrocortisone (normal endogenous morning levels) 4-30 μg/mL

Test Interactions Skin tests

Patient Information Limit caffeine; avoid alcohol; do not decrease dose or discontinue without physician's approval; avoid exposure to measles or chicken pox, advise physician immediately if exposed

Additional Information A variety of salt forms are available and can lead to confusion in prescribing, dispensing, and administration; please use the appropriate salt/dosage form for the following indications:

Acetate: For intra-articular, intrasynovial, intrabursal, intralesional, or soft tissue injection only (use **Cortisone** acetate for I.M. use)

Cypionate: Oral suspension

Sodium phosphate: For general I.V. use

Sodium succinate: For general I.V. use, I.V. use in patients allergic to sodium phosphate salt, I.V. for shock and for intrathecal use (must reconstitute with a preservative free diluent or use a preservative free product)

To facilitate retention of enema, prior antidiarrheal medication or sedation may be required (especially when beginning therapy)

Dosage Forms

Hydrocortisone **acetate**:
  Aerosol, rectal (Cortifoam®): 10% [90 mg/applicatorful] 20 g
  Cream: Hydrocortisone acetate, USP: 2.5%
    CaldeCORT®, Corticaine®, Cortaid® with Aloe, Cortef® Feminine Itch, Gynecort-5®, Lanacort-5®: 0.5% (15 g, 22.5 g, 30 g)
    CaldeCORT®, Clocort® Maximum Strength, Cortaid® Maximum Strength, Dermarest Dricort®, U-Cort™: 1% (15 g, 30 g, 120 g)
  Ointment, topical:
    Cortaid® with Aloe, Lanacort-5®: 0.5% (15 g, 30 g)
    Cortaid® Maximum Strength, Gynecort® 10, Lanacort® 10: 1% (15 g, 30 g)
  Injection, suspension: 25 mg/mL (10 mL); 50 mg/mL (10 mL)
    Hydrocortone® Acetate: 25 mg/mL (5 mL); 50 mg/mL (5 mL)
  Suppository, rectal (Cort-Dome® High Potency, Anusol-HC®): 25 mg
  Paste (Orabase® HCA): 0.5% (5 g)
Hydrocortisone **base**:
  Aerosol, topical:
    Aeroseb-HC®, CaldeCORT® Anti-Itch Spray, Cortaid®: 0.5% (45 g, 58 g)
    Cortaid® Maximum Strength: 1% (45 mL)
  Cream: 0.5% (15 g, 30 g, 120 g, 454 g); 1% (20 g, 30 g, 120 g, 454 g); 2.5% (20 g, 30 g, 454 g)
    Bactine® Hydrocortisone, Cort-Dome®, Cortizone®-5, DermiCort®, Dermolate®, Dermtex® HC with Aloe, HydroSKIN®, Hydro-Tex®: 0.5% (15 g, 30 g)
    Ala-Cort®, Cort-Dome®, Delcort®, Dermacort®, DermiCort®, Eldecort®, Hi-Cor 1.0®, Hycort®, Hytone®, Nutracort®, Penecort®, Synacort®: 1% (15 g, 20 g, 30 g)
    Anusol®-HC 2.5%, Eldecort®, Hi-Cor-2.5®, Hydrocort®, Hytone®, Synacort®: 2.5% (15 g, 20 g, 30 g, 60 g)
    Rectal (Proctocort™): 1% (30 g)
  Gel:
    CortaGel®: 0.5% (15 g, 30 g)
    CortaGel® Extra Strength: 1% (15 g, 30 g)
  Lotion: 0.5% (30 mL, 60 mL, 120 mL); 1% (120 mL)
    Cetacort®: 0.25% (120 mL)
    Cetacort®, DermiCort®, HydroSKIN®, S-T Cort®: 0.5% (60 mL, 120 mL)
    Acticort 100®, Ala-Cort®, Cetacort®, Cortizone-10®, Dermacort®, HydroSKIN® Maximum Strength, Hytone®, LactiCare-HC®, Nutracort®: 1% (60 mL, 120 mL)
    Ala-Scalp®: 2% (30 mL)
    Hytone®, LactiCare-HC®, Nutracort®: 2.5% (60 mL, 120 mL)
  Ointment, topical: 0.5% (30 g); 1% (20 g, 30 g, 120 g); 2.5% (20 g)
    Cortizone®-5, HydroSKIN®: 0.5% (30 g)
    Cortizone®-10, Hycort®, HydroSKIN®, Hydro-Tex®, Hytone®, Tegrin®-HC: 1% (15 g, 20 g, 30 g, 60 g, 120 g, 240 g, 454 g)
    Hytone®: 2.5% (30 g)
  Solution, rectal (Colocort™): 100 mg/60 mL (7s)
  Solution, topical (Penecort®, Scalpicin®, Texacort®): 1% (30 mL, 60 mL)
  Suspension, rectal (Cortenema®): 100 mg/60 mL (7s)
  Tablet: 10 mg, 20 mg
    Cortef®: 5 mg, 10 mg, 20 mg
    Hydrocortone®: 10 mg, 20 mg
Hydrocortisone **butyrate** (Locoid®):
  Cream: 0.1%
  Ointment, topical: 0.1%
  Solution, rectal (Colocort™): 100 mg/60 mL (7s)
  Solution, topical: 0.1% (20 mL, 60 mL)
Hydrocortisone **cypionate**:
  Suspension, oral (Cortef®): 10 mg/5 mL (120 mL)
Hydrocortisone **sodium phosphate**:
  Injection (Hydrocortone® Phosphate): 50 mg/mL (2 mL, 10 mL)
Hydrocortisone **sodium succinate**:
  Injection (A-hydroCort®, Solu-Cortef®): 100 mg, 250 mg, 500 mg, 1000 mg
Hydrocortisone **valerate** (Westcort®):
  Cream: 0.2% (15 g, 45 g, 60 g)
(Continued)

Hydrocortisone *(Continued)*

Ointment, topical: 0.2% (15 g, 45 g, 60 g, 120 g)

♦ **Hydrocortisone Acetate** *see* Hydrocortisone *on page 486*
♦ **Hydrocortisone Butyrate** *see* Hydrocortisone *on page 486*
♦ **Hydrocortisone Cypionate** *see* Hydrocortisone *on page 486*
♦ **Hydrocortisone, Neomycin, (Bacitracin), and Polymyxin B** *see* Neomycin, (Bacitracin) Polymyxin B, and Hydrocortisone *on page 679*
♦ **Hydrocortisone Sodium Phosphate** *see* Hydrocortisone *on page 486*
♦ **Hydrocortisone Sodium Succinate** *see* Hydrocortisone *on page 486*
♦ **Hydrocortisone Valerate** *see* Hydrocortisone *on page 486*
♦ **Hydrocortone® Acetate Injection** *see* Hydrocortisone *on page 486*
♦ **Hydrocortone® Oral** *see* Hydrocortisone *on page 486*
♦ **Hydrocortone® Phosphate Injection** *see* Hydrocortisone *on page 486*
♦ **Hydrocort® Topical** *see* Hydrocortisone *on page 486*
♦ **Hydro-Crysti-12®** *see* Hydroxocobalamin *on page 492*
♦ **HydroDIURIL®** *see* Hydrochlorothiazide *on page 483*
♦ **Hydrodolasetron** *see* Dolasetron *on page 337*
♦ **Hydrogen Dioxide** *see* Hydrogen Peroxide *on page 490*

Hydrogen Peroxide (HYE droe jen per OKS ide)

Brand Names Peroxyl®
Synonyms H_2O_2; Hydrogen Dioxide; Peroxide
Therapeutic Category Antibacterial, Otic; Antibacterial, Topical; Antibiotic, Oral Rinse
Generic Available Yes
Use Cleanse wounds, suppurating ulcers, and local infections; used in the treatment of inflammatory conditions of the external auditory canal and as a mouthwash or gargle; hydrogen peroxide concentrate (30%) has been used as a hair bleach and as a tooth bleaching agent
Contraindications Should not be used in abscesses
Warnings Hydrogen peroxide concentrate (30%) is a caustic liquid; it should not be tasted since it is strongly irritating to skin or mucous membranes
Precautions Repeat use as a mouthwash or gargle may produce irritation of the buccal mucous membrane or "hairy tongue"; bandages should not be applied too quickly after its use
Adverse Reactions
Dermatologic: Bleaching effect on hair, irritating burn
Gastrointestinal: Rupture of the colon, proctitis, ulcerative colitis, gas embolism, hairy tongue
Local: Irritation of the buccal mucous membrane
Stability Protect from light and heat; decomposes upon standing, upon repeated agitation, or when in contact with oxidizing or reducing substances
Mechanism of Action Antiseptic oxidant that slowly releases oxygen and water upon contact with serum or tissue catalase
Pharmacodynamics Duration of action: Only while bubbling action occurs
Usual Dosage Children and Adults:
Mouthwash or gargle: Dilute the 3% solution with an equal volume of water; swish around in the mouth over the affected area for at least 1 minute and then expel; use up to 4 times/day (after meals and at bedtime)
Topical:
1.5% to 3% solution for cleansing wounds
1.5% gel for cleansing wounds or mouth/gum irritations: Apply a small amount to the affected area for at least 1 minute, then expectorate; use up to 4 times/day (after meals and at bedtime)
Administration Topical: Do not inject or instill into closed body cavities from which released oxygen cannot escape; strong solutions (30.5%) of hydrogen peroxide should not be applied undiluted to tissues
Dosage Forms
Gel, oral: 1.5% (15 g)
Solution:
Concentrate: 30.5% (480 mL)
Topical: 3% (120 mL, 480 mL)

♦ **Hydrogesic®** *see* Hydrocodone and Acetaminophen *on page 485*

Hydromorphone (hye droe MOR fone)

Related Information

Laboratory Detection of Drugs in Urine *on page 1204*
Narcotic Analgesics Comparison *on page 1035*
Overdose and Toxicology *on page 1191*

Brand Names Dilaudid® Cough Syrup; Dilaudid-HP® Injection; Dilaudid® Injection; Dilaudid® Oral; Dilaudid® Suppository; PMS-Hydromorphone (Canada)

Available Salts Hydromorphone Hydrochloride

Therapeutic Category Analgesic, Narcotic; Antitussive; Cough Preparation

Generic Available Yes

Use Management of moderate to severe pain; antitussive at lower doses

Restrictions C-II

Pregnancy Risk Factor C

Contraindications Hypersensitivity to hydromorphone or any component

Warnings Some injectable formulations contain benzyl alcohol; tablet and syrup contain tartrazine which may cause allergic reactions

Precautions Use with caution in patients with hypersensitivity reactions to other phenanthrene derivative opioid agonists (morphine, hydrocodone, levorphanol, oxycodone, oxymorphone, codeine) or significant respiratory disease

Adverse Reactions

Cardiovascular: Palpitations, hypotension, bradycardia, peripheral vasodilation
Central nervous system: CNS depression, increased intracranial pressure, drowsiness, dizziness, sedation
Dermatologic: Pruritus
Endocrine & metabolic: Antidiuretic hormone release
Gastrointestinal: Nausea, vomiting, constipation, biliary tract spasm
Genitourinary: Urinary tract spasm
Ocular: Miosis
Respiratory: Respiratory depression
Miscellaneous: Histamine release, physical and psychological dependence with prolonged use

Drug Interactions CNS depressants, alcohol, phenothiazines, tricyclic antidepressants may potentiate the adverse effects of hydromorphone

Stability Protect tablets from light; do not store intact ampuls in refrigerator; a slight yellow discoloration has not been associated with a loss of potency

Mechanism of Action Binds to opiate receptors in the CNS, causing inhibition of ascending pain pathways, altering the perception of and response to pain; causes cough suppression by direct central action in the medulla; produces generalized CNS depression

Pharmacodynamics Analgesic effects: Oral:
Onset of action: Within 15-30 minutes
Peak effect: Within 30-90 minutes
Duration: 4-5 hours

Pharmacokinetics

Metabolism: Primarily in the liver
Bioavailability: 62%
Half-life: 1-3 hours
Elimination: In urine, principally as glucuronide conjugates

Usual Dosage

Antitussive: Oral:
Children 6-12 years: 0.5 mg every 3-4 hours as needed
Children >12 years and Adults: 1 mg every 3-4 hours as needed
Pain: Doses should be titrated to appropriate analgesic effects; when changing routes of administration, note that oral doses are less than one-half as effective as parenteral doses (may be only $^1/_5$ as effective):
Young children:
Oral: 0.03-0.08 mg/kg/dose every 4-6 hours as needed; maximum dose: 5 mg/dose
I.V.: 0.015 mg/kg/dose every 4-6 hours as needed
Older Children and Adults: Oral, I.M., I.V., S.C.: 1-4 mg/dose every 4-6 hours as needed; usual adult dose: 2 mg/dose

Administration

Oral: Administer with food or milk to decrease GI upset
Parenteral: I.V.: Administer via slow I.V. injection over at least 2-3 minutes

Monitoring Parameters Pain relief, respiratory rate, blood pressure

Patient Information Avoid alcohol; may cause drowsiness and impair ability to perform hazardous activities requiring mental alertness; may be habit-forming
(Continued)

491

Hydromorphone *(Continued)*

Additional Information Equianalgesic doses: Morphine 10 mg I.M. = hydromorphone 1.5 mg I.M.

Dosage Forms
Injection, as hydrochloride: 1 mg/mL (1 mL); 2 mg/mL (1 mL, 20 mL); 3 mg/mL (1 mL); 4 mg/mL (1 mL); 10 mg/mL (1 mL, 2 mL, 5 mL)
Solution, as hydrochloride: 5 mg/5 mL (480 mL)
Suppository, rectal, as hydrochloride: 3 mg (6s)
Syrup: Hydromorphone 1 mg with guaifenesin 100 mg per 5 mL
Tablet, as hydrochloride: 2 mg, 4 mg, 8 mg

♦ **Hydromorphone Hydrochloride** *see* Hydromorphone *on page 491*
♦ **Hydro-Par®** *see* Hydrochlorothiazide *on page 483*
♦ **Hydro-Tex® Topical [OTC]** *see* Hydrocortisone *on page 486*

Hydroxocobalamin *(hye droks oh koe BAL a min)*
Brand Names Hydro-Cobex®; Hydro-Crysti-12®; LA-12®
Synonyms Vitamin B$_{12}$
Therapeutic Category Nutritional Supplement; Vitamin, Water Soluble
Generic Available No
Use Treatment of pernicious anemia and other vitamin B$_{12}$ deficiency states; dietary supplement particularly in conditions of increased requirements (eg, pregnancy, thyrotoxicosis, hemorrhage, malignancy, liver or kidney disease)
Pregnancy Risk Factor C
Contraindications Hypersensitivity to cyanocobalamin or any component, cobalt
Warnings Parenteral injections may contain preservatives, avoid use in neonates; anaphylactic shock has occurred after parenteral vitamin B$_{12}$ administration; intradermal skin testing may be used prior to administration in individuals sensitive to cobalt
Precautions Serum potassium concentrations should be monitored early as severe hypokalemia has occurred after the conversion of megaloblastic anemia to normal erythropoiesis; the increase in nucleic acid degradation produced by administration of hydroxocobalamin to deficient patients may result in gout in susceptible individuals; use of hydroxocobalamin in folic acid deficient individuals may improve folate-deficient megaloblastic anemia and obscure the true diagnosis
Adverse Reactions
Cardiovascular: Peripheral vascular thrombosis
Dermatologic: Itching, exanthema, urticaria
Endocrine & metabolic: Hypokalemia
Gastrointestinal: Diarrhea
Local: Pain at injection site
Miscellaneous: Hypersensitivity reactions
Drug Interactions Decreased absorption of hydroxocobalamin from GI tract by aminoglycoside antibiotics, colchicine, extended release potassium products, aminosalicylic acid, excessive alcohol use, phenytoin, and phenobarbital; antagonism of hematopoietic response to hydroxocobalamin when administered with chloramphenicol
Stability Protect from light
Mechanism of Action Coenzyme for various metabolic functions, including fat and carbohydrate metabolism and protein synthesis, used in cell replication and hematopoiesis
Pharmacodynamics
Onset: I.M.:
Megaloblastic anemia:
Conversion of megaloblastic to normoblastic erythroid hyperplasia within bone marrow: 8 hours
Increased reticulocytes: 2-5 days
Complicated vitamin B$_{12}$ deficiency:
Psychiatric sequelae: 24 hours
Thrombocytopenia: 10 days
Granulocytopenia: 2 weeks
Pharmacokinetics
Distribution: Principally stored in the liver; also stored in the kidneys and adrenals
Protein binding: Bound to transcobalamin II
Metabolism: Converted in the tissues to active coenzymes methylcobalamin and deoxyadenosylcobalamin
Time to peak serum concentration: 2 hours
Elimination: 50% to 98% unchanged in the urine

Usual Dosage I.M.:

Schilling test (diagnostic for vitamin B_{12} deficiency): Children and Adults: 1000 mcg once

Congenital transcobalamin deficiency: Neonates: 1000 mcg twice weekly

Vitamin B_{12} deficiency or pernicious anemia: Varying regimens:

Uncomplicated disease:

Children: Initial: 100 mcg/day for 10-15 days (total dose: 1-5 mg); maintenance: 60 mcg/month

or as an alternative: 30-50 mcg/day for at least 2 weeks (total dose: 1-5 mg); maintenance: 100 mcg/month

Adults: Initial: 30 mcg/day for 5-10 days; maintenance: 100-200 mcg/monthly

or as an alternative: 1000 mcg/day for 5-10 days, followed by 100-200 mcg/month

or as an alternative: 100 mcg/day for 1 week, followed by 100 mcg every other day for 2 weeks; maintenance: 100 mcg/month

Complicated disease (eg, severe anemia with heart failure, thrombocytopenia with bleeding, granulocytopenia with infection, severe neurologic damage): Adults: 1000 mcg plus folic acid 15 mg once, followed by 100 mcg/day plus oral folic acid 5 mg/day for 1 week; maintenance dosing as above

Dosage interval in hepatic or renal impairment: A decrease in the interval between injections may be required

Administration Parenteral: I.M. injection only; do not administer S.C.

Monitoring Parameters Serum potassium, erythrocyte and reticulocyte counts, hemoglobin, hematocrit

Reference Range Normal: 200-900 pg/mL; vitamin B_{12} deficiency: <200 pg/mL; megaloblastic anemia: <100 pg/mL

Patient Information Life-long therapy is required in patients with pernicious anemia or other absorption defects; do not discontinue therapy without consulting your physician

Additional Information Cyanocobalamin is preferred over hydroxocobalamin due to reports of antibody formation to the hydroxocobalamin-transcobalamin complex

Dosage Forms Injection: 1000 mcg/mL (10 mL, 30 mL)

♦ **Hydroxy-1,4-naphthoquinone** see Atovaquone on page 103

Hydroxychloroquine (hye droks ee KLOR oh kwin)

Brand Names Plaquenil® Sulfate

Available Salts Hydroxychloroquine Sulfate

Therapeutic Category Antimalarial Agent; Antirheumatic, Disease Modifying

Generic Available No

Use Suppression or chemoprophylaxis of malaria caused by susceptible *P. vivax, P. ovale, P. malariae,* and some strains of *P. falciparum* (not active against pre-erythrocytic or exoerythrocytic tissue stages of *Plasmodium*); treatment of systemic lupus erythematosus (SLE) and rheumatoid arthritis

Pregnancy Risk Factor C

Contraindications Retinal or visual field changes; hypersensitivity to hydroxychloroquine, 4-aminoquinoline derivatives, or any component; patients with porphyria or psoriasis

Warnings Long-term use in children is **not** recommended; daily dose >6-6.5 mg/kg/day in patients with abnormal hepatic or renal function may be associated with an increased risk of retinal toxicity

Precautions Use with caution in patients with hepatic disease and G-6-PD deficiency

Adverse Reactions

Central nervous system: Insomnia, nervousness, nightmares, psychosis, headache, confusion, agitation, ataxia

Dermatologic: Lichenoid dermatitis, bleaching of the hair, pruritus, hyperpigmentation

Gastrointestinal: GI irritation, anorexia, nausea, vomiting, diarrhea

Hematologic: Bone marrow suppression, thrombocytopenia

Hepatic: Hepatic failure

Neuromuscular & skeletal: Muscle weakness, peripheral neuropathy

Ocular: Visual field defects, blindness, retinitis, macular degeneration, decreased night vision

Drug Interactions Increases digoxin serum levels

Food Interactions Food increases bioavailability

Stability Protect from light

(Continued)

Hydroxychloroquine *(Continued)*

Mechanism of Action Interferes with digestive vacuole function within sensitive malarial parasites by increasing the pH and interfering with lysosomal degradation of hemoglobin; inhibits locomotion of neutrophils and chemotaxis of eosinophils; impairs complement-dependent antigen-antibody reactions

Pharmacodynamics Onset of action for JRA: 2-4 months, up to 6 months

Pharmacokinetics

Absorption: Highly variable (31% to 100%)

Distribution: Extensive distribution to most body fluids and tissues; excreted into breast milk; crosses the placenta

Metabolism: In the liver

Bioavailability: Increased when administered with food

Elimination: Metabolites and unchanged drug slowly excreted in the urine

Usual Dosage Oral:

Children:

Chemoprophylaxis of malaria: 5 mg/kg **(base)** once weekly; should not exceed the recommended adult dose; begin 1-2 weeks before exposure; continue for 4 weeks after leaving endemic area

Uncomplicated acute attack of malaria: 10 mg/kg **(base)** initial dose; followed by 5 mg/kg **(base)** in 6-8 hours on day 1; 5 mg/kg **(base)** as a single dose on day 2 and on day 3

JRA or SLE: 3-5 mg/kg/day **(as sulfate)** divided 1-2 times/day to a maximum of 400 mg/day **(as sulfate)**; not to exceed 7 mg/kg/day

Adults:

Chemoprophylaxis of malaria: 310 mg **(base)** once weekly on same day each week; begin 1-2 weeks before exposure; continue for 4 weeks after leaving endemic area

Uncomplicated acute attack of malaria: 620 mg **(base)** first dose day 1; 310 mg **(base)** in 6-8 hours day 1; 310 mg **(base)** as a single dose day 2; and 310 mg **(base)** as a single dose on day 3

Rheumatoid arthritis: 400-600 mg/day **(as sulfate)** once daily to start; increase dose until optimum response level is reached; usually after 4-12 weeks dose should be reduced by 50% and a maintenance dose given of 200-400 mg/day **(as sulfate)** divided 1-2 times/day

Lupus erythematosus: 400 mg **(as sulfate)** every day or twice daily for several weeks depending on response; 200-400 mg/day **(as sulfate)** for prolonged maintenance therapy

Administration Oral: Administer with food or milk to decrease GI distress

Monitoring Parameters Ophthalmologic examination, CBC; check for muscular weakness with prolonged therapy

Patient Information Wear sunglasses in bright sunlight; notify physician if blurring of vision, vision change, emotional change, or unusual skin rashes occur; may cause dizziness and vision changes, so exercise caution when driving; avoid alcohol; contraindicated during breast-feeding

Dosage Forms Tablet, as sulfate: 200 mg [base 155 mg]

Extemporaneous Preparations A 25 mg/mL hydroxychloroquine sulfate suspension is made by removing the coating off of fifteen 200 mg hydroxychloroquine sulfate tablets with a towel moistened with alcohol; tablets are ground to a fine powder and levigated to a paste with 15 mL of Ora-Plus® suspending agent; add an additional 45 mL of suspending agent and levigate until a uniform mixture is obtained; qs ad to 120 mL with sterile water for irrigation; a 30 day expiration date is recommended, although stability testing has not been performed

Pesko LJ, "Compounding: Hydroxychloroquine," *Am Druggist*, 1993, 207:57.

References

Emery H, "Clinical Aspects of Systemic Lupus Erythematosus in Childhood," *Pediatr Clin North Am*, 1986, 33(5):1177-90.

Giannini EH and Cawkwell GD, "Drug Treatment in Children With Juvenile Rheumatoid Arthritis. Past, Present, and Future," *Pediatr Clin North Am*, 1995, 42(5):1099-125.

"Guidelines for the Management of Rheumatoid Arthritis. American College of Rheumatology Ad Hoc Committee on Clinical Guidelines," *Arthritis Rheum*, 1996, 39(5):713-22.

- ♦ **Hydroxychloroquine Sulfate** *see* Hydroxychloroquine *on page 493*
- ♦ **Hydroxydaunomycin** *see* Doxorubicin *on page 346*
- ♦ **Hydroxyethyl Starch** *see* Hetastarch *on page 474*
- ♦ **Hydroxynorephedrine** *see* Metaraminol *on page 612*

Hydroxyurea *(hye droks ee yoor EE a)*

Related Information

Adult and Adolescent HIV *on page 1133*

Emetogenic Potential of Single Chemotherapeutic Agents *on page 1095*

Brand Names Droxia™; Hydrea®

Therapeutic Category Antineoplastic Agent, Miscellaneous

Generic Available Yes

Use Treatment of chronic myelocytic leukemia (CML), melanoma, and ovarian carcinoma; used with radiation in treatment of tumors of the head and neck; adjunct in the management of sickle cell patients; combination therapy with didanosine for treatment of HIV infection

Pregnancy Risk Factor D

Contraindications Severe anemia, severe bone marrow suppression; WBC <2500/mm³ or platelet count <100,000/mm³; hypersensitivity to hydroxyurea or any component

Warnings The FDA currently recommends that procedures for proper handling and disposal of antineoplastic agents be considered; hydroxyurea is presumed to be a human carcinogen; secondary leukemia and skin cancer have been reported in patients receiving long-term hydroxyurea therapy. Hydroxyurea is embryotoxic and causes fetal malformations.

Precautions Use with caution and modify dose in patients with renal impairment

Adverse Reactions

Central nervous system: Dizziness, disorientation, hallucinations, seizures, headache, fever

Dermatologic: Maculopapular rash, facial erythema, thinning of the skin

Endocrine & metabolic: Hyperuricemia

Gastrointestinal: Nausea, vomiting, diarrhea, constipation, anorexia, stomatitis

Genitourinary: Dysuria

Hematologic: Myelosuppression (leukopenia, thrombocytopenia), megaloblastic anemia,

Hepatic: Elevated hepatic enzymes

Renal: Renal tubular function impairment, elevated BUN, elevated serum creatinine

Drug Interactions Fluorouracil, cytarabine (increases cytarabine activity)

Stability Store in a tightly sealed container since the drug is degraded by moisture; store at room temperature

Mechanism of Action Interferes with synthesis of DNA during the S-phase of cell division without interfering with RNA synthesis; inhibits ribonucleoside diphosphate reductase preventing conversion of ribonucleotides to deoxyribonucleotides; hydroxyurea also inhibits the incorporation of thymidine into DNA; in sickle cell patients, hydroxyurea increases the production of fetal hemoglobin

Pharmacodynamics Peak response for sickle cell disease: 6-18 months

Pharmacokinetics

Absorption: Readily from the GI tract

Distribution: Readily crosses the blood-brain barrier and the placenta; distributes into peritoneal or pleural effusions; excreted in breast milk

Metabolism: In the liver

Half-life: 3-4 hours

Time to peak serum concentration: Within 2 hours

Elimination: 50% of drug excreted unchanged in urine; renal excretion of urea (metabolite) and respiratory excretion of CO_2 (metabolic end product)

Usual Dosage Oral (refer to individual protocols): Base dosage on ideal body weight:

Children:

Treatment of pediatric astrocytoma, medulloblastoma, and primitive neuroectodermal tumors: No FDA approved dosage regimens have been established. Dosages of 1500-3000 mg/m² as a single dose in combination with other agents, followed by a second course 2 weeks later with subsequent courses every 4-6 weeks have been used (eight-in-1 regimen).

CML: Initial: 10-20 mg/kg/day once daily; adjust dose according to hematologic response

Children and Adults: Sickle cell anemia: Initial dose: 15 mg/kg/day (range: 10-20 mg/kg/day) once daily; increase dose in increments of 5 mg/kg/day every 12 weeks to a maximum dose of 35 mg/kg/day; reduced dosage of hydroxyurea alternating with erythropoietin may decrease myelotoxicity and increase levels of fetal hemoglobin in patients who have not been helped by hydroxyurea alone

Adults:

Solid tumors:

Intermittent therapy: 80 mg/kg as a single dose every third day

Continuous therapy: 20-30 mg/kg/day given as a single dose/day

(Continued)

Hydroxyurea *(Continued)*

Concomitant therapy with irradiation: 80 mg/kg as a single dose every third day starting at least 7 days before initiation of irradiation

Resistant chronic myelocytic leukemia: 20-30 mg/kg/day once daily

HIV infection: 500 mg twice daily (15 mg/kg/day divided twice daily) in combination with didanosine 200 mg twice daily

Dosing adjustment in renal impairment: Dose should be reduced 50% in patients with a GFR <10 mL/minute

Administration Oral: Administer with water on an empty stomach; for patients unable to swallow capsules, contents of capsule may be emptied into a glass of water if administered immediately

Monitoring Parameters CBC with differential and platelet count, hemoglobin, renal function and liver function tests, serum uric acid

Test Interactions False-negative triglyceride measurement by a glycerol oxidase method

Patient Information Inform physician if fever, sore throat, bruising, or bleeding develops; advise women of childbearing potential to avoid becoming pregnant while taking hydroxyurea

Additional Information Myelosuppressive effects:

WBC: Moderate

Platelets: Moderate

Onset (days): 7

Nadir (days): 10

Recovery (days): 21

Dosage Forms Capsule: 200 mg, 300 mg, 400 mg, 500 mg

References

Geyer JR, Finlay JL, Boyett JM, et al, "Survival of Infants With Malignant Astrocytomas. A Report From the Childrens Cancer Group," *Cancer*, 1995, 75(4):1045-50.

Geyer JR, Pendergrass TW, Milstein JM, et al, "Eight Drugs in One Day Chemotherapy in Children With Brain Tumors: A Critical Toxicity Appraisal," *J Clin Oncol*, 1988, 6(6):996-1000.

Maier-Redelsperger M, de Montalembert M, Flahault A, et al, "Fetal Hemoglobin and F-Cell Responses to Long-Term Hydroxyurea Treatment in Young Sickle Cell Patients. The French Study Group on Sickle Cell Disease," *Blood*, 1998, 91(12):4472-9.

Montaner JS, Zala C, Conway B, et al, "A Pilot Study of Hydroxyurea Among Patients With Advanced Human Immunodeficiency Virus (HIV) Disease Receiving Chronic Didanosine Therapy: Canadian HIV Trials Network Protocol 080," *J Infect Dis*, 1997, 175(4):801-6.

Rodgers GP, Dover GJ, Noguchi CT, et al, "Hematologic Responses of Patients With Sickle Cell Disease to Treatment With Hydroxyurea," *N Engl J Med*, 1990, 322(15):1037-45.

Rodgers GP, Dover GJ, Uyesaka N, et al, "Augmentation by Erythropoietin of the Fetal-Hemoglobin Response to Hydroxyurea in Sickle Cell Disease," *N Engl J Med*, 1993, 328(2):73-80.

Hydroxyzine *(hye DROKS i zeen)*

Related Information

Carbohydrate and Alcohol Content of Liquid Medications for Use in Patients Receiving Ketogenic Diets *on page 1228*

Compatibility of Medications Mixed in a Syringe *on page 1208*

Brand Names Anxanil® Oral; Apo®-Hydroxyzine (Canada); Atarax® Oral; Atozine® Oral; Durrax® Oral; Hy-Pam® Oral; Hyzine-50® Injection; Multipax® (Canada); Neucalm-50® Injection; Novo-Hydroxyzine® (Canada); PMS-Hydroxyzine (Canada); Quiess® Injection; Vamate® Oral; Vistacon-50® Injection; Vistaquel® Injection; Vistaril® Injection; Vistaril® Oral; Vistazine® Injection

Available Salts Hydroxyzine Hydrochloride; Hydroxyzine Pamoate

Therapeutic Category Antianxiety Agent; Antiemetic; Antihistamine; Sedative

Generic Available Yes

Use Treatment of anxiety; preoperative sedative; antipruritic; antiemetic

Pregnancy Risk Factor C

Contraindications Hypersensitivity to hydroxyzine or any component

Warnings Subcutaneous, intra-arterial and I.V. administration **not** recommended since thrombosis and digital gangrene can occur; extravasation can result in sterile abscess and marked tissue induration

Precautions Injection may contain benzyl alcohol; use with caution in patients with narrow-angle glaucoma, prostatic hypertrophy, bladder neck obstruction, asthma, or COPD

Adverse Reactions

Cardiovascular: Hypotension

Central nervous system: Drowsiness, dizziness, headache, ataxia

Gastrointestinal: Xerostomia

Genitourinary: Urinary retention

Local: Pain at injection site

Neuromuscular & skeletal: Weakness

Miscellaneous: Anticholinergic effects

Drug Interactions Hydroxyzine may potentiate other CNS depressants, alcohol, or anticholinergics, and can antagonize the vasopressor effects of epinephrine

Stability Protect from light

Mechanism of Action Competes with histamine for H_1-receptor sites on effector cells in the gastrointestinal tract, blood vessels, and respiratory tract

Pharmacodynamics
Onset of effects: Within 15-30 minutes
Duration: 4-6 hours

Usual Dosage
Children:
Oral: 2 mg/kg/day divided every 6-8 hours
I.M.: 0.5-1 mg/kg/dose every 4-6 hours as needed
Adults:
Antiemetic: I.M.: 25-100 mg/dose every 4-6 hours as needed
Anxiety: Oral: 25-100 mg 4 times/day; maximum dose: 600 mg/day
Preoperative sedation:
Oral: 50-100 mg
I.M.: 25-100 mg
Management of pruritus: Oral: 25 mg 3-4 times/day

Administration Parenteral: For I.M. administration in children, injections should be made into the midlateral muscles of the thigh; hydroxyzine has been administered slow I.V. to oncology patients via central venous lines without problems

Monitoring Parameters Relief of symptoms, mental status

Patient Information Avoid alcohol; may cause dry mouth; may cause drowsiness and impair ability to perform hazardous activities requiring mental alertness

Additional Information Atarax® syrup contains sucrose, spearmint, peppermint oil, and sodium benzoate; Vistaril® suspension contains sorbitol, lemon #78 flavoring

Dosage Forms
Hydroxyzine **hydrochloride:**
Injection:
Vistaril®: 25 mg/mL (1 mL, 2 mL, 10 mL)
Hydroxacen®, Hyzine-50®, Neucalm®, Quiess®, Vistacon-50®, Vistaquel®, Vistaril®, Vistazine®: 50 mg/mL (1 mL, 2 mL, 10 mL)
Syrup (Atarax®): 10 mg/5 mL (120 mL, 480 mL, 4000 mL)
Tablet:
Anxanil®: 25 mg
Atarax®: 10 mg, 25 mg, 50 mg, 100 mg
Atozine®: 10 mg, 25 mg, 50 mg
Durrax®: 10 mg, 25 mg
Hydroxyzine **pamoate:**
Capsule:
Hy-Pam®: 25 mg, 50 mg
Vamate®: 25 mg, 50 mg, 100 mg
Vistaril®: 25 mg, 50 mg, 100 mg
Suspension, oral (Vistaril®:) 25 mg/5 mL (120 mL, 480 mL)

References
Berde C, Ablin A, Glazer J, et al, "American Academy of Pediatrics Report of the Subcommittee on Disease-Related Pain in Childhood Cancer," *Pediatrics,* 1990, 86(5 Pt 2):818-25.

♦ **Hydroxyzine Hydrochloride** *see* Hydroxyzine *on page 496*
♦ **Hydroxyzine Pamoate** *see* Hydroxyzine *on page 496*
♦ **Hyoscine** *see* Scopolamine *on page 860*

Hyoscyamine (hye oh SYE a meen)

Brand Names Anaspaz®; A-Spas® S/L; Cystospaz®; Cystospaz-M®; Donnamar®; ED-SPAZ®; Gastrosed™; Levbid®; Levsin®; Levsinex®; Levsin/SL®

Available Salts Hyoscyamine Sulfate

Therapeutic Category Anticholinergic Agent; Antispasmodic Agent, Gastrointestinal

Generic Available Yes

Use Treatment of GI tract disorders caused by spasm; adjunctive therapy for peptic ulcers and hypermotility disorders of lower urinary tract; infant colic

Pregnancy Risk Factor C

Contraindications Hypersensitivity to hyoscyamine or any component; narrow-angle glaucoma, GI and GU obstruction, paralytic ileus, severe ulcerative colitis, myasthenia gravis
(Continued)

Hyoscyamine *(Continued)*

Warnings Low doses may cause a paradoxical decrease in heart rate; some commercial products contain sodium metabisulfite which may cause allergic reactions in susceptible individuals; heat prostration may occur in hot weather

Precautions Use with caution in patients with hyperthyroidism, CHF, cardiac arrhythmias, prostatic hypertrophy, autonomic neuropathy, chronic lung disease, biliary tract disease, children with spastic paralysis

Adverse Reactions

Cardiovascular: Tachycardia or palpitations, bradycardia (with very low doses), orthostatic hypotension

Central nervous system: Headache, lightheadedness, short-term memory loss, fatigue, delirium, restlessness, ataxia, dizziness, insomnia, psychosis, euphoria, nervousness, confusion, insomnia, fever

Dermatologic: Dry skin, photosensitivity, rash, urticaria

Gastrointestinal: Xerostomia, nausea, vomiting, constipation, dysphagia, dysgeusia, dry throat

Genitourinary: Difficult urination, urinary retention

Local: Irritation at injection site

Neuromuscular & skeletal: Weakness, tremor

Ocular: Blurred vision, photophobia, mydriasis, anisocoria, cycloplegia, increased intraocular pressure

Respiratory: Dry nose

Miscellaneous: Decreased diaphoresis

Drug Interactions Decreased absorption when given with antacids; increased anticholinergic activity with amantadine, antimuscarinics, haloperidol, phenothiazines, tricyclic antidepressants, antihistamines; MAO inhibitors

Mechanism of Action Blocks the action of acetylcholine at parasympathetic sites in smooth muscle, secretory glands, and the CNS; specific anticholinergic responses are dose-related; increases cardiac output, dries secretions, antagonizes histamine and serotonin

Pharmacodynamics

Onset of action:

Oral: 20-30 minutes

Sublingual: 5-20 minutes

I.V.: 2-3 minutes

Duration: 4-6 hours

Pharmacokinetics

Absorption: Well absorbed from the GI tract

Distribution: Crosses the placenta; small amounts appear in breast milk

Protein binding: 50%

Metabolism: In the liver

Half-life: 3.5 hours

Elimination: 30% to 50% eliminated unchanged in urine within 12 hours

Usual Dosage

GI tract disorders:

Infants <2 years: Oral: The following table lists the hyoscyamine dosage using the drop formulation; hyoscyamine drops are dosed every 4 hours as needed

Hyoscyamine Drops Dosage

Weight (kg)	Dose (drops)	Maximum Daily Dose (drops)
2.3	3	18
3.4	4	24
5	5	30
7	6	36
10	8	48
15	11	66

Oral, S.L.:

Children 2-12 years: 0.0625-0.125 mg every 4 hours as needed; maximum daily dosage 0.75 mg

Children >12 years to Adults: 0.125-0.25 mg every 4 hours as needed; maximum daily dosage 1.5 mg **or** using timed release 0.375-0.75 mg every 12 hours; maximum daily dosage 1.5 mg

I.V., I.M., S.C.: Children >12 years to Adults: 0.25-0.5 mg at 4-hour intervals for 1-4 doses

Adjunct to anesthesia: I.M., I.V., S.C.: Children >2 years to Adults: 5 mcg/kg given 30-60 minutes prior to induction of anesthesia

Hypermotility of lower urinary tract: Oral, S.L.: Adults: 0.15-0.3 mg four times daily; using timed release formulation: 0.375 mg every 12 hours

Reversal of neuromuscular blockage: I.V., I.M., S.C.: 0.2 mg for every 1 mg neostigmine or equivalent dose of physostigmine

Administration

Oral: Administer before meals; timed release tablets are scored and may be cut for easier dosage titration; S.L.: Place under the tongue

Parenteral: May be administered I.M., I.V., and S.C.; no information is available for I.V. administration rate or dilution

Monitoring Parameters Pulse, anticholinergic effects, urine output, GI symptoms

Patient Information Maintain good oral hygiene habits, because lack of saliva may increase chance of cavities; notify physician if skin rash, flushing or eye pain occurs, or if difficulty in urinating, constipation, or sensitivity to light becomes severe or persists; may cause dizziness or blurred vision; may cause drowsiness and impair ability to perform hazardous activities requiring mental alertness or physical coordination

Dosage Forms

Capsule, timed release, as sulfate (Cystospaz-M®, Levsinex®): 0.375 mg

Elixir, as sulfate (Levsin®): 0.125 mg/5 mL with alcohol 20% (480 mL)

Injection, as sulfate (Levsin®): 0.5 mg/mL (1 mL, 10 mL)

Solution, oral drops, as sulfate (Gastrosed™, Levsin®): 0.125 mg/mL with 5% alcohol (15 mL)

Tablet, as sulfate:

Anaspaz®, Gastrosed™, Levsin®, Neoquess®: 0.125 mg

Cystospaz®: 0.15 mg

Tablet, extended release, as sulfate: 0.375 mg

Tablet, sublingual, as sulfate: 0.125 mg

Hyoscyamine, Atropine, Scopolamine, and Phenobarbital

(hye oh SYE a meen, A troe peen, skoe POL a meen & fee noe BAR bi tal)

Brand Names Barbidonna®; Barophen®; Donnamor®; Donnapine®; Donna-Sed®; Donnatal®; Donphen®; Hyosophen®; Kinesed®; Malatal®; Relaxadon®; Spaslin®; Spasmolin®; Spasmophen®; Spasquid®; Susano®

Available Salts Hyoscyamine Sulfate, Atropine Sulfate, Scopolamine Hydrobromide, and Phenobarbital

Synonyms Atropine, Hyoscyamine, Scopolamine, and Phenobarbital; Phenobarbital, Hyoscyamine, Atropine, and Scopolamine; Scopolamine, Hyoscyamine, Atropine, and Phenobarbital

Therapeutic Category Anticholinergic Agent; Antispasmodic Agent, Gastrointestinal

Generic Available Yes

Use Adjunct in treatment of peptic ulcer disease, irritable bowel, spastic colitis, spastic bladder, and renal colic

Pregnancy Risk Factor C

Contraindications Hypersensitivity to hyoscyamine, atropine, scopolamine, phenobarbital, or any component; narrow-angle glaucoma, tachycardia, GI and GU obstruction, myasthenia gravis, asthma

Warnings Heat prostration can occur in the presence of high environmental temperature

Precautions Use with caution in patients with hepatic or renal disease, hyperthyroidism, cardiovascular disease, hypertension, prostatic hypertrophy, autonomic neuropathy

Adverse Reactions

Cardiovascular: Tachycardia, palpitations, bradycardia (with very low doses of atropine)

Central nervous system: Headache, drowsiness, nervousness, confusion, insomnia, fever

Gastrointestinal: Xerostomia, nausea, vomiting, constipation, dysphagia, paralytic ileus, dysgeusia

Genitourinary: Impotence, urinary retention

Neuromuscular & skeletal: Weakness

Ocular: Blurred vision, photophobia, mydriasis, cycloplegia, increased intraocular pressure

(Continued)

Hyoscyamine, Atropine, Scopolamine, and Phenobarbital *(Continued)*

Respiratory: Nasal congestion

Miscellaneous: Hypersensitivity reactions, decreased diaphoresis

Drug Interactions Additive CNS depression with CNS depressants, antihistamines, phenothiazines, tricyclic antidepressants; additive anticholinergic activity with antihistamines, phenothiazines, amantadine

Mechanism of Action Anticholinergic agents (hyoscyamine, atropine, and scopolamine) inhibit the muscarinic actions of acetylcholine at the postganglionic parasympathetic neuroeffector sites including smooth muscle, secretory glands, and CNS sites; specific anticholinergic responses are dose-related

Pharmacokinetics Absorption: Well absorbed from the GI tract

Usual Dosage Oral:

Children 2-12 years: Kinesed® dose: 0.5-1 tablet 3-4 times/day

Children: Donnatal®: 0.1 mL/kg/dose every 4 hours; maximum dose: 5 mL **or** see table for alternative.

Donnatal® Dosage

Weight (kg)	Dose (mL)	
	Every 4 Hours	Every 6 Hours
4.5	0.5	0.75
10	1	1.5
14	1.5	2
23	2.5	3.8
34	3.8	5
≥45	5	7.5

Adults:

Kinesed® or Spasmophen®: 1-2 tablets 3-4 times/day

Donnatal®: 1-2 tablets 3-4 times/day **or** 5-10 mL 3-4 times/day **or** 1 sustained release tablet every 12 hours

Barbidonna®: 1-2 tablets 3 times/day

Barophen®: 5-10 mL 3-4 times/day

Administration Oral: Do not crush or chew extended release tablets

Patient Information Maintain good oral hygiene habits because lack of saliva may increase chance of cavities. Notify physician if skin rash, flushing or eye pain occurs, or if difficulty in urinating, constipation, or sensitivity to light becomes severe or persists; observe caution while driving or performing other tasks requiring alertness, as may cause drowsiness, dizziness, or blurred vision

Dosage Forms

Capsule (Donnatal®, Spasmolin®): Hyoscyamine sulfate 0.1037 mg, atropine sulfate 0.0194 mg, scopolamine hydrobromide 0.0065 mg, and phenobarbital 16.2 mg

Elixir (Barophen®, Donna-Sed®, Donnatal®, Hyosophen®, Spasmophen®, Spasquid®, Susano®): Hyoscyamine sulfate 0.1037 mg, atropine sulfate 0.0194 mg, scopolamine hydrobromide 0.0065 mg, and phenobarbital 16.2 mg per 5 mL (120 mL, 480 mL, 4000 mL)

Tablet:

Barbidonna®: Hyoscyamine hydrobromide 0.1286 mg, atropine sulfate 0.025 mg, scopolamine hydrobromide 0.0074 mg, and phenobarbital 16 mg

Barbidonna® No. 2: Hyoscyamine hydrobromide 0.1286 mg, atropine sulfate 0.025 mg, scopolamine hydrobromide 0.0074 mg, and phenobarbital 32 mg

Chewable (Kinesed®): Hyoscyamine hydrobromide 0.12 mg, atropine sulfate 0.12 mg, scopolamine hydrobromide 0.007 mg, and phenobarbital 16 mg

Donnapine®, Donnatal®, Hyosophen®, Malatal®, Relaxadon®, Spaslin®, Susano®: Hyoscyamine sulfate 0.1037 mg, atropine sulfate 0.0194 mg, scopolamine hydrobromide 0.0065 mg, and phenobarbital 16.2 mg

Donnatal® No. 2: Hyoscyamine sulfate 0.1037 mg, atropine sulfate 0.0194 mg, scopolamine hydrobromide 0.0065 mg, and phenobarbital 32.4 mg

Donphen®: Hyoscyamine sulfate 0.1 mg, atropine sulfate 0.02 mg, scopolamine hydrobromide 0.006 mg, and phenobarbital 15 mg

Long-acting (Donnatal®): Hyoscyamine sulfate 0.3111 mg, atropine sulfate 0.0582 mg, scopolamine hydrobromide 0.0195 mg, and phenobarbital 48.6 mg

Spasmophen®: Hyoscyamine sulfate 0.1037 mg, atropine sulfate 0.0194 mg, scopolamine hydrobromide 0.0065 mg, and phenobarbital 15 mg

♦ **Hyoscyamine Sulfate** see Hyoscyamine on page 497
♦ **Hyoscyamine Sulfate, Atropine Sulfate, Scopolamine Hydrobromide, and Phenobarbital** see Hyoscyamine, Atropine, Scopolamine, and Phenobarbital on page 499
♦ **Hyosophen®** see Hyoscyamine, Atropine, Scopolamine, and Phenobarbital on page 499
♦ **Hy-Pam® Oral** see Hydroxyzine on page 496
♦ **Hyperstat® I.V.** see Diazoxide on page 310
♦ **Hy-Phen®** see Hydrocodone and Acetaminophen on page 485
♦ **HypRho®-D** see Rh₀(D) Immune Globulin, Intramuscular on page 840
♦ **HypRho®-D (Canada)** see Rh₀(D) Immune Globulin, Intramuscular on page 840
♦ **HypRho®-D Mini-Dose** see Rh₀(D) Immune Globulin, Intramuscular on page 840
♦ **Hyrexin-50® Injection** see Diphenhydramine on page 327
♦ **Hyskon® (Canada)** see Dextran on page 299
♦ **Hytakerol®** see Dihydrotachysterol on page 321
♦ **Hytinic®** see Iron Supplements, Oral/Enteral on page 530
♦ **Hytone® Topical** see Hydrocortisone on page 486
♦ **Hytuss® [OTC]** see Guaifenesin on page 464
♦ **Hytuss-2X® [OTC]** see Guaifenesin on page 464
♦ **Hyzine-50® Injection** see Hydroxyzine on page 496
♦ **Ibenzmethyzin** see Procarbazine on page 802
♦ **Ibidomide** see Labetalol on page 548
♦ **Ibuprin® [OTC]** see Ibuprofen on page 501

Ibuprofen (eye byoo PROE fen)

Related Information
Carbohydrate and Alcohol Content of Liquid Medications for Use in Patients Receiving Ketogenic Diets on page 1228
Overdose and Toxicology on page 1191

Brand Names Aches-N-Pain® [OTC]; Actiprofen® (Canada); Advil® [OTC]; Advil® Migraine Liqui-Gels; Apo®-Ibuprofen (Canada); Children's Advil® Suspension; Children's Motrin® Suspension [OTC]; Excedrin® IB [OTC]; Genpril® [OTC]; Haltran® [OTC]; Ibuprin® [OTC]; Ibuprohm® [OTC]; Ibu-Tab®; Infants' Advil® Concentrated Drops; Medipren® [OTC]; Menadol® [OTC]; Midol® IB [OTC]; Motrin®; Motrin® IB [OTC]; Motrin® Migraine Pain; Novo-Profen® (Canada); Nu-Ibuprofen® (Canada); Nuprin® [OTC]; Pamprin IB® [OTC]; Pedia-Profen™; Rufen®; Saleto-200® [OTC]; Saleto-400®; Strength Motrin® [OTC]; Trendar® [OTC]; Uni-Pro® [OTC]

Synonyms p-Isobutylhydratropic Acid

Therapeutic Category Analgesic, Non-narcotic; Anti-inflammatory Agent; Antipyretic; Nonsteroidal Anti-inflammatory Drug (NSAID), Oral

Generic Available Yes

Use Inflammatory diseases and rheumatoid disorders including juvenile rheumatoid arthritis (JRA); mild to moderate pain; migraine pain; fever; dysmenorrhea; gout

Pregnancy Risk Factor B (D if used in the 3rd trimester)

Contraindications Hypersensitivity to ibuprofen, any component, aspirin, or other NSAIDs; active GI bleeding, ulcer disease

Precautions Use with caution in patients with CHF, hypertension, decreased renal or hepatic function, dehydration, history of GI disease (bleeding or ulcers), or those receiving anticoagulants

Adverse Reactions
Cardiovascular: Edema
Central nervous system: Dizziness, drowsiness, fatigue, headache
Dermatologic: Rash, urticaria
Gastrointestinal: Dyspepsia, heartburn, nausea, vomiting, abdominal pain, peptic ulcer, GI bleed, GI perforation
Hematologic: Neutropenia, anemia, agranulocytosis, inhibition of platelet aggregation
Hepatic: Hepatitis
Ocular: Vision changes
Otic: Tinnitus
Renal: Acute renal failure

Drug Interactions Cytochrome P-450 isoenzyme CYP2C8 and CYP2C9 substrate
May increase digoxin, methotrexate and lithium serum concentrations; aspirin may decrease ibuprofen serum concentrations; other GI irritants (eg, NSAIDs, oral (Continued)

Ibuprofen *(Continued)*

potassium) may increase adverse GI effects; effects of antihypertensive agents, furosemide, thiazides may be decreased

Food Interactions Food may decrease the rate but not the extent of oral absorption

Mechanism of Action Inhibits prostaglandin synthesis by decreasing the activity of the enzyme, cyclo-oxygenase, which results in decreased formation of prostaglandin precursors

Pharmacodynamics

Fever reduction:

Onset (single dose 8 mg/kg):

Infants ≤1 year: Mean ± SD: 69 ± 22 minutes

Children ≥6 years: 109 ± 64 minutes

Peak effect: 2-4 hours

Duration: 6-8 hours (dose-related)

Pharmacokinetics

Absorption: Oral: Rapid (80%)

Protein binding: 90% to 99%

Metabolism: Oxidized in the liver

Half-life:

Children: 1-2 hours; children 3 months to 10 years: Mean: 1.6 hours

Adults: 2-4 hours

Time to peak serum concentration: Tablets: 2 hours; suspension: 1 hour

Elimination: ~1% excreted as unchanged drug and 14% as conjugated ibuprofen in urine; 45% to 80% eliminated in urine as metabolites; some biliary excretion

Usual Dosage Oral:

Infants and Children:

Analgesic: 4-10 mg/kg/dose every 6-8 hours

Antipyretic: 6 months to 12 years: Temperature <102.5°F (39°C): 5 mg/kg/dose; temperature ≥102.5°F: 10 mg/kg/dose; give every 6-8 hours; maximum daily dose: 40 mg/kg/day

Juvenile rheumatoid arthritis: 6 months to 12 years: 30-50 mg/kg/day in 4 divided doses; start at lower end of dosing range and titrate; maximum dose: 2.4 g/day

OTC pediatric labeling (analgesic, antipyretic): 2-11 years: 7.5 mg/kg/dose every 6-8 hours; maximum daily dose: 30 mg/kg

Cystic fibrosis: Ibuprofen when taken chronically (for 4 years) in doses to achieve peak plasma concentrations of 50-100 mcg/mL has been shown to slow the progression of lung disease in mild cystic fibrosis patients >5 years of age, and especially in patients who started therapy when <13 years of age. Doses administered twice daily ranged from 16.2-31.6 mg/kg/dose with 90% of patients requiring 20-30 mg/kg/dose (mean dose: ~25 mg/kg/dose), but individual patient's dose requirements were not predictable. Patients did not take pancreatic enzymes nor eat for 2 hours after the dose (Konstan, 1995); further studies are needed.

Adolescents and Adults:

Inflammatory disease: 400-800 mg/dose 3-4 times/day; maximum dose: 3.2 g/day

Pain/fever/dysmenorrhea: 200-400 mg/dose every 4-6 hours; maximum daily dose: 1.2 g

Administration Oral: Administer with food or milk to decrease GI upset; shake suspension well before use

Monitoring Parameters CBC, occult blood loss, liver enzymes; urine output, serum BUN, and creatinine in patients receiving diuretics, those with decreased renal function, or in patients on chronic therapy; patients receiving long-term therapy for JRA should receive periodic ophthalmological exams

Reference Range Plasma concentrations >200 µg/mL may be associated with severe toxicity

Patient Information Avoid alcohol; may cause dizziness or drowsiness and impair ability to perform tasks requiring mental alertness; notify physician if changes in vision occur

OTC (pediatrics): Do not administer to children for >3 days unless recommended by physician or other health care professional; notify physician if child's condition does not improve or if worsens within 24 hours

Additional Information Each 5 mL of suspension contains 2.5 g of sucrose; OTC suspension (Children's Motrin®) is an alcohol-free berry-flavored liquid; nystagmus, dizziness, hypotension, apnea and coma have been reported with overdose

Note: A study comparing the short-term use of acetaminophen and ibuprofen in 84,192 children (6 months to 12 years of age) found no significant difference in the rates of hospitalization for acute GI bleeding, acute renal failure, anaphylaxis or Reye's syndrome. (Four of 55,785 children in the ibuprofen group and zero of 28,130 children in the acetaminophen group were hospitalized with acute GI bleeding). A low WBC occurred more frequently in the ibuprofen group (8 vs 0).

There is currently no scientific evidence to support alternating acetaminophen with ibuprofen in the treatment of fever (see Mayoral, 2000)

Dosage Forms
Caplet: 100 mg

Capsule: 200 mg [OTC]

Capsule, liqui-gel: 200 mg [OTC] (Advil® Migraine Liqui-Gel, solubolized ibuprofen)

Drops, oral (berry flavor): 40 mg/mL (15 mL)

Suspension, oral: 100 mg/5 mL (60 mL, 120 mL, 240 mL, 480 mL) (Children's Motrin® [OTC])

Suspension, oral, **drops**: 40 mg/mL [OTC] (Infants' Advil® Concentrated Drops)

Tablet: 100 mg [OTC], 200 mg [OTC], 300 mg, 400 mg, 600 mg, 800 mg

Tablet, chewable: 50 mg, 100 mg

References
Berde C, Ablin A, Glazer J, et al, "American Academy of Pediatrics Report of the Subcommittee on Disease-Related Pain in Childhood Cancer," *Pediatrics*, 1990, 86(5 Pt 2):818-25.

Brewer EJ, "Nonsteroidal Anti-inflammatory Agents," *Arthritis Rheum*, 1977, 20(2):513-25.

Kauffman RE and Nelson MV, "Effect of Age on Ibuprofen Pharmacokinetics and Antipyretic Response," *J Pediatr*, 1992, 121(6):969-73.

Konstan MW, Byard PJ, Hoppel CL, et al, "Effect of High-Dose Ibuprofen in Patients With Cystic Fibrosis," *N Engl J Med*, 1995, 332(13):848-54.

Lesko SM and Mitchell AA, "An Assessment of the Safety of Pediatric Ibuprofen. A Practitioner-Based Randomized Clinical Trial," *JAMA*, 1995, 273(12):929-33.

Mayoral CE, Marino RV, Rosenfeld, W, et al, "Alternating Antipyretics: Is This an Alternative?" *Pediatrics*, 2000, 105(5):1009-12.

♦ **Ibuprohm® [OTC]** *see* Ibuprofen *on page 501*

♦ **Ibu-Tab®** *see* Ibuprofen *on page 501*

♦ **ICN-1299** *see* Ribavirin *on page 843*

♦ **IDA** *see* Idarubicin *on page 503*

♦ **Idamycin®** *see* Idarubicin *on page 503*

Idarubicin (eye da ROO bi sin)

Related Information
Emetogenic Potential of Single Chemotherapeutic Agents *on page 1095*

Brand Names Idamycin®

Available Salts Idarubicin Hydrochloride

Synonyms 4-Demethoxydaunorubicin; 4-DMDR; IDA

Therapeutic Category Antineoplastic Agent, Anthracycline; Antineoplastic Agent, Antibiotic

Generic Available No

Use Used in combination with other antineoplastic agents for treatment of acute myelogenous leukemia (AML) in adults and acute lymphocytic leukemia (ALL) in children

Pregnancy Risk Factor D

Contraindications Hypersensitivity to idarubicin or any component; patients with pre-existing bone marrow suppression unless the benefit warrants the risk; severe CHF, cardiomyopathy

Warnings The FDA currently recommends that procedures for proper handling and disposal of antineoplastic agents be considered; I.V. use only, severe local tissue necrosis will result if extravasation occurs; pre-existing heart disease and previous therapy with anthracyclines at high cumulative doses increase risk of idarubicin-induced cardiac toxicity (manifested by potentially fatal CHF, life-threatening arrhythmias, or cardiomyopathies); the maximum lifetime anthracycline dose for idarubicin is approximately 137.5 mg/m^2; severe myelosuppression occurs in all patients given a therapeutic dose and is the dose-limiting adverse effect associated with idarubicin

Precautions Use with caution and reduce dose in patients with impaired hepatic or renal function

Adverse Reactions
Cardiovascular: Arrhythmias, EKG changes, cardiomyopathy, CHF

Dermatologic: Alopecia, rash, urticaria

Endocrine & metabolic: Hyperuricemia

Gastrointestinal: Nausea, vomiting, diarrhea, stomatitis, anorexia

(Continued)

Idarubicin *(Continued)*

Hematologic: Leukopenia (nadir: 8-29 days), thrombocytopenia (nadir: 10-15 days), anemia

Hepatic: Elevated liver enzymes or bilirubin

Local: Tissue necrosis upon extravasation, erythematous streaking

Stability Store vials at room temperature; reconstituted solutions are chemically stable for 7 days when refrigerated or 72 hours at room temperature; reconstitution with a bacteriostatic diluent is not recommended; incompatible with acyclovir, ceftazidime, furosemide, hydrocortisone, sodium bicarbonate and heparin; inactivated by alkaline solutions

Mechanism of Action Intercalates with DNA causing strand breakage and affects topoisomerase II activity resulting in inhibition of chain elongation and inhibition of DNA and RNA synthesis

Pharmacokinetics

Distribution:

V_d: Large volume of distribution due to extensive tissue binding; distributes into CSF

V_{dss}: 1700 L/m^2

Protein binding:

Idarubicin: 97%

Idarubicinol: 97%

Metabolism: In the liver to idarubicinol (active metabolite)

Half-life:

Children: 18.7 hours (range: 2.5-22.4 hours)

Adults: 19 hours (range: 10.5-34.7 hours)

Idarubicinol: 45 hours

Elimination: Primarily by biliary excretion; 2.3% to 6.5% of a dose is eliminated renally

Usual Dosage I.V. (refer to individual protocols):

Children:

Leukemia: 10-12 mg/m^2 once daily for 3 days of treatment course

Solid tumors: 5 mg/m^2 once daily for 3 days of treatment course

Adults: 8-12 mg/m^2 once daily for 3 days of treatment course; reduce dose by 25% if severe mucositis is present

Dosing adjustment in hepatic and/or renal impairment:

Serum creatinine ≥2 mg/dL: Reduce dose by 25%

Bilirubin >2.5 mg/dL: Reduce dose by 50%

Bilirubin >5 mg/dL: **Do not administer**

Administration Parenteral: I.V.: Administer by I.V. intermittent infusion over 10-30 minutes into a free flowing I.V. solution of NS or D$_5$W; administer at a final concentration of 1 mg/mL

Monitoring Parameters CBC with differential, platelet count, ECHO, EKG, serum electrolytes, creatinine, uric acid, ALT, AST, bilirubin, signs of extravasation

Patient Information Notify physician if fever, sore throat, bleeding, or bruising occur

Nursing Implications Local erythematous streaking along the vein may indicate too rapid a rate of administration; care should be taken to avoid extravasation; the manufacturer recommends that topical ice packs be placed over the area of extravasation immediately for 30 minutes, then apply for 30 minutes 4 times/day for 3 days and elevate the affected extremity; alternative therapy includes topical application of dimethylsulfoxide

Dosage Forms Powder for injection, lyophilized, as hydrochloride: 5 mg, 10 mg

References

Reid JM, Pendergrass TW, Krailo MD, et al, "Plasma Pharmacokinetics and Cerebrospinal Fluid Concentrations of Idarubicin and Idarubicinol in Pediatric Leukemia Patients: A Children's Cancer Study Group Report," *Cancer Res*, 1990, 50(20):6525-8.

♦ **Idarubicin Hydrochloride** *see* Idarubicin *on page 503*

♦ **Ifex®** *see* Ifosfamide *on page 504*

♦ **IFLrA** *see* Interferon Alfa-2a *on page 522*

♦ **IFN** *see* Interferon Alfa-2a *on page 522*

♦ **IFN-α-2** *see* Interferon Alfa-2b *on page 524*

Ifosfamide *(eye FOSS fa mide)*

Related Information

Emetogenic Potential of Single Chemotherapeutic Agents *on page 1095*

Brand Names Ifex®

Therapeutic Category Antineoplastic Agent, Alkylating Agent

Generic Available No

Use In combination with other antineoplastics in treatment of lung cancer, Hodgkin's and non-Hodgkin's lymphoma, breast cancer, acute and chronic lymphocytic leukemia, ovarian cancer, testicular cancer, and sarcomas

Pregnancy Risk Factor D

Contraindications Hypersensitivity to ifosfamide or any component; patients with severely depressed bone marrow function

Warnings The FDA currently recommends that procedures for proper handling and disposal of antineoplastic agents be considered. May require therapy cessation if confusion or coma occurs; monitor for hemorrhagic cystitis and severe myelosuppression; carcinogenic in rats

Precautions Use with caution in patients with impaired renal function or those with compromised bone marrow reserve

Adverse Reactions
Cardiovascular: Cardiotoxicity
Central nervous system: Somnolence, confusion, depressive psychoses, hallucinations, dizziness, seizures, fever, ataxia
Dermatologic: Alopecia
Gastrointestinal: Nausea, vomiting, stomatitis, diarrhea
Genitourinary: Dysuria, hemorrhagic cystitis
Hematologic: Myelosuppression (leukocyte nadir: 7-14 days)
Hepatic: Elevated liver enzymes
Local: Phlebitis
Neuromuscular & skeletal: Polyneuropathy
Renal: Renal tubular acidosis, hematuria, elevated BUN, elevated serum creatinine

Drug Interactions Phenobarbital, phenytoin, chloral hydrate may increase the conversion of ifosfamide to active metabolites and increase toxicity; cisplatin may increase ifosfamide renal damage

Stability Reconstituted solution is stable for 7 days at room temperature and 21 days when refrigerated

Mechanism of Action Causes cross-linking of DNA strands by binding with nucleic acids and other intracellular structures; inhibits protein synthesis and DNA synthesis

Pharmacokinetics
Dose-dependent pharmacokinetics: Beta phase half-life: 11-15 hours with high-dose (3800-5000 mg/m^2) or 4-7 hours with lower doses (1800 mg/m^2)
Distribution: Unchanged ifosfamide penetrates the blood-brain barrier
Metabolism: Requires biotransformation by the cytochrome P-450 enzyme system in the liver before it can act as an alkylating agent; following hydroxylation, the metabolite breaks down to acrolein (bladder irritant) and ifosfamide mustard (active drug)
Elimination: 60% to 80% of a dose is excreted in urine as unchanged drug and metabolites

Usual Dosage I.V. (refer to individual protocols):
Children: 1200-1800 mg/m^2/day for 5 days every 21-28 days or 5000 mg/m^2 as a single 24-hour infusion or 3 g/m^2/day for 2 days
Adults: 700-2000 mg/m^2/day for 5 days or 2400 mg/m^2/day for 3 days every 21-28 days; 5000 mg/m^2 as a single dose over 24 hours

Administration Parenteral: Administer as a slow I.V. intermittent infusion over at least 30 minutes at a final concentration for administration not to exceed 40 mg/mL (usual concentration for administration is between 0.6-20 mg/mL), or administer as a 24-hour infusion

Monitoring Parameters CBC with differential and platelet count, urine output, urinalysis, liver function and renal function tests

Nursing Implications Maintain adequate patient hydration

Additional Information Usually used in combination with mesna, an agent used to prevent hemorrhagic cystitis

Dosage Forms Powder for injection: 1 g, 3 g

References
Ninane J, Baurain R, and de Kraker J, "Alkylating Activity in Serum, Urine, and CSF Following High-Dose Ifosfamide in Children," *Cancer Chemother Pharmacol*, 1989, 24(Suppl 1):S2-6.
Pinkerton CR, Rogers H, James C, et al, "A Phase II Study of Ifosfamide in Children With Recurrent Solid Tumors," *Cancer Chemother Pharmacol*, 1985, 15(3):258-62.

♦ **IGIV** see Immune Globulin, Intravenous *on page 510*
♦ **IL-2** see Aldesleukin *on page 42*
♦ **Iletin® (Canada)** see Insulin Preparations *on page 518*
♦ **Iletin® II Pork (Canada)** see Insulin Preparations *on page 518*

- Ilosone® *see* Erythromycin *on page 379*
- Ilosone® **Pulvules®** *see* Erythromycin *on page 379*
- Ilotycin® *see* Erythromycin *on page 379*
- Ilotycin® **(Canada)** *see* Erythromycin *on page 379*
- Ilozyme® *see* Pancrelipase *on page 724*
- **Imidazole Carboxamide** *see* Dacarbazine *on page 278*

Imiglucerase (imi GLOO ser ase)

Brand Names Cerezyme®

Therapeutic Category Enzyme, Glucocerebrosidase; Gaucher's Disease, Treatment Agent

Generic Available No

Use Long-term enzyme replacement therapy for patients with Type 1 Gaucher's disease

Pregnancy Risk Factor C

Contraindications Hypersensitivity to imiglucerase or any component

Warnings During clinical trials, 16% of patients developed IgG antibodies reactive with imiglucerase; no serious symptoms of hypersensitivity were reported, however, close observation for hypersensitivity reactions over long-term usage is recommended

Adverse Reactions
Cardiovascular: Hypertension (mild)
Central nervous system: Headache, dizziness
Dermatologic: Rash, pruritus
Gastrointestinal: Nausea, abdominal discomfort
Genitourinary: Decreased urinary frequency

Drug Interactions No information available at this time

Stability Store in refrigerator 2°C to 8°C (36°F to 46°F); after reconstitution, stable for 24 hours refrigerated

Mechanism of Action Imiglucerase, produced by recombinant DNA technology, is an analog of glucocerebrosidase; it acts by replacing the missing enzyme associated with Gaucher's disease; Gaucher's disease is an inherited metabolic disorder caused by the defective activity of beta-glucosidase and the resultant accumulation of glucosyl ceramide laden macrophages in the liver, bone, and spleen; this results in one or more of the following conditions: anemia, thrombocytopenia, bone disease, hepatomegaly, splenomegaly; the disease affects an estimated 10,000-15,000 people in the U.S., primarily of eastern European Jewish descent, with up to 5000 being symptomatic and requiring treatment

Pharmacodynamics
Onset of significant improvement in symptoms:
Hepatosplenomegaly and hematologic abnormalities: Within 6 months
Improvement in bone mineralization: Noted at 80-104 weeks of therapy

Pharmacokinetics
Distribution: V_d: 0.09-0.15 L/kg
Half-life, elimination: 3.6-10.4 minutes
Clearance: 9.8-20.3 mL/minute/kg

Usual Dosage I.V.:
Children and Adults:
Initial: Dosage dependent upon disease severity: Usual: 60 units/kg every 2 weeks; range in dosage: 2.5 units/kg 3 times/week to 60 units/kg once weekly to every 4 weeks
Maintenance: After patient response is well established a reduction in dosage may be attempted; progressive reductions may be made at intervals of 3-6 months

Administration Parenteral: Reconstitution with 5.1 mL sterile water results in 40 units/mL concentration; further dilute 5 mL (200 units) in 100-200 mL NS; infuse over 1-2 hours or a maximum of 1 unit/kg/minute

Monitoring Parameters CBC, platelets, liver function tests

Dosage Forms Powder for injection, preservative free (lyophilized): 212 units [equivalent to a withdrawal dose of 200 units]

- **Imipemide** *see* Imipenem and Cilastatin *on page 506*

Imipenem and Cilastatin (i mi PEN em & sye la STAT in)

Brand Names Primaxin®

Available Salts Cilastatin Sodium

Synonyms Cilastatin and Imipenem; Imipemide

Therapeutic Category Antibiotic, Carbapenem

Generic Available No

Use Treatment of documented multidrug-resistant gram-negative infection due to organisms proven or suspected to be susceptible to imipenem/cilastatin; treatment of multiple organism infection in which other agents have an insufficient spectrum of activity or are contraindicated due to toxic potential; therapeutic alternative for treatment of gram-negative sepsis in immunocompromised patients

Pregnancy Risk Factor C

Contraindications Hypersensitivity to imipenem/cilastatin or any component

Warnings Serious and occasionally fatal hypersensitivity reactions have been reported in patients receiving beta-lactam therapy; careful inquiry should be made concerning previous hypersensitivity reactions to penicillins, cephalosporins, or other beta-lactams before initiating imipenem. Seizures have been reported with imipenem therapy in children with meningitis. Pseudomembranous colitis has been reported in patients receiving imipenem; prolonged use may result in superinfection.

Precautions Use with caution in patients with history of seizures or who are predisposed and in patients with a history of hypersensitivity to penicillins; use with caution and adjust dose in patients with impaired renal function

Adverse Reactions

Cardiovascular: Hypotension, tachycardia

Central nervous system: Seizures, hallucinations, altered effect, confusion, fever, dizziness

Dermatologic: Rash, pruritus

Gastrointestinal: Nausea, vomiting, diarrhea, pseudomembranous colitis

Genitourinary: Discoloration of urine, anuria, oliguria

Hematologic: Eosinophilia, neutropenia

Hepatic: Transient elevation in liver enzymes

Local: Phlebitis, irritation at injection site

Miscellaneous: Emergence of resistant strains of *P. aeruginosa*

Drug Interactions Beta-lactam antibiotics, probenecid; ganciclovir (increased risk of seizures)

Stability When reconstituted suspension is further diluted with NS, it is stable for 10 hours at room temperature or 48 hours under refrigeration; when reconstituted suspension is further diluted with a compatible solution other than NS, it is stable for 4 hours at room temperature and 24 hours under refrigeration; incompatible with TPN; inactivated at alkaline or acidic pH

Mechanism of Action Inhibits cell wall synthesis by binding to all of the penicillin-binding proteins with greatest affinity for PBP 1 and PBP 2; cilastatin prevents renal metabolism of imipenem by competitive inhibition of dehydropeptidase along the brush border of the proximal renal tubules

Pharmacokinetics

Distribution: Imipenem appears in breast milk; crosses the placenta; only low concentrations penetrate into CSF

Protein binding:

Imipenem: 13% to 21%

Cilastatin: 40%

Metabolism: Imipenem is metabolized in the kidney by dehydropeptidase; cilastatin is partially metabolized in the kidneys

Half-life, both: Prolonged with renal insufficiency

Neonates: 1.5-3 hours

Infants and Children: 1-1.4 hours

Adults: 1 hour

Elimination: When imipenem is given with cilastatin, urinary excretion of unchanged imipenem increases to 70%; 70% to 80% of a cilastatin dose is excreted unchanged in the urine

Moderately dialyzable (20% to 50%)

Usual Dosage Dosage recommendation based on imipenem component for non-CNS infections: I.V. infusion: (I.M. is limited to mild-moderate infections):

Neonates:

0-4 weeks, <1200 g: 20 mg/kg/dose every 18-24 hours

Postnatal age ≤7 days, 1200-1500 g: 40 mg/kg/day divided every 12 hours

Postnatal age ≤7 days, >1500 g: 50 mg/kg/day divided every 12 hours

Postnatal age >7 days, 1200-1500 g: 40 mg/kg/day divided every 12 hours

Postnatal age >7 days, >1500 g: 75 mg/kg/day divided every 8 hours

Infants 4 weeks to 3 months: 100 mg/kg/day divided every 6 hours

Infants ≥3 months and Children: 60-100 mg/kg/day divided every 6 hours; maximum dose: 4 g/day

(Continued)

Imipenem and Cilastatin *(Continued)*

Adults:

Serious infections: 2-4 g/day divided every 6 hours

Mild to moderate infections: 1-2 g/day in 3-4 divided doses

Dosing adjustment in renal impairment: Imipenem doses should be reduced in patients with Cl_{cr} <30-70 mL/minute/1.73 m²: See table.

Creatinine Clearance (mL/min/1.73 m²)	Frequency	% Decrease in Daily Maximum Dose
30-70	Every 6 hours	50
20-30	Every 8 hours	63
<20	Every 12 hours	75

Administration

I.M.: Administer suspension by deep I.M. injection into a large muscle mass; the I.M. powder for suspension should be reconstituted with lidocaine hydrochloride 1% injection (without epinephrine)

I.V.: Administer by I.V. intermittent infusion; final concentration should not exceed 5 mg/mL; in fluid-restricted patients, a final concentration of 7 mg/mL has been administered; doses ≤500 mg may be infused over 15-30 minutes; doses >500 mg should be infused over 40-60 minutes

Monitoring Parameters Periodic renal, hepatic, and hematologic function tests

Test Interactions Interferes with urinary glucose determination using Clinitest®; Positive Coombs' [direct]

Nursing Implications If nausea and/or vomiting occur during administration, decrease the rate of I.V. infusion

Additional Information Sodium content of 1 g: 3.2 mEq

Dosage Forms Powder for injection, as sodium:

I.M.:

Imipenem 500 mg and cilastatin 500 mg

Imipenem 750 mg and cilastatin 750 mg

I.V.:

Imipenem 250 mg and cilastatin 250 mg

Imipenem 500 mg and cilastatin 500 mg

References

Ahonkhai VI, Cyhan GM, Wilson SE, et al, "Imipenem-Cilastatin in Pediatric Patients: An Overview of Safety and Efficacy in Studies Conducted in the United States," *Pediatr Infect Dis J,* 1989, 8(11):740-4.

Overturf GD, "Use of Imipenem-Cilastatin in Pediatrics," *Pediatr Infect Dis J,* 1989, 8(11):792-4.

Wong VK, Wright HT Jr, Ross LA, et al, "Imipenem/Cilastatin Treatment of Bacterial Meningitis in Children," *Pediatr Infect Dis J,* 1991, 10(2):122-5.

Imipramine *(im IP ra meen)*

Related Information

Comparison of Adverse Effects of Antidepressants *on page 1030*

Comparison of Usual Adult Dosage and Mechanism of Action of Antidepressants *on page 1029*

Drugs and Breast-Feeding *on page 1213*

Overdose and Toxicology *on page 1191*

Brand Names Apo®-Imipramine (Canada); Janimine®; Novo-Pramine® (Canada); PMS-Imipramine (Canada); Tofranil®; Tofranil-PM®

Available Salts Imipramine Hydrochloride; Imipramine Pamoate

Therapeutic Category Antidepressant, Tricyclic

Generic Available Yes: Tablet

Use Treatment of various forms of depression, often in conjunction with psycho-therapy; enuresis in children; analgesic for certain chronic and neuropathic pain

Pregnancy Risk Factor D

Contraindications Hypersensitivity to imipramine (cross-sensitivity with other tricyclics may occur) or any component; patients receiving MAO inhibitors within past 14 days; narrow-angle glaucoma

Warnings Do not discontinue abruptly in patients receiving long-term high-dose therapy; some oral preparations contain tartrazine and injection contains sulfites both of which can cause allergic reactions

Precautions Use with caution in patients with cardiovascular disease, conduction disturbances, seizure disorders, urinary retention, anorexia, hyperthyroidism or those receiving thyroid replacement

Adverse Reactions Less sedation and anticholinergic effects than amitriptyline

Cardiovascular: Arrhythmias, hypotension (especially orthostatic)

Central nervous system: Drowsiness, sedation, confusion, dizziness, fatigue, anxiety, nervousness, sleep disorders, seizures

Dermatologic: Rash, photosensitivity

Gastrointestinal: Nausea, vomiting, constipation, xerostomia, decreased appetite

Genitourinary: Urinary retention

Hematologic: Blood dyscrasias

Hepatic: Hepatitis

Ocular: Blurred vision, increased intraocular pressure

Neuromuscular & skeletal: Weakness

Miscellaneous: Hypersensitivity reactions

Drug Interactions Cytochrome P-450 isoenzyme CYP1A2 (demethylation), CYP2C9 (demethylation), CYP2C19 (demethylation), CYP2D6 (hydroxylation), and CYP3A3/4 substrate

May decrease or reverse effects of guanethidine and clonidine; may increase effects of CNS depressants, alcohol, adrenergic agents, anticholinergic agents; with MAO inhibitors, fever, tachycardia, hypertension, seizures, and death may occur; similar interactions as with other tricyclics may occur

Food Interactions Riboflavin dietary requirements may be increased; food does not alter bioavailability

Mechanism of Action Increases the synaptic concentration of serotonin and/or norepinephrine in the central nervous system by inhibition of their reuptake by the presynaptic neuronal membrane

Pharmacodynamics Maximum antidepressant effects usually occur after ≥ 2 weeks

Pharmacokinetics

Absorption: Oral: Well absorbed

Distribution: Crosses the placenta; distributes into breast milk

V_d: Children: 14.5 L/kg; Adults: ~17 L/kg

Protein binding: >90% (primarily to alpha$_1$ acid glycoprotein and lipoproteins; to a lesser extent albumin)

Metabolism: In the liver by microsomal enzymes to desipramine (active) and other metabolites; significant first-pass effect

Bioavailability: 20% to 80%

Half-life: Adults: Range: 6-18 hours

Mean: Children: 11 hours; Adults: 16-17 hours

Desipramine (active metabolite): Adults: 22-28 hours

Time to peak serum concentration: Within 1-2 hours

Elimination: In the urine

Usual Dosage

Children: Oral:

Depression: 1.5 mg/kg/day with dosage increments of 1 mg/kg every 3-4 days to a maximum dose of 5 mg/kg/day in 1-4 divided doses; monitor carefully especially with doses ≥ 3.5 mg/kg/day

Enuresis: ≥ 6 years: Initial: 10-25 mg at bedtime, if inadequate response still seen after 1 week of therapy, increase by 25 mg/day; dose should not exceed 2.5 mg/kg/day or 50 mg at bedtime if 6-12 years of age or 75 mg at bedtime if ≥ 12 years of age

Adjunct in the treatment of cancer pain: Initial: 0.2-0.4 mg/kg at bedtime; dose may be increased by 50% every 2-3 days up to 1-3 mg/kg/dose at bedtime

Adolescents: Oral: Initial: 25-50 mg/day; increase gradually; maximum dose: 200 mg/day in single or divided doses

Adults:

Oral: Initial: 25 mg 3-4 times/day, increase dose gradually, total dose may be given at bedtime; maximum dose: 300 mg/day

I.M.: Initial: Up to 100 mg/day in divided doses; change to oral as soon as possible

Administration Oral: May administer with food to decrease GI distress

Monitoring Parameters EKG, CBC, supine and standing blood pressure (especially in children), liver enzymes

Reference Range

Therapeutic: Imipramine and desipramine 150-250 ng/mL (SI: 530-890 nmol/L); desipramine 150-300 ng/mL (SI: 560-1125 nmol/L)

Potentially toxic: >300 ng/mL (SI: >1070 nmol/L)

Toxic: >1000 ng/mL (SI: >3570 nmol/L)

Patient Information Limit caffeine; avoid alcohol; may cause drowsiness and impair ability to perform hazardous activities requiring mental alertness; may cause dry mouth

(Continued)

Imipramine *(Continued)*

Additional Information Place in therapy: Considered to be first drug of choice for depression in adolescents, significantly overweight children, or those with a family history of "depressive spectrum biogeny"

Dosage Forms

Capsule, as pamoate (Tofranil-PM®): 75 mg, 100 mg, 125 mg, 150 mg

Injection, as hydrochloride (Tofranil®): 12.5 mg/mL (2 mL)

Tablet, as hydrochloride (Janimine®, Tofranil®): 10 mg, 25 mg, 50 mg

References

Berde C, Ablin A, Glazer J, et al, "American Academy of Pediatrics Report of the Subcommittee on Disease-Related Pain in Childhood Cancer," *Pediatrics*, 1990, 86(5 Pt 2):818-25.

Levy HB, Harper CR, and Weinberg WA, "A Practical Approach to Children Failing in School," *Pediatr Clin North Am*, 1992, 39(4):895-928.

♦ **Imipramine Hydrochloride** *see* Imipramine *on page 508*

♦ **Imipramine Pamoate** *see* Imipramine *on page 508*

♦ **Imitrex®** *see* Sumatriptan *on page 897*

♦ **Immune Globulin, Intramuscular** *see page 1138*

Immune Globulin, Intravenous

(i MYUN GLOB yoo lin, IN tra VEE nus)

Brand Names Gamimune® N; Gammagard S/D®; Gammar®-IV; Iveegam®; Polygam S/D®; Sandoglobulin®; Venoglobulin®-S

Synonyms IGIV; IVIG

Therapeutic Category Immune Globulin

Generic Available Yes

Use Immunodeficiency syndrome, idiopathic thrombocytopenic purpura (ITP) and B-cell chronic lymphocytic leukemia (CLL); used in conjunction with appropriate anti-infective therapy to prevent or modify acute bacterial or viral infections in patients with iatrogenically-induced or disease-associated immunodepression; autoimmune neutropenia, bone marrow transplantation patients, Kawasaki disease, pediatric HIV infection, HIV-associated thrombocytopenia, Guillain-Barré syndrome, dermatomyositis, polymyositis, demyelinating polyneuropathies

Pregnancy Risk Factor C

Contraindications Hypersensitivity to immune globulin, blood products, or any component, IgA deficiency (except with the use of Gammagard® or Polygam®)

Intravenous Immune Globulin Product Comparison

	Gamimune® N	Gammagard® S/D	Gammar-P® IV	Iveegam®
FDA indication	Primary immuno-deficiency, ITP, bone marrow transplantation, pediatric HIV infection	Primary immuno-deficiency, ITP, CLL prophylaxis	Primary immuno-deficiency	Primary immuno-deficiency, Kawasaki syndrome
Contraindication	IgA deficiency	None (caution with IgA deficiency)	IgA deficiency	IgA deficiency
IgA content	270 mcg/mL	1.2 mcg/mL	<25 mcg/mL	<10 mcg/mL
Adverse reactions	5.2%	6%	16%	1%
Plasma source	>2000 paid donors	10,000 paid donors	>1000 paid donors	>6000 paid donors
Half-life	21 d	24 d	21-24 d	26-29 d
IgG subclass (%)				
IgG$_1$ (60-70)	60	67 (66.8)[1]	69	64.1[2]
IgG$_2$ (19-31)	29.4	25 (25.4)	23	30.3
IgG$_3$ (5-8.4)	6.5	5 (7.4)	6	4
IgG$_4$ (0.7-4)	4.1	3 (0.3)	2	1.5
Monomers	>90%	>96.4%	>90%	93.8%
Gammaglobulin	>98%	>90%	>98%	100%
Storage	Refrigerate	Room temp	Room temp	Refrigerate
Recommended initial infusion rate	0.01-0.02 mL/kg/min	0.5 mL/kg/h	0.01-0.02 mL/kg/min	1 mL/min
Maximum infusion rate	0.08 mL/kg/min	4 mL/kg/h	0.06 mL/kg/min	2 mL/min
Maximum concentration for infusion	10%	5%	5%	5%

Adverse Reactions

Cardiovascular: Flushing of the face, hypotension, tachycardia

Central nervous system: Dizziness, fever, headache, chills, anxiety, lightheadedness

Gastrointestinal: Nausea, vomiting

Neuromuscular & skeletal: Myalgia

Respiratory: Tightness in the chest

Miscellaneous: Hypersensitivity reactions, diaphoresis

Drug Interactions Live virus vaccines (measles, mumps, rubella)

Stability Do not mix with other drugs; see tables for storage

Mechanism of Action Replacement therapy for primary and secondary immunodeficiencies; interference with F_c receptors on the cells of the reticuloendothelial system for autoimmune cytopenias and ITP

Pharmacokinetics Half-life: 21-29 days; see tables pages 510 and 511.

Usual Dosage Children and Adults: I.V.:

Immunodeficiency syndrome: 200-400 mg/kg/dose every 3-4 weeks; maintain trough IgG concentration of 500 mg/dL

Chronic lymphocytic leukemia (CLL): 400 mg/kg/dose every 3 weeks

Idiopathic thrombocytopenic purpura: 400-1000 mg/kg/day for 2-5 consecutive days; maintenance dose: 400-1000 mg/kg/dose every 3-6 weeks based on clinical response and platelet count

Pediatric HIV infection: 400 mg/kg/dose every 4 weeks in those patients with hypogammaglobulinemia (IgG concentration <250 mg/dL), those with recurrent serious bacterial infections (2 or more infections in a 1-year period), those who fail to form antibodies to common antigens such as measles vaccine, and those living in areas where measles is prevalent and have not developed an antibody response after 2 doses of MMR

HIV-associated thrombocytopenia: 500-1000 mg/kg/day for 3-5 days

Kawasaki disease: 2 g/kg as a single dose or 400 mg/kg/day for 4 days

Congenital and acquired immunodeficiency syndrome: 100-400 mg/kg/dose every 3-4 weeks

Adjuvant in severe cytomegalovirus infection: 500 mg/kg/dose every other day for 7 doses

Bone marrow transplant: 400-500 mg/kg/dose every week for 3 months and then once every month

(Continued)

	Polygam® S/D	Sandoglobulin®	Venoglobulin®-S
FDA indication	Primary immuno-deficiency, ITP, CLL	Primary immuno-deficiency, ITP	Primary immuno-deficiency, ITP, Kawasaki disease
Contraindication	None (caution with IgA deficiency)	IgA deficiency	IgA deficiency
IgA content	0.74±0.33 mcg/mL	720 mcg/mL	5% (15.1 mcg/mL) 10% (20-50 mcg/mL)
Adverse reactions	6%	2.5%-6.6%	5.8%-14.8%
Plasma source	50,000 voluntary donors	>16,000 voluntary donors	>10,000 paid donors
Half-life	24 d	21-23 d	33.5 d
IgG subclass (%)			
IgG₁ (60-70)	67	60.5 (55.3)[1]	65.7-67.2
IgG₂ (19-31)	25	30.2 (35.7)	23.7-25.3
IgG₃ (5-8.4)	5	6.6 (6.3)	5.7-5.9
IgG₄ (0.7-4)	3	2.6 (2.6)	3-3.4
Monomers	>96.4%	92%	>95%
Gammaglobulin	>90%	>96%	>99%
Storage	Room temp	Room temp	5% Room temp 10% Refrigerate
Recommended **initial** infusion rate	0.5 mL/kg/h	0.01-0.03 mL/kg/min	0.01-0.02 mL/kg/min
Maximum infusion rate	4 mL/kg/h	2.5 mL/min	0.04 mL/kg/min
Maximum concentration for infusion	10%	12%	10%

[1]Skvaril F and Gardi A, "Differences Among Available Immunoglobulin Preparations for Intravenous Use," *Pediatr Infect Dis J,* 1988, 7:543-48.

[2]Roomer J, Morgenthaler JJ, Scherz R, et al, "Characterization of Various Immunoglobulin Preparations for Intravenous Application," *Vox Sang,* 1982, 42:62-73.

Reference: ASHP Commission on Therapeutics, "ASHP Therapeutic Guidelines for Intravenous Immune Globulin," *Clin Pharm,* 1992, 11:117-36.

Immune Globulin, Intravenous *(Continued)*

Guillain-Barré syndrome: 400 mg/kg/day for 4 days **or** 1 g/kg/day for 2 days **or** 2 g/kg as a single dose

Refractory dermatomyositis: 2 g/kg/dose every month for 3-4 doses

Refractory polymyositis: 1 g/kg/day for 2 days every month for 4 doses

Chronic inflammatory demyelinating polyneuropathy: 400 mg/kg/day for 5 days once each month **or** 1 g/kg/day for 2 days once each month

Severe systemic viral and bacterial infections:

Neonates: 500 mg/kg/day for 2 days then once weekly

Children: 500-1000 mg/kg/week

Prevention of gastroenteritis: Infants and Children: Oral: 50 mg/kg/day divided every 6 hours

Administration I.V. use only; for initial treatment, a lower concentration and/or a slower infusion rate should be used; if an adverse reaction occurs, reduce I.V. infusion rate to previously tolerated rate; see tables on pages 510 and 511.

Monitoring Parameters Platelet count, blood pressure, vital signs, Quantitative Immunoglobulins (QUIGS)

Nursing Implications Appropriate agents for treatment of a hypersensitivity reaction (eg, epinephrine) should be readily available; patients may need to be pretreated with an antipyretic, antihistamine, and/or corticosteroid to prevent chills and fever; adverse reactions may also be alleviated by decreasing the rate or the concentration of infusion or utilizing a different IGIV preparation

Dosage Forms

Injection: Gamimune® N:

5% [50 mg/mL] with maltose 10% (0.5 g, 2.5 g, 5 g, 10 g)

10% (1 g, 2.5 g, 5 g, 10 g, 20 g)

Powder for injection, lyophilized:

Gammagard® S/D: 0.5 g, 2.5 g, 5 g, 10 g

Gammar®-P IV: 1 g, 2.5 g, 5 g, 10 g

Iveegam®: 0.5 g, 1 g, 2.5 g, 5 g

Polygam® S/D: 2.5 g, 5 g, 10 g

Sandoglobulin®: 1 g, 3 g, 6 g, 12 g

Venoglobulin®-S:

5%: 2.5 g, 5 g, 10 g

10%: 5 g, 10 g, 20 g

References

ASHP Commission on Therapeutics, "ASHP Therapeutic Guidelines for Intravenous Immune Globulin," *Am J Hosp Pharm*, 1992, 49(3):652-4.

Blanchette VS, Luke B, Andrew M, et al, "A Prospective Randomized Trial of High-Dose Intravenous Immune Globulin G Therapy, Oral Prednisone Therapy, and No Therapy in Childhood Acute Immune Thrombocytopenic Purpura," *J Pediatr*, 1993, 123(6):989-95.

NIH Consensus Conference, "Intravenous Immunoglobulin, Prevention and Treatment of Disease," *JAMA*, 1990, 264(24):3189-93.

"University Hospital Consortium Expert Panel for Off-Label Use of Polyvalent Intravenously Administered Immunoglobulin Preparations Consensus Statement," *JAMA*, 1995, 273(23):1865-70.

♦ **Immunization Guidelines** *see page 1138*

♦ **Imodium®** *see Loperamide on page 580*

♦ **Imodium® A-D [OTC]** *see Loperamide on page 580*

♦ **Imodium® Advanced** *see Loperamide on page 580*

♦ **Imuran®** *see Azathioprine on page 112*

Inamrinone *(eye NAM ri none)*

Related Information

Adult ACLS Algorithm, Hypotension, Shock *on page 1016*

Brand Names Inocor®

Available Salts Inamrinone Lactate

Synonyms Amrinone

Therapeutic Category Phosphodiesterase Enzyme Inhibitor

Generic Available Yes

Use Short-term treatment of low cardiac output states (sepsis, CHF); adjunctive therapy of pulmonary hypertension

Pregnancy Risk Factor C

Contraindications Hypersensitivity to inamrinone lactate, any component, or sulfites (contains sodium metabisulfite)

Precautions Monitor for hypotension, thrombocytopenia, hepatotoxicity, and GI effects; discontinue inamrinone if significant increase in liver enzymes with symptoms of idiosyncratic hypersensitivity reaction (ie, eosinophilia) occurs; monitor fluids and electrolytes. Diuresis may result from improvement in cardiac output and may require dosage reduction of diuretics.

Adverse Reactions

Cardiovascular: Hypotension (1.3% incidence), ventricular and supraventricular arrhythmias (3% incidence); may be related to infusion rate

Gastrointestinal: Nausea (1.7%), vomiting (0.9%), abdominal pain (0.4%), anorexia (0.4%); GI effects may be due to an increase in gastric acid secretion and intestinal motility, secondary to phosphodiesterase inhibition

Hematologic: Thrombocytopenia (2.4% incidence), may be dose-related; in one study, 8 of 16 children (1.5 months to 11.2 years of age) developed thrombocytopenia (mean count 66 x 10^9 platelets/L). Inamrinone bolus doses ranged from 1.2-3 mg/kg given in 4 divided doses over 1 hour and were followed by continuous infusions of 5-10 mcg/kg/minute. Thrombocytopenia developed 19-71 hours after starting inamrinone (mean $\pm$ SD = 51 $\pm$ 25 hours). Resolution of thrombocytopenia occurred 54 $\pm$ 15 hours after therapy was discontinued; thrombocytopenia developed in patients with a higher total dose, longer duration of infusion, higher plasma concentrations of N-acetylamrinone (major metabolite of inamrinone), and higher plasma ratios of N-acetylamrinone to inamrinone.

Hepatic: Hepatotoxicity (0.2% incidence)

Drug Interactions Disopyramide may increase hypotension (one case report; use with caution); diuretics may cause significant hypovolemia (dosage reduction of diuretic may be required)

Stability Do not directly dilute with dextrose-containing solutions, chemical interaction occurs; may be administered I.V. into running dextrose infusions. Furosemide forms a precipitate when injected in I.V. lines containing inamrinone; incompatible with sodium bicarbonate; use diluted solutions of inamrinone (1-3 mg/mL) within 24 hours.

Mechanism of Action Inhibits phosphodiesterase III (PDE III), the major PDE in cardiac and vascular tissues. Inhibition of PDE III increases cyclic adenosine monophosphate (cAMP) which potentiates the delivery of calcium to myocardial contractile systems and results in a positive inotropic effect. Inhibition of PDE III in vascular tissue results in relaxation of vascular muscle and vasodilatation.

Pharmacodynamics

Onset of action: I.V.: Within 2-5 minutes

Peak effect: Within 10 minutes

Duration: Dose dependent with low doses lasting ~30 minutes and higher doses lasting ~2 hours

Pharmacokinetics

Distribution: V_d:

Neonates: 1.8 L/kg

Infants: 1.6 L/kg

Adults: 1.2 L/kg

Protein binding: 10% to 49%

Metabolism: In the liver to several metabolites (N-acetate, N-glycolyl, N-glucuronide, and O-glucuronide)

Half-life:

Neonates, 1-2 weeks of age: 22.2 hours

Infants 6-38 weeks of age: 6.8 hours; negative correlation of age with half-life in infants 4-38 weeks of age

Infants and Children (1 month to 15 years of age): 2.2-10.5 hours

Adults, normal volunteers: 3.6 hours

Adults with CHF: 5.8 hours

Elimination: Excreted in urine as metabolites and unchanged drug; 10% to 40% as unchanged drug in the urine within 24 hours

Usual Dosage I.V.: **Note:** Dose should not exceed 10 mg/kg/24 hours; doses of 18 mg/kg/day have been used in adults for a short duration; titrate infusion based on patient clinical response and adverse effects

Neonates: 0.75 mg/kg I.V. bolus over 2-3 minutes followed by maintenance infusion 3-5 mcg/kg/minute; I.V. bolus may need to be repeated in 30 minutes; see Additional Information

Infants and Children: 0.75 mg/kg I.V. bolus over 2-3 minutes followed by maintenance infusion 5-10 mcg/kg/minute; I.V. bolus may need to be repeated in 30 minutes; see Additional Information

Adults: 0.75 mg/kg I.V. bolus over 2-3 minutes followed by maintenance infusion of 5-10 mcg/kg/minute; I.V. bolus may need to be repeated in 30 minutes

Administration Parenteral:

I.V. bolus: Infuse over 2-3 minutes; may be administered undiluted

(Continued)

Inamrinone *(Continued)*

Continuous infusion: Dilute with NS or ½NS to final concentration of 1-3 mg/mL; use controlled infusion device (eg, I.V. pump)

Monitoring Parameters Blood pressure, heart rate, platelet count, liver enzymes, fluid status, intake and output, body weight, serum electrolytes; if Swan-Ganz catheter is present, monitor cardiac index, stroke volume, systemic vascular resistance, pulmonary vascular resistance

Reference Range Proposed: Adults: 3 μg/mL; linear correlation with cardiac index observed from 0.5-7 μg/mL

Nursing Implications Do **not** administer furosemide I.V. push via "Y" site into inamrinone solutions as precipitate will occur; monitor patients closely (see Monitoring Parameters)

Additional Information Preliminary pharmacokinetic studies estimate that total initial bolus doses of 3-4.5 mg/kg given in divided doses to neonates and infants are required to obtain serum concentrations similar to therapeutic adult levels. The use of these higher doses has been reported in a small number of infants and children. Some centers use a total loading dose of 3 mg/kg (administered as 4 doses of 0.75 mg/kg/dose given every 15 minutes); each of the 0.75 mg/kg doses is given over 5 minutes. Further pharmacodynamic studies are needed to define pediatric inamrinone dosing guidelines.

Use of inamrinone in controlled trials did not extend beyond 48 hours; due to potential serious adverse effects and limited experience, inamrinone should only be used in patients who have not responded to other therapies (ie, digoxin, diuretics, vasodilators). Inamrinone has not been shown to be safe or effective for long-term treatment of CHF.

Effective July 1, 2000, the nonproprietary name of the drug (amrinone) was officially changed by the U.S. Pharmacopeia (USP) Nomenclature Committee and the U.S. Adopted Names (USAN) Council to inamrinone to prevent confusion with amiodarone; other countries will still use the name amrinone

Dosage Forms Injection, as lactate: 5 mg/mL (20 mL)

References

Allen-Webb EM, Ross MP, Pappas JB, et al, "Age-Related Amrinone Pharmacokinetics in a Pediatric Population," *Crit Care Med*, 1994, 22(6):1016-24.

Lawless S, Burckart G, Diven W, et al, "Amrinone in Neonates and Infants After Cardiac Surgery," *Crit Care Med*, 1989, 17(8):751-4.

Lawless ST, Zaritsky A, and Miles MV, "The Acute Pharmacokinetics and Pharmacodynamics of Amrinone in Pediatric Patients," *J Clin Pharmacol*, 1991, 31(9):800-3.

Lynn AM, Sorensen GK, and Williams GD, "Hemodynamic Effects of Amrinone and Colloid Administration in Children Following Cardiac Surgery," *J Cardiothorac Vasc Anesth*, 1993, 7(5):560-5.

Ross MP, Allen-Webb EM, Pappas JB, et al, "Amrinone-Associated Thrombocytopenia: Pharmacokinetic Analysis," *Clin Pharmacol Ther*, 1993, 53(6):661-7.

♦ **Inamrinone Lactate** *see* Inamrinone *on page 512*

♦ **I-Naphline® Ophthalmic** *see* Naphazoline *on page 671*

♦ **Inapsine®** *see* Droperidol *on page 351*

♦ **Inderal®** *see* Propranolol *on page 816*

♦ **Inderal® LA** *see* Propranolol *on page 816*

Indinavir *(in DIN a veer)*

Related Information

Adult and Adolescent HIV *on page 1133*
Pediatric HIV *on page 1129*

Brand Names Crixivan®

Synonyms L-735,524; MK-639

Therapeutic Category Antiretroviral Agent; HIV Agents (Anti-HIV Agents); Protease Inhibitor

Use Treatment of HIV infection in combination with other antiretroviral agents; **(Note:** Current preferred HIV regimens consist of three antiretroviral agents); postexposure chemoprophylaxis following occupational exposure to HIV

Pregnancy Risk Factor C

Contraindications Hypersensitivity to indinavir or any component

Warnings Cases of nephrolithiasis and nephrolithiasis associated with renal insufficiency or acute renal failure have been reported. If signs and symptoms of nephrolithiasis occur (flank pain with or without hematuria), interrupt or discontinue therapy. Due to potential serious and life-threatening drug interactions, the following drugs should not be coadministered with indinavir: terfenadine, astemizole, cisapride, ergot alkaloid derivatives, triazolam, and midazolam. Concomitant use with rifampin is contraindicated since rifampin may markedly reduce indinavir concentrations. Spontaneous bleeding episodes have been reported in patients with hemophilia A and B. New onset diabetes mellitus, exacerbation of diabetes and hyperglycemia have been reported in HIV-infected patients receiving protease inhibitors. Redistribution or accumulation of body fat may occur in patients taking protease inhibitors.

Precautions Use with caution in patients with hepatic impairment; modify dose in patients with impaired liver function

Adverse Reactions

Central nervous system: Insomnia, dizziness, headache, somnolence, asthenia, depression

Dermatologic: Rash, dry skin, urticaria, pruritus, paronychia

Endocrine & metabolic: Rare: Hyperglycemia, diabetes, ketoacidosis

Gastrointestinal: Nausea (10%), vomiting, diarrhea, abdominal pain, dyspepsia, metallic taste, pancreatitis

Genitourinary: Dysuria

Hematologic: Hemolytic anemia, spontaneous bleeding episodes in hemophiliacs (rare)

Hepatic: Hyperbilirubinemia (10%), elevated liver function tests, jaundice, liver cirrhosis

Neuromuscular & skeletal: Arthralgia

Renal: Nephrolithiasis (4%), hematuria, proteinuria, renal failure, interstitial nephritis

Respiratory: Dry throat, pharyngitis

Drug Interactions Coadministration with didanosine will decrease indinavir absorption; coadministration with rifampin will greatly reduce indinavir levels; indinavir increases rifabutin concentrations (decrease daily rifabutin dose by 50%); ketoconazole and itraconazole increase indinavir concentrations (dosage reduction of indinavir is recommended); ritonavir and other protease inhibitors decrease the metabolism of indinavir; coadministration with nevirapine may decrease indinavir concentrations; efavirenz decreases indinavir concentrations (indinavir dosage increase is recommended); delavirdine increases indinavir concentrations (dosage reduction of indinavir is recommended); (see Warnings related to potentially serious and life-threatening drug interactions)

Food Interactions Decreased absorption when administered with high amounts of protein or fatty foods; 26% decrease in AUC when administered with grapefruit juice

Stability Store capsules at room temperature in original container with desiccant since capsules are sensitive to moisture

Mechanism of Action A protease inhibitor which acts on an enzyme late in the HIV replication process after the virus has entered into the cell's nucleus preventing cleavage of the gag-pol protein precursors resulting in the production of immature, noninfectious virions; cross-resistance with other protease inhibitors is possible

Pharmacokinetics

Absorption: Rapid; presence of food decreases the extent of absorption

Protein binding: 60%

Metabolism: In the liver by CYP3A4 system to inactive metabolites

Bioavailability: Wide interpatient variability in children: 15% to 50%

Half-life: 1.8-2 hours

Time to peak serum concentration: 0.8-1 hour

Elimination: 83% in feces as unabsorbed drug and metabolites; 10% excreted in urine as unchanged drug

Usual Dosage Oral:

Neonates: Should not be administered to neonates until further studies are performed due to side effect of hyperbilirubinemia

Children: Under study in clinical trials: 500 mg/m^2/dose every 8 hours; maximum dose: 800 mg/dose every 8 hours

Adolescents and Adults: 800 mg/dose every 8 hours

Chemoprophylaxis after high-risk occupational exposure to HIV: 800 mg/dose every 8 hours in combination with zidovudine and lamivudine

Dosage adjustment in mild to moderate hepatic impairment: Reduce dose by 25%

Administration Administer with water on an empty stomach or with a light snack 1 hour before or 2 hours after a meal; may administer with other liquids (ie, skim milk, apple juice) or a light snack (ie, dry toast or cornflakes with skim milk); if coadministered with didanosine, give at least 1 hour apart on an empty stomach

Monitoring Parameters Serum bilirubin, liver function tests, urinalysis, blood glucose levels, CD4 cell count, plasma levels of HIV RNA

(Continued)

515

Indinavir (Continued)

Patient Information If dose is missed, the dose should be omitted and the next dose taken at the usual scheduled time; do not double the next dose

Nursing Implications Ensure adequate patient hydration to minimize the risk of nephrolithiasis

Dosage Forms Capsule: 200 mg, 333 mg, 400 mg

References

CDC and the National Foundation for Infectious Disease, "Update: Provisional Public Health Service Recommendations for Chemoprophylaxis After Occupational Exposure to HIV," *MMWR Morb Mortal Wkly Rep*, 1996, 45(22):468-80.

Mueller BU, Smith S, Sleasman J, et al, "A Phase I/II Study of the Protease Inhibitor Indinavir (MK-0639) in Children With HIV Infection," *Eleventh International Conference on AIDS*, Vancouver, Canada, 1996.

Stein DS, Fish DG, Bilello JA, et al, "A 24-Week Open-Label Phase I/II Evaluation of the HIV Protease Inhibitor MK-639 (Indinavir)," *AIDS*, 1996, 10(5):485-92.

Working Group on Antiretroviral Therapy and Medical Management of HIV-Infected Children, "Guidelines for the Use of Antiretroviral Agents in Pediatric HIV Infection," January 7, 2000, http://www.hivatis.org.

♦ **Indocin® I.V. Injection** *see* Indomethacin *on page 516*

♦ **Indocin® Oral** *see* Indomethacin *on page 516*

♦ **Indocin® SR Oral** *see* Indomethacin *on page 516*

♦ **Indocollyre® (Canada)** *see* Indomethacin *on page 516*

Indomethacin (in doe METH a sin)

Related Information

Overdose and Toxicology *on page 1191*

Brand Names Apo®-Indomethacin (Canada); Indocin® I.V. Injection; Indocin® Oral; Indocin® SR Oral; Indocollyre® (Canada); Indotec (Canada); Novo-Methacin® (Canada); Nu-Indo® (Canada); Pro-Indo® (Canada)

Available Salts Indomethacin Sodium Trihydrate

Therapeutic Category Analgesic, Non-narcotic; Anti-inflammatory Agent; Antipyretic; Nonsteroidal Anti-inflammatory Drug (NSAID), Oral; Nonsteroidal Anti-inflammatory Drug (NSAID), Parenteral

Generic Available Yes, except injection

Use Management of inflammatory diseases and rheumatoid disorders; moderate pain; acute gouty arthritis; I.V. form used as alternative to surgery for closure of patent ductus arteriosus (PDA) in neonates

Pregnancy Risk Factor B (D if used longer than 48 hours or after 34 weeks gestation)

Contraindications Hypersensitivity to indomethacin, any component, aspirin, or other NSAIDs; active GI bleeding, ulcer disease; premature neonates with necrotizing enterocolitis, impaired renal function (eg, neonates with urine output <0.6 mL/kg/hour or serum creatinine ≥1.8 mg/dL), IVH, active bleeding, thrombocytopenia

Precautions Use with caution in patients with cardiac dysfunction, hypertension, renal or hepatic impairment, epilepsy, patients receiving anticoagulants and for treatment of JRA in children (fatal hepatitis has been reported)

Adverse Reactions

Cardiovascular: Hypertension, edema

Central nervous system: Somnolence, fatigue, depression, confusion, dizziness, headache

Dermatologic: Rash

Endocrine & metabolic: Hyperkalemia, dilutional hyponatremia (I.V.), hypoglycemia (I.V.)

Gastrointestinal: Nausea, vomiting, epigastric pain, abdominal pain, anorexia, GI bleeding, ulcers, perforation

Hematologic: Hemolytic anemia, bone marrow suppression, agranulocytosis, thrombocytopenia, inhibition of platelet aggregation

Hepatic: Hepatitis

Ocular: Corneal opacities

Otic: Tinnitus

Renal: Renal failure, oliguria

Miscellaneous: Hypersensitivity reactions

Drug Interactions Cytochrome P-450 isoenzyme CYP2C9 substrate

Indomethacin may increase serum concentrations of digoxin, methotrexate, lithium, and aminoglycosides (reported with I.V. use in neonates); may increase nephrotoxicity of cyclosporin; may decrease antihypertensive and diuretic effects of furosemide and thiazides; may increase serum potassium with potassium-sparing diuretics; may decrease antihypertensive effects of beta-blockers, hydralazine, and captopril; aspirin may decrease and probenecid may increase indomethacin serum concentrations; other GI irritants (eg, potassium supplements, NSAIDs) may increase GI adverse effects

Food Interactions Food may decrease the rate but not the extent of absorption

Stability

Oral suspension: Store below 86°F; do not freeze

I.V. product: Protect from light; not stable in alkaline solution; reconstitute just prior to administration; discard any unused portion; do not use preservative-containing diluents for reconstitution; will precipitate if reconstituted with solutions at pH <6 (product is not buffered)

Mechanism of Action Inhibits prostaglandin synthesis by decreasing the activity of the enzyme, cyclo-oxygenase, which results in decreased formation of prostaglandin precursors

Pharmacokinetics

Absorption: Oral:

Neonates: Incomplete, nonuniform

Adults: Rapid and well absorbed

Distribution:

Neonates: PDA: 0.36 L/kg

Post-PDA closure: 0.26 L/kg

Adults: 0.34-1.57 L/kg

Protein binding: 99%

Metabolism: In the liver via glucuronide conjugation and other pathways

Bioavailability: Oral:

Neonates, premature: 13% to 20%

Adults: ~100%

Half-life:

Neonates:

Postnatal age (PNA) <2 weeks: ~20 hours

PNA >2 weeks: ~11 hours

Adults: 2.6-11.2 hours

Elimination: Significant enterohepatic recycling; 33% excreted in feces as demethylated metabolites with 1.5% as unchanged drug; 60% in urine as drug and metabolites

Usual Dosage

Patent ductus arteriosus:

Neonates: I.V.: Initial: 0.2 mg/kg, followed by 2 doses depending on postnatal age (PNA):

PNA **at time of first dose** <48 hours: 0.1 mg/kg at 12- to 24-hour intervals

PNA **at time of first dose** 2-7 days: 0.2 mg/kg at 12- to 24-hour intervals

PNA **at time of first dose** >7 days: 0.25 mg/kg at 12- to 24-hour intervals

In general, may use 12-hour dosing interval if urine output >1 mL/kg/hour after prior dose; use 24-hour dosing interval if urine output is <1 mL/kg/hour but >0.6 mL/kg/hour; doses should be withheld if patient has oliguria (urine output <0.6 mL/kg/hour) or anuria

Inflammatory/rheumatoid disorders:

Oral:

Children: 1-2 mg/kg/day in 2-4 divided doses; maximum dose: 4 mg/kg/day; not to exceed 150-200 mg/day

Adults: 25-50 mg/dose 2-3 times/day; maximum dose: 200 mg/day; extended release capsule should be given on a 1-2 times/day schedule

Rectal: Adults: Persistent night pain and/or morning stiffness: 50-100 mg at bedtime (as part of total daily dose maximum of 200 mg/day)

Administration

Oral: Administer with food, milk, or antacids to decrease GI adverse effects; extended release capsules must be swallowed whole, do not crush or chew

Parenteral: I.V.: Administer over 20-30 minutes at a concentration of 0.5-1 mg/mL in preservative free sterile water for injection or preservative free NS

Note: Do **not** administer via I.V. bolus or I.V. infusion via an umbilical catheter into vessels near the superior mesenteric artery, as these may cause vasoconstriction and can compromise blood flow to the intestines. Do not administer intra-arterially.

Rectal: Insert into rectum and retain

Monitoring Parameters BUN, serum creatinine, liver enzymes, CBC with differential; in addition, in neonates treated for PDA: heart rate, heart murmur, blood pressure, urine output, echocardiogram, serum sodium, platelet count, and serum concentrations of concomitantly administered drugs which are renally eliminated (eg, aminoglycosides, digoxin); periodic ophthalmic exams with chronic use

Patient Information Avoid alcohol; may cause dizziness

(Continued)

Indomethacin *(Continued)*

Additional Information Indomethacin may mask signs and symptoms of infections; fatalities in children have been reported, due to unrecognized overwhelming sepsis; drowsiness, lethargy, nausea, vomiting, seizures, paresthesia, headache, dizziness, tinnitus, GI bleeding, cerebral edema, and cardiac arrest have been reported with overdoses

Dosage Forms

Capsule: 25 mg, 50 mg

Capsule, sustained release: 75 mg

Powder for injection, as sodium trihydrate: 1 mg

Suppository, rectal: 50 mg

Suspension, oral (pineapple-coconut-mint flavor): 25 mg/5 mL (5 mL, 10 mL, 237 mL, 500 mL)

References

Coombs RC, Morgan ME, Durbin GM, et al, "Gut Blood Flow Velocities in the Newborn: Effects of Patent Ductus Arteriosus and Parenteral Indomethacin," *Arch Dis Child*, 1990, 65(10 Spec No):1067-71.

Gersony WM, Peckham GJ, Ellison RC, et al, "Effects of Indomethacin in Premature Infants With Patent Ductus Arteriosus: Results of a National Collaborative Study," *J Pediatr*, 1983, 102(6):895-906.

Kraus DM and Hatzopoulos FK, "Neonatal Therapy," *Applied Therapeutics: The Clinical Use of Drugs*, 6th ed, Young LY, Koda-Kimble MA, eds, Vancouver, WA: Applied Therapeutics, Inc, 1995.

Indomethacin Sodium Trihydrate *see* Indomethacin *on page 516*

Indotec (Canada) *see* Indomethacin *on page 516*

Infants' Advil® Concentrated Drops *see* Ibuprofen *on page 501*

Infasurf® *see* Calfactant *on page 161*

Infectrol® Ophthalmic *see* Dexamethasone, Neomycin, and Polymyxin B *on page 297*

InFed™ *see* Iron Dextran Complex *on page 528*

Inflamase® Forte Ophthalmic *see* Prednisolone *on page 791*

Inflamase® Mild Ophthalmic *see* Prednisolone *on page 791*

Influenza Virus Vaccine *see page 1138*

Infumorph® Injection *see* Morphine Sulfate *on page 657*

INH *see* Isoniazid *on page 534*

Innovar® *see* Droperidol and Fentanyl *on page 352*

Inocor® *see* Inamrinone *on page 512*

Insta-Char® [OTC] *see* Charcoal *on page 202*

Insta-Glucose® [OTC] *see* Dextrose *on page 305*

Insulin Lente® L *see* Insulin Preparations *on page 518*

Insulin Preparations *(IN su lin prep a RAY shuns)*

Brand Names Humalog®; Humalog® Mix 50/50™; Humalog® Mix 75/25™; Humulin® 50/50; Humulin® 70/30; Humulin® L; Humulin® N; Humulin® R; Humulin® U; Iletin® (Canada); Iletin® II Pork (Canada); Insulin Lente® L; Lantus®; Lente®; Lente® Iletin® I; Lente® Iletin® II; Novolin® 70/30; Novolin® ge (Canada); Novolin® L; Novolin® N; Novolin-Pen® II, -3 (Canada); Novolin® R; NovoLog™; NPH Iletin® I; NPH Insulin; NPH-N; Pork NPH; Pork Regular Iletin® II; Regular Iletin® I; Regular [Concentrated] Iletin® II U-500; Regular Insulin; Regular Purified Pork Insulin; Velosulin®; Velosulin® BR Human (Buffered)

Therapeutic Category Antidiabetic Agent

Generic Available Yes

Use Treatment of insulin-dependent diabetes mellitus, also noninsulin-dependent diabetes mellitus unresponsive to treatment with diet and/or oral hypoglycemics; to assure proper utilization of glucose and reduce glucosuria in nondiabetic patients receiving parenteral nutrition whose glucosuria cannot be adequately controlled with infusion rate adjustments or those who require assistance in achieving optimal caloric intakes; treatment of hyperkalemia (use with glucose to shift potassium into cells to lower serum potassium levels)

Pregnancy Risk Factor B

Contraindications Hypoglycemia; only regular insulin may be given intravenously; hypersensitivity to the insulin source (eg, beef or pork) or any components

Warnings Any change of insulin should be made cautiously; changing manufacturers, type and/or method of manufacture, may result in the need for a change of dosage; human insulin differs from animal-source insulin; hypoglycemia may result from increased work or exercise without eating

Adverse Reactions Primarily symptoms of hypoglycemia

Cardiovascular: Palpitations, tachycardia, pallor

Central nervous system: Fatigue, mental confusion, loss of consciousness, headache, hypothermia

Dermatologic: Urticaria, redness

Endocrine & metabolic: Hypoglycemia, hypokalemia

Gastrointestinal: Hunger, nausea, numbness of mouth

Local: Itching, redness, edema, stinging, or warmth at injection site, atrophy or hypertrophy of S.C. fat tissue

Neuromuscular & skeletal: Muscle weakness, tremors, tingling of fingers

Ocular: Transient presbyopia or blurred vision

Miscellaneous: Diaphoresis, anaphylaxis

Drug Interactions See tables.

Drug Interactions With Insulin

Decrease Hypoglycemic Effects	Increase Hypoglycemic Effects
Acetazolamide	ACE inhibitors
Antiretrovirals	Alcohol
Asparaginase	Alpha-blockers
Calcitonin	Anabolic steroids
Contraceptives, oral	Beta blockers, nonselective
Corticosteroids	Calcium
Cyclophosphamide	Chloroquine
Diazoxide	Clofibrate
Diltiazem	Guanethidine
Dobutamine	Lithium
Epinephrine	MAO inhibitors
Estrogens	Mebendazole
Ethacrynic acid	Octreotide
Isoniazid	Oral antidiabetic agents
Lithium	(oral hypoglycemic agents)
Morphine	Pentamidine
Niacin	Phenylbutazone
Phenothiazines	Pyridoxine
Phenytoin	Salicylates
Nicotine	Sulfinpyrazone
Thiazide diuretics	Sulfonamides
Thyroid hormone	Tetracyclines

Stability

Newer neutral formulations of insulin are stable at room temperature up to 1 month and 3 months refrigerated; cold (freezing) causes more damage to insulin than room temperatures up to 100°F; avoid direct sunlight; cold injections should be avoided

Insulin Mixture Compatibility

Insulin Preparations	Compatible Mixed With
Rapid-Acting Insulin injection (regular)	All (except Velosulin® BR and Lantus®)
Prompt insulin zinc suspension (Semilente®)	Lente®
Lispro insulin solution (Humalog®)	Ultralente®, NPH
Intermediate-Acting Isophane insulin suspension (NPH)	Regular and Humalog®
Insulin zinc suspension (Lente®)	Regular and Semilente®
Extended insulin zinc suspension (Ultralente®)	Regular, Semilente®, Humalog®

(Continued)

Insulin Preparations *(Continued)*

When mixing with NPH insulin in any proportion, the excess protamine may combine with regular insulin and may reduce or delay activity of regular insulin (does not appear to be clinically significant); phosphate-buffered regular insulins bind with Lente® insulins forming short-acting insulin

Stability of parenteral admixture of regular insulin in NS or 1/2 NS at room temperature (25°C) and at refrigeration temperature (4°C): 24 hours; all bags should be prepared fresh; tubing should be flushed 30 minutes prior to administration to allow adsorption as time permits

Mechanism of Action The principal hormone required for proper glucose utilization in normal metabolic processes; it is obtained from beef or pork pancreas or a biosynthetic process converting pork insulin to human insulin; insulins are categorized into 3 groups related to promptness, duration, and intensity of action

Pharmacodynamics Onset and duration of hypoglycemic effects depend upon the route of administration, site of injection, volume and concentration of injection, and the preparation administered; see table.

Pharmacodynamics of Insulin Preparations

Insulin Preparations	Onset (h)	Peak (h)	Duration (h)
Rapid-Acting			
Insulin aspart (NovoLog™)	0.25	1-3	3-5
Insulin injection (regular)	0.5-1	2-3	5-7
Prompt insulin zinc suspension (Semilente®)	1-1.5	5-10	12-16
Lispro insulin (Humalog®)	0.25	0.5-1.5	6-8
Intermediate-Acting			
Isophane insulin suspension (NPH)	1-1.5	4-12	24
Insulin zinc suspension (Lente®)	1-2.5	7-15	24
Long-Acting			
Extended insulin zinc suspension (Ultralente®)	4-8	10-30	>36

Usual Dosage Dose requires continuous medical supervision; only regular insulin may be given I.V. The daily dose should be divided up depending upon the product used and the patient's response (see table) (eg, regular insulin every 4-6 hours; NPH insulin every 8-12 hours).

Children and Adults: S.C.: 0.5-1 unit/kg/day in divided doses

Adolescents (during growth spurt) S.C.: 0.8-1.2 units/kg/day in divided doses

Diabetic ketoacidosis: Children: I.V. loading dose: 0.1 unit/kg, then maintenance continuous infusion: 0.1 unit/kg/hour (range: 0.05-0.2 unit/kg/hour depending upon the rate of decrease of serum glucose). Decreasing the serum glucose level too rapidly may lead to cerebral edema; optimum rate of decrease (serum glucose): 80-100 mg/dL/hour

> **Note:** Newly diagnosed patients with juvenile onset diabetes mellitus presenting in DKA and patients with blood sugars <800 mg/dL may be relatively "sensitive" to insulin and should receive loading and initial maintenance doses approximately 1/2 of those indicated above.

Sliding scale: Use only for brief transitional periods of treatment; newly diagnosed patients with juvenile onset diabetes may be "sensitive" to exogenous insulin and should be treated with the lower end of these ranges; see table.

Insulin Dosing Sliding Scale

Urine Glucose	Insulin Dose (units/kg)	
	Urine Ketones (-)	Urine Ketones (+)
0-1/2%	0	0
3/4%	0.03-0.1	0.05-0.12
1%	0.07-0.2	0.1-0.25
2%	0.15-0.4	0.2-0.5

To optimize caloric intake in neonates while on parenteral nutrition:
  Continuous infusion: I.V.: Neonates: 0.01-0.1 unit/kg/hour; neonates are very sensitive to insulin; start at low end of infusion rate and monitor closely
  Treatment of hyperkalemia (after treatment with I.V. calcium gluconate and NaHCO$_3$):
    Children: Dextrose 0.5-1 g/kg (using 25% or 50%) combined with insulin 1 unit for every 4-5 g dextrose; infuse over 2 hours or dextrose 0.5-1 g/kg infused over 15-30 minutes followed by 0.1 unit/kg insulin S.C. or I.V.
    Adults: 50% dextrose at 0.5-1 mL/kg and insulin 1 unit for every 4-5 g dextrose given

Dosing adjustment in renal impairment: Children and Adults:
  Cl$_{cr}$ 10-50 mL/minute: Administer 75% of recommended dose
  Cl$_{cr}$ <10 mL/minute: Administer 25% to 50% of recommended dose (follow blood sugar closely)

Administration
Parenteral: S.C., I.M. S.C.: Administration is usually made into the thighs, arms, buttocks, or abdomen, with sites rotated; when mixing regular insulin with other preparations of insulin, regular insulin should be drawn into syringe first; insulin lispro and insulin aspart (when used as "meal-time" insulin, due to a rapid onset of effect) should be administered 15 minutes before meals; regular insulin should be administered 30-60 minutes before meals; do not mix Velosulin® BR or Lantus® with other insulins; to achieve complete suspension, insulin pens should be tipped at least 20 times before injection

I.V. (**only regular insulin** may be administered I.V.) infusion (requires use of an infusion pump): To minimize adsorption problems to I.V. solution bag and tubing:
  If new tubing is **not** needed: Wait a minimum of 30 minutes between the preparation of the solution and the initiation of the infusion
  If new tubing is needed: After receiving the insulin drip solution, the administration set should be attached to the I.V. container and the line should be flushed with the insulin solution. The nurse should then wait 30 minutes, then flush the line again with the insulin solution prior to initiating the infusion.

Because of adsorption, the actual amount of insulin being administered could be substantially less than the apparent amount. Therefore, adjustment of the insulin drip rate should be based on effect and not solely on the apparent insulin dose. Furthermore, the apparent I.V. infusion dose should not be used as the basis for determining the subsequent insulin dose upon discontinuing the insulin drip. Dosage adjustment requires continuous medical supervision.

Monitoring Parameters Urine sugar and acetone, blood sugar, serum electrolytes

Patient Information Do not change insulins without physician's approval; patients should be counseled by someone experienced in diabetes education regarding signs and symptoms of hyper- and hypoglycemia, exercise and diet, blood glucose monitoring, and other related topics

Additional Information The term "purified" refers to insulin preparations containing no more than 10 ppm proinsulin (purified and human insulins are less immunogenic); buffering agent in Velosulin® BR may alter the activity of other insulin products

Dosage Forms All insulins are 100 units/mL (10 mL) except where indicated:
RAPID-ACTING:
Insulin aspart (rDNA origin): NovoLog™ (10 mL; 3 mL PenFill cartridges)
Insulin lispro rDNA origin: Humalog® [Lilly] (1.5 mL, 10 mL)
Insulin Injection (Regular Insulin)
  Beef and pork: Regular Iletin® I [Lilly]
  Human:
    rDNA: Humulin® R [Lilly], Novolin® R [Novo Nordisk], Novolin® R PenFill [Novo Nordisk], Novolin® R Prefilled [Novo Nordisk]
    rDNA, Buffered: Velosulin® BR
    Semisynthetic: Velosulin® Human [Novo Nordisk]
  Pork: Regular Insulin [Novo Nordisk]
  Purified pork:
    Pork Regular Iletin® II [Lilly], Regular Purified Pork Insulin [Novo Nordisk]
    Regular (Concentrated) Iletin® II U-500 (Lilly): 500 units/mL

INTERMEDIATE-ACTING:
Insulin Zinc Suspension (Lente)
  Beef and pork: Lente® Iletin® I [Lilly]
  Human, rDNA: Humulin® L [Lilly], Novolin® L [Novo Nordisk]
  Purified pork: Lente® Iletin® II [Lilly], Lente® L [Novo Nordisk]

Isophane Insulin Suspension (NPH)
  Beef and pork: NPH Iletin® I [Lilly]
(Continued)

Insulin Preparations *(Continued)*

Human, rDNA: Humulin® N [*Lilly*], Novolin® N [*Novo Nordisk*], Novolin® N PenFill [*Novo Nordisk*], Novolin® N Prefilled [*Novo Nordisk*]

Purified pork: Pork NPH Iletin® II [*Lilly*], NPH-N [*Novo Nordisk*]

LONG-ACTING:

Insulin zinc suspension, extended (Ultralente®)

Human, rDNA: Humulin® U [Lilly]

COMBINATIONS:

Isophane Insulin Suspension and Insulin Injection

Isophane insulin suspension (50%) and insulin injection (50%) human (rDNA): Humulin® 50/50 [*Lilly*]

Isophane insulin suspension (70%) and insulin injection (30%) human (rDNA): Humulin® 70/30 [*Lilly*], Novolin® 70/30 [*Novo Nordisk*], Novolin® 70/30 PenFill [*Novo Nordisk*], Novolin® 70/30 Prefilled [*Novo Nordisk*]

Insulin Lispro Protamine Suspension and Insulin Lispro Injection

Insulin lispro protamine suspension (75%) and insulin lispro injection (25%) Humalog® Mix 75/25™ [*Lilly*]

Insulin lispro protamine suspension (50%) and insulin lispro injection (50%) Humalog® Mix 50/50™ [*Lilly*]

HIGH POTENCY:

Insulin injection, concentrated (Regular insulin): Pork: Iletin® II [*Lilly*]: 500 units/mL

References

Simeon PS, Geffner ME, Levin SR, et al, "Continuous Insulin Infusions in Neonates: Pharmacologic Availability of Insulin in Intravenous Solutions," *J Pediatr*, 1994, 124(5 Pt 1):818-20.

Insulin Reaction [OTC] *see* Dextrose *on page 305*

Intal® *see* Cromolyn *on page 260*

α-2-interferon *see* Interferon Alfa-2b *on page 524*

Interferon Alfa-2a *(in ter FEER on AL fa too aye)*

Brand Names Roferon-A®

Synonyms IFLrA; IFN; rIFN-α

Therapeutic Category Antineoplastic Agent, Miscellaneous; Biological Response Modulator; Interferon

Generic Available No

Use FDA approved in patients >18 years of age: Hairy cell leukemia, AIDS-related Kaposi's sarcoma, Philadelphia chromosome-positive chronic myelogenous leukemia, hemangiomas of infancy; multiple unlabeled uses

Pregnancy Risk Factor C

Contraindications Hypersensitivity to alpha interferon or any component

Warnings The FDA currently recommends that procedures for proper handling and disposal of antineoplastic agents be considered; safety and efficacy in children <18 years of age have not been established; injection contains benzyl alcohol which may be toxic to newborns in high doses

Precautions Use with caution in patients with seizure disorders, brain metastases, multiple sclerosis, compromised CNS, and patients with pre-existing cardiac disease, myelosuppression, or severe renal/hepatic impairment

Adverse Reactions Flu-like symptoms (fever, fatigue/malaise, myalgia, chills, headache, arthralgia, rigors) begin about 2-6 hours after the dose is given and may persist as long as 24 hours; usually patient can build up a tolerance to side effects

Cardiovascular: Tachycardia, arrhythmias, hypotension, edema, chest pain

Central nervous system: Fatigue/malaise, dizziness, depression, confusion, sensory neuropathy, psychiatric effects, fever, headache, EEG abnormalities, chills

Dermatologic: Partial alopecia, rash, dry skin

Endocrine & metabolic: Increased uric acid level, thyroid dysfunction

Gastrointestinal: Anorexia, xerostomia, nausea, vomiting, diarrhea, abdominal cramps, dysgeusia, weight loss, stomatitis

Hematologic: Leukopenia (mainly neutropenia); anemia; thrombocytopenia; decreased hemoglobin, hematocrit, platelets; neutralizing antibodies

Hepatic: Increased ALT and AST

Local: Burning, pain, erythema, rash at the site of injection

Neuromuscular & skeletal: Myalgia, arthralgia, rigors, leg cramps

Ocular: Blurred vision

Renal: Proteinuria, elevated BUN, elevated serum creatinine

Respiratory: Coughing, nasal congestion

Miscellaneous: Diaphoresis

Drug Interactions
Interferon Alfa-2b: Possible competitive binding to same receptors
Acyclovir: Possible synergistic effects
Theophylline: Clearance of theophylline is reduced
Vinblastine: May increase interferon toxicity; increased neurotoxicity
Zidovudine: Possible additive myelosuppression

Stability Store in refrigerator; do not shake; after reconstitution stable at room temperature for 24 hours; do not store in syringes for prolonged periods

Mechanism of Action Inhibits cellular growth, alters the state of cellular differentiation, interferes with oncogene expression, alters cell surface antigen expression, increases phagocytic activity of macrophages and augments cytotoxicity of lymphocytes for target cells

Pharmacokinetics
Absorption: I.M., S.C.: >80%
Metabolism: In the kidney, filtered, and absorbed at the renal tubule
Half-life:
   I.M., I.V.: 2 hours
   S.C.: 3 hours
Time to peak serum concentration: Within 3-8 hours

Usual Dosage Refer to individual protocols
Infants and Children:
   Hemangiomas of infancy, pulmonary hemangiomatosis: S.C.: 1-3 million units/m^2/day once daily
   Philadelphia chromosome-positive CML: I.M., S.C.: 2.5-5 million units/m^2 daily
Children >18 years and Adults: I.M., S.C.:
   Hairy cell leukemia: Induction dose is 3 million units/day for 16-24 weeks; maintenance: 3 million units 3 times/week
   AIDS-related Kaposi's sarcoma: Induction dose: 36 million units/day for 10-12 weeks; maintenance: 36 million units 3 times/week (may begin with dose escalation from 3 to 9 to 18 million units each day over 3 consecutive days followed by 36 million units/day for the remainder of the 10-12 weeks of induction); **or** 20 million units/m^2 daily for 4 weeks, then if responding, 20 million units/m^2 3 times/week
   CML: 9 million units daily
   Hepatitis C: Initial: 6 million units once daily for 3 weeks followed by 3 million units 3 times/week for 6 months
   Melanoma: 12 million units/m^2 3 times/week for 3 months

Administration Parenteral: S.C. (rather than I.M.) administration is suggested for those patients who are at risk for bleeding or are thrombocytopenic; rotate S.C. injection site

Monitoring Parameters Baseline EKG, CBC with differential and platelet count, electrolytes, liver and renal function tests, weight

Patient Information Do not change brands as changes in dosage may result; possible mental status changes may occur while on therapy

Nursing Implications Patient should be well hydrated; pretreatment with NSAIDs or acetaminophen can decrease fever and its severity and alleviate headache

Additional Information Indications and dosage regimens are specific for a particular brand of interferon; other brands of interferon (ie, Intron® A) have different indications and dosage guidelines; do not change brands of interferon as changes in dosage may result

Dosage Forms
Injection: 3 million units/mL (1 mL); 6 million units/mL (3 mL); 36 million units/mL (1 mL)
Powder for injection: 6 million units/mL when reconstituted

References
Ezekowitz RAB, Mulliken JB, and Folkman J, "Interferon Alfa-2a Therapy for Life-Threatening Hemangiomas of Infancy," N Engl J Med, 1992, 326(22):1456-63.

(Continued)

Interferon Alfa-2a *(Continued)*

White CW, Sondheimer HM, Crouch EC, et al, "Treatment of Pulmonary Hemangiomatosis With Recombinant Interferon Alfa-2a," *N Engl J Med*, 1989, 320(18):1197-200.

Interferon Alfa-2b (in ter FEER on AL fa too bee)

Brand Names Intron® A

Synonyms IFN-α-2; α-2-interferon; rIFN-α2

Therapeutic Category Antineoplastic Agent, Miscellaneous; Biological Response Modulator; Interferon

Generic Available No

Use Induce hairy cell leukemia remission; treatment of AIDS-related Kaposi's sarcoma; condylomata acuminata; chronic hepatitis C; chronic hepatitis B

Pregnancy Risk Factor C

Contraindications Hypersensitivity to interferon alfa-2b or any component

Warnings The FDA currently recommends that procedures for proper handling and disposal of antineoplastic agents be considered; safety and efficacy in children <18 years of age have not been established; injection contains benzyl alcohol which may be toxic to newborns in high doses

Precautions Use with caution in patients with seizure disorders, brain metastases, compromised CNS, multiple sclerosis, and patients with pre-existing cardiac disease, severe renal or hepatic impairment, or myelosuppression

Adverse Reactions Flu-like symptoms (fever, fatigue/malaise, myalgia, chills, headache, arthralgia, rigors) begin about 2-6 hours after the dose is given and may persist as long as 24 hours; usually patient can build up a tolerance to side effects

Cardiovascular: Tachycardia, arrhythmias, hypotension, edema, chest pain

Central nervous system: Fatigue/malaise, dizziness, depression, confusion, sensory neuropathy, psychiatric effects, fever, headache, EEG abnormalities, chills

Dermatologic: Partial alopecia, rash

Endocrine & metabolic: Increased uric acid level, thyroid dysfunction

Gastrointestinal: Anorexia, xerostomia, nausea, vomiting, diarrhea, abdominal cramps, dysgeusia, weight loss

Hematologic: Leukopenia (mainly neutropenia); anemia; thrombocytopenia; decreased hemoglobin, hematocrit, platelets; neutralizing antibodies

Hepatic: Elevated ALT and AST

Local: Burning, pain, erythema, rash at the site of injection

Neuromuscular & skeletal: Myalgia, arthralgia, rigors

Ocular: Blurred vision

Renal: Proteinuria, elevated BUN and serum creatinine

Respiratory: Coughing, nasal congestion

Miscellaneous: Diaphoresis

Drug Interactions

Interferon Alfa-2a: May competitively bind to same receptors

Acyclovir: Possible synergistic effect

Theophylline: Clearance of theophylline is reduced

Vinblastine: May increase interferon toxicity; increased neurotoxicity

Zidovudine: Possible additive myelosuppression

Stability Refrigerate; reconstituted solution is stable for 1 month when refrigerated

Mechanism of Action Inhibits cellular growth, alters the state of cellular differentiation, interferes with oncogene expression, alters cell surface antigen expression, increases phagocytic activity of macrophages, and augments cytotoxicity of lymphocytes for target cells

Pharmacokinetics

Metabolism: Majority of dose is thought to be metabolized in the kidney, filtered and absorbed at the renal tubule

Half-life, elimination:

I.M., I.V.: 2 hours

S.C.: 3 hours

Time to peak serum concentration: I.M., S.C.: ~6-8 hours

Usual Dosage Adults (refer to individual protocols):

Hairy cell leukemia: I.M., S.C.: 2 million units/m² 3 times/week

AIDS-related Kaposi's sarcoma: I.M., S.C.: 30 million units/m² 3 times/week or 50 million units/m² I.V. 5 days/week every other week

Condylomata acuminata: Intralesionally: 1 million units/lesion 3 times/week for 3 weeks; not to exceed 5 million units per treatment (maximum dose: 5 lesions at one time) (use only the 10 million units vial)

Chronic hepatitis B: I.M., S.C.: 5 million units given once daily **or** 10 million units given 3 times/week for 4 months

Chronic hepatitis C: I.M., S.C.: 3 million units 3 times/week for approximately a 6-month course; relapse of hepatitis has occurred after treatment was stopped

Administration Parenteral: S.C. (rather than I.M.) administration is suggested for those patients who are at risk for bleeding or are thrombocytopenic; rotate S.C. injection site

Monitoring Parameters Baseline EKG, CBC with differential and platelet count, liver function tests, electrolytes, weight, chest x-ray

Patient Information Do not change brands of interferon as changes in dosage may result; do not operate heavy machinery while on therapy since changes in mental status may occur

Nursing Implications Patient should be well hydrated; may pretreat with NSAID or acetaminophen to decrease fever and its severity and to alleviate headache

Additional Information Myelosuppressive effects:
WBC: Mild
Platelets: Mild
Onset (days): 7-10
Nadir (days): 14
Recovery (days): 21

Dosage Forms Powder for injection, lyophilized: 3 million units, 5 million units, 10 million units, 18 million units, 25 million units, 50 million units

References
Davis GL, Balart LA, Schiff ER, et al, "Treatment of Chronic Hepatitis C With Recombinant Interferon Alfa. A Multicenter Randomized, Controlled Trial. Hepatitis Interventional Therapy Group," *N Engl J Med*, 1989, 321(22):1501-6.
Perrillo RP, "Interferon in the Management of Chronic Hepatitis B," *Dig Dis Sci*, 1993, 38(4):577-93.

- **Interleukin-2** see Aldesleukin on page 42
- **Intralipid®** see Fat Emulsion on page 403
- **Intravenous Fat Emulsion** see Fat Emulsion on page 403
- **Intron® A** see Interferon Alfa-2b on page 524
- **Intropin®** see Dopamine on page 339
- **Invirase®** see Saquinavir on page 857
- **Iobid DM®** see Guaifenesin and Dextromethorphan on page 466

Iodine (EYE oh dyne)

Related Information
Drugs and Breast-Feeding on page 1213

Therapeutic Category Topical Skin Product

Generic Available Yes

Use Used topically as an antiseptic in the management of minor, superficial skin wounds and has been used to disinfect the skin preoperatively

Pregnancy Risk Factor D

Contraindications Hypersensitivity to iodide preparations or any component; neonates

Warnings May be highly toxic if ingested

Adverse Reactions
Local: Skin irritation, discoloration, and burns
Miscellaneous: Hypersensitivity, allergic reactions

Mechanism of Action Free iodine oxidizes microbial protoplasm making it effective against bacteria, fungi, yeasts, protozoa, and viruses; complexes with amino groups in tissue compounds to form iodophors from which the iodine is slowly released causing a sustained action

Usual Dosage Apply topically as necessary to affected areas of skin

Administration Topical: Apply to affected areas; avoid tight bandages because iodine may cause burns on occluded skin

Patient Information May stain skin and clothing

Additional Information Sodium thiosulfate inactivates iodine and is an effective chemical antidote for iodine poisoning; solutions of sodium thiosulfate may be used to remove iodine stains from skin and clothing

Dosage Forms
Solution: 2%
Tincture: 2%

- **Iodine Sodium** see Trace Metals on page 940
- **Iodochlorhydroxyquin** see Clioquinol on page 239
- **Iodopen®** see Trace Metals on page 940

Iodoquinol (eye oh doe KWIN ole)

Brand Names Diodoquin® (Canada); Yodoxin®

Synonyms Diiodohydroxyquin

Therapeutic Category Amebicide

Generic Available No

Use Treatment of acute and chronic intestinal amebiasis due to *Entamoeba histolytica*; asymptomatic cyst passers; *Blastocystis hominis* infections; iodoquinol alone is ineffective for amebic hepatitis or hepatic abscess

Pregnancy Risk Factor C

Contraindications Hypersensitivity to iodine, iodoquinol, or any component; hepatic or renal damage; pre-existing optic neuropathy

Precautions Use with caution in patients with thyroid disease or neurological disorders

Adverse Reactions

Central nervous system: Agitation, retrograde amnesia, fever, chills, headache, ataxia

Dermatologic: Anal pruritus, rash, acne

Endocrine & metabolic: Enlargement of the thyroid

Gastrointestinal: Nausea, vomiting, diarrhea, gastritis, anorexia, constipation

Neuromuscular & skeletal: Weakness, peripheral neuropathy, myalgia

Ocular: Optic neuritis, optic atrophy, visual impairment

Mechanism of Action Contact amebicide that works in the lumen of the intestine by an unknown mechanism

Pharmacokinetics

Absorption: Oral: Poor and irregular

Metabolism: In the liver

Elimination: In feces; metabolites appear in urine

Usual Dosage Oral:

Children: 30-40 mg/kg/day in 3 divided doses for 20 days; not to exceed 1.95 g/day

Adults: 650 mg 3 times/day after meals for 20 days; not to exceed 2 g/day

Administration Oral: Administer medication after meals; tablets may be crushed and mixed with applesauce or chocolate syrup

Monitoring Parameters Ophthalmologic exam

Test Interactions May increase protein-bound serum iodine concentrations reflecting a decrease in iodine 131 uptake; false-positive ferric chloride test for phenylketonuria

Patient Information Notify physician if rash occurs

Dosage Forms

Powder: 25 g

Tablet: 210 mg, 650 mg

♦ **Ionil-T® Plus (Canada)** see Coal Tar on page 247

♦ **I-Paracaine®** see Proparacaine on page 811

Ipecac Syrup (IP e kak SIR up)

Therapeutic Category Antidote, Emetic

Generic Available Yes

Use Treatment of acute oral drug overdosage and certain poisonings; use only in alert conscious patients who have ingested potentially toxic amounts of substance

Pregnancy Risk Factor C

Contraindications Do not use in unconscious patients, patients with absent gag reflex or seizures; ingestion of strong bases or acids, other corrosive substances, volatile oils, hydrocarbons with high potential for aspiration

Warnings Avoid use in patients with coagulopathy or bleeding problems (risk of gastroesophageal hemorrhage) and in patients receiving calcium channel blockers, beta-blockers, clonidine, or digitalis glycosides (risk of exaggerated vagal stimulation with gagging, resulting in severe bradycardia); do not confuse ipecac syrup with ipecac fluid extract; fluid extract is 14 times more potent than syrup

Precautions Use with caution in patients with cardiovascular disease and bulimics

Adverse Reactions

Cardiovascular: Cardiotoxicity

Central nervous system: Lethargy, drowsiness

Gastrointestinal: Protracted vomiting, diarrhea; Mallory-Weiss syndrome, gastric rupture

Neuromuscular & skeletal: Myopathy

Respiratory: Aspiration (can be fatal)

Drug Interactions Activated charcoal may decrease effectiveness

Food Interactions Milk, carbonated beverages may decrease effectiveness

Mechanism of Action Irritates the gastric mucosa and stimulates the medullary chemoreceptor trigger zone to induce vomiting

Pharmacodynamics
Onset of vomiting after oral dose: Within 15-30 minutes; usual: 20 minutes
Duration: 20-25 minutes; can last longer, up to 1-2 hours

Usual Dosage Oral:
Children:
<6 months: Not recommended
6-12 months: 5-10 mL followed by 10-20 mL/kg or 120-240 mL of water; repeat dose one time if vomiting does not occur within 20-30 minutes
1-12 years: 15 mL followed by 10-20 mL/kg or 120-240 mL of water; repeat dose one time if vomiting does not occur within 20-30 minutes
Adolescents and Adults: 30 mL followed by 240 mL of water; repeat dose one time if vomiting does not occur within 20-30 minutes

Administration Oral: Administer within 60 minutes of ingestion; follow administration with water; do not administer with milk or carbonated beverages

Nursing Implications Do **not** administer to unconscious patients

Additional Information Patients should be kept active and moving following administration of ipecac; if vomiting does not occur after second dose, gastric lavage may be considered to remove ingested substance

The Position Statement of The American Academy of Clinical Toxicology and The European Association of Poisons Centres and Clinical Toxicologists does not recommend routine administration of ipecac syrup to poisoned patients; scientific literature does not support that ipecac improves patient outcome; this paper states that the **routine** administration of ipecac syrup in the emergency room should be abandoned. Also, scientific literature cannot support or exclude giving ipecac syrup soon after toxic ingestions; administration of ipecac syrup may delay the administration or decrease the effectiveness of activated charcoal, oral antidotes, or whole bowel irrigation; its use should be considered only if it can be given within 60 minutes after ingestion of poison.

Dosage Forms Syrup: 70 mg/mL (15 mL, 30 mL, 473 mL, 4000 mL)

References
"Position Statement: Ipecac Syrup. American Academy of Clinical Toxicology; European Association of Poisons Centres and Clinical Toxicologists," *J Toxicol Clin Toxicol*, 1997, 35(7):699-709.
Shannon M, "Ingestion of Toxic Substances by Children," *N Engl J Med*, 2000, 342(3):186-91.

♦ **I-Pentolate®** *see* Cyclopentolate *on page 266*
♦ **I-Phrine® Ophthalmic Solution** *see* Phenylephrine *on page 758*
♦ **I-Picamide®** *see* Tropicamide *on page 959*

Ipratropium (i pra TROE pee um)

Related Information
Asthma Guidelines *on page 1178*

Brand Names Atrovent® Aerosol Inhalation; Atrovent® Inhalation Solution; Atrovent® Nasal Spray

Available Salts Ipratropium Bromide

Therapeutic Category Antiasthmatic; Anticholinergic Agent; Bronchodilator

Generic Available No

Use Anticholinergic bronchodilator used in bronchospasm associated with asthma, COPD, bronchitis, and emphysema; symptomatic relief of rhinorrhea associated with allergic and nonallergic rhinitis

Pregnancy Risk Factor B

Contraindications Hypersensitivity to ipratropium, atropine, or its derivatives; history of hypersensitivity to soya lecithin or related food products such as soy bean and peanut

Warnings Not indicated for the initial treatment of acute episodes of bronchospasm

Precautions Use with caution in patients with narrow-angle glaucoma, bladder neck obstruction, or prostatic hypertrophy

Adverse Reactions
Note: Ipratropium is poorly absorbed from the lung, so systemic effects are rare

Cardiovascular: Palpitations, tachycardia, flushing, hypotension, hypertension
Central nervous system: Nervousness, dizziness, headache, fatigue, drowsiness, insomnia
Dermatologic: Rash, pruritus, alopecia
Gastrointestinal: Nausea, xerostomia, constipation
Genitourinary: Dysuria
Ocular: Blurred vision
(Continued)

Ipratropium *(Continued)*

Respiratory: Cough, hoarseness, dry secretions, epistaxis (with nasal spray)

Drug Interactions Additive effects with anticholinergics or drugs with anticholinergic properties

Stability Compatible for 1 hour when mixed with albuterol or metaproterenol in a nebulizer

Mechanism of Action Blocks the action of acetylcholine at parasympathetic sites in bronchial smooth muscle causing bronchodilation; inhibits secretions from the serous and seromucous glands lining the nasal mucosa

Pharmacodynamics

Onset of bronchodilation: 1-3 minutes after administration

Peak effect: Maximal effect within 1.5-2 hours

Duration: Bronchodilation persists for up to 4-6 hours

Pharmacokinetics

Absorption: Not readily absorbed into the systemic circulation from the surface of the lung or from the GI tract

Distribution: Following inhalation, 15% of dose reaches the lower airways

Half-life: 2 hours

Usual Dosage

Neonates: Nebulization: 25 mcg/kg/dose 3 times/day

Infants and Children: Nebulization: 125-250 mcg 3 times/day

Children 3-12 years: Metered inhaler: 1-2 inhalations 3 times/day, up to 6 inhalations/24 hours

Children ≥12 years and Adults:

Nebulization: 500 mcg 3-4 times/day

Metered inhaler: 2 inhalations 4 times/day, up to 12 inhalations/24 hours

Nasal spray:

Children >6 years and Adults: 0.03%: 2 sprays in each nostril 2-3 times/day

Children >5 years and Adults: 0.06%: 2 sprays in each nostril 3-4 times/day

Administration

Nasal spray: Pump must be primed before usage by 7 actuations into the air away from the face; if not used for >24 hours, pump must be reprimed with 2 actuations; if not used >7 days, reprime with 7 actuations

Nebulization: May be administered with or without dilution in NS

Oral Inhalation: Shake well before use; use spacer device in children <8 years

Dosage Forms Solution, as bromide:

Inhalation, oral: 18 mcg/actuation (14 g)

Nasal spray: 0.03% (30 mL); 0.06% (15 mL)

Nebulizing: 0.02% (2.5 mL)

References

Henry RI, Hiller EG, Milner AD, et al, "Nebulised Ipratropium Bromide and Sodium Cromoglycate in the First 2 Years of Life," *Arch Dis Child*, 1984, 59(1):54-7.

Mann NP and Hiller RG, "Ipratropium Bromide in Children With Asthma," *Thorax*, 1982, 37(1):72-4.

Schuh S, Johnson DW, Callahan S, et al, "Efficacy of Frequent Nebulized Ipratropium Added to Frequent High-Dose Albuterol Therapy in Severe Childhood Asthma," *J Pediatr*, 1995, 126(4):639-45.

Schuh S, Johnson D, Canny G, et al, "Efficacy of Adding Nebulized Ipratropium Bromide to Nebulized Albuterol Therapy in Acute Bronchiolitis," *Pediatrics*, 1992, 90(6): 920-3.

Wang EE, Milner R, Allen U, et al, "Bronchodilators for Treatment of Mild Bronchiolitis: A Factorial Randomized Trial," *Arch Dis Child*, 1992, 67(3):289-93.

Wilkie RA and Bryan MH, "Effect of Bronchodilators on Airway Resistance in Ventilator-dependent Neonates With Chronic Lung Disease," *J Pediatr*, 1987, 111(2):278-82.

♦ **Ipratropium Bromide** *see* Ipratropium *on page 527*

♦ **Iproveratril** *see* Verapamil *on page 974*

♦ **Ircon® [OTC]** *see* Iron Supplements, Oral/Enteral *on page 530*

Iron Dextran Complex (EYE ern DEKS tran KOM pleks)

Brand Names Dexferrum®; InFed™

Therapeutic Category Iron Salt, Parenteral; Mineral, Parenteral

Generic Available Yes

Use Treatment of microcytic, hypochromic anemia resulting from iron deficiency when oral iron administration is infeasible or ineffective

Pregnancy Risk Factor C

Contraindications Hypersensitivity to iron dextran or any component; anemias that are not associated with iron deficiency, hemochromatosis, hemolytic anemia

Warnings Deaths associated with parenteral administration following anaphylactic-type reactions have been reported; use only in patients where the iron deficient state is not amenable to oral iron therapy

Precautions Use with caution in patients with histories of significant allergies, asthma, hepatic impairment, rheumatoid arthritis; not recommended in infants <4 months of age; treatments for anaphylactic reactions (eg, epinephrine, steroids, diphenhydramine) should be immediately available; a test dose is recommended; hypotension in conjunction with flushing, lightheadedness, malaise, fatigue, weakness, or chest, back, groin, or flank pain has been associated with rapid intravenous administration

Adverse Reactions

Anaphylactoid reactions: Respiratory difficulties and cardiovascular collapse have been reported and occur most frequently within the first several minutes of administration

Cardiovascular: Cardiovascular collapse, hypotension, flushing

Central nervous system: Dizziness, fever, headache, chills, shivering

Dermatologic: Urticaria

Gastrointestinal: Nausea, vomiting, diarrhea, metallic taste

Genitourinary: Discoloration of urine

Hematologic: Leukocytosis

Local: Pain, staining of skin at the site of I.M. injection, phlebitis

Neuromuscular & skeletal: Arthralgia, arthritic reactivation in patients with quiescent arthritis, backache, paresthesia

Renal: Hematuria

Respiratory: Respiratory difficulty

Miscellaneous: Lymphadenopathy, diaphoresis

Note: Sweating, urticaria, arthralgia, fever, chills, dizziness, headache, and nausea may be delayed 24-48 hours after I.V. administration or 3-4 days after I.M. administration

Stability Store at room temperature; the manufacturers state iron dextran should not be mixed with other medications or in parenteral nutrition solutions

Mechanism of Action Iron is released from the plasma and eventually replenishes the depleted iron stores in the bone marrow where it is incorporated into hemoglobin

Pharmacodynamics

Onset of action: Hematologic response to either oral or parenteral iron salts is essentially the same; red blood cell form and color changes within 3-10 days

Peak effect: Peak reticulocytosis occurs in 5-10 days, and hemoglobin values increase within 2-4 weeks

Pharmacokinetics

Absorption: I.M.: 60% absorbed after 3 days; 90% after 1-3 weeks, the balance is slowly absorbed over months

Following I.V. doses, the uptake of iron by the reticuloendothelial system appears to be constant at about 10-20 mg/hour

Elimination: By the reticuloendothelial system and excreted in urine and feces (via bile)

Usual Dosage I.M., I.V.:

A 0.5 mL (25 mg) test dose (0.25 mL, 12.5 mg in infants) should be given 1 hour prior to starting iron dextran therapy

Total replacement dosage of iron dextran for iron deficiency anemia (mL) = 0.0476 x LBW (kg) x (Hb_n - Hb_o) + 1 mL/per 5 kg LBW (up to maximum of 14 mL)

LBW = Lean body weight

Hb_n = desired hemoglobin (g/dL) = 12 if <15 kg or 14.8 if >15 kg

Hb_o = measured hemoglobin (g/dL)

Total iron replacement dosage for acute blood loss: Assumes 1 mL of normocytic, normochromic red cells = 1 mg elemental iron: Iron dextran (mL) = 0.02 x blood loss (mL) x hematocrit (expressed as a decimal fraction)

Note: Total dose infusions have been used safely and are the preferred method of administration

Maximum daily dose: I.M.: Injected in daily or less frequent increments:

Infants <5 kg: 25 mg

Children 5-10 kg: 50 mg

Children >10 kg and Adults: 100 mg

Administration Parenteral:

I.M.: Use Z-track technique for I.M. administration (deep into the upper outer quadrant of buttock)

I.V.: Infuse test dose over at least 5 minutes; dilute replacement dose in NS (50-100 mL), maximum concentration 50 mg/mL and infuse over 1-6 hours at a maximum rate of 50 mg/minute; avoid dilution in dextrose due to an increased incidence of local pain and phlebitis

(Continued)

Iron Dextran Complex *(Continued)*

Monitoring Parameters Reticulocyte count, serum ferritin, hemoglobin, serum iron concentrations, and TIBC may not be meaningful for 3 weeks after administration, especially after large I.V. doses

Reference Range

Serum iron:
Newborns: 110-270 µg/dL
Infants: 30-70 µg/dL
Children: 55-120 µg/dL
Adults: Male: 75-175 µg/dL; Female: 65-165 µg/dL
Total iron binding capacity:
Newborns: 59-175 µg/dL
Infants: 100-400 µg/dL
Children and Adults: 230-430 µg/dL
Transferrin: 204-360 mg/dL
Percent transferrin saturation: 20% to 50%
Iron levels >300 µg/dL may be considered toxic; should be treated as an over-dosage
Ferritin: 13-300 ng/mL

Test Interactions May cause falsely elevated values of serum bilirubin and falsely decreased values of serum calcium

Additional Information Iron storage may lag behind the appearance of normal red blood cell morphology; use periodic hematologic determination to assess therapy

Dosage Forms Expressed as mg of elemental iron: Injection: 50 mg/mL (1 mL, 2 mL, 10 mL)

References

Auerbach M, Witt D, and Toler W, "Clinical Use of the Total Dose Intravenous Infusion of Iron Dextran," *J Lab Clin Med*, 1988, 111(5):566-70.

Benito RP and Guerrero TC, "Response to a Single Intravenous Dose Versus Multiple Intramuscular Administration of Iron Dextran Complex: A Comparative Study," *Curr Ther Res Clin Exp*, 1973, 15(7):373-82.

♦ **Iron Sulfate (Ferrous Sulfate)** *see* Iron Supplements, Oral/Enteral *on page 530*

Iron Supplements, Oral/Enteral (EYE ern SUP la ments)

Related Information

Carbohydrate and Alcohol Content of Liquid Medications for Use in Patients Receiving Ketogenic Diets *on page 1228*
Overdose and Toxicology *on page 1191*

Brand Names Apo®-Ferrous Gluconate (Canada); Apo®-Ferrous Sulfate (Canada); Femiron® [OTC]; Feosol® [OTC]; Feostat® [OTC]; Feratab® [OTC]; Fergon® [OTC]; Fer-In-Sol® [OTC]; Fer-Iron® [OTC]; Fero-Gradumet® [OTC]; Ferospace® [OTC]; Ferralet® [OTC]; Ferralyn® Lanacaps® [OTC]; Ferra-TD® [OTC]; Ferro-Sequels® [OTC]; Fumasorb® [OTC]; Fumerin® [OTC]; Hemocyte® [OTC]; Hytinic®; Ircon® [OTC]; Mol-Iron® [OTC]; Nephro-Fer™ [OTC]; Niferex®; Niferex® 150; Nu-Iron®; Nu-Iron® 150; Palafer® (Canada); PMS-Ferrous Sulfate (Canada); Simron® [OTC]; Slow FE® [OTC]; Span-FF® [OTC]

Available Salts Ferrous Fumarate; Ferrous Gluconate; Ferrous Sulfate

Synonyms FeSO₄ (Ferrous Sulfate); Iron Sulfate (Ferrous Sulfate)

Therapeutic Category Iron Salt; Mineral, Oral

Generic Available Yes

Use Prevention and treatment of iron deficiency anemias; supplemental therapy for patients receiving epoetin alfa

Pregnancy Risk Factor A

Contraindications Hemochromatosis, hemolytic anemia; hypersensitivity to iron salts

Warnings Avoid use in premature infants until the vitamin E stores, deficient at birth, are replenished

Precautions Avoid using for longer than 6 months, except in patients with conditions that require prolonged therapy; avoid in patients with peptic ulcer, enteritis, or ulcerative colitis; avoid in patients receiving frequent blood transfusions

Adverse Reactions

Gastrointestinal: GI irritation, epigastric pain, nausea, diarrhea, dark stools, constipation
Genitourinary: Discoloration of urine (black or dark)
Miscellaneous: Liquid preparations may temporarily stain the teeth

Drug Interactions Absorption of oral preparation of iron and tetracyclines are decreased when both of these drugs are given together; concurrent administration of antacids and cimetidine may decrease iron absorption; iron may decrease absorption of penicillamine, levothyroxine, methyldopa, and levodopa when given at the same time; response to iron therapy may be delayed in patients receiving chloramphenicol; concurrent administration ≥200 mg vitamin C per 30 mg elemental iron increases absorption of oral iron; absorption of quinolones may be decreased due to formation of a ferric ion-quinolone complex

Food Interactions Milk, cereals, dietary fiber, tea, coffee, or eggs decrease absorption of iron

Mechanism of Action Iron is released from the plasma and eventually replenishes the depleted iron stores in the bone marrow where it is incorporated into hemoglobin

Pharmacodynamics

Onset of action: Hematologic response to either oral or parenteral iron salts is essentially the same; red blood cell form and color changes within 3-10 days

Peak effect: Peak reticulocytosis occurs in 5-10 days, and hemoglobin values increase within 2-4 weeks

Pharmacokinetics

Absorption: Oral: Iron is absorbed in the duodenum and upper jejunum; in persons with normal iron stores 10% of an oral dose is absorbed, this is increased to 20% to 30% in persons with inadequate iron stores; food and achlorhydria will decrease absorption

Elimination: Iron is largely bound to serum transferrin and excreted in the urine, sweat, sloughing of intestinal mucosa, and by menses

Usual Dosage Note: Multiple salt forms of iron exist; close attention must be paid to the salt form when ordering and administering iron; incorrect selection or substitution of one salt for another without proper dosage adjustment may result in serious over- or underdosing.

Oral (dose expressed in terms of **elemental** iron):

Recommended Daily Allowance, see table

Recommended Daily Allowance of Iron
(dosage expressed as elemental iron)

Age	RDA (mg)
<5 mo	5
5 mo to 10 y	10
Male	
11-18 y	12
>18 y	10
Female	
11-50 y	15
>50 y	10

Premature neonates: 2-4 mg elemental iron/kg/day divided every 12-24 hours (maximum dose: 15 mg/day)

Infants and Children:

Severe iron deficiency anemia: 4-6 mg elemental iron/kg/day in 3 divided doses

Mild to moderate iron deficiency anemia: 3 mg elemental iron/kg/day in 1-2 divided doses

Prophylaxis: 1-2 mg elemental iron/kg/day up to a maximum of 15 mg elemental iron/day

Elemental Iron Content of Iron Salts

Iron Salt	Elemental Iron Content (% of salt form)	Approximate Equivalent Doses (mg of iron salt)
Ferrous fumarate	33	197
Ferrous gluconate	11.6	560
Ferrous sulfate	20	324
Ferrous sulfate, exsiccated	30	217

(Continued)

Iron Supplements, Oral/Enteral *(Continued)*

Adults:

Iron deficiency: 2-3 mg/kg/day or 60-100 mg elemental iron twice daily up to 60 mg elemental iron 4 times/day, or 50 mg elemental iron (extended release) 1-2 times/day

Prophylaxis: 60-100 mg elemental iron/day; see table on previous page.

Administration Oral: Do not chew or crush sustained release preparations; administer with water or juice between meals for maximum absorption; may administer with food if GI upset occurs; do not administer with milk or milk products

Monitoring Parameters Serum iron, total iron binding capacity, reticulocyte count, hemoglobin, ferritin

Reference Range

Serum iron:

Newborns: 110-270 µg/dL

Infants: 30-70 µg/dL

Children: 55-120 µg/dL

Adults: Male: 75-175 µg/dL; Female: 65-165 µg/dL

Total iron binding capacity:

Newborns: 59-175 µg/dL

Infants: 100-400 µg/dL

Children and Adults: 230-430 µg/dL

Transferrin: 204-360 mg/dL

Percent transferrin saturation: 20% to 50%

Iron levels >300 µg/dL may be considered toxic; should be treated as an overdosage

Ferritin: 13-300 ng/mL

Test Interactions False-positive for blood in stool by the guaiac test

Patient Information May color the stools and urine black; do not take within 2 hours of tetracyclines or fluoroquinolones, do not take with milk or antacids; keep out of reach of children

Additional Information When treating iron deficiency anemias, treat for 3-4 months after hemoglobin/hematocrit return to normal in order to replenish total body stores; elemental iron dosages as high as 15 mg/kg/day have been used to supplement neonates receiving concomitant epoetin alpha in the treatment of anemia of prematurity

Dosage Forms Amount of **elemental** iron is listed in brackets; most commonly used formulations are bolded

Ferrous fumarate:

Capsule, controlled release (Span-FF®): 325 mg [106 mg]

Drops (Feostat®): 45 mg/0.6 mL [15 mg/0.6 mL] (60 mL)

Suspension, oral (Feostat®): 100 mg/5 mL [33 mg/5 mL] (240 mL)

Tablet: 325 mg [106 mg]

Femiron®: 63 mg [20 mg]

Fumerin®: 195 mg [64 mg]

Fumasorb®, Ircon®: 200 mg [66 mg]

Hemocyte®: 324 mg [106 mg]

Nephro-Fer™: 350 mg [115 mg]

Tablet, chewable (chocolate flavor): Feostat®: 100 mg [33 mg]

Tablet, timed release:

Ferro-Sequels®: 150 mg [50 mg] with docusate sodium 100 mg

Ferrous gluconate:

Capsule, soft gelatin (Simron®): 86 mg [10 mg]

Elixir (Fergon®): 300 mg/5 mL [34 mg/5 mL] with alcohol 7% (480 mL)

Tablet: **300 mg [34 mg]**; 325 mg [38 mg]

Fergon®, Ferralet®: 320 mg [37 mg]

Sustained release (Ferralet® Slow Release): 320 mg [37 mg]

Ferrous sulfate:

Capsule:

Exsiccated (Fer-In-Sol®): 190 mg [60 mg]

Exsiccated, timed release (Feosol®): 159 mg [50 mg]

Exsiccated, timed release (Ferralyn® Lanacaps®, Ferra-TD®): 250 mg [50 mg]

Ferospace®: 250 mg [50 mg]

Drops, oral:

Fer-In-Sol®: **75 mg/0.6 mL [15 mg/0.6 mL]** (50 mL)

Fer-Iron®: 125 mg/mL [25 mg/mL] (50 mL)

Elixir (Feosol®): 220 mg/5 mL [44 mg/5 mL] with alcohol 5% (473 mL, 4000 mL)

Syrup (Fer-In-Sol®): **90 mg/5 mL [18 mg/5 mL]** with alcohol 5% (480 mL)

Tablet:
324 mg [65 mg]
Exsiccated (Feosol®) 200 mg [65 mg]
Exsiccated, timed release (Slow FE®): 160 mg [50 mg]
Feratab®: **300 mg [60 mg]**
Mol-Iron®: 195 mg [39 mg]
Timed release (Fero-Gradumet®): 525 mg [105 mg]
Lysaccharide - iron complex:
Capsule (Hytinic®, Niferex®-150, Nu-Iron®-150): 150 mg
Elixir (Hytinic®, Niferex®, Nu-Iron®): 100 mg/5 mL
Tablet (Niferex®): 50 mg

♦ **Isoamyl Nitrite** see Amyl Nitrite on page 84

Isoetharine (eye soe ETH a reen)

Related Information
Asthma Guidelines on page 1178

Brand Names Arm-a-Med®; Bronkosol® Inhalation Solution; Dey-Lute® Isoetharine; Isoetharine Bronkometer® Aerosol

Available Salts Isoetharine Hydrochloride; Isoetharine Mesylate

Therapeutic Category Adrenergic Agonist Agent; Antiasthmatic; Bronchodilator; Sympathomimetic

Generic Available Yes

Use Bronchodilator used in asthma and for the reversible bronchospasm occurring with bronchitis and emphysema

Pregnancy Risk Factor C

Contraindications Hypersensitivity to isoetharine, any component, or other sympathomimetics

Warnings Isoetharine hydrochloride solution contains sulfites which may cause allergic reactions in some patients

Precautions Excessive, prolonged use may lead to decreased effectiveness; use with caution in patients with hyperthyroidism, hypertension, acute coronary artery disease, cerebral arteriosclerosis

Adverse Reactions
Cardiovascular: Tachycardia, hypertension, palpitations
Central nervous system: Anxiety, dizziness, restlessness, excitement, headache, nervousness, insomnia, lightheadedness
Gastrointestinal: Nausea, vomiting, xerostomia
Neuromuscular & skeletal: Tremor, weakness

Drug Interactions Additive effects when used in combination with other sympathomimetics; decreased effect with beta-blocking agents

Mechanism of Action Relaxes bronchial smooth muscle and peripheral vasculature by action on beta$_2$-receptors with little effect on heart rate

Pharmacodynamics
Peak effect: Following inhaler administration, within 5-15 minutes
Duration: 1-4 hours

Pharmacokinetics
Metabolism: In many tissues including the liver and lungs
Elimination: Renal, primarily (90%) as metabolites

Usual Dosage Treatments are usually not repeated more often than every 4 hours, except in severe cases

Nebulizer:
Children: 0.01 mL/kg (0.1 mg/kg) of 1% solution; minimum dose 0.1 mL (1 mg); maximum dose: 0.5 mL (5 mg)
Adults: 0.5-1 mL (2.5-5 mg) of a 0.5% solution or equivalent dosages using 0.125%, 0.2%, 0.25%, or 1% solutions
Inhalation: Adults: 1-2 inhalations every 4 hours as needed

Administration
Nebulization: Dilute dosage of 0.5% or 1% solutions in 2-3 mL NS; 0.125%, 0.2%, and 0.25% solutions may be administered without dilution
Oral inhalation: Shake well before use; use spacer device in children <8 years of age

Monitoring Parameters Heart rate, blood pressure, respiratory rate

Dosage Forms
Aerosol, oral, as mesylate: 340 mcg/metered spray
Solution, inhalation, as hydrochloride: 0.062% (4 mL); 0.08% (3.5 mL); 0.1% (2.5 mL, 5 mL); 0.125% (4 mL); 0.167% (3 mL); 0.17% (3 mL); 0.2% (2.5 mL); 0.25% (2 mL, 3.5 mL); 0.5% (0.5 mL); 1% (0.5 mL, 0.25 mL, 10 mL, 14 mL, 30 mL)
(Continued)

Isoetharine *(Continued)*

References
Rachelefsky GS and Siegel SC, "Asthma in Infants and Children - Treatment of Childhood Asthma: Part 11," *J Allergy Clin Immunol*, 1985, 76(3):409-25.

♦ **Isoetharine Bronkometer® Aerosol** *see* Isoetharine *on page 533*
♦ **Isoetharine Hydrochloride** *see* Isoetharine *on page 533*
♦ **Isoetharine Mesylate** *see* Isoetharine *on page 533*

Isoniazid (eye soe NYE a zid)
Related Information
Overdose and Toxicology *on page 1191*
Brand Names Laniazid® Oral; Nydrazid® Injection; PMS-Isoniazid (Canada)
Synonyms INH; Isonicotinic Acid Hydrazide
Therapeutic Category Antitubercular Agent
Generic Available Yes
Use Treatment of susceptible mycobacterial infection due to *M. tuberculosis* and prophylactically to those individuals exposed to tuberculosis
Pregnancy Risk Factor C
Contraindications Acute liver disease; hypersensitivity to isoniazid or any component; previous history of hepatic damage during isoniazid therapy
Warnings Severe and sometimes fatal hepatitis may occur or develop even after many months of treatment; the administration of isoniazid in combination with rifampin is associated with an increased incidence of hepatotoxicity if isoniazid dose is >10 mg/kg/day; patients must report any prodromal symptoms of hepatitis such as fatigue, weakness, malaise, anorexia, nausea, vomiting, dark urine, or yellowing of eyes
Precautions Use with caution in patients with renal impairment and chronic liver disease
Adverse Reactions
Central nervous system: Seizure, stupor, dizziness, agitation, euphoria, psychosis, fever, ataxia
Dermatologic: Skin eruptions, rash, acne
Endocrine & metabolic: Hyperglycemia, metabolic acidosis, pellagra
Gastrointestinal: Nausea, vomiting, epigastric distress; diarrhea (associated with administration of syrup formulation)
Hematologic: Agranulocytosis, hemolytic anemia, aplastic anemia, thrombocytopenia, eosinophilia, leukopenia
Hepatic: Hepatitis, 3% to 10% of children experience transient elevated liver transaminase levels
Local: Irritation at I.M. injection site
Neuromuscular & skeletal: Peripheral neuropathy
Ocular: Optic neuritis
Otic: Tinnitus
Drug Interactions May increase serum concentrations of phenytoin, carbamazepine, diazepam; aluminum salts may decrease isoniazid absorption; prednisolone may increase isoniazid metabolism; cycloserine ethionamide (additive CNS toxicity)
Food Interactions Rate and extent of isoniazid absorption may be reduced when administered with food; avoid foods with histamine or tyramine (cheese, broad beans, dry sausage, salami, nonfresh meat, liver pate, soya bean, liquid and powdered protein supplements, wine); increase dietary intake of folate, niacin, magnesium, and pyridoxine; the American Academy of Pediatrics recommends that pyridoxine supplementation (1-2 mg/kg/day) should be administered to malnourished patients, children or adolescents on meat or milk-deficient diets, breast-feeding infants, and those predisposed to neuritis to prevent peripheral neuropathy
Stability Protect from light and excessive heat; avoid freezing
Mechanism of Action Inhibits mycolic acid synthesis resulting in disruption of the bacterial cell wall
Pharmacokinetics
Absorption: Oral, I.M.: Rapid and complete
Distribution: Crosses the placenta; appears in breast milk; distributes into most body tissues and fluids including the CSF
Protein binding: 10% to 15%
Metabolism: By the liver to acetylisoniazid with decay rate determined genetically by acetylation phenotype; undergoes further hydrolysis to isonicotinic acid and acetylhydrazine

Half-life: May be prolonged in patients with impaired hepatic function or severe renal impairment
  Fast acetylators: 30-100 minutes
  Slow acetylators: 2-5 hours
Time to peak serum concentration: Oral: Within 1-2 hours
Elimination: 75% to 95% excreted in urine as unchanged drug and metabolites; small amounts excreted in feces and saliva
Dialyzable (50% to 100%)

Usual Dosage Oral, I.M.:
Infants and Children:
  Treatment: 10-20 mg/kg/day in 1-2 divided doses; maximum dose: 300 mg/day
  Prophylaxis: 10 mg/kg/day given once daily, not to exceed 300 mg/day
Adults:
  Treatment: 5 mg/kg/day given daily (usual dose: 300 mg)
  Disseminated disease: 10 mg/kg/day in 1-2 divided doses
  Prophylaxis: 300 mg/day given daily
American Thoracic Society and CDC currently recommend twice weekly therapy as part of a short-course regimen which follows 1-2 months of daily treatment for uncomplicated pulmonary tuberculosis in **compliant** patients
  Children: 20-40 mg/kg/dose (up to 900 mg/dose) twice weekly
  Adults: 15 mg/kg/dose (up to 900 mg/dose) twice weekly
Duration of therapy:
  Asymptomatic infection (positive skin test):
    Isoniazid susceptible: 9 months of isoniazid
    Isoniazid resistant: 9 months of rifampin
  Pulmonary, hilar adenopathy, and extrapulmonary infection other than meningitis, bone/joint, or disseminated infection:
    6 months which includes 2-month therapy of isoniazid, rifampin, and pyrazinamide daily followed by 4 months of isoniazid and rifampin daily **or** 2 months of isoniazid, rifampin, and pyrazinamide daily, followed by 4 months of isoniazid and rifampin twice weekly under direct observation
    alternatively
    9 months of isoniazid and rifampin daily **or** 1 month of isoniazid and rifampin daily followed by 8 months of isoniazid and rifampin twice weekly under direct observation; if isoniazid resistance is identified, rifampin and ethambutol should be continued for a maximum of 12 months
    Note: If drug resistance is possible, ethambutol or streptomycin should be added to the initial therapy regimen until susceptibility is determined
  Meningitis, bone/joint, and disseminated infection:
    12 months which includes 2 months of isoniazid, rifampin, pyrazinamide, and streptomycin daily followed by 10 months of isoniazid and rifampin daily **or** 2 months of isoniazid, rifampin, pyrazinamide, and streptomycin daily followed by 10 months of isoniazid and rifampin twice weekly under direct observation

Administration
Oral: Administer 1 hour before or 2 hours after meals with water; administration of isoniazid syrup has been associated with diarrhea
Parenteral: I.M.: Administer I.M. when oral therapy is not possible

Monitoring Parameters
Periodic liver function tests; monitoring for prodromal signs of hepatitis; ophthalmologic exam

Test Interactions
False-positive urinary glucose with Clinitest®

Patient Information
Report any prodromal symptoms of hepatitis (fatigue, weakness, nausea, vomiting, dark urine, or yellowing of eyes) or any burning, tingling, or numbness in the extremities; avoid alcohol

Dosage Forms
Injection: 100 mg/mL (10 mL)
Syrup (orange flavor): 50 mg/5 mL (473 mL)
Tablet: 50 mg, 100 mg, 300 mg

References
Ad Hoc Committee of the Scientific Assembly on Microbiology, Tuberculosis, and Pulmonary Infections, "Treatment of Tuberculosis and Tuberculosis Infection in Adults and Children," *Clin Infect Dis*, 1995, 21:9-27.
American Academy of Pediatrics, Committee on Infectious Diseases, "Chemotherapy for Tuberculosis in Infants and Children," *Pediatrics*, 1992, 89(1):161-5.
Starke JR, "Modern Approach to the Diagnosis and Treatment of Tuberculosis in Children," *Pediatr Clin North Am*, 1988, 35(3):441-64.
Starke JR, "Multidrug Therapy for Tuberculosis in Children," *Pediatr Infect Dis J*, 1990, 9(11):785-93.
Van Scoy RE and Wilkowske CJ, "Antituberculous Agents: Isoniazid, Rifampin, Streptomycin, Ethambutol, and Pyrazinamide," *Mayo Clin Proc*, 1983, 58(4):233-40.

♦ **Isonicotinic Acid Hydrazide** see Isoniazid on page 534

♦ **Isonipecaine** *see* Meperidine *on page 602*

♦ **Isoprenaline** *see* Isoproterenol *on page 536*

Isoproterenol (eye soe proe TER e nole)

Related Information
Adult ACLS Algorithm, Bradycardia *on page 1012*
Asthma Guidelines *on page 1178*
Emergency Pediatric Drip Calculations *on page 1000*

Brand Names Arm-a-Med® Isoproterenol; Dey-Dose® Isoproterenol; Dispos-a-Med® Isoproterenol; Isuprel® Injection; Medihaler-Iso® Inhalation Aerosol; Norisodrine®

Available Salts Isoproterenol Hydrochloride; Isoproterenol Sulfate

Synonyms Isoprenaline

Therapeutic Category Adrenergic Agonist Agent; Antiasthmatic; $Beta_1$ & $Beta_2$-Adrenergic Agonist Agent; Bronchodilator; Sympathomimetic

Generic Available Yes

Use Asthma or COPD (reversible airway obstruction); ventricular arrhythmias due to A-V nodal block; hemodynamically compromised bradyarrhythmias or atropine-resistant bradyarrhythmias, temporary use in third degree A-V block until pacemaker insertion; low cardiac output or vasoconstrictive shock states

Pregnancy Risk Factor C

Contraindications Angina, pre-existing cardiac arrhythmias (ventricular); tachycardia or A-V block caused by cardiac glycoside intoxication; allergy to sulfites or isoproterenol or other sympathomimetic amines; narrow-angle glaucoma

Warnings Tolerance may occur with prolonged use; when discontinuing an isoproterenol continuous infusion used for bronchodilation, the infusion **must** be gradually tapered over a 24- to 48-hour period to prevent rebound bronchospasm

Precautions Use with caution in diabetics, renal or cardiovascular disease, hyperthyroidism, prostatic hypertrophy

Adverse Reactions
Cardiovascular: Flushing of the face or skin, ventricular arrhythmias, tachycardia, hypotension, chest pain, palpitations, hypertension
Central nervous system: Nervousness, restlessness, anxiety, dizziness, headache, vertigo, insomnia
Endocrine & metabolic: Parotid glands swelling
Gastrointestinal: Heartburn, GI distress, nausea, vomiting, dry throat, pinkish-red saliva (after inhalation), xerostomia
Neuromuscular & skeletal: Tremor, weakness, trembling
Respiratory: Cough, dyspnea, bronchitis (after inhalation therapy)
Miscellaneous: Diaphoresis

Drug Interactions Additive effects and increased cardiotoxicity when administered concomitantly with other sympathomimetic amines; beta-adrenergic blocking agents may decrease effectiveness due to beta blockade; may increase theophylline elimination

Mechanism of Action Stimulates $beta_1$- and $beta_2$-receptors resulting in relaxation of bronchial, GI, and uterine smooth muscle; increased heart rate and contractility; vasodilation of peripheral vasculature

Pharmacodynamics
Onset of action:
Oral inhalation: 2-5 minutes
I.V.: Immediately
S.L.: ~30 minutes
Duration:
Oral inhalation: 30 minutes to 2 hours
I.V. (single dose): Few minutes
S.L. or S.C.: Up to 2 hours

Pharmacokinetics
Metabolism: By conjugation in many tissues including the liver and lungs
Half-life: 2.5-5 minutes
Elimination: In urine principally as sulfate conjugates

Usual Dosage
Neonates, Infants, and Children: I.V. infusion: 0.05-2 mcg/kg/minute; rate (mL/hour) = dose (mcg/kg/minute) x weight (kg) x 60 minutes/hour divided by concentration (mcg/mL)
Children:
Oral inhalation: 1-2 metered doses up to 6 times/day

Nebulization: 0.01 mL/kg (0.1 mg/kg) of 1% solution; minimum dose: 0.1 mL (1 mg); maximum dose: 0.5 mL (5 mg); or equivalent doses using 0.25% and 0.5% solutions

S.L.: 5-10 mg every 3-4 hours (maximum dose: 30 mg/day)

Adults:

Oral inhalation: 1-2 metered doses 4-6 times/day

Nebulization: 0.25-0.5 mL (2.5-5 mg) of a 1% solution or equivalent doses using 0.25% or 0.5% solutions

S.L.: 10-20 mg every 3-4 hours (maximum dose: 60 mg/day)

I.V. infusion: 2-20 mcg/minute

Administration

Nebulization: Dilute dosage from 1% solution in 2-3 mL NS; other solutions at concentrations <1% may be administered without dilution

Oral: Do not swallow sublingual tablets, allow to dissolve under the tongue

Oral inhalation: Shake well before use; use spacer device in children <8 years of age

Parenteral: May be administered undiluted by direct I.V. injection; for continuous infusions, dilute in dextrose or NS to a maximum concentration of 20 mcg/mL; concentrations as high as 64 mcg/mL have been used safely and with efficacy in situations of extreme fluid restriction

Monitoring Parameters Heart rate, blood pressure, respiratory rate, arterial blood gases, central venous pressure, EKG

Patient Information After inhalation therapy, may cause saliva to turn pinkish-red; do not exceed recommended dosage; wait at least 3-5 minutes between metered dose inhalations (if more than 1 inhalation per dose)

Additional Information Hypotension is more common in hypovolemic patients

Dosage Forms

Inhalation, as sulfate: Aerosol: 0.2% [2 mg/mL = 1:500] (15 mL, 22.5 mL); 0.25% [2.5 mg/mL = 1:400] (15 mL)

Injection, as hydrochloride: 0.02% [0.2 mg/mL = 1:5000] (1 mL, 5 mL, 10 mL)

Solution for nebulization, as hydrochloride: 0.031% (4 mL); 0.062% (4 mL); 0.25% (0.5 mL, 30 mL); 0.5% (0.5 mL, 10 mL, 60 mL); 1% (10 mL)

Tablet, sublingual, as hydrochloride: 10 mg, 15 mg

References

Rachelefsky GS and Siegel SC, "Asthma in Infants and Children - Treatment of Childhood Asthma: Part 1I," J Allergy Clin Immunol, 1985, 76(3):409-25.

♦ **Isoproterenol Hydrochloride** see Isoproterenol on page 536
♦ **Isoproterenol Sulfate** see Isoproterenol on page 536
♦ **Isoptin®** see Verapamil on page 974
♦ **Isoptin® SR** see Verapamil on page 974
♦ **Isopto® Atropine Ophthalmic** see Atropine on page 107
♦ **Isopto® Carpine Ophthalmic** see Pilocarpine on page 770
♦ **Isopto® Eserine** see Physostigmine on page 768
♦ **Isopto® Frin Ophthalmic Solution** see Phenylephrine on page 758
♦ **Isopto® Homatropine** see Homatropine on page 477
♦ **Isopto® Hyoscine** see Scopolamine on page 860

Isotretinoin (eye soe TRET i noyn)

Brand Names Accutane®; Isotrex® (Canada)

Synonyms 13-cis-Retinoic Acid

Therapeutic Category Acne Products; Retinoic Acid Derivative; Vitamin A Derivative

Generic Available No

Use Treatment of severe recalcitrant cystic and/or conglobate acne unresponsive to conventional therapy; used investigationally for the treatment of children with high-risk neuroblastoma that does not respond to conventional therapy

Pregnancy Risk Factor X

Contraindications Sensitivity to parabens, vitamin A or other retinoids; patients who are pregnant or intend to become pregnant during treatment

Warnings Risk of isotretinoin teratogenesis is ~20%; it can cause fetal defects in the CNS, ears, and cardiovascular system; not to be used in women of child-bearing potential unless woman is capable of complying with effective contraceptive measures; therapy is normally begun on the second or third day of next normal menstrual period; effective contraception must be used for at least 1 month before beginning therapy, during therapy, and for 1 month after discontinuation of therapy

Precautions Use with caution in patients with diabetes mellitus or hypertriglyceridemia

(Continued)

Isotretinoin *(Continued)*

Adverse Reactions

Central nervous system: Fatigue, headache, dizziness, pseudotumor cerebri, mental depression, suicide ideation

Dermatologic: Pruritus, alopecia, cheilitis, photosensitivity, rash

Endocrine & metabolic: Hypertriglyceridemia, hyperuricemia, hyperglycemia, hypercalcemia

Gastrointestinal: Xerostomia, anorexia, nausea, vomiting, inflammatory bowel syndrome

Hematologic: Increase in erythrocyte sedimentation rate, decrease in hemoglobin and hematocrit

Hepatic: Hepatitis; elevated AST, ALT, and alkaline phosphatase

Neuromuscular & skeletal: Bone pain, arthralgia, myalgia

Ocular: Conjunctivitis, corneal opacities, cataracts, blurred vision

Renal: Hematuria, proteinuria

Respiratory: Epistaxis

Drug Interactions Increased clearance of carbamazepine; vitamin A supplements increase toxic effects; alcohol may potentiate an increase in serum triglycerides

Food Interactions Food or milk increases isotretinoin bioavailability

Stability Protect from light

Mechanism of Action Reduces sebaceous gland size and reduces sebum production; regulates cell proliferation and differentiation

Pharmacokinetics

Absorption: Oral: Demonstrates biphasic absorption

Distribution: Crosses the placenta; appears in breast milk, bile

Protein binding: 99% to 100%

Metabolism: In the liver; major metabolite: 4-oxo-isotretinoin (active); undergoes enterohepatic circulation

Half-life, terminal: 10-20 hours for isotretinoin, and 11-50 hours for its metabolite

Time to peak serum concentration: Within 3 hours

Elimination: Excreted in feces as unchanged drug and in urine as metabolites

Usual Dosage Oral:

Children: Maintenance therapy for neuroblastoma: 160 mg/m^2/day in 2 divided doses for 14 consecutive days in a 28-day cycle has been used investigationally

Children and Adults: Acne: 0.5-2 mg/kg/day in 2 divided doses (dosages as low as 0.05 mg/kg/day have been reported to be beneficial) for 15-20 weeks or until the total cyst count decreases by 70%, whichever is sooner

Administration Oral: Capsules can be swallowed or chewed and swallowed; the capsule may be opened with a large needle and the contents placed on apple sauce or ice cream for patients unable to swallow the capsule; administer with meals

Monitoring Parameters CBC with differential, platelet count, baseline ESR, serum triglyceride, liver enzymes, ophthalmologic exam

Patient Information Do not take vitamin supplements containing vitamin A; use caution when driving at night since decreased night vision can develop suddenly; patients who wear contact lenses may experience decreased tolerance to the lenses; avoid alcohol; avoid exposure to direct sunlight; notify physician of any abdominal pain, rectal bleeding, or severe diarrhea

Dosage Forms Capsule: 10 mg, 20 mg, 40 mg

References

American Academy of Pediatrics Committee on Drugs, "Retinoid Therapy for Severe Dermatological Disorders," *Pediatrics*, 1992, 90(1 Pt 1):119-20.

DiGiovanna JJ and Peck GL, "Oral Synthetic Retinoid Treatment in Children," *Pediatr Dermatol*, 1983, 1(1):77-88.

Matthay KK, Villablanca JG, Seeger RC, et al, "Treatment of High-Risk Neuroblastoma With Intensive Chemotherapy, Radiotherapy, Autologous Bone Marrow Transplantation, and 13-cis-Retinoic Acid. Children's Cancer Group," *N Engl J Med*, 1999, 341:1165-73.

Reynolds CP, Kane DJ, Einhorn PA, et al, "Response of Neuroblastoma to Retinoic Acid *In Vitro*, and *In Vivo*," *Prog Clin Biol Res*, 1991, 366:203-11

♦ **Isotrex® (Canada)** *see* Isotretinoin *on page 537*

♦ **Isoxazolyl Penicillin** *see* Oxacillin *on page 711*

♦ **I-Sulfacet®** *see* Sulfacetamide *on page 888*

♦ **Isuprel® Injection** *see* Isoproterenol *on page 536*

Itraconazole *(i tra KOE na zole)*

Brand Names Sporanox®

Therapeutic Category Antifungal Agent, Systemic

Generic Available No

Use Treatment of susceptible systemic fungal infections in immunocompromised and nonimmunocompromised patients including blastomycosis, coccidioidomycosis, paracoccidioidomycosis, histoplasmosis, and aspergillosis in patients who do not respond to or cannot tolerate amphotericin B

Oral solution: Treatment of oropharyngeal or esophageal candidiasis

Pregnancy Risk Factor C

Contraindications Hypersensitivity to itraconazole or any component; concomitant administration with terfenadine, astemizole, or cisapride

Warnings Itraconazole has induced bone defects (decreased bone plate activity, thinning of the zona compacta of large bones, increased bone fragility) and change in tooth appearance in rats; severe cardiovascular effects including Q-T interval prolongation, ventricular tachycardia, ventricular fibrillation, cardiac arrest, palpitations, syncope, and death have occurred in patients receiving itraconazole concomitantly with terfenadine, astemizole, or cisapride; do not use concurrently with terfenadine, astemizole, or cisapride; **itraconazole solution and capsules should not be used interchangeably**

Precautions Use with caution in patients with hypersensitivity to other azole antifungal agents and in patients with hepatic impairment; discontinue if signs and symptoms of liver disease develop

Adverse Reactions
  Cardiovascular: Hypertension, ventricular fibrillation, edema
  Central nervous system: Headache, dizziness, somnolence, fever, fatigue
  Dermatologic: Rash, pruritus, urticaria, angioedema, toxic epidermal necrolysis
  Endocrine & metabolic: Hypokalemia, adrenal insufficiency, gynecomastia
  Gastrointestinal: Nausea, vomiting, diarrhea, abdominal pain, anorexia
  Hepatic: Elevated liver enzymes, hepatitis
  Otic: Tinnitus
  Renal: Albuminuria

Drug Interactions
  Decreased effect of itraconazole with rifampin, carbamazepine, isoniazid, phenytoin, and phenobarbital (increases itraconazole's metabolism); H_2 antagonists, omeprazole, antacids, didanosine (decreases absorption)
  Increased effect of cyclosporine, tacrolimus (interferes with clearance); digoxin, warfarin, indinavir, and hypoglycemic agents (decreased metabolism)
  Increased toxicity of terfenadine, astemizole, triazolam, oral midazolam, cisapride, lovastatin, vinca alkaloids

Food Interactions Presence of food increases bioavailability of capsule formulation

Mechanism of Action Inhibits ergosterol synthesis in fungal cell membranes by inhibiting fungal cytochrome P-450

Pharmacokinetics
  Absorption: Rapid and complete when capsule is given immediately after a meal (bioavailability: 100%); decreased absorption reported when administered via nasogastric tube
  Distribution: High affinity for tissues (liver, lung, kidney, adipose tissue, brain, vagina, dermis, epidermis); poor penetration into CSF, eye fluid, saliva; distributes into breast milk, bronchial exudate, and sputum
  Protein binding: 99%
  Metabolism: Saturable hepatic metabolism to active and inactive metabolites
  Bioavailability: Capsules:
    Fasted state: 40%
    Fed state: Dose administered immediately after a meal: 100%
  Half-life: 17-30 hours
  Elimination: Metabolites are excreted in urine (35%) and bile (55%)
  Nondialyzable

Usual Dosage Oral:
  Children: Efficacy of itraconazole has not been established; a limited number of children have been treated with itraconazole using doses of 3-5 mg/kg/day once daily; doses as high as 5-10 mg/kg/day have been used in 32 patients with chronic granulomatous disease for prophylaxis against *Aspergillus* infection; doses of 6-8 mg/kg/day have been used in the treatment of disseminated histoplasmosis
    Prophylaxis for first episode of *Cryptococcus neoformans* or *Histoplasma capsulatum* in HIV-infected infants and children: 2-5 mg/kg/dose every 12-24 hours
    Prophylaxis for recurrence of opportunistic disease in HIV-infected infants and children:
      Cryptococcus neoformans: 2-5 mg/kg/dose every 12-24 hours
      Histoplasma capsulatum: 2-5 mg/kg/dose every 12-48 hours
(Continued)

Itraconazole *(Continued)*

Adults:

Blastomycosis and nonmeningeal histoplasmosis: Initial: 200 mg once daily; if poor response, increase dose in 100 mg increments to a maximum of 400 mg/day in 2 divided doses

Life-threatening infection and aspergillosis: Initial loading dose can be administered as follows: 600 mg/day in 3 divided doses for the first 3-4 days; maintenance dose: 200-400 mg/day in 2 divided doses; maximum dose: 600 mg/day in 3 divided doses

Esophageal candidiasis: Vigorously swish 10 mL in the mouth for several seconds and then swallow daily

Oropharyngeal candidiasis: Vigorously swish 10 mL in the mouth for several seconds at a time once daily (20 mL total daily dose), or 10 mL twice daily in patients refractory to oral fluconazole

Administration Oral:

Capsules: Administer with food

Solution: Administer on an empty stomach

Monitoring Parameters Periodic liver function tests, serum potassium; monitor for prodromal signs of hepatitis

Reference Range Therapeutic blood level: >250 ng/mL

Patient Information Report any prodromal symptoms of hepatitis (fatigue, weakness, nausea, vomiting, dark urine, or yellowing of eyes)

Nursing Implications Do not administer with antacids or H_2 antagonists

Dosage Forms

Capsule: 100 mg

Solution, oral: 100 mg/10 mL (150 mL)

References

Cowie F, Meller ST, Cushing P, et al, "Chemoprophylaxis for Pulmonary Aspergillosis During Intensive Chemotherapy," *Arch Dis Child*, 1994, 70(2):136-8.

Mouy R, Veber F, Blanche S, et al, "Long-Term Itraconazole Prophylaxis Against *Aspergillus* Infections in Thirty-Two Patients With Chronic Granulomatous Disease," *J Pediatr*, 1994, 125(6 Pt 1):998-1003.

Tobon AM, Franco L, Espinal D, et al, "Disseminated Histoplasmosis in Children: The Role of Itraconazole Therapy," *Pediatr Infect Dis J*, 1996; 15:1002-8.

"1997 USPHS/IDSA Guidelines for the Prevention of Opportunistic Infections in Persons Infected With Human Immunodeficiency Virus. USPHS/IDSA Prevention of Opportunistic Infections Working Group," *MMWR Morb Mortal Wkly Rep*, 1997, 46(RR-12):1-46.

+ **I-Tropine® Ophthalmic** *see* Atropine *on page 107*
+ **Iveegam®** *see* Immune Globulin, Intravenous *on page 510*
+ **IVIG** *see* Immune Globulin, Intravenous *on page 510*
+ **Jaa Amp® [Trihydrate] (Canada)** *see* Ampicillin *on page 78*
+ **Jaa-Prednisone® (Canada)** *see* Prednisone *on page 794*
+ **Janimine®** *see* Imipramine *on page 508*
+ **Jenamicin®** *see* Gentamicin *on page 452*
+ **K+® 8** *see* Potassium Supplements *on page 786*
+ **K+® 10** *see* Potassium Supplements *on page 786*
+ **Kabikinase®** *see* Streptokinase *on page 881*
+ **Kadian® Capsule** *see* Morphine Sulfate *on page 657*
+ **Kala [OTC]** *see* Lactobacillus acidophilus and Lactobacillus bulgaricus *on page 550*
+ **Kalcinate® Cal Plus®** *see* Calcium Supplements *on page 157*
+ **Kaochlor®** *see* Potassium Supplements *on page 786*
+ **Kaochlor-Eff** *see* Potassium Supplements *on page 786*
+ **Kaodene® [OTC]** *see* Kaolin and Pectin *on page 540*

Kaolin and Pectin (KAY oh lin & PEK tin)

Related Information

Carbohydrate and Alcohol Content of Liquid Medications for Use in Patients Receiving Ketogenic Diets *on page 1228*

Brand Names Donnagel®-MB (Canada); Kaodene® [OTC]; Kao-Spen® [OTC]; Kapectolin® [OTC]

Synonyms Pectin and Kaolin

Therapeutic Category Antidiarrheal

Generic Available Yes

Use Treatment of uncomplicated diarrhea

Pregnancy Risk Factor C

Contraindications Hypersensitivity to kaolin, pectin, or any component

Warnings Not to be used for self-medication of diarrhea for >48 hours or in presence of high fever in infants and children <3 years of age; do not use for diarrhea associated with pseudomembraneous enterocolitis or in diarrhea caused by toxigenic bacteria

Precautions Some products have added bismuth subsalicylate; use these products with caution in patients with bleeding disorders, salicylate sensitivity; do not use the subsalicylate-containing products in children <16 years of age who have chickenpox or flu symptoms due to the association with Reye's syndrome

Drug Interactions Kaolin and pectin may decrease absorption of quinidine, chloroquine, lincomycin, and digoxin (tablets only)

Usual Dosage Adequate controlled clinical studies documenting the efficacy of these combination products are lacking. Their usage and dosage have been primarily empiric; the following table describes the products available and the manufacturer's recommended dosage if stated.

Kaolin and Pectin Dosage*
(*mL/dose after each bowel movement)

Product	Content (per 30 mL)		Dosage (by age)		
	Kaolin	Pectin	3-6 y	6-12 y	>12 y to adult
Kao-Spen®	5.2 g	260 mg	—	—	60-120 mL
Kaolin w/pectin (Kapectolin®)	90 g	2 g	15-30 mL	30-60 mL	60-120 mL
Kaodene® (bismuth subsalicylate added)	3.9 g	194.4 mg	15 mL	22.5 mL	45 mL

Administration May be administered without regard to meals

Dosage Forms Suspension, oral: Kaolin 975 mg and pectin 22 mg per 5 mL

Ketamine (KEET a meen)

Related Information

Adult ACLS Algorithm, Electrical Conversion *on page 1014*
Preprocedure Sedatives in Children *on page 1169*

Brand Names Ketalar®

Therapeutic Category General Anesthetic

Generic Available No

Use Anesthesia, short surgical procedures, dressing changes

Restrictions C-III

Pregnancy Risk Factor D

Contraindications Elevated intracranial pressure; patients with hypertension, aneurysms, thyrotoxicosis, CHF, angina, psychotic disorders; hypersensitivity to ketamine or any component

Warnings Use only by or under the direct supervision of physicians experienced in administering general anesthetics. Resuscitative equipment should be available for use. Postanesthetic emergence reactions which can manifest as vivid dreams, hallucinations and/or frank delirium occur in 12% of patients; these reactions are less common in pediatric patients; emergence reactions may occur up to 24 hours postoperatively and may be reduced by minimization of verbal, tactile, and visual patient stimulation during recovery, or by pretreatment with a benzodiazepine.

Precautions Use with caution in patients with gastroesophageal reflux; use with caution and decrease the dose in patients with hepatic dysfunction; use with caution in patients with a full stomach, patients should fast (ie, be NPO) for an appropriate time before being sedated for elective procedures

Adverse Reactions

Cardiovascular: Hypertension, tachycardia, increased cardiac output, paradoxical direct myocardial depression, hypotension, bradycardia, increases cerebral blood flow

Central nervous system: Tonic-clonic movements, increased intracranial pressure, hallucinations

Endocrine & metabolic: Increased metabolic rate

Gastrointestinal: Hypersalivation, vomiting, postoperative nausea

Neuromuscular & skeletal: Increased skeletal muscle tone, tremor, purposeless movement, fasciculations

Ocular: Diplopia, nystagmus, increased intraocular pressure

Respiratory: Increased airway resistance, cough reflex may be depressed, decreased bronchospasm; respiratory depression or apnea with large doses or rapid infusions, laryngospasm; increased bronchial mucous gland secretion

Miscellaneous: Emergence reactions

Drug Interactions Barbiturates, narcotics, hydroxyzine prolong recovery from anesthesia

Stability Do not mix with barbiturates or diazepam as precipitation may occur

Mechanism of Action Produces dissociative anesthesia by direct action on the cortex and limbic system

Pharmacodynamics

Duration of action: Following single dose:

Anesthesia:
I.M.: 12-25 minutes
I.V.: 5-10 minutes
Analgesia: I.M.: 15-30 minutes
Recovery:
I.M.: 3-4 hours
I.V.: 1-2 hours

Usual Dosage

Children:

Oral: 6-10 mg/kg for 1 dose (mixed in cola or other beverage) given 30 minutes before the procedure

I.M.: 3-7 mg/kg

I.V.: Range: 0.5-2 mg/kg, use smaller doses (0.5-1 mg/kg) for sedation for minor procedures; usual induction dosage: 1-2 mg/kg

Continuous I.V. infusion: Sedation: 5-20 mcg/kg/minute; start at lower dosage listed and titrate to effect

Adults:

I.M.: 3-8 mg/kg

I.V.: Range: 1-4.5 mg/kg; usual induction dosage: 1-2 mg/kg

Children and Adults: Maintenance: Supplemental doses of 1/3 to 1/2 of initial dose

Administration
Oral: Use 100 mg/mL I.V. solution and mix the appropriate dose in 0.2-0.3 mL/kg of cola or other beverage

Parenteral: I.V.: Administer slowly, do not exceed 0.5 mg/kg/minute; do not administer faster than 60 seconds; do not exceed final concentration of 2 mg/mL

Monitoring Parameters Cardiovascular effects, heart rate, blood pressure, respiratory rate, transcutaneous O_2 saturation

Nursing Implications Resuscitative equipment should be available for use

Additional Information Used in combination with anticholinergic agents to decrease hypersalivation; should not be used for sedation for procedures that require a total lack of movement (eg, MRI, radiation therapy) due to association with purposeless movements

Dosage Forms Injection: 10 mg/mL (20 mL, 25 mL, 50 mL); 50 mg/mL (10 mL); 100 mg/mL (5 mL)

References
Cote CJ, "Sedation for the Pediatric Patient: A Review," *Pediatr Clin North Am*, 1994, 41(1):31-58.

Gutstein HB, Johnson KL, Heard MN, et al, "Oral Ketamine Premedication in Children," *Anesthesiology*, 1992, 76(1):28-33.

Tobias JD, Phipps S, Smith B, et al, "Oral Ketamine Premedication to Alleviate the Distress of Invasive Procedures in Pediatric Oncology Patients," *Pediatrics*, 1992, 90(4):537-41.

Tobias JD and Rasmussen GE, "Pain Management and Sedation in the Pediatric Intensive Care Unit," *Pediatr Clin North Am*, 1994, 41(6):1269-92.

Ketoconazole (kee toe KOE na zole)

Brand Names Nizoral®

Therapeutic Category Antifungal Agent, Systemic; Antifungal Agent, Topical

Generic Available No

Use Treatment of susceptible fungal infections, including candidiasis, oral thrush, blastomycosis, histoplasmosis, paracoccidioidomycosis, chronic mucocutaneous candidiasis, as well as certain recalcitrant cutaneous dermatophytoses; used topically for treatment of tinea corporis, tinea cruris, tinea versicolor, and cutaneous candidiasis; shampoo is used for dandruff

Pregnancy Risk Factor C

Contraindications Hypersensitivity to ketoconazole or any component; single agent in the treatment of CNS fungal infections (due to poor CNS penetration); concomitant administration of astemizole, terfenadine, or cisapride

Warnings Has been associated with hepatotoxicity, including some fatalities; perform periodic liver function tests; high doses of ketoconazole may depress adrenocortical function and decrease serum testosterone concentrations; risk of serious cardiac arrhythmias in patients receiving ketoconazole and astemizole, terfenadine, or cisapride; do not use concurrently with astemizole, terfenadine, or cisapride

Precautions Gastric acidity is necessary for the dissolution and absorption of ketoconazole; avoid concomitant (within 2 hours) administration of antacids, H_2-blockers, anticholinergics; use with caution in patients with impaired hepatic function

Adverse Reactions
Central nervous system: Lethargy, nervousness, headache, dizziness, somnolence, fever, chills, bulging fontanelles

Dermatologic: Pruritus, rash, dry skin

Endocrine & metabolic: Adrenocortical insufficiency, gynecomastia, decreased libido

Gastrointestinal: Nausea, vomiting, abdominal discomfort, GI bleeding, diarrhea

Genitourinary: Oligospermia

Hematologic: Leukopenia, thrombocytopenia, hemolytic anemia

Hepatic: Hepatotoxicity; elevated AST, ALT, and alkaline phosphatase; jaundice

Local: Irritation, stinging

Miscellaneous: Anaphylaxis

Drug Interactions Cytochrome P-450 isoenzyme CYP3A3/4 substrate; CYP1A2, CYP2C, CYP2C9 (weak), CYP2C19 (weak), CYP3A3/4, and CYP3A5-7 isoenzyme inhibitor

Drugs that decrease ketoconazole absorption (raise gastric pH) such as antacids, didanosine, sodium bicarbonate, omeprazole, H_2-receptor blockers; drugs that decrease serum concentrations of ketoconazole (rifampin, isoniazid); drug concentrations that are increased by ketoconazole (phenytoin, astemizole, cisapride, digoxin, cyclosporine, corticosteroids, terfenadine, indinavir, saquinavir, warfarin); drugs that cause hepatotoxicity; alcohol may cause disulfiram-like reactions; increased trough concentrations of delavirdine if given with ketoconazole (see Warnings)

(Continued)

Ketoconazole (Continued)

Food Interactions Food may increase ketoconazole absorption

Mechanism of Action Alters the permeability of the cell wall; inhibits fungal biosynthesis of triglycerides and phospholipids; inhibits several fungal enzymes that results in a build-up of toxic concentrations of hydrogen peroxide

Pharmacokinetics

Absorption: Oral: Rapid (~75%)

Distribution: Minimal penetration into the CNS; distributes to bile, saliva, urine, sweat, synovial fluid, lungs, liver, kidney and bone marrow

Protein binding: 84% to 99%

Metabolism: Partially in the liver by enzymes to inactive compounds

Bioavailability: Decreases as pH of the gastric contents increase

Half-life, biphasic:

Initial: 2 hours

Terminal: 8 hours

Time to peak serum concentration: Within 1-2 hours

Elimination: Primarily in feces (57%) with smaller amounts excreted in urine (~13%)

Not dialyzable (0% to 5%)

Usual Dosage

Infants and Children: Oral: 3.3-6.6 mg/kg/day once daily

Prophylaxis for recurrence of mucocutaneous candidiasis with HIV infection: 5-10 mg/kg/day divided every 12-24 hours; maximum: 800 mg/day divided twice daily

Adults: Oral: 200-400 mg/day as a single daily dose; maximum: 800 mg/day divided twice daily

Children and Adults:

Shampoo: Shampoo twice weekly (at least 3 days should elapse between each shampoo) for 4 weeks

Topical: Apply once daily to twice daily

Administration

Oral: May administer with or without food or with juice; administer with food to decrease nausea and vomiting; administer 2 hours prior to antacids, didanosine, proton pump inhibitors, or H_2-receptor antagonists to prevent decreased ketoconazole absorption; shake suspension well before using

Shampoo: Apply to wet hair and massage over entire scalp for 1 minute; rinse hair thoroughly and reapply shampoo for 3 minutes; rinse

Topical: Apply a sufficient amount and rub gently into the affected and surrounding area

Monitoring Parameters Liver function tests, signs of adrenal dysfunction

Patient Information Cream is for topical application to the skin only; avoid contact with the eye; notify physician of unusual fatigue, weakness, vomiting, dark urine, or yellowing of eyes; avoid alcohol

Additional Information Cream contains sodium sulfite

Dosage Forms

Cream: 2% (15 g, 30 g, 60 g)

Shampoo: 2% (120 mL)

Tablet: 200 mg

Extemporaneous Preparations A 20 mg/mL suspension may be made by pulverizing twelve 200 mg ketoconazole tablets to a fine powder; add 40 mL Ora-Plus® in small portions with thorough mixing; incorporate Ora-Sweet® to make a final volume of 120 mL and mix thoroughly; shake well before using; protect from light; stable for 60 days when stored without light at 5°C and 25°C

Allen LV and Erickson MA, "Stability of Ketoconazole, Metolazone, Metronidazole, Procainamide, Hydrochloride, and Spironolactone in Extemporaneously Compounded Oral Liquids," *AM J Health-Syst Pharm*, 1996, 53:2073-8.

References

Como JA and Dismukes WE, "Oral Azole Drugs as Systemic Antifungal Therapy," *N Engl J Med*, 1994, 330(4):263-72.

Ginsburg AM, McCracken GH Jr, and Olsen K, "Pharmacology of Ketoconazole Suspension in Infants and Children," *Antimicrob Agents Chemother*, 1983, 23(5):787-9.

Herrod HG, "Chronic Mucocutaneous Candidiasis in Childhood and Complications of non-*Candida* Infection: A Report of the Pediatric Immunodeficiency Collaborative Study Group," *J Pediatr*, 1990, 116(3):377-82.

Ketorolac (KEE toe role ak)

Brand Names Acular® Ophthalmic; Toradol® Injection; Toradol® Oral

Available Salts Ketorolac Tromethamine

Therapeutic Category Analgesic, Non-narcotic; Anti-inflammatory Agent; Anti-pyretic; Nonsteroidal Anti-inflammatory Drug (NSAID), Ophthalmic; Nonsteroidal Anti-inflammatory Drug (NSAID), Oral; Nonsteroidal Anti-inflammatory Drug (NSAID), Parenteral

Generic Available Yes: Injection, tablet

Use

Oral, I.M., I.V.,: Short-term (≤5 days) management of moderate to severe pain, including postoperative pain, visceral pain associated with cancer, pain associated with trauma, acute renal colic

Ophthalmic: Ocular itch associated with seasonal allergic conjunctivitis

Pregnancy Risk Factor C (D if used in 3rd trimester)

Contraindications Hypersensitivity to ketorolac, any component, or in patients with nasal polyps, angioedema, or bronchospastic reactions to aspirin or other NSAIDs; patients with active peptic ulcer disease (PUD), recent GI bleeding or perforation, or history of PUD or GI bleeding; advanced renal dysfunction; patients at risk for renal failure due to hypovolemia; women in labor and delivery or breast-feeding; preoperative or intraoperative use; patients with cerebrovascular bleeding, incomplete hemostasis, hemorrhagic diathesis, or at high risk of bleeding; contraindicated for epidural or intrathecal use due to alcohol content; do not administer with aspirin, NSAIDs, or probenecid

Precautions Use with caution and reduce dose in patients with decreased renal function; hepatic impairment; CHF; patients in whom prolongation of bleeding time would cause adverse effects; not recommended after plastic or neurosurgery due to increased risk of bleeding

Adverse Reactions

Cardiovascular: Edema (4%)

Central nervous system: Somnolence, drowsiness (6%), dizziness (7%), headache (17%), insomnia, euphoria, hallucinations, malaise (<1%)

Dermatologic: Purpura, urticaria

Gastrointestinal: Dyspepsia (12%), nausea (12%), diarrhea (7%), GI pain, peptic ulcer, melena, rectal bleeding, constipation (<1%)

Genitourinary: Urinary frequency

Hematologic: Inhibits platelet aggregation, may prolong bleeding time

Hepatic: Elevated liver enzymes

Local: Pain at injection site (2%)

Ocular: Blurred vision

Renal: Oliguria, interstitial nephritis, acute renal failure (rare)

Respiratory: Dyspnea, wheezing

Miscellaneous: Anaphylaxis, hypersensitivity reactions

Drug Interactions Warfarin, heparin, lithium, methotrexate, salicylates, NSAIDs, GI irritants (eg, potassium supplements), probenecid (significantly increases ketorolac half-life and plasma levels), furosemide, phenytoin, carbamazepine

Food Interactions High-fat meals may delay time to peak (by ~1 hour) and decrease peak concentrations

Stability Protect from light; color change indicates degradation; do not administer in same syringe with narcotics; ketorolac will precipitate if mixed with morphine, meperidine, promethazine, or hydroxyzine

Mechanism of Action Inhibits prostaglandin synthesis by decreasing the activity of the enzyme, cyclo-oxygenase, which results in decreased formation of prostaglandin precursors

Pharmacodynamics Analgesia:

Onset:

Oral: 30-60 minutes

I.M., I.V.: ~30 minutes

Peak:

Oral: 1.5-4 hours

I.M., I.V.: 1-2 hours

Duration: 4-6 hours

Pharmacokinetics

Absorption:

Oral: Well absorbed

I.M.: Rapid and complete

Distribution: Crosses placenta, crosses into breast milk, poor penetration into CSF; follows two-compartment model

V_d beta: Adults: 0.11-0.33 L/kg (mean: 0.18 L/kg)

Protein binding: 99%

(Continued)

Ketorolac *(Continued)*

Metabolism: In the liver; undergoes hydroxylation and glucuronide conjugation; in children 4-8 years, V_{dss} and plasma clearance were twice as high as adults, but terminal half-life was similar

Bioavailability: Oral, I.M.: 100%

Half-life, terminal:

Children 4-8 years: ~6 hours; range: 3.5-10 (n=10)

Adults: Mean: ~5 hours; range: 4-9 hours

With renal impairment: S_{cr} 1.9-5 mg/dL: Mean: ~11 hours; range: 4-19 hours

Renal dialysis patients: Mean: ~14 hours; range: 8-40 hours

Time to peak serum concentration:

Oral: ~45 minutes

I.M.: 30-45 minutes

I.V.: 1-3 minutes

Elimination: Renal excretion, 58% to 61% in urine as unchanged drug

Usual Dosage Note: The use of ketorolac in children <16 years of age is outside of product labeling

Children 2-16 years: Dosing guidelines are not established; **do not exceed adult doses**; see Additional Information

Single-dose treatment:

I.M., I.V.: 0.4-1 mg/kg as a single dose; **Note:** Limited information exists. Single I.V. doses of 0.5 mg/kg, 0.75 mg/kg, 0.9 mg/kg and 1 mg/kg have been studied in children 2-16 years of age for postoperative analgesia. One study (Maunuksela, 1992) used a titrating dose starting with 0.2 mg/kg up to a total of 0.5 mg/kg (median dose required: 0.4 mg/kg).

Oral: One study used 1 mg/kg as a single dose for analgesia in 30 children (mean ± SD age: 3 ± 2.5 years) undergoing bilateral myringotomy

Multiple-dose treatment: I.M., I.V., Oral: No pediatric studies exist; one report (Buck, 1994) of the clinical experience with ketorolac in 112 children, 6 months to 19 years of age (mean: 9 years), described usual I.V. maintenance doses of 0.5 mg/kg every 6 hours (mean dose: 0.52 mg/kg; range: 0.17-1 mg/kg)

Children >16 years and >50 kg and Adults <65 years:

Single-dose treatment:

I.M.: 60 mg as a single dose

I.V.: 30 mg as a single dose

Multiple-dose treatment:

I.M., I.V.: 30 mg every 6 hours; maximum dose: 120 mg/day

Oral: Initial: 20 mg, then 10 mg every 4-6 hours; maximum dose: 40 mg/day

Adults ≥65 years, renally impaired, or <50 kg:

Single-dose treatment:

I.M.: 30 mg as a single dose

I.V.: 15 mg as a single dose

Multiple-dose treatment:

I.M., I.V.: 15 mg every 6 hours; maximum dose: 60 mg/day

Oral: 10 mg every 4-6 hours; maximum dose: 40 mg/day

Adults: Ophthalmic: Instill 1 drop in eye(s) 4 times/day for up to 7 days

Administration

Oral: May administer with food or milk to decrease GI upset

Parenteral:

I.M.: Administer slowly and deeply into muscle; 60 mg/2 mL Tubex® is for I.M. use only

I.V. bolus: Administer over at least 15 seconds; I.V. ketorolac has been infused over 1-5 minutes in children

Monitoring Parameters Signs of pain relief (eg, increased appetite and activity); BUN, serum creatinine, liver enzymes, occult blood loss, urinalysis

Reference Range Serum concentration:

Therapeutic: 0.3-5 µg/mL

Toxic: >5 µg/mL

Patient Information Avoid alcohol; may cause drowsiness or dizziness and may impair ability to perform activities requiring mental alertness or physical coordination; do not exceed 5 days total use (I.M., I.V., oral)

Additional Information 30 mg provides analgesia comparable to 12 mg of morphine or 100 mg of meperidine; ketorolac may possess an opioid-sparing effect; diarrhea, pallor, vomiting, and labored breathing may occur with overdose

Note: A single I.V. dose of ketorolac (0.75 mg/kg) in 21 children (2.5-9 years of age) undergoing outpatient strabismus surgery was associated with less postoperative emesis than morphine plus metoclopramide (Munro, 1994). However, a single dose of I.V. ketorolac (1 mg/kg) in 25 children (2-15 years of age) undergoing tonsillectomy was associated with an increase in surgical bleeding, more patients requiring extra hemostatic measures (eg, synthetic collagen, extra Neo-Synephrine® packing), and a higher estimated blood loss compared to rectal acetaminophen (Rusy, 1995); further studies are needed.

Dosage Forms

Injection, as tromethamine: 15 mg/mL (1 mL); 30 mg/mL (1 mL, 2 mL, 10 mL)

Solution, ophthalmic, as tromethamine: 0.5% (5 mL)

Tablet, as tromethamine: 10 mg

References

Buck ML, "Clinical Experience With Ketorolac in Children," *Ann Pharmacother*, 1994, 28(9):1009-13.

Maunuksela E, Kokki H, and Bullingham RES, "Comparison of Intravenous Ketorolac With Morphine for Postoperative Pain in Children," *Clin Pharmacol Ther*, 1992, 52(4):436-43.

Munro HM, Reigger LQ, Reynolds PI, et al, "Comparison of the Analgesic and Emetic Properties of Ketorolac and Morphine for Paediatric Outpatient Strabismus Surgery," *Br J Anaesth*, 1994, 72(6):624-8.

Rusy LM, Houck CS, Sullivan LJ, et al, "A Double-Blind Evaluation of Ketorolac Tromethamine Versus Acetaminophen in Pediatric Tonsillectomy: Analgesia and Bleeding," *Anesth Analg*, 1995, 80(2):226-9.

Watcha MF, Jones MB, Laguereula RG, et al, "Comparison of Ketorolac and Morphine as Adjuvants During Pediatric Surgery," *Anesthesiology*, 1992, 76(3):368-72.

- ◆ Kytril™ Injection *see* Granisetron *on page 462*
- ◆ L-3-Hydroxytyramine *see* Levodopa *on page 565*
- ◆ L-735,524 *see* Indinavir *on page 514*
- ◆ LA-12® *see* Hydroxocobalamin *on page 492*

Labetalol (la BET a lole)

Related Information
  Overdose and Toxicology *on page 1191*
Brand Names Normodyne®; Trandate®
Available Salts Labetalol Hydrochloride
Synonyms Ibidomide
Therapeutic Category Alpha-/Beta- Adrenergic Blocker; Antihypertensive Agent
Generic Available Yes
Use Treatment of mild to severe hypertension; I.V. for hypertensive emergencies
Pregnancy Risk Factor C
Contraindications Asthma, obstructive airway disease, cardiogenic shock, uncompensated CHF, bradycardia, pulmonary edema, or heart block; history of asthma or obstructive airway disease
Warnings Orthostatic hypotension may occur with I.V. administration; patient should remain supine during and for up to 3 hours after I.V. administration; use with extreme caution when reducing severely elevated blood pressure; cerebral and cardiac adverse effects (infarction/ischemia) may occur if blood pressure is decreased too rapidly; blood pressure should be lowered over as long a period of time that is compatible with the status of the patient
Precautions Paradoxical increase in blood pressure has been reported with treatment of pheochromocytoma or clonidine withdrawal syndrome; use with extreme caution in patients with hyper-reactive airway disease, CHF, diabetes mellitus, hepatic dysfunction

Adverse Reactions
  Cardiovascular: Orthostatic hypotension especially with I.V. administration, edema, CHF, A-V conduction disturbances (but less than with propranolol), bradycardia
  Central nervous system: Drowsiness, fatigue, dizziness, behavior disorders, headache
  Dermatologic: Rash, tingling in scalp or skin (transient with initiation of therapy)
  Gastrointestinal: Nausea, xerostomia
  Genitourinary: Sexual dysfunction, urinary problems
  Neuromuscular & skeletal: Reversible myopathy has been reported in 2 children, paresthesia
  Respiratory: Bronchospasm, nasal congestion
Drug Interactions Cytochrome P-450 isoenzyme; CYP2D6 substrate and inhibitor
  Cimetidine may potentiate labetalol action; additive hypotensive effects with other hypotensive drugs; halothane may cause synergistic hypotension; tricyclic antidepressants; beta agonists; nitroglycerin; calcium antagonists
Food Interactions Avoid natural licorice (causes sodium and water retention and increases potassium loss); food may increase bioavailability
Stability
  Injection: Stable in D_5W, saline for 24 hours; incompatible with sodium bicarbonate, furosemide; most stable in pH of 2-4; store at room temperature; do not freeze; protect from light
  Tablets: Store at room temperature; protect unit dose boxes from excessive moisture
Mechanism of Action Blocks alpha-, beta$_1$- and beta$_2$-adrenergic receptor sites; elevated renins are reduced
Pharmacodynamics
  Onset of action:
    Oral: 20 minutes to 2 hours
    I.V.: 2-5 minutes
  Peak effect:
    Oral: 1-4 hours
    I.V.: 5-15 minutes
  Duration:
    Oral: 8-24 hours (dose dependent)
    I.V.: 2-4 hours
Pharmacokinetics
  Distribution: Crosses the placenta; small amounts in breast milk
    V_d: Adults: 3-16 L/kg; mean: 9.4 L/kg
  Protein-binding: 50%

Metabolism: In the liver primarily via glucuronide conjugation; extensive first-pass effect

Bioavailability: Oral: 25%; increased bioavailability with liver disease, elderly

Half-life: 5-8 hours

Elimination: Possible decreased clearance in neonates/infants; <5% excreted in urine unchanged

Usual Dosage

Children: **Note:** Limited information regarding labetalol use in pediatric patients is currently available in the literature; labetalol should be initiated cautiously in pediatric patients (using the lower doses listed) with careful dosage adjustment and blood pressure monitoring

Oral: Some centers recommend initial oral doses of 4 mg/kg/day in 2 divided doses. (Reported oral doses have started at 3 mg/kg/day and 20 mg/kg/day and have increased up to 40 mg/kg/day.)

I.V., intermittent bolus doses: Initial doses of 0.2-0.5 mg/kg/dose with a range of 0.2-1 mg/kg/dose have been suggested; maximum dose: 20 mg/dose

Treatment of pediatric hypertensive emergencies: Initial continuous infusions of 0.4-1 mg/kg/hour with a maximum of 3 mg/kg/hour have been used; one study used initial bolus dose of 0.2-1 mg/kg (maximum dose: 20 mg, mean: 0.5 mg/kg) followed by a continuous infusion of 0.25-1.5 mg/kg/hour (mean: 0.78 mg/kg/hour)

Adults:

Oral: Initial: 100 mg twice daily, may increase as needed every 2-3 days by 100 mg until desired response is obtained; usual dose: 200-400 mg twice daily; not to exceed 2.4 g/day

I.V.: Initial: 20 mg; may give 40-80 mg at 10-minute intervals, up to 300 mg total dose

I.V. infusion: Initial: 2 mg/minute; titrate to response

Administration

Oral: May administer with food but should be administered in a consistent manner with regards to meals

Parenteral:

I.V. bolus: Administer over 2-3 minutes; do not administer faster than 2 mg/minute; maximum concentration: 5 mg/mL

I.V. continuous infusion: Dilute to 1 mg/mL; undiluted labetalol injection (5 mg/mL) has been administered to a very small number of adult patients who were extremely fluid restricted

Monitoring Parameters Blood pressure, heart rate, pulse, EKG

Test Interactions False-positive urine catecholamines, VMA if measured by fluorometric or photometric methods; use HPLC or specific catecholamine radioenzymatic technique

Patient Information Limit alcohol; may cause drowsiness, dizziness and impair ability to perform activities requiring mental alertness; do not stop medication abruptly

Nursing Implications Instruct patient regarding compliance; do **not** abruptly withdraw medication in patients with ischemic heart disease; labetalol may mask other signs and symptoms of diabetes mellitus, but sweating can still occur

Dosage Forms

Injection, as hydrochloride: 5 mg/mL (20 mL, 40 mL, 60 mL)

Tablet, as hydrochloride: 100 mg, 200 mg, 300 mg

Extemporaneous Preparations

A 40 mg/mL oral liquid preparation made from tablets and 3 different vehicles (cherry syrup, a 1:1 mixture of Ora-Sweet® and Ora-Plus®, or a 1:1 mixture of Ora-Sweet® SF and Ora-Plus®) was stable for 60 days when stored in amber plastic prescription bottles in the dark at room temperature (25°C) or under refrigeration (5°C); grind sixteen 30 mg tablets in a mortar into a fine powder; add 20 mL of the vehicle and mix well to form a uniform paste; mix while adding the vehicle in geometric proportions to **almost** 120 mL; transfer to a calibrated bottle and qsad with vehicle to make 120 mL; label "shake well" and "protect from light" (Allen, 1996).

Extemporaneously prepared solutions (approximate concentrations 7-10 mg/mL) prepared in distilled water, simple syrup, apple juice, grape juice, and orange juice were stable for 4 weeks when stored in amber glass or plastic prescription bottles at 23°C and 4°C (Nahata, 1991).

Allen LV and Erickson MA, "Stability of Labetalol Hydrochloride, Metoprolol Tartrate, Verapamil Hydrochloride, and Spironolactone With Hydrochlorothiazide in Extemporaneously Compounded Oral Liquids," *Am J Health Syst Pharm*, 1996, 53(19):2304-9.

(Continued)

Labetalol *(Continued)*

Nahata MC, "Stability of Labetolol Hydrochloride in Distilled Water, Simple Syrup, and Three Fruit Juices," *DICP*, 1991, 25(5):465-9.

References

Bunchman TE, Lynch RE, and Wood EG, "Intravenously Administered Labetalol for Treatment of Hypertension in Children," *J Pediatr*, 1992, 120(1):140-4.

Farine M, and Arbus GS, "Management of Hypertensive Emergencies in Children," *Pediatr Emerg Care*, 1989, 5(1):51-5.

Ishisaka DY, Yonan CD, Housel BF, "Labetalol for Treatment of Hypertension in a Child," *Clin Pharm*, 1991, 10(7):500-1 (case report).

Jones SE, "Coarctation in Children. Controlled Hypotension Using Labetalol and Halothane," *Anaesthesia*, 1979, 34(10):1052-5.

Jureidini KF, "Oral Labetalol in a Child With Phaeochromocytoma and Five Children With Renal Hypertension," *N Z Med J*, 1980, 10:479 (abstract).

Mueller JB and Solhaug MJ, "Labetalol in Pediatric Hypertensive Emergencies," *Pediatr Res*, 1988, 23(Pt 2):543A (abstract).

Wesley AG, Hariparsad D, Pather M, et al, "Labetalol in Tetanus. The Treatment of Sympathetic Nervous System Overactivity," *Anaesthesia*, 1983, 38(3):243-9.

♦ **Labetalol Hydrochloride** *see* Labetalol *on page 548*
♦ **Laboratory Detection of Drugs in Urine** *see page 1204*
♦ **Lacri-Lube® SOP [OTC]** *see* Ocular Lubricant *on page 704*
♦ **LactiCare-HC® Topical** *see* Hydrocortisone *on page 486*
♦ **Lactinex® [OTC]** *see* Lactobacillus acidophilus and Lactobacillus bulgaricus *on page 550*

Lactobacillus acidophilus and Lactobacillus bulgaricus

(lak toe ba SIL us as i DOF fil us & lak toe ba SIL us bul GAR i cus)

Brand Names Bacid® [OTC]; Fermalac® (Canada); Kala [OTC]; Lactinex® [OTC]; More-Dophilus® [OTC]; Pro-Bionate® [OTC]; Superdophilus® [OTC]

Therapeutic Category Antidiarrheal

Generic Available No

Use Uncomplicated diarrhea particularly that caused by antibiotic therapy; re-establish normal physiologic and bacterial flora of the intestinal tract

Contraindications Allergy to milk or lactose

Warnings Discontinue if high fever present

Adverse Reactions Gastrointestinal: Intestinal flatus

Stability Store in the refrigerator

Mechanism of Action Creates an environment unfavorable to potentially pathogenic fungi or bacteria through the production of lactic acid, and favors establishment of an aciduric flora, thereby suppressing the growth of pathogenic microorganisms; helps re-establish normal intestinal flora

Pharmacokinetics
Absorption: Not orally absorbed
Distribution: Locally, primarily in the colon
Elimination: In feces

Usual Dosage Children and Adults: Oral:
Capsule: 1-2 capsules 2-4 times/day
Granules: 1 packet added to or taken with cereal, food, milk, fruit juice, or water, 3-4 times/day
Powder: $1/4$-1 teaspoon 1-3 times/day with liquid
Tablet, chewable: 4 tablets 3-4 times/day; may follow each dose with a small amount of milk, fruit juice, or water
Recontamination protocol for BMT unit: 1 packet 3 times/day for 6 doses for those patients who refuse yogurt

Administration Oral: Granules or contents of capsules may be added to or administered with cereal, food, milk, fruit juice, or water

Dosage Forms
Capsule: 50s, 100s
Granules: 1 g/packet (12 packets/box)
Powder: 37.5 g, 52.5 g, 75 g, 90 g, 120 g, 135 g
Tablet: 100s, 250s, 500s
Tablet, chewable: 50s

♦ **Lactoflavin** *see* Riboflavin *on page 844*
♦ **Lactulax (Canada)** *see* Lactulose *on page 550*

Lactulose (LAK tyoo lose)

Related Information

Carbohydrate and Alcohol Content of Liquid Medications for Use in Patients Receiving Ketogenic Diets *on page 1228*

Brand Names Acilac (Canada); Cephulac®; Cholac®; Chronulac®; Comalose-R (Canada); Constilac®; Constulose®; Duphalac®; Enulose®; Evalose®; Gen-Lac (Canada); Heptalac®; Kristalose®; Lactulax (Canada); Lactulose PSE®; Laxilose (Canada); PMS-Lactulose (Canada)

Therapeutic Category Ammonium Detoxicant; Hyperammonemia Agent; Laxative, Miscellaneous

Generic Available Yes

Use Adjunct in the prevention and treatment of portal-systemic encephalopathy (PSE); treatment of chronic constipation

Pregnancy Risk Factor B

Contraindications Patients with galactosemia

Warnings Accumulation of hydrogen gas in intestine could result in an explosion if the patient were to undergo electrocautery procedure

Precautions Use with caution in patients with diabetes mellitus; do not use with other laxatives especially when initiating PSE treatment as increased loose stools may falsely suggest adequate lactulose dosage

Adverse Reactions Gastrointestinal: Flatulence, abdominal discomfort, diarrhea, nausea, vomiting

Drug Interactions Oral antibiotics may interfere with desired degradation of lactulose by eliminating key GI bacteria; nonabsorbable antacids may eliminate desired lactulose-induced decreased GI tract pH

Food Interactions Contraindicated in patients on galactose-restricted diet

Mechanism of Action The bacterial degradation of lactulose resulting in an acidic pH inhibits the diffusion of NH_3 into the blood by causing the conversion of NH_3 to NH_4+; also enhances the diffusion of NH_3 from the blood into the gut where conversion to NH_4+ occurs; produces an osmotic effect in the colon with resultant distention promoting peristalsis and elimination of NH_4+ from the body

Pharmacokinetics

Absorption: Oral: Not absorbed appreciably

Metabolism: By colonic flora to lactic acid and acetic acid

Elimination: Primarily in feces and urine (~3%)

Usual Dosage

Prevention and treatment of portal systemic encephalopathy (PSE): Oral:

Infants: 2.5-10 mL/day divided 3-4 times/day, adjust dosage to produce 2-3 soft stools per day

Children: 40-90 mL/day divided 3-4 times/day, adjust dosage to produce 2-3 soft stools per day

Adults:

Oral:

Acute episodes of PSE: 30-45 mL (20-30 g) at 1- to 2-hour intervals until laxative effect observed, then adjust dosage to produce 2-3 soft stools per day

Chronic therapy: 30-45 mL/dose (20-30 g/dose) 3-4 times/day; titrate dose every 1-2 days to produce 2-3 soft stools per day

Rectal: 300 mL diluted with 700 mL of water or NS, and given via a rectal balloon catheter and retained for 30-60 minutes; may give every 4-6 hours

Constipation: Oral:

Children: 7.5 mL/day (5 g/day) after breakfast

Adults: 15-30 mL/day (10-20 g/day); increase to a maximum of 60 mL/day (40 g/day) if needed

Administration

Oral: Administer with juice, milk, or water; dissolve crystals in 4 ounces of water or juice

Rectal: See Usual Dosage

Monitoring Parameters Serum ammonia, serum potassium, fluid status, stool output

Additional Information Upon discontinuation of therapy, allow 24-48 hours for resumption of normal bowel movements

Dosage Forms

Crystals (Kristalose®): 10 g, 20 g (packets)

Syrup: 10 g/15 mL (15 mL, 30 mL, 237 mL, 473 mL, 946 mL, 1890 mL)

♦ **Lactulose PSE®** *see Lactulose on page 550*

♦ **L-AmB** *see Amphotericin B Liposome on page 77*

♦ **Lamictal®** *see Lamotrigine on page 554*

Lamivudine (la MI vyoo deen)

Related Information
Adult and Adolescent HIV *on page 1133*
Pediatric HIV *on page 1129*

Brand Names Epivir®; Epivir-HBV®; 3TC® (Canada)

Synonyms 2'-Deoxy-3'-Thiacytidine; 3TC

Therapeutic Category Antiretroviral Agent; HIV Agents (Anti-HIV Agents); Nucleoside Reverse Transcriptase Inhibitor (NRTI)

Generic Available No

Use Treatment of HIV infection in combination with other antiretroviral agents. (**Note:** Current preferred HIV regimens consist of **three** antiretroviral agents); chemoprophylaxis after occupational exposure to HIV; management of chronic hepatitis B infection associated with evidence of hepatitis B viral replication and active liver inflammation

Pregnancy Risk Factor C

Contraindications Hypersensitivity to lamivudine or any component

Warnings The major clinical toxicity of lamivudine in pediatric patients is pancreatitis which has occurred in 14% of patients in one open-label, uncontrolled study; discontinue lamivudine therapy if clinical signs, symptoms, or laboratory abnormalities suggestive of pancreatitis occur. Lactic acidosis and severe hepatomegaly with steatosis have been reported with the use of lamivudine. A majority of these cases have been in women. Obesity and prolonged nucleoside exposure may be risk factors. Discontinue lamivudine if clinical or laboratory abnormalities suggestive of lactic acidosis or pronounced hepatotoxicity occur.

Precautions Use with extreme caution and only if there is no satisfactory alternative therapy in pediatric patients with a history of pancreatitis or other significant risk factors for the development of pancreatitis; reduce dosage in patients with impaired renal function; mothers should not breast-feed if they are receiving lamivudine

Adverse Reactions
Central nervous system: Headache (6% to 11%), fatigue, insomnia, psychomotor disorders (11% to 15%)
Dermatologic: Rash, pruritus, urticaria, alopecia
Endocrine & metabolic: Lactic acidosis, hyperglycemia
Gastrointestinal: Nausea, feeding problem (12% to 19%), abdominal discomfort (10% to 12%), pancreatitis (14%), diarrhea, vomiting, anorexia
Hematologic: Neutropenia
Hepatic: Elevated ALT, AST, bilirubin, and amylase; hepatic steatosis
Neuromuscular & skeletal: Paresthesias, peripheral neuropathy, musculoskeletal pain (8% to 11%), gait disorder, myalgia, muscle weakness, rhabdomyolysis, elevated CPK
Respiratory: Cough

Drug Interactions Coadministration with trimethoprim/sulfamethoxazole increases the AUC of lamivudine (significance is unknown); when used with zidovudine, may prevent emergence of zidovudine resistance

Stability Store tablets and oral solution at room temperature in tightly closed bottles

Mechanism of Action A synthetic nucleoside analogue that is converted intracellularly to the active triphosphate metabolite which inhibits reverse transcription via viral DNA chain termination after incorporation of the nucleoside analogue. Lamivudine triphosphate is a weak inhibitor of DNA polymerase alpha- and beta-mitochondrial DNA polymerase.

Pharmacokinetics
Distribution: Into extravascular spaces; CSF concentration ranged from 5.6% to 30.9% of the simultaneous serum concentration
Protein binding: <36%
Metabolism: Converted intracellularly to the active triphosphate form
Bioavailability:
Children 4.8 months to 16 years: 70%
Adolescents and Adults: 82%
Half-life, elimination:
Children 4 months to 14 years: 1.7 hours
Adults with normal renal function: 2.5 hours
Time to peak serum concentration:
Fasting state: 0.9 hours
Fed state: 3.2 hours
Elimination: 70% of dose eliminated unchanged in urine

Usual Dosage Oral:
Neonates <30 days: 2 mg/kg/dose twice daily is being studied in clinical trials

Children: 4 mg/kg/dose twice daily; maximum dose: 150 mg/dose every 12 hours

Adolescents and Adults, body weight <50 kg: 2 mg/kg/dose twice daily

Adolescents (in later puberty: Tanner V) and Adults, body weight ≥50 kg: 150 mg/dose twice daily

Chemoprophylaxis after occupational exposure to HIV: 150 mg/dose twice daily in combination with zidovudine 200 mg 3 times/day and indinavir 800 mg 3 times/day are first-line agents after exposures for which prophylaxis is recommended.

Adolescents ≥16 years and Adults: Chronic hepatitis B infection: 100 mg/dose once daily

Dosing adjustment in renal impairment for HIV: Adults:

Cl$_{cr}$ 30-49 mL/minute: 150 mg once daily

Cl$_{cr}$ 15-29 mL/minute: 150 mg first dose, then 100 mg once daily

Cl$_{cr}$ 5-14 mL/minute: 150 mg first dose, then 50 mg once daily

Cl$_{cr}$ <5 mL/minute: 50 mg first dose, then 25 mg once daily

Dosing adjustment in renal impairment for chronic hepatitis B: Adults:

Cl$_{cr}$ 30-49 mL/minute: 100 mg first dose, then 50 mg once daily

Cl$_{cr}$ 15-29 mL/minute: 100 mg first dose, then 25 mg once daily

Cl$_{cr}$ 5-14 mL/minute: 35 mg first dose, then 15 mg once daily

Cl$_{cr}$ <5 mL/minute: 35 mg first dose, then 10 mg once daily

Dosing adjustment in hepatic impairment: No data

Administration Oral: Administer with or without food

Monitoring Parameters CBC with differential, hemoglobin, ALT, AST, serum amylase, bilirubin, CD4 cell count, HIV RNA plasma levels; signs and symptoms of pancreatitis, lactic acidosis, and pronounced hepatotoxicity

Patient Information Lamivudine is not a cure; notify physician if persistent severe abdominal pain, nausea, vomiting, numbness, or tingling occur; avoid alcohol

Dosage Forms

Solution: 5 mg/mL (240 mL); 10 mg/mL (240 mL)

Tablet: 100 mg, 150 mg

References

CDC and the National Foundation for Infectious Disease, "Update: Provisional Public Health Service Recommendations for Chemoprophylaxis After Occupational Exposure to HIV," *MMWR Morb Mortal Wkly Rep*, 1996, 45(22):468-80.

Eron JJ, Benoit SL, Jemsek J, et al, "Treatment With Lamivudine, Zidovudine, or Both in HIV-Positive Patients With 200 to 500 CD4+ Cells Per Cubic Millimeter," *N Engl J Med*, 1995, 333(25):1662-9.

Lai CL, Chien RN, Leung NW, et al, "A One-Year Trial of Lamivudine for Chronic Hepatitis B," *N Engl J Med*, 1998, 339(2):61-8.

Lewis LL, Mueller B, Schock R, et al, "A Phase I/II Study to Evaluate the Safety, Toxicity, and Preliminary Efficacy of Combinations of Lamivudine (3TC), Zidovudine (AZT) and Didanosine (ddl) in Children With HIV Infection," Natl Conf Hum Retroviruses Relat Infect (2nd), 1995, Jan 29-Feb 2:103.

Lewis LL, Venzon D, Church J, et al, "Lamivudine in Children With Human Immunodeficiency Virus Infection: A Phase I/II Study," *J Infect Dis*, 1996, 174(1):16-25.

Working Group on Antiretroviral Therapy and Medical Management of HIV-Infected Children, "Guidelines for the Use of Antiretroviral Agents in Pediatric HIV Infection," January 7, 2000, http://www.hivatis.org.

Lamivudine and Zidovudine (la MI vyoo deen & zye DOE vyoo deen)

Brand Names Combivir®

Synonyms AZT and 3TC; 3TC and AZT; 3TC and ZDV; Zidovudine and Lamivudine; ZVD and 3TC

Therapeutic Category Antiretroviral Agent; HIV Agents (Anti-HIV Agents); Nucleoside Reverse Transcriptase Inhibitor (NRTI)

Generic Available No

Use Treatment of HIV-1 infection in combination with at least one other antiretroviral agent; **(Note**: HIV regimens consisting of **three** antiretroviral agents are strongly recommended)

Pregnancy Risk Factor C

Contraindications Hypersensitivity to lamivudine, zidovudine, or any component

Warnings This product contains lamivudine and zidovudine as a fixed-dose combination; ordinarily, concomitant use of Combivir® with either lamivudine or zidovudine is not recommended. The major clinical toxicity of lamivudine in pediatric patients is pancreatitis; discontinue therapy if clinical signs, symptoms, or laboratory abnormalities suggestive of pancreatitis occur. Zidovudine is associated with hematologic toxicity including granulocytopenia and severe anemia requiring transfusions; use with caution in patients with ANC <1000 cells/mm^3 or hemoglobin <9.5 g/dL; discontinue treatment in children with an ANC <500 cells/mm^3 until marrow recovery is observed; use of erythropoietin, filgrastim, or reduced zidovudine dosage may be necessary in some patients; prolonged use of zidovudine may cause myositis and myopathy; zidovudine has been shown to be carcinogenic in rats and mice.

(Continued)

Lamivudine and Zidovudine *(Continued)*

Cases of lactic acidosis, severe hepatomegaly with steatosis, and death have been reported with the use of lamivudine, zidovudine and other antiretroviral agents; most of these cases have been in women; prolonged nucleoside use, obesity, and prior liver disease may be risk factors; use with extreme caution in patients with other risk factors for liver disease; discontinue therapy in patients who develop laboratory or clinical evidence of lactic acidosis or pronounced hepatotoxicity.

Precautions Always use Combivir® in combination with another antiretroviral agent; use with extreme caution and only if there is no satisfactory alternative therapy in pediatric patients with a history of pancreatitis or other significant risk factors for pancreatitis; use with caution in patients with bone marrow compromise or in patients with impaired renal or hepatic function. The dose of lamivudine should be reduced in patients with renal dysfunction; the dose of zidovudine should be reduced or therapy interrupted in patients with anemia, granulocytopenia, myopathy, renal or hepatic impairment; use of the fixed-dose combination product (Combivir®) is not recommended for patients who need a dosage reduction (use individual antiretroviral agents to appropriately adjust dosages).

Adverse Reactions See Lamivudine *on page 552* and Zidovudine *on page 990*

Drug Interactions See Lamivudine *on page 552* and Zidovudine *on page 990*

Food Interactions Food does not affect the extent of of absorption

Mechanism of Action See Lamivudine *on page 552* and Zidovudine *on page 990*

Pharmacokinetics One Combivir® tablet is bioequivalent to one lamivudine 150 mg tablet plus one zidovudine 300 mg tablet; see Lamivudine *on page 552* and Zidovudine *on page 990*

Usual Dosage Oral: Adolescents ≥12 years and Adults: One tablet twice daily
Dosage adjustment in renal impairment: Cl_{cr} ≤50 mL/minute: Not recommended (use individual antiretroviral agents to reduce dosage)

Administration Oral: May be administered without regard to meals

Monitoring Parameters CBC with differential, hemoglobin, MCV, reticulocyte count, liver enzymes, serum amylase, bilirubin, CD4 cell count, HIV RNA plasma levels, renal and hepatic function tests; signs and symptoms of pancreatitis, lactic acidosis, pronounced hepatotoxicity, anemia, and bone marrow suppression

Patient Information Avoid alcohol; Combivir® is not a cure; notify physician if persistent severe abdominal pain, nausea, or vomiting occurs; take Combivir® every day as prescribed; do not change dose or discontinue without physician's advice. If a dose is missed, take it as soon as possible, then return to normal dosing schedule; if a dose is skipped, do **not** double the next dose

Dosage Forms Tablet: Lamivudine 150 mg and zidovudine 300 mg

Lamotrigine *(la MOE tri jeen)*

Related Information

Antiepileptic Drugs *on page 1176*
Carbohydrate and Alcohol Content of Liquid Medications for Use in Patients Receiving Ketogenic Diets *on page 1228*

Brand Names Lamictal®

Synonyms BW-430C; LTG

Therapeutic Category Anticonvulsant, Miscellaneous

Generic Available No

Use Adjunctive treatment of partial seizures in adults (with or without secondary generalized seizures) and generalized seizures of Lennox-Gastaut syndrome in pediatric and adult patients; monotherapy of partial seizures in adults who are converted from a single enzyme-inducing AED

Note: Preliminary investigations have shown potential efficacy as add-on therapy for absence, atypical absence, generalized tonic-clonic, atonic, tonic, and myoclonic seizures; and as monotherapy in adults and adolescents for partial seizures and idiopathic generalized tonic-clonic seizures; additional studies are underway

Pregnancy Risk Factor C

Contraindications Hypersensitivity to lamotrigine or any component

Warnings Skin rash may occur (10%) and can be serious enough to require hospitalization or discontinuation of drug; rash usually appears in the first 4-8 weeks of therapy; a higher incidence is seen in children and in patients receiving valproic acid, high initial doses, or with rapid dosage increases; Stevens-Johnson syndrome has been reported. **Note:** Benign rashes may occur, but one cannot predict which rashes will become serious or life-threatening; the manufacturer recommends (ordinarily) discontinuation of lamotrigine at the first sign of rash (unless rash is clearly not drug related); discontinuation of lamotrigine may not prevent rash from becoming life-threatening or permanently disfiguring or disabling

Precautions Use with caution and decrease the dose in patients with renal or moderate to severe hepatic dysfunction; do not abruptly discontinue; when discontinuing therapy, gradually reduce the dose by ~50% per week and taper over at least 2 weeks unless safety concerns require a more rapid withdrawal. Long-term ophthalmologic effects are unknown; lamotrigine binds to melanin and may possibly accumulate in the eye and other tissues rich in melanin

Adverse Reactions

Central nervous system: Dizziness, sedation, headache, agitation, ataxia, fever; exacerbation of seizures has been reported

Dermatologic: Rash (especially in children, with valproic acid, with high initial doses, or with rapid dosage increases), angioedema, Stevens-Johnson syndrome, photosensitivity

Gastrointestinal: Nausea, vomiting

Ocular: Diplopia, amblyopia, nystagmus

Drug Interactions Acetaminophen may increase the clearance of lamotrigine; when administered at the same time, carbamazepine may increase adverse effects such as dizziness, diplopia, ataxia (space administration of drugs by at least 1 hour); valproic acid may increase incidence of rash and increases half-life and serum concentrations of lamotrigine; enzyme-inducing drugs (eg, carbamazepine, phenytoin) decrease lamotrigine's half-life by ~50%; lamotrigine may increase the clearance of valproic acid

Food Interactions Absorption is not affected by food

Stability Store at room temperature in a dry place away from heat and light

Mechanism of Action A triazine derivative which affects voltage-sensitive sodium channels and inhibits presynaptic release of glutamate and aspartate (excitatory amino acid CNS neurotransmitters)

Pharmacokinetics

Absorption: Oral: Rapid, 97.6% absorbed

Distribution: V_d: Adults: 1.1 L/kg; range: 0.9-1.3 L/kg; crosses into breast milk

Protein binding: 55% (primarily albumin)

Metabolism: >75% metabolized in the liver via glucuronidation; autoinduction may occur

Bioavailability: 98%

Half-life:

Children:

With enzyme-inducing AEDs (eg, phenytoin, carbamazepine): ~7-10 hours

With enzyme inducer and valproic acid (VPA): ~15-27 hours

With VPA: ~44-94 hours

Adults:

Normal: Single dose: 33 hours; multiple dose: ~25 hours

With enzyme-inducing AEDs: ~13-14 hours (range: 8-33 hours)

With enzyme inducer and VPA: ~27 hours

With VPA: 59 hours (range: 30-89 hours)

Hepatic dysfunction: Child-Pugh classification:

Grade A: 36 hours

Grade B: 60 hours

Grade C: 110 hours

Renal dysfunction (Cl_{cr} 13 mL/minute): ~43 hours

Severe renal dysfunction (Cl_{cr} <10 mL/minute): 57.4 hours

During dialysis: 13 hours

Time to peak serum concentration: Oral: ~2 hours (range: 1.4-4.8 hours); select patients may have second peak at 4-6 hours due to enterohepatic recirculation

Elimination: 75% to 90% excreted as glucuronide metabolites and 10% as unchanged drug

Dialysis: ~20% is removed during 4-hour hemodialysis period

Usual Dosage Note: Dosage depends on patient's concomitant medications, ie, valproic acid and enzyme-inducing AEDs (such as phenytoin, phenobarbital, carbamazepine, and primidone) (see Additional Information)

Adjunctive (add-on) therapy:

Children <17 kg: Not recommended; therapy cannot be initiated using the dosing guidelines (smallest available strength is 5 mg chewable, dispersible tablet)

Children 2-12 years: **Note:** Children 2-6 years will likely require maintenance doses at the higher end of recommended range

(Continued)

Lamotrigine *(Continued)*

Patients receiving AED regimens containing valproic acid:
Weeks 1 and 2: 0.15 mg/kg/day in 1-2 divided doses; round dose down to the nearest 5 mg; use 5 mg every other day if the initial calculated dose is 2.5-5 mg
Weeks 3 and 4: 0.3 mg/kg/day in 1-2 divided doses; round dose down to the nearest 5 mg
Maintenance dose: Titrate dose to effect; after week 4, increase dose every 1-2 weeks by a calculated increment; calculate increment as 0.3 mg/kg/day rounded down to the nearest 5 mg; add this amount to the previously administered daily dose; usual maintenance: 1-5 mg/kg/day in 1-2 divided doses; maximum: 200 mg/day

Patients receiving **enzyme-inducing** AED regimens **without** valproic acid:
Weeks 1 and 2: 0.6 mg/kg/day in 2 divided doses; round dose down to the nearest 5 mg
Weeks 3 and 4: 1.2 mg/kg/day in 2 divided doses; round dose down to the nearest 5 mg
Maintenance dose: Titrate dose to effect; after week 4, increase dose every 1-2 weeks by a calculated increment; calculate increment as 1.2 mg/kg/day rounded down to the nearest 5 mg; add this amount to the previously administered daily dose; usual maintenance: 5-15 mg/kg/day in 2 divided doses; maximum: 400 mg/day

Children >12 years and Adults:
Patients receiving AED regimens containing valproic acid:
Weeks 1 and 2: 25 mg every other day
Weeks 3 and 4: 25 mg every day
Maintenance dose: Titrate dose to effect; after week 4, increase dose every 1-2 weeks by 25-50 mg/day; usual maintenance: 100-400 mg/day in 1-2 divided doses; usual maintenance in patients adding lamotrigine to valproic acid **alone**: 100-200 mg/day

Patients receiving **enzyme-inducing** AED regimens **without** valproic acid:
Weeks 1 and 2: 50 mg/day
Weeks 3 and 4: 100 mg/day in 2 divided doses
Maintenance dose: Titrate dose to effect; after week 4, increase dose every 1-2 weeks by 100 mg/day; usual maintenance: 300-500 mg/day in 2 divided doses; doses as high as 700 mg/day in 2 divided doses have been used

Conversion from single enzyme-inducing AED to lamotrigine monotherapy: **Note:** First add lamotrigine and titrate it to the recommended maintenance monotherapy dose, while maintaining the enzyme-inducing AED at a fixed level; then gradually withdraw the enzyme-inducing AED over a 4-week period
Children ≥16 years and Adults:
Weeks 1 and 2: 50 mg/day
Weeks 3 and 4: 100 mg/day in 2 divided doses
Maintenance dose: After week 4, increase dose every 1-2 weeks by 100 mg/day; recommended maintenance monotherapy dose: 500 mg/day in 2 divided doses

Dosage adjustment in hepatic impairment:
Moderate impairment, Child-Pugh Grade B: Reduce initial, escalation, and maintenance doses by ~50%
Severe impairment, Child-Pugh Grade C: Reduce initial, escalation, and maintenance doses by ~75%
Note: Adjust escalation and maintenance doses by clinical response

Administration Oral: May be administered without regard to food
Regular tablet: Do not chew, as a bitter taste may result
Chewable, dispersible tablet: Only whole tablets should be administered; may swallow whole, chew, or disperse in water or diluted fruit juice; if chewed, administer a small amount of water or diluted fruit juice to help in swallowing. To disperse, add tablets to a small amount of liquid (~1 teaspoon or enough to cover the medication); when the tablets are completely dispersed (in about 1 minute), swirl the solution and administer the entire amount immediately. Do not attempt to administer partial quantities of dispersed tablets.

Monitoring Parameters Seizure frequency, duration, and severity
Reference Range Clinical value of serum concentrations not well established; proposed therapeutic range: 1-5 µg/mL
Patient Information Report any rash, fever, or swelling of glands to the physician immediately

Additional Information Low water solubility. Does **not** induce P-450 microsomal enzymes. The effect of AEDs (other than enzyme-inducing AEDs and valproic acid) on the metabolism of lamotrigine cannot be predicted and no specific dosing guidelines are recommended. Prudence dictates conservative initial doses and titration (as with regimens containing valproic acid); expected maintenance dosing would fall between maintenance doses with valproic acid and maintenance doses of enzyme-inducing AED regimens without valproic acid.

Dosage Forms
Tablet: 25 mg, 100 mg, 150 mg, 200 mg
Tablet, chewable, dispersible: 5 mg, 25 mg

Extemporaneous Preparations A 1 mg/mL oral suspension made from tablets and 2 different vehicles (a 1:1 mixture of Ora-Sweet® and Ora-Plus®, or a 1:1 mixture of Ora-Sweet® SF and Ora-Plus®) was stable for 91 days when stored in amber plastic prescription bottles at room temperature (25°C) or under refrigeration (4°C); grind one 100 mg tablet in a mortar into a fine powder; add a small amount of the vehicle and mix well to form a uniform paste; mix while adding the vehicle in geometric proportions to **almost** 100 mL; transfer the mixture to a graduated cylinder and qsad with vehicle to make 100 mL; label "shake well" and "protect from light" (Nahata, 1999)

Nahata MC, Morosco RS, and Hipple TF, "Stability of Lamotrigine in Two Extemporaneously Prepared Oral Suspensions at 4°C and 25°C," *Am J Health Syst Pharm*, 1999, 56(3):240-2.

References
Battino D, Estienne M, and Avanzini G, "Clinical Pharmacokinetics of Antiepileptic Drugs in Paediatric Patients: Part II. Phenytoin, Carbamazepine, Sulthiame, Lamotrigine, Vigabatrin, Oxcarbazepine, and Felbamate," *Clin Pharmacokinet*, 1995, 29(5):341-69.
Besag FM, Wallace SJ, Dulac O, et al, "Lamotrigine for the Treatment of Epilepsy in Childhood," *J Pediatr*, 1995, 127(6):991-7.
Burstein AH, "Lamotrigine," *Pharmacotherapy*, 1995, 15(2):129-43.
Dooley J, Camfield P, Gordon K, et al, "Lamotrigine-Induced Rash in Children," *Neurology*, 1996, 46(1):240-2.
Fitton A, and Goa KL, "Lamotrigine: An Update of its Pharmacology and Therapeutic Use in Epilepsy," *Drugs*, 1995, 50(4):691-713.
Messenheimer JA, "Lamotrigine," *Epilepsia*, 1995, 36(Suppl 2):S87-94.
Messenheimer JA, Giorgi L, and Risner ME, "The Tolerability of Lamotrigine in Children," *Drug Saf*, 2000, 22(4):303-12.
Nahata MC, Morosco RS, and Hipple RT, "Stability of Lamotrigine in Two Extemporaneously Prepared Oral Suspensions at 4°C and 25°C," *Am J Health Syst Pharm*, 1999, 56(93):240-2.

♦ **Lamprene®** see Clofazimine on page 239
♦ **Lanacane® [OTC]** see Benzocaine on page 124
♦ **Lanacort® Topical [OTC]** see Hydrocortisone on page 486
♦ **Laniazid® Oral** see Isoniazid on page 534
♦ **Lanophyllin®** see Theophylline on page 910
♦ **Lanoxicaps®** see Digoxin on page 318
♦ **Lanoxin®** see Digoxin on page 318

Lansoprazole (lan SOE pra zole)

Brand Names Prevacid®
Therapeutic Category Gastric Acid Secretion Inhibitor; Gastrointestinal Agent; Gastric or Duodenal Ulcer Treatment; Proton Pump Inhibitor
Generic Available No
Use Short-term treatment (up to 4 weeks) for healing and symptomatic relief of active duodenal ulcer; short-term treatment (up to 8 weeks) for healing and symptomatic relief of all grades of erosive esophagitis; maintenance of healed erosive esophagitis; pathological hypersecretory conditions, including Zollinger-Ellison syndrome; adjuvant therapy in the treatment of *Helicobacter pylori*-associated antral gastritis; short-term treatment of symptomatic gastroesophageal reflux disease (GERD)
Pregnancy Risk Factor B
Contraindications Hypersensitivity to lansoprazole or any component
Warnings Long-term effects are not known; enterochromaffin (ECF)-like hyperplasia and subsequent carcinoids have developed in rats following lifetime exposure to high doses (150 mg/kg/day)
Precautions Symptomatic response to therapy does not preclude the presence of gastric malignancy; use with caution in patients with liver disease, dosage reduction should be considered
Adverse Reactions
Cardiovascular: Angina, hypertension, hypotension, palpitations
Central nervous system: Fatigue, dizziness, headache
Dermatologic: Rash
(Continued)

Lansoprazole *(Continued)*

Gastrointestinal: Abdominal pain, nausea, melena, anorexia, cholelithiasis, xerostomia, dyspepsia, eructation, discoloration of feces, flatulence, hypergastrinemia, increased appetite, diarrhea

Hepatic: Increased serum transaminases

Otic: Tinnitus

Renal: Proteinuria

Drug Interactions Due to profound and long-lasting inhibition of gastric acid secretion, potential for interfering with the absorption of drugs where acid pH is important exists (such as ketoconazole, ampicillin, iron salts, and digoxin); sucralfate delays and decreases lansoprazole absorption by 30%; lansoprazole increases theophylline clearance mildly (~10%)

Food Interactions Food decreases lansoprazole's bioavailability by 50%

Stability Lansoprazole is unstable in acidic media (eg, stomach contents) and is, therefore, administered as enteric coated granules in capsule form

Mechanism of Action Suppresses gastric acid secretion by selectively inhibiting the parietal cell membrane enzyme (H+, K+)-ATPase or proton pump; demonstrates antimicrobial activity against *Helicobacter pylori*

Pharmacodynamics

Duration of antisecretory activity: >24 hours

Relief of symptoms:

Gastric or duodenal ulcers: 1 week

Reflux esophagitis: 1-4 weeks

Ulcer healing:

Duodenal: 2 weeks

Gastric: 4 weeks

Pharmacokinetics

Absorption: Extremely acid labile and will degrade in acid pH of stomach; enteric coated granules improve bioavailability (80%)

Protein binding: 97%

Metabolism: Extensive by the liver to inactive metabolites; in acid media of gastric parietal cell, lansoprazole is transformed to active sulfanilamide metabolite

Half-life: Plasma: 1.3-1.7 hours

Time to peak serum concentration: 1.7 hours

Elimination: 14% to 25% in urine as metabolites; <1% as unchanged drug; biliary excretion is major route of elimination

Usual Dosage Oral:

Children: Limited data in single dose studies in children 3 months to 14 years; dosing range used: 0.5-1.6 mg/kg:

<10 kg: 7.5 mg

10-20 kg: 15 mg

≥20 kg: 30 mg

Children ≥12 years and Adults:

Duodenal ulcer: 15 mg once daily for 4 weeks; maintenance therapy: 15 mg once daily

Gastric ulcer: 30 mg once daily for up to 8 weeks

Erosive esophagitis: 30 mg once daily for up to 8 weeks; additional 8 weeks may be tried in those patients who failed to respond or for a recurrence of esophagitis; maintenance: 15 mg once daily

GERD: 15 mg once daily for up to 8 weeks

Pathological hypersecretory conditions: Initial: 60 mg daily; adjust dosage based upon patient response; doses of 90 mg twice daily have been used; administer doses >120 mg/day in divided doses

Reflux esophagitis: 30-60 mg daily for 8 weeks

Helicobacter pylori-associated antral gastritis: 30 mg twice daily for 2 weeks (in combination with 1 g amoxicillin and 500 mg clarithromycin given twice daily for 14 days). Alternatively, in patients allergic to or intolerant of clarithromycin or in whom resistance to clarithromycin is known or suspected, lansoprazole 30 mg every 8 hours and amoxicillin 1 g every 8 hours may be given for 2 weeks

Administration Oral: Administer before eating; capsules may be opened and mixed with small amount of applesauce prior to administration without affecting the bioavailability; do not chew granules; for nasogastric tube administration, the capsules can be opened, the granules mixed (not crushed) with 40 mL of apple, cranberry, grape, orange, pineapple, prune, tomato, and V-8® vegetable juice, and then injected through the NG tube into the stomach; granules remain intact when mixed and stored for up to 30 minutes

Monitoring Parameters Patients with Zollinger-Ellison syndrome should be monitored for gastric acid output, which should be maintained at 10 mEq/hour or less during the last hour before the next lansoprazole dose; lab monitoring should include CBC, liver function, renal function, and serum gastrin levels

Reference Range Plasma levels do not correlate with pharmacologic activity

Dosage Forms Capsule, delayed release: 15 mg, 30 mg

Extemporaneous Preparations A 3 mg/mL suspension of lansoprazole is prepared by emptying the contents of ten 30 mg capsules and adding 100 mL 8.4% sodium bicarbonate solution; stir for 30 minutes; protect from light; stable for 8 hours at room temperature and for 14 days refrigerated (DiGiacinto, 2000). **Note:** The same formulation was studied by Phillips, et al. A 2-week stability at room temperature and 4-week stability under refrigeration were reported.

DiGiacinto JL, Olsen KM, Bergman KL, et al, "Stability of Suspension Formulations of Lansoprazole and Omeprazole Stored in Amber-Colored Plastic Oral Syringes," *Ann Pharmacother*, 2000, 34(5):600-4.

Phillips JO, Metzler MH, and Olsen K, "The Stability of Simplified Lansoprazole Suspension (SLS)," *Gastroen*, 1999, 116:A89.

References
Chun AH, Eason CJ, Shi HH, et al, "Lansoprazole: An Alternative Method of Administration of a Capsule Dosage Formulation," *Clin Ther*, 1995, 17(3):441-7.

Oderda G, Chiorboli E, Haitink AR, "Inhibition of Hastric ACidity in Children by Lansoprazole Granules," *Gastroent*, 1998, 114(4pt2):A295.

Tran X, et al, "Pharmacokinetics/Pharmacodynamics Study of Oral Lansoprazole in Children," *Fundam Clin Pharmacol*, 1996, 10:A221.

- **Lansoyl® [also sugar-free] (Canada)** *see* Mineral Oil *on page 649*
- **Lantus®** *see* Insulin Preparations *on page 518*
- **Lanvis® (Canada)** *see* Thioguanine *on page 918*
- **Largactil® (Canada)** *see* Chlorpromazine *on page 215*
- **Larodopa®** *see* Levodopa *on page 565*
- **Lasix® Injection** *see* Furosemide *on page 447*
- **Lasix® Oral** *see* Furosemide *on page 447*
- **Lasix® Special (Canada)** *see* Furosemide *on page 447*
- **Lassar's Zinc Paste** *see* Zinc Oxide *on page 993*
- **Lavacol® [OTC]** *see* Ethyl Alcohol *on page 394*
- **Laxilose (Canada)** *see* Lactulose *on page 550*
- **LazerSporin-C® Otic** *see* Neomycin, (Bacitracin) Polymyxin B, and Hydrocortisone *on page 679*
- **L-Bunolol** *see* Levobunolol *on page 564*
- **L-carnitine** *see* Carnitine *on page 173*
- **LCD** *see* Coal Tar *on page 247*
- **LCR** *see* Vincristine *on page 979*
- **L-Dopa** *see* Levodopa *on page 565*
- **Ledercillin® VK** *see* Penicillin V Potassium *on page 743*
- **Legatrin® [OTC]** *see* Quinine *on page 832*
- **Lenoltec® No.1, 2, 3, 4 (Canada)** *see* Acetaminophen and Codeine *on page 27*
- **Lente®** *see* Insulin Preparations *on page 518*
- **Lente® Iletin® I** *see* Insulin Preparations *on page 518*
- **Lente® Iletin® II** *see* Insulin Preparations *on page 518*

Leucovorin (loo koe VOR in)

Brand Names Wellcovorin®

Available Salts Calcium Leucovorin; Leucovorin Calcium

Synonyms Citrovorum Factor; Folinic Acid; 5-Formyl Tetrahydrofolate

Therapeutic Category Antidote, Methotrexate; Folic Acid Derivative

Generic Available Yes

Use Diminish toxicity and counteract the effects of impaired methotrexate elimination and of inadvertent overdosages of folic acid antagonists; treatment of folate deficient megaloblastic anemias of infancy, sprue, pregnancy; nutritional deficiency when oral folate therapy is not possible; adjunctive treatment with sulfadiazine and pyrimethamine to prevent hematologic toxicity

Pregnancy Risk Factor C

Contraindications Pernicious anemia and other megaloblastic anemias secondary to the lack of vitamin B_{12}

Warnings Administer promptly; when the time interval between administration of folic acid antagonists and leucovorin rescue increases, its effectiveness in treatment of toxicity diminishes

(Continued)

Leucovorin (Continued)

Adverse Reactions
Dermatologic: Rash, pruritus, erythema, urticaria
Hematologic: Thrombocytosis
Respiratory: Wheezing
Miscellaneous: Anaphylactoid reactions

Drug Interactions Leucovorin enhances the toxicity of fluorouracil; high doses of leucovorin may reduce the efficacy of intrathecally administered methotrexate

Stability When powder for injection is reconstituted with bacteriostatic water for injection, stability is 7 days at room temperature; protect from light; when doses >10 mg/m^2 are used, prepare leucovorin with preservative free sterile water to decrease the amount of benzyl alcohol intake; do not mix in the same solution with 5-fluorouracil as precipitation occurs

Mechanism of Action A derivative of tetrahydrofolic acid, a reduced form of folic acid; does not require a reduction by dihydrofolate reductase for activation; allows for purine and thymidine synthesis, a necessity for normal erythropoiesis; leucovorin supplies the necessary cofactor blocked by methotrexate, enters the cells via the same active transport system as methotrexate

Pharmacodynamics Onset of action:
Oral: Within 30 minutes
I.V.: Within 5 minutes

Pharmacokinetics
Absorption: Oral, I.M.: Rapid
Metabolism: Rapidly converted to (5MTHF) 5-methyl-tetrahydrofolate (active) in the intestinal mucosa and by the liver
Bioavailability:
Oral absorption is saturable in doses >25 mg; apparent bioavailability:
Tablet, 25 mg: 97%
Tablet, 50 mg: 75%
Tablet, 100 mg: 37%
Injection solution, when administered orally, provides equivalent bioavailability
Half-life:
Leucovorin: 15 minutes
5MTHF: 33-35 minutes
Elimination: Primarily in urine (80% to 90%) with small losses appearing in feces (5% to 8%)

Usual Dosage Children and Adults:
Treatment of folic acid antagonist overdosage (eg, pyrimethamine, trimethoprim): Oral: 2-15 mg/day for 3 days or until blood counts are normal or 5 mg every 3 days; doses of 6 mg/day are needed for patients with platelet counts <100,000/mm^3
Folate deficient megaloblastic anemia: I.M.: 1 mg/day
Megaloblastic anemia secondary to congenital deficiency of dihydrofolate reductase: I.M.: 3-6 mg/day
Rescue dose: I.V.: 10 mg/m^2 to start, then 10 mg/m^2 every 6 hours orally for 72 hours; if serum creatinine 24 hours after methotrexate is elevated ≥50% **or** the serum methotrexate concentration is >5 x 10^{-6} M (see graph), increase dose to 100 mg/m^2/dose every 3 hours until serum methotrexate level is less than 1 x 10^{-8} M
Adjunctive treatment with sulfadiazine to prevent hematologic toxicity (for toxoplasmosis): Infants, Children, and Adults: Oral, I.V.: 5-10 mg every 3 days (see Sulfadiazine *on page 889*)
Adjunctive treatment with pyrimethamine to prevent hematologic toxicity (*Pneumocystis carinii*): Adolescents and Adults: Oral, I.V.: 25 mg once weekly
Investigational: Post I.T. methotrexate: Oral, I.V.: 12 mg/m^2 as a single dose; post high-dose methotrexate: 100-1000 mg/m^2/dose until the serum methotrexate level is less than 1 x 10^{-7} molar

Administration
Oral: **This drug should be given parenterally instead of orally in patients with GI toxicity, nausea, vomiting, and when individual doses are >25 mg.**
Parenteral: Reconstitute 50 mg or 100 mg powder for injection vials with 5-10 mL sterile water (350 mg vial requires 17 mL diluent resulting in 20 mg/mL final concentration); infuse at a maximum rate of 160 mg/minute.

Monitoring Parameters CBC with differential; plasma methotrexate concentration as a therapeutic guide to high-dose methotrexate therapy with leucovorin factor rescue. Leucovorin is continued until the plasma methotrexate level is less than 1 x 10^{-7} molar. Each dose of leucovorin is increased if the plasma methotrexate concentration is excessively high (see graph). With 4- to 6-hour high-dose methotrexate infusions, plasma drug values in excess of 5 x 10^{-5} and 10^{-6} molar at 24 and 48 hours after starting the infusion, respectively, are often predictive of delayed methotrexate clearance; see graph.

LEUCOVORIN RESCUE DOSE
(Determined by Plasma Methotrexate Level and Time After Start of Methotrexate Infusion)

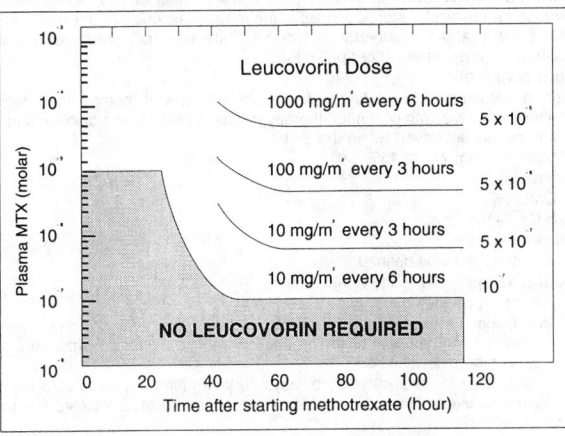

Dosage Forms
Injection, as calcium: 3 mg/mL (1 mL); 10 mg/mL (30 mL, 50 mL)
Powder for injection, as calcium: 50 mg, 100 mg, 200 mg, 350 mg
Tablet, as calcium: 5 mg, 15 mg, 25 mg

♦ **Leucovorin Calcium** see Leucovorin on page 559
♦ **Leukeran®** see Chlorambucil on page 206
♦ **Leukine™** see Sargramostim on page 858

Leuprolide (loo PROE lide)
Brand Names Lupron®; Lupron Depot®; Lupron Depot-3® Month; Lupron Depot-4® Month; Lupron Depot-Ped™
Available Salts Leuprolide Acetate
Synonyms Leuprorelin
Therapeutic Category Antineoplastic Agent, Hormone (Gonadotropin Hormone-Releasing Antigen); Luteinizing Hormone-Releasing Hormone Analog
Generic Available No
Use Treatment of precocious puberty; palliative treatment of advanced prostate carcinoma
Pregnancy Risk Factor X
Contraindications Pernicious anemia; hypersensitivity to leuprolide or any component; pregnancy
Warnings The FDA currently recommends that procedures for proper handling and disposal of antineoplastic agents be considered; gonadotropin-releasing hormone (GnRH) analog treatment of rodents has shown an increased incidence of pituitary tumors; urinary tract obstruction may occur upon initiation of therapy
Precautions Use with caution in patients with hypersensitivity to benzyl alcohol; long-term safety of leuprolide in children has not been established
Adverse Reactions
Cardiovascular: Edema, cardiac arrhythmias
Central nervous system: Dizziness, lethargy, insomnia, headache, pain
Dermatologic: Rash
Endocrine & metabolic: Estrogenic effects (gynecomastia, breast tenderness), hot flashes
Gastrointestinal: Nausea, vomiting, diarrhea, GI bleeding, constipation, anorexia
Hematologic: Decreased hemoglobin and hematocrit
Neuromuscular & skeletal: Myalgia, paresthesia, bone pain, weakness
Ocular: Blurred vision
Miscellaneous: Diaphoresis
(Continued)

Leuprolide *(Continued)*

Stability Refrigerate leuprolide acetate injection; leuprolide (Depot®) powder for suspension and its diluent may be stored at room temperature; upon reconstitution, the suspension is stable for 24 hours; protect from light and heat; do not freeze vials

Mechanism of Action Continuous daily administration results in suppression of ovarian and testicular steroidogenesis due to decreased levels of LH and FSH so that puberty and the pubertal growth spurt are arrested; produces a "medical castration" in prostate cancer patients

Pharmacokinetics

Serum testosterone levels first increase within 3 days of therapy, then decrease after 2-4 weeks with continued therapy; requires parenteral administration since it is rapidly destroyed within the GI tract

Protein binding: 7% to 15%

Bioavailability:

Oral: 0%

S.C.: 94%

Half-life: 3 hours

Elimination: Not well defined

Usual Dosage Refer to individual protocol

Children: Precocious puberty:

I.M. (Depot®) formulation: 0.15-0.3 mg/kg/dose given every 28 days; minimum dose: 7.5 mg; younger children generally require higher dosages on a mg/kg basis than older children

Initial dose for girls <8 years or boys <9 years (titrate dose in 3.75 mg increments every 4 weeks until clinical or laboratory tests indicate no disease progression):

<25 kg: 7.5 mg every 4 weeks

25-37.5 kg: 11.25 mg every 4 weeks

>37.5 kg: 15 mg every 4 weeks

S.C.: 35-50 mcg/kg once daily

Adults: Advanced prostatic carcinoma:

I.M. (Depot® formulation): 7.5 mg/dose given monthly **or** 22.5 mg once every 3 months

S.C.: 1 mg/day

Administration

Parenteral: Do not administer I.V.:

I.M.: For the Depot® formulation, diluent is added to the vial to form a milky suspension

Subcutaneous: 5 mg/mL solution is administered undiluted into areas on the arm, thigh, or abdomen

Monitoring Parameters Precocious puberty: Height, weight, bone age, Tanner staging test, GnRH testing (blood LH and FSH levels), testosterone in males and estradiol in females; closely monitor patients with prostatic carcinoma for plasma testosterone, acid phosphatase, and signs of weakness, paresthesias, and urinary tract obstruction during the first few weeks of therapy

Patient Information Female patients should be informed that menstruation or spotting may occur for the first 2 months of therapy; notify physician if vaginal bleeding continues after 2 months of drug therapy

Nursing Implications Rotate S.C. and I.M. injection sites periodically

Dosage Forms

Injection, as acetate: 5 mg/mL (2.8 mL)

Powder for injection (depot), as acetate:

Depot®: 3.75 mg, 7.5 mg

Depot-3® Month: 11.25 mg, 22.5 mg

Depot-4® Month: 30 mg

Depot-Ped™: 7.5 mg, 11.25 mg, 15 mg

References

Kappy MS, Stuart T, and Perelman A, "Efficacy of Leuprolide Therapy in Children With Central Precocious Puberty," *Am J Dis Child*, 1988, 142(10):1061-4.

Lee PA and Page JG, "Effects of Leuprolide in the Treatment of Central Precocious Puberty," *J Pediatr*, 1989, 114(2):321-4.

♦ **Leuprolide Acetate** *see* Leuprolide *on page 561*

♦ **Leuprorelin** *see* Leuprolide *on page 561*

♦ **Leurocristine** *see* Vincristine *on page 979*

♦ **Leustatin™** *see* Cladribine *on page 232*

Levalbuterol (leve al BYOO ter ole)

Brand Names Xopenex™

Available Salts Levalbuterol Hydrochloride

Synonyms Levosalbutamol; R-albuterol; R-salbutamol

Therapeutic Category Adrenergic Agonist Agent; Antiasthmatic; Beta$_2$-Adrenergic Agonist Agent; Bronchodilator; Sympathomimetic

Generic Available No

Use Treatment and prevention of bronchospasm in patients with reversible obstructive airway disease

Pregnancy Risk Factor C

Contraindications Hypersensitivity to levalbuterol, any component, albuterol, or adrenergic amine

Warnings Paradoxical bronchospasm may occur, especially with the first use

Precautions Use with caution in patients with hyperthyroidism, hypokalemia, diabetes mellitus, cardiovascular disorders including coronary insufficiency, hypertension, or history of arrhythmias; excessive or prolonged use can lead to tolerance

Adverse Reactions

Cardiovascular: Tachycardia, hypertension, hypotension, syncope, EKG abnormalities, chest pain

Central nervous system: Nervousness, dizziness, anxiety, headache, insomnia

Endocrine & metabolic: Hyperglycemia, hypokalemia

Gastrointestinal: Dyspepsia, diarrhea, xerostomia, dry throat, gastroenteritis, nausea

Neuromuscular & skeletal: Leg cramps, pain, tremor

Ocular: Eye itching

Respiratory: Cough, rhinitis, sinusitis, turbinate edema, paradoxical bronchospasm

Miscellaneous: Hypersensitivity reactions, flu-like syndrome

Drug Interactions Action of levalbuterol is antagonized by beta-adrenergic blocking agents such as propranolol; cardiovascular effects are potentiated in patients also receiving MAO inhibitors or tricyclic antidepressants; concomitant administration of sympathomimetics may result in enhanced cardiovascular effects

Food Interactions Caffeinated beverages may increase side effects of levalbuterol

Stability Store at room temperature; protect from light; after the foil covering is removed, use within 2 weeks; discard vial if solution is not colorless

Mechanism of Action R-enantiomer of racemic albuterol; relaxes bronchial smooth muscle by action on beta$_2$-receptors with little effect on heart rate

Pharmacodynamics

Onset of action: 10-17 minutes

Peak effect: 1.5 hours

Duration of action: 5-6 hours

Pharmacokinetics Nebulization:

Distribution: V_d: Adults: 1900 L

Metabolism: In the liver to an inactive sulfate

Half-life: 3.3-4.0 hours

Time to peak serum concentration: 0.2-1.8 hours

Elimination: 3% to 6% excreted unchanged in urine

Usual Dosage Inhalation by nebulization (**dosage expressed in terms of mg levalbuterol**):

Children 2-11 years: Limited data; in a randomized, double-blind, single dose, crossover study (Gawchik et al), doses ranging from 0.16-1.25 mg were used safely with clinically significant improvements in pulmonary function tests

Children ≥12 years and Adults: 0.63 mg 3 times/day, every 6-8 hours; may be increased to 1.25 mg 3 times/day

Administration Inhalation: By nebulization only; no dilution required

Monitoring Parameters Serum potassium, heart rate, asthma symptoms, pulmonary function tests, respiratory rate; arterial or capillary blood gases (if patient's condition warrants)

Patient Information Do not exceed recommended dosage; rinse mouth with water following each inhalation to help with dry throat and mouth; if more than one inhalation is necessary, wait at least 1 full minute between inhalations; notify physician if palpitations, tachycardia, chest pain, muscle tremors, dizziness, or headache occur, or if breathing difficulty persists; limit caffeinated beverages

Additional Information 0.63 mg levalbuterol comparable to 2.5 mg albuterol

Dosage Forms Solution, for inhalation: 0.63 mg (0.73 mg levalbuterol hydrochloride) (3 mL); 1.25 mg (1.44 mg levalbuterol hydrochloride) (3 mL)

(Continued)

Levalbuterol *(Continued)*

References
Gawchik SM, Saccar CL, Noonan M, et al, "The Safety and Efficacy of Nebulized Levalbuterol Compared With Racemic Albuterol and Placebo in the Treatment of Asthma in Pediatric Patients," *J Allergy Clin Immunol*, 1999, 103(4):615-21.

♦ **Levalbuterol Hydrochloride** *see* Levalbuterol *on page 563*

♦ **Levarterenol** *see* Norepinephrine *on page 695*

♦ **Levate® (Canada)** *see* Amitriptyline *on page 67*

♦ **Levbid®** *see* Hyoscyamine *on page 497*

Levobunolol *(lee voe BYOO noe lole)*

Brand Names AKBeta® Ophthalmic; Betagan® Liquifilm® Ophthalmic; Optho-Bunolol® (Canada)

Available Salts Levobunolol Hydrochloride

Synonyms *L*-Bunolol

Therapeutic Category Beta-Adrenergic Blocker, Ophthalmic

Generic Available Yes

Use To lower intraocular pressure in chronic open-angle glaucoma or ocular hypertension

Pregnancy Risk Factor C

Contraindications Hypersensitivity to levobunolol or any component; asthma, severe COPD, sinus bradycardia, second or third degree A-V block, cardiogenic shock

Warnings Contains metabisulfite; avoid use in susceptible individuals; use only in combination with miotic for patients with angle closure glaucoma

Precautions Use with caution in patients with CHF, diabetes mellitus, hyperthyroidism, myasthenia gravis

Adverse Reactions
Cardiovascular: Bradycardia, arrhythmias, hypotension, palpitations, cerebral ischemia, cerebral vascular accident, syncope, heart block, CHF
Central nervous system: Dizziness, headache, depression, ataxia, cerebral ischemia
Dermatologic: Rash, alopecia, itching
Endocrine & metabolic: Masked symptoms of hypoglycemia in diabetics
Gastrointestinal: Nausea, heartburn, diarrhea
Ocular: Stinging, burning, erythema, itching, blepharoconjunctivitis, keratitis, ptosis, decreased visual acuity, conjunctivitis, tearing
Respiratory: Bronchospasm

Drug Interactions May have additive toxicity with systemic beta-adrenergic blocking drugs; ophthalmic epinephrine decreases effectiveness

Mechanism of Action A nonselective beta-adrenergic blocking agent that lowers intraocular pressure by reducing aqueous humor production

Pharmacodynamics
Onset of action: Following ophthalmic instillation, decreases in intraocular pressure can be noted within 1 hour
Peak effect: Within 2-6 hours
Maximal effectiveness: 2-3 weeks
Duration: 1-7 days

Pharmacokinetics
Absorption: May be absorbed systemically and produce systemic side effects
Metabolism: Extensively metabolized into several metabolites; primary metabolite (active) dihydrolevobunolol
Elimination: Not well defined

Usual Dosage Adults: 1-2 drops of 0.5% solution in eye(s) once daily or 1-2 drops of 0.25% solution twice daily; may increase to 1 drop of 0.5% solution twice daily

Administration Intraocular: Apply drops into conjunctival sac of affected eye(s); avoid contacting bottle tip with skin; apply gentle pressure to lacrimal sac during and immediately following instillation (1-2 minutes) to decrease systemic absorption; see manufacturer's information regarding proper usage of C Cap (compliance cap)

Monitoring Parameters Intraocular pressure

Dosage Forms Solution, ophthalmic, as hydrochloride: 0.25% [2.5 mg/mL] (5 mL, 10 mL, 15 mL); 0.5% [5 mg/mL] (2 mL, 5 mL, 10 mL, 15 mL)

♦ **Levobunolol Hydrochloride** *see* Levobunolol *on page 564*

♦ **Levocarnitine** *see* Carnitine *on page 173*

Levodopa (lee voe DOE pa)

Related Information
Serotonin Syndrome *on page 1217*

Brand Names Dopar®; Larodopa®

Synonyms *L*-3-Hydroxytyramine; *L*-Dopa

Therapeutic Category Anti-Parkinson's Agent; Diagnostic Agent, Growth Hormone Function

Generic Available No

Use Diagnostic agent for growth hormone deficiency; treatment of Parkinson's disease

Pregnancy Risk Factor C

Contraindications Hypersensitivity to levodopa or any component; narrow-angle glaucoma, MAO inhibitor therapy, melanomas, or any undiagnosed skin lesions

Warnings GI hemorrhage has occurred in patients with a history of peptic ulcer disease; some products contain tartrazine which may cause hypersensitivity reactions in susceptible individuals

Precautions Use cautiously in patients with severe cardiovascular disease or pulmonary disease, asthma, occlusive cerebrovascular disease, renal, hepatic, or endocrine disease, affective disorders, major psychoses, cardiac arrhythmias, and chronic wide-angle glaucoma

Adverse Reactions
Cardiovascular: Orthostatic hypotension, palpitations, cardiac arrhythmias, hypertension
Central nervous system: Memory loss, nervousness, anxiety, insomnia, fatigue, hallucinations, dystonic movements, ataxia, headache, confusion
Gastrointestinal: Nausea, vomiting, GI bleeding, constipation, anorexia, xerostomia
Hematologic: Hemolytic anemia
Neuromuscular & skeletal: Muscle twitching
Ocular: Blurred vision, eyelid spasms
Miscellaneous: Discoloration of sweat

Drug Interactions Antacids increase bioavailability of levodopa; benzodiazepines, hydantoins, methionine, papaverine, and pyridoxine decrease levodopa's effectiveness; iron salts and anticholinergics decrease GI absorption of levodopa; MAO inhibitors may increase hypertensive reaction; levodopa may decrease metoclopramide's effects; methyldopa may have additive hypotensive effects

Food Interactions High protein diets may decrease the efficacy of levodopa when used for parkinsonism via competition with amino acids in crossing the blood-brain barrier; avoid foods high in pyridoxine content such as liver, fish, whole grain cereals, peas, and beans

Mechanism of Action Increases dopamine levels in the brain; stimulates dopaminergic receptors in the basal ganglia to improve the balance between cholinergic and dopaminergic activity

Pharmacokinetics
Metabolism: Majority of drug is peripherally decarboxylated to dopamine; small amounts of levodopa reach the brain where it is also decarboxylated to active dopamine
Half-life: 1.2-2.3 hours
Time to peak serum concentration: Oral: Within 1-2 hours
Elimination: Primarily in urine (80%) as dopamine, norepinephrine, and homovanillic acid

Usual Dosage
Children: Oral (given as a single dose to evaluate growth hormone deficiency)
0.5 g/m^2 **or**
<30 lb: 125 mg
30-70 lb: 250 mg
>70 lb: 500 mg
Adults: Parkinson's disease: 500-1000 mg/day in divided doses every 6-12 hours; increase by 100-750 mg/day every 3-7 days until response or total dose of 8000 mg is reached

Administration Oral: Administer with food

Monitoring Parameters Growth hormone level

Test Interactions False-positive reaction for urinary glucose with Clinitest®; false-negative reaction using Clinistix®; false-positive urine ketones with Acetest®, Ketostix®, Labstix®; false-positive Coombs' test; false increase in uric acid with colorimetric method

Dosage Forms
Capsule: 100 mg, 250 mg, 500 mg
(Continued)

Levodopa *(Continued)*

Tablet: 100 mg, 250 mg, 500 mg

References

Cara JF and Johanson HJ, "Growth Hormone for Short Stature Not Due to Classic Growth Hormone Deficiency," *Pediatr Clin North Am*, 1990, 37(6):1229-54.

♦ **Levophed®** *see* Norepinephrine *on page 695*

♦ **Levosalbutamol** *see* Levalbuterol *on page 563*

♦ **Levo-T™** *see* Levothyroxine *on page 566*

♦ **Levothroid® Injection** *see* Levothyroxine *on page 566*

♦ **Levothroid® Oral** *see* Levothyroxine *on page 566*

Levothyroxine *(lee voe thye ROKS een)*

Brand Names Eltroxin®; Eltroxin® (Canada); Levo-T™; Levothroid® Injection; Levothroid® Oral; Levoxyl™; PMS-Levothyroxine Sodium (Canada); Synthroid® Injection; Synthroid® Oral

Available Salts Levothyroxine Sodium

Synonyms *L*-Thyroxine; T_4 Thyroxine

Therapeutic Category Thyroid Product

Generic Available Yes

Use Replacement or supplemental therapy in hypothyroidism; management of nontoxic goiter, chronic lymphocytic thyroiditis, as adjunctive therapy with antithyroid agents in thyrotoxicosis to prevent goitrogenesis and hypothyroidism

Pregnancy Risk Factor A

Contraindications Hypersensitivity to levothyroxine sodium or any component; recent MI or thyrotoxicosis; uncorrected adrenal insufficiency

Warnings High doses may produce serious or even life-threatening toxic effects particularly when used with some anorectic drugs; use with extreme caution in patients with cardiovascular disease, adrenal insufficiency, hypertension or coronary artery disease; patients with diabetes mellitus and insipidus may have their symptoms exaggerated or aggravated

Adverse Reactions

Cardiovascular: Palpitations, tachycardia, cardiac arrhythmias, angina, CHF, hypertension

Central nervous system: Nervousness, insomnia, fever, headache

Dermatologic: Alopecia

Gastrointestinal: Diarrhea, abdominal cramps, increased appetite, weight loss

Neuromuscular & skeletal: Tremor

Miscellaneous: Diaphoresis

Drug Interactions Cholestyramine resin, iron salts, sodium polystyrene sulfonate, aluminum hydroxide, and sucralfate decrease absorption; antidiabetic drug requirements are increased; estrogens increase thyroid requirements; levothyroxine increases effect of oral anticoagulants; phenytoin may decrease levothyroxine levels

Food Interactions Limit intake of goitrogenic foods (asparagus, cabbage, peas, turnip greens, broccoli, spinach, brussel sprouts, lettuce, soybeans); soybean-based formulas may decrease absorption

Stability I.V. form must be prepared immediately prior to administration

Mechanism of Action Primary active compound is T_3 (triiodothyronine), which may be converted from T_4 (thyroxine); exact mechanism of action is unknown; however, it is believed the thyroid hormone exerts its many metabolic effects through control of DNA transcription and protein synthesis; involved in normal metabolism, growth, and development; promotes gluconeogenesis, increases utilization and mobilization of glycogen stores, and stimulates protein synthesis, increases basal metabolic rate

Pharmacodynamics

Onset of action:

Oral: 3-5 days for therapeutic effects

I.V.: Within 6-8 hours

Pharmacokinetics

Absorption: Oral: Erratic (48% to 79%)

Metabolism: In the liver to triiodothyronine (active)

Half-life: 6-7 days

Time to peak serum concentration: Within 2-4 hours

Elimination: In feces and urine

Usual Dosage

Neonates, Infants, and Children: Daily dosage:

Oral:

0-6 months: 8-10 mcg/kg or 25-50 mcg
6-12 months: 6-8 mcg/kg or 50-75 mcg
1-5 years: 5-6 mcg/kg or 75-100 mcg
6-12 years: 4-5 mcg/kg or 100-150 mcg
>12 years: 2-3 mcg/kg or ≥150 mcg
Growth and puberty complete: 1.6 mcg/kg

I.V., I.M.: 50% to 75% of the oral dose

Adults:

Oral: 12.5-50 mcg/day to start, then increase by 25-50 mcg/day at intervals of 2-4 weeks; average adult dose: 100-200 mcg/day

I.V., I.M.: 50% of the oral dose

Myxedema coma or stupor: I.V.: 300-500 mcg one time, then 75-100 mcg daily; begin oral therapy as soon as tolerated

Thyroid suppression therapy: Oral: 2-6 mcg/kg/day for 7-10 days

Administration

Oral: Administer on an empty stomach

Parenteral: Dilute vial with 5 mL NS; use immediately after reconstitution; administer by direct I.V. infusion over 2- to 3-minute period; may administer I.M.

Monitoring Parameters T_4, TSH, heart rate, blood pressure, clinical signs of hypo- and hyperthyroidism; TSH is the most reliable guide for evaluating adequacy of thyroid replacement dosage. TSH may be elevated during the first few months of thyroid replacement despite patients being clinically euthyroid. In cases where T_4 remains low and TSH is within normal limits, an evaluation of "free" (unbound) T_4 is needed to evaluate further increase in dosage

Reference Range See normal values in Normal Laboratory Values for Children on page 1155

Test Interactions Many drugs may have effects on thyroid function tests: para-aminosalicylic acid, aminoglutethimide, amiodarone, barbiturates, carbamazepine, chloral hydrate, clofibrate, colestipol, corticosteroids, danazol, diazepam, estrogens, ethionamide, fluorouracil, I.V. heparin, insulin, lithium, methadone, methimazole, mitotane, nitroprusside, oxyphenbutazone, phenylbutazone, PTU, perphenazine, phenytoin, propranolol, salicylates, sulfonylureas, and thiazides

Patient Information Do not change brands without physician's knowledge; report immediately to physician any chest pain, increased pulse, palpitations, heat intolerances, excessive sweating; do not discontinue without notifying physician

Additional Information Levothroid® tablets contain lactose; 15-37.5 mcg liothyronine = 50-60 mcg levothyroxine = 60 mg thyroid USP = 45 mg Thyroid Strong® = 60 mg thyroglobulin = 50-60 mcg liotrix

Dosage Forms

Powder for injection, as sodium, lyophilized: 0.2 mg/vial (6 mL, 10 mL); 0.5 mg/vial (6 mL, 10 mL)

Tablet, as sodium: 0.025 mg, 0.05 mg, 0.075 mg, 0.088 mg, 0.1 mg, 0.112 mg, 0.125 mg, 0.15 mg, 0.137 mg, 0.175 mg, 0.2 mg, 0.3 mg

Extemporaneous Preparations A 25 mcg/mL extemporaneous suspension may be compounded by crushing twenty-five 0.1 mg tablets; measure 40 mL glycerol; triturate powder into a pourable suspension with a small amount of glycerol and transfer to a calibrated 100 mL amber bottle; rinse the mortar with about 10 mL of the glycerol and pour into the bottle; repeat until the glycerol is used up; add water to bring the oral liquid to a total volume of 100 mL; label "shake well" and "refrigerate". The suspension is stable 8 days refrigerated.

Boulton DV, Fawcett JP, and Woods DJ, "Stability of an Extemporaneously Compounded Levothyroxine Sodium Oral Liquid," *Am J Health-Syst Pharm*, 1996; 53:1157-61.

Lidocaine (LYE doe kane)

Related Information

Adult ACLS Algorithm, Tachycardia *on page 1010*
Adult ACLS Algorithm, V. Fib and Pulseless V. Tach *on page 1004*
CPR Pediatric Drug Dosages *on page 999*
Emergency Pediatric Drip Calculations *on page 1000*
Pediatric ALS Algorithm, Asystole and Pulseless Arrest *on page 1002*

Brand Names Anestacon® Topical Solution; Dilocaine® Injection; Duo-Trach® Injection; Lidodan® (Canada); Lidoderm® Patch; LidoPen® I.M. Injection Auto-Injector; Nervocaine® Injection; PMS-Lidocaine Viscous (Canada); Solarcaine® Topical; Xylocaine® 2%, 4%, 5% (Canada); Xylocaine® HCl I.V. Injection for Cardiac Arrhythmias; Xylocaine® Oral; Xylocaine® Topical Ointment; Xylocaine® Topical Solution; Xylocaine® Topical Spray; Xylocard® (Canada)

Available Salts Lidocaine Hydrochloride

Synonyms Lignocaine

Therapeutic Category Analgesic, Topical; Antiarrhythmic Agent, Class I-B; Local Anesthetic, Injectable; Local Anesthetic, Topical

Generic Available Yes

Use Drug of choice for ventricular ectopy, ventricular tachycardia (VT), ventricular fibrillation (VF); for pulseless VT or VF preferably give **after** defibrillation and epinephrine; control of premature ventricular contractions, wide-complex PSVT; local anesthetic; pain relief of postherpetic neuralgia

Pregnancy Risk Factor B

Contraindications Hypersensitivity to lidocaine, amide-type local anesthetics, or any component; patients with Adams-Stokes syndrome or with severe degree of S-A, A-V, or intraventricular heart block (without a pacemaker)

Warnings Decrease dose in patients with decreased cardiac output or hepatic disease; do not use lidocaine solutions containing epinephrine for treatment of arrhythmias; do not use preservative-containing solution for I.V. use; do not apply patch to larger areas or for longer than recommended (toxicities may result)

Precautions Hepatic disease, heart failure, marked hypoxia, severe respiratory depression, hypovolemia or shock; incomplete heart block or bradycardia, atrial fibrillation

Adverse Reactions

Cardiovascular: Bradycardia, hypotension, heart block, arrhythmias, cardiovascular collapse
Central nervous system: Lethargy, coma, agitation, slurred speech, seizures, anxiety, euphoria, hallucinations
Gastrointestinal: Nausea, vomiting
Local: Thrombophlebitis; with patch: Erythema, edema, abnormal sensation
Neuromuscular & skeletal: Paresthesia, muscle twitching
Ocular: Blurred vision, diplopia
Respiratory: Respiratory depression or arrest
Miscellaneous: Allergic and anaphylactoid reactions (rare)

Drug Interactions Cytochrome P-450 isoenzyme CYP 3A3/4 substrate
Cimetidine or beta-blockers may increase lidocaine serum concentration and toxicity; Class I antiarrhythmic agents (mexiletine, tocainide) may increase adverse or toxic effects

Mechanism of Action Class IB antiarrhythmic; suppresses automaticity of conduction tissue by increasing electrical stimulation threshold of ventricle, HIS-Purkinje system, and spontaneous depolarization of the ventricles during diastole by a direct action on the tissues; blocks both the initiation and conduction of nerve impulses by decreasing the neuronal membrane's permeability to sodium ions, which results in inhibition of depolarization with resultant blockade of conduction

Pharmacodynamics

Antiarrhythmic effect:
Onset of action (single I.V. bolus dose): 45-90 seconds
Duration: 10-20 minutes
Local anesthetic effect: Duration: 1-2 hours

Pharmacokinetics

Distribution: V_d alterable by many patient factors; decreased V_d in CHF and liver disease
Protein binding: 60% to 80%; binds to alpha$_1$-acid glycoprotein
Metabolism: 90% in the liver; active metabolites monoethylglycinexylidide (MEGX) and glycinexylidide (GX) can accumulate and may cause CNS toxicity
Half-life, biphasic:
Alpha: 7-30 minutes

Beta, terminal:
Infants, premature: 3.2 hours
Adults: 1.5-2 hours
CHF, liver disease, shock, severe renal disease: Prolonged half-life
Elimination: <10% excreted unchanged in urine
Dialyzable (0% to 5%)

Usual Dosage
Children and Adults:
Topical: Apply to affected area as needed; maximum dose: 3 mg/kg/dose; do not repeat within 2 hours
Injectable local anesthetic: Dose varies with procedure, degree of anesthesia needed, vascularity of tissue, duration of anesthesia required, and physical condition of patient; maximum dose: 4.5 mg/kg/dose; do not repeat within 2 hours
Children: I.V., I.O., E.T.: (Note: For use in pulseless VT or VF, give after defibrillation and epinephrine): Loading dose: 1 mg/kg; may repeat if needed in 10-15 minutes times 2 doses; after loading dose, start I.V. continuous infusion 20-50 mcg/kg/minute. Use 20 mcg/kg/minute in patients with shock, hepatic disease, cardiac arrest, mild CHF; moderate to severe CHF may require ½ loading dose and lower infusion rates to avoid toxicity.
Adults (decrease the dose in patients with CHF, acute MI, shock, or hepatic disease):
I.V.:
Initial bolus: 1-1.5 mg/kg; may repeat doses of 0.5-1.5 mg/kg every 5-10 minutes if needed to a total of 3 mg/kg
Continuous infusion: 2-4 mg/minute
Ventricular fibrillation (after defibrillation and epinephrine): Initial dose: 1.5 mg/kg, may repeat boluses as above; follow with continuous infusion after return of perfusion
Prevention of ventricular fibrillation: I.V.: Initial bolus: 0.5 mg/kg; repeat every 5-10 minutes to a total dose of 2 mg/kg
Refractory ventricular fibrillation: Repeat 1.5 mg/kg bolus may be given 3-5 minutes after initial dose
E.T.: 2-2.5 times the I.V. bolus dose
I.M.: Prehospital post-MI antiarrhythmic prophylaxis: 300 mg
Lidoderm® patch: Postherpetic neuralgia: Apply patch to most painful areas; up to 3 patches may be applied per application; patch may remain in place for up to 12 hours in any 24-hour period

Administration
Endotracheal: Children: Dilute to 1-2 mL with NS prior to E.T. administration
Parenteral: I.V.: Solutions of 40-200 mg/mL must be diluted for I.V. use; final concentration not to exceed 20 mg/mL for I.V. push or 8 mg/mL for I.V. infusion; I.V. push rate of administration should not exceed 0.7 mg/kg/minute or 50 mg/minute, whichever is less; I.V. continuous infusion must be administered with a calibrated infusion device
Transdermal: Apply patch to intact skin so most painful area is covered; do not apply to broken or inflamed skin; patch may be cut to appropriate size; remove immediately if burning sensation occurs; wash hands after applying patch; avoid eye contact; keep out of the reach of children; dispose of used patch properly (see Additional Information)

Monitoring Parameters
Monitor EKG continuously; serum concentrations with continuous infusion; I.V. site (local thrombophlebitis may occur with prolonged infusions)

Reference Range
Therapeutic: 1.5-5 µg/mL (SI: 6-21 µmol/L)
Potentially toxic: >6 µg/mL (SI: >26 µmol/L)
Toxic: >9 µg/mL (SI: >38 µmol/L)

Nursing Implications
Multiple products and concentrations exist; use of an I.V. fluid filter is recommended where possible

Additional Information
Transdermal patches (both used and unused) may cause toxicities in children; used patches still contain large amounts of lidocaine; store and dispose patches out of the reach of children

Dosage Forms
Injection, as hydrochloride: 0.5% [5 mg/mL] (50 mL); 1% [10 mg/mL] (2 mL, 5 mL, 10 mL, 20 mL, 30 mL, 50 mL); 1.5% [15 mg/mL] (20 mL); 2% [20 mg/mL] (2 mL, 5 mL, 10 mL, 20 mL, 30 mL, 50 mL); 4% [40 mg/mL] (5 mL); 10% [100 mg/mL] (10 mL); 20% [200 mg/mL] (10 mL pin-top vial)
Injection, as hydrochloride:
I.M. use: 10% [100 mg/mL] (3 mL, 5 mL)
(Continued)

Lidocaine *(Continued)*

Direct I.V.: 1% [10 mg/mL] (5 mL, 10 mL); 20 mg/mL (5 mL)

I.V. admixture, preservative free: 4% [40 mg/mL] (25 mL, 30 mL); 10% [100 mg/mL] (10 mL); 20% [200 mg/mL] (5 mL, 10 mL)

I.V. infusion, in D$_5$W: 0.2% [2 mg/mL] (500 mL); 0.4% [4 mg/mL] (250 mL, 500 mL, 1000 mL); 0.8% [8 mg/mL] (250 mL, 500 mL)

Jelly, topical, as hydrochloride: 2% (30 mL)

Liquid, topical, as hydrochloride: 2.5% (10 mL) [OTC]

Liquid, viscous, as hydrochloride: 2% (20 mL, 100 mL)

Ointment, topical, as hydrochloride: 2.5% [OTC], 5% (35 g)

Solution, topical, as hydrochloride: 2% [20 mg/mL] (15 mL, 240 mL); 4% [40 mg/mL] (50 mL)

Transdermal patch: 5%

References

Emergency Cardiac Care Committee and Subcommittees, American Heart Association, "Guidelines for Cardiopulmonary Resuscitation and Emergency Cardiac Care, III: Adult Advanced Cardiac Life Support" and "VI: Pediatric Advanced Life Support," *JAMA*, 1992, 268(16):2199-241 and 2262-75.

Lidocaine and Epinephrine (LYE doe kane & ep i NEF rin)

Brand Names Octocaine® Injection; Xylocaine® (Canada); Xylocaine® With Epinephrine

Available Salts Lidocaine Hydrochloride and Epinephrine

Synonyms Epinephrine and Lidocaine

Therapeutic Category Local Anesthetic, Injectable

Generic Available Yes

Use Local infiltration anesthesia

Pregnancy Risk Factor B

Contraindications Hypersensitivity to epinephrine, lidocaine, amide-type local anesthetics, or any component

Warnings Some products contain sulfites which may cause allergic reactions

Precautions Do not use solutions in distal portions of the body (digits, nose, ears, penis); do not use large doses in patients with conduction defects (ie, heart block)

Adverse Reactions

Cardiovascular: Hypotension, bradycardia

Central nervous system: Lightheadedness, nervousness, confusion, dizziness, drowsiness, convulsions

Dermatologic: Urticaria

Neuromuscular & skeletal: Tremor

Ocular: Blurred vision

Otic: Tinnitus

Mechanism of Action Lidocaine blocks both the initiation and conduction of nerve impulses via decreased permeability of sodium ions; epinephrine increases the duration of action of lidocaine by causing vasoconstriction (via alpha effects) which slows the vascular absorption of lidocaine

Pharmacodynamics

Peak effect: Within 5 minutes

Duration: 2-6 hours, dependent on dose and anesthetic procedure

Usual Dosage Dosage varies with the anesthetic procedure

Children: Use lidocaine concentrations of 0.5% or 1% (or even more dilute) to decrease possibility of toxicity; lidocaine dose (when using combination product of lidocaine and epinephrine) should not exceed 7 mg/kg/dose; do not repeat within 2 hours

Administration Local injection: Before injecting, withdraw syringe plunger to make sure that injection is not into vein or artery; do not administer I.V. or intra-arterially

Additional Information Use preservative free solutions for epidural or caudal use

Dosage Forms Injection with epinephrine:

1:200,000: Lidocaine hydrochloride 0.5% [5 mg/mL] (50 mL); 1% [10 mg/mL] (30 mL); 1.5% [15 mg/mL] (5 mL, 10 mL, 30 mL); 2% [20 mg/mL] (20 mL)

1:100,000: Lidocaine hydrochloride 1% [10 mg/mL] (20 mL, 50 mL); 2% [20 mg/mL] (1.8 mL, 20 mL, 50 mL)

1:50,000: Lidocaine hydrochloride 2% [20 mg/mL] (1.8 mL)

Lidocaine and Prilocaine (LYE doe kane & PRIL oh kane)

Brand Names EMLA®

Available Salts Lidocaine Hydrochloride and Prilocaine

Synonyms Eutectic Mixture of Lidocaine and Prilocaine; Prilocaine and Lidocaine

Therapeutic Category Analgesic, Topical; Antipruritic, Topical; Local Anesthetic, Topical

Generic Available No

Use Topical anesthetic for use on normal intact skin to provide local analgesia for minor procedures such as I.V. cannulation or venipuncture; topical anesthetic for superficial minor surgery of genital mucous membranes and as an adjunct for local infiltration anesthesia in genital mucous membranes; has also been used for painful procedures such as lumbar puncture and skin graft harvesting

Pregnancy Risk Factor B

Contraindications Hypersensitivity to lidocaine, prilocaine, amide-type local anesthetics, or any component; patients with congenital or idiopathic methemoglobinemia, neonates <37 weeks gestation, infants <12 months of age who are receiving concurrent treatment with methemoglobin-inducing agents (ie, sulfas, acetaminophen, benzocaine, chloroquine, dapsone, nitrofurantoin, nitroglycerin, nitroprusside, phenobarbital, phenytoin, primaquine, quinine)

Precautions Use with caution in patients with severe hepatic disease, patients with G-6-PD deficiency, and patients taking drugs associated with drug-induced methemoglobinemia; adjust dosage by using smaller areas for application in small children (especially infants <3 months of age) or patients with impaired renal or hepatic function

Adverse Reactions

Cardiovascular: Bradycardia, hypotension, shock, angioedema

Central nervous system: Nervousness, euphoria, confusion, dizziness, drowsiness, convulsions, CNS excitation, alteration in temperature sensation

Dermatologic: Rash, urticaria

Hematologic: Methemoglobinemia

Local: Blanching, itching, erythema, edema

Neuromuscular & skeletal: Tremor

Ocular: Blurred vision

Otic: Tinnitus

Respiratory: Respiratory depression, bronchospasm

Drug Interactions Class IB antiarrhythmic drugs (tocainide, mexiletine): toxic effects are additive; drugs known to induce methemoglobinemia (see Contraindications)

Stability Store at room temperature

Mechanism of Action Local anesthetic action occurs by stabilization of neuronal membranes and inhibiting the ionic fluxes required for the initiation and conduction of impulses

Pharmacodynamics

Onset of action: 1 hour for sufficient dermal analgesia

Peak effect: 2-3 hours

Duration: 1-2 hours after removal of the cream

Pharmacokinetics

Absorption: Topical: Related to the duration of application and to the area over which it is applied

3-hour application: 3.6% lidocaine and 6.1% prilocaine were absorbed

24-hour application: 16.2% lidocaine and 33.5% prilocaine were absorbed

Distribution: Both cross the blood-brain barrier; lidocaine and probably prilocaine are excreted in breast milk; V_d:

Lidocaine: 1.1-2.1 L/kg

Prilocaine: 0.7-4.4 L/kg

Protein binding:

Lidocaine: 70%

Prilocaine: 55%

Metabolism:

Lidocaine: Metabolized by the liver to inactive and active metabolites

Prilocaine: Metabolized in both the liver and kidneys

Half-life:

Lidocaine: 65-150 minutes, prolonged with cardiac or hepatic dysfunction

Prilocaine: 10-150 minutes, prolonged in hepatic or renal dysfunction

Usual Dosage Topical:

Newborns ≥37 weeks gestation, Children, and Adults: For minor procedures, apply 2.5 g/site for at least 60 minutes; for painful procedures, apply 2 g/10 cm^2 of skin and leave on for at least 2 hours; see table on following page.

Adult male genital skin as an adjunct prior to local anesthetic infiltration: Apply 1 g/10 cm^2 to skin surface for 15 minutes followed immediately by local anesthetic infiltration after removal of EMLA® cream

(Continued)

571

Lidocaine and Prilocaine *(Continued)*

EMLA® Cream Maximum Recommended Dose and Application Area* for Infants and Children Based on Application to Intact Skin

Age and Body Weight Requirements	Maximum Total Dose of EMLA®	Maximum Application Area	Maximum Application Time
Birth to 3 mo or <5 kg	1 g	10 cm²	1 h
3-12 mo and >5 kg	2 g	20 cm²	4 h
1-6 y and >10 kg	10 g	100 cm²	4 h
7-12 y and >20 kg	20 g	200 cm²	4 h

Preliminary results in a study of 30 preterm neonates (n=30) using a single 0.5 g dose of EMLA® applied to the heel for 1 hour resulted in no measurable changes in methemoglobin levels

Administration Topical: Do not use on mucous membranes or the eyes; apply a thick layer of cream to intact skin and cover with an occlusive dressing

Patient Information Not for ophthalmic use; for external use only. EMLA® may block sensation in the treated skin.

Nursing Implications In small infants and children, an occlusive bandage should be placed over the EMLA® cream to prevent the child from placing the cream in his/ her mouth or smearing the cream on the eyes

Dosage Forms
Cream: Lidocaine 2.5% and prilocaine 2.5% [2 Tegaderm® dressings] (5 g, 30 g)
Disc, anesthetic: 1 g

References
Broadman LM, Soliman IE, Hannallah RS, et al, "Analgesic Efficacy of Eutectic Mixture of Local Anesthetics (EMLA®) vs Intradermal Infiltration Prior to Venous Cannulation in Children," *Am J Anaesth*, 1987, 34:S56.

Halperin DL, Koren G, Attias D, et al, "Topical Skin Anesthesia for Venous Subcutaneous Drug Reservoir and Lumbar Puncture in Children," *Pediatrics*, 1989, 84(2):281-4.

Robieux I, Kumar R, Radhakrishnan S, et al, "Assessing Pain and Analgesia With a Lidocaine-Prilo- caine Emulsion in Infants and Toddlers During Venipuncture," *J Pediatr*, 1991, 118(6):971-3.

Taddio A, Shennan AT, Stevens B, et al, "Safety of Lidocaine-Prilocaine Cream in the Treatment of Preterm Neonates," *J Pediatr*, 1995, 127(6):1002-5.

♦ **Lidocaine Hydrochloride** *see* Lidocaine *on page 568*
♦ **Lidocaine Hydrochloride and Epinephrine** *see* Lidocaine and Epinephrine *on page 570*
♦ **Lidocaine Hydrochloride and Prilocaine** *see* Lidocaine and Prilocaine *on page 570*
♦ **Lidodan® (Canada)** *see* Lidocaine *on page 568*
♦ **Lidoderm® Patch** *see* Lidocaine *on page 568*
♦ **LidoPen® I.M. Injection Auto-Injector** *see* Lidocaine *on page 568*
♦ **Lignocaine** *see* Lidocaine *on page 568*
♦ **Linctus Codeine Blac (Canada)** *see* Codeine *on page 249*
♦ **Linctus With Codeine Phosphate (Canada)** *see* Codeine *on page 249*

Lindane *(LIN dane)*

Brand Names G-well®; Hexit® (Canada); Kwell®; Kwellada™ (Canada); PMS- Lindane (Canada); Scabene®

Synonyms Benzene Hexachloride; Gamma Benzene Hexachloride; Hexachlorocy- clohexane

Therapeutic Category Antiparasitic Agent, Topical; Pediculocide; Scabicidal Agent; Shampoos

Generic Available Yes

Use Alternative treatment of scabies (*Sarcoptes scabiei*), *Pediculus capitis* (head lice), and *Pediculus pubis* (crab lice); (the AAP and CDC consider permethrin 5% to be the scabicide of choice due to its safety and efficacy profile; many clinicians no longer recommend lindane as initial therapy for pediculosis due to reports of resistance and neurotoxicity)

Pregnancy Risk Factor B

Contraindications Hypersensitivity to lindane or any component; premature neonates; pregnant or lactating women; acutely inflamed skin or raw, weeping surfaces

Warnings Avoid contact with the face, eyes, mucous membranes, and urethral meatus

Precautions Use with caution in infants, small children and patients with pre- existing seizure disorders due to its potential for neurologic toxicity; if used in young children, cover hands to prevent accidental lindane ingestion from thumb-sucking; **consider alternative therapy for the treatment of scabies in infants and young children <2 years of age (ie, permethrin)**

Adverse Reactions

Cardiovascular: Cardiac arrhythmia

Central nervous system: Dizziness, restlessness, seizures, headache, ataxia

Dermatologic: Eczematous eruptions, contact dermatitis, rash

Gastrointestinal: Nausea, vomiting

Hematologic: Aplastic anemia

Hepatic: Hepatitis

Local: Burning and stinging

Ocular: Conjunctivitis

Renal: Hematuria

Respiratory: Pulmonary edema

Mechanism of Action Directly absorbed by parasites and ova through the exoskeleton; stimulates the nervous system resulting in seizures and death of parasitic arthropods

Pharmacokinetics

Absorption: Topical: Up to 13% absorbed systemically (absorption is greater when applied to damaged skin, face, scalp, neck, or scrotum)

Distribution: Stored in body fat and accumulates in the brain; skin and adipose tissue may act as repositories

Metabolism: By the liver

Half-life, children: 17-22 hours

Time to peak serum concentration: Children: Topical: 6 hours

Elimination: In urine and feces

Usual Dosage Children and Adults: Topical:

Scabies: Apply a thin layer of lotion and massage it on skin from the neck to the toes (head to toe in infants).

Infants: Wash off 6 hours after application

Children: Wash off 6-8 hours after application

Adults: Bathe and remove drug 8-12 hours after application

Do not reapply sooner than 1 week later if live mites appear

Pediculosis: 15-30 mL of shampoo is applied and lathered for 4 minutes; rinse hair thoroughly and comb with a fine tooth comb to remove nits; repeat treatment in 7 days if lice or nits are still present

Pediculosis of the eyelashes: Do not treat with lindane; instead, apply an occlusive ophthalmic ointment like petrolatum to the eyelid margins twice daily for 10 days

Administration

For topical use only; do not apply to face; avoid getting in eyes; do **not** apply lotion immediately after a hot, soapy bath; lotion should be applied to dry, cool skin

Before applying lindane shampoo, wash hair with a plain shampoo, then dry

Patient Information Clothing and bedding should be washed in hot water or by dry cleaning to kill the scabies mite; combs and brushes may be washed with lindane shampoo then thoroughly rinsed with water

Nursing Implications

Children <6 years: ~30 mL lotion is sufficient volume for one application

Children ≥6 years and Adults: ~30-60 mL lotion is sufficient volume for one application

Pruritus associated with scabies or pediculosis may persist for longer than 1 week following treatment with drug. Oral antihistamine and/or topical corticosteroid may be used to help relieve pruritus.

Additional Information Excessive absorption may result in overdose with signs and symptoms which include nausea, vomiting, seizures, headaches, arrhythmias, apnea, pulmonary edema, hematuria, hepatitis, coma, and even death

Dosage Forms

Lotion: 1% (60 mL, 473 mL, 4000 mL)

Shampoo: 1% (60 mL, 473 mL, 4000 mL)

References

Eichenfield LF, Honig PJ, "Blistering Disorders in Childhood," *Pediatr Clin North Am*, 1991, 38(4):959-76.

Hogan DJ, Schachner L, Tanglertsampan C, "Diagnosis and Treatment of Childhood Scabies and Pediculosis," *Pediatr Clin North Am*, 1991, 38(4):941-57.

Pramanik AK and Hansen RC, "Transcutaneous Gamma Benzene Hexachloride Absorption and Toxicity in Infants and Children," *Arch Dermatol*, 1979, 115(10):1224-5.

♦ **Lioresal®** see Baclofen on page 119

Liothyronine (lye oh THYE roe neen)

Brand Names Cytomel® Oral; Triostat™ Injection

Available Salts Liothyronine Sodium

Synonyms L-Triiodothyronine; T₃

Therapeutic Category Thyroid Product

Generic Available Yes

Use Replacement or supplemental therapy in hypothyroidism, management of nontoxic goiter, chronic lymphocytic thyroiditis, as an adjunct in thyrotoxicosis and as a diagnostic aid; levothyroxine is recommended for chronic therapy; (if rapid correction of thyroid is needed, T₃ is preferred, but use cautiously and with lower recommended doses)

Pregnancy Risk Factor A

Contraindications Recent MI or thyrotoxicosis; hypersensitivity to liothyronine sodium or any component; uncorrected adrenal insufficiency

Warnings Patients with diabetes mellitus and insipidus may have their symptoms exaggerated or aggravated. Ineffective for weight reduction; high doses may produce serious or even life-threatening toxic effects particularly when used with some anorectic drugs. Short duration of action permits more rapid assessment of dosage changes and rapid diminution of adverse effects upon discontinuation.

Precautions Use with extreme caution in patients with cardiovascular disease, adrenal insufficiency, or coronary artery disease

Adverse Reactions

Cardiovascular: Palpitations, tachycardia, cardiac arrhythmias, angina, CHF, hypertension

Central nervous system: Nervousness, insomnia, fever, headache

Dermatologic: Alopecia, dermatitis herpetiformis

Gastrointestinal: Diarrhea, abdominal cramps, increased appetite, weight loss

Local: Phlebitis with parenteral form

Neuromuscular & skeletal: Tremor

Miscellaneous: Diaphoresis

Drug Interactions Cholestyramine resin, iron salts, sodium polystyrene sulfonate, aluminum hydroxide, and sucralfate decrease absorption; antidiabetic drug requirements are increased; estrogens increase thyroid requirements; liothyronine increases effect of oral anticoagulants

Food Interactions Limit intake of goitrogenic foods (asparagus, cabbage, peas, turnip greens, broccoli, spinach, brussel sprouts, lettuce, soybeans)

Stability Store parenteral solution at temperatures between 2°C and 8°C (36°F to 46°F); I.V. form must be prepared immediately prior to administration

Mechanism of Action Primary active compound is T₃ (triiodothyronine), which may be converted from T₄ (thyroxine); exact mechanism of action is unknown, however it is believed the thyroid hormone exerts its many metabolic effects through control of DNA transcription and protein synthesis; involved in normal metabolism, growth, and development; promotes gluconeogenesis, increases utilization and mobilization of glycogen stores, and stimulates protein synthesis; increases basal metabolic rate

Pharmacodynamics

Onset of effect: Within a few hours

Maximum effect: Within 48-72 hours

Duration: Up to 72 hours

Pharmacokinetics

Absorption: Oral: Well absorbed (~85% to 90%)

Metabolism: In the liver to inactive compounds

Half-life: 25 hours (range: 16-49 hours); hypothyroid 1.4 days; hyperthyroid 0.6 days

Elimination: 76% to 83% In urine

Usual Dosage

Congenital hypothyroidism (Cretinism): Neonates, Infants, and Children <3 years: Oral: 5 mcg/day; increase by 5 mcg every 3 days to a maximum dosage of 20 mcg/day for neonates and infants, 50 mcg/day for children 1-3 years of age

Hypothyroidism:

Children: Oral: 5 mcg/day increase by 5 mcg increments every 1-2 weeks; usual maintenance dose 15-20 mcg/day

Adults: Oral: 25 mcg/day increase by 12.5-25 mcg/day every 1-2 weeks to a maximum of 100 mcg/day

Goiter, nontoxic:
Children: Oral: 5 mcg/day increase by 5 mcg increments every 1-2 weeks; usual maintenance dose 15-20 mcg/day
Adults: Oral: 5 mcg/day; increase by 5-10 mcg/day every 1-2 weeks; when 25 mcg is reached, increase dosage by 12.5-25 mcg every 1-2 weeks; usual maintenance dosage: 75 mcg/day
T_3 suppression test: Adults: Oral: 75-100 mcg/day for 7 days
Myxedema coma: Adults: I.V.: 25-50 mcg
Patients with known or suspected cardiovascular disease: 10-20 mcg
Note: Normally, at least 4 hours should be allowed between I.V. doses to adequately assess therapeutic response and no more than 12 hours should elapse between doses to avoid fluctuations in hormone levels. Oral therapy should be resumed as soon as the clinical situation has been stabilized and the patient is able to take oral medication. If levothyroxine rather than liothyronine sodium is used in initiating oral therapy, there is a delay of several days before the onset of levothyroxine activity and I.V. liothyronine sodium therapy should be discontinued gradually.

Administration
Oral: Administer on an empty stomach
Parenteral: I.V.: Dilute 200 mcg/mL vial with 2 mL of NS injection and shake well until a clear solution is obtained; use immediately after reconstitution; should not be admixed with other solutions

Monitoring Parameters T_3, TSH, heart rate, blood pressure, clinical signs of hypo- and hyperthyroidism; TSH is the most reliable guide for evaluating adequacy of thyroid replacement dosage. TSH may be elevated during the first few months of thyroid replacement despite patients being clinically euthyroid.

Reference Range See normal values in Normal Laboratory Values for Children *on page 1155*

Test Interactions Many drugs may have effects on thyroid function tests (ie, para-aminosalicylic acid, aminoglutethimide, amiodarone, barbiturates, carbamazepine, chloral hydrate, clofibrate, colestipol, corticosteroids, danazol, diazepam, estrogens, ethionamide, fluorouracil, I.V. heparin, insulin, lithium, methadone, methimazole, mitotane, nitroprusside, oxyphenbutazone, phenylbutazone, PTU, perphenazine, phenytoin, propranolol, salicylates, sulfonylureas, and thiazides)

Patient Information Do not change brands without physician's knowledge; report immediately to physician any chest pain, increased pulse, palpitations, heat intolerance, excessive sweating; do not discontinue without notifying physician

Additional Information 15-37.5 mcg liothyronine = 50-60 mcg levothyroxine = 60 mg thyroid USP = 45 mg Thyroid Strong® = 60 mg thyroglobulin = 50-60 mcg liotrix

Dosage Forms
Injection, as sodium: 10 mcg/mL (1 mL)
Tablet, as sodium: 5 mcg, 25 mcg, 50 mcg

♦ **Liothyronine Sodium** *see* Liothyronine *on page 574*
♦ **Lipancreatin** *see* Pancrelipase *on page 724*
♦ **Lipid Emulsion** *see* Fat Emulsion *on page 403*
♦ **Liposyn®** *see* Fat Emulsion *on page 403*
♦ **Liquaemin®** *see* Heparin *on page 471*
♦ **Liquibid® Malotuss® [OTC]** *see* Guaifenesin *on page 464*
♦ **Liqui-Char® [OTC]** *see* Charcoal *on page 202*
♦ **Liquid Antidote** *see* Charcoal *on page 202*
♦ **Liquid Paraffin** *see* Mineral Oil *on page 649*
♦ **Liquid Pred®** *see* Prednisone *on page 794*
♦ **Liquiprin® [OTC]** *see* Acetaminophen *on page 26*

Lisinopril (lyse IN oh pril)
Related Information
Carbohydrate and Alcohol Content of Liquid Medications for Use in Patients Receiving Ketogenic Diets *on page 1228*
Brand Names Prinivil®; Zestril®
Therapeutic Category Angiotensin-Converting Enzyme (ACE) Inhibitor; Antihypertensive Agent
Generic Available No
Use Management of hypertension; adjunctive treatment of CHF; adjunctive therapy in hemodynamically stable post MI patients to improve survival
Pregnancy Risk Factor C (1st trimester); D (may cause injury and death to the developing fetus when used during the 2nd and 3rd trimesters of pregnancy)
(Continued)

Lisinopril *(Continued)*

Contraindications Hypersensitivity to lisinopril, any component, or other ACE inhibitors; patients with idiopathic or hereditary angioedema or a history of angioedema with previous ACE inhibitor use

Precautions Use with caution and modify dosage in patients with renal impairment (especially renal artery stenosis), hyponatremia, hypovolemia, severe CHF, left ventricular outflow tract obstruction, or with coadministered diuretic therapy. Severe hypotension may occur in patients who are sodium and/or volume depleted; initiate lower doses and monitor closely when starting therapy in these patients.

Adverse Reactions

Cardiovascular: Hypotension, chest discomfort, orthostatic hypotension

Central nervous system: Dizziness, headache, fatigue

Dermatologic: Rash, angioedema. **Note:** The relative risk of angioedema with ACE inhibitors is higher within the first 30 days of use (compared to >1 year of use), for Black Americans (compared to Whites), for lisinopril or enalapril (compared to captopril), and for patients previously hospitalized within 30 days (Brown, 1996).

Endocrine & metabolic: Hyperkalemia

Gastrointestinal: Diarrhea, nausea, vomiting, ageusia

Hematologic: Neutropenia, agranulocytosis

Renal: Elevated BUN, elevated serum creatinine

Respiratory: Cough, dyspnea, eosinophilic pneumonitis

Neuromuscular & skeletal: Weakness

Drug Interactions Use with potassium-sparing diuretics may result in an additive hyperkalemic effect; diuretics and other antihypertensive agents may increase hypotensive effect; indomethacin may decrease hypotensive effect; lisinopril may increase lithium levels; use with NSAIDs in patients with renal impairment may further decrease renal function (usually reversible)

Food Interactions Food does not effect oral absorption; limit salt substitutes or potassium-rich diet; avoid natural licorice (causes sodium and water retention and increases potassium loss)

Mechanism of Action Competitive inhibitor of angiotensin-converting enzyme (ACE); prevents conversion of angiotensin I to angiotensin II, a potent vasoconstrictor; results in lower levels of angiotensin II which causes an increase in plasma renin activity and a reduction in aldosterone secretion

Pharmacodynamics

Onset of action (decrease in blood pressure): 1 hour

Peak effect: 6-8 hours

Duration of action: 24 hours

Pharmacokinetics

Absorption: Oral: 25%

Protein binding: 25%

Half-life: 11-13 hours; half-life increases with renal dysfunction

Elimination: Excreted in urine as unchanged drug

Usual Dosage Dosage must be titrated according to patient's response; use lower doses (~1/2 of those listed) for patients with hyponatremia, hypovolemia, severe CHF, decreased renal function, or in those receiving diuretics

Children: Currently, no pediatric dosing information is available

Adults:

Hypertension: Initial: 10 mg/day given once daily; increase dose by 5-10 mg/day at 1- to 2-week intervals; usual dose 20-40 mg/day; doses up to 80 mg/day have been used, but do not appear to have a greater effect

CHF: Initial: 5 mg once daily; usual: 5-20 mg/day given once daily

Discontinue diuretics 2-3 days prior to initiating lisinopril, if possible; restart diuretic, if needed, after blood pressure is stable

Dosing adjustment in renal impairment:

Cl_{cr} 10-30 mL/minute: Administer 50% of normal dose

Cl_{cr} <10 mL/minute: Administer 25% of normal dose

Administration Oral: May be administered without regard to food

Monitoring Parameters Blood pressure, BUN, serum creatinine, renal function, WBC, and serum potassium

Patient Information Limit alcohol; notify physician if vomiting, diarrhea, excessive perspiration, or dehydration occurs or if swelling of face, lips, tongue or difficulty in breathing occurs; do not use a salt substitute (potassium-containing) without physician advice

Nursing Implications Discontinue if angioedema occurs; observe closely for hypotension after the first dose or initiation of a new higher dose (keep in mind that maximum effect on blood pressure occurs at 6-8 hours)

Dosage Forms Tablet: 2.5 mg, 5 mg, 10 mg, 20 mg, 30 mg, 40 mg

References

Brown NJ, Ray WA, Snowden M, et al, "Black Americans Have an Increased Rate of Angiotension-Converting Enzyme Inhibitor-Associated Angioedema," *Clin Pharmacol Ther*, 1996, 60(1):8-13.

Chase SL and Sutton JD, "Lisinopril: A New Angiotensin-Converting Enzyme Inhibitor," *Pharmacotherapy*, 1989, 9(3):120-30.

Raia JJ Jr, Barone JA, Byerly WG, et al, "Angiotensin-Converting Enzymes Inhibitors: A Comparative Review," *DICP*, 1990, 24(5):506-25.

♦ **Listermint® with Fluoride [OTC]** *see* Fluoride *on page 427*

♦ **Lithane®** *see* Lithium *on page 577*

Lithium (LITH ee um)

Related Information

Carbohydrate and Alcohol Content of Liquid Medications for Use in Patients Receiving Ketogenic Diets *on page 1228*

Drugs and Breast-Feeding *on page 1213*

Serotonin Syndrome *on page 1217*

Brand Names Carbolith™ (Canada); Duralith® (Canada); Eskalith®; Lithane®; Lithobid®; Lithonate®; Lithotabs®

Available Salts Lithium Carbonate; Lithium Citrate

Therapeutic Category Antimanic Agent

Generic Available Yes

Use Management of acute manic episodes, bipolar disorders, and depression

Pregnancy Risk Factor D

Contraindications Hypersensitivity to lithium or any component; severe cardiovascular or renal disease

Warnings Lithium toxicity is closely related to serum levels and can occur at therapeutic doses; serum lithium determinations are required to monitor therapy; some preparations may contain tartrazine

Precautions Use with caution in patients with cardiovascular or thyroid disease, patients receiving thiazide diuretics (monitor lithium levels, lithium dosage reduction may be required)

Adverse Reactions

Cardiovascular: Arrhythmias, sinus node dysfunction

Central nervous system: Sedation, confusion, somnolence, seizures, fatigue, headache, vertigo

Dermatologic: Rash

Endocrine & metabolic: Nephrogenic diabetes insipidus (thirst, polyuria, polydipsia), goiter, hypothyroidism

Gastrointestinal: Nausea, diarrhea, vomiting, xerostomia

Hematologic: Leukocytosis

Neuromuscular & skeletal: Muscle hyperirritability, muscle weakness, tremor

Drug Interactions Thiazide diuretics or NSAIDs may decrease lithium renal excretion and enhance lithium toxicity; iodide salts (or iodine) may increase hypothyroid effects

Food Interactions Avoid changes in sodium content of diet (reduction in sodium intake can increase lithium toxicity); syrup may precipitate in tube feedings

Mechanism of Action Alters cation transport across cell membrane in nerve and muscle cells and influences reuptake of serotonin and/or norepinephrine

Pharmacokinetics

Distribution: Crosses the placenta; appears in breast milk at 35% to 50% of the concentrations in serum

Adults:

V_d: Initial: 0.3-0.4 L/kg

V_{dss}: 0.7-1 L/kg

Half-life, terminal: Adults: 18-24 hours, can increase to more than 36 hours in elderly or patients with renal impairment

Time to peak serum concentrations (nonsustained release product): Within 0.5-2 hours

Elimination: 90% to 98% of a dose is excreted in the urine as unchanged drug; other excretory routes include feces (1%) and sweat (4% to 5%)

Dialyzable (50% to 100%)

Usual Dosage Oral: Monitor serum concentrations and clinical response (efficacy and toxicity) to determine proper dose

(Continued)

Lithium *(Continued)*

Children: 15-60 mg/kg/day in 3-4 divided doses; dose not to exceed usual adult dosage; initiate at lower dose and adjust dose weekly based on levels

Adolescents: 600-1800 mg/day in 3-4 divided doses for regular tablets or 2 divided doses for sustained release tablets

Adults: 300 mg 3-4 times/day; usual maximum maintenance dose: 2.4 g/day or 450-900 mg of sustained release tablets twice daily

Dosing adjustment in renal impairment:
Cl_{cr} 10-50 mL/minute: Administer 50% to 75% of normal dose
Cl_{cr} <10 mL/minute: Administer 25% to 50% of normal dose

Administration Oral: Administer with meals to decrease GI upset; do not crush or chew slow- or extended-release dosage form, swallow whole

Monitoring Parameters Serum lithium every 3-4 days during initial therapy; obtain lithium serum concentrations 8-12 hours postdose; renal, hepatic, thyroid and cardiovascular function; CBC with differential, urinalysis, serum sodium, calcium, potassium

Reference Range
Therapeutic: Acute mania: 0.6-1.5 mEq/L (SI: 0.6-1.5 mmol/L); protection against future episodes in most patients with bipolar disorder: 0.8-1 mEq/L (SI: 0.8-1 mmol/L). A higher rate of relapse is described in subjects who are maintained <0.4 mEq/L (SI: <0.4 mmol/L)
Toxic: >2 mEq/L (SI: >2 mmol/L)

Patient Information Limit caffeine; limit alcohol; avoid tasks requiring psychomotor coordination until CNS effects are known

Nursing Implications Avoid dehydration

Dosage Forms
Capsule, as carbonate: 150 mg, 300 mg, 600 mg
Syrup, as citrate: 300 mg/5 mL (5 mL, 10 mL, 480 mL)
Tablet, as carbonate: 300 mg
Tablet:
Controlled release, as carbonate: 450 mg
Slow release, as carbonate: 300 mg

References
Levy HB, Harper CR, and Weinberg WA, "A Practical Approach to Children Failing in School," *Pediatr Clin North Am*, 1992, 39(4):895-928.

Lomustine *(loe MUS teen)*

Related Information
Emetogenic Potential of Single Chemotherapeutic Agents *on page 1095*

Brand Names CeeNU®

Synonyms CCNU

Therapeutic Category Antineoplastic Agent, Alkylating Agent (Nitrosourea)

Generic Available No

Use Treatment of brain tumors, Hodgkin's and non-Hodgkin's lymphomas, melanoma, renal carcinoma, lung cancer, colon cancer

Pregnancy Risk Factor D

Contraindications Hypersensitivity to lomustine or any component

Warnings The FDA currently recommends that procedures for proper handling and disposal of antineoplastic agents be considered. Bone marrow suppression, notably thrombocytopenia and leukopenia, may lead to bleeding and overwhelming infections in an already compromised patient; nadir: ~6 weeks; do not give courses more frequently than every 6 weeks because the toxicity is cumulative; lomustine has been found to be mutagenic, teratogenic, and carcinogenic in animals.

Precautions Use with caution in patients with depressed platelet, leukocyte or erythrocyte counts; reduce dosage by 25% when platelet nadirs are 50,000-74,999/mm^3; reduce dosage by 50% when platelet nadirs are 25,000-49,999/mm^3; reduce dosage by 75% when platelet nadirs are <25,000/mm^3

Adverse Reactions

Central nervous system: Disorientation, lethargy, ataxia

Dermatologic: Alopecia

Gastrointestinal: Nausea, vomiting, stomatitis, anorexia, diarrhea

Hematologic: Anemia, thrombocytopenia, leukopenia, myelosuppression (occurs 4-6 weeks after a dose and may persist 1-2 weeks)

Hepatic: Hepatotoxicity, elevation of hepatic enzymes

Neuromuscular & skeletal: Dysarthria

Ocular: Blindness

Renal: Renal failure, interstitial nephritis

Respiratory: Pulmonary fibrosis with total cumulative dose >1 g/m^2

Drug Interactions Phenobarbital may increase metabolism and reduce activity of lomustine; cimetidine may decrease metabolism and increase myelotoxicity of lomustine

Food Interactions Avoid concurrent administration of food/drugs that cause vomiting

Stability Avoid exposure to excessive heat (>40°C) and prolonged exposure to moisture

Mechanism of Action Inhibits DNA and RNA synthesis through DNA alkylation and DNA cross-linking; carbamoylates amine groups on proteins; inhibits DNA polymerase activity, RNA and protein synthesis

Pharmacokinetics

Absorption: Rapid and complete absorption from the GI tract (30-60 minutes)

Distribution: Lomustine and/or its metabolites penetrate into the CNS; metabolites are present in breast milk

Protein binding: >90%

Metabolism: Rapid conversion to 4-hydroxy metabolites (active) partially by liver microsomal enzymes during first pass through the liver

Half-life, terminal (active metabolite): 1.3-2 days

Time to peak serum concentrations (of active metabolite): Within 3 hours

Elimination: Excreted primarily in urine as metabolites; <5% fecal excretion

Usual Dosage Oral (refer to individual protocol):

Children: 75-150 mg/m^2 as a single dose every 6 weeks; subsequent doses are readjusted after initial treatment according to platelet and leukocyte counts (see Precautions)

Adults: 100-130 mg/m^2 as a single dose every 6 weeks; readjust after initial treatment according to platelet and leukocyte counts (see Precautions)

With compromised marrow function: Initial dose: 100 mg/m^2 as a single dose every 6 weeks

Administration Oral: Administer with fluids on an empty stomach; do not administer food or drink for 2 hours after lomustine administration to decrease incidence of nausea and vomiting

Monitoring Parameters CBC with differential and platelet count, hepatic and renal function tests, pulmonary function tests

Patient Information Notify physician if fever, sore throat, bleeding, or bruising occur; avoid alcohol for short periods after taking lomustine

Dosage Forms

Capsule: 10 mg, 40 mg, 100 mg

Dose Pack: 10 mg (2s); 100 mg (2s); 40 mg (2s)

References

Berg SL, Griseli DL, DeLaney TF, et al, "Principles of Treatment of Pediatric Solid Tumors," *Pediatr Clin North Am*, 1991, 38(2):249-67.

Pendergrass TW, Milstein JM, Geyer JR, et al, "Eight Drugs in One Day Chemotherapy for Brain Tumors: Experience in 107 Children and Rationale for Preradiation Chemotherapy," *J Clin Oncol*, 1987, 5(8):1221-31.

♦ **Loniten® Oral** see Minoxidil on page 650

♦ **Lonox®** see Diphenoxylate and Atropine on page 329

Loperamide (loe PER a mide)

Related Information
Carbohydrate and Alcohol Content of Liquid Medications for Use in Patients Receiving Ketogenic Diets *on page 1228*

Brand Names Diar-aid® [OTC]; Imodium®; Imodium® A-D [OTC]; Imodium® Advanced; Kaopectate® II [OTC]; Pepto® Diarrhea Control [OTC]; PMS-Loperamine (Canada)

Available Salts Loperamide Hydrochloride

Therapeutic Category Antidiarrheal

Generic Available Yes

Use Treatment of acute diarrhea and chronic diarrhea associated with inflammatory bowel disease; chronic functional diarrhea (idiopathic), chronic diarrhea caused by bowel resection or organic lesions; to decrease the volume of ileostomy discharge

Pregnancy Risk Factor B

Contraindications Hypersensitivity to loperamide or any component; patients who must avoid constipation; infectious diarrhea resulting from organisms that penetrate the intestinal mucosa (eg, *Shigella*, *Salmonella*); patients with pseudomembranous colitis; bloody diarrhea

Precautions If clinical improvement in acute diarrhea is not observed in 48 hours, discontinue use; monitor patients with hepatic dysfunction closely for CNS toxicity

Adverse Reactions
Central nervous system: Sedation, fatigue, dizziness
Dermatologic: Rash
Gastrointestinal: Nausea, vomiting, constipation, abdominal cramping, xerostomia
Miscellaneous: Hypersensitivity reactions

Drug Interactions Additive CNS toxicity with CNS depressants, phenothiazines, tricyclic antidepressants, alcohol

Mechanism of Action Acts directly on intestinal muscles to inhibit peristalsis and prolong transit time

Pharmacodynamics Onset of action: Within 30-60 minutes

Pharmacokinetics
Absorption: Oral: 40%
Protein binding: 97%
Metabolism: Hepatic (>50%) to inactive compounds
Half-life: 9-14 hours
Time to peak serum concentration:
Capsules: 5 hours
Liquid: 2.5 hours
Elimination: Fecal and urinary (1%) excretion of metabolites and unchanged drug (30% to 40%)

Usual Dosage Oral:
Acute diarrhea:
Children: Initial doses (in first 24 hours):
2-5 years: 1 mg 3 times/day
6-8 years: 2 mg twice daily
8-12 years: 2 mg 3 times/day
After initial dosing, 0.1 mg/kg doses after each loose stool but not exceeding initial dosage
Adults: 4 mg (2 capsules) initially, followed by 2 mg after each loose stool, up to 16 mg/day (8 capsules)
Traveler's diarrhea: Treat for no more than 2 days
6-8 years: 1 mg after first loose stool followed by 1 mg after each subsequent stool; maximum dose: 4 mg/day
9-11 years: 2 mg after first loose stool followed by 1 mg after each subsequent stool; maximum dose: 6 mg/day
12 years to Adults: 4 mg after first loose stool followed by 2 mg after each subsequent stool; maximum dose: 8 mg/day
Chronic diarrhea: Children: 0.08-0.24 mg/kg/day divided 2-3 times/day, maximum dose: 2 mg/dose

Administration Oral: Drink plenty of fluids to help prevent dehydration

Patient Information Do not exceed maximum daily dosage; may cause drowsiness and impair ability to perform hazardous tasks requiring mental alertness; if acute diarrhea lasts longer than 48 hours; consult physician

Dosage Forms
Caplet, as hydrochloride: 2 mg
Capsule, as hydrochloride: 2 mg
Liquid, oral, as hydrochloride: 1 mg/5 mL (60 mL, 90 mL, 120 mL)

Tablet, as hydrochloride: 2 mg
Tablet, chewable, as hydrochloride (Imodium® Advanced): 2 mg with simethicone 125 mg

♦ **Loperamide Hydrochloride** see Loperamide on page 580
♦ **Lopremone** see Protirelin on page 821
♦ **Lopressor®** see Metoprolol on page 633
♦ **Lorabid™** see Loracarbef on page 581

Loracarbef (lor a KAR bef)

Related Information
Carbohydrate and Alcohol Content of Liquid Medications for Use in Patients Receiving Ketogenic Diets on page 1228

Brand Names Lorabid™

Therapeutic Category Antibiotic, Carbacephem

Generic Available No

Use Treatment of mild to moderate community-acquired infections of the respiratory tract, skin and skin structure, and urinary tract that are caused by susceptible *S. pneumoniae*, *H. influenzae*, *M. catarrhalis*, *S. aureus*, *S. pyogenes*, and *E. coli*

Pregnancy Risk Factor B

Contraindications Hypersensitivity to loracarbef, any component, or cephalosporins

Warnings Prolonged use may result in superinfection or pseudomembranous colitis

Precautions Use with caution in patients with a previous history of hypersensitivity to other beta-lactam antibiotics (eg, penicillins, cephalosporins); use with caution in patients with impaired renal function and patients with a history of colitis; modify dosage in patients with renal impairment

Adverse Reactions
Cardiovascular: Vasodilation
Central nervous system: Headache, somnolence, nervousness, dizziness, insomnia
Gastrointestinal: Diarrhea, nausea, vomiting, abdominal pain, anorexia
Dermatologic: Skin rashes, urticaria, pruritus, erythema multiforme, Stevens-Johnson syndrome
Genitourinary: Candidal vaginitis
Hematologic: Transient thrombocytopenia, leukopenia, eosinophilia
Hepatic: Transient elevations of ALT, AST, alkaline phosphatase; cholestasis
Renal: Transient elevation of BUN and serum creatinine
Respiratory: Rhinitis
Miscellaneous: Anaphylaxis

Drug Interactions Probenecid inhibits renal excretion and increases the serum concentration of loracarbef

Food Interactions Administration with food decreases and delays the peak plasma concentration

Stability After reconstitution, suspension may be stored at room temperature for 14 days

Mechanism of Action Inhibits bacterial cell wall synthesis by binding to one or more of the penicillin binding proteins; inhibits the final transpeptidation step of peptidoglycan synthesis in bacterial cell walls, thus inhibiting cell wall biosynthesis. Upon exposure to beta-lactam antibiotics, bacteria eventually lyse due to ongoing activity of cell wall autolytic enzymes (autolysins and murein hydrolases) while cell wall assembly is arrested.

Pharmacokinetics
Absorption: Oral: Rapid; 90% absorbed from the GI tract
Distribution: Loracarbef middle-ear fluid concentration approximates 48% of the plasma concentration 2 hours after a dose in pediatric patients
Protein binding: 25%
Bioavailability: 90%
Half-life, elimination:
Children (suspension): ~0.78-0.85 hours
Adults, normal renal function: ~1 hour
Time to peak serum concentration: 0.5-1 hour after administration
Elimination: Primarily by the kidneys as unchanged drug in the urine

Usual Dosage Oral:
Children 6 months to 12 years:
Acute otitis media: 30 mg/kg/day divided every 12 hours for 10 days (should be treated with the **suspension** which results in higher peak plasma concentrations than the capsule)
(Continued)

Loracarbef *(Continued)*

Acute maxillary sinusitis: 30 mg/kg/day divided every 12 hours for 10 days
Pharyngitis/tonsillitis/skin and skin structure infections: 15 mg/kg/day divided every 12 hours

Adults:

Pneumonia, chronic bacterial bronchitis, sinusitis: 400 mg every 12 hours
Acute bacterial bronchitis: 200-400 mg every 12 hours
Uncomplicated urinary tract infections: 200 mg once daily for 7 days
Skin and skin structure: 200 mg every 12 hours
Uncomplicated pyelonephritis: 400 mg every 12 hours for 14 days

Dosing adjustment in renal impairment:

Cl_{cr} 10-49 mL/minute: 50% of usual dose at usual interval or usual dose given half as often

Cl_{cr} <10 mL/minute: Give usual dose every 3-5 days

Hemodialysis: Removed by hemodialysis; postdialysis dose should be administered when appropriate

Administration Oral: Administer on an empty stomach at least 1 hour before or 2 hours after meals

Monitoring Parameters Observe patient for diarrhea; with prolonged therapy, monitor renal function periodically

Dosage Forms

Capsule: 200 mg, 400 mg
Suspension, oral: 100 mg/5 mL (50 mL, 100 mL); 200 mg/5 mL (50 mL, 75 mL, 100 mL)

References

Force RW and Nahata MC, "Loracarbef: A New Orally Administered Carbacephem Antibiotic," *Ann Pharmacother*, 1993, 27(3):321-9.

Foshee WS, "Loracarbef (LY163892) Versus Amoxicillin-Clavulanate in the Treatment of Acute Otitis Media With Effusion," *J Pediatr*, 1992, 120(6):980-6.

Nelson JD, Shelton S, and Kusmiesz H, "Pharmacokinetics of LY163892 in Infants and Children," *Antimicrob Agents Chemother*, 1988, 32(11):1738-9.

Loratadine *(lor AT a deen)*

Brand Names Claritin®; Claritin® RediTab®

Therapeutic Category Antihistamine

Generic Available No

Use Symptomatic relief of nasal and non-nasal symptoms of allergic rhinitis

Pregnancy Risk Factor B

Contraindications Hypersensitivity to loratadine or any component

Warnings Use with caution and adjust dosage in patients with severe liver impairment

Precautions Use cautiously in patients who are also taking ketoconazole, itraconazole, fluconazole, erythromycin, clarithromycin, or other drugs which may impair loratadine's hepatic metabolism; although increased plasma levels of loratadine have been observed, no adverse effects with concomitant administration have been reported including Q-T interval prolongation which has occurred when similar antihistamines, terfenadine, and astemizole were combined with these agents; while less sedating than other antihistamines, loratadine may cause drowsiness and impair ability to perform hazardous activities requiring mental alertness
Use cautiously in breast-feeding women as breast milk levels of loratadine are equivalent to serum levels

Adverse Reactions

Cardiovascular: Hypotension, hypertension, palpitations, tachycardia, chest pain, syncope

Central nervous system: Headache, somnolence, fatigue, anxiety, depression, dizziness, fever, migraine, agitation

Dermatologic: Alopecia, dermatitis, dry skin, rash, pruritus, photosensitivity

Gastrointestinal: Xerostomia, nausea, vomiting, gastritis

Endocrine & metabolic: Breast pain and enlargement (rare), menorrhagia, dysmenorrhea

Neuromuscular & skeletal: Hyperkinesia, arthralgias, myalgias, leg cramps

Ophthalmic: Blurred vision, altered lacrimation, eye pain, conjunctivitis

Genitourinary: Discoloration of urine

Respiratory: Nasal dryness, pharyngitis, dyspnea, nasal congestion

Miscellaneous: Diaphoresis

Drug Interactions Increased plasma concentrations and AUC of loratadine and its active metabolite with ketoconazole, erythromycin, and cimetidine; no change in Q-T_c interval or cardiac arrhythmias have been seen (see Warnings); a prolonged Q-T interval was reported in one patient who was receiving quinidine and loratadine;

LORAZEPAM

additive CNS depression with other CNS depressants, alcohol, and procarbazine; prolonged anticholinergic effects with MAO inhibitors

Food Interactions Administration with food increases loratadine's bioavailability by 40%

Mechanism of Action Long-acting tricyclic antihistamine with selective peripheral histamine H_1 receptor antagonistic properties

Pharmacodynamics
Onset of Action: Within 1-3 hours
Peak effect: 8-12 hours
Duration: >24 hours

Pharmacokinetics
Absorption: Rapid; food increases total bioavailability (AUC) by 40%
Distribution: Binds preferentially to peripheral nervous system H1 receptors; no appreciable entry into CNS; loratadine and metabolite pass easily into breast milk and achieve concentrations equivalent to plasma levels; breast milk to plasma ratio: 1.17
Protein binding: 97% (loratadine), 73% to 77% (metabolite)
Metabolism: Extensive first-pass metabolism by cytochrome P-450 system to an active metabolite (descarboethoxyloratadine)
Half-life: 8.4 hours (loratadine), 28 hours (metabolite)
Elimination: 80% eliminated via urine & feces as metabolic products

Usual Dosage Oral:
Children ≥3 years and Adults:
<30 kg: 5 mg once daily
>30 kg: 10 mg once daily
Dosing interval in renal (GFR <30 mL/minute) or hepatic impairment: Administer dosage every other day

Administration Oral: Administer on an empty stomach or before meals; place Claritin® RediTab® (rapidly disintegrating tablet) on the tongue; tablet disintegration occurs rapidly; may administer with or without water

Monitoring Parameters Improvement in signs and symptoms of allergic rhinitis

Reference Range Therapeutic serum levels (not used clinically): Loratadine: 2.5-100 ng/mL; active metabolite: 0.5-100 ng/mL

Test Interactions Antigen skin testing

Patient Information Drink plenty of water; may cause dry mouth; may color urine; may cause drowsiness and impair ability to perform hazardous tasks requiring mental alertness or physical coordination; avoid prolonged exposure to sunlight; notify physician if fainting episode occurs

Dosage Forms
Syrup: 1 mg/mL (16 oz)
Tablet: 10 mg
Tablet, rapid-disintegrating (Claritin® RediTab®): 10 mg

References
Lin CC, Radwanski E, Affrime M, et al, "Pharmacokinetics of Loratadine in Pediatric Subjects," *Am J Therapeut*, 1995, 2:504-8.
Luck JC and Evrard HM, "Atrial Fibrillation Associated With Loratadine Use," *J Allergy Clin Immunol*, 1995, 95(2):282.
Lutsky BN, Klose P, Melon J, et al, "A Comparative Study of the Efficacy and Safety of Loratadine Syrup and Terfenadine Suspension in the Treatment of 3 to 6 Year Old Children With Seasonal Allergic Rhinitis," *Clin Ther*, 1993, 15(5):855-65.

Lorazepam (lor A ze pam)

Related Information
Carbohydrate and Alcohol Content of Liquid Medications for Use in Patients Receiving Ketogenic Diets *on page 1228*
Drugs and Breast-Feeding *on page 1213*
Overdose and Toxicology *on page 1191*
Preprocedure Sedatives in Children *on page 1169*

Brand Names Apo®-Lorazepam (Canada); Ativan®; Novo-Lorazepam® (Canada); Nu-Loraz® (Canada); PMS-Lorazepam (Canada); Pro-Lorazepam® (Canada)

Therapeutic Category Antianxiety Agent; Anticonvulsant, Benzodiazepine; Antiemetic; Benzodiazepine; Hypnotic; Sedative

Generic Available Yes

Use Management of anxiety; status epilepticus; preoperative sedation and amnesia

Restrictions C-IV

Pregnancy Risk Factor D

Contraindications Hypersensitivity to lorazepam or any component; there may be a cross-sensitivity with other benzodiazepines; do not use in a comatose patient, (Continued)

Lorazepam *(Continued)*

those with pre-existing CNS depression, narrow-angle glaucoma, severe uncontrolled pain, severe hypotension

Warnings Dilute injection prior to I.V. use with equal volume of compatible diluent; do not inject intra-arterially, arteriospasm and gangrene may occur; injection contains benzyl alcohol 2%, polyethylene glycol and propylene glycol, which may be toxic to newborns in high doses

Precautions Use with caution in neonates, especially in preterm infants (several cases of neurotoxicity and myoclonus have been reported); use with caution in patients with renal or hepatic impairment, compromised pulmonary function, or those receiving other CNS depressants

Adverse Reactions

Cardiovascular: Bradycardia, circulatory collapse, hypertension, or hypotension

Central nervous system: Confusion, CNS depression, sedation, drowsiness, lethargy, hangover effect, dizziness, transitory hallucinations, ataxia, rhythmic myoclonic jerking in preterm infants

Gastrointestinal: Constipation, xerostomia, nausea, vomiting

Genitourinary: Urinary incontinence or retention

Local: Pain with injection

Ocular: Diplopia, nystagmus

Respiratory: Respiratory depression, apnea

Miscellaneous: Physical and psychological dependence with prolonged use

Drug Interactions Other CNS or respiratory depressants may increase adverse effects

Stability Do not use if injection is discolored or contains precipitate; protect from light; refrigerate injectable form and oral solution; injection is stable at room temperature for 8 weeks

Mechanism of Action Depresses all levels of the CNS, including the limbic and reticular formation, by binding to the benzodiazepine site on the gamma-aminobutyric acid (GABA) receptor complex and modulating GABA, which is a major inhibitory neurotransmitter in the brain

Pharmacodynamics Sedation:

Onset of effect:

Oral: Within 60 minutes

I.M.: 30-60 minutes

I.V.: 15-30 minutes

Duration: 8-12 hours

Pharmacokinetics

Absorption: Oral, I.M.: Rapid, complete

Distribution: Crosses into placenta; crosses into breast milk

V_d:

Neonates: 0.76 L/kg

Adults: 1.3 L/kg

Protein binding: ~85%

Metabolism: Primarily by glucuronide conjugation in the liver

Bioavailability: Oral: 90% to 93%

Half-life:

Full-term neonates: 40.2 hours; range: 18-73 hours

Older Children: 10.5 hours; range: 6-17 hours

Adults: 12.9 hours; range: 10-16 hours

Elimination: In urine primarily as the glucuronide conjugate

Usual Dosage

Adjunct to antiemetic therapy: Children: I.V.: 0.04-0.08 mg/kg/dose (maximum dose: 4 mg) every 6 hours as needed

Anxiety/sedation:

Infants and Children: Oral, I.V.: Usual: 0.05 mg/kg/dose (maximum dose: 2 mg/dose) every 4-8 hours; range: 0.02-0.1 mg/kg

Adults: Oral: 1-10 mg/day in 2-3 divided doses; usual dose: 2-6 mg/day in divided doses

Insomnia: Adults: Oral: 2-4 mg at bedtime

Operative amnesia: Adults: I.V.: up to 0.05 mg/kg; maximum dose: 4 mg/dose

Preoperative: Adults: I.M.: 0.05 mg/kg administered 2 hours before surgery; maximum dose: 4 mg/dose; I.V.: 0.044 mg/kg 15-20 minutes before surgery; usual maximum dose: 2 mg/dose

Sedation (preprocedure): Infants and Children:

Oral, I.M., I.V.: Usual: 0.05 mg/kg; range: 0.02-0.09 mg/kg

I.V.: may use smaller doses (eg, 0.01-0.03 mg/kg) and repeat every 20 minutes, as needed to titrate to effect

Status epilepticus: I.V.:
Neonates: 0.05 mg/kg over 2-5 minutes; may repeat in 10-15 minutes (see warning regarding benzyl alcohol)
Infants and Children: 0.1 mg/kg slow I.V. over 2-5 minutes, do not exceed 4 mg/single dose; may repeat second dose of 0.05 mg/kg slow I.V. in 10-15 minutes if needed
Adolescents: 0.07 mg/kg slow I.V. over 2-5 minutes; maximum dose: 4 mg/dose; may repeat in 10-15 minutes
Adults: 4 mg/dose given slowly over 2-5 minutes; may repeat in 10-15 minutes; usual total maximum dose per 12-hour period: 8 mg

Administration
Oral: May administer with food to decrease GI distress; oral solution may be diluted in water, juice, soda, or semisolid food (eg, applesauce, pudding)
Parenteral: I.V.: Do not exceed 2 mg/minute or 0.05 mg/kg over 2-5 minutes; dilute I.V. dose with equal volume of compatible diluent (D_5W, NS, SWI); administer I.V. using repeated aspiration with slow I.V. injection, to make sure the injection is not intra-arterial and that perivascular extravasation has not occurred

Monitoring Parameters Respiratory rate, blood pressure, heart rate; CBC with differential and liver function with long-term use

Patient Information Avoid alcohol; limit caffeine; may be habit-forming; may cause drowsiness and impair ability to perform activities requiring mental alertness or physical coordination

Additional Information Single oral doses >0.09 mg/kg produced increased ataxia without increasing sedative benefit vs lower doses; since both strengths of injection contain 2% benzyl alcohol, Neofax® recommends using the 4 mg/mL strength for dilution with preservative free sterile water to make a 0.4 mg/mL dilution for I.V. use in neonates (in order to decrease the amount of benzyl alcohol delivered to the neonate); however, the stability of this dilution has not been studied. Diarrhea in a 9 month old infant receiving high-dose oral lorazepam was attributed to the lorazepam oral solution that contained polyethylene glycol and propylene glycol (both are osmotically active); diarrhea resolved when crushed tablets were substituted for the oral solution (see Marshall, 1995).

Dosage Forms
Injection: 2 mg/mL (1 mL, 10 mL); 4 mg/mL (1 mL, 10 mL)
Solution, oral concentrated, alcohol and dye free: 2 mg/mL (30 mL)
Tablet: 0.5 mg, 1 mg, 2 mg

References
Crawford TO, Mitchell WG, and Snodgrass SR, "Lorazepam in Childhood Status Epilepticus and Serial Seizures: Effectiveness and Tachyphylaxis," *Neurology*, 1987, 37(2):190-5.
Deshmukh A, Wittert W, Schnitzler E, et al, "Lorazepam in the Treatment of Refractory Neonatal Seizures: A Pilot Study," *Am J Dis Child*, 1986, 140(10):1042-4.
Henry DW, Burwinkle JW, and Klutman NE, "Determination of Sedative and Amnestic Doses of Lorazepam in Children," *Clin Pharm*, 1991, 10(8):625-9.
Lee DS, Wong HA, and Knoppert DC, "Myoclonus Associated With Lorazepam Therapy in Very-Low-Birth-Weight Infants," *Biol Neonate*, 1994, 66(6):311-5.
Marshall JD, Farrar HC, and Kearns GL, "Diarrhea Associated With Enteral Benzodiazepine Solutions," *J Pediatr*, 1995, 126(4):657-9.
McDermott CA, Kowalczyk AL, Schnitzler ER, et al, "Pharmacokinetics of Lorazepam in Critically Ill Neonates With Seizures," *J Pediatr*, 1992, 120(3):479-83.

- **Luminal®** *see* Phenobarbital *on page 754*
- **Lupron®** *see* Leuprolide *on page 561*
- **Lupron Depot®** *see* Leuprolide *on page 561*
- **Lupron Depot-3® Month** *see* Leuprolide *on page 561*
- **Lupron Depot-4® Month** *see* Leuprolide *on page 561*
- **Lupron Depot-Ped™** *see* Leuprolide *on page 561*
- **Luride®** *see* Fluoride *on page 427*
- **Luride®-SF** *see* Fluoride *on page 427*
- **Lutrepulse®** *see* Gonadorelin *on page 461*
- **Luxiq™** *see* Betamethasone *on page 130*
- **Lyderm® (Canada)** *see* Fluocinonide *on page 426*

Lymphocyte Immune Globulin (LIM foe site i MYUN GLOB yoo lin)

Brand Names Atgam®

Synonyms Antithymocyte Globulin (equine); ATG; Horse Antihuman Thymocyte Gamma Globulin

Therapeutic Category Immunosuppressant Agent

Generic Available No

Use Prevention and/or treatment of allograft rejection; treatment of moderate to severe aplastic anemia in patients not considered suitable candidates for bone marrow transplantation; prevention of graft-vs-host disease following bone marrow transplantation

Pregnancy Risk Factor C

Contraindications Hypersensitivity to ATG, thimerosal, any component, or other equine gamma globulins; severe, unremitting leukopenia and/or thrombocytopenia

Warnings Should only be used by physicians experienced in immunosuppressive therapy or management of renal transplant patients; adequate laboratory and supportive medical resources must be readily available in the facility for patient management

Adverse Reactions

Cardiovascular: Hypotension, hypertension, tachycardia, edema

Central nervous system: Seizures, fever, headache, chills

Dermatologic: Rash, pruritus, urticaria

Gastrointestinal: Diarrhea, nausea, stomatitis

Hematologic: Leukopenia, thrombocytopenia, hemolysis, anemia

Local: Thrombophlebitis

Neuromuscular & skeletal: Arthralgia; pain in the chest, flank, or back; weakness

Renal: Acute renal failure

Respiratory: Dyspnea

Miscellaneous: Lymphadenopathy, serum sickness, night sweats; anaphylaxis may be indicated by hypotension or respiratory distress

Stability Store in refrigerator; dilute in $\frac{1}{2}$NS or NS; when diluted to concentrations up to 4 mg/mL, ATG infusion solution is stable for 24 hours; use of dextrose solutions is not recommended; precipitation can occur in solutions with a low salt concentration (ie, D_5W)

Mechanism of Action May involve elimination of antigen-reactive T-lymphocytes (killer cells) in peripheral blood or alteration of T-cell function

Pharmacokinetics

Distribution: Poor into lymphoid tissues

Binds to circulating lymphocytes, granulocytes, platelets, bone marrow cells

Half-life, plasma: 1.5-12 days

Elimination: ~1% of dose excreted in urine

Usual Dosage Intradermal skin test is recommended prior to administration of the initial dose of ATG; use 0.1 mL of a 1:1000 dilution of ATG in NS; observe the skin test every 15 minutes for 1 hour; a local reaction ≥10 mm diameter with a wheal or erythema or both should be considered a positive skin test

I.V.:

Children:

Aplastic anemia protocol: 10-20 mg/kg/day for 8-14 days, or 40 mg/kg/day once daily over 4 hours for 4 days; then give 10-30 mg/kg/dose every other day for 7 more doses

Cardiac allograft: 10 mg/kg/day for 7 days or as per protocol

Renal allograft: 5-25 mg/kg/day or as per protocol

Children and Adults:
Rejection prevention: 15 mg/kg/day for 14 days, then give every other day for 7 more doses; initial dose should be administered within 24 hours before or after transplantation
Rejection treatment: 10-15 mg/kg/day for 14 days, then give every other day for 7 more doses

Administration Parenteral: Administer via central line; use of high flow veins will minimize the occurrence of phlebitis and thrombosis; administer by slow I.V. infusion through a 0.2-1 micron in-line filter over 4-8 hours at a final concentration not to exceed 4 mg ATG/mL

Monitoring Parameters Lymphocyte profile; CBC with differential and platelet count, vital signs during administration, renal function test

Nursing Implications Patient may need to be pretreated with an antipyretic, antihistamine, and/or corticosteroid to prevent chills and fever

Dosage Forms Injection: 50 mg/mL (5 mL)

References
Rosenfeld SJ, Kimball J, Vining D, et al, "Intensive Immunosuppression With Antithymocyte Globulin and Cyclosporine as Treatment for Severe Acquired Aplastic Anemia," *Blood*, 1995, 85(11):3058-65.
Whitehead B, James I, Helms P, et al, "Intensive Care Management of Children Following Heart and Heart-Lung Transplantation," *Intensive Care Med*, 1990, 16(7):426-30.

♦ **Lymphocyte Mitogenic Factor** *see* Aldesleukin *on page 42*
♦ **Lyphocin® Injection** *see* Vancomycin *on page 969*
♦ **Maalox® [OTC]** *see* Antacid Preparations *on page 86*
♦ **Maalox Anti-Gas® [OTC]** *see* Simethicone *on page 868*
♦ **Maalox® Plus Extra Strength [OTC]** *see* Antacid Preparations *on page 86*
♦ **Macrobid®** *see* Nitrofurantoin *on page 689*
♦ **Macrodantin®** *see* Nitrofurantoin *on page 689*
♦ **Macrodex®** *see* Dextran *on page 299*

Mafenide (MA fe nide)

Brand Names Sulfamylon®
Available Salts Mafenide Acetate
Therapeutic Category Antibiotic, Topical
Generic Available No
Use Adjunct in the treatment of second and third degree burns to prevent septicemia caused by susceptible organisms such as *Pseudomonas aeruginosa*
Pregnancy Risk Factor C
Contraindications Hypersensitivity to mafenide, sulfites, or any component
Warnings Superinfection with nonsusceptible organisms has occurred in burn wounds treated with mafenide
Precautions Use with caution in patients with renal impairment and in patients with G-6-PD deficiency
Adverse Reactions
Dermatologic: Erythema, rash, pruritus, urticaria
Endocrine & metabolic: Hyperchloremia, metabolic acidosis
Hematologic: Bone marrow suppression, hemolytic anemia, bleeding, porphyria, eosinophilia
Local: Burning sensation, excoriation, pain, swelling
Respiratory: Hyperventilation, tachypnea
Miscellaneous: Hypersensitivity reactions, facial edema
Stability Prepared topical solution is stable for 48 hours at room temperature
Mechanism of Action Interferes with bacterial cellular metabolism and bacterial folic acid synthesis through competitive inhibition of para-aminobenzoic acid
Pharmacokinetics
Absorption: Diffuses through devascularized areas and is rapidly absorbed from burned surface
Metabolism: To para-carboxybenzene sulfonamide which is a carbonic anhydrase inhibitor
Time to peak serum concentration: Topical: 2-4 hours
Elimination: In urine as metabolites
Usual Dosage Children ≥3 months and Adults: Topical
Cream: Apply once or twice daily; apply to a thickness of approximately 16 mm; the burned area should be covered with cream at all times
Solution: Irrigate dressing every 4 hours or as needed to keep gauze moistened
Administration Topical:
Cream: Apply to cleansed, debrided, burned area with a sterile-gloved hand
(Continued)

Mafenide *(Continued)*

Solution: Reconstitute 50 g powder by adding to 1 liter sterile water or 1 liter NS for irrigation; mix until completely dissolved; filter solution through a 0.22 micron filter before use; cover area with gauze and the dressing wetted with mafenide solution; wound dressing may be left undisturbed for up to 5 days

Monitoring Parameters Acid base balance, improvement of wound healing

Patient Information Inform physician if rash, blisters, or swelling appear

Nursing Implications For external use only

Dosage Forms

Cream, topical, as acetate: 85 mg/g (56.7 g, 113.4 g, 411 g)

Powder, topical: 5% (50 g)

- ◆ **Mafenide Acetate** *see Mafenide on page 587*
- ◆ **Mag-200** *see Magnesium Supplements on page 588*
- ◆ **Magaldrate** *see Antacid Preparations on page 86*
- ◆ **Mag-Carb™** *see Magnesium Supplements on page 588*
- ◆ **Magnesia Magma (Magnesium Hydroxide)** *see Magnesium Supplements on page 588*
- ◆ **Magnesium Carbonate** *see Magnesium Supplements on page 588*
- ◆ **Magnesium Chloride** *see Magnesium Supplements on page 588*
- ◆ **Magnesium Citrate** *see Magnesium Supplements on page 588*
- ◆ **Magnesium Gluconate** *see Magnesium Supplements on page 588*
- ◆ **Magnesium Hydroxide** *see Magnesium Supplements on page 588*
- ◆ **Magnesium Hydroxide and Mineral Oil Emulsion** *see Magnesium Supplements on page 588*
- ◆ **Magnesium Lactate** *see Magnesium Supplements on page 588*
- ◆ **Magnesium Oxide** *see Magnesium Supplements on page 588*
- ◆ **Magnesium Sulfate** *see Magnesium Supplements on page 588*

Magnesium Supplements *(mag NEE zee um SUP la ments)*

Related Information

Adult ACLS Algorithm, V. Fib and Pulseless V. Tach *on page 1004*

Brand Names Almora®; Evac-Q-Mag®; Haley's M-O®; Mag-200; Mag-Carb™; Magonate®; Mag-Ox 400®; Mag-Tab SR®; Magtrate; Maox®; Phillips'® Milk of Magnesia; Slow-Mag®; Uro-Mag®

Available Salts Magnesium Carbonate; Magnesium Chloride; Magnesium Citrate; Magnesium Gluconate; Magnesium Hydroxide; Magnesium Hydroxide and Mineral Oil Emulsion; Magnesium Lactate; Magnesium Oxide; Magnesium Sulfate

Synonyms Citrate of Magnesia (Magnesium Citrate); Epsom Salts (Magnesium Sulfate); Magnesia Magma (Magnesium Hydroxide); Milk of Magnesia (Magnesium Hydroxide); MOM (Magnesium Hydroxide)

Therapeutic Category Antacid; Anticonvulsant, Miscellaneous; Electrolyte Supplement, Oral; Electrolyte Supplement, Parenteral; Laxative, Osmotic; Magnesium Salt

Generic Available Yes

Use

Treatment and prevention of hypomagnesemia **(magnesium chloride, magnesium lactate, magnesium carbonate, magnesium sulfate, magnesium gluconate, and magnesium oxide)**

Treatment of hypertension **(magnesium sulfate)**

Treatment of encephalopathy and seizures associated with acute nephritis **(magnesium sulfate)**

Short-term treatment of constipation **(magnesium citrate, magnesium hydroxide, magnesium sulfate, and magnesium oxide)**

Treatment of hyperacidity symptoms **(magnesium hydroxide and magnesium oxide)**

Adjunctive treatment in moderate to severe acute asthma **(magnesium sulfate)**

Pregnancy Risk Factor B

Contraindications Serious renal impairment, myocardial damage, heart block; patients with colostomy or ileostomy, intestinal obstruction, impaction, or perforation, appendicitis, abdominal pain

Precautions Use with caution in patients with impaired renal function (accumulation of magnesium may lead to magnesium intoxication); use with caution in digitalized patients (may alter cardiac conduction leading to heart block)

Adverse Reactions Adverse effects with magnesium therapy are related to the magnesium serum level

>3 mg/dL: Depressed CNS, blocked peripheral neuromuscular transmission leading to anticonvulsant effects

>5 mg/dL: Depressed deep tendon reflexes, flushing, somnolence

>12 mg/dL: Respiratory paralysis, complete heart block

Other effects:
  Cardiovascular: Hypotension
  Endocrine & metabolic: Hypermagnesemia
  Gastrointestinal: Diarrhea, abdominal cramps, gas formation
  Neuromuscular & skeletal: Muscle weakness

Drug Interactions Magnesium salts, when given orally, may decrease the absorption of the following: H_2 antagonists, phenytoin, iron salts, penicillamine, tetracycline, ciprofloxacin, benzodiazepines, chloroquine, steroids, and glyburide; systemic magnesium may enhance the effects of calcium channel blockers and neuromuscular blockers; may share additive CNS depressant effects with CNS depressants; if sufficient alkalinization of the urine by magnesium salts occurs, the excretion of salicylates is enhanced and the tubular reabsorption of quinidine is enhanced (increased effect)

Mechanism of Action Magnesium is important as a cofactor in many enzymatic reactions in the body. There are at least 300 enzymes which are dependent upon magnesium for normal functioning. Actions on lipoprotein lipase have been found to be important in reducing serum cholesterol. Magnesium is necessary for the maintaining of serum potassium and calcium levels due to its effect on the renal tubule. In the heart, magnesium acts as a calcium channel blocker. It also activates sodium potassium ATPase in the cell membrane to promote resting polarization and produce arrhythmias. Promotes bowel evacuation by causing osmotic retention of fluid which distends the colon and produces increased peristaltic activity when taken orally. To reduce stomach acidity, it reacts with hydrochloric acid in the stomach to form magnesium chloride.

Pharmacodynamics
Onset of action:
  Anticonvulsant:
    I.M.: 60 minutes
    I.V.: Immediately
  Laxative: Oral: 4-8 hours
Duration: Anticonvulsant:
  I.M.: 3-4 hours
  I.V.: 30 minutes

Pharmacokinetics
Absorption: Oral: Up to 30%
Elimination: Renal with unabsorbed drug excreted in feces

Usual Dosage Note: Multiple salt forms of magnesium exist; close attention must be paid to the salt form when ordering and administering magnesium; incorrect selection or substitution of one salt for another without proper dosage adjustment may result in serious over- or underdosing.

Recommended daily allowance of magnesium: See table.

Magnesium - Recommended Daily Allowance (RDA) and Estimated Average Requirement (EAR) (in terms of elemental magnesium)

Age	RDA (mg/day)	EAR (mg/day)
<6 mo	40	30*
6-12 mo	60	75*
1-3 y	80	65
4-8 y	130	110
Male		
9-13 y	240	200
14-18 y	410	340
19-30 y	400	330
Female		
9-13 y	240	200
14-18 y	360	300
19-30 y	310	255

*Adequate intake (AI)

(Continued)

Magnesium Supplements *(Continued)*

HYPOMAGNESEMIA:

Neonates: I.V.:

Magnesium sulfate: 25-50 mg/kg/dose (0.2-0.4 mEq/kg/dose) every 8-12 hours for 2-3 doses

Magnesium chloride: 0.2-0.4 mEq/kg/dose every 8-12 hours for 2-3 doses

Children:

I.M., I.V.:

Magnesium sulfate: 25-50 mg/kg/dose (0.2-0.4 mEq/kg/dose) every 4-6 hours for 3-4 doses; maximum single dose: 2000 mg (16 mEq)

Magnesium chloride: 0.2-0.4 mEq/kg/dose every 4-6 hours for 3-4 doses; maximum single dose 16 mEq

Oral:

Magnesium chloride, gluconate, lactate, carbonate, oxide, or sulfate salts: 10-20 mg/kg **elemental magnesium** per dose 4 times/day

Adults:

Magnesium gluconate: Oral: 500-1000 mg 3 times/day

Magnesium sulfate:

I.M., I.V.: 1 g every 6 hours for 4 doses, or 250 mg/kg over a 4-hour period; for severe hypomagnesemia: 8-12 g/day in divided doses has been used

Oral: 3 g every 6 hours for 4 doses

DAILY MAINTENANCE MAGNESIUM: I.V.:

Magnesium sulfate or magnesium chloride:

Neonates, Infants, and Children ≤45 kg: 0.25-0.5 mEq/kg/day

Adolescents >45 kg and Adults: 0.2-0.5 mEq/kg/day or 3-10 mEq/1000 kcal/day (maximum 8-16 mEq/day)

MANAGEMENT OF SEIZURES AND HYPERTENSION: I.M., I.V.:

Magnesium sulfate:

Children: 20-100 mg/kg/dose every 4-6 hours as needed; in severe cases doses as high as 200 mg/kg/dose have been used

Adults: 1 g every 6 hours for 4 doses as needed

BRONCHODILATION (adjunctive treatment in moderate to severe acute asthma; unlabeled use): I.V.:

Magnesium sulfate:

Children: 25 mg/kg/dose (maximum dose 2 g) as a single dose

Adults: 2 g as a single dose

Note: Literature evaluating magnesium sulfate's efficacy in the relief of bronchospasm has utilized single dosages in patient's with acute symptomatology who have received aerosol β-agonist therapy (see References).

CATHARTIC: Oral:

Magnesium citrate (Citrate of magnesia):

<6 years: 2-4 mL/kg given once or in divided doses

6-12 years: 100-150 mL

≥12 years and Adults: 150-300 mL

Magnesium hydroxide (Milk of magnesia, MOM):

<2 years: 0.5 mL/kg/dose

2-5 years: 5-15 mL/day once or in divided doses

6-11 years: 15-30 mL/day once or in divided doses

≥12 years and adults: 30-60 mL/day once or in divided doses

Magnesium hydroxide and mineral oil (Haley's M-O) (pediatric dosage to provide equivalent dosage of magnesium hydroxide)

<2 years: 0.6 mL/kg/dose

2-5 years: 6-18 mL/day once or in divided doses

6-11 years: 18-36 mL/day once or in divided doses

≥12 years and Adults: 30-45 mL once or in divided doses

Magnesium sulfate:

Children: 0.25 g/kg/dose once or in divided doses

Adults: 10-30 g

Magnesium oxide: Adults: 2-4 g at bedtime with full glass of water

ANTACID Oral:

Magnesium hydroxide:

Children: Liquid: 2.5-5 mL/dose, up to 4 times/day

Adults:

Liquid: 5-15 mL/dose, up to 4 times/day

Liquid concentrate: 2.5-7.5 mL/dose, up to 4 times/day

Tablet: 622-1244 mg/dose, up to 4 times/day

Magnesium oxide: Adults: 140 mg 3-4 times/day or 400-840 mg/day

Dosing in renal impairment: Patients in severe renal failure should not receive magnesium due to toxicity from accumulation. Patients with a Cl_{cr} <25 mL/minute receiving magnesium should have serum magnesium levels monitored.

Elemental Magnesium Content of Magnesium Salts

Magnesium Salt	Elemental Magnesium (mg per 500 mg salt)	mEq Magnesium per 500 mg salt
Magnesium carbonate	140	11.7
Magnesium chloride	59	4.9
Magnesium gluconate	27	2.4
Magnesium lactate	50	4.2
Magnesium oxide	302	25
Magnesium sulfate	49.3	4.1

Administration

Oral:

Solution: Mix with water and administer on an empty stomach; chill **magnesium citrate** prior to administration to improve palatability

Tablet: Take with full glass of water; chew **magnesium hydroxide** chewable tablets thoroughly; do not chew or crush sustained release formulations

Parenteral: Intermittent infusion: Dilute to a concentration of 0.5 mEq/mL (60 mg/mL of **magnesium sulfate**) (maximum concentration: 1.6 mEq/mL, 200 mg/mL of **magnesium sulfate**) and infuse over 2-4 hours; do not exceed 1 mEq/kg/hour (125 mg/kg/hour of **magnesium sulfate**); in severe circumstances, half of the dosage to be administered may be infused over the first 15-20 minutes; for I.M. administration, dilute **magnesium sulfate** to a maximum concentration of 200 mg/mL prior to injection

Monitoring Parameters Serum magnesium, deep tendon reflexes, respiratory rate, renal function, blood pressure, stool output (laxative use)

Reference Range

Neonates and Infants: 1.5-2.3 mEq/L

Children: 1.5-2.0 mEq/L

Adults: 1.4-2.0 mEq/L

Additional Information 1 g elemental magnesium = 83.3 mEq = 41.1 mmol

Dosage Forms Amount of magnesium salt is listed with **elemental** magnesium content in brackets

Magnesium, amino acid chelate: Tablet: 500 mg [100 mg]

Magnesium carbonate: Capsule, gelatin (Mag-Carb™): 250 mg [5.8 mEq; 70 mg]

Magnesium chloride:

Injection: 20% [1.97 mEq/mL] (50 mL)

Tablet, sustained release: 535 mg [5.2 mEq; 63 mg]

Magnesium citrate: Solution: 3.85-4.71 mEq/5mL (300 mL)

Magnesium gluconate:

Solution: 1000 mg/5 mL [4.8 mEq; 54 mg]

Tablet: 500 mg [2.4 mEq; 27 mg]

Magnesium hydroxide:

Liquid: 390 mg/5 mL (10 mL, 15 mL, 20 mL, 30 mL, 100 mL, 120 mL, 180 mL, 360 mL, 720 mL); 400 mg/5 mL; 800 mg/5 mL

Liquid, concentrate: 10 mL equivalent to 30 mL milk of magnesia USP

Suspension, oral: 2.5 g/30 mL (10 mL, 15 mL, 30 mL)

Tablet, chewable: 311 mg

Magnesium hydroxide and mineral oil:

Suspension (Haley's M-O®): Each 30 mL contains magnesium hydroxide 24 mL and mineral oil 6 mL

Magnesium lactate: Caplet, sustained release (Mag-Tab SR®): 835 mg [7 mEq; 84 mg]

Magnesium oxide:

Capsule: 140 mg [7 mEq; 84 mg]

Tablet: 400 mg [20 mEq; 242 mg], 420 mg [21 mEq; 254 mg], 500 mg [25 mEq; 302 mg]

Magnesium sulfate:

Granules: ~40 mEq magnesium/5 g (240 g)

Injection: 100 mg/mL (20 mL); 125 mg/mL (8 mL); 250 mg/mL (150 mL); 500 mg/mL (2 mL, 5 mL, 10 mL, 30 mL, 50 mL)

Solution, oral: 50% 500 mg/mL (30 mL) [4.1 mEq/mL; 49.3 mg]

(Continued)

Magnesium Supplements *(Continued)*

References

Bloch H, Silverman R, Mancherje N, et al, "Intravenous Magnesium Sulfate as an Adjunct in the Treatment of Acute Asthma," *Chest*, 1995, 107(6):1576-81.

Chernow B, Smith J, Rainey TG, et al, "Hypomagnesemia: Implications for the Critical Care Specialist," *Crit Care Med*, 1982, 10(3):193-6.

Ciarallo L, Sauer AH, and Shannon MW, "Intravenous Magnesium Therapy for Moderate to Severe Pediatric Asthma: Results of a Randomized, Placebo-Controlled Trial," *J Pediatr*, 1996, 129(6):809-14.

"Dietary Reference Intakes for Calcium, Phosphorus, Magnesium, Vitamin D, and Fluoride. Standing Committee on the Scientific Evaluation of Dietary Reference Intakes, Food and Nutrition Board, Institute of Medicine," National Academy of Sciences, Washington, DC: National Academy Press, 1997.

Engel J, "Normal Laboratory Values," *Pocket Guide to Pediatric Assessment*, St Louis, MO: CV Mosby, 1989, 259.

♦ **Magonate®** *see* Magnesium Supplements *on page 588*

♦ **Mag-Ox 400®** *see* Magnesium Supplements *on page 588*

♦ **Mag-Tab SR®** *see* Magnesium Supplements *on page 588*

♦ **Magtrate** *see* Magnesium Supplements *on page 588*

♦ **Ma Huang** *see* Ephedrine *on page 369*

♦ **Maigret-50** *see* Phenylpropanolamine *on page 761*

♦ **Malatal®** *see* Hyoscyamine, Atropine, Scopolamine, and Phenobarbital *on page 499*

♦ **Mallamint® [OTC]** *see* Calcium Supplements *on page 157*

♦ **Mallergan-VC® With Codeine** *see* Promethazine, Phenylephrine, and Codeine *on page 809*

Malt Soup Extract *(malt soop EKS trakt)*

Brand Names Maltsupex® [OTC]

Therapeutic Category Laxative, Bulk-Producing

Generic Available No

Use Short-term treatment of constipation

Contraindications Hypersensitivity to barley malt extract or any component

Warnings Do not use when abdominal pain, nausea, or vomiting are present

Adverse Reactions Gastrointestinal: Abdominal cramps, diarrhea, rectal obstruction

Mechanism of Action Holds water in stool, reduces fecal pH

Pharmacodynamics Onset of action: Effect is usually apparent in 12-24 hours

Pharmacokinetics Hydrolyzed in the colon, metabolized by the liver

Usual Dosage Oral:

Infants >1 month:

Breast-fed:

Liquid: 1-2 teaspoonfuls in 2-4 oz of water or fruit juice 1-2 times/day for 3-4 days

Powder: 4 g in 2-4 oz of water or fruit juice daily for 3-4 days

Bottle-fed:

Liquid: $^1/_2$ to 2 tablespoonfuls/day in formula for 3-4 days, then 1-2 teaspoonfuls/day

Powder: 8-16 g/day in formula for 3-4 days, then 4-8 g/day

Children:

2-6 years:

Liquid: 7.5 mL 1-2 times/day for 3-4 days

Powder: 8 g twice daily for 3-4 days

6-12 years:

Liquid: 15-30 mL 1-2 times/day for 3-4 days

Powder: Up to 16 g/day for 3-4 days

Children ≥12 years and Adults:

Liquid: 30 mL twice daily for 3-4 days, then 15-30 mL at bedtime

Powder: Up to 32 g twice daily for 3-4 days, then 16-32 g at bedtime

Tablets: 4 tablets 4 times/day (maximum dose: 64 g/day)

Administration Oral: Add to warm water and stir; then add milk, formula, water, or fruit juice until dissolved

Dosage Forms

Liquid: Nondiastatic barley malt extract 16 g/15 mL

Powder: Nondiastatic barley malt extract 16 g/tablespoonful

Tablet: Nondiastatic barley malt extract 750 mg

♦ **Maltsupex® [OTC]** *see* Malt Soup Extract *on page 592*

♦ **Mandelamine®** *see* Methenamine *on page 615*

♦ **Mandelamine® (Canada)** *see* Methenamine *on page 615*

♦ **Manganese Chloride** *see* Trace Metals *on page 940*
♦ **Manganese Sulfate** *see* Trace Metals *on page 940*

Mannitol (MAN i tole)

Brand Names Osmitrol® Injection; Resectisol® Irrigation Solution

Synonyms *D*-Mannitol

Therapeutic Category Diuretic, Osmotic

Generic Available Yes

Use Reduction of increased intracranial pressure (ICP) associated with cerebral edema; promotion of diuresis in the prevention and/or treatment of oliguria or anuria due to acute renal failure; reduction of increased intraocular pressure; promotion of urinary excretion of toxic substances

Pregnancy Risk Factor C

Contraindications Hypersensitivity to mannitol or any component; severe renal disease, dehydration, active intracranial bleeding, severe pulmonary edema, or congestion

Adverse Reactions
Cardiovascular: Circulatory overload, CHF (due to inadequate urine output and overexpansion of extracellular fluid)
Central nervous system: Convulsions, headache
Endocrine & metabolic: Fluid and electrolyte imbalance, hyponatremia or hypernatremia, hypokalemia or hyperkalemia, water intoxication, dehydration and hypovolemia secondary to rapid diuresis
Gastrointestinal: Xerostomia
Local: Tissue necrosis
Respiratory: Pulmonary edema
Miscellaneous: Allergic reactions

Drug Interactions Lithium

Stability Store at room temperature (15°C to 30°C); protect from freezing; crystallization may occur at low temperatures; do not use solutions that contain crystals; heating in a hot water bath and vigorous shaking may be utilized for resolubilization of crystals; cool solutions to body temperature before using; incompatible with strongly acidic or alkaline solutions; potassium chloride or sodium chloride may cause precipitation of mannitol 20% or 25% solution

Mechanism of Action Increases the osmotic pressure of glomerular filtrate, which inhibits tubular reabsorption of water and electrolytes and increases urinary output

Pharmacodynamics After I.V. injection:
Diuresis: Onset of action: Within 1-3 hours
Reduction in ICP:
Onset of action: Within 15 minutes
Duration: 3-6 hours

Pharmacokinetics
Distribution: Remains confined to extracellular space; does not penetrate blood-brain barrier (except in very high concentrations or with acidosis)
Metabolism: Minimal amounts in the liver to glycogen
Half-life: 1.1-1.6 hours
Elimination: Primarily unchanged in urine by glomerular filtration

Usual Dosage I.V.:
Children:
Test dose (to assess adequate renal function): 200 mg/kg (maximum dose: 12.5 g) over 3-5 minutes to produce a urine flow of at least 1 mL/kg/hour for 1-3 hours
Initial: 0.5-1 g/kg
Maintenance: 0.25-0.5 g/kg every 4-6 hours
Adults:
Test dose: 12.5 g (200 mg/kg) over 3-5 minutes to produce a urine flow of at least 30-50 mL of urine per hour over the next 2-3 hours
Initial: 0.5-1 g/kg
Maintenance: 0.25-0.5 g/kg every 4-6 hours

Administration Parenteral: In-line filter set (≤5 micron) should always be used for mannitol infusion with concentrations ≥20%; administer test dose (for oliguria) I.V. push over 3-5 minutes; for cerebral edema or elevated ICP, administer over 20-30 minutes

Monitoring Parameters Renal function, daily fluid intake and output, serum electrolytes, serum and urine osmolality; for treatment of elevated intracranial pressure, maintain serum osmolality 310-320 mOsm/kg

Nursing Implications Avoid extravasation; crenation and agglutination of red blood cells may occur if administered with whole blood
(Continued)

Mannitol *(Continued)*

Additional Information Approximate osmolarity: Mannitol 20%: 1100 mOsm/L; mannitol 25%: 1375 mOsm/L

Dosage Forms

Injection: 5% [50 mg/mL] (1000 mL); 10% [100 mg/mL] (500 mL, 1000 mL); 15% [150 mg/mL] (150 mL, 500 mL); 20% [200 mg/mL] (150 mL, 250 mL, 500 mL); 25% [250 mg/mL] (50 mL)

Solution, urogenital: 0.54% [5.4 mg/mL] (2000 mL)

- ♦ **Maox®** *see* Magnesium Supplements *on page 588*
- ♦ **Mapap®** **[OTC]** *see* Acetaminophen *on page 26*
- ♦ **Maranox®** **[OTC]** *see* Acetaminophen *on page 26*
- ♦ **Marbaxin®** *see* Methocarbamol *on page 619*
- ♦ **Marcaine®** *see* Bupivacaine *on page 148*
- ♦ **Marcillin®** *see* Ampicillin *on page 78*
- ♦ **Margesic® H** *see* Hydrocodone and Acetaminophen *on page 485*
- ♦ **Marinol®** *see* Dronabinol *on page 350*
- ♦ **Marmine® Injection** *see* Dimenhydrinate *on page 325*
- ♦ **Marmine® Oral [OTC]** *see* Dimenhydrinate *on page 325*
- ♦ **Matulane®** *see* Procarbazine *on page 802*
- ♦ **Maxair™ Autohaler™** *see* Pirbuterol *on page 776*
- ♦ **Maxair™ Inhalation Aerosol** *see* Pirbuterol *on page 776*
- ♦ **Maxeran® (Canada)** *see* Metoclopramide *on page 630*
- ♦ **Maxidex® Ophthalmic** *see* Dexamethasone *on page 294*
- ♦ **Maximum Strength Nytol® [OTC]** *see* Diphenhydramine *on page 327*
- ♦ **Maxipime®** *see* Cefepime *on page 179*
- ♦ **Maxitrol® Ophthalmic** *see* Dexamethasone, Neomycin, and Polymyxin B *on page 297*
- ♦ **Maxivate® Topical** *see* Betamethasone *on page 130*
- ♦ **Maxolon®** *see* Metoclopramide *on page 630*
- ♦ **Mazepine® (Canada)** *see* Carbamazepine *on page 165*
- ♦ **MCT Oil® [OTC]** *see* Medium Chain Triglycerides *on page 598*
- ♦ **Measles and Rubella Vaccines, Combined** *see page 1138*
- ♦ **Measles, Mumps, and Rubella Vaccines, Combined** *see page 1138*
- ♦ **Measles Virus Vaccine, Live, Attenuated** *see page 1138*
- ♦ **Measurin® [OTC]** *see* Aspirin *on page 99*
- ♦ **Mebaral®** *see* Mephobarbital *on page 605*

Mebendazole *(me BEN da zole)*

Brand Names Vermox®

Therapeutic Category Anthelmintic

Generic Available Yes

Use Treatment of enterobiasis (pinworm infection), trichuriasis (whipworm infection), ascariasis (roundworm infection), and hookworm infections caused by *Necator americanus* or *Ancylostoma duodenale*; drug of choice in the treatment of capillariasis

Pregnancy Risk Factor C

Contraindications Hypersensitivity to mebendazole or any component

Warnings Pregnancy and children <2 years of age are relative contraindications since safety has not been established

Adverse Reactions

Central nervous system: Dizziness, fever, headache

Dermatologic: Rash, pruritus, alopecia

Gastrointestinal: Diarrhea, abdominal pain, nausea, vomiting

Hematologic: Neutropenia, anemia, leukopenia

Hepatic: Transient abnormalities in liver function tests

Otic: Tinnitus

Renal: Hematuria

Drug Interactions Anticonvulsants such as carbamazepine and phenytoin may increase metabolism of mebendazole

Food Interactions Food increases mebendazole absorption

Mechanism of Action Selectively and irreversibly blocks uptake of glucose and other nutrients in susceptible intestine-dwelling helminths

Pharmacokinetics

Absorption: Oral: 2% to 10% of a dose is absorbed

Distribution: To Liver, fat, muscle, plasma, and hepatic cysts
Protein binding: 95%
Metabolism: Extensive in the liver
Half-life: 2.8-9 hours
Time to peak serum concentration: Variable (0.5-7 hours)
Elimination: Primarily in feces as inactive metabolites with 5% to 10% eliminated in urine
Not dialyzable

Usual Dosage Children and Adults: Oral:
Pinworms: Single chewable tablet (100 mg); may need to repeat after 2 weeks
Whipworms, roundworms, hookworms: 100 mg twice daily, morning and evening on 3 consecutive days; if patient is not cured within 3-4 weeks, a second course of treatment may be administered
Capillariasis: 200 mg twice daily for 20 days

Administration Oral: Administer with food; tablet can be crushed and mixed with food, swallowed whole, or chewed

Monitoring Parameters For treatment of trichuriasis, ascariasis, hookworm, or mixed infections, check for helminth ova in the feces within 3-4 weeks following the initial therapy

Dosage Forms Tablet, chewable: 100 mg

References
Hotez PJ, "Hookworm Disease in Children," *Pediatr Infect Dis J*, 1989, 8(8):516-20.

Mechlorethamine (me klor ETH a meen)

Related Information
Emetogenic Potential of Single Chemotherapeutic Agents *on page 1095*
Extravasation Treatment *on page 1050*

Brand Names Mustargen® Hydrochloride

Available Salts Mechlorethamine Hydrochloride

Synonyms HN_2; Mustine; Nitrogen Mustard

Therapeutic Category Antineoplastic Agent, Alkylating Agent (Nitrogen Mustard)

Generic Available No

Use Combination therapy of Hodgkin's disease, brain tumors, non-Hodgkin's lymphoma, and malignant lymphomas; palliative treatment of lung, breast, and ovarian carcinoma; sclerosing agent in intracavitary therapy of pleural, pericardial, and other malignant effusions

Pregnancy Risk Factor D

Contraindications Hypersensitivity to mechlorethamine or any component; pre-existing profound myelosuppression

Warnings The FDA currently recommends that procedures for proper handling, administration, and disposal of mechlorethamine powder and solution be followed. Avoid inhalation of dust or vapors and contact with skin or mucous membranes. Mechlorethamine is potentially carcinogenic, teratogenic, and mutagenic. It may cause permanent sterility and birth defects. Extravasation of the drug into subcutaneous tissues results in painful inflammation, erythema, and induration; sloughing may occur; promptly infiltrate the area with sterile isotonic sodium thiosulfate (1/6 molar) and apply a cold compress for 6-12 hours. See Extravasation Treatment *on page 1050*

Precautions Use with caution in patients with myelosuppression; patients with lymphoma should receive adequate hydration, alkalinization of the urine and/or prophylactic allopurinol to prevent complications such as uric acid nephropathy and hyperuricemia

Adverse Reactions
Cardiovascular: Thrombosis
Central nervous system: Vertigo, fever, headache, drowsiness, encephalopathy (high dose)
Dermatologic: Rash, alopecia
Endocrine & metabolic: Amenorrhea, impaired spermatogenesis, hyperuricemia
Gastrointestinal: Nausea, vomiting, anorexia, diarrhea, metallic taste, mucositis
Hematologic: Myelosuppression (leukopenia, thrombocytopenia), hemolytic anemia
Local: Thrombophlebitis
Neuromuscular & skeletal: Weakness
Ocular: Lacrimation
Otic: Tinnitus, deafness
Miscellaneous: Hypersensitivity reactions, diaphoresis

Stability Highly unstable in neutral or alkaline solutions; use immediately after reconstitution; discard any unused drug after 60 minutes (although manufacturer
(Continued)

Mechlorethamine *(Continued)*

reports only 15 minutes of stability after reconstitution, other studies indicate it is stable longer)

Mechanism of Action Alkylating agent that inhibits DNA and RNA synthesis via formation of carbonium ions which can attach to nucleic acids at the N^7 position of guanine; cross-links strands of DNA causing miscoding, breakage, and failure of replication

Pharmacokinetics

Absorption: Incomplete after intracavitary administration secondary to rapid deactivation by body fluids

Distribution: Following I.V. administration, drug undergoes rapid hydrolysis to a highly reactive alkylating intermediate; unchanged drug is undetectable in the blood within a few minutes

Half-life: <1 minute

Elimination: <0.01% of unchanged drug is recovered in urine

Usual Dosage Refer to individual protocols

Children:

Lymphoma: MOPP regimen: Mustargen® (mechlorethamine), Oncovin® (vincristine), procarbazine, and prednisone: I.V.: 6 mg/m^2 on days 1 and 8 of a 28-day cycle

Brain tumors: MOPP regimen: I.V.: 3 mg/m^2 on days 1 and 8 of a 28-day cycle

Adults:

I.V.: 0.4 mg/kg or 12-16 mg/m^2 as a single monthly dose or divided into 0.1 mg/kg/day once daily for 4 days, repeated at 4- to 6-week intervals

Intracavitary: 10-30 mg or 0.2-0.4 mg/kg

Administration

Intracavitary: Dilute dose in up to 100 mL NS; paracentesis is performed to remove most of the fluid from the cavity prior to administration; inject drug slowly with frequent aspiration to ensure that a free flow of fluid is present; change patient's position every 5-10 minutes for 1 hour following injection to distribute drug uniformly throughout the cavity

Parenteral: Administer I.V. push through a side port of an established I.V. line over 1-3 minutes at a concentration not to exceed 1 mg/mL

Monitoring Parameters CBC with differential and platelet count, hemoglobin

Patient Information Report to physician any pain or irritation at the site of injection, fever, sore throat, bruising, bleeding, shortness of breath, itching, or wheezing

Nursing Implications Avoid extravasation, inhalation of vapors, or contact with skin, mucous membranes, and eyes since mechlorethamine is a potent vesicant. If accidental eye contact occurs, copious irrigation for at least 15 minutes with NS or a balanced salt ophthalmic irrigating solution should be instituted immediately followed by prompt ophthalmologic consultation. If accidental skin contact occurs, irrigate the affected area with copious amounts of water for at least 15 minutes while removing contaminated clothing, followed by application of a 2% sodium thiosulfate solution; contaminated clothing should be destroyed. Medical attention should be sought immediately. A $^1/_6$ molar sodium thiosulfate solution can be instilled for nitrogen mustard extravasations; $^1/_6$ molar sodium thiosulfate solution can be prepared by diluting 4 mL of 10% sodium thiosulfate injection with 6 mL of sterile water for injection; Dorr recommends to inject 2 mL of the $^1/_6$ molar solution into site for each milligram of mechlorethamine extravasated

Additional Information Myelosuppressive effects:

WBC: Severe

Platelets: Severe

Onset (days): 4-7

Nadir (days): 14

Recovery (days): 21

Dosage Forms Powder for injection, as hydrochloride: 10 mg

References

Ater JL, van Eys J, Woo SY, et al, "MOPP Chemotherapy Without Irradiation as Primary Postsurgical Therapy for Brain Tumors in Infants and Young Children," *J Neurooncol*, 1997, 32(3):243-52.

Berg SL, Grisell DL, DeLaney TF, et al, "Principles of Treatment of Pediatric Solid Tumors," *Pediatr Clin North Am*, 1991, 38(2):249-67.

Dorr RT, Soble M, and Alberts DS, "Efficacy of Sodium Thiosulfate as a Local Antidote to Mechlorethamine Skin Toxicity in the Mouse," *Cancer Chemother Pharmacol*, 1988, 22(4):299-302.

Krischer JP, Ragab AH, Kun L, et al, "Nitrogen Mustard, Vincristine, Procarbazine, and Prednisone as Adjuvant Chemotherapy in the Treatment of Medulloblastoma. A Pediatric Oncology Group Study," *J Neurosurg*, 1991, 74(6):905-9.

♦ **Mechlorethamine Hydrochloride** *see* Mechlorethamine *on page 595*

♦ **Meclastine** *see* Clemastine *on page 236*

Meclizine (MEK li zeen)

Related Information
Overdose and Toxicology *on page 1191*

Brand Names Antivert®; Antrizine®; Bonamine® (Canada); Bonine® [OTC]; Dizmiss® [OTC]; Dramamine® II [OTC]; Meni-D®; Nico-Vert® [OTC]; Ru-Vert-M®; Vergon® [OTC]

Available Salts Meclizine Hydrochloride

Synonyms Meclozine

Therapeutic Category Antiemetic; Antihistamine

Generic Available Yes

Use Prevention and treatment of motion sickness; management of vertigo

Pregnancy Risk Factor B

Contraindications Hypersensitivity to meclizine or any component

Precautions Use with caution in patients with angle-closure glaucoma or obstructive diseases of the GI or GU tract

Adverse Reactions
Cardiovascular: Hypotension, palpitations, tachycardia

Central nervous system: Drowsiness, fatigue, auditory and visual hallucinations, restlessness, excitation, insomnia, nervousness

Dermatologic: Urticaria, rash

Gastrointestinal: Xerostomia, anorexia, nausea, vomiting, diarrhea, constipation, appetite increase, weight gain

Hepatic: Cholestatic jaundice, hepatitis

Neuromuscular & skeletal: Myalgia, tremor, paresthesia

Ocular: Blurred vision, diplopia

Otic: Tinnitus

Respiratory: Bronchospasm, epistaxis

Drug Interactions Additive sedation with CNS depressants (eg, sedatives, alcohol, antihistamines)

Mechanism of Action Has central anticholinergic action and CNS depressant activity; decreases excitability of the middle ear labyrinth and blocks conduction in the middle ear vestibular-cerebellar pathways

Pharmacodynamics
Onset of action: Oral: 30-60 minutes

Duration: 12-24 hours

Pharmacokinetics
Metabolism: In the liver

Half-life: 6 hours

Elimination: As metabolites in urine and as unchanged drug in feces

Usual Dosage Children >12 years and Adults: Oral:

Motion sickness: 25-50 mg 1 hour before travel, repeat dose every 24 hours if needed

Vertigo: 25-100 mg/day in divided doses

Administration Oral: Administer with food to decrease GI distress

Patient Information May cause drowsiness and impair ability to perform hazardous activities requiring mental alertness or physical coordination

Dosage Forms
Capsule, as hydrochloride: 25 mg, 30 mg

Tablet, as hydrochloride: 12.5 mg, 25 mg, 50 mg

Tablet, as hydrochloride:

Chewable: 25 mg

Film coated: 25 mg

♦ **Meclizine Hydrochloride** *see* Meclizine *on page 597*
♦ **Mecloprodin** *see* Clemastine *on page 236*
♦ **Meclozine** *see* Meclizine *on page 597*
♦ **Meda-Cap® [OTC]** *see* Acetaminophen *on page 26*
♦ **Meda® Tab [OTC]** *see* Acetaminophen *on page 26*
♦ **Medicinal Carbon** *see* Charcoal *on page 202*
♦ **Medicinal Charcoal** *see* Charcoal *on page 202*
♦ **Medihaler-Epi® [OTC]** *see* Epinephrine *on page 371*
♦ **Medihaler-Iso® Inhalation Aerosol** *see* Isoproterenol *on page 536*
♦ **Medimet® (Canada)** *see* Methyldopa *on page 625*
♦ **Mediplast® Plaster [OTC]** *see* Salicylic Acid *on page 854*
♦ **Medipren® [OTC]** *see* Ibuprofen *on page 501*

♦ **Medi-Quick® Topical Ointment [OTC]** *see* Neomycin, Polymyxin B, and Bacitracin *on page 680*

♦ **Medi-Tuss® [OTC]** *see* Guaifenesin *on page 464*

Medium Chain Triglycerides (mee DEE um chane trye GLIS er ides)

Brand Names MCT Oil® [OTC]

Synonyms Triglycerides, Medium Chain

Therapeutic Category Caloric Agent; Nutritional Supplement

Generic Available No

Use Nutritional supplement for those who cannot digest long chain fats; malabsorption associated with disorders such as pancreatic insufficiency, bile salt deficiency, and bacterial overgrowth of the small bowel; induce ketosis as a prevention for seizures (akinetic, clonic, and petit mal)

Pregnancy Risk Factor C

Contraindications Hypersensitivity to any component; should not be used in patients with hepatic encephalopathy due to earlier observations which report that short chain fatty acids may have a narcotic effect on the central nervous system and inhibit oxidative phosphorylation

Warnings Patients with cirrhosis demonstrate higher concentrations of medium chain fatty acids in the serum and CSF than normal individuals; this results from impaired hepatic clearance of medium chain fatty acids due to parenchymal dysfunction of medium chain fatty acid oxidation, portal systemic shunt, and impaired protein binding of fatty acid which enhances the passive diffusion of medium chain fatty acids into the CSF

Precautions Use with caution in patients with hepatic cirrhosis and complications such as portacaval shunts or encephalopathy

Adverse Reactions
Central nervous system: Sedation, narcosis, coma (cirrhotics)
Endocrine & metabolic: Ketosis
Gastrointestinal: Nausea, vomiting, abdominal pain, diarrhea, borborygmi

Mechanism of Action A semisynthetic class of lipids; medium chain triglycerides (MCT) are composed of fatty acids with chain length varying from 6-12 carbon atoms; preparations contain approximately 75% octanoic (caprylic), 20% to 25% decanoic (capric), 1% hexanoic (caproic), and 1% dodecanoic (lauric) acids

Hydrolyzed in the stomach and in the small intestine by pancreatic lipase to medium chain fatty acids; the medium chain fatty acids are incorporated into bile salts for more rapid solubilization and entrance into the mucosal cell for passage into the portal venous blood; can be absorbed unchanged as a triglyceride into the mucosal cell without chemical or physical alteration; medium chain fatty acids presented to the liver are minimally converted to hepatic lipid and are rapidly oxidized to carbon dioxide, ketones, and acetate; the medium chain fatty acids are esterified to long chain triglycerides

Pharmacodynamics Onset of action: Octanoic acid appeared in each subject by 30 minutes following ingestion; effect on seizures in children: Within 6 weeks

Pharmacokinetics
Absorption: Up to 30% of dose can be absorbed unchanged as a triglyceride in the mucosal cell
Metabolism: Almost entirely oxidized by the liver to acetyl CoA fragments and to carbon dioxide; little deposited in adipose tissue or elsewhere
Elimination: As much as 20% of oral dose of MCT, recovered in expired CO_2 in 50 minutes; <10% elimination of medium chain fatty acids in feces

Usual Dosage Oral:
Infants: Nutritional supplement: Initial: 0.5 mL every other feeding, then advance to every feeding, then increase in increments of 0.25-0.5 mL/feeding at intervals of 2-3 days as tolerated
Children: Seizures: About 40 mL with each meal or 50% to 70% (800-1120 kcal) of total calories (1600 kcal) as the oil will induce the ketosis necessary for seizure control
Children and Adults: Cystic fibrosis: 3 tablespoons/day in divided doses
Adults: Malabsorption syndromes: 15 mL 3-4 times/day

Administration Oral:
Dilute with at least an equal volume of water or mix with some other vehicle such as fruit juice (should not be cold; flavoring may be added); mixture should be sipped slowly; administer no more than 15-20 mL at any one time (up to 100 mL may be administered in divided doses in a 24-hour period)
Possible gastrointestinal side effects from medication can be prevented if therapy is initiated with small supplements at meals and gradually increased according to patient's tolerance

Patient Information GI symptoms may occur during the first few days of administration and then disappear; it is important to continue therapy with at least the
smallest dose

Additional Information Does not provide any essential fatty acids; only saturated
fats are contained; supplementation with safflower, corn oil, or other polyunsaturated vegetable oil must be given to provide the patient with the essential fatty
acids; caloric content: 8.3 calories/g; 115 calories/15 mL

Dosage Forms Oil: 14 g/15 mL (960 mL)

♦ **Medralone® Injection** *see* Methylprednisolone *on page 629*

♦ **Medrol® Oral** *see* Methylprednisolone *on page 629*

♦ **Medrol® Veriderm® Cream (Canada)** *see* Methylprednisolone *on page 629*

Medroxyprogesterone (me DROKS ee proe JES te rone)

Brand Names Amen® Oral; Curretab® Oral; Cycrin® Oral; Depo-Provera® Injection;
Provera® Oral

Available Salts Medroxyprogesterone Acetate

Synonyms Acetoxymethylprogesterone; Methylacetoxyprogesterone

Therapeutic Category Contraceptive, Progestin Only; Progestin

Generic Available Yes

Use Secondary amenorrhea or abnormal uterine bleeding due to hormonal imbalance; prevention of pregnancy

Pregnancy Risk Factor X

Contraindications Thrombophlebitis; hypersensitivity to medroxyprogesterone or
any component; cerebral apoplexy, undiagnosed vaginal bleeding, liver dysfunction, thromboembolic disorders, breast cancer, pregnancy (known or suspected)

Warnings Discontinue if there is a sudden partial or complete loss of vision, proptosis, diplopia, migraine, if papilledema or retinal vascular lesions are present, or
any other symptom of a thromboembolic event

Precautions Use with caution in patients with mental depression, diabetes,
epilepsy, asthma, migraines, renal or cardiac dysfunction

Adverse Reactions
Cardiovascular: Edema, thromboembolic disorders
Central nervous system: Depression, dizziness, nervousness, fever, insomnia
Dermatologic: Melasma, chloasma, urticaria, acne, photosensitivity, alopecia,
hirsutism
Endocrine & metabolic: Menstrual irregularities, amenorrhea, breakthrough
bleeding, breast tenderness
Gastrointestinal: Weight gain or loss, anorexia
Hepatic: Cholestatic jaundice
Local: Pain at injection site, thrombophlebitis
Neuromuscular & skeletal: Weakness

Drug Interactions Aminoglutethimide depresses serum concentrations of medroxyprogesterone acetate

Mechanism of Action Inhibits secretion of pituitary gonadotropins, which prevents
follicular maturation and ovulation, transforms a proliferative endometrium into a
secretory one

Pharmacokinetics
Absorption: I.M.: Slow
Bioavailability: 0.6% to 10%
Protein binding: 90%
Metabolism: In the liver
Half-life: 30 days
Elimination: Oral: In urine and feces

Usual Dosage Adolescents and Adults:
Amenorrhea: Oral: 5-10 mg/day for 5-10 days or 2.5 mg/day
Abnormal uterine bleeding: Oral: 5-10 mg for 5-10 days starting on day 16 or day
21 of menstrual cycle
Contraception: I.M.: 150 mg every 3 months; first dose to be given only during first
5 days of normal menstrual period; only within 5 days postpartum if not breast-
feeding, or only at sixth postpartum week if exclusively breast-feeding

Administration
Oral: Administer with food
Parenteral: I.M. only; not for I.V. use; shake well before drawing into syringe

Test Interactions Altered thyroid and liver function tests, prothrombin time, factors
VII, VIII, IX, X, metyrapone test

Patient Information Notify physician if sudden loss of vision or migraine headache
occurs; may cause photosensitivity, wear protective clothing or sunscreen
(Continued)

Medroxyprogesterone *(Continued)*

Additional Information I.M. dosing is recommended only for contraceptive purposes or in the treatment of endometrial or renal carcinoma

Dosage Forms
Injection, suspension, as acetate: 100 mg/mL (5 mL); 150 mg/mL (1 mL); 400 mg/mL (1 mL, 2.5 mL, 10 mL)
Tablet, as acetate: 2.5 mg, 5 mg, 10 mg

♦ **Medroxyprogesterone Acetate** *see Medroxyprogesterone on page 599*

Medrysone *(ME dri sone)*

Brand Names HMS Liquifilm®

Therapeutic Category Anti-inflammatory Agent, Ophthalmic; Corticosteroid, Ophthalmic

Generic Available No

Use Treatment of allergic conjunctivitis, vernal conjunctivitis, episcleritis, ophthalmic epinephrine sensitivity reaction

Pregnancy Risk Factor C

Contraindications Hypersensitivity to medrysone or any component; ocular fungal, viral, or tuberculosis infections; acute superficial herpes simplex

Warnings Effectiveness and safety have not been established in children

Precautions Prolonged use has been associated with the development of corneal or scleral perforation and posterior subcapsular cataracts; may mask or enhance the establishment of acute purulent untreated infections of the eye; dose should be tapered to avoid disease exacerbation

Adverse Reactions
Local: Stinging, burning
Ocular: Corneal thinning, increased intraocular pressure, glaucoma, damage to the optic nerve, defects in visual activity, cataracts
Miscellaneous: Hypersensitivity reactions

Mechanism of Action Inhibits inflammatory response by suppression of migration of polymorphonuclear leukocytes and reversal of increased capillary permeability

Pharmacokinetics
Absorption: Through aqueous humor
Metabolism: In the liver
Elimination: By the kidneys and feces

Usual Dosage Children and Adults: Ophthalmic: Instill 1 drop in conjunctival sac 2-4 times/day up to every 4 hours; may use every 1-2 hours during first 1-2 days

Administration Ophthalmic: Shake well before use; do not touch dropper to the eye or skin; finger pressure should be applied to lacrimal sac during and for 1-2 minutes after instillation to decrease risk of absorption and systemic reactions

Monitoring Parameters With prolonged use monitor intraocular pressure and periodic examination of lens

Additional Information Medrysone is a synthetic corticosteroid; structurally related to progesterone; if no improvement after several days of treatment, discontinue medrysone and institute other therapy; duration of therapy: 3-4 days to several weeks dependent on type and severity of disease

Dosage Forms Solution, ophthalmic: 1% (5 mL, 10 mL)

♦ **Mefoxin®** *see Cefoxitin on page 186*
♦ **Megacillin® Susp (Canada)** *see Penicillin G Benzathine on page 739*
♦ **Mellaril®** *see Thioridazine on page 920*
♦ **Mellaril-S®** *see Thioridazine on page 920*

Melphalan *(MEL fa lan)*

Related Information
Emetogenic Potential of Single Chemotherapeutic Agents *on page 1095*

Brand Names Alkeran®

Synonyms L-PAM; L-Sarcolysin; Phenylalanine Mustard

Therapeutic Category Antineoplastic Agent, Alkylating Agent (Nitrogen Mustard)

Generic Available No

Use Palliative treatment of multiple myeloma and nonresectable epithelial ovarian carcinoma; neuroblastoma, rhabdomyosarcoma, breast cancer, sarcoma; I.V. formulation: Use in patients in whom oral therapy is not appropriate

Pregnancy Risk Factor D

Contraindications Hypersensitivity to melphalan or any component; severe bone marrow suppression; patients whose disease was resistant to prior therapy

Warnings The FDA currently recommends that procedures for proper handling and disposal of antineoplastic agents be considered; potentially mutagenic, carcinogenic, and teratogenic; long-term oral dosing can increase the chance of developing secondary leukemia; produces amenorrhea

Precautions Reduce dosage or discontinue therapy if leukocyte count is <3000/mm^3 or platelet count is <100,000/mm^3; use with caution in patients with bone marrow suppression and impaired renal function; dosage reduction may be necessary in patients with impaired renal function

Adverse Reactions

Cardiovascular: Vasculitis, chest pain; hypotension, diaphoresis, and cardiac arrest have been reported following I.V. administration

Dermatologic: Alopecia, rash, pruritus, vesiculation of skin

Endocrine & metabolic: Amenorrhea

Gastrointestinal: Nausea, vomiting, diarrhea, stomatitis

Genitourinary: Bladder irritation, hemorrhagic cystitis

Hematologic: Leukopenia, thrombocytopenia, anemia, agranulocytosis, hemolytic anemia

Hepatic: Hepatic veno-occlusive disease

Local: Burning, discomfort, and skin ulceration at injection site

Respiratory: Pulmonary fibrosis, interstitial pneumonitis

Drug Interactions Cyclosporine (development of severe renal failure); nalidixic acid (increases incidence of severe hemorrhagic necrotic enterocolitis); cimetidine decreases bioavailability of oral melphalan

Food Interactions Food interferes with oral absorption

Stability Protect tablets from light and store at room temperature; reconstituted 5 mg/mL solution for injection is stable 90 minutes at room temperature; do not refrigerate since it may precipitate; once reconstituted solution is further diluted for I.V. infusion, administration must be completed within 1 hour

Mechanism of Action Alkylating agent that inhibits DNA and RNA synthesis via formation of carbonium ions; cross-links strands of DNA

Pharmacokinetics

Absorption: Oral: Variable and incomplete

Distribution: Distributes throughout total body water; V_{dss}: 0.5 L/kg

Protein binding: 60% to 90%

Metabolism: Nonenzymatic hydrolysis to mono- or dihydroxy products; some conjugation to glutathione

Bioavailability: Ranges from 49% to 95% depending on the presence of food

Half-life, terminal: 75-90 minutes

Time to peak serum concentration: Oral: Within 2 hours

Elimination: 10% to 15% of dose excreted unchanged in urine; after oral administration, 20% to 50% excreted in stool

Usual Dosage Refer to individual protocols

Children:

I.V.:

Pediatric rhabdomyosarcoma: 10-35 mg/m^2/dose every 21-28 days

High-dose melphalan with bone marrow transplantation for neuroblastoma: 70-100 mg/m^2/day on day 7 and 6 before BMT; or 140-220 mg/m^2 single dose before BMT; or 50 mg/m^2/day for 4 days; or 70 mg/m^2/day for 3 days

Oral: 4-20 mg/m^2/day for 1-21 days

Adults:

Multiple myeloma:

Oral: 6 mg/day once daily initially adjusted as indicated or 0.15 mg/kg/day for 7 days or 0.25 mg/kg/day for 4 days, repeat at 4- to 6-week intervals

I.V.: 16 mg/m^2/dose every 2 weeks for 4 doses, then repeat monthly as per protocol for multiple myeloma

Ovarian carcinoma: Oral: 0.2 mg/kg/day for 5 days, repeat in 4-5 weeks

Dosing adjustment in renal impairment:

BUN >30 mg/dL: Reduce dose by 50%

Serum creatinine >1.5 mg/dL: Reduce dose by 50%

Administration

Oral: Administer on an empty stomach

Parenteral: Reconstitute 50 mg vial for injection with special diluent to yield a 5 mg/mL solution; filter through a 0.45 μM Millex-HV filter; dilute the reconstituted solution with NS to a final concentration not to exceed 2 mg/mL for I.V. central line administration or 0.45 mg/mL for peripheral I.V. administration; administer by I.V. infusion over 15-30 minutes at a rate not to exceed 10 mg/minute but total infusion should be administered within 1 hour

(Continued)

Melphalan *(Continued)*

Monitoring Parameters CBC with differential and platelet count, serum electrolytes, serum uric acid, hemoglobin

Test Interactions Positive Coombs' [direct]

Patient Information Notify physician if fever, shortness of breath, persistent cough, sore throat, bleeding, or bruising occurs

Nursing Implications Ensure adequate patient hydration

Additional Information Myelosuppressive effects:
- WBC: Moderate
- Platelets: Moderate
- Onset (days): 7
- Nadir (days): 14-21
- Recovery (days): 42-50

Dosage Forms
- Powder for injection: 50 mg
- Tablet: 2 mg

References

Berg SL, Grisell DL, DeLaney TF, et al, "Principles of Treatment of Pediatric Solid Tumors," *Pediatr Clin North Am*, 1991, 38(2):249-67.

Pole JG, Casper J, Elfenbein G, et al, "High-Dose Chemoradiotherapy Supported by Marrow Infusions for Advanced Neuroblastoma: A Pediatric Oncology Group Study," *J Clin Oncol*, 1991, 9(1):152-8.

Schroeder H, Pinkerton CR, Powles RL, et al, "High-Dose Melphalan and Total Body Irradiation With Autologous Marrow Rescue in Childhood Acute Lymphoblastic Leukemia After Relapse," *Bone Marrow Transplant*, 1991, 7(1):11-15.

♦ **Menadol® [OTC]** *see* Ibuprofen *on page 501*

♦ **Meni-D®** *see* Meclizine *on page 597*

♦ **Meningococcal Polysaccharide Vaccine, Groups A, C, Y, and W-135** *see page 1138*

Meperidine *(me PER i deen)*

Related Information
Adult ACLS Algorithm, Electrical Conversion *on page 1014*
Compatibility of Medications Mixed in a Syringe *on page 1208*
Narcotic Analgesics Comparison *on page 1035*
Overdose and Toxicology *on page 1191*
Preprocedure Sedatives in Children *on page 1169*
Serotonin Syndrome *on page 1217*

Brand Names Demerol®

Available Salts Meperidine Hydrochloride

Synonyms Isonipecaine; Pethidine

Therapeutic Category Analgesic, Narcotic

Generic Available Yes

Use Management of moderate to severe pain; adjunct to anesthesia and preoperative sedation

Restrictions C-II

Pregnancy Risk Factor B (D if used for prolonged periods or in high doses at term)

Contraindications Hypersensitivity to meperidine or any component; patients receiving MAO inhibitors presently or in the past 14 days

Warnings Some preparations contain sulfites which may cause allergic reaction

Precautions Use with caution in patients with pulmonary, hepatic, or renal disorders; use with caution in patients with tachycardias, biliary, colic, increased intracranial pressure, seizure disorders or those receiving high-dose meperidine because normeperidine (an active metabolite and CNS stimulant) may accumulate and precipitate twitches, tremors, or seizures; decrease the dose in patients with renal or hepatic impairment

Adverse Reactions
- Cardiovascular: Palpitations, hypotension, bradycardia, peripheral vasodilation, tachycardia
- Central nervous system: CNS depression, dizziness, drowsiness, sedation, increased intracranial pressure; active metabolite (normeperidine) may precipitate twitches, tremors, or seizures
- Dermatologic: Pruritus
- Endocrine & metabolic: Antidiuretic hormone release
- Gastrointestinal: Nausea, vomiting, constipation, biliary tract spasm
- Genitourinary: Urinary tract spasm
- Local: Induration, irritation (repeated S.C. use)
- Ocular: Miosis

Respiratory: Respiratory depression

Miscellaneous: Physical and psychological dependence, histamine release

Drug Interactions Cytochrome P-450 isoenzyme CYP2D6 substrate

May aggravate the adverse effects of isoniazid; MAO inhibitors greatly potentiate the effects of meperidine (acute opioid overdosage symptoms can be seen, including severe toxic reactions); CNS depressants, alcohol, tricyclic antidepressants, phenothiazines may potentiate the effects of meperidine; phenytoin may decrease the analgesic effects; concurrent use of meperidine with ritonavir is not recommended

Stability Incompatible with aminophylline, heparin, phenobarbital, phenytoin, and sodium bicarbonate

Mechanism of Action Binds to opiate receptors in the CNS, causing inhibition of ascending pain pathways, altering the perception of and response to pain; produces generalized CNS depression

Pharmacodynamics Analgesia:

Onset of action:

Oral, I.M., S.C.: Within 10-15 minutes

I.V.: Within 5 minutes

Peak effect:

Oral, I.M., S.C.: Within 1 hour

I.V.: 5-7 minutes

Duration:

Oral, I.M., S.C.: 2-4 hours

I.V.: 2-3 hours

Pharmacokinetics

Distribution: Crosses the placenta; appears in breast milk

V_{dss}:

Neonates: Preterm 1-7 days: 8.8 L/kg; term 1-7 days: 5.6 L/kg

Infants: 1 week to 2 months: 8 L/kg; 3-18 months: 5 L/kg; 5-8 years: 2.8 L/kg

Adults: 3-4 L/kg

Protein binding: (to alpha$_1$-acid glycoprotein)

Neonates: 52%

Infants: 3-18 months: 85%

Adults: ~60% to 80%

Metabolism: In the liver via hydrolysis and N-demethylation

Bioavailability: ~50% to 60%, increased bioavailability with liver disease

Half-life, terminal:

Preterm infants 3.6-65 days of age: 11.9 hours (range: 3.3-59.4 hours)

Term infants:

0.3-4 days of age: 10.7 hours (range: 4.9-16.8 hours)

26-73 days of age: 8.2 hours (range: 5.7-31.7 hours)

Neonates: 23 hours (range: 12-39 hours)

Infants 3-18 months: 2.3 hours

Children 5-8 years: 3 hours

Adults: 2.5-4 hours

Adults with liver disease: 7-11 hours

Normeperidine (active metabolite): Neonates: 30-85 hours; Adults: 8-16 hours; normeperidine half-life is dependent on renal function and can accumulate with high doses or in patients with decreased renal function; normeperidine may precipitate tremors or seizures

Elimination: ~5% meperidine eliminated unchanged in urine

Usual Dosage Doses should be titrated to appropriate analgesic effect; when changing route of administration, note that oral doses are about half as effective as parenteral dose

Children:

Oral, I.M., I.V., S.C.: Usual: 1-1.5 mg/kg/dose every 3-4 hours as needed; 1-2 mg/kg as a single dose preoperative medication may be used; maximum dose: 100 mg/dose

I.V. continuous infusion: Loading dose: 0.5-1 mg/kg followed by initial rate: 0.3 mg/kg/hour; titrate dose to effect; may require 0.5-0.7 mg/kg/hour

Adults: Oral, I.M., I.V.: S.C.: 50-150 mg/dose every 3-4 hours as needed

Dosing adjustment in renal impairment:

Cl_{cr} 10-50 mL/minute: Administer 75% of normal dose

Cl_{cr} <10 mL/minute: Administer 50% of normal dose

Administration

Oral: Administer with water; dilute syrup in water prior to use (use 4 oz water for adults)

(Continued)

Meperidine *(Continued)*

Parenteral:

Slow I.V. push: Do not administer rapid I.V., administer over at least 5 minutes and dilute to ≤10 mg/mL

Intermittent infusion: Dilute to 1 mg/mL and administer over 15-30 minutes

Monitoring Parameters Respiratory and cardiovascular status; relief of pain, level of sedation

Patient Information Avoid alcohol; may be habit-forming; may cause drowsiness and impair ability to perform activities requiring mental alertness or physical coordination

Additional Information Equianalgesic doses: morphine 10 mg I.M. = meperidine 75-100 mg I.M.; Demerol® syrup also contains glucose, saccharin, artificial banana flavoring, and benzoic acid. **Note**: Although meperidine has been used in combination with chlorpromazine and promethazine as a premedication ("Lytic Cocktail"), this combination may have a higher rate of adverse effects compared to alternative sedatives and analgesics (See American Academy of Pediatrics Committee on Drugs, 1995)

Dosage Forms

Injection, as hydrochloride:

Multiple-dose vials: 50 mg/mL (30 mL); 100 mg/mL (20 mL)

Single dose: 10 mg/mL (5 mL, 10 mL, 30 mL); 25 mg/dose (0.5 mL, 1 mL); 50 mg/dose (1 mL); 75 mg/dose (1 mL, 1.5 mL); 100 mg/dose (1 mL)

Syrup, as hydrochloride (banana flavor): 50 mg/5 mL (500 mL)

Tablet, as hydrochloride: 50 mg, 100 mg

References

American Academy of Pediatrics Committee on Drugs, "Reappraisal of Lytic Cocktail/Demerol®, Phenergan®, and Thorazine® (DPT) for the Sedation of Children," *Pediatrics*, 1995, 95(4):598-602.

Cole TB, Sprinkle RH, Smith SJ, et al, "Intravenous Narcotic Therapy for Children With Severe Sickle Cell Pain Crisis," *Am J Dis Child*, 1986, 140(12):1255-9.

Olkkola KT, Hamunen K, and Maunuksela EL, "Clinical Pharmacokinetics and Pharmacodynamics of Opioid Analgesics in Infants and Children," *Clin Pharmacokinet*, 1995, 28(5):385-404.

Pokela ML, Olkkola KT, Koivisto ME, et al, "Pharmacokinetics and Pharmacodynamics of Intravenous Meperidine in Neonates and Infants," *Clin Pharmacol Ther*, 1992, 52(4):342-9.

♦ **Meperidine Hydrochloride** *see* Meperidine *on page 602*

Mephenytoin *(me FEN i toyn)*

Related Information

Overdose and Toxicology *on page 1191*

Brand Names Mesantoin®

Synonyms Methoin; Methylphenylethylhydantoin; Phenantoin

Therapeutic Category Anticonvulsant, Hydantoin

Generic Available No

Use Treatment of tonic-clonic and partial seizures in patients who are uncontrolled with less toxic anticonvulsants

Pregnancy Risk Factor C

Contraindications Hypersensitivity to mephenytoin or any component

Warnings Fatal irreversible aplastic anemia has occurred

Precautions Abrupt withdrawal may precipitate seizures

Adverse Reactions

Central nervous system: Insomnia, slurred speech, dizziness, lethargy, confusion, coma, sedation, nervousness, ataxia

Dermatologic: Rash, erythema multiforme, alopecia

Gastrointestinal: Nausea, vomiting, weight gain

Hematologic: Neutropenia, leukopenia, thrombocytopenia, agranulocytosis, anemia, Hodgkin's disease-like syndrome; fatal aplastic anemia has occurred

Hepatic: Hepatitis

Neuromuscular & skeletal: Tremor

Ocular: Nystagmus, blurred vision, diplopia, photophobia

Miscellaneous: Serum sickness

Mechanism of Action Stabilizes neuronal membranes and decreases seizure activity by increasing efflux or decreasing influx of sodium ions across cell membranes in the motor cortex during generation of nerve impulses; prolongs effective refractory period and suppresses ventricular pacemaker automaticity, shortens action potential in the heart

Usual Dosage Oral:

Children: 3-15 mg/kg/day in 3 divided doses; usual maintenance dose: 100-400 mg/day in 3 divided doses

Adults: Initial dose: 50-100 mg/day given daily; increase by 50-100 mg at weekly intervals; usual maintenance dose: 200-600 mg/day in 3 divided doses; maximum dose: 800 mg/day

Administration Oral: Administer with food

Monitoring Parameters CBC with differential, platelet count

Reference Range Total mephenytoin (mephenytoin plus 5-ethyl - 5-phenylhydantoin) = 25-40 µg/mL

Patient Information Avoid alcohol; may cause drowsiness and impair ability to perform activities requiring mental alertness or physical coordination

Additional Information Usually used in combination with other anticonvulsants; **Note:** The company that makes Mesantoin® has **discontinued manufacturing**; the drug is currently available from Novartis under a transition program; small quantities may be obtained while transitioning patients to other antiepileptic agents.

Dosage Forms Tablet: 100 mg

Mephobarbital (me foe BAR bi tal)

Brand Names Mebaral®

Synonyms Methylphenobarbital

Therapeutic Category Anticonvulsant, Barbiturate; Barbiturate; Sedative

Generic Available No

Use Treatment of generalized tonic-clonic and simple partial seizures

Restrictions C-IV

Pregnancy Risk Factor D

Contraindications Hypersensitivity to mephobarbital or any component; pre-existing CNS depression; respiratory depression; severe uncontrolled pain; history of porphyria

Precautions Use with caution in patients with hepatic or renal impairment or respiratory diseases

Adverse Reactions
Central nervous system: Drowsiness, lethargy, paradoxical excitement (especially in children)
Dermatologic: Rash, including Stevens-Johnson syndrome or erythema multiforme
Gastrointestinal: Nausea, vomiting
Hematologic: Agranulocytosis, thrombocytopenic purpura
Miscellaneous: Psychological and physical dependence

Drug Interactions Cytochrome P-450 isoenzyme CYP2C, CYP2C8, and CYP2C19 substrate
Mephobarbital is expected to have similar drug interactions as phenobarbital, since mephobarbital is metabolized in the liver to phenobarbital (see Phenobarbital *on page 754*)

Food Interactions High doses of pyridoxine may decrease drug effect; barbiturates may increase the metabolism of vitamin D & K; dietary requirements of vitamin D, K, C, B_{12}, folate and calcium may be increased with long-term use

Mechanism of Action Increases seizure threshold in the motor cortex; depresses monosynaptic and polysynaptic transmission in the CNS; depresses CNS activity by binding to barbiturate site at GABA-receptor complex enhancing GABA activity; depresses reticular activating system; higher doses may be gabamimetic

Pharmacokinetics
Absorption: Oral: ~50%
Protein binding: 58% to 68%
Metabolism: In the liver to phenobarbital
Half-life: 30-70 hours

Usual Dosage Epilepsy: Oral:
Children: 4-10 mg/kg/day in 2-4 divided doses
Adults: 200-600 mg/day in 2-4 divided doses

Administration Oral: Administer with water, milk, or juice

Monitoring Parameters Phenobarbital serum concentrations; CBC with differential, platelet count, hepatic and renal function

Reference Range Phenobarbital level should be in the range of 15-40 µg/mL (SI: 65-172 µmol/L)

Patient Information May cause drowsiness and impair ability to perform activities requiring mental alertness or physical coordination; do not discontinue abruptly; avoid alcohol; limit caffeine

Additional Information Sometimes used in specific patients who have excessive sedation or hyperexcitability from phenobarbital

Dosage Forms Tablet: 32 mg, 50 mg, 100 mg

♦ **Mephyton®** *see* Phytonadione *on page 769*

♦ **Mepron®** *see* Atovaquone *on page 103*

Mercaptopurine (mer kap toe PYOOR een)
Related Information
Emetogenic Potential of Single Chemotherapeutic Agents *on page 1095*
Brand Names Purinethol®
Synonyms 6-Mercaptopurine; 6-MP
Therapeutic Category Antineoplastic Agent, Antimetabolite; Antineoplastic Agent, Purine
Generic Available No
Use Treatment of acute leukemias (ALL, AML, CML); non-Hodgkin's lymphoma
Pregnancy Risk Factor D
Contraindications Hypersensitivity to mercaptopurine or any component; severe liver disease; severe bone marrow suppression; patients whose disease showed prior resistance to mercaptopurine or thioguanine
Warnings The FDA currently recommends that procedures for proper handling and disposal of antineoplastic agents be considered; mercaptopurine may cause birth defects; potentially carcinogenic
Precautions Use with caution and adjust dosage in patients with renal impairment or hepatic failure; patients who receive allopurinol concurrently should have the mercaptopurine dose reduced by 66% to 75%
Adverse Reactions
Central nervous system: Drug fever
Dermatologic: Rash, hyperpigmentation
Endocrine & metabolic: Hyperuricemia
Gastrointestinal: Mild nausea or vomiting, diarrhea, stomatitis, anorexia
Hematologic: Myelosuppression (leukopenia, thrombocytopenia, anemia), eosinophilia
Hepatic: Hepatotoxicity, hyperbilirubinemia, jaundice, elevation of liver enzymes
Renal: Renal toxicity (oliguria, hematuria)
Drug Interactions Allopurinol may potentiate the effect of bone marrow suppression (blocks metabolism of **orally** administered mercaptopurine by inhibiting xanthine oxidase); mercaptopurine decreases anticoagulant effect of warfarin; doxorubicin, hepatotoxic drugs (may potentiate liver toxicity)
Food Interactions Food decreases bioavailability
Stability Intact vials and tablets should be stored at room temperature and protected from light; reconstitute 500 mg vial with 49.8 mL sterile water; the 10 mg/mL solution is stable for 24 hours
Mechanism of Action Prodrug incorporated into DNA and RNA; blocks purine synthesis and inhibits DNA and RNA synthesis
Pharmacokinetics
Absorption: Oral: Variable and incomplete (16% to 50%)
Distribution: Distributed throughout total body water; penetrates into CSF at low concentrations
Protein binding: 19%
Metabolism: Undergoes first-pass metabolism in the GI mucosa and liver; metabolized in the liver to sulfate conjugates, 6-thiouric acid, and other inactive compounds
Bioavailability: <20% (variable)
Half-life: Age dependent
  Children: <60 minutes
  Adults: 36-90 minutes
Time to peak serum concentration: Oral: Within 2 hours
Elimination: 20% excreted unchanged in urine
Usual Dosage Refer to individual protocols
Children:
  Oral:
    Induction: 2.5-5 mg/kg/day given once daily, or 70-100 mg/m^2/day once daily
    Maintenance: 1.5-2.5 mg/kg/day given once daily
  I.V. continuous infusion (investigational; distributed under the auspices of the NCI for authorized studies): 50 mg/m^2/hour for 24-48 hours, or 1000 mg/m^2/day for 24 hours
Adults: Oral:
  Induction: 2.5-5 mg/kg/day given once daily, or 80-100 mg/m^2/day given once daily
  Maintenance: 1.5-2.5 mg/kg/day given once daily
Dosing adjustment in renal impairment: Children and Adults:
  Cl_{cr} <50 mL/minute: Administer every 48 hours

Administration
Oral: Do not administer with meals
Parenteral: Administer by slow I.V. push over several minutes or by slow I.V. continuous infusion to reduce the incidence of vein irritation; further dilute the 10 mg/mL reconstituted solution in NS or D_5W to a final concentration for administration of 1-2 mg/mL

Monitoring Parameters CBC with differential and platelet count, liver function tests, uric acid, urinalysis

Patient Information Report to physician if fever, sore throat, bleeding, bruising, shortness of breath, or painful urination occurs; avoid alcohol

Nursing Implications Avoid extravasation

Additional Information Myelosuppressive effects:
WBC: Moderate
Platelets: Moderate
Onset (days): 7-10
Nadir (days): 14
Recovery (days): 21

Dosage Forms
Injection (investigational use only): 500 mg vial
Tablet: 50 mg

Extemporaneous Preparations A 50 mg/mL oral suspension was made by crushing the tablets, mixing with a volume of Cologel® suspending agent equal to $\frac{1}{3}$ the final volume, and adding a 2:1 mixture of simple syrup and cherry syrup to make the final volume; stable for 14 days when stored in an amber glass bottle at room temperature
Dressman JB and Poust RI, "Stability of Allopurinol and of Five Antineoplastics in Suspension," *Am J Hosp Pharm*, 1983, 40:616-8.

References
Zimm S, Ettinger LJ, Holcenberg JS, et al, "Phase I and Clinical Pharmacological Study of Mercaptopurine Administered as a Prolonged Intravenous Infusion," *Cancer Res*, 1988, 45(4):1869-73.

♦ **6-Mercaptopurine** *see* Mercaptopurine *on page 606*
♦ **Merlenate® Topical [OTC]** *see* Undecylenic Acid and Derivatives *on page 962*

Meropenem (mer oh PEN em)
Brand Names Merrem®
Available Salts Meropenem Trihydrate
Synonyms SM-7338
Therapeutic Category Antibiotic, Carbapenem
Use Treatment of multidrug-resistant gram-negative and gram-positive aerobic and anaerobic pathogens documented or suspected to be susceptible to meropenem; used in treatment of meningitis, lower respiratory tract infections, urinary tract infections, intra-abdominal infections, skin and skin structure infections and sepsis caused by susceptible *S. aureus*, group A *Streptococcus*, *S. pneumoniae*, *H. influenzae*, *M. catarrhalis*, *E. coli*, *Klebsiella*, *Enterobacter*, *Serratia*, *P. aeruginosa*, and *B. fragilis*

Pregnancy Risk Factor B

Contraindications Hypersensitivity to meropenem, any component, other carbapenems, or in patients who have experienced anaphylactic reactions to beta-lactams

Warnings Safety and efficacy in children <3 months of age have not been established; pseudomembranous colitis has been reported with the use of meropenem; prolonged use may result in superinfection

Precautions Use with caution in patients with a history of seizures, CNS disease, CNS infection, and/or compromised renal function; dosage adjustment required in patients with renal impairment

Adverse Reactions
Cardiovascular: Hypotension
Central nervous system: Seizures (<0.38%), headache, pain, insomnia, dizziness, agitation
Dermatologic: Rash (1.4%), pruritus
Gastrointestinal: Nausea, vomiting (1%), diarrhea (4.3%), melena, constipation, oral moniliasis
Hematologic: Leukopenia, neutropenia
Hepatic: Elevation in AST, ALT, alkaline phosphatase, LDH, and bilirubin
Local: Phlebitis (1.2%), inflammation at the injection site
Renal: Elevated BUN, elevated serum creatinine
Respiratory: Dyspnea

Drug Interactions Probenecid inhibits renal excretion of meropenem
(Continued)

Meropenem (Continued)

Stability Meropenem solution reconstituted with sterile water for injection is stable for up to 2 hours at room temperature or for up to 12 hours when refrigerated; when reconstituted with NS at a final concentration between 2.5-50 mg/mL, the solution is stable for up to 2 hours at room temperature or 18 hours when refrigerated; when reconstituted with D_5W at a final concentration between 2.5-50 mg/mL, the solution is stable for up to 1 hour at room temperature or 8 hours when refrigerated; solutions prepared for infusion in plastic I.V. bags with NS at concentrations ranging from 2.5-20 mg/mL are stable for 4 hours at room temperature or 24 hours when refrigerated

Mechanism of Action Inhibits cell wall synthesis by binding to penicillin-binding proteins (PBPs) with its strongest affinities for PBPs 2, 3 and 4 of *E. coli* and *P. aeruginosa* and PBPs 1, 2 and 4 of *S. aureus*

Pharmacokinetics

Distribution: Penetrates into most tissues and body fluids including CSF, urinary tract, peritoneal fluid, bile, lung, bronchial mucosa, muscle tissue, and heart valves

Protein binding: 2%

Metabolism: 20% is hydrolyzed in plasma to an inactive metabolite

Half-life:

Premature newborns: 3 hours

Full-term newborns: 2 hours

Infants 3 months to 2 years: 1.4 hours

Children 2-12 years and Adults: 1 hour

Elimination: Cleared by the kidney with 70% excreted unchanged in urine

Usual Dosage I.V.:

Children ≥3 months: 60 mg/kg/day divided every 8 hours; meningitis: 120 mg/kg/day divided every 8 hours; maximum dose: 6 g/day

Adults:

Mild to moderate infection: 1.5-3 g/day divided every 8 hours

Meningitis: 6 g/day divided every 8 hours

Dosage adjustment in renal impairment:

Cl_{cr} 26-50 mL/minute: Standard dose every 12 hours

Cl_{cr} 10-25 mL/minute: One-half dose every 12 hours

Cl_{cr} <10 mL/minute: One-half dose every 24 hours

Administration Administer by I.V. push or I.V. intermittent infusion; final concentration for administration should not exceed 50 mg/mL; infuse I.V. push injection over 3-5 minutes; intermittent infusion dose should be administered over 15-30 minutes

Monitoring Parameters Periodic renal, hepatic, and hematologic function tests

Test Interactions Positive Coombs' [direct]

Additional Information Sodium content 1 g: 3.92 mEq

Dosage Forms Injection, as trihydrate: 500 mg, 1 g

References

Blummer JL, Reed MD, Kearns GL, et al, "Sequential, Single-Dose Pharmacokinetic Evaluation of Meropenem in Hospitalized Infants and Children," *Antimicrob Agents Chemother*, 1995, 39(8):1721-5.

Bradley, JS, "Meropenem: A New, Extremely Broad Spectrum Beta-lactam Antibiotic for Serious Infections in Pediatrics," *Pediatr Infect Dis J*, 1997, 16:263-8.

Wiseman LR, Wagstaff AJ, Brogden RN, et al, "Meropenem. A Review of its Antibacterial Activity, Pharmacokinetic Properties and Clinical Efficacy," *Drugs*, 1995, 50(1):73-101.

♦ **Meropenem Trihydrate** *see* Meropenem *on page 607*

♦ **Merrem®** *see* Meropenem *on page 607*

Mesalamine (me SAL a meen)

Related Information

Drugs and Breast-Feeding *on page 1213*

Brand Names Asacol® Oral; Pentasa® Oral; Rowasa® Rectal

Synonyms 5-Aminosalicylic Acid; 5-ASA; Fisalamine; Mesalazine

Therapeutic Category 5-Aminosalicylic Acid Derivative; Anti-inflammatory Agent; Anti-inflammatory Agent, Rectal

Generic Available No

Use Treatment of ulcerative colitis (UC), proctosigmoiditis, and proctitis

Pregnancy Risk Factor B

Contraindications Hypersensitivity to mesalamine, any component, sulfites, or salicylates

Warnings Pericarditis should be considered in patients with chest pain (has occurred rarely with mesalamine containing products); pancreatitis should be considered in any patient with new abdominal complaints; has been implicated in the production of an acute intolerance syndrome or exacerbation of colitis (<3%)

Precautions Use with caution in patients with hypersensitivity to sulfasalazines

Adverse Reactions

Cardiovascular: Pericarditis, chest pain, myocarditis, T-wave abnormalities, edema

Central nervous system: Chills, dizziness, fever, headache, insomnia, malaise, anxiety, depression

Dermatologic: Psoriasis, dry skin, urticaria, pyoderma gangrenosum, erythema nodosum, photosensitivity, lichen planus, alopecia

Endocrine & metabolic: Amenorrhea, menorrhagia, breast pain

Gastrointestinal: Abdominal pain, cramps, flatulence, bloody diarrhea, anal irritation, anorexia, pancreatitis, gastritis, dyspepsia, eructation, vomiting, hemorrhoids, constipation, dysgeusia

Genitourinary: Epididymitis, dysuria, discoloration of urine (yellow-brown)

Hematologic: Agranulocytosis, thrombocytopenia

Hepatic: Elevated liver enzymes, jaundice, cholestatic jaundice, liver necrosis/failure

Neuromuscular & skeletal: Weakness

Renal: Interstitial nephritis, renal papillary necrosis, nephrotic syndrome

Respiratory: Interstitial pneumonitis, pulmonary infiltrates, sinusitis, asthma exacerbation

Miscellaneous: Kawasaki-like syndrome

Drug Interactions Decreased digoxin bioavailability

Stability Unstable in presence of water or light; once foil has been removed, unopened bottles have an expiration of 1 year following the date of manufacture

Mechanism of Action Mesalamine (5-aminosalicylic acid) is the active component of sulfasalazine; the specific mechanism of action of mesalamine is unknown; however, it is thought that it modulates local chemical mediators of the inflammatory response, especially leukotrienes; action appears topical rather than systemic

Pharmacokinetics

Absorption:

Capsule: 20% to 30%

Rectal: ~15%; variable and dependent upon retention time, underlying GI disease, and colonic pH

Tablet: 28%

Distribution: Breast milk to plasma ratio:

5-ASA: 0.27

Acetyl 5-ASA: 5.1

Metabolism: In the liver by acetylation to acetyl-5-aminosalicylic acid (acetyl-5-ASA-active metabolite) and to glucuronide conjugates; intestinal metabolism may also occur

Half-life:

5-ASA: 0.5-1.5 hours

Acetyl 5-ASA: 5-10 hours

Time to peak serum concentration: Oral, Rectal: Within 4-7 hours

Elimination: Most metabolites are excreted in urine with <2% appearing in feces

Usual Dosage Oral (usual course of therapy is 3-6 weeks):

(Oral products are formulated to slowly release therapeutic quantities of drug throughout the GI tract):

Capsule (ethylcellulose-coated, controlled release):

Children: 50 mg/kg/day divided every 6-12 hours

Adults: 1 g 4 times/day for up to 8 weeks

Tablet (coated with acrylic-based resin; drug released after reaches terminal ileum):

Children: 50 mg/kg/day divided every 8-12 hours

Adults: Treatment: 800 mg 3 times/day; maintenance for remission of UC: 1.6 g daily in divided doses up to 6 months

Retention enema: Adults: 60 mL (4 g) at bedtime, retained overnight, approximately 8 hours for 3-6 weeks

Rectal suppository: Adults: Insert 1 suppository (500 mg) in rectum twice daily, retained for 1-3 hours, for 3-6 weeks

Administration

Oral: Administer with food; swallow tablets whole, do not break outer coating

Rectal: Retain enema for 8 hours or as long as practical; shake rectal suspension well before use

Patient Information May discolor urine yellow-brown

Dosage Forms

Capsule, controlled release (Pentasa®): 250 mg

(Continued)

Mesalamine *(Continued)*

Suppository, rectal (Rowasa®): 500 mg
Suspension, rectal (Rowasa®): 4 g/60 mL (7s)
Tablet, enteric coated (Asacol®): 400 mg

References

Grand RJ, Ramakrishna J, and Calenda KA, "Inflammatory Bowel Disease in the Pediatric Patient," *Gastroenterol Clin North Am*, 1995, 24(3):613-32.

♦ **Mesalazine** *see* Mesalamine *on page 608*
♦ **Mesantoin®** *see* Mephenytoin *on page 604*
♦ **M-Eslon® (Canada)** *see* Morphine Sulfate *on page 657*

Mesna *(MES na)*

Brand Names Mesnex™

Synonyms Sodium 2-Mercaptoethane Sulfonate

Therapeutic Category Antidote, Cyclophosphamide-induced Hemorrhagic Cystitis; Antidote, Ifosfamide-induced Hemorrhagic Cystitis

Generic Available No

Use Detoxifying agent used as a protectant against hemorrhagic cystitis induced by ifosfamide and cyclophosphamide

Pregnancy Risk Factor B

Contraindications Hypersensitivity to mesna, other thiol compounds, or any component

Precautions Examine morning urine specimen for hematuria prior to ifosfamide or cyclophosphamide treatment; if hematuria develops, reduce the ifosfamide/cyclophosphamide dose or discontinue the drug and consider increasing the mesna dosage; for children less than 2 years of age, use **preservative free** mesna to decrease the amount of benzyl alcohol delivered to the infant

Adverse Reactions

Cardiovascular: Hypotension
Central nervous system: Malaise, headache
Dermatologic: Skin rash
Gastrointestinal: Diarrhea, nausea, vomiting, dysgeusia
Neuromuscular & skeletal: Limb pain

Stability Diluted solutions in D_5W, D_5 and sodium chloride, NS, or LR are chemically and physically stable for 48 hours at room temperature; compatible with solutions containing ifosfamide or cyclophosphamide; incompatible with cisplatin

Mechanism of Action In the urinary bladder, mesna binds with and detoxifies acrolein and other urotoxic metabolites of ifosfamide and cyclophosphamide via an active sulfhydryl group on mesna

Pharmacokinetics

Distribution: No tissue penetration; following glomerular filtration, mesna disulfide is reduced in the renal tubules back to mesna and delivered to the bladder in the active form
Bioavailability: Oral: 50%
Half-life: 24 minutes (mesna); after I.V. administration, mesna is rapidly oxidized intravascularly to mesna disulfide (half-life: 72 minutes)
Elimination: Unchanged drug and metabolite are excreted primarily in the urine; time for maximum urinary mesna excretion: 1 hour after I.V. and 2-3 hours after an oral mesna dose

Usual Dosage Children and Adults (refer to individual protocols): **Mesna dose depends on dose of antineoplastic agent used:**

When used with ifosfamide: I.V.: Mesna dose is 20% w/w of ifosfamide dose 15 minutes before and 4 and 8 hours later or combined with ifosfamide administration; for high-dose ifosfamide, mesna has been administered at a dose of 20% w/w 15 minutes before and every 3 hours for 3-6 doses or combined with ifosfamide administration; **(Note:** In clinical protocols, total daily mesna dose ranged between 60% to 160% w/w of the daily ifosfamide dose)

When used with cyclophosphamide: I.V.: Mesna dose is 20% w/w of cyclophosphamide dose 15 minutes before and every 3 hours for 3-4 doses or combined with cyclophosphamide administration; **(Note:** In clinical protocols, total daily mesna dose ranged between 60% to 160% w/w of the daily cyclophosphamide dose)

I.V. continuous infusion: Mesna doses equivalent to 60% to 100% of the ifosfamide or cyclophosphamide dose have been used

Oral: Mesna dose is 40% w/w of the antineoplastic agent dose in 3 doses at 4-hour intervals or 20 mg/kg/dose every 4 hours x 3 (oral mesna is not recommended for the first dose before ifosfamide or cyclophosphamide)

Administration

Oral: Dilute mesna solution before oral administration to decrease sulfur odor; mesna can be diluted 1:1 to 1:10 in carbonated cola drinks, fruit juices (grape, apple, tomato, and orange juice) or in plain or chocolate milk (most palatable in chilled grape juice)

Parenteral: Administer by I.V. infusion over 15-30 minutes, or by continuous I.V. infusion, or per protocol; mesna may be diluted in D_5W or NS to a final concentration of 1-20 mg/mL; may be added to solutions containing ifosfamide or cyclophosphamide

Monitoring Parameters Urinalysis

Test Interactions False-positive urinary ketones with Chemstrip®, Multistix®, or Labstix®

Nursing Implications Used concurrently with and/or following high-dose ifosfamide or cyclophosphamide; ensure adequate patient hydration; report vomiting within 1 hour of an oral mesna dose to physician so that I.V. mesna can be administered

Additional Information pH of the commercial 100 mg/mL solution: 6.5-8.5

Dosage Forms

Injection: 100 mg/mL (10 mL)

Injection, preservative free: 100 mg/mL (2 mL, 4 mL)

References

Ben Yehuda A, Heyman A and Steiner Salz D, "False Positive Reaction for Urinary Ketones With Mesna," *Drug Intell Clin Pharm*, 1987, 21(6): 547-8.

Brock N and Pohl J, "The Development of Mesna for Regional Detoxification," *Cancer Treat Rev*, 1983, 10(Suppl A):33-43.

"Cancer Chemotherapy," *Med Lett Drugs Ther*, 1989, 31(793):49-56.

Schoenike SE and Dana WJ, "Ifosfamide and Mesna," *Clin Pharm*, 1990, 9(3):179-91.

◆ **Mesnex™** *see* Mesna *on page 610*
◆ **Mestatin® (Canada)** *see* Nystatin *on page 701*
◆ **Mestinon® Injection** *see* Pyridostigmine *on page 826*
◆ **Mestinon® Oral** *see* Pyridostigmine *on page 826*
◆ **Metacortandralone** *see* Prednisolone *on page 791*
◆ **Metadate™ ER** *see* Methylphenidate *on page 627*
◆ **Metamucil® [OTC]** *see* Psyllium *on page 823*
◆ **Metamucil® Instant Mix [OTC]** *see* Psyllium *on page 823*
◆ **Metaprel®** *see* Metaproterenol *on page 611*

Metaproterenol (met a proe TER e nol)

Related Information

Asthma Guidelines *on page 1178*

Carbohydrate and Alcohol Content of Liquid Medications for Use in Patients Receiving Ketogenic Diets *on page 1228*

Brand Names Alupent®; Arm-a-Med® Metaproterenol; Dey-Dose® Metaproterenol; Metaprel®; Prometa®

Available Salts Metaproterenol Sulfate

Synonyms Orciprenaline

Therapeutic Category Adrenergic Agonist Agent; Antiasthmatic; $Beta_2$-Adrenergic Agonist Agent; Bronchodilator; Sympathomimetic

Generic Available Yes: Except inhaler

Use Bronchodilator in reversible airway obstruction due to asthma or COPD

Pregnancy Risk Factor C

Contraindications Hypersensitivity to metaproterenol or any component; preexisting cardiac arrhythmias associated with tachycardia; narrow-angle glaucoma

Warnings Excessive use may result in cardiac arrest and death; do not use concurrently with other sympathomimetic bronchodilators

Precautions Use with caution in patients with ischemic heart disease, hypertension, hyperthyroidism, seizure disorders, CHF, cardiac arrhythmias, and diabetes mellitus

Adverse Reactions

Cardiovascular: Tachycardia, palpitations, hypertension

Central nervous system: Nervousness, dizziness, headache, fatigue, vertigo

Gastrointestinal: Nausea, vomiting, diarrhea, GI distress, xerostomia, dysgeusia, throat irritation

Neuromuscular & skeletal: Tremor, weakness, muscle cramps

Respiratory: Exacerbation of asthma, hoarseness, cough, nasal congestion

(Continued)

Metaproterenol *(Continued)*

Drug Interactions Beta-adrenergic blockers (eg, propranolol) may antagonize metaproterenol's effects; sympathomimetics may increase adverse effects if administered concomitantly; MAO inhibitors may cause hypertensive crisis

Stability Protect from light

Mechanism of Action Relaxes bronchial smooth muscle and peripheral vasculature by action on beta$_2$-receptors

Pharmacodynamics
Onset of bronchodilation:
Oral: Within 30 minutes
Inhalation: Within 60 seconds
Peak effect: Oral: Within 1 hour
Duration: (approximately 1-5 hours) regardless of route administered

Pharmacokinetics
Absorption: Oral: Well absorbed
Metabolism: Extensive first-pass in the liver (~40% of oral dose is available)
Elimination: Mainly as glucuronic acid conjugates

Usual Dosage
Oral:
Children:
<2 years: 0.4 mg/kg/dose given 3-4 times/day; in infants, the dose can be given every 8-12 hours
2-6 years: 1.3-2.6 mg/kg/day divided every 6-8 hours
6-9 years: 10 mg/dose given 3-4 times/day
Children >9 years and Adults: 20 mg/dose given 3-4 times/day
Inhalation: Children >12 years and Adults: 2-3 inhalations every 3-4 hours, up to 12 inhalations in 24 hours
Nebulizer:
Infants and Children: 0.01-0.02 mL/kg (0.5-1 mg/kg) of 5% solution; minimum dose: 0.1 mL (5 mg); maximum dose: 0.3 mL (15 mg) every 4-6 hours (may be given more frequently according to need); equivalent doses using more dilute solutions may be administered at the same frequency
Adolescents and Adults: 0.2 to 0.3 mL (10-15 mg) of 5% metaproterenol every 4-6 hours (can be given more frequently according to need); equivalent doses using more dilute solutions may be administered at the same frequency

Administration
Nebulization: Dilute 5% solution in 2-3 mL NS; more dilute solutions may be used without dilution
Oral: Administer with food to decrease GI distress

Monitoring Parameters Heart rate, respiratory rate, blood pressure, arterial or capillary blood gases if applicable, pulmonary function tests

Dosage Forms
Aerosol, oral, as sulfate: 0.65 mg/dose (5 mL, 10 mL)
Solution for inhalation, preservative free, as sulfate: 0.4% [4 mg/mL] (2.5 mL); 0.6% [6 mg/mL] (2.5 mL); 5% [50 mg/mL] (10 mL, 30 mL)
Syrup, as sulfate: 10 mg/5 mL (480 mL)
Tablet, as sulfate: 10 mg, 20 mg

♦ **Metaproterenol Sulfate** *see* Metaproterenol *on page 611*
♦ **Metaradrine** *see* Metaminol *on page 612*

Metaraminol *(met a RAM i nole)*

Brand Names Aramine®

Available Salts Metaraminol Bitartrate

Synonyms Hydroxynorephedrine; Metaradrine

Therapeutic Category Adrenergic Agonist Agent; Alpha-Adrenergic Agonist; Sympathomimetic

Generic Available Yes

Use Prevention and treatment of an acute hypotensive state occurring with spinal anesthesia; treatment of shock which persists after adequate fluid volume replacement

Pregnancy Risk Factor C

Contraindications Hypersensitivity to metaraminol or any component; use with cyclopropane or halothane anesthesia

Warnings Contains sulfites, avoid in sensitive individuals; extravasant; may cause tissue necrosis and sloughing of surrounding skin if I.V. infiltration occurs; see Extravasation Treatment *on page 1050*; use of MAO inhibitors may result in potentiation of its pressor effects

Precautions Blood/volume depletion should be corrected, if possible, before meta-raminol therapy; use with caution in patients with heart or thyroid disease, hypertension, diabetes mellitus, and cirrhosis; because of its prolonged action, a cumulative effect is possible resulting in a prolonged elevation of blood pressure despite discontinuation of therapy; may provoke a relapse in patients with a history of malaria

Adverse Reactions
Cardiovascular: Tachycardia, bradycardia, hypertension, cardiac arrhythmias, palpitations, cardiac arrest
Central nervous system: Headache, dizziness, apprehension
Gastrointestinal: Nausea
Local: Tissue necrosis, sloughing at injection site, abscess formation
Neuromuscular & skeletal: Tremors
Miscellaneous: Diaphoresis

Drug Interactions Atropine may block the reflex bradycardia caused by metaraminol and enhance the pressor response; tricyclic antidepressants, MAO inhibitors, and ergot alkaloids may potentiate the effects of metaraminol; ectopic arrhythmias with concurrent use of digoxin; phentolamine and other alpha-adrenergic blocking agents will reduce metaraminol's effects

Stability Stable at room temperature; stable when diluted in D_5W, NS, Ringer's injection, LR injection, Normosol®-R, and Normosol®-M in 5% dextrose; use diluted solutions within 24 hours

Mechanism of Action Predominantly stimulates alpha-adrenergic receptors resulting in vasoconstriction and increased systemic blood pressure; it also stimulates $beta_1$-adrenergic receptors causing increased contractility and heart rate; clinically the chronotropic effect (increased heart rate) is overcome by increased vagal activity occurring as a reflex to increased arterial blood pressure; bradycardia usually results; metaraminol also has an indirect effect by releasing norepinephrine from storage sites

Pharmacodynamics
Onset:
I.V.: 1-2 minutes
I.M.: 10 minutes
S.C.: 5-20 minutes
Duration: 20-90 minutes depending upon the route of administration

Usual Dosage Use the lowest effective dosage for the shortest possible time:
Prevention of hypotension: I.M., S.C.:
Children: 0.1 mg/kg or 3 mg/m^2; repeat as needed, after at least 10 minutes
Adults: 2-10 mg; repeat as needed, after at least 10 minutes
Adjunctive treatment of shock: I.V.:
Children: 0.01 mg/kg or 0.3 mg/m^2; may follow with infusion of 0.4 mg/kg or 12 mg/m^2 at a rate adjusted to maintain the desired blood pressure
Adults: 0.5-5 mg; may follow with infusion of 15-100 mg at a rate adjusted to maintain the desired blood pressure

Administration Parenteral: Although approved for S.C., use only if other routes are unavailable due to potentially severe tissue irritation; may administer single doses without dilution by direct I.V. infusion slowly; for continuous infusion, dilute 15-100 mg in 500 mL of D_5W or NS; concentrations as high as 1 mg/mL have been used; administer I.V. infusions in large peripheral veins or use central venous access

Monitoring Parameters Blood pressure, heart rate, urine output, peripheral perfusion

Nursing Implications Monitor I.V. site closely for signs of infiltration/extravasation

Dosage Forms Injection, as bitartrate: 10 mg/mL (10 mL)

♦ **Metaraminol Bitartrate** see Metaraminol on page 612

Methadone (METH a done)

Related Information
Narcotic Analgesics Comparison on page 1035
Overdose and Toxicology on page 1191

Brand Names Dolophine®; Methadose® (Canada)

Available Salts Methadone Hydrochloride

Therapeutic Category Analgesic, Narcotic

Generic Available Yes

Use Management of severe pain, used in narcotic detoxification maintenance programs and for the treatment of iatrogenic narcotic dependency

Restrictions C-II

(Continued)

Methadone *(Continued)*

Pregnancy Risk Factor B (D if used for prolonged periods or in high doses at term)

Contraindications Hypersensitivity to methadone or any component

Warnings Tablets are to be used only for oral administration and **must not** be used for injection

Precautions Due to the cumulative effects of methadone, the dose and frequency of administration need to be reduced with repeated use; use with caution in patients with respiratory diseases; methadone's effect on respiration lasts longer than analgesic effects

Adverse Reactions

Cardiovascular: Hypotension, bradycardia, peripheral vasodilation

Central nervous system: CNS depression, increased intracranial pressure, drowsiness, dizziness, sedation (marked sedation seen after repeated administration)

Endocrine & metabolic: Antidiuretic hormone release

Gastrointestinal: Nausea, vomiting, constipation, xerostomia, biliary tract spasm

Genitourinary: Urinary tract spasm

Ocular: Miosis

Respiratory: Respiratory depression

Miscellaneous: Histamine release, physical and psychological dependence with prolonged use

Drug Interactions Cytochrome P-450 isoenzyme CYP1A2, CYP2D6, CYP3A3/4 substrate; CYP2D6 isoenzyme inhibitor

CNS depressants, alcohol, phenothiazines, tricyclic antidepressants may potentiate the adverse effects of methadone; barbiturates, carbamazepine, phenytoin, primidone, nevirapine, and rifampin may increase the metabolism of methadone and may precipitate withdrawal (monitor patients, larger doses of methadone may be required)

Mechanism of Action Binds to opiate receptors in the CNS, causing inhibition of ascending pain pathways, altering the perception of and response to pain; produces generalized CNS depression

Pharmacodynamics Analgesia:

Onset of action:

Oral: Within 30-60 minutes

Parenteral: Within 10-20 minutes

Peak action: Parenteral: 1-2 hours

Duration: Oral: 6-8 hours; after repeated doses, duration increases to 22-48 hours

Pharmacokinetics

Distribution: Crosses the placenta; appears in breast milk

V_d: (Mean ± SD)

Children: 7.1 ± 2.5 L/kg

Adults: 6.1 ± 2.4 L/kg

Protein binding: 80% to 85%

Metabolism: N-demethylated in the liver

Half-life: May be prolonged with alkaline pH

Children: 19 ± 14 hours (range: 4-62 hours)

Adults: 35 ± 22 hours (range: 9-87 hours)

Elimination: In urine (<10% as unchanged drug); increased renal excretion with urine pH <6

Usual Dosage Doses should be titrated to appropriate effects:

Neonatal abstinence syndrome: Oral, I.V.: Initial: 0.05-0.2 mg/kg/dose given every 12-24 hours or 0.5 mg/kg/day divided every 8 hours; individualize dose and tapering schedule to control symptoms of withdrawal; usually taper dose by 10% to 20% per week over 1 to 1½ months. **Note:** Due to long elimination half-life, tapering is difficult; consider alternate agent.

Children:

Analgesia:

I.V.: Initial: 0.1 mg/kg/dose every 4 hours for 2-3 doses, then every 6-12 hours as needed; maximum dose: 10 mg/dose

Oral, I.M., S.C.: Initial: 0.1 mg/kg/dose every 4 hours for 2-3 doses, then every 6-12 hours as needed or 0.7 mg/kg/24 hours divided every 4-6 hours as needed; maximum dose: 10 mg/dose

Iatrogenic narcotic dependency: Oral: Controlled studies have not been conducted; several clinically used dosing regimens have been reported. Methadone dose **must be individualized** and will depend upon patient's previous narcotic dose and severity of opioid withdrawal; patients who have received higher doses of narcotics will require higher methadone doses.

General guidelines: Initial: 0.05-0.1 mg/kg/dose every 6 hours; increase by 0.05 mg/kg/dose until withdrawal symptoms are controlled; after 24-48 hours, the dosing interval can be lengthened to every 12-24 hours; to taper dose, wean by 0.05 mg/kg/day; if withdrawal symptoms recur, taper at a slower rate

Adults:
  Analgesia: Oral, I.M., I.V., S.C.: 2.5-10 mg every 3-8 hours as needed, up to 5-20 mg every 6-8 hours
  Detoxification: Oral: 15-40 mg/day
  Maintenance of opiate dependence: Oral: 20-120 mg/day
Dosing adjustment in renal impairment: Children and Adults:
  Cl_{cr} <10 mL/minute: Administer 50% to 75% of normal dose

Administration Oral: Administer with juice or water; dispersible tablet should be completely dissolved before administration; oral dose for detoxification and maintenance may be administered in Tang®, Kool-Aid®, apple juice, grape Crystal Light®

Monitoring Parameters Respiratory, cardiovascular, and mental status, pain relief (if used for analgesia)

Patient Information Avoid alcohol; may be habit-forming; may cause drowsiness and impair ability to perform activities requiring mental alertness or physical coordination

Additional Information Methadone accumulates with repeated doses and dosage may need to be adjusted downward after 3-5 days to prevent toxic effects. Some patients may benefit from every 8- to 12-hour dosing interval (pain control).

Methadone 10 mg I.M. = morphine 10 mg I.M.

Dosage Forms
Injection, as hydrochloride: 10 mg/mL (1 mL, 10 mL, 20 mL)
Solution, as hydrochloride:
  Oral: 5 mg/5 mL (5 mL, 500 mL); 10 mg/5 mL (500 mL)
  Oral, concentrate: 10 mg/mL (30 mL)
Tablet, as hydrochloride: 5 mg, 10 mg
Tablet, dispersible, as hydrochloride: 40 mg

References
Anand KJ and Arnold JH, "Opioid Tolerance and Dependence in Infants and Children," *Crit Care Med*, 1994, 22(2):334-42.
Berde C, Ablin A, Glazer J, et al, "American Academy of Pediatrics Report of the Subcommittee on Disease-Related Pain in Childhood Cancer," *Pediatrics*, 1990, 86(5 Pt 2):818-25.
Lauriault G, LeBelle MJ, Lodge BA, et al, "Stability of Methadone in Four Vehicles for Oral Administration," *Am J Hosp Pharm*, 1991, 48(6):1252-6.
Olkkola KT, Hamunen K, and Maunuksela EL, "Clinical Pharmacokinetics and Pharmacodynamics of Opioid Analgesics in Infants and Children," *Clin Pharmacokinet*, 1995, 28(5):385-404.

♦ **Methadone Hydrochloride** *see* Methadone *on page 613*
♦ **Methadose® (Canada)** *see* Methadone *on page 613*

Methenamine (meth EN a meen)

Brand Names Dehydral™ (Canada); Hiprex®; Mandelamine®; Mandelamine® (Canada); Urasal® (Canada); Urex®

Available Salts Methenamine Hippurate; Methenamine Mandelate

Synonyms Hexamethylenetetramine

Therapeutic Category Antibiotic, Miscellaneous

Generic Available Yes

Use Prophylaxis or suppression of recurrent urinary tract infections

Pregnancy Risk Factor C

Contraindications Severe dehydration, renal insufficiency (methenamine is ineffective in patients with renal impairment), hepatic insufficiency in patients receiving hippurate salt; hypersensitivity to methenamine, tartrazine dye (Hiprex® tablets), or any component

Warnings Dosage of 8 g/day has been associated with bladder irritation, albuminuria, and hematuria

Precautions Use with caution in patients with hepatic impairment

Adverse Reactions
Central nervous system: Headache
Dermatologic: Rash, pruritus, urticaria
Gastrointestinal: Nausea, vomiting, diarrhea, abdominal cramping, anorexia, stomatitis
Genitourinary: Bladder irritation, painful and frequent micturition, dysuria, crystalluria
Hepatic: Elevation in AST and ALT (with hippurate formulation)
Otic: Tinnitus
(Continued)

Methenamine *(Continued)*

Renal: Hematuria

Respiratory: Lipoid pneumonitis (with mandelate suspension), dyspnea

Drug Interactions Sulfamethizole (precipitates in acid urine); sodium bicarbonate, acetazolamide (decrease effect of methenamine)

Food Interactions Foods/diets which alkalinize urine pH >5.5 decrease activity of methenamine; cranberry juice can be used to acidify urine and increase activity of methenamine

Stability Protect from excessive heat

Mechanism of Action Methenamine is hydrolyzed to formaldehyde and ammonia in acidic urine; formaldehyde has nonspecific bactericidal action

Pharmacokinetics

Absorption: Readily from the GI tract; 10% to 30% of the drug will be hydrolyzed by gastric juices unless it is protected by an enteric coating

Distribution: Distributes into breast milk; crosses the placenta

Metabolism: ~10% to 25% in the liver

Half-life: 3-6 hours

Elimination: Excretion occurs via glomerular filtration and tubular secretion with ~70% to 90% of dose excreted unchanged in urine within 24 hours

Usual Dosage Oral:

Children 6-12 years:

Hippurate: 25-50 mg/kg/day divided every 12 hours; maximum dose: 2 g/day

Mandelate: 75 mg/kg/day divided every 12 hours; maximum dose: 4 g/day

Adults:

Hippurate: 1 g twice daily

Mandelate: 1 g 4 times/day after meals and at bedtime

Administration Oral: Administer with food to minimize GI upset; patient should drink plenty of fluids to ensure adequate urine flow; administer with cranberry juice, ascorbic acid, or ammonium chloride to acidify urine and avoid intake of alkalinizing agents (sodium bicarbonate, antacids)

Monitoring Parameters Urinary pH, urinalysis, periodic liver function tests in patients receiving hippurate salt

Test Interactions Formaldehyde interferes with fluorometric procedures causing falsely increased results for catecholamines and VMA (U); falsely decreased urine estriol concentration with tests using acid hydrolysis

Nursing Implications Urine should be acidic, pH <5.5 for maximum effect

Additional Information Should not be used to treat infections outside of the lower urinary tract (ie, pyelonephritis)

Dosage Forms

Suspension, as mandelate: 250 mg/5 mL (coconut flavor), 500 mg/5 mL (cherry flavor)

Tablet, as hippurate (Hiprex®, Urex®): 1 g (Hiprex® contains tartrazine dye)

Tablet, as mandelate, enteric coated (Mandelamine®): 250 mg, 500 mg, 1 g

References

"Practice Parameter: The Diagnosis, Treatment, and Evaluation of the Initial Urinary Tract Infection in Febrile Infants and Young Children. American Academy of Pediatrics. Committee on Quality Improvement. Subcommittee on Urinary Tract Infection," *Pediatrics,* 1999, 103(4 Pt 1):843-52.

♦ **Methenamine Hippurate** *see* Methenamine *on page 615*

♦ **Methenamine Mandelate** *see* Methenamine *on page 615*

Methicillin *(meth i SIL in)*

Brand Names Staphcillin®

Available Salts Methicillin Sodium

Synonyms Dimethoxyphenyl Penicillin

Therapeutic Category Antibiotic, Penicillin (Antistaphylococcal)

Generic Available No

Use Treatment of susceptible bacterial infections such as osteomyelitis, septicemia, endocarditis, and CNS infections due to penicillinase-producing strains of *Staphylococcus*

Pregnancy Risk Factor B

Contraindications Hypersensitivity to methicillin, penicillins, or any component

Warnings Elimination rate will be decreased in neonates; acute interstitial nephritis manifested by fever, macular rash, eosinophilia, oliguria, hematuria and proteinuria may occur 5 days to 5 weeks after starting methicillin; it occurs more frequently in patients receiving prolonged therapy or at doses >200 mg/kg/day

Precautions Use with caution and modify dosage in patients with renal impairment

Adverse Reactions

Central nervous system: Fever, seizures

Dermatologic: Rash, pruritus

Gastrointestinal: Hairy tongue, stomatitis

Genitourinary: Hemorrhagic cystitis

Hematologic: Eosinophilia, anemia, leukopenia, neutropenia, thrombocytopenia

Hepatic: Elevated AST and ALT

Local: Phlebitis

Renal: Nephrotoxicity (interstitial nephritis), hematuria

Miscellaneous: Serum sickness-like reactions

Drug Interactions Probenecid (increases serum concentration of methicillin)

Stability Reconstituted solution containing methicillin 500 mg/mL is stable for 24 hours at room temperature and 4 days when refrigerated; incompatible with aminoglycosides and tetracyclines

Mechanism of Action Inhibits bacterial cell wall synthesis by binding to one or more of the penicillin-binding proteins; inhibits the final transpeptidation step of peptidoglycan synthesis in bacterial cell walls

Pharmacokinetics

Distribution: Crosses the placenta; distributes into breast milk; distributes into synovial, pleural, and pericardial fluids, bone and bile; low concentrations attained in CSF when meninges are uninflamed

Protein binding: 40%

Metabolism: 20% to 30%

Half-life:

Neonates:

$\leq$2 weeks: 2-3.9 hours

>2 weeks: 0.9-3.3 hours

Infants and Children: 0.8-1.2 hours

Children 2-16 years: 0.8 hours

Adults: 0.5-0.8 hours with normal renal function

Time to peak serum concentration: I.M.: Within 30-60 minutes

Elimination: ~60% to 70% of dose eliminated unchanged in urine within 4 hours by tubular secretion and glomerular filtration

Not dialyzable (0% to 5%)

Usual Dosage I.M., I.V.:

Neonates:

0-4 weeks, <1200 g: 50 mg/kg/day divided every 12 hours; meningitis: 100 mg/kg/day divided every 12 hours

$\leq$7 days:

1200-2000 g: 50 mg/kg/day divided every 12 hours; meningitis: 100 mg/kg/day divided every 12 hours

>2000 g: 75 mg/kg/day divided every 8 hours; meningitis: 150 mg/kg/day divided every 8 hours

>7 days:

1200-2000 g: 75 mg/kg/day divided every 8 hours; meningitis: 150 mg/kg/day divided every 8 hours

>2000 g: 100 mg/kg/day divided every 6 hours; meningitis: 200 mg/kg/day divided every 6 hours

Children: 150-200 mg/kg/day divided every 6 hours; 200-400 mg/kg/day divided every 4-6 hours has been used for treatment of severe infections; maximum dose: 12 g/day; **Note:** Acute interstitial nephritis occurs more frequently in patients receiving doses >200 mg/kg/day

Adults: 4-12 g/day in divided doses every 4-6 hours

Dosing interval in renal impairment:

Cl_{cr} <10 mL/minute: Administer every 8-12 hours

Administration Parenteral:

I.M.: Administer deep I.M. into a large muscle mass (ie, gluteus maximus) using a solution with a final concentration of 500 mg/mL

I.V.: May administer IVP at a rate not to exceed 200 mg/minute or intermittent infusion over 15-30 minutes; final concentration for administration should not exceed 20 mg/mL; in fluid-restricted patients, a final concentration for administration of 100 mg/mL has been used

Monitoring Parameters Urinalysis, BUN, serum creatinine, CBC with differential, and periodic liver function tests

Test Interactions Positive Coombs' [direct], false increase in serum uric acid concentration when the copper-chelate method is used

Additional Information Sodium content of 1 g: 2.9 mEq

Dosage Forms Powder for injection, as sodium: 1 g, 4 g, 6 g, 10 g

(Continued)

Methicillin *(Continued)*

References
Prober CG, Stevenson DK, and Benitz WE, "The Use of Antibiotics in Neonates Weighing Less Than 1200 Grams," *Pediatr Infect Dis J*, 1990, 9(2):111-21.

Yow MD, Taber LH, Barrett FF, et al, "A Ten-Year Assessment of Methicillin-Associated Side Effects," *Pediatrics*, 1976, 58(3):329-34.

♦ **Methicillin Sodium** *see* Methicillin *on page 616*

Methimazole *(meth IM a zole)*
Brand Names Tapazole®
Synonyms Thiamazole
Therapeutic Category Antithyroid Agent
Generic Available No
Use Palliative treatment of hyperthyroidism, to return the hyperthyroid patient to a normal metabolic state prior to thyroidectomy, and to control thyrotoxic crisis that may accompany thyroidectomy

Pregnancy Risk Factor D

Contraindications Hypersensitivity to methimazole or any component, nursing mothers per manufacturer, however, expert analysis and the American Academy of Pediatrics state this drug may be used with caution in nursing mothers (see Drugs and Breast-Feeding *on page 1213*)

Precautions Use with extreme caution in patients receiving other drugs known to cause agranulocytosis

Adverse Reactions
Cardiovascular: Edema, periarteritis
Central nervous system: Drowsiness, vertigo, headache, CNS stimulation, neuropathies, CNS depression, fever, dizziness
Endocrine & metabolic: Goiter
Dermatologic: Rash, urticaria, pruritus, alopecia, skin pigmentation, exfoliative dermatitis
Gastrointestinal: Ageusia, nausea, vomiting, epigastric distress, splenomegaly, constipation, weight gain
Hematologic: Agranulocytosis, hypoprothrombinemia
Hepatic: Cholestatic jaundice, hepatitis
Neuromuscular & skeletal: Arthralgia, myalgia, paresthesia, neuritis
Renal: Nephritis
Respiratory: Interstitial pneumonitis
Miscellaneous: Lupus-like syndrome, lymphadenopathy, insulin autoimmune syndrome

Drug Interactions Lithium and potassium iodide may potentiate hypothyroid effects; potentiates warfarin's anticoagulant effects

Mechanism of Action Inhibits the synthesis of thyroid hormones by blocking the oxidation of iodine in the thyroid gland, blocking iodine's ability to combine with tyrosine to form thyroxine (T_4) and triiodothyronine (T_3)

Pharmacodynamics Antithyroid effect:
Onset: 12-18 hours
Duration: 36-72 hours

Pharmacokinetics
Distribution: Found in high concentrations in breast milk; breast milk to plasma ratio: 1.0
Bioavailability: 80% to 95%
Half-life: 5-13 hours
Time to peak serum concentration: 1 hour
Elimination: <12% excreted in urine

Usual Dosage Oral:
Children:
Initial: 0.4 mg/kg/day in 3 divided doses; maintenance: 0.2 mg/kg/day in 3 divided doses
or
Initial: 0.5-0.7 mg/kg/day or 15-20 mg/m²/day in 3 divided doses
Maintenance: 1/3 to 2/3 of initial dose; maximum dose: 30 mg/day
Adults: Initial: 5 mg every 8 hours; 10 mg every 8 hours for moderately severe disease and up to 20 mg every 8 hours for severe hyperthyroidism; maintenance: 5-15 mg/day

Administration Oral: Administer with meals

Monitoring Parameters CBC with differential, liver function (baseline and as needed); serum thyroxine, free thyroxine index, prothrombin time

Patient Information Notify physician of fever, sore throat, unusual bleeding or bruising, headache, rash, or yellowing of skin

Dosage Forms Tablet: 5 mg, 10 mg

References

Raby C, Lagorce JF, Jambut-Absil AC, et al, "The Mechanism of Action of Synthetic Antithyroid Drugs: Iodine Complexation During Oxidation of Iodide," *Endocrinology*, 1990, 126(3):1683-91.

Methocarbamol (meth oh KAR ba mole)

Brand Names Delaxin®; Marbaxin®; Robaxin®; Robomol®

Therapeutic Category Skeletal Muscle Relaxant, Nonparalytic

Generic Available Yes

Use Treatment of muscle spasm associated with acute painful musculoskeletal conditions; supportive therapy in tetanus

Pregnancy Risk Factor C

Contraindications Hypersensitivity to methocarbamol or any component

Warnings Solution is hypertonic, avoid extravasation; avoid using injection in patients with impaired renal function because the polyethylene glycol vehicle may be irritating to the kidneys

Precautions Use injectable form cautiously in patients with suspected or known seizure disorders

Adverse Reactions
Cardiovascular: Syncope, bradycardia, hypotension
Central nervous system: Drowsiness, dizziness, lightheadedness, headache, fever, vertigo, seizures
Dermatologic: Urticaria, pruritus
Gastrointestinal: Nausea, metallic taste, GI upset, vomiting
Genitourinary: Discoloration of urine (brown, black, or green)
Hematologic: Leukopenia
Local: Pain and phlebitis at injection site, thrombophlebitis
Ocular: Blurred vision, conjunctivitis, nystagmus, diplopia
Respiratory: Nasal congestion
Miscellaneous: Hypersensitivity reactions

Stability Injection when diluted to 4 mg/mL in sterile water, D_5W, or NS is stable for 6 days at room temperature; do **not** refrigerate after dilution

Mechanism of Action Central nervous system depressant with sedative and skeletal muscle relaxant effects; exact mechanism of action is unknown

Pharmacodynamics Onset of action: 30 minutes

Pharmacokinetics Oral:
Metabolism: Extensive in the liver
Half-life: 0.9-1.8 hours
Time to peak serum concentration: Within ~1-2 hours

Usual Dosage
Tetanus: I.V.:
Children (recommended **only** for use in tetanus): 15 mg/kg/dose or 500 mg/m²/dose, may repeat every 6 hours if needed; maximum dose: 1.8 g/m²/day for 3 days only
Adults: 1-2 g by direct I.V. injection followed by additional 1-2 g (maximum dose: 3 g total); repeat with 1-2 g every 6 hours until NG tube or oral therapy possible; total daily dose of up to 24 g may be needed
Muscle spasm: Adults:
Oral: 1.5 g 3-4 times/day or 750 mg every 4 hours for 2-3 days, then decrease to 4-4.5 g/day in 3-6 divided doses
I.M., I.V.: 1 g every 8 hours if oral not possible; maximum dose: 3 g/day for 3 consecutive days (except when treating tetanus); may be reinstituted after 2 drug-free days

Dosing adjustment in renal impairment: Do not administer parenteral formulation to patients with renal dysfunction

Administration
Parenteral: I.V.: May be injected directly I.V. without dilution at a maximum rate of 180 mg/m²/minute but not >3 mL/minute; may also be diluted in NS or D_5W to a concentration of 4 mg/mL and infused more slowly; patient should be in the recumbent position during and for 10-15 minutes after I.V. administration
I.M.: Do not inject more than 3 mL per site; not recommended for S.C. administration

Test Interactions 5-hydroxyindoleacetic acid (5-HIAA) and vanillylmandelic acid (VMA)
(Continued)

Methocarbamol *(Continued)*

Patient Information May cause drowsiness and impair ability to perform hazardous activities requiring mental alertness or physical coordination; urine may darken to brown, black, or green

Nursing Implications Avoid infiltration, extremely irritating to tissues

Dosage Forms
Injection: 100 mg/mL in polyethylene glycol 50% (10 mL)
Tablet: 500 mg, 750 mg

Methohexital *(meth oh HEKS i tal)*

Related Information
Adult ACLS Algorithm, Electrical Conversion *on page 1014*
Preprocedure Sedatives in Children *on page 1169*

Brand Names Brevital® Sodium; Brietal Sodium® (Canada)

Available Salts Methohexital Sodium

Therapeutic Category Barbiturate; General Anesthetic; Sedative

Generic Available No

Use Induction and maintenance of general anesthesia for short procedures; induction of hypnotic state

Restrictions C-IV

Pregnancy Risk Factor B

Contraindications Porphyria; hypersensitivity to methohexital, barbiturates, or any component; patients in whom general anesthesia is contraindicated

Warnings Continuously monitor respiratory function, pulse oximetry, and cardiac function. Resuscitative drugs, ventilation and intubation equipment, and trained personnel should be immediately available. For deep sedation, a designated individual (other than the person performing the procedure) should be present to continuously monitor the patient.

Precautions Use with extreme caution in patients with liver impairment, asthma, cardiovascular instability; may precipitate seizures in patients with history of convulsions, especially partial seizure disorders; prolonged administration may result in increased CNS, respiratory, and cardiovascular effects; use with caution in patients with obstructive pulmonary disease, severe hypertension or hypotension, myocardial disease, CHF, severe anemia, extreme obesity, renal impairment, or endocrine disorders

Adverse Reactions
Cardiovascular: Hypotension, peripheral vascular collapse, tachycardia (following induction)
Central nervous system: Seizures, headache, somnolence, unconsciousness
Gastrointestinal: Nausea, vomiting
Local: Pain on I.M. injection, thrombophlebitis
Neuromuscular & skeletal: Twitching, rigidity, tremor, involuntary muscle movement
Respiratory: Apnea, respiratory depression, laryngospasm, coughing
Miscellaneous: Hiccups

Drug Interactions CNS depressants may increase effects; prior chronic use of phenytoin, barbiturates, or other enzyme inducing agents may decrease effect of methohexital; methohexital may affect absorption or elimination of phenytoin, anticoagulants, corticosteroids, halothane, ethanol, propylene glycol containing solutions

Stability Do not dilute with solutions containing bacteriostatic agents; acceptable diluents: D_5W, NS, SWI, or accompanying diluent (for 500 mg vial to make a 1% solution); SWI is the preferred diluent except for making the 0.2% solution for I.V. continuous infusion (use of SWI to make the 0.2% solution will result in extreme hypotonicity; D_5W or NS should be used). Do not use I.V./I.M. solutions if not clear and colorless. Solutions are alkaline (pH 9.5-11) and incompatible with acids (eg, atropine sulfate, succinylcholine chloride); incompatible with phenol-containing solutions, silicone, and LR

Mechanism of Action Ultra short-acting I.V. barbiturate anesthetic; depresses CNS activity by binding to barbiturate site at GABA-receptor complex enhancing GABA activity; depresses reticular activating system; higher doses may be gabamimetic

Pharmacodynamics
Onset of Effect
I.M. (pediatric patients): 2-10 minutes
I.V.: 1 minute
Rectal (pediatric patients): 5-15 minutes

Duration:
  I.M.: 1-1.5 hours
  I.V.: 7-10 minutes
  Rectal: 1-1.5 hours

Pharmacokinetics
  Metabolism: In the liver via demethylation and oxidation
  Bioavailability: Rectal: 17%
  Elimination: Through the kidney via glomerular filtration

Usual Dosage Doses must be titrated to effect
  Manufacturer's recommendations:
    Infants <1 month: Safety and efficacy not established
    Infants ≥1 month and Children:
      I.M.: Induction: 6.6-10 mg/kg of a 5% solution
      Rectal: Induction: Usual: 25 mg/kg of a 1% solution
  Alternative pediatric dosing:
    Children 3-12 years:
      I.M.: Preoperative: 5-10 mg/kg/dose
      I.V.: Induction: 1-2 mg/kg/dose (additional studies are needed)
      Rectal: Preoperative/induction: 20-35 mg/kg/dose; usual: 25 mg/kg/dose; maximum dose: 500 mg/dose; give as 10% aqueous solution

  Adults: I.V.:
    Induction: Range: 50-120 or 1-1.5 mg/kg; usual: 70 mg (**Note:** This provides anesthesia for 5-7 minutes)
    Maintenance: Intermittent I.V. bolus injection: 20-40 mg (2-4 mL of a 1% solution) every 4-7 minutes **OR** Continuous infusion: Average dose: 6 mg/minute (eg, 3 mL/minute of a 0.2% solution); titrate to effect; reduce administration rate gradually for longer surgical procedures

Administration
  Parenteral:
    I.M.: Reconstitute with NS to a maximum concentration of 50 mg/mL (5% solution)
    I.V.: Adults:
      Bolus: Dilute with SWI (preferred), NS, or D_5W to a maximum concentration of 10 mg/mL (1% solution); for induction, infuse a 1% solution at a rate of 1 mL/ 5 seconds
      Continuous infusion: Dilute with D_5W or NS to prepare a 0.2% solution (see Usual Dosage)
    Rectal: Dilute with acceptable diluent to a recommended concentration of 10 mg/ mL (1% solution)

Monitoring Parameters Blood pressure, heart rate, respiratory rate, oxygen saturation, pulse oximetry

Patient Information May cause drowsiness and impair ability to perform activities requiring mental alertness or physical coordination; do not drive a motor vehicle or operate machinery until 8-12 hours after medication was administered, or until normal functions return (whichever is longer)

Nursing Implications Check catheter placement prior to I.V. injection; avoid extravasation; avoid intra-arterial administration (thrombosis, necrosis, and gangrene may occur)

Additional Information Does not possess analgesic properties; Brevital® has FDA-approved labeling for I.V. use in adults, and for rectal and I.M. use only in pediatric patients >1 month of age; 100 pediatric patients (3 months to 5 years of age) received rectal methohexital (25 mg/kg) for sedation prior to computed tomography (CT) scan; sedation was adequate in 95% of patients; mean time for full sedation = 8.2 ± 3.9 minutes; mean duration of action = 79.3 ± 30.9 minutes; 10% of patients had transient side effects (see Pomeranz, 2000)

Dosage Forms Injection, as sodium: 500 mg, 2.5 g, 5 g

References
Cote' CJ, "Sedation for the Pediatric Patient," *Pediatr Clin North Am*, 1994, 41(1):31-58.
Pomeranz ES, Chudnofsky CR, Deegan TJ, et al, "Rectal Methohexital Sedation for Computed Tomography Imaging of Stable Pediatric Emergency Department Patients," *Pediatrics*, 2000, 105(5):1110-4.

♦ **Methohexital Sodium** *see* Methohexital *on page 620*
♦ **Methoin** *see* Mephenytoin *on page 604*

Methotrexate (meth oh TREKS ate)

Related Information
  Drugs and Breast-Feeding *on page 1213*
  Emetogenic Potential of Single Chemotherapeutic Agents *on page 1095*
  Brand Names Rheumatrex® Oral
  (Continued)

Methotrexate *(Continued)*

Available Salts Methotrexate Sodium

Synonyms Amethopterin; MTX

Therapeutic Category Antineoplastic Agent, Antimetabolite; Antirheumatic, Disease Modifying

Generic Available Yes

Use Treatment of trophoblastic neoplasms, leukemias, histiocytoses, osteosarcoma, non-Hodgkin's lymphoma; psoriasis; children with severe polyarticular juvenile rheumatoid arthritis who have failed to respond to other agents

Pregnancy Risk Factor D

Contraindications Hypersensitivity to methotrexate or any component; severe renal or hepatic impairment; pre-existing profound bone marrow suppression; high-dose methotrexate (>1 g/m^2) should not be administered to patients with a creatinine clearance of <50% to 75% of normal

Warnings The FDA currently recommends that procedures for proper handling and disposal of antineoplastic agents be considered. Due to the possibility of severe toxic reactions, fully inform patient of the risks involved; do not use in women of childbearing age unless benefit outweighs risks; may cause hepatotoxicity, fibrosis and cirrhosis, along with marked bone marrow suppression; death from intestinal perforation may occur.

Precautions Use with caution in patients with peptic ulcer disease, ulcerative colitis, pre-existing bone marrow suppression; use with caution and reduce dosage in patients with renal or hepatic impairment, ascites, and pleural effusion

Adverse Reactions

Cardiovascular: Vasculitis

Central nervous system: Malaise, fatigue, dizziness, encephalopathy, seizures, confusion, fever, headache, chills

Dermatitis: Alopecia, rash, depigmentation or hyperpigmentation of skin, photosensitivity, pruritus, urticaria

Endocrine & metabolic: Hyperuricemia

Gastrointestinal: Nausea, vomiting, diarrhea, anorexia, stomatitis, enteritis

Genitourinary: Cystitis

Hematologic: Myelosuppression, leukopenia, thrombocytopenia, anemia, hemorrhage

Hepatic: Hepatotoxicity, elevation in liver enzymes, hyperbilirubinemia

Neuromuscular & skeletal: Arthralgia

Ocular: Blurred vision

Renal: Nephropathy (azotemia, hematuria, renal failure)

Respiratory: Interstitial pneumonitis

Miscellaneous: Anaphylaxis

Drug Interactions Salicylates may delay MTX's clearance; sulfonamides, phenytoin displace MTX from protein binding sites; live virus vaccines, pyrimethamine, 5-FU; NSAIDs increase toxicity of MTX by elevating serum MTX concentrations; penicillins may decrease renal clearance of MTX; probenecid decreases the renal elimination of MTX

Food Interactions Milk-rich foods may decrease MTX absorption; folate may decrease drug response

Stability Protect from light; incompatible with fluorouracil, cytarabine, prednisolone, and sodium phosphate

Mechanism of Action An antimetabolite that binds to dihydrofolate reductase blocking the reduction of dihydrofolate to tetrahydrofolic acid; depletion of tetrahydrofolic acid leads to depletion of DNA precursors and inhibition of DNA and purine synthesis

Pharmacodynamics Approximate time to benefit in treatment of rheumatoid arthritis: 1-2 months

Pharmacokinetics

Absorption:

Oral: Average: 30%; variable absorption at low doses (<30 mg/m^2); incomplete absorption after large doses

I.M.: Completely absorbed

Distribution: Small amounts excreted into breast milk; crosses the placenta; does not achieve therapeutic concentrations in the CSF; sustained concentrations are retained in the kidney and liver

Metabolism: In the liver to 7-hydroxymethotrexate

Protein binding: 50% to 60%

Time to peak serum concentration:

Oral: 0.5-4 hours

Parenteral: 0.5-2 hours

Half-life: 8-12 hours

Elimination: Small amounts in feces; primarily excreted unchanged in urine (90%) via glomerular filtration and active secretion by the renal tubule; 1% to 11% of a dose is excreted as the 7-hydroxy metabolite

Usual Dosage Refer to individual protocols:

Children:

Dermatomyositis: Oral: 15-20 mg/m^2/week as a single dose once weekly or 0.3-1 mg/kg/dose once weekly

Juvenile rheumatoid arthritis: Oral, I.M., S.C.: 5-15 mg/m^2/week as a single dose or in 3 divided doses given 12 hours apart; folic acid 1 mg daily or folinic acid ≤5 mg weekly are often used to prevent folate depletion from methotrexate

Antineoplastic dosage range:

Oral:, I.M.: 7.5-30 mg/m^2/week or every 2 weeks

I.V.: 10 mg to 33,000 mg/m^2 bolus dosing or continuous infusion over 6-42 hours

Antineoplastic dosing schedules (adapted from Dorr RT and Von Hoff DD, *Cancer Chemotherapy Handbook*, 2nd ed, 1994): See table.

Methotrexate Dosing Schedules

	Dose	Route	Frequency
Conventional dose	15-20 mg/m^2	Oral	Twice weekly
	30-50 mg/m^2	Oral, I.V.	Weekly
	15 mg/day for 5 days	Oral, I.M.	Every 2-3 weeks
Intermediate dose	50-150 mg/m^2	I.V. push	Every 2-3 weeks
	240 mg/m^{2*}	I.V. infusion	Every 4-7 days
	0.5-1 g/m^{2*}	I.V. infusion	Every 2-3 weeks
High dose	1-12 g/m^{2*}	I.V. infusion	Every 1-3 weeks

*Followed with leucovorin rescue

Pediatric solid tumors:

<12 years: 12 g/m^2 (dosage range: 12-18 g)

≥12 years: 8 g/m^2 (maximum dose: 18 g)

Meningeal leukemia: I.T.: 10-15 mg/m^2 (maximum: 15 mg) by protocol **or**

≤3 months: 3 mg dose

4-11 months: 6 mg dose

1 year: 8 mg dose

2 years: 10 mg dose

≥3 years: 12 mg dose

I.T. doses are administered at 2- to 5-day intervals until CSF counts return to normal followed by a dose once weekly for 2 weeks then monthly thereafter

ALL (high dose): I.V.: Loading dose: 200 mg/m^2 followed by a 24-hour infusion of 1200 mg/m^2/day

ANLL: I.V.: 7.5 mg/m^2/day on days 1-5 of treatment course

Resistant ANLL: I.V.: 100 mg/m^2/dose on day 1 of treatment course

Non-Hodgkin's lymphoma: I.V.: 200-500 mg/m^2; repeat every 28 days

Induction of remission in acute lymphoblastic leukemias: Oral: 3.3 mg/m^2/day for 4-6 weeks

Remission maintenance: Oral, I.M.: 20-30 mg/m^2 2 times/week

Adults:

Trophoblastic neoplasms: Oral, I.M.: 15-30 mg/day for 5 days, repeat in 7 days for 3-5 courses

Head and neck cancer: Oral, I.M. I.V.: 25-50 mg/m^2 once weekly

Rheumatoid arthritis: Oral: 7.5 mg once weekly or 2.5 mg every 12 hours for 3 doses/week; not to exceed 20 mg/week

Psoriasis: Oral: 2.5-5 mg/dose every 12 hours for 3 doses/week given once weekly

or

Oral, I.M.: 10-25 mg given once weekly

Dosing adjustment in renal impairment:

Cl$_{cr}$ 61-80 mL/minute: Decrease dose by 25%

Cl$_{cr}$ 51-60 mL/minute: Decrease dose by 33%

Cl$_{cr}$ 10-50 mL/minute: Decrease dose by 50% to 70%

Administration Parenteral:

Methotrexate may be administered I.V. push, I.V. intermittent infusion, or I.V. continuous infusion at a concentration <25 mg/mL; doses >100-300 mg/m^2 are (Continued)

623

Methotrexate (Continued)

usually administered by I.V. continuous infusion and are followed by a course of leucovorin rescue

For intrathecal use, mix methotrexate without preservatives with NS, Elliotts B solution, or LR to a concentration not greater than 2 mg/mL

Monitoring Parameters CBC with differential and platelet count, creatinine clearance, serum creatinine, BUN, hepatic function tests, serum electrolytes, urinalysis, plasma MTX concentrations (see leucovorin rescue graph *on page 561* to evaluate plasma MTX concentration versus leucovorin rescue dose)

Reference Range Serum levels >1 x 10^{-7} mol/L for more than 40 hours are toxic

Patient Information Report to physician any fever, sore throat, bleeding or bruising, shortness of breath, painful urination; avoid alcohol

Nursing Implications Intensive hydration should be administered and urine should be alkalinized prior to high doses to enhance methotrexate solubility

Additional Information Myelosuppressive effects:

WBC: Mild
Platelets: Moderate
Onset (days): 7
Nadir (days): 10
Recovery (days): 21

Dosage Forms

Injection, as sodium: 2.5 mg/mL (2 mL); 25 mg/mL (2 mL, 4 mL, 8 mL, 10 mL)
Injection, preservative free, as sodium: 25 mg (2 mL, 4 mL, 8 mL, 10 mL)
Powder for injection, as sodium: 20 mg, 25 mg, 50 mg, 100 mg, 250 mg, 1 g
Tablet, as sodium: 2.5 mg
Tablet, as sodium, dose pack: 2.5 mg (4 cards with 2, 3, 4, 5, or 6 tablets each)

References

Berg SL, Grisell DL, DeLaney TF, et al, "Principles of Treatment of Pediatric Solid Tumors," *Pediatr Clin North Am*, 1991, 38(2):249-67.

Bleyer WA, "Clinical Pharmacology of Intrathecal Methotrexate II. An Approved Dosage Regimen Derived From Age-Related Pharmacokinetics," *Cancer Treat Rep*, 1977, 61(8):1419-25.

Crom WR, Glynn-Barnhart AM, Rodman JH, et al, "Pharmacokinetics of Anticancer Drugs in Children," *Clin Pharmacokinet*, 1987, 12(3):168-213.

Giannini EH, Brewer EJ, Kuzmina N, et al, "Methotrexate in Resistant Juvenile Rheumatoid Arthritis. Results of the USA-USSR Double-Blind, Placebo-Controlled Trial," *N Engl J Med*, 1992, 326(16):1043-9.

Greaves MW and Weinstein GD, "Treatment of Psoriasis," *N Engl J Med*, 1995, 332(9):581-8.

Rose CD, Singsen BH, and Eichenfield AH, "Safety and Efficacy of Methotrexate Therapy for Juvenile Rheumatoid Arthritis," *J Pediatr*, 1990, 117(4):653-9.

♦ **Methotrexate Sodium** *see* Methotrexate *on page 621*

Methsuximide (meth SUKS i mide)

Related Information

Antiepileptic Drugs *on page 1176*

Brand Names Celontin®; Celontin® (Canada)

Therapeutic Category Anticonvulsant, Succinimide

Generic Available No

Use Control of absence (petit mal) seizures; useful adjunct in refractory, partial complex (psychomotor) seizures

Pregnancy Risk Factor C

Contraindications Hypersensitivity to methsuximide or any component

Precautions Use with caution in patients with hepatic or renal disease; avoid abrupt withdrawal

Adverse Reactions

Central nervous system: Dizziness, drowsiness, lethargy, euphoria, nervousness, hallucinations, insomnia, mental confusion, headache, ataxia
Dermatologic: Rash, urticaria, Stevens-Johnson syndrome
Gastrointestinal: Nausea, vomiting, anorexia, diarrhea, abdominal pain
Hematologic: Leukopenia, thrombocytopenia, eosinophilia, pancytopenia, monocytosis
Ocular: Periorbital edema
Miscellaneous: Hiccups

Stability Protect from high temperature

Mechanism of Action Increases the seizure threshold and suppresses paroxysmal spike-and-wave pattern in absence seizures; depresses nerve transmission in the motor cortex

Pharmacokinetics

Metabolism: Rapidly demethylated in the liver to N-desmethylmethsuximide (active metabolite)

Half-life: 2-4 hours
N-desmethylmethsuximide:
  Children: 26 hours
  Adults: 28-80 hours
Time to peak serum concentration: Within 1-3 hours
Elimination: <1% in urine as unchanged drug

Usual Dosage Oral:
Children: Initial: 10-15 mg/kg/day in 3-4 divided doses; increase weekly up to maximum of 30 mg/kg/day; mean dose required:
  <30 kg: 20 mg/kg/day
  >30 kg: 14 mg/kg/day
Adults: 300 mg/day for the first week; may increase by 300 mg/day at weekly intervals up to 1.2 g in 2-4 divided doses/day

Administration Oral: Administer with food

Monitoring Parameters CBC with differential, liver enzymes, urinalysis; measure trough serum levels for efficacy and 3-hour postdose concentrations for toxicity

Reference Range Measure N-desmethylmethsuximide concentrations:
  Therapeutic: 10-40 µg/mL (SI: 53-212 µmol/L)
  Toxic: >40 µg/mL (SI: >212 µmol/L)

Patient Information May cause drowsiness and impair ability to perform activities requiring mental alertness or physical coordination; do not discontinue abruptly

Dosage Forms Capsule: 150 mg, 300 mg

References
Miles MV, Tennison MB, and Greenwood RS, "Pharmacokinetics of N-desmethylmethsuximide in Pediatric Patients," *J Pediatr*, 1989, 114(4 Pt 1):647-50.
Tennison MB, Greenwood RS, Miles MV, "Methsuximide for Intractable Childhood Seizures," *Pediatrics*, 1991, 87(2):186-9.

♦ **Methylacetoxyprogesterone** *see* Medroxyprogesterone *on page 599*

Methyldopa (meth il DOE pa)

Brand Names Aldomet®; Apo®-Methyldopa (Canada); Dopamet® (Canada); Medimet® (Canada); Novo-Medopa® (Canada); Nu-Medopa® (Canada)

Available Salts Methyldopate Hydrochloride

Therapeutic Category Alpha-Adrenergic Inhibitors, Central; Antihypertensive Agent

Generic Available Yes

Use Management of moderate to severe hypertension

Pregnancy Risk Factor B

Contraindications Hypersensitivity to methyldopa or any component; liver disease, pheochromocytoma

Warnings Oral suspension contains benzoic acid (avoid use in neonates) and sodium bisulfite, injection contains sodium bisulfite which may cause allergic reactions

Precautions Use with caution and adjust dose in patients with renal dysfunction; active metabolite may accumulate in uremia

Adverse Reactions
Cardiovascular: Orthostatic hypotension, bradycardia, edema
Central nervous system: Drowsiness, sedation, vertigo, headache, depression, memory lapse, fever
Dermatologic: Rash
Endocrine & metabolic: Gynecomastia, sexual dysfunction, sodium retention
Gastrointestinal: Nausea, vomiting, diarrhea, xerostomia, "black" tongue
Genitourinary: Discoloration of urine (red or brown)
Hematologic: Hemolytic anemia, positive Coombs' test, leukopenia
Hepatic: Hepatitis, increased liver enzymes, jaundice, cirrhosis
Neuromuscular & skeletal: Weakness
Respiratory: Nasal congestion

Drug Interactions May increase lithium toxicity; concomitant oral administration of iron salts may decrease oral absorption of methyldopa and result in an increase in blood pressure, spacing drugs 2 hours apart may decrease this effect

Food Interactions Avoid natural licorice (causes sodium and water retention and increases potassium loss); dietary requirements for vitamin B_{12} and folate may be increased with high doses of methyldopa

Mechanism of Action Stimulates inhibitory alpha-adrenergic receptors via alpha-methylnorepinephrine (false transmitter); this results in a decreased sympathetic outflow to the heart, kidneys, and peripheral vasculature; may decrease plasma renin activity
(Continued)

Methyldopa *(Continued)*

Pharmacodynamics Hypotensive effects:
Peak effect: Oral, I.V.: Single-dose: Within 3-6 hours; multiple-dose: 2-3 days
Duration:
Oral: Single-dose: 12-24 hours; multiple-dose: 1-2 days
I.V.: 10-16 hours

Pharmacokinetics
Absorption: Oral: ~50%
Distribution: Crosses placenta; appears in breast milk
Protein binding: <15%
Metabolism: In the intestine and the liver
Half-life: Elimination:
Neonates: 10-20 hours
Adults: 1-3 hours
Elimination: ~70% of systemic dose eliminated in urine as drug and metabolites
Slightly dialyzable (5% to 20%)

Usual Dosage
Children:
Oral: Initial: 10 mg/kg/day in 2-4 divided doses; increase every 2 days as needed to maximum dose of 65 mg/kg/day; do not exceed 3 g/day
I.V.: Initial: 2-4 mg/kg/dose; if response is not seen within 4-6 hours, may increase to 5-10 mg/kg/dose; administer doses every 6-8 hours; maximum daily dose: 65 mg/kg or 3 g, whichever is less
Adults:
Oral: Initial: 250 mg 2-3 times/day; increase every 2 days as needed; usual dose 500 mg to 2 g daily in 2-4 divided doses; maximum dose: 3 g/day
I.V.: 250-1000 mg every 6-8 hours; maximum dose: 4 g/day
Dosing interval in renal impairment: Children and Adults:
Cl_{cr} >50 mL/minute: Administer normal dose every 8 hours
Cl_{cr} 10-50 mL/minute: Administer normal dose every 8-12 hours
Cl_{cr} <10 mL/minute: Administer normal dose every 12-24 hours

Administration
Oral: Administer new dosage increases in the evening to minimize sedation; shake suspension well before use
Parenteral: I.V.: Infuse I.V. dose slowly over 30-60 minutes at a concentration ≤10 mg/mL

Monitoring Parameters Blood pressure, CBC with differential, hemoglobin, hematocrit, Coombs' test [direct], liver enzymes

Test Interactions Urinary uric acid, serum creatinine (alkaline picrate method), AST (colorimetric method), and urinary catecholamines (falsely high levels)

Patient Information Avoid alcohol; may cause sedation and drowsiness and impair ability to perform activities requiring mental alertness or physical coordination; rise slowly from prolonged sitting or lying position; may cause urine to turn red or brown; notify physician of unexplained prolonged general tiredness, fever, or jaundice

Nursing Implications Transient sedation or depression may occur for first 72 hours of therapy, or when doses are increased

Additional Information Most effective if used with diuretic; titrate dose to optimal blood pressure control with minimal side effects

Dosage Forms
Injection, as methyldopate hydrochloride: 50 mg/mL (5 mL, 10 mL)
Suspension, oral: 250 mg/5 mL (5 mL, 473 mL)
Tablet: 125 mg, 250 mg, 500 mg

♦ **Methyldopate Hydrochloride** *see Methyldopa on page 625*

Methylene Blue (METH i leen bloo)

Brand Names Urolene Blue® Oral
Therapeutic Category Antidote, Cyanide; Antidote, Drug-induced Methemoglobinemia
Generic Available Yes
Use Antidote for cyanide poisoning and drug-induced methemoglobinemia, indicator dye, bacteriostatic genitourinary antiseptic
Pregnancy Risk Factor C (D if injected intra-amniotically)
Contraindications Renal insufficiency; hypersensitivity to methylene blue or any component
Warnings Do not inject subcutaneously or intrathecally as necrotic abscesses (S.C.) and neural damage (I.T.) including paraplegia have occurred

Precautions Use with caution in patients with G-6-PD deficiency; continued use can cause profound anemia

Adverse Reactions
Cardiovascular: Hypertension, cyanosis, large I.V. doses have been associated with precordial pain
Central nervous system: Dizziness, mental confusion, headache, fever
Dermatologic: Stains skin
Gastrointestinal: Nausea, vomiting, abdominal pain, diarrhea, discoloration of feces (blue-green)
Genitourinary: Bladder irritation, discoloration of urine (blue-green)
Hematologic: Formation of methemoglobin
Miscellaneous: Diaphoresis

Mechanism of Action Weak germicide; in low concentrations hastens the conversion of methemoglobin to hemoglobin; has opposite effect at high concentrations by converting ferrous iron of reduced hemoglobin to ferric iron to form methemoglobin; in cyanide toxicity, it combines with cyanide to form cyanmethemoglobin preventing the interference of cyanide with the cytochrome system

Pharmacokinetics
Absorption: Well absorbed from GI tract
Elimination: In bile, feces, and urine

Usual Dosage
Methemoglobinemia: Children and Adults: I.V.: 1-2 mg/kg or 25-50 mg/m²; may be repeated after 1 hour if necessary
Chronic methemoglobinemia: Adults: Oral: 100-300 mg/day
NADPH-methemoglobin reductase deficiency: Children: Oral: 1-1.5 mg/kg/day (maximum dose: 300 mg/day) given with 5-8 mg/kg/day ascorbic acid
Genitourinary antiseptic: Adults: Oral: 65-130 mg 3 times/day; maximum dose: 390 mg/day
Chronic urolithiasis: Adults: Oral: 65 mg 3 times/day

Administration
Parenteral: Administer undiluted by direct I.V. injection over several minutes
Oral: Administer after meals with a full glass of water

Patient Information May discolor urine and feces blue-green; may discolor skin on contact

Additional Information Has been used topically (0.1% solutions) in conjunction with polychromatic light to photoinactivate viruses such as herpes simplex (this is an unlabeled indication); has been used alone or in combination with vitamin C for the management of chronic urolithiasis; skin stains may be removed using a hypochlorite solution

Dosage Forms
Injection: 10 mg/mL (1 mL, 10 mL)
Tablet: 65 mg

♦ **Methylmorphine** see Codeine on page 249

Methylphenidate (meth il FEN i date)

Brand Names Metadate™ ER; PMS-Methylphenidate (Canada); Ritalin®; Ritalin-SR®

Available Salts Methylphenidate Hydrochloride

Therapeutic Category Central Nervous System Stimulant, Nonamphetamine

Generic Available Yes

Use Attention-deficit/hyperactivity disorder (ADHD); narcolepsy

Restrictions C-II

Pregnancy Risk Factor C

Contraindications Hypersensitivity to methylphenidate or any component; glaucoma; motor tics; Tourette's syndrome (diagnosis or family history); patients with marked agitation, tension, and anxiety

Warnings Suppression of growth may occur with long-term use in children (monitor carefully); may exacerbate symptoms of thought disorder and behavior disturbance in psychotic children; do not use for severe depression or normal fatigue states; may lower seizure threshold; EKG abnormalities and 4 cases of sudden cardiac death have been reported in children receiving clonidine with methylphenidate; reduce dose of methylphenidate by 40% when used concurrently with clonidine; consider EKG monitoring

Precautions Use with caution in patients with hypertension, seizures, acute stress reactions, emotional instability, patients with history of drug dependence
(Continued)

Methylphenidate *(Continued)*

Adverse Reactions

Cardiovascular: Tachycardia, hypertension, hypotension, palpitations, cardiac arrhythmias

Central nervous system: Nervousness, insomnia, dizziness, drowsiness, movement disorders, precipitation of Tourette's syndrome; fever, headache, toxic psychosis (rare); neuroleptic malignant syndrome (very rare and usually in patients receiving medications associated with the syndrome; one case with concurrent first dose of venlafaxine has been reported)

Dermatologic: Rash

Endocrine & metabolic: Growth retardation

Gastrointestinal: Anorexia, nausea, abdominal pain, weight loss

Hematologic: Thrombocytopenia

Ocular: Visual disturbances (rare), blurred vision, problems with accommodation

Miscellaneous: Hypersensitivity reactions; physical and psychological dependence

Drug Interactions Use with clonidine may potentially increase EKG effects (see Warnings); methylphenidate increases serum concentrations of tricyclic antidepressants, warfarin, phenytoin, phenobarbital and primidone; MAO inhibitors may potentiate effects of methylphenidate; effects of guanethidine, bretylium may be antagonized by methylphenidate

Food Interactions Food may increase oral absorption

Mechanism of Action Blocks the reuptake mechanism of dopaminergic neurons, appears to act at the cerebral cortex and subcortical structures

Pharmacodynamics Cerebral stimulation:

Peak effect:

Immediate release tablet: Within 2 hours

Sustained release tablet: Within 4-7 hours

Duration:

Immediate release tablet: 3-6 hours

Sustained release tablet: 8 hours

Pharmacokinetics

Absorption: From the GI tract, slow and incomplete

Protein binding: 15%

Metabolism: In the liver via hydroxylation to ritolinic acid

Half-life: 2-4 hours

Elimination: In urine as metabolites and unchanged drug; 45% to 50% excreted in feces via bile

Usual Dosage Oral:

Children ≥6 years: ADHD: Initial: 0.3 mg/kg/dose or 2.5-5 mg/dose given before breakfast and lunch; increase by 0.1 mg/kg/dose or by 5-10 mg/day at weekly intervals; usual dose: 0.3-1 mg/kg/day; maximum dose: 2 mg/kg/day or 60 mg/day; specific patients may require 3 doses/day (ie, additional dose at 4 PM)

Adults: Narcolepsy: 10 mg 2-3 times/day; maximum dose: 60 mg/day

Note: Sustained release and extended release tablets (duration of action ~8 hours) may be given in place of regular tablets, once the daily dose is titrated using the regular tablets and the titrated 8-hour dosage corresponds to sustained release tablet size

Administration Oral: Administer on an empty stomach ~30-45 minutes before meals; do not crush or chew sustained or extended release dosage form, swallow whole; to avoid insomnia, last daily dose should be administered several hours before retiring

Monitoring Parameters CBC with differential, platelet count, blood pressure, height, weight, heart rate

Patient Information Avoid caffeine; may be habit forming; may cause dizziness or drowsiness and impair ability to perform activities requiring mental alertness or physical coordination

Additional Information Treatment with methylphenidate should include "drug holidays" or periodic discontinuation in order to assess the patient's requirements, decrease tolerance and limit suppression of linear growth and weight

Dosage Forms

Tablet, as hydrochloride: 5 mg, 10 mg, 20 mg

Tablet, extended release, as hydrochloride (Metadate™ ER): 10 mg, 20 mg

Tablet, sustained release, as hydrochloride (Ritalin-SR®): 20 mg

References

Greenhill LL, "Pharmacologic Treatment of Attention Deficit Hyperactivity Disorder," *Psychiatr Clin North Am*, 1992, 15(1):1-27.

Kelly DP and Aylward GP, "Attention Deficits in School-Aged Children and Adolescents," *Pediatr Clin North Am*, 1992, 39(3):487-512.

Wilens TE and Biederman J, "The Stimulants," *Psychiatr Clin North Am*, 1992, 15(1):191-222.

- **Methylphenidate Hydrochloride** *see Methylphenidate on page 627*
- **Methylphenobarbital** *see Mephobarbital on page 605*
- **Methylphenyl** *see Oxacillin on page 711*
- **Methylphenylethylhydantoin** *see Mephenytoin on page 604*
- **Methylphytyl Napthoquinone** *see Phytonadione on page 769*

Methylprednisolone (meth il pred NIS oh lone)
Related Information
Asthma Guidelines *on page 1178*
Corticosteroids Comparison, Systemic *on page 1032*
Brand Names Adlone® Injection; A-methaPred® Injection; depMedalone® Injection; Depoject® Injection; Depo-Medrol® Injection; Depopred® Injection; D-Med® Injection; Duralone® Injection; Medralone® Injection; Medrol® Oral; Medrol® Veriderm® Cream (Canada); M-Prednisol® Injection; Solu-Medrol® Injection
Available Salts Methylprednisolone Acetate; Methylprednisolone Sodium Succinate
Synonyms 6-α-Methylprednisolone
Therapeutic Category Adrenal Corticosteroid; Antiasthmatic; Anti-inflammatory Agent; Corticosteroid, Systemic; Glucocorticoid
Generic Available Yes
Use Anti-inflammatory or immunosuppressant agent in the treatment of a variety of diseases including those of hematologic, allergic, inflammatory, neoplastic, and autoimmune origin
Pregnancy Risk Factor C
Contraindications Hypersensitivity to methylprednisolone or any component; administration of live virus vaccines; systemic fungal infections
Warnings May retard bone growth; methylprednisolone **acetate** I.M. injection (multiple-dose vial) and the diluent for methylprednisolone **sodium succinate** injection contain benzyl alcohol as a preservative; avoid use of benzyl alcohol products in neonates, especially premature neonates (benzyl alcohol may cause the gasping syndrome)
Precautions Use with caution in patients with hypothyroidism, cirrhosis, hypertension, CHF, ulcerative colitis, thromboembolic disorders
Adverse Reactions
Cardiovascular: Edema, hypertension
Central nervous system: Vertigo, seizures, psychoses, pseudotumor cerebri, headache
Dermatologic: Acne, skin atrophy, impaired wound healing
Endocrine & metabolic: Cushing's syndrome, pituitary-adrenal axis suppression, growth suppression, glucose intolerance, hypokalemia, alkalosis
Gastrointestinal: Peptic ulcer, nausea, vomiting
Hematologic: Transient leukocytosis
Neuromuscular & skeletal: Muscle weakness, osteoporosis, fractures
Ocular: Cataracts, glaucoma
Miscellaneous: Infections
Drug Interactions Cytochrome P-450 isoenzyme CYP3A3/4 inducer
Barbiturates, phenytoin, rifampin may increase the clearance of methylprednisolone; salicylates; toxoids; methylprednisolone may increase cyclosporine and tacrolimus serum concentrations; live virus vaccines (increase risk of viral infection); vaccines may have decreased effects
Food Interactions Systemic use of corticosteroids may require a diet with increased potassium, vitamins A, B_6, C, D, folate, calcium, zinc and phosphorus and decreased sodium
Mechanism of Action Decreases inflammation by suppression of migration of polymorphonuclear leukocytes and reversal of increased capillary permeability
Pharmacodynamics The time of peak effects and the duration of these effects is dependent upon the route of administration. See table.

Route	Peak Effect	Duration
Oral	1-2 h	30-36 h
I.M. (acetate)	4-8 d	1-4 wk
Intra-articular	1 wk	1-5 wk

(Continued)

Methylprednisolone *(Continued)*

Usual Dosage Note: Only sodium succinate salt may be given I.V.

Children:

Anti-inflammatory or immunosuppressive: Oral, I.M., I.V.: 0.5-1.7 mg/kg/day or 5-25 mg/m^2/day in divided doses every 6-12 hours

"Pulse" therapy: 15-30 mg/kg/dose over ≥30 minutes given once daily for 3 days

Status asthmaticus: I.V.: Loading dose: 2 mg/kg/dose, then 0.5-1 mg/kg/dose every 6 hours

Lupus nephritis: I.V.: 30 mg/kg over ≥30 minutes every other day for 6 doses

Acute spinal cord injury: I.V.: 30 mg/kg over 15 minutes followed in 45 minutes by a continuous infusion of 5.4 mg/kg/hour for 23 hours

Adults:

Oral: 2-60 mg/day in 1-4 divided doses

High-dose therapy: I.V.: 30 mg/kg over ≥30 minutes; repeat as needed every 4-6 hours for 48-72 hours

I.M. (acetate): 10-80 mg/day once daily

I.V.: 40-250 mg every 4-6 hours

Lupus nephritis: High-dose "pulse" therapy: I.V.: 1 g/day for 3 days

Intra-articular, intralesional: 4-40 mg, up to 80 mg for large joints every 1-5 weeks

Administration

Oral: Administer after meals or with food or milk

Parenteral: I.V.: Succinate: Low dose (eg, ≤1.8 mg/kg or ≤125 mg/dose): I.V. push over 3-15 minutes; moderate dose (eg, ≥2 mg/kg or 250 mg/dose): administer over 15-30 minutes; high dose (eg, 15 mg/kg or ≥500 mg/dose): administer over ≥30 minutes; doses >15 mg/kg or ≥1 g: administer over 1 hour. Do **not** administer high-dose I.V. push; hypotension, cardiac arrhythmia, and sudden death have been reported in patients given high-dose methylprednisolone I.V. push over <20 minutes; administer intermittent infusion over 15-60 minutes; maximum concentration: I.V. push: 125 mg/mL; I.V. infusion: 2.5 mg/mL.

Monitoring Parameters Blood pressure, serum glucose, and electrolytes

Test Interactions Interferes with skin tests

Patient Information Avoid alcohol; limit caffeine; do not decrease or discontinue dose without physician's approval

Nursing Implications Do **not** give acetate form I.V.

Additional Information Sodium content of 1 g sodium succinate injection: 2.01 mEq; methylprednisolone sodium succinate 53 mg = methylprednisolone base 40 mg

Dosage Forms

Injection, as acetate: 20 mg/mL (5 mL, 10 mL); 40 mg/mL (1 mL, 5 mL, 10 mL); 80 mg/mL (1 mL, 5 mL)

Powder for injection, as sodium succinate: 40 mg (1 mL, 3 mL); 125 mg (2 mL, 5 mL); 500 mg (1 mL, 4 mL, 8 mL, 20 mL); 1000 mg (1 mL, 8 mL, 50 mL); 2000 mg (30.6 mL)

Tablet: 2 mg, 4 mg, 8 mg, 16 mg, 24 mg, 32 mg

Tablet, dose pack: 4 mg (21s)

- **6-α-Methylprednisolone** *see* Methylprednisolone *on page 629*
- **Methylprednisolone Acetate** *see* Methylprednisolone *on page 629*
- **Methylprednisolone Sodium Succinate** *see* Methylprednisolone *on page 629*
- **4-Methylpyrazole** *see* Fomepizole *on page 440*
- **Methylrosaniline Chloride** *see* Gentian Violet *on page 455*
- **Meticorten®** *see* Prednisone *on page 794*

Metoclopramide *(met oh kloe PRA mide)*

Related Information

Carbohydrate and Alcohol Content of Liquid Medications for Use in Patients Receiving Ketogenic Diets *on page 1228*

Compatibility of Medications Mixed in a Syringe *on page 1208*

Drugs and Breast-Feeding *on page 1213*

Brand Names Apo®-Metoclop (Canada); Clopra®; Maxeran® (Canada); Maxolon®; Octamide®; Reglan®

Available Salts Metoclopramide Hydrochloride

Therapeutic Category Antiemetic; Gastrointestinal Agent, Prokinetic

Generic Available Yes

Use Gastroesophageal reflux; prevention of nausea and vomiting associated with chemotherapy; prevention of postoperative nausea and vomiting; facilitates intubation of the small intestine and symptomatic treatment of diabetic gastric stasis

Pregnancy Risk Factor B

Contraindications Hypersensitivity to metoclopramide or any component; GI obstruction, pheochromocytoma, history of seizure disorder or patients receiving drugs likely to cause extrapyramidal reactions

Warnings Some formulations contain sulfite

Precautions Use with caution and reduce dosage in patients with renal impairment, hypertension, or depression

Adverse Reactions Extrapyramidal reactions occur most frequently in children and young adults and following I.V. administration of high doses, usually within 24-48 hours after starting therapy

Cardiovascular: Hypertension, hypotension, SVT, bradycardia, A-V block

Central nervous system: Drowsiness, fatigue, restlessness, anxiety, agitation, depression, tardive dyskinesia, dystonia, seizures, hallucinations, neuroleptic malignant syndrome

Endocrine & metabolic: Gynecomastia, amenorrhea, galactorrhea, hyperprolactinemia

Gastrointestinal: Constipation, diarrhea

Genitourinary: Urinary frequency, impotence

Hematologic: Methemoglobinemia, neutropenia, leukopenia, agranulocytosis

Hepatic: Porphyria

Ocular: Visual disturbances

Miscellaneous: Hypersensitivity reactions

Drug Interactions Decreased cimetidine and digoxin GI absorption; increased cyclosporine GI absorption; levodopa decreases metoclopramide effects; increases hypertensive episodes with MAO inhibitors; increased neuromuscular blocking effects of succinylcholine; anticholinergics and narcotic analgesics antagonize GI motility effects of metoclopramide; metoclopramide may increase tacrolimus serum levels

Stability Stable for 48 hours at room temperature when admixed with ascorbic acid, cimetidine (in NS only), cytarabine, dexamethasone sodium phosphate, diphenhydramine, doxorubicin, heparin, benztropine, dexamethasone hydrochloride, hydrocortisone sodium phosphate, lidocaine, magnesium sulfate, mannitol, potassium acetate, potassium chloride, and potassium phosphate; stable for 24 hours at room temperature when admixed with clindamycin (in NS only) and cyclophosphamide; incompatible with cephalothin, chloramphenicol, and sodium bicarbonate

Mechanism of Action Potent dopamine receptor antagonist; blocks dopamine receptors in chemoreceptor trigger zone of the CNS, preventing emesis; accelerates gastric emptying and intestinal transit time without stimulating gastric, biliary, or pancreatic secretions

Pharmacodynamics

Onset of action:

Oral: Within 30-60 minutes

I.M.: Within 10-15 minutes

I.V.: Within 1-3 minutes

Duration: Therapeutic effects persist for 1-2 hours, regardless of route administered

Pharmacokinetics

Distribution: V_d: 3.5 L/kg; crosses the placenta; appears in breast milk; breast milk to plasma ratio: 0.5-4.06

Protein binding: 30%

Bioavailability: Oral: $80 \pm 15.5\%$

Half-life: 2.5-6 hours (half-life and clearance may be dose-dependent)

Elimination: Primarily as unchanged drug in the urine and feces

Usual Dosage

Intubation of small intestine to facilitate radiographic examination of upper GI tract:

I.V.:

Children:

<6 years: 0.1 mg/kg

6-14 years: 2.5-5 mg

Children >14 years and Adults: 10 mg

Gastroesophageal reflux: Oral, I.M., I.V.:

Neonates, Infants and Children: 0.4-0.8 mg/kg/day in 4 divided doses

Adults: 10-15 mg 4 times/day

Postoperative nausea and vomiting: I.V.:

Children: 0.1-0.2 mg/kg/dose; repeat every 6-8 hours as needed

(Continued)

Metoclopramide *(Continued)*

Children >14 years and Adults: 10 mg; repeat every 6-8 hours as needed

Antiemetic **(chemotherapy-induced emesis):** Oral, I.V.:

Children and Adults: 1-2 mg/kg/dose every 2-4 hours; pretreatment with diphenhydramine will decrease risk of extrapyramidal reactions to this dosage

Diabetic gastroparesis: Adults: Oral, I.V.: 10 mg before each meal and at bedtime for 2-8 weeks

Dosing adjustment in renal impairment: Children and Adults:

Cl_{cr} 40-50 mL/minute: Administer 75% of recommended dose

Cl_{cr} 10-40 mL/minute: Administer 50% of recommended dose

Cl_{cr} <10 mL/minute: Administer 25% to 50% of recommended dose

Administration

Oral: Administer 30 minutes before meals and at bedtime

Parenteral: Dilute to 0.2 mg/mL (maximum concentration: 5 mg/mL) and infuse over 15-30 minutes (maximum rate of infusion: 5 mg/minute); rapid I.V. administration is associated with a transient but intense feeling of anxiety and restlessness, followed by drowsiness

Monitoring Parameters Renal function

Patient Information Causes drowsiness and may impair ability to perform hazardous activities requiring mental alertness or physical coordination

Dosage Forms

Injection, as hydrochloride: 5 mg/mL (2 mL, 10 mL, 30 mL, 50 mL, 100 mL)

Solution, oral, concentrated, as hydrochloride: 10 mg/mL (10 mL, 30 mL)

Syrup, sugar free, as hydrochloride: 5 mg/5 mL (10 mL, 480 mL)

Tablet, as hydrochloride: 5 mg, 10 mg

♦ **Metoclopramide Hydrochloride** *see* Metoclopramide *on page 630*

Metolazone *(me TOLE a zone)*

Brand Names Mykrox®; Zaroxolyn®

Therapeutic Category Antihypertensive Agent; Diuretic, Miscellaneous

Generic Available No

Use Management of mild to moderate hypertension and impaired renal function (Zaroxolyn® only); treatment of edema in CHF, nephrotic syndrome, and impaired renal function

Pregnancy Risk Factor B

Contraindications Anuria; hypersensitivity to metolazone, any component, other thiazide diuretics, or sulfonamide-derived drugs; patients with hepatic coma

Warnings Mykrox® is **not** therapeutically equivalent to Zaroxolyn® and should not be interchanged for one another

Precautions Use with caution in patients with severe renal disease, impaired hepatic function, gout, lupus erythematosus, diabetes mellitus, moderate-high cholesterol concentrations, and/or high triglycerides

Adverse Reactions

Cardiovascular: Palpitations, chest pain, orthostatic hypotension, precordial pain

Central nervous system: Vertigo, headache, chills, drowsiness

Dermatologic: Rash, dry skin, photosensitivity

Endocrine & metabolic: Hypokalemia, hyponatremia, hypochloremia, metabolic alkalosis, hyperglycemia, hyperuricemia, hypomagnesemia

Gastrointestinal: Abdominal bloating, GI irritation, bitter taste, nausea, vomiting, anorexia

Hematologic: Blood dyscrasias, aplastic anemia, hemolytic anemia, leukopenia, agranulocytosis, thrombocytopenia

Hepatic: Hepatitis

Neuromuscular & skeletal: Arthralgia, back pain, paresthesias

Ocular: Eye itching

Otic: Tinnitus

Renal: Polyuria, prerenal azotemia, uremia

Respiratory: Cough, sinus congestion, epistaxis

Drug Interactions Increased digoxin toxicity (due to potassium and magnesium depletion); increased lithium toxicity; additive potassium losses with amphotericin B and steroids; salicylates and NSAIDs decrease antihypertensive effects; allopurinol increases hypersensitivity reactions; rare occurrence of hemolytic anemia with methyldopa; cholestyramine and colestipol decrease metolazone absorption

Food Interactions Avoid natural licorice (causes sodium and water retention and increases potassium loss)

Mechanism of Action Inhibits sodium reabsorption in the cortical diluting site and proximal convoluted tubules causing increased excretion of sodium and water as well as potassium and hydrogen ions

Pharmacodynamics
Onset of action: 1 hour
Maximal effect (Mykrox®): Hypertension: 2 weeks
Duration: 12-24 hours

Pharmacokinetics
Absorption: Oral: Rate and extent vary with the preparation
Protein binding: 95%
Half-life: 6-20 hours
Elimination: Enterohepatic recycling; 70% to 95% excreted unchanged in urine

Usual Dosage Oral (dosage based on Zaroxolyn®, lower dosages may be used with Mykrox®):

Children: 0.2-0.4 mg/kg/day divided every 12-24 hours
Adults:
Edema: 5-10 mg/dose every 24 hours
Edema associated with renal disease or cardiac failure: 5-20 mg/dose every 24 hours
Hypertension:
Zaroxolyn®: 2.5-5 mg/dose every 24 hours
Mykrox®: 0.5 mg/day; increase to a maximum of 1 mg/day, if needed

Administration Oral: Administer with food to decrease GI distress

Monitoring Parameters Serum electrolytes, renal function, blood pressure

Dosage Forms Tablet:
Zaroxolyn®: 2.5 mg, 5 mg, 10 mg
Mykrox®: 0.5 mg

Extemporaneous Preparations A 1 mg/mL suspension may be made by crushing one 10 mg Zaroxolyn® tablet; add simple syrup to total volume of 10 mL. Label "shake well"; stable 3 months refrigerated
Nahata MC and Hipple TF, *Pediatric Drug Formulations*, 3rd ed, Cincinnati, OH: Harvey Whitney Books Co, 1997.

References
Arnold WC, "Efficacy of Metolazone and Furosemide in Children With Furosemide-Resistant Edema," *Pediatrics*, 1984, 74(5):872-5.
Wells TG, "The Pharmacology and Therapeutics of Diuretics in the Pediatric Patient," *Pediatr Clin North Am*, 1990, 37(2):463-504.

Metoprolol (me toe PROE lole)

Brand Names Apo®-Metoprolol (Type L) (Canada); Betaloc® (Canada); Betaloc® Durules® (Canada); Lopressor®; Novo-Metoprolol (Canada); Nu-Metop (Canada); Toprol XL®

Available Salts Metoprolol Succinate; Metoprolol Tartrate

Therapeutic Category Antianginal Agent; Antiarrhythmic Agent, Class II; Antihypertensive Agent; Antimigraine Agent; Beta-Adrenergic Blocker

Generic Available Yes: Injection, tablets (nonsustained release)

Use Management of hypertension, angina pectoris, and arrhythmias (such as multifocal atrial tachycardia); prevention of MI and migraine headaches

Pregnancy Risk Factor C

Contraindications Hypersensitivity to metoprolol or any component; sinus bradycardia; heart block greater then first degree (except in patients with a functioning artificial pacemaker); cardiogenic shock; uncompensated CHF

Warnings May depress myocardial activity and precipitate CHF, use with caution and monitor closely, especially in patients with compensated heart failure. In patients with coronary artery disease, exacerbation of angina and, in some cases, MI may occur following abrupt discontinuation of therapy. Beta-blockers should generally be avoided in patients with bronchospastic disease; metoprolol, with relative beta$_1$ selectivity, should be used with caution and closely monitored in patients with bronchospastic disease; beta$_2$ stimulants and the lowest possible dose of metoprolol should be used in these patients. Metoprolol may block hypoglycemia-induced tachycardia and blood pressure changes; use with caution in patients with diabetes mellitus. May mask signs of thyrotoxicosis. Use with caution with verapamil, diltiazem, or anesthetic agents that decrease myocardial function.

Precautions Use with caution in patients with hepatic dysfunction. Patients who have a history of severe anaphylactic hypersensitivity reactions to various substances may be more reactive while receiving beta-blockers; these patients may not be responsive to the normal doses of epinephrine used to treat hypersensitivity reactions
(Continued)

Metoprolol *(Continued)*

Adverse Reactions

Cardiovascular: Bradycardia, reduced peripheral circulation, palpitations, CHF, hypotension, peripheral edema, worsening of AV conduction disturbances

Central nervous system: Dizziness, tiredness, depression, mental confusion, insomnia

Dermatologic: Rash, pruritus, worsening of psoriasis

Gastrointestinal: Diarrhea, nausea, abdominal pain, dry mouth, constipation

Hematologic (potential): Agranulocytosis, thrombocytopenia

Hepatic: Hepatitis, hepatic dysfunction, jaundice; rare: elevated transaminase, alkaline phosphatase, LDH

Respiratory: Bronchospasm, wheezing, dyspnea

Drug Interactions Cytochrome P-450 isoenzyme CYP 2D6 substrate

Catecholamine-depleting drugs, such as reserpine, may have additive effects (hypotension, bradycardia); hypotensive agents, diuretics, cardiac glycosides, amiodarone, calcium channel blockers, agents that slow AV conduction, and myocardial depressant general anesthetics may have additive effects with beta-blockers; verapamil may significantly increase the oral bioavailability of metoprolol (avoid concomitant use or reduce metoprolol dose and monitor closely); cimetidine, ciprofloxacin, fluoxetine, hydralazine, oral contraceptives, propoxyphene, and quinidine may increase metoprolol serum concentrations and effects. Abrupt withdrawal of clonidine while receiving beta-blockers may result in an exaggerated hypertensive crisis; NSAIDs may decrease the antihypertensive effects of beta-blockers; barbiturates and rifampin may increase the metabolism of metoprolol and decrease metoprolol serum concentrations; metoprolol may increase lidocaine serum concentrations

Food Interactions

Metoprolol tartrate: Food may enhance the extent of oral absorption

Metoprolol succinate (extended release tablets): Food does not significantly affect bioavailability

Stability

Tablets and extended release tablets: Store at controlled room temperature 15°C to 30°C (59°F to 86°F)

Tablets: Protect from moisture and dispense in tight, light-resistant container

Injection: Do not store above 30°C (86°F); protect from light

Mechanism of Action Selective inhibitor of beta$_1$-adrenergic receptors at lower doses; competitively blocks beta$_1$ adrenergic receptors with little or no effect on beta$_2$-receptors at doses in adults <100 mg/day; inhibits beta$_2$- receptors at higher doses; does not exhibit membrane stabilizing or intrinsic sympathomimetic activity

Pharmacodynamics

Beta blockade:

Onset: Oral: Metoprolol tartrate tablets: Within 1 hour

Maximum effect: I.V.: 20 minutes

Duration: Dose dependent

Antihypertensive effect:

Onset: Oral: Metoprolol tartrate tablets: Within 15 minutes

Maximum effect: Oral (multiple dosing): After 1 week

Duration: Oral: Metoprolol tartrate tablets (single dose): 6 hours; metoprolol succinate (extended release tablets): Up to 24 hours

Pharmacokinetics

Absorption: Rapid and complete, with large first-pass effect

Distribution: Crosses the blood brain barrier; CSF concentrations are 78% of plasma concentrations

Protein binding: 12% bound to albumin

Metabolism: Significant first-pass metabolism; extensive metabolism in the liver

Bioavailability: Oral: 50%

Half-Life:

Neonates: 5-10 hours

Adults: 3-7 hours

Adults with chronic renal failure: Similar to normal adults

Elimination: 10% of an I.V. dose and <5% of an oral dose is excreted unchanged in the urine

Usual Dosage (See Additional Information)

Oral: Hypertension:

Children: No pediatric studies are available

Adolescents: Limited information is available. Sixteen hypertensive adolescents (≥13 years of age) were treated with an initial dose of 50 mg twice daily;

patients were seen every 4-6 weeks and doses were increased to 100 mg twice daily if blood pressure was not controlled (see Falkner, 1982)

Adults:

Tablets (nonsustained release): Initial: 100 mg/day in single or divided doses, increase at weekly intervals to desired effect; usual dosage range: 100-450 mg/day; doses >450 mg/day have not been studied

Note: Lower once-daily dosing (especially 100 mg/day) may not control blood pressure for 24 hours; larger or more frequent dosing may be needed. Patients with bronchospastic diseases should receive the lowest possible daily dose; dose should initially be divided into 3 doses per day (to avoid high plasma concentrations).

Tablets, extended release: Initial: 50-100 mg/day as a single dose; increase at weekly intervals to desired effect; doses >400 mg/day have not been studied.

Administration Oral:

Metoprolol tartrate tablets: Administer with food or immediately after meals

Metoprolol succinate extended release tablets: May be administered without regard to meals

Monitoring Parameters Blood pressure, heart rate, respirations, circulation in extremities

Additional Information Do not abruptly discontinue therapy, taper dosage gradually over 1-2 weeks. Beta-blockers without intrinsic sympathomimetic activity (such as metoprolol) have been shown to decrease morbidity and mortality when initiated in the acute treatment of MI and continued long term; metoprolol injection is used for early treatment of definitive or suspected MI; consult adult reference for further information. Oral to I.V. ratio of approximately 2.5 to 1 provides equivalent maximal beta-blocking activity (ie, 50 mg oral is equivalent to 20 mg I.V.).

Limited pediatric dosing information is available in the literature; in one case report, oral metoprolol (2 mg/kg/day in 3 divided doses) helped control paroxysmal supraventricular tachycardia in a 6 month old infant receiving digoxin (see Hepner, 1983). Low dose oral metoprolol (initial: 0.1 mg/kg/dose given twice daily, then increased slowly as needed to a maximum of 0.9 ± 0.7 mg/kg/day) was used to treat severe CHF that failed conventional therapy in 4 children (mean age: 7.8 years) with cardiomyopathy who were under consideration for heart transplantation (see Shaddy, 1998). Two studies (Muller, 1993; O'Marcaigh, 1994) assessed metoprolol for unexplained syncope in children at I.V. doses of 0.1 to 0.2 mg/kg for tilt table testing; in both studies, oral metoprolol was given after tilt table testing to select patients; initial oral doses of 0.8-2.8 mg/kg/day were used in 15 patients (8-20 years of age), but treatment was discontinued in 3 patients receiving 1.8-2.8 mg/kg/day due to adverse effects (Muller, 1993); oral doses of 1 to 2 mg/kg/day, rounded to the nearest 25 mg/day and divided into 2 doses daily were used in 19 patients (7-18 years of age) with unexplained syncope; the mean effective dose was 1.5 mg/kg/day (O'Marcaigh, 1994). High-dose beta-blocker therapy has been recommended to treat childhood hypertrophic cardiomyopathy (see Ostman-Smith 1999). Further pediatric studies are required before these doses can be recommended.

Dosage Forms

Injection, as tartrate: 1 mg/mL (5 mL)

Tablet, as tartrate: 50 mg, 100 mg

Tablet, as succinate, extended release: 50 mg, 100 mg, 200 mg

Extemporaneous Preparations A 10 mg/mL metoprolol tartrate oral liquid preparation made with twelve 100 mg tablets and qsad to 120 mL with 3 different vehicles (a 1:1 mixture of Ora-Sweet® and Ora-Plus®, a 1:1 mixture of Ora-sweet® SF and Ora-Plus®, or cherry syrup) was found to be stable for 60 days when stored in amber plastic bottles in the dark at 5°C and 25°C. Microbial growth was not determined. Label "shake well" and "protect from light".

Allen LV and Erickson MA, "Stability of Labetalol Hydrochloride, Metoprolol Tartrate, Verapamil Hydrochloride, and Spironolactone With Hydrochlorothiazide in Extemporaneously Compounded Oral Liquids," *Am J Health Syst Pharm*, 1996, 53(19):2304-9.

References

Falkner B, Lowenthal DT, and Affrime MB, "The Pharmacodynamic Effectiveness of Metoprolol in Adolescent Hypertension," *Pediatr Pharmacol (New York)*, 1982, 2(1):49-55.

Hepner SI, and Davoli E, "Successful Treatment of Supraventricular Tachycardia With Metoprolol, a Cardioselective Beta Blocker," *Clin Pediatr (Phila)*, 1983, 22(7):522-3.

Morselli PL, Boutroy MJ, Bianchetti G, et al, "Pharmacokinetics of Antihypertensive Drugs in the Neonatal Period," *Dev Pharmacol Ther*, 1989, 13(2-4):190-8.

Muller G, Deal BJ, Strasburger JF, et al, "Usefulness of Metoprolol for Unexplained Syncope and Positive Response to Tilt Testing in Young Persons," *Am J Cardiol*, 1993, 71(7):592-5.

(Continued)

Metoprolol *(Continued)*

O'Marcaigh AS, MacLellan-Tobert SG, and Porter CJ, "Tilt-Table Testing and Oral Metoprolol Therapy in Young Patients With Unexplained Syncope," *Pediatrics*, 1994, 93(2):278-83.

Ostman-Smith I, Wettrell G, and Riesenfield T, "A Cohort Study of Childhood Hypertrophic Cardiomyopathy: Improved Survival Following High-Dose Beta-Adrenoceptor Antagonist Treatment," *J Am Coll Cardiol*, 1999, 34(6):1813-22.

Shaddy RE, "Beta-Blocker Therapy in Young Children With Congestive Heart Failure Under Consideration for Heart Transplantation," *Am Heart J*, 1998, 136(1):19-21.

♦ **Metoprolol Succinate** *see Metoprolol on page 633*

♦ **Metoprolol Tartrate** *see Metoprolol on page 633*

♦ **Metreton® Ophthalmic** *see Prednisolone on page 791*

♦ **Metrocream™ (Canada)** *see Metronidazole on page 636*

♦ **MetroGel® Topical** *see Metronidazole on page 636*

♦ **MetroGel®-Vaginal** *see Metronidazole on page 636*

♦ **Metro I.V.® Injection** *see Metronidazole on page 636*

Metronidazole *(me troe NI da zole)*

Related Information
Drugs and Breast-Feeding *on page 1213*

Brand Names Apo®-Metronidazole (Canada); Flagyl® Oral; Metrocream™ (Canada); MetroGel® Topical; MetroGel®-Vaginal; Metro I.V.® Injection; Nidagel™ (Canada); Noritate® (Canada); Novo-Nidazol® (Canada); Protostat® Oral; TriKacide® (Canada)

Available Salts Metronidazole Hydrochloride

Therapeutic Category Amebicide; Antibiotic, Anaerobic; Antibiotic, Topical; Antiprotozoal

Generic Available Yes

Use Treatment of susceptible anaerobic bacterial and protozoal infections in the following conditions: amebiasis (liver abscess, dysentery), giardiasis, symptomatic and asymptomatic trichomoniasis; skin and skin structure infections, CNS infections, intra-abdominal infections, and systemic anaerobic bacterial infections; topically for the treatment of acne rosacea; treatment of antibiotic-associated pseudomembranous colitis (AAPC) caused by *C. difficile*; bacterial vaginosis

Pregnancy Risk Factor B

Contraindications Hypersensitivity to metronidazole or any component; 1st trimester of pregnancy

Warnings Has been shown to be carcinogenic in rodents

Precautions Use with caution in patients with liver impairment, blood dyscrasias, CNS disease; metronidazole injection should be used with caution in patients receiving corticosteroids or patients predisposed to edema (injection contains 28 mEq of sodium/g metronidazole); reduce dosage in patients with severe liver impairment; dosage adjustment is not necessary in patients with moderate to severe renal insufficiency

Adverse Reactions
Central nervous system: Dizziness, confusion, seizures, headache, insomnia, hallucinations, paresthesias
Dermatologic: Rash
Endocrine & Metabolic: Disulfiram-type reaction with alcohol
Gastrointestinal: Metallic taste, nausea, xerostomia, diarrhea, furry tongue, vomiting
Genitourinary: Urethral burning, discoloration of urine (dark or reddish brown)
Hematologic: Leukopenia, neutropenia
Local: Thrombophlebitis
Neuromuscular & skeletal: Peripheral neuropathy

Drug Interactions Disulfiram (psychotic episodes); phenobarbital and rifampin (may increase metabolism of metronidazole); increased levels/toxicity of phenytoin, lithium, warfarin; alcohol may cause disulfiram-like reactions

Food Interactions Peak concentration is decreased and delayed when administered with food

Stability Do not refrigerate neutralized solution because precipitation may occur; reconstituted vials are chemically stable for 96 hours when stored at room temperature; protect from light

Mechanism of Action Reduced to a product which interacts with DNA to cause a loss of helical DNA structure and strand breakage resulting in inhibition of protein synthesis and cell death in susceptible organisms

Pharmacokinetics
Absorption: Oral: Well absorbed

Distribution: Excreted in breast milk; widely distributed into body tissues, fluids including bile, liver, bone, pleural fluid, vaginal secretions, CSF, erythrocytes, and hepatic abscesses

Protein binding: <20%

Metabolism: 30% to 60% in the liver to hydroxylated metabolite (60% to 80% bioactive), acetic acid metabolites, glucuronide, and sulfated conjugates

Half-life (increases with hepatic impairment):
 Neonates: 25-75 hours
 Children and Adults:
  Metronidazole: 6-12 hours
  Hydroxymetronidazole: 9.5-20 hours

Time to peak serum concentration: Within 1-2 hours

Elimination: Excreted via the urine (20% as unchanged drug) and feces (6% to 15%)

Extensively removed by hemodialysis and peritoneal dialysis

Usual Dosage
Neonates: Anaerobic infections: Oral, I.V.:
 0-4 weeks, <1200 g: 7.5 mg/kg every 48 hours
 Postnatal age ≤7 days:
  1200-2000 g: 7.5 mg/kg/day given every 24 hours
  >2000 g: 15 mg/kg/day in divided doses every 12 hours
 Postnatal age >7 days:
  1200-2000 g: 15 mg/kg/day in divided doses every 12 hours
  >2000 g: 30 mg/kg/day in divided doses every 12 hours

Infants and Children:
 Amebiasis: Oral: 35-50 mg/kg/day in divided doses every 8 hours
 Other parasitic infections: Oral: 15-30 mg/kg/day in divided doses every 8 hours
 Anaerobic infections: Oral, I.V.: 30 mg/kg/day in divided doses every 6 hours; maximum dose: 4 g/day
 AAPC: Oral: 30 mg/kg/day divided every 6 hours for 7-10 days
 Helicobacter pylori infection (has been used in combination with amoxicillin and bismuth subsalicylate): Oral: 15-20 mg/kg/day in 2 divided doses for 4 weeks

Adults:
 Amebiasis: Oral: 500-750 mg every 8 hours
 Other parasitic infections: Oral: 250 mg every 8 hours or 2 g as a single dose
 Anaerobic infections: Oral, I.V.: 30 mg/kg/day in divided doses every 6 hours; not to exceed 4 g/day
 AAPC: Oral: 250-500 mg 3-4 times/day for 10-14 days
 Helicobacter pylori infection: Oral: 250-500 mg 3 times/day in combination with at least one other agent active against *H. pylori*
 STD prophylaxis for acute sexual assault: Oral: 2 g in a single dose in combination with ceftriaxone and doxycycline
 Topical: Apply a thin film twice daily to affected areas
 Vaginal: One applicatorful (5 g) intravaginally 2 times/day for 5 days

Dosing adjustment in hepatic impairment: 50% to 67% decrease in dosage

Administration
Intravaginal: Use only **vaginal gel** intravaginally; do not apply to the eye

Oral: Administer on an empty stomach; may administer with food if GI upset occurs

Parenteral: Administer I.V. by slow intermittent infusion over 30-60 minutes at a final concentration for administration of 5-8 mg/mL

Topical: Wash affected areas with a mild cleanser; wait 15-20 minutes, then apply a thin film of drug to the affected area and rub in. Do not apply to the eye.

Monitoring Parameters WBC count

Test Interactions May cause falsely decreased AST and ALT levels

Patient Information May discolor urine dark or reddish brown; avoid alcohol; do not take alcohol for at least 48 hours after the last dose

Nursing Implications Avoid contact between the drug and aluminum in the infusion set

Additional Information Sodium content of 500 mg ready-to-use vial: 14 mEq

Dosage Forms
Gel, topical: 0.75% (30 g)

Gel, vaginal: 0.75% (70 g)

Injection, ready to use, in NS: 5 mg/mL (100 mL)

Powder for injection, as hydrochloride: 500 mg

Tablet: 250 mg, 500 mg

Extemporaneous Preparations To prepare metronidazole suspension 50 mg/mL, pulverize ten 250 mg tablets; levigate with a small amount of distilled water; add 10 mL Cologel® and levigate; add sufficient quantity of cherry syrup to total 50 (Continued)

Metronidazole *(Continued)*

mL and levigate until a uniform mixture is obtained; stable for 30 days if refrigerated

Committee on Extemporaneous Formulations, ASHP Special Interest Group (SIG) on Pediatric Pharmacy Practice, *Handbook on Extemporaneous Formulations*, 1987.

References

Committee on Adolescence, American Academy of Pediatrics, "Sexual Assault and the Adolescent," *Pediatrics*, 1994, 94(5):761-5.

Israel DM and Hassall E, "Treatment and Long-Term Follow-up of *Helicobacter pylori*-Associated Duodenal Ulcer Disease in Children," *J Pediatr*, 1993, 123(1):53-8.

Kelly CP, Pothoulakis C, and LaMont JT, "*Clostridium difficile* Colitis," *N Engl J Med*, 1994, 330(4):257-62.

Oldenburg B and Speck WT, "Metronidazole," *Pediatr Clin North Am*, 1983, 30(1):71-5.

♦ **Metronidazole Hydrochloride** *see* Metronidazole *on page 636*

Metyrapone (me TEER a pone)

Available Salts Metyrapone Tartrate

Therapeutic Category Diagnostic Agent, Hypothalamic-Pituitary ACTH Function

Generic Available No

Use Diagnostic test for hypothalamic-pituitary ACTH function

Pregnancy Risk Factor C

Contraindications Adrenal cortical insufficiency; hypersensitivity to metyrapone or any component

Warnings All corticosteroid therapy should be discontinued prior to and during the metyrapone test

Precautions The test may be abnormal in the presence of thyroid dysfunction; demonstrate the ability of the adrenals to respond to exogenous ACTH before using metyrapone

Adverse Reactions

Cardiovascular: Hypotension, tachycardia

Central nervous system: Dizziness, headache, sedation

Dermatologic: Rash

Gastrointestinal: Abdominal discomfort, nausea

Hematologic: Bone marrow suppression

Drug Interactions Phenytoin, chlorpromazine, amitriptyline, cyproheptadine, estrogens, phenobarbital may reduce test effectiveness

Stability Protect from light

Mechanism of Action Reduces cortisol and corticosterone production by inhibition of 11-beta-hydroxylation of precursors in the adrenal cortex. Continued inhibition stimulates increased ACTH production by the pituitary; increased precursor levels have a weak suppressive activity on ACTH release. Elevated levels of precursor metabolites (17-hydroxycorticosteroids [17-OHCS] or 17-ketogenic steroids [17-KGS]) appear in the urine which can easily serve as an index of pituitary ACTH responsiveness. Production of aldosterone may also be suppressed by metyrapone. The adrenal cortex must have the ability to respond to ACTH before metyrapone is employed to test the capacity of the pituitary to respond to a decreased concentration of plasma cortisol.

Pharmacodynamics Peak effect: Peak excretion of steroid during the first 24 hours after administration

Pharmacokinetics

Absorption: Oral: Well absorbed

Half-life, elimination: 1-2.5 hours (average)

Elimination: 5.3% of dose excreted in urine unchanged

Usual Dosage Oral:

Children: 15 mg/kg/dose or 300 mg/m^2/dose every 4 hours for 6 doses; minimum: 250 mg/dose **or as an alternative** 30 mg/kg as a single dose (maximum: 3 g) given at midnight the night before the test

Adults: 750 mg every 4 hours for 6 doses **or as an alternative** 3 g as a single dose given at midnight the night before the test

Administration Oral: May administer with food or milk to reduce GI irritation

Reference Range Normal response to metyrapone produces a 2-4 times increase in 17-OHCS or 2 times increase in 17-KGS

Patient Information Arise slowly from prolonged sitting or lying position

Dosage Forms Capsule, as tartrate: 250 mg

♦ **Metyrapone Tartrate** *see* Metyrapone *on page 638*

♦ **Meval® (Canada)** *see* Diazepam *on page 307*

Mexiletine (MEKS i le teen)
Brand Names Mexitil®
Therapeutic Category Antiarrhythmic Agent, Class I-B
Generic Available Yes
Use Management of serious ventricular arrhythmias; suppression of premature ventricular contractions; diabetic neuropathy
Pregnancy Risk Factor C
Contraindications Cardiogenic shock, second or third degree heart block; hypersensitivity to mexiletine or any component
Warnings Exercise extreme caution in patients with pre-existing sinus node dysfunction; mexiletine can worsen bradycardias and other arrhythmias
Precautions Use with caution in patients with seizure disorders, severe CHF, hypotension
Adverse Reactions
Cardiovascular: Palpitations, bradycardia, chest pain, syncope, hypotension, atrial or ventricular arrhythmias
Central nervous system: Dizziness, confusion, ataxia
Dermatologic: Rash
Gastrointestinal: Nausea, vomiting, diarrhea
Hematologic: Rarely thrombocytopenia
Hepatic: Hepatitis
Neuromuscular & skeletal: Paresthesia, tremor
Ocular: Diplopia
Otic: Tinnitus
Respiratory: Dyspnea
Miscellaneous: Positive antinuclear antibody
Drug Interactions Cytochrome P-450 isoenzyme CYP2D6 substrate; CYP1A2 isoenzyme inhibitor
Phenobarbital, phenytoin, rifampin, and other hepatic enzyme inducers may lower mexiletine plasma levels; cimetidine may increase mexiletine levels; antacids, narcotics, or anticholinergics may decrease rate of absorption; metoclopramide may increase rate of absorption; drugs which affect urine pH can increase or decrease excretion of mexiletine; mexiletine may increase the serum concentrations of theophylline and caffeine
Food Interactions Food may decrease the rate, but not the extent of oral absorption; diets which affect urine pH can increase or decrease excretion of mexiletine; avoid dietary changes that alter urine pH
Mechanism of Action Class IB antiarrhythmic; structurally related to lidocaine; may cause increase in systemic vascular resistance and decrease in cardiac output; no significant negative inotropic effect
Pharmacodynamics Onset after oral dose: 30-120 minutes
Pharmacokinetics
Distribution: V_d: 5-7 L/kg; found in breast milk in similar concentrations as plasma
Protein-binding: 50% to 70%
Metabolism: Extensive in the liver (some minor active metabolites)
Bioavailability: Oral: 88%
Half-life, adults: 10-14 hours; increase in half-life with hepatic or heart failure
Elimination: 10% to 15% excreted unchanged in urine; urinary acidification increases excretion
Usual Dosage Oral:
Children: Range: 1.4-5 mg/kg/dose (mean: 3.3 mg/kg/dose) given every 8 hours; start with lower initial dose and increase according to effects and serum concentrations
Adults: Initial: 200 mg every 8 hours (may load with 400 mg if necessary); adjust dose every 2-3 days; usual dose: 200-300 mg every 8 hours; some patients may respond to the same daily dose divided every 12 hours; maximum dose: 1.2 g/day
Dosing adjustment in renal impairment: Children and Adults: Cl_{cr} <10 mL/minute: Administer 50% to 75% of normal dose
Dosing adjustment in hepatic disease: Children and Adults: Administer 25% to 30% of normal dose; patients with severe liver disease may require even lower doses, monitor closely
Administration Oral: Administer with food or milk to decrease GI upset
Monitoring Parameters Liver enzymes, EKG, heart rate, serum concentrations
Reference Range
Therapeutic range: 0.5-2 µg/mL
Potentially toxic: >2 µg/mL
(Continued)

Mexiletine (Continued)

Patient Information Limit caffeine; may cause dizziness; notify physician if persistent abdominal pain, nausea, vomiting, yellowing of the eyes or skin, pale stools, dark urine, fever, sore throat, bleeding, or bruising occurs

Additional Information I.V. form under investigation

Dosage Forms Capsule: 150 mg, 200 mg, 250 mg

Extemporaneous Preparations A 10 mg/mL oral suspension can be made using capsules and distilled water or sorbitol USP; grind the contents of eight 150 mg capsules to a powder in a mortar and pestle; then add a small amount of distilled water or sorbitol; mix to make a uniform paste; add distilled water or sorbitol in geometric amounts (while mixing) to almost 120 mL; transfer to a graduated cylinder and qsad 120 mL while mixing; suspension made with sorbitol is stable in plastic prescription bottles for 2 weeks at room temperature (25°C) and 4 weeks if refrigerated (4°C); suspension made with distilled water is stable in plastic prescription bottles for 7 weeks at room temperature (25°C) and 13 weeks if refrigerated (4°C); extended storage at 4°C is recommended to minimize microbial contamination; shake well before use

> Nahata MC, Morosco RS, and Hipple TF, "Stability of Mexiletine in Two Extemporaneous Liquid Formulations Stored Under Refrigeration and at Room Temperature," *J Am Pharm Assoc*, 2000, 40(2):257-9.

References

Moak JP, Smith RT, and Garson A Jr, "Mexiletine: An Effective Antiarrhythmic Drug for Treatment of Ventricular Arrhythmias in Congenital Heart Disease," *J Am Coll Cardiol*, 1987, 10(4):824-9.

♦ **Mexitil®** see Mexiletine on page 639

♦ **Mezlin®** see Mezlocillin on page 640

Mezlocillin (mez loe SIL in)

Brand Names Mezlin®

Available Salts Mezlocillin Sodium

Therapeutic Category Antibiotic, Penicillin (Antipseudomonal)

Generic Available No

Use Treatment of infections caused by susceptible gram-negative aerobic bacilli (*Klebsiella*, *Proteus*, *Escherichia coli*, *Enterobacter*, *Pseudomonas aeruginosa*, *Serratia*) involving the skin and skin structure, bone and joint, respiratory tract, urinary tract, gastrointestinal tract, as well as septicemia

Pregnancy Risk Factor B

Contraindications Hypersensitivity to mezlocillin, any component, or penicillins

Warnings If bleeding occurs during therapy, mezlocillin should be discontinued

Precautions Use with caution in patients with renal impairment or biliary obstruction; dosage modification required in patients with impaired renal function

Adverse Reactions

Central nervous system: Seizures, dizziness, fever, headache

Dermatologic: Rash, exfoliative dermatitis

Endocrine & metabolic: Hypokalemia, hypernatremia

Gastrointestinal: Diarrhea

Hematologic: Eosinophilia, hemolytic anemia, neutropenia, leukopenia, thrombocytopenia, prolonged bleeding time

Hepatic: Elevated liver enzymes

Local: Thrombophlebitis

Renal: Interstitial nephritis, elevated BUN, elevated serum creatinine

Miscellaneous: Serum sickness-like reaction

Drug Interactions Aminoglycosides, probenecid (increases serum concentration of mezlocillin), vecuronium (prolongs neuromuscular blockade)

Stability Reconstituted solution is stable for 48 hours at room temperature and 7 days when refrigerated; incompatible with aminoglycosides

Mechanism of Action Inhibits bacterial cell wall synthesis by binding to one or more of the penicillin-binding proteins; inhibits the final transpeptidation step of peptidoglycan synthesis in bacterial cell walls

Pharmacokinetics

Absorption: I.M.: 63%

Distribution: Into bile, heart, peritoneal fluid, sputum, bone; does not cross the blood-brain barrier well unless meninges are inflamed; crosses the placenta; distributes into breast milk at low concentrations

Protein binding: 30%

Metabolism: 5% to 10%

Half-life:
  Neonates:
    ≤7 days: 3.7-4.4 hours
    >7 days: 2.5 hours
  Infants and Children: 0.5-1 hour
  Children 2-19 years: 0.9 hours
  Adults: 0.5-0.75 hours (dose dependent); half-life prolonged in renal impairment
Time to peak serum concentration:
  I.M.: Within 45-90 minutes
  I.V. infusion: Within 5 minutes
Elimination: Principally as unchanged drug in urine, also excreted via bile
Moderately dialyzable (20% to 50%)

Usual Dosage I.M., I.V.:
  Neonates:
    0-4 weeks, <1200 g: 150 mg/kg/day divided every 12 hours
    Postnatal age ≤7 days, ≥1200 g: 150 mg/kg/day divided every 12 hours
    Postnatal age >7 days, ≥1200 g: 225 mg/kg/day divided every 8 hours
  Children: 200-300 mg/kg/day divided every 4-6 hours; doses as high as 300-450 mg/kg/day divided every 4-6 hours have been used in acute pulmonary exacerbations of cystic fibrosis; maximum dose: 24 g/day
  Adults:
    Uncomplicated urinary tract infection: 1.5-2 g every 6 hours; serious infections: 3-4 g every 4-6 hours
Dosing interval in renal impairment:
  Cl$_{cr}$ 10-30 mL/minute: Administer every 6-8 hours
  Cl$_{cr}$ <10 mL/minute: Administer every 8-12 hours

Administration Parenteral:
  I.M.: Administer deep I.M. into a large muscle mass (ie, gluteus maximus) over 12-15 seconds
  I.V.: Administer IVP over 3-5 minutes at a final concentration for administration not to exceed 100 mg/mL or administer by I.V. intermittent infusion over 15-30 minutes at a concentration of 10-20 mg/mL; maximum concentration for administration in a fluid-restricted patient: 178 mg/mL

Monitoring Parameters Serum electrolytes; periodic renal, hepatic, and hematologic function tests

Test Interactions Positive Coombs' [direct]; false-positive urinary and serum protein

Nursing Implications If the patient is on concurrent aminoglycoside therapy, administration of both agents should be separated by at least 30-60 minutes

Additional Information Sodium content of 1 g: 1.8 mEq

Dosage Forms Powder for injection, as sodium: 1 g, 2 g, 3 g, 4 g, 20 g

References
Odio C, Threlkeld N, Thomas ML, et al, "Pharmacokinetic Properties of Mezlocillin in Newborn Infants," *Antimicrob Agents Chemother*, 1984, 25(5):556-9.

Prober CG, Stevenson DK, and Benitz WE, "The Use of Antibiotics in Neonates Weighing Less Than 1200 Grams," *Pediatr Infect Dis J*, 1990, 9(2):111-21.

♦ **Mezlocillin Sodium** *see* Mezlocillin *on page 640*

♦ **Miacalcin®** *see* Calcitonin *on page 154*

♦ **Miacalcin® Nasal Spray** *see* Calcitonin *on page 154*

♦ **Micatin® Topical [OTC]** *see* Miconazole *on page 641*

Miconazole (mi KON a zole)

Brand Names Breezee® Mist Antifungal [OTC]; Fungoid® Creme; Fungoid® Tincture; Micatin® Topical [OTC]; Monistat-Derm™ Topical; Monistat i.v.™ Injection; Monistat™ Vaginal

Available Salts Miconazole Nitrate

Therapeutic Category Antifungal Agent, Systemic; Antifungal Agent, Topical; Antifungal Agent, Vaginal

Generic Available Yes

Use
  I.V.: Treatment of severe systemic fungal infections and fungal meningitis due to susceptible *Cryptococcus neoformans*, *Candida albicans*, *Candida tropicalis*, *Candida parapsilosis*, *Coccidioides immitis*, and *Histoplasma capsulatum* that are refractory to standard treatment
  Topical: Treatment of vulvovaginal candidiasis; topical treatment of superficial fungal infections

Pregnancy Risk Factor C
(Continued)

Miconazole *(Continued)*

Contraindications Hypersensitivity to miconazole, polyoxyl 35 castor oil, or any component

Warnings The safety of miconazole in infants <1 year of age has not been established

Precautions I.V.: Use with caution in patients with hepatic insufficiency

Adverse Reactions

Cardiovascular: Tachycardia, arrhythmias

Central nervous system: Arachnoiditis and 12th cranial nerve palsy (I.T.); headache, fever, dizziness, confusion, hallucinations, seizures (rare)

Dermatologic: Maceration, urticaria, rash, pruritus

Endocrine & metabolic: Hyperlipidemia (may be due to the Cremophor EL® vehicle), hyponatremia

Gastrointestinal: Nausea, vomiting, diarrhea

Genitourinary: Pelvic cramps

Hematologic: Transient anemia, thrombocytopenia, thrombocytosis

Local: Irritation, burning, itching, phlebitis

Neuromuscular & skeletal: Tremors

Miscellaneous: Anaphylactoid reactions

Drug Interactions Enhanced hypoprothrombinemia with warfarin; oral sulfonylureas (severe hypoglycemia); may be antagonistic with amphotericin B; inhibits cisapride metabolism

Stability Further dilution of miconazole injection with NS or D_5W is stable for 24 hours at room temperature

Mechanism of Action Inhibits biosynthesis of ergosterol, damaging the fungal cell wall membrane which increases permeability and causes leaking of nutrients

Pharmacokinetics

Distribution: Into body tissues, joints, and fluids; poor penetration into sputum, saliva, urine, and CSF

Protein binding: 91% to 93%

Metabolism: In the liver

Half-life: Multiphasic degradation:

Initial: 40 minutes

Secondary: 126 minutes

Terminal: 24 hours

Elimination: ~50% excreted in feces and <1% in urine as unchanged drug

Usual Dosage

Neonates: I.V.: 5-15 mg/kg/day divided every 8-24 hours

Infants and Children:

Topical: Apply twice daily

I.V.: 20-40 mg/kg/day divided every 8 hours

Adolescents and Adults:

Vaginal: Insert contents of 1 applicator of vaginal cream or 100 mg vaginal suppository at bedtime for 7 days, or 200 mg vaginal suppository at bedtime for 3 days

Topical: Apply twice daily

I.T.: 20 mg every 1-2 days (using undiluted miconazole injection)

I.V.: Initial: 200 mg, then 1.2-3.6 g/day divided every 8 hours

Bladder irrigation: Dilute 200 mg in 250 mL NS; instill into the bladder 2-4 times/day or by continuous irrigation

Administration

Parenteral:

I.V.: Administer by slow I.V. intermittent infusion over 1-2 hours at a final concentration not to exceed 6 mg/mL

Intrathecal or intraventricular: When necessary the undiluted I.V. formulation may be used

Topical: Apply sparingly to the cleansed, dry affected area; if intertriginous areas are involved, rub cream gently into the skin

Monitoring Parameters Hematocrit, hemoglobin, serum electrolytes and lipids

Patient Information Avoid contact with the eyes

Nursing Implications I.V. administration over 2 hours may minimize the potential for arrhythmias or anaphylactoid reactions; diphenhydramine may help to reduce pruritus; an antihistamine or antiemetic prior to miconazole administration, or dosage reduction, or slowing the I.V. rate and avoiding administration at mealtime may decrease nausea and vomiting

Dosage Forms
Cream:
  Topical, as nitrate: 2% (15 g, 30 g, 56.7 g, 85 g)
  Vaginal, as nitrate: 2% (45 g is equivalent to 7 doses)
Injection: 1% [10 mg/mL] (20 mL) - **product discontinued in 1998**
Powder, topical, as nitrate: 2% (45 g, 90 g, 113 g)
Solution, topical, as nitrate: 2% with alcohol (7.39 mL, 29.57 mL)
Spray, topical, as nitrate: 2% (105 mL)
Suppository, vaginal, as nitrate: 100 mg (7s); 200 mg (3s)

♦ **Miconazole Nitrate** see Miconazole on page 641
♦ **MICRhoGAM™** see Rh₀(D) Immune Globulin, Intramuscular on page 840
♦ **Micro-K®** see Potassium Supplements on page 786
♦ **Micro-K® LS** see Potassium Supplements on page 786
♦ **microNefrin® [OTC]** see Epinephrine on page 371
♦ **Micronor®** see Norethindrone on page 696
♦ **Microzide®** see Hydrochlorothiazide on page 483
♦ **Midamor®** see Amiloride on page 58

Midazolam (MID aye zoe lam)
Related Information
Adult ACLS Algorithm, Electrical Conversion on page 1014
Compatibility of Medications Mixed in a Syringe on page 1208
Drugs and Breast-Feeding on page 1213
Overdose and Toxicology on page 1191
Preprocedure Sedatives in Children on page 1169
Brand Names Versed®
Available Salts Midazolam Hydrochloride
Therapeutic Category Anticonvulsant, Benzodiazepine; Benzodiazepine; Hypnotic; Sedative
Generic Available Yes: Injection
Use Sedation, anxiolysis, amnesia prior to procedure or before induction of anesthesia; conscious sedation prior to diagnostic or radiographic procedures; continuous I.V. sedation of intubated and mechanically ventilated patients; status epilepticus
Restrictions C-IV
Pregnancy Risk Factor D
Contraindications Hypersensitivity to midazolam, any component, or cherries (syrup); cross-sensitivity with other benzodiazepines may occur; uncontrolled pain; existing CNS depression; shock; narrow-angle glaucoma
Warnings Midazolam may cause respiratory depression/arrest; deaths and hypoxic encephalopathy have resulted when these were not promptly recognized and treated appropriately; dose must be individualized and patients must be appropriately monitored; serious respiratory adverse events occur most often when midazolam is used in combination with other CNS depressants; personnel and equipment needed for standard respiratory resuscitation should be immediately available during midazolam use; a dedicated individual (other than the one performing the procedure) should monitor the deeply sedated pediatric patient throughout the procedure
Precautions Use with caution in patients with CHF, renal impairment, pulmonary disease, hepatic dysfunction; injection contains benzyl alcohol and syrup contains sodium benzoate; use with caution in neonates especially premature neonates; several cases of myoclonus have been reported in premature infants; benzodiazepine withdrawal may occur if abruptly discontinued in patients receiving prolonged I.V. continuous infusions; doses should be tapered slowly with prolonged use; do not administer by rapid I.V. injection (especially in neonates where severe hypotension and seizures have occurred after rapid I.V. administration)
Adverse Reactions
Cardiovascular: Cardiac arrest, hypotension, bradycardia
Central nervous system: Drowsiness, sedation, amnesia, dizziness, paradoxical excitement, hyperactivity, combativeness, headache, ataxia, rhythmic myoclonic jerking in preterm infants (~8% incidence), nystagmus
Gastrointestinal: Nausea, vomiting
Local:
  I.M., I.V.: Pain and local reactions at injection site (severity less than diazepam)
  Nasal: Burning, irritation, discomfort
Neuromuscular & skeletal: Tonic/clonic movements, muscle tremor
Ocular: Blurred vision, diplopia, lacrimation
(Continued)

Midazolam *(Continued)*

Respiratory: Respiratory depression, oxygen desaturation, apnea, laryngospasm, bronchospasm, cough

Miscellaneous: Physical and psychological dependence with prolonged use, hiccups

Drug Interactions Cytochrome P-450 isoenzyme CYP3A3/4 substrate

CNS depressants, alcohol may increase sedation and respiratory depression; narcotic agents may increase hypotension (especially in neonates); doses of anesthetic agents should be reduced when used in conjunction with midazolam; cimetidine, ranitidine, erythromycin, diltiazem, verapamil, fluconazole, ketoconazole, itraconazole may increase midazolam serum concentrations; theophylline may antagonize the sedative effects of midazolam; rifampin reduces the plasma concentration of oral midazolam by >90%; carbamazepine and phenytoin may increase hepatic metabolism of midazolam; protease inhibitors (indinavir, nelfinavir, ritonavir, saquinavir) and delavirdine may potentially decrease midazolam's metabolism and increase midazolam serum concentrations; concurrent use of midazolam with protease inhibitors or delavirdine is not recommended

Food Interactions Grapefruit juice delays the absorption and significantly increases bioavailability of oral midazolam

Stability Stable at a concentration of 0.5 mg/mL for 24 hours in D_5W or NS and for 4 hours in LR

Mechanism of Action Depresses all levels of the CNS, including the limbic and reticular formation, by binding to the benzodiazepine site on the gamma-aminobutyric acid (GABA) receptor complex and modulating GABA, which is a major inhibitory neurotransmitter in the brain

Pharmacodynamics Sedation:

Onset:

Oral: Children: Within 10-20 minutes

I.M.:

Children: Within 5 minutes

Adults: Within 15 minutes

I.V.: Within 1-5 minutes

Intranasal: Within 5 minutes

Peak:

I.M.:

Children: 15-30 minutes

Adults: 30-60 minutes

I.V.: 5-7 minutes

Intranasal: 10 minutes

Duration:

I.M.: Mean: 2 hours, up to 6 hours

I.V.: 20-30 minutes

Intranasal: 30-60 minutes

Note: Full recovery may take more than 24 hours

Pharmacokinetics

Absorption: Oral, nasal: Rapid

Distribution: V_d:

Infants and Children 6 months to 16 years: 1.24-2.02 L/kg

Adults: 1-3.1 L/kg

Increased V_d with CHF and chronic renal failure; widely distributed in body including CSF and brain; crosses placenta; enters fetal circulation; crosses into breast milk

Protein binding: Children >1 year and Adults: 97%; primarily to albumin

Metabolism: Extensive in the liver via cytochrome P-450 CYP3A4 enzyme; undergoes hydroxylation and then glucuronide conjugation; primary metabolite (alpha-hydroxy-midazolam) is active and equipotent to midazolam

Bioavailability: Oral: 15% to 45% (syrup: 36%); I.M.: >90%; intranasal: ~60%; rectal: ~40% to 50%

Half-life, elimination: Increased half-life with cirrhosis, CHF, obesity, elderly, and acute renal failure

Neonates: 4-12 hours; seriously ill neonates: 6.5-12 hours

Children: I.V.: 2.9-4.5 hours; syrup: 2.2-6.8 hours

Adults: 3 hours (range: 1.8-6.4 hours)

Elimination: 63% to 80% excreted as alpha-hydroxy-midazolam glucuronide in urine; ~2% to 10% in feces, <1% eliminated as unchanged drug in the urine

Mean clearance:

Neonates <39 weeks gestational age (GA): 1.17 mL/minute/kg

Neonates >39 weeks GA: 1.84 mL/minute/kg

Seriously ill neonates: 1.2-2 mL/minute/kg
Infants >3 months: 9.1 mL/minute/kg
Children >1 year: 3.2-13.3 mL/minute/kg
Healthy adults: 4.2-9 mL/minute/kg
Adults with acute renal failure: 1.9 mL/minute/kg

Usual Dosage Dosage must be individualized and based on patient's age, underlying diseases, concurrent medications, and desired effect; decrease dose (by ~30%) if narcotics or other CNS depressants are administered concomitantly; use multiple small doses and titrate to desired sedative effect; allow 3-5 minutes between doses to decrease the chance of oversedation

Neonates: Conscious sedation during mechanical ventilation: I.V. continuous infusion:
<32 weeks: Initial: 0.03 mg/kg/hour (0.5 mcg/kg/minute)
>32 weeks: Initial: 0.06 mg/kg/hour (1 mcg/kg/minute)
Note: Do not use I.V. loading doses in neonates; for faster achievement of sedation, infuse the continuous infusion at a faster rate for the first several hours; use the smallest dose possible

Infants >2 months and Children: Status epilepticus refractory to standard therapy: I.V.: Loading dose: 0.15 mg/kg followed by a continuous infusion of 1 mcg/kg/minute; titrate dose upward every 5 minutes until clinical seizure activity is controlled; mean infusion rate required in 24 children was 2.3 mcg/kg/minute with a range of 1-18 mcg/kg/minute (Rivera, 1993)

Infants ≥6 months and Children: Sedation, anxiolysis, and amnesia prior to procedure or before induction of anesthesia: Oral: Single dose; 0.25-0.5 mg/kg, depending on patient status and desired effect; usual: 0.5 mg/kg; maximum dose: 20 mg;
Patient status-specific dosing:
Infants 6 months to <6 years, and less cooperative patients: Higher doses (up to 1 mg/kg) may be required
Children 6 to ≥16 years, or cooperative patients (especially if intensity and duration of sedation is less critical): 0.25 mg/kg may suffice
High risk pediatric patients (respiratory or cardiac compromised, concomitant CNS depressants, higher risk surgical patients): 0.25 mg/kg should be considered

Children:
Preoperative sedation or conscious sedation for procedures:
I.M.: Usual: 0.1-0.15 mg/kg 30-60 minutes before surgery or procedure; range: 0.05-0.15 mg/kg; doses up to 0.5 mg/kg have been used in more anxious patients; maximum total dose: 10 mg
I.V.:
Infants <6 months: Limited information is available in nonintubated infants; dosing recommendations are unclear; infants <6 months are at higher risk for airway obstruction and hypoventilation; titrate dose with small increments to desired clinical effect; monitor carefully
Infants 6 months to Children 5 years: Initial: 0.05-0.1 mg/kg; titrate dose carefully; total dose of 0.6 mg/kg may be required; usual total dose maximum dose: 6 mg
Children 6-12 years: Initial: 0.025-0.05 mg/kg; titrate dose carefully; total doses of 0.4 mg/kg may be required; usual total dose maximum: 10 mg
Children 12-16 years: Dose as adults; usual total dose maximum: 10 mg
Intranasal: Usual: 0.2 mg/kg; may repeat in 5-15 minutes; range: 0.2-0.3 mg/kg/dose
Conscious sedation during mechanical ventilation: I.V.: Continuous infusion: Loading dose: 0.05-0.2 mg/kg given slow I.V. over 2-3 minutes, then follow with initial continuous infusion: 0.06-0.12 mg/kg/hour (1-2 mcg/kg/minute); titrate to the desired effect; range: 0.4-6 mcg/kg/minute

Adults:
Preoperative sedation: I.M.: 0.07-0.08 mg/kg 30-60 minutes presurgery; usual dose: 5 mg
Conscious sedation: I.V.: Titrate dose slowly to desired effect; administer slowly over at least 2 minutes and wait another 2 or more minutes to evaluate effect. Some adults may respond to doses as low as 1 mg; do not give more than 2.5 mg over a period of 2 minutes. Titrate as needed, using small increments every 2-3 minutes. Usual total dose: 2.5-5 mg; total dose >5 mg is generally not needed; maintenance doses may be given by slow titration, if needed, in increments of 25% of the original dose used to reach sedative endpoint.
Conscious sedation during mechanical ventilation: I.V.: Optional loading dose: 0.01-0.05 mg/kg (~0.5-4 mg/dose); may repeat at 10- to 15-minute intervals until patient is adequately sedated, then begin continuous infusion

(Continued)

Midazolam (Continued)

Continuous infusion: Initial: 0.02-0.1 mg/kg/hour (1-7 mg/hour); use lowest doses listed for patients receiving other sedatives, or opioids, or having residual anesthetic effects; titrate the infusion to achieve adequate level of sedation; use lowest effective dose

Administration

Intranasal: Administer using a 1 mL needleless syringe into the nares over 15 seconds; use the 5 mg/mL injection; ½ of the dose may be administered to each nare

Oral: Administer on empty stomach (feeding is usually contraindicated prior to sedation for procedures)

Parenteral: I.V.: Administer by slow I.V. injection over at least 2-5 minutes at a concentration of 1-5 mg/mL or by I.V. infusion; avoid extravasation; do not administer intra-arterially

Monitoring Parameters Level of sedation, respiratory rate, heart rate, blood pressure, oxygen saturation (ie, pulse, oximetry)

Nursing Implications Abrupt discontinuation after prolonged use may result in withdrawal symptoms

Additional Information Sodium content of injection: 0.14 mEq/mL; for Neonates: Since both concentrations of the injection contain 1% benzyl alcohol, use the 5 mg/mL injection and dilute to 0.5 mg/mL with SWI without preservatives to decrease the amount of benzyl alcohol delivered to the neonate; with continuous infusion, midazolam may accumulate in peripheral tissues; use lowest effective infusion rate to reduce accumulation effects; midazolam is 3-4 times as potent as diazepam; paradoxical reactions associated with midazolam use in children (eg, agitation, restlessness, combativeness) have been successfully treated with flumazenil (see Massanari, 1997)

Dosage Forms

Injection, as hydrochloride: 1 mg/mL (2 mL, 5 mL, 10 mL); 5 mg/mL (1 mL, 2 mL, 5 mL, 10 mL)

Syrup, as hydrochloride (cherry flavor): 2 mg/mL (118 mL)

References

Adrian ER, "Intranasal Versed®: The Future of Pediatric Conscious Sedation," *Pediatr Nurs*, 1994, 20(3):287-92.

Booker PD, Beechey A, and Lloyd-Thomas AR, "Sedation of Children Requiring Artificial Ventilation Using an Infusion of Midazolam," *Br J Anaesth*, 1986, 58(10):1104-8.

Burtin P, Jacqz-Aigrain E, Girard P, et al, "Population Pharmacokinetics of Midazolam in Neonates," *Clin Pharmacol Ther*, 1994, 56(6 Pt 1):615-25.

Jacqz-Aigrain E, Daoud P, Burtin P, et al, "Placebo-Controlled Trial of Midazolam Sedation in Mechanically Ventilated Newborn Babies," *Lancet*, 1994, 344(8923):646-50.

Kupietzky A and Houpt MI, "Midazolam: A Review of Its Use for Conscious Sedation of Children," *Pediatr Dent*, 1993, 15(4):237-41.

Lugo RA, Fishbein M, Nahata MC, et al, "Complication of Intranasal Midazolam," *Pediatrics*, 1993, 92(4):638.

Magny JF, Zupan V, Dehan M, et al, "Midazolam and Myoclonus in Neonate," *Eur J Pediatr*, 1994, 153(5):389-90.

Malinovsky JM, Populaire C, Cozian A, et al, "Premedication With Midazolam in Children, Effect of Intranasal, Rectal and Oral Routes on Plasma Midazolam Concentrations," *Anaesthesia*, 1995, 50(4):351-4.

Massanari M, Novitsky J, and Reinstein LJ, "Paradoxical Reactions in Children Associated With Midazolam Use During Endoscopy," *Clin Pediatr*, 1997, 36(12):681-4.

Riva J, Lejbusiewicz G, Papa M, et al, "Oral Premedication With Midazolam in Paediatric Anaesthesia. Effects on Sedation and Gastric Contents," *Paediatr Anaesth*, 1997, 7(3):191-6.

Rivera R, Segnini M, Baltodano A, et al, "Midazolam in the Treatment of Status Epilepticus in Children," *Crit Care Med*, 1993, 21(7):991-4.

Silvasi DL, Rosen DA, and Rosen KR, "Continuous Intravenous Midazolam Infusion for Sedation in the Pediatric Intensive Care Unit," *Anesth Analg*, 1988, 67(3):286-8.

♦ **Midazolam Hydrochloride** see Midazolam *on page 643*

♦ **Midol® IB [OTC]** see Ibuprofen *on page 501*

♦ **Miles Nervine® Caplets [OTC]** see Diphenhydramine *on page 327*

♦ **Milkinol® [OTC]** see Mineral Oil *on page 649*

♦ **Milk of Magnesia (Magnesium Hydroxide)** see Magnesium Supplements *on page 588*

Milrinone (MIL ri none)

Brand Names Primacor®

Available Salts Milrinone Lactate

Therapeutic Category Phosphodiesterase Enzyme Inhibitor

Generic Available No

Use Short-term treatment of acute decompensated heart failure

Pregnancy Risk Factor C

Contraindications Hypersensitivity to milrinone, any component, or inamrinone (amrinone)

Warnings Longer treatment of heart failure (>48 hours) has not been shown to be safe and effective (there are no controlled trials using milrinone infusions for >48 hours); long-term oral use for heart failure was associated with no improvement in symptoms, increased risk of hospitalization, and increased risk of sudden death; monitor EKG continuously to promptly detect and manage ventricular arrhythmias

Precautions Avoid use in patients with severe obstructive aortic or pulmonic valvular disease; use in patients with hypertrophic subaortic stenosis may increase outflow tract obstruction; use with caution in patients with a history of ventricular arrhythmias, atrial fibrillation, or atrial flutter; use with caution and modify dosage in patients with impaired renal function

Adverse Reactions

Central nervous system: Headaches (mild to moderate, 2.9%)

Cardiovascular: Ventricular arrhythmias (12.1%) including ventricular ectopic activity (8.5%), nonsustained ventricular tachycardia (2.8%), sustained ventricular tachycardia (1%), and ventricular fibrillation (0.2%); supraventricular arrhythmias (3.8%); hypotension (2.9%); angina/chest pain (1.2%)

Endocrine & metabolic: Hypokalemia (0.6%)

Hematologic: Thrombocytopenia (0.4%)

Neuromuscular & skeletal: Tremor (0.4%)

Respiratory: Bronchospasm (rare)

Stability Incompatible with furosemide (a precipitate forms when furosemide is injected into I.V. lines containing milrinone); compatible with $\frac{1}{2}$NS, NS, and D_5W

Mechanism of Action Inhibits phosphodiesterase III (PDE III), the major PDE in cardiac and vascular tissues. Inhibition of PDE III increases cyclic adenosine monophosphate (cAMP) which potentiates the delivery of calcium to myocardial contractile systems and results in a positive inotropic effect. Inhibition of PDE III in vascular tissue results in relaxation of vascular muscle and vasodilatation.

Pharmacodynamics Onset (improved hemodynamic function): Within 5-15 minutes

Pharmacokinetics

Distribution: V_d beta

Infants (after cardiac surgery): 0.9 ± 0.4 L/kg

Children (after cardiac surgery): 0.7 ± 0.2 L/kg

Adults:

After cardiac surgery: 0.3 ± 0.1 L/kg

CHF (with single injection): 0.38 L/kg

CHF (with infusion): 0.45 L/kg

Protein binding: 70%

Half-life:

Infants (after cardiac surgery): 3.15 ± 2 hours

Children (after cardiac surgery): 1.86 ± 2 hours

Adults:

After cardiac surgery: 1.69 ± 0.18 hours

CHF: 2.3-2.4 hours

Renal impairment: Prolonged half-life

Elimination: Excreted in the urine as unchanged drug (83%) and glucuronide metabolite (12%)

Clearance:

Infants (after cardiac surgery): 3.8 ± 1 mL/kg/minute

Children (after cardiac surgery): 5.9 ± 2 mL/kg/minute

Children (with septic shock): 10.6 ± 5.3 mL/kg/minute

Adults:

After cardiac surgery: 2 ± 0.7 mL/kg/minute

CHF: 2.2-2.3 mL/kg/minute

Renal impairment: Decreased clearance

Usual Dosage I.V.:

Neonates, Infants, and Children: A limited number of studies have used different dosing schemes (see Additional Information). Two recent pharmacokinetic studies propose per kg doses for pediatric patients with septic shock that are greater than those recommended for adults (Lindsay, 1998) and in infants and children after cardiac surgery (Ramamoorthy, 1998). Further pharmacodynamic studies are needed to define pediatric milrinone guidelines. Several centers are using the following guidelines:

Loading dose: 50 mcg/kg administered over 15 minutes followed by a continuous infusion of 0.5 mcg/kg/minute; range: 0.25-0.75 mcg/kg/minute; titrate dose to effect

(Continued)

Milrinone *(Continued)*

Adults: Loading dose: 50 mcg/kg slow I.V. over 10 minutes, followed by a continuous infusion of 0.5 mcg/kg/minute; range: 0.375-0.75 mcg/kg/minute; titrate does to effect; maximum daily dose: 1.13 mg/kg/day

Dosing adjustment in renal impairment: For continuous infusion:

Cl_{cr} 50 mL/minute/1.73 m^2: Administer 0.43 mcg/kg/minute

Cl_{cr} 40 mL/minute/1.73 m^2: Administer 0.38 mcg/kg/minute

Cl_{cr} 30 mL/minute/1.73 m^2: Administer 0.33 mcg/kg/minute

Cl_{cr} 20 mL/minute/1.73 m^2: Administer 0.28 mcg/kg/minute

Cl_{cr} 10 mL/minute/1.73 m^2: Administer 0.23 mcg/kg/minute

Cl_{cr} 5 mL/minute/1.73 m^2: Administer 0.2 mcg/kg/minute

Administration

Loading dose: Administer slow I.V. push over 15 minutes for pediatric patients and over 10 minutes in adults; loading dose may be given as undiluted solution, but may dilute to 10-20 mL (in adults) for ease of administration.

I.V. continuous infusion: Dilute with ½NS, NS, or D_5W and administer via infusion pump or syringe pump; usual concentration: ≤200 mcg/mL; 250 mcg/mL in NS has been used (see Barton, 1996)

Monitoring Parameters Blood pressure, heart rate, cardiac output, CI, SVR, PVR, CVP, EKG, platelet count, serum potassium, renal function; clinical signs and symptoms of CHF

Nursing Implications Do not administer furosemide I.V. push via "Y" site into milrinone solutions as precipitate will occur; decrease the infusion rate if significant hypotension occurs

Additional Information Dosing schemes and proposed dosing based on pharmacokinetic data:

Neonates: A loading dose of 50 mcg/kg administered over 15 minutes, followed by a continuous infusion of 0.5 mcg/kg/minute for 30 minutes in 10 neonates (3-27 days old, median age 5 days) improved hemodynamic parameters and was well tolerated (see Chang, 1995). Further neonatal studies of longer duration are needed.

Infants and children with septic shock: Twelve patients (9 months to 15 years of age) were administered a loading dose of 50 mcg/kg, followed by a continuous infusion of 0.5 mcg/kg/minute. At 1 hour after the loading dose, if patients did not respond (defined as a ≥20% increase in CI or an improvement in peripheral perfusion), an additional loading dose of 25 mcg/kg was given and the infusion rate was increased to 0.75 mcg/kg/minute. Nine of 12 patients required the additional loading dose and increased rate of infusion (see Barton 1996). A subsequent pharmacokinetic analysis of these patients recommended larger loading doses of 75 mcg/kg and infusion rates of 0.75-1 mcg/kg/minute. However, these doses were based on a one-compartment pharmacokinetic model and are higher then the mean infusion rate of 0.69 mcg/kg/minute used in the study (see Lindsay 1998). Further studies are needed.

Infants and Children after open heart surgery: Group A: Eleven patients received a loading dose of 25 mcg/kg given over 5 minutes followed by an infusion of 0.25 mcg/kg/minute; 30 minutes later, a second 25 mcg/kg loading dose was given and the infusion was increased to 0.5 mcg/kg/minute. Group B: 8 patients received a loading dose of 50 mcg/kg given over 10 minutes followed by an infusion of 0.5 mcg/kg/minute; 30 minutes later, a second loading dose of 25 mcg/kg was given and the infusion was increased to 0.75 mcg/kg/minute. Patients in both groups received a third loading dose of 25 mcg/kg if needed. A two-compartment model and NONMEM pharmacokinetic analyses were performed. Based on the NONMEM analysis, the authors propose the following doses: Infants: Loading dose: 104 mcg/kg and continuous infusion of 0.49 mcg/kg/minute; children: loading dose: 67 mcg/kg and continuous infusion of 0.61 mcg/kg/minute. Further studies are needed before these proposed doses can routinely be used in the pediatric population.

Dosage Forms

Infusion, as lactate, in D_5W: 200 mcg/mL (100 mL, 200 mL)

Injection, as lactate: 1 mg/mL (5 mL, 10 mL, 20 mL)

References

Barton P, Garcia J, Kouatli A, et al, "Hemodynamic Effects of I.V. Milrinone Lactate in Pediatric Patients With Septic Shock. A Prospective Double-Blinded, Randomized, Placebo-Controlled, Interventional Study," *Chest*, 1996, 109(5):1302-12.

Chang AC, Atz AM, Wernovsky G, et al, "Milrinone: Systemic and Pulmonary Hemodynamic Effects in Neonates After Cardiac Surgery," *Crit Care Med*, 1995, 23(11):1907-14.

Lindsay CA, Barton P, Lawless S, et al, "Pharmacokinetics and Pharmacodynamics of Milrinone Lactate in Pediatric Patients With Septic Shock," *J Pediatr*, 1998, 132(2):329-34.

Ramamoorthy C, Anderson GD, Williams GD, et al, "Pharmacokinetics and Side Effects of Milrinone in Infants and Children After Open Heart Surgery," *Anesth Analg*, 1998, 86(2):283-9.

♦ **Milrinone Lactate** *see* Milrinone *on page 646*

Mineral Oil (MIN er al oyl)

Brand Names Agoral® Plain [OTC]; Fleet® Mineral Oil Enema [OTC]; Kondremul® [OTC]; Lansoyl® [also sugar-free] (Canada); Milkinol® [OTC]; Neo-Cultol® [OTC]; Zymenol® [OTC]

Synonyms Heavy Mineral Oil; Liquid Paraffin; White Mineral Oil

Therapeutic Category Laxative, Lubricant

Generic Available Yes

Use Temporary relief of constipation, to relieve fecal impaction, preparation for bowel studies or surgery

Pregnancy Risk Factor C

Contraindications Patients with a colostomy or an ileostomy, appendicitis, ulcerative colitis, diverticulitis

Warnings Oral form should be avoided in children <4 years of age and bedtime doses should be avoided because of the risk of aspiration

Adverse Reactions

Gastrointestinal: Nausea, vomiting, diarrhea, abdominal cramps, anal itching, anal seepage

Respiratory: Lipid pneumonitis with aspiration

Drug Interactions May impair absorption of fat-soluble vitamins, oral contraceptives, coumarin; increased absorption with docusate

Food Interactions May decrease absorption of fat-soluble vitamins, carotene, calcium, and phosphorus

Mechanism of Action Eases passage of stool by decreasing water absorption and lubricating the intestine

Pharmacodynamics Onset of action: ~6-8 hours

Pharmacokinetics

Absorption: Minimal following oral or rectal administration

Distribution: Into intestinal mucosa, liver, spleen, and mesenteric lymph nodes

Elimination: In feces

Usual Dosage

Children:

Oral: 5-11 years: 5-15 mL once daily or in divided doses; should not be used for longer than 1 week

Rectal: 2-11 years: 30-60 mL as a single dose

Children ≥12 years and Adults:

Oral: 15-45 mL/day once daily or in divided doses; should not be used for longer than 1 week

Rectal: Retention enema, contents of one enema (range 60-150 mL)/day as a single dose

Administration

Oral: Nonemulsified mineral oil may be administered at bedtime on an empty stomach, or administer 2 hours before or after food or meals; emulsified mineral oil should be shaken before using; may be administered with meals (more palatable than nonemulsified mineral oil)

Rectal: Gently insert enema tip into rectum with a slight side-to-side movement with tip pointing toward the navel; have patient bear down

Patient Information Do not take if experiencing abdominal pain, nausea, or vomiting; do not take at bedtime. Rectal enema: Do not take if experiencing rectal bleeding

Dosage Forms

Emulsion, oral: Dosage of mineral oil emulsion is expressed in terms of its mineral oil content: 1.4 g/5 mL (480 mL); 2.5 mL/5 mL (420 mL); 2.75 mL/5 mL (480 mL); 4.75 mL/5 mL (240 mL)

Jelly, oral: 2.75 mL/5 mL (180 mL)

Liquid:

Oral: 30 mL, 180 mL, 500 mL, 1000 mL, 4000 mL

Rectal: 133 mL

♦ **Mini-Gamulin® Rh** *see* Rh₀(D) Immune Globulin, Intramuscular *on page 840*
♦ **Minims® Pilocarpine (Canada)** *see* Pilocarpine *on page 770*
♦ **Minipress®** *see* Prazosin *on page 790*
♦ **Minitran® Patch** *see* Nitroglycerin *on page 690*

Minoxidil (mi NOKS i dil)

Brand Names Apo®-Gain (Canada); Gen-Minoxidil (Canada); Loniten® Oral; Mlnoxigaine™ (Canada); Rogaine® Topical

Therapeutic Category Antihypertensive Agent; Vasodilator

Generic Available Yes

Use Management of severe hypertension; topically for management of alopecia or male pattern alopecia

Pregnancy Risk Factor C

Contraindications Pheochromocytoma; hypersensitivity to minoxidil or any component

Precautions Use with caution in patients with coronary artery disease or with recent MI, pulmonary hypertension, significant renal dysfunction, CHF

Adverse Reactions

Cardiovascular: Edema, CHF, tachycardia, angina, pericardial effusion and tamponade, EKG changes

Central nervous system: Dizziness, fatigue, headache

Dermatologic: Hypertrichosis (commonly occurs within 1-2 months of therapy), coarsening facial features, dermatologic reactions, rash, Stevens-Johnson syndrome, photosensitivity

Endocrine & metabolic: Sodium and water retention

Gastrointestinal: Weight gain

Respiratory: Pulmonary hypertension, pulmonary edema

Drug Interactions Concurrent administration with guanethidine may cause profound orthostatic hypotensive effects; additive hypotensive effects with other hypotensive agents or diuretics

Food Interactions Avoid natural licorice (causes sodium and water retention and increases potassium loss)

Mechanism of Action Produces vasodilation by directly relaxing arteriolar smooth muscle, with little effect on veins; effects may be mediated by cyclic AMP; stimulation of hair growth is secondary to vasodilation, increased cutaneous blood flow and stimulation of resting hair follicles

Pharmacodynamics Hypotensive effects:

Onset of action: Oral: Within 30 minutes

Peak effect: Within 2-8 hours

Duration: Up to 2-5 days

Pharmacokinetics

Metabolism: 88% primarily via glucuronidation

Protein-binding: None

Bioavailability: Oral: 90%

Half-life, adults: 3.5-4.2 hours

Elimination: 12% excreted unchanged in urine

Dialyzable (50% to 100%)

Usual Dosage

Children <12 years: Hypertension: Oral: Initial: 0.1-0.2 mg/kg once daily; maximum dose: 5 mg/day; increase gradually every 3 days; usual dosage: 0.25-1 mg/kg/day in 1-2 divided doses; maximum dose: 50 mg/day

Children >12 years and Adults:

Hypertension: Oral: Initial: 5 mg once daily, increase gradually every 3 days; usual dose: 10-40 mg/day in 1-2 divided doses; maximum dose: 100 mg/day

Alopecia: Apply twice daily

Administration Oral: May be administered without regard to food

Monitoring Parameters Fluids and electrolytes, body weight, blood pressure

Patient Information May cause dizziness; rise slowly from prolonged lying or sitting position

Additional Information Usually used with a beta-blocker (to treat minoxidil-induced tachycardia) and a diuretic (for treatment of water retention/edema); may take 1-6 months for hypertrichosis to totally reverse after minoxidil therapy is discontinued

Dosage Forms

Solution, topical: 2% [20 mg/metered dose] (60 mL); 5% [50 mg/metered dose] (60 mL)

Tablet: 2.5 mg, 10 mg

♦ Mlnoxigaine™ (Canada) *see* Minoxidil *on page 650*

♦ Mintezol® *see* Thiabendazole *on page 915*

♦ Minute-Gel® *see* Fluoride *on page 427*

♦ Miocarpine® (Canada) *see* Pilocarpine *on page 770*

♦ **Miochol-E®** see Acetylcholine on page 31

♦ **MiraLax™** see Polyethylene Glycol-Electrolyte Solution on page 782

Misoprostol (mye soe PROST ole)

Brand Names Cytotec®

Therapeutic Category Gastrointestinal Agent, Gastric or Duodenal Ulcer Treatment; Prostaglandin

Use Prevention of NSAID-induced gastric ulcers; short term treatment of duodenal and gastric ulcers (up to 8 weeks); improvement in fat absorption in cystic fibrosis patients when used in conjunction with pancreatic enzyme supplements (unlabeled use)

Pregnancy Risk Factor X

Contraindications Hypersensitivity to misoprostol or any component, pregnancy

Warnings Not to be used in pregnant women or women of childbearing potential unless woman is capable of complying with effective contraceptive measures; women should have a negative serum pregnancy test within 2 weeks prior to initiating therapy with therapy begun on the second or third day of next menstrual period

Precautions Use with caution in patients with inflammatory bowel disease and renal impairment

Adverse Reactions

Central nervous system: Headache

Gastrointestinal: Nausea, vomiting, constipation, flatulence, diarrhea, abdominal pain

Genitourinary: Uterine stimulation, vaginal bleeding, menstrual irregularities

Drug Interactions Magnesium containing antacids enhance diarrhea associated with misoprostol

Mechanism of Action Misoprostol, a gastric antisecretory agent, is a synthetic prostaglandin E_1 analog that replaces the protective prostaglandins consumed with prostaglandin-inhibiting therapies (eg, NSAIDs) resulting in reduction of acid secretion from the gastric parietal cell and stimulation of bicarbonate production from the gastric and duodenal mucosa

Pharmacodynamics Inhibition of gastric acid secretion:

Onset of action: 30 minutes

Peak effect: 60-90 minutes

Duration of action: 3 hours

Pharmacokinetics

Absorption: Rapid

Protein binding (misoprostol acid): 80% to 90%

Metabolism: Extensive "first pass" de-esterification to misoprostol acid (active metabolite)

Bioavailability: 88%

Half-life (parent and metabolite combined): 1.5 hours

Time to peak serum concentrations (active metabolite): Within 15-30 minutes

Elimination: In urine (64% to 73% in 24 hours) and feces (15% in 24 hours)

Usual Dosage Oral:

Prevention of NSAID-induced ulcers: Adults: 200 mcg 4 times/day; if not tolerated, may decrease dose to 100 mcg 4 times/day or 200 mcg twice daily

Gastric or duodenal ulcers: Adults: 100-200 mcg four times daily or 400 mcg twice daily for 4-8 weeks

Improvement of fat malabsorption in cystic fibrosis (limited data available in children): Children 8-16 years: 100 mcg four times daily

Administration Oral: Administer after meals and at bedtime

Patient Information May cause diarrhea when first being used; avoid taking with magnesium-containing antacids

Nursing Implications Incidence of diarrhea may be lessened by having patient take dose right after meals

Dosage Forms Tablet: 100 mcg, 200 mcg

References

Cleghorn GJ, Shepherd RW, and Holt TL, "The Use of a Synthetic Prostaglandin E1 Analogue (Misoprostol) as an Adjunct to Pancreatic Enzyme Replacement in Cystic Fibrosis," Scand J Gastroenterol Suppl, 1988, 143:142-7.

Robinson PJ, Smith AL, and Sly PD, "Duodenal pH in Cystic Fibrosis and Its Relationship to Fat Malabsorption," Dig Dis Sci, 1990, 35(10):1299-304.

♦ **Mithracin®** see Plicamycin on page 778

♦ **Mithramycin** see Plicamycin on page 778

Mitomycin (mye toe MYE sin)

Related Information
Emetogenic Potential of Single Chemotherapeutic Agents *on page 1095*

Brand Names Mutamycin®

Synonyms Mitomycin-C; MTC

Therapeutic Category Antineoplastic Agent, Antibiotic

Generic Available No

Use Therapy of disseminated adenocarcinoma of stomach, colon, or pancreas in combination with other approved chemotherapeutic agents; bladder cancer, breast cancer

Pregnancy Risk Factor C

Contraindications Platelet counts <75,000/mm³; leukocyte counts <3000/mm³ or serum creatinine >1.7 mg/dL; coagulation disorders; hypersensitivity to mitomycin or any component

Warnings The FDA currently recommends that procedures for proper handling and disposal of antineoplastic agents be considered. Bone marrow suppression, notably thrombocytopenia and leukopenia, may contribute to the development of a secondary infection; hemolytic uremic syndrome, a serious and often fatal syndrome has occurred in patients receiving long-term therapy; the risk of hemolytic uremic syndrome increases with a total cumulative dose >50 mg/m²; mitomycin is potentially mutagenic and teratogenic.

Precautions Use with caution in patients with myelosuppression, impaired renal or hepatic function; modify dosage in patients with myelosuppression or renal impairment

Adverse Reactions
Central nervous system: Fever

Dermatologic: Alopecia, pruritus

Gastrointestinal: Nausea, vomiting, mouth ulcers, diarrhea, anorexia

Hematologic: Bone marrow suppression (leukopenia, thrombocytopenia), microangiopathic hemolytic anemia

Hepatic: Veno-occlusive disease

Local: Thrombophlebitis

Neuromuscular & skeletal: Paresthesia, weakness

Renal: Hemolytic uremic syndrome, nephrotoxicity

Respiratory: Pulmonary toxicity, interstitial pneumonia

Drug Interactions Anthracyclines (may enhance cardiotoxicity)

Stability Reconstitute solution with sterile water at a concentration of 0.5 mg/mL; the reconstituted solution must be protected from light if not used within 24 hours; stable for 7 days at room temperature and 14 days when refrigerated; I.V. infusion in D_5W is stable for 3 hours at room temperature; in NS solution is stable for 12 hours at room temperature; physically compatible with ondansetron for 4 hours

Mechanism of Action Inhibits DNA and RNA synthesis by alkylating and crosslinking the strands of DNA

Pharmacokinetics
Distribution: Into bile and ascites fluid

Half-life, terminal: 50 minutes

Elimination: Primarily by hepatic metabolism followed by urinary excretion (<10% as unchanged drug) and to a small extent biliary excretion

Usual Dosage Children and Adults: I.V. (refer to individual protocols): 10-20 mg/m²/dose every 6-8 weeks, or 3 mg/m²/day for 5 days every 4-6 weeks; subsequent doses should be adjusted to platelet and leukocyte response; see table.

Nadir After Prior Dose/mm³		% of Prior Dose to Be Given
Leukocytes	Platelets	
4000	>100,000	100
3000-3999	75,000-99,999	100
2000-2999	25,000-74,999	70
2000	<25,000	50

Very high doses (40-50 mg/m² as a single dose) have been administered by hepatic artery infusion followed by autologous bone marrow transplantation.

Dosing adjustment in renal impairment: Cl_{cr} <10 mL/minute: Administer 75% of normal dose

Administration Parenteral: Administer by short I.V. infusion over 30-60 minutes or by slow I.V. push over 5-10 minutes through a Y-site of a running I.V.; short I.V. infusions are usually administered at a final concentration of 20-40 mcg/mL (in 50-

250 mL of D$_5$W or NS); I.V. slow push can be administered at a concentration not to exceed 0.5 mg/mL

Monitoring Parameters Platelet count, CBC with differential, hemoglobin, prothrombin time, renal and pulmonary function tests

Patient Information Notify physician if fever, sore throat, bruising, bleeding, shortness of breath, or painful urination occur

Nursing Implications Care should be taken to avoid extravasation since ulceration and tissue sloughing can occur; mitomycin extravasation has been treated using a 99% (w/v) solution of dimethylsulfoxide (DMSO); apply 1.5 mL to the site every 6 hours for 14 days; allow to air-dry; do not cover

Additional Information Myelosuppressive effects:
WBC: Moderate
Platelets: Severe
Onset (days): 21
Nadir (days): 36
Recovery (days): 42-56

Dosage Forms Powder for injection: 5 mg, 20 mg, 40 mg

References
Alberts DS and Dorr RT, "Case Report: Topical DMSO for Mitomycin C-Induced Skin Ulceration," *Oncol Nurs Forum*, 1991, 18(4):693-5.

♦ **Mitomycin-C** *see* Mitomycin *on page 652*

Mitoxantrone (mye toe ZAN trone)

Related Information
Emetogenic Potential of Single Chemotherapeutic Agents *on page 1095*

Brand Names Novantrone®

Available Salts Mitoxantrone Hydrochloride

Synonyms DHAD

Therapeutic Category Antineoplastic Agent, Anthracycline; Antineoplastic Agent, Antibiotic

Generic Available No

Use FDA approved for remission-induction therapy of acute nonlymphocytic leukemia (ANLL); mitoxantrone is also active against other various leukemias, lymphoma, and breast cancer, and moderately active against pediatric sarcoma

Pregnancy Risk Factor D

Contraindications Hypersensitivity to mitoxantrone or any component

Warnings Avoid in patients with pre-existing myelosuppression; mitoxantrone is less cardiotoxic than anthracyclines. The predisposing factors for mitoxantrone-induced cardiotoxicity include prior anthracycline therapy, prior cardiovascular disease, and mediastinal irradiation. The risk of developing cardiotoxicity is <3% when the cumulative dose is <100-120 mg/m^2 in patients with predisposing factors and <160 mg/m^2 in patients with no predisposing factors; interstitial pneumonitis has been reported in patients receiving combination chemotherapy that included mitoxantrone; extravasation can result in tissue necrosis with resultant need for debridement and skin grafting; the FDA currently recommends that procedures for proper handling and disposal of antineoplastic agents be considered. In general, intrathecal administration is not recommended since local nerve demyelinization and paraplegia have been reported with this route.

Precautions Dosage should be reduced in patients with pre-existing bone marrow suppression, previous treatment with cardiotoxic agents, and patients with impaired hepatobiliary function

Adverse Reactions
Cardiovascular: Cardiotoxicity (arrhythmias, CHF), hypotension, tachycardia
Central nervous system: Seizures, headache
Dermatologic: Alopecia, pruritus, skin desquamation, rash, blue staining of skin
Gastrointestinal: Nausea, diarrhea, vomiting, stomatitis (occurs more frequently with "daily times 3 day" regimens than once every 3 week schedules), mucositis
Genitourinary: Discoloration of urine (blue-green)
Hematologic: Myelosuppression (leukopenia, pancytopenia), mild anemia, thrombocytopenia
Hepatic: Transient elevation of liver enzymes, jaundice
Local: Phlebitis
Respiratory: Interstitial pneumonitis

Drug Interactions High-dose cytarabine (therapeutic synergy)

Stability After penetration of the stopper, undiluted mitoxantrone solution is stable for 7 days at room temperature or 14 days when refrigerated; incompatible with heparin; physically compatible with ondansetron for at least 4 hours
(Continued)

Mitoxantrone *(Continued)*

Mechanism of Action Inhibits DNA and RNA synthesis by intercalating with DNA and causing template disordering and steric obstruction; replication is decreased by binding to DNA topoisomerase II (enzyme responsible for DNA helix supercoiling); active throughout entire cell cycle

Pharmacokinetics

Distribution: Distributes into thyroid, liver, pancreas, spleen, heart, bone marrow, and red blood cells; prolonged retention in tissues; excreted in breast milk

Protein binding: 78%

Half-life, terminal: 23-215 hours and may be prolonged with liver impairment

Elimination: Slowly excreted in urine (6% to 11%) and bile as unchanged drug and metabolites

Usual Dosage I.V. (refer to individual protocols):

Leukemias:

Children ≤2 years: 0.4 mg/kg/day once daily for 3-5 days

Children >2 years and Adults: 12 mg/m^2/day once daily for 2-3 days; acute leukemia in relapse: 8-12 mg/m^2/day once daily for 4-5 days; ANLL: 10 mg/m^2/day once daily for 3-5 days

Solid tumors:

Children: 18-20 mg/m^2 once every 3-4 weeks

Adults: 12-14 mg/m^2 once every 3-4 weeks

Dosing adjustment in hepatic impairment: Although official dosage adjustment recommendations have not been established, dosage reduction of 50% in patients with serum bilirubin of 1.5-3 mg/dL and dosage reduction of 75% in patients with serum bilirubin >3 mg/dL have been recommended

Administration Parenteral: I.V.: Do **not** administer I.V. bolus over <3 minutes; may administer by I.V. bolus over >3 minutes, I.V. intermittent infusion over 15-60 minutes or I.V. continuous infusion at a concentration of 0.02-0.5 mg/mL in D$_5$W or NS

Monitoring Parameters CBC with differential, serum uric acid, liver function tests, echocardiogram

Patient Information May discolor skin, sclera, tears, sweat, and urine to a blue-green color

Nursing Implications Mitoxantrone is a nonvesicant; if extravasation occurs, the drug should be discontinued and restarted in another vein; extravasation may result in erythema, swelling, pain, burning, and/or a blue discoloration of the skin

Additional Information Myelosuppression (leukocyte nadir: 10-14 days; recovery: 21 days); injection contains 0.14 mEq of sodium/mL

Dosage Forms Injection, as hydrochloride: 2 mg of mitoxantrone base/mL (10 mL, 12.5 mL, 15 mL)

References

Koeller J and Eble M, "Mitoxantrone: A Novel Anthracycline Derivative," *Clin Pharm*, 1988, 7(8):574-81.

LeMaistre CF and Herzig R, "Mitoxantrone: Potential for Use in Intensive Therapy," *Semin Oncol*, 1990, 17(1 Suppl 3):43-8.

Pratt CB, Vietti TJ, Etcubanas E, et al, "Novantrone® for Childhood Malignant Solid Tumors. A Pediatric Oncology Group Phase II Study," *Invest New Drugs*, 1986, 4(1):43-8.

Stevens RF, Hann IM, Wheatley K, et al, "Marked Improvements in Outcome With Chemotherapy Alone in Paediatric Acute Myeloid Leukemia: Results of the United Kingdom Medical Research Council's 10th AML Trial. MRC Childhood Leukaemia Working Party," *Br J Haematol*, 1998, 101(1):130-40.

♦ **Mitoxantrone Hydrochloride** *see Mitoxantrone on page 653*

♦ **Mivacron®** *see Mivacurium on page 654*

♦ **Mivacron® (Canada)** *see Mivacurium on page 654*

Mivacurium *(mye va KYOO ree um)*

Brand Names Mivacron®; Mivacron® (Canada)

Available Salts Mivacurium Chloride

Therapeutic Category Neuromuscular Blocker Agent, Nondepolarizing; Skeletal Muscle Relaxant, Paralytic

Generic Available No

Use Short-acting nondepolarizing neuromuscular blocking agent; an adjunct to general anesthesia; facilitates endotracheal intubation; provides skeletal muscle relaxation during surgery or mechanical ventilation

Pregnancy Risk Factor C

Contraindications Hypersensitivity to mivacurium chloride, any component, or other benzylisoquinolinium agents

Warnings Avoid use of multidose vials in neonates as contains benzyl alcohol

Precautions Use cautiously in patients with reduced plasma cholinesterase activity, asthma, severe cardiovascular disease

Adverse Reactions

Cardiovascular: Hypotension, bradycardia, tachycardia, flushing, cardiac arrhythmias

Central nervous system: Dizziness

Dermatologic: Cutaneous erythema, rash

Neuromuscular & skeletal: Muscle spasms

Local: Injection site reaction

Respiratory: Bronchospasm, wheezing

Miscellaneous: Endogenous histamine release

Drug Interactions See table.

Potential Drug Interactions

Potentiation	Antagonism
Anesthetics	Calcium
Desflurane, sevoflurane, enflurane and isoflurane > halothane > nitrous oxide	Carbamazepine
	Phenytoin
	Steroids (chronic administration)
Antibiotics	Theophylline
Aminoglycosides, polymyxins, clindamycin, vancomycin	Anticholinesterases*
Magnesium sulfate	Neostigmine, pyridostigmine, edrophonium, echothiophate
Antiarrhythmics	ophthalmic solution
Quinidine, procainamide, bretylium, and possibly lidocaine	Caffeine
Diuretics	Azathioprine
Furosemide, mannitol	
Amphotericin B (secondary to hypokalemia)	
Local anesthetics	
Dantrolene (directly depresses skeletal muscle)	
Beta blockers	
Calcium channel blockers	
Ketamine	
Lithium	
Succinylcholine (when administered prior to nondepolarizing neuromuscular-blocking agent)	
Cyclosporine	

*Can prolong the effects of acetylcholine

Stability Store at room temperature; stable in D_5W, D_5/LR, NS for 24 hours; avoid exposure to direct ultraviolet light; incompatible with alkaline solutions; compatible with Y-site administration with sufentanil, fentanyl, alfentanil, midazolam, droperidol

Mechanism of Action Mivacurium is a short-acting, nondepolarizing, neuromuscular-blocking agent. Like other nondepolarizing drugs, mivacurium antagonizes acetylcholine by competitively binding to cholinergic sites on motor endplates in skeletal muscle.

Pharmacodynamics

Peak neuromuscular blockade effect: I.V.: Within 2-3 minutes

Duration of action: Short due to rapid hydrolysis by plasma cholinesterases; recovery from muscular paralysis occurs within 15-30 minutes

Pharmacokinetics Mivacurium exists as a mixture of isomers; the most potent are the trans-trans and cis-trans isomers

Distribution: V_d: Trans-trans isomer: 0.15 L/kg; cis-trans isomer: 0.27 L/kg

Metabolism: Enzymatic hydrolysis by plasma cholinesterase

Half-life: Trans-trans isomer: 2.3 minutes (range: 1.4-3.6); cis-trans isomer: 2.1 minutes (range: 0.8-4.8)

Clearance: Trans-trans isomer: 53 mL/minute/kg; cis-trans isomer: 99 mL/minute/kg

Usual Dosage Children require higher doses mg/kg than adults and more frequent maintenance doses; I.V.:

Children 2-12 years: 0.2 mg/kg; continuous infusion: 10-14 mcg/kg/minute; doses
(Continued)

Mivacurium *(Continued)*

as high as 31 mcg/kg/minute have been used
Adults: 0.15-0.2 mg/kg; for prolonged neuromuscular block, continuous infusion: 9-10 mcg/kg/minute

Administration Parenteral: Administer undiluted by rapid I.V. injection; infusions diluted in D_5W to a maximum concentration of 0.5 mg/mL

Monitoring Parameters Assisted ventilation status, heart rate, blood pressure, peripheral nerve stimulator measuring twitch response

Nursing Implications Does not alter the patient's state of consciousness; addition of sedation is recommended

Dosage Forms
Infusion, as chloride, in D_5W: 0.5 mg/mL (50 mL, 100 mL)
Injection, as chloride:
Preservative free: 2 mg/mL (5 mL, 10 mL)
With benzyl alcohol: 2 mg/mL (20 mL, 50 mL)

+ **Mivacurium Chloride** *see* Mivacurium *on page 654*
+ **MK-639** *see* Indinavir *on page 514*
+ **Modane® Bulk [OTC]** *see* Psyllium *on page 823*
+ **Modane® Soft [OTC]** *see* Docusate *on page 336*
+ **Mol-Iron® [OTC]** *see* Iron Supplements, Oral/Enteral *on page 530*
+ **Mollifene® Ear Wax Removing Formula [OTC]** *see* Carbamide Peroxide *on page 167*
+ **Molypen®** *see* Trace Metals *on page 940*
+ **MOM (Magnesium Hydroxide)** *see* Magnesium Supplements *on page 588*
+ **Monafed®** *see* Guaifenesin *on page 464*
+ **Monistat-Derm™ Topical** *see* Miconazole *on page 641*
+ **Monistat i.v.™ Injection** *see* Miconazole *on page 641*
+ **Monistat™ Vaginal** *see* Miconazole *on page 641*
+ **Monoclate-P®** *see* Antihemophilic Factor (Human) *on page 89*
+ **Monoclonal Antibody** *see* Muromonab-CD3 *on page 661*
+ **Monodox®** *see* Doxycycline *on page 348*

Montelukast *(mon te LOO kast)*

Related Information
Asthma Guidelines *on page 1178*

Brand Names Singulair®

Available Salts Montelukast Sodium

Therapeutic Category Antiasthmatic; Leukotriene Receptor Antagonist

Generic Available No

Use Prophylaxis and chronic treatment of asthma

Pregnancy Risk Factor B

Contraindications Hypersensitivity to montelukast or any component

Warnings Montelukast is not indicated for use in the reversal of bronchospasm in acute asthma attacks, including status asthmaticus; it is not indicated as monotherapy for the treatment and management of exercise-induced bronchospasm; therapy with montelukast can be continued during acute exacerbations of asthma; chewable tablet contains phenylalanine and should be avoided in patients with phenylketonuria

Precautions Phenobarbital reduces the AUC of montelukast ~40% following a single 10 mg dosage; no dosage adjustment of montelukast is indicated, however, appropriate clinical monitoring is indicated when potent cytochrome P-450 enzyme inducers, such as phenobarbital or rifampin, are coadministered with montelukast

Adverse Reactions
Central nervous system: Headache, fever, dizziness, drowsiness, irritability, restlessness, dream abnormalities
Dermatologic: Rash
Gastrointestinal: Diarrhea, nausea, abdominal pain, dyspepsia
Hepatic: Elevated liver enzymes, hepatic eosinophilic infiltration
Otic: Otitis
Respiratory: Sinusitis, laryngitis, nasal congestion, cough
Miscellaneous: Viral infection, influenza, hypersensitivity reactions

Drug Interactions Phenobarbital (see Precautions)

Stability Store at room temperature; protect from light

Mechanism of Action Montelukast is a selective leukotriene receptor antagonist that inhibits the cysteinyl leukotriene CysLT₁ receptor. This activity produces inhibition of the effects of this leukotriene on bronchial smooth muscle resulting in the attenuation of bronchoconstriction and decreased vascular permeability, mucosal edema, and mucus production.

Pharmacokinetics
Absorption: Rapid
Distribution: V_d: Adults: 8-11 L
Protein binding: 99%
Metabolism: Extensive by cytochrome P-450 3A4 and 2C9
Bioavailability: Tablet:
5 mg: 73%
10 mg: 64%
Time to peak serum concentration: Tablet:
5 mg: 2-2.5 hours
10 mg: 3-4 hours
Elimination: Exclusively via bile; <0.2% excreted in urine

Usual Dosage Oral:
Children
2-5 years: 4 mg/day
6-14 years: 5 mg/day
Adolescents >14 years and Adults: 10 mg/day
Note: None of the clinical trials evaluated the safety and efficacy of therapy with morning dosing; the pharmacokinetics of montelukast are similar whether dosed in the morning or evening

Administration Oral: Administer in the evening without regard to time of meals

Monitoring Parameters Pulmonary function tests (FEV-1), improvement in asthma symptoms

Patient Information Take regularly as prescribed, even during symptom-free periods. Do not use to treat acute episodes of asthma. Do not decrease the dose or stop taking any other asthma medications unless instructed by a physician.

Dosage Forms
Tablet, as sodium: 10 mg
Tablet, chewable (cherry), as sodium: 4 mg, 5 mg

♦ **Montelukast Sodium** see Montelukast on page 656
♦ **More-Dophilus® [OTC]** see Lactobacillus acidophilus and Lactobacillus bulgaricus on page 550
♦ **Morphine-HP® (Canada)** see Morphine Sulfate on page 657

Morphine Sulfate (MOR feen SUL fate)

Related Information
Adult ACLS Algorithm, Electrical Conversion on page 1014
Adult ACLS Algorithm, Hypotension, Shock on page 1016
Compatibility of Medications Mixed in a Syringe on page 1208
Laboratory Detection of Drugs in Urine on page 1204
Narcotic Analgesics Comparison on page 1035
Overdose and Toxicology on page 1191
Preprocedure Sedatives in Children on page 1169

Brand Names Astramorph/PF™ Injection; Duramorph® Injection; Epimorph® (Canada); Infumorph® Injection; Kadian® Capsule; M-Eslon® (Canada); Morphine-HP® (Canada); MS Contin® Oral; MS-IR® (Canada); MSIR® Oral; OMS® Oral; Oramorph SR® Oral; RMS® Rectal; Roxanol™ Oral; Roxanol SR™ Oral; Statex® (Canada)

Synonyms MS

Therapeutic Category Analgesic, Narcotic

Generic Available Yes

Use Relief of moderate to severe acute and chronic pain; pain of MI; relieves dyspnea of acute left ventricular failure and pulmonary edema; preanesthetic medication

Restrictions C-II

Pregnancy Risk Factor B (D if used for prolonged periods or in high doses at term)

Contraindications Hypersensitivity to morphine sulfate or any component; increased intracranial pressure; severe respiratory depression; severe liver or renal insufficiency
(Continued)

Morphine Sulfate *(Continued)*

Warnings Some preparations contain sulfites which may cause allergic reactions; neonates and infants <3 months of age are more susceptible to respiratory depression, use with caution and in reduced doses in this age group; use only preservative free injections for epidural or intrathecal administration and in neonates

Precautions Use with caution in patients with hypersensitivity reactions to other phenanthrene derivative opioid agonists (codeine, hydrocodone, hydromorphone, levorphanol, oxycodone, oxymorphone)

Adverse Reactions

Cardiovascular: Palpitations, hypotension, bradycardia, peripheral vasodilation

Central nervous system: CNS depression, drowsiness, dizziness, sedation, increased intracranial pressure

Dermatologic: Pruritus (more common with epidural or intrathecal administration)

Endocrine & metabolic: Antidiuretic hormone release

Gastrointestinal: Nausea, vomiting, constipation, biliary tract spasm

Genitourinary: Urinary tract spasm (may be more common with epidural or intrathecal administration), urinary retention

Ocular: Miosis

Respiratory: Respiratory depression

Miscellaneous: Physical and psychological dependence, histamine release

Drug Interactions Cytochrome P-450 isoenzyme CYP2D6 substrate

CNS depressants, alcohol, phenothiazines, tricyclic antidepressants may potentiate the adverse effects of morphine

Food Interactions Food may increase bioavailability of oral morphine solution

Stability Refrigerate suppositories; do not freeze; degradation depends on pH and presence of oxygen; relatively stable in pH ≤4; darkening of solutions indicate degradation

Mechanism of Action Binds to opiate receptors in the CNS, causing inhibition of ascending pain pathways, altering the perception of and response to pain; produces generalized CNS depression

Pharmacodynamics See table.

Dosage Form/Route	Analgesia	
	Peak	Duration
Tablets	1 h	3-5 h
Oral solution	1 h	3-5 h
Epidural	1 h	12-20 h
Extended release tablets	3-4 h	8-12 h
Suppository	20-60 min	3-7 h
Subcutaneous injection	50-90 min	3-5 h
I.M. injection	30-60 min	3-5 h
I.V. injection	20 min	3-5 h

Pharmacokinetics

Absorption: Oral: Variable

Protein binding:

Premature Infants: <20%

Adults: ~35%

Metabolism: In the liver via glucuronide conjugation to morphine-6-glucuronide (active) and morphine-3-glucuronide (inactive)

Half-life:

Preterm: 10-20 hours

Neonates: 4.5-13.3 hours (mean: 7.6 hours)

Infants 1-3 months: 6.2 hours (range: 5-10 hours)

Children 6 months to 2.5 years: 2.9 hours (range: 1.4-7.8 hours)

Preschool Children: 1-2 hours

Children 6-19 years with sickle cell disease: Mean ~1.3 hours

Adults: 2-4 hours

Elimination: Excreted unchanged in urine

Neonates: 3% to 15%

Adults: 6% to 10%

Clearance:

Preterm: 0.5-3 mL/minute/kg

Neonates: 5 mL/minute/kg

Children 6 months to 2.5 years: 22 mL/minute/kg
Preschool Children: 20-40 mL/minute/kg
Children 6-19 years with sickle cell disease: Mean ~36 mL/minute/kg (range: 6-59 mL/minute/kg)
Adults: 10-20 mL/minute/kg

Usual Dosage Doses should be titrated to appropriate effect; when changing routes of administration in chronically treated patients, please note that oral doses are approximately one-half as effective as parenteral dose

Neonates (see Warnings; use preservative free formulation):
I.M., I.V., S.C.: Initial: 0.05 mg/kg every 4-8 hours; titrate carefully to effect; maximum dose: 0.1 mg/kg/dose
I.V. continuous infusion: Initial: 0.01 mg/kg/hour (10 mcg/kg/hour); do **not** exceed infusion rates of 0.015-0.02 mg/kg/hour due to decreased elimination, increased CNS sensitivity, and adverse effects

Infants and Children:
Oral: Tablet and solution (prompt release): 0.2-0.5 mg/kg/dose every 4-6 hours as needed; tablet (controlled release): 0.3-0.6 mg/kg/dose every 12 hours
I.M., I.V., S.C.: 0.1-0.2 mg/kg/dose every 2-4 hours as needed; may initiate at 0.05 mg/kg/dose; usual maximum dose: 15 mg/dose
I.V., S.C. continuous infusion:
Sickle cell or cancer pain: Range: 0.025-2.6 mg/kg/hour (median dose, cancer pain: 0.04-0.07 mg/kg/hour)
Postoperative pain: 0.01-0.04 mg/kg/hour
Sedation/analgesia for procedures: I.V.: 0.05-0.1 mg/kg 5 minutes before the procedure
Epidural (use preservative free): 0.03-0.05 mg/kg (30-50 mcg/kg); maximum dose: 0.1 mg/kg (100 mcg/kg) or 5 mg/24 hours

Adolescents >12 years: Sedation/analgesia for procedures: I.V.: 3-4 mg; may repeat in 5 minutes if necessary

Adults:
Oral: Prompt release: 10-30 mg every 4 hours as needed; controlled release: 15-30 mg every 8-12 hours
I.M., I.V., S.C.: 2.5-20 mg/dose every 2-6 hours as needed; usual: 10 mg/dose every 4 hours as needed
I.V., S.C. continuous infusion: 0.8-10 mg/hour; may increase depending on pain relief/adverse effects; usual range up to 80 mg/hour
Epidural (use preservative free): Initial: 5 mg in lumbar region; if inadequate pain relief within 1 hour, give 1-2 mg, maximum dose: 10 mg/24 hours
Intrathecal ($^{1}/_{10}$ of epidural dose, use preservative free): 0.2-1 mg/dose; repeat doses **not** recommended

Dosing adjustment in renal impairment: Children and Adults:
Cl_{cr} 10-50 mL/minute: Administer 75% of normal dose
Cl_{cr} <10 mL/minute: Administer 50% of normal dose

Administration
Oral: Administer with food; swallow extended release products whole, do not chew or crush
Parenteral:
I.V. push: Administer over at least 5 minutes at a final concentration of 0.5-5 mg/mL (rapid I.V. administration may increase adverse effects)
Intermittent infusion: Administer over 15-30 minutes
Continuous I.V. infusion: 0.1-1 mg/mL in D_5W
Epidural and intrathecal: Use only preservative free injections

Monitoring Parameters Respiratory and cardiovascular status, oxygen saturation, pain relief (if used for analgesia), level of sedation

Patient Information Avoid alcohol; may cause drowsiness and impair ability to perform hazardous duties requiring mental alertness or physical coordination

Nursing Implications Do not administer rapidly I.V.

Additional Information Less adverse effects are associated with epidural compared to intrathecal route of administration; equianalgesic doses: Codeine: 120 mg I.M. = morphine 10 mg I.M. = single dose oral morphine 60 mg **or** chronic dosing oral morphine 15-25 mg

Dosage Forms
Capsule, sustained release (Kadian®): 20 mg, 50 mg, 100 mg
Epidural or intrathecal infusion preparation (for administration via microinfusion device), preservative free (Infumorph®): 10 mg/mL (20 mL); 25 mg/mL (20 mL)
Injection: 0.5 mg/mL (10 mL); 1 mg/mL (10 mL, 30 mL, 60 mL); 2 mg/mL (1 mL, 2 mL, 60 mL); 3 mg/mL (50 mL); 4 mg/mL (1 mL, 2 mL); 5 mg/mL (1 mL, 30 mL); 8
(Continued)

Morphine Sulfate *(Continued)*

mg/mL (1 mL, 2 mL); 10 mg/mL (1 mL, 2 mL, 10 mL); 15 mg/mL (1 mL, 2 mL, 20 mL)

Injection, preservative free:

Astramorph/PF™, 0.5 mg/mL (2 mL, 10 mL); 1 mg/mL (2 mL, 10 mL)

Duramorph®: 0.5 mg/mL (10 mL); 1 mg/mL (10 mL)

I.V. via PCA pump: 1 mg/mL (10 mL, 30 mL, 60 mL); 5 mg/mL (30 mL)

I.V. infusion preparation: 25 mg/mL (4 mL, 10 mL, 20 mL)

Solution, oral: 10 mg/5 mL (5 mL, 10 mL, 100 mL, 120 mL, 500 mL); 20 mg/5 mL (5 mL, 100 mL, 120 mL, 500 mL); 20 mg/mL (30 mL)

Suppository, rectal: 5 mg, 10 mg, 20 mg, 30 mg

Tablet: 15 mg, 30 mg

Tablet:

Controlled release: 15 mg, 30 mg, 60 mg, 100 mg, 200 mg

Soluble: 10 mg, 15 mg, 30 mg

Sustained release: 30 mg, 60 mg, 100 mg

References

Berde C, Ablin A, Glazer J, et al, "American Academy of Pediatrics Report of the Subcommittee on Disease-Related Pain in Childhood Cancer," *Pediatrics*, 1990, 86(5 Pt 2):818-25.

Dampier CD, Setty BN, Logan J, et al, "Intravenous Morphine Pharmacokinetics in Pediatric Patients With Sickle Cell Disease," *J Pediatr*, 1995, 126(3):461-7.

Henneberg SW, Hole P, Madsen de Haas I, et al, "Epidural Morphine for Postoperative Pain Relief in Children," *Acta Anaesthesiol Scand*, 1993, 37(7):664-7.

McRorie TI, Lynn AM, Nespeca MK, et al, "The Maturation of Morphine Clearance and Metabolism," *Am J Dis Child*, 1992, 147(8):972-6.

Olkkola KT, Hamunen K, and Maunuksela EL, "Clinical Pharmacokinetics and Pharmacodynamics of Opioid Analgesics in Infants and Children," *Clin Pharmacokinet*, 1995, 28(5):385-404.

- **Motrin®** *see* Ibuprofen *on page 501*
- **Motrin® IB [OTC]** *see* Ibuprofen *on page 501*
- **Motrin® Migraine Pain** *see* Ibuprofen *on page 501*
- **4-MP** *see* Fomepizole *on page 440*
- **6-MP** *see* Mercaptopurine *on page 606*
- **M-Prednisol® Injection** *see* Methylprednisolone *on page 629*
- **MS** *see* Morphine Sulfate *on page 657*
- **MS Contin® Oral** *see* Morphine Sulfate *on page 657*
- **MSD® Enteric Coated ASA (Canada)** *see* Aspirin *on page 99*
- **MS-IR® (Canada)** *see* Morphine Sulfate *on page 657*
- **MSIR® Oral** *see* Morphine Sulfate *on page 657*
- **MTC** *see* Mitomycin *on page 652*
- **M.T.E.-4®** *see* Trace Metals *on page 940*
- **M.T.E.-5®** *see* Trace Metals *on page 940*
- **M.T.E.-6®** *see* Trace Metals *on page 940*
- **MTX** *see* Methotrexate *on page 621*
- **Muco-Fen-DM®** *see* Guaifenesin and Dextromethorphan *on page 466*
- **Muco-Fen-LA®** *see* Guaifenesin *on page 464*
- **Mucomyst®** *see* Acetylcysteine *on page 32*
- **Mucosil™** *see* Acetylcysteine *on page 32*
- **Multe-Pak-4®** *see* Trace Metals *on page 940*
- **Multipax® (Canada)** *see* Hydroxyzine *on page 496*
- **Multiple Trace Metals** *see* Trace Metals *on page 940*
- **Multiple Vitamin Products** *see page 1034*
- **Mumps Virus Vaccine, Live, Attenuated** *see page 1138*

Mupirocin *(myoo PEER oh sin)*

Brand Names Bactroban®

Synonyms Pseudomonic Acid A

Therapeutic Category Antibiotic, Topical

Generic Available No

Use Topical treatment of impetigo caused by *Staphylococcus aureus* and *Streptococcus pyogenes*; also effective for the topical treatment of folliculitis, furunculosis, minor wounds, burns, and ulcers caused by susceptible organisms; used as a prophylactic agent applied to intravenous catheter exit sites; used for eradication of *S. aureus* from nasal and perineal carriage sites

Pregnancy Risk Factor B

Contraindications Hypersensitivity to mupirocin, polyethylene glycol, or any component

Warnings Potentially toxic amounts of polyethylene glycol (PEG) contained in the vehicle may be absorbed percutaneously in patients with extensive burns or open wounds; the PEG vehicle may irritate mucous membranes and increase nasal secretions if applied intranasally; prolonged use may result in overgrowth of nonsusceptible organisms

Precautions Use with caution in patients with impaired renal function and in burn patients

Adverse Reactions
Dermatologic: Pruritus, rash, erythema, dry skin
Local: Burning, stinging, pain, tenderness, local edema

Stability Do not mix with Aquaphor®, coal tar solution, or salicylic acid

Mechanism of Action Binds to bacterial isoleucyl transfer-RNA synthetase preventing isoleucine incorporation resulting in the inhibition of protein and RNA synthesis

Pharmacokinetics
Absorption: Following topical administration, penetrates the outer layers of the skin; systemic absorption is minimal through intact skin
Protein binding: 95%
Metabolism: Extensive in the liver and skin to monic acid
Half-life: 17-36 minutes
Elimination: Metabolite is excreted in urine

Usual Dosage Children and Adults:
Intranasal (eliminate nasal carriage of *S. aureus*): Apply small amount 2-4 times/day for 5-14 days
Topical: Apply small amount 3-5 times/day for 5-14 days

Administration For topical use only; do not apply into the eye

Additional Information Contains polyethylene glycol vehicle

Dosage Forms Ointment, topical: 2% (15 g)

References
Blumer JL, Lemon E, O'Horo J, et al, "Changing Therapy for Skin and Soft Tissue Infections in Children: Have We Come Full Circle?" *Pediatr Infect Dis J*, 1987, 6(1):117-22.
Britton JW, Fajardo JE, and Krafte-Jacobs B, "Comparison of Mupirocin and Erythromycin in the Treatment of Impetigo," *J Pediatr*, 1990, 117(5):827-9.
Goldfarb J, Crenshaw D, O'Horo J, et al, "Randomized Clinical Trial of Topical Mupirocin Versus Oral Erythromycin for Impetigo," *Antimicrob Agents Chemother*, 1988, 32(12):1780-3.

♦ **Murine® Ear Drops [OTC]** *see* Carbamide Peroxide *on page 167*

♦ **Muro-128™ (Canada)** *see* Sodium Chloride *on page 871*

♦ **Muro 128® Ophthalmic [OTC]** *see* Sodium Chloride *on page 871*

Muromonab-CD3 (myoo roe MOE nab see dee three)

Brand Names Orthoclone OKT®3

Synonyms Monoclonal Antibody; OKT3

Therapeutic Category Immunosuppressant Agent

Generic Available No

Use Treatment of acute allograft rejection in renal transplant patients; effective in reversing acute hepatic, cardiac, and bone marrow transplant rejection episodes resistant to conventional treatment

Pregnancy Risk Factor C

Contraindications Hypersensitivity to OKT3 or any Murine® product; patients in fluid overload or those with >3% weight gain within 1 week prior to start of OKT3

Warnings May result in an increased susceptibility to infection; severe pulmonary edema has occurred in patients with fluid overload; first-dose effect (flu-like symptoms, anaphylactic-type reaction) may occur within 30 minutes to 6 hours, up to 24 hours after the first dose. Cardiopulmonary resuscitation may be needed. Methylprednisolone sodium succinate given prior to first OKT3 dose and I.V. hydrocortisone sodium succinate given 30 minutes after administration are strongly recommended to decrease the incidence of reactions to the first dose.

Precautions Dosage of concomitant immunosuppressants should be reduced by 50%, and cyclosporine discontinued or decreased by 50% during OKT3 therapy (see Additional Information); maintenance immunosuppression and cyclosporine should be resumed about 3 days before stopping OKT3 to protect against rebound rejection

Adverse Reactions
Cardiovascular: Tachycardia, hypertension, hypotension, perioral and peripheral cyanosis
Central nervous system: Aseptic meningitis, seizures, headache, pyrexia, confusion
Dermatologic: Pruritus, rash
(Continued)

Muromonab-CD3 *(Continued)*

Gastrointestinal: Diarrhea, nausea, vomiting

Neuromuscular & skeletal: Arthralgia, tremor, myalgia

Ocular: Photophobia

Renal: Elevated BUN, elevated serum creatinine

Respiratory: Dyspnea, chest pain, tightness, wheezing, pulmonary edema

Miscellaneous: Flu-like symptoms (ie, fever, chills), anaphylactic-type reactions

Stability Store in refrigerator; do not freeze or shake; OKT3 left out of the refrigerator for more than 4 hours must not be used

Mechanism of Action Coats the circulating T lymphocytes subjecting these cells to opsonization by the reticuloendothelial system; modulates the T lymphocyte antigen receptor CD3 complex which results in the removal of all CD3 molecules from the cell surface so that the cell lacks the ability to function as a T lymphocyte

Pharmacodynamics

Distribution: V_d is closely related to the apparent volume of distribution for albumin

Half-life: 18 hours

Elimination: Binds to T lymphocytes with resultant opsonization and removal by the reticuloendothelial system

Usual Dosage I.V. (refer to individual protocols):

Note: Children and Adults: Methylprednisolone sodium succinate 1 mg/kg I.V. given 2-6 hours prior to first OKT3 administration and I.V. hydrocortisone sodium succinate 50-100 mg given 30 minutes after administration are strongly recommended to decrease the incidence of reactions to the first dose; patient temperature should not exceed 37.8°C (100°F) at time of administration

Children <12 years: 0.1 mg/kg/day once daily for 10-14 days **or** patients ≤30 kg: 2.5 mg once daily for 10-14 days; patients >30 kg: 5 mg once daily for 10-14 days

Children ≥12 years and Adults: 5 mg/day once daily for 10-14 days

Administration Parenteral: Filter each dose through a low protein-binding 0.22 micron filter (Millex GV) before administration; administer I.V. push over 1 minute at a final concentration of 1 mg/mL

Monitoring Parameters Chest x-ray, weight gain, CBC with differential, vital signs (blood pressure, temperature, pulse, respiration) and immunologic monitoring of T cells, serum levels of OKT3, CD3+ cell count

Reference Range Mean serum trough levels rise during the first 3 days, then average 0.9 µg/mL on days 3-14; if serum trough OKT3 concentrations are maintained at 1 µg/mL, then CD3 counts remain low

Nursing Implications Inform patient of expected first dose effects which may include fever, chills, chest tightness, wheezing, nausea, vomiting, and diarrhea; first-dose reaction usually starts 40-60 minutes after the injection and lasts for several hours; first-dose effects are markedly reduced with subsequent doses; monitor patient closely for 48 hours after the first dose; corticosteroids are recommended; acetaminophen and antihistamines can be given concomitantly with OKT3 to reduce early reactions

Additional Information Recommend decreasing dose of prednisone to 0.5 mg/kg, azathioprine to 0.5 mg/kg (approximate 50% decrease in dose), and discontinuing cyclosporine or decreasing cyclosporine dose by 50% while patient is receiving OKT3

Dosage Forms Injection: 5 mg/5 mL

References

Ettenger RB, Marik JL, Rosenthal JT, et al, "OKT3 for Rejection Reversal in Pediatric Renal Transplantation," *Clin Transpl,* 1988, 2:180-4.

Hooks MA, Wade CS, and Millikan WJ Jr, "Muromonab CD-3: A Review of Its Pharmacology, Pharmacokinetics, and Clinical Use in Transplantation," *Pharmacotherapy,* 1991, 11(1):26-37.

Niaudet P, Murcia I, Jean G, et al, "A Comparative Trial of OKT3 and Antilymphocyte Serum in the Preventive Treatment of Rejection After Kidney Transplantation in Children," *Ann Pediatr Paris,* 1990, 37(2):83-5.

Todd PA and Brogden RN, "Muromonab CD3 A Review of Its Pharmacology and Therapeutic Potential," *Drugs,* 1989, 37(6):871-99.

♦ **Muroptic-5®** [OTC] *see* Sodium Chloride *on page 871*

♦ **Muse® Pellet** *see* Alprostadil *on page 51*

♦ **Mustargen® Hydrochloride** *see* Mechlorethamine *on page 595*

♦ **Mustine** *see* Mechlorethamine *on page 595*

♦ **Mutamycin®** *see* Mitomycin *on page 652*

♦ **Myambutol®** *see* Ethambutol *on page 391*

♦ **Myapap®** [OTC] *see* Acetaminophen *on page 26*

♦ **Mycelex®-G Topical** *see* Clotrimazole *on page 245*

♦ **Mycelex®-G Vaginal** [OTC] *see* Clotrimazole *on page 245*

- **Mycelex® Troche** *see Clotrimazole on page 245*
- **Mycifradin® Sulfate** *see Neomycin on page 677*
- **Myciguent® (Canada)** *see Neomycin on page 677*
- **Mycinettes® [OTC]** *see Benzocaine on page 124*
- **Mycitracin® Topical [OTC]** *see Neomycin, Polymyxin B, and Bacitracin on page 680*
- **Myclo-Derm® (Canada)** *see Clotrimazole on page 245*
- **Myclo-Gyne® (Canada)** *see Clotrimazole on page 245*
- **Mycobutin®** *see Rifabutin on page 845*

Mycophenolate (mye koe FEN oh late)

Brand Names CellCept®
Available Salts Mycophenolate Mofetil; Mycophenolate Mofetil Hydrochloride
Synonyms RS61443
Therapeutic Category Immunosuppressant Agent
Generic Available No
Use Immunosuppressant agent used in conjunction with other immunosuppressive therapies (eg, cyclosporine and corticosteroids with or without antithymocyte induction) for the prophylaxis of organ rejection in patients receiving allogeneic renal transplants or allogeneic cardiac transplants; add-on immunosuppressant agent that is typically used in place of azathioprine in combination regimens for the treatment of refractory acute kidney graft rejection. The use of mycophenolate is also being studied in liver and bone marrow transplant patients.
Pregnancy Risk Factor C
Contraindications Hypersensitivity to mycophenolate mofetil, mycophenolic acid, polysorbate 80 (I.V. formulation), or any component
Warnings Immunosuppression with mycophenolate may result in an increased susceptibility to infection and an increased risk of developing lymphomas and other malignancies, particularly of the skin. Mycophenolate has been shown to have teratogenic effects in animals; in women of childbearing potential, effective contraception must be initiated before starting mycophenolate therapy and continued for 6 weeks after it has been discontinued.
Precautions Use with caution in patients with active serious digestive disease and in patients with renal impairment; modify dosage in patients with severe chronic renal impairment (GFR <25 mL/minute/1.73 m² outside of the immediate post-transplant period) and in patients with neutropenia
Adverse Reactions
Cardiovascular: Hypertension
Central nervous system: Insomnia, dizziness, fever, headache
Dermatologic: Rash, acne
Endocrine & metabolic: Hypercholesteremia, hypophosphatemia, hypokalemia, hyperkalemia, hyperglycemia
Gastrointestinal: Diarrhea, constipation, nausea, vomiting, oral moniliasis, dyspepsia, GI tract hemorrhage
Hematologic: Leukopenia, neutropenia, anemia, thrombocytopenia
Local: Phlebitis, thrombosis
Neuromuscular & skeletal: Tremor, back pain, myalgia
Renal: Renal tubular necrosis, hematuria
Respiratory: Dyspnea, cough, pharyngitis
Miscellaneous: 1% incidence of lymphoproliferative disease
Drug Interactions Aluminum- and magnesium-containing antacids decrease mycophenolate absorption; cholestyramine decreases mycophenolate bioavailability by 40% (interrupts enterohepatic recirculation of mycophenolic acid); acyclovir and ganciclovir may compete with mycophenolic acid glucuronide (MPAG) for renal tubular secretion resulting in increased concentrations of both drugs; drugs which inhibit renal tubular secretion (probenecid) increase mycophenolate and MPAG concentrations
Food Interactions Presence of food decreases mycophenolate peak concentration by 40%
Stability Store at room temperature
Mechanism of Action Hydrolyzed to form mycophenolic acid (MPA), the active metabolite, which is a potent, noncompetitive reversible inhibitor of inosine monophosphate dehydrogenase (IMPDH) in the purine biosynthesis pathway; inhibition of IMPDH results in a depletion of guanosine triphosphate and deoxyguanosine triphosphate, thereby inhibiting T- and B-cell proliferation, cytotoxic T-cell generation and antibody secretion.
(Continued)

Mycophenolate *(Continued)*

Pharmacokinetics

Absorption: Rapid and extensive

Distribution: Mean V_d (adults): 4 L/kg

Protein binding:
Mycophenolate: 97%
Mycophenolate glucuronide: 82%

Metabolism: Mycophenolate mofetil undergoes hydrolysis to mycophenolic acid (MPA is the active metabolite); MPA is metabolized to mycophenolic acid glucuronide (MPAG is inactive)

Bioavailability: 94% based on MPA; enterohepatic recirculation contributes to MPA concentration

Half-life: 17.9 hours

Time to peak serum concentration: 0.8-1.3 hours

Elimination: 93% of dose recovered in urine, 6% in feces; 87% of dose recovered as MPAG in urine; <1% of dose excreted as MPA in urine

Usual Dosage

Oral:

Children: 600 mg/m²/dose twice daily. **Note:** Limited information regarding mycophenolate use in pediatric patients is currently available in the literature: 32 pediatric patients (14 underwent living donor and 18 receiving cadaveric donor renal transplants) received mycophenolate 8-30 mg/kg/dose orally twice daily with cyclosporine, prednisone, and Atgam® induction. However, pharmacokinetic studies suggest that doses of mycophenolate adjusted to body surface area resulted in AUCs which better approximated those of adults versus doses adjusted for body weight which resulted in lower AUCs in pediatric patients.

Adults: 2000 mg/day divided twice daily in combination with corticosteroids and cyclosporine; dosages as high as 3-3.5 g/day were used in clinical trials, but no efficacy advantage could be established with the higher doses.

I.V. infusion (administer within 24 hours following transplantation; can be given for up to 14 days; patients should be switched to oral formulation as soon as oral medication is tolerated):

Adults:

Renal transplant: 1 g twice daily

Cardiac transplant: 1.5 g twice daily

Administration

Oral: Administer on an empty stomach; one center has mixed the contents of the capsule in chocolate syrup

I.V.: Reconstitute and dilute to a final concentration of 6 mg/mL using D_5W. Administer by slow I.V. infusion over a period of no less than 2 hours. Administration of the infusion solution should be within 4 hours from reconstitution and dilution of the drug.

Monitoring Parameters CBC

Nursing Implications

Mycophenolate capsules should not be opened or crushed; avoid inhalation or direct contact of the capsule contents with skin or mucous membranes

Dosage Forms

Capsule, as mofetil: 250 mg

Powder for injection, as mofetil hydrochloride: 500 mg

Tablet, as mofetil: 500 mg

Extemporaneous Preparations

A 50 mg/mL suspension can be prepared in a vertical flow hood by emptying six 250 mg mycophenolate mofetil capsules into a mortar wetted and triturated with 7.5 mL Ora-Plus® to a smooth paste. Add 15 mL of cherry syrup and triturate to make a final volume of 30 mL. The suspension is stable for 210 days when stored at 5°C, stable for 28 days when stored at 37°C or 25°C, and stable for 11 days when stored at 45°C.

Venkataramanan R, McCombs JR, Zudarnan S, et al, "Stability of Mycophenolate Mofetil as an Extemporaneous Suspension," *Ann Pharmacother*, 1998, 32:755-7.

References

Ettenger R, Warshaw B, Menster M, et al, "Mycophenolate Mofetil in Pediatric Renal Transplantation: A Report of the Ped MMF Study Group." Abstract: 1996, Annual Meeting, ASTP.

Sollinger HW, "Mycophenolate Mofetil for the Prevention of Acute Rejection in Primary Cadaveric Renal Allograft Recipients. U.S. Renal Transplant Mycophenolate Mofetil Study Group," *Transplantation*, 1995, 60:225-32.

♦ **Mycophenolate Mofetil** *see* Mycophenolate *on page 663*

♦ **Mycophenolate Mofetil Hydrochloride** *see* Mycophenolate *on page 663*

- ♦ **Mycostatin**® *see* Nystatin *on page 701*
- ♦ **Mydfrin**® **Ophthalmic Solution** *see* Phenylephrine *on page 758*
- ♦ **Mydriacyl**® *see* Tropicamide *on page 959*
- ♦ **Mykrox**® *see* Metolazone *on page 632*
- ♦ **Mylanta**® **[OTC]** *see* Antacid Preparations *on page 86*
- ♦ **Mylanta Gas**® **[OTC]** *see* Simethicone *on page 868*
- ♦ **Mylanta**®-**II [OTC]** *see* Antacid Preparations *on page 86*
- ♦ **Mylanta**® **Soothing Antacids [OTC]** *see* Calcium Supplements *on page 157*
- ♦ **Myleran**® *see* Busulfan *on page 150*
- ♦ **Mylicon**® **[OTC]** *see* Simethicone *on page 868*
- ♦ **Myochrysine**® *see* Gold Sodium Thiomalate *on page 460*
- ♦ **Myotonachol**™ *see* Bethanechol *on page 132*
- ♦ **Myphetapp**® **[OTC]** *see* Brompheniramine and Phenylpropanolamine *on page 143*
- ♦ **Mysoline**® *see* Primidone *on page 796*
- ♦ **Mytussin**® **[OTC]** *see* Guaifenesin *on page 464*
- ♦ **Mytussin**® *see* Guaifenesin and Codeine *on page 465*
- ♦ **Mytussin**® **DM [OTC]** *see* Guaifenesin and Dextromethorphan *on page 466*
- ♦ *N*-**Acetylcysteine** *see* Acetylcysteine *on page 32*
- ♦ *N*-**Acetyl-L-Cysteine** *see* Acetylcysteine *on page 32*
- ♦ **N-Acetyl-P-Aminophenol** *see* Acetaminophen *on page 26*
- ♦ **NaCl** *see* Sodium Chloride *on page 871*

Nadolol (nay DOE lole)

Related Information
Adult ACLS Algorithm, Tachycardia *on page 1010*
Overdose and Toxicology *on page 1191*

Brand Names Apo®-Nadol (Canada); Corgard®; Syn-Nadolol® (Canada)

Therapeutic Category Antianginal Agent; Antiarrhythmic Agent, Class II; Antihypertensive Agent; Antimigraine Agent; Beta-Adrenergic Blocker

Generic Available Yes

Use Treatment of hypertension and angina pectoris; prophylaxis of migraine headaches

Pregnancy Risk Factor C

Contraindications Uncompensated CHF, cardiogenic shock, bradycardia or heart block, bronchial asthma, bronchospasms

Precautions Therapy should not be discontinued abruptly; reduce dosage gradually over a period of 1-2 weeks; increase dosing interval in patients with renal dysfunction; use with caution in patients with diabetes mellitus

Adverse Reactions
Cardiovascular: Persistent bradycardia, orthostatic hypotension, Raynaud's syndrome, CHF, edema
Central nervous system: Fatigue, dizziness
Dermatological: Rash
Gastrointestinal: GI discomfort
Respiratory: Bronchospasm

Drug Interactions Other hypotensive agents, diuretics and phenothiazines may increase hypotensive effects of nadolol; nadolol may enhance neuromuscular blocking agents and will antagonize beta-sympathomimetic drugs; other drug interactions similar to propranolol may occur

Food Interactions Avoid natural licorice (causes sodium and water retention and increases potassium loss)

Mechanism of Action Competitively blocks response to beta-adrenergic stimulation; nonselective beta-blocker

Pharmacodynamics Duration of effect: 24 hours

Pharmacokinetics
Absorption: Oral: 30% to 40%
Distribution: Concentration in human breast milk is 4.6 times higher than serum
Protein-binding: 28%
Half-life, elimination:
Increased half-life with decreased renal function
Infants 3-22 months (n=3): 3.2-4.3 hours
Children 10 years (n=1): 15.7 hours
Children ~15 years (n=1): 7.3 hours
Adults: 10-24 hours
Moderately dialyzable (20% to 50%)
(Continued)

Nadolol *(Continued)*

Usual Dosage Oral:

Children: Very limited information (ie, one study) regarding pediatric dosage currently available in literature: The study used oral nadolol to control supraventricular tachycardia (SVT) in 26 children 3 months to 15 years of age. SVT was well controlled in 23 out of 26 children; recommended initial dose: 0.5-1 mg/kg once daily; monitor carefully, gradually increase dose; median dose required: 1 mg/kg/day; maximum dose: 2.5 mg/kg/day.

Adults: Initial: 40 mg once daily; increase gradually; usual dosage: 40-80 mg/day; may need up to 240-320 mg/day; doses as high as 640 mg/day have been used

Dosage adjustment in adults with renal impairment:

Cl_{cr} 10-50 mL/minute: Administer 50% of normal dose

Cl_{cr} <10 mL/minute: Administer 25% of normal dose

Administration Oral: May administer without regard to meals

Monitoring Parameters Blood pressure, heart rate, fluid intake and output, weight

Patient Information Limit alcohol; do not abruptly discontinue; may mask symptoms of hypoglycemia, but sweating may still occur

Dosage Forms Tablet: 20 mg, 40 mg, 80 mg, 120 mg, 160 mg

References

Devlin RG and Duchin KL, "Nadolol in Human Serum and Breast Milk," *Br J Clin Pharmacol,* 1981, 12(3).393-6.

Mehta AV and Chidambaram B, "Efficacy and Safety of Intravenous and Oral Nadolol for Supraventricular Tachycardia in Children," *J Am Coll Cardiol,* 1992, 19(3):630-5.

Mehta AV and Chidambaram B, and Rice PJ, "Pharmacokinetics of Nadolol in Children With Supraventricular Tachycardia," *J Clin Pharmacol,* 1992, 32(1):1023-7.

- ♦ **Nadopen-V® (Canada)** *see* Penicillin V Potassium *on page 743*
- ♦ **Nadostine® (Canada)** *see* Nystatin *on page 701*
- ♦ **Nafazair® Ophthalmic** *see* Naphazoline *on page 671*
- ♦ **Nafcil™ Injection** *see* Nafcillin *on page 666*

Nafcillin *(naf SIL in)*

Related Information

Extravasation Treatment *on page 1050*

Brand Names Nafcil™ Injection; Nallpen® Injection; Unipen® Injection; Unipen® Oral

Available Salts Nafcillin Sodium

Synonyms Ethoxynaphthamido Penicillin

Therapeutic Category Antibiotic, Penicillin (Antistaphylococcal)

Generic Available Yes

Use Treatment of bacterial infections such as osteomyelitis, septicemia, endocarditis, and CNS infections due to susceptible penicillinase-producing strains of *Staphylococcus*

Pregnancy Risk Factor B

Contraindications Hypersensitivity to nafcillin, any component, or penicillins

Warnings Elimination rate will be decreased in neonates; avoid using in neonates during the first 2 weeks of life

Precautions Extravasation of I.V. infusions should be avoided; modification of dosage is necessary in patients with both severe renal and hepatic impairment; use with caution in patients with cephalosporin hypersensitivity

Adverse Reactions

Central nervous system: Fever

Dermatologic: Skin rash

Endocrine & metabolic: Hypokalemia

Gastrointestinal: Nausea, diarrhea

Hematologic: Neutropenia, anemia, eosinophilia

Hepatic: Elevations in AST

Local: Pain, thrombophlebitis

Renal: Acute interstitial nephritis (rare), hematuria

Miscellaneous: Hypersensitivity reactions

Drug Interactions Probenecid (decreases rate of nafcillin elimination), oral anticoagulants (may decrease half-life of warfarin), may increase hepatic metabolism of cyclosporine

Food Interactions Presence of food decreases GI absorption

Stability Refrigerate oral suspension after reconstitution, discard after 7 days. Reconstituted nafcillin 250 mg/mL solution for injection is stable for 3 days at room temperature and 7 days when refrigerated; when diluted for I.V. intermittent infusion in D_5W or NS, solution is stable for 24 hours at room temperature and 96 hours when refrigerated; incompatible with aminoglycosides

Mechanism of Action Interferes with bacterial cell wall synthesis during active multiplication by binding to one or more of the penicillin-binding proteins; inhibits the final transpeptidation step of peptidoglycan synthesis causing cell wall death and resultant bactericidal activity against susceptible bacteria

Pharmacokinetics

Absorption: Oral: Poor and erratic

Distribution: Distributes into bile, synovial, pleural, and pericardial fluids and into bone and liver; CSF penetration is poor unless meninges are inflamed; crosses the placenta

Protein binding: 90%

Metabolism: 70% to 90%

Half-life:

Neonates:

<3 weeks: 2.2-5.5 hours

4-9 weeks: 1.2-2.3 hours

Children 1 month to 14 years: 0.75-1.9 hours

Adults with normal renal and hepatic function: 0.5-1.5 hours

Time to peak serum concentration:

Oral: Within 2 hours

I.M.: Within 30-60 minutes

Elimination: Primarily in bile and 10% to 30% in urine as unchanged drug; undergoes enterohepatic recycling

Not dialyzable (0% to 5%)

Usual Dosage

Neonates: I.M., I.V.:

0-4 weeks, <1200 g: 50 mg/kg/day in divided doses every 12 hours

≤7 days:

1200-2000 g: 50 mg/kg/day in divided doses every 12 hours

>2000 g: 75 mg/kg/day in divided doses every 8 hours

>7 days:

1200-2000 g: 75 mg/kg/day in divided doses every 8 hours

>2000 g: 100 mg/kg/day in divided doses every 6 hours

Children:

I.M., I.V.:

Mild to moderate infections: 50-100 mg/kg/day in divided doses every 6 hours

Severe infections: 100-200 mg/kg/day in divided doses every 4-6 hours

Maximum dose: 12 g/day

Oral: 50-100 mg/kg/day divided every 6 hours

Adults:

Oral: 250-500 mg every 4-6 hours, up to 1 g every 4-6 hours for more severe infections

I.M.: 500 mg every 4-6 hours

I.V.: 500-2000 mg every 4-6 hours

Dosing adjustment in patients with both severe renal/hepatic impairment: Use lower range of usual dose or reduce dose 33% to 50%

Administration

Oral: Administer on an empty stomach with water 1 hour before or 2 hours after meals

Parenteral:

I.M.: Administer deep I.M. into a large muscle (ie, gluteus maximus) using a solution containing 250 mg/mL

I.V.: Nafcillin may be administered by I.V. push over 5-10 minutes or by I.V. intermittent infusion over 15-60 minutes at a final concentration not to exceed 40 mg/mL; in fluid-restricted patients, a maximum concentration of 100 mg/mL may be administered

Monitoring Parameters Periodic CBC with differential, urinalysis, BUN, serum creatinine, AST, and ALT

Test Interactions False-positive urinary and serum proteins

Nursing Implications Extravasation may cause tissue sloughing and necrosis; hyaluronidase infiltration may help avoid injury

Additional Information Sodium content of 1 g injection: 2.9 mEq

Dosage Forms

Capsule, as sodium: 250 mg

Powder for injection, as sodium: 500 mg, 1 g, 2 g, 4 g, 10 g

Solution, as sodium: 250 mg/5 mL (100 mL)

Tablet, as sodium: 500 mg

References

Banner W Jr, Gooch WM 3d, Burckart G, et al, "Pharmacokinetics of Nafcillin in Infants With Low Birth Weights," *Antimicrob Agents Chemother*, 1980, 17(4):691-4.

(Continued)

Nafcillin (Continued)

Zenk KE, Dungy CL, and Greene CR, "Nafcillin Extravasation Injury: Use of Hyaluronidase as an Antidote," *Am J Dis Child*, 1981, 135(12):1113-4.

♦ **Nafcillin Sodium** *see Nafcillin on page 666*
♦ **NaHCO₃** *see Sodium Bicarbonate on page 870*

Nalbuphine (NAL byoo feen)

Brand Names Nubain®
Available Salts Nalbuphine Hydrochloride
Therapeutic Category Analgesic, Narcotic; Opiate Partial Agonist
Generic Available Yes
Use Relief of moderate to severe pain
Pregnancy Risk Factor B (D if used for prolonged periods or in high doses at term)
Contraindications Hypersensitivity to nalbuphine or any component
Warnings Some products may contain sulfites; abrupt discontinuation after prolonged use may result in narcotic withdrawal; administration to patients receiving chronic opiates may precipitate narcotic withdrawal
Precautions Reduce dose with hepatic impairment; use with caution in patients with impaired respiration, recent MI, biliary tract surgery, or sulfite sensitivity; may produce respiratory depression; use with caution in patients with a history of drug dependence, head trauma or increased intracranial pressure, decreased hepatic or renal function, pregnancy, or patients suspected to be opioid dependent
Adverse Reactions
Cardiovascular: Hypotension, tachycardia, bradycardia, peripheral vasodilation
Central nervous system: CNS depression, drowsiness, headache, dizziness, sedation, increased ICP
Dermatologic: Urticaria, pruritus, rash
Gastrointestinal: Anorexia, nausea, vomiting, xerostomia, biliary tract spasm
Genitourinary: Urinary tract spasm, urinary retention
Ocular: Blurred vision, miosis
Respiratory: Respiratory depression
Miscellaneous: Histamine release, physical and psychological dependence, narcotic withdrawal in patients receiving opiate agonists chronically
Drug Interactions CNS depressants, alcohol, phenothiazine, tricyclic antidepressants may potentiate adverse effects
Mechanism of Action Binds to opiate receptors in the CNS, causing inhibition of ascending pain pathways, altering the perception of and response to pain; produces generalized CNS depression; opiate antagonistic effect may result from competitive inhibition at the opiate mu receptor
Pharmacodynamics
Onset of action:
I.M., S.C.: Within 15 minutes
I.V.: 2-3 minutes
Peak effect:
I.M.: 30 minutes
I.V.: 1-3 minutes
Duration: 3-6 hours
Pharmacokinetics
Metabolism: In the liver; extensive first-pass metabolism
Protein binding: ~50%
Half-life, terminal:
Children 1-8 years: 0.9 hours
Adults 23-32 years: ~2 hours; range: 3.5-5 hours
Adults 65-90 years: 2.3 hours
Time to peak serum concentration:
I.M.: 30 minutes
I.V.: 1-3 minutes
Elimination: Metabolites primarily in feces (via bile) and in urine; 4% to 7% eliminated unchanged in the urine
Usual Dosage I.M., I.V., S.C.:
Children 1-14 years: Premedication: 0.2 mg/kg; maximum dose: 20 mg/dose
Children: Analgesia: 0.1-0.15 mg/kg every 3-6 hours as needed
Adults: 10 mg/70 kg every 3-6 hours as needed; maximum single-dose: 20 mg; maximum daily dose: 160 mg
Administration Parenteral: I.V.: Administer over 5-10 minutes; larger doses should be administered over 10-15 minutes

Monitoring Parameters Relief of pain, respiratory and mental status, blood pressure

Patient Information Avoid alcohol; may cause drowsiness and impair ability to perform activities requiring mental alertness or physical coordination; may impair judgment; may be habit-forming; will cause withdrawal in patients currently dependent on narcotics

Nursing Implications Observe patient for excessive sedation, respiratory depression, implement safety measures, assist with ambulation; observe for narcotic withdrawal (nausea, vomiting, abdominal cramps, lacrimation, rhinorrhea, piloerection, anxiety, restlessness, increased temperature)

Additional Information Analgesic potency: 1 mg nalbuphine ~1 mg morphine

Dosage Forms Injection, as hydrochloride: 10 mg/mL (1 mL, 10 mL); 20 mg/mL (1 mL, 10 mL)

References
Jaillon P, Gardin ME, Lecocq B, et al, "Pharmacokinetics of Nalbuphine in Infants, Young Healthy Volunteers, and Elderly Patients," *Clin Pharmacol Ther*, 1989, 46(2):226-33.

♦ **Nalbuphine Hydrochloride** *see* Nalbuphine *on page 668*
♦ **Naldecon® Senior DX [OTC]** *see* Guaifenesin and Dextromethorphan *on page 466*
♦ **Naldecon® Senior EX [OTC]** *see* Guaifenesin *on page 464*

Nalidixic Acid (nal i DIKS ik AS id)

Brand Names NegGram®

Synonyms Nalidixinic Acid

Therapeutic Category Antibiotic, Quinolone

Generic Available Yes

Use Lower urinary tract infections due to susceptible gram-negative organisms including *E. coli*, *Enterobacter*, *Klebsiella*, and *Proteus* (inactive against *Pseudomonas*)

Pregnancy Risk Factor B

Contraindications History of convulsive disorders; hypersensitivity to nalidixic acid or any component; infants <3 months of age; should not be used to treat UTI in febrile infants and young children in whom renal involvement is present

Warnings Has been shown to cause cartilage degeneration in immature animals; usefulness may be limited by the emergence of bacterial resistance to nalidixic acid during treatment

Precautions Use with caution in patients with impaired hepatic or renal function, prepubertal children, patients with G-6-PD deficiency, severe cerebral arteriosclerosis, or respiratory insufficiency

Adverse Reactions
Central nervous system: Malaise, drowsiness, vertigo, confusion, toxic psychosis, convulsions, fever, headache, increased intracranial pressure, chills, depression, insomnia
Dermatologic: Rash, urticaria, pruritus, photosensitivity
Endocrine & metabolic: Metabolic acidosis (in premature infants)
Gastrointestinal: Nausea, vomiting, diarrhea, abdominal pain
Hematologic: Leukopenia, thrombocytopenia, eosinophilia, hemolytic anemia
Hepatic: Hepatotoxicity, cholestatic jaundice
Neuromuscular & skeletal: Myalgia, weakness, arthralgia with joint stiffness, peripheral neuritis
Ocular: Visual disturbances, nystagmus

Drug Interactions Warfarin (increases anticoagulant effect due to displacement of warfarin from albumin binding sites), antacids (decrease nalidixic acid absorption)

Mechanism of Action Inhibits DNA topoisomerase in susceptible organisms resulting in inhibition of DNA polymerization at late stages of chromosomal replication and promotion of double-stranded DNA breakage

Pharmacokinetics
Absorption: Rapid and complete from the GI tract
Distribution: Crosses the placenta; appears in breast milk; negligible amounts enter CSF; achieves significant antibacterial concentrations only in the urinary tract
Protein binding: 90%
Metabolism: Partial in the liver to hydroxynalidixic acid (active metabolite)
Half-life: 6-7 hours (increases significantly with renal impairment)
Time to peak serum concentration: 1-2 hours
Elimination: In urine as unchanged drug and 80% as metabolites; small amounts appear in feces

Usual Dosage Oral:
Children >3 months: 55 mg/kg/day divided every 6 hours
(Continued)

Nalidixic Acid *(Continued)*

Prophylaxis of UTI: 30 mg/kg/day divided every 12 hours

Adults: 1 g 4 times/day for 2 weeks; then suppressive therapy of 500 mg 4 times/day

Administration Oral: Administer 1 hour before meals; may administer with food to minimize GI upset

Monitoring Parameters Urinalysis, urine culture; CBC, renal and hepatic function tests

Test Interactions False-positive urine glucose with Clinitest®, false increase in urinary VMA

Patient Information Avoid undue exposure to direct sunlight

Additional Information In a study of 31 case-control pairs, short treatment periods (1-2 weeks) with nalidixic acid in children <15 years of age did not cause arthropathies or hamper growth

Dosage Forms

Suspension, oral (raspberry flavor): 250 mg/5 mL (473 mL)

Tablet: 250 mg, 500 mg, 1 g

References

Nuutinen M, Turtinen J, and Uhari M, "Growth and Joint Symptoms in Children Treated With Nalidixic Acid," *Pediatr Infect Dis J*, 1994, 13(9):798-800.

"Practice Parameter: The Diagnosis, Treatment, and Evaluation of the Initial Urinary Tract Infection in Febrile Infants and Young Children. American Academy of Pediatrics. Committee on Quality Improvement. Subcommittee on Urinary Tract Infection," *Pediatrics*,1999, 103(4 Pt 1):843-52.

Stutman HR and Marks MI, "Review of Pediatric Antimicrobial Therapies," *Semin Pediatr Infect Dis*, 1991, 2:3-17.

- ♦ **Nalidixinic Acid** *see* Nalidixic Acid *on page 669*
- ♦ **Nallpen® Injection** *see* Nafcillin *on page 666*
- ♦ **N-allylnoroxymorphine** *see* Naloxone *on page 670*

Naloxone *(nal OKS one)*

Related Information

CPR Pediatric Drug Dosages *on page 999*

Brand Names Narcan®

Available Salts Naloxone Hydrochloride

Synonyms *N*-allylnoroxymorphine

Therapeutic Category Antidote for Narcotic Agonists

Generic Available Yes

Use Reverses CNS and respiratory depression in suspected narcotic overdose; neonatal opiate depression; coma of unknown etiology; used investigationally for shock, phencyclidine, and alcohol ingestion

Pregnancy Risk Factor B

Contraindications Hypersensitivity to naloxone or any component

Warnings May precipitate withdrawal symptoms (hypertension, sweating, agitation, irritability, shrill cry, failure to feed) in patients with physical dependence to opiates (including newborns of narcotic dependent mothers)

Precautions Use with caution in patients with chronic cardiac or pulmonary disease or coronary artery disease. Following the use of narcotics during surgery, naloxone may reverse analgesia and increase blood pressure; use with caution and administer in smaller increments to patients suspected to be opioid dependent and in postoperative patients (to avoid large cardiovascular changes)

Adverse Reactions

Cardiovascular: Hypertension, hypotension, tachycardia, ventricular arrhythmias, cardiac arrest

Gastrointestinal: Nausea, vomiting

Miscellaneous: Increased diaphoresis

Stability Protect from light; stable in NS and D_5W at 4 mcg/mL for 24 hours; do not mix with alkaline solutions

Mechanism of Action Competes and displaces narcotics at narcotic receptor sites

Pharmacodynamics

Onset of action:

E.T., I.M., S.C.: Within 2-5 minutes

I.V.: Within 2 minutes

Duration: (20-60 minutes) is shorter than that of most opioids; therefore, repeated doses are usually needed

Pharmacokinetics

Distribution: Crosses the placenta

Metabolism: Primarily by glucuronidation in the liver

Half-life:
Neonates: 1.2-3 hours
Adults: 0.5-1.5 hours (mean: ~1 hour)
Elimination: In urine as metabolites

Usual Dosage I.M., I.V. (preferred), E.T. (preferred if I.V. route not available), S.C.:
Note: The dose for pediatric postoperative narcotic reversal is **one-tenth** of the dose used for opiate intoxication:

Opiate intoxication:
Birth (including premature infants) to 5 years or <20 kg: 0.1 mg/kg; repeat every 2-3 minutes if needed; may need to repeat doses every 20-60 minutes
>5 years or ≥20 kg: 2 mg/dose; if no response, repeat every 2-3 minutes; may need to repeat doses every 20-60 minutes
Children and Adults: I.V. continuous infusion: If continuous infusion is required, calculate the initial dosage/hour based on the effective intermittent dose used and duration of adequate response seen; titrate dose; a range of: 2.5-160 mcg/kg/hour has been reported; taper continuous infusion gradually to avoid relapse
Adults: 0.4-2 mg every 2-3 minutes as needed; may need to repeat doses every 20-60 minutes; **Note:** Use 0.1-0.2 mg increments in patients who are opioid dependent and in postoperative patients to avoid large cardiovascular changes
Postanesthesia narcotic reversal: Infants and Children: **0.01 mg/kg**; may repeat every 2-3 minutes as needed based on response

Administration
Endotracheal: Dilute to 1-2 mL with NS
Parenteral:
I.V. continuous infusion: Dilute to 4 mcg/mL in D_5W or NS
I.V. push: Administer over 30 seconds as undiluted preparation
Note: I.M. or S.C. administration in hypotensive patients or patients with peripheral vasoconstriction or hypoperfusion may result in erratic or delayed absorption

Monitoring Parameters Respiratory rate, heart rate, blood pressure

Nursing Implications Use of neonatal naloxone (0.02 mg/mL) is no longer recommended because unacceptably high fluid volumes will result, especially in small neonates; the 0.4 mg/mL preparation is available and can be accurately dosed with appropriately sized syringes (1 mL)

Additional Information Contains methyl and propylparabens

Dosage Forms
Injection, as hydrochloride: 0.4 mg/mL (1 mL, 2 mL, 10 mL); 1 mg/mL (2 mL, 10 mL)
Injection, neonatal, as hydrochloride: 0.02 mg/mL (2 mL)

References

American Academy of Pediatrics Committee on Drugs, "Naloxone Dosage and Route of Administration for Infants and Children: Addendum to Emergency Drug Doses for Infants and Children," *Pediatrics*, 1990, 86(3):484-5.
Chamberlain JM and Klein BL, "A Comprehensive Review of Naloxone for the Emergency Physician," *Am J Emerg Med*, 1994, 12(6):650-60.

♦ **Naloxone Hydrochloride** *see* Naloxone *on page 670*

Naphazoline (naf AZ oh leen)

Brand Names AK-Con® Ophthalmic; Albalon® Liquifilm® Ophthalmic; Allerest® Eye Drops [OTC]; Clear Eyes® [OTC]; Comfort® Ophthalmic [OTC]; Degest® 2 Ophthalmic [OTC]; Estivin® II Ophthalmic [OTC]; I-Naphline® Ophthalmic; Nafazair® Ophthalmic; Naphcon Forte® Ophthalmic; Naphcon® Ophthalmic [OTC]; Opcon® Ophthalmic; Privine® Nasal [OTC]; Red Away® (Canada); VasoClear® Ophthalmic [OTC]; Vasocon Regular® Ophthalmic

Available Salts Naphazoline Hydrochloride

Therapeutic Category Adrenergic Agonist Agent, Ophthalmic; Decongestant, Nasal; Nasal Agent, Vasoconstrictor; Ophthalmic Agent, Vasoconstrictor

Generic Available Yes

Use Topical ocular vasoconstrictor (to soothe, refresh, moisturize, and relieve redness due to minor eye irritation); temporarily relieves nasal congestion associated with rhinitis, sinusitis, hay fever, or the common cold

Pregnancy Risk Factor C

Contraindications Hypersensitivity to naphazoline or any component; narrow-angle glaucoma; prior to peripheral iridectomy (in patients susceptible to angle block)

Warnings Excessive dosage may cause marked sedation in children, particularly infants; some products contain sulfites which may cause hypersensitivity reactions in susceptible individuals
(Continued)

Naphazoline *(Continued)*

Precautions Rebound congestion may occur with extended use (use no longer than 3-5 days); use with caution in the presence of hypertension, diabetes mellitus, hyperthyroidism, heart disease, coronary artery disease, cerebral arteriosclerosis, or long-standing asthma

Adverse Reactions

Cardiovascular: Systemic cardiovascular stimulation (rare), pallor

Central nervous system: Dizziness, headache, nervousness, anxiety, tenseness, drowsiness, hallucinations, convulsions, CNS depression, prolonged psychosis

Gastrointestinal: Nausea, vomiting

Local: Transient stinging, nasal mucosa irritation, dryness

Ocular: Mydriasis, increased intraocular pressure, blurring of vision, blepharospasm

Respiratory: Respiratory difficulty, sneezing, rebound nasal congestion

Miscellaneous: Diaphoresis

Drug Interactions Anesthetics (discontinue naphazoline prior to use of anesthetics that sensitize the myocardium to sympathomimetics, ie, cyclopropane, halothane); MAO inhibitors, methyldopa, tricyclic antidepressants increase hypertensive response

Mechanism of Action Stimulates alpha-adrenergic receptors in the arterioles of the conjunctiva and the nasal mucosa to produce vasoconstriction

Pharmacodynamics

Onset of action: Following topical administration, decongestion occurs within 10 minutes

Duration: 2-6 hours

Pharmacokinetics Elimination: Not well defined

Usual Dosage

Nasal: Intranasal not recommended for use in children <6 years of age (especially in infants) due to CNS depression; therapy should not exceed 3-5 days

Children 6-12 years: 0.05%, 1 drop or spray every 6 hours if needed

Children >12 years to Adults: 0.05%, 1-2 drops or sprays every 3-6 hours if needed

Ophthalmic: Therapy should generally not exceed 3-4 days; not recommended for use in children <6 years of age due to CNS depression (especially in infants)

Children >6 years and Adults (0.01% to 0.1%): Instill 1-2 drops every 3-4 hours

Administration

Ophthalmic: Instill drops into conjunctival sac of affected eye; finger pressure should be applied to lacrimal sac during and for 1-2 minutes after instillation to decrease risk of absorption and systemic reactions; avoid contact of bottle tip with skin or eye

Nasal: Spray or drop medication into one nostril while gently occluding the other; then reverse procedure

Patient Information Discontinue eye drops if visual changes or ocular pain occur

Dosage Forms Solution, as hydrochloride:

Nasal:

Drops: 0.05% (20 mL)

Spray: 0.05% (15 mL)

Ophthalmic: 0.012% (7.5 mL, 30 mL); 0.02% (15 mL); 0.03% (15 mL); 0.1% (15 mL)

♦ **Naphazoline Hydrochloride** *see* Naphazoline *on page 671*

♦ **Naphcon Forte® Ophthalmic** *see* Naphazoline *on page 671*

♦ **Naphcon® Ophthalmic [OTC]** *see* Naphazoline *on page 671*

♦ **Naprelan®** *see* Naproxen *on page 672*

♦ **Naprosyn®** *see* Naproxen *on page 672*

Naproxen *(na PROKS en)*

Related Information

Carbohydrate and Alcohol Content of Liquid Medications for Use in Patients Receiving Ketogenic Diets *on page 1228*

Overdose and Toxicology *on page 1191*

Brand Names Aleve® [OTC]; Anaprox®; Apo®-Naproxen (Canada); EC-Naprosyn®; Naprelan®; Naprosyn®; Naxen® (Canada); Novo-Naprox® (Canada); Nu-Naprox® (Canada); Synflex® (Canada)

Available Salts Naproxen Sodium

Therapeutic Category Analgesic, Non-narcotic; Anti-inflammatory Agent; Antipyretic; Nonsteroidal Anti-inflammatory Drug (NSAID), Oral

Generic Available Yes

Use Management of inflammatory disease and rheumatoid disorders (including juvenile rheumatoid arthritis); acute gout; mild to moderate pain; dysmenorrhea; fever

Pregnancy Risk Factor B (D in 3rd trimester)

Contraindications Hypersensitivity to naproxen, any component, aspirin, or other NSAIDs

Precautions Use with caution in patients with GI disease, cardiac disease, renal or hepatic impairment, and patients receiving anticoagulants

Adverse Reactions

Cardiovascular: Edema

Central nervous system: Fatigue, drowsiness, vertigo, headache

Dermatologic: Pruritus, rash; pseudoporphyria (ie, increased skin fragility and blistering with scarring in sun-exposed skin), incidence: 12% in naproxen-treated children with JRA (discontinue therapy if this occurs)

Gastrointestinal: Abdominal discomfort, nausea, heartburn, constipation, vomiting, GI bleed, ulcers, perforation

Hematologic: Thrombocytopenia, inhibits platelet aggregation, prolongs bleeding time, agranulocytosis

Hepatic: Hepatitis

Ocular: Visual disturbances

Otic: Tinnitus

Renal: Renal dysfunction

Drug Interactions Cytochrome P-450 isoenzyme CYP2C8 (5-hydroxylation), CYP2C9 (5-hydroxylation), and CYP2C18 substrate

Naproxen may increase serum concentrations of methotrexate and decrease the effects of furosemide; aspirin may decrease and probenecid may increase naproxen serum concentrations; drug interactions similar to other NSAIDs may also occur; other GI irritants (eg, oral potassium supplements) may increase GI adverse effects

Mechanism of Action Inhibits prostaglandin synthesis by decreasing the activity of the enzyme, cyclo-oxygenase, which results in decreased formation of prostaglandin precursors

Pharmacokinetics

Absorption: Oral: Almost 100%

Distribution: Crosses the placenta; ~1% distributed into breast milk

Protein binding: 99%

Metabolism: In the liver

Half-life, elimination: Children: Range: 8-17 hours

Children 8-14 years: 8-10 hours

Adults: 10-20 hours

Time to peak serum concentration: Within 1-2 hours for naproxen sodium; within 2-4 hours for naproxen

Elimination: 10% excreted unchanged in the urine

Usual Dosage Oral as naproxen:

Children >2 years:

Analgesia: 5-7 mg/kg/dose every 8-12 hours

Inflammatory disease: Usual: 10-15 mg/kg/day in 2 divided doses; range: 7-20 mg/kg/day; maximum dose: 1000 mg/day

Adults:

Rheumatoid arthritis, osteoarthritis, and ankylosing spondylitis: 500-1000 mg/day in 2 divided doses

Acute gout: 250 mg every 8 hours

Mild to moderate pain or dysmenorrhea: Initial: 500 mg, then 250 mg every 6-8 hours; maximum dose: 1250 mg/day

Administration Oral: Administer with food, milk, or antacids to decrease GI adverse effects; shake suspension before use

Monitoring Parameters CBC, BUN, serum creatinine, liver enzymes, occult blood loss, periodic ophthalmologic exams, hemoglobin

Patient Information Avoid alcohol; may cause drowsiness and impair ability to perform activities requiring mental alertness or physical coordination; children with JRA: Protect skin from sun; use sunscreen, wide-brimmed hats, etc

Additional Information Naproxen sodium 220 mg = 200 mg base; naproxen sodium 550 mg = 500 mg base; naproxen sodium 275 mg = 250 mg base

Dosage Forms Sodium content is in brackets

Suspension, oral: 125 mg/5 mL [0.34 mEq/mL] (15 mL, 30 mL, 480 mL)

Tablet (Naprosyn®): 250 mg, 375 mg, 500 mg

Tablet, delayed release, enteric coated (EC-Naprosyn®): 375 mg, 500 mg

Tablet, as sodium

(Continued)

Naproxen *(Continued)*

Aleve®: 220 mg [0.87 mEq] (200 mg base)

Anaprox®: 275 mg [1 mEq] (250 mg base); 550 mg [2 mEq] (500 mg base)

Tablet, as sodium, extended release: 375 mg, 500 mg, 750 mg

Naprelan®: 421.5 mg (375 mg base); 550 mg (500 mg base)

References

Berde C, Ablin A, Glazer J, et al, "American Academy of Pediatrics Report of the Subcommittee on Disease-Related Pain in Childhood Cancer," *Pediatrics*, 1990, 86(5 Pt 2):818-25.

Lang BA and Finlayson LA, "Naproxen-Induced Pseudoporphyria in Patients With Juvenile Rheumatoid Arthritis," *J Pediatr*, 1994, 124(4):639-42.

Wells TG, Mortensen ME, Dietrich A, et al, "Comparison of the Pharmacokinetics of Naproxen Tablets and Suspension in Children," *J Clin Pharmacol*, 1994, 34(1):30-3.

♦ **Naproxen Sodium** *see Naproxen on page 672*

♦ **Narcan®** *see Naloxone on page 670*

♦ **Narcotic Analgesics Comparison** *see page 1035*

♦ **Nasacort®** *see Triamcinolone on page 946*

♦ **Nasacort® AQ** *see Triamcinolone on page 946*

♦ **Nasahist B®** *see Brompheniramine on page 142*

♦ **NaSal™ [OTC]** *see Sodium Chloride on page 871*

♦ **Nasalcrom® [OTC]** *see Cromolyn on page 260*

♦ **Nasalide® Nasal Spray** *see Flunisolide on page 423*

♦ **Nasal Moist® [OTC]** *see Sodium Chloride on page 871*

♦ **Nasarel® Nasal Spray** *see Flunisolide on page 423*

♦ **Natulan® (Canada)** *see Procarbazine on page 802*

♦ **Natural Lung Surfactant** *see Beractant on page 128*

♦ **Navane®** *see Thiothixene on page 923*

♦ **Naxen® (Canada)** *see Naproxen on page 672*

♦ **ND-Stat®** *see Brompheniramine on page 142*

♦ **Nebcin® Injection** *see Tobramycin on page 931*

♦ **NebuPent™ Inhalation** *see Pentamidine on page 745*

Nedocromil *(ne doe KROE mil)*

Related Information

Asthma Guidelines *on page 1178*

Brand Names Alocril™; Tilade® Inhalation Aerosol

Available Salts Nedocromil Sodium

Therapeutic Category Antiallergic, Ophthalmic; Antiasthmatic; Inhalation, Miscellaneous

Generic Available No

Use

Aerosol: Maintenance therapy in patients with mild to moderate asthma

Ophthalmic: Treatment of itching associated with allergic conjunctivitis

Pregnancy Risk Factor B

Contraindications Hypersensitivity to nedocromil or any component

Warnings If systemic or inhaled steroid therapy is at all reduced, monitor patients carefully; nedocromil is **not** a bronchodilator and, therefore, should not be used for reversal of acute bronchospasm

Precautions Refrain from wearing contact lenses while exhibiting the signs and symptoms of allergic conjunctivitis

Adverse Reactions

Cardiovascular: Chest pain

Central nervous system: Dizziness, dysphonia, headache, fatigue

Dermatologic: Rash

Gastrointestinal: Nausea, vomiting, dyspepsia, diarrhea, abdominal pain, xerostomia, dysgeusia, unpleasant taste

Hepatic: Increased ALT

Neuromuscular and skeletal: Arthritis, tremor

Ocular: Burning, irritation, stinging, conjunctivitis, eye redness, photophobia

Respiratory: Cough, pharyngitis, rhinitis, bronchitis, upper respiratory infection, bronchospasm, increased sputum production, pneumonitis with eosinophilia (PIE syndrome)

Stability Store at room temperature; do not freeze

Mechanism of Action Inhibits the activation of and mediator release from a variety of inflammatory cell types associated with asthma including eosinophils, neutrophils, macrophages, mast cells, monocytes, and platelets; it inhibits the release of histamine, leukotrienes, and slow-reacting substance of anaphylaxis; it inhibits the development of early and late bronchoconstriction responses to inhaled antigen

Pharmacodynamics Inhalation: Duration of effect: 2 hours; maximum therapeutic benefit is seen after at least 1 week of therapy

Pharmacokinetics
Absorption: Systemic: Inhalation: 7% to 9%; ophthalmic: <4%
Protein binding, plasma: 89%
Elimination: Excreted unchanged in urine 70%; feces 30%

Usual Dosage
Inhalation: Children ≥6 years and Adults: 2 inhalations 4 times/day; may reduce dosage to 2-3 times/day once desired clinical response to initial dose is observed
Ophthalmic: Children ≥3 years and Adults: 1-2 drops in each eye twice daily throughout the period of exposure to allergen

Administration
Oral inhalation: Shake well before use; must be primed by 3 actuations prior to first use; if canister remains unused for >7 days, reprime with 3 actuations; discard canister after 104 actuations
Ophthalmic: Instill drops into conjunctival sac; avoid contact of bottle tip with skin or eye

Additional Information Has no known therapeutic systemic activity when delivered by inhalation

Dosage Forms
Aerosol, as sodium: 1.75 mg/activation (16.2 g)
Solution as sodium, ophthalmic: 2% (5 mL)

♦ **Nedrocromil Sodium** see Nedocromil on page 674
♦ **NegGram®** see Nalidixic Acid on page 669

Nelfinavir (nel FIN a veer)

Related Information
Adult and Adolescent HIV on page 1133
Pediatric HIV on page 1129

Brand Names Viracept®

Therapeutic Category Antiretroviral Agent; HIV Agents (Anti-HIV Agents); Protease Inhibitor

Use Treatment of HIV infection in combination with other antiretroviral agents. (**Note:** Current preferred HIV regimens consist of **three** antiretroviral agents)

Pregnancy Risk Factor B

Contraindications Hypersensitivity to nelfinavir or any component

Warnings Avoid use of powder formulation in patients with phenylketonuria since it contains 11.2 mg phenylalanine per gram of powder; due to potential serious and life-threatening drug interactions, the following drugs should not be coadministered with nelfinavir: terfenadine, astemizole, cisapride, triazolam, midazolam, ergot derivatives, amiodarone, or quinidine; concurrent use with some anticonvulsants may significantly limit nelfinavir's effectiveness; spontaneous bleeding episodes have been reported in patients with hemophilia A and B; new onset diabetes mellitus, exacerbations of diabetes and hyperglycemia have been reported in HIV-infected patients receiving protease inhibitors

Precautions Use caution in patients with hepatic insufficiency since nelfinavir is metabolized in the liver and excreted predominantly in the feces

Adverse Reactions
Cardiovascular: Hypertension
Central nervous system: Decreased concentration, anxiety, depression, dizziness, emotional lability, hyperkinesia, insomnia, migraine, seizures, sleep disorder, somnolence, suicide ideation, fever, headache, asthenia, malaise
Dermatologic: Rash, pruritus, urticaria, diaphoresis
Endocrine & metabolic: Hyperlipemia, hyperuricemia; rare: hyperglycemia, diabetes, ketoacidosis; changes in the distribution of body fat
Gastrointestinal: Diarrhea (30%), nausea, flatulence, abdominal pain, anorexia, dyspepsia, epigastric pain, mouth ulceration, GI bleeding, pancreatitis, vomiting
Genitourinary: Kidney calculus, sexual dysfunction
Hematologic: Anemia, leukopenia, thrombocytopenia; rare: spontaneous bleeding episodes in hemophiliacs
Hepatic: Hepatitis, elevated liver function tests
Neuromuscular & skeletal: Weakness, arthralgia, arthritis, cramps, myalgia, myasthenia, myopathy, paresthesia, back pain
Ocular: Acute iritis
Respiratory: Dyspnea, pharyngitis, rhinitis, sinusitis
(Continued)

Nelfinavir *(Continued)*

Drug Interactions Nelfinavir inhibits the metabolism and increases the levels of cisapride, terfenadine, astemizole, amiodarone, quinidine, cyclosporine, tacrolimus, sildenafil, ergot derivatives, midazolam, and triazolam; nelfinavir increases rifabutin plasma AUC by 207% so reduce rifabutin dose by 50% when coadministering with nelfinavir; rifampin decreases nelfinavir plasma AUC by ~82% (concurrent use not recommended); phenobarbital, phenytoin, and carbamazepine decrease nelfinavir concentration; ketoconazole, indinavir, and ritonavir increase nelfinavir concentration; nelfinavir decreases hormone levels of oral contraceptives (ethinyl estradiol, norethindrone); nelfinavir increases levels of saquinavir and indinavir; coadministration with delavirdine increases nelfinavir concentrations by twofold and decreases delavirdine concentrations by 50%; if coadministered with didanosine, administer nelfinavir 2 hours before or 1 hour after didanosine

Food Interactions Administer with food to increase absorption; do not administer with acidic food or juice (ie, orange juice, apple juice, applesauce) since the combination may result in a bitter taste

Stability Store at room temperature

Mechanism of Action A protease inhibitor which acts on an enzyme late in the HIV replication process after the virus has entered into the cell's nucleus preventing cleavage of the gag-pol protein precursors resulting in the production of immature, noninfectious virions; cross-resistance with other protease inhibitors is possible

Pharmacokinetics

Absorption: AUC is two- to threefold higher under fed conditions versus fasting

Distribution: V_d: 2-7 L/kg

Protein binding: 98%

Metabolism: Via multiple cytochrome P-450 isoforms including CYP3A4 to inactive and an active metabolite which has comparable activity to the parent drug

Half-life: 3.5-5 hours

Time to peak serum concentration: 2-4 hours

Elimination: 98% to 99% excreted in feces (78% as metabolites and 22% as unchanged nelfinavir); 1% to 2% excreted in urine

Usual Dosage Oral:

Neonates: Investigational, under study in PACTG 353: 40 mg/kg/dose twice daily

Children and Adolescents (early puberty, Tanner I-II): 20-30 mg/kg/dose 3 times/day (some experts administer a minimum dose of 30 mg/kg/dose 3 times/day); maximum dose: 750 mg/dose 3 times/day

Adolescents (late puberty, Tanner V) and Adults: 750 mg 3 times/day or 1250 mg/dose twice daily

Administration Administer with a meal or light snack to optimize absorption; do not mix with any acidic food or juice because of resulting bitter taste; if patient is unable to swallow tablets, consider using oral powder formulation mixed in small amount of water, milk, formula, dietary supplementation, ice cream, or pudding; do not store mixture for more than 6 hours; tablet can be readily dissolved in water to produce a dispersion that can be mixed with milk or chocolate milk or tablets can be crushed and administered with pudding; if coadministered with didanosine, nelfinavir should be administered 2 hours before or 1 hour after didanosine

Monitoring Parameters Liver function tests, blood glucose levels, CBC with diff, CD4 cell count, plasma levels of HIV RNA

Patient Information Use an alternative method of contraception to birth control pills during nelfinavir therapy. If a nelfinavir dose is missed, take the dose as soon as possible and then return to the normal schedule. However, if a dose is skipped, the patient should not double the next dose.

Nursing Implications Do not add water to bottles of oral powder; a special scoop is provided with powder for measuring purposes. If diarrhea occurs, it may be treated with an antimotility agent like loperamide

Dosage Forms

Powder for oral suspension (200 mg per 1 level teaspoon): 50 mg/g or 50 mg per 1 level scoop (144 g), contains 11.2 mg phenylalanine/g powder

Tablet: 250 mg

References

McDonald CK and Kuritzkes DR, "Human Immunodeficiency Virus Type I Protease Inhibitors," *Arch Intern Med*, 1997, 157(9):951-9.

Working Group on Antiretroviral Therapy and Medical Management of HIV-Infected Children, "Guidelines for the Use of Antiretroviral Agents in Pediatric HIV Infection," January 7, 2000, http://www.hivatis.org.

♦ **Nembutal**® *see* Pentobarbital *on page 748*

- ◆ **Neo-Calglucon®** [OTC] *see* Calcium Supplements *on page 157*
- ◆ **Neo-Codema® (Canada)** *see* Hydrochlorothiazide *on page 483*
- ◆ **Neo-Cultol®** [OTC] *see* Mineral Oil *on page 649*
- ◆ **Neofed®** [OTC] *see* Pseudoephedrine *on page 822*
- ◆ **Neo-fradin®** *see* Neomycin *on page 677*
- ◆ **Neoloid®** [OTC] *see* Castor Oil *on page 175*
- ◆ **Neomixin® Topical** *see* Neomycin, Polymyxin B, and Bacitracin *on page 680*

Neomycin (nee oh MYE sin)

Related Information
Emetogenic Potential of Single Chemotherapeutic Agents *on page 1095*
Overdose and Toxicology *on page 1191*

Brand Names Mycifradin® Sulfate; Myciguent® (Canada); Neo-fradin®; Neo-Tabs®

Available Salts Neomycin Sulfate

Therapeutic Category Ammonium Detoxicant; Antibiotic, Aminoglycoside; Antibiotic, Topical; Hyperammonemia Agent

Generic Available Yes

Use Administered orally to prepare GI tract for surgery; treat minor skin infections; treat diarrhea caused by *E. coli*; adjunct in the treatment of hepatic encephalopathy

Pregnancy Risk Factor C

Contraindications Hypersensitivity to neomycin or any component; patients with intestinal obstruction

Warnings Neomycin is more toxic than other aminoglycosides when given parenterally; **do not administer parenterally**; topical neomycin is a contact sensitizer with sensitivity occurring in 5% to 15% of patients treated with the drug; systemic absorption can occur when neomycin is utilized for irrigation of wounds or surgical sites

Precautions Use with caution in patients with renal impairment, pre-existing hearing impairment, neuromuscular disorders; modify dosage in patients with renal impairment

Adverse Reactions
Dermatologic: Contact dermatitis, erythema, rash, urticaria
Gastrointestinal: Nausea, vomiting, diarrhea, colitis, malabsorption
Local: Burning
Neuromuscular & skeletal: Neuromuscular blockade
Ocular: Contact conjunctivitis
Otic: Ototoxicity
Renal: Nephrotoxicity
Miscellaneous: Candidiasis

Drug Interactions Oral neomycin may potentiate the effects of oral anticoagulants; may decrease GI absorption of digoxin and methotrexate; synergistic effects seen with penicillins; increase adverse effects with other neurotoxic, ototoxic or nephrotoxic drugs

Stability Reconstituted neomycin solution is stable for 7 days when refrigerated

Mechanism of Action Interferes with bacterial protein synthesis by binding to 30S ribosomal subunits

Pharmacokinetics
Absorption: Poor orally (3%) or percutaneously; readily absorbed through denuded or abraded skin and body cavities
Distribution: V_d: 0.36 L/kg
Half-life: 2-3 hours (age and renal function dependent)
Time to peak serum concentration:
I.M.: Within 2 hours
Oral: 1-4 hours
Elimination: In urine (30% to 50% as unchanged drug); 97% of an oral dose eliminated unchanged in feces
Dialyzable (50% to 100%)

Usual Dosage
Neonates: Oral: Diarrhea: 50 mg/kg/day divided every 6 hours
Children: Oral: 50-100 mg/kg/day in divided doses every 6-8 hours
Preoperative bowel antisepsis: 90 mg/kg/day divided every 4 hours for 2 days; or 25 mg/kg at 1, 2, and 11 PM on the day preceding surgery as an adjunct to mechanical cleansing of the intestine and in combination with erythromycin base
Hepatic coma: 2.5-7 g/m^2/day divided every 4-6 hours for 5-6 days not to exceed 12 g/day

(Continued)

Neomycin *(Continued)*

Diarrhea caused by enteropathogenic *E. coli*: 50 mg/kg/day divided every 6 hours for 2-3 days

Children and Adults: Topical: Apply ointment 1-3 times/day; topical solutions containing 0.1% to 1% neomycin have been used for irrigation

Adults: Oral: 500-2000 mg every 6-8 hours

Preoperative bowel antisepsis: 1 g each hour for 4 doses then 1 g every 4 hours for 5 doses; or 1 g at 1 PM, 2 PM, and 11 PM with oral erythromycin on day preceding surgery as an adjunct to mechanical cleansing of the bowel; or 6 g/day divided every 4 hours for 2-3 days

Hepatic coma: 4-12 g/day divided every 4-6 hours

Diarrhea caused by enteropathogenic *E. coli*: 3 g/day divided every 6 hours

Monitoring Parameters Renal function tests

Patient Information Notify physician if ringing in the ears, hearing impairment, or dizziness occurs

Dosage Forms

Cream, as sulfate: 0.5% (15 g)

Ointment, topical, as sulfate: 0.5% (15 g, 30 g, 120 g)

Powder, micronized, as sulfate: For prescription compounding

Solution, oral, as sulfate: 125 mg/5 mL (480 mL)

Tablet, as sulfate: 500 mg

References

Feigin RD and Cherry JD, *Textbook of Pediatric Infectious Diseases*, 4th ed, Philadelphia, PA: WB Saunders Co, 1997.

Neomycin and Polymyxin B (nee oh MYE sin & pol i MIKS in bee)

Brand Names Neosporin® Cream [OTC]; Neosporin® G.U. Irrigant

Available Salts Neomycin Sulfate and Polymyxin B Sulfate

Synonyms Polymyxin B and Neomycin

Therapeutic Category Antibiotic, Topical; Antibiotic, Urinary Irrigation; Genitourinary Irrigant

Generic Available Yes

Use Short-term use as a continuous irrigant or rinse in the urinary bladder to prevent bacteriuria and gram-negative rod septicemia associated with the use of indwelling catheters; to help prevent infection in minor cuts, scrapes, and burns

Pregnancy Risk Factor C (D if used as GU irrigant)

Contraindications Hypersensitivity to neomycin, polymyxin B, or any component; ophthalmic use; irrigation should be avoided in patients with defects in the bladder mucosa or wall

Warnings Topical neomycin is a contact sensitizer

Precautions Use with caution in patients with impaired renal function, dehydrated patients, burn patients, and patients receiving a high dose for prolonged treatment; use topical cream with caution in infants with diaper rash involving large area of abraded skin

Adverse Reactions

Dermatologic: Contact dermatitis, erythema, rash, urticaria

Genitourinary: Bladder irritation

Local: Burning

Neuromuscular & skeletal: Neuromuscular blockade

Otic: Ototoxicity

Renal: Nephrotoxicity

Stability Store irrigant solution in the refrigerator

Mechanism of Action Neomycin inhibits bacterial protein synthesis by binding to the 30S ribosomal subunits; polymyxin B interacts with phospholipid components in the cytoplasmic membranes of susceptible bacteria disrupting the osmotic integrity of the cell membrane

Pharmacokinetics Absorption: Not absorbed following topical application to intact skin; absorbed through denuded or abraded skin, peritoneum, wounds, or ulcers

Usual Dosage Children and Adults:

Bladder irrigation: 1 mL is added to 1 L of NS with administration rate adjusted to patient's urine output; usually administered via a 3-way catheter (approximately 40 mL/hour); continuous irrigation or rinse of the urinary bladder should not exceed 10 days

Topical: Apply cream 1-4 times/day

Administration

Bladder irrigant: Do not inject irrigant solution; concentrated irrigant solution must be diluted in 1 liter NS before administration; connect irrigation container to the inflow lumen of a 3-way catheter to permit continuous irrigation of the urinary bladder

Topical: Apply a thin layer to the cleansed, dry affected area; may cover with a sterile bandage

Monitoring Parameters Urinalysis

Patient Information Notify physician if condition worsens or if rash/irritation develops

Additional Information GU irrigant contains methylparaben

Dosage Forms

Cream: Neomycin sulfate 3.5 mg and polymyxin B sulfate 10,000 units per g (0.94 g, 15 g)

Solution, GU irrigant: Neomycin sulfate 40 mg and polymyxin B sulfate 200,000 units per mL (1 mL, 20 mL)

Neomycin, (Bacitracin) Polymyxin B, and Hydrocortisone

(nee oh MYE sin, bas i TRAY sin, pol i MIKS in bee, & hye droe KOR ti sone)

Brand Names AK-Spore H.C.® Otic; AntibiOtic® Otic; Bacticort® Otic; Cortatrigen® Otic; Cortisporin® Ophthalmic Suspension; Cortisporin® Otic; Cortisporin® Topical Cream; Drotic® Otic; LazerSporin-C® Otic; Octicair® Otic; Ocutricin® HC Otic; Otocort® Otic; Otomycin-HPN® Otic; Otosporin® Otic; PediOtic® Otic

Available Salts Neomycin Sulfate, (Bacitracin) Polymyxin B Sulfate, and Hydrocortisone

Synonyms Bacitracin, Neomycin, Polymyxin B, and Hydrocortisone; Hydrocortisone, Neomycin, (Bacitracin), and Polymyxin B; Polymyxin B, Neomycin, (Bacitracin), and Hydrocortisone

Therapeutic Category Antibacterial, Otic; Antibiotic, Ophthalmic; Antibiotic, Otic; Antibiotic, Topical; Corticosteroid, Ophthalmic; Corticosteroid, Otic; Corticosteroid, Topical

Generic Available Yes

Use Steroid-responsive inflammatory condition for which a corticosteroid is indicated and where bacterial infection or a risk of bacterial infection exists

Pregnancy Risk Factor C

Contraindications Hypersensitivity to hydrocortisone, polymyxin B sulfate, bacitracin, neomycin sulfate, or any component; in herpes simplex, vaccinia and varicella; otic use: perforated tympanic membrane

Warnings Neomycin may cause cutaneous and conjunctival sensitization; children are more susceptible to topical corticosteroid-induced hypothalamic pituitary-adrenal axis suppression and Cushing's syndrome

Precautions Use with caution in patients with chronic otitis media and when the integrity of the tympanic membrane is in question

Adverse Reactions

Dermatologic: Contact dermatitis

Local: Itching, pain, stinging, burning, local edema

Ocular: Elevation of intraocular pressure, glaucoma, cataracts, conjunctival erythema

Otic: Ototoxicity

Miscellaneous: Sensitization to neomycin, secondary infections

Usual Dosage

Children: Otic: Solution and suspension: 3 drops into affected ear 3-4 times/day

Adults: Otic: Solution and suspension: 4 drops into affected ear 3-4 times/day

Children and Adults:

Topical ointment: Apply thin layer to affected area 2-4 times/day

Ophthalmic:

Ointment: Apply ½" ribbon to inside of lower lid every 3-4 hours until improvement occurs then 1-3 times/day

Suspension: Instill 1-2 drops in the affected eye every 3-4 hours

Administration

Ophthalmic: Avoid contamination of the tip of the eye dropper or ointment tube

Otic: Drops can be instilled directly into the affected ear, or a cotton wick may be saturated with suspension and inserted in ear canal. Keep wick moist with suspension every 4 hours; wick should be replaced every 24 hours.

Topical: Apply a thin layer to the cleansed, dry affected area; may cover with a sterile bandage

Patient Information Ophthalmic: May cause sensitivity to bright light; may cause temporary blurring of vision or stinging following administration

(Continued)

Neomycin, (Bacitracin) Polymyxin B, and Hydrocortisone *(Continued)*

Additional Information Otic **suspension** is the preferred otic preparation; otic **suspension** can be used for the treatment of infections of mastoidectomy and fenestration cavities caused by susceptible organisms; otic **solution** is used **only** for superficial infections of the external auditory canal (ie, swimmer's ear)

Dosage Forms

Ointment: Neomycin sulfate 5 mg, bacitracin 400 units, polymyxin B sulfate 5000 units and hydrocortisone 10 mg per g (15 g)

Ointment, ophthalmic: Neomycin sulfate 5 mg, bacitracin 400 units, polymyxin B sulfate and hydrocortisone 10 mg per g (3.5 g)

Solution, otic: Neomycin sulfate 5 mg, polymyxin B sulfate 10,000 units, and hydrocortisone 10 mg per mL (10 mL)

Suspension:

Ophthalmic: Neomycin sulfate 5 mg, polymyxin B sulfate 10,000 units and hydrocortisone 10 mg per mL (7.5 mL)

Otic: Neomycin sulfate 5 mg, polymyxin B sulfate 10,000 units and hydrocortisone 10 mg per mL (10 mL)

♦ **Neomycin, Dexamethasone, and Polymyxin B Polymyxin B, Dexamethasone, and Neomycin** *see Dexamethasone, Neomycin, and Polymyxin B on page 297*

Neomycin, Polymyxin B, and Bacitracin

(nee oh MYE sin, pol i MIKS in bee, & bas i TRAY sin)

Brand Names AK-Spore® Ophthalmic Ointment; Medi-Quick® Topical Ointment [OTC]; Mycitracin® Topical [OTC]; Neomixin® Topical; Neosporin® Ophthalmic Ointment; Neosporin® Topical Ointment [OTC]; Neotopic® (Canada); Ocutricin® Topical Ointment; Septa® Topical Ointment [OTC]; Triple Antibiotic® Topical

Available Salts Neomycin Sulfate, Polymyxin B Sulfate, and Bacitracin Zinc

Synonyms Bacitracin. Neomycin, and Polymyxin B; Polymyxin B, Neomycin, and Bacitracin

Therapeutic Category Antibiotic, Ophthalmic; Antibiotic, Topical

Generic Available Yes

Use Help prevent infection in minor cuts, scrapes and burns; short-term treatment of superficial external ocular infections caused by susceptible organisms

Pregnancy Risk Factor C

Contraindications Hypersensitivity to neomycin, polymyxin B, zinc bacitracin, or any component

Warnings Symptoms of neomycin sensitization include itching, reddening, edema, failure to heal; ophthalmic ointments may retard corneal healing

Precautions Prolonged use may result in overgrowth of nonsusceptible organisms

Adverse Reactions

Local: Rash and hypersensitivity reactions ranging from generalized itching, local edema, and erythema have been reported

Ocular: Conjunctival sensitization

Usual Dosage Children and Adults:

Ophthalmic ointment: Instill into the conjunctival sac 1 or more times daily every 3-4 hours for 7-10 days

Topical: Apply 1-3 times/day

Administration

Ophthalmic: Avoid contamination of the tip of the ointment tube

Topical: Apply a thin layer to the cleansed affected area; may cover with a sterile bandage

Patient Information Ophthalmic: May cause sensitivity to bright light; may cause temporary blurring of vision or stinging following administration

Dosage Forms Ointment:

Ophthalmic: Bacitracin 400 units, neomycin sulfate 3.5 mg, and polymyxin B sulfate 10,000 units per g (3.5 g)

Topical: Bacitracin 400 units, neomycin sulfate 3.5 mg, and polymyxin B sulfate 5000 units per g (0.94 g, 2.4 g, 9.6 g, 14.2 g, 15 g, 28.3 g, 30 g)

Neomycin, Polymyxin B, and Prednisolone

(nee oh MYE sin, pol i MIKS in bee, & pred NIS oh lone)

Brand Names Poly-Pred® Liquifilm®

Available Salts Neomycin Sulfate, Polymyxin B Sulfate, and Prednisolone

Synonyms Polymyxin B, Neomycin, and Prednisolone; Prednisolone, Neomycin, and Polymyxin B

Therapeutic Category Antibiotic, Ophthalmic; Corticosteroid, Ophthalmic

Generic Available Yes

Use Used for steroid-responsive inflammatory ocular condition in which bacterial infection or a risk of bacterial ocular infection exists

Pregnancy Risk Factor C

Contraindications Hypersensitivity to neomycin, polymyxin B, prednisolone, or any component; dendritic keratitis, viral disease of the cornea and conjunctiva, mycobacterial infection of the eye, fungal disease of the ocular structure, or after uncomplicated removal of a corneal foreign body

Warnings Symptoms of neomycin sensitization include itching, reddening, edema, or failure to heal

Precautions Prolonged use may result in overgrowth of nonsusceptible organisms, glaucoma, damage to the optic nerve, defects in visual acuity, and cataract formation

Adverse Reactions
Dermatologic: Cutaneous sensitization, skin rash, delayed wound healing
Ocular: Increased intraocular pressure, glaucoma, optic nerve damage, cataracts, conjunctival sensitization

Usual Dosage Children and Adults:
Ophthalmic: Instill 1-2 drops every 3-4 hours; acute infections may require every 30-minute instillation initially with frequency of administration reduced as the infection is brought under control
To treat the eye lids: Instill 1-2 drops every 3-4 hours, close the eye and rub the excess on the lids and lid margins.

Administration Ophthalmic: Avoid contamination of the dropper tip

Patient Information Ophthalmic: May cause sensitivity to bright light; may cause temporary blurring of vision or stinging following administration

Nursing Implications Shake suspension before using

Dosage Forms Suspension, ophthalmic: Neomycin sulfate 0.35%, polymyxin B sulfate 10,000 units and prednisolone acetate 0.5% per mL (5 mL, 10 mL)

♦ **Neomycin Sulfate** *see* Neomycin *on page 677*

♦ **Neomycin Sulfate and Polymyxin B Sulfate** *see* Neomycin and Polymyxin B *on page 678*

♦ **Neomycin Sulfate, (Bacitracin) Polymyxin B Sulfate, and Hydrocortisone** *see* Neomycin, (Bacitracin) Polymyxin B, and Hydrocortisone *on page 679*

♦ **Neomycin Sulfate, Polymyxin B Sulfate, and Bacitracin Zinc** *see* Neomycin, Polymyxin B, and Bacitracin *on page 680*

♦ **Neomycin Sulfate, Polymyxin B Sulfate, and Prednisolone** *see* Neomycin, Polymyxin B, and Prednisolone *on page 680*

♦ **Neonatal Trace Metals** *see* Trace Metals *on page 940*

♦ **Neopap® [OTC]** *see* Acetaminophen *on page 26*

♦ **Neoral®** *see* Cyclosporine *on page 270*

♦ **Neosar®** *see* Cyclophosphamide *on page 268*

♦ **Neosporin® Cream [OTC]** *see* Neomycin and Polymyxin B *on page 678*

♦ **Neosporin® G.U. Irrigant** *see* Neomycin and Polymyxin B *on page 678*

♦ **Neosporin® Ophthalmic Ointment** *see* Neomycin, Polymyxin B, and Bacitracin *on page 680*

♦ **Neosporin® Topical Ointment [OTC]** *see* Neomycin, Polymyxin B, and Bacitracin *on page 680*

Neostigmine (nee oh STIG meen)

Related Information
Overdose and Toxicology *on page 1191*

Brand Names Prostigmin®

Available Salts Neostigmine Bromide; Neostigmine Methylsulfate

Therapeutic Category Antidote, Neuromuscular Blocking Agent; Cholinergic Agent; Diagnostic Agent, Myasthenia Gravis

Generic Available Yes

Use Treatment of myasthenia gravis; prevention and treatment of postoperative bladder distention and urinary retention; reversal of the effects of nondepolarizing neuromuscular blocking agents after surgery

Pregnancy Risk Factor C

Contraindications Hypersensitivity to neostigmine, bromides, or any component; GI or GU obstruction, peritonitis

Warnings Does **not** antagonize, and may prolong the phase I block of depolarizing muscle relaxants (eg, succinylcholine); adequate facilities should be available for
(Continued)

Neostigmine *(Continued)*

cardiopulmonary resuscitation when testing and adjusting dose for myasthenia gravis; have atropine and epinephrine ready to treat hypersensitivity reactions; anticholinesterase insensitivity can develop for brief or prolonged periods

Precautions Use with caution in patients with epilepsy, asthma, bradycardia, hyperthyroidism, cardiac arrhythmias, peptic ulcer, vagotonia, or recent coronary occlusion

Adverse Reactions

Cardiovascular: Bradycardia, hypotension, asystole, A-V block, nodal rhythms, flushing, syncope

Central nervous system: Restlessness, agitation, seizures, dysphonia, dizziness, drowsiness, headache

Dermatologic: Rash, urticaria

Gastrointestinal: Hyperperistalsis, nausea, vomiting, diarrhea, dysphagia, flatulence, abdominal cramps; increased salivary, gastric, and intestinal secretions

Genitourinary: Urinary frequency and incontinence

Local: Thrombophlebitis

Neuromuscular & skeletal: Weakness, muscle cramps, arthralgia, tremor, dysarthria

Ocular: Miosis, lacrimation, diplopia, conjunctival hyperemia

Respiratory: Bronchoconstriction, increased secretions, laryngospasm, dyspnea, respiratory arrest, bronchospasm, respiratory paralysis

Miscellaneous: Allergic reactions, diaphoresis

Drug Interactions Antagonizes effects of nondepolarizing muscle relaxants (eg, pancuronium, tubocurarine); atropine and magnesium antagonize the muscarinic effects of neostigmine; corticosteroids may decrease neostigmine effects; prolongs effects of depolarizing muscle relaxants (eg, succinylcholine)

Mechanism of Action Competitively inhibits the hydrolysis of acetylcholine by acetylcholinesterase facilitating transmission of impulses across the myoneural junction and producing cholinergic activity

Pharmacodynamics

Onset of action:

Oral: 45-75 minutes

I.M.: Within 20-30 minutes

I.V.: Within 1-20 minutes

Duration:

Oral: 2-4 hours

I.M.: 2-4 hours

I.V.: 1-2 hours

Pharmacokinetics

Absorption: Oral: Poor (~1% to 2%)

Metabolism: In the liver

Half-life: 0.5-2.1 hours

Elimination: 50% excreted renally as unchanged drug

Usual Dosage

Myasthenia gravis:

Diagnosis: I.M. (all cholinesterase medications should be discontinued at least 8 hours before; atropine should be administered I.V. immediately prior to or I.M. 30 minutes before neostigmine):

Children: 0.025-0.04 mg/kg as a single dose

Adults: 0.022 mg/kg as a single dose

Treatment (dosage requirements are variable; adjust dosage so patient takes larger doses at times of greatest fatigue):

Children:

Oral: 0.333 mg/kg/dose or 10 mg/m^2/dose 6 times/day

I.M., I.V., S.C.: 0.01-0.04 mg/kg every 2-4 hours

Adults:

Oral: Initial: 15 mg/dose 3 times/day, gradually increase every 1-2 days; usual daily range: 15-375 mg

I.M., I.V., S.C.: 0.5-2.5 mg every 1-3 hours up to 10 mg/24 hours maximum

Reversal of nondepolarizing neuromuscular blockade after surgery in conjunction with atropine or glycopyrrolate: I.V.:

Infants: 0.025-0.1 mg/kg/dose

Children: 0.025-0.08 mg/kg/dose

Adults: 0.5-2 mg; total dose not to exceed 5 mg

Bladder atony: Adults: I.M., S.C.:

Prevention: 0.25 mg every 4-6 hours for 2-3 days

Treatment: 0.5-1 mg every 3 hours for 5 doses after bladder has emptied

Dosing adjustment in renal impairment:
Cl_{cr} 10-50 mL/minute: Administer 50% of normal dose
Cl_{cr} <10 mL/minute: Administer 25% of normal dose

Administration
Parenteral: May be administered undiluted by slow I.V. injection over several minutes; may be administered I.M. or S.C.
Oral: Divide dosages so patient receives larger doses at times of greatest fatigue; may be administered with or without food

Monitoring Parameters Muscle strength, heart rate, respiratory rate

Patient Information The side effects are generally due to exaggerated pharmacologic effects; the most common side effects are salivation and muscle fasciculations; notify physician if nausea, vomiting, muscle weakness, severe abdominal pain, or difficulty breathing occurs

Dosage Forms
Injection, as methylsulfate: 0.25 mg/mL (1 mL); 0.5 mg/mL (1 mL, 10 mL); 1 mg/mL (10 mL)
Tablet, as bromide: 15 mg

- **Neostigmine Bromide** see Neostigmine on page 681
- **Neostigmine Methylsulfate** see Neostigmine on page 681
- **Neo-Synephrine® 12 Hour Nasal Solution [OTC]** see Oxymetazoline on page 718
- **Neo-Synephrine® Nasal Solution [OTC]** see Phenylephrine on page 758
- **Neo-Synephrine® Ophthalmic Solution** see Phenylephrine on page 758
- **Neo-Tabs®** see Neomycin on page 677
- **Neotopic® (Canada)** see Neomycin, Polymyxin B, and Bacitracin on page 680
- **Neotrace-4®** see Trace Metals on page 940
- **Nephro-Calci® [OTC]** see Calcium Supplements on page 157
- **Nephrocaps®** see page 1034
- **Nephro-Fer™ [OTC]** see Iron Supplements, Oral/Enteral on page 530
- **Nephronex® (Canada)** see Nitrofurantoin on page 689
- **Nephrovite** see page 1034
- **Nervocaine® Injection** see Lidocaine on page 568
- **Nestrex®** see Pyridoxine on page 827
- **Neucalm-50® Injection** see Hydroxyzine on page 496
- **Neupogen®** see Filgrastim on page 411
- **Neurontin®** see Gabapentin on page 448
- **Neut® Injection** see Sodium Bicarbonate on page 870
- **Neutra-Phos®-K** see Phosphate Supplements on page 765
- **Neutrogena® Acne Mask [OTC]** see Benzoyl Peroxide on page 126
- **Neutrogena® T/Derm** see Coal Tar on page 247

Nevirapine (ne VYE ra peen)

Related Information
Adult and Adolescent HIV on page 1133
Pediatric HIV on page 1129

Brand Names Viramune®

Therapeutic Category Antiretroviral Agent; HIV Agents (Anti-HIV Agents); Non-nucleoside Reverse Transcriptase Inhibitor (NNRTI)

Generic Available No

Use Treatment of HIV infection in combination with other antiretroviral agents. **(Note:** Current preferred HIV regimens consist of **three** antiretroviral agents)

Pregnancy Risk Factor C

Contraindications Hypersensitivity to nevirapine or any component

Warnings Severe and life-threatening skin reactions (eg, Stevens-Johnson syndrome) have occurred in patients receiving nevirapine. Discontinue nevirapine in patients who develop a severe rash or rash accompanied by fever, blistering, oral lesions, conjunctivitis, swelling, muscle or joint aches, or malaise. Majority of skin reactions occur within the first 6 weeks of therapy. Initiating therapy at a lower dose for the first 14 days of therapy has been shown to reduce the frequency of rash. Nevirapine induces hepatic cytochrome P-450 3A and has the potential for interacting with numerous drugs; drugs having suspected interactions and that should only be used with careful monitoring include rifampin, rifabutin, triazolam, midazolam, oral contraceptives, oral anticoagulants, digoxin, phenytoin, and theophylline.
(Continued)

Nevirapine *(Continued)*

Precautions Use caution in patients with either renal or hepatic dysfunction; discontinue therapy in patients experiencing liver function test abnormalities until tests return to baseline values; permanently discontinue therapy if liver function abnormalities recur on rechallenge

Adverse Reactions

Central nervous system: Headache, fever, sedation

Dermatologic: Rash (usually maculopapular erythematous cutaneous eruptions with or without pruritus, located on the trunk, face, and extremities; 19% of pediatric patients developed rash), Stevens-Johnson syndrome (see Warnings)

Gastrointestinal: Nausea, diarrhea

Hepatic: Elevated liver enzymes, hepatitis (rare)

Neuromuscular & skeletal: Myalgia

Drug Interactions Cimetidine, macrolides increase nevirapine plasma concentrations; rifabutin, rifampin decrease nevirapine plasma concentrations; nevirapine decreases indinavir and saquinavir concentrations; may decrease plasma concentration of ritonavir; decreases hormonal contraceptive efficacy; decreases metabolism of triazolam, midazolam, oral anticoagulants, digoxin, phenytoin, theophylline

Stability Store at room temperature

Mechanism of Action A non-nucleoside reverse transcriptase inhibitor which specifically binds to HIV-1 reverse transcriptase blocking the RNA-dependent and DNA-dependent DNA polymerase activity and disrupting the virus' life cycle. Nevirapine does not inhibit HIV-2 reverse transcriptase or human DNA polymerase.

Pharmacokinetics

Absorption: Rapid and readily absorbed

Distribution: V_d: 1.21 L/kg; widely distributed; crosses the placenta; excreted in breast milk; 45% of the plasma concentration in CSF

Metabolism: Metabolized by cytochrome P-450 isozymes from the CYP3A family to hydroxylated metabolites; autoinduction of metabolism occurs in 2-4 weeks with a 1.5-2 times increase in clearance; nevirapine is more rapidly metabolized in pediatric patients than in adults

Protein binding, plasma: 60%

Bioavailability: 91% to 93%

Half-life: Single dose (45 hours); multiple dosing (25-30 hours)

Time to peak serum concentration: 4 hours

Elimination: 81.3% in urine as metabolites, 10.1% in feces; <3% of the total dose is eliminated in urine as parent drug

Usual Dosage Oral:

Neonates to 3 months (Investigational, under study in PACTG 356): 5 mg/kg/dose once daily for 14 days, followed by 120 mg/m^2/dose every 12 hours for 14 days, followed by 200 mg/m^2/dose every 12 hours

Children 2 months to 8 years: Initial: 4 mg/kg/dose once daily for 14 days; increase dose to every 12 hours if no rash or other adverse effects occur; maintenance dose: 7 mg/kg/dose every 12 hours; maximum dose: 200 mg/dose every 12 hours

Children ≥8 years: Initial: 4 mg/kg/dose once daily for 14 days; increase dose to 4 mg/kg/dose every 12 hours if no rash or other adverse effects occur; maximum dose: 200 mg/dose every 12 hours

Adolescents and Adults: Initial: 200 mg/dose once daily for the first 14 days; increase to full dose if no rash or other adverse effects occur; maintenance dose: 200 mg every 12 hours

Administration Oral: May be administered with or without food; may be administered with an antacid or didanosine; shake suspension gently prior to administration

Monitoring Parameters Clinical chemistry tests including liver function tests, CD4 cell count, plasma levels of HIV RNA

Patient Information Inform physician immediately of any rash; use an alternative method of contraception from birth control pills during nevirapine therapy; if a dose is missed, take the next dose as soon as possible, however, if a dose is skipped, do not double the next dose

Dosage Forms

Suspension, oral: 10 mg/mL

Tablet: 200 mg

References

D'Aquila RT, Hughes MD, Johnson VA, et al, "Nevirapine, Zidovudine, and Didanosine Compared With Zidovudine and Didanosine in Patients With HIV-1 Infection. A Randomized, Double-Blind, Placebo-

Controlled Trial. National Institute of Allergy and Infectious Diseases AIDS Clinical Trials Group Protocol 241 Investigators," *Ann Intern Med*, 1996, 124(12):1019-30.

Mueller BU, Sei S, Anderson B, et al, "Comparison of Virus Burden in Blood and Sequential Lymph Node Biopsy Specimens From Children Infected With Human Immunodeficiency Virus," *J Pediatr*, 1996, 129(3):410-8.

Working Group on Antiretroviral Therapy and Medical Management of HIV-Infected Children, "Guidelines for the Use of Antiretroviral Agents in Pediatric HIV Infection," March 1, 1999, http://www.hivatis.org.

♦ **NH₄Cl** *see* Ammonium Chloride *on page 69*

♦ **Niacels™ [OTC]** *see* Niacin *on page 685*

Niacin (NYE a sin)

Brand Names Niacels™ [OTC]; Niaspan®; Nicobid® [OTC]; Nicolar® [OTC]; Nicotinex [OTC]; Slo-Niacin® [OTC]

Synonyms Nicotinic Acid; Vitamin B₃

Therapeutic Category Antilipemic Agent; Nutritional Supplement; Vitamin, Water Soluble

Generic Available Yes

Use Adjunctive treatment of hyperlipidemias; peripheral vascular disease and circulatory disorders; treatment of pellagra; dietary supplement

Pregnancy Risk Factor A (C if used in doses greater than RDA suggested doses)

Contraindications Liver disease, peptic ulcer, severe hypotension, arterial hemorrhaging; hypersensitivity to niacin or any component; GERD (relative contraindication)

Warnings Hepatotoxicity may occur and may be more common if extended release product is substituted for immediate release product at same dosage; some products may contain tartrazine

Precautions May elevate uric acid levels, use with caution in patients predisposed to gout; large doses should be administered with caution to patients with gallbladder disease, jaundice, liver disease, diabetes, or renal dysfunction

Adverse Reactions
Cardiovascular: Flushing, hypotension, tachycardia, syncope, vasovagal attacks
Central nervous system: Dizziness, headache
Dermatologic: Pruritus, increased sebaceous gland activity, tingling skin, burning, acanthosis nigricans (reversible)
Endocrine & metabolic: Hyperuricemia, hyperglycemia
Gastrointestinal: GI upset, nausea, vomiting, heartburn, diarrhea, anorexia
Hepatic: Abnormal liver function tests, jaundice, chronic liver damage, hepatitis
Ocular: Blurred vision

Drug Interactions May inhibit uricosuric effects of sulfinpyrazone and probenecid; adrenergic blocking agents may cause additive vasodilating effect and postural hypotension; use with lipid-lowering agents will enhance anti-lipid effects

Mechanism of Action Component of two coenzymes necessary for tissue respiration, lipid metabolism, and glycogenolysis; inhibits the synthesis of very low density lipoproteins

Pharmacodynamics Vasodilation:
Onset of action: Within 20 minutes
Extended release: Within 1 hour
Duration: 20-60 minutes
Extended release: 8-10 hours

Pharmacokinetics
Distribution: Crosses into breast milk
Metabolism: Niacin in smaller doses is converted to niacinamide which is metabolized in the liver
Half-life: 45 minutes
Elimination: In urine, with ~33% as unchanged drug; with larger doses, a greater percentage is excreted unchanged in urine

Usual Dosage Oral (preferred), I.M., I.V., S.C. (**Note:** Parenteral routes of administration are for treatment of vitamin deficiencies only, not for hyperlipidemia)

Children:
Hyperlipidemia: Initial: 100-250 mg/day (maximum dose: 10 mg/kg/day) in 3 divided doses with meals; increase weekly by 100 mg/day or increase every 2-3 weeks by 250 mg/day as tolerated; evaluate efficacy and adverse effects with laboratory tests at 20 mg/kg/day or 1000 mg/day (whichever is less); continue to increase if needed and as tolerated; re-evaluate at each 500 mg increment; doses up to 2250 mg/day have been used; **Note:** Routine use in children and adolescents is not recommended due to limited safety and efficacy information
Pellagra: 50-100 mg/dose 3 times/day
(Continued)

Niacin *(Continued)*

Recommended daily allowances:
  0-0.5 years: 5 mg/day
  0.5-1 year: 6 mg/day
  1-3 years: 9 mg/day
  4-6 years: 12 mg/day
  7-10 years: 13 mg/day
  Male:
    11-14 years: 17 mg/day
    15-18 years: 20 mg/day
    19-24 years: 19 mg/day
  Female: 11-24 years: 15 mg/day

Adults:
  Hyperlipidemia:
    Immediate release products: Initial: 50-100 mg twice daily for 1 week; increase slowly over 1 month (by doubling daily dose every week) to 1-1.5 g/day divided in 2-3 doses; assess therapy at 4 and 8 weeks of therapy; if needed, dose may be increased slowly to 3 g/day or until desired result is attained; maximum dose: 3 g/day in 3 divided doses; **Note:** Some patients may require a slower dose titration
    Extended release products: Initial: 500 mg/day divided in 2 doses for 1 week; increase to 500 mg twice daily for 3 weeks; if needed, dose may be increased to 2 g/day or until desired result is attained; maximum dose: 2 g/day

  Niacin deficiency: 10-20 mg/day, maximum dose: 100 mg/day
  Pellagra: 50-100 mg 3-4 times/day, maximum dose: 500 mg/day
  Recommended daily allowances:
    Male:
      25-50 years: 19 mg/day
      >51 years: 15 mg/day
    Female:
      25-50 years: 15 mg/day
      >51 years: 13 mg/day

Administration

Oral: Administer with food or milk to decrease GI upset; swallow timed release tablet and capsule whole; do not chew or crush; to minimize flushing, administer dose at bedtime, take aspirin (adults: 325 mg) 30 minutes before niacin, and avoid alcohol or hot drinks around the time of administration

Parenteral: I.V.: Slow I.V. injection

Monitoring Parameters Blood glucose; serum uric acid, periodic liver function tests (with large doses or prolonged therapy); Treatment of hyperlipidemias: Baseline: Liver enzymes, uric acid, fasting glucose, and minimum of 2 fasting lipid profiles; repeat 4-6 weeks after dose is stabilized; once LDL-C goal is reached, repeat every 2-3 months for first year and then every 6-12 months if no sign of toxicity develops and dose remains stable

Test Interactions False elevations in some fluorometric determinations of urinary catecholamines; false-positive urine glucose (Benedict's reagent)

Patient Information Transient flushing of the skin and a sensation of warmth (especially of face and upper body), itching, tingling or headache may occur; if dizziness occurs, avoid sudden changes in posture and notify physician; notify physician if taking vitamins or other products that contain niacin or nicotinamide; do not change brands once dosage is stabilized; report signs and symptoms of hepatotoxicity (nausea, vomiting, loss of appetite, yellow skin, dark urine, general feeling of weakness) to physician

Additional Information Discontinue use if liver enzymes increase to ≥3 times the upper limit of normal

Dosage Forms

Capsule, timed release: 125 mg, 250 mg, 300 mg, 400 mg, 500 mg
Elixir: 50 mg/5 mL (473 mL, 4000 mL)
Injection: 100 mg/mL (30 mL)
Tablet: 25 mg, 50 mg, 100 mg, 250 mg, 500 mg
Tablet, extended release: 375 mg, 500 mg, 750 mg, 1000 mg
Tablet, timed release: 150 mg, 250 mg, 500 mg, 750 mg

References

"ASHP Therapeutic Position Statement on the Safe Use of Niacin in the Management of Dyslipidemias. American Society of Health-System Pharmacists," *Am J Health Syst Pharm*, 1997, 54(24):2815-9.

Colletti RB, Neufeld EJ, Roff NK, et al, "Niacin Treatment of Hypercholesterolemia in Children," *Pediatrics*, 1993, 92(1):78-82.

Schuna AA, "Safe Use of Niacin," *Am J Health Syst Pharm*, 1997, 54(24):2803.

♦ **Niaspan®** see Niacin on page 685
♦ **N'ice®** see Ascorbic Acid on page 96
♦ **Niclocide®** see Niclosamide on page 687

Niclosamide (ni KLOE sa mide)

Brand Names Niclocide®
Therapeutic Category Anthelmintic
Generic Available No
Use Treatment of *Taenia saginata* (beef tapeworm), *Diphyllobothrium latum* (fish tapeworm), *Dipylidium caninum* (dog and cat tapeworm), and *Hymenolepis nana* (dwarf tapeworm) infections
Pregnancy Risk Factor B
Contraindications Hypersensitivity to niclosamide or any component; treatment of cysticercosis (niclosamide is only active against intestinal cestodes)
Adverse Reactions
　Central nervous system: Drowsiness, dizziness, fever, headache
　Dermatologic: Rash, pruritus, alopecia
　Gastrointestinal: Mild abdominal pain, bloating, nausea, vomiting, diarrhea, anorexia, rectal bleeding, dysgeusia, constipation
　Miscellaneous: Diaphoresis
Stability Protect from light; avoid freezing
Mechanism of Action Inhibits the synthesis of ATP through inhibition of oxidative phosphorylation in the mitochondria of cestodes
Pharmacokinetics
　Absorption: Oral: Unabsorbed from the GI tract
　Elimination: In feces
Usual Dosage Oral:
　Beef and fish tapeworm:
　　Children: 40 mg/kg as a single dose one time; maximum dose: 2 g/dose
　　Adults: 2 g (4 tablets) in a single dose
　　May repeat treatment 7 days later if proglottids and/or eggs are still present in stool
　Dwarf tapeworm:
　　Children: 40 mg/kg/day once every 24 hours for 7 days, maximum dose: 2 g/day
　　Adults: 2 g (4 tablets) in a single dose daily for 7 days
Administration Oral: Administer after a light meal (ie, breakfast); have patient chew tablets thoroughly and swallow with a small amount of water; tablets can be pulverized and mixed with water to form a paste for administration to children
Monitoring Parameters Stool for proglottids and eggs
Nursing Implications Can administer laxative 1-4 hours after the niclosamide dose if treating *Taenia solium* infections to prevent the development of cysticercosis
Dosage Forms Tablet, chewable (vanilla flavor): 500 mg

♦ **Nicobid® [OTC]** see Niacin on page 685
♦ **Nicolar® [OTC]** see Niacin on page 685
♦ **Nicotinex [OTC]** see Niacin on page 685
♦ **Nicotinic Acid** see Niacin on page 685
♦ **Nico-Vert® [OTC]** see Meclizine on page 597
♦ **Nidagel™ (Canada)** see Metronidazole on page 636

Nifedipine (nye FED i peen)

Brand Names Adalat®; Adalat® CC; Adalat PA® (Canada); Apo®-Nifed (Canada); Gen-Nifedipine (Canada); Novo-Nifedin® (Canada); Nu-Nifedin® (Canada); Procardia®; Procardia XL®
Therapeutic Category Antianginal Agent; Antihypertensive Agent; Calcium Channel Blocker
Generic Available Yes, except sustained-release tablet
Use Angina, hypertrophic cardiomyopathy, hypertension
Pregnancy Risk Factor C
Contraindications Hypersensitivity to nifedipine or any component
Precautions May increase frequency, duration, and severity of angina during initiation of therapy; use with caution in patients with CHF or aortic stenosis (especially with concomitant beta-blocker)
Adverse Reactions
　Cardiovascular: Flushing, hypotension, tachycardia, palpitations, syncope, peripheral edema
　(Continued)

Nifedipine *(Continued)*

Central nervous system: Dizziness, fever, headache, chills
Dermatologic: Dermatitis, urticaria, purpura
Gastrointestinal: Nausea, diarrhea, constipation, gingival hyperplasia
Hematologic: Thrombocytopenia, leukopenia, anemia
Neuromuscular & skeletal: Joint stiffness, arthritis with increased ANA
Ocular: Blurred vision, transient blindness
Respiratory: Shortness of breath
Miscellaneous: Diaphoresis

Drug Interactions Cytochrome P-450 isoenzyme CYP3A3/4 and CYP3A5-7 substrate

Beta-blockers may increase cardiovascular adverse effects; anesthetic doses of fentanyl may cause hypotension; cimetidine may increase nifedipine serum concentration; nifedipine may increase phenytoin, cyclosporine, and possibly digoxin serum concentrations; combined use of nifedipine with cyclosporine may significantly increase gingival hyperplasia; delavirdine may decrease the metabolism of nifedipine and increase nifedipine levels; concurrent use of delavirdine and nifedipine is not recommended; saquinavir may increase nifedipine levels

Food Interactions Capsule is rapidly absorbed orally if it is administered without food but may result in vasodilator side effects; administration with low-fat meals may decrease flushing; grapefruit juice may increase the oral bioavailability of nifedipine tablets; food may decrease the rate but not the extent of absorption of Procardia XL®

Mechanism of Action Inhibits calcium ion from entering the "slow channels" or select voltage-sensitive areas of vascular smooth muscle and myocardium during depolarization, producing a relaxation of coronary vascular smooth muscle and coronary vasodilation; increases myocardial oxygen delivery in patients with vasospastic angina

Pharmacodynamics
Onset:
S.L. or "bite and swallow": Within 1-5 minutes
Oral: Within 20-30 minutes
Duration: 4-6 hours

Pharmacokinetics
Protein-binding: 92% to 98% (concentration-dependent)
Metabolism: In the liver to inactive metabolites
Bioavailability:
Capsules: 45% to 75%
Sustained release: 65% to 86%
Half-life:
Normal adults: 2-5 hours
Cirrhosis: 7 hours
Elimination: In urine

Usual Dosage Oral, S.L. or "bite and swallow" (eg, patient bites capsule to release liquid contents and then swallows): **Note:** Doses are usually titrated upward at 7- to 14-day intervals; may increase every 3 days if clinically necessary:

Children:
Hypertensive emergencies: 0.25-0.5 mg/kg/dose; maximum dose: 10 mg/dose; may repeat if needed every 4-6 hours; monitor carefully; maximum dose: 1-2 mg/kg/day
Hypertrophic cardiomyopathy: 0.6-0.9 mg/kg/24 hours in 3-4 divided doses
Adolescents and Adults: Initial: 10 mg 3 times/day (capsules) or 30-60 mg once daily (sustained release tablet); maintenance: 10-30 mg 3-4 times/day (capsules); maximum dose: 180 mg/24 hours (capsules) or 120 mg/day (sustained release)

Administration Oral: Administer with food; do not administer with grapefruit juice; swallow sustained release tablets whole, do not crush, break, or chew; liquid-filled capsule may be punctured and drug solution administered sublingually or orally; when measuring smaller doses from the liquid-filled capsules, consider the following concentrations (for Adalat® and Procardia®) 10 mg capsule = 10 mg/0.34 mL; 20 mg capsule = 20 mg/0.45 mL

Note: When nifedipine is administered sublingually, only a small amount is absorbed sublingually; the observed effects are actually due to swallowing of the drug with subsequent rapid oral absorption

Monitoring Parameters Blood pressure

Patient Information Avoid alcohol; rise slowly from prolonged sitting or lying position

Dosage Forms

Capsule, liquid-filled (Adalat®, Procardia®): 10 mg, 20 mg

Tablet, extended release (Adalat® CC): 30 mg, 60 mg, 90 mg

Tablet, sustained release (Procardia XL®): 30 mg, 60 mg, 90 mg

References

Dilmen U, Çağlar MK, Senses A, et al, "Nifedipine in Hypertensive Emergencies of Children," *Am J Dis Child*, 1983, 137(12):1162-5.

Lopez-Herce J, Albajara L, Cagigas P, et al, "Treatment of Hypertensive Crisis in Children With Nifedipine," *Intensive Care Med*, 1988, 14(5):519-21.

Rosen WJ and Johnson CE, "Evaluation of Five Procedures for Measuring Nonstandard Doses of Nifedipine Liquid," *Am J Hosp Pharm*, 1989, 46(11):2313-7.

♦ **Niferex®** *see* Iron Supplements, Oral/Enteral *on page 530*

♦ **Niferex® 150** *see* Iron Supplements, Oral/Enteral *on page 530*

♦ **Nilstat®** *see* Nystatin *on page 701*

♦ **Nimbex®** *see* Cisatracurium *on page 228*

♦ **Nitro-Bid® I.V. Injection** *see* Nitroglycerin *on page 690*

♦ **Nitro-Bid® Ointment** *see* Nitroglycerin *on page 690*

♦ **Nitrodisc® Patch** *see* Nitroglycerin *on page 690*

♦ **Nitro-Dur® Patch** *see* Nitroglycerin *on page 690*

♦ **Nitroferricyanide** *see* Nitroprusside *on page 692*

Nitrofurantoin (nye troe fyoor AN toyn)

Related Information

Carbohydrate and Alcohol Content of Liquid Medications for Use in Patients Receiving Ketogenic Diets *on page 1228*

Brand Names Apo®-Nitrofurantoin (Canada); Furadantin®; Furalan®; Furan®; Furanite®; Macrobid®; Macrodantin®; Nephronex® (Canada); Novo-Furan® (Canada)

Therapeutic Category Antibiotic, Miscellaneous

Generic Available Yes: Tablet and suspension

Use Prevention and treatment of urinary tract infections caused by susceptible gram-negative and some gram-positive organisms including *E. coli*, *Klebsiella*, *Enterobacter*, enterococci, and *S. aureus*; *Pseudomonas*, *Serratia*, and most species of *Proteus* are generally resistant to nitrofurantoin

Pregnancy Risk Factor B; contraindicated in pregnant women at term and during labor (due to possible hemolytic anemia in the neonate)

Contraindications Hypersensitivity to nitrofurantoin or any component; renal impairment; infants <1 month of age (due to the possibility of hemolytic anemia); pregnant patients at term; should not be used to treat UTI in febrile infants and young children in whom renal involvement is likely

Warnings Therapeutic concentrations of nitrofurantoin are not attained in the urine of patients with renal insufficiency (Cl_{cr} <40 mL/minute, anuria, or oliguria)

Precautions Use with caution in patients with G-6-PD deficiency, patients with anemia, vitamin B deficiency, diabetes mellitus, or electrolyte abnormalities

Adverse Reactions

Central nervous system: Dizziness, headache, chills, fever

Dermatologic: Rash, exfoliative dermatitis, urticaria

Gastrointestinal: Nausea, vomiting, anorexia, pancreatitis

Genitourinary: Discoloration of urine (dark yellow or brown)

Hematologic: Hemolytic anemia, eosinophilia, leukopenia, granulocytopenia, thrombocytopenia, megaloblastic anemia

Hepatic: Hepatotoxicity, cholestatic jaundice, hepatitis

Neuromuscular & skeletal: Arthralgia, peripheral neuropathy, muscle weakness

Respiratory: Interstitial pneumonitis and/or fibrosis

Drug Interactions Probenecid decreases renal excretion of nitrofurantoin, antacids decrease extent and rate of absorption of nitrofurantoin; drugs which delay gastric emptying increase the extent of nitrofurantoin absorption

Food Interactions Food increases the total amount absorbed; cranberry juice and other urinary acidifiers may enhance the action of nitrofurantoin; ensure diet is adequate in protein and vitamin B complex

Stability Protect from light

Mechanism of Action Inhibits several bacterial enzyme systems including acetyl coenzyme A; reduced by bacterial enzymes to active intermediates that may alter ribosomal proteins resulting in inhibition of protein, DNA, RNA, and cell wall synthesis

(Continued)

Nitrofurantoin *(Continued)*

Pharmacokinetics

Absorption: Well absorbed from the GI tract; macrocrystalline form is absorbed more slowly due to slower dissolution, but causes less GI distress than formulations containing microcrystals of the drug

Distribution: V_d: 0.8 L/kg; crosses the placenta; appears in breast milk and bile

Protein binding: ~40%

Metabolism: Partially in the liver

Bioavailability: Presence of food increases bioavailability

Half-life: 20-60 minutes and is prolonged with renal impairment

Elimination: As metabolites and unchanged drug (40%) in the urine and small amounts in the bile; renal excretion is via glomerular filtration and tubular secretion

Usual Dosage Oral:

Children: 5-7 mg/kg/day divided every 6 hours; maximum dose: 400 mg/day
  Prophylaxis of UTI: 1-2 mg/kg/day as a single daily dose; maximum dose: 100 mg/day

Adults: 50-100 mg/dose every 6 hours
  Prophylaxis of UTI: 50-100 mg/dose at bedtime

Administration Oral: Administer with food or milk; suspension may be mixed with water, milk, fruit juice, or infant formula

Monitoring Parameters Signs of pulmonary reaction; signs of numbness or tingling of the extremities; periodic liver and renal function tests

Test Interactions Causes false-positive urine glucose with Clinitest®

Patient Information May discolor urine to a dark yellow or brown color; avoid alcohol

Dosage Forms

Capsule: 50 mg, 100 mg
Capsule:
  Extended release: 100 mg
  Macrocrystal: 25 mg, 50 mg, 100 mg
  Macrocrystal/monohydrate: 100 mg
Suspension, oral: 25 mg/5 mL (470 mL)

References

Brendstrup L, Hjelt K, Petersen KE, et al, "Nitrofurantoin Versus Trimethoprim Prophylaxis in Recurrent Urinary Tract Infections in Children," *Acta Paediatr Scand,* 1990, 79(12):1225-34.

Coraggio MJ, Gross TP, and Roscelli JD, "Nitrofurantoin Toxicity in Children," *Pediatr Infect Dis J,* 1989, 8(3):163-6.

"Practice Parameter: The Diagnosis, Treatment, and Evaluation of the Initial Urinary Tract Infection in Febrile Infants and Young Children. American Academy of Pediatrics. Committee on Quality Improvement. Subcommittee on Urinary Tract Infection," *Pediatrics,* 1999, 103(4 Pt 1):843-52.

♦ **Nitrogard® Buccal** *see* Nitroglycerin *on page 690*

♦ **Nitrogen Mustard** *see* Mechlorethamine *on page 595*

Nitroglycerin *(nye troe GLI ser in)*

Related Information

Adult ACLS Algorithm, Hypotension, Shock *on page 1016*

Brand Names Deponit® Patch; Minitran® Patch; Nitro-Bid® I.V. Injection; Nitro-Bid® Ointment; Nitrodisc® Patch; Nitro-Dur® Patch; Nitrogard® Buccal; Nitroglyn® Oral; Nitrolingual® Translingual Spray; Nitrol® Ointment; Nitrong® Oral Tablet; Nitrong® SR (Canada); Nitrostat® Sublingual; Transdermal-NTG® Patch; Transderm-Nitro® Patch; Tridil® Injection

Synonyms Glyceryl Trinitrate; Nitroglycerol; NTG

Therapeutic Category Antianginal Agent; Antihypertensive Agent; Nitrate; Vasodilator; Vasodilator, Coronary

Generic Available Yes

Use Angina pectoris; I.V. for CHF (especially when associated with acute MI); pulmonary hypertension; hypertensive emergencies occurring perioperatively (especially during cardiovascular surgery)

Pregnancy Risk Factor C

Contraindications Hypersensitivity to nitroglycerin, organic nitrates, or any component (including adhesives in transdermal patches); glaucoma; severe anemia; increased ICP; concurrent use with sildenafil (see Drug Interactions); I.V. product is also contraindicated in hypotension, uncontrolled hypokalemia, pericardial tamponade, or constrictive pericarditis

Warnings May cause severe hypotension; use with caution in hypovolemia, hypotension, and right ventricular infarctions; do not chew or swallow sublingual dosage form

NITROGLYCERIN

Adverse Reactions
Cardiovascular: Flushing, hypotension, pallor, reflex tachycardia, cardiovascular collapse; severe hypotension, bradycardia, and acute coronary vascular insufficiency with abrupt withdrawal

Central nervous system: Dizziness, restlessness, headache

Dermatologic: Allergic contact dermatitis, exfoliative dermatitis

Endocrine & metabolic: Alcohol intoxication from one I.V. formulation

Gastrointestinal: Nausea, vomiting

Miscellaneous: Perspiration

Drug Interactions I.V. nitroglycerin may antagonize the anticoagulant effect of heparin, monitor closely, may need to decrease heparin dosage when nitroglycerin is discontinued; alcohol, beta-blockers, calcium channel blockers may enhance nitroglycerin's hypotensive effect; sildenafil may increase vasodilatory effects and result in severe hypotension

Stability Nitroglycerin adsorbs to plastics; I.V. must be prepared in glass bottles and special administration sets intended for nitroglycerin (nonpolyvinyl chloride) must be used; do not mix with other drugs; store sublingual tablets and ointment in tightly closed container; store at 15°C to 30°C

Mechanism of Action Reduces cardiac oxygen demand by decreasing left ventricular end diastolic pressure and systemic vascular resistance; dilates coronary arteries and improves collateral flow to ischemic regions; vasodilates veins more than arteries

Pharmacodynamics Onset and duration of action is dependent upon dosage form administered; see table.

Nitroglycerin*

Dosage Form	Onset (min)	Duration
I.V.	1-2	3-5 min
Sublingual	1-3	30-60 min
Translingual spray	2	30-60 min
Buccal, extended release	2-3	3-5 h
Oral, sustained release	40	4-8 h
Topical ointment	20-60	2-12 h
Transdermal	40-60	18-24 h

*Hemodynamic and antianginal tolerance often develops within 24-48 h of continuous nitrate administration.

Adapted from Corwin S and Reiffel, JA, "Nitrate Therapy for Angina Pectoris," Arch Intern Med, 1985, 145:538-43 and Franciosa JA, "Nitroglycerin and Nitrates in Congestive Heart Failure," Heart and Lung, 1980, 9(5):873-82.

Pharmacokinetics
Protein binding: 60%

Metabolism: Extensive first-pass

Half-life: 1-4 minutes

Elimination: Excretion of inactive metabolites in urine

Usual Dosage Tolerance to the hemodynamic and antianginal effects can develop within 24-48 hours of continuous use

Children: I.V. continuous infusion: Initial: 0.25-0.5 mcg/kg/minute; titrate by 0.5-1 mcg/kg/minute every 3-5 minutes as needed; usual dose: 1-3 mcg/kg/minute; usual maximum dose: 5 mcg/kg/minute; doses up to 20 mcg/kg/minute may be used

Adults:

Oral: 2.5-9 mg every 8-12 hours

I.V. continuous infusion: Initial: 5 mcg/minute, increase by 5 mcg/minute every 3-5 minutes to 20 mcg/minute, then increase as needed by 10 mcg/minute every 3-5 minutes, up to 200 mcg/minute

Sublingual: 0.2-0.6 mg every 5 minutes for maximum of 3 doses in 15 minutes

Ointment: 1" to 2" every 8 hours

Patch, transdermal: Initial: 0.2-0.4 mg/hour, titrate to 0.4-0.8 mg/hour; use a "patch-on" period of 12-14 hours per day and a "patch-off" period of 10-12 hours per day to minimize tolerance

Lingual: 1-2 sprays into mouth onto or under tongue every 3-5 minutes for maximum of 3 sprays in 15 minutes; may administer 5-10 minutes before activities that may precipitate angina

Buccal: Initial: 1 mg every 5 hours while awake (3 times/day); titrate dosage upward if angina occurs with tablet in place

(Continued)

Nitroglycerin *(Continued)*

Administration

Oral:

Buccal tablet: Place in buccal pouch and allow to dissolve; do not swallow, chew, or crush

Lingual spray: Do not shake container; spray onto or under tongue with container as close to mouth as possible; do not inhale spray; avoid swallowing immediately after spray; do not expectorate or rinse mouth for 5-10 minutes after use

Sublingual tablet: Place under tongue and allow to dissolve, do not swallow, chew, or crush; do not eat or drink while tablet dissolves

Regular or sustained release capsule/tablet: Administer with a full glass of water on an empty stomach; swallow sustained release capsules/tablets whole, do not crush or chew

Parenteral: I.V. continuous infusion: Dilute in D_5W or NS to 50-100 mcg/mL; maximum concentration not to exceed 400 mcg/mL; rate of infusion (mL/hour) = dose (mcg/kg/minute) x weight (kg) x 60 minutes/hour divided by the concentration (mcg/mL); administer via controlled infusion device

Transdermal: Place on hair-free area of skin; rotate patch sites; **Note:** Some products are a membrane-controlled system (eg, Transderm-Nitro®); do **not** cut these patches to deliver partial doses; rate of drug delivery, reservoir contents, and adhesion may be affected; if partial dose is needed, surface area of patch can be blocked proportionally using adhesive bandage (see Lee, 1997 and see specific product labeling)

Monitoring Parameters Blood pressure, heart rate (continuously with I.V. use)

Patient Information Avoid alcohol; may cause dizziness, headache; if no relief of chest pains after 3 sublingual doses, seek emergency care immediately

Nursing Implications Transdermal patches are now labeled as mg/hour (rates of release used to be described as mg/24 hours)

Additional Information I.V. preparations contain alcohol and/or propylene glycol; may need to use nitrate-free interval (10-12 hours/day) to avoid tolerance development; tolerance may possibly be reversed with acetylcysteine; gradually decrease dose in patients receiving NTG for prolonged period to avoid withdrawal reaction; lingual spray contains 20% alcohol, do not spray toward flames

Dosage Forms

Capsule, sustained release: 2.5 mg, 6.5 mg, 9 mg

Injection: 0.5 mg/mL (10 mL); 0.8 mg/mL (10 mL); 5 mg/mL (1 mL, 5 mL, 10 mL, 20 mL); 10 mg/mL (5 mL, 10 mL)

Ointment, topical (Nitrol®): 2% [20 mg/g] (30 g, 60 g)

Patch, transdermal, topical: Systems designed to deliver 0.1 mg/hour (2.5 mg/24 hours); 0.2 mg/hour (5 mg/24 hours); 0.4 mg/hour (10 mg/24 hours); 0.6 mg/hour (15 mg/24 hours); 0.8 mg/hour (20 mg/24 hours)

Spray, translingual: 400 mcg/metered spray [5.7 g (75 metered sprays); 12 g (200 metered sprays)]

Tablet:

Buccal, controlled release: 1 mg, 2 mg, 3 mg

Sublingual (Nitrostat®): 0.3 mg, 0.4 mg, 0.6 mg

Sustained release: 2.6 mg, 6.5 mg, 9 mg

References

Elkayam U, "Tolerance to Organic Nitrates: Evidence, Mechanisms, Clinical Relevance, and Strategies for Prevention," *Ann Intern Med*, 1991, 114(8):667-77.

Lee HA and Anderson PO, "Giving Partial Doses of Transdermal Patches," *Am J Health Syst Pharm*, 1997, 54(15):1759-60.

♦ **Nitroglycerol** *see* Nitroglycerin *on page 690*
♦ **Nitroglyn® Oral** *see* Nitroglycerin *on page 690*
♦ **Nitrolingual® Translingual Spray** *see* Nitroglycerin *on page 690*
♦ **Nitrol® Ointment** *see* Nitroglycerin *on page 690*
♦ **Nitrong® Oral Tablet** *see* Nitroglycerin *on page 690*
♦ **Nitrong® SR (Canada)** *see* Nitroglycerin *on page 690*
♦ **Nitropress®** *see* Nitroprusside *on page 692*

Nitroprusside *(nye troe PRUS ide)*

Related Information

Adult ACLS Algorithm, Hypotension, Shock *on page 1016*

Brand Names Nitropress®

Available Salts Nitroprusside Sodium; Sodium Nitroprusside

Synonyms Nitroferricyanide

Therapeutic Category Antihypertensive Agent; Vasodilator

Generic Available Yes

Use Management of hypertensive crises; CHF; used for controlled hypotension during anesthesia

Pregnancy Risk Factor C

Contraindications Hypersensitivity to nitroprusside or any component; decreased cerebral perfusion; arteriovenous shunt or coarctation of the aorta (ie, compensatory hypertension)

Warnings Use only as an infusion with D_5W; continuously monitor patient's blood pressure; excessive amounts of nitroprusside can cause cyanide toxicity (usually in patients with decreased liver function) or thiocyanate toxicity (usually in patients with decreased renal function, or in patients with normal renal function but prolonged nitroprusside use)

Precautions Use with caution in patients with severe renal impairment, hepatic failure, hypothyroidism, hyponatremia, increased intracranial pressure

Adverse Reactions
Cardiovascular: Excessive hypotensive response, palpitations, substernal distress
Central nervous system: Restlessness, disorientation, psychosis, headache, increased intracranial pressure
Endocrine & metabolic: Thyroid suppression
Gastrointestinal: Nausea, vomiting
Hematologic: Thiocyanate toxicity
Neuromuscular & skeletal: Weakness
Miscellaneous: Diaphoresis, cyanide toxicity

Stability Discard solution 24 hours after reconstitution and dilution; discard highly colored solutions

Mechanism of Action Causes peripheral vasodilation by direct action on venous and arteriolar smooth muscle, thus reducing peripheral resistance; will increase cardiac output by decreasing afterload; reduces aortal and left ventricular impedance

Pharmacodynamics Hypotensive effects:
Onset of action: Within 2 minutes
Duration: 1-10 minutes

Pharmacokinetics
Half-life: <10 minutes
Thiocyanate: 2.7-7 days
Metabolism: Converted to cyanide by erythrocyte and tissue sulfhydryl group interactions; cyanide is converted in the liver by the enzyme rhodanase to thiocyanate
Elimination: Thiocyanate is excreted in the urine

Usual Dosage Children and Adults: I.V. continuous infusion: Start 0.3-0.5 mcg/kg/minute, titrate to effect; usual dose: 3 mcg/kg/minute; rarely need >4 mcg/kg/minute; maximum dose: 8-10 mcg/kg/minute

Rate (mL/hour) = dose (mcg/kg/minute) x weight (kg) x 60 minutes/hour divided by concentration (mcg/mL)

Administration Parenteral: I.V. continuous infusion only via controlled infusion device; not for direct injection; dilute in plain dextrose solutions only (eg, D_5W); solution should be protected from light, but not necessary to wrap administration set or I.V. tubing. Final concentration for administration: Usual maximum: 200 mcg/mL; in fluid restricted patients a final maximum concentration of 1000 mcg/mL in D_5W has been used. Do not add other medications to nitroprusside solutions.

Monitoring Parameters Blood pressure, heart rate; monitor for cyanide and thiocyanate toxicity; monitor acid-base status as acidosis can be the earliest sign of cyanide toxicity; monitor thiocyanate levels if requiring prolonged infusion (>3 days) or dose ≥4 mcg/kg/minute or patient has renal dysfunction; monitor cyanide blood levels in patients with decreased hepatic function

Reference Range
Thiocyanate:
Toxic: 35-100 μg/mL
Fatal: >200 μg/mL
Cyanide:
Normal <0.2 μg/mL
Normal (smoker): <0.4 μg/mL
Toxic: >2 μg/mL
Potentially lethal: >3 μg/mL

Additional Information Thiocyanate toxicity includes psychoses, blurred vision, confusion, weakness, tinnitus, seizures; cyanide toxicity includes metabolic acidosis, tachycardia, pink skin, decreased pulse, decreased reflexes, altered consciousness, coma, almond smell on breath, methemoglobinemia, dilated pupils
(Continued)

Nitroprusside *(Continued)*

Dosage Forms Injection, as sodium: 10 mg/mL (5 mL); 25 mg/mL (2 mL)

- ♦ **Nitroprusside Sodium** *see* Nitroprusside *on page 692*
- ♦ **Nitrostat® Sublingual** *see* Nitroglycerin *on page 690*
- ♦ **Nix™ Creme Rinse** *see* Permethrin *on page 752*

Nizatidine (ni ZA ti deen)

Brand Names Axid®; Axid® AR Acid Reducer [OTC]

Therapeutic Category Gastrointestinal Agent, Gastric or Duodenal Ulcer Treatment; Histamine H_2 Antagonist

Generic Available No

Use Treatment and maintenance therapy of duodenal ulcer; treatment of active benign gastric ulcer; esophagitis; gastroesophageal reflux disease (GERD); over-the-counter (OTC) formulation for use in the relief of heartburn, acid indigestion, and sour stomach; adjunctive therapy in the treatment of *Helicobacter pylori*-associated duodenal ulcer

Pregnancy Risk Factor C

Contraindications Hypersensitivity to nizatidine, H_2 antagonists or any component

Warnings Use with caution and modify dosage in patients with impaired renal function

Adverse Reactions

Cardiovascular: Chest pain, ventricular tachycardia (short, asymptomatic episodes)

Central nervous system: Headache, fever, dizziness, insomnia, somnolence, anxiety, nervousness

Dermatologic: Rash, pruritus

Endocrine & metabolic: Hyperuricemia

Gastrointestinal: Nausea, vomiting, diarrhea, flatulence, dyspepsia, constipation, dry mouth, anorexia, abdominal pain

Genitourinary: Impotence

Hematologic: Anemia, thrombocytopenia, eosinophilia, leukopenia

Hepatic: Elevated liver enzymes, jaundice, hepatitis

Neuromuscular & skeletal: Back pain, asthenia, myalgia

Ocular: Amblyopia

Respiratory: Rhinitis, pharyngitis, sinusitis, cough

Miscellaneous: Hypersensitivity reactions, serum sickness

Drug Interactions May increase salicylate serum concentration (high-dose salicylate therapy); decreases absorption of itraconazole, delavirdine, and ketoconazole

Food Interactions Limit xanthine-containing foods and beverages

Stability Nizatidine is stable for 48 hours at room temperature when the contents of a capsule are mixed in Gatorade® lemon-lime, Cran-Grape® grape-cranberry drink, V8®, apple juice, or aluminum- and magnesium hydroxide suspension (approximate concentration 2.5 mg/mL)

Mechanism of Action Competitive inhibition of histamine at H_2-receptors of the gastric parietal cells, which inhibits gastric acid secretion

Pharmacodynamics Peak response: Duodenal ulcer: 4 weeks

Pharmacokinetics

Distribution: V_d: 0.8-1.5 L/kg (adults)

Protein binding: 35%

Bioavailability: Oral: 70%

Half-life, elimination: 2.1 hours; anuric: 3.5-11 hours

Time to peak concentration: 0.5-3 hours

Elimination: 60% excreted unchanged in urine

Usual Dosage Oral:

Infants 6 months to Children 11 years: Limited information available: 6-10 mg/kg/day divided twice daily (see References)

Adults:

Active duodenal and gastric ulcers: 300 mg once daily at bedtime or 150 mg twice daily for 6-8 weeks

Maintenance of healed duodenal ulcer: 150 mg once daily at bedtime for up to 1 year

GERD, esophagitis: 150 mg twice daily for up to 12 weeks

Relief of heartburn, acid indigestion, sour stomach (OTC use): 75 mg 30-60 minutes before meals; no more than 2 tablets/day

Helicobacter pylori-associated duodenal ulcer (limited information): 300 mg twice daily for 4 weeks (combined with clarithromycin and bismuth formulation; followed by 300 mg/day)

Dosage adjustment in renal impairment: Adults:
Active duodenal or gastric ulcer:
Cl_{cr} 20-50 mL/min: 150 mg/day
Cl_{cr} <20 mL/min: 150 mg every other day
Maintenance therapy:
Cl_{cr} 20-50 mL/min: 150 mg every other day
Cl_{cr} <20 mL/min: 150 mg every 3 days
Administration Oral: May administer with or without food; see Stability
Test Interactions False-positive urobilinogen with Multistix®
Patient Information Avoid excessive amounts of caffeinated beverages and aspirin; with self medication, if the symptoms of heartburn, acid indigestion, or sour stomach persist after 2 weeks of continuous use of the drug, consult clinician
Dosage Forms
Capsule: 150 mg, 300 mg
Tablet: 75 mg
References
Mikawa K, Nishina K, Maekawa N, et al, "Effects of Oral Nizatidine on Preoperative Gastric Fluid pH and Volume in Children," *Br J Anaesth*, 1994, 73(5):600-4.
Simeone D, Caria MC, Miele E, et al, "Treatment of Childhood Peptic Esophagitis: A Double-Blind Placebo-Controlled Trial of Nizatidine," *J Pediatr Gastroenterol Nur*, 1997, 25(1):51-5.

♦ **Nizoral®** *see* Ketoconazole *on page 543*
♦ **No Pain-HP® [OTC]** *see* Capsaicin *on page 162*
♦ **Noradrenaline Acid Tartrate** *see* Norepinephrine *on page 695*
♦ **Norcet®** *see* Hydrocodone and Acetaminophen *on page 485*
♦ **Norcuron®** *see* Vecuronium *on page 972*
♦ **Nordeoxyguanosine** *see* Ganciclovir *on page 450*
♦ **Norditropin® Injection** *see* Human Growth Hormone *on page 478*
♦ **Nordryl® Injection** *see* Diphenhydramine *on page 327*
♦ **Nordryl® Oral** *see* Diphenhydramine *on page 327*

Norepinephrine (nor ep i NEF rin)
Related Information
Adult ACLS Algorithm, Hypotension, Shock *on page 1016*
Extravasation Treatment *on page 1050*
Brand Names Levophed®
Available Salts Norepinephrine Bitartrate
Synonyms Levarterenol; Noradrenaline Acid Tartrate
Therapeutic Category Adrenergic Agonist Agent; Alpha-Adrenergic Agonist; Sympathomimetic
Generic Available No
Use Treatment of shock which persists after adequate fluid volume replacement; severe hypotension; cardiogenic shock
Pregnancy Risk Factor C
Contraindications Hypersensitivity to norepinephrine, any component, or sulfites
Warnings Potent drug; must be diluted prior to use; monitor hemodynamic status
Precautions Blood/volume depletion should be corrected, if possible, before norepinephrine therapy; extravasation may cause severe tissue necrosis; do **not** give to patients with peripheral or mesenteric vascular thrombosis because ischemia may be increased and the area of infarct extended; use with caution during cyclopropane or halothane anesthesia and in patients with occlusive vascular disease
Adverse Reactions
Cardiovascular: Cardiac arrhythmias, palpitations, bradycardia, tachycardia, hypertension, chest pain, pallor
Central nervous system: Anxiety, headache
Endocrine & metabolic: Uterine contractions
Gastrointestinal: Vomiting
Local: Organ ischemia (due to vasoconstriction of renal and mesenteric arteries), ischemic necrosis and sloughing of superficial tissue after extravasation
Ocular: Photophobia
Respiratory: Respiratory distress
Miscellaneous: Diaphoresis
Drug Interactions Atropine sulfate may block the reflex bradycardia caused by norepinephrine and enhance the pressor response; tricyclic antidepressants, MAO inhibitors, antihistamines (diphenhydramine, tripelennamine), guanethidine, ergot alkaloids, and methyldopa may potentiate the effect of norepinephrine
Stability Readily oxidized, do not use if brown coloration; dilute with D_5W or $D_5W/$ NS; not recommended for dilution in NS; not stable with alkaline solutions
(Continued)

Norepinephrine *(Continued)*

Mechanism of Action Stimulates beta₁-adrenergic receptors and alpha-adrenergic receptors causing increased contractility and heart rate as well as vasoconstriction, thereby increasing systemic blood pressure and coronary blood flow; clinically alpha effects (vasoconstriction) are greater than beta effects (inotropic and chronotropic effects)

Pharmacodynamics
Onset of action: Very rapid
Duration: Limited duration following I.V. injection

Pharmacokinetics
Metabolism: By catechol-o-methyltransferase (COMT) and monoamine oxidase (MAO)
Elimination: In urine (84% to 96% as inactive metabolites)

Usual Dosage I.V. (dose stated in terms of **norepinephrine base**):
Children: Initial: 0.05-0.1 mcg/kg/minute, titrate to desired effect; maximum dose: 1-2 mcg/kg/minute
Rate (mL/hour) = dose (mcg/kg/minute) x weight (kg) x 60 minutes/hour divided by concentration (mcg/mL)
Adults: 8-12 mcg/minute as an infusion; initiate at 4 mcg/minute and titrate to desired response; ACLS dosing range: 0.5-30 mcg/minute

Administration Parenteral: Administer into large vein to avoid potential extravasation; standard concentration: 4 mcg/mL but 16 mcg/mL has been used safely and with efficacy in situations of extreme fluid restriction

Monitoring Parameters Blood pressure, heart rate, urine output, peripheral perfusion

Additional Information Treat extravasations with local injections of phentolamine (see Extravasation Treatment *on page 1050*)

Dosage Forms Injection, as bitartrate: 1 mg/mL norepinephrine base (4 mL)

♦ **Norepinephrine Bitartrate** *see* Norepinephrine *on page 695*

Norethindrone *(nor eth IN drone)*
Related Information
Oral Contraceptives *on page 1052*
Brand Names Aygestin®; Micronor®; NOR-Q.D.®
Available Salts Norethindrone Acetate
Synonyms Norethisterone
Therapeutic Category Contraceptive, Oral; Contraceptive, Progestin Only; Progestin
Generic Available No
Use Treatment of amenorrhea, abnormal uterine bleeding, endometriosis, oral contraceptive
Pregnancy Risk Factor X
Contraindications Hypersensitivity to norethindrone or any component; thromboembolic disorders, severe hepatic disease, breast cancer, cerebral hemorrhage, undiagnosed vaginal bleeding
Warnings Use of any progestin during the first 4 months of pregnancy is not recommended; discontinue if sudden partial or complete loss of vision, proptosis, diplopia, or migraine occur; **there is a higher rate of failure with progestin only contraceptives**; progestin-induced withdrawal bleeding occurs within 3-7 days after discontinuation of drug
Precautions Use with caution in patients with asthma, diabetes, seizure disorder, migraine, cardiac or renal dysfunction, psychic depression; may affect lipid and carbohydrate metabolism; women with diabetes or hyperlipidemias should be monitored closely
Adverse Reactions
Cardiovascular: Edema, thromboembolic disorders, hypertension
Central nervous system: Mental depression, nervousness, dizziness, fatigue, headache
Dermatologic: Hirsutism, rash, melasma or chloasma, photosensitivity
Endocrine & metabolic: Breakthrough bleeding, spotting, changes in menstrual flow
Gastrointestinal: Weight gain or loss
Hepatic: Cholestatic jaundice
Drug Interactions Rifampin decreases pharmacologic effect of norethindrone
Food Interactions High-dose vitamin C (1 g/day) may increase adverse effects; increase dietary intake of folate and pyridoxine

Mechanism of Action Inhibits secretion of pituitary gonadotropin (LH) which prevents follicular maturation and ovulation; in the presence of adequate endogenous estrogen, transforms a proliferative endometrium to a secretory one

Pharmacokinetics
Protein binding: 80%
Metabolism: In the liver
Half-life: 5-14 hours
Time to peak serum concentration: 0.5-4 hours

Usual Dosage Adolescents and Adults: Oral:
Amenorrhea and abnormal uterine bleeding: Norethindrone acetate 2.5-10 mg/day for 5-10 days beginning during the latter half of the menstrual cycle
Endometriosis: Norethindrone acetate 5 mg/day for 14 days; increase at increments of 2.5 mg/day every 2 weeks up to 15 mg/day
Contraception: Progesterone only: Norethindrone 0.35 mg every day of the year starting on first day of menstruation; if one dose is missed take as soon as remembered, then next tablet at regular time; if two doses are missed, take one of the missed doses, discard the other, and take daily dose at usual time; if three doses are missed, use another form of birth control until menses appear or pregnancy is ruled out

Administration Oral: Administer with food

Test Interactions Thyroid function test, metyrapone test, liver function tests, coagulation tests (prothrombin time, factors VII, VIII, IX, X)

Patient Information Progestin-induced withdrawal bleeding occurs within 3-7 days after discontinuation of the drug; limit caffeine

Dosage Forms
Tablet: 0.35 mg
Tablet, as acetate: 5 mg

♦ **Norethindrone Acetate** *see* Norethindrone *on page 696*

♦ **Norethisterone** *see* Norethindrone *on page 696*

♦ **Norisodrine®** *see* Isoproterenol *on page 536*

♦ **Noritate® (Canada)** *see* Metronidazole *on page 636*

♦ **Normal Human Serum Albumin** *see* Albumin *on page 39*

♦ **Normal Laboratory Values for Children** *see page 1155*

♦ **Normal Saline** *see* Sodium Chloride *on page 871*

♦ **Normal Serum Albumin (Human)** *see* Albumin *on page 39*

♦ **Normodyne®** *see* Labetalol *on page 548*

♦ **Norpace®** *see* Disopyramide *on page 333*

♦ **Norpace® CR** *see* Disopyramide *on page 333*

♦ **Norpramin®** *see* Desipramine *on page 291*

♦ **NOR-Q.D.®** *see* Norethindrone *on page 696*

♦ **Nor-tet® Oral** *see* Tetracycline *on page 908*

♦ **North and South American Antisnake-bite Serum** *see* Antivenin (*Crotalidae*) Polyvalent *on page 91*

Nortriptyline (nor TRIP ti leen)

Related Information
Comparison of Adverse Effects of Antidepressants *on page 1030*
Comparison of Usual Adult Dosage and Mechanism of Action of Antidepressants *on page 1029*

Brand Names Aventyl® Hydrochloride; Pamelor®

Available Salts Nortriptyline Hydrochloride

Therapeutic Category Antidepressant, Tricyclic

Generic Available Yes

Use Treatment of various forms of depression, often in conjunction with psychotherapy; nocturnal enuresis

Pregnancy Risk Factor D

Contraindications Hypersensitivity to nortriptyline or amitriptyline (cross-sensitivity with other tricyclics may occur) or any component; angle-closure glaucoma, patients receiving MAO inhibitors within the past 14 days

Warnings Do not discontinue abruptly in patients receiving high doses chronically; use with extreme caution with renal or hepatic impairment

Precautions Use with caution in patients with cardiac conduction disturbances, cardiovascular disease, seizure disorder, history of urinary retention, hyperthyroidism, or those receiving thyroid hormone replacement

Adverse Reactions Nortriptyline has lower anticholinergic and sedative effects compared to amitriptyline
(Continued)

Nortriptyline *(Continued)*

Cardiovascular: Postural hypotension, arrhythmias, tachycardia, sudden death

Central nervous system: Sedation, fatigue, anxiety, impaired cognitive function, seizures

Dermatologic: Photosensitivity

Endocrine & metabolic: Rarely SIADH

Gastrointestinal: Xerostomia, constipation, increased appetite, weight gain

Genitourinary: Urinary retention

Hematologic: Rarely agranulocytosis, leukopenia, eosinophilia

Hepatic: Cholestatic jaundice, elevated liver enzymes

Neuromuscular & skeletal: Tremor, weakness

Ocular: Blurred vision, increased intraocular pressure

Miscellaneous: Allergic reactions

Drug Interactions Cytochrome P-450 isoenzyme CYP1A2 and CYP2D6 substrate

Nortriptyline may decrease the effects of guanethidine and clonidine (use with clonidine may result in possible hypertensive crisis); nortriptyline may increase the effects of other CNS depressants (including alcohol), adrenergic agents (epinephrine, isoproterenol), anticholinergic agents and warfarin

With MAO inhibitors, hyperpyrexia, hypertension, tachycardia, confusion, seizures, and death have been reported

Cimetidine, fluoxetine, and methylphenidate may decrease the metabolism and phenobarbital may increase the metabolism of nortriptyline

Food Interactions Riboflavin dietary requirements may be increased

Stability Protect from light

Mechanism of Action Increases the synaptic concentration of serotonin and/or norepinephrine in the central nervous system by inhibition of their reuptake by the presynaptic neuronal membrane

Pharmacodynamics Onset of action: Therapeutic antidepressant effects begin in 7-21 days; maximum effects may not occur for ≥2-3 weeks

Pharmacokinetics

Absorption: Oral: Rapid; well absorbed

Distribution: V_d: 14-22 L/kg; crosses placenta; enters breast milk

Protein binding: 93% to 95%

Metabolism: Undergoes significant first-pass metabolism; primarily detoxified in the liver via hydroxylation followed by glucuronide conjugation

Half-life:

Children (mean ± SD): 18 ± 4 hours

Adults (mean ± SD): 46 ± 24 hours

Time to peak serum concentration: Oral: Within 7-8.5 hours

Elimination: Metabolites and small amounts of unchanged drug excreted in urine; small amounts of biliary elimination occur

Not Dialyzable

Usual Dosage Oral:

Nocturnal enuresis: Children (give dose 30 minutes before bedtime):

6-7 years (20-25 kg): 10 mg/day

8-11 years (25-35 kg): 10-20 mg/day

>11 years (35-54 kg): 25-35 mg/day

Depression:

Children 6-12 years: 1-3 mg/kg/day or 10-20 mg/day in 3-4 divided doses

Adolescents: 1-3 mg/kg/day or 30-50 mg/day in 3-4 divided doses; usual maximum dose: 150 mg/day

Adults: 25 mg 3-4 times/day up to 150 mg/day

Dosing adjustment in hepatic impairment: Use lower doses and slower titration; individualization of dosage is recommended

Administration Oral: May administer with food to decrease GI upset; dilute oral solution in water, milk, or fruit juice immediately before use; do not dilute in grape juice or carbonated beverages

Monitoring Parameters Heart rate, blood pressure, mental status, weight, plasma concentrations

Reference Range Therapeutic: 50-150 ng/mL (SI: 190-570 nmol/L)

Patient Information Avoid alcohol; limit caffeine; do not discontinue medication abruptly; may cause drowsiness and impair ability to perform activities requiring mental alertness or physical coordination

Nursing Implications Treatment of nocturnal enuresis is usually ≤3 months

Additional Information Place in therapy: Nortriptyline is a second-line agent for depression in children and adolescents; solution contains 4% alcohol

Dosage Forms
Capsule, as hydrochloride: 10 mg, 25 mg, 50 mg, 75 mg
Solution, as hydrochloride: 10 mg/5 mL (473 mL)

References
Levy HB, Harper CR, and Weinberg WA, "A Practical Approach to Children Failing in School," *Pediatr Clin North Am*, 1992, 39(4):895-928

- **Nortriptyline Hydrochloride** *see Nortriptyline on page 697*
- **Norvir®** *see Ritonavir on page 849*
- **Norzine®** *see Thiethylperazine on page 917*
- **Nōstrilla® [OTC]** *see Oxymetazoline on page 718*
- **Nostril® Nasal Solution [OTC]** *see Phenylephrine on page 758*
- **Novahistine® (Canada)** *see Phenylephrine on page 758*
- **Novamoxin® (Canada)** *see Amoxicillin on page 70*
- **Novantrone®** *see Mitoxantrone on page 653*
- **Nova Rectal® (Canada)** *see Pentobarbital on page 748*
- **Novasen (Canada)** *see Aspirin on page 99*
- **Novo-Aloprazol® (Canada)** *see Alprazolam on page 50*
- **Novo-Atenol® (Canada)** *see Atenolol on page 102*
- **Novo-AZT® (Canada)** *see Zidovudine on page 990*
- **Novo-Captopril® (Canada)** *see Captopril on page 163*
- **Novo-Carbamaz® (Canada)** *see Carbamazepine on page 165*
- **Novo-Chlorhydrate® (Canada)** *see Chloral Hydrate on page 204*
- **Novo-Chlorpromazine® (Canada)** *see Chlorpromazine on page 215*
- **Novo-Cimetidine® (Canada)** *see Cimetidine on page 222*
- **Novo-Clonidine® (Canada)** *see Clonidine on page 242*
- **Novo-Clopate® (Canada)** *see Clorazepate on page 244*
- **Novo-Cloxin® (Canada)** *see Cloxacillin on page 246*
- **Novo-Cromolyn® (Canada)** *see Cromolyn on page 260*
- **Novo-Cycloprine® (Canada)** *see Cyclobenzaprine on page 265*
- **Novo-Difenac® (Canada)** *see Diclofenac on page 312*
- **Novo-Difenac-SR® (Canada)** *see Diclofenac on page 312*
- **Novo-Digoxin® (Canada)** *see Digoxin on page 318*
- **Novo-Diltazem® (Canada)** *see Diltiazem on page 323*
- **Novo-Dipam® (Canada)** *see Diazepam on page 307*
- **Novo-Dipiradol® (Canada)** *see Dipyridamole on page 331*
- **Novo-Doxepin® (Canada)** *see Doxepin on page 345*
- **Novo-Doxylin® (Canada)** *see Doxycycline on page 348*
- **Novo-Famotidine® (Canada)** *see Famotidine on page 401*
- **Novo-Flupam® (Canada)** *see Flurazepam on page 434*
- **Novo-Flurprofen® (Canada)** *see Flurbiprofen on page 435*
- **Novo-Folacid® (Canada)** *see Folic Acid on page 439*
- **Novo-Furan® (Canada)** *see Nitrofurantoin on page 689*
- **Novo-Gesic-C8® (Canada)** *see Acetaminophen and Codeine on page 27*
- **Novo-Gesic-C15® (Canada)** *see Acetaminophen and Codeine on page 27*
- **Novo-Gesic-C30® (Canada)** *see Acetaminophen and Codeine on page 27*
- **Novo-Hexidyl® (Canada)** *see Trihexyphenidyl on page 952*
- **Novo-Hydrazide® (Canada)** *see Hydrochlorothiazide on page 483*
- **Novo-Hydroxyzine® (Canada)** *see Hydroxyzine on page 496*
- **Novo-Hylazin® (Canada)** *see Hydralazine on page 482*
- **Novo-Lexin® (Canada)** *see Cephalexin on page 196*
- **Novolin® 70/30** *see Insulin Preparations on page 518*
- **Novolin® ge (Canada)** *see Insulin Preparations on page 518*
- **Novolin® L** *see Insulin Preparations on page 518*
- **Novolin® N** *see Insulin Preparations on page 518*
- **Novolin-Pen® II, -3 (Canada)** *see Insulin Preparations on page 518*
- **Novolin® R** *see Insulin Preparations on page 518*
- **NovoLog™** *see Insulin Preparations on page 518*
- **Novo-Lorazepam® (Canada)** *see Lorazepam on page 583*
- **Novo-Medopa® (Canada)** *see Methyldopa on page 625*
- **Novo-Methacin® (Canada)** *see Indomethacin on page 516*
- **Novo-Metoprolol (Canada)** *see Metoprolol on page 633*

- Novo-Mucilax® **(Canada)** *see* Psyllium *on page 823*
- Novo-Naprox® **(Canada)** *see* Naproxen *on page 672*
- Novo-Nidazol® **(Canada)** *see* Metronidazole *on page 636*
- Novo-Nifedin® **(Canada)** *see* Nifedipine *on page 687*
- Novo-Pen-VK® **(Canada)** *see* Penicillin V Potassium *on page 743*
- Novo-Piroxicam® **(Canada)** *see* Piroxicam *on page 777*
- Novo-Pramine® **(Canada)** *see* Imipramine *on page 508*
- Novo-Prazin® **(Canada)** *see* Prazosin *on page 790*
- Novo-Prednisolone® **(Canada)** *see* Prednisolone *on page 791*
- Novo-Prednisone® **(Canada)** *see* Prednisone *on page 794*
- Novo-Profen® **(Canada)** *see* Ibuprofen *on page 501*
- Novo-Propoxyn® **(Canada)** *see* Propoxyphene *on page 814*
- Novo-purol® **(Canada)** *see* Allopurinol *on page 48*
- Novo-Ranidine® **(Canada)** *see* Ranitidine *on page 835*
- Novo-Ridazine® **(Canada)** *see* Thioridazine *on page 920*
- Novo-Rythro Encap **(Canada)** *see* Erythromycin *on page 379*
- Novo-Salmol® **(Canada)** *see* Albuterol *on page 40*
- Novo-Secobarb® **(Canada)** *see* Secobarbital *on page 861*
- Novo-Semide® **(Canada)** *see* Furosemide *on page 447*
- Novo-Soxazole® **(Canada)** *see* Sulfisoxazole *on page 894*
- Novo-Spiroton® **(Canada)** *see* Spironolactone *on page 877*
- Novo-Sucralate® **(Canada)** *see* Sucralfate *on page 886*
- Novo-Sundac® **(Canada)** *see* Sulindac *on page 896*
- Novo-Tetra® **(Canada)** *see* Tetracycline *on page 908*
- Novo-Timol® **(Canada)** *see* Timolol *on page 929*
- Novo-Tolmetin® **(Canada)** *see* Tolmetin *on page 935*
- Novo-Trimel® **(Canada)** *see* Co-Trimoxazole *on page 258*
- Novo-Triolam® **(Canada)** *see* Triazolam *on page 950*
- Novo-Tryptin® **(Canada)** *see* Amitriptyline *on page 67*
- Novo-Veramil® **(Canada)** *see* Verapamil *on page 974*
- Novo-Zolamide® **(Canada)** *see* Acetazolamide *on page 29*
- NP-27® **[OTC]** *see* Tolnaftate *on page 936*
- NPH Iletin® I *see* Insulin Preparations *on page 518*
- NPH Insulin *see* Insulin Preparations *on page 518*
- NPH-N *see* Insulin Preparations *on page 518*
- NS *see* Sodium Chloride *on page 871*
- ½NS *see* Sodium Chloride *on page 871*
- NSC-373364 *see* Aldesleukin *on page 42*
- NTG *see* Nitroglycerin *on page 690*
- NTZ® Long Acting Nasal Solution **[OTC]** *see* Oxymetazoline *on page 718*
- Nu-Alprax® **(Canada)** *see* Alprazolam *on page 50*
- Nu-Amoxi® **(Canada)** *see* Amoxicillin *on page 70*
- Nu-Ampi® **[Trihydrate] (Canada)** *see* Ampicillin *on page 78*
- Nu-Atenol® **(Canada)** *see* Atenolol *on page 102*
- Nubain® *see* Nalbuphine *on page 668*
- Nu-Capto® **(Canada)** *see* Captopril *on page 163*
- Nu-Carbamazepine® **(Canada)** *see* Carbamazepine *on page 165*
- Nu-Cephalex® **(Canada)** *see* Cephalexin *on page 196*
- Nu-Cimet® **(Canada)** *see* Cimetidine *on page 222*
- Nu-Clonidine® **(Canada)** *see* Clonidine *on page 242*
- Nu-Cloxi® **(Canada)** *see* Cloxacillin *on page 246*
- Nu-Cotrimox® **(Canada)** *see* Co-Trimoxazole *on page 258*
- Nu-Diclo® **(Canada)** *see* Diclofenac *on page 312*
- Nu-Diltiaz® **(Canada)** *see* Diltiazem *on page 323*
- Nu-Doxycycline® **(Canada)** *see* Doxycycline *on page 348*
- Nu-Famotidine® **(Canada)** *see* Famotidine *on page 401*
- Nu-Flurprofen® **(Canada)** *see* Flurbiprofen *on page 435*
- Nu-Hydral® **(Canada)** *see* Hydralazine *on page 482*
- Nu-Ibuprofen® **(Canada)** *see* Ibuprofen *on page 501*
- Nu-Indo® **(Canada)** *see* Indomethacin *on page 516*
- Nu-Iron® *see* Iron Supplements, Oral/Enteral *on page 530*

- **Nu-Iron® 150** *see* Iron Supplements, Oral/Enteral *on page 530*
- **Nu-Loraz® (Canada)** *see* Lorazepam *on page 583*
- **NuLYTELY®** *see* Polyethylene Glycol-Electrolyte Solution *on page 782*
- **Nu-Medopa® (Canada)** *see* Methyldopa *on page 625*
- **Nu-Metop (Canada)** *see* Metoprolol *on page 633*
- **Numzitdent® [OTC]** *see* Benzocaine *on page 124*
- **Numzit Teething® [OTC]** *see* Benzocaine *on page 124*
- **Nu-Naprox® (Canada)** *see* Naproxen *on page 672*
- **Nu-Nifedin® (Canada)** *see* Nifedipine *on page 687*
- **Nu-Pen-VK® (Canada)** *see* Penicillin V Potassium *on page 743*
- **Nupercainal® [OTC]** *see* Dibucaine *on page 311*
- **Nupercainal®** *see* Hemorrhoidal Preparations *on page 470*
- **Nu-Pirox® (Canada)** *see* Piroxicam *on page 777*
- **Nu-Prazo® (Canada)** *see* Prazosin *on page 790*
- **Nuprin® [OTC]** *see* Ibuprofen *on page 501*
- **Nu-Prochlor® (Canada)** *see* Prochlorperazine *on page 803*
- **Nu-Propranolol® (Canada)** *see* Propranolol *on page 816*
- **Nu-Ranit® (Canada)** *see* Ranitidine *on page 835*
- **Nuromax® Injection** *see* Doxacurium *on page 342*
- **Nu-Tetra® (Canada)** *see* Tetracycline *on page 908*
- **Nu-Timolol® (Canada)** *see* Timolol *on page 929*
- **Nutracort® Topical** *see* Hydrocortisone *on page 486*
- **Nu-Triazo® (Canada)** *see* Triazolam *on page 950*
- **Nutrilipid®** *see* Fat Emulsion *on page 403*
- **Nutropin® AQ Injection** *see* Human Growth Hormone *on page 478*
- **Nutropin® Depot™** *see* Human Growth Hormone *on page 478*
- **Nutropin® Injection** *see* Human Growth Hormone *on page 478*
- **Nu-Verap® (Canada)** *see* Verapamil *on page 974*
- **Nyaderm (Canada)** *see* Nystatin *on page 701*
- **Nydrazid® Injection** *see* Isoniazid *on page 534*

Nystatin (nye STAT in)
Related Information
Carbohydrate and Alcohol Content of Liquid Medications for Use in Patients Receiving Ketogenic Diets *on page 1228*

Brand Names Candistatin® (Canada); Mestatin® (Canada); Mycostatin®; Nadostine® (Canada); Nilstat®; Nyaderm (Canada); Nystat-Rx®; Nystex®; O-V Staticin®; PMS-Nystatin (Canada)

Therapeutic Category Antifungal Agent, Oral Nonabsorbed; Antifungal Agent, Topical; Antifungal Agent, Vaginal

Generic Available Yes

Use Treatment of susceptible cutaneous, mucocutaneous, oral cavity and vaginal fungal infections normally caused by the *Candida* species

Pregnancy Risk Factor B

Contraindications Hypersensitivity to nystatin or any component

Adverse Reactions
Dermatologic: Contact dermatitis, Stevens-Johnson syndrome
Gastrointestinal: Nausea, vomiting, diarrhea
Local: Irritation

Stability Store vaginal inserts in refrigerator; protect from moisture and light

Mechanism of Action Binds to sterols in fungal cell membrane, changing the cell wall permeability allowing for leakage of cellular contents

Pharmacodynamics Onset of symptomatic relief from candidiasis: Within 24-72 hours

Pharmacokinetics
Absorption: Not absorbed through mucous membranes or intact skin; poorly absorbed from the GI tract
Elimination: In feces as unchanged drug

Usual Dosage
Oral candidiasis:
Neonates: 100,000 units 4 times/day or 50,000 units to each side of mouth 4 times/day
Infants: 200,000 units 4 times/day or 100,000 units to each side of mouth 4 times/day
(Continued)

Nystatin *(Continued)*

Children and Adults: 400,000-600,000 units 4 times/day; troche: 200,000-400,000 units 4-5 times/day

Cutaneous candidal infections: Children and Adults: Topical: Apply 2-4 times/day

Intestinal infections: Adults: Oral: 500,000-1,000,000 units every 8 hours

Vaginal infections: Adolescents and Adults: Vaginal tablets: Insert 1 tablet/day at bedtime for 2 weeks

Administration

Oral: Suspension should be swished about the mouth and retained in the mouth for as long as possible (several minutes) before swallowing. For neonates and infants, paint nystatin suspension into recesses of the mouth. Troches must be allowed to dissolve slowly and should not be chewed or swallowed whole.

Topical:

Cream or ointment: Gently massage formulation into the skin

Intravaginal: Insert vaginal tablet high in the vagina

Powder: Dust in shoes, in stockings, and on feet for treatment of candidal infection of the feet; also used on very moist lesions

Patient Information Inform physician if irritation or sensitization occur during therapy

Dosage Forms

Cream: 100,000 units/g (15 g, 30 g)

Ointment, topical: 100,000 units/g (15 g, 30 g)

Powder, for preparation of oral suspension: 50 million units, 1 billion units, 2 billion units, 5 billion units

Powder, topical: 100,000 units/g (15 g)

Suspension, oral: 100,000 units/mL (5 mL, 60 mL, 480 mL)

Tablet:

Oral: 500,000 units

Vaginal: 100,000 units (15 and 30/box with applicator)

Troche: 200,000 units

References

Dismukes WE, Wade JS, Lee JY, et al, "A Randomized, Double-Blind Trial of Nystatin Therapy for the Candidiasis Hypersensitivity Syndrome," *N Engl J Med*, 1990, 323(25):1717-23.

♦ **Nystat-Rx®** *see* Nystatin *on page 701*

♦ **Nystex®** *see* Nystatin *on page 701*

♦ **Nytol® Oral [OTC]** *see* Diphenhydramine *on page 327*

♦ **Occlucort® (Canada)** *see* Betamethasone *on page 130*

♦ **Occlusal-HP Liquid** *see* Salicylic Acid *on page 854*

♦ **Ocean Nasal Mist [OTC]** *see* Sodium Chloride *on page 871*

♦ **OCL®** *see* Polyethylene Glycol-Electrolyte Solution *on page 782*

♦ **Octamide®** *see* Metoclopramide *on page 630*

♦ **Octicair® Otic** *see* Neomycin, (Bacitracin) Polymyxin B, and Hydrocortisone *on page 679*

♦ **Octocaine® Injection** *see* Lidocaine and Epinephrine *on page 570*

♦ **Octostim® (Canada)** *see* Desmopressin *on page 292*

Octreotide Acetate *(ok TREE oh tide AS e tate)*

Brand Names Sandostatin®; Sandostatin LAR® Depot

Therapeutic Category Antidiarrheal; Antisecretory Agent; Somatostatin Analog

Generic Available No

Use Control of symptoms in patients with metastatic carcinoid, vasoactive intestinal peptide-secreting tumors (VIPomas), and secretory diarrhea; acromegaly

Unlabeled uses: AIDS-associated secretory diarrhea, control of bleeding of esophageal varices, breast cancer, cryptosporidiosis, Cushing's syndrome, insulinomas, small bowel fistulas, postgastrectomy dumping syndrome, chemotherapy-induced diarrhea, GVHD-induced diarrhea, Zollinger-Ellison syndrome

Pregnancy Risk Factor B

Contraindications Hypersensitivity to octreotide or any component

Warnings Dosage adjustment may be required to maintain symptomatic control; insulin requirements may be reduced as well as sulfonylurea requirements

Precautions Patients must be monitored closely for biliary tract abnormalities (including biliary obstruction, cholecystitis, and cholelithiasis), hypothyroidism, and glucose tolerance; use with caution in patients with renal impairment

Adverse Reactions

Cardiovascular: Flushing, edema, chest pain, hypertension, palpitations, CHF, orthostatic hypotension, syncope, bradycardia

Central nervous system: Dizziness, fatigue, anxiety, headache, depression, insomnia, fever, chills, seizures, vertigo, hyperesthesia, Bell's palsy

Dermatologic: Erythema, alopecia, bruising, pruritus, rash

Endocrine & metabolic: Hypoglycemia, hyperglycemia, galactorrhea, hypothyroidism

Gastrointestinal: Nausea, diarrhea, abdominal pain, vomiting, constipation, flatulence, fat malabsorption, GI bleeding (rare), xerostomia, dyspepsia, steatorrhea, cholelithiasis, biliary sludge, pancreatitis

Genitourinary: Prostatitis

Hepatic: Hepatitis, jaundice, increased liver enzymes

Local: Injection site pain, thrombophlebitis

Neuromuscular & skeletal: Weakness, increased CPK, backache, muscle spasm, muscle cramps, arthralgia, tremor, numbness

Ocular: Visual disturbance, ocular burning

Renal: Oliguria, urinary hyperosmolarity

Respiratory: Shortness of breath, rhinorrhea

Drug Interactions Decreased effect: Cyclosporine (case report of a transplant rejection due to reduction of serum cyclosporine levels) possibly due to decreased bioavailability

Food Interactions Schedule injections between meals to decrease GI effects; may decrease vitamin B_{12} levels and decrease absorption of dietary fats

Stability Store in refrigerator; Sandostatin® injection is stable 14 days at room temperature if protected from light; stable in D_5W or NS for 4 days at room temperature; not compatible in TPN solutions due to glycosyl octreotide conjugate which may have decreased activity; Sandostatin LAR® Depot must be used immediately after reconstitution

Mechanism of Action A synthetic polypeptide which mimics natural somatostatin by inhibiting serotonin release, and the secretion of gastrin, vasoactive intestinal peptide (VIP), insulin, glucagon, secretin, motilin, and pancreatic polypeptide; in animals, also a potent inhibitor of growth hormone

Pharmacodynamics Duration of action: 6-12 hours

Pharmacokinetics

Absorption:

S.C.: Rapid

I.M.(Sandostatin LAR® Depot): 60% to 63% when compared with S.C. immediate release formulation

Distribution: V_d: 13.6 L/kg (adults)

Metabolism: Extensive by the liver

Half-life: 60-110 minutes

Elimination: 32% excreted unchanged in urine

Note: When using Sandostatin LAR® Depot formulation, steady state levels are achieved after 3 injections (3 months of therapy)

Usual Dosage Dosage should be individualized according to the patient's response

Sandostatin®:

Diarrhea:

Infants and Children: I.V., S.C.: Doses of 1-10 mcg/kg every 12 hours have been used in children beginning at the low end of the range and increasing by 0.3 mcg/kg/dose at 3-day intervals; suppression of growth hormone (animal data) is of concern when used as long-term therapy

Adults:

S.C.: Initial: 50 mcg 1-2 times/day

I.V.: Initial: 50-100 mcg every 8 hours; increase by 100 mcg/dose at 48-hour intervals; maximum dose: 500 mcg every 8 hours

The following are effective dosing ranges for specific therapies: Adults: S.C., I.V.:

Carcinoid: 100-600 mcg/day in 2-4 divided doses

VIPomas: 200-300 mcg/day in 2-4 divided doses

Esophageal varices bleeding: I.V. bolus: 25-50 mcg followed by continuous I.V. infusion of 25-50 mcg/hour

Acromegaly: 50 mcg 3 times/day; increase as needed (usual requirement: 100 mcg 3 times/day); maximum dose: 500 mcg 3 times/day; hold dose for 4 weeks per year (8 weeks if Sandostatin LAR® Depot) in patients who have been irradiated, to assess disease activity; resume therapy if growth hormone or somatomedin C (IGF-I) levels increase and signs and symptoms recur

(Continued)

Octreotide Acetate *(Continued)*

Sandostatin LAR® Depot: May be used in patients who have responded to the immediate release formulation; Adults: I.M.:

Acromegaly: Initial: 20 mg at 4-week intervals for 3 months; dosage may be adjusted based upon the following:

Maintain same dosage **IF:** Growth hormone level <2.5 ng/mL, IGF-I normal, and clinical symptoms controlled

Increase dosage to 30 mg **IF:** Growth hormone level >2.5 ng/mL, IGF-I elevated, and clinical symptoms uncontrolled

Reduce dosage to 10 mg **IF:** Growth hormone level ≤1 ng/mL, IGF-I normal, and clinical symptoms controlled

(May increase dosage to maximum 40 mg every 4 weeks if 30 mg dosage ineffective; it is not recommended to administer dosage at intervals >4 weeks)

VIPomas, carcinoid: Initial: 20 mg at 4-week intervals; due to the need for serum octreotide to reach therapeutically effective levels following initial injection for Sandostatin LAR® Depot, subcutaneous Sandostatin® injection should be continued at the current dosage **at the same time** for at least the first 2 weeks of therapy (some patients may require 3 or 4 weeks of such therapy). Adjust Sandostatin LAR® Depot dosage after 2 months of therapy depending upon patient response; doses >30 mg are not recommended

Administration Parenteral: Only Sandostatin® injection may be administered I.V., I.M., and S.C.; Sandostatin LAR® Depot may only be administered I.M.

I.V. infusion: Dilute Sandostatin® injection in 50-200 mL NS or D$_5$W and infuse over 15-30 minutes; in emergency situations, may be administered undiluted by direct I.V. push over 3 minutes; see Stability for compatibility information; allow solution to come to room temperature before administration

I.M. administration: Reconstitute with provided diluent; use immediately after reconstitution; administer into gluteal area only (avoid deltoid injections due to significant pain and discomfort at injection site)

Monitoring Parameters Baseline and periodic ultrasound evaluations for cholelithiasis, blood sugar, baseline and periodic thyroid function tests, fluid and electrolyte balance, fecal fat, and serum carotene determinations; for carcinoid, monitor urinary 5-hydroxyindole acetic acid (5-HIAA), plasma serotonin, plasma substance P; for VIPoma, monitor VIP; vitamin B$_{12}$ levels (chronic therapy); for acromegaly: growth hormone levels, IGF-I (somatomedin C)

Reference Range Vasoactive intestinal peptide (VIP): <75 ng/L; levels vary considerably between laboratories; growth hormone level: <5 ng/mL; IGF-I (somatomedin C): males: <1.9 units/mL, females: <2.2 units/mL

Dosage Forms

Injection: 0.05 mg/mL (1 mL); 0.1 mg/mL (1 mL); 0.2 mg/mL (5 mL); 0.5 mg/mL (1 mL); 1 mg/mL (1 mL)

Injection, microspheres for suspension (Sandostatin LAR® Depot): 10 mg, 20 mg, 30 mg

References

Couper RT, Berzen A, Berall G, et al, "Clinical Response to the Long-Acting Somatostatin Analogue SMS 201-995 in a Child With Congenital Microvillus Atrophy," *Gut*, 1989, 30(7):1020-4.

Jaros W, Biller J, Greer S, et al, "Successful Treatment of Idiopathic Secretory Diarrhea of Infancy With the Somatostatin Analogue SMS 201-995," *Gastroenterology*, 1988, 94(1):189-93.

Katz MD and Erstad BL, "Octreotide, A New Somatostatin Analogue," *Clin Pharm*, 1989, 8(4):255-73.

♦ **Ocu-Carpine® Ophthalmic** *see* Pilocarpine *on page 770*
♦ **OcuClear® Ophthalmic [OTC]** *see* Oxymetazoline *on page 718*
♦ **Ocufen® Ophthalmic** *see* Flurbiprofen *on page 435*
♦ **Ocugram® (Canada)** *see* Gentamicin *on page 452*

Ocular Lubricant *(OK yoo lar LOO bri kant)*

Brand Names Duratears® [OTC]; Lacri-Lube® SOP [OTC]

Therapeutic Category Lubricant, Ocular; Ophthalmic Agent, Miscellaneous

Generic Available Yes

Use Ocular lubricant

Contraindications Hypersensitivity to any component

Warnings Discontinue if eye pain, vision change, redness or eye irritation occurs or if condition worsens or persists >72 hours

Adverse Reactions Ocular: Temporary blurring of vision, irritation

Stability Store away from heat

Mechanism of Action Forms an occlusive film on the surface of the eye to lubricate and protect the eye from drying

Usual Dosage Children and Adults: Ophthalmic: Apply ¼" of ointment to the inside of the lower lid as needed

Administration Ophthalmic: Do not use with contact lenses; to avoid contamination, do not touch tip of container to any surface

Additional Information Contains petrolatum, mineral oil, chlorobutanol and lanolin alcohols

Dosage Forms Ointment, ophthalmic: 3.5 g

Olsalazine (ole SAL a zeen)

Brand Names Dipentum®

Available Salts Olsalazine Sodium

Therapeutic Category 5-Aminosalicylic Acid Derivative; Anti-inflammatory Agent

Generic Available No

Use Maintenance of remission of ulcerative colitis in patients intolerant to sulfasalazine

Pregnancy Risk Factor C

Contraindications Hypersensitivity to olsalazine, salicylates, or any component

Warnings Diarrhea is a common adverse effect of olsalazine

Precautions Use with caution in patients with hypersensitivity to sulfasalazine, salicylates, or mesalamine

Adverse Reactions

Cardiovascular: Pericarditis, heart block, hypertension, orthostatic hypotension, edema, chest pain, tachycardia

Central nervous system: Headache, fatigue, drowsiness, depression, insomnia, vertigo, fever

Dermatologic: Erythema nodosum, photosensitivity

Gastrointestinal: Diarrhea, cramps, nausea, dyspepsia, bloating, vomiting, pancreatitis, rectal bleeding, xerostomia

Genitourinary: Urinary frequency, dysuria

Hematologic: Leukopenia, neutropenia, lymphopenia, eosinophilia, thrombocytopenia

Hepatic: Mild cholestatic hepatitis, increased AST and ALT

Neuromuscular & skeletal: Arthralgia, tremor, paresthesia

Ocular: Blurred vision, dry eyes

Renal: Hematuria, proteinuria

Respiratory: Bronchospasm, respiratory infection

Mechanism of Action Olsalazine is a sodium salt of a salicylate compound that is effectively bioconverted to 5-aminosalicylic acid (5-ASA). The exact mechanism of action appears to be topical rather than systemic. It may diminish colonic inflammation by blocking cyclo-oxygenase and inhibiting colon prostaglandin production in the bowel mucosa.

Pharmacokinetics

Absorption: <3%; very little intact olsalazine is systemically absorbed

Protein binding: High

Metabolism: Mostly by colonic bacteria to the active drug, 5-aminosalicylic acid

Bioavailability: 2.4%

Half-life, elimination: 56 minutes (in serum)

Elimination: Primarily in feces

Usual Dosage Adults: Oral: 1 g/day in 2 divided doses

Administration Oral: Administer with food in evenly divided doses

Patient Information Contact physician if diarrhea occurs

Dosage Forms Capsule, as sodium: 250 mg

♦ **Olsalazine Sodium** *see* Olsalazine *on page 705*

Omeprazole (oh ME pray zol)

Brand Names Losec® (Canada); Prilosec®

Therapeutic Category Gastric Acid Secretion Inhibitor; Gastrointestinal Agent, Gastric or Duodenal Ulcer Treatment; Proton Pump Inhibitor

Generic Available No

Use Treatment and maintenance of healing of severe erosive esophagitis (grade 2 or above) diagnosed by endoscopy; short-term treatment (4-8 weeks) of active duodenal ulcer; short-term treatment of active benign gastric ulcers; short-term treatment of symptomatic gastroesophageal reflux disease (GERD) poorly responsive to customary medical treatment; pathological hypersecretory conditions; peptic ulcer disease; adjunctive treatment of duodenal ulcers associated with *Helicobacter pylori*

Pregnancy Risk Factor C

Contraindications Hypersensitivity to omeprazole or any component

Warnings In long-term (2-year) studies in rats, omeprazole produced a dose-related increase in gastric carcinoid tumors. While available endoscopic evaluations and histologic examinations of biopsy specimens from human stomachs have not detected a risk from short-term exposure to omeprazole, further human data on the effect of sustained hypochlorhydria and hypergastrinemia are needed to rule out the possibility of an increased risk for the development of tumors in humans receiving long-term therapy.

Adverse Reactions

Cardiovascular: Chest pain, tachycardia, bradycardia, palpitations

Central nervous system: Headache, dizziness, vertigo, insomnia, anxiety, hemifacial dysesthesia, nervousness, fever

Dermatologic: Rash, dry skin

Endocrine & metabolic: Hypoglycemia

Gastrointestinal: Diarrhea, nausea, abdominal pain, vomiting, constipation, flatulence, discoloration of feces, irritable colon, xerostomia, anorexia, dysgeusia, abdominal pain

Genitourinary: Urinary frequency

Hematologic: Agranulocytosis, pancytopenia, thrombocytopenia, anemia, leukocytosis

Hepatic: Hepatitis, increased liver function tests, jaundice

Neuromuscular & skeletal: Muscle cramps, myalgia, arthralgia, leg pain, paresthesia, back pain

Otic: Tinnitus

Renal: Hematuria, pyuria, proteinuria, glycosuria

Respiratory: Pharyngeal pain, cough, epistaxis

Drug Interactions Omeprazole inhibits oxidative metabolism; the full potential related to specific drugs remains to be determined; decreases absorption of ketoconazole, itraconazole, iron salts, ampicillin esters; increases half-life (decreased clearance) of diazepam, phenytoin, and warfarin; may increase absorption of digoxin and didanosine

Stability Omeprazole stability is a function of pH; it is rapidly degraded in acidic media, but has acceptable stability under alkaline conditions. Prilosec® is supplied as capsules for oral administration; each capsule of omeprazole contains enteric coated granules to prevent omeprazole degradation by gastric acidity.

Mechanism of Action Suppresses gastric acid secretion by inhibiting the parietal cell membrane enzyme (H^+/K^+)-ATPase or proton pump; demonstrates antimicrobial activity against *Helicobacter pylori*

Pharmacodynamics

Onset of action: 1 hour

Peak effect: 2 hours

Duration: 72 hours

Maximum secretory inhibition: 4 days

Pharmacokinetics

Protein binding: 95%

Metabolism: Extensive first-pass metabolism in the liver

Bioavailability: 30% to 40%; improves slightly with repeated administration; also increased in the elderly

Half-life: 0.5-1 hour

Usual Dosage Oral:

Children: Dosage not established, but a starting dose of 0.6-0.7 mg/kg/day in the morning is recommended; a second dose 12 hours later may be given if necessary; range of effective dosages in the literature: 0.3-3.3 mg/kg/day

Adults:
  Active duodenal ulcer: 20 mg/day for 4-8 weeks
  GERD or severe erosive esophagitis: 20 mg/day for 4-8 weeks
  Pathological hypersecretory conditions: 60 mg/day to start; doses up to 120 mg 3 times/day have been administered; administer daily doses >80 mg in divided doses
  Adjunctive therapy of duodenal ulcers associated with *Helicobacter pylori*: 20 mg twice daily, or 40 mg/day (in combination with antibiotic therapy)
  Gastric ulcers: 40 mg/day for 4-8 weeks
Administration Oral: Administer before food or meals; capsule should be swallowed whole, do not chew or crush; because the enteric coating of granules will dissolve in alkaline pH, administration via NG tube should be in acidic juice (eg, apple juice or cranberry juice); stable 30 minutes after mixing; to administer via jejunostomy tube, crush the granules and dissolve in a mixture of water to which a crushed 650 mg sodium bicarbonate tablet has been added
Dosage Forms Capsule, delayed release: 10 mg, 20 mg, 40 mg
Extemporaneous Preparations Omeprazole 2 mg/mL suspension may be made by adding 100 mL 8.4% sodium bicarbonate solution to the contents of ten 20 mg omeprazole capsules; stir for 30 minutes; protect from light; stable 14 days at room temperature and 45 days refrigerated
  DiGiacinto JL, Olsen KM, Bergman KL, et al, "Stability of Suspension Formulations of Lansoprazole and Omeprazole Stored in Amber-colored Plastic Oral Syringes," *Ann Pharmacother*, 2000, 34(5):600-4.

References
Gunasekaran TS and Hassall EG, "Efficacy and Safety of Omeprazole for Severe Gastroesophageal Reflux in Children," *J Pediatr*, 1993, 123(1):148-54.

Kane DL, "Administration of Omeprazole (Prilosec®) in the Atypical Patient," *Int J Pharm Compounding*, 1997, 1(1):13.

Kato S, Ebina K, Fujii K, et al, "Effect of Omeprazole in the Treatment of Refractory Acid-Related Diseases in Childhood: Endoscopic Healing and Twenty-Four Hour Intragastric Acidity," *J Pediatr*, 1996, 128(3):415-21.

♦ **Omnipen®** *see* Ampicillin *on page 78*

♦ **Omnipen®-N** *see* Ampicillin *on page 78*

♦ **OMS® Oral** *see* Morphine Sulfate *on page 657*

♦ **Oncaspar®** *see* Pegaspargase *on page 735*

♦ **Oncovin®** *see* Vincristine *on page 979*

Ondansetron (on DAN se tron)
Brand Names Zofran®; Zofran® ODT
Therapeutic Category Antiemetic
Generic Available No
Use Prevention of nausea and vomiting associated with highly emetogenic cancer chemotherapy and prevention of postoperative nausea and vomiting
Pregnancy Risk Factor B
Contraindications Hypersensitivity to ondansetron or any component
Warnings Zofran® ODT tablets contain aspartame; avoid use in phenylketonuric patients
Adverse Reactions
  Cardiovascular: Tachycardia, bradycardia, angina, syncope
  Central nervous system: Lightheadedness, seizures, headache, dizziness, drowsiness, sedation, fatigue, fever, shivers
  Dermatologic: Rash, local injection site reaction
  Endocrine & metabolic: Hypokalemia
  Gastrointestinal: Constipation, diarrhea, abdominal pain, xerostomia
  Hepatic: Transient elevations in liver enzymes
  Neuromuscular & skeletal: Weakness, musculoskeletal pain, tremor, twitching, ataxia
  Ocular: Blurred vision
  Respiratory: Bronchospasm
  Miscellaneous: Hypersensitivity reactions
Drug Interactions No documented drug interactions; however, ondansetron does contain the same imidazole nucleus as cimetidine and omeprazole; patients receiving concurrent theophylline, phenytoin, or warfarin should be followed closely; ondansetron is metabolized by the cytochrome P-450 enzyme system, inducers or inhibitors of this system may affect ondansetron's elimination
Stability
  Compatible for 7 days at room temperature when diluted in saline or dextrose solutions; Y-site injection compatibility with bleomycin, carboplatin, carmustine,
(Continued)

Ondansetron *(Continued)*

chlorpromazine, cisplatin, cyclophosphamide, cytarabine, dacarbazine, dactino-mycin, daunorubicin, dexamethasone, diphenhydramine, doxorubicin, droper-idol, etoposide, fludarabine, ifosfamide, mechlorethamine, methotrexate, mesna, metoclopramide, mitoxantrone, prochlorperazine, promethazine, teniposide, vinblastine, and vincristine

Incompatible with acyclovir, ampicillin, aminophylline, furosemide, ganciclovir, lorazepam, methylprednisolone, and piperacillin

Mechanism of Action Selective 5-HT$_3$ receptor antagonist, blocking serotonin, both peripherally on vagal nerve terminals and centrally in the chemoreceptor trigger zone

Pharmacokinetics

Absorption: Oral: 100%; nonlinear absorption occurs with increasing oral doses; Zofran® ODT tablets are bioequivalent to Zofran® tablets; absorption does not occur via oral mucosa

Distribution: V_d: Children: 1.6-1.7 L/kg; Adults: 1.9 L/kg

Protein binding, plasma: 70% to 76%

Metabolism: Extensive first-pass metabolism; primarily by hydroxylation, followed by glucuronidation and sulfate conjugation

Bioavailability: Oral: 50% to 70% due to significant first-pass metabolism; in cancer patients (adult) 85% to 87% bioavailability possibly related to changes in metabolism

Half-life:

Children: 3-7 years: 2.6 hours; 7-12 years: 3.1 hours

Adults: 4-5 hours

Elimination: In urine and feces; <5% of the parent drug is recovered unchanged in urine

Clearance:

Children: 3-7 years: 0.5 L/hour/kg; 7-12 years: 0.39 L/hour/kg

Adults: 25-50.7 L/hour (normal); 16-32 L/hour (cancer)

Usual Dosage

Prevention of chemotherapy-induced nausea and vomiting:

Oral (all doses given 30 minutes before chemotherapy and repeated at 8-hour intervals):

Children <4 years: No FDA-approved oral dosage; however, the following dosages based upon body surface area have been used:

<0.3 m^2: 1 mg 3 times/day

0.3-0.6 m^2: 2 mg 3 times/day

0.6-1 m^2: 3 mg 3 times/day

>1 m^2: 4 mg 3 times/day

or

Children 4-11 years: 4 mg 3 times/day

Children >11 years and Adults: 8 mg 3 times/day

Adults: Total body irradiation: 8 mg 1-2 hours before each fraction of radio-therapy administered each day

Single high-dose fraction radiotherapy to abdomen: 8 mg 1-2 hours before irradiation, then 8 mg every 8 hours after first dose for 1-2 days after completion of radiotherapy

Daily fractionated radiotherapy to abdomen: 8 mg 1-2 hours before irradia-tion, then 8 mg every 8 hours after first dose for each day of radio-therapy

I.V.:

Children >3 years: 0.15 mg/kg/dose infused 30 minutes before the start of emetogenic chemotherapy, with subsequent doses administered 4 and 8 hours after the first dose; decreased effectiveness has been reported when administered for prolonged therapy (eg, more than 3 doses)

Adults: 0.15 mg/kg/dose infused 30 minutes before the start of emetogenic chemotherapy with subsequent doses administered 4 and 8 hours after the first dose **or as an alternative,** a single dose as follows: 45-80 kg: 8 mg, >80 kg: 12 mg; a few studies have evaluated a single 8 mg loading dose followed by a continuous 1 mg/hour infusion

Prevention of postoperative nausea and vomiting: I.V.: Give immediately before induction of anesthesia, or postoperatively if the patient is symptomatic:

Children ≥2 years <40 kg: 0.1 mg/kg

Children >40 kg and Adults: 4 mg

Note: Repeating a second ondansetron dose in patients who did not achieve adequate control of postoperative nausea and vomiting after a single dose will not provide additional control.

Dosing adjustment in severe hepatic impairment: Adults: Once daily dosage; maximum 8 mg per dose

Administration

Oral: May administer without regard to meals; Zofran® ODT tablet: Place tablet on tongue, it will disintegrate immediately; may also swallow with fluids as whole tablet

Parenteral: I.V.: Dilute in 50 mL I.V. fluid (maximum concentration: 1 mg/mL) and infuse over 15 minutes; single doses for prevention of postoperative nausea/vomiting may be administered I.V. undiluted over 2-5 minutes or I.M.

Dosage Forms

Injection: 2 mg/mL (2 mL, 20 mL); 32 mg (single-dose vials)

Solution: 4 mg/5 mL

Tablet: 4 mg, 8 mg, 24 mg

Tablet, orally disintegrating, as ondansetron base (Zofran® ODT): 4 mg, 8 mg

References

Carden PA, Mitchell SL, Waters KD, et al, "Prevention of Cyclophosphamide/Cytarabine-Induced Emesis With Ondansetron in Children With Leukemia," *J Clin Oncol*, 1990, 8(9):1531-5.

Marty M, Pouillart P, Scholl S, et al, "Comparison of the 5-hydroxytryptamine 3 (Serotonin) Antagonist Ondansetron (GR 38032F) With High-Dose Metoclopramide in the Control of Cisplatin-Induced Emesis," *N Engl J Med*, 1990, 322(12):816-21.

Pinkerton CR, Williams D, Wootton C, et al, "5-HT₃ Antagonist Ondansetron - An Effective Outpatient Antiemetic in Cancer Treatment," *Arch Dis Child*, 1990, 65(8):822-5.

Roila F and Del Favero A, "Ondansetron Clinical Pharmacokinetics," *Clin Pharmacokinet*, 1995, 29(2):95-109.

Seynaeve C, Schuller J, Buser K, et al, "Comparison of the Anti-emetic Efficacy of Different Doses of Ondansetron, Given as Either a Continuous Infusion or a Single Intravenous Dose, in Acute Cisplatin-Induced Emesis," *Br J Cancer* 1992, 66(1):192-7.

Spahr-Schopfer IA, Lerman J, Sikich N, et al, "Pharmacokinetics of Intravenous Ondansetron in Healthy Children Undergoing Ear, Nose, and Throat Surgery," *Clin Pharmacol Ther*, 1995, 58(3):316-21.

♦ **Opcon® Ophthalmic** *see Naphazoline on page 671*

♦ **Ophthacet®** *see Sulfacetamide on page 888*

♦ **Ophthaine®** *see Proparacaine on page 811*

♦ **Ophthalgan® Ophthalmic** *see Glycerin on page 457*

♦ **Ophthetic®** *see Proparacaine on page 811*

♦ **Ophthochlor® Ophthalmic** *see Chloramphenicol on page 207*

♦ **Ophtho-tate® (Canada)** *see Prednisolone on page 791*

Opium Tincture (OH pee um TING chur)

Related Information

Overdose and Toxicology *on page 1191*

Synonyms Deodorized Opium Tincture; DTO; Tincture of Opium

Therapeutic Category Analgesic, Narcotic; Antidiarrheal

Generic Available Yes

Use Treatment of diarrhea or relief of pain; **a 25-fold dilution with water** (final concentration 0.4 mg/mL morphine) can be used to treat neonatal abstinence syndrome (opiate withdrawal)

Restrictions C-II

Pregnancy Risk Factor B (D if used for prolonged periods or in high doses at term)

Contraindications Hypersensitivity to opium, morphine, or any component; diarrhea caused by poisoning until the toxic material has been removed; increased intracranial pressure, severe respiratory depression, severe liver or renal insufficiency

Warnings Do not confuse opium tincture with paregoric; opium tincture is 25 times as potent as paregoric; opium shares the toxic potential of opiate agonists, usual precautions of opiate agonist therapy should be observed; some preparations contain sulfites which may cause allergic reactions; opium may mask dehydration by producing fluid retention in the bowel; monitor patients with prolonged or severe diarrhea carefully

Precautions Use with caution in patients with respiratory, hepatic, or renal dysfunction, severe prostatic hypertrophy, or history of narcotic abuse; infants <3 months of age are more susceptible to respiratory depression, use with caution and in reduced doses in this age group

Adverse Reactions

Cardiovascular: Hypotension, bradycardia, peripheral vasodilation

Central nervous system: CNS depression, increased intracranial pressure, drowsiness, dizziness, sedation

Dermatologic: Pruritus

Endocrine & metabolic: Antidiuretic hormone release

(Continued)

Opium Tincture *(Continued)*

Gastrointestinal: Nausea, vomiting, constipation
Genitourinary: Urinary tract spasm, urinary retention
Hepatic: Biliary tract spasm
Ocular: Miosis
Respiratory: Respiratory depression
Miscellaneous: Physical and psychological dependence, histamine release

Drug Interactions CNS depressants (eg, alcohol, narcotics, benzodiazepines, tricyclic antidepressants, MAO inhibitors, phenothiazines) may increase effects/toxicity

Stability Protect from light and excessive heat; do not refrigerate, decreased solubility and precipitation may occur

Mechanism of Action Contains many narcotic alkaloids including morphine; gastric motility inhibition is primarily due to morphine content; decreases digestive secretions, increases GI muscle tone, and reduces GI propulsion

Pharmacodynamics Duration of effect: 4-5 hours

Pharmacokinetics
Absorption: Variable from GI tract
Metabolism: In the liver
Elimination: In urine and bile

Usual Dosage Oral:
Neonates (full-term): Neonatal abstinence syndrome (opiate withdrawal): **Use a 25-fold dilution of opium tincture** (final concentration: 0.4 mg/mL morphine); Initial: Give 0.1 mL/kg or 2 drops/kg of the 25-fold dilution per dose with feedings every 3-4 hours; increase as needed by 0.1 mL/kg or 2 drops/kg of the 25-fold dilution every 3-4 hours until withdrawal symptoms are controlled; usual dose: 0.2-0.5 mL of the 25-fold dilution per dose given every 3-4 hours; it is rare to exceed 0.7 mL of the 25-fold dilution per dose; stabilize withdrawal symptoms for 3-5 days, then gradually decrease the dosage (keeping the same dosage interval) over a 2- to 4- week period
Children:
Diarrhea: 0.005-0.01 mL/kg/dose every 3-4 hours for a maximum of 6 doses/24 hours
Analgesia: 0.01-0.02 mL/kg/dose every 3-4 hours
Adults:
Diarrhea: Usual: 0.6 mL/dose; range: 0.3-1 mL/dose every 3-6 hours to maximum of 6 mL/24 hours
Analgesia: 0.6-1.5 mL/dose every 3-4 hours; usual maximum dose: 6 mL/24 hours

Administration Oral: May administer with food to decrease GI upset; for neonatal abstinence syndrome (opiate withdrawal), use a 25-fold dilution of opium tincture

Monitoring Parameters Respiratory rate, blood pressure, heart rate, resolution of diarrhea or pain, mental status; if using a 25-fold dilution to treat neonatal abstinence syndrome, monitor for resolution of withdrawal symptoms (such as irritability, high-pitched cry, stuffy nose, rhinorrhea, vomiting, poor feeding, diarrhea, sneezing, yawning etc), and signs of overtreatment (such as bradycardia, lethargy, hypotonia, irregular respirations, respiratory depression etc). An abstinence scoring system (eg, Finnegan abstinence scoring system) can be used to more objectively assess neonatal opiate withdrawal symptoms and the need for dosage adjustment. Monitor fluid and electrolyte balance in young children being treated for prolonged or severe diarrhea.

Patient Information Avoid alcohol; may cause drowsiness and impair ability to perform activities requiring mental alertness or physical coordination; may be habit-forming

Nursing Implications Observe patient for excessive sedation, respiratory depression; implement safety measures; assist with ambulation; do not abruptly discontinue after prolonged use

Additional Information Opium tincture contains 10 mg/mL morphine and 17% to 21% alcohol; for treatment of neonatal abstinence syndrome, a 25-fold dilution of opium tincture (final concentration: 0.4 mg/mL morphine) is preferred over paregoric; the 25-fold dilution of opium tincture contains the same morphine concentration as paregoric, but without the high amount of alcohol or additives of paregoric

Dosage Forms Liquid: 10% [0.6 mL equivalent to morphine 6 mg]

References
Kraus DM and Hatzopoulos FK, "Neonatal Therapy," *Applied Therapeutics: The Clinical Use of Drugs,* 6th ed, Young LY and Koda-Kimble MA, eds, Vancouver, WA: Applied Therapeutics, Inc, 1995.
Levy M and Spino M, "Neonatal Withdrawal Syndrome: Associated Drugs and Pharmacologic Management," *Pharmacotherapy,* 1993, 13(3):202-11.
"Neonatal Drug Withdrawal. American Academy of Pediatrics Committee on Drugs," *Pediatrics,* 1998, 101(6):1079-88.

- **Optho-Bunolol® (Canada)** *see Levobunolol on page 564*
- **Optho-Dipivefrin™ (Canada)** *see Dipivefrin on page 330*
- **Opticrom®** *see Cromolyn on page 260*
- **Opticrom® (Canada)** *see Cromolyn on page 260*
- **Optimyxin® (Canada)** *see Polymyxin B on page 782*
- **Optivar™** *see Azelastine on page 113*
- **Orabase®-B [OTC]** *see Benzocaine on page 124*
- **OrabaseGel® [OTC]** *see Benzocaine on page 124*
- **Orabase® HCA Topical** *see Hydrocortisone on page 486*
- **Orabase®-O [OTC]** *see Benzocaine on page 124*
- **Oracit®** *see Citrate and Citric Acid on page 231*
- **Orajel® Brace-Aid Oral Anesthetic [OTC]** *see Benzocaine on page 124*
- **Orajel® Maximum Strength [OTC]** *see Benzocaine on page 124*
- **Orajel® Mouth-Aid [OTC]** *see Benzocaine on page 124*
- **Orajel® Perioseptic [OTC]** *see Carbamide Peroxide on page 167*
- **Oral Contraceptives** *see page 1052*
- **Oraminic® II** *see Brompheniramine on page 142*
- **Oramorph SR® Oral** *see Morphine Sulfate on page 657*
- **Orasept® [OTC]** *see Benzocaine on page 124*
- **Orasol® [OTC]** *see Benzocaine on page 124*
- **Orasone®** *see Prednisone on page 794*
- **Orastect® [OTC]** *see Benzocaine on page 124*
- **Orazinc® [OTC]** *see Zinc Supplements on page 994*
- **Orbenin® (Canada)** *see Cloxacillin on page 246*
- **Orciprenaline** *see Metaproterenol on page 611*
- **Oretic®** *see Hydrochlorothiazide on page 483*
- **ORF17070** *see Histrelin on page 476*
- **Organidin NR®** *see Guaifenesin on page 464*
- **ORG NC 45** *see Vecuronium on page 972*
- **Ormazine®** *see Chlorpromazine on page 215*
- **Oro-Clense (Canada)** *see Chlorhexidine Gluconate on page 209*
- **Ortho-Chloram® (Canada)** *see Chloramphenicol on page 207*
- **Orthoclone OKT®3** *see Muromonab-CD3 on page 661*
- **Or-Tyl® Injection** *see Dicyclomine on page 314*
- **Os-Cal® 500 [OTC]** *see Calcium Supplements on page 157*
- **Osmitrol® Injection** *see Mannitol on page 593*
- **Osmoglyn® Ophthalmic** *see Glycerin on page 457*
- **Osteocalcin®** *see Calcitonin on page 154*
- **Ostoforte®(Canada)** *see Ergocalciferol on page 377*
- **OTC Cough & Cold Preparations, Pediatric** *see page 1037*
- **Oto®** *see Antipyrine and Benzocaine on page 90*
- **Otocalm® Ear** *see Antipyrine and Benzocaine on page 90*
- **Otocort® Otic** *see Neomycin, (Bacitracin) Polymyxin B, and Hydrocortisone on page 679*
- **Otomycin-HPN® Otic** *see Neomycin, (Bacitracin) Polymyxin B, and Hydrocortisone on page 679*
- **Otosporin® Otic** *see Neomycin, (Bacitracin) Polymyxin B, and Hydrocortisone on page 679*
- **Overdose and Toxicology** *see page 1191*
- **Ovol® (Canada)** *see Simethicone on page 868*
- **O-V Staticin®** *see Nystatin on page 701*

Oxacillin (oks a SIL in)

Brand Names Bactocill®; Prostaphlin®
Available Salts Oxacillin Sodium
Synonyms Isoxazolyl Penicillin; Methylphenyl
Therapeutic Category Antibiotic, Penicillin (Antistaphylococcal)
Generic Available Yes
Use Treatment of bacterial infections such as osteomyelitis, septicemia, endocarditis, and CNS infections due to susceptible penicillinase-producing strains of *Staphylococcus*
(Continued)

Oxacillin *(Continued)*

Pregnancy Risk Factor B

Contraindications Hypersensitivity to oxacillin, other penicillins, or any component

Warnings Elimination rate will be decreased in neonates

Precautions Use with caution in patients with hypersensitivity to cephalosporins, severe renal impairment; dosage modification required in patients with renal impairment

Adverse Reactions

Central nervous system: Fever

Dermatologic: Rash

Gastrointestinal: Diarrhea, nausea, vomiting, *C. difficile* colitis

Hematologic: Mild leukopenia, agranulocytosis, thrombocytopenia, eosinophilia

Hepatic: Elevated AST, hepatotoxicity

Local: Thrombophlebitis

Renal: Acute interstitial nephritis; hematuria and azotemia have occurred in neonates and infants receiving high-dose oxacillin; albuminuria

Miscellaneous: Hypersensitivity reactions, serum sickness-like reactions

Drug Interactions Probenecid (decreases oxacillin elimination rate)

Food Interactions Presence of food decreases GI absorption of oxacillin

Stability Reconstituted oxacillin 250 mg/1.5 mL solution for injection is stable for 3 days at room temperature or 7 days when refrigerated; reconstituted oxacillin oral solution is stable for 3 days at room temperature or 14 days when refrigerated; potentially incompatible with aminoglycosides and tetracyclines

Mechanism of Action Interferes with bacterial cell wall synthesis during active multiplication by binding to one or more of the penicillin-binding proteins; inhibits the final transpeptidation step of peptidoglycan synthesis causing cell wall death and resultant bactericidal activity against susceptible bacteria

Pharmacokinetics

Absorption: Oral: ~35% to 67%

Distribution: Distributes into bile, pleural, synovial, and pericardial fluids and into lungs and bone; penetrates the blood-brain barrier only when meninges are inflamed; crosses the placenta; appears in breast milk

Protein binding: 90% to 95%

Metabolism: In the liver to active and inactive metabolites

Half-life (prolonged with reduced renal function):

Neonates 8-15 days: 1.6 hours

Children 1 week to 2 years: 0.9-1.8 hours

Adults: 0.3-0.8 hours

Time to peak serum concentration:

Oral: Within 30-120 minutes

I.M.: Within 30-60 minutes

Elimination: By the kidneys and to small degree via bile as parent drug and metabolites

Not dialyzable (0% to 5%)

Usual Dosage

Neonates: I.M., I.V.:

Postnatal age ≤7 days:

≤2000 g: 50 mg/kg/day in divided doses every 12 hours

>2000 g: 75 mg/kg/day in divided doses every 8 hours

Postnatal age >7 days:

<1200 g: 50 mg/kg/day in divided doses every 12 hours

1200-2000 g: 75 mg/kg/day in divided doses every 8 hours

>2000 g: 100 mg/kg/day in divided doses every 6 hours

Infants and Children: I.M., I.V.:

Mild to moderate infections: 100-150 mg/kg/day in divided doses every 6 hours

Severe infections: 150-200 mg/kg/day in divided doses every 4-6 hours; maximum dose: 12 g/day

Children: Oral: 50-100 mg/kg/day divided every 6 hours

Adults:

Oral: 500-1000 mg every 4-6 hours

I.M., I.V.: 250 mg to 2 g/dose every 4-6 hours

Dosing interval in renal impairment: Cl_{cr} <10 mL/minute: Use lower range of the usual dosage

Administration

Oral: Administer on an empty stomach with water 1 hour before or 2 hours after meals

Parenteral:

I.V. push: Administer over 10 minutes at a maximum concentration of 100 mg/mL

I.V. intermittent infusion: Administer over 15-30 minutes at a final concentration ≤40 mg/mL

Monitoring Parameters Periodic CBC with differential, urinalysis, BUN, serum creatinine, AST and ALT

Test Interactions False-positive urinary and serum proteins

Additional Information Sodium content:
1 g injection: 2.8-3.1 mEq
250 mg capsule: 0.7 mEq
250 mg/5 mL oral solution: 0.8 mEq/5 mL

Dosage Forms
Capsule, as sodium: 250 mg, 500 mg
Powder for injection, as sodium: 250 mg, 500 mg, 1 g, 2 g, 4 g, 10 g
Powder for oral solution, as sodium: 250 mg/5 mL (100 mL)

References
Olans RN and Weiner LB, "Reversible Oxacillin Hepatotoxicity," *J Pediatr*, 1976, 89(5):835-8.
Prober CG, Stevenson DK, and Benitz WE, "The Use of Antibiotics in Neonates Weighing Less Than 1200 Grams," *Pediatr Infect Dis J*, 1990, 9(2):111-21.

♦ Oxacillin Sodium *see* Oxacillin *on page 711*

Oxcarbazepine (ox car BAZ e peen)

Brand Names Trileptal®

Therapeutic Category Anticonvulsant, Miscellaneous

Generic Available No

Use Adjunctive treatment of partial seizures in pediatric and adult patients; monotherapy of partial seizures in adults

Pregnancy Risk Factor C

Contraindications Hypersensitivity to oxcarbazepine or any component

Warnings Significant hyponatremia may occur; a serum sodium <125 mEq/L has been reported in 2.5% of patients; consider monitoring serum sodium especially in patients who receive other drugs that may cause hyponatremia and in patients with symptoms of hyponatremia (eg, nausea, headache, malaise, confusion, lethargy, or obtundation). Do not abruptly discontinue therapy, withdraw gradually to lessen chance for increased seizure frequency (unless a more rapid withdrawal is required due to safety concerns). Cross-hypersensitivity reactions with carbamazepine may occur (incidence: 25% to 30%); discontinue oxcarbazepine immediately if signs or symptoms of hypersensitivity develop

Precautions CNS adverse effects may occur including somnolence, fatigue, coordination abnormalities (ataxia and gait disturbances), and cognitive symptoms (difficulty concentrating, speech or language problems, and psychomotor slowing); these effects may be more common when oxcarbazepine is used as add-on therapy versus monotherapy. Use with caution and modify dose in patients with renal impairment. Multiple drug interactions may occur (see Drug Interactions).

Adverse Reactions
Central nervous system: Headache, dizziness, somnolence, fatigue, ataxia, tremor, insomnia, cognitive symptoms (psychomotor slowing, difficulty concentrating, speech or language problems), vertigo, anxiety, nervousness, emotional lability
Dermatologic: Rash; rare: Stevens-Johnson syndrome, erythema multiforme, toxic epidermal necrolysis
Endocrine and Metabolic: Hyponatremia (incidence: 2.5%; usually occurs within the first 3 months of therapy, but has been reported in patients more than 1 year after starting medication; serum sodium returns towards normal after discontinuation, reduction of dose, or with conservative treatment such as fluid restriction); reduction in T_4 levels
Gastrointestinal: Nausea, vomiting, abdominal pain, dyspepsia
Neuromuscular & skeletal: Abnormal gait
Ocular: Diplopia, abnormal vision, nystagmus
Miscellaneous: Hypersensitivity reactions; a rare, multi-organ hypersensitivity reaction with rash, lymphadenopathy, fever, eosinophilia, abnormal liver function tests, and arthralgia has also been reported

Drug Interactions Cytochrome P-450 isoenzyme CYP2C19 inhibitor; CYP3A4 and CYP3A5 inducer
Oxcarbazepine may inhibit hepatic metabolism and increase the serum concentrations of phenobarbital (by 14%) and phenytoin (by 40% with high-dose oxcarbazepine; dosage reduction of phenytoin may be needed); may induce hepatic metabolism and decrease serum concentrations of felodipine, lamotrigine, and oral contraceptives such as ethinyl estradiol and levonorgestrel (alternative methods of contraception are recommended)
(Continued)

Oxcarbazepine *(Continued)*

P-450 enzyme inducers such as carbamazepine, phenobarbital, and phenytoin, may significantly decrease MHD concentrations by 25% to 40%; valproic acid decreases MHD concentrations by 18% and verapamil decreases MHD concentrations by 20%

Food Interactions Food does not affect rate or extent of absorption

Stability Store at controlled room temperature (25°C); dispense in tight container

Mechanism of Action Active 10-monohydroxy metabolite (MHD) is primarily responsible for anticonvulsant activity; exact mechanism unknown; both MHD and oxcarbazepine are thought to decrease the spread of seizure activity by blockade of sodium channels; also increases conductance of potassium and modulates activity of high-voltage activated calcium channels

Pharmacokinetics

Absorption: Oral: Complete

Distribution: MHD: V_d (apparent): Adults: 49 L

Protein binding: Oxcarbazepine: 67%; MHD: 40%, primarily to albumin; parent drug and metabolite do not bind to alpha-1-acid glycoprotein

Metabolism: Oxcarbazepine is extensively metabolized in the liver to its active 10-monohydroxy metabolite (MHD); MHD undergoes further metabolism via glucuronide conjugation; 4% of dose is oxidized to the 10,11-dihydroxy metabolite (DHD) (inactive); 70% of serum concentration appears as MHD, 2% as unchanged oxcarbazepine, and the rest as minor metabolites; **Note:** Unlike carbamazepine, autoinduction of metabolism has not been observed and biotransformation of oxcarbazepine does not result in an epoxide metabolite

Half-life:

Adults:

Oxcarbazepine: 2 hours

MHD: 9 hours

Adults with renal impairment (Cl_{cr} <30 mL/minute): MHD: 19 hours

Time to peak serum concentration: Adults: 3-13 hours (median: 4.5 hours)

Elimination: >95% of dose is excreted in the urine with <1% as unchanged parent drug, 27% as unchanged MHD, 49% as MHD glucuronides, 3% as DHD (inactive), and 13% as conjugate of oxcarbazepine and MHD; <4% excreted in feces

Clearance:

Children <8 years: Increased by 30% to 40% compared to children >8 years and adults

Children >8 years: Values approach adult clearance

Hepatic impairment: Mild to moderate: No effect on pharmacokinetics; Severe: Not studied

Usual Dosage Oral:

Neonates, Infants, and Children <4 years: Not approved for use; controlled trials in children <2 years have not been conducted

Children 4-16 years: Adjunctive therapy: Initial: 8-10 mg/kg/day given in 2 divided doses (usual maximum: 600 mg/day); increase dose slowly over 2 weeks to weight-dependent target maintenance dose:

20-29 kg: 900 mg/day in 2 divided doses

29.1-39 kg: 1200 mg/day in 2 divided doses

>39 kg: 1800 mg/day in 2 divided doses

Note: Use of these pediatric target maintenance doses in one clinical trial resulted in doses ranging from 6-51 mg/kg/day (median dose: 31 mg/kg/day)

Adults:

Adjunctive therapy: Initial: 300 mg twice daily; increase if needed by no more than 600 mg/day at approximately weekly intervals; recommended maintenance dose: 600 mg twice daily; **Note:** Doses >1200 mg/day may have greater efficacy, but most patients are not able to tolerate 2400 mg/day (mostly due to CNS effects); monitor patient closely and measure concentrations of concomitant antiepileptic agents during dosage titration and especially with oxcarbazepine doses >1200 mg/day

Conversion to monotherapy: Initial: 300 mg twice daily with a simultaneous initial reduction of the dose of concomitant antiepileptic drugs (AEDs); withdraw concomitant AEDs completely over 3-6 weeks, while increasing oxcarbazepine dose as needed by no more than 600 mg/day at approximately weekly intervals; recommended oxcarbazepine dose (1200 mg twice daily) should be reached in about 2-4 weeks; **Note:** A lower dose (1200 mg/day) was effective in one study in patients who initiated oxcarbazepine monotherapy

Initiation of monotherapy: Initial: 300 mg twice daily; increase by 300 mg/day every third day to 1200 mg/day; a higher dose (2400 mg/day) was effective in patients who were converted from other AEDs to oxcarbazepine monotherapy.

Dosing adjustment in renal impairment: Cl_{cr} <30 mL/minute: Initial dose: Administer 50% of the normal starting dose; slowly increase the dose if needed, using a slower dosage titration than normal

Dosing adjustment in hepatic impairment:
Mild to moderate hepatic impairment: No dosage adjustment recommended
Severe hepatic impairment: Not evaluated

Administration Oral: May be taken without regard to meals

Monitoring Parameters Seizure frequency, duration and severity; symptoms of CNS depression (dizziness, headache, somnolence) and allergic reaction; consider monitoring serum sodium (particularly during first three months of therapy) especially in patients who receive other drugs that may cause hyponatremia and in patients with symptoms of hyponatremia (eg, nausea, headache, malaise, confusion, lethargy, or obtundation)

Patient Information Inform prescriber if allergic to carbamazepine; do not abruptly discontinue, an increase in seizure activity may result; report excessive somnolence or allergic reactions to physician immediately; report unusual symptoms such as nausea, headache, malaise, confusion, lethargy, or obtundation to physician immediately; blood test for serum sodium may be needed; avoid alcohol; may cause drowsiness and impair ability to perform activities that require mental alertness or physical coordination

Additional Information Symptoms of overdose may include CNS depression (somnolence, ataxia, obtundation); treatment is symptomatic and supportive; consider general poisoning management (eg, gastric lavage, activated charcoal); largest reported overdose is 24 g; oxcarbazepine is a keto analogue of carbamazepine

Dosage Forms Tablet: 150 mg, 300 mg, 600 mg

References
Tecoma ES, "Oxcarbazepine," *Epilepsia*, 1999, 40(Suppl 5): S37-46.

♦ **Oxpentifylline** *see* Pentoxifylline *on page 750*
♦ **Oxy-5® Advanced Formula for Sensitive Skin [OTC]** *see* Benzoyl Peroxide *on page 126*
♦ **Oxy-5® Tinted [OTC]** *see* Benzoyl Peroxide *on page 126*
♦ **Oxy-10® Advanced Formula for Sensitive Skin [OTC]** *see* Benzoyl Peroxide *on page 126*
♦ **Oxy 10® Wash [OTC]** *see* Benzoyl Peroxide *on page 126*

Oxybutynin (oks i BYOO ti nin)

Related Information
Carbohydrate and Alcohol Content of Liquid Medications for Use in Patients Receiving Ketogenic Diets *on page 1228*

Brand Names Ditropan®; Ditropan® XL

Available Salts Oxybutynin Chloride

Therapeutic Category Antispasmodic Agent, Urinary

Generic Available Yes

Use Relief of bladder spasms associated with voiding in patients with uninhibited and reflex neurogenic bladder

Pregnancy Risk Factor B

Contraindications Glaucoma (angle-closure), myasthenia gravis, partial or complete GI obstruction, GU obstruction, ulcerative colitis; hypersensitivity to oxybutynin or any component; intestinal atony, megacolon, toxic megacolon

Precautions Use with caution in patients with hepatic or renal disease, heart disease, hyperthyroidism, reflux esophagitis, hypertension, prostatic hypertrophy, autonomic neuropathy

Adverse Reactions
Cardiovascular: Tachycardia, palpitations, vasodilation
Central nervous system: Drowsiness, dizziness, insomnia, fever, hallucinations
Dermatologic: Rash
Endocrine & metabolic: Hot flashes
Gastrointestinal: Xerostomia, nausea, vomiting, constipation, decreased GI motility
Genitourinary: Impotence, urinary hesitancy or retention
Neuromuscular & skeletal: Weakness
Ocular: Blurred vision, mydriasis, decreased lacrimation, amblyopia, cycloplegia
Miscellaneous: Hypersensitivity reactions, decreased diaphoresis

Drug Interactions Additive sedation with CNS depressants and alcohol; additive anticholinergic effects with antihistamines and anticholinergic agents; decreased haloperidol serum concentrations; may increase digoxin serum levels
(Continued)

Oxybutynin *(Continued)*

Mechanism of Action Direct antispasmodic effect on smooth muscle, also inhibits the action of acetylcholine on smooth muscle; does not block effects at skeletal muscle or at autonomic ganglia

Pharmacodynamics

Immediate release formulation:

Onset of action: Oral: Within 30-60 minutes

Peak effect: 3-6 hours

Duration: 6-10 hours

Extended release formulation: Maximum effects: 3 days

Pharmacokinetics

Absorption: Oral: Rapid and well absorbed

Metabolism: In the liver

Half-life: 1-2.3 hours

Time to peak serum concentration:

Immediate release: Within 60 minutes

Extended release: 12-13 hours

Elimination: In urine

Usual Dosage Oral:

Children:

1-5 years: 0.2 mg/kg/dose 2-4 times/day

>5 years: 5 mg twice daily, up to 5 mg 4 times/day

Adults: 5 mg 2-3 times/day up to 5 mg 4 times/day maximum **or** extended release tablet (Ditropan® XL) 5-10 mg once daily; maximum 30 mg once daily

Note: Should be discontinued periodically to determine whether the patient can manage without the drug and to minimize tolerance to the drug

Administration Oral: May administer with food or milk to decrease GI distress; extended release formulation may be administered with or without food; swallow extended release tablets whole; do not chew or crush

Patient Information Causes drowsiness and may impair ability to perform hazardous activities requiring mental alertness or physical coordination; avoid alcohol; nonabsorbable tablet shell may be seen in stool, but active drug has been released

Dosage Forms

Syrup, as chloride: 5 mg/5 mL (473 mL)

Tablet, as chloride: 5 mg

Tablet, extended release, as chloride (Ditropan® XL): 5 mg, 10 mg, 15 mg

♦ **Oxybutynin Chloride** *see Oxybutynin on page 715*

♦ **Oxycocet® (Canada)** *see Oxycodone and Acetaminophen on page 716*

♦ **Oxycodan® (Canada)** *see Oxycodone and Aspirin on page 717*

Oxycodone and Acetaminophen

(oks i KOE done & a seet a MIN oh fen)

Related Information

Narcotic Analgesics Comparison *on page 1035*

Overdose and Toxicology *on page 1191*

Brand Names Endocet® (Canada); Oxycocet® (Canada); Percocet 2.5/325™; Percocet 5/325™; Percocet 7.5/500™; Percocet 10/650™; Percocet®-Demi (Canada); Roxicet® 5/500; Roxilox®; Tylox®

Available Salts Oxycodone Hydrochloride and Acetaminophen

Synonyms Acetaminophen and Oxycodone

Therapeutic Category Analgesic, Narcotic

Generic Available Yes

Use Management of moderate to severe pain

Restrictions C-II

Pregnancy Risk Factor C

Contraindications Hypersensitivity to oxycodone, acetaminophen, or any component; severe respiratory depression, severe liver or renal insufficiency

Warnings Some preparations contain bisulfites which may cause allergies

Precautions Use with caution in patients with hypersensitivity to other phenanthrene derivative opioid agonists (morphine, codeine, hydrocodone, hydromorphone, oxymorphone, levorphanol)

Adverse Reactions

Cardiovascular: Hypotension, bradycardia, peripheral vasodilation

Central nervous system: CNS depression, increased intracranial pressure, drowsiness, sedation

Dermatologic: Pruritus
Endocrine & metabolic: Antidiuretic hormone release
Gastrointestinal: Nausea, vomiting, constipation, biliary tract spasm
Genitourinary: Urinary tract spasm
Ocular: Miosis
Respiratory: Respiratory depression
Miscellaneous: Physical and psychological dependence, histamine release

Drug Interactions CNS depressants, phenothiazines, tricyclic antidepressants may potentiate the effects of oxycodone; see also Acetaminophen *on page 26*

Food Interactions Rate of absorption of acetaminophen may be decreased when given with food high in carbohydrates

Pharmacodynamics
Onset of action: Within 10-15 minutes
Peak effect: Within 1 hour
Duration: 3-6 hours

Pharmacokinetics (Oxycodone); see also Acetaminophen *on page 26*
Protein binding: 38%
Distribution: V_{dss}
Children 2-10 years: Mean: 2.1 L/kg; range: 1.2-3.7 L/kg
Adults: 2.6 L/kg
Metabolism: In the liver primarily to oxymorphone and noroxycodone
Bioavailability: 40% to 60%
Half-life, (elimination):
Children 2-10 years: 1.8 hours; range: 1.2-3 hours
Adults: 3.7 hours
Elimination: In the urine as unchanged drug (~7%) and metabolites

Usual Dosage Oral (titrate dose to appropriate analgesic effects):
Children: Based on **oxycodone component**: 0.05-0.15 mg/kg/dose up to 5 mg/dose every 4-6 hours as needed
Adults: 1-2 tablets every 4-6 hours as needed for pain; maximum daily dose of acetaminophen: 4 g/day

Administration Oral: May administer with food or milk to decrease GI upset

Monitoring Parameters Pain relief, respiratory rate, mental status, blood pressure

Patient Information Avoid alcohol; may be habit-forming; may cause drowsiness and impair ability to perform hazardous activities requiring mental alertness or physical coordination

Dosage Forms
Caplet: Oxycodone hydrochloride 5 mg and acetaminophen 500 mg
Capsule: Oxycodone hydrochloride 5 mg and acetaminophen 500 mg
Solution, oral: Oxycodone hydrochloride 5 mg and acetaminophen 325 mg per 5 mL (5 mL, 500 mL)
Tablet:
Percocet 2.5/325™: Oxycodone hydrochloride 2.5 mg and acetaminophen 325 mg
Percocet 5/325™: Oxycodone hydrochloride 5 mg and acetaminophen 325 mg
Roxicet® 5/500: Oxycodone hydrochloride 5 mg and acetaminophen 500 mg
Percocet 7.5/500™: Oxycodone hydrochloride 7.5 mg and acetaminophen 500 mg
Percocet 10/650™: Oxycodone hydrochloride 10 mg and acetaminophen 650 mg

References
Olkkola KT, Hamunen K, and Maunuksela EL, "Clinical Pharmacokinetics and Pharmacodynamics of Opioid Analgesics in Infants and Children," *Clin Pharmacokinet*, 1995, 28(5):385-404.

Oxycodone and Aspirin (oks i KOE done & AS pir in)

Related Information
Overdose and Toxicology *on page 1191*

Brand Names Codoxy®; Endodan® (Canada); Oxycodan® (Canada); Percodan®; Percodan®-Demi; Roxiprin®

Available Salts Oxycodone Hydrochloride, Oxycodone Terephthalate, and Aspirin

Synonyms Aspirin and Oxycodone

Therapeutic Category Analgesic, Narcotic

Generic Available Yes

Use Relief of moderate to moderately severe pain

Restrictions C-II

Pregnancy Risk Factor D

Contraindications Hypersensitivity to oxycodone, aspirin, or any component; severe respiratory depression, severe liver, or renal insufficiency
(Continued)

Oxycodone and Aspirin *(Continued)*

Warnings Contains aspirin, do not use aspirin-containing products in children <16 years of age for chickenpox or flu symptoms due to the association with Reye's syndrome

Precautions Use with caution in patients with hypersensitivity to other phenanthrene derivative opioid agonists (morphine, codeine, hydrocodone, hydromorphone, oxymorphone, levorphanol); contains aspirin, use with caution in patients with impaired renal function, erosive gastritis, peptic ulcer, gout

Adverse Reactions
Cardiovascular: Hypotension, bradycardia, peripheral vasodilation
Central nervous system: CNS depression, increased intracranial pressure, drowsiness, sedation
Dermatologic: Pruritus, rash
Endocrine & metabolic: Antidiuretic hormone release
Gastrointestinal: Nausea, vomiting, constipation, biliary tract spasm, GI distress
Genitourinary: Urinary tract spasm
Hematologic: Inhibition of platelet aggregation (due to aspirin)
Hepatic: Hepatotoxicity (due to aspirin)
Ocular: Miosis
Respiratory: Respiratory depression
Miscellaneous: Histamine release, physical and psychological dependence

Drug Interactions CNS depressants, phenothiazines, tricyclic antidepressants may potentiate the effects of oxycodone; see also Aspirin *on page 99*

Food Interactions Aspirin may increase renal excretion of vitamin C and may decrease serum folate levels

Usual Dosage Oral: Based on **oxycodone-combined salt component**:
Children: 0.05-0.15 mg/kg/dose every 4-6 hours as needed; maximum dose: 5 mg/dose (1 tablet Percodan® or 2 tablets Percodan®-Demi/dose)
  or alternatively:
Percodan®-Demi:
  6-12 years: $1/4$ tablet every 6 hours as needed for pain
  >12 years: $1/2$ tablet every 6 hours as needed for pain
Adults: Percodan®: 1 tablet every 6 hours as needed for pain or Percodan®-Demi: 1-2 tablets every 6 hours as needed for pain

Administration Oral: May administer with food or milk to decrease GI upset

Monitoring Parameters Pain relief, respiratory rate, mental status, blood pressure

Patient Information Avoid alcohol; may cause drowsiness and impair ability to perform activities requiring mental alertness or physical coordination; may be habit-forming

Additional Information One tablet (Percodan®) contains ~5 mg oxycodone as combined salt

Dosage Forms Tablet:
Percodan®: Oxycodone hydrochloride 4.5 mg, oxycodone terephthalate 0.38 mg, and aspirin 325 mg
Percodan®-Demi: Oxycodone hydrochloride 2.25 mg, oxycodone terephthalate 0.19 mg, and aspirin 325 mg

♦ **Oxycodone Hydrochloride and Acetaminophen** *see* Oxycodone and Acetaminophen *on page 716*

♦ **Oxycodone Hydrochloride, Oxycodone Terephthalate, and Aspirin** *see* Oxycodone and Aspirin *on page 717*

♦ **Oxyderm™ 5%, 10%, 20% (Canada)** *see* Benzoyl Peroxide *on page 126*

Oxymetazoline *(oks i met AZ oh leen)*

Related Information
OTC Cough & Cold Preparations, Pediatric *on page 1037*

Brand Names Afrin® Children's Nose Drops [OTC]; Afrin® Nasal Solution [OTC]; Allerest® 12 Hour Nasal Solution [OTC]; Chlorphed®-LA Nasal Solution [OTC]; Dristan® Long Lasting Nasal Solution [OTC]; Drixoral® Nasal (Canada); Duramist Plus® [OTC]; Duration® Nasal Solution [OTC]; Neo-Synephrine® 12 Hour Nasal Solution [OTC]; Nōstrilla® [OTC]; NTZ® Long Acting Nasal Solution [OTC]; OcuClear® Ophthalmic [OTC]; Sinarest® 12 Hour Nasal Solution; Sinex® Long-Acting [OTC]; Twice-A-Day® Nasal Solution [OTC]; Visine® L.R. Ophthalmic [OTC]; 4-Way® Long Acting Nasal Solution [OTC]

Available Salts Oxymetazoline Hydrochloride

Therapeutic Category Adrenergic Agonist Agent; Decongestant, Nasal; Nasal Agent, Vasoconstrictor; Vasoconstrictor, Nasal; Vasoconstrictor, Ophthalmic

Generic Available Yes

Use Symptomatic relief of nasal mucosal congestion associated with acute or chronic rhinitis, the common cold, sinusitis, hay fever, or other allergies

Pregnancy Risk Factor C

Contraindications Hypersensitivity to oxymetazoline or any component; patients on MAO inhibitor therapy

Warnings Use for periods exceeding 3 days may result in severe rebound nasal congestion; excessive dosage in children may cause profound CNS depression

Precautions Use with caution in patients with hyperthyroidism, heart disease, hypertension, diabetes mellitus, increased intraocular pressure, or prostatic hypertrophy

Adverse Reactions

Cardiovascular: Hypertension, palpitations, reflex bradycardia, pallor

Central nervous system: Nervousness, dizziness, insomnia, headache, anxiety, tenseness, drowsiness, CNS depression, convulsions, hallucinations

Gastrointestinal: Nausea, vomiting

Ocular: Stinging to eye, mydriasis, increased intraocular pressure, blurred vision

Respiratory: Sneezing, respiratory difficulty, rebound congestion with prolonged use, dryness of nasal mucosa

Miscellaneous: Diaphoresis

Drug Interactions Anesthetics (discontinue oxymetazoline prior to use of anesthetics that sensitize the myocardium to sympathomimetics, ie, cyclopropane, halothane); MAO inhibitors, methyldopa, tricyclic antidepressants increase hypertensive response

Mechanism of Action Stimulates alpha-adrenergic receptors in the arterioles of the nasal mucosa and arterioles of the conjunctiva to produce vasoconstriction

Pharmacodynamics

Intranasal: Onset of action: Within 5-10 minutes

Duration: 5-6 hours

Pharmacokinetics Metabolic fate is unknown

Usual Dosage

Nasal: Therapy should not exceed 3-5 days; avoid use of 0.05% solution in children <6 years of age

Children 2-5 years: 0.025% solution: 2-3 drops in each nostril twice daily

Children ≥6 years and Adults: 0.05% solution: 2-3 drops or 2-3 sprays or 1-2 metered sprays (Nōstrilla®) into each nostril twice daily

Ophthalmic: Children ≥6 years and Adults: Instill 1-2 drops into the affected eye(s) 2-4 times/day (≥6 hours apart)

Administration

Nasal: Spray or apply drops into each nostril while gently occluding the other

Ophthalmic: Instill drops into conjunctival sac of affected eye(s); avoid contact of bottle tip with skin or eye; finger pressure should be applied to lacrimal sac during and for 1-2 minutes after instillation to decrease the risk of absorption and systemic reactions

Dosage Forms

Nasal, solution, as hydrochloride:

Drops:

Afrin® Children's Nose Drops: 0.025% (20 mL)

Afrin®, NTZ® Long Acting Nasal Solution: 0.05% (15 mL, 20 mL)

Spray (Afrin®, Allerest® 12 Hours, Chlorphed®-LA, Dristan® Long Lasting, Duration®, 4-Way® Long Acting, Neo-Synephrine® 12 Hour, Nōstrilla®, NTZ® Long Acting Nasal Solution, Sinex® Long-Acting, Twice-A-Day®): 0.05% (15 mL, 30 mL)

Ophthalmic solution, as hydrochloride (OcuClear®, Visine® L.R.): 0.025% (15 mL, 30 mL)

♦ **Oxymetazoline Hydrochloride** *see* Oxymetazoline *on page 718*

♦ **Oyst-Cal 500 [OTC]** *see* Calcium Supplements *on page 157*

♦ **Oystercal® 500** *see* Calcium Supplements *on page 157*

♦ **P-071** *see* Cetirizine *on page 201*

♦ **Pacerone®** *see* Amiodarone *on page 63*

Paclitaxel (PAK li taks el)

Brand Names Taxol®

Therapeutic Category Antineoplastic Agent, Antimicrotubular

Generic Available No

Use Treatment of advanced metastatic breast cancer, metastatic ovarian cancer, and AIDS-related Kaposi's sarcoma that is refractory to conventional therapy; (Continued)

Paclitaxel *(Continued)*

active in lung cancer, head and neck cancer, bladder cancer, malignant melanoma, and other refractory solid tumors, and leukemias

Pregnancy Risk Factor D

Contraindications Hypersensitivity to paclitaxel, Cremophor® EL (polyoxyethylated castor oil) or any component

Warnings The FDA currently recommends that procedures for proper handling and disposal of antineoplastic agents be considered. Anaphylaxis and severe hypersensitivity reactions have occurred in 2% of patients receiving paclitaxel in clinical trials during first or subsequent infusions. **All patients should be premedicated with a corticosteroid, diphenhydramine, and an H$_2$-receptor antagonist to prevent hypersensitivity reactions.** Patients who experience severe hypersensitivity reactions to paclitaxel should not be rechallenged with the drug. Be prepared to treat a severe hypersensitivity reaction with epinephrine, I.V. fluids, diphenhydramine and a corticosteroid.

CNS toxicity has been reported in pediatric patients receiving high doses of paclitaxel (350-420 mg/m^2 as a 3-hour infusion) which may have resulted from the ethanol contained in the formulation. Severe bone marrow suppression (primarily neutropenia) with resulting infection may occur. In general, do not administer paclitaxel to patients with baseline neutrophil counts <1500/mm^3.

Precautions Use with caution in patients with moderate or severe hepatic impairment; dosage adjustment may be necessary in patients with hepatic impairment, severe neutropenia, or peripheral neuropathy

Adverse Reactions

Cardiovascular: Hypotension or hypertension, bradycardia, arrhythmias, flushing, syncope, edema

Central nervous system: Seizures, ataxia

Dermatologic: Alopecia, rash, changes in nail pigmentation

Endocrine & metabolic: Elevations in serum triglyceride levels

Gastrointestinal: Mild to moderate nausea/vomiting, diarrhea, mucositis

Hematologic: Severe neutropenia (dose-limiting toxicity), leukopenia, thrombocytopenia, anemia

Hepatic: Elevated AST, alkaline phosphatase, bilirubin

Local: Erythema, tenderness, swelling at the injection site

Neuromuscular & skeletal: Peripheral neuropathy (dose-dependent, characterized by paresthesia with numbness and tingling in a stocking-and-glove distribution), myalgia, muscle weakness, motor dysfunction, arthralgia

Ocular: Loss of visual acuity

Renal: Elevated serum creatinine

Respiratory: Dyspnea

Miscellaneous: Anaphylactoid reactions (dyspnea, bronchospasm, hypotension, generalized urticaria), ethanol intoxication

Drug Interactions Paclitaxel clearance decreases approximately 33% when administered following cisplatin. Since paclitaxel is metabolized by cytochrome P-450 3A4 and 2C8 isozymes, potential drug interactions can occur with agents that are isoenzyme inducers which reduce plasma paclitaxel concentration (ie, phenytoin) or inhibitors (ie, ketoconazole, verapamil, diazepam, cyclosporine, vincristine, etoposide, dexamethasone) which may increase plasma paclitaxel concentration; opiate, antihistamines, or other CNS depressants may potentiate CNS depression caused by ethanol in the paclitaxel formulation

Stability Refrigerate intact vials or store at room temperature; undiluted vials of paclitaxel may precipitate upon refrigeration, but will redissolve at room temperature with no loss in potency; dilution of paclitaxel in NS or D$_5$W is stable for up to 27 hours at room temperature; incompatible with amphotericin B, chlorpromazine, hydroxyzine, methylprednisolone, and mitoxantrone

Mechanism of Action An antimicrotubule agent that promotes the assembly of microtubules from tubulin dimers and stabilizes microtubules by preventing depolymerization; results in the inhibition of mitotic cellular functions and cell replication by blocking cells in the late G2 phase and M phase of the cell cycle

Pharmacokinetics

Distribution: Biphasic with initial rapid distribution to the peripheral compartment; later phase is a slow efflux of paclitaxel from the peripheral compartment V$_d$: 227-688 L/m^2

Protein binding: 89% to 98%

Metabolism: Cytochrome P-450 hepatic isoenzymes metabolize paclitaxel to 6 alpha-hydroxypaclitaxel

Half-life: 20-53 hours (varies with dose and infusion duration)

Elimination: Urinary recovery of unchanged drug: 1.3% to 12.6%

Hemodialysis: No significant drug removal

Usual Dosage I.V. infusion (refer to individual protocols):

Children:

Treatment for refractory leukemia is still undergoing investigation: 250-360 mg/m²/dose infused over 24 hours every 14 days

Recurrent Wilms' tumor: 250-350 mg/m²/dose infused over 24 hours every 3 weeks

Adults:

Ovarian carcinoma: 135-175 mg/m²/dose infused over 1-24 hours every 3 weeks

Metastatic breast cancer: 175 mg/m²/dose infused over 3 hours every 3 weeks (protocols have used dosages ranging between 135-250 mg/m²/dose over 1-24 hours every 3 weeks)

Kaposi's sarcoma: 135 mg/m²/dose infused over 3 hours every 3 weeks, or 100 mg/m²/dose infused over 3 hours every 2 weeks

Dosage adjustment in renal impairment: None

Dosage adjustment in hepatic impairment:

Total bilirubin ≤1.5 mg/dL and AST >2x normal limits: Total dose <135 mg/m²

Total bilirubin 1.6-3.0 mg/dL: Total dose ≤75 mg/m²

Total bilirubin ≥3.1 mg/dL: Total dose ≤50 mg/m²

Administration Parenteral: I.V.: Patients should be premedicated with a corticosteroid, diphenhydramine and an H₂-receptor antagonist 30-60 minutes prior to paclitaxel administration. To minimize patient exposure to the plasticizer diethylhexylphthalate (DEHP) from polyoxyl 35 castor oil-induced leaching of polyvinyl chloride-containing I.V. infusion bags and administration sets, prepare paclitaxel infusions in glass or polypropylene bottles or in polypropylene or polyolefin bags and administer through polyethylene lined administration sets with a 0.22 micron in-line filter. Paclitaxel can be further diluted in D₅W, NS, D₅/NS or D₅ in Ringer's injection to a final concentration of 0.3-1.2 mg/mL. Paclitaxel has been infused over short (1-3 hours) and long periods (24, 72, and 96 hours to 14 days continuous infusion)

Monitoring Parameters CBC with differential, platelet count, vital signs, ECG, liver function test; observe I.V. injection site for extravasation

Patient Information Avoid alcohol; may cause drowsiness and impair ability to perform hazardous activities requiring mental alertness

Dosage Forms Injection: 30 mg/5 mL vial

References

Woo MH, Gregornik D, Shearer PD, et al, "Pharmacokinetics of Paclitaxel in an Anephric Patient," Cancer Chemother Pharmacol, 1999, 43(1):92-6.

♦ **Palafer® (Canada)** *see* Iron Supplements, Oral/Enteral *on page 530*

Palivizumab (pah li VIZ u mab)

Brand Names Synagis®

Therapeutic Category Monoclonal Antibody

Use Prevention of serious lower respiratory tract disease caused by respiratory syncytial virus (RSV) in infants and children <2 years of age with chronic lung disease who have required medical therapy for their chronic lung disease within 6 months before the anticipated RSV season; prevention of serious RSV disease in patients with a history of prematurity (≤28 weeks gestation) up to 12 months of age or infants born at 29-32 weeks of gestation up to 6 months of age; prophylaxis of infants with severe immune deficiency exposed to RSV

Pregnancy Risk Factor C

Contraindications History of severe prior reaction to palivizumab or any component; not recommended for children with cyanotic congenital heart disease

Warnings Anaphylactoid reactions have not been observed following palivizumab administration, but can occur following the administration of proteins. If anaphylaxis or severe allergic reaction occurs, administer epinephrine (1:1000) and provide supportive care as required.

Precautions Use with caution in patients with thrombocytopenia or any coagulation disorder. Safety and efficacy have not been demonstrated for treatment of established RSV disease.

Adverse Reactions

Dermatologic: Rash

Gastrointestinal: Diarrhea, vomiting

Hepatic: Elevation in SGOT

Local: Injection site reaction, erythema, induration

Respiratory: Upper respiratory infection, otitis media, rhinitis, pharyngitis, cough

(Continued)

Palivizumab *(Continued)*

Drug Interactions No formal drug interaction studies have been conducted. Note: No interference with measles, mumps, and rubella vaccines (combined) and varicella vaccine occurs

Stability Store in refrigerator at a temperature between 2°C to 8°C (35.6°F to 46.4°F) in original container; do not freeze; the single-use vial does not contain a preservative

Reconstitute single-use vial with 1 mL of sterile water for injection; swirl vial gently for 30 seconds to avoid foaming. Do not shake vial. Allow solution to stand at room temperature for 20 minutes until it clears; solution should be administered within 6 hours of reconstitution.

Mechanism of Action Humanized monoclonal antibody directed to an epitope in the A antigenic site of the respiratory syncytial virus F protein resulting in neutralizing and fusion-inhibitory activity against RSV

Pharmacokinetics
Half-life:
Children <24 months: 20 days
Adults: 18 days
Time to achieve adequate serum antibody titers: 48 hours

Usual Dosage Children: I.M.: 15 mg/kg once monthly during RSV season

Administration Parenteral: Administer I.M., preferably in the anterolateral aspect of the thigh; gluteal muscle should not be used routinely as an injection site because of the risk of damage to the sciatic nerve; injection volume over 1 mL should be given as a divided dose

Monitoring Parameters Observe for anaphylactic or severe allergic reactions

Additional Information RSV prophylaxis should be initiated at the onset of the RSV season. In most areas of the United States, onset of RSV outbreaks is October to December, and termination is March to May, but regional differences occur.

Dosage Forms Injection, lyophilized: 100 mg

References
"Palivizumab, a Humanized Respiratory Syncytial Virus Monoclonal Antibody, Reduces Hospitalization From Respiratory Syncytial Virus Infection in High-Risk Infants. The IMpact-RSV Study Group, ," *Pediatrics,* 1998, 102(3 Pt 1):531-7.
"Prevention of Respiratory Syncytial Virus Infections: Indications for the Use of Palivizumab and Update on the Use of RSV-IGIV. American Academy of Pediatrics Committee on Infectious Diseases and Committee on Fetus and Newborn," *Pediatrics,* 1998, 102(5):1211-6.

♦ **Palmitate-A® 5000 [OTC]** *see* Vitamin A *on page 981*

♦ **2-PAM** *see* Pralidoxime *on page 788*

♦ **Pamelor®** *see* Nortriptyline *on page 697*

Pamidronate *(pa mi DROE nate)*

Brand Names Aredia™

Available Salts Pamidronate Disodium

Synonyms Aminohydroxypropylidene Diphosphonate; APD

Therapeutic Category Antidote, Hypercalcemia; Bisphosphonate Derivative

Generic Available No

Use Symptomatic treatment of moderate to severe Paget's disease; hypercalcemia associated with malignancy; treatment of osteolytic bone lesions associated with multiple myeloma or metastatic breast cancer
Investigation use: Inhibit bone resorption in severe osteogenesis imperfecta

Pregnancy Risk Factor C

Contraindications Hypersensitivity to pamidronate or any component

Warnings Leukopenia has been observed with oral pamidronate; monitoring of white blood cell counts is suggested; vein irritation and thrombophlebitis may occur with I.V. infusions

Precautions Use with caution in patients with renal impairment; maintain adequate hydration and urinary output during treatment

Adverse Reactions
Cardiovascular: Tachycardia, hypertension, syncope
Central nervous system: Malaise, fever, fatigue, somnolence, insomnia, seizures
Dermatologic: Rash
Endocrine & metabolic: Hypocalcemia, hypophosphatemia, hypothyroidism, hypokalemia, hypomagnesemia, fluid overload
Gastrointestinal: Nausea, anorexia, constipation, GI hemorrhage, abdominal pain, occult blood in stools, abnormal taste
Hematologic: Leukopenia, anemia

Local: Vein irritation, thrombophlebitis
Neuromuscular & skeletal: Bone pain
Ocular: Scleritis, uveitis, conjunctivitis
Respiratory: Rales, rhinitis
Miscellaneous: Moniliasis (associated with 90 mg dosage)

Stability Reconstituted solution stable for 24 hours at room temperature or refrigerated; incompatible with calcium-containing I.V. fluids (ie, Ringer's solution)

Mechanism of Action Pamidronate, a biphosphonate, lowers serum calcium concentrations by binding to bone and inhibiting osteoclast-mediated calcium resorption; this agent does not appear to produce any significant effect on renal tubular calcium handling

Pharmacodynamics
Onset of hypocalcemic effect: 24-48 hours
Maximum effect: 5-7 days

Pharmacokinetics
Absorption: Poorly from the GI tract; pharmacokinetic studies are lacking
Distribution half-life: 1.6 hours
Bone half-life: 300 days
Half-life, unmetabolized: 2.5 hours
Elimination: Biphasic; ~50% excreted unchanged in urine within 72 hours

Usual Dosage
Hypercalcemia: I.V.:
Children (limited experience): 0.5-1 mg/kg
Adults: Dosage based upon serum calcium measurement:
Serum calcium 12-13.5 mg/dL: 60-90 mg
Serum calcium >13.5 mg/dL: 90 mg
Consider retreatment if the serum calcium becomes elevated again; allow a minimum of 7 days between each treatment to allow for a full response to the initial treatment
Osteogenesis imperfecta:
Children (limited experience): 0.5-1 mg/kg/day for 3 days; may repeat in 4- to 6-month intervals
Osteolytic bone lesions of breast cancer or multiple myeloma: Adults: 90 mg/month
Paget's disease: Adults: 30 mg for 3 consecutive days

Administration Dilute in 250-500 mL D_5W, ½NS, or NS; infuse over 2-4 hours; in treatment of hypercalcemia, 90 mg doses should be infused over 24 hours

Monitoring Parameters Serum calcium, phosphate, potassium, magnesium, creatinine, hemoglobin, hematocrit, CBC with differential; in addition (Paget's disease) serum alkaline phosphatase, urinary hydroxyproline excretion

Dosage Forms Powder for injection, lyophilized, as disodium: 30 mg, 60 mg, 90 mg

References
Glorieux FH, Bishop NH, Plotkin H, et al, "Cyclic Administration of Pamidronate in Children With Severe Osteogenesis Imperfecta," *N Engl J Med*, 1998, 339(14):947-52.
Lteif AN and Zimmerman D, "Biphosphonates for Treatment of Childhood Hypercalcemia," *Pediatrics*, 1998, 102(4 Pt 1):990-3.

♦ **Pamidronate Disodium** *see* Pamidronate *on page 722*

♦ **Pamprin IB® [OTC]** *see* Ibuprofen *on page 501*

♦ **Panadol® [OTC]** *see* Acetaminophen *on page 26*

♦ **Pancrease®** *see* Pancrelipase *on page 724*

♦ **Pancrease® MT** *see* Pancrelipase *on page 724*

Pancreatin (PAN kree a tin)

Brand Names Creon®; Donnazyme®; Entozyme®; Hi-Vegi-Lip®
Therapeutic Category Enzyme, Pancreatic; Pancreatic Enzyme
Generic Available No
Use Replacement therapy in symptomatic treatment of malabsorption syndrome caused by pancreatic enzyme insufficiency
Pregnancy Risk Factor C
Contraindications Hypersensitivity to pancreatin, any component, or to bovine or pork protein; acute pancreatitis; acute exacerbations of chronic pancreatic diseases
Warnings Pancreatin is inactivated by acids; use microencapsulated products whenever possible, since these products permit better dissolution of enzymes in the duodenum and protect the enzyme preparations from acid degradation in the stomach; these products are not bioequivalent, do not substitute without consulting a physician or pharmacist
Precautions Do not spill powder on hands as is a skin irritant; inhalation of powder may produce an asthmatic attack
(Continued)

Pancreatin *(Continued)*

Adverse Reactions
Dermatologic: Rash
Endocrine & metabolic: Hyperuricemia
Gastrointestinal: Nausea, abdominal cramps, constipation, diarrhea, colonic strictures, mouth irritation
Ocular: Lacrimation
Renal: Hyperuricosuria
Respiratory: Sneezing, bronchospasm
Miscellaneous: Hypersensitivity reactions

Drug Interactions Calcium carbonate, magnesium hydroxide may decrease effectiveness of enzymes; pancreatin may decrease the response to oral iron therapy; H_2-antagonists (eg, ranitidine, cimetidine) increase effectiveness of pancreatic enzymes

Mechanism of Action Replaces endogenous pancreatic enzymes to assist in digestion of protein, starch and fats

Pharmacokinetics
Absorption: Not absorbed, acts locally in the GI tract
Elimination: In feces

Usual Dosage Oral: The following dosage recommendations are only an approximation for initial dosages; the actual dosage will depend on the digestive requirements of the individual patient

Infants: 2000-4000 lipase units/120 mL (4 ounce) formula
Children ≤4 years: 1000 lipase units/kg/meal (maximum: 2500 lipase units/kg), with ½ dose with each snack
Children >4 years and Adults: 400-500 lipase units/kg/meal (maximum: 2500 lipase units/kg), with ½ dose with each snack

Administration Oral: Swallow capsules/tablets whole; retention in the mouth before swallowing may cause mucosal irritation and stomatitis; administer before or with meals; when administering to infants, may open capsule and spread over acidic foods (applesauce, mashed fruits, rice cereal) in a rubber-tipped teaspoon (use mixture immediately, do not make ahead of time). Place mixture onto the middle of the infant's tongue and then give bottle or breast. As an alternative, the parent may dip a clean finger into the food/enzyme mixture and then place finger into the infant's mouth and allow infant to suck on. Check infant's mouth after eating for lodged enzyme beads and remove.

Monitoring Parameters Stool fat content

Additional Information Concomitant administration of conventional pancreatin enzymes with an H_2-receptor antagonist has been used to decrease acid inactivation of enzyme activity. Colonic strictures have been reported in several pediatric patients. There is a possible association between the development of strictures and a high lipase intake (mean >16,000 units/kg/meal). Patients receiving doses >2500 lipase units/kg/meal or 4000 lipase units/g fat/day should be re-evaluated or titrated downward to lowest effective dose

Dosage Forms See table.

Pancreatin

Product	Dosage Form	Lipase USP Units	Amylase USP Units	Protease USP Units	Pancreatin mg
Creon®	Capsule, delayed release	8000	30,000	13,000	300
Donnazyme®	Tablet	1000	12,500	12,500	500
Entozyme®	Tablet	600	7500	7500	300
Hi-Vegi-Lip®	Tablet	4800	60,000	60,000	2400

References
Pettei MJ, Leonidas JC, Levinne JJ, et al, "Pancolonic Disease in Cystic Fibrosis and High-Dose Pancreatic Enzyme Therapy," *J Pediatr*, 1994, 125(4):587-9.
Taylor CJ, "Colonic Strictures in Cystic Fibrosis," *Lancet*, 1994, 343(8898):615-6.

♦ **Pancrecarb®** see Pancrelipase on page 724

Pancrelipase *(pan kre LI pase)*
Related Information
Pancreatin on page 723

Brand Names Cotazym®; Cotazym-S®; Creon® 10; Creon® 20; Digess®8000 (Canada); Ilozyme®; Ku-Zyme® HP; Pancrease®; Pancrease® MT; Pancrecarb®; Protilase®; Ultrase® MT; Viokase®; Zymase®

Synonyms Lipancreatin

Therapeutic Category Enzyme, Pancreatic; Pancreatic Enzyme

Generic Available Yes

Use Replacement therapy in symptomatic treatment of malabsorption syndrome caused by pancreatic enzyme insufficiency

Pregnancy Risk Factor C

Contraindications Hypersensitivity to pancrelipase, any component, or to pork protein; acute pancreatitis; acute exacerbations of chronic pancreatic diseases

Warnings Pancrelipase is inactivated by acids; use microencapsulated products whenever possible, since these products permit better dissolution of enzymes in the duodenum and protect the enzyme preparations from acid degradation in the stomach; products are not bioequivalent, do not substitute without consulting a physician or pharmacist

Precautions Do not spill powder on hands as is skin irritant; inhalation of powder may produce an asthmatic attack

Adverse Reactions

Dermatologic: Rash

Endocrine & metabolic: Hyperuricemia

Gastrointestinal: Nausea, abdominal cramps, constipation, diarrhea, colonic strictures, mouth irritation

Ocular: Lacrimation

Renal: Hyperuricosuria

Respiratory: Sneezing, bronchospasm

Miscellaneous: Hypersensitivity reactions

Drug Interactions Calcium carbonate, magnesium hydroxide may decrease effectiveness of enzymes; may decrease the response to oral iron therapy; H_2-antagonists (eg, ranitidine, cimetidine) may increase effectiveness of pancreatic enzymes

Mechanism of Action Replaces endogenous pancreatic enzymes to assist in digestion of protein, starch and fats

Pharmacokinetics

Absorption: Not absorbed, acts locally in the GI tract

Elimination: In feces

Usual Dosage The following dosage recommendations are only an approximation for initial dosages. The actual dosage will depend on the digestive requirements of the individual patient. Oral:

Infants: 2000-4000 lipase units/120 mL (4 ounce) formula

Children ≤4 years: 1000 lipase units/kg/meal (maximum: 2500 lipase units/kg), with ½ dose with each snack

Children >4 years and Adults: 400-500 lipase units/kg/meal (maximum: 2500 lipase units/kg), with ½ dose with each snack

Occluded feeding tubes: Children and Adults: One tablet of Viokase® crushed with one 325 mg tablet of sodium bicarbonate (to activate the Viokase®) in 5 mL of water can be instilled into the nasogastric tube and clamped for 5 minutes; then flushed with 50 mL of water

Administration Oral: Swallow tablets and capsules whole; do not chew the microspheres or microtablets; retention in the mouth before swallowing may cause mucosal irritation and stomatitis; administer before or with meals; when administering to infants, may open capsule and spread over acidic foods (applesauce, mashed fruits, rice cereal) in a rubber-tipped teaspoon (use mixture immediately, do not make ahead of time). Place mixture onto the middle of the infant's tongue and then give bottle or breast. As an alternative, the parent may dip a clean finger into the food/enzyme mixture and then place finger into the infant's mouth and allow infant to suck on. Check infant's mouth after eating for lodged enzyme beads and remove.

Monitoring Parameters Stool fat content

Additional Information Concomitant administration of conventional pancreatin enzymes with an H_2-receptor antagonist has been used to decrease acid inactivation of enzyme activity. Colonic strictures have been reported in several pediatric patients. There is a possible association between the development of strictures and a high lipase intake (mean >16,000 units/kg/meal). Patients receiving doses >2500 lipase units/kg/meal or 4000 lipase units/g fat/day should be re-evaluated or titrated downward to lowest effective dose

Dosage Forms See table on following page.

(Continued)

Pancrelipase *(Continued)*

Pancrelipase

Product	Dosage Form	Lipase USP Units	Amylase USP Units	Protease USP Units
Cotazym® Ku-Zyme® HP	Capsule	8000	30,000	30,000
Cotazym®-S	Capsule, enteric coated spheres	5000	20,000	20,000
Creon® 5	Capsule, delayed release	5000	16,600	18,750
Creon® 10	Capsule, delayed release	10,000	33,200	37,500
Creon® 20	Capsule, delayed release	20,000	66,400	75,000
Entolase®, Pancrease® Protilase®	Capsule, delayed release	4000	20,000	25,000
Entolase HP®	Enteric coated microbeads	8000	40,000	50,000
Festal® II	Tablet, delayed release	6000	30,000	20,000
Ilozyme®	Tablet	11,000	30,000	30,000
Lipram®-PN 16	Capsule	16,000	48,000	48,000
Lipram®-PN 10	Capsule	10,000	30,000	30,000
Lipram®-CR 20	Capsule	20,000	66,400	75,000
Lipram®-UL 12	Capsule	12,000	39,000	39,000
Lipram®-UL 18	Capsule	18,000	58,500	58,500
Lipram®-UL 20	Capsule	20,000	65,000	65,000
Pancrease®		4500	20,000	25,000
Pancrease® MT	Capsule, enteric coated microtablets	4000	12,000	12,000
MT 10		10,000	30,000	30,000
MT 16		16,000	48,000	48,000
MT 20		20,000	56,000	44,000
Pancrecarb® MS-8	Buffered, enteric-coated microspheres	8000	40,000	45,000
Ultrase® MT	Capsule, enteric coated microspheres	4500	20,000	25,000
MT 12		12,000	39,000	39,000
MT 18		18,000	58,500	58,500
MT 20		20,000	65,000	65,000
Viokase®	Powder	16,800 (per 0.7 g)	70,000 (per 0.7 g)	70,000 (per 0.7 g)
	Tablet	8000	30,000	30,000
Zymase®	Capsule, enteric coated spheres	12,000	24,000	24,000

References

Pettei MJ, Leonidas JC, Levinne JJ, et al, "Pancolonic Disease in Cystic Fibrosis and High-Dose Pancreatic Enzyme Therapy," *J Pediatr*, 1994, 125(4):587-9.

Taylor CG, "Colonic Strictures in Cystic Fibrosis," *Lancet*, 1994, 343(8898):615-6.

Pancuronium *(pan kyoo ROE nee um)*

Brand Names Pavulon®

Available Salts Pancuronium Bromide

Therapeutic Category Neuromuscular Blocker Agent, Nondepolarizing; Skeletal Muscle Relaxant, Paralytic

Generic Available Yes

Use Produces skeletal muscle relaxation during surgery after induction of general anesthesia, increases pulmonary compliance during assisted mechanical respiration, facilitates endotracheal intubation

Pregnancy Risk Factor C

Contraindications Hypersensitivity to pancuronium, bromide, or any component

Warnings Ventilation must be supported during neuromuscular blockade; electrolyte imbalance alters blockade

Precautions Use with caution and decrease dose in patients with decreased renal function; many clinical conditions may affect the response to neuromuscular blockade, see table.

Clinical Conditions Affecting Neuromuscular Blockade

Potentiation	Antagonism
Electrolyte abnormalities	Alkalosis
Severe hyponatremia	Hypercalcemia
Severe hypocalcemia	Demyelinating lesions
Severe hypokalemia	Peripheral neuropathies
Hypermagnesemia	Diabetes mellitus
Neuromuscular diseases	
Acidosis	
Acute intermittent porphyria	
Renal failure	
Hepatic failure	

Adverse Reactions Most frequent adverse reactions are related to prolongation of pharmacologic actions

Cardiovascular: Tachycardia, hypertension
Dermatologic: Rash, erythema
Gastrointestinal: Excessive salivation
Local: Burning sensation along the vein
Neuromuscular & skeletal: Muscle weakness
Respiratory: Wheezes, bronchospasm
Miscellaneous: Hypersensitivity reactions

Drug Interactions See table.

Potential Drug Interactions

Potentiation	Antagonism
Anesthetics	Calcium
Desflurane, sevoflurane, enflurane and	Carbamazepine
isoflurane > halothane > nitrous	Phenytoin
oxide	Steroids (chronic administration)
Antibiotics	Theophylline
Aminoglycosides, polymyxins,	Anticholinesterases*
clindamycin, vancomycin	Neostigmine, pyridostigmine,
Magnesium sulfate	edrophonium, echothiophate
Antiarrhythmics	ophthalmic solution
Quinidine, procainamide, bretylium, and	Caffeine
possibly lidocaine	Azathioprine
Diuretics	
Furosemide, mannitol	
Amphotericin B (secondary to hypokalemia)	
Local anesthetics	
Dantrolene (directly depresses skeletal muscle)	
Beta blockers	
Calcium channel blockers	
Ketamine	
Lithium	
Succinylcholine (when administered prior to nondepolarizing neuromuscular-blocking agent)	
Cyclosporine	

*Can prolong the effects of acetylcholine

Stability Refrigerate; however, stable for up to 6 months at room temperature; compatible with D_5W, NS, D_5NS, and LR injections

Mechanism of Action Nondepolarizing neuromuscular blocker which blocks acetylcholine from binding to receptors on motor endplate thus inhibiting depolarization
(Continued)

Pancuronium *(Continued)*

Pharmacodynamics
Peak effect: I.V. injection: Within 2-3 minutes
Duration: 40-60 minutes (dose dependent)

Pharmacokinetics
Protein binding: 87%
Metabolism: 30% to 40% metabolized in liver
Half-life: 110 minutes
Elimination: Primarily in urine (55% to 70%) as unchanged drug

Usual Dosage Neonates, Infants, Children, and Adults: I.V.: 0.04-0.1 mg/kg every 30-60 minutes as needed or as continuous infusion of 0.1 mg/kg/hour

Dosing adjustment in renal impairment:
Cl_{cr} 10-50 mL/minute: Administer 50% of normal dose
Cl_{cr} <10 mL/minute: Do not use

Administration Parenteral: May be administered undiluted by rapid I.V. injection; for continuous infusion, dilute to 0.01-0.8 mg/mL in D_5NS, D_5W, LR, or NS.

Monitoring Parameters Heart rate, blood pressure, assisted ventilation status, peripheral nerve stimulator measuring twitch response

Nursing Implications Does not alter the patient's state of consciousness; addition of sedation and analgesia are recommended

Additional Information Patients with hepatic and biliary disease have a larger V_d which may result in a higher total initial dose and possibly a slower onset of effect; due to decreased clearance, the duration of neuromuscular blocking effects may be prolonged

Dosage Forms Injection, as bromide: 1 mg/mL (10 mL); 2 mg/mL (2 mL, 5 mL)

♦ **Pancuronium Bromide** see Pancuronium *on page 726*
♦ **Panmycin® Oral** see Tetracycline *on page 908*
♦ **PanOxyl®-AQ** see Benzoyl Peroxide *on page 126*
♦ **PanOxyl® Bar [OTC]** see Benzoyl Peroxide *on page 126*
♦ **Panscol® Lotion [OTC]** see Salicylic Acid *on page 854*
♦ **Panscol® Ointment [OTC]** see Salicylic Acid *on page 854*

Papaverine *(pa PAV er een)*

Brand Names Genabid®; Pavabid®; Pavatine®
Available Salts Papaverine Hydrochloride
Therapeutic Category Antimigraine Agent; Vasodilator
Generic Available Yes
Use Relief of peripheral and cerebral ischemia associated with arterial spasm; investigationally for prophylaxis of migraine headache; intracavernosal injection for impotence
Pregnancy Risk Factor C
Contraindications Complete atrioventricular block; Parkinson's disease
Precautions Use with caution in patients with glaucoma; administer I.V. slowly and with caution since arrhythmias and apnea may occur with rapid I.V. use
Adverse Reactions
Cardiovascular: Flushing of the face, tachycardia, hypotension, arrhythmias with rapid I.V. use
Central nervous system: Depression, dizziness, vertigo, drowsiness, sedation, lethargy, headache
Dermatologic: Pruritus
Gastrointestinal: Xerostomia, nausea, constipation
Hepatic: Hepatic hypersensitivity
Local: Thrombosis at the I.V. administration site
Respiratory: Apnea with rapid I.V. use
Miscellaneous: Diaphoresis
Drug Interactions Cytochrome P-450 isoenzyme CYP2D6 substrate
Additive effects with CNS depressants or morphine; papaverine decreases the effects of levodopa
Stability Protect from heat or freezing; do not refrigerate injection; solutions should be clear to pale yellow; precipitates with LR
Mechanism of Action Smooth muscle spasmolytic producing a generalized smooth muscle relaxation including vasodilatation, gastrointestinal sphincter relaxation, bronchiolar muscle relaxation, and potentially a depressed myocardium
Pharmacodynamics Onset of action: Oral: Rapid
Pharmacokinetics
Protein binding: 90%

Metabolism: Rapid in the liver
Bioavailability: Oral: ~54%
Half-life: 30-120 minutes
Elimination: Primarily as metabolites in urine

Usual Dosage
Children: I.M., I.V.: 1.5 mg/kg 4 times/day
Migraine prophylaxis: 6-15 years: Oral: Initial: 5 mg/kg/day given once daily; range: 5-10 mg/kg/day divided into 2-3 doses/day
Adults:
Oral: 75-300 mg 3-5 times/day
Oral, sustained release: 150-300 mg every 12 hours
I.M., I.V.: 30-120 mg every 3 hours as needed

Administration
Oral: Administer after or with meals, milk or antacids to decrease nausea; swallow sustained release capsule whole, do not crush or chew
Parenteral: Rapid I.V. administration may result in arrhythmias and fatal apnea; administer slow I.V. over 1-2 minutes

Monitoring Parameters Liver enzymes; intraocular pressure in glaucoma patients

Patient Information May cause dizziness, flushing, headache; may cause drowsiness and impair ability to perform hazardous activities requiring mental alertness or physical coordination

Additional Information Evidence of therapeutic value of systemic use for relief of peripheral and cerebral ischemia related to arterial spasm is lacking

Note: The manufacturer (Eli Lilly) is limiting the distribution of the injectable form to hospitals and similar settings to discourage its use for the treatment of impotence

Further studies are needed to determine the benefit of adding papaverine (60 mg/ 500 mL) to arterial catheter infusions containing NS or ½NS and heparin 1 unit/mL. One investigation showed a lower risk of arterial catheter failure and longer duration of arterial catheter function in patients 7 months to 5.5 years of age who received papaverine in their arterial catheter solutions; these results should be verified by additional studies before the addition of papaverine to arterial catheter solutions can be recommended; also, papaverine should **not** be used in neonates due to the increased risk of drug-induced cerebral vasodilation and possibility of an intracranial bleed.

Dosage Forms
Capsule, sustained release, as hydrochloride: 150 mg
Injection, as hydrochloride: 30 mg/mL (2 mL, 10 mL)

References
Heulitt MJ, Farrington EA, O'Shea TM, et al, "Double-Blind, Randomized, Controlled Trial of Papaverine-Containing Infusions to Prevent Failure of Arterial Catheters in Pediatric Patients," Crit Care Med, 1993, 21(6):825-9.
Sillanpää M and Koponen M, "Papaverine in the Prophylaxis of Migraine and Other Vascular Headache in Children," Acta Paediatr Scand, 1978, 67(2):209-12.

♦ **Papaverine Hydrochloride** see Papaverine on page 728
♦ **Parabromdylamine** see Brompheniramine on page 142
♦ **Paracetaldehyde** see Paraldehyde on page 729
♦ **Paracetamol** see Acetaminophen on page 26
♦ **Paraflex®** see Chlorzoxazone on page 218
♦ **Parafon Forte™ DSC** see Chlorzoxazone on page 218
♦ **Paral®** see Paraldehyde on page 729

Paraldehyde (par AL de hyde)
Brand Names Paral®
Synonyms Paracetaldehyde
Therapeutic Category Anticonvulsant, Miscellaneous; Hypnotic; Sedative
Generic Available Yes
Use Treatment of status epilepticus and tetanus-induced seizures; has been used as a sedative/hypnotic and in the treatment of alcohol withdrawal symptoms
Restrictions C-IV
Pregnancy Risk Factor C
Contraindications Severe hepatic insufficiency, respiratory disease, GI inflammation or ulceration
Warnings Do not abruptly discontinue in patients receiving chronic therapy
Precautions May need to decrease dose in patients with liver disease
Adverse Reactions
Dermatologic: Erythematous rash
Endocrine & metabolic: Metabolic acidosis
(Continued)

Paraldehyde *(Continued)*

Gastrointestinal: Gastric irritation, corrosion of the stomach or rectum
Hepatic: Hepatitis
Respiratory: Coughing, strong and unpleasant breath, pulmonary edema
Miscellaneous: Psychological and physical dependence with prolonged use

Drug Interactions Barbiturates and alcohol may enhance CNS depression

Stability Decomposes with exposure to air and light to acetaldehyde which then oxidizes to acetic acid; store in tightly closed containers; protect from light

Mechanism of Action Unknown mechanism of action; causes depression of CNS, including the ascending reticular activating system to provide sedation/hypnosis and anticonvulsant activity

Pharmacodynamics Hypnosis: Oral:
Onset of action: Within 10-15 minutes
Duration: 6-8 hours

Pharmacokinetics
Distribution: Crosses the placenta
Metabolism: ~70% to 80% in the liver
Half-life:
Neonates: 10 hours
Adults: 3.5-10 hours
Elimination: 30% excreted as unchanged drug in expired air via the lungs; trace amounts are excreted in urine unchanged

Usual Dosage See table.

Paraldehyde

	Sedative	Hypnotic	Seizures
Neonates Rectal			0.3 mL/kg; may repeat once if needed in 4-6 h
Children Oral, rectal	0.15 mL/kg	0.3 mL/kg	0.3 mL/kg every 2-4 h; maximum dose is 5 mL
Adults Oral, rectal	5-10 mL	10-30 mL	

Administration
Oral: Dilute in milk or iced fruit juice
Rectal: Mix paraldehyde 2:1 with oil (cottonseed, olive, or mineral oil)

Do **not** use any plastic equipment for administration, use glass syringes and rubber tubing (paraldehyde will dissolve plastic)

Patient Information Avoid alcohol; causes sedation and impairs ability to perform hazardous activities requiring mental alertness or physical coordination

Nursing Implications Discard unused contents of any container which has been opened for more than 24 hours; do **not** use discolored solution or solutions with strong smell of acetic acid (vinegar); outdated preparations can be toxic

Additional Information Parenteral dosage form is no longer available in the United States

Dosage Forms Liquid, oral or rectal: 1 g/mL (30 mL)

♦ **Paraplatin®** *see* Carboplatin *on page 170*

Paregoric *(par e GOR ik)*

Related Information
Carbohydrate and Alcohol Content of Liquid Medications for Use in Patients Receiving Ketogenic Diets *on page 1228*
Overdose and Toxicology *on page 1191*

Synonyms Camphorated Tincture of Opium

Therapeutic Category Analgesic, Narcotic; Antidiarrheal

Generic Available Yes

Use Treatment of diarrhea or relief of pain; neonatal abstinence syndrome (neonatal opiate withdrawal)

Restrictions C-III

Pregnancy Risk Factor B (D when used for long-term or in high-doses)

Contraindications Hypersensitivity to opium or any component (see Additional Information); diarrhea caused by poisoning until the toxic material has been removed

Warnings Some commercial preparations contain sulfites which may cause allergic reactions

Precautions Use with caution in patients with respiratory, hepatic or renal dysfunction, severe prostatic hypertrophy, or history of narcotic abuse; opium shares the toxic potential of opiate agonists, usual precautions of opiate agonist therapy should be observed; infants <3 months of age are more susceptible to respiratory depression, use with caution and in reduced doses in this age group

Adverse Reactions
Cardiovascular: Hypotension, bradycardia, vasodilation
Central nervous system: CNS depression, increased intracranial pressure, drowsiness, dizziness, sedation
Endocrine & metabolic: Antidiuretic hormone release
Gastrointestinal: Nausea, vomiting, constipation, biliary tract spasm
Genitourinary: Urinary tract spasm, urinary retention
Ocular: Miosis
Respiratory: Respiratory depression
Miscellaneous: Physical and psychological dependence, histamine release

Drug Interactions CNS depressants (eg, alcohol, narcotics, benzodiazepines, tricyclic antidepressants, MAO inhibitors, phenothiazines) may increase effects/toxicity

Stability Store in light-resistant, tightly closed container; protect from freezing

Mechanism of Action Increases smooth muscle tone in GI tract, decreases motility and peristalsis, diminishes digestive secretions

Pharmacokinetics
Metabolism: Opium is metabolized in the liver
Elimination: In urine, primarily as morphine glucuronide conjugates and as parent compound (morphine, codeine, papaverine, etc)

Usual Dosage Oral:
Neonates (full term): Neonatal abstinence syndrome (opiate withdrawal): Initial: 0.1 mL/kg or 2 drops/kg with feedings every 3-4 hours; increase dosage by 0.1 mL/kg or 2 drops/kg every 3-4 hours until withdrawal symptoms are controlled; it is rare to exceed 0.7 mL/dose. Stabilize withdrawal symptoms for 3-5 days, then gradually decrease the dosage (keeping the same dosing interval) over a 2- to 4-week period.
Children: 0.25-0.5 mL/kg 1-4 times/day
Adults: 5-10 mL 1-4 times/day

Administration Oral: May administer with food to decrease GI upset; shake well before use

Monitoring Parameters Respiratory rate, blood pressure, heart rate, level of sedation; neonatal abstinence syndrome (opiate withdrawal): Monitor for resolution of withdrawal symptoms (such as irritability, high-pitched cry, stuffy nose, rhinorrhea, vomiting, poor feeding, diarrhea, sneezing, yawning, etc) and signs of over treatment (such as bradycardia, lethargy, hypotonia, irregular respirations, respiratory depression, etc); an abstinence scoring system (eg, Finnegan abstinence scoring system) can be used to more objectively assess neonatal opiate withdrawal symptoms and the need for dosage adjustment

Patient Information Avoid alcohol; may cause drowsiness and impair ability to perform hazardous tasks requiring mental alertness; may be habit-forming

Additional Information Do **not** confuse this product with opium tincture which is 25 times **more** potent; each 5 mL of paregoric contains 2 mg morphine equivalent, 0.02 mL anise oil, 20 mg benzoic acid, 20 mg camphor, 0.2 mL glycerin and alcohol; final alcohol content 45%; paregoric also contains papaverine and noscapine; because all of these additives may be harmful to neonates, **a 25-fold dilution of opium tincture** is often preferred for treatment of neonatal abstinence syndrome (opiate withdrawal); see Opium Tincture *on page 709*

Dosage Forms Liquid: 2 mg morphine equivalent/5 mL [equivalent to 20 mg opium powder] (5 mL, 60 mL, 473 mL, 4000 mL)

References
Kraus DM and Hatzopoulos FK, "Neonatal Therapy," *Applied Therapeutics: The Clinical Use of Drugs*, 6th ed, Young LY and Koda-Kimble MA, eds, Vancouver, WA: Applied Therapeutics, Inc., 1995.
Levy M and Spino M, "Neonatal Withdrawal Syndrome: Associated Drugs and Pharmacologic Management," *Pharmacotherapy*, 1993, 13(3):202-11.
"Neonatal Drug Withdrawal. American Academy of Pediatrics Committee on Drugs," *Pediatrics*, 1998, 101(6):1079-88.

♦ **Parenteral Nutrition (PN)** *see page 1072*
♦ **Parepectolin®** *see* Attapulgite *on page 109*

Paromomycin (par oh moe MYE sin)
Brand Names Humatin®
Available Salts Paromomycin Sulfate
Therapeutic Category Amebicide
Generic Available No
Use Treatment of acute and chronic intestinal amebiasis due to susceptible *Entamoeba histolytica* (not effective in the treatment of extraintestinal amebiasis); tapeworm infestations; adjunctive management of hepatic coma; treatment of cryptosporidial diarrhea
Pregnancy Risk Factor C
Contraindications Hypersensitivity to paromomycin or any component; intestinal obstruction
Warnings May result in overgrowth of nonsusceptible organisms
Precautions Use with caution in patients with impaired GI motility or possible or proven ulcerative bowel lesions; use with caution in patients with impaired renal function
Adverse Reactions
Central nervous system: Headache, vertigo
Dermatologic: Exanthema, rash, pruritus ani
Endocrine & metabolic: Hypocholesterolemia
Gastrointestinal: Diarrhea, abdominal cramps, nausea, vomiting, anorexia, steatorrhea, secondary enterocolitis, pancreatitis
Hematologic: Eosinophilia
Otic: Ototoxicity
Renal: Hematuria
Drug Interactions May decrease digoxin level; increased effect of oral anticoagulants
Food Interactions Paromomycin may cause malabsorption of xylose, sucrose, and fats
Mechanism of Action Acts directly on ameba in the intestinal lumen; interferes with bacterial protein synthesis by binding to 30S ribosomal subunit of susceptible bacteria
Pharmacokinetics
Absorption: Poor from the GI tract
Elimination: Excreted unchanged in feces; portion of oral dose that may be absorbed is excreted in urine
Usual Dosage Oral:
Children:
Intestinal amebiasis (*Entamoeba histolytica*): 25-35 mg/kg/day divided every 8 hours for 7 days
Dientamoeba fragilis infection: 25-30 mg/kg/day divided every 8 hours for 7 days
Tapeworm:
T. saginata, T. solium, D. latum: 11 mg/kg/dose every 15 minutes for 4 doses
H. nana: 45 mg/kg/day once daily for 5-7 days
Adults:
Intestinal amebiasis (*Entamoeba histolytica*): 25-35 mg/kg/day divided every 8 hours for 7 days
Dientamoeba fragilis infection: 25-30 mg/kg/day divided every 8 hours for 7 days
Tapeworm:
T. saginata, T. solium, D. latum: 1 g every 15 minutes for 4 doses
H. nana: 45 mg/kg/day once daily for 5-7 days
Hepatic coma: 4 g/day in 2-4 divided doses for 5-6 days
Cryptosporidial diarrhea: 1.5-2 g/day in 3-4 divided doses for 10-14 days
Administration Oral: Administer with or after meals
Monitoring Parameters Periodic urinalysis and renal function tests; be alert to ototoxicity
Patient Information Notify physician if ringing in ears, hearing loss, or dizziness occurs
Additional Information With the treatment of cestodiasis caused by *T. solium*, paromomycin may cause disintegration of worm segments and release of viable eggs resulting in an increased risk for the development of cysticercosis
Dosage Forms Capsule, as sulfate: 250 mg
References
Danziger LH, Kanyok TP, and Novak RM, "Treatment of Cryptosporidial Diarrhea in an AIDS Patient With Paromomycin," *Ann Pharmacother*, 1993, 27(12):1460-2.
Liu LX and Weller PF, "Antiparasitic Drugs," *N Engl J Med*, 1996, 334(18):1178-84.

♦ **Paromomycin Sulfate** *see* Paromomycin *on page 732*

Paroxetine (pa ROKS e teen)

Related Information

Comparison of Adverse Effects of Antidepressants *on page 1030*
Comparison of Usual Adult Dosage and Mechanism of Action of Antidepressants *on page 1029*
Serotonin Syndrome *on page 1217*

Brand Names Paxil®; Paxil® CR™

Available Salts Paroxetine Hydrochloride

Therapeutic Category Antidepressant, Serotonin Reuptake Inhibitor

Generic Available No

Use Treatment of depression, obsessive compulsive disorder, panic disorder, and social anxiety disorder

Pregnancy Risk Factor C

Contraindications Hypersensitivity to paroxetine or any component; patients receiving MAO inhibitors currently or in past 2 weeks

Warnings Avoid abrupt discontinuation; taper dosage gradually in patients receiving >20 mg/day as withdrawal symptoms (sweating, dizziness, confusion, and tremor) have been reported following abrupt discontinuation

Precautions Use with caution in patients with a history of seizures, mania, renal disease, cardiac disease, or hepatic disease and in suicidal patients, children, or during breast-feeding in lactating women; modify dosage in patients with renal or hepatic impairment; may cause hyponatremia, use with caution in patients with volume depletion or diuretic use; may cause abnormal bleeding (eg, ecchymosis, purpura); use with caution in patients with impaired platelet aggregation; no clinical studies have assessed the combined use of paroxetine and electroconvulsive therapy

Adverse Reactions

Cardiovascular: Palpitations, tachycardia, vasodilation, postural hypotension, bradycardia, hypotension

Central nervous system: Headache, somnolence, dizziness, insomnia, nervousness, agitation, anxiety, migraine

Dermatologic: Alopecia, purpura, ecchymosis

Endocrine & metabolic: Hyponatremia (elderly or volume-depleted patients), SIADH, sexual dysfunction

Gastrointestinal: Nausea, xerostomia, constipation, vomiting, diarrhea, anorexia, flatulence, gastritis

Hematologic: Anemia, leukopenia

Neuromuscular & skeletal: Weakness, tremor, arthritis, paresthesia, asthenia

Ocular: Eye pain

Otic: Ear pain

Respiratory: Asthma

Miscellaneous: Diaphoresis, thirst, bruxism, akinesia

Drug Interactions Cytochrome P-450 isoenzyme CYP2D6 substrate (minor); CYP2D6 and CYP1A2 (high dose) (weak) isoenzyme inhibitor; CYP3A3/4 isoenzyme inhibitor (weak)

Decreased effect with phenobarbital, phenytoin (may also decrease phenytoin levels)

Increased effect/toxicity with alcohol, cimetidine, ritonavir, MAO inhibitors (potential fatal serotonin syndrome: hypertension, hyperthermia, mental status change, myoclonus, hyperpyrexic crisis), dextromethorphan (serotonin syndrome); phenothiazines, type 1C antiarrhythmics

Increased effect/toxicity of tricyclic antidepressants, fluoxetine, sertraline, theophylline, warfarin

Cyproheptadine may decrease or antagonize effects of paroxetine; use with sumatriptan may cause weakness, incoordination, and hyper-reflexia; paroxetine may decrease the AUC of digoxin by 15%; tryptophan, which can be metabolized to serotonin, may increase serious serotonin side effects and its use is **not** recommended; the combination of paroxetine and pimozide resulted in an oculogyric crisis in a 9-year old boy (Horrigan, 1994); paroxetine may increase or worsen lysergic acid diethylamide (LSD) flashbacks

Food Interactions Food or milk does not affect absorption; tryptophan supplements may increase serious side effects

Mechanism of Action Paroxetine is a selective serotonin reuptake inhibitor (SSRI), chemically unrelated to tricyclic, tetracyclic, or other antidepressants; the inhibition of serotonin reuptake from CNS neuronal synapses potentiates serotonin activity in the brain

Pharmacodynamics

Onset of action: Antidepressant effects: Within 1-4 weeks
(Continued)

Paroxetine *(Continued)*

Anti-obsessional and antipanic effects: Up to several weeks

Pharmacokinetics

Absorption: Oral: Well absorbed

Distribution: V_d (adults): Mean: 8.7 L/kg; range: 3-28 L/kg

Protein binding: 95%

Metabolism: Extensive by cytochrome P-450 enzymes via oxidation and methyla-tion followed by glucuronide and sulfate conjugation; nonlinear kinetics may be seen with higher doses and longer duration of therapy due to saturation of P-450 2D6 (CYP2D6), an enzyme partially responsible for metabolism

Bioavailability: Tablet and oral suspension have equal bioavailability

Half-life: Adults: Mean: 21 hours; range: 3-65 hours

Elimination: Metabolites are excreted in urine and bile; 2% of drug excreted unchanged in urine

Usual Dosage Oral:

Children: Limited information is available

Depression: Paroxetine was shown to be effective and well tolerated in an open label clinical trial in 45 children <14 years of age (mean age: 10.7 ± 2 years) with major depression (Rey-Sanchoz, 1997). Doses were initiated at 10 mg/day and adjusted upward on an individual basis with a mean dose of 16.2 mg/day used for an average of 8.4 months. Further studies are needed.

Self-injurious behavior: A 15-year old autistic male with self-injurious behavior was successfully treated with paroxetine 20 mg/day (Snead, 1994). Further studies are needed.

Adults:

Depression: Initial: 20 mg/day given once daily preferably in the morning; increase if needed by 10 mg/day increments at intervals of at least 1 week; maximum dose: 50 mg/day

Obsessive compulsive disorder: Initial: 20 mg/day given once daily preferably in the morning; increase by 10 mg/day increments at intervals of at least 1 week; recommended dose: 40 mg/day; range: 20-60 mg/day; maximum dose: 60 mg/day

Panic disorder: Initial: 10 mg/day given once daily preferably in the morning; increase by 10 mg/day increments at intervals of at least 1 week; recom-mended dose: 40 mg/day; range: 10-60 mg/day; maximum dose: 60 mg/day

Social anxiety disorder: Initial: 20 mg/day given once daily preferably in the morning; recommended dose: 20 mg/day; range: 20-60 mg/day; doses >20 mg may not have additional benefit

Severe hepatic or renal impairment: Adults: Initial: 10 mg/day; increase if needed by 10 mg/day increments at intervals of at least 1 week; maximum dose: 40 mg/day

Administration May be administered without regard to meals; administration with food may decrease GI side effects; shake suspension well before use

Monitoring Parameters Blood pressure, heart rate, liver and renal function

Patient Information Avoid alcohol and tryptophan; may cause drowsiness or dizzi-ness and impair ability to perform activities requiring mental alertness or physical coordination; may cause dry mouth; avoid abrupt discontinuation; inform physician if taking or planning to take other medications

Additional Information Paroxetine is more potent and more selective than other SSRIs (eg, fluoxetine, fluvoxamine, sertraline, and clomipramine) in the inhibition of serotonin reuptake

Dosage Forms

Suspension, oral, as hydrochloride (orange flavor): 10 mg/5 mL (250 mL)

Tablet, as hydrochloride: 10 mg, 20 mg, 30 mg, 40 mg

Tablet, controlled release, as hydrochloride (Paxil® CR™): 12.5 mg, 25 mg

References

Horrigan JP and Barnhill LJ, "Paroxetine-Pimozide Drug Interactions," *J Am Acad Child Adolesc Psychiatry*, 1994, 33(7):1060-1.

Markel H, Lee A, Holmes RD, et al, "LSD Flashback Syndrome Exacerbated by Selective Serotonin Reuptake Inhibitor Antidepressants in Adolescents," *J Pediatr*, 1994, 125(5 Pt 1):817-9.

Rey-Sanchez F and Guitierrez-Cassares JR, "Paroxetine in Children With Major Depressive Disorder: An Open Trial," *J Am Acad Child Adolesc Psychiatry*, 1997, 36(10):1443-7.

Snead RW, Boon F, and Presberg J, "Paroxetine for Self-Injurious Behavior," *J Am Acad Child Adolesc Psychiatry*, 1994, 33(6):909-10.

♦ **Paroxetine Hydrochloride** see Paroxetine *on page 733*

♦ **Parvolex® (Canada)** see Acetylcysteine *on page 32*

♦ **Pathocil®** see Dicloxacillin *on page 313*

♦ **Pavabid®** see Papaverine *on page 728*

- **Pavatine®** *see* Papaverine *on page 728*
- **Paveral Stanley Syrup With Codeine Phosphate (Canada)** *see* Codeine *on page 249*
- **Pavulon®** *see* Pancuronium *on page 726*
- **Paxil®** *see* Paroxetine *on page 733*
- **Paxil® CR™** *see* Paroxetine *on page 733*
- **Pazo® Hemorrhoid [OTC]** *see* Hemorrhoidal Preparations *on page 470*
- **PCA** *see* Procainamide *on page 799*
- **PCE®** *see* Erythromycin *on page 379*
- **Pectin and Kaolin** *see* Kaolin and Pectin *on page 540*
- **PediaCare® Oral** *see* Pseudoephedrine *on page 822*
- **Pediaflor®** *see* Fluoride *on page 427*
- **PediaPatch Transdermal Patch [OTC]** *see* Salicylic Acid *on page 854*
- **Pediapred® Oral** *see* Prednisolone *on page 791*
- **Pedia-Profen™** *see* Ibuprofen *on page 501*
- **Pediatric ALS Algorithm, Asystole and Pulseless Arrest** *see page 1002*
- **Pediatric ALS Algorithm, Bradycardia** *see page 1001*
- **Pediatric HIV** *see page 1129*
- **Pediatrix® (Canada)** *see* Acetaminophen *on page 26*
- **Pediazole®** *see* Erythromycin and Sulfisoxazole *on page 382*
- **Pedi-Boro® [OTC]** *see* Aluminum Acetate *on page 53*
- **Pedi-Dent™ (Canada)** *see* Fluoride *on page 427*
- **Pedi-Dri Topical** *see* Undecylenic Acid and Derivatives *on page 962*
- **PediOtic® Otic** *see* Neomycin, (Bacitracin) Polymyxin B, and Hydrocortisone *on page 679*
- **Pedi-Pro Topical [OTC]** *see* Undecylenic Acid and Derivatives *on page 962*
- **Pedte-Pak-5®** *see* Trace Metals *on page 940*
- **Pedtrace-4®** *see* Trace Metals *on page 940*

Pegaspargase (peg AS par jase)

Related Information
Emetogenic Potential of Single Chemotherapeutic Agents *on page 1095*

Brand Names Oncaspar®

Synonyms PEG-L-Asparaginase

Therapeutic Category Antineoplastic Agent, Miscellaneous

Generic Available No

Use Induction treatment of acute lymphoblastic leukemia in combination with other chemotherapeutic agents in patients who have developed hypersensitivity to native forms of L-asparaginase derived from *E. coli* and/or *Erwinia chrysanthemia*; treatment of lymphoma

Pregnancy Risk Factor C

Contraindications Pancreatitis; patients who have had significant hemorrhagic events associated with prior L-asparaginase therapy; patients who have had previous serious allergic reactions to pegaspargase

Warnings The FDA currently recommends that procedures for proper handling and disposal of antineoplastic agents be considered; inhalation of vapors and contact with skin, eyes, or mucous membranes must be avoided; be prepared to treat anaphylaxis at each administration

Precautions Use with caution in patients receiving anticoagulation therapy, aspirin, or NSAIDs; use with caution in patients with hepatic dysfunction or in patients receiving hepatotoxic agents

Adverse Reactions
Cardiovascular: Hypotension, chest pain, tachycardia

Central nervous system: Somnolence, confusion, seizures, fever, chills, headache, dizziness, malaise, coma, mental status changes

Dermatologic: Rash, pruritus, urticaria

Endocrine & metabolic: Hyperglycemia, transient diabetes mellitus, hyperammonemia, hyperuricemia

Gastrointestinal: Protracted nausea and vomiting, abdominal pain, diarrhea, anorexia, pancreatitis

Genitourinary: Hemorrhagic cystitis

Hematologic: Leukopenia; prolonged prothrombin, thrombin and partial thromboplastin times; decreased fibrinogen; thrombosis; hemorrhage

Hepatic: Hepatotoxicity

Neuromuscular & skeletal: Paresthesia, weakness

(Continued)

Pegaspargase *(Continued)*

Renal: Elevated BUN, elevated serum creatinine, renal failure
Respiratory: Cough, bronchospasm, epistaxis
Miscellaneous: Anaphylaxis

Drug Interactions Methotrexate (decreases antineoplastic effect if given immediately prior to MTX); vincristine (increases toxicity if given concomitantly); prednisone (increases hyperglycemic effect); may increase toxicity of highly protein bound drugs; may increase bleeding in patients receiving warfarin, heparin, aspirin, NSAID, or dipyridamole

Stability Store vials in refrigerator; do not freeze; do not administer if there is any indication that the drug has been frozen; avoid excessive agitation, do not shake; do not use if cloudy or if precipitate is present; use of a 0.2 micron filter may result in some loss of potency

Mechanism of Action Hydrolyzes asparagine to aspartic acid and ammonia depleting the exogenous asparagine supply needed by leukemic cells for protein synthesis

Pharmacokinetics
Absorption: Not absorbed from the GI tract; therefore, requires parenteral administration
Distribution: Apparent V_d: Plasma volume
Half-life: 5.73 days; patients who have had a hypersensitivity reaction to asparaginase have a decreased half-life
Elimination: Clearance is unaffected by age, renal function, or hepatic function; not detected in urine

Usual Dosage Refer to individual protocols; Children and Adults:
I.M., I.V.: 2500 units/m²/dose every 14 days; for children with BSA <0.6 m²: 82.5 units/kg every 14 days

Administration
I.M.: Preferred route of administration due to the lower incidence of hepatotoxicity, coagulopathy, and GI and renal disorders compared to the I.V. route; for I.M. administration, limit the volume at a single injection site to 2 mL; if the volume to be administered is >2 mL, use multiple injection sites
I.V.: Infusion in 100 mL of D_5W or NS over a period of 1-2 hours

Monitoring Parameters Vital signs during administration, CBC, urinalysis, serum amylase, liver enzymes, bilirubin, prothrombin time, renal function tests, urine glucose, blood glucose

Patient Information Notify physician if fever, sore throat, painful/burning urination, bruising, bleeding, or shortness of breath occurs

Nursing Implications Patients should be observed for 1 hour following injection; appropriate agents for maintenance of an adequate airway and treatment of a hypersensitivity reaction (antihistamine, epinephrine, oxygen, I.V. corticosteroids) should be readily available

Dosage Forms Injection, preservative free: 750 units/mL

References
Asselin BL, Whitin JC, Cappola DJ, et al, "Comparative Pharmacokinetic Studies of Three Asparaginase Preparations," *J Clin Oncol*, 1993, 11(9):1780-6.
Capizzi RL, "Asparaginase Revisited," *Leuk Lymphoma*, 1993, 10(Suppl):147-50.

♦ **PEG-L-Asparaginase** *see* Pegaspargase *on page 735*
♦ **Peglyte™ (Canada)** *see* Polyethylene Glycol-Electrolyte Solution *on page 782*

Pemoline *(PEM oh leen)*

Related Information
Carbohydrate and Alcohol Content of Liquid Medications for Use in Patients Receiving Ketogenic Diets *on page 1228*

Brand Names Cylert®

Synonyms Phenylisohydantoin

Therapeutic Category Central Nervous System Stimulant, Nonamphetamine

Generic Available Yes

Use Attention-deficit/hyperactivity disorder (ADHD) (not first-line therapy, see Warnings); narcolepsy

Restrictions C-IV

Pregnancy Risk Factor B

Contraindications Liver disease; hypersensitivity to pemoline or any component; children <6 years of age; Tourette's syndrome

Warnings Life-threatening acute hepatic failure may occur; 15 cases of acute hepatic failure were reported to the FDA since 1975; this is 4 to 17 times the expected rate; 12 of the 15 cases resulted in death or liver transplantation; therefore, pemoline is not considered as first-line drug therapy for ADHD. Initiate pemoline only in patients without liver dysfunction/disease and only with normal baseline liver function tests; monitor serum ALT (SGPT) at baseline and every 2 weeks; discontinue drug if serum ALT increases ≥2 times the upper limit of normal, or to a clinically significant level, or if patient develops signs and symptoms of liver failure. Written informed consent (consent form provided by manufacturer; 847-937-7302) should be obtained prior to starting therapy; therapy should be withdrawn if no significant clinical benefit is seen within 3 weeks after completion of dose titration

Precautions Use with caution in patients with renal dysfunction, hypertension, or history of drug abuse; may cause growth suppression in children (monitor carefully); may decrease seizure threshold; may exacerbate thought disorder and behavior disturbance in psychotic children

Adverse Reactions
Central nervous system: Insomnia, seizures, precipitation of Tourette's syndrome, dizziness, hallucinations, headache
Dermatologic: Skin rashes
Endocrine & metabolic: Suppression of linear growth
Gastrointestinal: Stomach ache, nausea, diarrhea, anorexia, weight loss
Hematologic: Aplastic anemia (rare)
Hepatic: Elevated liver enzymes (usually reversible upon discontinuation), jaundice, fatal hepatic failure
Neuromuscular & skeletal: Movement disorders
Miscellaneous: Physical and psychological dependence

Drug Interactions CNS stimulants, CNS depressants, sympathomimetics; may alter insulin requirements in diabetics

Mechanism of Action Blocks the reuptake mechanism of dopaminergic neurons, appears to act at the cerebral cortex and subcortical structures; CNS and respiratory stimulant with weak sympathomimetic effects

Pharmacodynamics
Peak effect: 4 hours; significant benefit on hyperactivity may not be evident until 3rd or 4th week of administration
Duration: 8 hours

Pharmacokinetics
Protein binding: 50%
Metabolism: In the liver
Half-life:
Children: 7-8.6 hours
Adults: 12 hours
Elimination: 43% to 50% excreted unchanged in the urine

Usual Dosage Children ≥6 years: Oral: Initial: 37.5 mg given once daily in the morning, increase by 18.75 mg/day at weekly intervals; effective dose range: 56.25-75 mg/day; maximum dose: 112.5 mg/day; dosage range: 0.5-3 mg/kg/24 hours

Administration Oral: Administer medication in the morning

Monitoring Parameters Liver enzymes; for ADHD: Height, weight

Patient Information Avoid alcohol; avoid caffeine; chewable tablet should be chewed; may cause dizziness; may be habit-forming; do not abruptly discontinue; drug may cause liver failure; inform physician immediately of any signs of liver dysfunction such as dark urine, yellow skin, lack of appetite, GI complaints, general feeling of weakness; comply with blood testing of liver function

Additional Information Treatment of ADHD should include "Drug Holidays" or periodic discontinuation of stimulant medication in order to assess the patient's requirements, to decrease tolerance, and limit suppression of linear growth and weight

Dosage Forms
Tablet: 18.75 mg, 37.5 mg, 75 mg
Tablet, chewable: 37.5 mg

References
Adcock KG, MacElroy DE, Wolford ET, et al, "Pemoline Therapy Resulting in Liver Transplantation," *Ann Pharmacother*, 1998, 32(4):422-5.
Marotta PJ and Roberts EA, "Pemoline Hepatotoxicity in Children," *J Pediatr*, 1998, 132(5):894-7.
Rosh JR, Dellert SF, Narkewicz M, et al, "Four Cases of Severe Hepatotoxicity Associated With Pemoline: Possible Autoimmune Pathogenesis," *Pediatrics*, 1998, 101(5):921-3.

♦ **Penbritin® (Canada)** *see* Ampicillin *on page 78*
♦ **Penecort® Topical** *see* Hydrocortisone *on page 486*
♦ **Pen G** *see* Penicillin G, Parenteral, Aqueous *on page 741*

Penicillamine (pen i SIL a meen)

Related Information

Overdose and Toxicology *on page 1191*

Brand Names Cuprimine®; Depen®

Synonyms D-3-Mercaptovaline; β,β-Dimethylcysteine; D-Penicillamine

Therapeutic Category Antidote, Copper Toxicity; Antidote, Lead Toxicity; Chelating Agent, Oral

Generic Available No

Use Treatment of Wilson's disease, cystinuria, adjunct in the treatment of severe rheumatoid arthritis; lead poisoning, primary biliary cirrhosis (as adjunctive therapy following initial treatment with calcium EDTA or BAL)

Pregnancy Risk Factor D

Contraindications Hypersensitivity to penicillamine, any component, and possibly penicillin; patients with renal insufficiency; patients with previous penicillamine-related aplastic anemia or agranulocytosis; concomitant administration with other hematopoietic-depressant drugs (eg, gold, immunosuppressants, antimalarials, phenylbutazone), pregnancy, breast-feeding

Warnings Penicillamine has been associated with fatalities due to agranulocytosis, aplastic anemia, thrombocytopenia, Goodpasture's syndrome, and myasthenia gravis; patients should be warned to promptly report any symptoms suggesting toxicity; interruption of continuous therapy for Wilson's disease or cystinuria even for a few days has been associated with sensitivity reactions upon reinstitution of therapy; approximately 33% of patients will experience an allergic reaction

Precautions Patients on penicillamine for Wilson's disease or cystinuria should receive pyridoxine supplementation 25-50 mg/day; when treating rheumatoid arthritis, daily pyridoxine supplementation is also recommended

Adverse Reactions

Cardiovascular: Edema of the face, feet, or lower legs

Central nervous system: Fever, chills, myasthenic syndrome, fatigue

Dermatologic: Rash, pruritus, pemphigus, increased friability of the skin, exfoliative dermatitis, alopecia, angioedema

Endocrine & metabolic: Iron deficiency, hypoglycemia, thyroiditis

Gastrointestinal: Oral lesions, nausea, vomiting (in children with doses >60 mg/kg/day), epigastric pain, colitis, dysgeusia, ageusia, pancreatitis, sore throat, weight gain

Genitourinary: Urinary incontinence, bloody or cloudy urine

Hematologic: Leukopenia, thrombocytopenia, eosinophilia, aplastic anemia, agranulocytosis, hemolytic anemia

Hepatic: Hepatic dysfunction

Neuromuscular & skeletal: Arthralgia, dermatomyositis, polymyositis, peripheral neuropathy

Ocular: Optic neuritis

Otic: Tinnitus

Renal: Nephrotic syndrome, renal vasculitis, Goodpasture's syndrome, proteinuria, hematuria

Respiratory: Obliterative bronchiolitis, pulmonary fibrosis, interstitial pneumonitis, coughing, wheezing

Miscellaneous: Lymphadenopathy, allergic reactions, SLE-like syndrome, white spots on lips or mouth

Drug Interactions Gold, antimalarials, immunosuppressants, phenylbutazone are associated with similar serious hematologic reactions; iron salts, zinc salts, and antacids decrease penicillamine absorption; decreases serum digoxin levels

Food Interactions Do not administer with milk or food; iron and zinc may decrease drug action; increase dietary intake of pyridoxine; for Wilson's disease, decrease copper in diet and omit chocolate, nuts, shellfish, mushrooms, liver, raisins, broccoli, and molasses; for lead poisoning, decrease calcium in diet

Mechanism of Action Chelates with lead, copper, mercury, iron, and other heavy metals to form stable, soluble complexes that are excreted in the urine; depresses circulating IgM rheumatoid factor levels and *in vitro*, depresses T-cell but not B-cell activity; combines with cystine to form a more soluble compound which prevents the formation of cystine calculi

Pharmacokinetics

Absorption: 40% to 70%

Protein binding: 80% bound to albumin

Metabolism: In the liver

Half-life: 1.7-3.2 hours

Time to peak serum concentration: Within 1-2 hours

Elimination: Primarily (30% to 60%) in urine as unchanged drug

Usual Dosage Oral:

Rheumatoid arthritis:

Children: Initial: 3 mg/kg/day (≤250 mg/day) for 3 months, then 6 mg/kg/day (≤500 mg/day) in 2 divided doses for 3 months to a maximum of 10 mg/kg/day (≤1-1.5 g/day) in 3-4 divided doses

Adults: 125-250 mg/day, may increase dose at 1- to 3-month intervals up to 1-1.5 g/day; doses >500 mg/day should be given in divided doses

Wilson's disease (doses titrated to maintain urinary copper excretion >1 mg/day):

Infants and Children: 20 mg/kg/day in 2-4 doses; maximum dose: 1 g/day

Adults: 1 g/day in 4 divided doses; maximum dose: 2 g/day

Cystinuria (doses titrated to maintain urinary cystine excretion at <100-200 mg/day):

Children: 30 mg/kg/day in 4 divided doses; maximum dose: 4 g/day

Adults: Initial: 2 g/day divided every 6 hours (range: 1-4 g/day)

Lead poisoning (continue until blood lead level is <60 µg/dL; treatment duration varies from 4-12 weeks):

Children: 20-30 mg/kg/day in 3-4 divided doses; initiating treatment at 25% of this dose and gradually increasing to the full dose over 2-3 weeks may minimize adverse reactions; maximum dose: 1.5 g/day

Adults: 1-1.5 g/day in 3-4 divided doses; initiating treatment at 25% of this dose and gradually increasing to the full dose over 2-3 weeks may minimize adverse reactions

Primary biliary cirrhosis: Adults: 250 mg/day to start, increase by 250 mg every 2 weeks up to a maintenance dose of 1 g/day, as 250 mg 4 times/day

Dosing adjustment in renal impairment: Cl_{cr} <50 mL/minute: Avoid use

Administration Oral: Administer on an empty stomach 1 hour before or 2 hours after meals; patients unable to swallow capsules may mix contents of capsule with fruit juice or chilled pureed fruit; patients with cystinuria should drink copious amounts of water

Monitoring Parameters Urinalysis, CBC with differential, hemoglobin, platelet count, liver function tests; weekly measurements of urinary and blood concentrations of the intoxicating metal is indicated (3 months has been tolerated); annual x-ray for renal stones; Wilson's disease: 24-hour urinary copper excretion; quantitative 24-hour urine protein at 1- to 2-week intervals initially (first 2-3 months); urinalysis

Patient Information Possible severe allergic reaction if patient allergic to penicillin; notify physician if unusual bleeding or bruising, or persistent fever, sore throat, or fatigue occur. Report any unexplained cough, shortness of breath, or rash; loss of taste may occur; do not skip or miss doses or discontinue without notifying physician.

Dosage Forms

Capsule: 125 mg, 250 mg

Tablet: 250 mg

Extemporaneous Preparations A 50 mg/mL suspension may be made by mixing sixty 250 mg capsules with 3 g carboxymethylcellulose, 150 g sucrose, 300 mg citric acid, parabens (methylparaben 120 mg, propylparaben 12 mg, propylene glycol qsad to 100 mL), and purified water to a total volume of 300 mL; cherry flavor may be added. Stability is 30 days refrigerated.

DeCastro FJ, Jaeger RQ, and Rolfe UT, "An Extemporaneously Prepared Penicillamine Suspension Used to Treat Lead Intoxication," *Hosp Pharm*, 1977, 2:446-8.

Penicillin G Benzathine (pen i SIL in jee BENZ a theen)

Brand Names Bicillin® L-A; Megacillin® Susp (Canada); Permapen®

Synonyms Benzathine Benzylpenicillin; Benzathine Penicillin G; Benzylpenicillin Benzathine

Therapeutic Category Antibiotic, Penicillin

Generic Available No

Use Active against most gram-positive organisms and some spirochetes; used only for the treatment of mild to moderately severe infections (ie, *Streptococcus* pharyngitis) caused by organisms susceptible to low concentrations of penicillin G, or for prophylaxis of infections caused by these organisms such as rheumatic fever prophylaxis

Pregnancy Risk Factor B

Contraindications Hypersensitivity to penicillin or any component

Precautions Use with caution in patients with impaired renal function, impaired cardiac function, pre-existing seizure disorder, or hypersensitivity to cephalosporins

(Continued)

Penicillin G Benzathine *(Continued)*

Adverse Reactions

Central nervous system: Convulsions, confusion, lethargy, fever, dizziness

Dermatologic: Rash

Hematologic: Hemolytic anemia

Local: Pain at injection site

Neuromuscular & skeletal: Myoclonus

Renal: Interstitial nephritis

Miscellaneous: Jarisch-Herxheimer reaction, hypersensitivity reactions, anaphylaxis

Drug Interactions Probenecid increases serum concentration of penicillin; antibacterial activity with aminoglycosides is synergistic; tetracyclines, chloramphenicol, and erythromycin may antagonize the activity of penicillin

Stability Store in the refrigerator; avoid freezing

Mechanism of Action Inhibits bacterial cell wall synthesis by binding to one or more of the penicillin-binding proteins; inhibits the final transpeptidation step of peptidoglycan synthesis in bacterial cell wall

Pharmacokinetics

Absorption: I.M.: Slow

Distribution: Minimal concentrations attained in CSF with inflamed or uninflamed meninges

Time to peak serum concentration: Within 12-24 hours; serum levels are usually detectable for 1-4 weeks depending on the dose; larger doses result in more sustained levels rather than higher levels

Elimination: Penicillin G is detected in urine for up to 12 weeks after a single I.M. injection; renal clearance is delayed in neonates, young infants, and patients with impaired renal function

Usual Dosage I.M. (dosage frequency depends on infection being treated):

Neonates >1200 g: Asymptomatic congenital syphilis: 50,000 units/kg for 1 dose

Infants and Children:

Group A streptococcal upper respiratory infection: 25,000-50,000 units/kg as a single dose; maximum dose: 1.2 million units/dose **or**

Children <27 kg: 300,000-600,000 units as a single dose

Children ≥27 kg: 900,000 units as a single dose

Prophylaxis of recurrent rheumatic fever: 25,000-50,000 units/kg every 3-4 weeks; maximum dose: 1.2 million units/dose

Congenital syphilis: 50,000 units/kg every week for 3 weeks; maximum dose: 2.4 million units/dose

Syphilis of more than 1-year duration: 50,000 units/kg every week for 3 successive weeks; maximum dose: 2.4 million units/dose

Adults:

Group A streptococcal upper respiratory infection: 1.2 million units as a single dose

Prophylaxis of recurrent rheumatic fever: 1.2 million units every 3-4 weeks or 600,000 units twice monthly

Early syphilis: 2.4 million units as a single dose in 2 injection sites

Syphilis of more than 1-year duration: 2.4 million units (in 2 injection sites) once weekly for 3 doses

Administration Parenteral: I.M.: Give undiluted injection; administer by deep I.M. injection in the upper outer quadrant of the buttock (adolescents and adults) or into the midlateral muscle of the thigh (infants and children); do **not** give I.V., intra-arterially or S.C.; inadvertent I.V. administration has resulted in thrombosis, severe neurovascular damage, cardiac arrest, and death

Monitoring Parameters CBC, urinalysis, renal function tests

Test Interactions Positive Coombs' [direct], false-positive urinary and/or serum proteins

Nursing Implications S.C. administration may cause pain and induration; avoid repeated I.M. injections into the anterolateral thigh in neonates and infants since quadriceps femoris fibrosis and atrophy may occur

Additional Information Use a penicillin G benzathine/penicillin G procaine combination (ie, Bicillin C-R®) to achieve early peak levels in acute infections

Dosage Forms Injection: 300,000 units/mL (10 mL); 600,000 units/mL (1 mL, 2 mL, 4 mL)

References

Kaplan EL, Berrios X, Speth J, et al, "Pharmacokinetics of Benzathine Penicillin G: Serum Levels During the 28 Days After Intramuscular Injection of 1,200,000 Units," *J Pediatr*, 1989, 115(1):146-50.

Paryani SG, Vaughn AJ, Crosby M, et al, "Treatment of Asymptomatic Congenital Syphilis: Benzathine Versus Procaine Penicillin G Therapy," *J Pediatr*, 1994, 125(3):471-5.

WHO Study Group, "Rheumatic Fever and Rheumatic Heart Disease," *World Health Organ Tech Rep Ser,* 1988, 764:1-58.

Penicillin G, Parenteral, Aqueous

(pen i SIL in jee, pa REN ter al, AYE kwee us)

Brand Names Pfizerpen®

Available Salts Penicillin G Potassium; Penicillin G Sodium

Synonyms Crystalline Penicillin; Pen G

Therapeutic Category Antibiotic, Penicillin

Generic Available Yes

Use Treatment of sepsis, meningitis, pericarditis, endocarditis, pneumonia, and other infections due to susceptible gram-positive organisms (except *Staphylococcus aureus*), some gram-negative organisms such as *Neisseria gonorrhoeae*, or *N. meningitidis* and some anaerobes and spirochetes

Pregnancy Risk Factor B

Contraindications Hypersensitivity to penicillin or any component

Precautions Use with caution in patients with renal impairment, hypersensitivity to cephalosporins, or pre-existing seizure disorder; dosage modification required in patients with renal impairment; further dosage reduction recommended in patients with impaired hepatic and renal function

Adverse Reactions

Central nervous system: Convulsions, confusion, lethargy, fever, dizziness

Dermatologic: Rash, urticaria

Endocrine & metabolic: Electrolyte imbalance

Gastrointestinal: Diarrhea

Hematologic: Hemolytic anemia, neutropenia

Local: Thrombophlebitis

Neuromuscular & skeletal: Myoclonus

Renal: Acute interstitial nephritis

Miscellaneous: Jarisch-Herxheimer reaction, hypersensitivity reactions, anaphylaxis

Drug Interactions Probenecid increases serum concentration of penicillin; antibacterial activity with aminoglycosides is synergistic; tetracyclines, chloramphenicol, and erythromycin may antagonize the activity of penicillin

Food Interactions Presence of food or milk decreases absorption

Stability Reconstituted parenteral solution is stable for 7 days when refrigerated; incompatible with aminoglycosides; inactivated in acidic or alkaline solutions

Mechanism of Action Inhibits bacterial cell wall synthesis by binding to one or more of the penicillin-binding proteins; inhibits the final transpeptidation step of peptidoglycan synthesis in bacterial cell wall

Pharmacokinetics

Absorption: Oral: <30%

Distribution: Penetration across the blood-brain barrier is poor with uninflamed meninges; crosses the placenta; appears in breast milk

Protein binding: 65%

Metabolism: In the liver (10% to 30%) to penicilloic acid

Half-life:

Neonates:

<6 days: 3.2-3.4 hours

7-13 days: 1.2-2.2 hours

>14 days: 0.9-1.9 hours

Infants and Children: 0.5-1.2 hours

Adults: 0.5-0.75 hours with normal renal function

Time to peak serum concentration:

Oral: Within 30-60 minutes

I.M.: Within 30 minutes

Elimination: Penicillin G and its metabolites are excreted in urine mainly by tubular secretion

Moderately dialyzable (20% to 50%)

Usual Dosage

Neonates: I.M., I.V.:

Postnatal age ≤7 days:

≤2000 g: 50,000 units/kg/day in divided doses every 12 hours

Meningitis: 100,000 units/kg/day in divided doses every 12 hours

>2000 g: 75,000 units/kg/day in divided doses every 8 hours

Meningitis: 150,000 units/kg/day in divided doses every 8 hours

Congenital syphilis: 100,000 units/kg/day in divided doses every 12 hours

(Continued)

Penicillin G, Parenteral, Aqueous *(Continued)*

Group B streptococcal meningitis: 250,000-450,000 units/kg/day in divided doses every 8 hours
Postnatal age >7 days:
<1200 g: 50,000 units/kg/day in divided doses every 12 hours
Meningitis: 100,000 units/kg/day in divided doses every 12 hours
1200-2000 g: 75,000 units/kg/day in divided doses every 8 hours
Meningitis: 150,000 units/kg/day in divided doses every 8 hours
>2000 g: 100,000 units/kg/day in divided doses every 6 hours
Meningitis: 200,000 units/kg/day in divided doses every 6 hours
Congenital syphilis: 150,000 units/kg/day in divided doses every 8 hours
Group B streptococcal meningitis: I.V.: 450,000 units/kg/day in divided doses every 6 hours
Infants and Children:
I.M., I.V.: 100,000 to 250,000 units/kg/day in divided doses every 4-6 hours
Severe infections: 250,000-400,000 units/kg/day in divided doses every 4-6 hours; maximum dose: 24 million units/day
Adults: I.M., I.V.: 2-24 million units/day in divided doses every 4-6 hours
Dosing interval in renal impairment:
Cl_{cr} 10-30 mL/minute: Administer normal dose every 8-12 hours
Cl_{cr} <10 mL/minute: Administer normal dose every 12-18 hours
Administration Parenteral: Administer by I.V. intermittent infusion over 15-60 minutes at a final concentration for administration of 100,000-500,000 units/mL. A final concentration of 50,000 units/mL infused over 15-30 minutes is recommended for neonates and infants. The potassium or sodium content of the dose should be considered when determining the infusion rate.
Monitoring Parameters Periodic serum electrolytes, renal and hematologic function tests
Test Interactions False-positive or negative urinary glucose determination using Clinitest®; positive Coombs' [direct]; false-positive urinary and/or serum proteins
Additional Information
Penicillin G potassium: 1.7 mEq of potassium and 0.3 mEq of sodium per 1 million units of penicillin G
Penicillin G sodium: 2 mEq of sodium per 1 million units of penicillin G
Dosage Forms
Injection, as sodium: 5 million units
Injection:
Frozen premixed, as potassium: 1 million units, 2 million units, 3 million units
Powder, as potassium: 1 million units, 5 million units, 10 million units, 20 million units
References
American Academy of Pediatrics Committee on Infectious Diseases, "Treatment of Bacterial Meningitis," *Pediatrics*, 1988, 81(6):904-7.
Prober CG, Stevenson DK, and Benitz WE, "The Use of Antibiotics in Neonates Weighing Less Than 1200 Grams," *Pediatr Infect Dis J*, 1990, 9(2):111-21.

♦ **Penicillin G Potassium** *see* Penicillin G, Parenteral, Aqueous *on page 741*

Penicillin G Procaine *(pen i SIL in jee PROE kane)*
Brand Names Ayercillin® (Canada); Crysticillin® A.S.; Pfizerpen®-AS; Wycillin®
Synonyms APPG; Aqueous Procaine Penicillin G; Procaine Benzylpenicillin; Procaine Penicillin G
Therapeutic Category Antibiotic, Penicillin
Generic Available Yes
Use Moderately severe infections due to *Treponema pallidum* and other penicillin G-sensitive microorganisms that are susceptible to low but prolonged serum penicillin concentrations
Pregnancy Risk Factor B
Contraindications Hypersensitivity to penicillin, procaine, or any component
Warnings Some formulations contain a sulfite that may cause allergic-type reactions
Precautions Use with caution in patients with renal impairment, hypersensitivity to cephalosporins, or history of seizures; modify dosage in patients with severe renal impairment
Adverse Reactions
Cardiovascular: Myocardial depression, vasodilation, conduction disturbances
Central nervous system: Seizures, confusion, lethargy, dizziness, disorientation, agitation, hallucinations
Hematologic: Hemolytic anemia

Local: Sterile abscess and pain at injection site
Neuromuscular & skeletal: Myoclonus
Renal: Interstitial nephritis
Miscellaneous: Pseudoanaphylactic reactions, Jarisch-Herxheimer reaction, hypersensitivity reactions

Drug Interactions Probenecid increases serum concentration of penicillin; antibacterial activity with aminoglycosides is synergistic; tetracyclines, chloramphenicol, and erythromycin may antagonize the activity of penicillin

Stability Store in refrigerator

Mechanism of Action Inhibits bacterial cell wall synthesis by binding to one or more of the penicillin-binding proteins; inhibits the final transpeptidation step of peptidoglycan synthesis in bacterial cell wall

Pharmacokinetics
Absorption: I.M.: Slow
Distribution: Penetration across the blood-brain barrier is poor, despite inflamed meninges; appears in breast milk
Time to peak serum concentration: Within 1-4 hours and can persist within the therapeutic range for 15-24 hours
Elimination: Renal clearance is delayed in neonates, young infants, and patients with impaired renal function
Moderately dialyzable (20% to 50%)

Usual Dosage I.M.:
Neonates ≥1200 g: Avoid using in this age group since sterile abscesses and procaine toxicity occur more frequently with neonates than older patients
Congenital syphilis: 50,000 units/kg/day once daily for 10 days; if more than 1 day of therapy is missed, the entire course should be restarted
Infants and Children: 25,000-50,000 units/kg/day in divided doses every 12-24 hours; not to exceed 4.8 million units/24 hours
Congenital syphilis: 50,000 units/kg/day once daily for 10 days; if more than 1 day of therapy is missed, the entire course should be restarted
Adults: 0.6-4.8 million units/day in divided doses every 12-24 hours
When used in conjunction with an aminoglycoside for the treatment of endocarditis caused by susceptible *S. viridans*: 1.2 million units every 6 hours for 2-4 weeks
Neurosyphilis: 2.4 million units once daily for 10 days with probenecid 500 mg every 6 hours

Administration Parenteral: Procaine suspension for deep I.M. injection only; inadvertent I.V. administration has resulted in neurovascular damage; in infants and children it is preferable to administer I.M. into the midlateral muscles of the thigh; in adults, administer into the gluteus maximus or into the midlateral muscles of the thigh

Monitoring Parameters Periodic renal and hematologic function tests with prolonged therapy

Test Interactions Positive Coombs' [direct], false-positive urinary and/or serum proteins

Nursing Implications Do **not** give I.V., intra-arterially, or S.C.; avoid repeated I.M. injections into the anterolateral thigh in neonates and infants since quadriceps femoris fibrosis and atrophy may occur

Dosage Forms Injection, suspension: 300,000 units/mL (10 mL); 500,000 units/mL (1.2 mL); 600,000 units/mL (1 mL, 2 mL, 4 mL)

References
Paryani SG, Vaughn AJ, Crosby M, et al, "Treatment of Asymptomatic Congenital Syphilis: Benzathine Versus Procaine Penicillin G Therapy," *J Pediatr*, 1994, 125(3):471-5.

♦ **Penicillin G Sodium** *see* Penicillin G, Parenteral, Aqueous *on page 741*

Penicillin V Potassium (pen i SIL in vee poe TASS ee um)

Related Information
Carbohydrate and Alcohol Content of Liquid Medications for Use in Patients Receiving Ketogenic Diets *on page 1228*

Brand Names Apo®-Pen VK (Canada); Beepen-VK®; Betapen®-VK; Ledercillin® VK; Nadopen-V® (Canada); Novo-Pen-VK® (Canada); Nu-Pen-VK® (Canada); Pen-Vee® (Canada); Pen.Vee® K; PVF® K (Canada); Robicillin® VK; V-Cillin K®; Veetids®

Synonyms Phenoxymethyl Penicillin

Therapeutic Category Antibiotic, Penicillin

Generic Available Yes

(Continued)

Penicillin V Potassium *(Continued)*

Use Treatment of mild to moderately severe susceptible bacterial infections involving the upper respiratory tract, skin, and urinary tract; prophylaxis of pneumococcal infections and rheumatic fever

Pregnancy Risk Factor B

Contraindications Hypersensitivity to penicillin or any component

Precautions Use with caution in patients with renal impairment, hypersensitivity to cephalosporins, or history of seizures; dosage adjustment may be necessary in patients with renal impairment

Adverse Reactions

Central nervous system: Convulsions, fever

Dermatologic: Rash

Gastrointestinal: Nausea, diarrhea, vomiting, black hairy tongue, pseudomembranous colitis

Hematologic: Hemolytic anemia

Renal: Acute interstitial nephritis

Miscellaneous: Hypersensitivity reactions, anaphylaxis

Drug Interactions Probenecid (higher, prolonged penicillin serum concentration)

Food Interactions Presence of food or milk decreases absorption

Stability Refrigerate suspension after reconstitution; discard after 14 days

Mechanism of Action Interferes with bacterial cell wall synthesis during active multiplication by binding to one or more of the penicillin-binding proteins; inhibits the final transpeptidation step of peptidoglycan synthesis causing cell wall death and resultant bactericidal activity against susceptible bacteria

Pharmacokinetics

Absorption: Oral: 60% to 73% from the GI tract

Distribution: Widely distributed to kidneys, liver, skin, tonsils, and into synovial, pleural, and pericardial fluids; appears in breast milk

Protein binding: 80%

Metabolism: 10% to 30%

Half-life: 30 minutes and is prolonged in patients with renal impairment

Time to peak serum concentration: Within 30-60 minutes

Elimination: Penicillin V and its metabolites are excreted in urine mainly by tubular secretion

Usual Dosage Oral:

Systemic infections:

Children <12 years: 25-50 mg/kg/day in divided doses every 6-8 hours; maximum dose: 3 g/day

Children ≥12 years and Adults: 125-500 mg every 6-8 hours

Prophylaxis of pneumococcal infections:

Children <5 years: 125 mg twice daily

Children ≥5 years and Adults: 250 mg twice daily

Prophylaxis of recurrent rheumatic fever:

Children <5 years: 125 mg twice daily

Children ≥5 years and Adults: 250 mg twice daily

Administration Oral: Administer with water on an empty stomach 1 hour before or 2 hours after meals; may be administered with food to decrease GI upset

Monitoring Parameters Periodic renal and hematologic function tests during prolonged therapy

Test Interactions False-positive or negative urinary glucose determination using Clinitest®; positive Coombs' [direct]; false-positive urinary and/or serum proteins

Additional Information 0.7 mEq of potassium/250 mg penicillin V; 250 mg = 400,000 units of penicillin

Dosage Forms

Powder for oral solution: 125 mg/5 mL (3 mL, 100 mL, 150 mL, 200 mL); 250 mg/5 mL (100 mL, 150 mL, 200 mL)

Tablet: 125 mg, 250 mg, 500 mg

References

Dajani AS, Bisno AL, Chung KJ, et al, "Prevention of Rheumatic Fever. A Statement for Health Professionals by the Committee on Rheumatic Fever, Endocarditis, and Kawasaki Disease of the Council on Cardiovascular Disease in the Young, The American Heart Association," *Pediatr Infect Dis J*, 1989, 8(5):263-6.

♦ **Penicilloyl-polylysine** *see* Benzylpenicilloyl-polylysine *on page 127*

♦ **Pentacef™** *see* Ceftazidime *on page 190*

♦ **Pentam-300® Injection** *see* Pentamidine *on page 745*

Pentamidine (pen TAM i deen)

Brand Names NebuPent™ Inhalation; Pentam-300® Injection

Available Salts Pentamidine Isethionate

Therapeutic Category Antibiotic, Miscellaneous; Antiprotozoal

Generic Available No

Use Treatment and prevention of pneumonia caused by *Pneumocystis carinii* in patients who cannot tolerate or who fail to respond to co-trimoxazole; treatment of African trypanosomiasis; treatment of visceral leishmaniasis caused by *L. donovani*

Pregnancy Risk Factor C

Contraindications Hypersensitivity to pentamidine isethionate or any component (inhalation and injection); do not use concomitantly with didanosine since both drugs can cause pancreatitis

Warnings Healthcare personnel who administer aerosolized pentamidine inhalation therapy, a cough-producing procedure, should be aware of the possibility of secondary exposure to tuberculosis or other infections from patients with undiagnosed pulmonary disease

Precautions Use with caution in patients with diabetes mellitus, renal or hepatic dysfunction, hypertension or hypotension; adjust dose in renal impairment

Adverse Reactions

Cardiovascular: Hypotension, tachycardia, cardiac arrhythmias

Central nervous system: Dizziness, fever, fatigue, delirium

Dermatologic: Rash, itching

Endocrine & metabolic: Hypoglycemia, hyperglycemia, hypocalcemia, hyperkalemia

Gastrointestinal: Nausea, vomiting, metallic taste, pancreatitis

Hematologic: Megaloblastic anemia, neutropenia, leukopenia, thrombocytopenia

Hepatic: Mild hepatic injury

Local: Pain at injection site, thrombophlebitis, sterile abscess, erythema

Renal: Nephrotoxicity, elevated BUN, elevated serum creatinine

With aerosolized pentamidine: Irritation of the airway, cough, transient arterial desaturation, bronchospasm, fatigue, conjunctivitis

Miscellaneous: Jarisch-Herxheimer-like reaction

Drug Interactions Aminoglycosides, amphotericin B, cisplatin and vancomycin (additive nephrotoxicity); didanosine (additive toxicity)

Stability Reconstituted solution is stable for 48 hours at room temperature when protected from light; do not refrigerate due to the possibility of crystallization

Mechanism of Action Interferes with RNA/DNA, phospholipids and protein synthesis through inhibition of oxidative phosphorylation and/or interference with incorporation of nucleotides and nucleic acids into RNA and DNA, in protozoa

Pharmacokinetics

Absorption: I.M.: Well absorbed; limited systemic absorption following pentamidine inhalation therapy

Distribution: Binds to tissues and plasma protein; high concentrations are found in the liver, kidney, adrenals, spleen, lungs and pancreas; poor penetration into CNS; following oral inhalation, high concentrations are found in bronchoalveolar fluid

Half-life, terminal: 6.4-9.4 hours; half-life may be prolonged in patients with severe renal impairment

Elimination: 33% to 66% in urine as unchanged drug

Not appreciably removed by hemodialysis or peritoneal dialysis

Usual Dosage

Children:

Treatment of *Pneumocystis carinii* pneumonia: I.M., I.V. (I.V. preferred): 4 mg/kg/day once daily for 14-21 days

Prophylaxis for *Pneumocystis carinii* pneumonia (See "Note" in Additional Information):

I.M., I.V.: 4 mg/kg/dose every 2-4 weeks **or**

Inhalation: Every month via Respirgard® II nebulizer

Infants <1 year: Aerosolized pentamidine is administered at doses adjusted for minute ventilation and weight

Infant dose = 2.27 mg/kg × nebulizer output (L/minute) × wt (kg) divided by alveolar ventilation (L/minute)

Children <5 years: Some institutions have used a dose of 8 mg/kg

Children ≥5 years: 300 mg/dose

Treatment of trypanosomiasis: I.M.: 4 mg/kg/day once daily for 10 days

Treatment of visceral leishmaniasis: I.M.: 2-4 mg/kg/day once daily or every 2 days for up to 15 doses

(Continued)

Pentamidine *(Continued)*

Adults:

Treatment: I.M., I.V. (I.V. preferred): 4 mg/kg/day once daily for 14 days

Prevention: Inhalation: 300 mg every 4 weeks via Respirgard® II nebulizer

Dosing adjustment in renal impairment:

Cl_{cr} 10-30 mL/min: Administer normal dose once every 36 hours

Cl_{cr} <10 mL/min: Administer normal dose once every 48 hours

Administration

Oral inhalation: Safe and effective administration via nebulization in children is dependent on patients wearing an appropriately sized pediatric face mask

Parenteral: May administer deep I.M. or by slow I.V. infusion; rapid I.V. administration can cause severe hypotension; infuse I.V. slowly over a period of at least 60 minutes at a final concentration for administration not to exceed 6 mg/mL

Monitoring Parameters Liver function tests, renal function tests, blood glucose, serum potassium and calcium, CBC with differential and platelet count, EKG, blood pressure

Patient Information Maintain adequate fluid intake; notify physician if fever, cough, or shortness of breath occurs; avoid alcohol

Nursing Implications Patients should receive parenteral pentamidine while lying down and blood pressure should be monitored closely during administration and after completion of the infusion until blood pressure is stabilized; if hypotension occurs due to rapid I.V. administration, slow infusion rate to administer dose over 1-2 hours

Additional Information

Note: Guidelines for prophylaxis of *Pneumocystis carinii* pneumonia: Initiate PCP prophylaxis for the following patients: All HIV-exposed children at 4-6 weeks of age and continue through the first year of life or until HIV infection has been reasonably excluded; children 1-5 years of age with CD4+ count <500 or CD4+ percentage <15%; children 6-12 years of age with CD4+ count <200 or CD4+ percentage <15%; for children who had a CD4+ count <750 or a CD4+ percentage <15% in the first year of life, prophylaxis should be continued until 2 years of age

1 mg pentamidine: 1.74 mg pentamidine isethionate

Dosage Forms

Inhalation, as isethionate: 300 mg

Powder for injection, as isethionate, lyophilized: 300 mg

References

Hand IL, Wiznia AA, Porricolo M, et al, "Aerosolized Pentamidine for Prophylaxis of *Pneumocystis carinii* Pneumonia in Infants With Human Immunodeficiency Virus Infection," *Pediatr Infect Dis J*, 1994, 13(2):100-4.

Hughes WT, "*Pneumocystis carinii* Pneumonia: New Approaches to Diagnosis, Treatment, and Prevention," *Pediatr Infect Dis J*, 1991, 10(5):391-9.

"1997 USPHS/IDSA Guidelines for the Prevention of Opportunistic Infections in Persons Infected With Human Immunodeficiency Virus," *MMWR Morb Mortal Wkly Rep*, 1997, 46(RR-12):1-46.

♦ **Pentamidine Isethionate** *see* Pentamidine *on page 745*

♦ **Pentamycetin® (Canada)** *see* Chloramphenicol *on page 207*

♦ **Pentasa® Oral** *see* Mesalamine *on page 608*

Pentazocine *(pen TAZ oh seen)*

Related Information

Compatibility of Medications Mixed in a Syringe *on page 1208*

Narcotic Analgesics Comparison *on page 1035*

Brand Names Talwin®; Talwin® NX

Available Salts Pentazocine Hydrochloride; Pentazocine Lactate

Synonyms Pentazocine and Naloxone

Therapeutic Category Analgesic, Narcotic; Opiate Partial Agonist; Sedative

Generic Available No

Use Relief of moderate to severe pain; a sedative prior to surgery; supplement to surgical anesthesia

Restrictions C-IV

Pregnancy Risk Factor B (D if used for prolonged periods or in high doses at term)

Contraindications Hypersensitivity to pentazocine or any component

Warnings Pentazocine may precipitate opiate withdrawal symptoms in patients who have been receiving opiates regularly; injection contains sulfites which may cause allergic reaction

Precautions Use with caution in seizure-prone patients, acute MI, patients undergoing biliary tract surgery, patients with renal and hepatic dysfunction, and patients with a history of prior opioid dependence or abuse; decrease dosage in patients with decreased hepatic or renal function

Adverse Reactions

Cardiovascular: Palpitations, hypotension, tachycardia, peripheral vasodilation

Central nervous system: CNS depression, drowsiness, sedation, dizziness, euphoria, lightheadedness (more frequently than morphine), hallucinations, confusion, disorientation, increased intracranial pressure; seizures may occur in seizure-prone patients especially with large I.V. doses

Dermatologic: Pruritus, rash

Endocrine & metabolic: Antidiuretic hormone release

Gastrointestinal: Nausea (more frequently than morphine), vomiting, constipation, biliary tract spasm

Genitourinary: Urinary tract spasm

Local: Tissue damage and irritation with I.M./S.C. use

Ocular: Miosis

Respiratory: Respiratory depression, laryngospasm

Miscellaneous: Physical and psychological dependence, histamine release

Drug Interactions Cytochrome P-450 isoenzyme CYP2D6 substrate

May potentiate or reduce analgesic effect of opiate agonist (ie, morphine), depending on patient's tolerance to opiates; additive effects seen with other CNS depressants; tripelennamine potentiates pentazocine effects and lethality and the two have been abused in combination (Ts and blues) I.V. to provide effects similar to heroin

Mechanism of Action Binds to opiate receptors in the CNS, causing inhibition of ascending pain pathways, altering the perception of and response to pain; produces generalized CNS depression

Pharmacodynamics

Onset:

Oral, I.M., S.C.: Within 15-30 minutes

I.V.: Within 2-3 minutes

Duration:

Oral: 4-5 hours

Parenteral: 2-3 hours

Pharmacokinetics

Protein binding: 60%

Metabolism: In the liver via oxidative and glucuronide conjugation pathways

Bioavailability: Oral: ~20% due to large first-pass effect; increased oral bioavailability to 60% to 70% in patients with cirrhosis

Half-life: Increased half-life with decreased hepatic function

Children 4-8 years (mean ± SD): 3 ± 1.5 hours

Adults: 2-3 hours

Elimination: Small amounts excreted unchanged in urine

Usual Dosage

Children <14 years: Limited information available:

I.M. doses of 15 mg for children 5-8 years of age and 30 mg for children 9-14 years of age to treat postoperative pain have been used (n=30) (Waterworth, 1974)

In 300 children (1-14 years) I.M. doses ranging from approximately 0.45-1.5 mg/kg in children <27 kg to 0.65-1.9 mg/kg in children >27 kg were used preoperatively (Rita, 1970)

I.V.: Intraoperative: Titrating doses of 0.5 mg/kg every 30-45 minutes as needed for analgesia have been given in 50 children 5-9 years of age; total dose required: 1-1.5 mg/kg (Ray, 1993)

Children >14 years and Adults: Oral: 50 mg every 3-4 hours; may increase to 100 mg/dose if needed; maximum dose: 600 mg/day

Adults:

I.M., S.C.: 30-60 mg every 3-4 hours

I.V.: 30 mg every 3-4 hours

Dosing adjustment in renal impairment: Children and Adults:

Cl_{cr} 10-50 mL/minute: Administer 75% of normal dose

Cl_{cr} <10 mL/minute: Administer 50% of normal dose

Administration

Oral: May be administered with food or milk to decrease GI upset

Parenteral: S.C. route not advised due to tissue damage; rotate injection site for I.M., S.C. use; avoid intra-arterial injection

Monitoring Parameters Respiratory and cardiovascular status; level of pain relief and sedation; blood pressure

(Continued)

Pentazocine *(Continued)*

Patient Information Avoid alcohol; may cause drowsiness and impair ability to perform hazardous activities requiring mental alertness or physical coordination; may be habit-forming; will cause narcotic withdrawal symptoms in patients currently dependent on narcotics

Additional Information Use only in patients who are not tolerant to or physically dependent upon narcotics

Talwin® NX tablet (pentazocine hydrochloride with naloxone) was formulated to decrease abuse potential of dissolving tablets in water and using as injection

Dosage Forms

Injection, as lactate: 30 mg/mL (1 mL, 1.5 mL, 2 mL, 10 mL)

Tablet, scored: Pentazocine hydrochloride 50 mg and naloxone hydrochloride 0.5 mg

References

Hanunen K, Olkkola KT, Seppala T, et al, "Pharmacokinetics and Pharmacodynamics of Pentazocine in Children," *Pharmacol Toxicol*, 1993, 73(2):120-3.

Ray AD and Gupta M, "Clinical Trial of Pentazocine as Analgesic in Pediatric Cases," *J Indian Med Assoc*, 1994, 92(3):77-9.

Rita L, Seleny FL, and Levin RM, "A Comparison of Pentazocine and Morphine for Pediatric Premedication," *Anesth Analg*, 1970, 49(3):377-82.

Waterworth TA, "Pentazocine (Fortal) as Postoperative Analgesic in Children," *Arch Dis Child*, 1974, 49(6):488-90.

- ♦ **Pentazocine and Naloxone** *see* Pentazocine *on page 746*
- ♦ **Pentazocine Hydrochloride** *see* Pentazocine *on page 746*
- ♦ **Pentazocine Lactate** *see* Pentazocine *on page 746*

Pentobarbital *(pen toe BAR bi tal)*

Related Information

Compatibility of Medications Mixed in a Syringe *on page 1208*

Laboratory Detection of Drugs in Urine *on page 1204*

Overdose and Toxicology *on page 1191*

Preprocedure Sedatives in Children *on page 1169*

Brand Names Nembutal®; Nova Rectal® (Canada)

Available Salts Pentobarbital Sodium

Therapeutic Category Anticonvulsant, Barbiturate; Barbiturate; General Anesthetic; Hypnotic; Sedative

Generic Available Yes

Use Short-term treatment of insomnia; preoperative sedation; high-dose barbiturate coma for treatment of increased intracranial pressure or status epilepticus unresponsive to other therapy

Restrictions C-II; C-III (suppositories)

Pregnancy Risk Factor D

Contraindications Marked liver function impairment or latent porphyria; chronic or acute pain; hypersensitivity to barbiturates or any component

Warnings Capsules may contain tartrazine which may cause allergic reactions; commercially available injection contains propylene glycol

Precautions Use with caution in patients with hypovolemic shock, CHF, or hepatic impairment

Adverse Reactions

Cardiovascular: Arrhythmias, bradycardia, hypotension

Central nervous system: Drowsiness, lethargy, CNS excitation or depression, impaired judgment, hypothermia

Dermatologic: Rash

Gastrointestinal: Nausea, vomiting

Local: Arterial spasm, gangrene with inadvertent intra-arterial injection, thrombophlebitis

Renal: Oliguria

Respiratory: Laryngospasm, respiratory depression, apnea (especially with rapid I.V. use)

Miscellaneous: Physical and psychological dependency with chronic use

Drug Interactions Barbiturates are enzyme inducers (monitor patient closely for decreased effect of concomitantly administered medications or increased effect when barbiturates are discontinued); carbamazepine, chloramphenicol, cimetidine, corticosteroids, CNS depressants, alcohol, doxycycline, warfarin, valproic acid

Food Interactions Food may decrease the rate but not the extent of oral absorption; high doses of pyridoxine may decrease drug effect; barbiturates may increase the metabolism of vitamins D and K; dietary requirements of vitamins D, K, C, B_{12}, folate, and calcium may be increased with long-term use

Stability Protect from light; aqueous solutions are not stable; low pH may cause precipitate; use only clear solution

Mechanism of Action Short-acting barbiturate with sedative, hypnotic, and anticonvulsant properties; depresses CNS activity by binding to barbiturate site at GABA-receptor complex enhancing GABA activity; depresses reticular activating system; higher doses may be gabamimetic

Pharmacodynamics

Onset:

Oral or rectal: 15-60 minutes

I.M.: Within 10-15 minutes

I.V.: Within 1 minute

Duration:

Oral, rectal: 1-4 hours

I.V.: 15 minutes

Pharmacokinetics

Absorption: Oral: ~95%

Distribution: V_d:

Children: 0.8 L/kg

Adults: 1 L/kg

Protein binding: 35% to 55%

Metabolism: Extensive in the liver via hydroxylation and oxidation pathways

Half-life, terminal:

Children: 25 hours

Normal adults: 22 hours; range: 35-50 hours

Elimination: <1% excreted unchanged renally

Usual Dosage

Children:

Sedative: Oral: 2-6 mg/kg/day divided in 3 doses; maximum dose: 100 mg/day

Hypnotic: I.M.: 2-6 mg/kg; maximum dose: 100 mg/dose

Rectal:

2 months to 1 year (10-20 lb): 30 mg

1-4 years (20-40 lb): 30-60 mg

5-12 years (40-80 lb): 60 mg

12-14 years (80-110 lb): 60-120 mg **or**

<4 years: 3-6 mg/kg/dose

>4 years: 1.5-3 mg/kg/dose

Preoperative/preprocedure sedation: ≥6 months:

Oral, I.M., rectal: 2-6 mg/kg; maximum dose: 100 mg/dose

I.V.: 1-3 mg/kg to a maximum of 100 mg until asleep

Conscious sedation prior to a procedure: Children >18 months: I.V.: Initial: 2 mg/kg, additional doses of 1-2 mg/kg may be given every 5-10 minutes until adequate sedation is achieved; maximum total dose: 6 mg/kg or 150-200 mg; mean total dose required (for CT scan sedation): 3.3-4.5 mg/kg

Adolescents: Conscious sedation: Oral, I.V.: 100 mg prior to a procedure

Children and Adults: Pentobarbital coma: I.V.:

Loading dose: 10-15 mg/kg given slowly over 1-2 hours; monitor blood pressure and respiratory rate

Maintenance infusion: Initial: 1 mg/kg/hour; may increase to 2-3 mg/kg/hour; maintain burst suppression on EEG

Adults·

Hypnotic:

Oral: 100-200 mg at bedtime

I.M.: 150-200 mg

I.V.: Initial: 100 mg, may repeat every 1-3 minutes up to 200-500 mg total

Rectal: 120-200 mg at bedtime

Preoperative sedation: I.M.: 150-200 mg

Administration

Oral: May administer with food to decrease GI upset

Parenteral: I.V.: Do not inject >50 mg/minute; rapid I.V. injection may cause respiratory depression, apnea, laryngospasm, bronchospasm, and hypotension; administer over 10-30 minutes; maximum concentration: 50 mg/mL for slow I.V. push

Monitoring Parameters Vital signs, respiratory status (includes pulse oximetry for conscious sedation), cardiovascular status, CNS status; monitor ICP and cerebral perfusion pressure (MAP - ICP) when using pentobarbital coma to reduce ICP

Reference Range Therapeutic:

Sedation: 1-5 µg/mL (SI: 4-22 µmol/L)

Sleep: 5-15 µg/mL (SI: 22-66 µmol/L)

Coma: 20-40 µg/mL (SI: 88-177 µmol/L)

(Continued)

Pentobarbital *(Continued)*

Patient Information Avoid alcohol; limit caffeine; may be habit-forming; do not abruptly discontinue; may cause drowsiness and impair ability to perform activities requiring mental alertness or physical coordination

Nursing Implications Suppositories should not be divided; parenteral solutions are very alkaline; avoid extravasation; avoid intra-arterial injection

Additional Information Tolerance to hypnotic effect can occur; do not use for >2 weeks to treat insomnia; taper dose to prevent withdrawal; **Note:** Loading doses of 15-35 mg/kg (given over 1-2 hours) have been utilized in pediatric patients for pentobarbital coma but these higher loading doses often cause hypotension requiring vasopressor therapy

I.V. continuous infusions of pentobarbital using initial bolus doses of 1-2 mg/kg followed by initial continuous infusions of 1-2 mg/kg/hour have been used for PICU sedation in six intubated, mechanically ventilated infants (age: 2-17 months) who "failed" sedation with fentanyl and midazolam infusions; doses were titrated to effect and supplemental boluses were administered as needed; further studies are needed (see Tobias, 1995)

Dosage Forms
Capsule, as sodium: 50 mg, 100 mg
Elixir: 18.2 mg/5 mL (473 mL, 4000 mL)
Injection, as sodium: 50 mg/mL (1 mL, 2 mL, 20 mL, 50 mL)
Suppository, rectal, as sodium (C-III): 30 mg, 60 mg, 120 mg, 200 mg

References

Fischer JH and Raineri DL, "Pentobarbital Anesthesia for Status Epilepticus," *Clin Pharm*, 1987, 6(8):601-2.

Hubbard AM, Markowitz RI, Kimmel B, et al, "Sedation for Pediatric Patients Undergoing CT and MRI," *J Comput Assist Tomogr*, 1992, 16(1):3-6.

Pereira JK, Burrows PE, Richards HM, et al, "Comparison of Sedation Regimens for Pediatric Outpatient CT," *Pediatr Radiol*, 1993, 23(5):341-4.

Schaible DH, Cupit GC, Swedlow DB, et al, "High-Dose Pentobarbital Pharmacokinetics in Hypothermic Brain-Injured Children," *J Pediatr*, 1982, 100(4):655-60.

Tobias JD, Deshpande JK, Pietsch JB, et al, "Pentobarbital Sedation for Patients in the Pediatric Intensive Care Unit," *South Med J*, 1995, 88(3):290-4.

♦ **Pentobarbital Sodium** *see* Pentobarbital *on page 748*

♦ **Pentothal® Sodium** *see* Thiopental *on page 919*

Pentoxifylline *(pen toks I fi leen)*

Brand Names Trental®

Synonyms Oxpentifylline

Therapeutic Category Blood Viscosity Reducer Agent

Generic Available Yes

Use Symptomatic management of peripheral vascular disease, mainly intermittent claudication

Investigational use: AIDS patients with increased tumor necrosis factor, cerebrovascular accidents, cerebrovascular diseases, new onset type I diabetes mellitus, diabetic atherosclerosis, diabetic neuropathy, gangrene, cutaneous polyarteritis nodosa, hemodialysis shunt thrombosis, cerebral malaria, septic shock, sepsis in premature neonates, sickle cell syndromes, vasculitis, Kawasaki disease, Raynaud's syndrome, cystic fibrosis, and persistent pulmonary hypertension of the newborn (case report)

Pregnancy Risk Factor C

Contraindications Hypersensitivity to pentoxifylline, any component, or other xanthine derivatives (eg, caffeine, theophylline, theobromine); recent cerebral or retinal hemorrhage

Warnings Use with caution in patients with renal or hepatic impairment, insulin-treated diabetics, chronic occlusive arterial disease of the limbs, recent surgery, or peptic ulcerations

Adverse Reactions
Cardiovascular: Mild hypotension, angina
Central nervous system: Headache, dizziness, agitation
Gastrointestinal: Dyspepsia, nausea, vomiting
Ocular: Blurred vision

Drug Interactions Cimetidine may increase plasma concentrations of pentoxifylline; pentoxifylline may increase the effect of antihypertensive agents, warfarin, heparin

Food Interactions Food may decrease rate but not extent of absorption

Mechanism of Action Mechanism of action remains unclear; is thought to reduce blood viscosity and improve blood flow by altering the rheology of red blood cells;

inhibits production of tumor necrosis factor-alpha; inhibits neutrophil activation and adhesion; increases tissue oxygen levels in patients with peripheral arterial disease; inhibits platelet aggregation

Pharmacodynamics Onset of action: 2-4 weeks with multiple doses

Pharmacokinetics
Absorption: Oral: Well absorbed
Metabolism: Undergoes first-pass in the liver, dose-related (nonlinear) pharmacokinetics
Half-life, apparent:
Parent drug: 24-48 minutes
Metabolites: 60-96 minutes
Time to peak serum concentration: Within 2-4 hours
Elimination: Metabolites excreted in urine; 0% eliminated unchanged in the urine

Usual Dosage Oral:
Children: Minimal information available; one investigation (Furukawa, 1994) found a lower incidence of coronary artery lesions in 22 children (mean age 2 years) treated for acute Kawasaki disease with versus without pentoxifylline 20 mg/kg/day (given in 3 divided doses); all patients received aspirin and I.V. gamma globulin therapy; a lower dose (10 mg/kg/day) was not effective; higher doses have been used investigationally for the treatment of cystic fibrosis (Aronoff 1994)
Adults: 400 mg 3 times/day with meals; decrease to 400 mg twice daily if CNS or GI side effects occur

Administration Oral: Administer with food or antacids to decrease GI upset; swallow extended release tablet whole, do not crush, break, or chew

Test Interactions False increase in theophylline levels

Patient Information Limit caffeine; if GI or CNS side effects continue, contact physician; while beneficial effects may be seen in 2-4 weeks, continue treatment for at least 8 weeks

Dosage Forms Tablet, extended release: 400 mg

References
Aronoff SC, Quinn FJ, Carpenter LS, et al, "Effects of Pentoxifylline on Sputum Neutrophil Elastase and Pulmonary Function in Patients With Cystic Fibrosis: Preliminary Observations," *J Pediatr*, 1994, 125(6 Pt 1):992-7.
Berman W Jr, Berman N, Pathak D, et al, "Effects of Pentoxifylline (Trental®) on Blood Flow, Viscosity, and Oxygen Transport in Young Adults With Inoperable Cyanotic Congenital Heart Disease," *Pediatr Cardiol*, 1994, 15(2):66-70.
Furukawa S, Matsubara T, Umezawa Y, et al, "Pentoxifylline and Intravenous Gamma Globulin Combination Therapy for Acute Kawasaki Disease," *Eur J Pediatr*, 1994, 153(9):663-7.
Lauterbach R, "Pentoxifylline Treatment of Persistent Pulmonary Hypertension of Newborn," *Eur J Pediatr*, 1993, 152(5):460. (I.V. use)
Lauterbach R, Pawlik D, Tomaszczyk B, et al, "Pentoxifylline Treatment of Sepsis of Premature Infants; Preliminary Clinical Observations," *Eur J Pediatr*, 1994, 153(9):672-4. (I.V. use)
MacDonald MJ, Shahidi NT, Allen DB, et al, "Pentoxifylline in the Treatment of Children With New-Onset Type I Diabetes Mellitus," *JAMA*, 1994, 271(1):27-8.

◆ **Periochip®** *see* Chlorhexidine Gluconate *on page 209*
◆ **PerioGard®** *see* Chlorhexidine Gluconate *on page 209*
◆ **Permapen®** *see* Penicillin G Benzathine *on page 739*

Permethrin (per METH rin)

Brand Names Elimite™ Cream; Nix™ Creme Rinse

Therapeutic Category Antiparasitic Agent, Topical; Pediculocide; Scabicidal Agent

Generic Available No

Use Single application treatment of infestation with *Pediculus humanus capitis* (head louse) and its nits; treatment of *Sarcoptes scabiei* (scabies)

Pregnancy Risk Factor B

Contraindications Hypersensitivity to pyrethroid, pyrethrin, any component, or to chrysanthemums

Precautions For external use only; do not use near the eyes or on mucous membranes such as inside the nose, mouth, or vagina

Adverse Reactions

Dermatologic: Pruritus, erythema, rash of the scalp

Local: Burning, stinging, pain, edema, tingling, numbness, scalp discomfort

Mechanism of Action Inhibits sodium ion influx through nerve cell membrane channels in parasites resulting in delayed repolarization, paralysis, and death of organism

Pharmacokinetics

Absorption: Topical: Minimal (<2%)

Metabolism: By ester hydrolysis to inactive metabolites

Usual Dosage Topical: Children >2 months and Adults:

Head lice: After hair has been washed with shampoo, rinsed with water and towel dried, apply a sufficient volume of creme rinse to saturate the hair and scalp; also apply behind the ears and at the base of the neck; leave on hair for 10 minutes before rinsing off with water; remove remaining nits. May repeat in 1 week if lice or nits still present; in areas of head lice resistance to 1% permethrin, 5% permethrin has been applied to clean, dry hair and left on overnight (8-14 hours) under a shower cap.

Scabies: Apply cream from head to toe; leave on for 8-14 hours before washing off with water; for infants, also apply on the hairline, neck, scalp, temple, and forehead; may reapply in 1 week if live mites appear. Permethrin 5% cream was shown to be safe and effective when applied to an infant <1 month of age with neonatal scabies; time of application was limited to 6 hours before rinsing with soap and water.

Administration Topical: Avoid contact with eyes during application; shake creme rinse well before using

Patient Information Clothing and bedding should be washed in hot water or by dry cleaning to kill the scabies mite

Nursing Implications

To remove nits: Comb hair with a fine-toothed nit comb and apply a damp towel to the scalp for 30-60 minutes

For infestation of eyelashes: Apply petroleum ointment to eyelashes 3-4 times/day for 8-10 days; remove nits mechanically from the eyelashes

For scabies: Itching may continue for several weeks despite successful treatment; oral antihistamines and/or topical corticosteroids may be helpful in relieving symptoms

Additional Information Topical cream formulation contains formaldehyde which is a contact allergen

Dosage Forms

Cream: 5% (60 g)

Creme rinse: 1% (60 mL with comb)

References

"Drugs for Head Lice," *Med Lett Drugs Ther*, 1997, 39(992):6-7.

Hogan DJ, Schachner L, Tanglertsampan C, "Diagnosis and Treatment of Childhood Scabies and Pediculosis," *Pediatr Clin North Am*, 1991, 38(4):941-57.

Krowchuk DP, Tunnessen WW Jr, and Hurwitz S, "Pediatric Dermatology Update," *Pediatrics*, 1992, 90(2 Pt 1):259-64.

Quarterman MJ and Lesher JL, "Neonatal Scabies Treated With Permethrin 5% Cream," *Pediatr Dermatol*, 1994, 11(3):264-6.

◆ **Pernox®** [OTC] *see* Sulfur and Salicylic Acid *on page 896*
◆ **Peroxide** *see* Hydrogen Peroxide *on page 490*
◆ **Peroxin A5®** *see* Benzoyl Peroxide *on page 126*
◆ **Peroxin A10®** *see* Benzoyl Peroxide *on page 126*

- **Peroxyl**® *see* Hydrogen Peroxide *on page 490*
- **Persa-Gel**® *see* Benzoyl Peroxide *on page 126*
- **Persantine**® *see* Dipyridamole *on page 331*
- **Pertussin**® **CS [OTC]** *see* Dextromethorphan *on page 304*
- **Pertussin**® **ES [OTC]** *see* Dextromethorphan *on page 304*
- **Pethidine** *see* Meperidine *on page 602*
- **PFA** *see* Foscarnet *on page 441*
- **Pfizerpen**® *see* Penicillin G, Parenteral, Aqueous *on page 741*
- **Pfizerpen**®**-AS** *see* Penicillin G Procaine *on page 742*
- **PGE₁** *see* Alprostadil *on page 51*
- **Phanatuss**® **[OTC]** *see* Guaifenesin and Dextromethorphan *on page 466*
- **Pharmaflur**® *see* Fluoride *on page 427*
- **Phazyme**® **[OTC]** *see* Simethicone *on page 868*
- **Phenadex**® **Senior [OTC]** *see* Guaifenesin and Dextromethorphan *on page 466*
- **Phenantoin** *see* Mephenytoin *on page 604*
- **Phenaphen**® **With Codeine** *see* Acetaminophen and Codeine *on page 27*
- **Phenazine**® **Injection** *see* Promethazine *on page 805*
- **Phenazo (Canada)** *see* Phenazopyridine *on page 753*

Phenazopyridine (fen az oh PEER i deen)

Brand Names Azo-Standard®; Baridium®; Geridium®; Phenazo (Canada); Prodium® [OTC]; Pyridiate®; Pyridium®; Pyronium® (Canada); Urodine®; Urogesic®; Vito Reins® (Canada)

Available Salts Phenazopyridine Hydrochloride

Synonyms Phenylazo Diamino Pyridine

Therapeutic Category Analgesic, Urinary; Local Anesthetic, Urinary

Generic Available Yes

Use Symptomatic relief of urinary burning, itching, frequency and urgency in association with urinary tract infection, or following urologic procedures

Pregnancy Risk Factor B

Contraindications Hypersensitivity to phenazopyridine or any component; liver or kidney disease (do not use in patients with Cl_cr <50 mL/minute)

Warnings Does not treat infection, acts only as an analgesic; drug should be discontinued if skin or sclera develop a yellow color

Precautions Use with caution in patients with renal impairment

Adverse Reactions
  Central nervous system: Vertigo, headache
  Dermatologic: Skin pigmentation, rash, pruritus
  Gastrointestinal: Stomach cramps
  Genitourinary: Discoloration of urine (orange or red)
  Hematologic: Methemoglobinemia, hemolytic anemia
  Hepatic: Hepatitis
  Renal: Transient acute renal failure

Mechanism of Action Exerts local topical anesthetic or analgesic action on urinary tract mucosa through an unknown mechanism

Pharmacokinetics
  Metabolism: In the liver and other tissues
  Elimination: In urine (where it exerts its action); renal excretion (as unchanged drug) is rapid and accounts for 65% of the drug's elimination

Usual Dosage Oral:
  Children: 12 mg/kg/day in 3 divided doses for 2 days if used concomitantly with an antibacterial agent for UTI
  Adults: 100-200 mg 3-4 times/day for 2 days if used concomitantly with an antibacterial agent for UTI
  Dosing interval in renal impairment:
    Cl_cr 50-80 mL/minute: Administer every 8-16 hours
    Cl_cr <50 mL/minute: Avoid use

Administration Oral: Administer with food to decrease GI distress

Test Interactions False-negative Clinistix®, Tes-Tape®, Ictotest®, Acetest®, Ketostix®, urinalysis based upon spectrometry or color reactions

Patient Information May discolor urine orange or red; may stain contact lenses and fabric

Dosage Forms Tablet, as hydrochloride:
  Azo-Standard®, Prodium® [OTC]: 95 mg
  Baridium®, Geridium®, Pyridiate®, Pyridium®, Urodine®, Urogesic®: 100 mg
  Geridium®, Pyridium®, Urodine®: 200 mg
  (Continued)

Phenazopyridine *(Continued)*

Extemporaneous Preparations A 10 mg/mL suspension may be made by crushing three 200 mg tablets. Mix with a small amount of distilled water or glycerin. Add 20 mL Cologel® and levigate until a uniform mixture is obtained. Add sufficient 2:1 simple syrup/cherry syrup mixture to make a final volume of 60 mL. Store in an amber container. Label "shake well". Stability is 60 days refrigerated.
Handbook on Extemporaneous Formulations, Bethesda MD: American Society of Hospital Pharmacists, 1987.

Phenobarbital *(fee noe BAR bi tal)*

Related Information

Antiepileptic Drugs *on page 1176*
Blood Level Sampling Time Guidelines *on page 1189*
Carbohydrate and Alcohol Content of Liquid Medications for Use in Patients Receiving Ketogenic Diets *on page 1228*
Drugs and Breast-Feeding *on page 1213*
Laboratory Detection of Drugs in Urine *on page 1204*
Overdose and Toxicology *on page 1191*

Brand Names Barbilixir® (Canada); Barbita®; Luminal®; Solfoton®

Available Salts Phenobarbital Sodium

Synonyms Phenobarbitone; Phenylethylmalonylurea

Therapeutic Category Anticonvulsant, Barbiturate; Barbiturate; Hypnotic; Sedative

Generic Available Yes

Use Management of generalized tonic-clonic (grand mal) and partial seizures; neonatal seizures; febrile seizures in children; sedation; may also be used for prevention and treatment of neonatal hyperbilirubinemia and lowering of bilirubin in chronic cholestasis

Restrictions C-IV

Pregnancy Risk Factor D

Contraindications Hypersensitivity to phenobarbital or any component; pre-existing CNS depression, severe uncontrolled pain, porphyria, severe respiratory disease with dyspnea or obstruction

Warnings Abrupt withdrawal may precipitate status epilepticus

Precautions Use with caution in patients with renal or hepatic impairment

Adverse Reactions

Cardiovascular: Hypotension, circulatory collapse
Central nervous system: Drowsiness, paradoxical excitement, hyperkinetic activity, cognitive impairment, defects in general comprehension, short-term memory deficits, decreased attention span, ataxia
Dermatologic: Skin eruptions, skin rash, exfoliative dermatitis
Hematologic: Megaloblastic anemia
Hepatic: Hepatitis
Respiratory: Respiratory depression, apnea (especially with rapid I.V. use)
Miscellaneous: Psychological and physical dependence

Drug Interactions Cytochrome P-450 isoenzyme CYP1A2, CYP2B6, CYP2C8, CYP3A3/4, and CYP3A5-7 inducer

Phenobarbital may decrease the serum concentration or effect of lamotrigine, ritonavir, saquinavir, delavirdine, ethosuximide, warfarin, oral contraceptives, chloramphenicol, griseofulvin, doxycycline, beta-blockers, theophylline, corticosteroids, tricyclic antidepressants, cyclosporin, quinidine, haloperidol, and phenothiazines

Valproic acid, methylphenidate, chloramphenicol, felbamate, and propoxyphene may inhibit the metabolism of phenobarbital with resultant increase in phenobarbital serum concentration; ritonavir may affect the metabolism of phenobarbital;

phenobarbital and benzodiazepines or other CNS depressants may increase CNS and respiratory depression (especially with I.V. loading doses of phenobarbital)

Food Interactions High doses of pyridoxine may decrease drug effect; barbiturates may increase the metabolism of vitamins D and K; dietary requirements of vitamins D, K, C, B_{12}, folate, and calcium may be increased with long-term use

Stability Protect elixir from light; not stable in aqueous solutions; use only clear solutions; do not add to acidic solutions, precipitation may occur

Mechanism of Action Depresses CNS activity by binding to barbiturate site at GABA-receptor complex enhancing GABA activity; depresses reticular activating system; higher doses may be gabamimetic

Pharmacodynamics Hypnosis:
Onset of action:
Oral: Within 20-60 minutes
I.V.: Within 5 minutes
Peak effect: I.V.: Within 30 minutes
Duration:
Oral: 6-10 hours
I.V.: 4-10 hours

Pharmacokinetics
Absorption: Oral: 70% to 90%
Distribution: V_d:
Neonates: 0.8-1 L/kg
Infants: 0.7-0.8 L/kg
Children: 0.6-0.7 L/kg
Protein binding: 35% to 50%, decreased protein binding in neonates
Metabolism: In the liver via hydroxylation and glucuronide conjugation
Half-life:
Neonates: 45-200 hours
Infants: 20-133 hours
Children: 37-73 hours
Adults: 53-140 hours
Time to peak serum concentration: Oral: Within 1-6 hours
Elimination: 20% to 50% excreted unchanged in urine; clearance can be increased with alkalinization of urine or with oral multiple-dose activated charcoal
Moderately dialyzable (20% to 50%)

Usual Dosage
Anticonvulsant: Status epilepticus: **Loading dose:** I.V.:
Neonates: 15-20 mg/kg in a single or divided dose
Infants, Children, and Adults: 15-18 mg/kg in a single or divided dose; usual maximum loading dose: 20 mg/kg
Note: In select patients, may give additional 5 mg/kg/dose every 15-30 minutes until seizure is controlled or a total dose of 30 mg/kg is reached; be prepared to support respirations
Anticonvulsant **maintenance dose:** Oral, I.V. (**Note:** Maintenance dose usually starts 12 hours after loading dose):
Neonates: 3-4 mg/kg/day given once daily; assess serum concentrations; increase to 5 mg/kg/day if needed (usually by second week of therapy)
Infants: 5-6 mg/kg/day in 1-2 divided doses
Children:
1-5 years: 6-8 mg/kg/day in 1-2 divided doses
5-12 years: 4-6 mg/kg/day in 1-2 divided doses
>12 years and adults: 1-3 mg/kg/day in 1-2 divided doses
Children:
Sedation: Oral: 2 mg/kg 3 times/day
Hypnotic: I.M., I.V., S.C.: 3-5 mg/kg at bedtime
Hyperbilirubinemia: <12 years: Oral: 3-8 mg/kg/day in 2-3 divided doses; doses up to 12 mg/kg/day have been used
Preoperative sedation: Oral, I.M., I.V.: 1-3 mg/kg 1-1.5 hours before procedure
Adults:
Sedation: Oral, I.M.: 30-120 mg/day in 2-3 divided doses
Hypnotic: Oral, I.M., I.V., S.C.: 100-320 mg at bedtime
Hyperbilirubinemia: Oral: 90-180 mg/day in 2-3 divided doses
Preoperative sedation: I.M.: 100-200 mg 1-1.5 hours before procedure

Administration
Oral: Administer elixir with water, milk, or juice
Parenteral: Do not inject I.V. faster than 1 mg/kg/minute with a maximum of 30 mg/minute for infants and children and 60 mg/minute for adults >60kg; do not
(Continued)

Phenobarbital *(Continued)*

administer intra-arterially; avoid extravasation; use only powder for injection for S.C. use, not solutions for injection

Monitoring Parameters CNS status, seizure activity, liver enzymes, CBC with differential, renal function, serum concentrations; I.V. use: Respiratory rate, heart rate, blood pressure; hyperbilirubinemia: bilirubin (total and direct)

Reference Range
Therapeutic: 15-40 µg/mL (SI: 65-172 µmol/L)
Potentially toxic: >40 µg/mL (SI: >172 µmol/L)
Coma: >50 µg/mL (SI: >215 µmol/L)
Potentially lethal: >80 µg/mL (SI: >344 µmol/L)

Patient Information Avoid alcohol; limit caffeine; may be habit-forming; may cause dizziness or drowsiness and impair ability to perform activities requiring mental alertness or physical coordination; do not abruptly discontinue

Nursing Implications Parenteral solutions are very alkaline

Additional Information Injectable solutions contain propylene glycol

Dosage Forms
Capsule: 16 mg
Elixir: 15 mg/5 mL (5 mL, 10 mL, 20 mL); **20 mg/5 mL** (3.75 mL, 5 mL, 7.5 mL, 120 mL, 473 mL, 946 mL, 4000 mL)
Injection, as sodium: 30 mg/mL (1 mL); 60 mg/mL (1 mL); 65 mg/mL (1 mL); 130 mg/mL (1 mL)
Powder for injection: 120 mg
Tablet: 8 mg, 15 mg, 16 mg, 30 mg, 32 mg, 60 mg, 65 mg, 100 mg

◆ **Phenobarbital, Hyoscyamine, Atropine, and Scopolamine** *see* Hyoscyamine, Atropine, Scopolamine, and Phenobarbital *on page 499*

◆ **Phenobarbital Sodium** *see* Phenobarbital *on page 754*

◆ **Phenobarbitone** *see* Phenobarbital *on page 754*

Phenoxybenzamine (fen oks ee BEN za meen)

Related Information
Overdose and Toxicology *on page 1191*

Brand Names Dibenzyline®

Available Salts Phenoxybenzamine Hydrochloride

Therapeutic Category Alpha-Adrenergic Blocking Agent, Oral; Antihypertensive Agent; Vasodilator

Generic Available No

Use Symptomatic management of hypertension and sweating in patients with pheochromocytoma

Pregnancy Risk Factor C

Contraindications Shock

Precautions Use with caution in patients with renal dysfunction, cerebral or coronary arteriosclerosis

Adverse Reactions
Cardiovascular: Postural hypotension, tachycardia, syncope, shock
Central nervous system: Lethargy, headache, dizziness
Gastrointestinal: Vomiting, nausea, diarrhea
Neuromuscular & skeletal: Weakness
Ocular: Miosis
Respiratory: Nasal congestion

Drug Interactions Antagonizes effects of alpha-adrenergic stimulating sympathomimetic agents

Mechanism of Action Produces long-lasting noncompetitive alpha-adrenergic blockade of postganglionic synapses in exocrine glands and smooth muscle

Pharmacodynamics Oral:
Onset of action: Within 2 hours
Peak effect: Within 4-6 hours
Duration: Effects can continue for up to 4 days

Pharmacokinetics
Absorption: Oral: ~20% to 30%
Distribution: Distributes to and may accumulate in adipose tissues
Half-life: Adults: 24 hours
Elimination: Primarily in urine and bile

Usual Dosage Oral:
Children: Initial: 0.2 mg/kg once daily; maximum dose: 10 mg/dose; increase every 4 days by 0.2 mg/kg/day increments; usual maintenance dose: 0.4-1.2 mg/kg/

day every 6-8 hours; maximum doses of up to 2-4 mg/kg/day have been recommended

Adults: Initial: 10 mg twice daily; increase dose every other day to usual dose of 10-40 mg every 8-12 hours; higher doses may be needed

Administration Oral: May administer with milk to decrease GI upset

Monitoring Parameters Blood pressure, orthostasis, heart rate

Patient Information Avoid alcohol; may cause dizziness; avoid sudden changes in posture; may cause nasal congestion and constricted pupils; avoid cough, cold, or allergy medications containing sympathomimetics

Dosage Forms Capsule, as hydrochloride: 10 mg

Extemporaneous Preparations

A 2 mg/mL oral liquid preparation made from capsules and with 1% propylene glycol and 0.15% citric acid in distilled water was stable for 7 days when stored in amber glass prescription bottles under refrigeration (4°C). The vehicle is made by dissolving 150 mg of citric acid in a minimal amount of distilled water; then 1 mL of propylene glycol is added and the solution is mixed well; qsad to 100 mL with distilled water. Grind the contents of two 10 mg capsules in a mortar into a fine powder; add a small amount of the vehicle and mix well; transfer to a graduated cylinder and qsad with vehicle to 10 mL; transfer to an amber glass prescription bottle with tight-fitting cap; label "shake well" and "refrigerate" (Lim, 1997).

A stock solution of 10 mg/mL in propylene glycol was stable for 30 days when stored under refrigeration (4°C); when this stock solution was diluted 1:4 (v/v) with syrup (66.7% sucrose) to 2 mg/mL, the preparation was stable for 1 hour at 4°C (see Lim, 1997). **Note:** Although the stock solution is stable for 30 days, it **must be diluted** before administration to decrease the amount of propylene glycol delivered to the patient.

Lim LY, Tan LL, Chan EW, et al "Stability of Phenoxybenzamine Hydrochloride in Various Vehicles," *Am J Health Syst Pharm*, 1997, 54(18):2073-8.

♦ **Phenoxybenzamine Hydrochloride** *see* Phenoxybenzamine *on page 756*

♦ **Phenoxymethyl Penicillin** *see* Penicillin V Potassium *on page 743*

Phentolamine (fen TOLE a meen)

Related Information

Extravasation Treatment *on page 1050*

Overdose and Toxicology *on page 1191*

Brand Names Regitine®; Rogitine® (Canada)

Available Salts Phentolamine Mesylate

Therapeutic Category Alpha-Adrenergic Blocking Agent, Parenteral; Antidote, Extravasation; Antihypertensive Agent; Diagnostic Agent, Pheochromocytoma; Vasodilator

Generic Available Yes

Use Diagnosis of pheochromocytoma; treatment of hypertension associated with pheochromocytoma or other causes of excess sympathomimetic amines; local treatment of dermal necrosis after extravasation of drugs with alpha-adrenergic effects (dobutamine, dopamine, epinephrine, metaraminol, norepinephrine, phenylephrine)

Pregnancy Risk Factor C

Contraindications Hypersensitivity to phentolamine or any component; renal impairment; coronary or cerebral arteriosclerosis; MI

Precautions Use with caution in patients with gastritis, peptic ulcer; history of cardiac arrhythmias; MI, cerebrovascular spasm, and cerebrovascular occlusion may occur

Adverse Reactions

Cardiovascular: Hypotension, tachycardia, angina, arrhythmias

Central nervous system: Dizziness, headache

Gastrointestinal: Nausea, vomiting, diarrhea, exacerbation of peptic ulcer

Neuromuscular & skeletal: Weakness

Respiratory: Nasal congestion

Stability Reconstituted solution is stable for 48 hours at room temperature and 1 week when refrigerated

Mechanism of Action Competitively blocks alpha-adrenergic receptors to produce brief antagonism of circulating epinephrine and norepinephrine; reduces hypertension caused by alpha effects of catecholamines; also has positive inotropic and chronotropic effects on the heart

(Continued)

Phentolamine *(Continued)*

Pharmacodynamics
Onset of action:
I.M.: Within 15-20 minutes
I.V.: Immediate
Peak effect:
I.M.: Within 20 minutes
I.V.: Within 2 minutes
Duration:
I.M.: 30-45 minutes
I.V.: Within 15-30 minutes

Pharmacokinetics
Metabolism: In the liver
Half-life: Adults: 19 minutes
Elimination: 10% to 13% excreted in urine as unchanged drug

Usual Dosage
Treatment of alpha-adrenergic drug extravasation: S.C.:
Neonates: Infiltrate area with a small amount (eg, 1 mL) of solution (made by diluting 2.5-5 mg in 10 mL of preservative free NS) within 12 hours of extravasation; do not exceed 0.1 mg/kg or 2.5 mg total
Infants, Children, and Adults: Infiltrate area with a small amount (eg, 1 mL) of solution (made by diluting 5-10 mg in 10 mL of NS) within 12 hours of extravasation; do not exceed 0.1-0.2 mg/kg or 5 mg total
Diagnosis of pheochromocytoma: I.M., I.V.:
Children: 0.05-0.1 mg/kg/dose, maximum single dose: 5 mg
Adults: 5 mg
Hypertension (prior to surgery for pheochromocytoma): I.M., I.V.:
Children: 0.05-0.1 mg/kg/dose given 1-2 hours before pheochromocytomectomy; repeat as needed to control blood pressure; maximum single dose: 5 mg
Adults: 5 mg given 1-2 hours before pheochromocytomectomy; repeat as needed to control blood pressure
Hypertensive crisis due to MAO inhibitor/sympathomimetic amine interaction: I.M., I.V.: Adults: 5-20 mg

Administration Parenteral: Treatment of extravasation: Infiltrate area of extravasation with multiple small injections of a diluted solution (see Usual Dosage); use 27- or 30-gauge needles and change needle between each skin entry; do not inject a volume such that swelling of the extremity or digit with resultant compartment syndrome occurs

Monitoring Parameters Blood pressure, heart rate, orthostasis; treatment of extravasation: site of extravasation, skin color, local perfusion

Nursing Implications When drugs with alpha-adrenergic effects extravasate, they cause local vasoconstriction which causes blanching of the skin and a pale, cold, hard appearance; S.C. phentolamine blocks the alpha-adrenergic receptors and reverses the vasoconstriction; the extravasation area should "pink up" and return to normal skin color; monitor the site of extravasation closely, as repeat doses of S.C. phentolamine may be needed

Additional Information Injection contains mannitol 25 mg/vial

Dosage Forms Injection, as mesylate: 5 mg/mL (1 mL)

♦ **Phentolamine Mesylate** *see* Phentolamine *on page 757*
♦ **Phenylalanine Mustard** *see* Melphalan *on page 600*
♦ **Phenylazo Diamino Pyridine** *see* Phenazopyridine *on page 753*
♦ **4-Phenylbutyric Acid Sodium** *see* Sodium Phenylbutyrate *on page 873*

Phenylephrine *(fen il EF rin)*

Related Information
Extravasation Treatment *on page 1050*
OTC Cough & Cold Preparations, Pediatric *on page 1037*
Promethazine and Phenylephrine *on page 808*

Brand Names Afrin® Allergy Nasal Spray; Afrin® Nasal Decongestant Children's Pump Mist; AK-Dilate® Ophthalmic Solution; AK-Nefrin® Ophthalmic Solution; Alconefrin® Nasal Solution [OTC]; Dionephrine (Canada); Doktors® Nasal Solution [OTC]; I-Phrine® Ophthalmic Solution; Isopto® Frin Ophthalmic Solution; Mydfrin® Ophthalmic Solution; Neo-Synephrine® Nasal Solution [OTC]; Neo-Synephrine® Ophthalmic Solution; Nostril® Nasal Solution [OTC]; Novahistine® (Canada); Prefrin® Liquifilm® (Canada); Prefrin™ Ophthalmic Solution; Relief® Ophthalmic Solution; Rhinall® Nasal Solution [OTC]; Sinarest® Nasal Solution [OTC]; St.

PHENYLEPHRINE

Joseph® Measured Dose Nasal Solution [OTC]; Vicks® Sinex® Nasal Solution [OTC]

Available Salts Phenylephrine Hydrochloride

Therapeutic Category Adrenergic Agonist Agent; Adrenergic Agonist Agent, Ophthalmic; Alpha-Adrenergic Agonist; Nasal Agent, Vasoconstrictor; Ophthalmic Agent, Mydriatic; Sympathomimetic

Generic Available Yes

Use Treatment of hypotension and vascular failure in shock; supraventricular tachycardia; as a vasoconstrictor in regional analgesia; symptomatic relief of nasal and nasopharyngeal mucosal congestion; as a mydriatic in ophthalmic procedures and treatment of wide-angle glaucoma

Pregnancy Risk Factor C

Contraindications Pheochromocytoma, severe hypertension, ventricular tachycardia; hypersensitivity to phenylephrine or any component; acute pancreatitis, hepatitis; peripheral or mesenteric vascular thrombosis, myocardial disease, severe coronary disease, narrow-angle glaucoma (ophthalmic preparation)

Warnings Injection may contain sulfites which may cause allergic reactions in some patients; do not use if solution turns brown or contains a precipitate

Precautions Pressor therapy is **not** a substitute for replacement of blood, plasma, and body fluids in shock; use with caution in patients with hyperthyroidism, bradycardia, partial heart block, myocardial disease, or severe arteriosclerosis; infuse into large veins to prevent extravasation which may cause severe necrosis

Adverse Reactions

Cardiovascular: Hypertension, angina, reflex severe bradycardia, arrhythmias, peripheral vasoconstriction

Central nervous system: Restlessness, excitability, headache, anxiety, nervousness, dizziness

Dermatologic: Pilomotor response, skin blanching

Local: Necrosis if extravasation occurs

Neuromuscular & skeletal: Tremor

Ocular: (Ophthalmic preparation): Transient stinging, browache, blurred vision, photophobia, lacrimation

Respiratory: Respiratory distress, rebound nasal congestion, sneezing, burning, stinging, dryness

Drug Interactions With alpha- and beta-adrenergic blocking agents, may see decreased actions; with oxytocic drugs, may see increased actions; with sympathomimetics and halogenated hydrocarbon anesthetics, tachycardia or arrhythmias may occur; with MAO inhibitors, guanethidine, and bretylium, actions may be potentiated

Stability Compatible when admixed with dextrose, dextrose-saline, Ringer's, LR, NS, and 1/6 M sodium lactate injection

Mechanism of Action Potent, direct-acting alpha-adrenergic stimulator with weak beta-adrenergic activity; causes vasoconstriction of the arterioles of the nasal mucosa and conjunctiva; activates the dilator muscle of the pupil to cause contraction; produces systemic arterial vasoconstriction

Pharmacodynamics

Onset of action:

I.M.: Within 10-15 minutes

I.V.: Following parenteral injection, effects occur immediately

S.C.: 10-15 minutes

Duration:

I.M.: 30 minutes to 2 hours

I.V.: 15-20 minutes

S.C.: 1 hour

Pharmacokinetics

Metabolism: In the liver and intestine by the enzyme monoamine oxidase

Half-life: 2.5 hours

Elimination: Metabolites, routes, and rates of excretion have not been identified

Usual Dosage

Ophthalmic procedures:

Infants <1 year: Instill 1 drop of 2.5% 15-30 minutes before procedures

Children and Adults: Instill 1 drop of 2.5% or 10% solution, may repeat in 10-60 minutes as needed

Nasal decongestant (therapy should not exceed 3-5 days):

Infants >6 months: 1-2 drops of 0.16% every 3 hours

Children:

1-6 years: 2-3 drops every 4 hours of 0.125% solution as needed

6-12 years: 2-3 drops every 4 hours of 0.25% solution as needed

(Continued)

759

Phenylephrine *(Continued)*

Children >12 years and Adults: 2-3 drops or 1-2 sprays every 4 hours of 0.25% to 0.5% solution as needed; 1% solution may be used in adults in cases of extreme nasal congestion

Hypotension/shock:

Children:

I.M., S.C.: 0.1 mg/kg/dose every 1-2 hours as needed (maximum dose: 5 mg)

I.V. bolus: 5-20 mcg/kg/dose every 10-15 minutes as needed

I.V. infusion: 0.1-0.5 mcg/kg/minute, titrate to desired effect

Adults:

I.M., S.C.: 2-5 mg/dose every 1-2 hours as needed (initial dose should not exceed 5 mg)

I.V. bolus: 0.1-0.5 mg/dose every 10-15 minutes as needed (initial dose should not exceed 0.5 mg)

I.V. infusion: 100-180 mcg/minute, titrate to desired effect; once stabilized, a maintenance rate of 40-60 mcg/minute is usually effective

Paroxysmal supraventricular tachycardia: I.V.:

Children: 5-10 mcg/kg over 20-30 seconds

Adults: 0.25-0.5 mg over 20-30 seconds

Administration

Intranasal: Spray or apply drops into each nostril while gently occluding the other

Ophthalmic: Instill drops into conjunctival sac of affected eye(s); avoid contact of bottle tip with skin or eye; finger pressure should be applied to the lacrimal sac during and for 1-2 minutes after instillation to decrease risk of absorption and systemic reactions

Parenteral: For direct I.V. administration, dilute to 1 mg/mL by adding 1 mL to 9 mL of sterile water, then administer dose over 20-30 seconds; continuous infusion concentrations are usually 20-60 mcg/mL by adding 5 mg to 250 mL I.V. solution (20 mcg/mL) or 15 mg to 250 mL (60 mcg/mL); rate of infusion (mL/hour) = dose (mcg/kg/minute) x weight (kg) x 60 minutes/hour divided by concentration (mcg/mL); administer into a large vein to prevent the possibility of extravasation; use infusion device to control rate of flow; administration into an umbilical arterial catheter is **not** recommended

Monitoring Parameters Heart rate, blood pressure, central venous pressure, arterial blood gases

Nursing Implications Extravasant; avoid I.V. infiltration; extravasation may be treated with local infiltration of phentolamine 5-10 mg diluted in 10-15 mL saline solution

Dosage Forms

Injection, as hydrochloride (Neo-Synephrine®): 1% [10 mg/mL] (1 mL)

Nasal solution, as hydrochloride:

Drops:

Alconefrin® 25, Neo-Synephrine®, Children's Nostril®, Rhinall®: 0.25% (15 mL, 30 mL, 40 mL)

Alconefrin®, Neo-Synephrine®: 0.5% (15 mL, 30 mL)

Spray:

Afrin® Nasal Decongestant Children's Pump Mist, Alconefrin® 25, Neo-Synephrine®, Rhinall®: 0.25% (15 mL, 30 mL, 40 mL)

Afrin® Allergy Nasal Spray, Neo-Synephrine®, Nostril®, Sinex®: 0.5% (15 mL, 30 mL)

Neo-Synephrine®: 1% (15 mL)

Ophthalmic solution, as hydrochloride:

AK-Nefrin®, Isopto® Frin, Prefrin™ Liquifilm®, Relief®: 0.12% (0.3 mL, 15 mL, 20 mL)

AK-Dilate®, Mydfrin®, Neo-Synephrine®, Phenoptic®: 2.5% (2 mL, 3 mL, 5 mL, 15 mL)

AK-Dilate®, Neo-Synephrine®, Neo-Synephrine® Viscous: 10% (1 mL, 2 mL, 5 mL, 15 mL)

♦ **Phenylephrine and Cyclopentolate** *see* Cyclopentolate and Phenylephrine *on page 267*

♦ **Phenylephrine and Promethazine** *see* Promethazine and Phenylephrine *on page 808*

♦ **Phenylephrine, Guaifenesin, and Phenylpropanolamine** *see* Guaifenesin, Phenylpropanolamine, and Phenylephrine *on page 467*

♦ **Phenylephrine Hydrochloride** *see* Phenylephrine *on page 758*

♦ **Phenylephrine, Promethazine, and Codeine** *see* Promethazine, Phenylephrine, and Codeine *on page 809*

♦ **Phenylethylmalonylurea** *see* Phenobarbital *on page 754*
♦ **Phenylisohydantoin** *see* Pemoline *on page 736*

Phenylpropanolamine (fen il proe pa NOLE a meen)

Brand Names Acutrim® Precision Release® [OTC]; BC® Cold Powder Non-Drowsy Formula (Cold-Sinus) [OTC]; Control® [OTC]; Dex-A-Diet® [OTC]; Dexatrim® [OTC]; Genex® [OTC]; Maigret-50; Prolamine® [OTC]; Propadrine; Propagest® [OTC]; Rhindecon® Rhinocaps® [OTC]; Stay Trim® Diet Gum [OTC]; St. Joseph® Aspirin-Free Cold Tablets for Children [OTC]; Westrim-I; Westrim® LA [OTC]

Available Salts Phenylpropanolamine Hydrochloride

Synonyms PPA

Therapeutic Category Adrenergic Agonist Agent; Anorexiant; Decongestant; Sympathomimetic

Use Nasal decongestant; anorexiant

Pregnancy Risk Factor C

Contraindications Hypersensitivity to phenylpropanolamine or any component

Warnings Do not use for more than 3 weeks for weight loss; prolonged use for nasal congestion may result in rebound nasal congestion; excessive dosing or chronic usage may result in hypertension

Precautions Use with caution in patients with hypertension, diabetes mellitus, hyperthyroidism, prostatic hypertrophy, glaucoma, cardiovascular disorders, pheochromocytoma, or arteriosclerosis

Adverse Reactions
Cardiovascular: Hypertension (dose-related), palpitations, tightness in chest, bradycardia, arrhythmias, angina
Central nervous system: Insomnia, restlessness, dizziness, severe headache, anxiety, nervousness
Gastrointestinal: Xerostomia, nausea
Genitourinary: Dysuria
Ocular: Mydriasis

Drug Interactions
Decreased effect of antihypertensives
Increased effect/toxicity with MAO inhibitors (hypertensive crisis), beta-blockers (increased pressor effects), other sympathomimetics, tricyclic antidepressants, ganglionic blocking agents, cyclopropane, or halogenated hydrocarbon general anesthetics (increased arrhythmias)

Mechanism of Action Releases tissue stores of norepinephrine producing alpha- and beta-adrenergic stimulation resulting in vasoconstriction of the nasal mucosa, increased heart rate, force of contraction, and cardiac output; it also appears to depress central appetite centers

Pharmacodynamics
Nasal decongestant: Onset of action: 15-30 minutes
Nasal decongestant: Duration of action: 3 hours (excluding timed release formulations)

Pharmacokinetics
Absorption: Well absorbed
V_d:
  Children: 2.5-2.8 L/kg
  Adults: 4.4 L/kg
Metabolism: In the liver to norephedrine
Bioavailability: Oral: 100%
Half-life:
  Children: 2.4-2.8 hours
  Adults: 4.6-6.6 hours
Elimination: in urine primarily as unchanged drug
  Clearance:
    Children: 13.3-13.6 mL/minute/kg
    Adults: 1.8-6.8 mL/minute/kg

Usual Dosage Oral:
Decongestant:
  Children 2-6 years: 6.25 mg every 4 hours; maximum daily dose 37.5 mg
  6-12 years: 10-12.5 mg every 4 hours; maximum daily dose 75 mg
  Children >12 years to Adults: 20-25 mg every 4 hours or 50 mg every 8 hours, or 75 mg (timed release) every 12 hours; maximum daily dose: 150 mg
Anorexic: Adults: 25 mg 3 times/day or 37.5 mg twice daily or 50-75 mg (timed release) once daily in the morning
(Continued)

Phenylpropanolamine *(Continued)*

Administration Oral: As anorectic: take 30 minutes before meals with 1-2 glassfuls of water; if timed release formula, take midmorning; swallow timed release formulation whole; do not crush or chew

Monitoring Parameters Blood pressure, heart rate, weight (if anorectic use)

Test Interactions False-positive test for amphetamines by EMIT assay

Patient Information Should not be used more than 3 consecutive weeks for weight loss; prolonged therapy for nasal congestion may result in rebound nasal congestion; contact physician for insomnia, tremor, or irregular heartbeat

Nursing Implications When used as an anorectic, administer dose early in day to prevent insomnia; observe for signs of nervousness, excitability

Dosage Forms

Capsule, as hydrochloride, timed release: 37.5 mg, 75 mg

Tablet, as hydrochloride: 25 mg, 50 mg

Tablet, timed release, as hydrochloride: 75 mg

Combinations: Capsule:

Genex®: 18 mg (with acetaminophen 325 mg)

Rhinocaps®: 20 mg (with acetaminophen 162 mg and aspirin 162 mg)

Solution, as hydrochloride (BC® Cold Powder Non-Drowsy Formula (Cold-Sinus)): 25 mg (with aspirin 650 mg) per packet

Tablet, chewable, as hydrochloride (St. Joseph® Aspirin-Free Cold Tablets for Children): 3.125 mg (with acetaminophen 80 mg)

♦ **Phenylpropanolamine and Brompheniramine** *see* Brompheniramine and Phenylpropanolamine *on page 143*

♦ **Phenylpropanolamine, Guaifenesin, and Phenylephrine** *see* Guaifenesin, Phenylpropanolamine, and Phenylephrine *on page 467*

♦ **Phenylpropanolamine Hydrochloride** *see* Phenylpropanolamine *on page 761*

Phenytoin *(FEN i toyn)*

Related Information

Antiepileptic Drugs *on page 1176*

Blood Level Sampling Time Guidelines *on page 1189*

Carbohydrate and Alcohol Content of Liquid Medications for Use in Patients Receiving Ketogenic Diets *on page 1228*

Fosphenytoin *on page 443*

Overdose and Toxicology *on page 1191*

Brand Names Dilantin®; Diphenylan Sodium®; Tremytoine® (Canada)

Available Salts Phenytoin Sodium

Synonyms Diphenylhydantoin; DPH

Therapeutic Category Antiarrhythmic Agent, Class I-B; Anticonvulsant, Hydantoin

Generic Available Yes

Use Management of generalized tonic-clonic (grand mal), simple partial and complex partial seizures; prevention of seizures following head trauma/neurosurgery; ventricular arrhythmias, including those associated with digitalis intoxication, prolonged Q-T interval and surgical repair of congenital heart diseases in children; epidermolysis bullosa

Pregnancy Risk Factor D

Contraindications Hypersensitivity to phenytoin or any component; heart block, sinus bradycardia

Precautions Use with caution in patients with porphyria; discontinue if rash or lymphadenopathy occurs; modify dosage in patients with hepatic or renal dysfunction

Adverse Reactions

Dose-related:

Central nervous system: Slurred speech, dizziness, drowsiness, lethargy, coma, ataxia, dyskinesias

Ocular: Nystagmus, blurred vision, diplopia

Cardiovascular: I.V.: Hypotension, bradycardia, arrhythmias, cardiovascular collapse (especially with rapid I.V. use)

Central nervous system: Fever, mood changes

Dermatologic: Hirsutism, coarsening of facial features, Stevens-Johnson syndrome, rash, exfoliative dermatitis

Endocrine & metabolic: Folic acid depletion, hyperglycemia

Gastrointestinal: Nausea, vomiting, gingival hyperplasia, gum tenderness

Hematologic: Blood dyscrasias, pseudolymphoma, lymphoma

Hepatic: Hepatitis

Local: Venous irritation and pain, thrombophlebitis

Neuromuscular & skeletal: Peripheral neuropathy, osteomalacia

Miscellaneous: Lymphadenopathy, SLE-like syndrome

Drug Interactions Cytochrome P-450 isoenzyme CYP2C9 and CYP2C19 substrate; CYP2Cs, CYP3A3/4, and CYP3A5-7 isoenzyme inducer

Phenytoin may decrease the serum concentration or effectiveness of lamotrigine, ritonavir, saquinavir, delavirdine, felbamate, valproic acid, ethosuximide, primidone, warfarin, oral contraceptives, corticosteroids, cyclosporin, theophylline, chloramphenicol, rifampin, doxycycline, quinidine, mexiletine, disopyramide, dopamine, or nondepolarizing skeletal muscle relaxants; protein binding of phenytoin can be affected by valproic acid or salicylates; serum phenytoin concentrations may be increased by cimetidine, chloramphenicol, felbamate, zidovudine, isoniazid, trimethoprim, or sulfonamides and decreased by rifampin, zidovudine, cisplatin, vinblastine, bleomycin, antacids (concurrent administration), folic acid, or continuous NG feeds; suspected interaction with nevirapine (monitor closely); ritonavir may affect the metabolism of phenytoin

Food Interactions Tube feedings decrease phenytoin bioavailability; to avoid decreased serum levels with continuous NG feeds, hold feedings for 2 hours prior to and 2 hours after phenytoin administration, if possible; phenytoin may increase the metabolism of vitamins D and K; dietary requirements of vitamins D, K, B$_{12}$, folate, and calcium may be increased with long-term use; high doses of folate may decrease bioavailability of phenytoin; avoid giving calcium or magnesium supplements at the same time as phenytoin, space administration by ≥ 2 hours

Stability Parenteral solution may be used as long as there is no precipitate and it is not hazy; slightly yellowed solution may be used; refrigeration may cause precipitate, sometimes the precipitate is resolved by allowing the solution to reach room temperature again; drug may precipitate with pH ≤ 11.5; do not mix with other medications; may dilute with NS for I.V. infusion, but must be diluted to a concentration <6 mg/mL

Mechanism of Action Stabilizes neuronal membranes and decreases seizure activity by increasing efflux or decreasing influx of sodium ions across cell membranes in the motor cortex during generation of nerve impulses; prolongs effective refractory period and suppresses ventricular pacemaker automaticity, shortens action potential in the heart

Pharmacokinetics

Absorption: Oral: Slow, variable; decreased in neonates

Distribution: V_d:

Neonates:

Premature: 1-1.2 L/kg

Full-term: 0.8-0.9 L/kg

Infants: 0.7-0.8 L/kg

Children: 0.7 L/kg

Adults: 0.6-0.7 L/kg

Protein binding: Adults: 90% to 95%; increased free fraction (decreased protein binding) in neonates (up to 20% free), infants (up to 15% free), and patients with hyperbilirubinemia, hypoalbuminemia, renal dysfunction, or uremia

Metabolism: Follows dose-dependent (Michaelis-Menten) pharmacokinetics; "apparent" or calculated half-life is dependent upon serum concentration, therefore, metabolism is best described in terms of K_m and V_{max}; V_{max} is increased in infants >6 months and children compared to adults; major metabolite (via oxidation) HPPA undergoes enterohepatic recycling and elimination in urine as glucuronides

Bioavailability: Formulation dependent

Time to peak serum concentration: Oral: Dependent upon formulation

Extended release capsule: Within 4-12 hours

Immediate release preparation: Within 2-3 hours

Elimination: <5% excreted unchanged in urine; increased clearance and decreased serum concentrations with febrile illness; highly variable clearance, dependent upon intrinsic hepatic function and dose administered

Usual Dosage

Status epilepticus: I.V.:

Loading dose:

Neonates: 15-20 mg/kg in a single or divided dose;

Infants, Children, and Adults: 15-18 mg/kg in a single or divided dose

Maintenance dose, anticonvulsant (**Note:** Maintenance dose usually starts 12 hours after the loading dose):

Neonates: Initial: 5 mg/kg/day in 2 divided doses; usual: 5-8 mg/kg/day in 2 divided doses; some patients may require dosing every 8 hours

(Continued)

Phenytoin *(Continued)*

Infants and Children: Initial: 5 mg/kg/day in 2-3 divided doses; usual doses:
0.5-3 years: 8-10 mg/kg/day
4-6 years: 7.5-9 mg/kg/day
7-9 years: 7-8 mg/kg/day
10-16 years: 6-7 mg/kg/day
Some patients require every 8 hours dosing due to fast apparent half-life
Adults: Usual: 300 mg/day or 4-6 mg/kg/day in 2-3 divided doses
Anticonvulsant: Infants, Children and Adults: Oral:
Loading dose: 15-20 mg/kg; based on phenytoin serum concentrations and recent dosing history; administer oral loading dose in 3 divided doses given every 2-4 hours to decrease GI adverse effects and to ensure complete oral absorption
Maintenance dose: Same as I.V. maintenance dose/day listed above. Divide daily dose into 3 doses/day when using suspension, chewable tablets or nonextended release preparations. Extended release preparations may be dosed in adults every 12 or 24 hours if patient is not receiving concomitant enzyme-inducing drugs and apparent half-life is sufficiently long.
Arrhythmias:
Children and Adults: Loading dose: I.V.: 1.25 mg/kg every 5 minutes, may repeat up to total loading dose: 15 mg/kg
Children: Maintenance dose: Oral, I.V.: 5-10 mg/kg/day in 2-3 divided doses
Adults: Loading dose: Oral: 250 mg 4 times/day for 1 day, 250 mg twice daily for 2 days, then maintenance at 300-400 mg/day in divided doses 1-4 times/day

Administration

Oral: May administer with food or milk to decrease GI upset; but to ensure consistent absorption, phenytoin should be administered at the same time with regards to meals; shake oral suspension well prior to each dose; separate administration of antacids or tube feedings and oral phenytoin by 2 hours
Parenteral: I.V.: Neonates: Do not exceed I.V. infusion rate of 0.5 mg/kg/minute; Infants, Children, Adults: Do not exceed I.V. infusion rate of 1-3 mg/kg/minute, maximum rate: 50 mg/minute; I.V. injections should be followed by NS flushes through the same needle or I.V. catheter to avoid local irritation of the vein; I.V. intermittent infusion: Dilute with NS to a concentration <6 mg/mL, use an in-line 0.22 micron filter; avoid extravasation; avoid I.M. use due to erratic absorption, pain on injection, and precipitation of drug at injection site

Monitoring Parameters Serum concentrations, CBC with differential, liver enzymes; blood pressure with I.V. use; free and total serum concentrations in patients with hyperbilirubinemia, hypoalbuminemia, renal dysfunction, or uremia

Reference Range

Neonates: Therapeutic: 8-15 µg/mL
Children and Adults:
Therapeutic: 10-20 µg/mL (SI: 40-79 µmol/L); toxicity is measured clinically, some patients require levels outside the suggested therapeutic range
Toxic: >20 µg/mL (SI: >79 µmol/L)
Lethal: >100 µg/mL (SI: >400 µmol/L)
Commonly accepted therapeutic free (unbound) concentration: 1-2 µg/mL

Patient Information Avoid alcohol; do not change brand or dosage without consulting physician; maintain good oral hygiene

Additional Information The 30 mg/5 mL oral suspension is no longer made; injection contains propylene glycol and benzyl alcohol; possible permanent cerebellum damage may occur with chronic toxic serum concentrations

Dosage Forms

Capsule, as sodium:
Extended: 30 mg, 100 mg
Prompt: 100 mg
Injection, as sodium: 50 mg/mL (2 mL, 5 mL)
Suspension, oral: 125 mg/5 mL (5 mL, 240 mL)
Tablet, chewable: 50 mg

References

Bauer LA and Blouin RA, "Phenytoin Michaelis-Menten Pharmacokinetics in Caucasian Pediatric Patients," *Clin Pharmacokinet*, 1983, 8(6):545-9.

Chiba K, Ishizaki T, Miura H, et al, "Michaelis-Menten Pharmacokinetics of Diphenylhydantoin and Application in the Pediatric Age Patient," *J Pediatr*, 1980, 96(3 Pt 1):479-84.

Suzuki Y, Mimaki T, Cox S, et al, "Phenytoin Age-Dose-Concentration Relationship in Children," *Ther Drug Monit*, 1994, 16(2):145-50.

♦ **Phenytoin Sodium** *see* Phenytoin *on page 762*
♦ **Pherazine® With Codeine** *see* Promethazine and Codeine *on page 807*

♦ **Phillips'® Milk of Magnesia** *see Magnesium Supplements on page 588*

♦ **pHisoHex®** *see Hexachlorophene on page 475*

♦ **Phos-Ex®** *see Calcium Supplements on page 157*

♦ **Phos-Flur®** *see Fluoride on page 427*

♦ **PhosLo®** *see Calcium Supplements on page 157*

Phosphate Supplements (FOS fate SUP la ments)

Brand Names Fleet® Enema [OTC]; Fleet® Phospho®-Soda [OTC]; K-Phos® M.F.; K-PHOS® Neutral; K-Phos® No. 2; K-Phos® Original; Neutra-Phos®-K; Uro-KP-Neutral®

Available Salts Potassium Acid Phosphate; Potassium Phosphate; Potassium Phosphate and Sodium Phosphate; Sodium Phosphate

Therapeutic Category Electrolyte Supplement, Oral; Electrolyte Supplement, Parenteral; Laxative, Saline; Phosphate Salt; Potassium Salt; Sodium Salt; Urinary Acidifying Agent

Generic Available Yes

Use Treatment and prevention of hypophosphatemia; short-term treatment of constipation (oral/rectal); evacuation of the colon for rectal and bowel exams; source of phosphate in large volume I.V. fluids; urinary acidifier (potassium acid phosphate) for reduction in formation of calcium stones

Pregnancy Risk Factor C

Contraindications Hyperphosphatemia, hyperkalemia (potassium salt form), hypocalcemia, hypomagnesemia, hypernatremia (sodium salt form), severe renal impairment, severe tissue trauma, heat cramps, CHF, abdominal pain (rectal forms), fecal impaction (rectal forms); patients with infected phosphate kidney stones

Warnings Parenteral **potassium** salt forms: should be administered only in patients with adequate urine flow; must be diluted before I.V. use and infused slowly (see Administration), and patients must be on a cardiac monitor during intermittent infusions

Precautions Use with caution in patients with renal impairment, patients receiving potassium-sparing drugs (potassium salt forms), patients with adrenal insufficiency, cirrhosis

Adverse Reactions

Cardiovascular: Hypotension, edema; **potassium salt form:** arrhythmias, heart block, cardiac arrest

Central nervous system: Tetany, mental confusion, seizures, dizziness, headache

Endocrine & metabolic: Hyperphosphatemia, hyperkalemia **(potassium salt form)**, hypocalcemia, hypernatremia **(sodium salt form)**

Gastrointestinal: Nausea, vomiting, diarrhea, flatulence (oral use)

Local: Phlebitis (parenteral forms)

Neuromuscular & skeletal: Paresthesia, bone and joint pain, arthralgia, weakness, muscle cramps

Renal: Acute renal failure

Drug Interactions Do not give orally at the same time as aluminum- and magnesium-containing antacids or sucralfate which can act as phosphate binders; use of potassium phosphate with potassium-sparing diuretics, ACE inhibitors, or salt substitutes may result in hyperkalemia

Food Interactions Avoid giving with oxalate (ie, berries, nuts, chocolate, beans, celery, tomatoes) or phytate-containing foods (ie, bran, whole wheat)

Stability Phosphate salts may precipitate when mixed with calcium salts; solubility is improved in amino acid parenteral nutrition solutions; check with a pharmacist to determine compatibility

Mechanism of Action Phosphorus participates in bone deposition, calcium metabolism, utilization of B complex vitamins, and as a buffer in acid-base equilibrium; as a laxative, exerts osmotic effect in the small intestine by drawing water into the lumen of the gut, producing distension, promoting peristalsis, and evacuation of the bowel

Pharmacodynamics Onset of action (catharsis):

Oral: 3-6 hours

Rectal: 2-5 minutes

Pharmacokinetics

Absorption: Oral: 1% to 20%

Elimination: Oral forms excreted in feces; I.V. forms are excreted in the urine with over 80% of dose reabsorbed by the kidney

(Continued)

Phosphate Supplements *(Continued)*

Usual Dosage Note: Phosphate supplements are either sodium or potassium salt forms. Consider the contribution of these electrolytes also when determining appropriate phosphate replacement.

Phosphorus: See table.

Phosphorus - Recommended Daily Allowance (RDA) and Estimated Average Requirement (EAR) (in terms of elemental magnesium)

Age	RDA (mmol/day)	EAR (mmol/day)
0-6 mo	–	3.2*
7-12 mo	–	8.9*
1-3 y	14.8	12.3
4-8 y	16.1	13.1
9-18 y	40.3	34
19-30 y	22.6	18.7

*Adequate intake (AI)

I.V. doses should be incorporated into the patient's maintenance I.V. fluids; intermittent I.V. infusion should be reserved for severe depletion situations; requires continuous cardiac monitoring (for potassium salts). **Note:** Doses listed as mmol of **phosphate**:

Hypophosphatemia: Intermittent I.V. infusion: Treatment: It is difficult to provide concrete guidelines for the treatment of severe hypophosphatemia because the extent of total body deficits and response to therapy are difficult to predict. Aggressive doses of phosphate may result in a transient serum elevation followed by redistribution into intracellular compartments or bone tissue. It is recommended that repletion of severe hypophosphatemia be done I.V. because large doses of oral phosphate may cause diarrhea and intestinal absorption may be unreliable

Children:

   Low dose: 0.08 mmol/kg over 6 hours; use if losses are recent and uncomplicated

   Intermediate dose: 0.16-0.24 mmol/kg over 4-6 hours; use if serum phosphorus level 0.5-1 mg/dL

   High dose: 0.36 mmol/kg over 6 hours; use if serum phosphorus <0.5 mg/dL

Adults: Varying dosages: 0.15-0.3 mmol/kg/dose over 12 hours; may repeat as needed to achieve desired serum level **or**

   15 mmol/dose over 2 hours; use if serum phosphorus <2 mg/dL **or**

   Low dose: 0.16 mmol/kg over 4-6 hours; use if serum phosphorus level 2.3-3 mg/dL

   Intermediate dose: 0.32 mmol/kg over 4-6 hours; use if serum phosphorus level 1.6-2.2 mg/dL

   High dose: 0.64 mmol/kg over 8-12 hours; use if serum phosphorus <1.5 mg/dL

Maintenance:

   Children:

      I.V.: 0.5-1.5 mmol/kg/day

      Oral: 2-3 mmol/kg/day in divided doses

   Adults:

      I.V.: 50-70 mmol/day

      Oral: 50-150 mmol/day in divided doses

Laxative: Oral

Neutra-Phos®, Neutra-Phos®-K, or Uro-KP-Neutral®:

   Children <4 years: 1 capsule or packet (250 mg phosphorus/8 mmol) 4 times/day; dilute as instructed

   Children >4 years and Adults: 1-2 capsules or packets (250-500 mg phosphorus/8-16 mmol) 4 times/day; dilute as instructed

Fleet® Phospho®-Soda:® Oral:

   Children 5-9 years: 5 mL as a single dose

   Children 10-12 years: 10 mL as a single dose

   Children ≥12 years and Adults: 20-30 mL as a single dose

Laxative: Rectal:

Fleet® Enema:

Children 2-11 years: Contents of one 2.25 oz pediatric enema as a single dose, may repeat

Children ≥12 years and Adults: Contents of one 4.5 oz enema as a single dose, may repeat

Urinary acidification: Adults: Oral (K-Phos® Original): 2 tablets 4 times/day

Administration

Oral: Administer with food to reduce the risk of diarrhea; do not swallow the capsule; contents of 1 capsule or packet should be diluted in 75 mL water before administration; administer tablets with a full glass of water; maintain adequate fluid intake; dilute oral solution with an equal volume of cool water; K-Phos® Original tablets (urinary acidifier) should be dissolved in 6-8 ounces of water before administration

Parenteral: For intermittent I.V. infusion: Peripheral line: Dilute to a maximum concentration of 0.05 mmol/mL; Central line: Dilute to a maximum concentration of 0.12 mmol/mL; maximum rate of infusion: 0.06 mmol/kg/hour; do **not** infuse with calcium containing I.V. fluids

Monitoring Parameters
Serum potassium (potassium salt forms), sodium (sodium salt forms), calcium, phosphorus, magnesium, renal function, reflexes; cardiac monitor (when intermittent infusion or high-dose I.V. replacement of potassium salts needed), stool output (laxative use)

Reference Range
Phosphorus:

Newborns: 4.2-9 mg/dL

6 weeks to 18 months: 3.8-6.7 mg/dL

18 months to 3 years: 2.9-5.9 mg/dL

3-15 years: 3.6-5.6 mg/dL

>15 years: 2.5-5 mg/dL

Dosage Forms

Capsule:

Neutra-Phos®-K: Phosphorus 250 mg [8 mmol] and **potassium** 556 mg [14.25 mEq] per capsule

Neutra-Phos®: Phosphorus 250 mg [8 mmol], **potassium** 278 mg [7.125 mEq], and **sodium** 164 mg [7.125 mEq] per capsule

Enema (Fleet® Enema): **Sodium** phosphate 6 g and sodium biphosphate 16 g per 100 mL (67.5 mL pediatric enema unit, 135 mL adult enema unit)

Injection:

Phosphate **(as potassium phosphate)** 3 mmol and **potassium** 4.4 mEq per mL (15 mL)

Phosphate **(as sodium phosphate)** 3 mmol and **sodium** 4 mEq per mL (15 mL)

Powder:

Neutra-Phos®-K: Phosphorus 250 mg [8 mmol] and **potassium** 556 mg [14.25 mEq] per packet

Neutra-Phos®: Phosphorus 250 mg [8 mmol], **potassium** 278 mg [7.125 mEq], and **sodium** 164 mg [7.125 mEq] per packet

Solution, oral (Fleet® Phospho®-Soda): Phosphate 4 mmol/mL; **sodium** phosphate 18 g and sodium biphosphate 48 g per 100 mL (30 mL, 45 mL, 90 mL, 237 mL) (96.4 mEq sodium/20 mL)

Tablet:

K-Phos® M.F.: Phosphorus 125.6 mg [4 mmol], **potassium** 44.5 mg [1.1 mEq], and **sodium** 67 mg [2.9 mEq]

K-Phos® Neutral: Phosphorus 250 mg [8 mmol], **potassium** 45 mg [1.1 mEq], and **sodium** 298 mg [13 mEq] per tablet

K-Phos® No. 2: Phosphorus 250 mg [8 mmol], **potassium** 88 mg [2.3 mEq], and **sodium** 134 mg [5.8 mEq]

K-Phos® Original: Phosphorus 114 mg [3.7 mmol] and **potassium** 144 mg [3.7 mEq] per tablet

Uro-KP-Neutral®: Phosphorus 250 mg [8 mmol], **potassium** 49.4 mg [1.27 mEq], and **sodium** 250.5 mg [10.9 mEq]

References

Clark CL, Sacks GS, Dickerson RN, et al, "Treatment of Hypophosphatemia in Patients Receiving Specialized Nutrition Support Using a Graduated Dosing Scheme: Results From a Prospective Clinical Trial," *Crit Care Med*, 1995, 23(9):1504-11.

"Dietary Reference Intakes for Calcium, Phosphorus, Magnesium, Vitamin D, and Fluoride. Standing Committee on the Scientific Evaluation of Dietary Reference Intakes, Food and Nutrition Board, Institute of Medicine," National Academy of Sciences, Washington, DC: National Academy Press, 1997.

Lentz RD, Brown BM, and Kjellstrand CM, "Treatment of Severe Hypophosphatemia," *Ann Intern Med*, 1978, 89(6):941-4.

Lloyd CW and Johnson CE, "Management of Hypophosphatemia," *Clin Pharm*, 1988, 7(2):123-8.

(Continued)

Phosphate Supplements *(Continued)*

Rosen GH, Boullata JI, O'Rangers EA, et al, "Intravenous Phosphate Repletion Regimen for Critically Ill Patients With Moderate Hypophosphatemia," *Crit Care Med*, 1995, 23(7):1204-10.

♦ **Phosphonoformate** *see* Foscarnet *on page 441*
♦ **3-Phosphoryloxymethyl Phenytoin Disodium** *see* Fosphenytoin *on page 443*
♦ ***p*-Hydroxyampicillin** *see* Amoxicillin *on page 70*
♦ **Phyllocontin®** *see* Aminophylline *on page 61*
♦ **Phylloquinone** *see* Phytonadione *on page 769*

Physostigmine *(fye zoe STIG meen)*

Related Information
Overdose and Toxicology *on page 1191*

Brand Names Antilirium® Injection; Isopto® Eserine

Available Salts Physostigmine Salicylate; Physostigmine Sulfate

Synonyms Eserine

Therapeutic Category Antidote, Anticholinergic Agent; Cholinergic Agent; Cholinergic Agent, Ophthalmic

Generic Available Yes: Ophthalmic

Use Reverse toxic CNS and cardiac effects caused by anticholinergics and tricyclic antidepressants; ophthalmic solution is used as a miotic in the treatment of open-angle glaucoma

Pregnancy Risk Factor C

Contraindications Hypersensitivity to physostigmine or any component; GI or GU obstruction, asthma, diabetes mellitus, gangrene, severe cardiovascular disease, active uveal inflammation or any inflammatory disease of the iris or ciliary body, glaucoma associated with iridocyclitis; patients receiving depolarizing neuromuscular blockers (eg, succinylcholine)

Warnings Because physostigmine has the potential for producing severe adverse effects, (ie, seizures, bradycardia), routine use as an antidote is controversial; atropine should be readily available to treat severe adverse effects; ophthalmic ointment may delay corneal healing, may cause loss of dark adaptation

Precautions Use with caution in patients with epilepsy, narrow-angle glaucoma, marked vagotonia, parkinsonism, bradycardia; injectable contains benzyl alcohol and bisulfites, avoid in sensitive individuals and neonates

Adverse Reactions
Cardiovascular: Palpitations, bradycardia
Central nervous system: Restlessness, hallucinations, seizures, nervousness
Dermatologic: Burning, redness
Gastrointestinal: Nausea, vomiting, epigastric pain, salivation, diarrhea
Neuromuscular & skeletal: Weakness, muscle twitching
Ocular: Miosis, lacrimation, stinging, burning, eye pain, browache
Respiratory: Dyspnea, bronchospasm, respiratory paralysis, pulmonary edema
Miscellaneous: Diaphoresis

Drug Interactions Additive cholinergic activity with bethanechol and methacholine; succinylcholine

Mechanism of Action Inhibits destruction of acetylcholine by acetylcholinesterase which prolongs the central and peripheral effects of acetylcholine

Pharmacodynamics
Onset of action:
Ophthalmic: Within 20-30 minutes
Parenteral: Within 3-8 minutes
Duration:
Ophthalmic: 12-36 hours
Parenteral: 30 minutes to 1 hour

Pharmacokinetics
Distribution: Widely distributed throughout the body; crosses into the CNS
Half-life: 1-2 hours
Elimination: Via hydrolysis by cholinesterases

Usual Dosage
Reversal of toxic anticholinergic effects:
Children: Reserve for life-threatening situations only: I.V.: 0.01-0.03 mg/kg/dose; may repeat after 15-20 minutes to a maximum total dose of 2 mg
Adults: I.M., I.V., S.C.: 0.5-2 mg initially, repeat every 20 minutes until response or adverse effect occurs; repeat 1-4 mg every 30-60 minutes as life-threatening signs (arrhythmias, seizures, deep come) recur

Preanesthetic reversal: Children and Adults:
   I.M., I.V.: Give twice the dose, on a weight basis, of the anticholinergic drug (atropine, scopolamine)
Ophthalmic: Children and Adults:
   Drops: Instill 1-2 drops of 0.25% or 0.5% solution every 4-8 hours (up to 4 times/day)
   Ointment: Apply small quantity at night or up to 3 times/day

Administration
Ophthalmic: Apply drops or ointment strip to affected eye(s); avoid contact of bottle tip with skin or eye; finger pressure should be applied to lacrimal sac during and for 1-2 minutes after instillation to decrease risk of absorption and systemic reaction

Parenteral: Infuse slowly I.V. without additional dilution at a maximum rate of 0.5 mg/minute in children or 1 mg/minute in adults

Monitoring Parameters Heart rate, respiratory rate

Patient Information Burning or stinging may occur with ophthalmic application; may cause loss of dark adaptation; use with caution while driving at night or performing hazardous tasks in poor light

Dosage Forms
Injection, as salicylate: 1 mg/mL (2 mL)
Ointment, ophthalmic, as sulfate: 0.25% (3.5 g)
Solution, ophthalmic, as sulfate: 0.25% (15 mL); 0.5% (2 mL, 15 mL)

♦ **Physostigmine Salicylate** see Physostigmine on page 768
♦ **Physostigmine Sulfate** see Physostigmine on page 768
♦ **Phytomenadione** see Phytonadione on page 769

Phytonadione (fye toe na DYE one)
Brand Names AquaMEPHYTON®; Konakion®; Mephyton®
Synonyms Methylphytyl Napthoquinone; Phylloquinone; Phytomenadione; Vitamin K_1
Therapeutic Category Nutritional Supplement; Vitamin, Fat Soluble
Generic Available No
Use Prevention and treatment of hypoprothrombinemia caused by vitamin K deficiency or anticoagulant-induced hypoprothrombinemia; hemorrhagic disease of the newborn
Pregnancy Risk Factor C
Contraindications Hypersensitivity to phytonadione or any component
Warnings Ineffective in hereditary hypoprothrombinemia and hypoprothrombinemia caused by severe liver disease; severe hemolytic anemia and hyperbilirubinemia has been reported rarely in neonates following large doses (10-20 mg) of phytonadione
Precautions Severe reactions resembling anaphylaxis or hypersensitivity have occurred rarely during or immediately after I.V. administration (even with proper dilution and rate of administration); restrict I.V. administration for emergency use only; injection contains benzyl alcohol 0.9% as preservative; safe in neonates when used in appropriate doses
Adverse Reactions See Warnings and Precautions
   Cardiovascular: Flushing, hypotension, cyanosis
   Central nervous system: Dizziness
   Gastrointestinal: GI upset, dysgeusia, hyperbilirubinemia (neonates)
   Hematologic: Hemolysis
   Local: Pain, edema, tenderness at injection site
   Miscellaneous: Anaphylactoid reactions, diaphoresis
   Respiratory: Dyspnea
Drug Interactions Antagonizes action of warfarin; mineral oil decreases phytonadione absorption
Mechanism of Action Cofactor in the liver synthesis of clotting factors (II, VII, IX, X)
Pharmacodynamics Onset of action: Blood coagulation factors increase within 6-12 hours after oral doses and within 1-2 hours following parenteral administration; after parenteral administration prothrombin time may become normal after 12-14 hours
Pharmacokinetics
   Absorption: Oral: From the intestines in the presence of bile
   Metabolism: Rapidly in the liver
   Elimination: In bile and urine
Usual Dosage I.V. route should be restricted for emergency use only
(Continued)

Phytonadione *(Continued)*

Hemorrhagic disease of the newborn: Neonates: I.M., S.C.:
Prophylaxis: 0.5-1 mg within 1 hour of birth; may repeat if necessary 6-8 hours later
Treatment: 1-2 mg/dose/day

Oral anticoagulant overdose:
Infants and Children:
No bleeding, rapid reversal needed, patient will require further oral anticoagulant therapy: I.V., S.C.: 0.5-2 mg
No bleeding, rapid reversal needed, patient will **not** require further oral anticoagulant therapy: I.V., S.C.: 2-5 mg
Significant bleeding, not life-threatening: I.V., S.C.: 0.5-2 mg
Significant bleeding, life-threatening: I.V.: 5 mg
Adults: I.V., S.C.: 2.5-10 mg/dose (rarely up to 25-50 mg has been used); may repeat in 6-8 hours if given by I.V., S.C. route; may repeat 12-48 hours after oral route

Vitamin K deficiency due to drugs, malabsorption, or decreased synthesis of vitamin K:
Infants and Children:
Oral: 2.5-5 mg/24 hours
I.M., I.V., S.C.: 1-2 mg/dose as a single dose
Adults:
Oral: 2.5-25 mg/24 hours
I.M., I.V., S.C.: 10 mg

Minimum daily requirement: Not well established
Infants: 1-5 mcg/kg/day
Adults: 0.03 mcg/kg/day

Administration
Oral: May be administered with or without food
Parenteral: Dilute in 5-10 mL I.V. fluid (D_5W or NS) (maximum concentration: 10 mg/mL); infuse over 15-30 minutes; maximum rate of infusion: 1 mg/minute

Monitoring Parameters PT

Additional Information Phytonadione is more effective and is preferred to other vitamin K preparations in the presence of impending hemorrhage; oral absorption depends on the presence of bile salts

Dosage Forms
Injection:
Aqueous colloidal: 2 mg/mL (0.5 mL); 10 mg/mL (1 mL, 2.5 mL, 5 mL)
Aqueous (I.M. only): 2 mg/mL (0.5 mL); 10 mg/mL (1 mL)
Tablet: 5 mg

Extemporaneous Preparations A 1 mg/mL suspension may be made by crushing six 5 mg tablets, add 5 mL purified water and 5 mL 1% methylcellulose, mix well, add 70% sorbitol to a total volume of 30 mL; shake well, refrigerate, expected stability: 3 days.
Nahata MC and Hipple TF, *Pediatric Drug Formulations*, 3rd ed, Cincinnati, OH: Harvey Whitney Books Co, 1997.

References
Michelson AD, Bovill E, Monagle P, et al, "Antithrombic Therapy in Children," *Chest*, 1998, 114(5 Suppl):748S-69S.

♦ **Pilagan® Ophthalmic** *see* Pilocarpine *on page 770*
♦ **Pilocar® Ophthalmic** *see* Pilocarpine *on page 770*

Pilocarpine *(pye loe KAR peen)*

Brand Names Adsorbocarpine® Ophthalmic; Akarpine® Ophthalmic; Diocarpine (Canada); Isopto® Carpine Ophthalmic; Minims® Pilocarpine (Canada); Miocarpine® (Canada); Ocu-Carpine® Ophthalmic; Ocusert Pilo-20® Ophthalmic; Ocusert Pilo-40® Ophthalmic; Pilagan® Ophthalmic; Pilocar® Ophthalmic; Pilopine HS® Ophthalmic; Piloptic® Ophthalmic; Pilostat® Ophthalmic; Salagen® Oral

Available Salts Pilocarpine Hydrochloride; Pilocarpine Nitrate

Therapeutic Category Cholinergic Agent; Cholinergic Agent, Ophthalmic; Ophthalmic Agent, Miotic

Generic Available Yes: Hydrochloride Solution

Use
Ophthalmic: Management of chronic simple glaucoma, chronic and acute angle-closure glaucoma; counter effects of cycloplegics

Oral: Symptomatic treatment of xerostomia caused by salivary gland hypofunction resulting from radiotherapy for cancer of the head and neck; and in Sjögren's syndrome

Pregnancy Risk Factor C

Contraindications Hypersensitivity to pilocarpine or any component; when cholinergic effects such as constriction are undesirable, eg, acute inflammatory disease of anterior chamber, acute iritis

Precautions Use with caution in patients with pre-existing retinal disease, CHF, asthma, peptic ulcer, urinary tract obstruction, Parkinson's disease, corneal abrasion, or those predisposed to retinal tears; may occasionally precipitate angle closure by increased resistance to aqueous flow from the posterior to anterior eye chamber

Adverse Reactions

Cardiovascular: Rare hypertension, tachycardia

Central nervous system: Headache

Gastrointestinal (rare): Nausea, vomiting, diarrhea, salivation

Genitourinary: Polyuria

Local: Stinging, burning

Ocular: Miosis, ciliary spasm, blurred vision, retinal detachment, photophobia, acute iritis, keratitis, corneal opacities, lacrimation, browache, conjunctival and ciliary congestion early in therapy

Miscellaneous: Hypersensitivity reactions, diaphoresis

Drug Interactions Topical NSAIDs may decrease pilocarpine effect; increased toxicities when combined with other parasympathomimetics; decreased effectiveness with anticholinergics

Mechanism of Action Directly stimulates cholinergic receptors in the eye causing miosis (by contraction of the iris sphincter), loss of accommodation (by constriction of ciliary muscle), and lowering of intraocular pressure (with decreased resistance to aqueous humor outflow)

Pharmacodynamics

Ophthalmic solution instillation: Miosis:

Onset of action: Within 10-30 minutes

Duration: 4-8 hours

Intraocular pressure reduction:

Onset of action: 1 hour

Duration: 4-12 hours

Ocusert® Pilo application: Miosis: Onset of effect: 10-30 minutes

Maximal effects: 1.5-2 hours

Duration: 7 days

Oral: Increased salivary flow

Onset of action: 20 minutes

Peak effect: 1 hour

Duration: 3-5 hours

Usual Dosage

Ophthalmic: Children and Adults:

Gel: 0.5" (1.3 cm) ribbon applied to lower conjunctival sac once daily at bedtime; adjust dosage as required to control elevated intraocular pressure

Nitrate solution: Instill 1-2 drops 2-4 times/day

Hydrochloride solution: Instill 1-2 drops up to 6 times/day; adjust the concentration and frequency as required to control elevated intraocular pressure

To counteract the mydriatic effects of sympathomimetic agents: Instill 1 drop of a 1% solution in the affected eye

Ocular systems: Systems are labeled in terms of the mean rate of release of pilocarpine over 7 days; begin with 20 mcg/hour at night; adjust based upon response

Oral: Adults: 5 mg 3 times/day, titration up to 10 mg 3 times/day may be considered for patients who have not responded adequately

Administration

Ointment: After topical instillation, close the eye for 1-2 minutes and instruct patient to roll the eyeball in all directions

Oral: May be administered with or without food

Solution: Shake well before use; after topical instillation, finger pressure should be applied to lacrimal sac to decrease drainage into the nose and throat and minimize possible systemic absorption

Monitoring Parameters Intraocular pressure, funduscopic exam, visual field testing

(Continued)

Pilocarpine *(Continued)*

Patient Information May sting on instillation; notify physician of sweating, urinary retention; usually causes difficulty in dark adaptation; use caution when driving at night or doing hazardous activities in poor light

Additional Information
Ocusert® 20 mcg is approximately equivalent to 0.5% or 1% drops
Ocusert® 40 mcg is approximately equivalent to 2% or 3% drops

Dosage Forms
Gel, ophthalmic, as hydrochloride (Pilopine HS®): 4% (3.5 g)
Ocular therapeutic system (Ocusert® Pilo): Releases 20 or 40 mcg per hour for 1 week (8s)
Solution, ophthalmic, as hydrochloride (Adsorbocarpine®, Akarpine®, Isopto®, Carpine®, Pilagan®, Pilocar®, Piloptic®, Pilostat®): 0.25% (15 mL); 0.5% (15 mL, 30 mL); 1% (1 mL, 2 mL, 15 mL, 30 mL); 2% (1 mL, 2 mL, 15 mL, 30 mL); 3% (15 mL, 30 mL); 4% (1 mL, 2 mL, 15 mL, 30 mL); 5% (15 mL); 6% (15 mL, 30 mL); 8% (2 mL); 10% (15 mL)
Solution, ophthalmic, as nitrate (Pilagan®): 1% (15 mL); 2% (15 mL); 4% (15 mL)
Tablet, as hydrochloride: 5 mg

♦ **Pilocarpine Hydrochloride** *see Pilocarpine on page 770*
♦ **Pilocarpine Nitrate** *see Pilocarpine on page 770*
♦ **Pilopine HS® Ophthalmic** *see Pilocarpine on page 770*
♦ **Piloptic® Ophthalmic** *see Pilocarpine on page 770*
♦ **Pilostat® Ophthalmic** *see Pilocarpine on page 770*
♦ **Pima®** *see Potassium Iodide on page 785*
♦ **Pink Bismuth® [OTC]** *see Bismuth on page 134*
♦ **Pin-Rid® [OTC]** *see Pyrantel Pamoate on page 824*
♦ **Pin-X® [OTC]** *see Pyrantel Pamoate on page 824*

Piperacillin *(pi PER a sil in)*

Brand Names Pipracil®
Available Salts Piperacillin Sodium
Therapeutic Category Antibiotic, Penicillin (Antipseudomonal)
Generic Available No
Use Treatment of serious infections caused by susceptible strains of gram-positive, gram-negative, and anaerobic bacilli; mixed aerobic-anaerobic bacterial infections or empiric antibiotic therapy in granulocytopenic patients. Primary use is in the treatment of serious carbenicillin-resistant or ticarcillin-resistant *Pseudomonas aeruginosa* infections susceptible to piperacillin.
Pregnancy Risk Factor B
Contraindications Hypersensitivity to piperacillin, penicillins, or any component
Warnings Superinfection has been reported in up to 6% to 8% of patients receiving an extended spectrum penicillin; piperacillin therapy has been associated with an increased incidence of fever and rash in cystic fibrosis patients
Precautions Use with caution in patients with hypersensitivity to cephalosporins; dosage modification required in patients with impaired renal function
Adverse Reactions
Central nervous system: Seizures, fever, headache, dizziness, confusion, drowsiness
Dermatologic: Rash, exfoliative dermatitis
Endocrine & metabolic: Hypokalemia
Gastrointestinal: Diarrhea, vomiting
Hematologic: Hemolytic anemia, eosinophilia, neutropenia, prolonged bleeding time, thrombocytopenia
Hepatic: Elevated liver enzymes, cholestatic hepatitis
Local: Thrombophlebitis
Neuromuscular & skeletal: Myoclonus
Renal: Acute interstitial nephritis
Miscellaneous: Hypersensitivity reactions, anaphylaxis, serum sickness-like reaction
Drug Interactions Aminoglycosides (antibacterial activity is synergistic), probenecid (increases serum concentration of piperacillin), vecuronium (prolongs neuromuscular blockade)
Stability Reconstituted piperacillin solution is stable for 24 hours at room temperature and 7 days when refrigerated; incompatible with aminoglycosides

Mechanism of Action Inhibits bacterial cell wall synthesis by binding to one or more of the penicillin-binding proteins; inhibits the final transpeptidation step of peptidoglycan synthesis in bacterial cell walls

Pharmacokinetics

Absorption: I.M.: 70% to 80%

Distribution: Crosses the placenta; distributes into breast milk at low concentrations; penetration across the blood-brain barrier is poor when meninges are uninflamed; good biliary concentration (30-60 times higher than serum concentration)

Protein binding: 22%

Metabolism: 5% to 10%

Half-life: Prolonged with moderately severe renal or hepatic impairment

Neonates:

1-5 days: 3.6 hours

>6 days: 2.1-2.7 hours

Children:

1-6 months: 0.5-1 hours

6 months to 12 years: 0.39-0.5 hours

Adults: 36-80 minutes (dose-dependent)

Time to peak serum concentration: I.M.: Within 30-50 minutes

Elimination: Principally in urine and partially in feces (via bile)

Dialyzable (20% to 50%)

Usual Dosage Not FDA approved for children <12 years of age

I.M., I.V.:

Neonates:

≤7 days: 150 mg/kg/day divided every 8 hours

>7 days: 200 mg/kg/day divided every 6 hours

Infants and Children: 200-300 mg/kg/day in divided doses every 4-6 hours; maximum dose: 24 g/day

Higher doses have been used in cystic fibrosis: 350-500 mg/kg/day in divided doses every 4 hours

Adults: 2-4 g/dose every 4-8 hours; maximum dose: 24 g/day

Dosing interval in renal impairment:

Cl_{cr} 20-40 mL/minute: Administer every 8 hours

Cl_{cr} <20 mL/minute: Administer every 12 hours

Administration Parenteral:

I.M.: Reconstitute each gram of piperacillin with at least 2 mL of sterile water, NS, or 0.5% or 1% lidocaine hydrochloride (without epinephrine) to make a 400 mg/mL solution; administer by deep I.M. injection into the gluteus maximus

I.V. push: Administer over 3-5 minutes at a maximum concentration of 200 mg/mL

I.V. intermittent infusion: Administer over 30-60 minutes at a final concentration ≤20 mg/mL; if the patient is on concurrent aminoglycoside therapy, separate piperacillin administration from the aminoglycoside by at least 30-60 minutes

Monitoring Parameters Serum electrolytes, bleeding time especially in patients with renal impairment; periodic tests of renal, hepatic and hematologic function

Test Interactions False-positive urinary and serum proteins, positive Coombs' [direct]

Additional Information Sodium content of 1 g: 1.85 mEq

Dosage Forms Powder for injection, as sodium: 2 g, 3 g, 4 g, 40 g

References

Placzek M, Whitelaw A, Want S, et al, "Piperacillin in Early Neonatal Infection," *Arch Dis Child*, 1983, 58(12):1006-9.

Prince AS and Neu HC, "Use of Piperacillin, A Semisynthetic Penicillin, in the Therapy of Acute Exacerbations of Pulmonary Disease in Patients With Cystic Fibrosis," *J Pediatr*, 1980, 97(1):148-51.

Thirumoorthi MC, Asmar BI, Buckley JA, et al, "Pharmacokinetics of Intravenously Administered Piperacillin in Preadolescent Children," *J Pediatr*, 1983, 102(6):941-6.

Piperacillin and Tazobactam (pi PER a sil in & ta zoe BAK tam)

Brand Names Tacozin® (Canada); Zosyn™

Available Salts Piperacillin Sodium and Tazobactam Sodium

Synonyms Tazobactam and Piperacillin

Therapeutic Category Antibiotic, Beta-lactam and Beta-lactamase Combination; Antibiotic, Penicillin (Antipseudomonal)

Generic Available No

Use Treatment of sepsis, gynecologic, intra-abdominal infections, and infections involving skin and skin structures, the lower respiratory tract, and urinary tract caused by piperacillin-resistant, beta-lactamase producing strains that are piperacillin/tazobactam susceptible. Tazobactam expands activity of piperacillin to

(Continued)

Piperacillin and Tazobactam *(Continued)*

include beta-lactamase producing strains of *S. aureus, H. influenzae, B. fragilis, Klebsiella, E. coli,* and *Acinetobacter.*

Pregnancy Risk Factor B

Contraindications Hypersensitivity to piperacillin, tazobactam, penicillins, or any component

Warnings Prolonged use may result in superinfection; abnormal platelet aggregation and prolonged bleeding have been reported in patients with renal failure; piperacillin therapy has been associated with an increased incidence of fever and rash in cystic fibrosis patients

Precautions Use with caution in patients with hypersensitivity to cephalosporins or other beta-lactamase inhibitors; use with caution in patients with renal impairment or pre-existing seizure disorder; dosage modification required in patients with impaired renal function

Adverse Reactions

Cardiovascular: Hypertension, hypotension, edema

Central nervous system: Insomnia, headache, dizziness, agitation, confusion, fever, convulsions

Dermatologic: Rash, pruritus, erythema multiforme

Endocrine & metabolism: Hypokalemia

Gastrointestinal: Diarrhea, constipation, nausea, vomiting, dyspepsia, melena, pseudomembranous colitis

Hematologic: Leukopenia, decrease in hemoglobin/hematocrit, eosinophilia, prolonged prothrombin time

Hepatic: Elevation of AST, ALT, bilirubin; cholestatic hepatitis

Local: Phlebitis, pain

Renal: Elevated BUN, elevated serum creatinine, interstitial nephritis

Miscellaneous: Hypersensitivity reactions, anaphylaxis

Drug Interactions Probenecid prolongs half-life of piperacillin/tazobactam; vecuronium (prolongs neuromuscular blockade); aminoglycosides (antibacterial activity is synergistic)

Stability Reconstituted piperacillin/tazobactam solution is stable for 24 hours at room temperature and 2 days when refrigerated; incompatible with LR solution and aminoglycosides

Mechanism of Action Inhibits bacterial cell wall synthesis by binding to one or more of the penicillin-binding proteins; inhibits the final transpeptidation step of peptidoglycan synthesis in bacterial cell walls; tazobactam prevents degradation of piperacillin by binding to beta-lactamases

Pharmacokinetics Both AUC and peak concentrations are dose proportional

Distribution: Widely distributed into tissues and body fluids including lungs, intestinal mucosa, female reproductive tissues, interstitial fluid, gallbladder, and bile; penetration into CSF is poor when meninges are uninflamed; piperacillin is excreted into breast milk

Protein binding:

Piperacillin: ~26% to 33%

Tazobactam: 31% to 32%

Metabolism:

Piperacillin: 6% to 9%

Tazobactam: ~22%

Bioavailability: I.M.:

Piperacillin: 71%

Tazobactam: 84%

Half-life:

Piperacillin:

Infants 2-5 months: 1.4 hours

Children 6-23 months: 0.9 hour

Children 2-12 years: 0.7 hour

Adults: 0.7-1.2 hours

Metabolite: 1-1.5 hours

Tazobactam:

Infants 2-5 months: 1.6 hours

Children 6-23 months: 1 hour

Children 2-12 years: 0.8-0.9 hour

Adults: 0.7-0.9 hour

Elimination: Piperacillin and tazobactam are both eliminated by renal tubular secretion and glomerular filtration

Piperacillin: 50% to 70% eliminated unchanged in urine

Tazobactam: Found in urine at 24 hours, with 22% as the inactive metabolite

Hemodialysis removes 30% to 40% of a piperacillin/tazobactam dose; peritoneal dialysis removes 21% of tazobactam and 6% of piperacillin; hepatic impairment does not affect the kinetics of piperacillin or tazobactam significantly

Usual Dosage Not FDA-approved for children <12 years of age

Infants <6 months of age: I.V.: 150-300 mg of piperacillin component/kg/day in divided doses every 6-8 hours

Infants and Children ≥6 months: I.V.: 240 mg of piperacillin component/kg/day in divided doses every 8 hours; higher doses have been used for serious pseudomonal infections: 300-400 mg of piperacillin component/kg/day in divided doses every 6 hours

Adults: I.V.: 3.375 g (3 g piperacillin/0.375 g tazobactam) every 6 hours

Dosing interval in renal impairment:

Cl$_{cr}$ 20-40 mL/minute: Decrease dose by 30% and administer every 6 hours

Cl$_{cr}$ <20 mL/minute: Decrease dose by 30% and administer every 8 hours

Hemodialysis: Adults: Administer 2.25 g every 8 hours with an additional dose of 0.75 g after each dialysis

Administration Parenteral: I.V. intermittent infusion: May administer over 30 minutes at a maximum concentration of 200 mg/mL (piperacillin component); however, concentrations ≤20 mg/mL are preferred. If the patient is on concurrent aminoglycoside therapy, separate piperacillin and tazobactam administration from the aminoglycoside by at least 30-60 minutes.

Monitoring Parameters Serum electrolytes, bleeding time especially in patients with renal impairment; periodic tests of renal, hepatic, and hematologic function

Test Interactions Positive Coombs' [direct], false-positive urinary and serum proteins; false-positive urine glucose using Clinitest®

Additional Information Sodium content of 1 g piperacillin component: 2.35 mEq

Dosage Forms Injection: Piperacillin sodium 2 g and tazobactam sodium 0.25 g; piperacillin sodium 3 g and tazobactam sodium 0.375 g; piperacillin sodium 4 g and tazobactam sodium 0.5 g (vials at an 8:1 ratio of piperacillin sodium to tazobactam sodium)

References

Bryson HM and Brogden RN, "Piperacillin/Tazobactam. A Review of its Antibacterial Activity, Pharmacokinetic Properties, and Therapeutic Potential," *Drugs*, 1994, 47(3):506-35.

Reed MD, Goldfarb J, Yamashita T, et al, "Single-Dose Pharmacokinetics of Piperacillin and Tazobactam in Infants and Children," *Antimicrob Agents Chemother*, 1994, 38(12):2817-26.

♦ **Piperacillin Sodium** *see* Piperacillin *on page 772*

♦ **Piperacillin Sodium and Tazobactam Sodium** *see* Piperacillin and Tazobactam *on page 773*

Piperazine (PI per a zeen)

Brand Names Vermizine®

Available Salts Piperazine Citrate

Therapeutic Category Anthelmintic

Generic Available Yes

Use Treatment of pinworm (*Enterobius vermicularis*) and roundworm (*Ascaris lumbricoides*) infections; used as an alternative to first-line agents mebendazole or pyrantel pamoate for the treatment of these infections

Pregnancy Risk Factor B

Contraindications Seizure disorders, liver or kidney impairment; hypersensitivity to piperazine or any component

Precautions Use with caution in patients with anemia or malnutrition or patients receiving chlorpromazine; avoid prolonged or repeated piperazine use in children due to potential neurotoxicity

Adverse Reactions

Central nervous system: Dizziness, vertigo, seizures, EEG changes, headache

Gastrointestinal: Nausea, vomiting, diarrhea, abdominal cramps

Hematologic: Hemolytic anemia

Neuromuscular & skeletal: Tremor, weakness

Ocular: Visual impairment, nystagmus

Respiratory: Cough

Miscellaneous: Hypersensitivity reactions (urticaria, erythema multiforme, photodermatitis, fever, arthralgia, bronchospasm)

Drug Interactions Pyrantel pamoate (antagonistic mode of action)

Mechanism of Action Causes muscle paralysis of the roundworm by blocking the effects of acetylcholine at the neuromuscular junction

Pharmacokinetics

Absorption: Well absorbed from the GI tract

Time to peak serum concentration: 1 hour

(Continued)

Piperazine *(Continued)*

Elimination: In urine as metabolites and unchanged drug

Usual Dosage Oral:

Pinworms: Children and Adults: 65 mg/kg/day as a single daily dose for 7 days; in severe infections, repeat course after a 1-week interval; not to exceed 2.5 g/day

Roundworms:

Children: 75 mg/kg/day as a single daily dose for 2 days; maximum dose: 3.5 g/day; in severe infections, repeat course after a 1-week interval

Adults: 3.5 g/day for 2 days (in severe infections, repeat course, after a 1-week interval)

Administration Oral: In the case of partial or complete intestinal obstruction due to a heavy roundworm load, administer dose as a solution through a gastrointestinal tube

Monitoring Parameters Stool exam for worms and ova

Nursing Implications Cure rates may be decreased with massive infections or in patients with hypermotility of the GI tract

Dosage Forms

Tablet, as citrate: 250 mg

♦ **Piperazine Citrate** *see Piperazine on page 775*

♦ **Pipracil®** *see Piperacillin on page 772*

Pirbuterol *(peer BYOO ter ole)*

Brand Names Maxair™ Autohaler™; Maxair™ Inhalation Aerosol

Available Salts Pirbuterol Acetate

Therapeutic Category Adrenergic Agonist Agent; Antiasthmatic; Beta$_2$-Adrenergic Agonist Agent; Bronchodilator; Sympathomimetic

Generic Available No

Use Prevention and treatment of bronchospasm in patients with reversible airway obstruction due to asthma or COPD

Pregnancy Risk Factor C

Contraindications Hypersensitivity to pirbuterol or or any component

Warnings Paradoxical bronchospasm may occur, especially with the first use of a new cannister

Precautions Use with caution in patients with hyperthyroidism, diabetes mellitus, cardiovascular disorders (including coronary insufficiency or hypertension); excessive or prolonged use can lead to tolerance

Adverse Reactions

Cardiovascular: Tachycardia, palpitations, hypertension, chest pain

Central nervous system: Nervousness, CNS stimulation, anxiety, syncope, hyperactivity, insomnia, dizziness, depression, lightheadedness, drowsiness, headache

Dermatologic: Rash, pruritus, alopecia

Endocrine & metabolic: Hypokalemia

Gastrointestinal: GI upset, xerostomia, glossitis, abdominal pain, vomiting, nausea, unusual taste, hoarseness

Neuromuscular & skeletal: Tremor, weakness, muscle cramping

Respiratory: Irritation of oropharynx, cough, paradoxical bronchospasm

Miscellaneous: Diaphoresis

Drug Interactions Action of pirbuterol is antagonized by beta-adrenergic blocking agents such as propranolol; cardiovascular effects are potentiated in patients also receiving MAO inhibitors or tricyclic antidepressants; concomitant administration of sympathomimetics may result in enhanced cardiovascular effects

Stability Store at room temperature

Mechanism of Action Relaxes bronchial smooth muscle by action on beta$_2$-adrenergic receptors with little effect on heart rate

Pharmacodynamics

Onset: 5 minutes

Peak action: 30-60 minutes

Duration: 5 hours

Pharmacokinetics

Metabolism: Liver (by sulfate conjugation)

Half-life: 2-3 hours

Elimination: 51% excreted in the urine as pirbuterol plus its sulfate conjugate

Usual Dosage Oral inhalation:

Children ≥12 years and Adults: 1-2 inhalations (0.2-0.4 mg) every 4-6 hours; do not exceed 12 inhalations/day

Administration Oral inhalation: Shake well before administration; Maxair™ Autohaler™ is breath activated; after sealing lips around mouthpiece, inhale deeply with steady, moderate force; inhalation triggers the release "puff" of medication; do not stop inhalation when puff occurs, but continue to take a deep, full breath; hold breath for 10 seconds, then exhale slowly

Monitoring Parameters Serum potassium, heart rate, pulmonary function tests, respiratory rate; arterial or capillary blood gases (if patient's condition warrants)

Patient Information Do not exceed recommended dosage; rinse mouth with water following each inhalation to help with dry throat and mouth; if more than one inhalation is necessary, wait at least 1 full minute between inhalations; notify physician if palpitations, tachycardia, chest pain, muscle tremors, dizziness, headache, flushing occur, or if breathing difficulty persists

Dosage Forms
Aerosol, oral
Maxair™ Inhaler: 0.2 mg/actuation [300 metered doses] (25.6 g)
Maxair™ Autohaler™: 0.2 mg/actuation [80 metered doses] (2.8 g); [400 metered doses] (14 g)

♦ **Pirbuterol Acetate** see Pirbuterol on page 776

Piroxicam (peer OKS i kam)

Related Information
Overdose and Toxicology on page 1191

Brand Names Apo®-Piroxicam (Canada); Feldene®; Novo-Piroxicam® (Canada); Nu-Pirox® (Canada); Pro-Piroxicam® (Canada)

Therapeutic Category Analgesic, Non-narcotic; Anti-inflammatory Agent; Nonsteroidal Anti-inflammatory Drug (NSAID), Oral

Generic Available Yes

Use Management of inflammatory diseases and rheumatoid disorders; dysmenorrhea

Pregnancy Risk Factor B (D if used in 3rd trimester)

Contraindications Hypersensitivity to piroxicam, any component, aspirin, or other NSAIDs; active GI bleeding

Precautions Use with caution in patients with impaired cardiac function, hypertension, impaired renal function, GI disease and patients receiving anticoagulants

Adverse Reactions
Cardiovascular: Edema
Central nervous system: Dizziness, headache
Dermatologic: Rash, phototoxic skin eruptions
Gastrointestinal: Nausea, epigastric distress, anorexia, abdominal discomfort, vomiting, GI bleeding, ulcers, perforation
Hematologic: Reduction in hemoglobin and hematocrit, inhibition of platelet aggregation
Hepatic: Hepatitis
Renal: Acute renal failure, elevated BUN, elevated serum creatinine

Drug Interactions Cytochrome P-450 isoenzyme CYP2C9 and CYP2C18 substrate
May increase serum concentrations of lithium; aspirin may decrease piroxicam serum concentrations; GI irritants (eg, potassium supplements) may increase GI adverse effects; drug interactions similar to other NSAIDs may also occur; concurrent use of piroxicam with ritonavir is not recommended

Food Interactions Food may decrease the rate but not the extent of absorption

Mechanism of Action Inhibits prostaglandin synthesis by decreasing the activity of the enzyme, cyclo-oxygenase, which results in decreased formation of prostaglandin precursors

Pharmacodynamics Analgesia:
Onset of action: Oral: Within 1 hour
Peak effect: 3-5 hours

Pharmacokinetics
Protein binding: 99%
Metabolism: In the liver
Half-life: 45-50 hours
Elimination: Excreted as metabolites and unchanged drug (~5% to 10%) in the urine; small amount excreted in feces

Usual Dosage Oral:
Children: 0.2-0.3 mg/kg/day once daily; maximum dose: 15 mg/day
Adults: 10-20 mg/day once daily; although associated with increase in GI adverse effects, doses >20 mg/day have been used (ie, 30-40 mg/day)
(Continued)

Piroxicam *(Continued)*

Administration Oral: May administer with food or milk to decrease GI upset

Monitoring Parameters CBC, BUN, serum creatinine, liver enzymes; periodic ophthalmologic exams with chronic use

Patient Information Avoid alcohol

Dosage Forms Capsule: 10 mg, 20 mg

♦ *p*-Isobutylhydratropic Acid *see Ibuprofen on page 501*

♦ **Pitressin®** *see Vasopressin on page 971*

♦ **Pitrex® (Canada)** *see Tolnaftate on page 936*

♦ **Plantago Seed** *see Psyllium on page 823*

♦ **Plantain Seed** *see Psyllium on page 823*

♦ **Plaquenil® Sulfate** *see Hydroxychloroquine on page 493*

♦ **Plasbumin®** *see Albumin on page 39*

♦ **Platinol®** *see Cisplatin on page 229*

♦ **Platinol®-AQ** *see Cisplatin on page 229*

Plicamycin *(plye kay MYE sin)*

Brand Names Mithracin®

Synonyms Mithramycin

Therapeutic Category Antidote, Hypercalcemia; Antineoplastic Agent, Antibiotic

Generic Available No

Use Malignant testicular tumors; treatment of hypercalcemia and hypercalciuria of malignancy not responsive to conventional treatment; chronic myelogenous leukemia in blast phase; Paget's disease

Pregnancy Risk Factor D

Contraindications Thrombocytopenia, bleeding diatheses, coagulation disorders, bone marrow function impairment, or hypocalcemia

Warnings The FDA currently recommends that procedures for proper handling and disposal of antineoplastic agents be considered. Discontinue therapy if bleeding or epistaxis occurs; plicamycin may cause permanent sterility and may cause birth defects.

Precautions Use with caution in patients with hepatic or renal impairment; reduce dosage in patients with renal impairment

Adverse Reactions

Cardiovascular: Facial flushing

Central nervous system: Fever, headache, malaise, dizziness

Endocrine & metabolic: Decreased serum calcium, phosphorus, and potassium

Gastrointestinal: Anorexia, stomatitis, nausea, vomiting, diarrhea

Hematologic: Thrombocytopenia, hemorrhagic diathesis (hematemesis, hemoptysis), leukopenia, increase in fibrinolytic activity

Hepatic: Hepatotoxicity, elevation in AST, ALT, and LDH

Local: Phlebitis

Renal: Nephrotoxicity (elevated serum creatinine, elevated BUN, elevated proteinuria)

Respiratory: Epistaxis

Drug Interactions Calcitonin, etidronate, glucagon, aspirin

Stability Refrigeration is recommended but drug remains stable for up to 3 months unrefrigerated; drug is unstable at a pH <4; reconstituted solution is stable for 24 hours at room temperature and 48 hours when refrigerated; chelates divalent cations (especially iron); incompatible with trace element solution

Mechanism of Action Forms a complex with DNA in the presence of magnesium or other divalent cations inhibiting DNA-directed RNA synthesis; may inhibit parathyroid hormone effect on osteoclasts lowering serum calcium concentrations; inhibits bone resorption

Pharmacodynamics

Onset of action for decreasing serum calcium: Within 24-48 hours

Peak effect on calcium levels: 48-72 hours

Duration: 3-15 days

Pharmacokinetics

Distribution: Crosses the blood-brain barrier

Protein-binding: 0%

Half-life, plasma: 1 hour

Elimination: 90% of dose excreted in urine within the first 24 hours

Usual Dosage Adults (dose based on ideal weight): I.V. (refer to individual protocols):

Testicular cancer: 25-30 mcg/kg/day once daily for 8-10 days

Blastic chronic granulocytic leukemia: 25 mcg/kg over 2-4 hours every other day for 3 weeks

Hypercalcemia: 15-25 mcg/kg/day once daily for 3-4 days or 25 mcg/kg every 48-72 hours; additional courses of therapy may be given at intervals of 1 week or more if the initial course is unsuccessful. Reduce dose to 12.5 mcg/kg in patients with pre-existing hepatic or renal impairment

Paget's disease: 15 mcg/kg/day once daily for 10 days

Dosing adjustment in renal impairment:

Cl_{cr} 10-50 mL/minute: Decrease dosage by 25%

Cl_{cr} <10 mL/minute: Decrease dosage by 50%

Administration Parenteral: Dose should be diluted in 1 L of D_5W or NS and administered as an I.V. infusion over 4-6 hours; bolus or short infusion over 30-60 minutes in 100-150 mL D_5W is an alternative method of administration; avoid rapid I.V. push injections

Monitoring Parameters Hepatic and renal function tests, CBC, platelet count, prothrombin time, serum electrolytes

Patient Information Notify physician if fever, sore throat, bleeding, bruising, shortness of breath, or painful urination occur

Nursing Implications Rapid I.V. infusion has been associated with an increased incidence of nausea and vomiting; an antiemetic given prior to and during plicamycin infusion may be helpful. Avoid extravasation since local irritation and cellulitis at the injection site may result; minimize tissue irritation by applying moderate heat to the extravasation site

Additional Information Treatment of hemorrhagic episodes should include transfusion of fresh whole blood or packed red blood cells and fresh frozen plasma, vitamin K, and corticosteroids

Myelosuppressive effects:
WBC: Moderate
Platelets: Moderate
Nadir (days): 7-12
Recovery (days): 21

Dosage Forms Powder for injection: 2.5 mg

References

Mutch RS, Hutson PR, and Lewinsky DB, "Plicamycin: Bolus or Infusion?" *DICP*, 1990, 24(9):885-6.
Ritch PS, "Treatment of Cancer-Related Hypercalcemia," *Semin Oncol*, 1990, 17(2 Suppl 5):26-33.
Stumpf JL, "Pharmacologic Management of Paget's Disease," *Clin Pharm*, 1989, 8(7):485-95.

- ◆ **PMS-Methylphenidate (Canada)** *see* Methylphenidate *on page 627*
- ◆ **PMS-Nystatin (Canada)** *see* Nystatin *on page 701*
- ◆ **PMS-Prochlorperazine (Canada)** *see* Prochlorperazine *on page 803*
- ◆ **PMS-Pseudoephedrine (Canada)** *see* Pseudoephedrine *on page 822*
- ◆ **PMS-Pyrazinamide (Canada)** *see* Pyrazinamide *on page 825*
- ◆ **PMS-Sodium Cromoglycate (Canada)** *see* Cromolyn *on page 260*
- ◆ **PMS-Sulfasalazine (Canada)** *see* Sulfasalazine *on page 893*
- ◆ **PMS-Thioridazine (Canada)** *see* Thioridazine *on page 920*
- ◆ **PMS-Trihexyphenidyl (Canada)** *see* Trihexyphenidyl *on page 952*
- ◆ **Pneumococcal Polysaccharide Vaccine, Polyvalent** *see* Pneumococcal Vaccine *on page 780*

Pneumococcal Vaccine (noo moe KOK al vak SEEN)

Brand Names Pneumovax® 23; Pnu-Imune® 23

Synonyms Pneumococcal Polysaccharide Vaccine, Polyvalent

Therapeutic Category Vaccine, Inactivated Bacteria

Use Immunocompetent patients 2-64 years of age with a chronic illness (CHF, sickle cell disease, cardiomyopathy, COPD, diabetes mellitus, chronic liver disease, or CSF leak) or with functional or anatomic asplenia; immunocompromised patients ≥2 years of age with the following conditions: HIV, leukemia, lymphoma, Hodgkin's disease, generalized malignancy, chronic renal failure, nephrotic syndrome or conditions associated with immunosuppression (ie, organ transplantation or long-term corticosteroid therapy); adults ≥65 years of age

Contraindications Hypersensitivity to the vaccine or thimerosal; acute febrile illness; children <2 years of age (antibody response to the vaccine is poor in this age group); pregnancy

Warnings Epinephrine injection (1:1000) must be immediately available in case of anaphylaxis; may cause relapse in patients with stable idiopathic thrombocytopenia purpura

Adverse Reactions

Central nervous system: Low grade fever, Guillain-Barré syndrome

Dermatologic: Rash, urticaria

Neuromuscular & skeletal: Arthralgia

Local: Soreness at the injection site, erythema

Drug Interactions Decreased effect with immunosuppressive agents, live vaccines, immunoglobulin; initiate vaccine at least 2 weeks prior to immunosuppressive therapy and avoid during chemotherapy or radiation therapy

Stability Refrigerate

Usual Dosage I.M., S.C.: Children ≥2 years and Adults: 0.5 mL; if an elective splenectomy is planned, administer dose 2 weeks prior to surgery

Revaccination schedule:

A. Persons 2-64 years of age with functional or anatomic asplenia or immunocompromised persons:

1. Patients >10 years of age: Single revaccination ≥5 years after the previous dose

2. Patients ≤10 years of age: Single revaccination 3-5 years after the previous dose

B. Patients ≥65 years of age: Single revaccination if first dose was ≥5 years ago and patient was <65 years at the time

Administration Do not inject I.V.; avoid intradermal administration; administer S.C. or I.M. into the deltoid muscle or lateral midthigh; pneumococcal vaccine may be given concurrently with other vaccines including MMR, DTP, poliovirus, *H. influenzae* type b, hepatitis B, or influenza vaccine

Patient Information Vaccination does not guarantee protection from fulminant pneumococcal disease in patient's with functional or anatomic asplenia

Nursing Implications Federal law requires that the date of administration, the vaccine manufacturer, lot number of the vaccine, and the administering person's name, title, and address be entered into the patient's permanent medical record

Dosage Forms Injection: 25 mcg of each type of capsular polysaccharide per 0.5 mL

References

Advisory Committee on Immunization Practices, "Prevention of Pneumococcal Disease," *MMWR Morb Mortal Wkly Rep*, 1997, 46(RR-8):1-31.

- ◆ **Pneumococcal Vaccine** *see page 1138*
- ◆ **Pneumomist®** *see* Guaifenesin *on page 464*
- ◆ **Pneumovax® 23** *see* Pneumococcal Vaccine *on page 780*

- **Pnu-Imune® 23** *see* Pneumococcal Vaccine *on page 780*
- **Pod-Ben-25®** *see* Podophyllum Resin *on page 781*
- **Podocon-25®** *see* Podophyllum Resin *on page 781*
- **Podofilm® (Canada)** *see* Podophyllum Resin *on page 781*
- **Podofin®** *see* Podophyllum Resin *on page 781*

Podophyllum Resin (po DOF fil um REZ in)

Brand Names Pod-Ben-25®; Podocon-25®; Podofilm® (Canada); Podofin®

Therapeutic Category Keratolytic Agent

Generic Available Yes

Use Topical treatment of benign growths including external genital and perianal warts (condylomata acuminata), papillomas, fibroids

Pregnancy Risk Factor X

Contraindications Not to be used on birthmarks, moles, or warts with hair growth; cervical, urethral, oral warts; not to be used by diabetic patients or patients with poor circulation; pregnant women; do not apply to normal tissue

Warnings Avoid contact with the eyes as it can cause severe corneal damage; 25% solution should not be applied to or near mucous membranes; podophyllum resin has caused teratogenic effects (skin tags, polyneuritis, limb malformations, septal heart defects) and fetal death when used during pregnancy

Precautions Topical application to large areas or in excessive amounts for prolonged periods should be avoided

Adverse Reactions
Central nervous system: Confusion, lethargy, hallucinations, ataxia, apnea, agitation, seizures
Dermatologic: Pruritus, erythema, scarring
Gastrointestinal: Nausea, vomiting, abdominal pain, diarrhea
Hematologic: Leukopenia, thrombocytopenia
Hepatic: Hepatotoxicity
Local: Pain, local edema
Neuromuscular & skeletal: Peripheral neuropathy, weakness
Renal: Renal failure

Stability Protect from light; avoid exposure to excessive heat

Mechanism of Action Directly affects epithelial cell metabolism by arresting mitosis through binding to a protein subunit of spindle microtubules (tubulin)

Usual Dosage Children and Adults: Topical: 10% to 25% solution in compound benzoin tincture; use 1 drop at a time allowing drying between drops until area is covered; total volume should be limited to <0.5 mL to an area <10 cm² for genital or perianal warts or <2 cm² for vaginal warts per treatment session; therapy may be repeated once weekly for up to 4 applications for the treatment of genital or perianal warts; use 10% solution when applied to or near mucous membranes

Verrucae: 25% solution is applied directly to the wart; remove drug from area of application within 6 hours

Administration Topical: Shake well before using; apply drug to dry surface of affected area

Patient Information Notify physician if undue skin irritation develops

Nursing Implications Solution should be washed off within 1-4 hours for genital and perianal warts and within 1-2 hours for accessible meatal warts; use protective occlusive dressing around warts to prevent contact with unaffected skin

Dosage Forms Liquid, topical: 25% in benzoin (5 mL, 7.5 mL, 30 mL)

References
Goldfarb MT, Gupta AK, Gupta MA, et al, "Office Therapy for Human Papillomavirus Infection in Nongenital Sites," *Dermatol Clin*, 1991, 9(2):287-96.
"1993 Sexually Transmitted Diseases Treatment Guidelines," *MMWR Morb Mortal Wkly Rep*, 1993, 42(RR-14):1-102.

- **Point-Two®** *see* Fluoride *on page 427*
- **Polaramine®** *see* Chlorpheniramine *on page 214*
- **Poliovirus Vaccine, Live, Inactivated** *see page 1138*
- **Poliovirus Vaccine, Live, Trivalent, Oral** *see page 1138*
- **Polycillin®** *see* Ampicillin *on page 78*
- **Polycillin-N®** *see* Ampicillin *on page 78*
- **Polycitra®** *see* Citrate and Citric Acid *on page 231*
- **Polycitra K®** *see* Citrate and Citric Acid *on page 231*
- **Polycitra-LC®** *see* Citrate and Citric Acid *on page 231*

Polyethylene Glycol-Electrolyte Solution
(pol i ETH i leen GLY kol ee LEK troe lite soe LOO shun)

Brand Names Co-Lav®; Colovage®; CoLyte®; CoLyte®-Flavored; Go-Evac®; GoLYTELY®; Klean-Prep® (Canada); MiraLax™; NuLYTELY®; OCL®; Peglyte™ (Canada)

Synonyms Colonic Lavage Solution; Electrolyte Lavage Solution

Therapeutic Category Laxative, Bowel Evacuant; Laxative, Osmotic

Generic Available No

Use Bowel cleansing prior to GI examination; treatment of occasional constipation (MiraLax™)

Pregnancy Risk Factor C

Contraindications Gastrointestinal obstruction, gastric retention, bowel perforation, toxic colitis, megacolon

Warnings Do not add flavorings as additional ingredients before use

Precautions May interfere with barium coating of intestinal wall using the double contrast technique; use with caution in patients with ulcerative colitis; use with caution in patients with impaired gag reflex or those who are otherwise prone to regurgitation or aspiration during administration; treatment duration for occasional constipation should not exceed 2 weeks

Adverse Reactions
Dermatologic: Irritative perineal rashes
Endocrine & metabolic: Mild metabolic acidosis with prolonged irrigation periods, electrolyte disturbances
Gastrointestinal: Nausea, cramps, vomiting, abdominal distention, bloating

Drug Interactions Increased peristalsis may decrease absorption of oral medications given within 1 hour of beginning lavage solution

Mechanism of Action Induces catharsis by strong electrolyte and osmotic effects

Pharmacodynamics Onset of action: Bowel cleansing: Within 1-2 hours; constipation: 2-4 days

Usual Dosage
Bowel cleansing: Patient should fast at least 2 hours (preferably 3-4 hours) prior to ingestion:
Children: Oral, nasogastric: 25-40 mL/kg/hour until rectal effluent is clear (usually in 4-10 hours)
Adults:
Oral: Drink 240 mL (8 oz) every 10 minutes until 4 liters are consumed or the rectal effluent is clear
Nasogastric: 20-30 mL/minute (1.2-1.8 L/hour) until 4 liters are administered
Occasional constipation: Adults: Oral: 17 g (~1 heaping tablespoon) daily

Administration Oral: Add tap water to "fill-line" for reconstitution of powder for solution; no solid foods for 2 hours prior to initiation of therapy; rapid drinking is preferred to drinking small amounts continuously; chilled solution often more palatable; do not add flavorings as additional ingredients before use; MiraLax™ 17 g (dose may be measured using bottle cap) added to 8 oz of water

Monitoring Parameters Electrolytes, BUN, serum glucose, urine osmolality

Patient Information Chilled solution is often more palatable

Nursing Implications First bowel movement should occur in 1 hour

Dosage Forms Powder, for oral solution:
PEG 3350 236 g, sodium sulfate 22.74 g, sodium bicarbonate 6.74 g, sodium chloride 5.86 g and potassium chloride 2.97 g (2000 mL, 4000 mL, 4800 mL, 6000 mL)
MiraLax™: PEG 3350 14 oz (255 g), 27 oz (527 g)

References
Sondheimer JM, Sokol RJ, Taylor SF, et al, "Safety, Efficacy and Tolerance of Intestinal Lavage in Pediatric Patients Undergoing Diagnostic Colonoscopy," *J Pediatr*, 1991, 119(1):148-52.
Tuggle DW, Hoelzer DJ, Tunell WP, et al, "The Safety and Cost-Effectiveness of Polyethylene Glycol Electrolyte Solution Bowel: Preparation in Infants and Children," *J Pediatr Surg*, 1987, 22(6):513-5.

♦ **Polygam S/D®** *see* Immune Globulin, Intravenous *on page 510*
♦ **Polymox®** *see* Amoxicillin *on page 70*

Polymyxin B (pol i MIKS in bee)
Brand Names Aerosporin® Injection; Optimyxin® (Canada)

Available Salts Polymyxin B Sulfate

Therapeutic Category Antibiotic, Ophthalmic; Antibiotic, Urinary Irrigation; Antibiotic, Miscellaneous

Generic Available Yes

Use Topically for wound irrigation and bladder irrigation against *Pseudomonas aeruginosa*; used occasionally for gut decontamination. Parenteral use of polymyxin B has mainly been replaced by less toxic antibiotics. Reserved for life-threatening infections caused by organisms resistant to the preferred drugs; used as inhalation therapy for gram-negative respiratory infections resistant to preferred drugs; used intrathecally for meningeal infections due to susceptible organisms which are resistant to less toxic antibiotics

Pregnancy Risk Factor B

Contraindications Hypersensitivity to polymyxin or any component

Warnings Polymixin B can cause serious nephrotoxicity and or neurotoxicity; neurotoxic reactions may be manifested by irritability, weakness, drowsiness, ataxia, perioral paresthesia, numbness of the extremities and blurring of vision. These reactions are usually associated with high serum levels found in patients with impaired renal function or nephrotoxicity. Avoid concurrent or sequential use of other nephrotoxic and neurotoxic drugs, particularly bacitracin, kanamycin, streptomycin, paromomycin, colistin, tobramycin, neomycin, gentamicin, and amikacin. The drug's neurotoxicity can result in respiratory paralysis from neuromuscular blockade, especially when the drug is given soon after anesthesia or muscle relaxants. Polymyxin B sulfate is toxic when given parenterally; **avoid parenteral use whenever possible**.

Precautions Use with caution in patients with myasthenia gravis, patients receiving neuromuscular blocking agents or anesthetics, and in patients with impaired renal function; modify dosage in patients with renal impairment; **I.M. use is not recommended in infants and children due to severe pain at injection site**

Adverse Reactions
Cardiovascular: Facial flushing
Central nervous system: Drowsiness, ataxia, fever, dizziness
Dermatologic: Rash, urticaria
Endocrine & metabolic: Hypocalcemia, hyponatremia, hypokalemia, hypochloremia
Local: Pain at injection site, thrombophlebitis
Neuromuscular & skeletal: Neuromuscular blockade, paresthesia
Ocular: Diplopia
Renal: Nephrotoxicity (hematuria, proteinuria, azotemia)
Respiratory: Respiratory arrest
Miscellaneous: Hypersensitivity reactions

Drug Interactions Neuromuscular blocking agents, anesthetics (increase skeletal muscle relaxation); aminoglycosides, colistin, sodium citrate, parenteral quinidine

Stability Protect from light; incompatible with calcium, magnesium, cephalothin, chloramphenicol, heparin, penicillins; inactivated by acidic or alkaline solutions

Mechanism of Action Binds to phospholipids, alters permeability and damages the bacterial cytoplasmic membrane permitting leakage of intracellular constituents

Pharmacokinetics
Absorption: Well absorbed from the peritoneum; minimal absorption (<10%) from the GI tract (except in neonates), from mucous membranes or intact skin
Distribution: Widely distributed to body tissues in the liver, kidneys, heart, muscle; does not penetrate into CSF or synovial fluid; does not cross the placenta
Half-life: 4.5-6 hours, increased with reduced renal function
Time to peak serum concentration: I.M.: Within 2 hours
Elimination: Primarily as unchanged drug (>60%) in urine via glomerular filtration
Not removed by hemodialysis

Usual Dosage
Infants <2 years:
I.M.: 25,000-40,000 units/kg/day divided every 6 hours
I.V.: 15,000-45,000 units/kg/day by continuous I.V. infusion or divided every 12 hours
Intrathecal: 20,000 units once daily for 3-4 days or 25,000 units once every other day; continue 25,000 units once every other day for at least 2 weeks after cultures of the CSF are negative
Children ≥2 years and Adults:
I.M.: 25,000-30,000 units/kg/day divided every 6 hours
I.V.: 15,000-25,000 units/kg/day divided every 12 hours or by continuous infusion; total daily dose should not exceed 2,000,000 units/day
Bladder irrigation: Continuous irrigation of the urinary bladder for up to 10 days using 20 mg (equal to 200,000 units) added to 1 L of NS; usually no more than 1 L of irrigant is used per day unless urine flow rate is high; administration rate is adjusted to patient's urine output

(Continued)

Polymyxin B *(Continued)*

Topical irrigation or topical solution: 0.1% to 0.3% solution used to irrigate infected wounds; should not exceed 2 million units/day in adults

Gut sterilization: Oral: 100,000-200,000 units/kg/day divided every 6-8 hours

Ophthalmic: A concentration of 0.1% to 0.25% is administered as 1-3 drops every hour, then increasing the interval as response indicates

Inhalation: 2-2.5 mg/kg/day divided every 6 hours; final concentration for administration should not exceed 10 mg/mL

Intrathecal: 50,000 units once daily for 3-4 days, then reduce to once every other day for at least 2 weeks after cultures of the CSF are negative

Dosing adjustment in renal impairment:

Cl_{cr} 5-20 mL/minute: Administer 50% of usual daily dose divided every 12 hours

Cl_{cr} <5 mL/minute: Administer 15% of the usual daily dose divided every 12 hours

Administration Parenteral (avoid parenteral use whenever possible):

I.M.: Not recommended for routine use in infants and children because of the severe pain which occurs with I.M. injection; administer I.M. injections deep into the upper outer quadrant of the gluteal muscles at a final concentration of 250,000 units/mL

I.V.: Infuse drug slowly over 60-90 minutes or by continuous infusion at a concentration of 1000-1667 units/mL in D_5W

Intrathecal: Reconstitute vial with 10 mL NS without preservatives to provide a final concentration of 50,000 units/mL

Monitoring Parameters WBC, serum electrolytes, renal function tests, serum drug concentration, urine output

Reference Range Serum concentration >5 µg/mL are toxic in adults

Additional Information 1 mg = 10,000 units; neuromuscular blockade may be reversed with calcium chloride

Dosage Forms

Injection, as sulfate: 500,000 units (20 mL)

Powder for solution, ophthalmic, as sulfate: 500,000 units (20-50 mL diluent)

- ♦ **Polymyxin B and Bacitracin** *see* Bacitracin and Polymyxin B *on page 119*
- ♦ **Polymyxin B and Neomycin** *see* Neomycin and Polymyxin B *on page 678*
- ♦ **Polymyxin B, Neomycin, and Bacitracin** *see* Neomycin, Polymyxin B, and Bacitracin *on page 680*
- ♦ **Polymyxin B, Neomycin, and Prednisolone** *see* Neomycin, Polymyxin B, and Prednisolone *on page 680*
- ♦ **Polymyxin B, Neomycin, (Bacitracin), and Hydrocortisone** *see* Neomycin, (Bacitracin) Polymyxin B, and Hydrocortisone *on page 679*
- ♦ **Polymyxin B Sulfate** *see* Polymyxin B *on page 782*
- ♦ **Poly-Pred® Liquifilm®** *see* Neomycin, Polymyxin B, and Prednisolone *on page 680*
- ♦ **Polysporin® Ophthalmic** *see* Bacitracin and Polymyxin B *on page 119*
- ♦ **Polysporin® Topical** *see* Bacitracin and Polymyxin B *on page 119*
- ♦ **Polytar® [OTC]** *see* Coal Tar *on page 247*
- ♦ **Polytopic® (Canada)** *see* Bacitracin and Polymyxin B *on page 119*
- ♦ **Polytracin® (Canada)** *see* Bacitracin and Polymyxin B *on page 119*
- ♦ **Poly-Vi-Sol®** *see page 1034*
- ♦ **Pontocaine®** *see* Tetracaine *on page 907*

Poractant Alfa *(por AKT ant AL fa)*

Brand Names Curosurf®

Synonyms Porcine Lung Surfactant

Therapeutic Category Lung Surfactant

Generic Available No

Use Treatment of respiratory distress syndrome (RDS) in premature infants

Warnings Rapidly affects oxygenation and lung compliance and should be restricted to a highly supervised use in a clinical setting with immediate availability of clinicians experienced with intubation and ventilatory management of premature infants; if transient episodes of bradycardia and decreased oxygen saturation occur, discontinue the dosing procedure and initiate measures to alleviate the condition; produces rapid improvements in lung oxygenation and compliance that may require immediate reductions in ventilator settings and FiO_2.

Precautions Correction of acidosis, hypotension, anemia, hypoglycemia, and hypothermia is recommended prior to administration

Adverse Reactions
Cardiovascular: Transient bradycardia, hypotension
Local: Endotracheal tube blockage
Respiratory: Oxygen desaturation

Stability Store in refrigerator; protect from light; prior to administration, allow to slowly warm to room temperature; artificial warming methods should **not** be used; unused, unopened vials warmed to room temperature may be returned to the refrigerator within 24 hours of warming only once

Mechanism of Action Poractant alfa, an extract of natural porcine lung surfactant, replaces deficient or ineffective endogenous lung surfactant in neonates with respiratory distress syndrome (RDS); surfactant prevents the alveoli from collapsing during expiration by lowering surface tension between air and alveolar surfaces

Usual Dosage Neonates: Intratracheal: Initial: 2.5 mL/kg/dose (200 mg/kg/dose); may repeat 1.25 mL/kg/dose (100 mg/kg/dose) at 12-hour intervals for up to 2 additional doses; maximum total dose: 5 mL/kg

Administration Intratracheal: For intratracheal administration only; suction infant prior to administration; inspect solution to verify complete mixing of the suspension; do not shake; gently turn vial upside-down to obtain uniform suspension; administer intratracheally by instillation through a 5-French end-hole catheter inserted into the infant's endotracheal tube; each dose should be administered as two aliquots, with each aliquot administered into one of the two main bronchi by positioning the infant with either the right or left side dependent

Monitoring Parameters Continuous heart rate and transcutaneous O_2 saturation should be monitored during administration; frequent ABG sampling is necessary to prevent postdosing hyperoxia and hypocarbia

Dosage Forms Suspension: 120 mg (1.5 mL); 240 mg (3 mL)

♦ **Porcine Lung Surfactant** *see* Poractant Alfa *on page 784*

♦ **Pork NPH** *see* Insulin Preparations *on page 518*

♦ **Pork Regular Iletin® II** *see* Insulin Preparations *on page 518*

♦ **Posterisan® [OTC]** *see* Hemorrhoidal Preparations *on page 470*

♦ **Posture® [OTC]** *see* Calcium Supplements *on page 157*

♦ **Potasalan®** *see* Potassium Supplements *on page 786*

♦ **Potassium Acetate** *see* Potassium Supplements *on page 786*

♦ **Potassium Acid Phosphate** *see* Phosphate Supplements *on page 765*

♦ **Potassium Bicarbonate** *see* Potassium Supplements *on page 786*

♦ **Potassium Chloride** *see* Potassium Supplements *on page 786*

♦ **Potassium Citrate** *see* Citrate and Citric Acid *on page 231*

♦ **Potassium Citrate** *see* Potassium Supplements *on page 786*

♦ **Potassium Gluconate** *see* Potassium Supplements *on page 786*

Potassium Iodide (poe TASS ee um EYE oh dide)
Related Information
Carbohydrate and Alcohol Content of Liquid Medications for Use in Patients Receiving Ketogenic Diets *on page 1228*

Brand Names Pima®; Potassium Iodide Enseals®; SSKI®; Thyro-Block®

Synonyms KI; Lugol's Solution; Strong Iodine Solution

Therapeutic Category Antithyroid Agent; Expectorant

Generic Available Yes

Use To facilitate bronchial drainage and cough; to reduce thyroid vascularity prior to thyroidectomy and management of thyrotoxic crisis; block thyroidal uptake of radioactive isotopes of iodine in a radiation emergency; treatment of cutaneous sporotrichosis

Pregnancy Risk Factor D

Contraindications Hypersensitivity to iodides; hyperkalemia, tuberculosis, acute bronchitis, hypothyroidism, Addison's disease, acute dehydration, heat cramps

Warnings Some commercially available products contain sulfites, avoid use in sensitive patients; prolonged use can lead to hypothyroidism

Precautions Use with caution in patients with cystic fibrosis (may have exaggerated susceptibility to goitrogenic effects); may cause flare-up of acne; use with caution in patients with a history of thyroid disease and in patients with cardiac disease or renal failure

Adverse Reactions
Cardiovascular: Arrhythmia
Central nervous system: Fever, headache, confusion
Dermatologic: Urticaria, acne, angioedema, cutaneous hemorrhage
(Continued)

Potassium Iodide *(Continued)*

Endocrine & metabolic: Goiter with hypothyroidism, thyroid adenoma, acute parotitis

Gastrointestinal: Metallic taste, GI upset, GI bleeding, soreness of teeth and gums, cutaneous and mucosal hemorrhage

Hematologic: Eosinophilia

Neuromuscular & skeletal: Arthralgia, numbness, paresthesia

Respiratory: Rhinitis

Miscellaneous: Lymph node enlargement

Drug Interactions Potassium-containing medications, ACE inhibitors, and potassium-sparing diuretics may increase serum potassium; lithium and antithyroid drugs may potentiate hypothyroid and goitrogenic effects

Stability Store at room temperature; cold temperatures result in crystallization; warming with shaking will redissolve crystals

Mechanism of Action Reduces viscosity of mucus by increasing respiratory tract secretions; inhibits the release and synthesis of thyroid hormone

Pharmacodynamics Antithyroid effects:

Onset of action: 24-48 hours

Peak effect: 10-15 days after continuous therapy

Duration: May persist up to 6 weeks

Usual Dosage Oral:

Expectorant:

Children: 60-250 mg 4 times/day; maximum single dose: 500 mg

Adults: 300-650 mg 3-4 times/day

Preoperative thyroidectomy: Children and Adults: Given 10-14 days before surgery: 50-250 mg (1-5 drops, 1 g/mL SSKI®) 3 times/day **or** 0.1-0.3 mL (3-5 drops) strong iodine (Lugol's solution) 3 times/day

Graves' disease in neonates: 1 drop strong iodine (Lugol's solution) 3 times/day

Thyrotoxic crisis:

Infants <1 year: 150-250 mg (3-5 drops, 1 g/mL SSKI®) 3 times/day

Children and Adults: 300-500 mg (6-10 drops 1 g/mL SSKI®) 3 times/day **or** 1 mL strong iodine (Lugol's solution) 3 times/day

Cutaneous Sporotrichosis: Oral:

Children: 250-500 mg (5-10 drops, 1 g/mL SSKI®) 3 times/day; increase gradually to a maximum of 1.25-2 g (25-40 drops SSKI®)

Adults: 250-500 mg (5-10 drops, 1 g/mL SSKI®) 3 times/day; increase gradually to a maximum of 2-2.5 g (40-50 drops SSKI®)

Note:Therapy is continued at the maximum tolerated dosage until the cutaneous lesions have resolved, usually 6-12 weeks

Administration Oral: Administer after meals with food or milk or dilute with a large quantity of water, fruit juice, milk, or broth

Monitoring Parameters Thyroid function tests

Additional Information 10 drops SSKI® = potassium iodide 500 mg

Dosage Forms

Solution, oral:

SSKI®: 1 g/mL (30 mL, 240 mL)

Lugol's Solution, strong iodine: Potassium iodide 100 mg and iodine 50 mg per mL (120 mL, 473 mL, 4000 mL)

Syrup: 325 mg/5 mL (473 mL, 4000 mL)

Tablet: 130 mg

♦ **Potassium Iodide Enseals®** *see* Potassium Iodide *on page 785*

♦ **Potassium Phosphate** *see* Phosphate Supplements *on page 765*

♦ **Potassium Phosphate and Sodium Phosphate** *see* Phosphate Supplements *on page 765*

Potassium Supplements *(poe TASS ee um SUP la ments)*

Related Information

Carbohydrate and Alcohol Content of Liquid Medications for Use in Patients Receiving Ketogenic Diets *on page 1228*

Brand Names Cena-K®; Gen-K®; K+® 8; K+® 10; Kaochlor®; Kaochlor-Eff; Kaon-Cl®; Kato®; Kay Ciel®; Kaylixir®; K+ Care®; K+ Care® ET; K-Dur®; K-Electrolyte®; K-G® Elixir; K-Gen®; K-Lease®; K-Lor™; Klor-Con® 10; Klor-Con® 20; Klor-Con/25®; Klorvess®; Klorvess Klyte/Cl; Klotrix®; K-lyte®; K-Lyte/Cl®; K-lyte DS; K-Norm®; Kolyum®; K-Tab®; Micro-K®; Micro-K® LS; Potasalan®; Rum-K®; S-F Kaon®; Slow-K®; Ten-K®; Tri-K®; Trikates®; Twin-K®

Available Salts Potassium Acetate; Potassium Bicarbonate; Potassium Chloride; Potassium Citrate; Potassium Gluconate

Synonyms KCl (Potassium Chloride)

Therapeutic Category Electrolyte Supplement, Oral; Electrolyte Supplement, Parenteral; Potassium Salt

Generic Available Yes

Use Potassium deficiency; treatment or prevention of hypokalemia

Pregnancy Risk Factor C

Contraindications Severe renal impairment, untreated Addison's disease, heat cramps, hyperkalemia, severe tissue trauma; solid oral dosage forms are contraindicated in patients in whom there is a structural, pathological, and/or pharmacologic cause for delay or arrest in passage through the GI tract; an oral liquid potassium preparation should be used in patients with esophageal compression or delayed gastric emptying time

Warnings Potassium injections should be administered only in patients with adequate urine flow; injection must be diluted before I.V. use and infused slowly (see Administration); some oral products contain the dye tartrazine (avoid use in sensitive individuals)

Precautions Use with caution in patients with cardiac disease, patients receiving potassium-sparing drugs; patients must be on a cardiac monitor during intermittent infusions

Adverse Reactions

Cardiovascular (with rapid I.V. administration): Arrhythmias and cardiac arrest, heart block, hypotension

Central nervous system: Mental confusion

Endocrine & metabolic: Hyperkalemia, metabolic alkalosis (acetate salt)

Gastrointestinal (with oral administration): Nausea, vomiting, diarrhea, abdominal pain, GI lesions, flatulence

Local: Pain at the site of injection, phlebitis

Neuromuscular & skeletal: Muscle weakness, paresthesia, flaccid paralysis

Drug Interactions Potassium-sparing diuretics, salt substitutes, captopril, and enalapril may result in increased serum potassium

Mechanism of Action Potassium is the major cation of intracellular fluid and is essential for the conduction of nerve impulses in heart, brain, and skeletal muscle; contraction of cardiac, skeletal, and smooth muscles; and maintenance of normal renal function, acid-base balance (acetate form), carbohydrate metabolism, and gastric secretion

Pharmacokinetics

Absorption: Well from upper GI tract; enters cells via active transport from extracellular fluid

Elimination: Largely by the kidneys

Usual Dosage I.V. doses should be incorporated into the patient's maintenance I.V. fluids; intermittent I.V. potassium administration should be reserved for severe depletion situations and requires EKG monitoring. Doses listed as mEq of **potassium**. When using microencapsulated or wax matrix formulations, use no more than 20 mEq as a single dose.

Normal daily requirement: Oral, I.V.:
Neonates and Infants: 2-6 mEq/kg/day
Children: 2-3 mEq/kg/day
Adults: 40-80 mEq/day

Prevention of hypokalemia during diuretic therapy: Oral:
Neonates, Infants, and Children: 1-2 mEq/kg/day in 1-2 divided doses
Adults: 20-40 mEq/day in 1-2 divided doses

Treatment of hypokalemia: Oral, I.V.:
Neonates, Infants, and Children: 2-5 mEq/kg/day in divided doses
Adults: 40-100 mEq/day in divided doses

Treatment of hypokalemia: I.V. intermittent infusion (must be diluted prior to administration):
Neonates, Infants, and Children: 0.5-1 mEq/kg/dose (maximum dose: 30 mEq) to infuse at 0.3-0.5 mEq/kg/hour (maximum dose: 1 mEq/kg/hour)
Adults: 10-20 mEq/dose (maximum dose: 40 mEq/dose) to infuse over 2-3 hours (maximum dose: 40 mEq over 1 hour)

Administration

Oral: Sustained release and wax matrix tablets should be swallowed whole, do not crush or chew; effervescent tablets must be dissolved in water before use; administer with food; granules can be diluted or dissolved in water or juice; do not administer liquid full strength, must be diluted in 2-6 parts of water or juice

Parenteral: Potassium must be diluted prior to parenteral administration; maximum recommended concentration (peripheral line): 80 mEq/L; maximum recommended concentration (central line): 150 mEq/L or 15 mEq/100 mL; in severely

(Continued)

Potassium Supplements *(Continued)*

fluid-restricted patients (with central lines): 200 mEq/L or 20 mEq/100 mL has been used; maximum rate of infusion, see Usual Dosage, I.V. intermittent infusion

Monitoring Parameters Serum potassium, glucose, chloride, pH, urine output (if indicated), cardiac monitor (if intermittent I.V. infusion or potassium I.V. infusion rates >0.25 mEq/kg/hour)

Dosage Forms

Potassium acetate: Injection: 2 mEq/mL

Potassium chloride:

Capsule, controlled release:

Micro-K®: 600 mg [8 mEq]

K-Lease®, K-Norm®, Micro-K® 10: 750 mg [10 mEq]

Injection, concentrate: 2 mEq/mL (5 mL, 10 mL, 20 mL, 50 mL, 100 mL)

Liquid:

Cena-K®, Kaochlor®, Kaochlor® SF, Kay Ciel®, Klorvess®, Potasalan®: 20 mEq/15 mL 10% (118 mL, 480 mL, 3840 mL)

Rum-K®: 30 mEq/15 mL 15% (480 mL, 3840 mL)

Cena-K®, Kaon-Cl®: 40 mEq/15 mL 20% (480 mL, 3840 mL)

Powder:

K + Care®: 15 mEq per packet

Gen-K®, Kato®, Kay Ciel®, K + Care®, K-Lor™, Klor-Con®, Micro-K® LS: 20 mEq per packet

K + Care®, Klor-Con/25®, K-Lyte/Cl®: 25 mEq per packet

Tablet, controlled release:

Kaon-Cl®: 500 mg [6.7 mEq]

Klor-Con® 8, K+® 8, Slow-K®: 600 mg [8 mEq]

K+® 10, Kaon-Cl® 10, K-Dur® 10, Klor-Con® 10, Klotrix®, K-Tab®, Ten-K®: 750 mg [10 mEq]

K-Dur® 20, Klor-Con® 20: 1500 mg [20 mEq]

Tablet, extended release: 750 mg [10 mEq]

Potassium gluconate:

Elixir: 20 mEq/15 mL (5 mL, 10 mL, 118 mL, 480 mL, 4000 mL) (K-G® Elixir, Kaon® Elixir)

Tablet: 500 mg, 595 mg

Potassium bicarbonate: Tablet for oral solution: 6.5 mEq potassium, 25 mEq bicarbonate (K+ Care®, K-Electrolyte®, K-Gen®, K-Lyte, Klor-Con/EF®); 25 mEq potassium (K+Care ET)

Potassium bicarbonate and potassium chloride:

Granules for solution: 20 mEq potassium per packet

Tablets for solution: 20 mEq potassium (Klorvess®), 25 mEq potassium (K-Lyte/CL), 50 mEq potassium (K-Lyte/CL® 50)

Potassium bicarbonate and potassium citrate: Tablet for solution: 50 mEq potassium (K-Lyte® DS)

Potassium chloride and potassium gluconate: Solution: 6.7 mEq potassium per 5 mL (Kolyum®)

Potassium citrate and potassium gluconate: Solution: 6.7 mEq potassium per 5 mL (Twin-K®)

Potassium bicarbonate, potassium chloride, and potassium citrate: Tablet for solution: 20 mEq potassium (Kaochlor-Eff®)

Potassium acetate, potassium bicarbonate, and potassium citrate: Solution: 15 mEq/5 mL (Tri-K®, Trikates®)

References

Hamill RJ, Robinson LM, Wexler HR, et al, "Efficacy and Safety of Potassium Infusion Therapy in Hypokalemic Critically Ill Patients," *Crit Care Med*, 1991, 19(5):694-9.

Khilnani P, "Electrolyte Abnormalities in Critically Ill Children," *Crit Care Med*, 1992, 20(2):241-50.

♦ **PPA** *see* Phenylpropanolamine *on page 761*

♦ **PPL** *see* Benzylpenicilloyl-polylysine *on page 127*

Pralidoxime *(pra li DOKS eem)*

Brand Names Protopam®

Available Salts Pralidoxime Chloride

Synonyms 2-PAM; 2-Pyridine Aldoxime Methochloride

Therapeutic Category Antidote, Anticholinesterase; Antidote, Organophosphate Poisoning

Generic Available No

Use Reverse muscle paralysis associated with toxic exposure to organophosphate anticholinesterase pesticides and chemicals; control of overdosage by anticholinesterase drugs used to treat myasthenia gravis (neostigmine, pyridostigmine)

Pregnancy Risk Factor C

Contraindications Hypersensitivity to pralidoxime or any component; poisonings due to phosphorus, inorganic phosphates, or organic phosphates without anticholinesterase activity

Warnings Not indicated as an antidote for carbamate classes of pesticides and may increase toxicity of carbaryl

Precautions Use with caution in patients with myasthenia gravis; dosage modification required in patients with impaired renal function; use with caution in patients receiving theophylline, succinylcholine, phenothiazines, respiratory depressants (eg, narcotic, barbiturates)

Adverse Reactions
Cardiovascular: Tachycardia (after rapid I.V. infusion), hypertension
Central nervous system: Dizziness, headache, drowsiness
Dermatologic: Rash
Gastrointestinal: Nausea
Local: Pain at injection site after I.M. use
Neuromuscular & skeletal: Muscular weakness, muscle rigidity (after rapid I.V. infusion), transient elevated CPK
Ocular: Blurred vision, diplopia
Respiratory: Hyperventilation, laryngospasm (after rapid I.V. administration)

Drug Interactions Barbiturates potentiated by anticholinesterases

Mechanism of Action Reactivates cholinesterase that had been inactivated by phosphorylation as a result of exposure to organophosphate pesticides; removes the phosphoryl group from the active site of the inactivated enzyme

Pharmacokinetics
Half-life: 0.8-2.7 hours
Time to peak concentration: I.V.: Within 5-15 minutes
Elimination: 80% to 90% excreted unchanged in urine 12 hours after administration

Usual Dosage
Organophosphate poisoning:
Children: I.M., I.V. (use in conjunction with atropine): 20-50 mg/kg/dose; repeat in 1-2 hours if muscle weakness has not been relieved, then at 10- to 12-hour intervals if cholinergic signs recur
Adults:
I.M., I.V. (use in conjunction with atropine): 1-2 g; repeat in 1-2 hours if muscle weakness has not been relieved, then at 10- to 12-hour intervals if cholinergic signs recur
Treatment of toxicity from medications used to treat myasthenia gravis: Adults: I.V.: 1-2 g followed by increments of 250 mg every 5 minutes

Administration Parenteral: Reconstitute with 20 mL sterile water (preservative free) resulting in 50 mg/mL solution; dilute in NS to 20 mg/mL and infuse over 15-30 minutes; if a more rapid onset of effect is desired or in a fluid-restricted situation, the maximum concentration is 50 mg/mL; the maximum rate of infusion is over 5 minutes and not exceeding 200 mg/minute

Monitoring Parameters Heart rate, respiratory rate, blood pressure, continuous EKG

Dosage Forms
Injection: 20 mL vial containing 1 g each pralidoxime chloride with one 20 mL ampul diluent, disposable syringe, needle, and alcohol swab
Injection, as chloride: 300 mg/mL (2 mL)

♦ **Pralidoxime Chloride** *see* Pralidoxime *on page 788*

Praziquantel (pray zi KWON tel)

Brand Names Biltricide®

Therapeutic Category Anthelmintic

Generic Available No

Use Treatment of all stages of schistosomiasis caused by *Schistosoma* species pathogenic to humans; also active in the treatment of clonorchiasis, opisthorchiasis, cysticercosis, and many intestinal tapeworm and trematode infections

Pregnancy Risk Factor B

Contraindications Ocular cysticercosis, spinal cysticercosis; hypersensitivity to praziquantel or any component

Precautions Use with caution in patients with severe hepatic disease and in patients with a history of seizures
(Continued)

Praziquantel *(Continued)*

Adverse Reactions
Central nervous system: Dizziness, drowsiness, fever, headache, vertigo, malaise, CSF reaction syndrome in patients being treated for neurocysticercosis (syndrome includes headache, seizures, intracranial hypertension, increased CSF protein concentrations, hyperthermia)

Dermatologic: Urticarial rash, itching

Gastrointestinal: Abdominal pain, nausea, vomiting, anorexia, diarrhea

Hematologic: Eosinophilia

Miscellaneous: Diaphoresis

Drug Interactions
Alcohol may increase CNS depression; phenytoin and carbamazepine may induce metabolism of praziquantel and decrease its activity; cimetidine increases praziquantel serum concentrations

Mechanism of Action
Increases the cell permeability to calcium in schistosomes; causes strong contractions and paralysis of worm musculature leading to detachment of suckers from the blood vessel walls and to dislodgment

Pharmacokinetics
Absorption: Oral: ~80%

Distribution: CSF concentration is 14% to 20% of plasma concentration; excreted in breast milk

Protein binding: ~80%

Metabolism: Extensive first-pass effect; metabolized by the liver to hydroxylated and conjugated metabolites

Half-life: 0.8-1.5 hours

Metabolites: 4.5 hours

Time to peak serum concentration: Within 1-3 hours

Elimination: Praziquantel and metabolites excreted mainly in urine (99% as metabolites)

Usual Dosage
Children and Adults: Oral:

Schistosomiasis:

S. mansoni, S. haematobium: 20 mg/kg/dose twice daily for 1 day

S. japonicum, S. mekongi: 20 mg/kg/dose 3 times/day for 1 day at 4- to 6-hour intervals

Flukes:

Liver, intestine: 75 mg/kg/day divided every 8 hours for 1 day

Lung: 75 mg/kg/day divided every 8 hours for 2 days

Nanophyetus salmincola: 60 mg/kg/day divided every 8 hours for 1 day

Cysticercosis: 50 mg/kg/day divided every 8 hours for 15 days (adjunctive therapy with dexamethasone is recommended for patients with numerous cysts and for those in whom neurologic symptoms or intracranial hypertension develops); for neurocysticercosis, steroids should be administered **prior** to starting praziquantel

Tapeworms: 5-10 mg/kg as a single dose (25 mg/kg for *H. nana*)

Administration
Oral: Administer with food; tablets can be halved or quartered; patient should not chew tablets due to bitter taste

Patient Information
Avoid alcohol (increased CNS depression); may cause drowsiness and impair ability to perform activities requiring mental alertness or physical coordination

Dosage Forms
Tablet, tri-scored: 600 mg

References
King CH and Mahmoud AA, "Drug Five Years Later: Praziquantel," *Ann Intern Med,* 1989, 110(4):290-6.

Liu LX and Weller PF, "Antiparasitic Drug," *N Engl J Med,* 1996, 334(18):1178-84.

Prazosin *(PRA zoe sin)*

Related Information
Overdose and Toxicology *on page 1191*

Brand Names
Apo®-Prazo (Canada); Minipress®; Novo-Prazin® (Canada); Nu-Prazo® (Canada)

Available Salts
Prazosin Hydrochloride

Synonyms
Furazosin

Therapeutic Category
Alpha-Adrenergic Blocking Agent, Oral; Antihypertensive Agent; Vasodilator

Generic Available
Yes

Use
Hypertension, severe CHF (in conjunction with diuretics and cardiac glycosides)

Pregnancy Risk Factor
C

Contraindications
Hypersensitivity to prazosin or any component

Precautions
Marked orthostatic hypotension, syncope, and loss of consciousness may occur with first dose ("first dose phenomenon"). This reaction is more likely to

occur in patients receiving beta-blockers, diuretics, low sodium diets or larger first doses (ie, >1 mg/dose in adults); avoid rapid increase in dose; use with caution in patients with renal impairment.

Adverse Reactions
Cardiovascular: Orthostatic hypotension, syncope, palpitations, tachycardia, edema
Central nervous system: Dizziness, lightheadedness, nightmares, drowsiness, headache, hypothermia
Dermatologic: Rash
Endocrine & metabolic: Fluid retention, sexual dysfunction
Gastrointestinal: Nausea, xerostomia
Genitourinary: Urinary frequency
Neuromuscular & skeletal: Weakness
Respiratory: Nasal congestion

Drug Interactions Diuretics and antihypertensive medications (especially beta-blockers) may increase prazosin's hypotensive effect

Food Interactions Avoid natural licorice (causes sodium and water retention and increases potassium loss); food has variable effects on absorption

Mechanism of Action Competitively inhibits postsynaptic alpha-adrenergic receptors which results in vasodilation of veins and arterioles and a decrease in total peripheral resistance and blood pressure

Pharmacodynamics Hypotensive effect:
Onset of action: Within 2 hours
Maximum decrease: 2-4 hours
Duration: 10-24 hours

Pharmacokinetics
Distribution: V_d: 0.5 L/kg (hypertensive adults)
Protein-binding: 92% to 97%
Metabolism: Extensive in the liver, metabolites may be active
Bioavailability, oral: 43% to 82%
Half-life, adults: 2-4 hours, increased half-life with CHF
Elimination: 6% to 10% excreted renally as unchanged drug

Usual Dosage Oral:
Children: Initial: 5 mcg/kg/dose (to assess hypotensive effects); usual dosing interval every 6 hours; increase dosage gradually up to 25 mcg/kg/dose every 6 hours; maximum daily dose: 15 mg or 0.4 mg/kg/day (400 mcg/kg/day); may be divided in 2 or 3 doses/day for treatment of hypertension
Adults: Initial: 1 mg/dose 2-3 times/day; usual maintenance dose: 3-15 mg/day in divided doses 2-4 times/day; maximum daily dose: 20 mg

Administration Oral: Administer in a consistent manner with respect to meals

Monitoring Parameters Blood pressure (standing and sitting or supine)

Patient Information Avoid alcohol; rise slowly from sitting or lying position; may cause dizziness

Nursing Implications Be aware of "first-dose phenomenon" (see Precautions); syncope may occur usually within 90 minutes of initial dose

Dosage Forms Capsule, as hydrochloride: 1 mg, 2 mg, 5 mg

References
Friedman WF and George BL, "New Concepts and Drugs in the Treatment of Congestive Heart Failure," *Pediatr Clin North Am*, 1984, 31(6):1197-227.
Sinaiko AR, "Pharmacologic Management of Childhood Hypertension," *Pediatr Clin North Am*, 1993, 40(1):195-212.

♦ **Prazosin Hydrochloride** see Prazosin on page 790
♦ **Predalone® 50 Injection** see Prednisolone on page 791
♦ **Pred Forte® Ophthalmic** see Prednisolone on page 791
♦ **Pred-G®** see Prednisolone and Gentamicin on page 793
♦ **Predicort-50®** see Prednisolone on page 791
♦ **Pred Mild® Ophthalmic** see Prednisolone on page 791
♦ **Prednicen-M®** see Prednisone on page 794

Prednisolone (pred NIS oh lone)

Related Information
Asthma Guidelines on page 1178
Carbohydrate and Alcohol Content of Liquid Medications for Use in Patients Receiving Ketogenic Diets on page 1228
Corticosteroids Comparison, Systemic on page 1032

Brand Names AK-Pred® Ophthalmic; Delta-Cortef® Oral; Econopred® Ophthalmic; Econopred® Plus Ophthalmic; Inflamase® Forte Ophthalmic; Inflamase® Mild Ophthalmic; Key-Pred® Injection; Key-Pred-SP® Injection; Metreton® Ophthalmic; (Continued)

Prednisolone *(Continued)*

Novo-Prednisolone® (Canada); Ophtho-tate® (Canada); Pediapred® Oral; Predalone® 50 Injection; Pred Forte® Ophthalmic; Predicort-50®; Pred Mild® Ophthalmic; Prednisol® TBA Injection; Prelone® Oral

Available Salts Prednisolone Acetate; Prednisolone Sodium Phosphate; Prednisolone Tebutate

Synonyms Deltahydrocortisone; Metacortandralone

Therapeutic Category Adrenal Corticosteroid; Antiasthmatic; Anti-inflammatory Agent; Anti-inflammatory Agent, Ophthalmic; Corticosteroid, Ophthalmic; Corticosteroid, Systemic; Glucocorticoid

Generic Available Yes

Use Treatment of endocrine disorders, rheumatic disorders, collagen diseases, dermatologic diseases, allergic states, ophthalmic diseases, respiratory diseases, hematologic disorders, neoplastic diseases, edematous states, and gastrointestinal diseases

Ophthalmic: Treatment of palpebral and bulbar conjunctivitis; corneal injury from chemical, radiation, thermal burns, or foreign body penetration

Pregnancy Risk Factor C

Contraindications Acute superficial herpes simplex keratitis; systemic fungal infections; varicella; hypersensitivity to prednisolone or any component

Warnings May retard bone growth

Precautions Use with caution in patients with hypothyroidism, cirrhosis, hypertension, CHF, ulcerative colitis, thromboembolic disorders

Adverse Reactions

Cardiovascular: Edema, hypertension

Central nervous system: Vertigo, seizures, psychoses, pseudotumor cerebri, headache

Dermatologic: Acne, skin atrophy

Endocrine & metabolic: Cushing's syndrome, pituitary-adrenal axis suppression, growth suppression, glucose intolerance, hypokalemia, alkalosis

Gastrointestinal: Peptic ulcer, nausea, vomiting

Neuromuscular & skeletal: Muscle weakness, osteoporosis, fractures

Ocular: Cataracts, glaucoma

Drug Interactions Cytochrome P-450 isoenzyme CYP3A3/4 substrate and inducer Barbiturates, phenytoin, rifampin, salicylates, toxoids, NSAIDs, diuretics (potassium depleting); caffeine and alcohol may increase risk for GI ulcer; live virus vaccines (increase risk of viral infection); vaccines may have decreased effects

Food Interactions Systemic use of corticosteroids may require a diet with increased potassium, vitamins A, B_6, C, D, folate, calcium, zinc, and phosphorus and decreased sodium

Stability May dilute sodium phosphate salt in dextrose or saline solutions for I.V. administration

Mechanism of Action Decreases inflammation by suppression of migration of polymorphonuclear leukocytes and reversal of increased capillary permeability; suppresses the immune system by reducing activity and volume of the lymphatic system

Pharmacokinetics

Absorption: Oral: Well absorbed

Protein binding: 70% to 90% (concentration dependent)

Metabolism: Primarily in the liver, but also metabolized in most tissues, to inactive compounds

Half-life (serum): Adults: 2-4 hours

Elimination: In urine, principally as glucuronide and sulfate-conjugated metabolites

Usual Dosage Dose depends upon condition being treated and response of patient; dosage for infants and children should be based on disease severity and patient response rather than by rigid adherence to dosage guidelines by age, weight, or body surface area. Consider alternate day therapy for long-term therapy. Discontinuation of long-term therapy requires gradual withdrawal by tapering the dose.

Children:

Acute asthma:

Oral: 1-2 mg/kg/day in divided doses 1-2 times/day for 3-5 days

I.V.: 2-4 mg/kg/day divided 3-4 times/day

Anti-inflammatory or immunosuppressive dose: Oral, I.V.: 0.1-2 mg/kg/day in divided doses 1-4 times/day

Nephrotic syndrome: Oral: First 3 episodes: Initial: 2 mg/kg/day or 60 mg/m²/day given every day (maximum dose: 80 mg/day) until urine is protein free for 3 consecutive days (maximum dose: 28 days); followed by 1-1.5 mg/kg/dose or 40 mg/m²/dose given every other day for 4 weeks

Frequent relapses (long-term maintenance dose): 0.5-1 mg/kg/dose given every other day for 3-6 months

Children and Adults: Ophthalmic suspension: Instill 1-2 drops into conjunctival sac every hour during day, every 2 hours at night until favorable response is obtained, then use 1 drop every 4 hours

Adults: Oral, I.V.: 5-60 mg/day

Administration

Oral: Administer after meals or with food or milk to decrease GI upset

Ophthalmic: Shake suspension well before use; instill drops into affected eye(s); avoid contact of container tip with skin or eye; apply finger pressure to lacrimal sac during and for 1-2 minutes after instillation to decrease risk of absorption and systemic effects

Parenteral: I.V. (**sodium phosphate salt only**): Administer via I.V. infusion; do not give acetate or tebutate salts I.V.

Monitoring Parameters Blood pressure, weight, electrolytes, serum glucose; children's height and growth

Test Interactions Skin tests

Patient Information Avoid alcohol; limit caffeine; do not decrease dose or discontinue without physician's approval

Dosage Forms

Prednisolone acetate:

Injection: 25 mg/mL (10 mL, 30 mL); 50 mg/mL (10 mL, 30 mL)

Key-Pred® 25: 25 mg/mL (10 mL, 30 mL)

Key-Pred® 50, Predalone 50, Predcor-50®, Predicort-50®: 50 mg/mL (10 mL, 30 mL)

Suspension, ophthalmic: 0.125% (5 mL, 10 mL)

Pred Mild®: 0.12% (5 mL, 10 mL)

Econopred®: 0.125% (5 mL, 10 mL)

Econopred® Plus, Pred Forte®: 1% (1 mL, 5 mL, 10 mL, 15 mL)

Prednisolone base:

Syrup (cherry flavor)(Prelone®): 15 mg/5 mL (240 mL)

Tablet (Delta-Cortef®): 5 mg

Prednisolone sodium phosphate:

Injection (Key-Pred-SP®): 20 mg/mL (2 mL, 5 mL, 10 mL)

Liquid, oral (raspberry flavor)(Pediapred®): 5 mg/5 mL (120 mL)

Solution, ophthalmic: 1% (5 mL, 15 mL)

AK-Pred®, Inflamase® Mild: 0.125% (5 mL, 10 mL, 15 mL)

AK-Pred®, Inflamase® Forte: 1% (5 mL, 10 mL, 15 mL)

Prednisolone tebutate:

Injection (Predalone® T.B.A., Prednisol®): 20 mg/mL (1 mL, 5 mL, 10 mL)

References

Report of a Workshop by the British Association for Paediatric Nephrology and Research Unit, Royal College of Physicians, "Consensus Statement on Management and Audit Potential for Steroid Responsive Nephrotic Syndrome," *Arch Dis Child*, 1994, 70(2):151-7.

♦ **Prednisolone Acetate** *see* Prednisolone *on page 791*

♦ **Prednisolone Acetate and Gentamicin Sulfate** *see* Prednisolone and Gentamicin *on page 793*

Prednisolone and Gentamicin (pred NIS oh lone & jen ta MYE sin)

Brand Names Pred-G®

Available Salts Prednisolone Acetate and Gentamicin Sulfate

Synonyms Gentamicin and Prednisolone

Therapeutic Category Antibiotic, Ophthalmic; Corticosteroid, Ophthalmic

Generic Available Yes

Use Treatment of steroid responsive inflammatory conditions and superficial ocular infections due to strains of microorganisms susceptible to gentamicin such as *Staphylococcus*, *E. coli*, *H. influenzae*, *Klebsiella*, *Neisseria*, *Pseudomonas*, *Proteus*, and *Serratia* species

Pregnancy Risk Factor C

Contraindications Hypersensitivity to prednisolone, gentamicin, or any component; dendritic keratitis, fungal diseases, vaccinia, varicella, most other viral infections, and mycobacterial infection of the eye. The product's use is contraindicated after uncomplicated removal of a corneal foreign body.

(Continued)

Prednisolone and Gentamicin *(Continued)*

Warnings Prolonged use may result in glaucoma, damage to the optic nerve, defects in visual acuity, posterior subcapsular cataract formation, and secondary ocular infections

Adverse Reactions

Local: Burning, stinging, redness

Ocular: Elevation of intraocular pressure, glaucoma, infrequent optic nerve damage, posterior subcapsular cataract formation, superficial punctate keratitis, increased lacrimation

Miscellaneous: Development of secondary infection, allergic sensitization, delayed wound healing

Mechanism of Action See individual monographs for Prednisolone *on page 791* and Gentamicin *on page 452*

Usual Dosage Children and Adults: Ophthalmic: Instill 1 drop 2-4 times/day; during the initial 24-48 hours, the dosing frequency may be increased if necessary, up to 1 drop every hour; or small amount (½" ribbon) of ointment can be applied into the conjunctival sac 1-3 times/day

Administration Suspension: Shake well before using; instill drop into affected eye; avoid contacting bottle tip with skin or eye

Monitoring Parameters With use >10 days, monitor intraocular pressure

Dosage Forms

Ointment, ophthalmic: Prednisolone acetate 0.6% and gentamicin sulfate 0.3% (3.5 g)

Suspension, ophthalmic: Prednisolone acetate 1% and gentamicin sulfate 0.3% (2 mL, 5 mL, 10 mL)

♦ **Prednisolone, Neomycin, and Polymyxin B** *see* Neomycin, Polymyxin B, and Prednisolone *on page 680*

♦ **Prednisolone Sodium Phosphate** *see* Prednisolone *on page 791*

♦ **Prednisolone Tebutate** *see* Prednisolone *on page 791*

♦ **Prednisol® TBA Injection** *see* Prednisolone *on page 791*

Prednisone *(PRED ni sone)*

Related Information

Antiepileptic Drugs *on page 1176*

Asthma Guidelines *on page 1178*

Carbohydrate and Alcohol Content of Liquid Medications for Use in Patients Receiving Ketogenic Diets *on page 1228*

Corticosteroids Comparison, Systemic *on page 1032*

Brand Names Apo®-Prednisone (Canada); Deltasone®; Jaa-Prednisone® (Canada); Liquid Pred®; Meticorten®; Novo-Prednisone® (Canada); Orasone®; Prednicen-M®; Sterapred®; Winpred (Canada)

Synonyms Deltacortisone; Deltadehydrocortisone

Therapeutic Category Adrenal Corticosteroid; Antiasthmatic; Anti-inflammatory Agent; Corticosteroid, Systemic; Glucocorticoid

Generic Available Yes

Use Management of adrenocortical insufficiency; used for its anti-inflammatory or immunosuppressant effects

Pregnancy Risk Factor C

Contraindications Serious infections, except septic shock or tuberculous meningitis; systemic fungal infections; hypersensitivity to prednisone or any component; varicella

Warnings May retard bone growth

Precautions Use with caution in patients with hypothyroidism, cirrhosis, hypertension, CHF, ulcerative colitis, thromboembolic disorders

Adverse Reactions

Cardiovascular: Edema, hypertension

Central nervous system: Vertigo, seizures, psychoses, pseudotumor cerebri, headache

Dermatologic: Acne, skin atrophy

Endocrine & metabolic: Cushing's syndrome, pituitary-adrenal axis suppression, growth suppression, glucose intolerance, hypokalemia, alkalosis

Gastrointestinal: Peptic ulcer, nausea, vomiting

Neuromuscular & skeletal: Muscle weakness, osteoporosis, fractures

Ocular: Cataracts, glaucoma

Drug Interactions Cytochrome P-450 isoenzyme CYP3A3/4 substrate and inducer

Barbiturates, phenytoin, rifampin, salicylates, toxoids, NSAIDs, diuretics (potassium depleting); caffeine and alcohol may increase risk for GI ulcer; live virus vaccines (increase risk of viral infection); vaccines may have decreased effects

Food Interactions Systemic use of corticosteroids may require a diet with increased potassium, vitamins A, B_6, C, D, folate, calcium, zinc, and phosphorus and decreased sodium

Mechanism of Action Decreases inflammation by suppression of migration of polymorphonuclear leukocytes and reversal of increased capillary permeability; suppresses the immune system by reducing activity and volume of the lymphatic system

Pharmacokinetics Converted rapidly in the liver to prednisolone (active)

Usual Dosage Dose depends upon condition being treated and response of patient; dosage for infants and children should be based on disease severity and patient response rather than by rigid adherence to dosage guidelines by age, weight, or body surface area. Consider alternate day therapy for long-term therapy. Discontinuation of long-term therapy requires gradual withdrawal by tapering the dose.

Children: Oral:
Anti-inflammatory or immunosuppressive: 0.05-2 mg/kg/day divided 1-4 times/day
Acute asthma: 1-2 mg/kg/day in divided doses 1-2 times/day for 3-5 days
Alternatively (for 3-5 day "burst"):
<1 year: 10 mg every 12 hours
1-4 years: 20 mg every 12 hours
5-13 years: 30 mg every 12 hours
>13 years: 40 mg every 12 hours
Asthma long-term therapy (alternative dosing by age):
<1 year: 10 mg every other day
1-4 years: 20 mg every other day
5-13 years: 30 mg every other day
>13 years: 40 mg every other day
Nephrotic syndrome: First 3 episodes: Initial: 2 mg/kg/day or 60 mg/m²/day given every day (maximum dose: of 80 mg/day) until urine is protein free for 3 consecutive days (maximum dose: 28 days); followed by 1-1.5 mg/kg/dose or 40 mg/m²/dose given every other day for 4 weeks
Frequent relapses (long-term maintenance dose): 0.5-1 mg/kg/dose given every other day for 3-6 months
Children and Adults: Physiologic replacement: Oral: 4-5 mg/m²/day
Adults: Oral: 5-60 mg/day in divided doses 1-4 times/day

Administration Oral: Administer after meals or with food or milk to decrease GI upset

Monitoring Parameters Blood pressure, weight, serum electrolytes, glucose; children's height and growth

Test Interactions Skin tests

Patient Information Avoid alcohol; limit caffeine; do not decrease dose or discontinue without physician's approval

Dosage Forms
Solution:
Concentrate: 5 mg/mL (5 mL, 30 mL)
Oral: 5 mg/5 mL (10 mL, 20 mL, 500 mL)
Syrup: 5 mg/5 mL (120 mL, 240 mL)
Tablet: 1 mg, 2.5 mg, 5 mg, 10 mg, 20 mg, 50 mg

References
Murphy CM, Coonce SL, and Simon PA, "Treatment of Asthma in Children," *Clin Pharm*, 1991, 10(9):685-703.
Report of a Workshop by the British Association for Paediatric Nephrology and Research Unit, Royal College of Physicians, "Consensus Statement on Management and Audit Potential for Steroid Responsive Nephrotic Syndrome," *Arch Dis Child*, 1994, 70(2):151-7.

- **Prepulsid® (Canada)** *see* Cisapride *U.S. - Available Via Limited-Access Protocol Only on page 226*
- **Pressyn® (Canada)** *see* Vasopressin *on page 971*
- **Pretz® [OTC]** *see* Sodium Chloride *on page 871*
- **Prevacid®** *see* Lansoprazole *on page 557*
- **Prevalite®** *see* Cholestyramine Resin *on page 219*
- **Prevex™ Baby Diaper Rash (Canada)** *see* Zinc Oxide *on page 993*
- **Prevex™ HC (Canada)** *see* Hydrocortisone *on page 486*
- **Prevident®** *see* Fluoride *on page 427*
- **Prilocaine and Lidocaine** *see* Lidocaine and Prilocaine *on page 570*
- **Prilosec®** *see* Omeprazole *on page 706*
- **Primacor®** *see* Milrinone *on page 646*

Primaquine (PRIM a kween)

Available Salts Primaquine Phosphate

Therapeutic Category Antimalarial Agent

Generic Available No

Use In conjunction with a blood schizonticidal agent to provide radical cure of *P. vivax* or *P. ovale* malaria after a clinical attack has been confirmed by blood smear or serologic titer; prevention of relapse of *P. ovale* or *P. vivax* malaria; malaria postexposure prophylaxis

Pregnancy Risk Factor C

Contraindications Acutely ill patients who have a tendency to develop granulocytopenia (rheumatoid arthritis, SLE); patients receiving other drugs capable of depressing the bone marrow; patients receiving quinacrine

Precautions Use with caution in patients with G-6-PD deficiency or NADH methemoglobin reductase deficiency

Adverse Reactions
  Cardiovascular: Arrhythmias, hypertension
  Central nervous system: Headache
  Dermatologic: Pruritus
  Gastrointestinal: Nausea, vomiting, abdominal cramps
  Hematologic: Hemolytic anemia, methemoglobinemia, leukocytosis, leukopenia, agranulocytosis
  Ocular: Interference with visual accommodation

Drug Interactions Quinacrine (increased toxicity of primaquine)

Stability Protect from light

Mechanism of Action Eliminates the primary tissue exoerythrocytic forms of *P. falciparum*, *P. malariae*, *P. ovale*, and *P. vivax*; interferes with plasmodial DNA

Pharmacokinetics
  Absorption: Oral: Well absorbed
  Metabolism: Liver metabolism to carboxyprimaquine, an active metabolite
  Half-life: 3.7-9.6 hours
  Time to peak serum concentration: Within 6 hours
  Elimination: Small amount of unchanged drug excreted in urine

Usual Dosage Oral:
  Children: 0.3 mg base/kg/day once daily for 14 days not to exceed 15 mg base/day, or 0.9 mg base/kg once weekly for 8 weeks not to exceed 45 mg base/week
  Adults: 15 mg/day (base) once daily for 14 days or 45 mg base once weekly for 8 weeks

Administration Oral: Administer with meals to decrease adverse GI effects; drug has a bitter taste

Monitoring Parameters Periodic CBC, visual color check of urine, hemoglobin

Patient Information Notify physician if a darkening of the urine occurs

Dosage Forms Tablet, as phosphate: 26.3 mg [15 mg base]

References
Lynk A and Gold R, "Review of 40 Children With Imported Malaria," *Pediatr Infect Dis J*, 1989, 8(11):745-50.

Wyler DJ, "Malaria Chemoprophylaxis for the Traveler," *N Engl J Med*, 1993, 329(1):31-7.

- **Primaquine Phosphate** *see* Primaquine *on page 796*
- **Primatene® Mist [OTC]** *see* Epinephrine *on page 371*
- **Primaxin®** *see* Imipenem and Cilastatin *on page 506*

Primidone (PRI mi done)

Related Information
  Antiepileptic Drugs *on page 1176*

Carbohydrate and Alcohol Content of Liquid Medications for Use in Patients Receiving Ketogenic Diets *on page 1228*
Drugs and Breast-Feeding *on page 1213*

Brand Names Apo®-Primidone (Canada); Mysoline®; Sertan® (Canada)

Therapeutic Category Anticonvulsant, Barbiturate; Barbiturate

Generic Available Yes: Tablet

Use Management of generalized tonic-clonic (grand mal), complex partial and simple partial (focal) seizures

Pregnancy Risk Factor D

Contraindications Hypersensitivity to primidone or any component; porphyria

Precautions Use with caution in patients with renal or hepatic impairment; abrupt discontinuation may precipitate status epilepticus

Adverse Reactions

Central nervous system: Drowsiness, vertigo, lethargy, behavior change, ataxia

Dermatologic: Rash

Gastrointestinal: Nausea, vomiting

Hematologic: Leukopenia, malignant lymphoma-like syndrome, megaloblastic anemia

Ocular: Diplopia, nystagmus

Miscellaneous: Systemic lupus-like syndrome

Drug Interactions Cytochrome P-450 isoenzyme CYP1A2, CYP2B6, CYP2C, CYP2C8, CYP3A3/4, and CYP3A5-7 inducer

Primidone may decrease serum concentrations of ethosuximide, valproic acid, griseofulvin; methylphenidate may increase primidone serum concentrations; phenytoin may decrease primidone serum concentrations; valproic acid may increase phenobarbital concentrations derived from primidone

Food Interactions May increase the metabolism of vitamins D and K; dietary requirements of vitamins D, K, B_{12}, folate, and calcium may be increased with long-term use

Mechanism of Action Decreases neuron excitability, raises seizure threshold similar to phenobarbital

Pharmacokinetics

Distribution: V_d: Adults: 2-3 L/kg

Protein-binding: 99%

Metabolism: In the liver to phenobarbital (active) and phenylethylmalonamide (PEMA)

Bioavailability: 60% to 80%

Half-life:

Primidone: 10-12 hours

PEMA: 16 hours

Phenobarbital: 52-118 hours (age-dependent)

Time to peak serum concentration: Oral: Within 4 hours

Elimination: Urinary excretion of both active metabolites and unchanged primidone (15% to 25%)

Usual Dosage Oral:

Neonates: 12-20 mg/kg/day in divided doses 2-4 times/day; start with lower dosage and titrate upward

Children <8 years: Initial: 50-125 mg/day given at bedtime; increase by 50-125 mg/day increments every 3-7 days; usual dose: 10-25 mg/kg/day in divided doses 3-4 times/day

Children >8 years and Adults: Initial: 125-250 mg/day at bedtime; increase by 125-250 mg/day every 3-7 days; usual dose: 750-1500 mg/day in divided doses 3-4 times/day with maximum dosage of 2 g/day

Administration Oral: Administer with food to decrease GI upset

Monitoring Parameters Serum primidone and phenobarbital concentrations; CBC with differential; neurological status, seizure frequency, duration, severity

Reference Range

Therapeutic: 5-12 µg/mL (SI: 23-55 µmol/L)

Toxic effects rarely present with levels <10 µg/mL (SI: 46 µmol/L) if phenobarbital concentrations are low

Toxic: >15 µg/mL (SI: >69 µmol/L); monitor both primidone and phenobarbital concentrations

Patient Information Avoid alcohol; limit caffeine; may cause drowsiness and impair ability to perform activities requiring mental alertness or physical coordination; do not abruptly discontinue or change dose without physician approval

Dosage Forms

Suspension, oral: 250 mg/5 mL (240 mL)

Tablet: 50 mg, 250 mg

- **Primsol® Solution** *see* Trimethoprim *on page 955*
- **Principen®** *see* Ampicillin *on page 78*
- **Prinivil®** *see* Lisinopril *on page 575*
- **Priscoline®** *see* Tolazoline *on page 934*
- **Pristinamycin** *see* Quinupristin/Dalfopristin *on page 834*
- **Privine® Nasal [OTC]** *see* Naphazoline *on page 671*
- **Pro-Amox® (Canada)** *see* Amoxicillin *on page 70*
- **Pro-Ampi® [Trihydrate] (Canada)** *see* Ampicillin *on page 78*
- **Probalan®** *see* Probenecid *on page 798*
- **Pro-Banthine®** *see* Propantheline *on page 810*

Probenecid (proe BEN e sid)

Brand Names Benemid® (Canada); Benuryl™ (Canada); Probalan®

Therapeutic Category Adjuvant Therapy, Penicillin Level Prolongation; Antigout Agent; Uric Acid Lowering Agent; Uricosuric Agent

Generic Available Yes

Use Prevention of gouty arthritis; hyperuricemia; prolong serum levels of penicillin/cephalosporin

Pregnancy Risk Factor B

Contraindications Hypersensitivity to probenecid or any component; high dose aspirin therapy; moderate to severe renal impairment (Cl_{cr} <10 mL/minute); children <2 years of age, blood dyscrasias, uric acid kidney stones

Precautions Use with caution in patients with peptic ulcer; hematuria, renal colic; formation of uric acid stones associated with the use of probenecid may be prevented by liberal fluid intake and alkalinization of urine; may not be effective when Cl_{cr} 10-30 mL/minute

Adverse Reactions

Cardiovascular: Flushing

Central nervous system: Dizziness, headache

Dermatologic: Rash

Gastrointestinal: Anorexia, nausea, vomiting, sore gums

Genitourinary: Urinary frequency

Hematologic: Anemia, leukopenia, aplastic anemia, hemolytic anemia (possibly related to G-6-PD deficiency)

Hepatic: Hepatic necrosis

Renal: Nephrotic syndrome, renal colic, uric acid stones

Miscellaneous: Hypersensitivity reactions

Drug Interactions Salicylates and probenecid inhibit the uricosuric actions of each other; probenecid may increase the plasma levels of acyclovir, penicillins, ciprofloxacin, ganciclovir, cephalosporins, methotrexate, dapsone, NSAIDs, and zidovudine; benzodiazepines and thiopental may have prolonged effects; sulfonylureas may have an increase in half-life; clofibrate may have an increased accumulation of its active metabolite; avoid concomitant use with ketorolac since its half-life is increased twofold and levels and toxicity are significantly increased; niacin may inhibit uricosuric effects of probenecid

Mechanism of Action Competitively inhibits the reabsorption of uric acid at the proximal convoluted tubule, thereby promoting its excretion and reducing serum uric acid levels; increases plasma levels of weak organic acids (penicillins, cephalosporins, or other beta-lactam antibiotics) by competitively inhibiting their renal tubular secretion

Pharmacodynamics Exerts maximal effects on penicillin levels after 2 hours; produces maximal renal clearance of uric acid in 30 minutes

Pharmacokinetics

Absorption: Rapid and complete from GI tract

Protein binding: 85% to 95%

Metabolism: In the liver

Half-life: 4-17 hours

Time to peak serum concentration: Within 2-4 hours

Usual Dosage Oral:

Prolongation of penicillin serum levels:

Children 2-14 years: Initial: 25 mg/kg/dose or 0.7 g/m²/dose as a single dose; maintenance: 40 mg/kg/day or 1.2 g/m²/day in 4 divided doses (maximum single dose: 500 mg)

Adults: 500 mg 4 times/day

Hyperuricemia: Adults: Initial: 250 mg twice daily for 1 week; increase to 500 mg twice daily; may increase in 500 mg increments every 4 weeks if needed to a maximum of 2-3 g/day; begin therapy 2-3 weeks after an acute gouty attack

Gonorrhea: Adults: 1 g 30 minutes before penicillin, ampicillin, or amoxicillin

Dosing adjustment in renal impairment: Cl_{cr} <50 mL/minute: Avoid use

Administration Oral: Administer with food or antacids to minimize GI effects

Monitoring Parameters Uric acid, renal function, CBC

Test Interactions False-positive glucosuria with Clinitest®; falsely elevated serum theophylline level (Schack & Waxler technique); inhibits renal excretion of phenosulfonphthalein (PSP), 17-ketosteroids, and sulfobromophthalein (BSP)

Patient Information Drink plenty of fluids to reduce the risk of uric acid stones; the frequency of acute gouty attacks may increase during the first 6-12 months of therapy; avoid taking large doses of aspirin or other salicylates; avoid alcohol

Dosage Forms Tablet: 500 mg

♦ **Pro-Bionate® [OTC]** see Lactobacillus acidophilus and Lactobacillus bulgaricus on page 550

Procainamide (proe kane A mide)

Related Information

Adult ACLS Algorithm, Tachycardia on page 1010
Adult ACLS Algorithm, V. Fib and Pulseless V. Tach on page 1004

Brand Names Apo®-Procainamide (Canada); Procan™ SR (Canada); Pronestyl®; Pronestyl-SR®

Available Salts Procainamide Hydrochloride

Synonyms PCA; Procaine Amide

Therapeutic Category Antiarrhythmic Agent, Class I-A

Generic Available Yes

Use Ventricular tachycardia, premature ventricular contractions, paroxysmal atrial tachycardia, and atrial fibrillation; to prevent recurrence of ventricular tachycardia, paroxysmal supraventricular tachycardia, atrial fibrillation or flutter

Pregnancy Risk Factor C

Contraindications Complete heart block; second or third degree heart block without pacemaker; "torsade de pointes" (twisting of the points), an unusual ventricular tachycardia; pre-existing Q-T prolongation; hypersensitivity to the procainamide, procaine, related drugs, or any component; myasthenia gravis; SLE

Warnings Long-term administration leads to the development of a positive antinuclear antibody (ANA) test in 50% of patients which may lead to a lupus erythematosus-like syndrome (in 20% to 30% of patients); assess relative benefits and risks if ANA titer becomes positive and consider alternative agent; discontinue procainamide if SLE symptoms develop and change to alternative agent; do not use sustained release preparation for initial therapy; some tablets contain tartrazine; injection may contain bisulfite; 100 mg/mL injection contains benzyl alcohol (use with caution in neonates)

Precautions Use with caution in patients with marked A-V conduction disturbances, bundle-branch block or severe cardiac glycoside intoxication, ventricular arrhythmias in patients with organic heart disease or coronary occlusion, supraventricular tachyarrhythmias unless digitalis glycoside levels are adequate to prevent marked increases in ventricular rates; drug may accumulate in patients with renal or hepatic dysfunction, dosage adjustment required

Adverse Reactions

Cardiovascular: Hypotension, tachycardia, arrhythmias, A-V block, Q-T prolongation, widening QRS complex

Central nervous system: Confusion, disorientation, drug fever

Gastrointestinal: Nausea, vomiting, GI complaints

Hematologic: Agranulocytosis, neutropenia

Hepatic: Hepatomegaly, increased liver enzymes

Miscellaneous: Lupus-like syndrome (arthralgia, positive Coombs' test, thrombocytopenia, rash, myalgia, fever, pericarditis, pleural effusion)

Drug Interactions Cimetidine, ranitidine, amiodarone, beta-blocking agents, trimethoprim may increase plasma procainamide and NAPA concentrations, procainamide dosage adjustment may be required; procainamide may potentiate skeletal muscle relaxants; anticholinergic drugs may have enhanced effects

Stability Use only clear or slightly yellow solutions; stability of parenteral admixture with D_5W at room temperature (25°C) is 24 hours but 7 days at refrigerated temperature (2°C to 8°C)

Mechanism of Action Class IA antiarrhythmic with anticholinergic and local anesthetic effects; decreases myocardial excitability and conduction velocity and depresses myocardial contractility, by increasing the electrical stimulation threshold of ventricle, His-Purkinje system and through direct cardiac effects

Pharmacodynamics Onset of action: I.M. 10-30 minutes

(Continued)

Procainamide *(Continued)*

Pharmacokinetics

Distribution: V_d (decreased with CHF or shock):
  Children: 2.2 L/kg
  Adults: 2 L/kg

Protein binding: 15% to 20%

Metabolism: By acetylation in the liver to produce N-acetyl procainamide (NAPA) (active metabolite)

Bioavailability, oral: 75% to 95%

Half-life:
  Procainamide (dependent upon hepatic acetylator phenotype, cardiac function, and renal function):
    Children: 1.7 hours
    Adults with normal renal function: 2.5-4.7 hours
  NAPA (dependent upon renal function):
    Children: 6 hours
    Adults with normal renal function: 6-8 hours

Time to peak serum concentration:
  Oral (capsule): Within 45 minutes to 2.5 hours
  I.M.: 15-60 minutes

Elimination: Urinary excretion (25% as NAPA)

Moderately dialyzable by hemodialysis (20% to 50%), but not dialyzable by peritoneal dialysis

Usual Dosage Must be titrated to patient's response

Children:
  Oral: 15-50 mg/kg/24 hours divided every 3-6 hours; maximum 4 g/24 hours
  I.M.: 20-30 mg/kg/24 hours divided every 4-6 hours; maximum 4 g/24 hours
  I.V.:
    Loading dose: 3-6 mg/kg/dose over 5 minutes, not to exceed 100 mg/dose; may repeat every 5-10 minutes to maximum of 15 mg/kg/load; do not exceed 500 mg in 30 minutes
    Maintenance: Continuous I.V. infusion: 20-80 mcg/kg/minute; maximum dose: 2 g/24 hours

Adults:
  Oral: 250-500 mg/dose every 3-6 hours **or** 500 mg to 1 g every 6 hours (sustained release); usual dose: 50 mg/kg/24 hours or 2-4 g/24 hours
  I.V.:
    Loading dose: 50-100 mg/dose, repeated every 5-10 minutes until patient controlled; or load with 15-18 mg/kg; maximum loading dose: 1-1.5 g
    Maintenance: Continuous I.V. infusion: 3-4 mg/minute; range: 1-6 mg/minute; monitor levels and do not exceed 3 mg/minute for >24 hours in patients with renal failure

ACLS guidelines: Adults:
  I.V.: Loading dose: Infuse 20 mg/minute until arrhythmia is controlled, hypotension occurs, QRS complex widens by 50% of its original width, or total of 17 mg/kg is given
  Refractory ventricular fibrillation:
    Loading dose: 30 mg/minute up to a total of 17 mg/kg
    I.V. maintenance infusion: 1-4 mg/minute; monitor levels and do not exceed 3 mg/minute for >24 hours in adults with renal failure

Dosing interval in renal dysfunction:

Cl_{cr} 10-50 mL/minute: Administer normal dose every 6-12 hours
Cl_{cr} <10 mL/minute: Administer normal dose every 8-24 hours

Administration

Oral: Administer with water on an empty stomach; if GI distress occurs may administer with food or milk to decrease GI upset; swallow sustained release tablets whole, do not chew or crush

Parenteral: I.V.: Do not administer faster than 20-30 mg/minute; severe hypotension can occur with rapid I.V. administration; administer I.V. push over at least 5 minutes; administer I.V. loading doses and intermittent infusions over 25-30 minutes; use concentration of 20-30 mg/mL for loading dose and 2-4 mg/mL for maintenance infusions; rate of infusion (mL/hour) = dose (mcg/kg/minute) x weight (kg) x 60 minutes/hour divided by the concentration

Monitoring Parameters

EKG, blood pressure, CBC with differential, platelet count, antinuclear antibody test (ANA); serum drug concentrations, procainamide and NAPA, especially in patients with renal failure or those receiving higher maintenance doses (eg, adults: >3 mg/minute) for >24 hours

Reference Range

Therapeutic:

Procainamide: 4-10 µg/mL (SI: 15-37 µmol/L)

Sum of procainamide and N-acetyl procainamide: 10-30 µg/mL (SI: <110 µmol/L)

Optimal ranges must be ascertained for individual patients, with EKG monitoring

Toxic (procainamide): >10-12 µg/mL (SI: >37-44 µmol/L)

Patient Information Limit alcohol; some sustained release tablets have a wax core that slowly releases the drug, this wax core is not absorbed and will be eliminated in the stool

Dosage Forms

Capsule, as hydrochloride: 250 mg, 375 mg, 500 mg

Injection, as hydrochloride: 100 mg/mL (10 mL); 500 mg/mL (2 mL)

Tablet, as hydrochloride: 250 mg, 375 mg, 500 mg

Tablet, sustained release, as hydrochloride: 250 mg, 500 mg, 750 mg, 1000 mg

Extemporaneous Preparations Note: Several formulations have been described, some being more complex; for all formulations, the pH must be 4-6 to prevent degradation; some preparations require adjustment of pH; **label all preparations "shake well before use"**

A 50 mg/mL oral liquid preparation made from the contents of capsules and 3 different vehicles (cherry syrup, a 1:1 mixture of Ora-Sweet® and Ora-Plus®, or a 1:1 mixture of Ora-Sweet® SF and Ora-Plus®) was stable for 60 days when stored in amber plastic prescription bottles in the dark at room temperature (25°C) or under refrigeration (5°C); empty the contents of twenty-four 250 mg capsules into a mortar; break up the powder and pulverize it; add 20 mL of the vehicle and mix well to form a uniform paste; mix while adding the vehicle in geometric proportions to **almost** 120 mL; transfer to a calibrated bottle and qsad with vehicle to 120 mL; label "protect from light" (Allen, 1996)

A suspension of 50 mg/mL can be made with the capsules, distilled water, and a 2:1 simple syrup/cherry syrup mixture; stability 2 weeks under refrigeration (ASHP, 1987)

Concentrations of 5, 50, and 100 mg/mL oral liquid preparations, (made with the capsules, sterile water for irrigation and cherry syrup) stored at 4°C to 6°C (pH 6) were stable for at least 6 months (Metras, 1992)

A sucrose-based syrup (procainamide 50 mg/mL) made with capsules, distilled water, simple syrup, parabens, and cherry flavoring had a calculated stability of 456 days at 25°C and measured stability of 42 days at 40°C (pH ~5) while a maltitol-based syrup (procainamide 50 mg/mL) made with capsules, distilled water, Lycasin® (a syrup vehicle with 75% w/w maltitol), parabens, sodium bisulfate, saccharin, sodium acetate, pineapple and apricot flavoring, FD & C yellow number 6, (pH adjusted to 5 with glacial acetic acid) had a calculated stability of 97 days at 25°C and a measured stability of 94 days at 40°C. The maltitol-based syrup was more stable than the sucrose-based syrup when temperature was >37°C, but the sucrose-based syrup was more stable at temperatures <37°C (Alexander, 1993)

Alexander KS, Pudipeddi M, and Parker GA, "Stability of Procainamide Hydrochloride Syrups Compounded From Capsules," *Am J Hosp Pharm*, 1993, 50(4):693-8.

Allen LV and Erickson MA, "Stability of Ketoconazole, Metolazone, Metronidazole, Procainamide Hydrochloride, and Spironolactone in Extemporaneously Compounded Oral Liquids," *Am J Health Syst Pharm*, 1996, 53(17):2073-8.

Handbook in Extemporaneous Formulations, Bethesda, MD: American Society of Hospital Pharmacists, 1987.

Metras JI, Swenson CF, and MacDermott MP, "Stability of Procainamide Hydrochloride in an Extemporaneously Compounded Oral Liquid," *Am J Hosp Pharm*, 1992, 49(7):1720-4.

Swenson CF, "Importance of Following Instructions When Compounding," *Am J Hosp Pharm*, 1993, 50(2):261.

References

American College of Cardiology, American Heart Association Task Force, "Adult Advanced Cardiac Life Support" and "Pediatric Advanced Life Support Guidelines," *JAMA*, 1992, 268(16):2199-241 and 2262-75.

Singh S, Gelband H, Mehta AV, et al, "Procainamide Elimination Kinetics in Pediatric Patients," *Clin Pharmacol Ther*, 1982, 32(5):607-11.

♦ **Procainamide Hydrochloride** *see* Procainamide *on page 799*

♦ **Procaine Amide** *see* Procainamide *on page 799*

♦ **Procaine Benzylpenicillin** *see* Penicillin G Procaine *on page 742*

♦ **Procaine Penicillin G** *see* Penicillin G Procaine *on page 742*

♦ **Pro-Cal-Sof® [OTC]** *see* Docusate *on page 336*

♦ **Procan™ SR (Canada)** *see* Procainamide *on page 799*

Procarbazine (proe KAR ba zeen)

Related Information
  Emetogenic Potential of Single Chemotherapeutic Agents *on page 1095*
Brand Names Matulane®; Natulan® (Canada)
Available Salts Procarbazine Hydrochloride
Synonyms Ibenzmethyzin
Therapeutic Category Antineoplastic Agent, Miscellaneous
Generic Available No
Use Treatment of Hodgkin's disease, non-Hodgkin's lymphoma, brain tumor, bronchogenic carcinoma
Pregnancy Risk Factor D
Contraindications Hypersensitivity to procarbazine or any component; pre-existing bone marrow aplasia
Warnings The FDA currently recommends that procedures for proper handling and disposal of antineoplastic agents be considered; procarbazine is a carcinogen which may cause a secondary acute nonlymphocytic leukemia; procarbazine may cause infertility and is potentially teratogenic
Precautions May potentiate CNS depression when used with phenothiazine derivatives, barbiturates, narcotics, alcohol, tricyclic antidepressants, methyldopa; use with caution in patients with pre-existing renal or hepatic impairment; reduce dosage in patients with marrow disorders, renal impairment (serum creatinine >2 mg/dL and/or a blood urea nitrogen >40 mg/dL), or decreased hepatic function (total bilirubin >3 mg/dL)
Adverse Reactions
  Central nervous system: CNS depression, somnolence, confusion, nervousness, irritability, cerebellar ataxia, hallucinations, seizures, nightmares, headache, chills, fever, dizziness
  Dermatologic: Dermatitis, alopecia, hypersensitivity rash, pruritus
  Endocrine & metabolic: Disulfiram-like reaction, amenorrhea
  Gastrointestinal: Nausea, vomiting, diarrhea, stomatitis, anorexia
  Genitourinary: Azoospermia, ovarian failure
  Hematologic: Myelosuppression, thrombocytopenia, pancytopenia, hemolysis
  Neuromuscular & skeletal: Arthralgia, myalgia, tremor, neuropathy, weakness
  Ocular: Nystagmus, diplopia, photophobia
  Miscellaneous: Flu-like syndrome
Drug Interactions Alcohol (disulfiram-like reaction with nausea, vomiting, headache, sedation, and visual disturbances); MAO inhibitors, tricyclic antidepressants, ephedrine, epinephrine, isoproterenol (hypertensive crisis, tremor, excitation, cardiac palpitations, angina); narcotics, phenothiazines, barbiturates, methyldopa (additive CNS depression); phenytoin, phenobarbital (increases cytotoxic activity of procarbazine)
Food Interactions Avoid food with high tyramine content (cheese, tea, dark beer, coffee, cola drinks, wine, bananas) as hypertensive crisis, tremor, excitation, cardiac palpitations, and angina may occur
Stability Unstable in water or aqueous solution; avoid contact of the drug with moisture
Mechanism of Action Inhibits DNA, RNA, and protein synthesis; may damage DNA directly via free-radical formation and suppress mitosis
Pharmacokinetics
  Absorption: Oral: Well absorbed
  Distribution: Crosses the blood-brain barrier and distributes into CSF, liver, kidney, intestine, and skin
  Metabolism: In the liver; first-pass conversion to cytotoxic metabolites
  Half-life: 10 minutes
  Time to peak serum concentration: Within 1 hour
  Elimination: In urine (<5% as unchanged drug) and 70% as metabolites
Usual Dosage Oral (refer to individual protocols; base dosage on ideal body weight):
  Children:
    Hodgkin's disease: 50-100 mg/m^2/day once daily for 10-14 days of a 28-day cycle
    BMT aplastic anemia conditioning regimen: 12.5 mg/kg/dose every other day for 4 doses
    Brain tumor: 75 mg/m^2 at hour 1 on day 1; repeat cycle every 2-4 weeks if tolerated; **or** 100 mg/m^2 on days 1-14 of a treatment course
    Neuroblastoma and medulloblastoma: Doses as high as 100-200 mg/m^2/day once daily have been used

Adults: Initial: 2-4 mg/kg/day in single or divided doses for 7 days then increase dose to 4-6 mg/kg/day until response is obtained or leukocyte count decreases to <4000/mm^3 or the platelet count decreases to <100,000/mm^3; maintenance: 1-2 mg/kg/day

Administration Oral: Administer with food or after meals; total daily dose may be administered at a single time or in divided doses throughout the day to minimize GI toxicity

Monitoring Parameters CBC with differential, platelet count, and reticulocyte count; urinalysis, liver function test, renal function test

Patient Information Notify physician of fever, sore throat, bleeding, or bruising; avoid alcohol (disulfiram-like reaction with nausea, vomiting, headache, sedation, and visual disturbances)

Additional Information Myelosuppressive effects:
WBC: Moderate
Platelets: Moderate
Onset (days): 14
Nadir (days): 21
Recovery (days): 28

Dosage Forms Capsule, as hydrochloride: 50 mg

References

Longo DL, Young RC, Wesley M, et al, "Twenty Years of MOPP Therapy for Hodgkin's Disease," *J Clin Oncol*, 1986, 4(9):1295-306.
Rodriguez LA, Prados M, Silver P, et al, "Re-evaluation of Procarbazine for the Treatment of Recurrent Malignant Central Nervous System Tumors," *Cancer*, 1989, 64(12):2420-3.

♦ **Procarbazine Hydrochloride** *see* Procarbazine *on page 802*
♦ **Procardia®** *see* Nifedipine *on page 687*
♦ **Procardia XL®** *see* Nifedipine *on page 687*

Prochlorperazine (proe klor PER a zeen)

Related Information
Carbohydrate and Alcohol Content of Liquid Medications for Use in Patients Receiving Ketogenic Diets *on page 1228*
Compatibility of Medications Mixed in a Syringe *on page 1208*
Overdose and Toxicology *on page 1191*

Brand Names Compazine®; Nu-Prochlor® (Canada); PMS-Prochlorperazine (Canada); Prorazin® (Canada); Stemetil® (Canada)

Available Salts Prochlorperazine Edisylate; Prochlorperazine Maleate

Therapeutic Category Antiemetic; Antipsychotic Agent; Phenothiazine Derivative

Generic Available Yes

Use Management of nausea and vomiting; acute and chronic psychosis

Pregnancy Risk Factor C

Contraindications Hypersensitivity to prochlorperazine or any component; cross-sensitivity with other phenothiazines may exist; avoid use in patients with narrow-angle glaucoma; bone marrow suppression; severe liver or cardiac disease, severe toxic CNS depression or coma

Warnings High incidence of extrapyramidal reactions especially in children, reserve use in children <5 years of age to those who are unresponsive to other antiemetics; incidence of extrapyramidal reactions is increased with acute illnesses such as chicken pox, measles, CNS infections, gastroenteritis, and dehydration; injection contains sulfites which may cause allergic reactions; lowers seizure threshold, use cautiously in patients with seizure history; some products contain tartrazine dye, avoid use in sensitive individuals; discontinue use at least 48 hours before myelography and do not resume until 24 hours post myelography

Precautions Safety and efficacy have not been established in children <9 kg or <2 years of age

Adverse Reactions Incidence of extrapyramidal reactions are higher with prochlorperazine than chlorpromazine
Cardiovascular: Hypotension (especially with I.V. use); orthostatic hypotension; tachycardia, arrhythmias, sudden death
Central nervous system: Sedation, drowsiness, restlessness, anxiety; extrapyramidal reactions which include dystonic reactions such as spasm of neck muscles, torticollis, extensor rigidity of back muscles, opisthotonos, trismus, and mandibular tics; pseudoparkinsonian signs and symptoms, tardive dyskinesia, neuroleptic malignant syndrome, seizures, altered central temperature regulation
Dermatologic: Hyperpigmentation, pruritus, rash, photosensitivity
Endocrine & metabolic: Amenorrhea, galactorrhea, gynecomastia, abnormal glucose tolerance
(Continued)

Prochlorperazine *(Continued)*

Gastrointestinal: GI upset, xerostomia, constipation, weight gain

Genitourinary: Impotence, urinary retention

Hematologic: Agranulocytosis, leukopenia (usually in patients with large doses for prolonged periods), thrombocytopenia, hemolytic anemia, eosinophilia

Hepatic: Cholestatic jaundice

Ocular: Retinal pigmentation, blurred vision

Miscellaneous: Anaphylactoid reactions

Drug Interactions

Phenothiazines inhibit the ability of bromocriptine to lower serum prolactin concentrations

Benztropine (and other anticholinergics) may inhibit the therapeutic response to prochlorperazine and excess anticholinergic effects may occur

Chloroquine may increase prochlorperazine concentrations

Cigarette smoking may enhance the hepatic metabolism of prochlorperazine. Larger doses may be required compared to a nonsmoker.

Concurrent use of prochlorperazine with an antihypertensive may produce additive hypotensive effects

Antihypertensive effects of guanethidine and guanadrel may be inhibited by prochlorperazine

Concurrent use with TCA may produce increased toxicity or altered therapeutic response

Prochlorperazine may inhibit the antiparkinsonian effect of levodopa; avoid this combination

Prochlorperazine plus lithium may rarely produce neurotoxicity

Barbiturates may reduce prochlorperazine concentrations

Propranolol may increase prochlorperazine concentrations

Sulfadoxine-pyrimethamine may increase prochlorperazine concentrations

prochlorperazine and possibly other low potency antipsychotics may reverse the pressor effects of epinephrine

Prochlorperazine and CNS depressants (ethanol, narcotics) may produce additive CNS depressant effects

Prochlorperazine and trazodone may produce additive hypotensive effects

Use with cisapride may increase the risk of malignant arrhythmias, concurrent use is contraindicated

Food Interactions Increase dietary intake of riboflavin

Stability Protect from light; clear or slightly yellow solutions may be used; incompatible with aminophylline, amphotericin B, ampicillin, calcium salts, cephalothin, foscarnet (Y-site), furosemide, hydrocortisone, hydromorphone, methohexital, midazolam, penicillin G, pentobarbital, phenobarbital, thiopental

Mechanism of Action Blocks postsynaptic mesolimbic dopaminergic receptors in the brain, including the medullary chemoreceptor trigger zone; exhibits a strong alpha-adrenergic blocking effect and depresses the release of hypothalamic and hypophyseal hormones

Pharmacodynamics

Onset of action:

Oral: 30-40 minutes

I.M.: Within 10-20 minutes

Rectal: Within 60 minutes

Duration:

I.M., oral extended release: 12 hours

Rectal, oral immediate release: 3-4 hours

Usual Dosage

Antiemetic:

Children >10 kg:

Oral, rectal: 0.4 mg/kg/day in 3-4 divided doses; **or**

9-14 kg: 2.5 mg every 12-24 hours as needed; maximum dose: 7.5 mg/day

14-18 kg: 2.5 mg every 8-12 hours as needed; maximum dose: 10 mg/day

18-39 kg: 2.5 mg every 8 hours or 5 mg every 12 hours as needed; maximum dose: 15 mg/day

I.M.: 0.1-0.15 mg/kg/dose; usual: 0.13 mg/kg/dose; change to oral as soon as possible

I.V.: Not recommended

Adults:

Oral: 5-10 mg 3-4 times/day; usual maximum dose: 40 mg/day

Oral, extended release: 10 mg twice daily or 15 mg once daily

I.M.: 5-10 mg every 3-4 hours; usual maximum dose: 40 mg/day

I.V.: 2.5-10 mg; maximum 10 mg/dose or 40 mg/day; may repeat dose every 3-4 hours as needed

Rectal: 25 mg twice daily

Treatment of psychoses:

Children 2-12 years:

Oral, rectal: 2.5 mg 2-3 times/day, increase dosage as needed to a maximum daily dose of 20 mg for 2-5 years and 25 mg for 6-12 years

I.M.: 0.13 mg/kg/dose, change to oral as soon as possible

Adults:

Oral: 5-10 mg 3-4 times/day, increase as needed to a daily maximum dose of 150 mg

I.M.: 10-20 mg every 4 hours as needed, change to oral as soon as possible

Administration

Oral: Administer with food or water

Parenteral: I.M. is preferred; avoid I.V. administration; if necessary, may be administered by direct I.V. injection at a maximum rate of 5 mg/minute; do not administer by S.C. route (tissue damage may occur)

Monitoring Parameters CBC with differential and periodic ophthalmic exams (if chronically used)

Test Interactions False-positives for phenylketonuria, urinary amylase, uroporphyrins, urobilinogen

Patient Information Limit caffeine; causes drowsiness and may impair ability to perform hazardous tasks requiring mental alertness or physical coordination

Nursing Implications Avoid skin contact with oral solution or injection, contact dermatitis has occurred

Additional Information Use lowest possible dose in pediatric patients to try to decrease incidence of extrapyramidal reactions

Dosage Forms

Capsule, sustained action, as maleate: 10 mg, 15 mg, 30 mg

Injection, as edisylate: 5 mg/mL (2 mL, 10 mL)

Suppository, rectal: 2.5 mg, 5 mg, 25 mg (12/box)

Syrup, as edisylate: 5 mg/5 mL (120 mL)

Tablet, as maleate: 5 mg, 10 mg, 25 mg

- ◆ **Prochlorperazine Edisylate** *see* Prochlorperazine *on page 803*
- ◆ **Prochlorperazine Maleate** *see* Prochlorperazine *on page 803*
- ◆ **Procrit®** *see* Epoetin Alfa *on page 373*
- ◆ **Proctocort™ Rectal** *see* Hydrocortisone *on page 486*
- ◆ **Proctofoam® [OTC]** *see* Hemorrhoidal Preparations *on page 470*
- ◆ **Procytox® (Canada)** *see* Cyclophosphamide *on page 268*
- ◆ **Prodiem® Plain (Canada)** *see* Psyllium *on page 823*
- ◆ **Prodium® [OTC]** *see* Phenazopyridine *on page 753*
- ◆ **Profasi® HP** *see* Chorionic Gonadotropin *on page 221*
- ◆ **Profilate® HP** *see* Antihemophilic Factor *on page 89*
- ◆ **Profilnine® Heat-Treated** *see* Factor IX Complex (Human) *on page 399*
- ◆ **Proglycem® Oral** *see* Diazoxide *on page 310*
- ◆ **Prograf®** *see* Tacrolimus *on page 901*
- ◆ **Pro-Indo® (Canada)** *see* Indomethacin *on page 516*
- ◆ **Prokine™** *see* Sargramostim *on page 858*
- ◆ **Prolamine® [OTC]** *see* Phenylpropanolamine *on page 761*
- ◆ **Proleukin®** *see* Aldesleukin *on page 42*
- ◆ **Proloprim®** *see* Trimethoprim *on page 955*
- ◆ **Pro-Lorazepam® (Canada)** *see* Lorazepam *on page 583*
- ◆ **Prometa®** *see* Metaproterenol *on page 611*

Promethazine *(proe METH a zeen)*

Related Information

Compatibility of Medications Mixed in a Syringe *on page 1208*

Overdose and Toxicology *on page 1191*

Promethazine and Phenylephrine *on page 808*

Brand Names Anergan® Injection; Histantil (Canada); Phenazine® Injection; Phenergan® Injection; Phenergan® Oral; Phenergan® Rectal; Prometh® Injection; Prorex® Injection

Available Salts Promethazine Hydrochloride

Therapeutic Category Antiemetic; Phenothiazine Derivative; Sedative

Generic Available Yes

(Continued)

Promethazine *(Continued)*

Use Symptomatic treatment of various allergic conditions and motion sickness; sedative and an antiemetic

Pregnancy Risk Factor C

Contraindications Hypersensitivity to promethazine or any component; narrow-angle glaucoma, severe toxic CNS depression or coma, prostatic hypertrophy, GI or GU obstruction

Warnings Do not give S.C. or intra-arterially, necrotic lesions may occur; injection may contain sulfites which may cause allergic reactions in some patients; rapid I.V. administration may produce a transient fall in blood pressure; slow I.V. administration may produce a slightly elevated blood pressure

Precautions Use with caution in patients with cardiovascular disease, impaired liver function, asthma, peptic ulcer, sleep apnea, seizures, hypertensive crisis; avoid in patients with suspected Reye's syndrome

Adverse Reactions
Cardiovascular: Tachycardia, bradycardia, hypotension (rapid I.V. administration), hypertension (slow I.V. administration), palpitations
Central nervous system: Sedation (pronounced), drowsiness, confusion, fatigue, excitation, extrapyramidal reactions, dystonia, tardive dyskinesia
Dermatologic: Photosensitivity, rash, angioedema
Gastrointestinal: Xerostomia, GI upset, increased appetite, weight gain, abdominal pain, diarrhea, nausea
Genitourinary: Urinary retention
Hematologic: Thrombocytopenia, leukopenia, agranulocytosis (rare)
Hepatic: Cholestatic jaundice, hepatitis
Ocular: Blurred vision
Neuromuscular & skeletal: Arthralgia, tremor, paresthesia, myalgia
Respiratory: Thickening of bronchial secretions, pharyngitis
Miscellaneous: Allergic reactions

Drug Interactions CYP2D6 enzyme substrate
Phenothiazines inhibit the ability of bromocriptine to lower serum prolactin concentrations
Benztropine (and other anticholinergics) may inhibit the therapeutic response to promethazine and excess anticholinergic effects may occur
Chloroquine may increase promethazine concentrations
Cigarette smoking may enhance the hepatic metabolism of promethazine. Larger doses may be required compared to a nonsmoker.
Concurrent use of promethazine with an antihypertensive may produce additive hypotensive effects
Antihypertensive effects of guanethidine and guanadrel may be inhibited by promethazine
Concurrent use with TCA may produce increased toxicity or altered therapeutic response
Promethazine may inhibit the antiparkinsonian effect of levodopa; avoid this combination
Promethazine plus lithium may rarely produce neurotoxicity
Barbiturates may reduce promethazine concentrations
Propranolol may increase promethazine concentrations
Sulfadoxine-pyrimethamine may increase promethazine concentrations
Promethazine and possibly other low potency antipsychotics may reverse the pressor effects of epinephrine
Promethazine and CNS depressants (ethanol, narcotics) may produce additive CNS depressant effects
Promethazine and trazodone may produce additive hypotensive effects
Use with cisapride may increase the risk of malignant arrhythmias; concurrent use is contraindicated

Food Interactions Increase dietary intake of riboflavin

Stability Protect from light; **compatible** (when comixed in the same syringe) with atropine, chlorpromazine, diphenhydramine, droperidol, fentanyl, glycopyrrolate, hydromorphone, hydroxyzine hydrochloride, meperidine, midazolam, nalbuphine, pentazocine, prochlorperazine, scopolamine; **incompatible** when mixed with aminophylline, cefoperazone (Y-site), chloramphenicol, dimenhydrinate (same syringe), foscarnet (Y-site), furosemide, heparin, hydrocortisone, methohexital, penicillin G, pentobarbital, phenobarbital, thiopental

Mechanism of Action Blocks postsynaptic mesolimbic dopaminergic receptors in the brain; exhibits a strong alpha-adrenergic blocking effect and depresses the release of hypothalamic and hypophyseal hormones; competes with histamine for the H_1-receptor

Pharmacodynamics

Onset of action:
Oral, I.M.: Within 20 minutes
I.V.: 3-5 minutes
Duration: 2-8 hours

Pharmacokinetics

Metabolism: In the liver
Elimination: Principally as inactive metabolites in the urine and in the feces

Usual Dosage

Children:
Antihistamine: Oral: 0.1 mg/kg/dose every 6 hours during the day and 0.5 mg/kg/dose at bedtime as needed
Antiemetic: Oral, I.M., I.V., rectal: 0.25-1 mg/kg 4-6 times/day as needed
Motion sickness: Oral: 0.5 mg/kg 30 minutes to 1 hour before departure, then every 12 hours as needed
Sedation: Oral, I.M., I.V., rectal: 0.5-1 mg/kg/dose every 6 hours as needed
Adults:
Antihistamine:
Oral, rectal: 12.5 mg 3 times/day and 25 mg at bedtime
I.M., I.V.: 25 mg, may repeat in 2 hours when necessary; switch to oral route as soon as feasible
Antiemetic: Oral, I.M., I.V., rectal: 12.5-25 mg every 4 hours as needed
Motion sickness: Oral: 25 mg 30 minutes to 1 hour before departure, then every 12 hours as needed
Sedation: Oral, I.M., I.V., rectal: 25-50 mg/dose; repeat every 4-6 hours if needed

Administration

Oral: Administer with food, water, or milk to decrease GI distress
Parenteral: I.M. administration is preferred; avoid I.V. use (see Warnings); in selected patients, promethazine has been administered I.V. diluted to a maximum concentration of 25 mg/mL and infused at a maximum rate of 25 mg/minute; avoid S.C. administration, promethazine is a chemical irritant which may produce necrosis

Test Interactions Alters the flare response in intradermal allergen tests; false negative and positive reactions with pregnancy tests relying on immunological reactions between hCG and anti-hCG

Patient Information Causes drowsiness and may impair ability to perform hazardous tasks which require mental alertness or physical coordination; may cause photosensitivity; avoid excessive sunlight; notify physician of involuntary movements or feelings of restlessness

Additional Information Although promethazine has been used in combination with meperidine and chlorpromazine as a premedication (lytic cocktail), this combination may have a higher rate of adverse effects compared to alternative sedative/analgesics

Dosage Forms

Injection, as hydrochloride: 25 mg/mL (1 mL, 10 mL); 50 mg/mL (1 mL, 10 mL)
Suppository, rectal, as hydrochloride: 12.5 mg, 25 mg, 50 mg
Syrup, as hydrochloride: 6.25 mg/5 mL (5 mL, 120 mL, 240 mL, 480 mL, 4000 mL); 25 mg/5 mL (120 mL, 480 mL, 4000 mL)
Tablet, as hydrochloride: 12.5 mg, 25 mg, 50 mg

Promethazine and Codeine (proe METH a zeen & KOE deen)

Brand Names Phenergan® With Codeine; Pherazine® With Codeine; Prothazine-DC®

Available Salts Promethazine Hydrochloride and Codeine Phosphate

Synonyms Codeine and Promethazine

Therapeutic Category Antitussive; Cough Preparation; Phenothiazine Derivative

Generic Available Yes

Use Temporary relief of coughs and upper respiratory symptoms associated with allergy or the common cold

Restrictions C-V

Pregnancy Risk Factor C

Contraindications Hypersensitivity to promethazine, codeine, or any component; lower respiratory tract symptoms, including asthma; concurrent use of MAO inhibitors, narrow-angle glaucoma

Precautions Use with caution in patients with cardiovascular disease, impaired liver function, impaired renal function, sleep apnea, seizures, hypertensive crisis, (Continued)

Promethazine and Codeine *(Continued)*

suspected Reye's syndrome; hypersensitivity reactions to morphine, hydrocodone, hydromorphone, levorphanol, oxycodone, oxymorphone

Adverse Reactions

Promethazine:

Cardiovascular: Tachycardia, bradycardia, palpitations

Central nervous system: Sedation (pronounced), confusion, drowsiness, restlessness, anxiety, extrapyramidal reactions, tardive dyskinesia, seizures

Dermatologic: Rash, photosensitivity

Endocrine & metabolic: Antidiuretic hormone release

Gastrointestinal: GI upset, xerostomia, constipation

Genitourinary: Urinary retention

Hematologic: Agranulocytosis, leukopenia (rare), thrombocytopenia

Hepatic: Cholestatic jaundice, hepatitis

Neuromuscular & skeletal: Arthralgia, tremor, paresthesia, myalgia

Ocular: Blurred vision

Respiratory: Thickening of bronchial secretions, pharyngitis

Miscellaneous: Allergic reactions

Codeine:

Cardiovascular: Palpitations, orthostatic hypotension, tachycardia or bradycardia, peripheral vasodilation

Central nervous system: CNS depression, dizziness, sedation, euphoria, hallucination, seizures

Dermatologic: Pruritus

Gastrointestinal: Nausea, vomiting, constipation, biliary tract spasm

Genitourinary: Urinary tract spasm

Ocular: Miosis

Respiratory: Respiratory depression

Miscellaneous: Physical and psychological dependence, histamine release, allergic reactions

Drug Interactions See Promethazine *on page 805* and Codeine *on page 249*

Food Interactions Increase fluids, fiber intake, and riboflavin in diet

Mechanism of Action See individual monographs for Codeine *on page 249* and Promethazine *on page 805*

Usual Dosage Oral (**in terms of codeine**):

Children: 1-1.5 mg/kg/day divided every 4 hours as needed; maximum dose: 30 mg/day **or**

2-6 years: 1.25-2.5 mL every 4-6 hours as needed or 2.5-5 mg/dose every 4-6 hours as needed; maximum dose: 30 mg codeine/day

6-12 years: 2.5-5 mL every 4-6 hours as needed or 5-10 mg/dose every 4-6 hours as needed; maximum dose: 60 mg codeine/day

Adults: 10-20 mg/dose every 4-6 hours as needed; maximum dose: 120 mg codeine/day; or 5-10 mL every 4-6 hours as needed

Administration Oral: Administer with food or water to decrease GI upset

Test Interactions Alters the flare response in intradermal allergen tests; false negative and positive reactions with pregnancy tests relying on immunological reactions between hCG and anti-hCG

Patient Information Causes drowsiness and may impair ability to perform hazardous activities which require mental alertness or physical coordination

Dosage Forms Syrup: Promethazine hydrochloride 6.25 mg and codeine phosphate 10 mg per 5 mL (120 mL, 180 mL, 473 mL)

Promethazine and Phenylephrine

(proe METH a zeen & fen il EF rin)

Brand Names Phenergan® VC; Promethazine VC Plain Syrup; Promethazine VC Syrup; Prometh VC Plain Liquid

Available Salts Promethazine Hydrochloride and Phenylephrine Hydrochloride

Synonyms Phenylephrine and Promethazine

Therapeutic Category Antihistamine/Decongestant Combination

Generic Available Yes

Use Temporary relief of upper respiratory symptoms associated with allergy or the common cold

Pregnancy Risk Factor C

Contraindications Hypersensitivity to promethazine, phenylephrine, or any component; asthma, peripheral vascular disease, narrow-angle glaucoma, severe hypertension, cardiovascular disease, liver disease, patients receiving MAO inhibitors

Precautions Use with caution in patients with cardiovascular disease, impaired liver function, asthma, peptic ulcer, sleep apnea, seizures, hypertensive crisis; avoid in patients with suspected Reye's syndrome

Adverse Reactions
Promethazine:
Cardiovascular: Hypertension, hypotension, tachycardia
Central nervous system: Sedation (pronounced), drowsiness, confusion, fatigue, excitation, extrapyramidal reactions, dystonia, tardive dyskinesia
Dermatologic: Photosensitivity, rash, angioedema
Gastrointestinal: Xerostomia, GI upset, increased appetite, weight gain, abdominal pain, diarrhea, nausea
Genitourinary: Urinary retention
Hematologic: Thrombocytopenia, leukopenia, agranulocytosis (rare)
Hepatic: Cholestatic jaundice, hepatitis
Ocular: Blurred vision
Neuromuscular & skeletal: Arthralgia, tremor, paresthesia, myalgia
Respiratory: Thickening of bronchial secretions, pharyngitis
Miscellaneous: Allergic reactions
Phenylephrine:
Cardiovascular: Hypertension, angina, reflex severe bradycardia, arrhythmias, peripheral vasoconstriction
Central nervous system: Restlessness, excitability, headache, anxiety, nervousness, dizziness
Dermatologic: Pilomotor response, skin blanching
Neuromuscular & skeletal: Tremor
Respiratory: Respiratory distress, rebound nasal congestion, sneezing, burning, stinging, dryness

Drug Interactions See Promethazine *on page 805* and Phenylephrine *on page 758*
Food Interactions Increase dietary intake of riboflavin
Usual Dosage Oral:
Children:
2-6 years: 1.25 mL every 4-6 hours, not to exceed 7.5 mL in 24 hours
6-12 years: 2.5 mL every 4-6 hours, not to exceed 15 mL in 24 hours
Children >12 years and Adults: 5 mL every 4-6 hours, not to exceed 30 mL in 24 hours
Administration Oral: Administer with food, water, or milk to decrease GI distress
Test Interactions Alters the flare response in intradermal allergen tests; false negative and positive reactions with pregnancy tests relying on immunological reactions between hCG and anti-hCG
Patient Information Causes drowsiness and may impair ability to perform hazardous activities requiring mental alertness or physical coordination
Dosage Forms Liquid: Promethazine hydrochloride 6.25 mg and phenylephrine hydrochloride 5 mg per 5 mL (120 mL, 180 mL, 240 mL, 480 mL, 4000 mL)

♦ **Promethazine Hydrochloride** see Promethazine *on page 805*
♦ **Promethazine Hydrochloride and Codeine Phosphate** see Promethazine and Codeine *on page 807*
♦ **Promethazine Hydrochloride and Phenylephrine Hydrochloride** see Promethazine and Phenylephrine *on page 808*
♦ **Promethazine Hydrochloride, Phenylephrine Hydrochloride, and Codeine Phosphate** see Promethazine, Phenylephrine, and Codeine *on page 809*

Promethazine, Phenylephrine, and Codeine
(proe METH a zeen, fen il EF rin, & KOE deen)
Brand Names Mallergan-VC® With Codeine; Phenergan® VC With Codeine
Available Salts Promethazine Hydrochloride, Phenylephrine Hydrochloride, and Codeine Phosphate
Synonyms Codeine, Promethazine, and Phenylephrine; Phenylephrine, Promethazine, and Codeine
Therapeutic Category Antihistamine/Decongestant Combination; Antitussive; Cough Preparation
Generic Available Yes
Use Temporary relief of coughs and upper respiratory symptoms including nasal congestion
Restrictions C-V
Pregnancy Risk Factor C
(Continued)

Promethazine, Phenylephrine, and Codeine *(Continued)*

Contraindications Hypersensitivity to promethazine, codeine, phenylephrine, or any component; asthma, peripheral vascular disease; patients receiving MAO inhibitors

Warnings See individual monographs for Promethazine *on page 805*, Phenylephrine *on page 758*, and Codeine *on page 249*

Precautions See individual monographs for Promethazine *on page 805*, Phenylephrine *on page 758*, and Codeine *on page 249*

Adverse Reactions See individual monographs for Promethazine *on page 805*, Phenylephrine *on page 758*, and Codeine *on page 249*

Drug Interactions See individual monographs for Promethazine *on page 805*, Phenylephrine *on page 758*, and Codeine *on page 249*

Food Interactions Increase fluids, fiber intake, and riboflavin in diet

Usual Dosage Oral: Not recommended for children <2 years of age

  Children (**dose expressed in terms of codeine**): 1-1.5 mg/kg/day divided every 4-6 hours, maximum dose: 30 mg/day **or**
  <6 years:
     Weight 25 lb: 1.25-2.5 mL every 4-6 hours, not to exceed 6 mL/24 hours
     Weight 30 lb: 1.25-2.5 mL every 4-6 hours, not to exceed 7 mL/24 hours
     Weight 35 lb: 1.25-2.5 mL every 4-6 hours, not to exceed 8 mL/24 hours
     Weight 40 lb: 1.25-2.5 mL every 4-6 hours, not to exceed 9 mL/24 hours
     6-11 years: 2.5-5 mL every 4-6 hours, not to exceed 15 mL/24 hours
  Children ≥12 years and Adults: 5 mL every 4-6 hours, not to exceed 30 mL/24 hours

Administration Oral: Administer with food or water to decrease GI upset

Dosage Forms Liquid: Promethazine hydrochloride 6.25 mg, phenylephrine hydrochloride 5 mg, and codeine phosphate 10 mg per 5 mL with alcohol 7% (120 mL, 240 mL, 480 mL, 4000 mL)

♦ **Promethazine VC Plain Syrup** *see* Promethazine and Phenylephrine *on page 808*

♦ **Promethazine VC Syrup** *see* Promethazine and Phenylephrine *on page 808*

♦ **Prometh® Injection** *see* Promethazine *on page 805*

♦ **Prometh VC Plain Liquid** *see* Promethazine and Phenylephrine *on page 808*

♦ **Pronestyl®** *see* Procainamide *on page 799*

♦ **Pronestyl-SR®** *see* Procainamide *on page 799*

♦ **Propacet®** *see* Propoxyphene and Acetaminophen *on page 815*

♦ **Propaderm® (Canada)** *see* Beclomethasone *on page 122*

♦ **Propadrine** *see* Phenylpropanolamine *on page 761*

♦ **Propagest® [OTC]** *see* Phenylpropanolamine *on page 761*

♦ **Propanthel™ (Canada)** *see* Propantheline *on page 810*

Propantheline *(proe PAN the leen)*

Brand Names Pro-Banthine®; Propanthel™ (Canada)

Available Salts Propantheline Bromide

Therapeutic Category Anticholinergic Agent; Antispasmodic Agent, Gastrointestinal; Antispasmodic Agent, Urinary

Generic Available Yes: 15 mg tablet

Use Adjunctive treatment of peptic ulcer, irritable bowel syndrome, pancreatitis, ureteral and urinary bladder spasm; to reduce duodenal motility during diagnostic radiologic procedures

Pregnancy Risk Factor C

Contraindications Narrow-angle glaucoma; hypersensitivity to propantheline or any component; ulcerative colitis; toxic megacolon; obstructive disease of the GI or urinary tract

Warnings Infants, blondes, patients with Down's syndrome, and children with spastic paralysis or brain damage may be hypersensitive to antimuscarinic effects

Precautions Use with caution in febrile patients, patients with hyperthyroidism, hepatic, cardiac, or renal disease, hypertension, GI infections, diarrhea, reflux esophagitis

Adverse Reactions

  Cardiovascular: Tachycardia, palpitations, flushing
  Central nervous system: Insomnia, drowsiness, dizziness, nervousness, headache
  Dermatologic: Rash, dry skin
  Endocrine & metabolic: Suppression of lactation
  Gastrointestinal: Xerostomia, nausea, vomiting, constipation, dry throat, dysphagia
  Genitourinary: Impotence, urinary retention

Ocular: Mydriasis, blurred vision
Neuromuscular & skeletal: Weakness
Respiratory: Dry nose
Miscellaneous: Allergic reactions, diaphoresis (decreased)

Drug Interactions May increase potential of potassium chloride wax-matrix preparations to cause intestinal lesions due to decreased peristalsis; increased effect/toxicity with anticholinergics, disopyramide, narcotic analgesics, bretylium, type I antiarrhythmics, antihistamines, phenothiazines, tricyclic antidepressants, corticosteroids (increased IOP), CNS depressants (sedation), adenosine, amiodarone, beta-blockers, amoxapine

Mechanism of Action Competitively blocks the action of acetylcholine at postganglionic parasympathetic receptor sites

Pharmacodynamics
Onset of action: Within 30-45 minutes
Duration: 4-6 hours

Pharmacokinetics
Metabolism: In the liver and GI tract
Elimination: In urine, bile, and other body fluids

Usual Dosage Oral:
Antisecretory:
Children: 1-2 mg/kg/day in 3-4 divided doses
Adults: 15 mg 3 times/day before meals or food and 30 mg at bedtime; for mild manifestations: 7.5 mg 3 times/day
Antispasmodic:
Children: 2-3 mg/kg/day in divided doses every 4-6 hours and at bedtime
Adults: 15 mg 3 times/day before meals or food and 30 mg at bedtime

Administration Oral: Administer 30 minutes before meals and at bedtime

Patient Information Causes drowsiness and may impair ability to perform hazardous tasks requiring mental alertness or physical coordination; notify physician if skin rash, flushing, or eye pain occurs; or if difficulty in urinating, constipation, or sensitivity to light becomes severe or persists; maintain good oral hygiene habits, because lack of saliva may increase chance of cavities

Dosage Forms Tablet, as bromide: 7.5 mg, 15 mg

♦ **Propantheline Bromide** see Propantheline on page 810

Proparacaine (proe PAR a kane)

Brand Names AK-Taine®; Alcaine®; Diocaine(Canada); I-Paracaine®; Ophthaine®; Ophthetic®

Available Salts Proparacaine Hydrochloride

Synonyms Proxymetacaine

Therapeutic Category Local Anesthetic, Ophthalmic

Generic Available Yes

Use Local anesthesia for tonometry, gonioscopy; suture removal from cornea; removal of corneal foreign body; cataract extraction, glaucoma surgery; short operative procedure involving the cornea and conjunctiva

Pregnancy Risk Factor C

Contraindications Hypersensitivity to proparacaine or any component

Precautions Use with caution in patients with cardiac disease, hyperthyroidism

Adverse Reactions
Dermatologic: Allergic contact dermatitis
Local: Irritation, stinging, sensitization
Ocular: Keratitis, iritis, erosion of the corneal epithelium, conjunctival congestion and hemorrhage, corneal opacification

Mechanism of Action Local anesthetic; prevents initiation and transmission of impulse at the nerve cell membrane by decreasing ion permeability

Pharmacodynamics
Onset of action: Within 20 seconds of instillation
Duration: 15-20 minutes

Usual Dosage Children and Adults:
Ophthalmic surgery: Instill 1 drop of 0.5% solution in eye every 5-10 minutes for 5-7 doses
Tonometry, gonioscopy, suture removal: Instill 1-2 drops of 0.5% solution in eye just prior to procedure

Administration Ophthalmic: Instill drops into affected eye(s); avoid contact of bottle tip with skin or eye

Patient Information Do not rub eye until anesthesia has worn off

Dosage Forms Ophthalmic, solution, as hydrochloride: 0.5% (2 mL, 15 mL)

- **Proparacaine Hydrochloride** *see Proparacaine on page 811*
- **Propine®** *see Dipivefrin on page 330*
- **Pro-Piroxicam® (Canada)** *see Piroxicam on page 777*
- **Proplex® SX-T** *see Factor IX Complex (Human) on page 399*
- **Proplex® T** *see Factor IX Complex (Human) on page 399*

Propofol (PROE po fole)

Brand Names Diprivan® Injection

Therapeutic Category General Anesthetic

Generic Available Yes

Use Induction or maintenance of anesthesia in children ≥3 years and adults; initiation and maintenance of monitored anesthesia care sedation in adults; continuous sedation of adult intensive care unit patient

Pregnancy Risk Factor B

Contraindications Hypersensitivity to propofol, sulfites (generic product contains sodium metabisulfite), disodium edetate (Diprivan® contains disodium edetate), or any component (eg, soybean oil, egg yolk phospholipid, or egg lecithin); patients who are not intubated or mechanically ventilated; other contraindications to general anesthesia or sedation apply

Warnings Not recommended for use in children <3 years of age; not recommended for monitored anesthesia care sedation in children; not recommended for sedation of PICU patients, especially at high doses or for prolonged periods of time; metabolic acidosis with fatal cardiac failure has occurred in several children (4 weeks to 11 years of age) who received propofol infusions at average rates of infusion of 4.5-10 mg/kg/hour for 66-115 hours (maximum rates of infusion 6.2-11.5 mg/kg/hour); see Parke, 1992; Strickland, 1995; and Bray, 1995. Patients require continuous monitoring and airway management; cardiovascular and respiratory resuscitation equipment should be available; decrease the dose in ASA III or IV, elderly, debilitated, or hypovolemic patients; not recommended for use in obstetrics, cesarean deliveries, lactating women, patients with increased ICP or impaired cerebral circulation. Abrupt discontinuation may result in rapid awakening, anxiety, agitation, and resistance to mechanical ventilation. Although products contain preservatives, rapid growth of micro-organisms can occur; failure to use aseptic technique can result in microbial contamination and fever, sepsis, infection, life-threatening illnesses, or death; discard I.V. tubing and unused portions after 12 hours; **do not use if microbial contamination is suspected.**

Propofol should be administered by qualified healthcare professionals trained in advanced cardiac life support and anesthetic drug use (when used for general anesthesia and monitored anesthesia care sedation) or management of critically ill patients (when used for sedation in intensive care patient).

Precautions Use with caution in patients with seizures or history of epilepsy, or severe cardiac or respiratory disease; I.V. injection may produce transient local pain; perioperative myoclonia may occur; decrease dose and rate of infusion for elderly, debilitated, or ASA III/IV patients.

Diprivan® contains disodium edetate which can chelate trace metals, including zinc; as much as 10 mg of elemented zinc may be lost per day when calcium disodium edetate is used in gram doses to treat heavy metal poisonings; no reports of zinc deficiency or low zinc levels have been reported with Diprivan®, however, the manufacturer recommends that Diprivan® not be infused for >5 days without giving a "drug holiday"; during this time off of Diprivan®, replacement of estimated or measured urine zinc losses is recommended. **Note:** The generic product does not contain disodium edetate, but contains metabisulfite as the preservative.

Adverse Reactions

Cardiovascular: Hypotension (dose related), bradycardia, myocardial depression, flushing

Central nervous system: Fever, headache, dizziness

Dermatologic: Rash, pruritus

Endocrine & metabolic: Hyperlipidemia; fatal metabolic acidosis has been reported

Gastrointestinal: Nausea, vomiting, abdominal cramping

Genitourinary: Discoloration of urine (green)

Local: Pain at injection site (especially when administered via small vein); **Note:** Dilution with D_5W or administration of lidocaine pretreatment may decrease local pain

Neuromuscular & skeletal: Myalgia, twitching, clonic/myoclonic movement

Respiratory: Respiratory acidosis, respiratory depression, apnea

Miscellaneous: Anaphylaxis, anaphylactoid reactions

Drug Interactions Theophylline may antagonize the CNS effects of propofol; propofol may increase serum concentrations of alfentanil; increased toxicity may occur with acetazolamide (cardiorespiratory instability), CNS depressants, atracurium (anaphylaxis), phenothiazines, fentanyl (increased concentration of propofol), guanabenz, MAO inhibitors, narcotic analgesics, vecuronium (increased neuromuscular blockade)

Stability Does not require refrigeration; protect from light; do not use if there is evidence of separation of phases of emulsion, particulate matter, or discoloration; discard unused portions at end of surgical procedure; ICU use: Discard tubing and unused portions after 12 hours; dilute with D_5W only; do not dilute to <2 mg/mL; diluted emulsion is more stable in glass; stability in plastic: 95% potency after 2 hours; may administer with D_5W, LR, D_5LR, $D_5/_{1/2}NS$, $D_5/_{1/4}NS$; do not administer with blood or blood products through the same I.V. catheter

Mechanism of Action Propofol is a hindered phenolic compound with intravenous general anesthetic properties. The drug is unrelated to any of the currently used barbiturate, opioid, benzodiazepine, arylcyclohexylamine, or imidazole intravenous anesthetic agents.

Pharmacodynamics
Onset of anesthesia: Within 30 seconds after bolus infusion
Duration: ~3-10 minutes depending on the dose, rate and duration of administration; with prolonged use (eg, 10 days ICU sedation), propofol accumulates in tissues and redistributes into plasma when the drug is discontinued, so that the time to awakening (duration of action) is increased; however, if dose is titrated on a daily basis, so that the minimum effective dose is utilized, time to awakening may be within 10-15 minutes even after prolonged use

Pharmacokinetics
Distribution: Large volume of distribution; highly lipophilic
V_d (apparent): Children 4-12 years: 5-10 L/kg
V_{dss}:
Adults: 170-350 L
Adults (10-day infusion): 60 L/kg
Protein binding: 97% to 99%
Metabolism: In the liver via glucuronide and sulfate conjugation
Half-life (three-compartment model):
Initial: 2-8 minutes
Second distribution: ~40 minutes
Terminal: ~200 minutes; range: 300-700 minutes
Terminal (after 10-day infusion): 1-3 days
Elimination: ~90% excreted in urine as metabolites and <1% as unchanged drug

Usual Dosage Dosage must be individualized based on total body weight and titrated to the desired clinical effect; wait at least 3-5 minutes between dosage adjustments to clinically assess drug effects; smaller doses are required when used with narcotics; the following are general dosing guidelines:

General anesthesia:
I.V. induction: (See "Symbols and Abbreviations Used in This Handbook" in front section of this book for explanation of ASA classes):
Children ≥3 years, ASA I or II: 2.5-3.5 mg/kg; use a lower dose for children ASA III or IV
Adults, ASA I or II, <55 years: 2-2.5 mg/kg (~40 mg every 10 seconds until onset of induction)
Elderly, debilitated, hypovolemic, or ASA III or IV: 1-1.5 mg/kg (~20 mg every 10 seconds until onset of induction)
Cardiac anesthesia: 0.5-1.5 mg/kg (~20 mg every 10 seconds until onset of induction)
Neurosurgical patients: 1-2 mg/kg (~20 mg every 10 seconds until onset of induction)
Maintenance: I.V. infusion:
Children ≥3 years, ASA I or II: Initial: 200-300 mcg/kg/minute; decrease dose after 30 minutes if clinical signs of light anesthesia are absent; usual infusion rate: 125-150 mcg/kg/minute; children ≤5 years may require larger infusion rates compared to older children
Adults, ASA I or II, <55 years: Initial: 150-200 mcg/kg/minute for 10-15 minutes; decrease by 30% to 50% during first 30 minutes of maintenance; usual infusion rate: 100-200 mcg/kg/minute
Elderly, debilitated, hypovolemic, ASA III or IV: 50-100 mcg/kg/minute
Cardiac anesthesia:
Low dose propofol with primary opioid: 50-100 mcg/kg/minute (see manufacturer's labeling)
(Continued)

Propofol (Continued)

Primary propofol with secondary opioid: 100-150 mcg/kg/minute

Neurosurgical patients: 100-200 mcg/kg/minute

Maintenance: I.V. intermittent bolus: Adults, ASA I or II, <55 years: 20-50 mg increments as needed

Monitored Anesthesia Care sedation:

Initiation:

Adults, ASA I or II, <55 years: Slow I.V. infusion: 100-150 mcg/kg/minute for 3-5 minutes; slow injection: 0.5 mg/kg over 3-5 minutes

Elderly, debilitated, neurosurgical, or ASA III or IV patients: Use similar doses to healthy adults; avoid rapid I.V. boluses

Maintenance:

Adults, ASA I or II, <55 years: I.V. infusion using variable rates (preferred over intermittent boluses): 25-75 mcg/kg/minute; incremental bolus doses: 10 mg or 20 mg

Elderly, debilitated, neurosurgical, or ASA III or IV patients: Use 80% of healthy adult dose; **do not** use rapid bolus doses (single or repeated)

ICU sedation in intubated mechanically ventilated patients: Avoid rapid bolus injection; individualize dose and titrate to response

Adults: Continuous infusion: Initial: 0.3 mg/kg/hour; increase by 0.3-0.6 mg/kg/hour every 5-10 minutes until desired sedation level is achieved; usual maintenance: 0.3-3 mg/kg/hour or higher; reduce dose by 80% in elderly, debilitated, and ASA III or IV patients; reduce dose after adequate sedation established and adjust to response (ie, evaluate frequently to use minimum dose for sedation)

Administration Parenteral: I.V.: Shake injection well before use; administer pediatric induction doses over 20-30 seconds; do not administer via filter with <5-micron pore size

Monitoring Parameters Respiratory rate, blood pressure, heart rate, oxygen saturation, ABGs, depth of sedation; serum lipids or triglycerides with use >24 hours

Nursing Implications May change urine color to green

Additional Information Due to poor water solubility, the I.V. formulation is an isotonic oil-in-water emulsion and contains soybean oil, glycerol, egg lecithin, and sodium hydroxide (for pH adjustment); the brand name and generic product differ in the preservative used; Diprivan® contains 0.005% disodium edetate, while the generic product contains sodium metabisulfite (0.25 mg/mL)

Dosage Forms Injection: 10 mg/mL (20 mL, 50 mL, 100 mL)

References

Bray RJ, "Fatal Myocardial Failure Associated With a Propofol Infusion in a Child," *Anaesthesia,* 1995, 50(1):94.

Parke TJ, Stevens JE, Rice ASC, et al, "Metabolic Acidosis and Fatal Myocardial Failure After Propofol Infusion in Children: Five Case Reports," *BMJ,* 1992, 305(6854):613-6.

Strickland RA and Murray MJ, "Fatal Metabolic Acidosis in a Pediatric Patient Receiving an Infusion of Propofol in the Intensive Care Unit: Is There a Relationship?" *Crit Care Med,* 1995, 23(2):405-9.

Propoxyphene (proe POKS i feen)

Related Information

Overdose and Toxicology *on page 1191*

Brand Names 642® (Canada); Darvon®; Darvon-N®; Dolene®; Novo-Propoxyn® (Canada)

Available Salts Propoxyphene Hydrochloride; Propoxyphene Napsylate

Synonyms Dextropropoxyphene

Therapeutic Category Analgesic, Narcotic

Generic Available Yes: Capsule

Use Management of mild to moderate pain

Restrictions C-IV

Pregnancy Risk Factor C

Contraindications Hypersensitivity to propoxyphene or any component

Warnings Do not exceed recommended dosage

Precautions Use with caution in patients with renal or hepatic dysfunction, or when substituting propoxyphene for opiates in narcotic dependent patients; reduce dose in patients with hepatic dysfunction; avoid use in patients with Cl_{cr} <10 mL/minute

Adverse Reactions

Central nervous system: Dizziness, lightheadedness, sedation, paradoxical excitement and insomnia, headache

Dermatologic: Rashes

Gastrointestinal: GI upset, nausea, vomiting, constipation

Hepatic: Increased liver enzymes

Neuromuscular & skeletal: Weakness

Miscellaneous: Psychologic and physical dependence

Drug Interactions Cytochrome P-450 isoenzyme CYP3A3/4 inhibitor
CNS depressants, alcohol, MAO inhibitors, may potentiate adverse effects; propoxyphene may inhibit the metabolism and increase the serum concentrations of carbamazepine, phenobarbital, tricyclic antidepressants, and warfarin; concurrent use of propoxyphene with ritonavir is not recommended

Food Interactions Food may decrease rate of absorption, but may slightly increase bioavailability

Mechanism of Action Binds to opiate receptors in the CNS, causing inhibition of ascending pain pathways, altering the perception of and response to pain; produces generalized CNS depression

Pharmacodynamics
Onset of effects: Oral: Within 30-60 minutes
Duration: 4-6 hours

Pharmacokinetics
Metabolism: In the liver to an active metabolite (norpropoxyphene) and inactive metabolites
Bioavailability: Oral: 30% to 70% due to first-pass effect
Half-life, adults: 8-24 hours (mean: ~15 hours)
Norpropoxyphene, adults: 34 hours
Not dialyzable (0% to 5%)

Usual Dosage Oral:
Children: Dose not well established; doses of propoxyphene hydrochloride of 2-3 mg/kg/day divided every 6 hours have been used
Adults:
Hydrochloride: 65 mg every 3-4 hours as needed for pain; maximum dose: 390 mg/day
Napsylate: 100 mg every 4 hours as needed for pain; maximum dose: 600 mg/day
Dosing adjustment in renal impairment: Cl_{cr} <10 mL/minute: Avoid use
Dosing adjustment in hepatic impairment: Reduced doses should be used

Administration Oral: May administer with food to decrease GI upset

Monitoring Parameters Pain relief, respiratory rate, blood pressure, mental status; liver enzymes with long-term use

Test Interactions False-positive methadone test

Patient Information Avoid alcohol; may be habit-forming; may cause dizziness or drowsiness and impair ability to perform activities requiring mental alertness or physical coordination

Additional Information Propoxyphene does not possess any anti-inflammatory or antipyretic actions; it possesses little, if any, antitussive effects; propoxyphene napsylate 100 mg is equivalent to 65 mg of propoxyphene hydrochloride; several cases utilizing propoxyphene in children for opioid detoxification have been reported (see References)

Dosage Forms
Capsule, as hydrochloride: 65 mg
Tablet, as napsylate: 100 mg

References
Hasday JD and Weintraub M, "Propoxyphene in Children With Iatrogenic Morphine Dependence," *Am J Dis Child*, 1983, 137(8):745-8.

Propoxyphene and Acetaminophen
(proe POKS i feen & a seet a MIN oh fen)

Related Information
Narcotic Analgesics Comparison *on page 1035*
Overdose and Toxicology *on page 1191*

Brand Names Darvocet-N®; Darvocet-N® 100; Genagesic®; Propacet®; Wygesic®

Available Salts Propoxyphene Hydrochloride and Acetaminophen; Propoxyphene Napsylate and Acetaminophen

Synonyms Acetaminophen and Propoxyphene

Therapeutic Category Analgesic, Narcotic

Generic Available Yes

Use Management of mild to moderate pain

Restrictions C-IV

Pregnancy Risk Factor C

Contraindications Hypersensitivity to propoxyphene, acetaminophen, or any component

Warnings Do not exceed recommended dosage
(Continued)

Propoxyphene and Acetaminophen *(Continued)*

Precautions Use with caution in patients with renal or hepatic dysfunction or when substituting propoxyphene for opiates in narcotic dependent patients

Adverse Reactions

Propoxyphene:

Central nervous system: Dizziness, lightheadedness, sedation, paradoxical excitement, insomnia, headache

Dermatologic: Rashes

Gastrointestinal: GI upset, nausea, vomiting, constipation

Hepatic: Increased liver enzymes

Neuromuscular & skeletal: Weakness

Miscellaneous: Psychologic and physical dependence

Acetaminophen:

Dermatologic: Rash

Hematologic: Blood dyscrasias (neutropenia, pancytopenia, leukopenia)

Hepatic: Hepatic necrosis with overdose

Renal: Renal injury with chronic use

Miscellaneous: Hypersensitivity reactions (rare)

Drug Interactions See Propoxyphene *on page 814* and Acetaminophen *on page 26*

Food Interactions Food may decrease rate of absorption of propoxyphene, but may slightly increase bioavailability; the rate of absorption of acetaminophen may be decreased when given with food high in carbohydrates

Pharmacodynamics See individual monographs for Propoxyphene *on page 814* and Acetaminophen *on page 26*

Pharmacokinetics See individual monographs for Propoxyphene *on page 814* and Acetaminophen *on page 26*

Usual Dosage Adults: Oral:

Darvocet-N®: 1-2 tablets every 4 hours as needed; maximum dose: 600 mg propoxyphene napsylate/day

Darvocet-N® 100 or Wygesic®: 1 tablet every 4 hours as needed; maximum dose: 600 mg propoxyphene napsylate/day

Administration Oral: Administer with water on an empty stomach; may administer with food to decrease GI upset

Monitoring Parameters Pain relief, respiratory rate, blood pressure, mental status; liver enzymes with long-term use

Test Interactions False-positive methadone test

Patient Information Avoid alcohol; may be habit-forming; may cause dizziness, drowsiness and impair ability to perform hazardous tasks requiring mental alertness

Additional Information Propoxyphene napsylate 100 mg is equivalent to 65 mg of propoxyphene hydrochloride

Dosage Forms Tablet:

Darvocet-N®: Propoxyphene napsylate 50 mg and acetaminophen 325 mg

Darvocet-N® 100: Propoxyphene napsylate 100 mg and acetaminophen 650 mg

Genagesic®, Wygesic®: Propoxyphene hydrochloride 65 mg and acetaminophen 650 mg

♦ **Propoxyphene Hydrochloride** *see* Propoxyphene *on page 814*

♦ **Propoxyphene Hydrochloride and Acetaminophen** *see* Propoxyphene and Acetaminophen *on page 815*

♦ **Propoxyphene Napsylate** *see* Propoxyphene *on page 814*

♦ **Propoxyphene Napsylate and Acetaminophen** *see* Propoxyphene and Acetaminophen *on page 815*

Propranolol *(proe PRAN oh lole)*

Related Information

Adult ACLS Algorithm, Tachycardia *on page 1010*

Carbohydrate and Alcohol Content of Liquid Medications for Use in Patients Receiving Ketogenic Diets *on page 1228*

Overdose and Toxicology *on page 1191*

Brand Names Apo®-Propranolol (Canada); Betachron®; Detensol® (Canada); Inderal®; Inderal® LA; Nu-Propranolol® (Canada)

Available Salts Propranolol Hydrochloride

Therapeutic Category Antianginal Agent; Antiarrhythmic Agent, Class II; Antihypertensive Agent; Antimigraine Agent; Beta-Adrenergic Blocker

Generic Available Yes

Use Management of hypertension, angina pectoris, pheochromocytoma, essential tremor, tetralogy of Fallot cyanotic spells, and arrhythmias (such as atrial fibrillation and flutter, A-V nodal re-entrant tachycardias, and catecholamine-induced arrhythmias); prevention of MI, migraine headache; symptomatic treatment of hypertrophic subaortic stenosis; short-term adjunctive therapy of thyrotoxicosis

Pregnancy Risk Factor C

Contraindications Hypersensitivity to propranolol or any component; uncompensated CHF, cardiogenic shock, bradycardia or heart block, asthma, hyperactive airway disease, chronic obstructive lung disease, Raynaud's syndrome

Warnings In patients with angina pectoris, exacerbation of angina and, in some cases, MI occurred following abrupt discontinuance of therapy

Precautions Propranolol may block hypoglycemia-induced tachycardia and blood pressure changes, use with caution in patients with diabetes mellitus; avoid I.V. use in patients receiving calcium channel blockers (eg, verapamil) (effects may be potentiated)

Adverse Reactions
Cardiovascular: Hypotension, impaired myocardial contractility, CHF, bradycardia, worsening of A-V conduction disturbances
Central nervous system: Lightheadedness, insomnia, vivid dreams, lethargy, depression
Endocrine & metabolic: Hypoglycemia [also blunts warning signs of hypoglycemia (eg, tachycardia)], hyperglycemia
Gastrointestinal: Nausea, vomiting, diarrhea, GI distress
Hematologic: Agranulocytosis
Neuromuscular & skeletal: Weakness
Respiratory: Bronchospasm
Miscellaneous: Cold extremities

Drug Interactions Cytochrome P-450 isoenzyme, CYP1A2, CYP2C18, CYP2C19, and CYP2D6 substrate
Phenobarbital, rifampin may increase propranolol clearance and may decrease its activity; cimetidine may reduce propranolol clearance and may increase its effects; aluminum-containing antacid may reduce GI absorption of propranolol; flecainide, hydralazine, quinidine, verapamil may increase cardiovascular adverse effects

Food Interactions Avoid natural licorice (causes sodium and water retention and increases potassium loss); protein-rich foods may increase bioavailability; a change in diet from high carbohydrate/low protein to low carbohydrate/high protein may result in increased oral clearance

Stability Injection is compatible in saline, incompatible with bicarbonate; protect injection from light

Mechanism of Action Nonselective beta-adrenergic blocker (class II antiarrhythmic); competitively blocks response to beta$_1$- and beta$_2$-adrenergic stimulation which results in decrease in heart rate, myocardial contractility, blood pressure, and myocardial oxygen demand

Pharmacodynamics Beta blockade: Oral:
Onset of action: Within 1-2 hours
Duration: ~6 hours

Pharmacokinetics
Distribution: V_d: Adults: 3.9 L/kg; crosses the placenta; small amounts appear in breast milk
Protein-binding (Alpha$_1$-acid glycoprotein and albumin):
Newborns: 60% to 68%
Adults: 93%
Metabolism: Extensive first-pass effect, metabolized in the liver to active and inactive compounds
Bioavailability: 30% to 40%; oral bioavailability may be increased in Down syndrome children
Half-life (prolonged with hepatic dysfunction):
Neonates and Infants: Possible increased half-life
Children: 3.9-6.4 hours
Adults: 4-6 hours
Elimination: Metabolites are excreted primarily in urine (96% to 99%); <1% excreted in urine as unchanged drug
Not dialyzable: (0% to 5%)

Usual Dosage
Neonates:
Oral: Initial: 0.25 mg/kg/dose every 6-8 hours; increase slowly as needed to maximum of 5 mg/kg/day

(Continued)

Propranolol *(Continued)*

I.V.: Initial: 0.01 mg/kg slow I.V. push over 10 minutes; may repeat every 6-8 hours as needed; increase slowly to maximum of 0.15 mg/kg/dose every 6-8 hours

Arrhythmias:

Oral:

Children: Initial: 0.5-1 mg/kg/day in divided doses every 6-8 hours; titrate dosage upward every 3-5 days; usual dose: 2-4 mg/kg/day; higher doses may be needed; do not exceed 16 mg/kg/day or 60 mg/day

Adults: Initial: 10-20 mg/dose every 6-8 hours, increase gradually; usual range: 40-320 mg/day

I.V.:

Children: 0.01-0.1 mg/kg slow I.V. over 10 minutes; maximum dose: 1 mg (infants); 3 mg (children)

Adults: 1 mg/dose slow I.V.; repeat every 5 minutes up to a total of 5 mg

Hypertension: Oral:

Children: Initial: 0.5-1 mg/kg/day in divided doses every 6-12 hours; increase gradually every 3-5 days; usual dose: 1-5 mg/kg/day; maximum dose: 8 mg/kg/day

Adults: Initial: 40 mg twice daily or 60-80 mg once daily as sustained release capsules; increase dosage every 3-5 days; usual dose: ≤320 mg divided in 2-3 doses/day or once daily as sustained release; maximum daily dose: 640 mg

Migraine headache prophylaxis: Oral:

Children: 0.6-1.5 mg/kg/day divided every 8 hours; maximum dose: 4 mg/kg/day
or
≤35 kg: 10-20 mg 3 times/day
>35 kg: 20-40 mg 3 times/day

Adults: Initial: 80 mg/day divided every 6-8 hours; increase by 20-40 mg/dose every 3-4 weeks to a maximum of 160-240 mg/day given in divided doses every 6-8 hours

Tetralogy spells: Infants and Children:

Oral: Usual: 1-2 mg/kg/dose every 6 hours, may initiate at ½ the usual dose; may increase by 1 mg/kg/day every 24 hours to maximum of 5 mg/kg/day; if refractory may increase slowly to a maximum of 10-15 mg/kg/day but must carefully monitor heart rate, heart size, and cardiac contractility (Garson, 1981).

I.V.: 0.15-0.25 mg/kg/dose slow I.V.; may repeat in 15 minutes

Thyrotoxicosis:

Neonates: Oral: 2 mg/kg/day in divided doses every 6-12 hours; occasionally higher doses may be required

Adolescents and Adults: Oral: 10-40 mg/dose every 6 hours

Adults: I.V.: 1-3 mg/dose slow I.V. as a single dose

Administration

Oral: Administer with food; do not chew or crush sustained action capsules, swallow whole; mix concentrated oral solution with water, fruit juice, liquid, or semisolid food before administration

Parenteral: I.V. administration should not exceed 1 mg/minute; administer slow I.V. over 10 minutes in children; maximum concentration for injection: 1 mg/mL

Monitoring Parameters EKG, blood pressure

Reference Range Therapeutic: 50-100 ng/mL (SI: 190-390 nmol/L) at end of dosing interval

Patient Information Avoid alcohol; do not discontinue abruptly; may mask fast heart rate of hypoglycemia, but sweating will still occur

Nursing Implications The I.V. dose is much smaller than oral dose

Additional Information Not indicated for hypertensive emergencies; do not abruptly discontinue therapy, taper dosage gradually over 2 weeks

Dosage Forms

Capsule, sustained action, as hydrochloride: 60 mg, 80 mg, 120 mg, 160 mg

Injection, as hydrochloride: 1 mg/mL (1 mL)

Solution, oral, as hydrochloride (strawberry-mint flavor): 4 mg/mL (5 mL, 500 mL); 8 mg/mL (5 mL, 500 mL)

Solution, oral, concentrate, as hydrochloride: 80 mg/mL (30 mL)

Tablet, as hydrochloride: 10 mg, 20 mg, 40 mg, 60 mg, 80 mg

References

Garson A Jr, Gillette PC, and McNamara DG, "Propranolol: The Preferred Palliation for Tetralogy of Fallot," *Am J Cardiol*, 1981, 47(5):1098-104.

Lai CW, Ziegler DK, Lansky LL, et al, "Hemiplegic Migraine in Childhood: Diagnostic and Therapeutic Aspects," *J Pediatr*, 1982, 101(5):696-9.

Pickoff AS, Zies L, Ferrer PL, et al, "High-Dose Propranolol Therapy in the Management of Supraventricular Tachycardia," *J Pediatr*, 1979, 94(1):144-6.

Rasoulpour M and Marinelli KA, "Systemic Hypertension," *Clin Perinatol*, 1992, 19(1):121-37.
Sinaiko AR, "Pharmacologic Management of Childhood Hypertension," *Pediatr Clin North Am*, 1993, 40(1):195-212.

♦ **Propranolol Hydrochloride** *see* Propranolol *on page 816*

♦ **Propulsid®** *see* Cisapride *U.S. - Available Via Limited-Access Protocol Only on page 226*

♦ **2-Propylpentanoic Acid** *see* Valproic Acid and Derivatives *on page 966*

Propylthiouracil (proe pil thye oh YOOR a sil)

Brand Names Propyl-Thyracil® (Canada)

Synonyms PTU

Therapeutic Category Antithyroid Agent

Generic Available Yes

Use Palliative treatment of hyperthyroidism; adjunct to ameliorate hyperthyroidism in preparation for surgical treatment or radioactive iodine therapy; management of thyrotoxic crisis

Pregnancy Risk Factor D

Contraindications Hypersensitivity to propylthiouracil or any component

Warnings May cause agranulocytosis, thyroid hyperplasia, thyroid carcinoma (usage >1 year)

Precautions Use with caution in patients receiving other drugs known to cause agranulocytosis

Adverse Reactions

Cardiovascular: Edema, cutaneous vasculitis

Central nervous system: Drowsiness, vertigo, dizziness, headache, drug fever

Dermatologic: Rash, urticaria, pruritus, exfoliative dermatitis, alopecia, skin pigmentation

Gastrointestinal: Nausea, vomiting, ageusia, sialadenopathy, constipation

Hematologic: Agranulocytosis, leukopenia, thrombocytopenia, bleeding, hypoprothrombinemia

Hepatic: Jaundice, hepatitis

Neuromuscular & skeletal: Arthralgia, paresthesia, neuritis

Renal: Nephritis

Respiratory: Interstitial pneumonitis

Miscellaneous: Lymphadenopathy

Drug Interactions Anticoagulants (enhanced anticoagulant activity)

Mechanism of Action Inhibits the synthesis of thyroid hormones by blocking the oxidation of iodine in the thyroid gland; blocks synthesis of thyroxine and triiodothyronine

Pharmacodynamics For significant therapeutic effects 24-36 hours are required; remission of hyperthyroidism usually does not occur before 4 months of continued therapy

Pharmacokinetics

Distribution: Breast milk to plasma ratio: 0.1

Protein binding: 75% to 80%

Metabolism: Hepatic

Bioavailability: 80% to 95%

Half-life: 1.5-5 hours

End-stage renal disease: 8.5 hours

Time to peak serum concentration: Oral: Within 1 hour; persists for 2-3 hours

Elimination: 35% excreted in urine

Usual Dosage Oral:

Neonates: 5-10 mg/kg/day in divided doses every 8 hours

Children: 5-7 mg/kg/day in divided doses every 8 hours **or**

6-10 years: 50-150 mg/day divided every 8 hours

≥10 years: 150-300 mg/day divided every 8 hours

Maintenance: $1/3$-$2/3$ of the initial dose in divided doses every 8-12 hours; this begins usually after 2 months on an effective initial dosage

Adults: Initial: 300-450 mg/day in divided doses every 8 hours (doses of 600-1200 mg/day are sometimes needed); maintenance: 100-150 mg/day in divided doses every 8-12 hours

Dosing adjustment in renal impairment: Adjustment is not necessary

Administration Oral: Administer with food

Monitoring Parameters CBC with differential, liver function tests, platelets, thyroid function tests (TSH, T_3, T_4), prothrombin time

Reference Range See normal values for thyroid function in Normal Laboratory Values for Children *on page 1155*

Dosage Forms Tablet: 50 mg

(Continued)

Propylthiouracil *(Continued)*

Extemporaneous Preparations A 5 mg/mL oral suspension may be made by crushing six 50 mg propylthiouracil tablets; add 30 mL 1.5% carboxymethylcellulose while mixing; qsad to 60 mL with simple syrup; label "refrigerate," "protect from light," "shake well"; expected stability: 10 days

Nahata MC and Hipple TF, *Pediatric Drug Formulations*, 3rd ed, Cincinnati, OH: Harvey Whitney Books Co, 1997.

References

Raby C, Lagorce JF, Jambut-Absil AC, et al, "The Mechanism of Action of Synthetic Antithyroid Drugs: Iodine Complexation During Oxidation of Iodide," *Endocrinology*, 1990, 126(3):1683-91.

♦ **Propyl-Thyracil® (Canada)** *see* Propylthiouracil *on page 819*
♦ **2-Propylvaleric Acid** *see* Valproic Acid and Derivatives *on page 966*
♦ **Prorazin® (Canada)** *see* Prochlorperazine *on page 803*
♦ **Prorex® Injection** *see* Promethazine *on page 805*
♦ **Pro-Sof® Plus [OTC]** *see* Docusate and Casanthranol *on page 337*
♦ **Prostaglandin E₁** *see* Alprostadil *on page 51*
♦ **Prostaphlin®** *see* Oxacillin *on page 711*
♦ **Prostigmin®** *see* Neostigmine *on page 681*
♦ **Prostin VR Pediatric® Injection** *see* Alprostadil *on page 51*

Protamine *(PROE ta meen)*

Available Salts Protamine Sulfate

Therapeutic Category Antidote, Heparin

Generic Available Yes

Use Treatment of heparin overdosage; neutralize heparin during surgery or dialysis procedures

Pregnancy Risk Factor C

Contraindications Hypersensitivity to protamine or any component

Warnings Heparin rebound associated with anticoagulation and bleeding has been reported to occur occasionally; symptoms typically occur 8-9 hours after protamine administration, but may occur as long as 18 hours later

Precautions Use with caution in patients allergic to fish, with prior history of vasectomy, patients receiving protamine-containing insulin or previous protamine therapy

Adverse Reactions

Cardiovascular: Hypotension, bradycardia, flushing, pulmonary hypertension
Central nervous system: Lassitude
Gastrointestinal: Nausea, vomiting
Neuromuscular & skeletal: Back pain
Respiratory: Dyspnea
Miscellaneous: Hypersensitivity reactions

Stability Refrigerate; stable for at least 2 weeks at room temperature

Mechanism of Action Combines with strongly acidic heparin to form a stable complex (salt) neutralizing the anticoagulant activity of both drugs

Pharmacodynamics Onset of action: Heparin neutralization occurs within 5 minutes following I.V. injection

Pharmacokinetics Elimination: Unknown

Usual Dosage I.V.: Protamine dosage is determined by the most recent dosage of heparin or low molecular weight heparin (LMWH); 1 mg of protamine neutralizes 90 USP units of heparin (lung), 115 USP units of heparin (intestinal), and 1 mg (100 units) LMWH; maximum dose: 50 mg

Heparin overdosage: Since blood heparin concentrations decrease rapidly **after** heparin administration, adjust the protamine dosage depending upon the duration of time since heparin administration as follows (see table):

Time Elapsed	Dose of Protamine (mg) to Neutralize 100 units of Heparin
Immediate	1-1.5
30-60 min	0.5-0.75
>2 h	0.25-0.375

If heparin is administered by deep S.C. injection, use 1-1.5 mg protamine per 100 units heparin; this may be done by administering a portion of the dose (eg, 25-50 mg) slowly I.V. followed by the remaining portion as a continuous infusion over 8-16 hours (the expected absorption time of the S.C. heparin dose)

LMWH overdosage: If most recent LMWH dose has been administered within the last 4 hours, use 1 mg protamine per 1 mg (100 units) LMWH; a second dose of 0.5 mg protamine per 1 mg (100 units) LMWH may be given if APTT remains prolonged 2-4 hours after the first dose

Administration Parenteral: Reconstitute vial with 5 mL sterile water; if using protamine in neonates, reconstitute with preservative free sterile water for injection; resulting solution equals 10 mg/mL; inject without further dilution over 10 minutes; maximum of 50 mg in any 10-minute period

Monitoring Parameters Coagulation tests, APTT or ACT, cardiac monitor, and blood pressure monitor required during administration

Dosage Forms Injection, as sulfate: 10 mg/mL (5 mL, 10 mL, 25 mL)

References
Michelson AD, Bovill E, Monagle P, et al, "Antithrombic Therapy in Children," *Chest*, 1998, 114(5 Suppl):748S-69S.

♦ **Protamine Sulfate** *see* Protamine *on page 820*

♦ **Prothazine-DC®** *see* Promethazine and Codeine *on page 807*

♦ **Protilase®** *see* Pancrelipase *on page 724*

Protirelin (proe TYE re lin)

Brand Names Combantrin® (Canada); Relefact® TRH; Thypinone®; Thyrel® TRH

Synonyms Lopremone

Therapeutic Category Diagnostic Agent, Thyroid Function

Generic Available No

Use Adjunct in the diagnostic assessment of thyroid function, and an adjunct to other diagnostic procedures in assessment of patients with pituitary or hypothalamic dysfunction; also causes release of prolactin from the pituitary and is used to detect defective control of prolactin secretion.

Pregnancy Risk Factor C

Contraindications Hypersensitivity to protirelin or any component

Warnings Due to transient changes in blood pressure (both increases and decreases), monitor blood pressure frequently during and at frequent intervals during first 15 minutes after administration; patient should be supine before, during, and immediately after administration

Adverse Reactions
Cardiovascular: Marked changes in blood pressure (hypotension or hypertension), flushing, chest tightness
Central nervous system: Lightheadedness, anxiety, seizures (rare), drowsiness
Endocrine & metabolic: Breast enlargement
Gastrointestinal: Nausea, dysgeusia, abdominal discomfort, xerostomia
Genitourinary: Urinary frequency
Miscellaneous: Diaphoresis

Drug Interactions Aspirin in therapeutic doses, pharmacologic doses of steroids, levodopa, and thyroid hormones reduce TSH response to protirelin

Mechanism of Action Increases release of thyroid stimulating hormone (TSH) from the anterior pituitary

Pharmacodynamics Peak TSH levels occur in 20-30 minutes; TSH returns to baseline after about 3 hours

Pharmacokinetics Mean plasma half-life: 5 minutes

Usual Dosage I.V.:
Infants and Children: 7 mcg/kg to a maximum dose of 500 mcg
Adults: 500 mcg (range 200-500 mcg)

Administration Parenteral: Administer undiluted direct I.V. over 15-30 seconds with the patient remaining supine for an additional 15 minutes (see Warnings)

Monitoring Parameters Blood pressure, prolactin, TSH, T_4, and T_3

Nursing Implications Keep patient supine during drug administration

Dosage Forms Injection: 500 mcg/mL (1 mL)

♦ **Protopam®** *see* Pralidoxime *on page 788*

♦ **Protostat® Oral** *see* Metronidazole *on page 636*

♦ **Pro-Trin® (Canada)** *see* Co-Trimoxazole *on page 258*

♦ **Protropin® Injection** *see* Human Growth Hormone *on page 478*

♦ **Proventil®** *see* Albuterol *on page 40*

♦ **Proventil® HFA** *see* Albuterol *on page 40*

♦ **Provera® Oral** *see* Medroxyprogesterone *on page 599*

♦ **Proxigel® Oral [OTC]** *see* Carbamide Peroxide *on page 167*

♦ **Proxymetacaine** *see* Proparacaine *on page 811*

♦ **Prozac®** *see* Fluoxetine *on page 431*

Pseudoephedrine (soo doe e FED rin)

Related Information

OTC Cough & Cold Preparations, Pediatric *on page 1037*

Brand Names Actifed® Allergy Tablet (Day) [OTC]; Afrinol® [OTC]; Balminil® Decongestant (Canada); Cenafed® [OTC]; Children's Silfedrine® [OTC]; Decofed® Syrup [OTC]; Drixoral® Non-Drowsy [OTC]; Efidac/24® [OTC]; Eltor® (Canada); Neofed® [OTC]; PediaCare® Oral; PMS-Pseudoephedrine (Canada); Robidrine® (Canada); Sudafed® [OTC]; Sudafed® 12 Hour [OTC]; Sufedrin® [OTC]; Triaminic® AM Decongestant Formula [OTC]

Available Salts Pseudoephedrine Hydrochloride; Pseudoephedrine Sulfate

Synonyms *d*-Isoephedrine

Therapeutic Category Adrenergic Agonist Agent; Decongestant; Sympathomimetic

Generic Available Yes

Use Temporary symptomatic relief of nasal congestion due to common cold, upper respiratory allergies, and sinusitis; also promotes nasal or sinus drainage

Pregnancy Risk Factor C

Contraindications Hypersensitivity to pseudoephedrine or any component; MAO inhibitor therapy, severe hypertension, severe coronary artery disease

Precautions Use with caution in patients with hyperthyroidism, diabetes mellitus, prostatic hypertrophy, mild-moderate hypertension, arrhythmias

Adverse Reactions

Cardiovascular: Tachycardia, palpitations, arrhythmias

Central nervous system: Nervousness, excitability, dizziness, insomnia, drowsiness, headache, seizures, hallucinations

Gastrointestinal: Nausea, vomiting

Neuromuscular & skeletal: Tremor, weakness

Miscellaneous: Diaphoresis

Drug Interactions Additive effects with other sympathomimetics; hypertensive crisis with MAO inhibitors; phenothiazines and tricyclic antidepressants potentiate pressor effects; propranolol (beta-blockers)

Mechanism of Action Directly stimulates alpha-adrenergic receptors of respiratory mucosa causing vasoconstriction; directly stimulates beta-adrenergic receptors causing bronchial relaxation, increased heart rate and contractility

Pharmacodynamics

Onset of action: Oral: Decongestant effects occur within 15-30 minutes

Duration: 4-6 hours (up to 12 hours with extended release formulation administration)

Pharmacokinetics

Distribution: Children: V_d: 2.4-2.6 L/kg; breast milk to plasma ratio: 2.6-3.3

Metabolism: Incomplete in the liver to inactive metabolite

Half-life:

Children 3.1 hours

Adults: 9-16 hours

Elimination: 55% to 75% of dose excreted unchanged in urine

Clearance:

Children: 9.2-10.3 mL/minute/kg

Adults: 7.3-7.6 mL/minute/kg

Usual Dosage Oral:

Children:

<2 years: 4 mg/kg/day in divided doses every 6 hours

2-5 years: 15 mg every 6 hours; maximum dose: 60 mg/24 hours

6-12 years: 30 mg every 6 hours; maximum dose: 120 mg/24 hours

Children >12 years and Adults: 60 mg every 6 hours; maximum dose: 240 mg/24 hours **or** extended release product: 120 mg every 12 hours

Administration Oral: Administer with water or milk to decrease GI distress; swallow timed release tablets or capsules whole, do not chew or crush

Test Interactions False-positive test for amphetamines by EMIT assay

Dosage Forms

Capsule, as hydrochloride: 60 mg

Capsule, timed release, as hydrochloride: 120 mg

Drops, oral, as hydrochloride: 7.5 mg/0.8 mL (15 mL)

Liquid, as hydrochloride: 15 mg/5 mL (120 mL); 30 mg/5 mL (120 mL, 240 mL, 473 mL)

Syrup, as hydrochloride: 15 mg/5 mL (118 mL)

Tablet, as hydrochloride: 30 mg, 60 mg

Tablet:
  Timed release, as hydrochloride: 120 mg
  Extended release, as sulfate: 120 mg, 240 mg

References
Simons FE, Gu X, Watson WT, et al, "Pharmacokinetics of the Orally Administered Decongestants Pseudoephedrine and Phenylpropanolamine in Children," *J Pediatr*, 1996, 129(5):729-34.

♦ **Pseudoephedrine and Carbinoxamine** *see* Carbinoxamine and Pseudoephedrine *on page 169*

♦ **Pseudoephedrine and Triprolidine** *see* Triprolidine and Pseudoephedrine *on page 957*

♦ **Pseudoephedrine Hydrochloride** *see* Pseudoephedrine *on page 822*

♦ **Pseudoephedrine Sulfate** *see* Pseudoephedrine *on page 822*

♦ **Pseudomonic Acid A** *see* Mupirocin *on page 660*

♦ **psoriGel® [OTC]** *see* Coal Tar *on page 247*

♦ **Psorion® Topical** *see* Betamethasone *on page 130*

♦ **P&S® Shampoo [OTC]** *see* Salicylic Acid *on page 854*

Psyllium (SIL i yum)

Brand Names Effer-Syllium® [OTC]; Fiberall® Powder [OTC]; Fiberall® Wafer [OTC]; Fibrepur® (Canada); Hydrocil® [OTC]; Konsyl® [OTC]; Konsyl-D® [OTC]; Metamucil® [OTC]; Metamucil® Instant Mix [OTC]; Modane® Bulk [OTC]; Novo-Mucilax® (Canada); Perdiem® Plain [OTC]; Prodiem® Plain (Canada); Reguloid® [OTC]; Serutan® [OTC]; Siblin® [OTC]; Syllact® [OTC]; V-Lax® [OTC]

Synonyms Plantago Seed; Plantain Seed; Psyllium Hydrophilic Mucilloid

Therapeutic Category Laxative, Bulk-Producing

Generic Available Yes

Use Treatment of chronic atonic or spastic constipation and in constipation associated with rectal disorders; management of irritable bowel syndrome; adjunctive treatment with low cholesterol and saturated fat diet to reduce risk of coronary artery disease

Pregnancy Risk Factor B

Contraindications Fecal impaction, GI obstruction; hypersensitivity to psyllium or any component

Warnings Products may contain aspartame; avoid use in phenylketonurics; inhalation of psyllium powder may produce allergic reactions in susceptible individuals

Precautions Use with caution in patients with esophageal strictures, ulcers, stenosis, or intestinal adhesions

Adverse Reactions
  Gastrointestinal: Esophageal or bowel obstruction, diarrhea, constipation, abdominal cramps
  Respiratory: Bronchospasm
  Miscellaneous: Rhinoconjunctivitis, anaphylaxis upon inhalation in susceptible individuals

Drug Interactions Decreased effect of warfarin, digitalis, potassium-sparing diuretics, salicylates, tetracyclines, nitrofurantoin

Mechanism of Action Adsorbs water in the intestine to form a viscous liquid which promotes peristalsis and reduces transit time

Pharmacodynamics
  Onset of action: 12-24 hours
  Peak effect: May take 2-3 days

Pharmacokinetics Absorption: Oral: Generally not absorbed; small amounts of grain extract present in the preparation have been reportedly absorbed following colonic hydrolysis

Usual Dosage Oral:
  Children 6-11 years: Approximately ½ the adult dose; ½-1 rounded teaspoonful in 4 oz glass of liquid 1-3 times/day
  Adults: 1-2 rounded teaspoonfuls or 1-2 packets or 1-2 wafers in 8 oz glass of liquid 1-4 times/day

Administration Oral: Granules and powder must be mixed in a glass of water or juice; drink a full glass of liquid with each dose

Patient Information Each dose must be taken with full glass of water; inadequate fluid intake may result in throat swelling and choking

Nursing Implications Inhalation of psyllium dust may cause sensitivity to psyllium (runny nose, watery eyes, wheezing)

Additional Information 3.4 g psyllium hydrophilic mucilloid/7 g powder is equivalent to a rounded teaspoonful or 1 packet

(Continued)

Psyllium *(Continued)*

Dosage Forms

Granules: 2.5 g per rounded teaspoon (480 g); 4.03 g per rounded teaspoon (100 g, 250 g)

Powder: Psyllium 50% and dextrose 50% (6.5 g, 325 g, 420 g, 480 g, 500 g)

Powder:

Effervescent:

Lemon-Lime (sugar free): 3.4 g/dose (single-dose packets)

Orange (sugar free): 3.4 g/dose (single-dose packets, 141 g, 261 g, 387 g, 621 g)

Psyllium hydrophilic: 3.4 g/per rounded teaspoon (210 g, 300 g, 420 g, 630 g)

Squares, chewable: 1.7 g, 3.4 g

Wafers: 3.4 g

- ♦ **Psyllium Hydrophilic Mucilloid** *see* Psyllium *on page 823*
- ♦ **P.T.E.-4®** *see* Trace Metals *on page 940*
- ♦ **P.T.E.-5®** *see* Trace Metals *on page 940*
- ♦ **Pteroylglutamic Acid** *see* Folic Acid *on page 439*
- ♦ **PTU** *see* Propylthiouracil *on page 819*
- ♦ **Pulmicort®, -Nebuamp®, -Turbuhaler® (Canada)** *see* Budesonide *on page 144*
- ♦ **Pulmicort® Turbuhaler®** *see* Budesonide *on page 144*
- ♦ **Pulmozyme®** *see* Dornase Alfa *on page 341*
- ♦ **Purge® [OTC]** *see* Castor Oil *on page 175*
- ♦ **Purinethol®** *see* Mercaptopurine *on page 606*
- ♦ **Purinol® (Canada)** *see* Allopurinol *on page 48*
- ♦ **PVF® K (Canada)** *see* Penicillin V Potassium *on page 743*

Pyrantel Pamoate *(pi RAN tel PAM oh ate)*

Brand Names Antiminth® [OTC]; Pin-Rid® [OTC]; Pin-X® [OTC]; Reese's® Pinworm Medicine [OTC]

Therapeutic Category Anthelmintic

Generic Available No

Use Roundworm (*Ascaris lumbricoides*), pinworm (*Enterobius vermicularis*), and hookworm (*Ancylostoma duodenale* and *Necator americanus*) infestations, and trichostrongyliasis

Pregnancy Risk Factor C

Contraindications Hypersensitivity to pyrantel pamoate or any component

Precautions Use with caution in patients with liver impairment, anemia, malnutrition

Adverse Reactions

Central nervous system: Dizziness, drowsiness, insomnia, headache, fever

Dermatologic: Rash

Gastrointestinal: Nausea, vomiting, anorexia, diarrhea, abdominal cramps, tenesmus

Hepatic: Elevated liver enzymes

Neuromuscular & skeletal: Weakness

Drug Interactions Piperazine (antagonist)

Stability Protect from light

Mechanism of Action Promotes release of acetylcholine and inhibits cholinesterase causing neuromuscular paralysis of susceptible helminths

Pharmacokinetics

Absorption: Oral: Poor

Metabolism: Undergoes partial hepatic metabolism

Time to peak serum concentration: Within 1-3 hours

Elimination: In feces (50% as unchanged drug) and urine (7% as unchanged drug)

Usual Dosage Children and Adults: Oral:

Roundworm, pinworm, or trichostrongyliasis: 11 mg/kg administered as a single dose; maximum dose: 1 g; dosage should be repeated after 2 weeks for pinworm infection

Hookworm: 11 mg/kg/day once daily for 3 days

Maximum daily dose: 1 g

Administration Oral: May mix drug with milk or fruit juice; may administer with or without food

Monitoring Parameters Stool for presence of eggs, worms, and occult blood; serum AST and ALT

Patient Information Hygienic precaution is essential to prevent reinfection

Nursing Implications Shake suspension well before pouring to assure accurate dosage; fasting or purgation is not required prior to administration

Dosage Forms
Capsule, as pamoate: 180 mg
Liquid, as pamoate: 50 mg/mL (30 mL); 144 mg/mL (30 mL)
Suspension, oral (caramel-currant flavor), as pamoate: 50 mg/mL (60 mL)

Pyrazinamide (peer a ZIN a mide)

Brand Names PMS-Pyrazinamide (Canada); Tebrazid (Canada)
Synonyms Pyrazinoic Acid Amide
Therapeutic Category Antitubercular Agent
Generic Available No
Use In combination with other antituberculosis agents in the treatment of *Mycobacterium* tuberculosis infection (especially useful in disseminated and meningeal tuberculosis); CDC currently recommends a 3 or 4 multidrug regimen which includes pyrazinamide, rifampin, INH, and at times ethambutol or streptomycin for the treatment of tuberculosis
Pregnancy Risk Factor C
Contraindications Severe hepatic damage; hypersensitivity to pyrazinamide or any component
Precautions Use with caution in patients with renal failure, gout, or diabetes mellitus
Adverse Reactions
Central nervous system: Malaise, fever
Dermatologic: Urticaria, rash, photosensitivity
Endocrine & metabolic: Gout, hyperuricemia
Gastrointestinal: Nausea, vomiting, anorexia
Hepatic: Hepatotoxicity (increased incidence with doses >30 mg/kg/day), jaundice
Neuromuscular & skeletal: Arthralgia
Drug Interactions Isoniazid (decreased INH serum levels)
Mechanism of Action Converted to pyrazinoic acid in susceptible strains of *Mycobacterium* which lowers the pH of the environment
Pharmacokinetics
Absorption: Oral: Well absorbed
Distribution: Widely distributed into body tissues and fluids including the liver, lung, and CSF
Protein binding: 50%
Metabolism: In the liver
Half-life: 9-10 hours, prolonged with reduced renal or hepatic function
Time to peak serum concentration: Within 2 hours
Elimination: In urine (4% as unchanged drug)
Usual Dosage Oral:
Infants, Children, and Adolescents: 20-40 mg/kg/day in divided doses every 12-24 hours for the first 2 months of active treatment; daily dose not to exceed 2 g; **or** daily pyrazinamide for 2 weeks followed by directly observed therapy of 50 mg/kg/dose twice weekly to a maximum of 2 g/dose for 6 weeks
Adults: 15-30 mg/kg/day in 1-4 divided doses for the first 2 months of active treatment; maximum daily dose: 2 g/day; or daily pyrazinamide for 2 weeks followed by directly observed therapy of 50-70 mg/kg/dose twice weekly to a maximum of 4 g/dose for 6 weeks
Monitoring Parameters Periodic liver function tests, serum uric acid
Patient Information Notify physician if fatigue, weakness, nausea, vomiting, or joint pain and swelling occur
Dosage Forms Tablet: 500 mg
Extemporaneous Preparations
Pyrazinamide suspension can be compounded with simple syrup or 0.5% methylcellulose with simple syrup at a concentration of 100 mg/mL; the suspension is stable for 2 months at 4°C or 25°C when stored in glass or plastic bottles
To prepare pyrazinamide suspension in 0.5% methylcellulose with simple syrup: Crush 200 pyrazinamide 500 mg tablets and mix with a suspension containing 500 mL of 1% methylcellulose and 500 mL simple syrup. Add to this a suspension containing 140 crushed pyrazinamide tablets in 350 mL of 1% methylcellulose and 350 mL of simple syrup to make 1.7 L of suspension containing pyrazinamide 100 mg/mL in 0.5% methylcellulose with simple syrup.
Nahata MC, Morosco RS, and Peritre SP, "Stability of Pyrazinamide in Two Suspensions," *Am J Health-Syst Pharm*, 1995, 52:1558-60.
(Continued)

Pyrazinamide *(Continued)*

References

Ad Hoc Committee of the Scientific Assembly on Microbiology, Tuberculosis and Pulmonary Infections, "Treatment of Tuberculosis and Tuberculosis Infection in Adults and Children," *Clin Infect Dis*, 1995, 21:9-27.

American Academy of Pediatrics, Committee on Infectious Diseases, "Chemotherapy for Tuberculosis in Infants and Children," *Pediatrics*, 1992, 89(1):161-5.

Starke JR, "Multidrug Therapy for Tuberculosis in Children," *Pediatr Infect Dis J*, 1990, 9(11):785-93.

Starke JR and Correa AG, "Management of Mycobacterial Infection and Disease in Children," *Pediatr Infect Dis J*, 1995, 14(6):455-70.

♦ **Pyrazinoic Acid Amide** *see* Pyrazinamide *on page 825*

♦ **Pyridiate®** *see* Phenazopyridine *on page 753*

♦ **2-Pyridine Aldoxime Methochloride** *see* Pralidoxime *on page 788*

♦ **Pyridium®** *see* Phenazopyridine *on page 753*

Pyridostigmine *(peer id oh STIG meen)*

Related Information
Overdose and Toxicology *on page 1191*

Brand Names Mestinon® Injection; Mestinon® Oral; Regonol® Injection

Available Salts Pyridostigmine Bromide

Therapeutic Category Antidote, Neuromuscular Blocking Agent; Cholinergic Agent

Generic Available No

Use Symptomatic treatment of myasthenia gravis by improving muscle strength; reversal of effects of nondepolarizing neuromuscular blocking agents

Pregnancy Risk Factor C

Contraindications Hypersensitivity to pyridostigmine, bromides, or any component; GI or GU obstruction

Warnings Overdosage may result in cholinergic crisis, this must be distinguished from myasthenic crisis; adequate facilities should be available for cardiopulmonary resuscitation when testing and adjusting dose for myasthenia gravis; have atropine and epinephrine ready to treat hypersensitivity reactions; injection contains benzyl alcohol; avoid use in neonates

Precautions Use with caution in patients with epilepsy, asthma, bradycardia, hyperthyroidism, arrhythmias, recent coronary occlusion, vagotonia, or peptic ulcer

Adverse Reactions
Cardiovascular: Bradycardia, hypotension, arrhythmias, A-V block, syncope
Central nervous system: Headache, convulsions, drowsiness, dizziness
Dermatologic: Rash
Gastrointestinal: Nausea, vomiting, diarrhea, increased peristalsis, abdominal cramps, dysphagia, salivation
Genitourinary: Urinary frequency
Local: Thrombophlebitis (after I.V. administration)
Neuromuscular & skeletal: Muscle cramps, weakness
Ocular: Miosis, lacrimation, diplopia, conjunctival hyperemia
Respiratory: Increased bronchial secretions, bronchospasm, laryngospasm, dyspnea
Miscellaneous: Diaphoresis

Drug Interactions Corticosteroids and magnesium may decrease effect of pyridostigmine; increases neuromuscular blocking effects of succinylcholine; atropine is direct antagonist

Stability Protect oral solution from light

Mechanism of Action Competitively inhibits destruction of acetylcholine by acetylcholinesterase which facilitates transmission of impulses across myoneural junction producing generalized cholinergic responses such as miosis, increased tonus of skeletal and intestinal musculature, bronchial and ureteral constriction, bradycardia, and increased salivary and sweat gland production

Pharmacodynamics
Onset of action:
Oral: 30-45 minutes
I.M.: <15 minutes
I.V.: Within 2-5 minutes
Duration:
Oral: 3-6 hours
I.M., I.V.: 2-3 hours

Pharmacokinetics

Absorption: Oral: Very poor (10% to 20%) from the GI tract; sustained release products may release up to $1/3$ of a dose immediately after ingestion and the remainder over 8-12 hours

Metabolism: In the liver and at tissue site by cholinesterases

Usual Dosage
Myasthenia gravis (dosage should be adjusted so patient takes larger doses prior to time of greatest fatigue)

Oral:
Neonates: 5 mg every 4-6 hours
Children: 7 mg/kg/day in 5-6 divided doses
Adults: Initial: 60 mg 3 times/day with maintenance dose ranging from 60 mg to 1.5 g/day (incremental increases every 48 hours or more if needed); sustained release formulation should be dosed every 12-24 hours; this formulation is preferably dosed at bedtime for patients who complain of morning weakness

I.M., I.V.:
Neonates and Children: 0.05-0.15 mg/kg/dose (maximum single dose: 10 mg)
Adults: 2 mg every 2-3 hours (or 1/30th of oral dose)
Reversal of nondepolarizing neuromuscular blocker: I.V.:
Children: 0.1-0.25 mg/kg/dose preceded by atropine or glycopyrrolate
Adults: 10-20 mg preceded by atropine or glycopyrrolate

Administration
Parenteral: Administer direct I.V. slowly over 2-4 minutes; patients receiving large parenteral doses should be pretreated with atropine
Oral: Swallow sustained release tablets whole, do not chew or crush

Monitoring Parameters
Muscle strength, heart rate, vital capacity

Dosage Forms
Injection, as bromide (with benzyl alcohol): 5 mg/mL (2 mL, 5 mL)
Syrup, as bromide (raspberry flavor): 60 mg/5 mL (480 mL)
Tablet, as bromide: 60 mg
Tablet, sustained release, as bromide: 180 mg

♦ **Pyridostigmine Bromide** *see* Pyridostigmine *on page 826*

Pyridoxine (peer i DOKS een)

Related Information
Antiepileptic Drugs *on page 1176*

Brand Names Nestrex®

Available Salts Pyridoxine Hydrochloride

Synonyms Vitamin B_6

Therapeutic Category Antidote, Cycloserine Toxicity; Antidote, Hydrazine Toxicity; Antidote, Mushroom Toxicity; Drug-induced Neuritis, Treatment Agent; Nutritional Supplement; Vitamin, Water Soluble

Generic Available Yes

Use Prevention and treatment of vitamin B_6 deficiency, pyridoxine-dependent seizures in infants; treatment of drug-induced deficiency (eg, isoniazid or hydralazine); treatment of acute intoxication of isoniazid, cycloserine, hydrazine, mushroom (genus *Gyromitra*)

Pregnancy Risk Factor A (C if dose exceeds RDA recommendation)

Contraindications Hypersensitivity to pyridoxine or any component

Adverse Reactions
Central nervous system: Sensory neuropathy (after chronic administration of large doses), seizures (following I.V. administration of very large doses), headache
Gastrointestinal: Nausea
Hematologic: Decreased serum folic acid concentration
Hepatic: Elevated AST
Local: Burning or stinging at injection site
Neuromuscular & skeletal: Paresthesia
Respiratory: Respiratory distress
Miscellaneous: Allergic reactions have been reported

Drug Interactions Decreases levodopa effectiveness when used without carbidopa; decreases serum levels of phenobarbital and phenytoin

Mechanism of Action Precursor to pyridoxal and pyridoxamine which function as cofactors in the metabolism of proteins, carbohydrates, and fats; also aids in the release of liver and muscle stored glycogen and in the synthesis of GABA (within the CNS) and heme

Pharmacokinetics
Absorption: Readily from the GI tract; primarily in jejunum
Metabolism: Converted to pyridoxal (active form in liver)
(Continued)

Pyridoxine *(Continued)*

Half-life, biologic: 15-20 days
Elimination: By liver metabolism

Usual Dosage
Adequate intake: Infants:
<6 months: 0.1 mg (0.01 mg/kg)
6-12 months: 0.3 mg (0.03 mg/kg)
Recommended daily allowance:
1-3 years: 0.5 mg
4-8 years: 0.6 mg
9-13 years: 1 mg
14-19 years:
Male: 1.3 mg
Female: 1.2 mg
20-50 years: 1.3 mg
>50 years:
Male: 1.7 mg
Female: 1.5 mg
Pyridoxine-dependent seizures: Oral, I.M., I.V.:
Neonates and Infants: Initial: 10-100 mg; maintenance: Oral: 50-100 mg/day
Dietary deficiency: Oral:
Children: 5-25 mg/day for 3 weeks, then 1.5-2.5 mg/day in multivitamin product
Adults: 2.5-10 mg/day until clinical signs are corrected, then 2-5 mg/day (dosage found in multivitamin products)
Drug-induced neuritis (eg, isoniazid, hydralazine, penicillamine, cycloserine): Oral:
Children:
Treatment: 10-50 mg/day
Prophylaxis: 1-2 mg/kg/day
Adults:
Cycloserine: Treatment 100-300 mg/day in divided doses
Isoniazid or penicillamine: Treatment: 100-200 mg/day for 3 weeks; prophylaxis: 25-100 mg/day
Acute intoxication:
Cycloserine: 300 mg daily
Hydrazine: 25 mg/kg: $^1/_3$ dose I.M. and $^2/_3$ dose I.V. infusion over 3 hours
Isoniazid: Dose equal to isoniazid ingested given as a first dose of 1-4 g I.V., followed by 1 g I.M. every 30 minutes until total dosage completed
Mushroom ingestion (genus *Gyromitra*): I.V.: 25 mg/kg; repeat as necessary to a maximum total dose of 15-20 g

Administration Parenteral: Administer slow I.V.

Monitoring Parameters When administering large I.V. doses, monitor respiratory rate, heart rate, and blood pressure

Reference Range 30-80 ng/mL

Test Interactions False positive urobilinogen spot test using Ehrlich's reagent

Dosage Forms
Injection, as hydrochloride: 100 mg/mL (10 mL, 30 mL)
Tablet, as hydrochloride: 25 mg, 50 mg, 100 mg, 200 mg, 250 mg, 500 mg
Tablet, extended release, as hydrochloride: 100 mg

Extemporaneous Preparations A 1 mg/mL oral solution has an expected stability of 30 days when refrigerated when compounded as follows: Withdraw 100 mg (1 mL of a 100 mg/mL injection) from a vial with a needle and syringe, add to 99 mL of simple syrup in an amber bottle; keep in refrigerator
Nahata MC and Hipple TF, *Pediatric Drug Formulations*, 3rd ed, Cincinnati, OH: Harvey Whitney Books Co, 1997.

♦ **Pyridoxine Hydrochloride** *see* Pyridoxine *on page 827*

Pyrimethamine *(peer i METH a meen)*

Brand Names Daraprim®

Therapeutic Category Antimalarial Agent

Generic Available No

Use Used in combination with sulfadiazine for treatment of toxoplasmosis; used in combination with dapsone as primary or secondary prophylaxis for *Pneumocystis carinii* in HIV-infected patients; pyrimethamine has been used for chemoprophylaxis of malaria, however, due to severe adverse reactions and reports of resistance to pyrimethamine, other antimalarial agents are now generally preferred

Pregnancy Risk Factor C

Contraindications Megaloblastic anemia; hypersensitivity to pyrimethamine, chloroguanide, or any component; resistant malaria and patients with seizure disorders

Precautions Use with caution in patients with impaired renal or hepatic function and in patients with possible folate deficiency

Adverse Reactions
Cardiovascular: Shock
Central nervous system: Seizures, fever, fatigue, ataxia, headache
Dermatologic: Rash, photosensitivity
Endocrine & metabolic: Folic acid deficiency
Gastrointestinal: Anorexia, abdominal cramps, vomiting, atrophic glossitis, diarrhea
Hematologic: Megaloblastic anemia, leukopenia, thrombocytopenia, agranulocytosis, pancytopenia, pulmonary eosinophilia
Neuromuscular & skeletal: Tremor
Renal: Hematuria
Respiratory: Respiratory failure

Drug Interactions Para-aminobenzoic acid, sulfonamides

Mechanism of Action Inhibits parasitic dihydrofolate reductase resulting in inhibition of tetrahydrofolic acid synthesis

Pharmacokinetics
Absorption: Oral: Well absorbed
Distribution: V_d: Adults: 2.9 L/kg; appears in breast milk; distributed to the kidneys, lung, liver, and spleen
Protein binding: 80% to 87%
Half-life: 111 hours (range: 54-148 hours)
Time to peak serum concentration: Within 2-6 hours
Elimination: Pyrimethamine and metabolites are excreted in urine

Usual Dosage Oral:
Toxoplasmosis (with sulfadiazine):
Newborns and Infants: Initial: 2 mg/kg/day divided every 12 hours for 2 days, then 1 mg/kg/day once daily given with sulfadiazine for the first 6 months; next 6 months: 1 mg/kg/day 3 times/week with sulfadiazine; oral folinic acid 5-10 mg 3 times/week should be administered to prevent hematologic toxicity
Children: 2 mg/kg/day divided every 12 hours for 3 days followed by 1 mg/kg/day (maximum: 25 mg/day) once daily or divided twice daily for 4 weeks given with sulfadiazine; oral folinic acid 5-10 mg 3 times/week should be administered to prevent hematologic toxicity
Adults: 50-75 mg/day together with 1-4 g of a sulfonamide plus oral folinic acid 5-10 mg 3 times/week for 1-3 weeks depending on patient's tolerance and response, then reduce dose by 50% and continue for 4-5 weeks or 25-50 mg/day for 3-4 weeks
Prophylaxis for first episode of *Toxoplasma gondii*:
Children ≥1 month of age: 1 mg/kg/day once daily with dapsone plus oral folinic acid 5 mg every 3 days
Adolescents and Adults: 50 mg once weekly with dapsone plus oral folinic acid 25 mg once weekly
Prophylaxis for recurrence of *Toxoplasma gondii*:
Children ≥1 month of age: 1 mg/kg/day once daily given with sulfadiazine or clindamycin, plus oral folinic acid 5 mg every 3 days
Adolescents and Adults: 25-75 mg once daily in combination with sulfadiazine or clindamycin, plus oral folinic acid 10-25 mg daily
Prophylaxis for first episode or recurrence of *Pneumocystis carinii*:
Adolescents and Adults: 50-75 mg once weekly in combination with dapsone plus oral folinic acid 25 mg once weekly

Administration Oral: Administer with meals to minimize vomiting

Monitoring Parameters CBC including platelet counts

Patient Information Notify physician if rash, sore throat, pallor, or glossitis occurs

Additional Information Folinic acid may be given in a dosage of 3-9 mg/day for 3 days, or 5 mg every 3 days, or as required to reverse symptoms or to prevent hematologic problems due to pyrimethamine-induced folic acid deficiency

Dosage Forms Tablet: 25 mg

Extemporaneous Preparations Pyrimethamine tablets may be crushed to prepare oral suspensions of the drug in a 1:1 mixture of simple syrup and 1% methylcellulose to yield a suspension with a pyrimethamine concentration of 2 mg/mL; stable for at least 91 days when stored in plastic or glass prescription bottles at 4°C or 25°C
Nahata MC, Morosco RS, and Hipple TF, "Stability of Pyrimethamine in a Liquid Dosage Formulation Stored for Three Months," *Am J Health-Syst Pharm*, 1997, 54:2714-6.

(Continued)

Pyrimethamine *(Continued)*

References
1997 USPHS/IDSA Guidelines for the Prevention of Opportunistic Infections in Persons Infected With Human Immunodeficiency Virus," *MMWR Morb Mortal Wkly Rep*, 1997, 46(RR-12):1-46.

Van Voorhis WC, "Therapy and Prophylaxis of Systemic Protozoan Infections," *Drugs*, 1990, 40(2):176-202.

♦ **Pyrimethamine and Sulfadoxine** *see* Sulfadoxine and Pyrimethamine *on page 890*

♦ **Pyronium® (Canada)** *see* Phenazopyridine *on page 753*

♦ **Quelicin®** *see* Succinylcholine *on page 884*

♦ **Questran®** *see* Cholestyramine Resin *on page 219*

♦ **Questran® Light** *see* Cholestyramine Resin *on page 219*

♦ **Quibron®-T** *see* Theophylline *on page 910*

♦ **Quibron®-T/SR** *see* Theophylline *on page 910*

♦ **Quick Dissolve Maalox® Maximum Strength** *see* Calcium Supplements *on page 157*

♦ **Quiess® Injection** *see* Hydroxyzine *on page 496*

♦ **Quinaglute® Dura-Tabs®** *see* Quinidine *on page 830*

♦ **Quinalan®** *see* Quinidine *on page 830*

♦ **Quinalbarbitone** *see* Secobarbital *on page 861*

♦ **Quinamm®** *see* Quinine *on page 832*

♦ **Quinidex® Extentabs®** *see* Quinidine *on page 830*

Quinidine *(KWIN i deen)*

Related Information
Adult ACLS Algorithm, Tachycardia *on page 1010*

Brand Names Biquin® Durules® (Canada); Cardioquin®; Quinaglute® Dura-Tabs®; Quinalan®; Quinidex® Extentabs®; Quinora®

Available Salts Quinidine Gluconate; Quinidine Polygalacturonate; Quinidine Sulfate

Therapeutic Category Antiarrhythmic Agent, Class I-A

Generic Available Yes

Use Prophylaxis after cardioversion of atrial fibrillation and/or flutter to maintain normal sinus rhythm; also used to prevent reoccurrence of paroxysmal supraventricular tachycardia, paroxysmal A-V junctional rhythm, paroxysmal ventricular tachycardia, paroxysmal atrial fibrillation, and atrial or ventricular premature contractions; also has activity against *Plasmodium falciparum* malaria

Pregnancy Risk Factor C

Contraindications Patients with complete A-V block with an A-V junctional or idioventricular pacemaker; patients with intraventricular conduction defects (marked widening of QRS complex); patients with cardiac glycoside-induced A-V conduction disorders; hypersensitivity to quinidine, any component, or cinchona derivatives

Warnings May cause syncope, most likely due to ventricular tachycardia or fibrillation; syncope may subside spontaneously, but occasionally may be fatal; discontinue quinidine if syncope occurs

Precautions Use with caution in patients with myocardial depression, sick sinus syndrome, incomplete A-V block, cardiac glycoside intoxication, hepatic and/or renal insufficiency, myasthenia gravis; hemolysis may occur in patients with G-6-PD deficiency; quinidine-induced hepatotoxicity, including granulomatous hepatitis, increased serum AST and alkaline phosphatase concentrations, and jaundice may occur; use with caution in nursing women; adjust dose with severe renal impairment

Adverse Reactions
Cardiovascular: Syncope, hypotension, tachycardia, heart block, ventricular fibrillation, vascular collapse, severe hypotension with rapid I.V. administration

Central nervous system: Fever, headache

Dermatologic: Angioedema, rash

Gastrointestinal: GI disturbances, nausea, vomiting, cramps

Hematologic: Blood dyscrasias, thrombotic thrombocytopenic purpura

Respiratory: Respiratory depression

Miscellaneous: Cinchonism (nausea, tinnitus, headache, impaired hearing or vision, vomiting, abdominal pain, vertigo, confusion, delirium, syncope)

Drug Interactions Cytochrome P-450 isoenzyme CYP3A3/4 and CYP3A5-7 substrate; CYP2D6 and CYP3A3/4 isoenzyme inhibitor

Quinidine potentiates nondepolarizing and depolarizing muscle relaxants; diltiazem, verapamil, delavirdine, saquinavir, amiodarone, alkalinizing agents, and cimetidine may increase quinidine serum concentrations; phenobarbital, phenytoin, and rifampin may decrease quinidine serum concentrations. Quinidine may increase plasma concentration of digoxin; closely monitor digoxin concentrations; digoxin dosage may need to be reduced (by one-half) when quinidine is initiated; new steady-state digoxin plasma concentrations occur in 5-7 days. Beta-blockers plus quinidine may increase bradycardia; quinidine may enhance coumarin anticoagulants; potential interaction with ritonavir, concurrent use is not recommended

Food Interactions Excessive intake of fruit juices or vitamin C may decrease urine pH and result in increased clearance of quinidine with decreased serum concentration; alkaline foods may result in increased quinidine serum concentrations; food has a variable effect on absorption of sustained release formulation; grapefruit juice significantly increases the AUC of 3-hydroxyquinidine (a metabolite of quinidine)

Stability Do not use discolored parenteral solution

Mechanism of Action Class IA antiarrhythmic with anticholinergic, local anesthetic, and mild negative inotropic effects; depresses phase 0 of the action potential; decreases myocardial excitability, conduction velocity, and myocardial contractility by decreasing sodium influx during depolarization and potassium efflux in repolarization; also reduces calcium transport across cell membrane

Pharmacokinetics

Distribution: V_d: Adults: 2-3.5 L/kg, decreased V_d with CHF, malaria; increased V_d with cirrhosis; crosses the placenta; appears in breast milk

Protein-binding:

Newborns: 60% to 70%

Adults: 80% to 90%

Decreased protein binding with cyanotic congenital heart disease, cirrhosis, or acute MI

Metabolism: Extensive in the liver (50% to 90%) to inactive compounds

Bioavailability:

Sulfate: 80%

Gluconate: 70%

Half-life, plasma (increased half-life with elderly, cirrhosis, and CHF):

Children: 2.5-6.7 hours

Adults: 6-8 hours

Elimination: In urine (15% to 25% as unchanged drug)

Slightly dialyzable (5% to 20%) by hemodialysis; not removed by peritoneal dialysis

Usual Dosage Note: Dose expressed in terms of the salt: 267 mg of quinidine gluconate = 275 mg of quinidine polygalacturonate = 200 mg of quinidine sulfate

Children: Test dose (for idiosyncratic reaction, intolerance, syncope, thrombocytopenia) (sulfate, oral or gluconate, I.M.): 2 mg/kg or 60 mg/m²

Oral (quinidine sulfate): Usual: 30 mg/kg/day or 900 mg/m²/day given in 5 daily doses or 6 mg/kg every 4-6 hours; range: 15-60 mg/kg/day in 4-5 divided doses

I.V. (quinidine gluconate): 2-10 mg/kg/dose every 3-6 hours as needed (I.V. route **not** recommended)

Adults: Test dose (for idiosyncratic reaction, intolerance, syncope, thrombocytopenia): 200 mg administered several hours before full dosage

Oral (sulfate): 100-600 mg/dose every 4-6 hours; begin at 200 mg/dose and titrate to desired effect

Oral (gluconate): 324-972 mg every 8-12 hours

Oral (polygalacturonate): 275 mg every 8-12 hours

I.M.: 400 mg/dose every 4-6 hours

I.V.: 200-400 mg/dose diluted and given at a rate ≤10 mg/minute

Dosing adjustment in renal impairment: Children and Adults: Cl_{cr} <10 mL/minute: Administer 75% of normal dose

Administration

Oral: Administer with water on an empty stomach, but may administer with food or milk to decrease GI upset; best to administer in a consistent manner with regards to meals; swallow sustained-release tablets whole, do not chew or crush

Parenteral: I.V.: Maximum rate of infusion: 10 mg/minute; maximum concentration: 16 mg/mL; I.V. tubing length should be minimized (quinidine may be significantly adsorbed to polyvinyl chloride tubing)

(Continued)

Quinidine (Continued)

Monitoring Parameters CBC with differential, platelet count, liver and renal function tests, and serum concentrations should be routinely performed during long-term administration

Reference Range Optimal therapeutic level is method dependent
Therapeutic: 2-7 µg/mL (SI: 6.2-15.4 µmol/L)
Toxic: >8 µg/mL (SI: >18 µmol/L)

Patient Information Notify physician if fever, rash, unusual bruising or bleeding, visual disturbances, or ringing in the ears occurs; avoid excessive intake of fruit juices or vitamin C

Additional Information Use of sustained release products is not recommended in children

Dosage Forms
Injection, as gluconate: 80 mg/mL (10 mL)
Tablet, as polygalacturonate: 275 mg
Tablet, as sulfate: 200 mg, 300 mg
Tablet:
Sustained action, as sulfate: 300 mg
Sustained release, as gluconate: 324 mg

Extemporaneous Preparations
A 10 mg/mL oral liquid preparation made from tablets and 3 different vehicles (cherry syrup, a 1:1 mixture of Ora-Sweet® and Ora-Plus®, or a 1:1 mixture of Ora-Sweet® SF and Ora-Plus®) was stable for 60 days when stored in amber plastic prescription bottles in the dark at room temperature (25°C) or under refrigeration (5°C); Grind six 200 mg tablets in a mortar into a fine powder; add 15 mL of the vehicle and mix well to form a uniform paste; mix while adding the vehicle in geometric proportions to **almost** 120 mL; transfer to a calibrated bottle and qsad to 120 mL; label "shake well" and "protect from light" (Allen 1998).

A 10 mg/mL quinidine sulfate solution made with six 200 mg capsules, 15 mL alcohol USP, and citric acid syrup USP qsad to a total amount of 120 mL is stable for 30 days under refrigeration (Nahata, 1997)

Allen LV and Erickson MA, "Stability of Bethanechol Chloride, Pyrazinamide, Quinidine Sulfate, Rifampin, and Tetracycline in Extemporaneously Compounded Oral Liquids," *Am J Health Syst Pharm*, 1998, 55(17):1804-9.

Nahata MC and Hipple TF, *Pediatric Drug Formulations*, 3nd ed, Cincinnati, OH: Harvey Whitney Books Co, 1997.

References
Pickoff AS, Singh S, and Gelband H, *The Medical Management of Cardiac Arrhythmias in Cardiac Arrhythmias in the Neonate, Infant and Child*, Roberts NK and Gelband H, ed, Norwalk, CT: Appleton-Century-Crofts, 1983.

Szefler SJ, Pieroni DR, Gingell RL, et al, "Rapid Elimination of Quinidine in Pediatric Patients," *Pediatrics*, 1982, 70(3):370-5.

♦ **Quinidine Gluconate** see Quinidine on page 830
♦ **Quinidine Polygalacturonate** see Quinidine on page 830
♦ **Quinidine Sulfate** see Quinidine on page 830

Quinine (KWYE nine)

Brand Names Legatrin® [OTC]; Quinamm®; Quiphile®; Q-vel®

Available Salts Quinine Sulfate

Therapeutic Category Antimalarial Agent; Skeletal Muscle Relaxant, Miscellaneous

Generic Available Yes

Use Suppression or treatment of chloroquine-resistant *P. falciparum* malaria (inactive against sporozoites, pre-erythrocytic or exoerythrocytic forms of plasmodia); treatment of *Babesia microti* infection; prevention and treatment of nocturnal recumbency leg muscle cramps

Pregnancy Risk Factor D

Contraindications Tinnitus, optic neuritis, G-6-PD deficiency; hypersensitivity to quinine or any component; history of black water fever; pregnancy

Precautions Use with caution in patients with cardiac arrhythmias (quinine has quinidine-like activity), in patients with myasthenia gravis, and in patients with impaired liver function

Adverse Reactions
Cardiovascular: Flushing of the skin, anginal symptoms, conduction disturbances, ventricular tachycardia
Central nervous system: Fever, headache, confusion
Dermatologic: Rash, pruritus
Endocrine & metabolic: Hypoglycemia

Gastrointestinal: Nausea, vomiting, epigastric pain

Hematologic: Hemolysis, thrombocytopenia

Hepatic: Hepatitis

Ocular: Visual disturbances

Otic: Tinnitus, impaired hearing

Miscellaneous: Hypersensitivity reactions, cinchonism (nausea, tinnitus, headache, impaired hearing or vision, vomiting, abdominal pain, vertigo, confusion, delirium, syncope)

Drug Interactions Quinine may decrease the clearance of digoxin or digitoxin leading to increased plasma concentrations of these cardiac glycosides; cimetidine (prolongs half-life of quinine), aluminum-containing antacids (decreases quinine absorption); quinine may potentiate the effects of neuromuscular blocking agents; oral anticoagulants, urinary alkalinizers (may increase quinine toxicity); mefloquine (additive cardiotoxicity)

Stability Protect from light

Mechanism of Action Depresses oxygen uptake and carbohydrate metabolism; intercalates into DNA, disrupting the parasite's replication and transcription; affects calcium distribution within muscle fibers and decreases the excitability of the motor end-plate region

Pharmacokinetics

Absorption: Oral: Readily absorbed, mainly from the upper small intestine

Distribution: Widely distributed to body tissues and fluids including small amounts into bile and CSF; crosses the placenta; excreted into breast milk

V_d (children): 0.8 L/kg

V_d (adults): 1.9 L/kg

Protein binding: 70% to 90%

Metabolism: Primarily in the liver via hydroxylation pathways

Half-life:

Children: 6-12 hours

Adults: 8-14 hours

Time to peak serum concentration: Within 1-3 hours

Elimination: In bile and saliva with <5% excreted unchanged in urine

Not effectively removed by peritoneal dialysis, removed by hemodialysis

Usual Dosage Oral:

Children:

Treatment of chloroquine-resistant malaria: 30 mg/kg/day in divided doses every 8 hours for 3-7 days in conjunction with another agent; maximum dose: 2 g/day

Babesiosis: 25 mg/kg/day, divided every 8 hours for 7 days; maximum dose: 650 mg/dose

Adults:

Treatment of chloroquine-resistant malaria: 650 mg every 8 hours for 3-7 days in conjunction with another agent

Suppression of malaria: 325 mg twice daily and continued for 6 weeks after exposure

Babesiosis: 650 mg every 6-8 hours for 7 days

Leg cramps: 200-300 mg at bedtime

Administration Oral: Do not crush tablets or capsule to avoid bitter taste

Monitoring Parameters CBC with platelet count, liver function tests, blood glucose, ophthalmologic examination

Patient Information Report to physician if tinnitus, hearing loss, rash, or visual disturbances occur during therapy

Additional Information Parenteral form of quinine (dihydrochloride) is no longer available from the CDC; quinidine gluconate should be used instead; the FDA has banned over-the-counter (OTC) drug products containing quinine sold for treatment and/or prevention of malaria, as well as, products labeled for treatment or prevention of nocturnal leg cramps

Dosage Forms

Capsule, as sulfate: 64.8 mg, 65 mg, 200 mg, 300 mg, 325 mg

Tablet, as sulfate: 162.5 mg, 260 mg

References

Schulbe DE, "Quinine Ban Signals Change for Pharmacists, APhA," *Pharmacy Today*, 1995, 1(12):6.

♦ **Quinine Sulfate** *see* Quinine *on page 832*

♦ **Quinora®** *see* Quinidine *on page 830*

♦ **Quinsana® Plus Topical [OTC]** *see* Undecylenic Acid and Derivatives *on page 962*

Quinupristin/Dalfopristin (kwi NYOO pris tin/dal FOE pris tin)
Brand Names Synercid®
Synonyms Pristinamycin; RP59500
Therapeutic Category Antibiotic, Streptogramin
Use Treatment of serious or life-threatening infections caused by vancomycin-resistant *Enterococcus faecium*; treatment of complicated skin and skin structure infections caused by *Staphylococcus aureus* (methcillin-susceptible and methcillin-resistant strains) or *Streptococcus pyogenes*
Pregnancy Risk Factor B
Contraindications Hypersensitivity to quinupristin, dalfopristin, other streptogramins (pristinamycin or virginiamycin), or to any component
Warnings Quinupristin/dalfopristin inhibit cytochrome P-450 3A4 metabolism of cyclosporine, midazolam, nifedipine, and terfenadine. There was a 77% increase in cyclosporine's half-life with a 63% increase in the AUC. Cyclosporine levels should be closely monitored in patients who are receiving quinupristin/dalfopristin therapy concomitantly. Coadministration of quinupristin/dalfopristin with cytochrome P-450 3A4 substrates with narrow therapeutic ranges require serum concentration monitoring of these drugs. Concurrent use with astemizole, terfenadine, and cisapride is not recommended. Superinfections and pseudomembranous colitis have been reported with the use of quinupristin/dalfopristin. Resistance to quinupristin/dalfopristin has been reported in a few cases of *Entercoccus faecium* infections.
Precautions Use with caution in patients with hepatic or renal dysfunction; dosage reduction may be necessary in patients with hepatic cirrhosis; may cause pain and phlebitis when infused through a peripheral line; episodes of severe arthralgia and myalgia have been reported which improve with a dose frequency reduction to "q12h" or discontinuation of quinupristin/dalfopristin
Adverse Reactions
Central nervous system: Headache
Dermatologic: Rash, pruritus, urticaria
Hepatic: Elevated AST, ALT, bilirubin
Local: Pain, edema, inflammation at infusion site; thrombophlebitis
Neuromuscular & skeletal: Arthralgia, myalgia
Miscellaneous: Superinfection
Drug Interactions Cytochrome P-450 isoenzyme CYP3A4 inhibitor
Quinupristin/dalfopristin may increase plasma concentration of cyclosporine, tacrolimus, astemizole, terfenadine, delavirdine, nevirapine, indinavir, ritonavir, vinca alkaloids, docetaxel, paclitaxel, midazolam, diazepam, dihydropyridines, verapamil, diltiazem, HMG-CoA reductase inhibitors, cisapride, methylprednisolone, carbamazepine, quinidine, lidocaine, disopyramide (see Warnings)
Stability Unopened vials should be stored in a refrigerator at 2°C to 8°C; reconstituted drug is stable for 1 hour at room temperature; infusion bag is stable for 5 hours at room temperature and for 54 hours if refrigerated at 2°C to 8°C; incompatible with NS and heparin; compatible with aztreonam, ciprofloxacin, fluconazole, haloperidol, metoclopramide, morphine, and potassium chloride during Y-site administration
Mechanism of Action Inhibits bacterial protein synthesis by binding to the 50S bacterial ribosomal subunit resulting in peptide chain elongation inhibition and peptidyl transferase inhibition
Pharmacokinetics
Distribution:
V_d: Quinupristin: 0.45 L/kg
V_d: Dalfopristin: 0.24 L/kg
Protein binding:
Quinupristin: 23% to 32%
Dalfopristin: 50% to 56%
Metabolism: Quinupristin is conjugated with glutathione and cysteine to active metabolites; dalfopristin is hydrolyzed to an active metabolite
Half-life:
Quinupristin: 0.85 hour
Dalfopristin: 0.7 hour
Elimination: 75% to 77% excreted in the bile and feces
Usual Dosage Dosage is expressed in terms of combined "mg" of quinupristin plus dalfopristin: I.V.:
Children: Limited information is available; quinupristin/dalfopristin has been used in a limited number of pediatric patients under a compassionate use protocol
Treatment of vancomycin-resistant *Enterococcus faecium* infection: 7.5 mg/kg/ dose every 8 hours

Treatment of vancomycin-resistant *Enterococcus faecium* CNS shunt infection: 7.5 mg/kg/dose every 8 hours (plus 1 mg intrathecal dose daily at the time of shunt tap was used in an 8-month old infant for 68 days in one case report; 1 or 2 mg doses every day for 5-33 days have been administered intrathecally in 6 patients)

Treatment of complicated skin and skin structure infection: 7.5 mg/kg/dose every 12 hours for at least 7 days

Adolescents ≥16 years and Adults:

Treatment of vancomycin-resistant *Enterococcus faecium* infection: 7.5 mg/kg/dose every 8 hours

Treatment of complicated skin and skin structure infection: 7.5 mg/kg/dose every 12 hours

Dosage adjustment in hepatic impairment: Dosage adjustment may be necessary, but exact recommendations cannot be made at this time

Administration Parenteral: Reconstitute vial by slowly adding 5 mL D_5W or sterile water for injection to make a 100 mg/mL solution; gently swirl the vial contents without shaking to minimize foam formation; further dilute the reconstituted solution with D_5W to a final maximum concentration for administration via peripheral line of 2 mg/mL; maximum concentration for administration via a central line is 5 mg/mL; if an injection site reaction occurs, the dose can be further diluted to a final concentration of <1 mg/mL; administer infusion over 60 minutes; following infusion of quinupristin/dalfopristin, the infusion line should be flushed with D_5W to minimize venous irritation; **DO NOT FLUSH** with saline or heparin solutions due to incompatibility

Monitoring Parameters CBC, liver function test; monitor infusion site closely

Nursing Implications If moderate to severe venous irritation occurs following peripheral quinupristin/dalfopristin administration, consider increasing the infusion volume, changing infusion sites, or establishing central venous access; administration of hydrocortisone or diphenhydramine did not decrease infusion site reactions

Dosage Forms Powder for injection: 500 mg vial (150 mg quinupristin and 350 mg dalfopristin)

References

Gransden WR, King A, Marossy D, et al, "Quinupristin/Dalfopristin in Neonatal *Enterococcus faecium* Meningitis," *Arch Dis Child Fetal Neonatal Ed*, 1998, 78(3):F235-6.

Gray JW, Darbyshire PJ, Beath SV, et al, "Experience With Quinupristin/Dalfopristin in Treating Infections With Vancomycin-Resistant *Enterococcus faecium* in Children," *Pediatr Infect Dis J*, 2000, 19(3):234-8.

Nachman SA, Verma R, and Egnor M, "Vancomycin-Resistant *Enterococcus faecium* Shunt Infection in an Infant: An Antibiotic Cure," *Microb Drug Resist*, 1995, 1(1):95-6

♦ **Quiphile®** *see* Quinine *on page 832*

♦ **Q-vel®** *see* Quinine *on page 832*

♦ **Rabies Immune Globulin, Human** *see page 1138*

♦ **Rabies Virus Vaccine, Human Diploid** *see page 1138*

♦ **Racemic Epinephrine** *see* Epinephrine *on page 371*

♦ **Radiostol® (Canada)** *see* Ergocalciferol *on page 377*

♦ **R-albuterol** *see* Levalbuterol *on page 563*

Ranitidine (ra NI ti deen)

Related Information

Carbohydrate and Alcohol Content of Liquid Medications for Use in Patients Receiving Ketogenic Diets *on page 1228*

Brand Names Apo®-Ranitidine (Canada); Novo-Ranidine® (Canada); Nu-Ranit® (Canada); Zantac®; Zantac® 75 [OTC]

Available Salts Ranitidine Hydrochloride

Therapeutic Category Gastrointestinal Agent, Gastric or Duodenal Ulcer Treatment; Histamine H_2 Antagonist

Generic Available Yes (except gel capsules, effervescent granules and tablets)

Use Short-term treatment of active duodenal ulcers and benign gastric ulcers; long-term prophylaxis of duodenal ulcer and gastric hypersecretory states; gastroesophageal reflux disease (GERD); recurrent postoperative ulcer; treatment and prophylaxis of erosive esophagitis; upper GI bleeding, prevention of acid-aspiration pneumonitis during surgery, and prevention of stress-induced ulcers; over-the-counter (OTC) formulation for use in the relief of heartburn, acid indigestion, and sour stomach

Pregnancy Risk Factor B

Contraindications Hypersensitivity to ranitidine or any component or other H_2 antagonists; patients with history of acute porphyria

(Continued)

835

Ranitidine *(Continued)*

Warnings Zantac® 150 EFFERdose® tablets and Zantac® 150 EFFERdose® granules contain phenylalamine and should be avoided in phenylketonurics

Precautions Use with caution in patients with liver and renal impairment; dosage modification required in patients with renal impairment

Adverse Reactions

Cardiovascular: Bradycardia, tachycardia

Central nervous system: Dizziness, sedation, malaise, mental confusion, headache, hallucinations, anxiety

Dermatologic: Rash, alopecia, erythema multiforme

Endocrine & metabolic: Gynecomastia

Gastrointestinal: Constipation, nausea, vomiting, abdominal discomfort, pancreatitis (rare)

Hematologic: Thrombocytopenia, aplastic anemia (rare), granulocytopenia, leukopenia

Hepatic: Hepatitis

Local: Transient pain at injection site

Neuromuscular & skeletal: Arthralgias

Renal: Elevated serum creatinine

Drug Interactions CYP2D6 and 3A3/4 enzyme inhibitor

Decreased effect: Variable effects on warfarin; antacids may decrease absorption of ranitidine; ketoconazole and itraconazole absorptions are decreased; may produce altered serum levels of procainamide and ferrous sulfate; decreased effect of nondepolarizing muscle relaxants, cefpodoxime, cyanocobalamin (decreased absorption), diazepam, oxaprozin

Decreased toxicity of atropine

Increased toxicity of cyclosporine (increased serum creatinine), gentamicin (neuromuscular blockade), glipizide, glyburide, midazolam, triazolam (increased concentrations), metoprolol, pentoxifylline, phenytoin, quinidine

Stability Protect injection from light; stable for 48 hours at room temperature or 30 days when frozen in D_5W or NS; stable for 24 hours in TPN solutions; stable for 24 hours in TPN with lipids

Mechanism of Action Competitive inhibition of histamine at H_2-receptors of the gastric parietal cells, which inhibits gastric acid secretion

Pharmacokinetics

Distribution: V_d: 1.4 L/kg; minimally penetrates the blood-brain barrier; breast milk to plasma ratio: 1.9-6.7

Protein binding: 15%

Metabolism: In the liver

Bioavailability: Oral: ~50%

Half-life:

Infants: 3.5 hours

Children 3.5-16 years: 1.8-2 hours

Adults:

Normal renal and hepatic function: 2-3 hours

Decreased renal function: 8.7 hours

Time to peak serum concentration: Oral: 1-3 hours

Elimination: 30% (oral) or 70% (I.V.) eliminated as unchanged drug in the urine and in feces

Hemodialysis: Slightly dialyzable (5% to 20%)

Usual Dosage

Premature and Term Infants <2 weeks:

Oral: 2 mg/kg/day divided every 12 hours

I.V.: 1.5 mg/kg/dose as loading dose, then 12 hours later maintenance dose of 1.5-2 mg/kg/day divided every 12 hours

Continuous infusion: 1.5 mg/kg/dose as loading dose followed by 0.04-0.08 mg/kg/hour infusion (or 1-2 mg/kg/day)

Children ≥1 month to 16 years:

Gastric/duodenal ulcer:

Oral:

Treatment: 2-4 mg/kg/day divided twice daily; maximum: 300 mg/day

Maintenance: 2-4 mg/kg/day divided twice daily; maximum: 150 mg/day

I.V.: 2-4 mg/kg/day divided every 6-8 hours; maximum: 150 mg/day

GERD and erosive esophagitis:

Oral: 4-10 mg/kg/day divided twice daily; maximum: GERD: 300 mg/day; erosive esophagitis: 600 mg/day

I.V.: 2-4 mg/kg/day divided every 6-8 hours; maximum: 150 mg/day **or as an alternative**

Continuous infusion: Initial: 1 mg/kg/dose for one dose followed by infusion of 0.08-0.17 mg/kg/hour or 2-4 mg/kg/day

Adults:

Treatment of duodenal or gastric ulcers, GERD, maintenance of erosive esophagitis: Oral: 150 mg/dose twice daily or 300 mg at bedtime

Prophylaxis of recurrent duodenal ulcer: Oral: 150 mg at bedtime

Gastric hypersecretory conditions:

Oral: 150 mg twice daily; maximum: 600 mg/day

I.M., I.V.: 50 mg/dose every 6-8 hours (dose not to exceed 400 mg/day)

Continuous I.V. infusion: Initial 50 mg I.V. followed by 6.25 mg/hour titrated to gastric pH >4.0 for prophylaxis or >7.0 for treatment; **continuous I.V. infusion is preferred in patients with active bleeding**

Erosive esophagitis: Oral: 150 mg 4 times/day

Pathologic hypersecretory conditions (eg, Zollinger-Ellison syndrome):

Continuous I.V. infusion: Initial 50 mg I.V. followed by 1 mg/kg/hour infusion; titrate dosage in 0.5 mg/kg/hour increments to maintain gastric acid output at <10 mEq/hour; doses up to 2.5 mg/kg/hour (220 mg/hour) have been used

Oral: 150 mg twice daily; more frequent administration may be indicated depending upon response; doses up to 6.3 g/day have been used in severe cases

Relief of heartburn, acid indigestion, sour stomach (OTC use): Oral: 75 mg 30-60 minutes before eating; no more than 2 tablets/day

Dosing interval in renal impairment:

Cl_{cr} 10-50 mL/minute: Administer at 75% of normal dose or administer every 18-24 hours

Cl_{cr} <10 mL/minute: Administer at 50% of normal dose or administer every 18-24 hours

Administration

Oral: Administer with meals and at bedtime; EFFERdose® tablets and granules must be dissolved in 6-8 ounces of water before use

Parenteral: Intermittent I.V. infusion preferred over direct injection to decrease risk of bradycardia; for intermittent infusion, infuse over 15-30 minutes, at a usual concentration of 0.5 mg/mL; for direct I.V. injection, administer over a period not less than 5 minutes at a final concentration not to exceed 2.5 mg/mL

Monitoring Parameters AST, ALT, serum creatinine; when used to prevent stress-related GI bleeding, measure the intragastric pH and try to maintain pH >4; gastric acid secretion (<10 mEq/hour)

Test Interactions False-positive urine protein using Multistix®; gastric acid secretion test, skin test allergen extracts

Patient Information Avoid excessive amounts of coffee and aspirin; when self-medicating, if symptoms of heartburn, acid indigestion, or sour stomach persist after 2 weeks of continuous use of the drug, consult a clinician.

Additional Information Causes fewer CNS adverse reactions and drug interactions compared to cimetidine; safety and efficacy of full-dose therapy extending beyond 8 weeks have not been determined

Dosage Forms

Capsule, as hydrochloride (GELdose™): 150 mg, 300 mg

Granules, effervescent, as hydrochloride (EFFERdose®): 150 mg

Infusion, preservative free, as hydrochloride, in NaCl 0.45%: 0.5 mg/mL (50 mL)

Injection, as hydrochloride: 25 mg/mL (2 mL, 10 mL, 40 mL)

Syrup, as hydrochloride, (peppermint flavor): 15 mg/mL (473 mL)

Tablet, as hydrochloride: 75 mg, 150 mg, 300 mg

Tablet, effervescent, as hydrochloride (EFFERdose®): 150 mg

References

Blumer JL, Rothstein FC, Kaplan BS, et al, "Pharmacokinetic Determination of Ranitidine Pharmacodynamics in Pediatric Ulcer Disease," *J Pediatr*, 1985, 107(2):301-6.

Eddleston JM, Booker PD, and Green JR, "Use of Ranitidine in Children Undergoing Cardiopulmonary Bypass," *Crit Care Med*, 1989, 17(1):26-9.

Fontana M, Massironi E, Rossi A, et al, "Ranitidine Pharmacokinetics in Newborn Infants," *Arch Dis Child*, 1993, 68(5 Spec No):602-3.

Lopez-Herce J, Albajara L, Codoceo R, et al, "Ranitidine Prophylaxis in Acute Gastric Mucosal Damage in Critically Ill Pediatric Patients," *Crit Care Med*, 1988, 16(6):591-93.

Morris DL, Markham SJ, Beechey A, et al, "Ranitidine-Bolus or Infusion Prophylaxis for Stress Ulcer," *Crit Care Med*, 1988, 16(3):229-32.

Roberts CJ, "Clinical Pharmacokinetics of Ranitidine," *Clin Pharmacokinet*, 1984, 9(3):211-21.

♦ **Ranitidine Hydrochloride** see Ranitidine *on page 835*

♦ **Reactine™ (Canada)** see Cetirizine *on page 201*

♦ **Recombinant Human Deoxyribonuclease** see Dornase Alfa *on page 341*

♦ **Rectal Medicone® [OTC]** see Hemorrhoidal Preparations *on page 470*

♦ **Rectocort (Canada)** see Hydrocortisone *on page 486*

- **Red Away® (Canada)** *see* Naphazoline *on page 671*
- **Redisol®** *see* Cyanocobalamin *on page 263*
- **Redoxon® (Canada)** *see* Ascorbic Acid *on page 96*
- **Redutemp® [OTC]** *see* Acetaminophen *on page 26*
- **Reese's® Pinworm Medicine [OTC]** *see* Pyrantel Pamoate *on page 824*
- **Regitine®** *see* Phentolamine *on page 757*
- **Reglan®** *see* Metoclopramide *on page 630*
- **Regonol® Injection** *see* Pyridostigmine *on page 826*
- **Regulace® [OTC]** *see* Docusate and Casanthranol *on page 337*
- **Regular Iletin® I** *see* Insulin Preparations *on page 518*
- **Regular [Concentrated] Iletin® II U-500** *see* Insulin Preparations *on page 518*
- **Regular Insulin** *see* Insulin Preparations *on page 518*
- **Regular Purified Pork Insulin** *see* Insulin Preparations *on page 518*
- **Regulax SS® [OTC]** *see* Docusate *on page 336*
- **Regulex® (Canada)** *see* Docusate *on page 336*
- **Reguloid® [OTC]** *see* Psyllium *on page 823*
- **Regutol® [OTC]** *see* Docusate *on page 336*
- **Relaxadon®** *see* Hyoscyamine, Atropine, Scopolamine, and Phenobarbital *on page 499*
- **Relefact® TRH** *see* Protirelin *on page 821*
- **Relief® Ophthalmic Solution** *see* Phenylephrine *on page 758*
- **Resectisol® Irrigation Solution** *see* Mannitol *on page 593*
- **Respa-DM®** *see* Guaifenesin and Dextromethorphan *on page 466*
- **Respa-GF®** *see* Guaifenesin *on page 464*
- **Respbid®** *see* Theophylline *on page 910*
- **RespiGam®** *see* Respiratory Syncytial Virus Immune Globulin (Intravenous) *on page 838*
- **Respinol-G®** *see* Guaifenesin, Phenylpropanolamine, and Phenylephrine *on page 467*

Respiratory Syncytial Virus Immune Globulin (Intravenous)

(RES peer rah tor ee sin SISH al VYE rus i MYUN GLOB yoo lin in tra VEE nus)

Brand Names RespiGam®

Synonyms RSV-IGIV; RSV-IVIG

Therapeutic Category Immune Globulin

Generic Available No

Use Prevention of serious lower respiratory tract infection caused by RSV in children <24 months of age with BPD who are receiving supplemental oxygen; history of prematurity (≤32 weeks gestation); prophylaxis of infants with severe immune deficiency exposed to RSV; prophylaxis of infants and children with severe immunosuppression (eg, BMT patient exposed to RSV)

Pregnancy Risk Factor C

Contraindications History of a severe reaction associated with the administration of RSV-IGIV or other human immunoglobulin preparations; patients with IgA deficiency; hypersensitivity to any component

Warnings Adverse reactions may be related to the rate of administration; loop diuretics should be available for the management of patients who are at risk for fluid overload; epinephrine and diphenhydramine should be available for treatment of acute hypersensitivity reactions. Aseptic meningitis syndrome (onset of several hours to 2 days following RSV-IGIV administration: Symptoms of severe headache, drowsiness, fever, photophobia, painful eye movements, muscle rigidity, nausea and vomiting with pleocytosis and elevated protein levels in CSF have occurred in 3 patients in the PREVENT trial); (see Additional Information)

Precautions Use with caution in patients with underlying pulmonary disease since these patients are sensitive to extra fluid volume; immunization with MMR and varicella vaccines should be deferred for 9 months after the last RSV-IGIV dose

Adverse Reactions

Cardiovascular: Tachycardia, hypertension, edema, hypotension, heart murmur, cyanosis

Central nervous system: Fever/pyrexia (6%), dizziness, anxiety, aseptic meningitis syndrome

Dermatologic: Rash, eczema, pruritus

Gastrointestinal: Vomiting (6%), diarrhea, gastroenteritis

Local: Injection site inflammation

Respiratory: Respiratory distress, wheezing, rales, hypoxia, tachypnea, cyanosis, cough, rhinorrhea, dyspnea

Drug Interactions Live virus vaccine (ie, MMR, measles, varicella) when given during or within 10 months after RSV-IGIV administration; antibody response to DPT, DTaP, OPV, and *H. influenzae* b vaccine may be lower

Stability Refrigerate; do not freeze; do not shake vials; compatible with dextrose 5% through dextrose 20% with or without sodium chloride

Pharmacokinetics Half-life: 22-28 days

Usual Dosage I.V. infusion: Infants and Young Children: 750 mg/kg once monthly during RSV season (starting November with the last infusion in April).

Administration Infusion should start within 6 hours and be completed by 12 hours after vial entry; an in-line filter is not necessary, but if one is used, the pore size should be larger than 15 µM; if dilution is needed, a dilution of no greater than 1:2 should be used.

The infusion schedule is as follows:

Initial infusion rate for the first 15 minutes: 1.5 mL/kg/hour, then increase infusion rate for the next 15 minutes to 3 mL/kg/hour

30 minutes to end of infusion: 6 mL/kg/hour

Maximum infusion rate: 6 mL/kg/hour

Monitoring Parameters Heart rate, blood pressure, temperature, respiratory rate; observe for retractions and rales

Additional Information PREVENT (Prophylaxis of RSV in elevated-risk neonates trial) was a multicenter, randomized, double-blind, placebo-controlled trial (n=250 RSV-IGIV, n=260 placebo) among infants ≤24 months, born prematurely (≤35 weeks gestation), or children with BPD and a requirement for supplemental oxygen within the past 6 months. Each patient received a monthly infusion from November through April. The trial showed that children treated with RSV-IGIV had less RSV hospitalizations (20 days vs. 35 days, p=0.047); fewer RSV hospital days per 100 days (60 days vs. 129 days, p=0.045); fewer RSV hospital days with supplemental oxygen (34 days vs. 85 days, p=0.007). There was no difference between the two groups for ICU admissions, RSV ICU days per 100 children, RSV mechanical ventilation or days of ventilation per 100 children. (Groothius, 1993)

RSV-IGIV is a sterile liquid without preservatives purified using Cohn-Oncley cold ethanol fractionation and further treatment with a solvent-detergent partitioning method; contains trace amounts of IgA and IgM, sucrose and albumin; sodium content: 20-30 mEq/L

Dosage Forms Injection, preservative free: 1000 mg, 2500 mg (50 mL)

References

American Academy of Pediatrics Committee on Infectious Diseases, Committee on Fetus and Newborn, "Respiratory Syncytial Virus Immune Globulin Intravenous: Indications for Use," *Pediatrics*, 1997, 99(4):645-50.

Ellenberg SS, Epstein JS, Fratantoni JC, et al, "A Trial of RSV Immune Globulin in Infants and Young Children: The FDA's View," *N Engl J Med*, 1994, 331(3):203-5.

Groothius JR, Simoes EA, Levin MJ, et al, "Prophylactic Administration of Respiratory Syncytial Virus Immune Globulin to High-Risk Infants and Young Children. The Respiratory Syncytial Virus Immune Globulin Study Group," *N Engl J Med*, 1993, 329(21):1524-30.

♦ **Retin-A™** *see* Tretinoin *on page 945*

♦ **Retinoic Acid** *see* Tretinoin *on page 945*

♦ **Retinova™ (Canada)** *see* Tretinoin *on page 945*

♦ **Retisol-A® (Canada)** *see* Tretinoin *on page 945*

♦ **Retrovir®** *see* Zidovudine *on page 990*

♦ **Reversol®** *see* Edrophonium *on page 359*

♦ **Revitalose C-1000® (Canada)** *see* Ascorbic Acid *on page 96*

♦ **R-Gel® [OTC]** *see* Capsaicin *on page 162*

♦ **R-Gene®** *see* Arginine *on page 95*

♦ **rGM-CSF** *see* Sargramostim *on page 858*

♦ **Rheaban® [OTC]** *see* Attapulgite *on page 109*

♦ **Rheomacrodex®** *see* Dextran *on page 299*

♦ **Rhesonativ®** *see* Rh₀(D) Immune Globulin, Intramuscular *on page 840*

♦ **Rheumatrex® Oral** *see* Methotrexate *on page 621*

♦ **Rhinalar® (Canada)** *see* Flunisolide *on page 423*

♦ **Rhinall® Nasal Solution [OTC]** *see* Phenylephrine *on page 758*

♦ **Rhinaris-F® (Canada)** *see* Flunisolide *on page 423*

♦ **Rhindecon® Rhinocaps® [OTC]** *see* Phenylpropanolamine *on page 761*

♦ **Rhinocort®** *see* Budesonide *on page 144*

♦ **Rhinocort® Aqua™** *see* Budesonide *on page 144*

♦ **Rhinocort® Turbuhaler® (Canada)** *see* Budesonide *on page 144*

♦ **Rhinosyn-DMX® [OTC]** *see* Guaifenesin and Dextromethorphan *on page 466*

Rh$_o$(D) Immune Globulin, Intramuscular

(ar aych oh (dee) i MYUN GLOB yoo lin)

Brand Names HypRho®-D; HypRho®-D (Canada); HypRho®-D Mini-Dose; MICRhoGAM™; Mini-Gamulin® Rh; Rhesonativ®; RhoGAM™; WinRho SD® (Canada)

Therapeutic Category Immune Globulin

Generic Available No

Use Prevention of isoimmunization in Rh-negative individuals exposed to Rh-positive blood during delivery of an Rh-positive infant, as a result of an abortion, following amniocentesis or abdominal trauma, or following a transfusion accident; prevention of hemolytic disease of the newborn if there is a subsequent pregnancy with an Rh-positive fetus

Pregnancy Risk Factor C

Contraindications Rh$_o$(D)-positive patient; hypersensitivity to immune globulins or to thimerosal; transfusion of Rh$_o$(D)-positive blood in previous 3 months; prior sensitization to Rh$_o$(D)

Warnings Do not inject I.V.; do not administer to the neonate

Precautions Use with caution in patients with thrombocytopenia or bleeding disorders, patients with IgA deficiency

Adverse Reactions
Central nervous system: Lethargy, fever
Gastrointestinal: Splenomegaly
Hepatic: Elevated bilirubin
Local: Pain at the injection site
Neuromuscular & skeletal: Myalgia

Drug Interactions Live virus vaccines (Rh$_o$(D) may interfere with immune response to measles, mumps, rubella)

Stability Refrigerate; may be stable for up to 30 days at room temperature; avoid freezing

Mechanism of Action Suppresses the immune response and antibody formation of Rh-negative individuals to Rh-positive red blood cells

Pharmacokinetics
Distribution: Appears in breast milk, however not absorbed by the nursing infant
Half-life: 23-26 days

Usual Dosage Adults: Administer to mother **NOT** to infant: I.M.:
Obstetrical usage: 1 vial (300 mcg) prevents maternal sensitization if fetal packed red blood cell volume that has entered the maternal circulation is <15 mL; if it is more, give additional vials. The number of vials = RBC volume of the calculated fetomaternal hemorrhage divided by 15 mL
Postpartum prophylaxis: 300 mcg within 72 hours of delivery
Antepartum prophylaxis: 300 mcg at approximately 26-28 weeks gestation; followed by 300 mcg within 72 hours of delivery if infant is Rh-positive
Following miscarriage, abortion, or termination of ectopic pregnancy at up to 13 weeks of gestation: 50 mcg ideally within 3 hours, but may be given up to 72 hours after; if pregnancy has been terminated at 13 or more weeks of gestation, administer 300 mcg within 72 hours

Administration Parenteral: Administer I.M. preferably in the anterolateral aspects of the upper thigh or the deltoid muscle of the upper arm. The total volume can be given in divided doses at different sites at one time or may be divided and given at intervals, provided the total dosage is given within 72 hours of the fetomaternal hemorrhage or transfusion.

Dosage Forms
Injection: Each vial contains one single dose 300 mcg of Rh$_o$(D) immune globulin
Injection, microdose: Each vial contains one single dose of microdose, 50 mcg of Rh$_o$(D) immune globulin

Rh$_o$(D) Immune Globulin, Intravenous

(ar aych oh (dee) i MYUN GLOB yoo lin, in tra VEE nus)

Brand Names WinRho SDF®

Synonyms Rh$_o$(D) Immune Human Globulin; Rh$_o$IGIV

Therapeutic Category Immune Globulin

Use Treatment of nonsplenectomized, Rh$_o$(D) positive children and adults with chronic idiopathic thrombocytopenic purpura (ITP), children with acute ITP, or children and adults with ITP secondary to HIV infection; prevention of isoimmunization in Rh-negative individuals exposed to Rh-positive blood during delivery of an Rh-positive infant, within 72 hours of an abortion, following amniocentesis or abdominal trauma, or following a transfusion accident; prevention of hemolytic disease of the newborn if there is a subsequent pregnancy with an Rh-positive infant

Pregnancy Risk Factor C

Contraindications Hypersensitivity to immune globulin, thimerosal, or any component; IgA deficiency

Warnings When used for ITP in a patient who is $Rh_o(D)$-positive, a decrease in hemoglobin concentration as a result of destruction of $Rh_o(D)$-positive red blood cells can be expected; reduce WinRho SDF® dosage in these patients to minimize risk of increasing the severity of anemia; these patients should be monitored for signs and/or symptoms of intravascular hemolysis, clinically compromising anemia, and renal insufficiency; when used for suppression of Rh isoimmunization, the drug is administered to the mother **not** the infant; use only the I.V. route when treating ITP; anaphylactic hypersensitivity reactions can occur; studies indicate that there is no discernible risk of transmitting HIV or hepatitis B

Precautions Use with caution in patients with thrombocytopenia or bleeding disorders or individuals with hemoglobin concentrations <8 g/dL

Adverse Reactions
Cardiovascular: Hypotension, vasodilation
Central nervous system: Fever, headache, chills, dizziness, somnolence
Dermatologic: Rash, pruritus
Local: Discomfort and swelling at injection site
Gastrointestinal: Abdominal pain, diarrhea
Genitourinary: Hemoglobinuria
Hematologic: Hemolysis (hemoglobin decrease of >2 g/dL in 5% to 10% of ITP patients)
Neuromuscular & skeletal: Back pain, myalgia, hyperkinesia
Miscellaneous: Hypersensitivity reactions

Drug Interactions May interfere with the immune response to live virus vaccines (allow 3 months after administration of vaccine)

Stability Refrigerate do not freeze; reconstituted powder is stable 12 hours at room temperature

Mechanism of Action The $Rh_o(D)$ antigen is responsible for most cases of Rh sensitization, which occurs when Rh-positive fetal RBCs enter the maternal circulation of an Rh-negative woman. Injection of anti-D globulin results in opsonization of the fetal RBCs, which are then phagocytized in the spleen, preventing immunization of the mother. Injection of anti-D into an Rh-positive patient with ITP coats the patient's own D-positive RBCs with antibody and, as they are cleared by the spleen, they saturate the capacity of the spleen to clear antibody-coated cells, sparing antibody-coated platelets. Other proposed mechanisms involve the generation of cytokines following the interaction between antibody-coated RBCs and macrophages.

Pharmacodynamics
Onset of effect:
Rh isoimmunization: I.V.: 8 hours
ITP: I.V.: 1-2 days
Peak response: ITP: 7-14 days
Duration of effect: ITP: (single dose) 30 days

Pharmacokinetics
Half-life, elimination:
I.M.: 5-10 days
I.V.: 24 days
Time to peak concentration:
I.M.: 5-10 days
I.V.: 2 hours

Usual Dosage
ITP: **I.V. only:** Children and Adults:
Initial:
Hemoglobin ≥10 g/dL: 50 mcg/kg (250 international units/kg) as single dose or divided into 2 doses given on separate days
Hemoglobin <10 g/dL: 25-40 mcg/kg (125-200 international units/kg) as single dose or divided into 2 doses given on separate days
Hemoglobin <8 g/dL: Use with caution (see Precautions and Warnings)
Maintenance (usage dependent upon clinical response, platelet count, hemoglobin, red blood cell counts, and reticulocyte levels)

(Continued)

Rh₀(D) Immune Globulin, Intravenous *(Continued)*

Response to initial dose: 25-60 mcg/kg (125-300 international units/kg) as single dose

Nonresponse to initial therapy:

Hemoglobin >10 g/dL: 50-60 mcg/kg (250-300 international units/kg) as single dose

Hemoglobin 8-10 g/dL: 25-40 mcg/kg (125-200 international units/kg) as single dose

Hemoglobin <8 g/dL: Use with caution (see Precautions and Warnings)

Suppression of Rh isoimmunization: Adult female: I.V. or I.M.: see table.

I.V. Rh₀D Immune Globulin Dosage in Pregnancy and Obstetrical Conditions

Condition	Dosage
28 weeks gestation	300 mcg (1500 international units); repeat every 12 weeks throughout pregnancy
Postpartum (if newborn Rh-positive)	120 mcg (600 international units) **as soon as possible,** preferrably <72 hours, after delivery; if baby's Rh status is not known by 72 hours, administer as soon as possible up to 28 days after delivery
Threatened abortion at any time	300 mcg (1500 international units) as soon as possible within 72 hours
Amniocentesis and chronic villus sampling before 34 weeks gestation	300 mcg (1500 international units) within 72 hours; repeat every 12 weeks throughout pregnancy
Abortion, amniocentesis, or any other manipulation after 34 weeks gestation	120 mcg (600 international units) within 72 hours

Treatment of exposure to incompatible blood transfusion or massive fetal hemorrhage; within 72 hours of event:

Exposed to Rh₀(D) positive whole blood:

I.M.: 12 mcg (60 international units)/mL blood; administer in 1200 mcg (6000 international units) aliquots every 12 hours until the total calculated dose is administered

I.V.: 9 mcg (45 international units)/mL blood; administer in 600 mcg (3000 international units) aliquots every 8 hours until the total calculated dose is administered

Exposed to Rh₀(D) positive red blood cells:

I.M.: 24 mcg (120 international units)/mL cells administer in 1200 mcg (6000 international units) aliquots every 12 hours until the total calculated dose is administered

I.V.: 18 mcg (90 international units)/mL cells; administer in 600 mcg (3000 international units) aliquots every 8 hours until the total calculated dose is administered

Administration Parenteral: WinRho SDF® is the only immune globulin product available that can be administered **both** I.M. and I.V.; however, **for the treatment of ITP, it must be administered I.V.**

I.M.: Reconstitute 120 mcg and 300 mcg vials with 1.25 mL NS and the 100 mcg vial with 8.5 mL NS; gently swirl vial; do not shake; administer into the deltoid muscle of upper arm or the anterolateral aspect of the upper thigh; the gluteal region is not recommended for routine administration due to the potential risk of sciatic nerve injury; if gluteal area is used, administer only in the upper, outer quadrant

I.V.: Reconstitute 120 mcg and 300 mcg vials with 2.5 mL NS and 8.5 mL NS for the 1000 mcg vial; gently swirl vial; do not shake; infuse over 3-5 minutes

Monitoring Parameters ITP: CBC, reticulocytes, UA, renal function

Additional Information WinRho SDF® 1 mcg ≈ 5 international units

Dosage Forms Injection, freeze dried: 120 mcg (600 international units); 300 mcg (1500 international units); 1000 mcg (5000 international units) [each vial is accompanied with NS diluent]

References

Gaines AR, "Acute Onset Hemoglobinemia and/or Hemoglobinuria and Sequela Following Rh(o)(D) Immune Globulin Intravenous Administration in Immune Thrombocytopenic Purpura Patients," *Blood,* 2000, 95(8):2523-9.

♦ **Rh₀(D) Immune Human Globulin** *see* Rh₀(D) Immune Globulin, Intravenous *on page 840*

♦ **RhoGAM™** *see* Rh₀(D) Immune Globulin, Intramuscular *on page 840*

♦ **Rh₀IGIV** *see* Rh₀(D) Immune Globulin, Intravenous *on page 840*

♦ **Rhoprolene®** **(Canada)** *see* Betamethasone *on page 130*

♦ **Rhoprosone®** **(Canada)** *see* Betamethasone *on page 130*

♦ **rHuEPO** *see* Epoetin Alfa *on page 373*

♦ **rHuEPO-α** *see* Epoetin Alfa *on page 373*

♦ **Rhulicaine® [OTC]** *see* Benzocaine *on page 124*

Ribavirin (rye ba VYE rin)

Brand Names Virazole®

Synonyms ICN-1299; RTCA; Tribavirin

Therapeutic Category Antiviral Agent, Inhalation Therapy

Generic Available No

Use Treatment of patients with RSV infections; specially indicated for treatment of severe lower respiratory tract RSV infections in patients with an underlying compromising condition (prematurity, BPD and other chronic lung conditions, congenital heart disease, immunodeficiency, immunosuppression), and recent transplant recipients; may also be used in other viral infections including influenza A and B and adenovirus

Pregnancy Risk Factor X

Contraindications Females of childbearing age

Warnings Ribavirin is potentially mutagenic, tumor-promoting, and gonadotoxic; there is evidence that ribavirin is teratogenic in small animals

Precautions Use with caution in patients requiring assisted ventilation because precipitation of the drug in the respiratory equipment may interfere with safe and effective patient ventilation; carefully monitor patients with COPD and asthma for deterioration of respiratory function

Adverse Reactions

    Cardiovascular: Hypotension, cardiac arrest

    Central nervous system: Headache

    Dermatologic: Rash, skin irritation

    Hematologic: Anemia

    Ocular: Conjunctivitis

    Respiratory: Mild bronchospasm, worsening of respiratory function, nasal and throat irritation

Drug Interactions Ribavirin antagonizes the antiviral activity of zidovudine and zalcitabine against HIV

Stability Reconstituted solution is stable for 24 hours at room temperature

Mechanism of Action Inhibits replication of RNA and DNA viruses; inhibits influenza virus RNA polymerase activity and interferes with the expression of messenger RNA resulting in inhibition of viral protein synthesis

Pharmacokinetics

    Absorption: Systemically absorbed from the respiratory tract following nasal and oral inhalation; absorption is dependent upon respiratory factors and method of drug delivery; maximal absorption occurs with the use of the aerosol generator via an endotracheal tube

    Distribution: Highest concentrations are found in the respiratory tract and erythrocytes

    Metabolism: Occurs intracellularly and may be necessary for drug action; metabolized by the liver to deribosylated ribavirin (active metabolite)

    Half-life:

        Respiratory tract secretions: ~2 hours

        Plasma:

            Children: 6.5-11 hours

            Adults: 24 hours; half-life is much longer in the erythrocyte (16-40 days), which can be used as a marker for intracellular metabolism

    Time to peak serum concentration: Aerosol inhalation: At the end of the inhalation period

    Elimination: Hepatic metabolism is the major route of elimination with 40% of the drug cleared renally as unchanged drug and metabolites

Usual Dosage Infants, Children, and Adults: Aerosol inhalation:

    Use with Viratek® small particle aerosol generator (SPAG-2) at a concentration of 20 mg/mL (6 g reconstituted with 300 mL of sterile water without preservatives); 6 g ribavirin vial has also been diluted with 300 mL of sterile NS solution rather than sterile water to achieve a near isotonic solution.

    Note: Dose actually delivered to the patient will depend on patient's minute ventilation

    Continuous aerosolization: 12-18 hours/day for 3 days, or up to 7 days in length

    Intermittent aerosolization (high-dose, short-duration aerosol): 2 g over 2 hours 3 times/day at a concentration of 60 mg/mL (6 g reconstituted with 100 mL of

(Continued)

Ribavirin *(Continued)*

sterile water without preservatives) in **non-mechanically ventilated** patients for 3-7 days has been used to permit easier accessibility for patient care and limit environmental exposure of healthcare worker. Due to apparent increased potential for crystallization of the high-dose 60 mg/mL solution around areas of turbulent flow such as bends in tubing or connector pieces, use of high-dose therapy in individuals with an endotracheal tube in place is **not** recommended.

Administration Ribavirin should be administered in well-ventilated rooms (at least 6 air changes/hour)

Mechanically ventilated patients: Ribavirin can potentially be deposited in the ventilator delivery system depending on temperature, humidity, and electrostatic forces; this deposition can lead to malfunction or obstruction of the expiratory valve, resulting in inadvertently high positive end-expiratory pressures. The use of one-way valves in the inspiratory lines, a breathing circuit filter in the expiratory line, and frequent monitoring and filter replacement have been effective in preventing these problems.

Monitoring Parameters Respiratory function, hemoglobin, reticulocyte count, CBC, I & O

Nursing Implications Healthcare workers who are pregnant or who may become pregnant should be advised of the potential risks of exposure and counseled about risk reduction strategies including alternate job responsibilities; limit contact by visitors with patients receiving ribavirin; ribavirin may adsorb to contact lenses

Additional Information RSV season is usually December to April; viral shedding period for RSV is usually 3-8 days

Dosage Forms Powder for aerosol: 6 g (100 mL)

References

American Academy of Pediatrics Committee on Infectious Diseases, "Reassessment of the Indications for Ribavirin Therapy in Respiratory Syncytial Virus Infections," *Pediatrics*, 1996, 97(1):137-40.

Englund JA, Piedra PA, Ahn Y-M, et al, "High-Dose, Short-Duration Ribavirin Aerosol Therapy Compared With Standard Ribavirin Therapy in Children With Suspected Respiratory Syncytial Virus Infection," *J Pediatr*, 1994, 125:635-41.

Janai HK, Marks MI, Zaleska M, et al, "Ribavirin: Adverse Drug Reactions 1986 to 1988," *Pediatr Infect Dis J*, 1990, 9(3):209-11.

Meert KL, Sarnaik AP, Gelmini MJ, et al, "Aerosolized Ribavirin in Mechanically Ventilated Children With Respiratory Syncytial Virus Lower Respiratory Tract Disease: A Prospective, Double-Blind, Randomized Trial," *Crit Care Med*, 1994, 22(4):566-72.

Smith DW, Frankel LR, Mathers LH, et al, "A Controlled Trial of Aerosolized Ribavirin in Infants Receiving Mechanical Ventilation for Severe Respiratory Syncytial Virus Infection," *N Engl J Med*, 1991, 325(1):24-9.

Riboflavin *(RYE boe flay vin)*

Brand Names Riobin®

Synonyms Lactoflavin; Vitamin B_2; Vitamin G

Therapeutic Category Nutritional Supplement; Vitamin, Water Soluble

Generic Available Yes

Use Prevention of riboflavin deficiency and treatment of ariboflavinosis; microcytic anemia associated with glutathione reductase deficiency

Pregnancy Risk Factor A (C if dose exceeds RDA recommendation)

Contraindications Hypersensitivity to riboflavin or any component

Adverse Reactions Genitourinary: Discoloration of urine (bright yellow) with large doses

Drug Interactions Probenecid

Food Interactions Food increases the extent of GI absorption

Stability Protect from light

Mechanism of Action Converted to coenzymes which act as hydrogen-carrier molecules, which are necessary for normal tissue respiration; also needed for activation of pyridoxine and conversion of tryptophan to niacin

Pharmacokinetics

Absorption: Readily via GI tract, however, food increases extent of GI absorption; GI absorption is decreased in patients with hepatitis, cirrhosis, or biliary obstruction

Metabolism: Metabolic fate unknown

Half-life, biologic: 66-84 minutes

Elimination: 9% eliminated unchanged in urine

Usual Dosage Oral:

Riboflavin deficiency:

Children: 3-10 mg/day in divided doses

Adults: 5-30 mg/day in divided doses

Adequate intake: Infants:
  <6 months: 0.3 mg (0.04 mg/kg)
  6-12 months: 0.4 mg (0.04 mg/kg)
Recommended daily allowance (RDA):
Children:
  1-3 years: 0.5 mg
  4-8 years: 0.6 mg
  9-13 years: 0.9 mg
  14-18 years:
    Male: 1.3 mg
    Female: 1 mg
  19-70 years:
    Male: 1.3 mg
    Female: 1.1 mg
Microcytic anemia associated with glutathione reductase deficiency: Adults: 10 mg daily for 10 days

Administration Oral: Administer with food

Monitoring Parameters CBC and reticulocyte counts (if anemic when treating deficiency)

Test Interactions Large doses may interfere with urinalysis based on spectrometry; may cause false elevations in fluorometric determinations of catecholamines and urobilinogen

Patient Information Large doses may cause bright yellow urine

Dosage Forms Tablet: 25 mg, 50 mg, 100 mg

♦ **Rid-A-Pain® [OTC]** *see* Benzocaine *on page 124*
♦ **Ridaura®** *see* Auranofin *on page 109*
♦ **Ridenol® [OTC]** *see* Acetaminophen *on page 26*

Rifabutin (rif a BYOO tin)

Brand Names Mycobutin®
Synonyms Ansamycin
Therapeutic Category Antibiotic, Miscellaneous; Antitubercular Agent
Generic Available No
Use Prevention of disseminated *Mycobacterium avium* complex (MAC) in patients with advanced HIV infection; utilized in multiple drug regimens for treatment of MAC
Pregnancy Risk Factor B
Contraindications Hypersensitivity to rifabutin, any component, or other rifamycin; rifabutin is contraindicated in patients with a WBC <1000/mm³ or a platelet count <50,000 mm³
Warnings Rifabutin as a single agent must not be administered to patients with active tuberculosis since its use may lead to the development of tuberculosis that is resistant to both rifabutin and rifampin; rifabutin should be discontinued in patients with AST >500 int. units/L or if total bilirubin is >3 mg/dL
Precautions Use with caution in patients with liver impairment
Adverse Reactions
Central nervous system: Fever, headache, seizures, confusion, insomnia
Dermatologic: Rash, staining of skin (brown-orange)
Gastrointestinal: Abdominal pain, diarrhea, dyspepsia, nausea, vomiting, dysgeusia, flatulence
Genitourinary: Discoloration of urine (brown-orange)
Hematologic: Thrombocytopenia, anemia, leukopenia, neutropenia
Hepatic: Elevated liver enzymes
Neuromuscular & skeletal: Arthralgia, myositis
Ocular: Uveitis
Miscellaneous: Discoloration of body fluids (brown-orange)
Drug Interactions May decrease the serum concentration or effect of dapsone, verapamil, methadone, ketoconazole, digoxin, theophylline, barbiturates, protease inhibitors, non-nucleoside reverse transcriptase inhibitors, anticoagulants, corticosteroids, zidovudine, cyclosporine, quinidine, and oral contraceptives (alternative form of contraception should be considered); indinavir and ritonavir increase rifabutin concentrations (decrease daily rifabutin dose by 50% if given with indinavir or decrease rifabutin adult dose to 150 mg 2-3 times per week if given with ritonavir); protease inhibitors, erythromycin, clarithromycin, ketoconazole, fluconazole, and itraconazole may increase serum concentration of rifabutin
Food Interactions High-fat meal may decrease the rate but not the extent of absorption
(Continued)

Rifabutin *(Continued)*

Mechanism of Action Inhibits DNA-dependent RNA polymerase at the beta subunit which prevents chain initiation

Pharmacokinetics

Absorption: Oral: Readily absorbed

Distribution: To body tissues including the lungs, liver, spleen, eyes, and kidneys

Protein binding: 85%

Metabolism: To active and inactive metabolites

Half life, terminal: 45 hours (range: 16-69 hours)

Time to peak serum concentration: 2-4 hours

Elimination: Renal and biliary clearance of unchanged drug is 10%; 30% excreted in feces

Usual Dosage Oral:

Children: Efficacy and safety of rifabutin have not been established in children; a limited number of HIV-positive children with MAC (n=22) have been given rifabutin for MAC prophylaxis; dosages of up to 75 mg/day have been given to children <4 years of age (~5-6 mg/kg/day)

Infants and Children: Prophylaxis for first episode of MAC in HIV-infected patients:

Children <6 years: 5 mg/kg once daily

Children ≥6 years: 300 mg once daily

Infants and Children: Prophylaxis for recurrence of MAC in HIV-infected patients: 5 mg/kg (maximum dose: 300 mg) once daily in combination with clarithromycin

Adolescents and Adults:

Prophylaxis for first episode of MAC in HIV-infected patient: 300 mg once daily; for patients who experience gastrointestinal upset, rifabutin can be administered 150 mg twice daily with food

Prophylaxis for recurrence of MAC in HIV-infected patient: 300 mg once daily as a component of a multiple drug regimen

Administration Oral: May administer with or without food or mix with applesauce; administer with food to decrease GI upset

Monitoring Parameters Periodic liver function tests, CBC with differential, platelet count, hemoglobin, hematocrit

Patient Information May discolor skin, urine, tears, perspiration, or other body fluids to a brown-orange color; soft contact lenses may be permanently stained

Dosage Forms Capsule: 150 mg

Extemporaneous Preparations A 20 mg/mL rifabutin suspension is made by placing the powder from eight 150 mg rifabutin capsules into a glass mortar, levigating with 20 mL of a 1:1 vehicle of Ora-Sweet® and Ora-Plus® and triturating the mixture to make a paste. Additional vehicle is added in geometric proportion levigating until a uniform mixture is obtained; qsad to 60 mL with vehicle. Stable for 12 weeks at 4°C, 25°C, 30°C, and 40°C. Label "shake well before using."

Haslam JL, Egodage KL, Chen Y, et al, "Stability of Rifabutin in Two Extemporaneously Compounded Oral Liquids," *Am J Health Syst Pharm*, 1999, 56(4):333-6.

References

1999 USPHS/IDSA Guidelines for the Prevention of Opportunistic Infections in Persons Infected With Human Immunodeficiency Virus, *MMWR Morb Mortal Wkly Rep*, 1999, 48(RR-10): 1-6 6.

Krause PJ, Hight DW, Schwartz AN, et al, "Successful Management of *Mycobacterium intracellulare* Pneumonia in a Child," *Pediatr Infect Dis*, 1986, 5(2):269-71.

Levin RH and Bolinger AM, "Treatment of Nontuberculous Mycobacterial Infections in Pediatric Patients," *Clin Pharm*, 1988, 7(7):545-51.

Starke JR and Correa AG, "Management of Mycobacterial Infection and Disease in Children," *Pediatr Infect Dis J*, 1995, 14(6):455-70.

♦ **Rifadin®** *see* Rifampin *on page 846*

♦ **Rifadin® (Canada)** *see* Rifampin *on page 846*

♦ **Rifampicin** *see* Rifampin *on page 846*

Rifampin *(RIF am pin)*

Brand Names Rifadin®; Rifadin® (Canada); Rimactane®; Rimactane® (Canada); Rofact™ (Canada)

Synonyms Rifampicin

Therapeutic Category Antibiotic, Miscellaneous; Antitubercular Agent

Generic Available No

Use Used in combination with other antitubercular drugs for the treatment of active tuberculosis; elimination of meningococci from asymptomatic carriers; prophylaxis in contacts of patients with *Haemophilus influenzae* type B infection; used in combination with other anti-infectives in the treatment of staphylococcal infections

Pregnancy Risk Factor C

Contraindications Hypersensitivity to rifampin or any component

Precautions Use with caution in patients with liver impairment; modification of dosage should be considered in patients with severe liver impairment

Adverse Reactions

Central nervous system: Drowsiness, fatigue, confusion, ataxia, fever, headache

Dermatologic: Rash, pruritus

Gastrointestinal: Nausea, vomiting, diarrhea, stomatitis, anorexia

Hematologic: Eosinophilia, blood dyscrasias (leukopenia, thrombocytopenia), hemolytic anemia

Hepatic: Hepatitis, cholestatic jaundice

Local: Irritation at the I.V. site

Neuromuscular & skeletal: Myalgias, arthralgia

Renal: Renal failure, interstitial nephritis

Miscellaneous: Flu-like syndrome; discoloration of body fluids (red-orange)

Drug Interactions Rifampin induces liver enzymes which may decrease the plasma concentration of the following drugs: verapamil, methadone, digoxin, cyclosporine, corticosteroids, oral anticoagulants, theophylline, barbiturates, chloramphenicol, ketoconazole, oral contraceptives (alternate form of contraception should be considered), and quinidine; halothane (additive hepatotoxic effects)

Food Interactions Food may delay and reduce the amount of rifampin absorbed

Stability Reconstituted I.V. solution is stable for 24 hours at room temperature; once the reconstituted I.V. solution is further diluted in D_5W (preferably) or NS, the I.V. infusion solution should be administered within 4 hours of preparation to avoid precipitation

Mechanism of Action Inhibits bacterial RNA synthesis by binding to the beta subunit of DNA-dependent RNA polymerase, blocking RNA transcription

Pharmacokinetics

Absorption: Oral: Well absorbed

Distribution: Highly lipophilic; crosses the blood-brain barrier and is widely distributed into body tissues and fluids such as the liver, lungs, gallbladder, bile, tears, and breast milk; distributes into CSF when meninges are inflamed

Protein binding: 80%

Metabolism: Undergoes enterohepatic recycling; metabolized in the liver to a deacetylated metabolite (active)

Half-life: 3-4 hours, prolonged with hepatic impairment

Time to peak serum concentration: Oral: Within 2-4 hours

Elimination: Principally in feces (60% to 65%) and urine (~30%)

Plasma rifampin concentrations are not significantly affected by hemodialysis or peritoneal dialysis

Usual Dosage Oral (I.V. infusion dose is the same as for the oral route):

Tuberculosis:

Children: 10-20 mg/kg/day in divided doses every 12-24 hours

Adults: 10 mg/kg/day administered once daily; maximum dose: 600 mg/day

American Thoracic Society and CDC currently recommend twice weekly therapy as part of a short-course regimen which follows 1-2 months of daily treatment of uncomplicated pulmonary tuberculosis in the compliant patient

Children: 10-20 mg/kg/dose (up to 600 mg) twice weekly under supervision to ensure compliance

Adults: 10 mg/kg (up to 600 mg) twice weekly

H. influenzae prophylaxis:

Neonates <1 month: 10 mg/kg/day every 24 hours for 4 days

Infants and Children: 20 mg/kg/day every 24 hours for 4 days, not to exceed 600 mg/dose

Adults: 600 mg every 24 hours for 4 days

Meningococcal prophylaxis:

<1 month: 10 mg/kg/day in divided doses every 12 hours for 2 days

Infants and Children: 20 mg/kg/day in divided doses every 12 hours for 2 days, not to exceed 600 mg/dose

Adults: 600 mg every 12 hours for 2 days

Nasal carriers of *Staphylococcus aureus*:

Children: 15 mg/kg/day divided every 12 hours for 5-10 days in combination with other antibiotics

Adults: 600 mg once daily for 5-10 days in combination with other antibiotics

(Continued)

Rifampin *(Continued)*

Administration

Oral: Administer 1 hour before or 2 hours after a meal on an empty stomach; may administer with food to decrease GI distress; may mix contents of capsule with applesauce or jelly

Parenteral: Do not administer I.M. or S.C.; administer I.V. preparation once daily by slow I.V. infusion over 30 minutes to 3 hours at a final concentration not to exceed 6 mg/mL

Monitoring Parameters Periodic monitoring of liver function (AST, ALT); bilirubin, CBC

Patient Information May discolor urine, tears, sweat, or other body fluids to a red-orange color; soft contact lenses may be permanently stained

Nursing Implications The compounded oral suspension must be shaken well before using

Dosage Forms

Capsule: 150 mg, 300 mg

Powder for injection: 600 mg (contains a sulfite)

Extemporaneous Preparations Rifampin oral suspension can be compounded with simple syrup or wild cherry syrup at a concentration of 10 mg/mL; the suspension is stable for 4 weeks at room temperature or in a refrigerator when stored in a glass amber prescription bottle. However, there are some experts who do not recommend using rifampin syrup formulated from capsules due to conflicting reports indicating that the product is unstable (14.5% to 68% of labeled potency after preparation). It may be preferable to perform trituration, rather than simple mixing in syrup when preparing rifampin oral suspension.

Nahata MC, Morosco RS, and Hipple TF, "Effect of Preparation Method and Storage on Rifampin Concentration in Suspensions," *Ann Pharmacother,* 1994, 28(2):182-5.

References

American Academy of Pediatrics Committee on Infectious Diseases, "Chemotherapy for Tuberculosis in Infants and Children," *Pediatrics,* 1992, 89(1):161-5.

Starke JR, "Modern Approach to the Diagnosis and Treatment of Tuberculosis in Children," *Pediatr Clin North Am,* 1988, 35(3):441-64.

Starke JR, "Multidrug Therapy for Tuberculosis in Children," *Pediatr Infect Dis J,* 1990, 9(11):785-93.

- ♦ **rIFN-α** *see* Interferon Alfa-2a *on page 522*
- ♦ **rIFN-α2** *see* Interferon Alfa-2b *on page 524*
- ♦ **Rimactane®** *see* Rifampin *on page 846*
- ♦ **Rimactane® (Canada)** *see* Rifampin *on page 846*

Rimantadine *(ri MAN ta deen)*

Brand Names Flumadine® Oral

Available Salts Rimantadine Hydrochloride

Therapeutic Category Antiviral Agent, Oral

Generic Available No

Use Prophylaxis (adults and children) and treatment (adults) of influenza A viral infection

Pregnancy Risk Factor C

Contraindications Hypersensitivity to rimantadine, amantadine, or any component

Precautions Use with caution in patients with liver disease, epilepsy, history of recurrent eczematoid dermatitis, uncontrolled psychosis, severe psychoneurosis, and in patients receiving CNS stimulant drugs; modify dosage in patients with renal impairment, severe hepatic dysfunction, or active seizure disorder

Adverse Reactions

Cardiovascular: Orthostatic hypotension, edema

Central nervous system: Dizziness, confusion, headache, insomnia, difficulty in concentrating, anxiety, restlessness, irritability, hallucinations; CNS adverse effects are less than with amantadine

Gastrointestinal: Nausea, vomiting, xerostomia

Genitourinary: Urinary retention

Drug Interactions Anticholinergic agents, CNS stimulants may possibly increase adverse effects

Food Interactions Food does not affect rate or extent of absorption

Mechanism of Action Blocks the uncoating of influenza A viral RNA and prevents penetration of the virus into host cell; inhibits M_2 protein in the assembly of progeny virions

Pharmacokinetics

Absorption: Oral: Well absorbed

Distribution: Adults: 17-25 L/kg
Protein binding: ~40%
Metabolism: Extensively in the liver via hydroxylation and glucuronidation
Half-life:
  Children 4-8 years: 13-38 hours
  Adults: 24-36 hours
Elimination: <25% excreted unchanged in the urine
Hemodialysis: Negligible effect

Usual Dosage Oral: (See Additional Information for duration of therapy)
Prophylaxis:
  Children <10 years: 5 mg/kg once daily; maximum dose: 150 mg/day
  Children >10 years and Adults: 100 mg twice daily (see Note)
Treatment: Adults: 100 mg twice daily (see Note)
Note: Patients with severe hepatic or renal dysfunction or elderly nursing home patients: 100 mg/day

Administration Oral: May administer with food

Patient Information May cause dizziness or confusion and may impair ability to perform activities requiring mental alertness or physical coordination

Additional Information Not active against influenza B; treatment or prophylaxis in immunosuppressed patients has not been fully evaluated
  Duration of treatment: 5-7 days; optimal duration not established
  Duration of prophylactic therapy: For at least 10 days after known exposure; usually for 6-8 weeks during influenza A season or local outbreak (or until vaccine produces sufficient antibody titers)
  Duration of fever and other symptoms can be reduced if rimantadine therapy is started within the first 48 hours of influenza A illness
  During an outbreak of influenza, administer rimantadine prophylaxis for 2-3 weeks after influenza vaccination until vaccine antibody titers are sufficient to provide protection

Dosage Forms
Syrup, as hydrochloride: 50 mg/5 mL (60 mL, 240 mL, 480 mL)
Tablet, as hydrochloride: 100 mg

♦ **Rimantadine Hydrochloride** *see* Rimantadine *on page 848*
♦ **Riobin®** *see* Riboflavin *on page 844*
♦ **Riopan® [OTC]** *see* Antacid Preparations *on page 86*
♦ **Ritalin®** *see* Methylphenidate *on page 627*
♦ **Ritalin-SR®** *see* Methylphenidate *on page 627*

Ritonavir (rye TON a veer)

Related Information
  Adult and Adolescent HIV *on page 1133*
  Pediatric HIV *on page 1129*

Brand Names Norvir®

Therapeutic Category Antiretroviral Agent; HIV Agents (Anti-HIV Agents); Protease Inhibitor

Use Treatment of HIV infection in combination with other antiretroviral agents. **(Note:** Current preferred HIV regimens consist of **three** antiretroviral agents)

Pregnancy Risk Factor B

Contraindications Hypersensitivity to ritonavir or any component

Warnings Ritonavir is a potent CYP3A enzyme inhibitor which interacts with numerous drugs. Due to potential serious and/or life-threatening drug interactions, the following drugs should not be coadministered with ritonavir: amiodarone, astemizole, bepridil, bupropion, cisapride, clozapine, dihydroergotamine, ergotamine, flecainide, encainide, meperidine, pimozide, piroxicam, propafenone, propoxyphene, quinidine, rifabutin, terfenadine, alprazolam, clorazepate, diazepam, estazolam, flurazepam, midazolam, triazolam, and zolpidem (see Drug Interactions). Spontaneous bleeding episodes have been reported in patients with hemophilia type A and B. New onset diabetes mellitus, exacerbation of diabetes, and hyperglycemia have been reported in HIV-infected patients receiving protease inhibitors.

Precautions Use caution in patients with hepatic insufficiency

Adverse Reactions
Central nervous system: Headache, confusion
Endocrine & metabolic: Elevated triglycerides and cholesterol, increased creatine phosphokinase; rare: hyperglycemia, diabetes, ketoacidosis
Gastrointestinal: Nausea, vomiting, diarrhea, taste perversion, abdominal pain, anorexia, pancreatitis
(Continued)

Ritonavir *(Continued)*

Hematologic: Rare: Spontaneous bleeding episodes in hemophiliacs

Hepatic: Elevated liver enzymes, hepatitis

Neuromuscular & skeletal: Circumoral and peripheral paresthesias, weakness

Miscellaneous: Allergic reaction (urticaria, rash, bronchospasm, angioedema)

Drug Interactions Increases plasma concentration of amiodarone, astemizole, warfarin (monitor anticoagulant effect), bepridil, bupropion, cisapride, clozapine, dihydroergotamine, encainide, ergotamine, flecainide, meperidine, pimozide, piroxicam, propafenone, propoxyphene, quinidine, rifabutin, and terfenadine; inhibits metabolism of alprazolam, clorazepate, diazepam, estazolam, flurazepam, midazolam, triazolam, and zolpidem resulting in profound and prolonged sedation; 77% increase in clarithromycin AUC (decrease clarithromycin dose in patients with renal impairment); 145% increase in desipramine AUC (consider dosage reduction); 13% decrease in didanosine AUC (if patient is on concurrent ritonavir and didanosine therapy, doses should be spaced 2.5 hours apart); 40% decrease in ethinyl estradiol AUC (consider alternative contraceptive measures); 43% decrease in theophylline AUC (monitor theophylline levels); metronidazole (disulfiram-like reaction); inhibits indinavir and saquinavir metabolism; coadministration with nelfinavir increases concentration of nelfinavir

Stability Refrigerate capsules; liquid formulation is stable for 30 days at room temperature; liquid formulation should be stored in the original container; protect from light

Mechanism of Action A protease inhibitor which acts on an enzyme late in the HIV replication process after the virus has entered into the cell's nucleus preventing cleavage of protein precursors essential for HIV infection of new cells and viral replication. Saquinavir- and zidovudine-resistant HIV isolates are generally susceptible to ritonavir but strains resistant to ritonavir are usually cross-resistant to indinavir and saquinavir.

Pharmacokinetics

Absorption: Well absorbed

Distribution: High concentrations in serum and lymph nodes

Protein binding: 98% to 99%

Time to peak serum concentration: 2-4 hours

Metabolism: In the liver by the cytochrome P-450 enzyme 3A (CYP3A) to an active and inactive metabolite

Half-life: 3-5 hours

Elimination: Renal clearance is negligible

Usual Dosage Oral:

Neonates: Under investigation in PACTG 354

Children ≤12 years: Initial: 250 mg/m²/dose twice daily; titrate upward by 50 mg/m²/dose twice daily increments over 5 days, up to 400 mg/m²/dose twice daily; dosage range: 350-400 mg/m²/dose twice daily (every 12 hours); maximum dose: 600 mg/dose twice daily

Adolescents and Adults: 600 mg twice daily; may use a dose titration schedule to reduce adverse events (nausea/vomiting) by initiating therapy at 300 mg twice daily; increase dose by 100 mg twice daily increments over 5 days up to a maximum dose of 600 mg twice daily

Administration Administer with food to increase absorption; consider reserving liquid formulation for use in patients receiving tube feeding due to its bad taste. May mix liquid formulation with milk, chocolate milk, vanilla or chocolate pudding or ice cream, or a liquid nutritional supplement. Other techniques used to increase tolerance in children include dulling the taste buds by chewing ice, giving popsicles or spoonfuls or partially frozen orange or grape juice concentrates before administration of ritonavir; coating the mouth with peanut butter to eat before the dose; administration of strong-tasting foods such as maple syrup, cheese, or strong-flavored chewing gum immediately after a dose.

Monitoring Parameters Liver function tests, blood glucose levels, CD4 cell count, plasma levels of HIV RNA

Patient Information If dose is missed, take the next dose as soon as possible; however, if a dose is skipped, do not double the next dose

Dosage Forms

Capsule: 100 mg (contains ethanol and polyoxyl 35 castor oil)

Solution: 80 mg/mL (240 mL) (contains ethanol and polyoxyl 35 castor oil)

References
Danner SA, Carr A, Leonard JM, et al, "A Short-Term Study of the Safety, Pharmacokinetics, and Efficacy of Ritonavir, an Inhibitor of HIV-1 Protease. European-Australian Collaborative Ritonavir Study Group," *N Engl J Med*, 1995, 333(23):1528-33.

Mueller BU, Zuckerman J, Nelson J, et al, "A Phase I/II Study of the Protease Inhibitor Ritonavir (ABT-538) in Children With HIV Infection," *Eleventh International Conference on AIDS*, Vancouver, Canada, 1996.

Working Group on Antiretroviral Therapy and Medical Management of HIV-Infected Children, "Guidelines for the Use of Antiretroviral Agents in Pediatric HIV Infection," April 15, 1999, http://www.hivatis.org.

- **Rivotril® (Canada)** *see* Clonazepam *on page 241*
- **RMS® Rectal** *see* Morphine Sulfate *on page 657*
- **Robafen DM® [OTC]** *see* Guaifenesin and Dextromethorphan *on page 466*
- **Robaxin®** *see* Methocarbamol *on page 619*
- **Robicillin® VK** *see* Penicillin V Potassium *on page 743*
- **Robidrine® (Canada)** *see* Pseudoephedrine *on page 822*
- **Robinul®** *see* Glycopyrrolate *on page 458*
- **Robinul® Forte** *see* Glycopyrrolate *on page 458*
- **Robitet® Oral** *see* Tetracycline *on page 908*
- **Robitussin® [OTC]** *see* Guaifenesin *on page 464*
- **Robitussin® A-C** *see* Guaifenesin and Codeine *on page 465*
- **Robitussin® Cough Calmers [OTC]** *see* Dextromethorphan *on page 304*
- **Robitussin®-DM [OTC]** *see* Guaifenesin and Dextromethorphan *on page 466*
- **Robitussin® Pediatric [OTC]** *see* Dextromethorphan *on page 304*
- **Robomol®** *see* Methocarbamol *on page 619*
- **Rocaltrol®** *see* Calcitriol *on page 155*
- **Rocephin®** *see* Ceftriaxone *on page 192*

Rocuronium (roe kyoor OH nee um)

Brand Names Zemuron®; Zemuron™ (Canada)

Available Salts Rocuronium Bromide

Therapeutic Category Neuromuscular Blocker Agent, Nondepolarizing; Skeletal Muscle Relaxant, Paralytic

Generic Available No

Use Produces skeletal muscle relaxation during surgery after induction of general anesthesia, increases pulmonary compliance during assisted mechanical respiration, facilitates endotracheal intubation

Pregnancy Risk Factor B

Contraindications Hypersensitivity to rocuronium or any component

Warnings Dosage adjustment needed in patients with severe hepatic disease; ventilation must be supported during neuromuscular blockade

Precautions Many clinical conditions may potentiate or antagonize neuromuscular blockade, see table.

Clinical Conditions Affecting Neuromuscular Blockade

Potentiation	Antagonism
Electrolyte abnormalities	Alkalosis
Severe hyponatremia	Hypercalcemia
Severe hypocalcemia	Demyelinating lesions
Severe hypokalemia	Peripheral neuropathies
Hypermagnesemia	Diabetes mellitus
Neuromuscular diseases	
Acidosis	
Acute intermittent porphyria	
Renal failure	
Hepatic failure	

Increased sensitivity in patients with myasthenia gravis, Eaton-Lambert syndrome; resistance to neuromuscular blockade in burn patients (>30% of body) for period of 5-70 days postinjury; resistance to neuromuscular blockade in patients with muscle trauma, denervation, immobilization, infection

Adverse Reactions Most frequent adverse reactions are associated with prolongation of its pharmacologic actions

Cardiovascular: Hypotension, hypertension, arrhythmias, tachycardia

Dermatologic: Rash, pruritus

Gastrointestinal: Vomiting

Local: Injection site edema

Neuromuscular & skeletal: Muscle weakness

(Continued)

Rocuronium *(Continued)*

Respiratory: Bronchospasm
Miscellaneous: Hiccups

Drug Interactions See table.

Potential Drug Interactions

Potentiation	Antagonism
Anesthetics	Calcium
Desflurane, sevoflurane, enflurane and	Carbamazepine
isoflurane > halothane > nitrous	Phenytoin
oxide	Steroids (chronic administration)
Antibiotics	Theophylline
Aminoglycosides, polymyxins,	Anticholinesterases*
clindamycin, vancomycin	Neostigmine, pyridostigmine,
Magnesium sulfate	edrophonium, echothiophate
Antiarrhythmics	ophthalmic solution
Quinidine, procainamide, bretylium, and	Caffeine
possibly lidocaine	Azathioprine
Diuretics	
Furosemide, mannitol	
Amphotericin B (secondary to hypokalemia)	
Local anesthetics	
Dantrolene (directly depresses skeletal muscle)	
Beta blockers	
Calcium channel blockers	
Ketamine	
Lithium	
Succinylcholine (when administered prior to nondepolarizing neuromuscular-blocking agent)	
Cyclosporine	

*Can prolong the effects of acetylcholine

Stability Refrigerate; unopened vials are stable 60 days at room temperature; open vials are stable for 30 days at room temperature; compatible with NS and D_5W; do not mix with alkaline solutions

Mechanism of Action Nondepolarizing neuromuscular blocking agent which blocks neural transmission at the myoneural junction by binding with cholinergic receptor sites

Pharmacodynamics
Peak effect:
Children: 30 seconds to 1 minute
Adults: 1-3.7 minutes
Duration:
Children: 30-40 minutes (dose-related)
Adults: 20-94 minutes (dose-related) (most prolonged in elderly ≥65 years of age)

Pharmacokinetics
Distribution: V_d:
Children: 0.21-0.36 L/kg
Adults: 0.22-0.26 L/kg
Hepatic dysfunction: 0.53 L/kg
Renal dysfunction: 0.34 L/kg
Protein binding: ~30%
Half-life:
Alpha elimination: 1-2 minutes
Beta elimination:
Children: 0.8-1.3 hours
Adults: 1.4-2.4 hours
Hepatic dysfunction: 4.3 hours
Renal dysfunction: 2.4 hours

Elimination: Primarily biliary excretion; up to 33% of dose excreted unchanged in urine

Usual Dosage Children and Adults:
I.V.: Initial: 0.6-1.2 mg/kg/dose with repeat doses of 0.2 mg/kg every 20-30 minutes
Continuous infusion: 10-12 mcg/kg/minute

Administration Parenteral: May be administered undiluted by rapid I.V. injection; for continuous infusion, dilute with NS, D_5W, or LR to a concentration of 0.5-1 mg/mL

Monitoring Parameters Peripheral nerve stimulator measuring twitch response, heart rate, blood pressure, assisted ventilation status

Nursing Implications Does not alter the patient's state of consciousness; addition of sedation and analgesia are recommended

Dosage Forms Injection, as bromide: 10 mg/mL (5 mL, 10 mL)

♦ **Rocuronium Bromide** *see* Rocuronium *on page 851*
♦ **Rofact™ (Canada)** *see* Rifampin *on page 846*
♦ **Roferon-A®** *see* Interferon Alfa-2a *on page 522*
♦ **Rogaine® Topical** *see* Minoxidil *on page 650*
♦ **Rogitine® (Canada)** *see* Phentolamine *on page 757*
♦ **Rolaids®** *see* Calcium Supplements *on page 157*
♦ **Romazicon® Injection** *see* Flumazenil *on page 421*
♦ **Rondec® Drops** *see* Carbinoxamine and Pseudoephedrine *on page 169*
♦ **Rondec® Filmtab®** *see* Carbinoxamine and Pseudoephedrine *on page 169*
♦ **Rondec® Syrup** *see* Carbinoxamine and Pseudoephedrine *on page 169*
♦ **Rondec-TR®** *see* Carbinoxamine and Pseudoephedrine *on page 169*
♦ **Roubac® (Canada)** *see* Co-Trimoxazole *on page 258*
♦ **Rowasa® Rectal** *see* Mesalamine *on page 608*
♦ **Roxanol™ Oral** *see* Morphine Sulfate *on page 657*
♦ **Roxanol SR™ Oral** *see* Morphine Sulfate *on page 657*
♦ **Roxicet® 5/500** *see* Oxycodone and Acetaminophen *on page 716*
♦ **Roxilox®** *see* Oxycodone and Acetaminophen *on page 716*
♦ **Roxiprin®** *see* Oxycodone and Aspirin *on page 717*
♦ **RP59500** *see* Quinupristin/Dalfopristin *on page 834*
♦ **RS61443** *see* Mycophenolate *on page 663*
♦ **R-salbutamol** *see* Levalbuterol *on page 563*
♦ **RSV-IGIV** *see* Respiratory Syncytial Virus Immune Globulin (Intravenous) *on page 838*
♦ **RSV-IVIG** *see* Respiratory Syncytial Virus Immune Globulin (Intravenous) *on page 838*
♦ **RTCA** *see* Ribavirin *on page 843*
♦ **Rubella Virus Vaccine, Live** *see page 1138*
♦ **Rubex®** *see* Doxorubicin *on page 346*
♦ **Rubidomycin** *see* Daunorubicin *on page 285*
♦ **Rubramin® (Canada)** *see* Cyanocobalamin *on page 263*
♦ **Rubramin-PC®** *see* Cyanocobalamin *on page 263*
♦ **Rufen®** *see* Ibuprofen *on page 501*
♦ **Rum-K®** *see* Potassium Supplements *on page 786*
♦ **Ru-Vert-M®** *see* Meclizine *on page 597*
♦ **RWJ17070** *see* Histrelin *on page 476*
♦ **Rynacrom® (Canada)** *see* Cromolyn *on page 260*
♦ **Rythmodan®, -LA (Canada)** *see* Disopyramide *on page 333*
♦ **Sabulin® (Canada)** *see* Albuterol *on page 40*

Sacrosidase (sak RO se dase)

Brand Names Sucraid®
Therapeutic Category Sucrase Deficiency, Treatment Agent
Generic Available No
Use Oral replacement therapy in congenital sucrase-isomaltase deficiency (CSID)
Pregnancy Risk Factor C
Contraindications Hypersensitivity to sacrosidase or any component, yeast and yeast products and glycerol
Warnings Hypersensitivity reactions to sacrosidase, including bronchospasm, have been reported; administer initial doses in a setting where acute hypersensitivity
(Continued)

Sacrosidase *(Continued)*

reactions may be treated within a few minutes; skin testing may be performed prior to administration to potentially identify patients at risk for hypersensitivity reactions.

Precautions Use with caution in CSID patients with diabetes, as Sucraid® will improve absorption of the products of sucrose hydrolysis (glucose and fructose); diet and/or insulin dosage may need to be adjusted

Adverse Reactions

Central nervous system: Insomnia, headache, nervousness

Endocrine & metabolic: Dehydration

Gastrointestinal: Abdominal pain, vomiting, nausea, diarrhea, constipation

Respiratory: Bronchospasm

Miscellaneous: Hypersensitivity reactions (see Warnings)

Drug Interactions None as yet have been identified

Food Interactions May be inactivated or denatured if administered with fruit juice, warm or hot food or liquids; since isomaltase deficiency is not affected by sacrosidase, adherence to a low-starch diet may be required to decrease symptomatology

Stability Refrigerate at 4°C to 8°C (36°F to 46°F); protect from light; discard 4 weeks after opening

Mechanism of Action Sacrosidase is a naturally occurring gastrointestinal enzyme which breaks down the disaccharide sucrose into its monosaccharide components; this hydrolysis is necessary to allow absorption of these nutrients

Pharmacokinetics Metabolism: Sacrosidase is metabolized in the gastrointestinal tract to individual amino acids which are systemically absorbed

Usual Dosage Oral:

Infants and Children ≤15 kg: 8500 international units (1 mL) per meal or snack

Children >15 kg and Adults: 17,000 international units (2 mL) per meal or snack

Administration Oral: Dilute in 2-4 ounces of water, milk, or formula; approximately ½ of the dose may be taken before, and the remainder of the dose at the completion of, each meal or snack; do not administer with fruit juices, warm or hot food or liquids (see Food Interactions)

Monitoring Parameters Breath hydrogen test, oral sucrose tolerance test, urinary disaccharides, intestinal disaccharidases (measured from small bowel biopsy)

CSID symptomatology: Diarrhea, abdominal pain, gas and bloating

Additional Information 1 mL = 22 drops from sacrosidase container tip

Dosage Forms Solution, oral: 8500 international units/mL (118 mL)

References

Treem WR, McAdams L, Stanford L, et al, "Sacrosidase Therapy for Congenital Sucrose-Isomaltase Deficiency," *J Pediatr Gastroenterol Nutr*, 1999, 28(2):137-42.

♦ **Safe Tussin® 30 [OTC]** *see* Guaifenesin and Dextromethorphan *on page 466*

♦ **Saizen® Injection** *see* Human Growth Hormone *on page 478*

♦ **Salac™ (Canada)** *see* Salicylic Acid *on page 854*

♦ **Salacid® Ointment** *see* Salicylic Acid *on page 854*

♦ **Sal-Acid® Plaster** *see* Salicylic Acid *on page 854*

♦ **Salagen® Oral** *see* Pilocarpine *on page 770*

♦ **Salazopyrin® (Canada)** *see* Sulfasalazine *on page 893*

♦ **Salazopyrin EN-Tabs® (Canada)** *see* Sulfasalazine *on page 893*

♦ **Salbutamol** *see* Albuterol *on page 40*

♦ **Saleto-200® [OTC]** *see* Ibuprofen *on page 501*

♦ **Saleto-400®** *see* Ibuprofen *on page 501*

♦ **Salicylazosulfapyridine** *see* Sulfasalazine *on page 893*

Salicylic Acid *(sal i SIL ik AS id)*

Brand Names Acnex® (Canada); Acnomel® (Canada); Clear Away® Disc [OTC]; Duoforte® 27 (Canada); Freezone® Solution [OTC]; Gordofilm® Liquid; Keralyt® (Canada); Mediplast® Plaster [OTC]; Occlusal-HP Liquid; Panscol® Lotion [OTC]; Panscol® Ointment [OTC]; PediaPatch Transdermal Patch [OTC]; P&S® Shampoo [OTC]; Salac™ (Canada); Salacid® Ointment; Sal-Acid® Plaster; Sebcur® (Canada); Soluver® (Canada); Trans-Plantar® (Canada); Trans-Plantar® Transdermal Patch [OTC]; Trans-Ver-Sal® (Canada); Trans-Ver-Sal® Transdermal Patch [OTC] Verukan® Solution; Vergogel® Gel [OTC]; X-Seb™ (Canada)

Therapeutic Category Keratolytic Agent

Generic Available Yes

Use Topically for its keratolytic effect in controlling seborrheic dermatitis or psoriasis of body and scalp, dandruff, and other scaling dermatoses; to remove warts, corns, calluses; also used in the treatment of acne

Pregnancy Risk Factor C

Contraindications Hypersensitivity to salicylic acid or any component; children <2 years of age

Warnings Should not be used systemically due to severe irritating effect on GI mucosa; prolonged use over large areas, especially in children, may result in salicylate toxicity; do not apply on irritated, reddened, or infected skin; do not use on moles, birthmarks, warts with hair growing from them, or genital warts

Precautions For external use only; avoid contact with eyes, face, and other mucous membranes

Adverse Reactions
Dermatologic: Facial scarring, erythema, scaling
Local: Irritation, burning

Mechanism of Action Produces desquamation of hyperkeratotic epithelium; increases hydration of the stratum corneum causing the skin to swell, soften, and desquamate

Pharmacokinetics
Absorption: Topical: Readily absorbed
Time to peak serum concentration: Within 5 hours when applied with an occlusive dressing
Elimination: Salicyluric acid (52%), salicylate glucuronides (42%), and salicylic acid (6%) are the major metabolites identified in urine after percutaneous absorption

Usual Dosage Children ≥2 years and Adults: Topical:
Lotion, cream, gel: Apply a thin layer to the affected area once or twice daily
Plaster: Cut to size that covers the corn or callus, apply and leave in place for 48 hours; do not exceed 5 applications over a 14-day period
Shampoo: Initial: Use daily or every other day; apply to wet hair and massage vigorously into the scalp; rinse hair thoroughly after shampooing; 1-2 treatments/week will usually maintain control
Solution: Apply a thin layer directly to wart using brush applicator once daily as directed for 1 week or until the wart is removed

Administration Topical: For external use only; when applying in concentrations >10%, protect surrounding normal tissue with petrolatum

Monitoring Parameters Signs and symptoms of salicylate toxicity: Nausea, vomiting, dizziness, tinnitus, loss of hearing, lethargy, diarrhea, psychic disturbances

Nursing Implications For warts: Before applying product, soak area in warm water for 5 minutes; dry area thoroughly, then apply medication

Dosage Forms
Cream: 2% (30 g); 2.5% (30 g); 10% (60 g)
Gel: 5% (60 g); 6% (30 g); 17% (7.5 g)
Liquid: 13.6% (9.3 mL); 17% (9.3 mL, 13.5 mL, 15 mL); 16.7% (15 mL)
Lotion: 2% (177 mL)
Ointment: 25% (60 g, 454 g); 40% (454 g); 60% (60 g)
Patch, transdermal: 15% (20 mm)
Plaster: 15% (6 mm, 12 mm); 40%
Pledgets: 0.5%; 2%
Shampoo: 2% (120 mL, 240 mL); 4% (120 mL)

♦ **Salicylic Acid and Sulfur** *see* Sulfur and Salicylic Acid *on page 896*

♦ **Saline from Otrivin® (Canada)** *see* Sodium Chloride *on page 871*

♦ **SalineX® [OTC]** *see* Sodium Chloride *on page 871*

Salmeterol (sal ME te role)

Related Information
Asthma Guidelines *on page 1178*

Brand Names Serevent®; Serevent® Diskus®

Available Salts Salmeterol Xinafoate

Therapeutic Category Adrenergic Agonist Agent; Antiasthmatic; Beta₂-Adrenergic Agonist Agent; Bronchodilator

Generic Available No

Use Maintenance treatment of asthma and COPD; prevention of bronchospasm in patients >4 years of age with reversible obstructive airway disease; prevention of exercise-induced bronchospasm in children >4 years of age and adults

Pregnancy Risk Factor C

Contraindications Hypersensitivity to salmeterol, adrenergic amines, or any component
(Continued)

Salmeterol *(Continued)*

Warnings Cardiovascular effects are not common with salmeterol when used in recommended doses. Salmeterol is not meant to relieve acute asthmatic symptoms. Acute episodes should be treated with short-acting beta$_2$ agonist. Do not increase the frequency of salmeterol use. Paroxysmal bronchospasm (which can be fatal) has been reported with this and other inhaled agents. If this occurs, discontinue treatment; most commonly occurs with first use of a new canister or vial

Precautions Use with caution in patients with cardiovascular disorders, convulsive disorders, thyrotoxicosis, or others who are sensitive to the effects of sympathomimetic amines

Adverse Reactions

Cardiovascular: Prolonged Q-T$_c$ interval (large doses), tachycardia, palpitations, arrhythmias

Central nervous system: Dizziness, headache, nervousness, hyperactivity, insomnia, malaise

Dermatologic: Rash, pruritus

Endocrine & metabolic: Hypokalemia

Gastrointestinal: GI upset, diarrhea, nausea

Neuromuscular & skeletal: Joint and back pain, tremors, muscle cramps

Respiratory: Respiratory arrest, cough, pharyngitis, paradoxical bronchospasm (see Warnings)

Miscellaneous: Hypersensitivity reactions, tachyphylaxis

Drug Interactions Additive effects with beta-adrenergic agents; MAO inhibitors and tricyclic antidepressants potentiate cardiovascular effects; beta-blocking agents antagonize effects; increased potassium losses with diuretics

Stability The therapeutic effect may decrease when the cannister is cold, therefore, the canister should remain at room temperature. Do not store at temperatures >120°F. Serevent® Diskus® is stable for 6 weeks after protective foil is removed.

Mechanism of Action Relaxes bronchial smooth muscle by selective action on beta$_2$-receptors with little effect on heart rate

Pharmacodynamics

Onset of effect: 10-20 minutes

Peak effect: 3 hours

Duration: Up to 12 hours

Pharmacokinetics

Protein binding: 94% to 95%

Metabolism: Extensive via hydroxylation

Half-life: 3-4 hours

Usual Dosage Children >4 years and Adults:

Maintenance and prevention of asthma, COPD

Inhalation, oral:

Serevent®: 42 mcg (2 actuations/puffs) twice daily, 12 hours apart

Serevent® Diskus®: 50 mcg (1 actuation/puff) twice daily, 12 hours apart

Prevention of exercise-induced asthma: Inhalation: Serevent® 42 mcg (2 actuations/puffs) 30-60 minutes prior to exercise; additional doses should not be used for 12 hours; patients who are using salmeterol twice daily should **not** use an additional dose prior to exercise; if twice daily use is not effective during exercise, consider other appropriate therapy

Administration Inhalation:

Serevent®: Shake well before use; before using inhaler for first time or if unused for more than 4 weeks, "test spray" 4 times into the air; use Serevent® with spacer device in children <8 years of age

Serevent® Diskus®: May not be used with a spacer

Monitoring Parameters Pulmonary function tests

Patient Information Do not use to treat acute symptoms; do not exceed the prescribed dose of salmeterol; do not stop using inhaled or oral corticosteroids without medical advice even if feeling better; avoid spraying in eyes; remove the cannister and rinse the plastic case and cap under warm water and dry daily. Store cannister with nozzle end down.

Additional Information When salmeterol is initiated patients should be instructed to discontinue the short-acting beta agonist which was used on a routine basis and to utilize this shorter-acting agent for symptomatic or acute episodes only. Although each puff delivers 25 mcg the amount delivered through the mouthpiece is actually 21 mcg per puff.

Dosage Forms
Aerosol, oral, as xinafoate (Serevent®): 21 mcg/actuation [60 inhalations] (6.5 g), [120 inhalations] (13 g)

Inhalation, powder, oral, as xinafoate (Serevent® Diskus®): 50 mcg/actuation (28 blisters, 60 blisters)

References
Meyer JM, Wenzel CL, and Kradjan WA, "Salmeterol: A Novel, Long-Acting Beta₂-Agonist," *Ann Pharmacother*, 1993, 27(12):1478-87.

♦ **Salmeterol Xinafoate** *see* Salmeterol *on page 855*
♦ **Salmonine®** *see* Calcitonin *on page 154*
♦ **Salt Poor Albumin** *see* Albumin *on page 39*
♦ **Sandimmune®** *see* Cyclosporine *on page 270*
♦ **Sandoglobulin®** *see* Immune Globulin, Intravenous *on page 510*
♦ **Sandostatin®** *see* Octreotide Acetate *on page 702*
♦ **Sandostatin LAR® Depot** *see* Octreotide Acetate *on page 702*
♦ **SangCya™** *see* Cyclosporine *on page 270*
♦ **Sani-Supp® Suppository [OTC]** *see* Glycerin *on page 457*

Saquinavir (sa KWIN a veer)

Related Information
Adult and Adolescent HIV *on page 1133*

Brand Names Fortovase®; Invirase®

Available Salts Saquinavir Mesylate

Therapeutic Category Antiretroviral Agent; HIV Agents (Anti-HIV Agents); Protease Inhibitor

Generic Available No

Use Treatment of HIV infection in combination with other antiretroviral agents; (**Note:** Current preferred HIV regimens consist of **three** antiretroviral agents); in a randomized, double-blind study of 297 patients, a triple drug combination of saquinavir, zalcitabine, and zidovudine reduced HIV-1 replication, increased CD4+ cell counts, and decreased levels of activation markers in serum more than did treatment with zidovudine and either saquinavir or zalcitabine; postexposure chemoprophylaxis following occupational exposure to HIV

Pregnancy Risk Factor B

Contraindications Hypersensitivity to saquinavir or any component

Warnings Spontaneous bleeding episodes have been reported in patients with hemophilia receiving an HIV protease inhibitor; new onset diabetes mellitus, exacerbation of diabetes and hyperglycemia have been reported in HIV-infected patients receiving protease inhibitors; do not administer concurrently with terfenadine, cisapride, astemizole, triazolam, midazolam, or ergot derivatives

Precautions Use with caution in patients with diabetes mellitus, hepatic impairment or in patients receiving drugs which induce or are substrates of cytochrome P-450 3A; interaction studies with saquinavir (metabolized by cytochrome P-450 3A) and terfenadine, astemizole, or cisapride have not been conducted; concurrent use with terfenadine, astemizole, or cisapride is not recommended

Adverse Reactions
Cardiovascular: Cyanosis, heart murmur, hypotension, hypertension, syncope
Central nervous system: Confusion, ataxia, headache, dizziness, seizures, fever, hallucinations, asthenia, agitation, fatigue
Dermatologic: Rash, photosensitivity reaction, acne
Endocrine & metabolic: Hypoglycemia, increased creatine phosphokinase; rare: hyperglycemia, diabetes, ketoacidosis
Gastrointestinal: Diarrhea, abdominal discomfort, nausea, vomiting, stomatitis
Hematologic: Hemolytic anemia, pancytopenia, thrombocytopenia, microhemorrhages; rare: spontaneous bleeding episodes in hemophiliacs
Hepatic: Elevated ALT, AST, bilirubin, and amylase
Neuromuscular & skeletal: Parethesias, peripheral neuropathy, tremor, arthralgia
Respiratory: Cough

Drug Interactions Rifampin decreases saquinavir concentrations by 80%; rifabutin, nevirapine, phenobarbital, phenytoin, dexamethasone, carbamazepine may decrease saquinavir concentrations; saquinavir may increase concentrations of calcium channel blockers, clindamycin, dapsone, quinidine, astemizole, terfenadine, cisapride, ergot alkaloid derivatives, midazolam, and triazolam; ketoconazole, delavirdine, clarithromycin, indinavir, nelfinavir, ritonavir may increase saquinavir levels

Food Interactions Presence of a high fat meal maximizes bioavailability of saquinavir; grapefruit juice may increase saquinavir levels
(Continued)

Saquinavir (Continued)

Stability

Fortovase®: Store capsules in refrigerator; stable for 3 months if stored at room temperature

Invirase®: Store at room temperature in tightly closed bottles

Mechanism of Action
Saquinavir is an HIV protease inhibitor which acts late in the life cycle of the virus inside the cell by blocking the cleavage of a polyprotein precursor into structural proteins required for the assembly of infectious virions in lymphocytes and monocytes

Pharmacokinetics

Distribution: CSF concentration is negligible when compared to concentrations from matched plasma samples; partitions into tissues

Protein binding: 98%

Metabolism: Extensive first-pass effect; hepatic metabolism by cytochrome P-450 3A system to inactive metabolites

Bioavailability:

Invirase®: 4% (increased in the presence of food)

Fortovase®: Relative to Invirase® is ~331%

Half-life: Adults: 13 hours

Elimination: 88% of dose eliminated in feces; 1% excreted in urine

Usual Dosage
Oral:

Children: Safety and efficacy in children and adolescents <16 years of age have not been established; some centers have utilized an initial dose of 350 mg/m^2/dose (Invirase®) or 700 mg/m^2/dose (Fortovase®) 3 times/day

Adults:

Invirase®: 600 mg 3 times/day; lower doses (<1800 mg/day) have not shown effective antiviral activity

Fortovase®: 1200 mg 3 times/day

Administration
Oral: Administer within 2 hours after a full meal to increase absorption

Monitoring Parameters
Liver function tests, triglyceride levels, blood glucose levels, CD4 cell count, plasma levels of HIV RNA

Patient Information
Saquinavir is not a cure for HIV infection; if a dose is missed, take the next dose as soon as possible; however, if a dose is skipped, do not double the next dose; notify physician if numbness, tingling, persistent severe abdominal pain, nausea, or vomiting occurs. Since sun exposure can cause photosensitivity reactions, use of sunscreen or protective clothing is recommended.

Dosage Forms

Capsule, as mesylate (Invirase®): 200 mg

Capsule, soft gelatin (Fortovase®): 200 mg

References

Collier AC, Coombs RW, Schoenfeld DA, et al, "Treatment of Human Immunodeficiency Virus Infection With Saquinavir, Zidovudine, and Zalcitabine," N Engl J Med, 1996, 334(16):1011-7.

Mueller BU, "Antiviral Chemotherapy," Curr Opin Pediatr, 1997, 9(2):178-83.

Working Group on Antiretroviral Therapy and Medical Management of HIV-Infected Children, "Guidelines for the Use of Antiretroviral Agents in Pediatric HIV Infection," January 7, 2000, http://www.hivatis.org.

♦ Saquinavir Mesylate see Saquinavir on page 857

♦ Sarafem™ see Fluoxetine on page 431

Sargramostim (sar GRAM oh stim)

Brand Names
Leukine™; Prokine™

Synonyms
GM-CSF; Granulocyte Macrophage Colony Stimulating Factor; rGM-CSF

Therapeutic Category
Colony-Stimulating Factor

Generic Available
No

Use
Accelerates myeloid recovery in patients undergoing autologous or allogeneic BMT; mobilize hematopoietic progenitor cells into peripheral blood for collection by leukapheresis; accelerate myeloid engraftment following autologous peripheral blood progenitor cell transplantation; increase neutrophil counts in patients with malignancies receiving myelosuppressive chemotherapy; increase leukocyte counts in patients with severe aplastic anemia

Pregnancy Risk Factor
C

Contraindications
Excessive leukemic myeloid blasts in bone marrow or peripheral blood ≥10%; history of idiopathic thrombocytopenic purpura; hypersensitivity to GM-CSF, yeast-derived products, or any component

Precautions Use with caution in patients with autoimmune or chronic inflammatory disease, hypertension, cardiovascular disease, pulmonary disease, or renal or hepatic impairment

Rapid increase in peripheral blood counts: If ANC is >20,000/mm^3 or platelets >500,000/mm^3, decrease dose by 50% or discontinue drug (counts will fall to normal within 3-7 days after discontinuing drug)

Growth factor potential: Caution with myeloid malignancies; do **not** administer within 24 hours prior to or after chemotherapy or 12 hours prior to or after radiation therapy

Adverse Reactions

Cardiovascular: Hypotension, tachycardia, flushing, pericardial effusion, fluid retention, venous thrombosis

Central nervous system: Malaise, fever, headache, chills

Dermatologic: Rash

Endocrine & metabolic: Polydipsia

Gastrointestinal: Nausea, vomiting, diarrhea, stomatitis, GI hemorrhage

Hepatic: Elevated liver function tests

Neuromuscular & skeletal: Bone pain, myalgia, rigors, weakness

Respiratory: Dyspnea

Miscellaneous: "First dose" reaction (fever, hypotension, tachycardia, rigors, flushing, nausea, vomiting, dyspnea)

Drug Interactions Lithium and corticosteroids may potentiate myeloproliferative effects of sargramostim

Stability Store vial in the refrigerator; stable after reconstitution for 6 hours at room temperature; use only NS to prepare I.V. infusion solution; GM-CSF at a concentration ≥10 mcg/mL is compatible with TPN during Y-site administration

Mechanism of Action Stimulates proliferation, differentiation and functional activity of neutrophils, eosinophils, monocytes and macrophages

Pharmacodynamics

Onset of action: Increase in WBC in 7-14 days

Duration: WBC will return to baseline within 1 week after discontinuing drug

Pharmacokinetics

Half-life: 2 hours

Time to peak serum concentration: S.C.: Within 3 hours

Usual Dosage I.V., S.C.:

Children (no dosing for children has been FDA approved): 250 mcg/m^2/day once daily for 21 days to begin 2-4 hours after the marrow infusion on day 0 of BMT or not less than 24 hours after chemotherapy. If significant adverse effects or "first dose" reaction is seen at this dose, discontinue the drug until toxicity resolves, then restart at a reduced dose of 125 mcg/m^2/day

Aplastic anemia: 8-32 mcg/kg/day once daily

Cancer chemotherapy recovery: 3-15 mcg/kg/day once daily for 14-21 days; maximum dose: 30 mcg/kg/day or 1500 mcg/m^2/day

Adults: 250 mcg/m^2/day once daily for 21 days to begin 2-4 hours after BMT, or not less than 24 hours after chemotherapy (to minimize first dose reaction, start with low doses and increase gradually)

Aplastic anemia: 15-480 mcg/m^2 once daily

Cancer chemotherapy recovery: 3-15 mcg/kg/day once daily for 10 days

Administration Parenteral:

I.V.: Administer as a 30-minute, 2-hour, or 6-hour I.V. infusion or by continuous I.V. infusion. Do not shake solution to avoid foaming. Dilute in NS; if the final concentration of GM-CSF in NS is <10 mcg/mL, then add 1 mg albumin per mL of I.V. fluid. Albumin acts as a carrier molecule to prevent drug adsorption to the I.V. tubing. Albumin should be added to the saline prior to addition of GM-CSF.

S.C.: Reconstituted 250 mcg/mL or 500 mcg/mL solution may be administered without further dilution; rotate injection sites

Monitoring Parameters CBC with differential, platelets; renal/liver function tests, especially with previous dysfunction; vital signs, weight; pulmonary function

Reference Range Excessive leukocytosis (WBC >50,000 cells/mm^3, ANC >20,000 cells/mm^3)

Patient Information Possible bone pain may occur

Nursing Implications Can premedicate with analgesics and antipyretics; control bone pain with non-narcotic analgesics

Additional Information Produced by recombinant DNA technology using a yeast-derived expression system

Dosage Forms Injection: 250 mcg, 500 mcg

(Continued)

Sargramostim *(Continued)*

References

Lieschke GJ and Burgess AW, "Granulocyte Colony-Stimulating Factor and Granulocyte-Macrophage Colony-Stimulating Factor," (1) *N Engl J Med*, 1992, 327(1):28-35.

Lieschke GJ and Burgess AW, "Granulocyte Colony-Stimulating Factor and Granulocyte-Macrophage Colony-Stimulating Factor," (2) *N Engl J Med*, 1992, 327(2):99-106.

Stute N, Furman WL, Schell M, et al, "Pharmacokinetics of Recombinant Human Granulocyte - Macrophage Colony - Stimulating Factor in Children After Intravenous and Subcutaneous Administration," *J Pharm Sci*, 1995, 84(7):824-8.

Trissel LA, Bready BB, Kwan JW, et al, "Visual Compatibility of Sargramostim With Selected Antineoplastic Agents, Anti-infectives, or Other Drugs During Simulated Y-Site Injection," *Am J Hosp Pharm*, 1992, 49(2):402-6.

♦ **S.A.S™ (Canada)** *see* Sulfasalazine *on page 893*

♦ **Sastid® Plain Therapeutic Shampoo and Acne Wash [OTC]** *see* Sulfur and Salicylic Acid *on page 896*

♦ **Scabene®** *see* Lindane *on page 572*

♦ **Scalpicin® Topical** *see* Hydrocortisone *on page 486*

Scopolamine *(skoe POL a meen)*

Related Information

Overdose and Toxicology *on page 1191*

Brand Names Isopto® Hyoscine; Transdermal-V® (Canada); Transderm Scop®

Available Salts Scopolamine Hydrobromide

Synonyms Hyoscine

Therapeutic Category Anticholinergic Agent; Anticholinergic Agent, Ophthalmic; Anticholinergic Agent, Transdermal; Ophthalmic Agent, Mydriatic

Generic Available Yes

Use Preoperative medication to produce amnesia and decrease salivary and respiratory secretions; to produce cycloplegia and mydriasis (ophthalmic formulation); treatment of iridocyclitis (ophthalmic formulation); prevention of motion sickness (transdermal formulation)

Pregnancy Risk Factor C

Contraindications Hypersensitivity to scopolamine or any component; patients hypersensitive to belladonna or barbiturates may be hypersensitive to scopolamine; narrow-angle glaucoma, GI or GU obstruction, thyrotoxicosis, tachycardia secondary to cardiac insufficiency, paralytic ileus, myasthenia gravis

Warnings Drug withdrawal symptoms such as nausea, vomiting, headache, dizziness, and equilibrium disturbance have been reported following removal of transdermal system, primarily in patients using the system for more than 3 days

Precautions Use with caution with hepatic or renal dysfunction since adverse CNS effects occur more often in these patients; use with caution in infants and children since they may be more susceptible to adverse effects of scopolamine

Adverse Reactions

Cardiovascular: Tachycardia, palpitations

Central nervous system: Disorientation, drowsiness, hallucinations, confusion, psychosis, delirium, excitement, restlessness

Gastrointestinal: Xerostomia, constipation, nausea, vomiting, dysphagia, dysgeusia

Genitourinary: Urinary retention

Ocular: Blurred vision, cycloplegia, mydriasis, photophobia, increased intraocular pressure

Miscellaneous: Anaphylaxis, allergic reactions

Note: Systemic adverse effects have been reported with both the topical and ophthalmic preparations

Drug Interactions Additive adverse effects with other anticholinergic agents and amantadine; GI absorption of the following drugs may be affected: acetaminophen, levodopa, ketoconazole, digoxin (tablets only), riboflavin, KCl wax-matrix preparations; additive CNS effects with other CNS depressants, alcohol

Stability Physically compatible when mixed in the same syringe with atropine, butorphanol, chlorpromazine, dimenhydrinate, diphenhydramine, droperidol, fentanyl, glycopyrrolate, hydromorphone, hydroxyzine, meperidine, metoclopramide, morphine, pentazocine, pentobarbital, perphenazine, prochlorperazine, promazine, promethazine, or thiopental

Mechanism of Action Blocks the action of acetylcholine at parasympathetic sites in smooth muscle, secretory glands and the CNS; antagonizes histamine and serotonin

Pharmacodynamics
Onset of effect:
 Oral, I.M.: 30 minutes to 1 hour
 I.V.: 10 minutes
 Transdermal: 4 hours
Duration of effect:
 Oral, I.M.: 4-6 hours
 I.V.: 2 hours
 Transdermal: 72 hours

Pharmacokinetics
Absorption: Well absorbed by all routes of administration
Metabolism: In the liver

Usual Dosage
Preoperatively and antiemetic: I.M., I.V., S.C.:
 Children: 6 mcg/kg/dose (maximum dose: 0.3 mg/dose); may be repeated every 6-8 hours
 Adults: 0.3-0.65 mg; may be repeated 3-4 times/day
Motion sickness: Transdermal:
 Children >12 years and Adults: Apply 1 disc behind the ear at least 4 hours prior to exposure every 3 days as needed
Ophthalmic:
 Refraction:
  Children: Instill 1 drop of 0.25% to eye(s) twice daily for 2 days before procedure
  Adults: Instill 1-2 drops of 0.25% to eye(s) 1 hour before procedure
 Iridocyclitis:
  Children: Instill 1 drop of 0.25% to eye(s) up to 3 times/day
  Adults: Instill 1-2 drops of 0.25% to eye(s) up to 3 times/day

Administration
Oral: May be administered without regard to food
Parenteral: I.V.: Dilute with an equal volume of sterile water and administer by direct I.V. injection over 2-3 minutes
Transdermal: Apply patch to hairless area behind one ear; wash hands before and after application; if becomes dislodged, replace with fresh patch
Ophthalmic: Instill drops to conjunctival sac of affected eye(s); avoid contact of bottle tip with skin or eye; finger pressure should be applied to lacrimal sac during and for 1-2 minutes after instillation to decrease risk of absorption and systemic reactions

Patient Information Causes drowsiness and may impair ability to perform hazardous activities requiring mental alertness or physical coordination; may cause blurred vision if contacts eye

Additional Information Transdermal disc is programmed to deliver *in vivo* 0.5 mg over 3 days

Dosage Forms
Disc, transdermal: 1.5 mg/disc (4s)
Injection, as hydrobromide: 0.3 mg/mL (1 mL); 0.4 mg/mL (0.5 mL, 1 mL); 0.86 mg/mL (0.5 mL); 1 mg/mL (1 mL)
Solution, ophthalmic, as hydrobromide: 0.25% (5 mL, 15 mL)

♦ **Scopolamine Hydrobromide** *see* Scopolamine *on page 860*
♦ **Scopolamine, Hyoscyamine, Atropine, and Phenobarbital** *see* Hyoscyamine, Atropine, Scopolamine, and Phenobarbital *on page 499*
♦ **Scot-Tussin® [OTC]** *see* Guaifenesin *on page 464*
♦ **Scot-Tussin DM® Cough Chasers [OTC]** *see* Dextromethorphan *on page 304*
♦ **Scot-Tussin® Senior Clear [OTC]** *see* Guaifenesin and Dextromethorphan *on page 466*
♦ **SeaMist® [OTC]** *see* Sodium Chloride *on page 871*
♦ **Sebcur® (Canada)** *see* Salicylic Acid *on page 854*
♦ **Sebulex® [OTC]** *see* Sulfur and Salicylic Acid *on page 896*

Secobarbital (see koe BAR bi tal)
Related Information
Laboratory Detection of Drugs in Urine *on page 1204*
Brand Names Novo-Secobarb® (Canada); Seconal®
Available Salts Secobarbital Sodium
Synonyms Quinalbarbitone
Therapeutic Category Barbiturate; Hypnotic; Sedative
Generic Available Yes
 (Continued)

Secobarbital *(Continued)*

Use Short-term treatment of insomnia; preanesthetic agent

Restrictions C-II

Pregnancy Risk Factor D

Contraindications Hypersensitivity to secobarbital or any component, pre-existing CNS depression, severe uncontrolled pain, porphyria, severe respiratory disease with dyspnea or obstruction

Precautions Use with caution in patients with hypovolemic shock, CHF, hepatic impairment, respiratory dysfunction or depression, previous addiction to the seda-tive/hypnotic group, chronic or acute pain, renal dysfunction; tolerance or psychological and physical dependence may occur with prolonged use

Adverse Reactions

Cardiovascular: Hypotension, cardiac arrhythmias, bradycardia

Central nervous system: Dizziness, lightheadedness, drowsiness, "hangover" effect, lethargy, impaired judgment, CNS depression or paradoxical excitation, hypothermia, nightmares, hallucinations

Dermatologic: Rash, exfoliative dermatitis, Stevens-Johnson syndrome

Gastrointestinal: Nausea, vomiting, constipation

Hematologic: Megaloblastic anemia, thrombocytopenia, agranulocytosis

Local: Pain at injection site, thrombophlebitis with I.V. use, arterial spasm and gangrene with inadvertent intra-arterial injection

Respiratory: Laryngospasm, respiratory depression, apnea (especially with rapid I.V. use)

Miscellaneous: Psychological and physical dependence with prolonged use

Drug Interactions Cytochrome P-450 isoenzyme CYP2C9, CYP3A3/4, and CYP3A5-7 inducer

Barbiturates are enzyme inducers (monitor patients closely for decreased effect of concomitantly administered medications or increased effect when barbiturates are discontinued)

Secobarbital may decrease the serum concentration or effect of ethosuximide, warfarin, oral contraceptives, chloramphenicol, griseofulvin, doxycycline, beta-blockers, cyclophosphamide, theophylline, corticosteroids, tricyclic antidepressants, quinidine, haloperidol, and phenothiazines

Secobarbital given with other CNS depressants may increase CNS and respiratory depression

Chloramphenicol, valproic acid, and chlorpropamide may inhibit the metabolism of secobarbital with a resultant increase in secobarbital serum concentration

Food Interactions High doses of pyridoxine may decrease drug effect; barbiturates may increase the metabolism of vitamins D and K

Stability Injection: Store under refrigeration; protect from light; secobarbital in Tubex cartridges is stable for 9 months at 25°C (room temperature); compatible with NS and Ringer's injection but incompatible with LR; do not dilute with solutions containing bacteriostatic agents; injection is alkaline (pH 9.5-10.5) and incompatible with acids; incompatible with cimetidine (same syringe), codeine, erythromycin, glycopyrrolate (same syringe), hydrocortisone, insulin, levorphanol, norepinephrine, phenytoin, sodium bicarbonate, tetracycline, vancomycin, succinylcholine, pancuronium, and atracurium

Mechanism of Action Depresses CNS activity by binding to barbiturate site at GABA-receptor complex enhancing GABA activity; depresses reticular activating system; higher doses may be gabamimetic

Pharmacodynamics

Onset: Hypnosis:

Oral: 15-30 minutes

I.V.: 1-3 minutes

I.M.: 7-10 minutes

Duration: Hypnosis:

Oral: 3-4 hours with 100 mg dose

I.V.: 15 minutes

Pharmacokinetics

Absorption: Oral: Well absorbed (90%)

Distribution: V_d: Adult: 1.5 L/kg; crosses the placenta; appears in breast milk

Protein binding: 45% to 60%

Metabolism: In the liver by the microsomal enzyme system

Half-life:

Children: 2-13 years: 2.7-13.5 hours

Adults: 15-40 hours; mean 28 hours

Time to peak serum concentration: Oral: Within 2-4 hours

Elimination: Renally as inactive metabolites and small amounts as unchanged drug

Hemodialysis: Slightly dialyzable (5% to 20%)

Usual Dosage

Neonates: Sedation for neonates receiving mechanical ventilation: Limited information is available; one study (Nahata, 1991) assessed secobarbital dosing and prolonged sedation (sedation >24 hours after the last dose) in 17 ventilated infants (GA 30-40 weeks; PNA 0-3 days) who received secobarbital 4-14 mg/kg/day I.V. for 1-10 days for sedation; duration of sedation after the last dose increased with higher daily doses and with the total cumulative dose; the authors recommend that initial daily doses should not exceed 7 mg/kg/day to avoid prolonged sedation; further studies are needed

Children:

Hypnotic:

I.M.: 3-5 mg/kg/dose; maximum dose: 100 mg/dose

I.V.: 1-2 mg/kg/dose; maximum dose: 50-100 mg/dose

Preoperative sedation:

Oral: 2-6 mg/kg (maximum dose: 100 mg/dose) 1-2 hours before procedure

Rectal: 4-5 mg/kg **or** <6 months: 30-60 mg; 6 months to 3 years: 60 mg; >3 years: 60-120 mg

Sedation: Oral: 6 mg/kg/day divided every 8 hours

Adults:

Hypnotic:

Oral: Usual: 100 mg/dose at bedtime; range 100-200 mg/dose

I.M.: 100-200 mg/dose

I.V.: 50-250 mg/dose

Preoperative sedation: Oral: 100-300 mg 1-2 hours before procedure

Administration

I.V.: Administer undiluted or diluted with SWI, NS, or Ringer's injection; maximum infusion rate: 50 mg/15 seconds; avoid intra-arterial injection

Rectal: Commercial rectal formulations are no longer available in the U.S.; the I.V. product has been diluted with water to a concentration of 10-15 mg/mL and administered rectally

Monitoring Parameters Blood pressure, heart rate, respiratory rate, pulse oximetry, CNS status

Patient Information Avoid alcohol and other CNS depressants; may be habit-forming; may cause dizziness or drowsiness and impair ability to perform activities requiring mental alertness or physical coordination; do not abruptly discontinue

Additional Information Injection contains polyethylene glycol 50% and phenol; effectiveness for insomnia decreases greatly after 2 weeks of use; alkalinization of urine does not significantly increase excretion; withdraw slowly over 5-6 days after prolonged use to avoid sleep disturbances and rapid eye movement (REM) rebound

Dosage Forms

Capsule: 100 mg

Injection, as sodium: 50 mg/mL (2 mL)

References

Levine HL, Cohen ME, Duffner PK, et al, "Rectal Absorption and Disposition of Secobarbital in Epileptic Children," *Pediatr Pharmacol (New York)*, 1982, 2(1):33-8.

Nahata MC, Starling S, and Edwards RC, "Prolonged Sedation Associated With Secobarbital in Newborn Infants Receiving Ventilatory Support," *Am J Perinatol*, 1991, 8(1):35-6.

Wolfert RR and Cox RM, "Room Temperature Stability of Drug Products Labeled for Refrigerated Storage," *Am J Hosp Pharm*, 1975, 32(6):585-7.

♦ **Secobarbital Sodium** *see* Secobarbital *on page 861*

♦ **Seconal**® *see* Secobarbital *on page 861*

Secretin (SEE kre tin)

Brand Names Secretin-Ferring

Therapeutic Category Diagnostic Agent, Pancreatic Exocrine Insufficiency; Diagnostic Agent, Zollinger-Ellison Syndrome and Pancreatic Exocrine Disease

Generic Available No

Use Diagnosis of Zollinger-Ellison syndrome, chronic pancreatic dysfunction, and some hepatobiliary diseases such as obstructive jaundice resulting from cancer or stones in the biliary tract

Pregnancy Risk Factor C

Contraindications Do not give to patients with acute pancreatitis until attack has subsided

Precautions Patients with a history of hypersensitivity, allergy or asthma should receive an I.V. test dose of 0.1-1 clinical units (CU); use with caution in patients who are highly nervous or have an excessive gag reflex

(Continued)

Secretin *(Continued)*

Adverse Reactions
Cardiovascular: Syncope, venous spasm
Miscellaneous: Hypersensitivity reactions

Stability Store in freezer (-20°C); stable in refrigerator up to 3 weeks; should be used immediately after reconstitution

Mechanism of Action Hormone normally secreted by duodenal mucosa and upper jejunal mucosa which increases the volume and bicarbonate content of pancreatic juice; stimulates the flow of hepatic bile with a high bicarbonate concentration, stimulates gastrin release in patients with Zollinger-Ellison syndrome

Pharmacodynamics
Peak output of pancreatic secretions: Within 30 minutes
Duration: At least 2 hours

Pharmacokinetics
Inactivated by proteolytic enzymes if administered orally
Metabolism: Metabolic fate is thought to be enzymatic inactivation in blood

Usual Dosage Adults: I.V.:
Pancreatic function: 1 CU/kg
Zollinger-Ellison: 2 CU/kg

Administration Parenteral: Reconstitute with 7.5 mL of NS; **do not shake**; use immediately by direct I.V. injection slowly over 1 minute

Monitoring Parameters Duodenal fluid volume and bicarbonate content; serum gastrin (Zollinger-Ellison syndrome)

Reference Range Normal adult response:
Gastric volume: 175-295 mL/hour
Gastric bicarbonate concentration: 94-134 mEq/L
Bicarbonate output: 0.295-0.577 mEq/kg/hour

Nursing Implications Patients should fast 12-15 hours before testing for Zollinger-Ellison syndrome

Additional Information Potency of secretin is expressed in terms of clinical units (CU)

Dosage Forms Powder for injection: 75 CU (10 mL)

♦ **Secretin-Ferring** *see* Secretin *on page 863*
♦ **Selax® (Canada)** *see* Docusate *on page 336*
♦ **Selenium** *see* Trace Metals *on page 940*

Selenium Sulfide *(se LEE nee um SUL fide)*

Brand Names Exsel® Shampoo; Selsun Blue® Shampoo [OTC]; Selsun® Shampoo; Versel™ (Canada)

Therapeutic Category Antiseborrheic Agent, Topical; Shampoos

Generic Available Yes

Use To treat itching and flaking of the scalp associated with dandruff; to control scalp seborrheic dermatitis; treatment of tinea versicolor

Pregnancy Risk Factor C

Contraindications Hypersensitivity to selenium or any component

Warnings Safety in infants has not been established; avoid use in children <2 years of age

Precautions Do not use on damaged skin to avoid any systemic toxicity

Adverse Reactions
Central nervous system: Lethargy
Dermatologic: Alopecia, discoloration of hair
Gastrointestinal: Vomiting following long-term use on damaged skin, abdominal pain, garlic breath
Local: Local irritation
Neuromuscular & skeletal: Tremor
Miscellaneous: Perspiration

Mechanism of Action May block the enzymes involved in growth of epithelial tissue

Pharmacokinetics Absorption: Not absorbed topically through intact skin, but can be absorbed topically through damaged skin

Usual Dosage Children ≥ 2 years and Adults: Topical:
Dandruff, seborrhea: Massage 5-10 mL into wet scalp, leave on scalp 2-3 minutes, rinse thoroughly and repeat application; alternatively, 5-10 mL of shampoo is applied and allowed to remain on scalp for 5-10 minutes before being rinsed off thoroughly without a repeat application; shampoo twice weekly for 2 weeks initially, then use once every 1-4 weeks as indicated depending upon control

Tinea versicolor: Apply the 2.5% lotion in a thin layer covering the body surface from the face to the knees; leave on skin for 30 minutes, then rinse thoroughly; apply every day for 7 days; then follow with monthly applications for 3 months to prevent recurrences

Administration Topical: For external use only; avoid contact with eyes or acutely inflamed skin

Patient Information Remove all jewelry before using the lotion; wash hands thoroughly following application of the lotion; may discolor hair

Dosage Forms Lotion, shampoo: 1% (120 mL, 210 mL, 240 mL, 330 mL); 2.5% (120 mL)

References
Lester RS, "Topical Formulary for the Pediatrician," *Pediatr Clin North Am*, 1983, 30(4):749-65.

- ♦ **Sele-Pak®** *see* Trace Metals *on page 940*
- ♦ **Selepen®** *see* Trace Metals *on page 940*
- ♦ **Selestoject® [Sodium Phosphate] (Canada)** *see* Betamethasone *on page 130*
- ♦ **Selestoject® Injection** *see* Betamethasone *on page 130*
- ♦ **Selsun Blue® Shampoo [OTC]** *see* Selenium Sulfide *on page 864*
- ♦ **Selsun® Shampoo** *see* Selenium Sulfide *on page 864*

Senna (SEN na)

Related Information
Carbohydrate and Alcohol Content of Liquid Medications for Use in Patients Receiving Ketogenic Diets *on page 1228*

Brand Names Black Draught® [OTC]; Glysennid® (Canada); Senna-Gen® [OTC]; Senokot® [OTC]; Senolax® [OTC]; X-Prep® Liquid [OTC]

Therapeutic Category Laxative, Stimulant

Generic Available Yes

Use Short-term treatment of constipation; evacuate the colon for bowel or rectal examinations

Pregnancy Risk Factor C

Contraindications Hypersensitivity to senna or any component; nausea and vomiting; undiagnosed abdominal pain, appendicitis, intestinal obstruction or perforation

Precautions Avoid prolonged use (>1 week); chronic use may lead to dependency, fluid and electrolyte imbalance, vitamin and mineral deficiencies

Adverse Reactions
Endocrine & metabolic: Electrolyte and fluid imbalance
Gastrointestinal: Nausea, vomiting, diarrhea, abdominal cramps, perianal irritation, discoloration of feces
Genitourinary: Discoloration of urine

Drug Interactions Docusate may enhance the absorption of senna

Mechanism of Action Active metabolite (aglycone) acts as a local irritant on the colon, stimulates Auerbach's plexus to produce peristalsis

Pharmacodynamics Onset of action:
Oral: Within 6-24 hours
Rectal: Evacuation occurs in 30 minutes to 2 hours

Pharmacokinetics
Metabolism: In the liver
Elimination: In the feces (via bile) and in urine

Usual Dosage
Children: Oral: 10-20 mg/kg/dose at bedtime; maximum daily dose: 872 mg
Granules: >27 kg: ½ teaspoon at bedtime to a maximum of 1 teaspoon twice daily
Tablet: >27 kg: 1 tablet at bedtime to a maximum of 2 tablets twice daily
Syrup:
1 month to 1 year: 1.25-2.5 mL at bedtime up to a maximum of 5 mL/day
1-5 years: 2.5-5 mL at bedtime to a maximum of 10 mL/day
5-15 years: 5-10 mL at bedtime to a maximum of 20 mL/day
Adults: Oral:
Granules: 1 teaspoonful at bedtime, not to exceed 2 teaspoonfuls twice daily
Syrup: 2-3 teaspoonfuls at bedtime, not to exceed 3 teaspoonfuls twice daily
Tablet: 2 tablets at bedtime, not to exceed 4 tablets twice daily
Rectal:
Children >27 kg: ½ suppository at bedtime
Adults: 1 suppository at bedtime; repeat in 2 hours if necessary

Administration Oral: Administer with water; syrup can be taken with juice or milk to mask taste

(Continued)

Senna *(Continued)*

Monitoring Parameters I & O, frequency of bowel movements, serum electrolytes if severe diarrhea occurs

Patient Information May discolor urine or feces; drink plenty of fluids

Dosage Forms
Granules: 326 mg/teaspoonful
Suppository, rectal: 652 mg
Syrup: 218 mg/5 mL (60 mL, 240 mL)
Tablet: 187 mg, 217 mg, 600 mg

References
Perkin JM, "Constipation in Childhood: A Controlled Comparison Between Lactulose and Standardized Senna," *Curr Med Res Opin*, 1977, 4(8):540-3.

♦ **Senna-Gen® [OTC]** *see* Senna *on page 865*
♦ **Senokot® [OTC]** *see* Senna *on page 865*
♦ **Senolax® [OTC]** *see* Senna *on page 865*
♦ **Sensorcaine®** *see* Bupivacaine *on page 148*
♦ **Sensorcaine-MPF®** *see* Bupivacaine *on page 148*
♦ **Septa® Topical Ointment [OTC]** *see* Neomycin, Polymyxin B, and Bacitracin *on page 680*
♦ **Septisol®** *see* Hexachlorophene *on page 475*
♦ **Septra®** *see* Co-Trimoxazole *on page 258*
♦ **Septra® DS** *see* Co-Trimoxazole *on page 258*
♦ **Serevent®** *see* Salmeterol *on page 855*
♦ **Serevent® Diskus®** *see* Salmeterol *on page 855*
♦ **Seromycin® Pulvules®** *see* Cycloserine *on page 269*
♦ **Serostim® Injection** *see* Human Growth Hormone *on page 478*
♦ **Serotonin Syndrome** *see page 1217*
♦ **Sertan® (Canada)** *see* Primidone *on page 796*
♦ **Serutan® [OTC]** *see* Psyllium *on page 823*
♦ **S-F Kaon®** *see* Potassium Supplements *on page 786*
♦ **Shohl's Solution, Modified** *see* Citrate and Citric Acid *on page 231*
♦ **Siblin® [OTC]** *see* Psyllium *on page 823*
♦ **Siladryl® Oral [OTC]** *see* Diphenhydramine *on page 327*
♦ **Silafed® [OTC]** *see* Triprolidine and Pseudoephedrine *on page 957*
♦ **Silain® [OTC]** *see* Simethicone *on page 868*
♦ **Silapap® [OTC]** *see* Acetaminophen *on page 26*
♦ **Silphen® Cough [OTC]** *see* Diphenhydramine *on page 327*
♦ **Silphen DM® [OTC]** *see* Dextromethorphan *on page 304*
♦ **Siltussin® [OTC]** *see* Guaifenesin *on page 464*
♦ **Siltussin DM® [OTC]** *see* Guaifenesin and Dextromethorphan *on page 466*
♦ **Silvadene®** *see* Silver Sulfadiazine *on page 867*

Silver Nitrate *(SIL ver NYE trate)*

Brand Names Dey-Drop® Ophthalmic Solution

Therapeutic Category Ophthalmic Agent, Miscellaneous; Topical Skin Product

Generic Available Yes

Use Prevention of gonococcal ophthalmia neonatorum; cauterization of wounds and sluggish ulcers, removal of granulation tissue and warts

Pregnancy Risk Factor C

Contraindications Not for use on broken skin or cuts; hypersensitivity to silver nitrate or any component

Warnings Do not use applicator sticks on the eyes; repeated applications of the ophthalmic solution into the eye can cause cauterization of the cornea and blindness; not effective for the prevention of neonatal chlamydial conjunctivitis

Adverse Reactions
Dermatologic: Staining of the skin
Hematologic: Methemoglobinemia
Local: Burning and skin irritation
Ocular: Cauterization of the cornea, blindness, chemical conjunctivitis

Drug Interactions Sulfacetamide eye preparations are incompatible with silver nitrate solutions

Stability Store applicator sticks in a dry place since moisture causes the oxidized film to dissolve; protect from light

Mechanism of Action Free silver ions precipitate bacterial proteins by combining with chloride in tissue forming silver chloride; coagulates cellular protein to form an eschar

Pharmacokinetics Absorption: Not readily absorbed from mucous membranes

Usual Dosage
Neonates: Ophthalmic: Instill 2 drops immediately after birth into conjunctival sac of each eye as a single dose; do not irrigate eyes following instillation of eye drops; silver nitrate prophylaxis should be administered immediately after delivery or no later than 1 hour after delivery

Children and Adults:
Sticks: Apply to mucous membranes and other moist skin surfaces only on area to be treated 2-3 times/week for 2-3 weeks
Topical solution: Apply a cotton applicator dipped in solution on the affected area 2-3 times/week for 2-3 weeks

Monitoring Parameters With prolonged use, monitor methemoglobin levels

Patient Information Discontinue topical preparation if redness or irritation develop; silver nitrate solution may stain skin

Nursing Implications Silver nitrate solutions stain skin and utensils

Dosage Forms
Applicator, topical: 75% with potassium nitrate 25% (6")
Ointment, topical: 10% (30 g)
Solution:
Ophthalmic: 1% (wax ampuls)
Topical: 10% (30 mL); 25% (30 mL); 50% (30 mL)

References
Cushing AH and Smith S, "Methemoglobinemia With Silver Nitrate Therapy of a Burn: Report of a Case," *J Pediatr*, 1969, 74(4):613-5.
Hammerschlag MR, Cummings C, Roblin PM, et al, "Efficacy of Neonatal Ocular Prophylaxis for the Prevention of Chlamydial and Gonococcal Conjunctivitis," *N Engl J Med*, 1989, 320(12):769-72.

Silver Sulfadiazine (SIL ver sul fa DYE a zeen)

Brand Names Dermazin™ (Canada); Flamazine® (Canada); Silvadene®; SSD® AF; SSD® Cream; Thermazene®

Therapeutic Category Antibiotic, Topical

Generic Available No

Use Adjunct in the prevention and treatment of infection in second and third degree burns

Pregnancy Risk Factor C

Contraindications Hypersensitivity to silver sulfadiazine or any component; premature infants or neonates <2 months of age since sulfas may displace bilirubin from protein binding sites and cause kernicterus

Precautions Use with caution in patients with G-6-PD deficiency and renal impairment; sulfadiazine may accumulate in patients with impaired hepatic or renal function

Adverse Reactions
Dermatologic: Itching, rash, erythema multiforme, discoloration of skin
Hematologic: Hemolytic anemia, leukopenia, agranulocytosis, aplastic anemia, thrombocytopenia
Hepatic: Hepatitis
Local: Pain, burning
Renal: Interstitial nephritis
Miscellaneous: Serum hyperosmolality (due to propylene glycol component in the cream), hypersensitivity reactions to sulfas

Drug Interactions Topical proteolytic enzymes (silver may inactivate enzymes)

Stability Discard if cream is darkened (reacts with heavy metals resulting in release of silver)

Mechanism of Action Acts upon the bacterial cell wall and cell membrane

Pharmacokinetics
Absorption: Significant percutaneous absorption of sulfadiazine can occur especially when applied to extensive burns
Half-life: 10 hours and is prolonged in patients with renal insufficiency
Time to peak serum concentration: Within 3-11 days of continuous topical therapy
Elimination: ~50% excreted unchanged in urine

Usual Dosage Children and Adults: Topical: Apply once or twice daily with a sterile gloved hand; apply to a thickness of 1/16"; burned area should be covered with cream at all times

Administration Topical: Apply to cleansed, debrided burned areas
(Continued)

Silver Sulfadiazine *(Continued)*

Monitoring Parameters Serum electrolytes, UA, renal function test, CBC in patients with extensive burns on long-term treatment

Patient Information For external use only; may discolor skin

Additional Information Contains methylparaben and propylene glycol

Dosage Forms Cream, topical: 1% [10 mg/g] (20 g, 50 g, 100 g, 400 g, 1000 g)

References

Kulick MI, Wong R, Okarma TB, et al, "Prospective Study of Side Effects Associated With the Use of Silver Sulfadiazine in Severely Burned Patients," *Ann Plast Surg*, 1985, 14(5):407-18.

Lockhart SP, Rushworth A, Azmy AA, et al, "Topical Silver Sulfadiazine: Side Effects and Urinary Excretion," *Burns Incl Therm Inj*, 1983, 10(1):9-12.

Simethicone (sye METH i kone)

Related Information

Carbohydrate and Alcohol Content of Liquid Medications for Use in Patients Receiving Ketogenic Diets *on page 1228*

Brand Names Degas® [OTC]; Flatulex® [OTC]; Gas-X® [OTC]; Maalox Anti-Gas® [OTC]; Mylanta Gas® [OTC]; Mylicon® [OTC]; Ovol® (Canada); Phazyme® [OTC]; Silain® [OTC]

Synonyms Activated Dimethicone; Activated Methylpolysiloxane

Therapeutic Category Antiflatulent

Generic Available Yes: Tablet

Use Relieve flatulence, functional gastric bloating, and postoperative gas pains

Pregnancy Risk Factor C

Food Interactions Avoid gas-forming foods

Mechanism of Action Spreads on surface of aqueous liquids forming a film of low surface tension which collapses foam bubbles; allows mucous-surrounded gas bubbles to coalesce and be expelled

Pharmacokinetics Elimination: In feces

Usual Dosage Oral:

Infants and Children <2 years: 20 mg 4 times/day

Children 2-12 years: 40 mg 4 times/day

Children >12 years and Adults: 40-125 mg after meals and at bedtime as needed, not to exceed 500 mg/day

Administration Oral: Administer after meals or at bedtime; chew tablets thoroughly before swallowing; shake suspension before using; mix with water, infant formula or other liquids

Patient Information Avoid carbonated beverages

Dosage Forms

Capsule: 125 mg

Drops, oral: 40 mg/0.6 mL (15 mL, 30 mL)

Tablet: 50 mg, 60 mg, 95 mg

Tablet, chewable: 40 mg, 80 mg, 125 mg

♦ **Sodium 2-Mercaptoethane Sulfonate** *see Mesna on page 610*
♦ **Sodium 4-Phenylbutyrate** *see Sodium Phenylbutyrate on page 873*

Sodium Acetate (SOW dee um AS e tate)
Therapeutic Category Alkalinizing Agent, Parenteral; Electrolyte Supplement, Parenteral; Sodium Salt
Generic Available Yes
Use Sodium salt replacement; correction of acidosis through conversion of acetate to bicarbonate
Pregnancy Risk Factor C
Contraindications Alkalosis, hypocalcemia, edema, cirrhosis, excessive chloride losses, hypernatremia
Warnings Avoid extravasation
Precautions Use with caution in patients with hepatic failure, CHF or other sodium-retaining conditions
Adverse Reactions
Cardiovascular: Thrombosis, hypervolemia, edema, cerebral hemorrhage
Endocrine & metabolic: Hypernatremia, hypokalemic metabolic alkalosis, hypocalcemia
Local: Extravasant, local cellulitis
Respiratory: Pulmonary edema
Stability Protect from light, heat, and from freezing; **incompatible** with acids, acidic salts, catecholamines, atropine
Mechanism of Action Sodium is the principal extracellular cation; functions in fluid and electrolyte balance, osmotic pressure control, and water distribution; acetate is metabolized to bicarbonate which neutralizes hydrogen ion concentration and raises blood and urinary pH
Usual Dosage Sodium acetate is metabolized to bicarbonate on an equimolar basis outside the liver; administer in large volume I.V. fluids as a sodium source. Dosage is dependent upon the clinical condition, fluid, electrolytes and acid-base balance of the patient.

Maintenance sodium requirements: I.V.:
Neonates, Infants, and Children: 3-4 mEq/kg/day; maximum dose: 100-150 mEq/day
Adults: 154 mEq/day
Metabolic acidosis: If sodium acetate is desired over sodium bicarbonate, the amount of acetate may be dosed utilizing the equation found in the sodium bicarbonate monograph as each mEq acetate is converted to a mEq of HCO_3; see Sodium Bicarbonate *on page 870*
Administration Parenteral: Must be diluted prior to I.V. administration; infuse hypertonic solutions (>154 mEq/L) via a central line; maximum rate of administration: 1 mEq/kg/hour
Monitoring Parameters Serum electrolytes including calcium, arterial blood gases (if indicated)
Additional Information Sodium and acetate content of 1 g: 7.3 mEq
Dosage Forms Injection: 2 mEq/mL (20 mL, 50 mL); 4 mEq/mL (50 mL)

♦ **Sodium Acid Carbonate** *see Sodium Bicarbonate on page 870*

Sodium Benzoate (SOW dee um BENZ oh ate)
Therapeutic Category Ammonium Detoxicant; Hyperammonemia Agent; Urea Cycle Disorder (UCD) Treatment Agent
Generic Available Yes
Use Adjunctive therapy for the prevention and treatment of hyperammonemia due to suspected or proven urea cycle defects
Precautions Use with caution in patients with Reye's syndrome, propionic or methylmalonic acidemia; use with caution in neonates with hyperbilirubinemia due to potential displacement of bilirubin from albumin binding sites
Adverse Reactions
Endocrine & metabolic: Metabolic acidosis
Gastrointestinal: Nausea, vomiting
Mechanism of Action Assists in lowering serum ammonia levels by activation of a nonurea cycle pathway (the benzoate-hippurate pathway); ammonia in the presence of benzoate will conjugate with glycine to form hippurate which is excreted by the kidney
Pharmacokinetics
Half-life: 0.75-7.4 hours
(Continued)

Sodium Benzoate *(Continued)*

Elimination: Clearance is largely attributable to metabolism with urinary excretion of hippurate, the major metabolite

Usual Dosage Investigational use (not FDA approved): Children: Oral, I.V.: 0.25 g/kg bolus followed by 0.25-0.5 g/kg/day as continuous infusion or divided every 6-8 hours

Monitoring Parameters Serum ammonia level

Additional Information Used to treat urea cycle enzyme deficiency in combination with arginine; not available commercially; oral solutions must be compounded using chemical powder form; I.V. solutions must also be compounded and tested for sterility and pyrogenicity prior to use

Dosage Forms Powder: 454 g

References

Batshaw ML, "Hyperammonemia," *Curr Probl Pediatr*, 1984, 14(11):1-69.

Batshaw ML and Brusilow SW, "Treatment of Hyperammonemic Coma Caused by Inborn Errors of Urea Synthesis," *J Pediatr*, 1980, 97(6):893-900.

Green TP, Marchessault RP, and Freese DK, "Disposition of Sodium Benzoate in Newborn Infants With Hyperammonemia," *J Pediatr*, 1983, 102(5):785-90.

Maestri NE, Hauser ER, Bartholomew D, et al, "Prospective Treatment of Urea Cycle Disorders," *J Pediatr*, 1991, 119(6):923-8.

Sodium Bicarbonate *(SOW dee um bye KAR bun ate)*

Related Information

Adult ACLS Algorithm, Asystole *on page 1008*
Adult ACLS Algorithm, Pulseless Electrical Activity *on page 1006*
Adult ACLS Algorithm, V. Fib and Pulseless V. Tach *on page 1004*
Antacid Preparations *on page 86*
CPR Pediatric Drug Dosages *on page 999*

Brand Names Neut® Injection

Synonyms Baking Soda; NaHCO₃; Sodium Acid Carbonate; Sodium Hydrogen Carbonate

Therapeutic Category Alkalinizing Agent, Oral; Alkalinizing Agent, Parenteral; Antacid; Electrolyte Supplement, Oral; Electrolyte Supplement, Parenteral; Sodium Salt

Generic Available Yes

Use Management of metabolic acidosis; antacid; alkalinization of urine; stabilization of acid base status in cardiac arrest (see Precautions) and treatment of life-threatening hyperkalemia

Pregnancy Risk Factor C

Contraindications Alkalosis, hypocalcemia, hypernatremia; unknown abdominal pain, inadequate ventilation during cardiopulmonary resuscitation; excessive chloride losses

Warnings Avoid extravasation, tissue necrosis can occur due to the hypertonicity of NaHCO₃; use of I.V. NaHCO₃ should be reserved for documented metabolic acidosis and for life-threatening hyperkalemia; routine use in cardiac arrest is not recommended

Precautions Use with caution in patients with CHF or other sodium-retaining conditions, renal insufficiency

Adverse Reactions

Cardiovascular: Edema, cerebral hemorrhage (especially with rapid injection of the hyperosmotic NaHCO₃ solution in infants)
Central nervous system: Tetany, intracranial acidosis
Endocrine & metabolic: Metabolic alkalosis, hypernatremia, hypokalemia, hypocalcemia, hyperosmolality
Gastrointestinal: Gastric distention, flatulence may occur with oral administration
Local: Tissue necrosis, ulceration after I.V. extravasation
Respiratory: Pulmonary edema

Drug Interactions Chlorpropamide, lithium, methotrexate, salicylates, and tetracycline have increased renal clearance with alkaline urine; anorexiants, flecainide, mecamylamine, quinidine, and sympathomimetics have decreased renal clearance with alkaline urine; concurrent doses with iron may decrease iron absorption

Stability Do not mix NaHCO₃ with calcium salts, catecholamines, atropine

Mechanism of Action Dissociates to provide bicarbonate ion which neutralizes hydrogen ion concentration and raises blood and urinary pH

Pharmacodynamics

Onset of action:
Oral, as antacid: 15 minutes
I.V.: Rapid

Duration:
  Oral: 1-3 hours
  I.V.: 8-10 minutes

Pharmacokinetics
  Absorption: Oral: Well absorbed
  Elimination: Reabsorbed by kidney and <1% is excreted in urine

Usual Dosage
  Cardiac arrest: See Precautions; patient should be adequately ventilated before administering $NaHCO_3$
    Infants: 1 mEq/kg slow IVP initially; may repeat with 0.5 mEq/kg in 10 minutes one time, or as indicated by the patient's acid-base status
    Children and Adults: 1 mEq/kg IVP initially; may repeat with 0.5 mEq/kg in 10 minutes one time, or as indicated by the patient's acid-base status
  Metabolic acidosis: Dosage should be based on the following formula if blood gases and pH measurements are available:
    Neonates, Infants and Children: $HCO_3^-(mEq) = 0.3$ x weight (kg) x base deficit (mEq/L) **or** $HCO_3^-(mEq) = 0.5$ x weight (kg) x [24 - serum $HCO_3^-(mEq/L)$]
    Adults: $HCO_3^-(mEq) = 0.2$ x weight (kg) x base deficit (mEq/L) **or** $HCO_3^-(mEq) = 0.5$ x weight (kg) x [24 - serum $HCO_3^-(mEq/L)$]
    If acid-base status is not available: Dose for older Children and Adults: 2-5 mEq/kg I.V. infusion over 4-8 hours; subsequent doses should be based on patient's acid-base status
  Prevention of hyperuricemia secondary to tumor lysis syndrome (urinary alkalinization) (refer to individual protocols):
    Infants and Children:
      I.V.: 120-200 mEq/m^2/day diluted in maintenance I.V. fluids of 3000 mL/m^2/day; titrate to maintain urine pH between 6-7
      Oral: 12 g/m^2/day divided into 4 doses; titrate to maintain urine pH between 6-7
  Chronic renal failure: Oral: Initiate when plasma HCO_3^- <15 mEq/L:
    Children: 1-3 mEq/kg/day in divided doses
    Adults: 20-36 mEq/day in divided doses
  Renal tubular acidosis: Oral:
    Distal:
      Children: 2-3 mEq/kg/day in divided doses
      Adults: 0.5-2 mEq/kg/day given in 4-5 divided doses
    Proximal: Children and Adults: Initial: 5-10 mEq/kg/day in divided doses; maintenance: Increase as required to maintain serum bicarbonate in the normal range
  Urine alkalinization: Oral:
    Children: 1-10 mEq (84-840 mg)/kg/day in divided doses; dose should be titrated to desired urinary pH
    Adults: 48 mEq (4 g) initially, then 12-24 mEq (1-2 g) every 4 hours; dose should be titrated to desired urinary pH; doses up to 16 g/day have been used
  Antacid: Oral: Adults: 325 mg to 2 grams 1-4 times/day

Administration
  Oral: Administer 1-3 hours after meals
  Parenteral: For direct I.V. administration: in neonates and infants, use the 0.5 mEq/mL solution or dilute the 1 mEq/mL solution 1:1 with **sterile water**; in children and adults, the 1 mEq/mL solution may be used; administer slowly (maximum rate in neonates and infants: 10 mEq/minute); for infusion, dilute to a maximum concentration of 0.5 mEq/mL in dextrose solution and infuse over 2 hours (maximum rate of administration: 1 mEq/kg/hour)

Monitoring Parameters Serum electrolytes including calcium, urinary pH, arterial blood gases (if indicated)

Additional Information 1 mEq $NaHCO_3$ is equivalent to 84 mg; each g of $NaHCO_3$ provides 12 mEq each of sodium and bicarbonate ions

Dosage Forms
  Injection: 4% [40 mg/mL = 2.4 mEq/5 mL] (5 mL); 4.2% [42 mg/mL = 5 mEq/10 mL] (10 mL); 7.5% [75 mg/mL = 8.92 mEq/10 mL] (10 mL, 50 mL); 8.4% [84 mg/mL = 10 mEq/10 mL] (10 mL, 50 mL)
  Powder: 120 g, 480 g
  Tablet: 300 mg [3.6 mEq]; 325 mg [3.8 mEq]; 520 mg [6.3 mEq]; 600 mg [7.3 mEq]; 650 mg [7.6 mEq]

Sodium Chloride (SOW dee um KLOR ide)
  Brand Names Adsorbonac® Ophthalmic [OTC]; Afrin® Saline Mist [OTC]; AK-NaCl® [OTC]; Ayr® Nasal [OTC]; Breathe Free® [OTC]; Dristan® Saline Spray [OTC]; HuMist® Nasal Mist [OTC]; Muro-128™ (Canada); Muro 128® Ophthalmic [OTC]; (Continued)

Sodium Chloride *(Continued)*

Muroptic-5® [OTC]; NaSal™ [OTC]; Nasal Moist® [OTC]; Ocean Nasal Mist [OTC]; Pretz® [OTC]; Saline from Otrivin® (Canada); SalineX® [OTC]; SeaMist® [OTC]

Synonyms NaCl; Normal Saline; NS; ½NS

Therapeutic Category Electrolyte Supplement, Oral; Electrolyte Supplement, Parenteral; Lubricant, Ocular; Sodium Salt

Generic Available Yes

Use Prevention of muscle cramps and heat prostration; restoration of sodium ion in hyponatremia; restores moisture to nasal membranes; reduction of corneal edema; source of electrolytes and water for expansion of the extracellular fluid compartment

Pregnancy Risk Factor C

Contraindications Hypersensitivity to sodium chloride or any component; hypertonic uterus, hypernatremia, fluid retention

Warnings Sodium toxicity is almost exclusively related to how fast a sodium deficit is corrected; both rate and magnitude of correction are extremely important

Precautions Use with caution in patients with CHF, renal insufficiency, cirrhosis, hypertension

Adverse Reactions
Cardiovascular: Edema, thrombosis, hypervolemia
Endocrine & metabolic: Hypernatremia, dilution of serum electrolytes, overhydration
Gastrointestinal: Nausea, vomiting (oral use)
Local: Phlebitis (with concentrations >0.9%)
Respiratory: Pulmonary edema

Mechanism of Action Principal extracellular cation; functions in fluid and electrolyte balance, osmotic pressure control and water distribution

Pharmacokinetics
Absorption: Oral, I.V.: Rapid
Distribution: Widely distributed
Elimination: Mainly in urine but also in sweat, tears, and saliva

Usual Dosage Dosage depends upon clinical condition, fluid, electrolyte and acid-base balance of patient; hypertonic solutions (>0.9%) should only be used for the initial treatment of acute serious symptomatic hyponatremia; see Fluid and Electrolyte Requirements in Children *on page 1068*

Maintenance sodium requirements: Oral, I.V.:
Premature neonates: 2-8 mEq/kg/day
Term neonates: 1-4 mEq/kg/day
Infants and Children: 3-4 mEq/kg/day; maximum dose: 100-150 mEq/day
Adults: 154 mEq/day
Nasal: Children and Adults: Use as often as needed
Heat cramps: Adults: Oral: 0.5-1 g, up to 5-10 times/day (5 g/day maximum)
Ophthalmic, ointment: Children and Adults: Apply once daily or more often as needed
To correct acute, serious hyponatremia: mEq sodium = [desired sodium (mEq/L) - actual sodium (mEq/L)] x 0.6 x wt (kg); for acute correction use 125 mEq/L as the desired serum sodium; acutely correct serum sodium in 5 mEq/L/dose increments; more gradual correction in increments of 10 mEq/L/day is indicated in the asymptomatic patient

Administration
Nasal: Spray into 1 nostril while gently occluding other
Ophthalmic: Apply to affected eye(s); avoid contact of bottle tip with eye or skin
Oral: Administer with full glass of water
Parenteral: Infuse hypertonic solutions (>0.9% saline) via central line only; maximum rate of administration: 1 mEq/kg/hour

Monitoring Parameters Serum sodium, chloride, I & O, weight

Reference Range Serum/plasma sodium levels:
Premature neonates: 132-140 mEq/L
Full-term neonates: 133-142 mEq/L
Infants ≥2 months to Adults: 135-145 mEq/L

Nursing Implications Bacteriostatic NS should not be used for diluting or reconstituting drugs for administration in neonates

Additional Information Normal saline (0.9%) = 154 mEq/L; 3% NaCl = 513 mEq/L; 5% NaCl = 855 mEq/L

Dosage Forms
Drops, nasal: 0.9% with dropper

Injection: 0.2% (3 mL); 0.45% (3 mL, 5 mL, 500 mL, 1000 mL); 0.9% (1 mL, 2 mL, 3 mL, 4 mL, 5 mL, 10 mL, 20 mL, 25 mL, 30 mL, 50 mL, 100 mL, 130 mL, 150 mL, 250 mL, 500 mL, 1000 mL); 3% (500 mL); 5% (500 mL); 20% (250 mL); 23.4% (30 mL, 100 mL)

Injection:
Admixtures: 50 mEq (20 mL); 100 mEq (40 mL); 625 mEq (250 mL)
Bacteriostatic: 0.9% (30 mL)
Concentrated: 14.6% (2.5 mEq/mL)(20 mL, 40 mL, 200 mL); 23.4% (4 mEq/mL) (10 mL, 20 mL, 30 mL)

Irrigation: 0.45% (500 mL, 1000 mL, 1500 mL); 0.9% (250 mL, 500 mL, 1000 mL, 1500 mL, 2000 mL, 3000 mL, 4000 mL)

Ointment, ophthalmic (Muro 128®): 5% (3.5 g)

Solution:
Irrigation: 0.9% (1000 mL, 2000 mL)
Nasal: 0.4% (15 mL, 50 mL); 0.6% (15 mL); 0.65% (20 mL, 45 mL, 50 mL)
Ophthalmic (Adsorbonac®): 2% (15 mL); 5% (15 mL, 30 mL)

Tablet: 650 mg (11.3 mEq), 1 g (17 mEq), 2.25 g (38.5 mEq)

Tablet:
Enteric coated: 1 g (17 mEq)
Slow release: 600 mg (10.3 mEq)

◆ **Sodium Citrate and Citric Acid** *see* Citrate and Citric Acid *on page 231*

◆ **Sodium Edetate** *see* Edetate Disodium *on page 358*

◆ **Sodium Etidronate** *see* Etidronate Disodium *on page 396*

◆ **Sodium Ferric Gluconate** *see* Ferric Gluconate *on page 410*

◆ **Sodium Ferric Gluconate Complex in Sucrose Injection** *see* Ferric Gluconate *on page 410*

◆ **Sodium Fluoride** *see* Fluoride *on page 427*

◆ **Sodium Hydrogen Carbonate** *see* Sodium Bicarbonate *on page 870*

◆ **Sodium Hyposulfate** *see* Sodium Thiosulfate *on page 875*

◆ **Sodium Nitroprusside** *see* Nitroprusside *on page 692*

Sodium Phenylbutyrate (SOW dee um fen il BYOO ti rate)

Brand Names Buphenyl®

Synonyms Ammonapse; 4-Phenylbutyric Acid Sodium; Sodium 4-Phenylbutyrate

Therapeutic Category Ammonium Detoxicant; Hyperammonemia Agent; Urea Cycle Disorder (UCD) Treatment Agent

Use Adjunctive therapy in the chronic management of patients with urea cycle disorder involving deficiencies of carbamoylphosphate synthetase, ornithine transcarbamylase, or argininosuccinic acid synthetase; provides an alternative pathway for waste nitrogen excretion

Pregnancy Risk Factor C

Contraindications Hypersensitivity to phenylbutyrate, or any component; patients with severe hypertension, heart failure or renal dysfunction; **phenylbutyrate is not indicated in the treatment of acute hyperammonemia**

Precautions Use cautiously in patients with renal or hepatic dysfunction and in patients who must maintain a low sodium diet as each gram of drug contains 125 mg sodium

Adverse Reactions
Cardiovascular: Edema, arrhythmias, syncope
Central nervous system: Headache, depression
Dermatologic: Rash
Endocrine & metabolic: Amenorrhea, menstrual dysfunction, acidosis, alkalosis, hyperchloremia, hyperuricemia, hypokalemia, hypernatremia, hyperphosphatemia
Gastrointestinal: Anorexia, abnormal taste, abdominal pain, nausea, vomiting, weight gain, gastritis; rare: peptic ulcer, rectal bleeding, pancreatitis
Hematologic: Anemia, leukopenia, leukocytosis, thrombocytopenia, aplastic anemia
Hepatic: Hypoalbuminemia, elevated liver enzymes, elevated bilirubin
Renal: Renal tubular acidosis
Miscellaneous: Offensive body odor

Drug Interactions Haloperidol, valproic acid and corticosteroids increase ammonia concentrations and may decrease effectiveness of sodium phenylbutyrate; probenecid may decrease urinary excretion

Food Interactions Avoid mixing with acidic-type beverages (eg, colas, lemonade, grape juice) since drug may precipitate
(Continued)

Sodium Phenylbutyrate *(Continued)*

Stability Store at room temperature (59°F to 86°F); after opening, containers should be kept tightly closed

Mechanism of Action Sodium phenylbutyrate is a prodrug that, when given orally, is rapidly converted to phenylacetate. Phenylacetate is conjugated with glutamine to form the active compound phenylacetyglutamine. Phenylacetyglutamine serves as a substitute for urea and is excreted in the urine carrying with it 2 moles nitrogen (equivalent to urea) per mole of phenylacetyglutamine thus assisting in the clearance of nitrogenous waste in patients with urea cycle disorders.

Pharmacokinetics

Distribution: V_d: 0.2 L/kg

Metabolism: conjugation to phenylacetylglutamine (active form); undergoes nonlinear Michaelis-Menten elimination kinetics

Half-life: 0.8 hours (parent compound); 1.2 hours (phenylacetate)

Time to peak serum concentration:

Powder: 1 hour

Tablet: 1.35 hours

Elimination: 80% of metabolite excreted in urine in 24 hours

Usual Dosage Oral:

Neonates, Infants, and Children <20 kg: 450-600 mg/kg/day divided four to six times daily; maximum daily dose 20 g/day

Children >20 kg and Adults: 9.9-13 $g/m^2/day$, divided four to six times daily; maximum daily dose 20 g/day

Administration Oral: Administer with meals or feedings; mix powder with food or drink; avoid mixing with acidic beverages (eg, most fruit juices or colas)

Monitoring Parameters Plasma ammonia and glutamine concentrations, serum electrolytes, proteins, hepatic and renal function tests, physical signs/symptoms of hyperammonemia (ie, lethargy, ataxia, confusion, vomiting, seizures, and memory impairment)

Patient Information It is important to follow the dietary restrictions required when treating this disorder, the medication must be taken in strict accordance with the prescribed regimen; avoid altering the dosage without the prescriber's knowledge; the powder formulation has a very salty taste

Additional Information Teaspoon and tablespoon measuring devices are provided with the powder; each 1 g powder contains 0.94 g sodium phenylbutyrate = 125 mg sodium; each tablet contains 0.5 g sodium phenylbutyrate = 62 mg sodium

Dosage Forms

Powder: 3.2 g [sodium phenylbutyrate 3 g] per **teaspoon or** 9.1 g [sodium phenylbutyrate 8.6 g] per **tablespoon**

Tablet: 500 mg

References

Brusilow SW, "Phenylacetylglutamine May Replace Urea as a Vehicle for Waste Nitrogen Excretion," *Pediatr Res*, 1991, 29(2):147-50.

Maestri NE, Brusilow SW, Clissold DB, et al, "Long-Term Treatment of Girls With Ornithine Trans-carbamylase Deficiency," *N Engl J Med*, 1996, 335(12):855-9.

♦ **Sodium Phosphate** *see* Phosphate Supplements *on page 765*

Sodium Polystyrene Sulfonate

(SOW dee um pol ee STYE reen SUL fon ate)

Related Information

Carbohydrate and Alcohol Content of Liquid Medications for Use in Patients Receiving Ketogenic Diets *on page 1228*

Brand Names Kayexalate®; Kionex®; SPS®

Therapeutic Category Antidote, Hyperkalemia

Generic Available Yes

Use Treatment of hyperkalemia

Pregnancy Risk Factor C

Contraindications Hypernatremia; intestinal obstruction or perforation (oral use)

Warnings Avoid using the commercially available liquid product in neonates due to the preservative content. Enema may be prepared with powder and diluted with sorbitol 10% solution or oral solution may be made by dilution with 25% sorbitol solution. Treatment with this drug alone may be insufficient to rapidly correct severe hyperkalemia; other more rapidly effective appropriate measures should be used; enema will reduce the serum potassium faster than oral administration, but the oral route will result in a greater reduction over several hours.

Precautions Use with caution in patients with severe CHF, hypertension, or edema; small amounts of magnesium and calcium may also be lost in binding

Adverse Reactions

Endocrine & metabolic: Hypokalemia, hypocalcemia, hypomagnesemia, hypernatremia

Gastrointestinal: Anorexia, nausea, vomiting, constipation, intestinal necrosis

Drug Interactions Cation-donating antacids (such as magnesium hydroxide or calcium carbonate)

Food Interactions Never mix in orange juice

Mechanism of Action Removes potassium by exchanging sodium ions for potassium ions in the intestine before the resin is passed from the body

Pharmacodynamics Onset of action: Within 2-24 hours

Pharmacokinetics Elimination: Remains in the GI tract to be completely excreted in the feces (primarily as potassium polystyrene sulfonate)

Usual Dosage

Children:

Oral: 1 g/kg/dose every 6 hours

Rectal: 1 g/kg/dose every 2-6 hours

Adults:

Oral: 15 g 1-4 times/day

Rectal: 30-50 g every 6 hours

Administration

Oral or NG: Administer as ~25% sorbitol solution; shake suspension well before use

Enema: See Warnings; retain enema in colon for at least 30-60 minutes or several hours, if possible

Monitoring Parameters Serum sodium, potassium, calcium, magnesium, EKG (if applicable)

Additional Information 1 g of resin binds ~1 mEq of potassium; 4.1 mEq sodium per g of powder

Dosage Forms Oral or rectal:

Powder for suspension: 454 g

Suspension: 1.25 g/5 mL with sorbitol 33% and alcohol 0.3% (60 mL, 120 mL, 200 mL, 500 mL)

♦ **Sodium Sulamyd®** *see* Sulfacetamide *on page 888*

♦ **Sodium Sulfacetamide** *see* Sulfacetamide *on page 888*

Sodium Thiosulfate (SOW dee um thye oh SUL fate)

Brand Names Tinver® [OTC]; Versiclear™

Synonyms Disodium Thiosulfate Pentahydrate; Sodium Hyposulfate; Thiosulfuric Acid

Therapeutic Category Antidote, Cisplatin; Antidote, Cyanide; Antidote, Extravasation; Antifungal Agent, Topical

Generic Available Yes

Use

Parenteral: Used alone or with sodium nitrite or amyl nitrite in cyanide poisoning or arsenic poisoning; reduce the risk of nephrotoxicity associated with cisplatin therapy; local infiltration (in diluted form) of selected chemotherapy extravasation

Topical: Treatment of tinea versicolor, acne

Pregnancy Risk Factor C

Contraindications Hypersensitivity to sodium thiosulfate or any component

Precautions Discontinue if irritation or sensitivity occurs; rapid I.V. infusion has caused transient hypotension and EKG changes in dogs

Adverse Reactions

Cardiovascular: Hypotension

Central nervous system: Coma, CNS depression secondary to thiocyanate intoxication, psychosis, confusion

Dermatologic: Contact dermatitis

Local: Local irritation

Neuromuscular & skeletal: Weakness

Otic: Tinnitus

Stability Stable diluted in NS or D_5W at concentrations of 1.5% and 9.76% sodium thiosulfate for 24 hours

Mechanism of Action

Prevention of cyanide toxicity: By providing an extra sulfur group to the enzyme rhodanase, it increases the rate of detoxification of cyanide

(Continued)

875

Sodium Thiosulfate *(Continued)*

Prevention of cisplatin nephrotoxicity: Complexes with cisplatin to form a compound that is nontoxic to either normal or cancerous cells

Pharmacokinetics
Half-life, elimination: 0.65 hours
Elimination: 28.5% excreted unchanged in the urine

Usual Dosage
Cyanide and nitroprusside antidote: I.V.:
Children <25 kg: 50 mg/kg after receiving 4.5-10 mg/kg sodium nitrite; one-half the dose of each may be repeated if necessary
Children >25 kg and Adults: 12.5 g after 300 mg of sodium nitrite; one-half the dose of each may be repeated if necessary
Prevention of cisplatin nephrotoxicity: Adults: I.V.: 12 g over 6 hours in association with cisplatin **or** 9 g/m^2 I.V. bolus then 1.2 g/m^2/hour for 6 hours; should be administered before or during cisplatin administration
Chemotherapy infiltration: Dilute 10% sodium thiosulfate 4-8 mL with 6 mL sterile water to make $1/6$ to $1/3$ molar solution; as local infiltration for the following chemotherapy agents:
Mechlorethamine: Use 2 mL for each mg infiltrated
Cis-platinum: 2 mL for each 100 mg infiltrated; use only for large infiltrates (>20 mL) and concentrations >0.5 mg/mL of cis-platinum
Topical use (antifungal, acne): Children and Adults: 25% solution: Apply thin film twice daily to affected areas for several weeks to months

Administration
Parenteral: I.V.: Inject slowly, over at least 10 minutes; rapid administration may cause hypotension
Topical: Do not apply topically to or near eyes; thoroughly cleanse and dry affects areas prior to application

Dosage Forms
Injection: 100 mg/mL (10 mL); 250 mg/mL (50 mL)
Lotion: 25% with salicylic acid 1% and isopropyl alcohol 10% (120 mL, 180 mL)

References
Hall AH and Rumack BH, "Hydroxocobalamin/Sodium Thiosulfate as a Cyanide Antidote," *J Emerg Med*, 1987, 5(2):115-21.
Naughton M, "Acute Cyanide Poisoning," *Anaesth Intensive Care*, 1974, 2(4):351-6.

- **Sodium Thiosulfate, Sodium Nitrite, and Amyl Nitrite** *see* Cyanide Antidote Kit *on page 262*
- **Soflax™ (Canada)** *see* Docusate *on page 336*
- **Softgels® [OTC]** *see* Vitamin E *on page 982*
- **Solarcaine® [OTC]** *see* Benzocaine *on page 124*
- **Solarcaine® Topical** *see* Lidocaine *on page 568*
- **Solfoton®** *see* Phenobarbital *on page 754*
- **Solganal®** *see* Aurothioglucose *on page 110*
- **Solu-Cortef® Injection** *see* Hydrocortisone *on page 486*
- **Solugel® 4, 8 (Canada)** *see* Benzoyl Peroxide *on page 126*
- **Solu-Medrol® Injection** *see* Methylprednisolone *on page 629*
- **Solurex® Injection** *see* Dexamethasone *on page 294*
- **Solurex L.A.® Injection** *see* Dexamethasone *on page 294*
- **Soluver® (Canada)** *see* Salicylic Acid *on page 854*
- **Somatrem** *see* Human Growth Hormone *on page 478*
- **Somatropin** *see* Human Growth Hormone *on page 478*
- **Sominex® Oral [OTC]** *see* Diphenhydramine *on page 327*
- **Somnol® (Canada)** *see* Flurazepam *on page 434*
- **Somophyllin®** *see* Aminophylline *on page 61*
- **Som Pam® (Canada)** *see* Flurazepam *on page 434*
- **Sopamycetin® (Canada)** *see* Chloramphenicol *on page 207*

Sorbitol *(SOR bi tole)*

Therapeutic Category Laxative, Hyperosmolar; Laxative, Osmotic
Generic Available Yes
Use Humectant; sweetening agent; hyperosmotic laxative; facilitates the passage of sodium polystyrene sulfonate or a charcoal-toxin complex through the intestinal tract
Contraindications Anuria

Adverse Reactions
Endocrine & metabolic: Fluid and electrolyte losses, lactic acidosis
Gastrointestinal: Diarrhea, abdominal distress, nausea, vomiting

Mechanism of Action
A polyalcoholic sugar with osmotic cathartic actions

Pharmacodynamics
Onset of action: Oral: Mean time to first stool in patients receiving a charcoal-sorbitol slurry:
Children (ingestions):
6.4 hours (dose: 1.5 g/kg in 4 patients)
8.48 hours (dose: 2 g/kg in 33 patients)
Adults:
Nonpoisoned volunteers: 1.6 hours (dose: 2 g/kg)
Ingestion: 7.2 hours (14 adults; dose not specified)

Pharmacokinetics
Absorption: Oral, rectal: Poor
Metabolism: Mainly in the liver to fructose

Usual Dosage
Hyperosmotic laxative (as single dose, at infrequent intervals):
Children 2-11 years:
Oral: 2 mL/kg (as 70% solution)
Rectal enema: 30-60 mL as 25% to 30% solution
Children ≥12 years and Adults:
Oral: 30-150 mL (as 70% solution)
Rectal enema: 120 mL as 25% to 30% solution
Adjunct to sodium polystyrene sulfonate: 15 mL as 70% solution orally until diarrhea occurs (10-20 mL/2 hours) or 20-100 mL as an oral vehicle for the sodium polystyrene sulfonate resin
When administered with charcoal: Oral:
Children: 4.3 mL/kg of 35% sorbitol with 1 g/kg of activated charcoal or maximum dose: 2 g/kg sorbitol with activated charcoal
Adults: 4.3 mL/kg of 70% sorbitol with 1 g/kg of activated charcoal

Monitoring Parameters
Serum electrolytes, I & O

Dosage Forms
Powder: 500 g
Solution, oral: 70% (480 mL)

References
Charney EB and Bodurtha JN, "Intractable Diarrhea Associated With the Use of Sorbitol," *J Pediatr*, 1981, 98:157-8.
James LP, Nichols MH, and King WD, "A Comparison of Cathartics in Pediatric Ingestions," *Pediatrics*, 1995, 96(2 Pt 1):235-8.
Kumar A, Weatherly MR, and Beaman DC, "Sweeteners, Flavorings, and Dyes in Antibiotic Preparations," *Pediatrics*, 1991, 87(3):352-60.

♦ **Soyacal®** *see* Fat Emulsion *on page 403*

♦ **Span-FF® [OTC]** *see* Iron Supplements, Oral/Enteral *on page 530*

♦ **Spaslin®** *see* Hyoscyamine, Atropine, Scopolamine, and Phenobarbital *on page 499*

♦ **Spasmoject® Injection** *see* Dicyclomine *on page 314*

♦ **Spasmolin®** *see* Hyoscyamine, Atropine, Scopolamine, and Phenobarbital *on page 499*

♦ **Spasmophen®** *see* Hyoscyamine, Atropine, Scopolamine, and Phenobarbital *on page 499*

♦ **Spasquid®** *see* Hyoscyamine, Atropine, Scopolamine, and Phenobarbital *on page 499*

♦ **Spec-T® [OTC]** *see* Benzocaine *on page 124*

♦ **Spectazole™** *see* Econazole *on page 356*

♦ **Spironazide®** *see* Hydrochlorothiazide and Spironolactone *on page 484*

Spironolactone (speer on oh LAK tone)
Brand Names Aldactone®; Novo-Spiroton® (Canada)
Therapeutic Category Antihypertensive Agent; Diuretic, Potassium Sparing
Generic Available Yes
Use Management of edema associated with excessive aldosterone excretion; hypertension; primary hyperaldosteronism; hypokalemia; treatment of hirsutism; cirrhosis of liver accompanied by edema or ascites
Pregnancy Risk Factor D
Contraindications Hypersensitivity to spironolactone or any component; renal failure, anuria, hyperkalemia
Warnings Spironolactone has been shown to be tumorigenic in toxicity studies using 25-250 times the usual human dose in rats
(Continued)

Spironolactone *(Continued)*

Precautions Use with caution in patients with dehydration, hyponatremia, impaired renal clearance (Cl_{cr} <50 mL/minute) or hepatic dysfunction; patients receiving other potassium-sparing diuretics or potassium supplements

Adverse Reactions

Cardiovascular: Arrhythmia

Central nervous system: Lethargy, headache, mental confusion, fever, ataxia

Dermatologic: Rash, urticaria

Endocrine & metabolic: Hyperkalemia, dehydration, hyponatremia, hyperchloremic metabolic acidosis, postmenopausal bleeding, amenorrhea, gynecomastia (in males); breast tenderness, deepening of voice, and increased hair growth (in females)

Gastrointestinal: Anorexia, nausea, vomiting, diarrhea, gastritis, cramping, gastric bleeding

Genitourinary: Dysuria

Hematologic: Agranulocytosis

Neuromuscular & skeletal: Weakness, numbness or paresthesia in hands, feet or lips, lower back or side pain

Renal: Decreased renal function (including renal failure)

Respiratory: Cough, shortness of breath, dyspnea, hoarseness

Drug Interactions Potassium, other potassium-sparing diuretics, and ACE inhibitors (eg, captopril) may additively increase the serum potassium; may decrease digoxin clearance and attenuate its inotropic effect; decreased hypoprothrombinemic effect of oral anticoagulants; salicylates may interfere with natriuretic action of spironolactone

Food Interactions Avoid natural licorice (causes sodium and water retention and increases potassium loss) and salt substitutes

Mechanism of Action Competes with aldosterone for receptor sites in the distal renal tubules, increasing sodium chloride and water excretion while conserving potassium and hydrogen ions; may block the effect of aldosterone on arteriolar smooth muscle as well

Pharmacokinetics

Distribution: V_d: Breast milk to plasma ratio: 0.51-0.72

Protein binding: 91% to 98%

Metabolism: In the liver to multiple metabolites, including canrenone (active)

Half-life:

Spironolactone: 78-84 minutes

Canrenone: 13-24 hours

Time to peak serum concentration: Within 1-3 hours (primarily as the active metabolite)

Elimination: Urinary and biliary

Usual Dosage Oral:

Neonates: Diuretic: 1-3 mg/kg/day every 12-24 hours

Children:

Diuretic, hypertension: 1.5-3.3 mg/kg/day or 60 mg/m²/day in divided doses every 6-24 hours

Diagnosis of primary aldosteronism: 100-400 mg/m²/day in divided doses

Adults:

Edema, hypertension, hypokalemia: 25-200 mg/day in 1-2 divided doses

Diagnosis of primary aldosteronism: 100-400 mg/day in 1-2 divided doses

Hirsutism in women: 50-200 mg/day in 1-2 divided doses

CHF: Patients with severe heart failure already using an ACE inhibitor and a loop diuretic ± digoxin: 25 mg/day, increase or reduce depending on individual response and evidence of hyperkalemia

Dosing interval in renal impairment:

Cl_{cr} 10-50 mL/minute: Administer every 12-24 hours

Cl_{cr} <10 mL/minute: Avoid use

Administration Oral: Administer with food

Monitoring Parameters Serum potassium, sodium, and renal function

Test Interactions May cause false elevation in serum digoxin concentrations measured by RIA

Patient Information May cause drowsiness and impair ability to perform hazardous tasks which require mental alertness or physical coordination

Dosage Forms Tablet: 25 mg, 50 mg, 100 mg

Extemporaneous Preparations

A 5 mg/mL suspension may be made by crushing tablets, levigating with a small amount of distilled water or glycerin; dilute with 1 part Cologel® and 2 parts simple syrup and/or cherry syrup to make the final concentration; stable 60 days when refrigerated (ASHP, 1987)

A 1 mg/mL suspension may be compounded by crushing ten 25 mg tablets, add a small amount of water and soak for 5 minutes; add 50 mL 1.5% carboxymethylcellulose, 100 mL syrup NF, and mix; use a sufficient quantity of purified water to a total volume of 250 mL; stable at room temperature or refrigerated for 3 months (Nahata, 1993)

A 25 mg/mL suspension may be made by crushing one-hundred twenty-five 25 mg tablets, add in geometric proportions a 1:1 mixture of Ora-Sweet® and Ora-Plus® or Ora-Sweet® SF and Ora-Plus® to a total volume of 120 mL; stable 60 days refrigerated stored in amber bottles; shake well (Allen, 1996)

Allen LV and Erickson MA, "Stability of Labetalol Hydrochloride, Metoprolol Tartrate, Verapamil Hydrochloride, and Spironolactone With Hydrochlorothiazide in Extemporaneously Compounded Oral Liquids," *Am J Health Syst Pharm*, 1996, 53(19):2304-9.

Handbook on Extemporaneous Formulations, Bethesda, MD: American Society of Hospital Pharmacists, 1987.

Nahata MC, Morosco RS, and Hipple TF, "Stability of Spironolactone in an Extemporaneously Prepared Suspension at Two Temperatures," *Ann Pharmacother*, 1993, 27:1198-9.

♦ **Spironolactone and Hydrochlorothiazide** *see Hydrochlorothiazide and Spironolactone on page 484*

♦ **Spirozide®** *see Hydrochlorothiazide and Spironolactone on page 484*

♦ **Sporanox®** *see Itraconazole on page 538*

♦ **SPS®** *see Sodium Polystyrene Sulfonate on page 874*

♦ **SSD® AF** *see Silver Sulfadiazine on page 867*

♦ **SSD® Cream** *see Silver Sulfadiazine on page 867*

♦ **SSKI®** *see Potassium Iodide on page 785*

♦ **Stagesic®** *see Hydrocodone and Acetaminophen on page 485*

♦ **Stannous Fluoride** *see Fluoride on page 427*

♦ **Staphcillin®** *see Methicillin on page 616*

♦ **Statex® (Canada)** *see Morphine Sulfate on page 657*

♦ **Staticin®** *see Erythromycin on page 379*

Stavudine (STAV yoo deen)

Related Information
Adult and Adolescent HIV *on page 1133*
Pediatric HIV *on page 1129*

Brand Names Zerit™

Synonyms d4T; 2',3'-didehydro-3'-deoxythymidine

Therapeutic Category Antiretroviral Agent; HIV Agents (Anti-HIV Agents); Nucleoside Reverse Transcriptase Inhibitor (NRTI)

Generic Available No

Use Treatment of HIV infection in combination with other antiretroviral agents. **(Note:** Current preferred IV regimens consist of **three** antiretroviral agents)

Pregnancy Risk Factor C

Contraindications Hypersensitivity to stavudine or any component

Warnings The major clinical toxicity of stavudine is peripheral neuropathy which has occurred in 15% to 21% of patients in controlled trials; lactic acidosis and severe hepatomegaly with steatosis is a rare but potentially life-threatening toxicity associated with the use of NRTIs

Precautions Use with caution in patients with a history of peripheral neuropathy, or hepatic or renal impairment; dosage adjustment required in patients with impaired renal function

Adverse Reactions
Central nervous system: Headache, fever, insomnia, malaise, dizziness, nervousness, increased energy, mania
Dermatologic: Rash, pruritus
Gastrointestinal: Abdominal pain, diarrhea, nausea, vomiting, anorexia, pancreatitis
Hepatic: Elevation in AST and ALT
Neuromuscular & skeletal: Peripheral neuropathy (tingling, burning, pain, numbness of hands or feet), weakness
Otic: Ear pain
Respiratory: Rhinitis, cough
(Continued)

Stavudine *(Continued)*

Drug Interactions Drugs associated with peripheral neuropathy (chloramphenicol, cisplatin, dapsone, ethionamide, gold, hydralazine, iodoquinol, isoniazid, lithium, metronidazole, nitrofurantoin, pentamidine, phenytoin, ribavirin, vincristine) may increase risk for stavudine peripheral neuropathy; drugs that decrease renal function could decrease clearance of stavudine; stavudine should not be administered in combination with zidovudine (poor antiretroviral effect)

Stability
Capsules: Store in tightly closed containers at room temperature
Oral solution: Reconstitute powder for oral solution according to manufacturer's instructions; keep refrigerated; solution is stable for 30 days

Mechanism of Action Antiviral activity is dependent on intracellular conversion of stavudine to the active metabolite d4-triphosphate; Inhibits replication of retroviruses by competing with thymidine triphosphate for viral RNA-directed DNA polymerase and incorporation into DNA

Pharmacokinetics
Distribution: Penetrates into the CSF achieving 16% to 97% of concomitant plasma concentrations; distributes into extravascular spaces
Metabolism: Converted intracellularly to active triphosphate form
Bioavailability: Children: 61% to 78%; adults: 80%
Half-life, elimination: Children: 1.1 hours; adults: 1.2-1.45 hours
Time to peak serum concentration: 0.5-0.75 hours
Elimination: 24% to 57% is excreted unchanged in the urine

Usual Dosage Oral:
Neonates: Under investigation in PACTG 332
Children <30 kg: 1 mg/kg/dose every 12 hours
Adolescent and Adults:
30-59 kg: 30 mg every 12 hours
≥60 kg: 40 mg every 12 hours
Dosing adjustment in renal impairment:
Cl_{cr} 26-50 mL/minute: Decrease dose by 50% (eg, ≥60 kg: administer 20 mg every 12 hours)
Cl_{cr} <10-25 mL/minute: Decrease dose by 75% (eg, ≥60 kg: administer 20 mg every 24 hours)
Dosing adjustment in hepatic impairment: no data

Administration Oral: Administer with or without food; shake solution well before using

Monitoring Parameters Periodic CBC with differential, hemoglobin, renal function, liver enzymes, serum amylase, CD4 cell count, HIV RNA plasma levels, signs/symptoms of peripheral neuropathy

Patient Information Avoid alcohol. Stavudine is not a cure; notify physician if tingling, burning, pain, or numbness of hands or feet occurs

Dosage Forms
Capsule: 15 mg, 20 mg, 30 mg, 40 mg
Powder for oral solution: 1 mg/mL

References
Kline MW, Dunkle LM, Church JA, et al, "A Phase I/II Evaluation of Stavudine (d4T) in Children With Human Immunodeficiency Virus Infection," *Pediatrics*, 1995, 96(2 Pt 1):247-52.
Working Group on Antiretroviral Therapy and Medical Management of HIV-Infected Children, "Guidelines for the Use of Antiretroviral Agents in Pediatric HIV Infection," April 15, 1999, http://www.hivatis.org.

- ♦ **Stay Trim® Diet Gum [OTC]** *see* Phenylpropanolamine *on page 761*
- ♦ **S-T Cort® Topical** *see* Hydrocortisone *on page 486*
- ♦ **Stemetil® (Canada)** *see* Prochlorperazine *on page 803*
- ♦ **Sterapred®** *see* Prednisone *on page 794*
- ♦ **Stieva-A® (Canada)** *see* Tretinoin *on page 945*
- ♦ **Stieva-A® Forte (Canada)** *see* Tretinoin *on page 945*
- ♦ **Stimate®** *see* Desmopressin *on page 292*
- ♦ **St. Joseph® Aspirin-Free Cold Tablets for Children [OTC]** *see* Phenylpropanolamine *on page 761*
- ♦ **St. Joseph® Cough Suppressant [OTC]** *see* Dextromethorphan *on page 304*
- ♦ **St. Joseph® Measured Dose Nasal Solution [OTC]** *see* Phenylephrine *on page 758*
- ♦ **Stop® [OTC]** *see* Fluoride *on page 427*
- ♦ **Strength Motrin® [OTC]** *see* Ibuprofen *on page 501*
- ♦ **Streptase®** *see* Streptokinase *on page 881*

Streptokinase (strep toe KYE nase)

Brand Names Kabikinase®; Streptase®

Therapeutic Category Thrombolytic Agent

Generic Available No

Use Thrombolytic agent used in treatment of recent severe or massive deep vein thrombosis, pulmonary emboli, MI, and occluded arteriovenous cannulas

Pregnancy Risk Factor C

Contraindications Hypersensitivity to streptokinase or any component; recent streptococcal infection; any internal bleeding, CVA (within 2 months); brain carcinoma, intracranial or intraspinal surgery

Warnings Avoid I.M. injections

Precautions Relative contraindications: major surgery within the last 10 days, GI bleeding, recent trauma, severe hypertension

Adverse Reactions
Cardiovascular: Hypotension, arrhythmias, flushing
Central nervous system: Fever
Dermatologic: Itching, urticaria, angioneurotic edema
Hematologic: Surface bleeding, internal bleeding, cerebral hemorrhage
Neuromuscular & skeletal: Musculoskeletal pain
Respiratory: Bronchospasm

Drug Interactions Anticoagulants, antiplatelet agents, antifibrinolytic agents

Stability Store unopened vials at room temperature; store reconstituted solutions in refrigerator and use within 24 hours

Mechanism of Action Promotes thrombolysis; activates the conversion of plasminogen to plasmin by forming a complex, exposing plasminogen-activating site, and cleaving a peptide bond that converts plasminogen to plasmin; plasmin degrades fibrin, fibrinogen and other procoagulant proteins into soluble fragments; effective both outside and within the formed thrombus/embolus

Pharmacodynamics
Onset of action: Activation of plasminogen: Almost immediate
Duration:
Fibrinolytic effects: Only a few hours
Anticoagulant effects: 12-24 hours

Pharmacokinetics
Half-life, biologic: 83 minutes
Elimination: By circulating antibodies and via the reticuloendothelial system

Usual Dosage
Children: Safety and efficacy not established; limited studies have used the following doses:
Thromboses: I.V.: *Chest*, 1998 recommendations: Initial (loading dose): 2000 units/kg followed by 2000 units/kg/hour for 6-12 hours **or** initial (loading dose): 3500-4000 units/kg over 30 minutes followed by I.V. continuous infusion: 1000-1500 units/kg/hour; dose should be individualized based on response
Clotted catheter: **Note**: Not recommended due to possibility of allergic reactions with repeated doses: 10,000-25,000 units diluted in NS to a final volume equivalent to catheter volume; instill into catheter and leave in place for 1 hour, then aspirate contents out of catheter and flush catheter with NS
Adults:
Thromboses: I.V.: 250,000 units to start, then 100,000 units/hour for 24-72 hours depending on location
Cannula occlusion: 250,000 units into cannula, clamp for 2 hours, then aspirate contents out of catheter and flush with NS

Administration Parenteral: I.V.: Dilute in NS (preferred) or D_5W; maximum concentration: 1.5 million units/50 mL

Monitoring Parameters For systemic therapy: Blood pressure, TT, PTT, APTT, fibrinogen level, fibrin/fibrinogen degradation products, D-dimers, platelet count, hemoglobin, hematocrit, signs of bleeding

Nursing Implications For intravenous or intracoronary use only; avoid I.M. injections

Additional Information Best results are realized if used within 5-6 hours of MI; antibodies to streptokinase remain for 3-6 months after initial dose, use another thrombolytic enzyme (ie, urokinase) if repeat thrombolytic therapy is indicated

Failure of thrombolytic agents in newborns/neonates may occur due to the low plasminogen concentrations (~50% to 70% of adult levels); streptokinase-induced clot lysis may be more impaired than urokinase or TPA in these patients; supplementing plasminogen (via administration of fresh frozen plasma) may possibly help
(Continued)

Streptokinase *(Continued)*

Dosage Forms Powder for injection: 250,000 units (5 mL, 6.5 mL); 600,000 units (5 mL); 750,000 units (6 mL, 6.5 mL); 1,500,000 units (6.5 mL, 10 mL, 50 mL)

References

Andrew M, Brooker L, Leaker M, et al,"Fibrin Clot Lysis by Thrombolytic Agents Is Impaired in Newborns Due to a Low Plasminogen Concentration," *Thromb Haemost*, 1992, 68(3):325-30.

David M and Andrew M, "Venous Thromboembolic Complications in Children," *J Pediatr*, 1993, 123(3):337-46.

Kothari SS, Varma S, and Wasir HS, "Thrombolytic Therapy in Infants and Children," *Am Heart J*, 1994, 127(3):651-7.

Michelson AD, Bovill E, Monagle P, et al, "Antithrombotic Therapy in Children," *Chest*, 1998, 114(5 Suppl):748S-69S.

Streptomycin (strep toe MYE sin)

Related Information

Overdose and Toxicology *on page 1191*

Available Salts Streptomycin Sulfate

Therapeutic Category Antibiotic, Aminoglycoside; Antitubercular Agent

Generic Available Yes

Use Combination therapy of active tuberculosis; used in combination with other agents for treatment of streptococcal or enterococcal endocarditis, mycobacterial infections, plague, tularemia, and brucellosis

Pregnancy Risk Factor D

Contraindications Hypersensitivity to streptomycin or any component

Warnings Aminoglycosides are associated with significant nephrotoxicity or ototoxicity; the ototoxicity is directly proportional to the amount of drug given and the duration of treatment; tinnitus or vertigo are indications of vestibular injury and impending bilateral irreversible deafness; renal damage is usually reversible

Precautions Use with caution in patients with pre-existing vertigo, tinnitus, hearing loss, neuromuscular disorders, or renal impairment; modify dosage in patients with renal impairment

Adverse Reactions

Cardiovascular: Myocarditis, cardiovascular collapse

Central nervous system: Dizziness, vertigo, headache, ataxia

Dermatologic: Toxic epidermal necrolysis

Gastrointestinal: Vomiting

Hematologic: Bone marrow suppression

Neuromuscular & skeletal: Neuromuscular blockade

Otic: Ototoxicity, hearing loss

Renal: Nephrotoxicity

Miscellaneous: Hypersensitivity reactions, serum sickness

Drug Interactions Additive nephrotoxicity with acyclovir, amphotericin B, cisplatin, vancomycin; additive ototoxicity with ethacrynic acid, furosemide, urea, mannitol; potentiates neuromuscular blocking action of succinylcholine, tubocurarine

Stability Streptomycin injection should be stored in the refrigerator

Mechanism of Action Inhibits bacterial protein synthesis by binding directly to the 30S ribosomal subunits causing faulty peptide sequence to form in the protein chain

Pharmacokinetics

Distribution: Distributes into most body tissues and fluids except the brain; small amounts enter the CSF only with inflamed meninges; crosses the placenta; small amounts appear in breast milk

Protein binding: 34%

Half-life (prolonged with renal impairment):

Newborns: 4-10 hours

Adults: 2-4.7 hours

Time to peak serum concentration: I.M.: Within 1-2 hours

Elimination: 30% to 90% of dose excreted as unchanged drug in urine, with small amount (1%) excreted in bile, saliva, sweat, and tears

Usual Dosage I.M. (I.V. in patients who cannot tolerate I.M. injections):

Newborns: 10-20 mg/kg/day once daily

Infants: 20-30 mg/kg/day in divided doses every 12 hours

Children:

Tuberculosis: 20-40 mg/kg/day once daily, not to exceed 1 g/day; **or** 20-40 mg/kg/dose twice weekly under direct observation, not to exceed 1.5 g/dose; usually discontinued after 2-3 months of therapy or as soon as isoniazid and rifampin susceptibility is established

Other infections: 20-40 mg/kg/day in combination with other antibiotics divided every 6-12 hours

Plague: 30 mg/kg/day divided every 8-12 hours

Adults:

Tuberculosis: 15 mg/kg/day once daily, not to exceed 1 g/day; **or** 25-30 mg/kg/dose twice weekly under direct observation, not to exceed 1.5 g/dose

Enterococcal endocarditis: 1 g every 12 hours for 2 weeks, then 500 mg every 12 hours for 4 weeks in combination with penicillin

Streptococcal endocarditis: 1 g every 12 hours for 1 week, then 500 mg every 12 hours for 1 week

Tularemia: 1-2 g/day in divided doses for 7-10 days or until patient is afebrile for 5-7 days

Plague: 2 g/day in divided doses until the patient is afebrile for at least 3 days

Dosing adjustment in renal impairment:

Cl_{cr} 50-80 mL/minute: Administer 7.5 mg/kg/dose every 24 hours

Cl_{cr} 10-50 mL/minute: Administer 7.5 mg/kg/dose every 24-72 hours

Cl_{cr} <10 mL/minute: Administer 7.5 mg/kg/dose every 72-96 hours

Administration Parenteral:

I.M.: Inject deep I.M. into a large muscle mass; administer at a concentration not to exceed 500 mg/mL; rotate injection sites

I.V.: I.V. infusion through a peripheral or central line; 12-15 mg/kg/dose is diluted in 100 mL of NS; infuse over 30-60 minutes

Monitoring Parameters Hearing (audiogram), BUN, creatinine; serum concentration of the drug should be monitored in patients with renal impairment; eighth cranial nerve damage is usually preceded by high-pitched tinnitus, roaring noises, sense of fullness in ears, or impaired hearing and may persist for weeks after drug is discontinued

Reference Range Therapeutic serum concentrations: Peak: 15-40 µg/mL; trough: <5 µg/mL

Test Interactions False-positive urine glucose with Benedict's solution

Additional Information For use by patients with active tuberculosis that is resistant to isoniazid and rifampin or patients with active tuberculosis in areas where resistance is common and whose drug susceptibility is not yet known. Pfizer will distribute streptomycin directly to physicians and health clinics at no charge. Call Pfizer at 1-800-254-4445.

Dosage Forms Injection, as sulfate: 400 mg/mL (2.5 mL)

References

Ad Hoc Committee of the Scientific Assembly on Microbiology, Tuberculosis, and Pulmonary Infections, "Treatment of Tuberculosis and Tuberculosis Infection in Adults and Children," *Clin Infect Dis*, 1995, 21:9-27.

American Academy of Pediatrics Committee on Infectious Diseases, "Chemotherapy for Tuberculosis in Infants and Children," *Pediatrics* 1992, 89(1):161-5.

Arguedas AG and Wehrle PP, "New Concepts for Antimicrobial Use in Central Nervous System Infections," *Semin Pediatr Infect Dis*, 1991, 2(1):36-42.

Lorin MI, Hsu KH, and Jacob SC, "Treatment of Tuberculosis in Children," *Pediatr Clin North Am*, 1983, 30(2):333-48.

♦ **Streptomycin Sulfate** *see* Streptomycin *on page 882*

♦ **Strong Iodine Solution** *see* Potassium Iodide *on page 785*

♦ **Sublimaze® Injection** *see* Fentanyl *on page 406*

Succimer (SUKS i mer)

Brand Names Chemet®

Synonyms DMSA

Therapeutic Category Antidote, Lead Toxicity; Chelating Agent, Oral

Generic Available No

Use Treatment of lead poisoning in children with blood levels >45 mcg/dL; not indicated for prophylaxis of lead poisoning in a lead-containing environment

Pregnancy Risk Factor C

Contraindications Hypersensitivity to succimer or any component

Warnings Elevated blood lead levels and associated symptoms may return rapidly after discontinuation due to redistribution of lead from bone stores to soft tissues and blood; monitor blood lead levels for "rebound" after therapy

Precautions Use with caution in patients with renal or hepatic impairment; adequate hydration should be maintained during therapy

Adverse Reactions The most common events attributable to succimer have been observed in about 10% of patients treated

Central nervous system: Headache, fatigue, dizziness

Dermatologic: Rash, pruritus

Gastrointestinal: Nausea, vomiting, diarrhea, appetite loss, metallic taste, hemorrhoidal symptoms, sulfurous odor to breath, sore throat

Hematologic: Thrombocytosis, eosinophilia, reversible neutropenia

(Continued)

Succimer *(Continued)*

Hepatic: Transiently elevated AST, ALT, alkaline phosphatase, and serum cholesterol

Neuromuscular & skeletal: Paresthesia, sensorimotor neuropathy, back, rib, kneecap, and leg pains

Ocular: Watery eyes, cloudy film in eye

Renal: Sulfurous odor to urine, decreased urination, proteinuria

Respiratory: Rhinorrhea, nasal congestion

Miscellaneous: Flu-like symptoms

Drug Interactions Not recommended to be used concomitantly with edetate calcium disodium or penicillamine

Mechanism of Action Forms stable water-soluble complexes with lead resulting in increased urinary excretion; also chelates other toxic heavy metals such as arsenic and mercury

Pharmacokinetics

Absorption: Oral: Rapid, variable

Metabolism: Extensive to mixed succimer-cysteine disulfides

Half-life, elimination: 2 days

Time to peak serum concentration: ~1-2 hours

Elimination: ~25% in urine with peak urinary excretion occurring between 2-4 hours after dosing; of the total amount of succimer eliminated in urine, 90% is eliminated as mixed succimer-cysteine disulfide conjugates; 10% is excreted unchanged; fecal excretion of succimer probably represents unabsorbed drug

Usual Dosage Oral: Children and Adults: 10 mg/kg/dose (or 350 mg/m^2/dose) every 8 hours for 5 days followed by 10 mg/kg/dose (or 350 mg/m^2/dose) every 12 hours for 14 days

Note: Concomitant iron therapy has been reported in a small number of children without the formation of a toxic complex with iron (as seen with dimercaprol); courses of therapy may be repeated if indicated by weekly monitoring of blood lead levels; lead levels should be stabilized to <15 mcg/dL; 2 weeks between courses is recommended unless more timely treatment is indicated by lead levels

Dosing adjustment in renal/hepatic impairment: Administer with caution and monitor closely

Administration Oral: Ensure adequate patient hydration; for patients who cannot swallow the capsule, sprinkle the medicated beads on a small amount of soft food or administer with a fruit juice to mask the odor

Monitoring Parameters Blood lead levels, serum aminotransferases

Test Interactions Falsely elevated serum creatine phosphokinase (CPK); false-positive urine ketones with Ketostix®, falsely decreased uric acid measurements

Dosage Forms Capsule: 100 mg

References

Mann KV and Travers JD, "Succimer, An Oral Lead Chelator," *Clin Pharm*, 1991, 10(12):914-22.

Succinylcholine (suks in il KOE leen)

Brand Names Anectine®; Anectine® Chloride; Flo-Pack®; Quelicin®

Available Salts Succinylcholine Chloride

Synonyms Suxamethonium

Therapeutic Category Neuromuscular Blocker Agent, Depolarizing; Skeletal Muscle Relaxant, Paralytic

Generic Available No

Use Used to produce skeletal muscle relaxation in procedures of short duration such as endotracheal intubation or endoscopic exams

Pregnancy Risk Factor C

Contraindications Hypersensitivity to succinylcholine chloride or any component; history of decreased concentrations and/or decreased activity of plasma pseudocholinesterase; malignant hyperthermia; myopathies associated with elevated serum creatinine values; narrow-angle glaucoma; penetrating eye injuries

Warnings Malignant hyperthermia may be triggered by succinylcholine use; monitor closely for signs/symptoms; some products contain benzyl alcohol; avoid use in neonates

Precautions As rare reports of acute rhabdomyolysis with hyperkalemia followed by ventricular dysrhythmias, cardiac arrest, and death have been reported in children with undiagnosed skeletal muscle myopathy, use with caution in patients recovering from severe trauma; use with caution in patients with pre-existing hyperkalemia, paraplegia, extensive or severe burns, extensive denervation of skeletal muscle because of disease or injury to the CNS or with degenerative or dystrophic neuromuscular disease

Adverse Reactions

Cardiovascular: Bradycardia, hypotension, cardiac arrhythmias, flushing, cardiac arrest, hypertension, tachycardia

Central nervous system: Malignant hyperthermia

Dermatologic: Rash

Endocrine & metabolic: Hyperkalemia, myoglobinemia

Gastrointestinal: Increased intragastric pressure, salivation

Neuromuscular & skeletal: Myalgia due to muscle fasciculations, muscle weakness

Ocular: Increased intraocular pressure

Renal: Myoglobinuria

Respiratory: Apnea, bronchospasm, respiratory depression

Drug Interactions Decreased neuromuscular blockade with diazepam; increased neuromuscular blockade with promazine, cyclophosphamide, oral contraceptives, glucocorticoids, MAO inhibitors, oxytocin, phenothiazines, quinidine, beta-blocking agents, procainamide, lidocaine, lithium, trimethaphan, furosemide, magnesium, chloroquine, acetylcholine, anticholinesterases, amphotericin B, and thiazide diuretics (due to electrolyte imbalances); cyclophosphamide, aminoglycosides, clindamycin may increase bradycardia; narcotic analgesics and inhalation anesthetics may increase the risk of sinus arrest; increased arrhythmias with digoxin (due to potassium changes)

Stability Both injections are incompatible with alkaline solutions

Liquid injection: Store in refrigerator; stable for 14 days at room temperature

Powder for injection: Store at room temperature; after reconstitution, chemical stability is maintained for 4 weeks refrigerated, 1 week at room temperature; due to lack of preservative, the manufacturer recommends using within 24 hours of reconstitution

Mechanism of Action Acts similarly to acetylcholine, produces depolarization of the motor endplate at the myoneural junction which causes sustained flaccid skeletal muscle paralysis

Pharmacodynamics

I.M.:

Onset of effect: 2-3 minutes

Duration: 10-30 minutes

I.V.:

Onset of action: Within 30-60 seconds

Duration: ~4-6 minutes

Pharmacokinetics

Metabolism: Succinylcholine is rapidly hydrolyzed by plasma pseudocholinesterase

Elimination: 10% excreted unchanged in urine

Usual Dosage

Children:

I.M.: 2.5-4 mg/kg (maximum dose: 150 mg)

I.V.: Initial: 1-2 mg/kg; maintenance: 0.3-0.6 mg/kg every 5-10 minutes as needed; because of the risk of malignant hyperthermia, use of continuous infusions is **not** recommended in infants and children

Adults: I.M., I.V.: 0.6 mg/kg (range: 0.3-1.1 mg/kg), up to 150 mg total dose; maintenance: 0.04-0.07 mg/kg every 5-10 minutes as needed

Continuous infusion: 2.5 mg/minute (range: 0.5-10 mg/minute)

Note: Pretreatment with atropine may reduce occurrence of bradycardia

Dosing adjustment in hepatic impairment: Dose should be decreased in patients with severe liver disease

Administration Parenteral: I.V.: May be administered by rapid I.V. injection without further dilution; I.M.: Injection should be made deeply

Monitoring Parameters Heart rate, serum potassium, assisted ventilator status, peripheral nerve stimulator measuring twitch response

Dosage Forms

Injection, as chloride: 20 mg/mL (10 mL); 50 mg/mL (10 mL); 100 mg/mL (5 mL, 10 mL, 20 mL)

Powder for injection, as chloride: 100 mg, 500 mg, 1 g

♦ **Succinylcholine Chloride** see Succinylcholine on page 884

♦ **Sucraid®** see Sacrosidase on page 853

Sucralfate (soo KRAL fate)

Related Information

Carbohydrate and Alcohol Content of Liquid Medications for Use in Patients Receiving Ketogenic Diets *on page 1228*

Brand Names Carafate®; Novo-Sucralate® (Canada); Sulcrate® (Canada); Sulcrate® Suspension Plus (Canada)

Synonyms Aluminum Sucrose Sulfate, Basic

Therapeutic Category Gastrointestinal Agent, Gastric or Duodenal Ulcer Treatment

Generic Available No

Use Short-term management of duodenal ulcers

Unlabeled uses: Gastric ulcers; suspension may be used topically for treatment of stomatitis due to cancer chemotherapy or other causes of esophageal and gastric erosions; treatment of NSAID mucosal damage; prevention of stress ulcers

Pregnancy Risk Factor B

Contraindications Hypersensitivity to sucralfate or any component

Warnings Because of the potential for sucralfate to alter the absorption of some drugs, separate administration times (administer other medications 2 hours before or after sucralfate) should be considered when alterations in bioavailability are believed to be critical

Precautions Use with caution in renal failure due to accumulation of aluminum

Adverse Reactions

Cardiovascular: Facial edema

Central nervous system: Dizziness, sleepiness, vertigo, headache

Dermatologic: Rash, pruritus, angioedema

Gastrointestinal: Constipation, diarrhea, nausea, gastric discomfort, indigestion, xerostomia, flatulence

Neuromuscular & skeletal: Back pain

Respiratory: Laryngospasm, rhinitis, respiratory difficulty

Drug Interactions Absorption of orally administered tetracycline, phenytoin, ketoconazole, quinidine, ranitidine, colistin, gentamicin, amphotericin B, sodium and potassium phosphate salts, digoxin, sustained release theophylline, quinolones, and cimetidine may be decreased (separate administration by 2 hours); aluminum-containing antacids may increase total body burden of aluminum; antacids, cimetidine, and ranitidine when administered concomitantly may decrease sucralfate's activity (gastric acidity is required for sucralfate to form its protective barrier)

Food Interactions Interferes with absorption of vitamin A, vitamin D, vitamin E, and vitamin K

Mechanism of Action Aluminum salt of sulfated sucrose which in the presence of acid pH (gastric acid) forms a complex, paste-like substance that adheres to the damaged mucosal area. This selectively forms a protective coating that protects the lining against peptic acid, pepsin, and bile salts.

Pharmacodynamics GI protection effect:

Onset of action: 1-2 hours

Duration: Up to 6 hours

Pharmacokinetics

Absorption: Oral: <5%

Metabolism: Not metabolized

Elimination: 90% excreted in stool; small amounts that are absorbed are excreted in the urine as unchanged compounds

Usual Dosage Oral:

Children: Dose not established; doses of 40-80 mg/kg/day divided every 6 hours have been used

Stomatitis: 5-10 mL (1 g/10 mL); swish and spit or swish and swallow 4 times/day

Adults:

Stress ulcer prophylaxis: 1 g 4 times/day

Stress ulcer treatment: 1 g every 4 hours

Duodenal ulcer:

Treatment: 1 g 4 times/day for 4-8 weeks, or alternatively 2 g twice daily; treatment is recommended for 4-8 weeks in adults

Maintenance: Prophylaxis: 1 g twice daily

Stomatitis: 1 g/10 mL suspension, swish and spit or swish and swallow 4 times/day

Dosage comment in renal impairment: Aluminum salt is minimally absorbed (<5%), however, may accumulate in renal failure

Administration Oral: Administer on an empty stomach 1 hour before meals and at bedtime (see Warnings); tablet may be broken or dissolved in water before ingestion; do not administer antacids within 30 minutes of administration; shake suspension well before use

Additional Information There is approximately 14-16 mEq acid neutralizing capacity per 1g sucralfate

Dosage Forms

Suspension, oral: 1 g/10 mL (420 mL)

Tablet: 1 g

♦ **Sucrets® [OTC]** *see Dyclonine on page 355*

♦ **Sucrets® Cough Calmers [OTC]** *see Dextromethorphan on page 304*

♦ **Sudafed® [OTC]** *see Pseudoephedrine on page 822*

♦ **Sudafed® 12 Hour [OTC]** *see Pseudoephedrine on page 822*

♦ **Sufedrin® [OTC]** *see Pseudoephedrine on page 822*

♦ **Sufenta® Injection** *see Sufentanil on page 887*

Sufentanil (soo FEN ta nil)

Related Information

Overdose and Toxicology *on page 1191*

Brand Names Sufenta® Injection

Available Salts Sufentanil Citrate

Therapeutic Category Analgesic, Narcotic; General Anesthetic

Generic Available No

Use Analgesia; analgesia adjunct; anesthetic agent

Restrictions C-II

Pregnancy Risk Factor C

Contraindications Hypersensitivity to sufentanil or any component; increased intracranial pressure; severe respiratory depression

Warnings May cause severe respiratory depression; rapid I.V. infusion may result in skeletal muscle and chest wall rigidity → impaired ventilation → respiratory distress, apnea, bronchoconstriction, laryngospasm, arrest; inject slowly over 3-5 minutes; nondepolarizing skeletal muscle relaxant may be required

Precautions Use with caution in patients with head injuries, hepatic impairment, pulmonary disease, or with use of MAO inhibitors within past 14 days; sufentanil shares the toxic potential of opiate agonists, precautions of opiate agonist therapy should be observed

Adverse Reactions

Cardiovascular: Bradycardia, hypotension, peripheral vasodilation

Central nervous system: CNS depression, drowsiness, dizziness, sedation

Dermatologic: Erythema, pruritus, rash

Endocrine & metabolic: ADH release

Gastrointestinal: Nausea, vomiting, constipation, biliary tract spasm

Genitourinary: Urinary tract spasm

Neuromuscular & skeletal: Skeletal and thoracic muscle rigidity, especially after rapid I.V. administration

Ocular: Miosis, blurred vision

Respiratory: Respiratory depression, apnea

Miscellaneous: Physical and psychological dependence with prolonged use

Drug Interactions Cytochrome P-450 isoenzyme CYP3A3/4 substrate

CNS depressants, phenothiazines, MAO inhibitors, tricyclic antidepressants may potentiate adverse effects of opiates; beta-blocker therapy may potentiate sufentanil bradycardia

Mechanism of Action Binds with stereospecific receptors at many sites within the CNS, increases pain threshold, alters pain reception, inhibits ascending pain pathways; ultra short-acting narcotic

Pharmacodynamics

Onset of action: 1-3 minutes

Duration: Dose dependent; anesthesia adjunct doses: 5 minutes

Pharmacokinetics

Distribution: V_{dss}:

Children 2-8 years: 2.9 ± 0.6 L/kg

Adults: 1.7 ± 0.2 L/kg

Protein binding (alpha$_1$-acid glycoprotein):

Neonates: 79%

Adults:

Male: 93%

Postpartum women: 91%

(Continued)

Sufentanil *(Continued)*

Metabolism: Primarily by the liver via demethylation and dealkylation

Half-life, elimination:
Neonates: 382-1162 minutes
Children 2-8 years: 97 ± 42 minutes
Adolescents 10-15 years: 76 ± 33 minutes
Adults: 164 ± 22 minutes

Elimination: ~2% excreted unchanged in the urine; 80% of dose excreted in urine (mostly as metabolites) within 24 hours

Clearance:
Children 2-8 years: 30.5 ± 8.8 mL/minute/kg
Adolescents: 12.8 ± 12 mL/minute/kg
Adults: 12.7 ± 0.8 mL/minute/kg

Usual Dosage Doses should be titrated to appropriate effects; wide range of doses, dependent upon desired degree of analgesia or anesthesia; use lean body weight to dose patients who are >20% above ideal body weight

Children <12 years: Anesthesia: I.V.: Initial: 10-25 mcg/kg; maintenance: Up to 25-50 mcg as needed

Adults: I.V.:
Adjunct to general anesthesia:
Low dose: Initial: 0.5-1 mcg/kg; maintenance: 10-25 mcg as needed
Moderate dose: Initial: 2-8 mcg/kg; maintenance: 10-50 mcg as needed
Anesthesia: Initial: 8-30 mcg/kg; maintenance: 10-50 mcg as needed

Administration Parenteral: I.V.: Slow I.V. injection or by infusion

Monitoring Parameters Respiratory rate, blood pressure, heart rate, oxygen saturation, neurological status (for degree of analgesia/anesthesia)

Nursing Implications Patient may develop rebound respiratory depression postoperatively

Dosage Forms Injection, as citrate: 50 mcg/mL (1 mL, 2 mL, 5 mL)

References

Guay J, Gaudreault P, Tang A, et al, "Pharmacokinetics of Sufentanil in Normal Children," *Can J Anaesth*, 1992, 39(1):14-20.

Seguin JH, Erenberg A, and Leff RD, "Safety and Efficacy of Sufentanil Therapy in the Ventilated Infant," *Neonatal Netw*, 1994, 13(4):37-40.

♦ **Sufentanil Citrate** *see Sufentanil on page 887*

♦ **Sulbactam and Ampicillin** *see Ampicillin and Sulbactam on page 81*

♦ **Sulcrate® (Canada)** *see Sucralfate on page 886*

♦ **Sulcrate® Suspension Plus (Canada)** *see Sucralfate on page 886*

♦ **Sulf-10®** *see Sulfacetamide on page 888*

Sulfacetamide *(sul fa SEE ta mide)*

Brand Names AK-Sulf®; Bleph®-10; Cetamide®; I-Sulfacet®; Ophthacet®; Sodium Sulamyd®; Sulf-10®; Sulfair®; Sulfex® 10% (Canada)

Available Salts Sodium Sulfacetamide; Sulfacetamide Sodium

Therapeutic Category Antibiotic, Ophthalmic; Antibiotic, Sulfonamide Derivative

Generic Available Yes

Use Treatment and prophylaxis of conjunctivitis, corneal ulcers, and other superficial ocular infections due to susceptible organisms; adjunctive treatment with systemic sulfonamides for therapy of trachoma

Pregnancy Risk Factor C

Contraindications Hypersensitivity to sulfacetamide, any component, or sulfonamides; infants <2 months of age; epithelial herpes simplex keratitis, vaccinia, varicella, and other viral diseases of the cornea and conjunctiva; fungal diseases of the ocular structures

Warnings Antibacterial activity may be decreased in the presence of purulent exudates containing para-aminobenzoic acid (PABA); nonsusceptible organisms such as fungi may proliferate with prolonged or repeated use of sulfonamide preparations; hemolysis may occur in patients with G-6-PD deficiency

Precautions Use with caution in patients with severe dry eye or G-6-PD deficiency

Adverse Reactions

Central nervous system: Headache, fever

Dermatologic: Stevens-Johnson syndrome, exfoliative dermatitis, toxic epidermal necrolysis, rash, photosensitivity

Hematologic: Bone marrow suppression

Local: Irritation, stinging and burning (especially with 30% solution), itching

Ocular: Blurred vision, transient epithelial keratitis, reactive hyperemia, conjunctival edema

Miscellaneous: Hypersensitivity reactions, syndrome resembling systemic lupus erythematosus

Drug Interactions Silver, gentamicin (antagonism)

Stability Protect from light; discolored or cloudy solutions should not be used; incompatible with silver and zinc sulfate; sulfacetamide is inactivated by blood or purulent exudates

Mechanism of Action Interferes with bacterial growth by inhibiting bacterial folic acid synthesis through competitive antagonism of PABA

Pharmacodynamics Onset of action: Improvement of conjunctivitis is usually seen within 3-6 days

Pharmacokinetics
Distribution: Excreted in breast milk
Half-life: 7-13 hours
Elimination: When absorbed, excreted primarily in urine as unchanged drug

Usual Dosage Children >2 months and Adults: Ophthalmic:
Ointment: Apply to lower conjunctival sac 1-4 times/day and at bedtime or apply ½" to 1" into the conjunctival sac at night in conjunction with the use of drops during the day
Solution: Instill 1-2 drops into the lower conjunctival sac every 1-3 hours according to severity of infection during the waking hours and less frequently at night; **Note:** 30% solution is used for more severe infections
Trachoma (30% solution): 2 drops every 2 hours (concomitant use of systemic sulfonamide therapy is recommended)

Administration Ophthalmic: Avoid contact of tube or bottle tip with skin or eye

Monitoring Parameters Response to therapy

Patient Information Eye drops may burn and sting when first instilled; may cause sensitivity to bright light

Dosage Forms Ophthalmic, as sodium:
Ointment: 10% (3.5 g, 3.75 g)
Solution: 10% (1 mL, 2 mL, 2.5 mL, 3.75 mL, 5 mL, 15 mL); 15% (2 mL, 5 mL, 15 mL); 30% (5 mL, 15 mL)

References
Lohr JA, Austin RD, Grossman M, et al, "Comparison of Three Topical Antimicrobials for Acute Bacterial Conjunctivitis," *Pediatr Infect Dis J*, 1988, 7(9):626-9.

♦ **Sulfacetamide Sodium** *see* Sulfacetamide *on page 888*

Sulfadiazine (sul fa DYE a zeen)

Brand Names Coptin® (Canada)

Therapeutic Category Antibiotic, Sulfonamide Derivative

Generic Available Yes

Use Adjunctive treatment in toxoplasmosis; treatment of urinary tract infections and nocardiosis; rheumatic fever prophylaxis in penicillin-allergic patient; uncomplicated attack of malaria

Pregnancy Risk Factor B (D at term)

Contraindications Porphyria; hypersensitivity to any sulfa drug or any component; infants <2 months of age due to competition with bilirubin for protein-binding sites (unless indicated for the treatment of congenital toxoplasmosis); pregnant women during third trimester

Precautions Use with caution in patients with impaired hepatic function or impaired renal function, urinary obstruction, blood dyscrasia, G-6-PD deficiency; dosage modification required in patients with renal impairment

Adverse Reactions
Cardiovascular: Vasculitis
Central nervous system: Dizziness, fever, headache
Dermatologic: Rash, exfoliative dermatitis, Stevens-Johnson syndrome, photosensitivity, urticaria
Gastrointestinal: Nausea, vomiting, abdominal pain
Genitourinary: Crystalluria
Hematologic: Granulocytopenia, leukopenia, thrombocytopenia, aplastic anemia, hemolytic anemia
Hepatic: Jaundice, hepatitis
Renal: Acute nephropathy, hematuria
Miscellaneous: Serum sickness-like reactions

Drug Interactions PABA, procaine; tetracaine antagonizes antibacterial action of sulfonamides; paraldehyde increases potential for crystalluria; displaces agents from protein binding sites: coumarin anticoagulants increase bleeding, MTX increases toxicity, sulfonylurea antidiabetic agents (hypoglycemia) (Continued)

Sulfadiazine *(Continued)*

Food Interactions Supplemental folinic acid should be administered to reverse symptoms or prevent problems due to folic acid deficiency; avoid large quantities of vitamin C or acidifying agents (cranberry juice) to prevent crystalluria

Stability Protect from light

Mechanism of Action Interferes with bacterial growth by inhibiting bacterial folic acid synthesis through competitive antagonism of PABA

Pharmacokinetics

Absorption: Oral: Well absorbed

Distribution: Excreted in breast milk; diffuses into CSF with higher concentrations reached when meninges are inflamed; distributed into most body tissues

Protein binding: 32% to 56%

Metabolism: Metabolized by N-acetylation

Half-life: 10 hours

Time to peak serum concentration: Within 4 hours

Elimination: In urine as metabolites (15% to 40%) and as unchanged drug (43% to 60%)

Usual Dosage Oral:

Congenital toxoplasmosis: Newborns: 100 mg/kg/day divided every 12 hours for 12 months in conjunction with pyrimethamine 1 mg/kg/day once daily and supplemental folinic acid 5 mg every 3 days for first 6 months, then pyrimethamine 1 mg/kg/day 3 times/week and folinic acid 10 mg 3 times/week for the next 6 months

Toxoplasmosis:

Children: 120-200 mg/kg/day divided every 6 hours in conjunction with pyrimethamine 2 mg/kg/day divided every 12 hours for 3 days followed by 1 mg/kg/day once daily (maximum dose: 25 mg/day) with supplemental folinic acid 5-10 mg every 3 days

Adults: 2-8 g/day divided every 6 hours in conjunction with pyrimethamine 25 mg/day and with supplemental folinic acid 5-10 mg every 3 days

Prophylaxis of recurrent rheumatic fever:

≤30 kg: 500 mg once daily

>30 kg: 1 g once daily

Administration Oral: Administer with water on an empty stomach

Monitoring Parameters CBC, renal function tests, urinalysis

Patient Information Drink plenty of fluids; avoid prolonged exposure to sunlight; limit alcohol; notify physician if rash, sore throat, fever, arthralgia, shortness of breath, or jaundice occurs

Dosage Forms Tablet: 500 mg

Extemporaneous Preparations Tablets may be crushed to prepare oral suspension of the drug in water or with a sucrose-containing solution; aqueous suspension with concentrations of 100 mg/mL should be stored in the refrigerator and used within 7 days

References

Frenkel JK, "Toxoplasmosis," *Pediatr Clin North Am*, 1985, 32(4):917-32.

Sulfadoxine and Pyrimethamine

(sul fa DOKS een & peer i METH a meen)

Brand Names Fansidar®

Synonyms Pyrimethamine and Sulfadoxine

Therapeutic Category Antimalarial Agent

Generic Available No

Use Treatment of *Plasmodium falciparum* malaria in patients in whom chloroquine resistance is suspected; malaria prophylaxis for travelers to areas where chloroquine-resistant malaria is endemic

Pregnancy Risk Factor C

Contraindications Hypersensitivity to any sulfa drug, pyrimethamine, or any component; porphyria, megaloblastic anemia, severe renal insufficiency; children <2 months of age due to competition with bilirubin for protein binding sites; pregnant women at term; do not use for treatment of malaria acquired in Southeast Asia or the Amazon Basin since resistance to sulfadoxine and pyrimethamine has been reported

Warnings Fatalities associated with sulfonamides, although rare, have occurred due to severe reactions including Stevens-Johnson syndrome, toxic epidermal necrolysis, hepatic necrosis, agranulocytosis, aplastic anemia and other blood dyscrasias; discontinue use at first sign of rash or any sign of adverse reaction; hemolysis may occur in patients with G-6-PD deficiency

Precautions Use with caution in patients with renal or hepatic impairment, patients with possible folate deficiency, patients with bronchial asthma, and patients with seizure disorders

Adverse Reactions

Cardiovascular: Vasculitis

Central nervous system: Seizures, headache, insomnia, ataxia, fatigue, hyperesthesia

Dermatologic: Erythema multiforme, Stevens-Johnson syndrome, toxic epidermal necrolysis, rash, photosensitivity, urticaria, pruritus

Endocrine & metabolic: Folic acid deficiency

Gastrointestinal: Anorexia, vomiting, gastritis, glossitis, diarrhea, abdominal cramps

Hematologic: Megaloblastic anemia, leukopenia, thrombocytopenia, pancytopenia, agranulocytosis, pulmonary eosinophilia

Hepatic: Hepatic necrosis; jaundice; elevated ALT, AST

Neuromuscular & skeletal: Tremor

Respiratory: Respiratory failure

Drug Interactions Para-aminobenzoic acid, folic acid

Stability Protect from light

Mechanism of Action Sulfadoxine interferes with bacterial folic acid synthesis and growth via competitive inhibition of para-aminiobenzoic acid; pyrimethamine inhibits microbial dihydrofolate reductase, resulting in inhibition of tetrahydrofolic acid synthesis

Pharmacokinetics

Absorption: Oral: Well absorbed

Distribution: Excreted in breast milk; pyrimethamine is distributed to kidneys, lungs, liver, and spleen; sulfadoxine is widely distributed in the body

Protein binding:

Pyrimethamine: 80% to 87%

Sulfadoxine: 90% to 95%

Half-life:

Pyrimethamine: 111 hours

Sulfadoxine: 169 hours

Time to peak serum concentration: Within 2-8 hours

Elimination: In urine as parent compounds and several unidentified metabolites

Usual Dosage Children ≥ 2 months and Adults: Oral:

Treatment of acute attack of malaria: A single dose of the following number of Fansidar® tablets is used in sequence with quinine on last day of quinine therapy:

2-11 months: $\frac{1}{4}$ tablet

1-3 years: $\frac{1}{2}$ tablet

4-8 years: 1 tablet

9-14 years: 2 tablets

>14 years: 3 tablets

Adults: 3 tablets on last day of quinine therapy

Malaria prophylaxis (for areas where chloroquine-resistant *P. falciparum* exists):

Short-term travel (≤3 weeks): Travelers should carry pyrimethamine-sulfadoxine for use as presumptive self-treatment if a febrile illness develops while taking chloroquine for prophylaxis. Take single dose in the event of febrile illness when medical attention is not immediately available:

2-11 months: $\frac{1}{4}$ tablet

1-3 years: $\frac{1}{2}$ tablet

4-8 years: 1 tablet

9-14 years: 2 tablets

>14 years and Adults: 3 tablets

Administration Oral: Administer with meals

Monitoring Parameters Liver function tests, CBC including platelet counts, renal function tests and urinalysis should be performed periodically

Patient Information Drink plenty of fluids; avoid prolonged exposure to the sun; notify physician if rash, sore throat, pallor, glossitis, fever, arthralgia, cough, shortness of breath, or jaundice occurs; limit alcohol

Additional Information Leucovorin should be administered to reverse signs and symptoms of folic acid deficiency

Dosage Forms Tablet: Sulfadoxine 500 mg and pyrimethamine 25 mg (25s)

References

Lynk A and Gold R, "Review of 40 Children With Imported Malaria," *Pediatr Infect Dis J*, 1989, 8(11):745-50.

Randall G and Seidel JS, "Malaria," *Pediatr Clin North Am*, 1985, 32(4):893-916.

- **Sulfair®** *see* Sulfacetamide *on page 888*
- **Sulfalax® [OTC]** *see* Docusate *on page 336*
- **Sulfamethoprim®** *see* Co-Trimoxazole *on page 258*

Sulfamethoxazole (sul fa meth OKS a zole)

Brand Names Apo®-Sulfamethoxazole (Canada); Gantanol®; Urobak®

Therapeutic Category Antibiotic, Sulfonamide Derivative

Generic Available Yes: Tablet

Use Treatment of urinary tract infections, nocardiosis, chlamydial infections, toxoplasmosis, acute otitis media, and acute exacerbations of chronic bronchitis due to susceptible organisms

Pregnancy Risk Factor B (D at term)

Contraindications Porphyria; hypersensitivity to sulfa drug or any component; infants <2 months of age (sulfas compete with bilirubin for protein binding sites which may result in kernicterus in newborns); pregnant women during third trimester

Warnings Should not be used for group A beta-hemolytic streptococcal infections

Precautions Maintain adequate fluid intake to prevent crystalluria; use with caution in patients with renal or hepatic impairment, patients with G-6-PD deficiency, and in patients with urinary obstruction

Adverse Reactions

Cardiovascular: Vasculitis

Central nervous system: Dizziness, fever, headache, vertigo, disorientation

Dermatologic: Rash, exfoliative dermatitis, Stevens-Johnson syndrome, photosensitivity

Gastrointestinal: Nausea, vomiting, anorexia, stomatitis, pseudomembranous colitis

Genitourinary: Crystalluria

Hematologic: Granulocytopenia, leukopenia, thrombocytopenia, aplastic anemia, hemolytic anemia, neutropenia

Hepatic: Jaundice, hepatitis

Renal: Acute nephropathy

Miscellaneous: Serum sickness-like reactions

Drug Interactions Warfarin, sulfonylurea antidiabetic agents, methotrexate, (displaces sulfonylureas, warfarin, and methotrexate from protein binding sites)

Food Interactions Avoid large quantities of vitamin C or acidifying agents (cranberry juice) to prevent crystalluria; presence of food delays but does not reduce absorption

Stability Protect from light

Mechanism of Action Interferes with bacterial growth by inhibiting bacterial folic acid synthesis through competitive antagonism of PABA

Pharmacokinetics

Absorption: Oral: 70% to 90%

Distribution: Crosses the placenta; widely distributed into most body tissues

Protein binding: 50% to 70%

Metabolism: Primarily in the liver to a N-acetylated metabolite (inactive but contributes to nephrotoxicity) and a N-glucuronide conjugate

Half-life: 7-12 hours, prolonged with renal impairment

Time to peak serum concentration: Within 3-4 hours

Elimination: Unchanged drug (20%) and its metabolites are excreted in urine Moderately dialyzable (20% to 50%)

Usual Dosage Oral:

Children ≥2 months: Initial: 50-60 mg/kg/dose one time, followed by 50-60 mg/kg/day divided every 12 hours, not to exceed 75 mg/kg/day or a maximum dose: 3 g/24 hours

Adults: 2 g stat, followed by 1 g 2-3 times/day; maximum dose: 3 g/24 hours

Dosing adjustment in renal impairment:

Cl$_{cr}$ 10-30 mL/minute: Decrease usual dose by 50%

Cl$_{cr}$ <10 mL/minute: Decrease usual dose by 75%

Administration Oral: Administer with a glass of water on an empty stomach; shake suspension well before use

Monitoring Parameters CBC, UA, renal function test

Patient Information Report to physician any sore throat, mouth sores, rash, jaundice, unusual bleeding or fever; drink plenty of fluids; avoid vitamin C products; avoid prolonged exposure to sunlight

Dosage Forms

Suspension, oral (cherry flavor): 500 mg/5 mL (480 mL)

Tablet: 500 mg

♦ **Sulfamethoxazole and Trimethoprim** *see* Co-Trimoxazole *on page 258*

♦ **Sulfamylon®** *see* Mafenide *on page 587*

Sulfasalazine (sul fa SAL a zeen)

Related Information

Drugs and Breast-Feeding *on page 1213*

Brand Names Apo®-Sulfasalazine (Canada); Azulfidine®; Azulfidine® EN-tabs®; PMS-Sulfasalazine (Canada); Salazopyrin® (Canada); Salazopyrin EN-Tabs® (Canada); S.A.S™ (Canada)

Synonyms Salicylazosulfapyridine

Therapeutic Category 5-Aminosalicylic Acid Derivative; Anti-inflammatory Agent

Generic Available Yes

Use Management of ulcerative colitis; treatment of active Crohn's disease and juvenile rheumatoid arthritis

Pregnancy Risk Factor B (D at term)

Contraindications Hypersensitivity to sulfasalazine, sulfa drugs, or any component; porphyria, GI or GU obstruction; hypersensitivity to salicylates; children <2 years of age

Precautions Use with caution in patients with renal impairment, G-6-PD deficiency, blood dyscrasias, or bronchial asthma

Adverse Reactions Incidence of adverse effects increase with dosage >4 g/day and in slow acetylators of sulfapyridine

Cardiovascular: Vasculitis

Central nervous system: Headache, fever, convulsions, vertigo, malaise, mood changes

Dermatologic: Rash, toxic epidermal necrolysis, urticaria, Stevens-Johnson syndrome, photosensitivity, staining of skin (orange-yellow)

Gastrointestinal: Nausea, vomiting, diarrhea, pancreatitis, anorexia

Genitourinary: Crystalluria, infertility (oligospermia), discoloration of urine (orange-yellow)

Hematologic: Hemolytic anemia, agranulocytosis, neutropenia, leukopenia

Hepatic: Elevated liver enzymes, jaundice, cholestatic jaundice, cirrhosis, liver necrosis/failure

Otic: Tinnitus

Renal: Nephrotoxicity

Respiratory: Fibrosing alveolitis, pulmonary eosinophilia

Miscellaneous: Serum sickness-like reaction

Drug Interactions

Decreased effect of iron, digoxin, folic acid, and PABA or PABA metabolites of drugs (ie, procaine, proparacaine, tetracaine)

Increased effect of oral anticoagulants, methotrexate, and oral hypoglycemic agents (as with other sulfa drugs)

Food Interactions Need to increase dietary intake of iron; since sulfasalazine impairs folate absorption, consider providing 1 mg/day folate supplement

Mechanism of Action Acts locally in the colon to decrease the inflammatory response and interfere with secretion by inhibiting prostaglandin synthesis; therapeutic effect may result from antibacterial action with change in intestinal flora

Pharmacodynamics

Onset for JRA: minimum trial of 3 months is necessary;

Onset for ulcerative colitis: >3-4 weeks

Pharmacokinetics

Absorption: Oral: 10% to 15% as unchanged drug from the small intestine; upon administration, the drug is split into sulfapyridine and 5-aminosalicylic acid (5-ASA) in the colon

Distribution: Breast milk to plasma ratio: 0.09-0.17

Metabolism: Both components are metabolized in the liver; slow acetylators have higher plasma sulfapyridine concentrations

Half-life:

Sulfasalazine:

Single dose: 5.7 hours

Multiple doses: 7.6 hours

Sulfapyridine:

Single dose: 8.4 hours

Multiple doses: 10.4 hours

Time to peak serum concentration:

Serum sulfasalazine: Within 1.5-6 hours

Serum sulfapyridine (active metabolite): Within 6-24 hours

(Continued)

Sulfasalazine *(Continued)*

Elimination: Primarily in urine (as unchanged drug, components, and acetylated metabolites); small amounts appear in feces

Usual Dosage Oral:

Children ≥2 years:

Ulcerative colitis:

Mild exacerbation: 40-50 mg/kg/day divided every 6 hours

Moderate-severe exacerbation: 50-75 mg/kg/day divided every 4-6 hours, not to exceed 6 g/day

Maintenance dose: 30-50 mg/kg/day divided every 4-8 hours; not to exceed 2 g/day

Juvenile rheumatoid arthritis (JRA): Initial: 10 mg/kg/day; increase weekly by 10 mg/kg/day; usual dose: 30-50 mg/kg/day in 2 divided doses; maximum dose: 2 g/day

Adults: 1 g 3-4 times/day divided every 4-6 hours, not to exceed 6 g/day; maintenance: 2 g/day divided every 6-12 hours

Administration Oral: Administer after meals or with food; do not administer with antacids

Monitoring Parameters Stool frequency, hematocrit, reticulocyte count, CBC, urinalysis, renal function tests, liver function tests

Patient Information Maintain adequate fluid intake; may cause orange-yellow discoloration of urine and skin; may stain soft contact lenses yellow; avoid prolonged exposure to sunlight

Additional Information Good response to sulfasalazine for JRA is most likely to occur in HLA B27-positive boys who are older than 9 years of age at onset of arthritis

Dosage Forms

Tablet: 500 mg

Tablet, enteric coated: 500 mg

References

American College of Rheumatology Ad Hoc Committee on Clinical Guidelines, "Guidelines for the Management of Rheumatoid Arthritis," *Arthritis Rheum*, 1996, 39(5):713-22.

Giannini EH and Cawkwell GD, "Drug Treatment in Children With Juvenile Rheumatoid Arthritis," *Pediatr Clin North Am*, 1995, 42(5):1099-125.

Kirschner BS, "Inflammatory Bowel Disease in Children," *Pediatr Clin North Am*, 1988, 35(1):189-208.

♦ **Sulfatrim®** *see* Co-Trimoxazole *on page 258*

♦ **Sulfatrim® DS** *see* Co-Trimoxazole *on page 258*

♦ **Sulfex® 10% (Canada)** *see* Sulfacetamide *on page 888*

♦ **Sulfimycin®** *see* Erythromycin and Sulfisoxazole *on page 382*

Sulfisoxazole *(sul fi SOKS a zole)*

Related Information

Carbohydrate and Alcohol Content of Liquid Medications for Use in Patients Receiving Ketogenic Diets *on page 1228*

Brand Names Gantrisin®; Novo-Soxazole® (Canada); Sulfizole® (Canada)

Available Salts Sulfisoxazole Acetyl; Sulfisoxazole Diolamine

Synonyms Sulphafurazole

Therapeutic Category Antibiotic, Sulfonamide Derivative

Generic Available Yes

Use Treatment of uncomplicated urinary tract infections, otitis media, *Chlamydia*; nocardiosis; treatment of acute pelvic inflammatory disease in prepubertal children

Pregnancy Risk Factor B (D at term)

Contraindications Hypersensitivity to any sulfa drug or any component; porphyria; infants <2 months of age (sulfas compete with bilirubin for protein binding sites which may result in kernicterus in newborns); patients with urinary obstruction; pregnant women during third trimester; nursing mothers

Precautions Use with caution in patients with G-6-PD deficiency (hemolysis may occur), hepatic or renal impairment; dosage modification required in patients with renal impairment; risk of crystalluria should be considered in patients with impaired renal function

Adverse Reactions

Cardiovascular: Vasculitis

Central nervous system: Dizziness, headache, fever, vertigo, disorientation

Dermatologic: Rash, Stevens-Johnson syndrome, photosensitivity, exfoliative dermatitis

Gastrointestinal: Nausea, vomiting, anorexia, stomatitis, pseudomembranous colitis

Genitourinary: Crystalluria (rare)

Hematologic: Thrombocytopenia, leukopenia, agranulocytosis, aplastic anemia, hemolytic anemia, neutropenia

Hepatic: Jaundice, hepatitis

Renal: Nephrotoxicity

Miscellaneous: Hypersensitivity reactions

Drug Interactions Methotrexate, tolbutamide, chlorpropamide, oral anticoagulants (displaced from protein binding sites); PABA (antagonizes the antibacterial activity of sulfas); thiopental (competes for plasma protein binding)

Food Interactions Interferes with folate absorption

Stability Protect from light

Mechanism of Action Interferes with bacterial growth by inhibiting bacterial folic acid synthesis through competitive antagonism of PABA

Pharmacokinetics

Absorption: Sulfisoxazole acetyl is hydrolyzed in the GI tract to sulfisoxazole which is readily absorbed

Distribution: Crosses the placenta; excreted into breast milk; distributes into extra-cellular space; CSF concentration ranges from 8% to 57% of blood concentration in patients with normal meninges

Protein binding: 85% to 88%

Metabolism: In the liver by acetylation and glucuronide conjugation to inactive compounds

Half-life: 4-8 hours, prolonged with renal impairment

Time to peak serum concentration: Within 2-4 hours

Elimination: Primarily in urine (95% within 24 hours), 40% to 60% as unchanged drug

>50% removed by hemodialysis

Usual Dosage

Infants ≥2 months and Children: Oral: Initial: 75 mg/kg for 1 dose, followed by 120-150 mg/kg/day in divided doses every 4-6 hours; not to exceed 6 g/day

Pelvic inflammatory disease: 100 mg/kg/day in divided doses every 6 hours; used in combination with ceftriaxone

Chlamydia trachomatis: 100 mg/kg/day divided every 6 hours; maximum dose: 2 g/day

Prophylaxis of UTI: 10-20 mg/kg/day divided every 12 hours

Adults: Oral: 2-4 g stat, followed by 4-8 g/day in divided doses every 4-6 hours

Children and Adults: Ophthalmic:

Ointment: Apply small amount to conjunctiva of affected eye 1-3 times/day and at bedtime

Solution: Instill 1-2 drops to conjunctiva of affected eye every 2-3 hours

Dosing interval in renal impairment:

Cl_{cr} 10-50 mL/minutes: Administer every 8-12 hours

Cl_{cr} <10 mL/minute: Administer every 12-24 hours

Administration

Ophthalmic: Avoid contact of tube or bottle tip with skin or eye; apply finger pressure to lacrimal sac during and for 1-2 minutes after instillation of drops to decrease risk of absorption and systemic effects

Oral: Administer with a glass of water on an empty stomach; shake suspension well before use

Monitoring Parameters CBC, urinalysis, renal function tests

Test Interactions False-positive protein in urine; false-positive urine glucose with Clinitest®

Patient Information Avoid prolonged exposure to sunlight; report to physician any sore throat, mouth sores, rash, unusual bleeding, or fever; limit alcohol

Nursing Implications Maintain adequate patient fluid intake

Dosage Forms

Solution, ophthalmic, as diolamine: 4% [40 mg/mL] (15 mL)

Suspension, oral, pediatric, as acetyl (raspberry flavor): 500 mg/5 mL (480 mL)

Syrup, as acetyl (chocolate flavor): 500 mg/5 mL (480 mL)

Tablet: 500 mg

References

"Practice Parameter: The Diagnosis, Treatment, and Evaluation of the Initial Urinary Tract Infection in Febrile Infants and Young Children. American Academy of Pediatrics. Committee on Quality Improvement. Subcommittee on Urinary Tract Infection," *Pediatrics*, 1999, 103(4 Pt 1):843-52.

Thoene DE and Johnson CE, "Pharmacotherapy of Otitis Media," *Pharmacotherapy*, 1991, 11(3):212-21.

♦ **Sulfisoxazole Acetyl** *see* Sulfisoxazole *on page 894*

♦ **Sulfisoxazole and Erythromycin** *see* Erythromycin and Sulfisoxazole *on page 382*

♦ **Sulfisoxazole Diolamine** see Sulfisoxazole *on page 894*

♦ **Sulfizole® (Canada)** see Sulfisoxazole *on page 894*

Sulfur and Salicylic Acid (SUL fur & sal i SIL ik AS id)

Brand Names Aveeno® Cleansing Bar [OTC]; Fostex® [OTC]; Pernox® [OTC]; Sastid® Plain Therapeutic Shampoo and Acne Wash [OTC]; Sebulex® [OTC]

Synonyms Salicylic Acid and Sulfur

Therapeutic Category Antiseborrheic Agent, Topical

Generic Available Yes

Use Therapeutic shampoo for dandruff and seborrheal dermatitis; acne skin cleanser

Contraindications Hypersensitivity to sulfur, salicylic acid, or any component

Warnings For external use only; avoid contact with eyes; discontinue use if skin irritation develops

Precautions Infants are more sensitive to sulfur than adults; do not use in children <2 years of age

Adverse Reactions Topical preparations containing 2% to 5% sulfur generally are well tolerated; concentration >15% is very irritating to the skin; higher concentrations (eg, 10% or higher) may cause systemic toxicity

Cardiovascular: Collapse (with sulfur concentration >10%)
Central nervous system: Dizziness, headache
Gastrointestinal: Vomiting
Local: Irritation
Neuromuscular & skeletal: Muscle cramps

Stability Preparations containing sulfur may react with metals including silver and copper, resulting in discoloration of the metal

Mechanism of Action Salicylic acid works synergistically with sulfur in its keratolytic action to break down keratin and promote skin peeling

Pharmacokinetics Absorption: 1% of topically applied sulfur is absorbed; sulfur is reduced to hydrogen sulfide

Usual Dosage Children ≥2 years and Adults: Topical:

Shampoo: Initial: Massage onto wet scalp; leave lather on scalp for 5 minutes, rinse, repeat application, then rinse thoroughly; use daily or every other day; 1-2 treatments/week will usually maintain control

Soap: Use daily or every other day

Administration Topical: Avoid contact with the eyes; for external use only

Patient Information Contact physician if condition worsens or rash or irritation develops

Dosage Forms

Cake: Sulfur 2% and salicylic acid 2% (123 g)
Cleanser: Sulfur 2% and salicylic acid 1.5% (60 mL, 120 mL)
Shampoo: Micropulverized sulfur 2% and salicylic acid 2% (120 mL, 240 mL)
Soap: Micropulverized sulfur 2% and salicylic acid 2% (113 g)
Wash: Sulfur 1.6% and salicylic acid 1.6% (75 mL)

Sulindac (sul IN dak)

Related Information

Overdose and Toxicology *on page 1191*

Brand Names Apo®-Sulin (Canada); Clinoril®; Novo-Sundac® (Canada)

Therapeutic Category Analgesic, Non-narcotic; Anti-inflammatory Agent; Nonsteroidal Anti-inflammatory Drug (NSAID), Oral

Generic Available Yes

Use Management of inflammatory disease, rheumatoid disorders; acute gouty arthritis

Pregnancy Risk Factor B (D in 3rd trimester or near delivery)

Contraindications Hypersensitivity to sulindac, any component, aspirin, or other NSAIDs

Precautions Use with caution in patients with peptic ulcer disease, GI bleeding, bleeding abnormalities, impaired renal or hepatic function, CHF, hypertension, and patients receiving anticoagulants

Adverse Reactions

Cardiovascular: Edema
Central nervous system: Dizziness, nervousness, headache
Dermatologic: Rash, pruritus
Gastrointestinal: Abdominal pain; GI bleeding, ulcer, perforation; nausea; vomiting; diarrhea; constipation

Hematologic: Thrombocytopenia, agranulocytosis, inhibition of platelet aggregation, bone marrow suppression

Hepatic: Hepatitis

Otic: Tinnitus

Renal: Renal impairment

Respiratory: Bronchospasm

Drug Interactions Sulindac may potentiate effects of warfarin; probenecid may increase serum concentration of sulindac; dimethyl sulfoxide or ASA may decrease sulindac serum concentration; sulindac may increase methotrexate serum concentrations and may increase cyclosporin nephrotoxicity; potassium supplements and other GI irritants may increase GI adverse effects; effects of antihypertensive agents, furosemide, thiazides may be decreased; drug interactions similar to other NSAIDs may also occur

Food Interactions Food may decrease rate and extent of absorption

Mechanism of Action Inhibits prostaglandin synthesis by decreasing the activity of the enzyme, cyclo-oxygenase, which results in decreased formation of prostaglandin precursors

Usual Dosage Oral:

Children: Dose not established; doses of 4 mg/kg/day divided in 2 doses have been used

Adults: 150-200 mg twice daily; not to exceed 400 mg/day

Administration Oral: Administer with food or milk to decrease GI upset

Monitoring Parameters Liver enzymes, BUN, serum creatinine, CBC with differential, platelet count; periodic ophthalmologic exams with chronic use

Patient Information Avoid alcohol; may cause dizziness; do not take with aspirin

Dosage Forms Tablet: 150 mg, 200 mg

♦ **Sulphafurazole** *see* Sulfisoxazole *on page 894*

Sumatriptan (SOO ma trip tan)

Related Information

Serotonin Syndrome *on page 1217*

Brand Names Imitrex®

Available Salts Sumatriptan Succinate

Therapeutic Category Antimigraine Agent

Generic Available No

Use

Injection, intranasal, and tablets: Acute treatment of migraine with or without aura

Injection: Acute treatment of cluster headaches

Pregnancy Risk Factor C

Contraindications I.V. administration (coronary vasospasm may occur); ischemic heart disease, Prinzmetal angina, cerebrovascular or peripheral vascular syndromes (eg, stroke, TIA, ischemic bowel disease), severe hepatic impairment, patients with signs or symptoms of ischemic heart disease, MI, silent MI, uncontrolled hypertension; concomitant use of ergotamine derivatives (within last 24 hours), vasoconstrictive drugs, methysergide, or MAO inhibitors; use of MAO inhibitors within past 2 weeks; hypersensitivity to sumatriptan or any component; management of hemiplegic or basilar migraine

Warnings Life-threatening or fatal hypersensitivity reactions may occur; rarely, serious coronary events including acute MI, life-threatening arrhythmias, and death, may occur; avoid use in patients with risk factors for coronary artery disease, unless cardiovascular disease can be ruled out; consider administering first dose under close supervision to patients at high risk for coronary disease; EKG should be performed if angina-like symptoms occur; periodically evaluate cardiovascular system in patients with risk factors for coronary artery disease

Precautions Temporary increases in peripheral vascular resistance and blood pressure may occur; use with caution in patients with impaired hepatic or renal function, epilepsy; cross-hypersensitivity to sulfonamides is possible; other potentially serious neurological conditions should be ruled out prior to acute migraine therapy; sumatriptan (given at five times the maximum oral single dose) has caused corneal opacities in dogs; other animal studies suggest it may bind to the melanin of the eye; human studies are not available

Adverse Reactions

Cardiovascular: Hypertension; flushing; chest tightness, pressure, pain; coronary artery vasospasm; vascular ischemia; colonic ischemia; rarely: acute MI, life-threatening arrhythmias

Central nervous system: Dizziness, drowsiness, headache

(Continued)

Sumatriptan *(Continued)*

Gastrointestinal: Nausea, vomiting, abdominal discomfort; bad or unusual taste (with intranasal use)

Local: Injection site reaction (59%), pain, redness at injection site

Neuromuscular & skeletal: Weakness, myalgia, neck pain with stiffness

Miscellaneous: Atypical sensations of tingling, heat, flushing, burning, heaviness, pressure, tightness, numbness; jaw, mouth, tongue discomfort; diaphoresis; rarely: hypersensitivity reactions (potentially fatal anaphylaxis or anaphylactoid reactions)

Drug Interactions Use with ergot-containing drugs may result in prolonged vasospasm reactions; vasoconstrictive drugs; methysergide; MAO inhibitors (MAO inhibitors may significantly increase sumatriptan serum concentrations; use of MAO inhibitors is contraindicated); selective serotonin reuptake inhibitors (may cause weakness, incoordination, hyperreflexia; monitor patients carefully)

Food Interactions Food slightly delays the rate but not the extent of oral absorption

Stability Store at 2°C to 20°C (36°F to 86°F); protect from light

Mechanism of Action Selective agonist for serotonin (5-HT$_1$) receptor in cranial arteries; causes vasoconstriction and reduces sterile inflammation associated with antidromic neuronal transmission correlating with relief of migraine

Pharmacodynamics Migraine pain relief:

Onset:

Oral: 1-1.5 hours

S.C.: 10 minutes to 2 hours

Maximum effect: Oral: 2-4 hours

Pharmacokinetics

Distribution: Adults:

V_d (central): 50 L;

V_d (apparent): 2.4 L/kg

Protein binding: 14% to 21%

Metabolism: In the liver to an indole acetic acid metabolite (inactive) which then undergoes ester glucuronide conjugation; may be metabolized by monoamine oxidase (MAO)

Bioavailability:

Oral: ~15%; may be significantly increased with liver disease

Intranasal: 17% (compared to S.C.)

S.C.: 97%

Half-life:

Distribution: 15 minutes

Terminal: 2 hours; range: 1-4 hours

Time to peak serum concentration:

Oral: Healthy adults: 2 hours; during migraine attacks: 2.5 hours

S.C.: Range: 5-20 minutes; mean: 12 minutes

Elimination: 60% of an oral dose is renally excreted (primarily as metabolites), 40% is eliminated via the feces, and only 3% as unchanged drug; 42% of an intranasal dose is excreted as the indole acetic acid metabolite with 3% excreted in the urine unchanged; 22% of a S.C. dose is excreted in urine unchanged and 38% as the indole acetic acid metabolite

Usual Dosage

Children and Adolescents <18 years: Use not recommended:

Oral: Efficacy of oral sumatriptan was **not** established in placebo-controlled trials in patients 12-17 years of age (n=701) with doses of 25-100 mg; adverse events were similar to adults; frequency of adverse events was dose- and age-dependent (increased frequency of adverse events in younger patients); postmarketing reports include the occurrence of MI in a 14-year-old male after oral sumatriptan with symptoms occurring within 1 day of drug use

S.C.: An open-labeled prospective trial in 17 children 6-16 years of age with juvenile migraine used S.C. doses of 6 mg in 15 children 30-70 kg, and 3 mg/dose in two children who weighed 22 kg and 30 kg (MacDonald, 1994); additional studies are needed

Adults:

Intranasal: Initial single dose: 5 mg, 10 mg, or 20 mg administered in one nostril, given as soon as possible after the onset of migraine; 10 mg dose may be administered as 5 mg in each nostril; may repeat after 2 hours; maximum: 40 mg/day

Oral: Initial single dose: 25 mg given as soon as possible after the onset of a migraine; range: 25-100 mg/dose; maximum single dose: 100 mg; may repeat after 2 hours; maximum: 200 mg/day

S.C.: 6 mg given as soon as possible after the onset of a migraine; a second injection (≤6 mg) may be administered at least 1 hour after the initial dose; maximum dose: 12 mg/24 hours

Dosing adjustment in hepatic dysfunction: Adults: Oral: Maximum single dose: 50 mg

Administration

Intranasal: Each nasal spray unit is preloaded with 1 dose; **do not** test the spray unit before use; remove unit from plastic pack when ready to use; while sitting down, gently blow nose to clear nasal passages; keep head upright and close one nostril gently with index finger; hold container with other hand, with thumb supporting bottom and index and middle fingers on either side of nozzle; insert nozzle into nostril about ¹/₂ inch; close mouth; take a breath through nose while releasing spray into nostril by pressing firmly on blue plunger; remove nozzle from nostril; keep head level for 10-20 seconds and gently breathe in through nose and out through mouth; **do not breathe deeply**

Oral: Administer with fluids

Parenteral: S.C. use only; do **not** administer I.M.; do **not** administer I.V. (may cause coronary vasospasm)

Patient Information If pain or tightness in chest or throat occurs, notify physician; females should avoid pregnancy; pain at injection site lasts <1 hour

Additional Information Safety of treating >4 headaches per month is not established; sumatriptan is **not** indicated for migraine prophylaxis

Dosage Forms

Injection, as succinate: 12 mg/mL (base) (0.5 mL, 2 mL)

Spray, intranasal: 5 mg (100 µL unit dose spray device); 20 mg (100 µL unit dose spray device)

Tablet, as succinate: 25 mg, 50 mg (base)

Extemporaneous Preparations A 5 mg/mL oral liquid preparation made from tablets and 3 different vehicles (Ora-Sweet®, Ora-Sweet® SF, or Syrpalta® syrups) was stable for 21 days when stored in amber glass bottles in the dark under refrigeration (4°C); **Note:** Preparations with Ora-Sweet® and Ora-Sweet® SF used Ora-Plus® as a suspending vehicle; grind nine 100 mg tablets in a mortar into a fine powder; add 40 mL of Ora-Plus® Suspending Vehicle, 5 mL at a time, and mix thoroughly between each addition; **Note:** The suspending vehicle helps to facilitate dispersion of the tablets and is used only if Ora-Sweet® or Ora-Sweet® SF is the vehicle to be used (ie, suspending vehicle is not used if preparation uses Syrpalta® syrup as the vehicle); transfer to a calibrated amber glass bottle; rinse mortar and pestle 5 times with 10 mL of Ora-Plus® suspension vehicle pouring into bottle each time; qsad with appropriate syrup (Ora-Sweet® or Ora-Sweet® SF) to 180 mL; label "shake well," "refrigerate," and "protect from light"; (**Note:** This study also tested microbial growth on days 0 and 28; no growth of bacteria or fungus occurred) (Fish, 1997)

Fish DN, Beall HD, Goodwin SD, et al, "Stability of Sumatriptan Succinate in Extemporaneously Prepared Oral Liquids," *Am J Health Syst Pharm*, 1997, 54(14):1619-22.

References

MacDonald JT, "Treatment of Juvenile Migraine With Subcutaneous Sumatriptan," *Headache*, 1994, 34(10):581-2.

Scott AK, "Sumatriptan Clinical Pharmacokinetics," *Clin Pharmacokinet*, 1994, 27(5):337-44.

Sutilains (SOO ti lains)

Brand Names Travase®
Therapeutic Category Enzyme, Topical Debridement
Generic Available No
Use Promote debridement of necrotic debris; adjunct in the treatment of second and third degree burns; decubitus ulcers
Pregnancy Risk Factor B
Contraindications Wounds communicating with major body cavities; wounds with exposed nerves; fungating neoplastic ulcers; hypersensitivity to sutilains or any component
Warnings A topical anti-infective agent should be used with sutilains
Precautions Should not be applied to more than 10% to 15% of the burned area at one time; safety and efficacy have not been established in children
Adverse Reactions
  Dermatologic: Dermatitis
  Local: Pain, bleeding, paresthesia
Drug Interactions Benzalkonium chloride, hexachlorophene, iodine, nitrofurazone, thimerosal, and silver nitrate decrease activity of sutilains
Stability Store in the refrigerator; activity is greatest at pH 6-6.8
Mechanism of Action Enzymatically converts denatured proteins (necrotic soft tissue, hemoglobin and purulent exudate) to peptides and amino acids
Pharmacodynamics
  Onset of action: Following topical application, within 60 minutes
  Peak effect: May not be seen until 5-7 days for burns or 8-12 days for decubital ulcers
  Duration: 8-12 hours
Usual Dosage Children and Adults: Topical: Apply ointment in a thin layer extending ¼" to ½" beyond the tissue being debrided; apply loose moist dressing; repeat 3-4 times/day
Administration Topical: Thoroughly cleanse and irrigate wound before applying ointment
Patient Information Discontinue use if bleeding or dermatitis occurs
Nursing Implications Avoid contact with the eyes; keep wound area moist for optimal activity
Dosage Forms Ointment: 82,000 casein units/g (14.2 g)

- **Suxamethonium** see Succinylcholine on page 884
- **Syllact® [OTC]** see Psyllium on page 823
- **Symadine®** see Amantadine on page 53
- **Symmetrel®** see Amantadine on page 53
- **Synacort® Topical** see Hydrocortisone on page 486
- **Synacthen** see Cosyntropin on page 257
- **Synacthen® Depot (Canada)** see Cosyntropin on page 257
- **Synagis®** see Palivizumab on page 721
- **Synalar-HP® Topical** see Fluocinolone on page 425
- **Synalar® Topical** see Fluocinolone on page 425
- **Syn-Captopril® (Canada)** see Captopril on page 163
- **Syn-Diltiazem® (Canada)** see Diltiazem on page 323
- **Synemol® Topical** see Fluocinolone on page 425
- **Synercid®** see Quinupristin/Dalfopristin on page 834
- **Synflex® (Canada)** see Naproxen on page 672
- **Syn-Flunisolide® (Canada)** see Flunisolide on page 423
- **Syn-Nadolol® (Canada)** see Nadolol on page 665
- **Synthetic Lung Surfactant** see Colfosceril on page 252
- **Synthroid® Injection** see Levothyroxine on page 566
- **Synthroid® Oral** see Levothyroxine on page 566
- **Syracol-CF® [OTC]** see Guaifenesin and Dextromethorphan on page 466
- **Sytobex®** see Cyanocobalamin on page 263
- **T_3** see Liothyronine on page 574
- **T_4 Thyroxine** see Levothyroxine on page 566
- **Tac™-3 Injection** see Triamcinolone on page 946
- **Tac™-40 Injection** see Triamcinolone on page 946
- **Tacozin® (Canada)** see Piperacillin and Tazobactam on page 773

Tacrolimus (ta KROE li mus)

Brand Names Prograf®

Synonyms FK506

Therapeutic Category Immunosuppressant Agent

Generic Available No

Use Immunosuppressant used with corticosteroids to prevent graft versus host disease in patients who have received organ transplants and are not responding to cyclosporine

Pregnancy Risk Factor C

Contraindications Hypersensitivity to tacrolimus, polyoxyl 60 hydrogenated castor oil, or any component

Warnings Avoid use with other immunosuppressants; immunosuppression with tacrolimus may result in increased susceptibility to infection and the possible development of lymphoma; adequate airway, supportive measures, and agents for treating anaphylaxis should be available when tacrolimus is administered I.V.

Precautions Use with caution and modify dosage in patients with hepatic or renal impairment

Adverse Reactions

Cardiovascular: Hypertension, peripheral edema

Central nervous system: Encephalopathy, headache, hallucinations, pain, fever, seizures, altered mental status, insomnia, dizziness

Dermatologic: Pruritus, rash

Endocrine & metabolic: Hyperkalemia, hyperglycemia, hypomagnesemia, hypophosphatemia

Gastrointestinal: Diarrhea, nausea, vomiting, constipation, dyspepsia

Hematologic: Anemia, thrombocytopenia, leukocytosis, eosinophilia

Hepatic: Hepatotoxicity; elevated AST, ALT, and LDH

Neuromuscular & skeletal: Tremor, paresthesia, back pain, arthralgia

Ocular: Abnormal vision

Otic: Tinnitus

Renal: Nephrotoxicity, elevated BUN and serum creatinine

Respiratory: Pleural effusion, respiratory distress

Miscellaneous: Increased susceptibility to infections, lymphoproliferative disorders, anaphylaxis (may be due to polyoxyl 60 hydrogenated castor oil injectable vehicle)

Drug Interactions Diltiazem, verapamil, nifedipine, fluconazole, itraconazole, ketoconazole, cimetidine, clarithromycin, erythromycin, methylprednisolone, isoniazid, metoclopramide, cyclosporine, and oral clotrimazole increase tacrolimus serum concentrations; antacids, cholestyramine, sodium polystyrene sulfonate, carbamazepine, phenobarbital, primidone, phenytoin, rifabutin, and rifampin decrease tacrolimus serum concentrations; additive nephrotoxicity when used with NSAIDs or cyclosporine

Food Interactions Food reduces the rate and extent of absorption by ~27%; grapefruit juice may increase tacrolimus blood concentration

Stability Reconstitution: Stable for 24 hours when mixed in D_5W or NS in glass or polyolefin containers; 24-hour stability in plastic syringes stored at 24°C; no need to protect from light; do not store in polyvinyl chloride containers since the polyoxyl 60 hydrogenated castor oil injectable vehicle may leach phthalates from polyvinyl chloride containers; polyvinyl-containing administration sets adsorb drug and may lead to a lower dose being delivered to the patient; tacrolimus is unstable in alkaline media; do not mix with acyclovir or ganciclovir

Mechanism of Action Binds to an intracellular protein forming a complex which inhibits phosphatase activity of calcineurin resulting in the inhibition of T-cell activation

Pharmacokinetics

Absorption: Erratic and incomplete oral absorption (5% to 67%)

Distribution: Distributes to erythrocytes, breast milk, lung, kidneys, pancreas, liver, placenta, heart, and spleen; V_d: 5-65 L/kg (V_d is increased in pediatric patients versus adults)

Protein binding: 75% to 97% to alpha-acid glycoprotein (some binding to albumin)

Metabolism: Hepatic metabolism through the cytochrome P-450 system

Bioavailability: Average: 27%

Half-life, elimination: 3.5-40.5 hours (mean: 8.7 hours)

Time to peak serum concentration: Oral: 1-4 hours

Elimination: Primarily in bile; <1% excreted unchanged in urine

Clearance: 7-103 mL/minute/kg (average: 30 mL/minute/kg); clearance may be higher in children

(Continued)

Tacrolimus *(Continued)*

Usual Dosage

Children:

Oral: 0.3 mg/kg/day divided every 12 hours; children generally require higher maintenance dosages on a mg/kg basis than adults

I.V. continuous infusion: 0.05-0.15 mg/kg/day

Adults:

Oral: 0.15-0.3 mg/kg/day divided every 12 hours

I.V. continuous infusion: 0.05-0.1 mg/kg/day

Dosing adjustment in renal or hepatic impairment: Patients with renal or hepatic impairment should receive the lowest dose in the dosage range

Administration

Oral: Administer on an empty stomach; use oral syringe or glass container (not plastic or foam cup) when administering this medication

Parenteral: May administer by I.V. continuous infusion; I.V. concentrate for injection must be diluted to 0.004-0.02 mg/mL in NS or D_5W prior to administration

Monitoring Parameters Liver enzymes, BUN, serum creatinine, glucose, potassium, magnesium, blood tacrolimus concentrations, CBC with differential; blood pressure, neurologic status

Reference Range Limited data correlating serum level to therapeutic efficacy/toxicity:

Trough (whole blood ELISA): 9.8-19.4 ng/mL

Trough (HPLC): 0.5-1.5 ng/mL

Patient Information Administer dose at the same time each day

Nursing Implications Patients receiving I.V. tacrolimus should be under continuous observation for at least the first 30 minutes following dosage initiation; adequate airway, supportive measures, and agents for treating anaphylaxis should be available when tacrolimus is administered I.V.

Additional Information Tacrolimus should be initiated no sooner than 6 hours after transplant; convert I.V. tacrolimus to oral form as soon as possible or within 2-3 days (the oral formulation should be started 8-12 hours after stopping the I.V. infusion); when switching a patient from cyclosporine to tacrolimus, allow at least 24 hours after discontinuing cyclosporine before initiating tacrolimus therapy to minimize the risk of nephrotoxicity

Dosage Forms

Capsule: 1 mg, 5 mg

Injection, with alcohol and polyoxyl 60 hydrogenated castor oil: 5 mg/mL (1 mL)

Extemporaneous Preparations A 0.5 mg/mL suspension has been prepared by mixing the contents of six 5 mg tacrolimus capsules with equal amounts of Ora-Plus® and Simple Syrup, NF to make a final volume of 60 mL. When compounding tacrolimus oral suspension, protect hands with latex gloves. The suspension is stable for 56 days when stored at room temperature in either glass or plastic amber prescription bottles. Label "shake well before using."

Jacobson PA, Johnson CE, West NJ, et al, "Stability of Tacrolimus in an Extemporaneously Compounded Oral Liquid," *Am J Health Sys Pharm* , 1997, 54(2):178-80.

References

Asante-Korang A, Boyle GJ, Webber SA, et al, "Experience of FK506 Immune Suppression in Pediatric Heart Transplantation: A Study of Long-Term Adverse Effects," *J Heart Lung Transplant*, 1996, 15(4):415-22.

McDiarmid SV, Colonna JO, Shaked A, et al, "Differences in Oral FK506 Dose Requirements Between Adults and Pediatric Liver Transplant Patients," *Transplantation*, 1993, 55(6):1328-32.

Menegaux F, Keeffe EB, Andrews BT, et al, "Neurological Complications of Liver Transplantation in Adult Versus Pediatric Patients," *Transplantation*, 1994, 58(4):447-50.

+ **Taro-Cloxacillin® (Canada)** *see* Cloxacillin *on page 246*
+ **Taro-Sone® (Canada)** *see* Betamethasone *on page 130*
+ **Tavist®** *see* Clemastine *on page 236*
+ **Tavist®-1 [OTC]** *see* Clemastine *on page 236*
+ **Taxol®** *see* Paclitaxel *on page 719*
+ **Tazicef®** *see* Ceftazidime *on page 190*
+ **Tazidime®** *see* Ceftazidime *on page 190*
+ **Tazobactam and Piperacillin** *see* Piperacillin and Tazobactam *on page 773*
+ **3TC** *see* Lamivudine *on page 552*
+ **3TC and AZT** *see* Lamivudine and Zidovudine *on page 553*
+ **3TC and ZDV** *see* Lamivudine and Zidovudine *on page 553*
+ **3TC® (Canada)** *see* Lamivudine *on page 552*
+ **T-Cell Growth Factor** *see* Aldesleukin *on page 42*
+ **TCGF** *see* Aldesleukin *on page 42*
+ **TCN** *see* Tetracycline *on page 908*
+ **Tebamide® Rectal** *see* Trimethobenzamide *on page 954*
+ **Tebrazid (Canada)** *see* Pyrazinamide *on page 825*
+ **Tega-Vert® Oral** *see* Dimenhydrinate *on page 325*
+ **Tegopen®** *see* Cloxacillin *on page 246*
+ **Tegretol®** *see* Carbamazepine *on page 165*
+ **Tegretol®-XR** *see* Carbamazepine *on page 165*
+ **Tegrin®-HC Topical [OTC]** *see* Hydrocortisone *on page 486*
+ **Telachlor® Oral** *see* Chlorpheniramine *on page 214*
+ **Teladar® Topical** *see* Betamethasone *on page 130*
+ **Teldrin® Oral [OTC]** *see* Chlorpheniramine *on page 214*
+ **Teline® Oral** *see* Tetracycline *on page 908*
+ **Tempra® [OTC]** *see* Acetaminophen *on page 26*
+ **Ten-K®** *see* Potassium Supplements *on page 786*
+ **Tenormin®** *see* Atenolol *on page 102*
+ **Tensilon®** *see* Edrophonium *on page 359*

Terbutaline (ter BYOO ta leen)

Related Information
Asthma Guidelines *on page 1178*

Brand Names Brethaire®; Brethine®; Bricanyl®

Available Salts Terbutaline Sulfate

Therapeutic Category Adrenergic Agonist Agent; Antiasthmatic; Beta$_2$-Adrenergic Agonist Agent; Bronchodilator; Sympathomimetic; Tocolytic Agent

Generic Available No

Use Bronchodilator for relief of reversible bronchospasm in patients with asthma, bronchitis, and emphysema

Pregnancy Risk Factor B

Contraindications Hypersensitivity to terbutaline or any component

Warnings Paradoxical bronchoconstriction may occur with excessive use; if it occurs, discontinue terbutaline immediately

Precautions Use with caution in patients with diabetes mellitus, hypertension, hyperthyroidism, history of seizures, or cardiac disease; excessive or prolonged use may lead to tolerance

Adverse Reactions
Cardiovascular: Tachycardia, hypertension, arrhythmias, flushing
Central nervous system: Drowsiness, headache, nervousness, seizures, dizziness
Gastrointestinal: Nausea, vomiting, dysgeusia
Neuromuscular & skeletal: Tremor
Otic: Tinnitus
Respiratory: Dyspnea, bronchospasm (with excessive use), pharyngitis, dry throat, chest tightness
Miscellaneous: Diaphoresis

Drug Interactions Additive effects with other sympathomimetics; increased pressor response with methyldopa, MAO inhibitors, oxytocic drugs, and tricyclic antidepressants

Mechanism of Action Relaxes bronchial smooth muscle and muscles of peripheral vasculature by action on beta$_2$-receptors with less effect on heart rate
(Continued)

903

Terbutaline *(Continued)*

Pharmacodynamics
Onset of action:
   Oral: 30 minutes
   Oral inhalation: 5-30 minutes
   S.C.: 6-15 minutes
Duration:
   Oral: 4-8 hours
   Oral inhalation: 3-6 hours
   S.C.: 1.5-4 hours

Pharmacokinetics
Absorption: 33% to 50%
Distribution: Breast milk to plasma ratio: <2.9
Metabolism: Possible first-pass metabolism after oral use
Half-life: 11-16 hours
Elimination: Primarily (60%) unchanged in urine after parenteral use

Usual Dosage
Children <12 years:
   Oral: Initial: 0.05 mg/kg/dose every 8 hours, increase gradually, up to 0.15 mg/kg/dose; maximum daily dose: 5 mg
   S.C.: 0.005-0.01 mg/kg/dose to a maximum of 0.4 mg/dose every 15-20 minutes for 2 doses
Children ≥12 years and Adults:
   Oral: 2.5-5 mg/dose every 6-8 hours; maximum daily dose:
      12-15 years: 7.5 mg
      >15 years: 15 mg
   S.C.: 0.25 mg/dose repeated in 15-30 minutes for one time only; a total dose of 0.5 mg should not be exceeded within a 4-hour period
   Note: Continuous I.V. infusion has been used successfully in children with asthma; a 2-10 mcg/kg loading dose followed by an 0.08-0.4 mcg/kg/minute continuous infusion; depending upon the clinical response, the dosage may require titration in increments of 0.1-0.2 mcg/kg/minute every 30 minutes; doses as high as 6 mcg/kg/minute have been used.
Inhalation: Children and Adults: 1-2 puffs every 4-6 hours
Nebulization: Children and Adults: 0.01-0.03 mL/kg (1 mg = 1 mL using injection); minimum dose: 0.1 mL; maximum dose: 2.5 mL diluted with 1-2 mL NS, every 4-6 hours

Administration
Oral: May administer with or without food
Oral Inhalation: Shake well; administer with spacer in children <8 years of age
Parenteral: May administer undiluted, direct I.V. over 5-10 minutes; for continuous infusion, dilute to a maximum concentration of 1 mg/mL

Monitoring Parameters Heart rate, blood pressure, respiratory rate, arterial or capillary blood gases (if applicable)

Dosage Forms
Aerosol, oral, as sulfate: 0.2 mg/actuation (10.5 g)
Injection, as sulfate: 1 mg/mL (1 mL)
Tablet, as sulfate: 2.5 mg, 5 mg

Extemporaneous Preparations A 1 mg/mL suspension made from terbutaline tablets in simple syrup NF is stable 30 days when refrigerated
   Horner RK and Johnson CE, "Stability of An Extemporaneously Compounded Terbutaline Sulfate Oral Liquid," *Am J Hosp Pharm*, 1991, 48(2):293-5.

References
Bohn D, Kalloghlian A, Jenkins J, et al, "Intravenous Salbutamol in the Treatment of Status Asthmaticus in Children," *Crit Care Med*, 1984, 12(10):892-6.

Canny GJ and Levison H, "Aerosols - Therapeutic Use and Delivery in Childhood Asthma," *Ann Allergy*, 1988, 60(1):11-9.

Fuglsang G, Pedersen S, and Borgstrom L, "Dose-Response Relationships of I.V. Administered Terbutaline in Children With Asthma," *J Pediatr*, 1989, 114(2):315-20.

Goldenhersh N and Rachelefsky GS, "Childhood Asthma: Management," *Pediatr Rev*, 1989, 10(9):259-67.

Expert Panel Report 2, "Guidelines for the Diagnosis and Management of Asthma," *Clinical Practice Guidelines*, National Institutes of Health, National Heart, Lung, and Blood Institute, NIH Publication No. 94-4051, April, 1997.

Rachelefsky GS and Siegel SC, "Asthma in Infants and Children - Treatment of Childhood Asthma: Part II," *J Allergy Clin Immunol*, 1985, 76(3):409-25.

Tipton WR and Nelson HS, "Frequent Parenteral Terbutaline in the Treatment of Status Asthmaticus in Children," *Ann Allergy*, 1987, 58(4):252-6.

♦ **Terbutaline Sulfate** *see* Terbutaline *on page 903*
♦ **Tesamone® Injection** *see* Testosterone *on page 905*

♦ **TESPA** *see* Thiotepa *on page 922*
♦ **Testoderm® Transdermal System** *see* Testosterone *on page 905*
♦ **Testoderm® TTS** *see* Testosterone *on page 905*
♦ **Testoderm® with Adhesive** *see* Testosterone *on page 905*
♦ **Testopel® Pellet** *see* Testosterone *on page 905*

Testosterone (tes TOS ter one)

Brand Names Androderm® Transdermal System; AndroGel™; Andro-L.A.® Injection; Andropository® Injection; Delatest® Injection; Delatestryl® Injection; depAndro® Injection; Depotest® Injection; Depo®-Testosterone Injection; Duratest® Injection; Durathate® Injection; Everone® Injection; Histerone® Injection; Tesamone® Injection; Testoderm® Transdermal System; Testoderm® TTS; Testoderm® with Adhesive; Testopel® Pellet

Available Salts Testosterone Cypionate; Testosterone Enanthate; Testosterone Propionate

Synonyms Aqueous Testosterone

Therapeutic Category Androgen

Generic Available Yes

Use Androgen replacement therapy in the treatment of delayed male puberty; male hypogonadism

Restrictions C-III

Pregnancy Risk Factor X

Contraindications Severe renal, hepatic, or cardiac disease; male patients with prostatic or breast cancer, hypercalcemia, pregnancy; hypersensitivity to testosterone or any component

Warnings May accelerate bone maturation without producing compensating gain in linear growth; perform radiographic examination of the hand and wrist every 6 months to determine the rate of bone maturation (when using in prepubertal children)

Precautions Use with caution in patients with hepatic, cardiac, or renal dysfunction

Adverse Reactions
Cardiovascular: Flushing, edema, hypertension, tachycardia
Central nervous system: Excitation, aggressive behavior, sleeplessness, anxiety, mental depression, headache, nervousness
Dermatologic: Acne, hirsutism, urticaria
Endocrine & metabolic: Gynecomastia, hypercalcemia, hypoglycemia, increased serum cholesterol, hyperlipemia, hyponatremia, increased or decreased libido
Gastrointestinal: Nausea, abdominal pain, diarrhea
Genitourinary: Epididymitis, priapism, bladder irritability
Hematologic: Leukopenia, suppression of clotting factors, polycythemia
Hepatic: Cholestatic hepatitis, peliosis hepatitis, hepatocellular carcinoma (high doses), increased liver function tests
Local: Inflammation and itching at injection site
Neuromuscular & skeletal: Myalgia

Drug Interactions Potentiates effects of oral anticoagulants; increases propranolol clearance

Mechanism of Action Principal endogenous androgen responsible for promoting the growth and development of the male sex organs and maintaining secondary sex characteristics in androgen-deficient males

Pharmacodynamics Duration of effect: Based upon the route of administration and which testosterone ester is used; the cypionate and enanthate esters have the longest duration, up to 2-4 weeks after I.M. administration; pellets 3-4 months

Pharmacokinetics
Protein binding: 98%
Metabolism: Inactivation in liver
Half-life: 10-100 minutes
Elimination: 90% excreted in urine as metabolites

Usual Dosage
Children: I.M.:
Male hypogonadism:
Initiation of pubertal growth: 40-50 mg/m²/dose (cypionate or enanthate ester) monthly until the growth rate falls to prepubertal levels
Terminal growth phase: 100 mg/m²/dose (cypionate or enanthate ester) monthly until growth ceases
Maintenance virilizing dose: 100 mg/m²/dose (cypionate or enanthate ester) twice monthly

(Continued)

Testosterone *(Continued)*

Delayed puberty: 40-50 mg/m²/dose monthly (cypionate or enanthate ester) for 6 months

Adults: Hypogonadism:

Testosterone or testosterone propionate: I.M.: 10-25 mg 2-3 times/week

Testosterone cypionate or enanthate:

I.M.: 50-400 mg every 2-4 weeks

Transdermal: 5-6 mg/day initially (use 4 mg/day if scrotal area cannot accommodate 6 mg/day system); adjust dosage in 3-4 weeks depending upon testosterone level

Testosterone pellets: S.C.: Dosage depends on the minimum daily requirements of testosterone propionate [each 25 mg testosterone propionate weekly equals 150 mg (2 pellets)]; usual dose (testosterone pellets): 150-450 mg (2-6 pellets) every 3 months

AndroGel™: Transdermal gel: Males >18 years: Initial: 5 g applied once daily (preferably in the morning); may increase as needed to a maximum of 10 g once daily

Adults: Postpubertal cryptorchism: Testosterone or testosterone propionate: I.M.: 10-25 mg 2-3 times/week

Administration

Parenteral: Administer deep I.M.; not for I.V. administration; pellets only are for S.C. administration

Topical: Apply Testoderm® or Testoderm® with Adhesive transdermal system to scrotum; apply Testoderm® TTS or Androderm® to skin on the arm back or upper buttocks; **do not** apply these two formulations (Testoderm® TTS and Androderm®) to the scrotum; skin should be clean and dry, scrotal hair should be dry-shaved; do not use chemical depilatories; apply transdermal system firmly for 10 seconds. If system should fall off <12 hours from initial application, it may be reapplied; if >12 hours, apply new system at the next scheduled time. Apply AndroGel™ to clean, dry, intact skin of the shoulder and upper arms and/or abdomen. Upon opening the packet(s), the entire contents should be squeezed into the palm of the hand and immediately applied to the application site(s). Application sites should be allowed to dry for a few minutes prior to dressing. Hands should be washed with soap and water after application. **Do not apply AndroGel® to the genitals**

Monitoring Parameters Periodic liver function tests, radiologic examination of wrist and hand every 6 months (when using in prepubertal children); hemoglobin, hematocrit, testosterone level

Reference Range Testosterone, Urine:

Male: 100-1500 ng/24 hours

Female: 100-500 ng/24 hours

Nursing Implications 0.1% triamcinolone cream may be applied to skin under Androderm® to decrease irritation

Additional Information Testosterone 5% cream, not available commercially (must be compounded), has been effective in the treatment of microphallus when applied topically for 21 days

Dosage Forms

Injection:

Aqueous suspension: 25 mg/mL (10 mL, 30 mL); 50 mg/mL (10 mL, 30 mL); 100 mg/mL (10 mL, 30 mL)

In oil, as cypionate: 100 mg/mL (1 mL, 10 mL); 200 mg/mL (1 mL, 10 mL)

In oil, as enanthate: 100 mg/mL (5 mL, 10 mL); 200 mg/mL (5 mL, 10 mL)

In oil, as propionate: 50 mg/mL (10 mL, 30 mL); 100 mg/mL (10 mL, 30 mL)

Pellets, for subcutaneous implantation: 75 mg

Transdermal gel: AndroGel™: 1%: 50 mg (5 g gel); 75 mg (7.5 g gel)

Transdermal system:

Androderm®: 2.5 mg/day, 5 mg/day

Testoderm®: 4 mg/day, 6 mg/day

Tesoderm® TTS: 5 mg/day

Testoderm® with Adhesive: 6 mg/day

♦ **Testosterone Cypionate** *see* Testosterone *on page 905*

♦ **Testosterone Enanthate** *see* Testosterone *on page 905*

♦ **Testosterone Propionate** *see* Testosterone *on page 905*

♦ **Tetanus Immune Globulin, Human** *see page 1138*

♦ **Tetanus Toxoid, Adsorbed** *see page 1138*

♦ **Tetanus Toxoid, Fluid** *see page 1138*

Tetracaine (TET ra kane)

Brand Names Pontocaine®; Supracaine® (Canada)

Available Salts Tetracaine Hydrochloride

Synonyms Amethocaine

Therapeutic Category Analgesic, Topical; Local Anesthetic, Injectable; Local Anesthetic, Ophthalmic; Local Anesthetic, Oral; Local Anesthetic, Topical

Generic Available Yes

Use Local anesthesia in the eye for various diagnostic and examination purposes; spinal anesthesia; topical anesthesia for local skin disorders; local anesthesia for mucous membranes

Pregnancy Risk Factor C

Contraindications Hypersensitivity to tetracaine or any component; ophthalmic secondary bacterial infection, patients with liver disease; CNS disease, meningitis (if used for epidural or spinal anesthesia); myasthenia gravis, impaired cardiac conduction

Warnings Parenteral form may contain sulfites which may cause severe hypersensitivity reactions in sensitive individuals

Precautions Use with caution in patients with cardiac disease and hyperthyroidism

Adverse Reactions

Cardiovascular: Cardiac arrest, bradycardia, myocardial depression, cardiac arrhythmias, hypotension

Central nervous system: Anxiety, apprehension, nervousness, disorientation, seizures, drowsiness, unconsciousness

Dermatologic: Urticaria, contact dermatitis with topical form

Gastrointestinal: Nausea, vomiting

Local: Stinging, burning at injection site

Ocular: Lacrimation, photophobia, corneal epithelial erosion, keratitis, corneal opacification, miosis

Otic: Tinnitus

Respiratory: Respiratory arrest

Drug Interactions Inhibits sulfonamide activity; enhances CNS depression of other CNS depressants

Mechanism of Action Blocks both the generation and conduction of sensory, motor, and autonomic nerve fibers by decreasing the neuronal membrane's permeability to sodium ions, which results in decreasing the rate of depolarization of the nerve membrane

Pharmacodynamics

Onset of action:

Ophthalmic instillation: Anesthetic effects occur within 60 seconds

Topical: Within 3 minutes when applied to mucous membranes

Duration: 1.5-3 hours

Pharmacokinetics

Metabolism: By the liver

Elimination: Metabolites are renally excreted

Usual Dosage

Children: Safety and efficacy have not been established

Adults:

Cream: Apply to affected area as needed

Injection: Dosage varies with the anesthetic procedure, the degree of anesthesia required, and the individual patient response; it is administered by subarachnoid injection for spinal anesthesia:

Perineal anesthesia: 5 mg

Perineal and lower extremities: 10 mg

Anesthesia extending up to the costal margin: 15-20 mg

Low spinal anesthesia (saddle block): 2-5 mg

Ophthalmic:

Ointment: Apply ½" to 1" to lower conjunctival fornix

Solution: Instill 1-2 drops

Administration

Ophthalmic: Apply drops or ointment to conjunctiva of affected eye(s); avoid contact of bottle tip with skin or eye; finger pressure should be applied to lacrimal sac during and for 1-2 minutes after instillation to decrease risk of absorption and systemic reactions

Parenteral: Subarachnoid administration by experienced individuals only

Patient Information Do not touch or rub eye until anesthesia (if ophthalmic) has worn off

Nursing Implications Not for prolonged use topically

(Continued)

Tetracaine *(Continued)*

Dosage Forms

Cream, as hydrochloride: 1% (28 g)

Injection, as hydrochloride: 1% [10 mg/mL] (2 mL)

Injection, as hydrochloride, with dextrose 6%: 0.2% [2 mg/mL] (2 mL); 0.3% [3 mg/mL] (5 mL)

Ointment, as hydrochloride:

Ophthalmic: 0.5% [5 mg/mL] (3.75 g)

Topical: 0.5% [5 mg/mL] (28 g)

Powder for injection, as hydrochloride: 20 mg

Solution, as hydrochloride:

Ophthalmic: 0.5% [5 mg/mL] (1 mL, 2 mL, 15 mL, 59 mL)

Topical: 2% [20 mg/mL] (30 mL, 118 mL)

♦ **Tetracaine Hydrochloride** *see* Tetracaine *on page 907*

♦ **Tetracap® Oral** *see* Tetracycline *on page 908*

♦ **Tetracosactide** *see* Cosyntropin *on page 257*

Tetracycline *(tet ra SYE kleen)*

Related Information

Carbohydrate and Alcohol Content of Liquid Medications for Use in Patients Receiving Ketogenic Diets *on page 1228*

Brand Names Achromycin® Ophthalmic; Achromycin® Topical; Achromycin® V Oral; Apo®-Tetra (Canada); Nor-tet® Oral; Novo-Tetra® (Canada); Nu-Tetra® (Canada); Panmycin® Oral; Robitet® Oral; Sumycin® Oral; Teline® Oral; Tetracap® Oral; Tetracyn® (Canada); Tetralan® Oral; Tetram® Oral; Topicycline® Topical

Available Salts Tetracycline Hydrochloride

Synonyms TCN

Therapeutic Category Acne Products; Antibiotic, Ophthalmic; Antibiotic, Tetracycline Derivative; Antibiotic, Topical

Generic Available Yes

Use

Children, Adolescents and Adults: Treatment of Rocky Mountain spotted fever caused by susceptible *Rickettsia* or brucellosis

Adolescents and Adults: Presumptive treatment of chlamydial infection in patients with gonorrhea

Older children, Adolescents and Adults: Treatment of moderate to severe inflammatory acne vulgaris, Lyme disease, mycoplasmal disease or *Legionella*

Pregnancy Risk Factor D; B (topical)

Contraindications Hypersensitivity to tetracycline or any component; pregnancy; children ≤8 years; use of tetracyclines during tooth development may cause permanent discoloration of the teeth, enamel hypoplasia and retardation of skeletal development and bone growth with risk being greatest for children <4 years and in those receiving high doses

Warnings Photosensitivity reaction may occur with this drug; avoid prolonged exposure to sunlight or tanning equipment; prolonged use may result in superinfection

Precautions Use with caution in patients with renal and liver impairment; dosage modification required in patients with renal impairment

Adverse Reactions

Central nervous system: Pseudotumor cerebri, fever

Dermatologic: Rash, exfoliative dermatitis, photosensitivity, angioedema, discoloration of nails

Gastrointestinal: Nausea, vomiting, diarrhea, stomatitis, glossitis, antibiotic-associated pseudomembranous colitis, esophagitis, oral candidiasis

Hematologic: Hemolytic anemia

Hepatic: Hepatotoxicity

Neuromuscular & skeletal: Injury to growing bones and teeth

Renal: Renal damage, Fanconi-like syndrome

Respiratory: Pulmonary infiltrates with eosinophilia

Miscellaneous: Hypersensitivity reactions, candidal superinfection

Drug Interactions Calcium-, magnesium- or aluminum-containing antacids; iron, zinc; kaolin-, pectin-, or bismuth-containing antidiarrheals decrease tetracycline absorption; tetracycline enhances the hypoprothrombinemic effect of warfarin; methoxyflurane increases chance of nephrotoxicity

Food Interactions Decreases absorption of magnesium, zinc, calcium, dairy products, iron, and amino acids; calcium, dairy products, iron supplements decrease tetracycline absorption

Stability Protect from light; outdated tetracyclines have caused a Fanconi-like syndrome

Mechanism of Action Inhibits bacterial protein synthesis by binding to the 30S and possibly the 50S ribosomal subunit(s) of susceptible bacteria preventing additions of amino acids to the growing peptide chain; may also cause alterations in the cytoplasmic membrane

Pharmacokinetics

Distribution: Widely distributed to most body fluids and tissues including ascitic, synovial and pleural fluids; bronchial secretions; appears in breast milk; poor penetration into CSF

Oral: 75%

I.M.: Poor, with less than 60% of dose absorbed

Protein binding: 30% to 60%

Half-life: 6-12 hours with normal renal function and is prolonged with renal impairment

Time to peak serum concentration: Within 2-4 hours

Elimination: Primary route is the kidney, with 60% of a dose excreted as unchanged drug in urine, small amounts appear in bile

Slightly dialyzable (5% to 20%)

Usual Dosage

Children >8 years:

Oral: 25-50 mg/kg/day in divided doses every 6 hours; not to exceed 3 g/day

Ophthalmic:

Ointment: Apply every 2-12 hours

Suspension: Instill 1-2 drops 2-4 times/day

Adolescents and Adults:

Oral: 250-500 mg/dose every 6-12 hours

Ophthalmic:

Ointment: Apply every 2-12 hours

Suspension: Instill 1-2 drops 2-4 times/day

Topical:

Ointment: Apply small amount of ointment to cleansed area 2-3 times daily

Solution: Acne: Apply each morning and evening

Administration

Oral: Administer 1 hour before or 2 hours after meals with adequate amounts of fluid; avoid taking antacids, calcium, iron, dairy products, or milk formulas within 3 hours of tetracyclines

Ophthalmic: Avoid contact of tube or bottle tip with skin or eye; instill ointment or drops in the lower conjunctival sac

Topical: Acne: Topical solution should be applied to cleansed affected area; reconstitute topical solution by inserting the plastic applicator unit containing the powder into the bottle containing the diluent; apply solution by tilting the bottle and rubbing applicator tip over the skin while gently applying pressure

Monitoring Parameters Renal, hepatic, and hematologic function tests

Test Interactions False-negative urine glucose with Clinistix®

Patient Information Avoid prolonged exposure to sunlight or sunlamps

Dosage Forms

Capsule, as hydrochloride: 100 mg, 250 mg, 500 mg

Ointment:

Ophthalmic: 1% [10 mg/mL] (3.5 g)

Topical, as hydrochloride: 3% [30 mg/mL] (14.2 g, 30 g)

Solution, topical, as hydrochloride: 2.2 mg/mL (70 mL)

Suspension:

Ophthalmic: 1% [10 mg/mL] (0.5 mL, 1 mL, 4 mL)

Oral, as hydrochloride: 125 mg/5 mL (60 mL, 480 mL)

Tablet, as hydrochloride: 250 mg, 500 mg

References
American Academy of Pediatrics. Committee on Drugs. "Requiem for Tetracyclines," *Pediatrics*, 1975, 55(1):142-3.

- ♦ **T/Gel® [OTC]** see Coal Tar *on page 247*
- ♦ **T-Gen® Rectal** see Trimethobenzamide *on page 954*
- ♦ **T-Gesic®** see Hydrocodone and Acetaminophen *on page 485*
- ♦ **THAM®** see Tromethamine *on page 958*
- ♦ **THAM-E®** see Tromethamine *on page 958*
- ♦ **THC** see Dronabinol *on page 350*
- ♦ **Theo-24®** see Theophylline *on page 910*
- ♦ **Theobid®** see Theophylline *on page 910*
- ♦ **Theochron®** see Theophylline *on page 910*
- ♦ **Theoclear-80®** see Theophylline *on page 910*
- ♦ **Theoclear® L.A.** see Theophylline *on page 910*
- ♦ **Theo-Dur®** see Theophylline *on page 910*
- ♦ **Theolair™** see Theophylline *on page 910*

Theophylline (thee OF i lin)
Related Information
Asthma Guidelines *on page 1178*
Blood Level Sampling Time Guidelines *on page 1189*
Carbohydrate and Alcohol Content of Liquid Medications for Use in Patients Receiving Ketogenic Diets *on page 1228*
Overdose and Toxicology *on page 1191*

Brand Names Accurbron®; Aerolate III®; Aerolate JR®; Aerolate SR® S; Aquaphyllin®; Asmalix®; Bronkodyl®; Elixomin®; Elixophyllin®; Lanophyllin®; Quibron®-T; Quibron®-T/SR; Respbid®; Slo-bid™; Slo-Phyllin®; Sustaire®; Theo-24®; Theobid®; Theochron®; Theoclear-80®; Theoclear® L.A.; Theo-Dur®; Theolair™; Theo-Sav®; Theospan®-SR; Theostat-80®; Theovent®; Theo-X®; T-Phyl®; Uni-Dur®; Uniphyl®

Therapeutic Category Antiasthmatic; Bronchodilator; Respiratory Stimulant; Theophylline Derivative

Generic Available Yes

Use Treatment of symptoms and reversible airway obstruction due to chronic asthma, chronic bronchitis, or COPD; treatment of idiopathic apnea of prematurity in neonates

Pregnancy Risk Factor C

Contraindications Hypersensitivity to theophylline or any component

Warnings If a patient develops signs and symptoms of theophylline toxicity (eg, persistent, repetitive vomiting), a serum theophylline level should be measured and subsequent doses held; due to potential saturation of theophylline clearance at serum levels in or (in some patients) less than the therapeutic range, dosage adjustment should be made in small increments (maximum dosage adjustment: 25%); due to wide interpatient variability, theophylline serum level measurements must be used to optimize therapy and prevent serious toxicity

Precautions Use with caution in patients with peptic ulcer, hyperthyroidism, seizure disorders, hypertension, and patients with cardiac arrhythmias (excluding bradyarrhythmias)

Adverse Reactions See table.

Theophylline Serum Levels (µg/mL)*	Adverse Reactions
15-25	GI upset, GE reflux, diarrhea, nausea, vomiting, abdominal pain, nervousness, headache, insomnia, agitation, dizziness, muscle cramp, tremor
25-35	Tachycardia, occasional PVC
>35	Ventricular tachycardia, frequent PVC, seizure

*Adverse effects do not necessarily occur according to serum levels. Arrhythmia and seizure can occur without seeing the other adverse effects.

Drug Interactions Decreases adenosine, esmolol, benzodiazepine, and pancuronium effects; increases lithium clearance; increases central nervous system side effects with ephedrine; increases risk of cardiac arrhythmias with halothane; decreases zafirlukast serum levels; for medications which alter theophylline clearance, see tables on following page.

Food Interactions Food does not appreciably affect the absorption of liquid, fast-release products and most sustained release products; however, food may induce a sudden release (dose-dumping) of once-daily sustained release products resulting in an increase in serum drug levels and potential toxicity; avoid excessive amounts of caffeine; avoid extremes of dietary protein and carbohydrate intake; limit charcoal-broiled foods and caffeinated beverages

Mechanism of Action Competitively inhibits two isoenzymes of the enzyme phosphodiesterase resulting in increased levels of cyclic adenine monophosphate (cAMP) which may be responsible for most of theophylline's effects; effects on the myocardium and neuromuscular transmission may be due to the intracellular translocation of ionized calcium; overall, theophylline produces the following effects: relaxation of the smooth muscle of the respiratory tract, suppression of the response of airways to stimuli, increases the force of contraction of diaphragmatic muscles; pulmonary, coronary, and renal artery dilation; CNS stimulation, diuresis, stimulation of catecholamine release, gastric acid secretion, and relaxation of biliary and GI smooth muscle

Clinical Factors Reported to Affect Theophylline Clearance

Decreased Theophylline Level	Increased Theophylline Level
Smoking (cigarettes, marijuana)	Acute pulmonary edema
High protein/low carbohydrate diet	Cessation of smoking (after chronic use)
Charcoal broiled beef	Cor pulmonale
	Congestive heart failure
	Hypothyroidism
	Fever (≥102° for 24 hours or more, or lesser temperature elevations for longer periods)
	Hepatic cirrhosis/acute hepatitis
	Renal failure in infants <3 mo of age
	Sepsis with multisystem organ failure
	Shock
	Viral illness

Medications Affecting Theophylline Clearance Resulting in Either Increased or Decreased Serum Levels

Decreased Theophylline Level	Increased Theophylline Level
Aminoglutethimide	Alcohol
Carbamazepine	Allopurinol (>600 mg/day)
Isoproterenol (I.V.)	Beta-blockers
Isoniazid*	Calcium channel blockers
Ketoconazole	Cimetidine
Loop diuretics*	Ciprofloxacin
Nevirapine	Clarithromycin
Phenobarbital	Corticosteroids
Phenytoin	Disulfiram
Rifampin	Ephedrine
Ritonavir	Erythromycin
Sulfinpyrazone	Esmolol
Sympathomimetics	Influenza virus vaccine
	Interferon, human recombinant alpha 2-a and 2-b
	Isoniazid*
	Loop diuretics*
	Methotrexate
	Mexiletine
	Oral contraceptives
	Propafenone
	Propranolol
	Tacrine
	Thiabendazole
	Thyroid hormones
	Troleandomycin (TAO®)
	Verapamil
	Zileuton

*Both increased and decreased theophylline levels have been reported.

Pharmacokinetics

Absorption: Oral: Rapid and complete with up to 100% absorption depending upon the formulation used

Distribution: V_d: 0.45 L/kg; distributes into breast milk; breast milk to plasma ratio: 0.67; crosses the placenta and into the CSF

(Continued)

Theophylline (Continued)

Protein binding: 40%; decreased protein binding in neonates (due to a greater percentage of fetal albumin), hepatic cirrhosis, uncorrected acidemia, women in third trimester of pregnancy, and geriatric patients

Metabolism: In the liver by demethylation and oxidation; theophylline is metabolized to caffeine (active); in neonates this theophylline-derived caffeine accumulates (due to decreased hepatic metabolism) and significant concentrations of caffeine may occur; a substantial decrease in serum caffeine concentrations occurs after 40 weeks postconceptional age

Half-life: See table.

Theophylline Clearance and Half-Life With Respect to Age and Altered Physiological States*

Patient Group	Mean Clearance (mL/kg/min)	Mean Half-life (h)
Premature infants		
postnatal age 3-15 d	0.29	30
postnatal age 25-57 d	0.64	20
Term infants		
postnatal age 1-2 d	Not reported†	25
postnatal age 3-30 wk‡	Not reported†	11
Children		
1-4 y	1.7	3.4
4-12 y	1.6	Not reported†
13-15 y	0.9	Not reported†
16-17 y	1.4	3.7 (range: 1.5-5.9)
Adults		
16-60 (nonsmoking)	0.65	8.2
>60 y (nonsmoking, healthy)	0.41	9.8
Acute pulmonary edema	0.33	19
Cystic fibrosis (14-28 y)	1.25	6
Liver disease		
acute hepatitis	0.35	19.2
cholestasis	0.65	14.4
cirrhosis	0.31	32
Sepsis with multiorgan failure	0.46	18.8
Hypothyroid	0.38	11.6
Hyperthyroid	0.8	4.5
COPD >60 y, nonsmoking >1 y	0.54	11

*From Hendels L, et al.

†Either not reported or not reported in a comparable format

‡Maturation of clearance in premature infants and term infants is most closely related to postconceptional age (PCA); adult clearance values are reached at approximately 55 weeks PCA and higher pediatric values at approximately 60 weeks PCA (Kraus, et al).

Elimination: In urine; children >3 months and adults excrete 10% in urine as unchanged drug; neonates excrete approximately 50% of the dose unchanged in urine

Usual Dosage Oral (see Aminophylline *on page 61* for I.V. doses):

Loading dose:

Neonates: Apnea of prematurity: 4 mg/kg/dose

Infants and Children: Treatment of acute bronchospasm: (to achieve a serum level of about 10 mcg/mL; loading doses should be given using a rapidly absorbed oral product **not** a sustained release product):

If no theophylline has been administered in the previous 24 hours: 5 mg/kg theophylline

If theophylline has been administered in the previous 24 hours: 2.5 mg/kg theophylline may be given in emergencies when serum levels are not available

A modified loading dose (mg/kg) may be calculated (when the serum level is known) by: [Blood level desired - blood level measured] divided by 2 (for every

1 mg/kg theophylline given, the blood level will rise by approximately 2 mcg/mL)

Maintenance dose: See table.

Maintenance Dose for Acute Symptoms

Population Group	Oral Theophylline (mg/kg/day)
Premature infant or newborn to 6 wk (for apnea/bradycardia)	4*
6 wk to 6 mo	10*
Infants 6 mo to 1 y	12-18*
Children 1-9 y	20-24
Children 9-12 y, adolescent daily smokers of cigarettes or marijuana, and otherwise healthy adult smokers <50 y	16
Adolescents 12-16 y (nonsmokers)	13
Otherwise healthy nonsmoking adults (including elderly patients)	10 (not to exceed 900 mg/day)
Cardiac decompensation, cor pulmonale, and/or liver dysfunction	5 (not to exceed 400 mg/day)
*Alternative dosing regimen for full-term infants <1 year of age: Total daily dose (mg) = [(0.2 x age in weeks) + 5] x weight (kg) Postnatal Age <26 weeks: Total daily dose divided every 8 hours Postnatal Age >26 weeks: Total daily dose divided every 6 hours	

These recommendations, based on mean clearance rates for age or risk factors, were calculated to achieve a serum level of 10 mcg/mL (5 mcg/mL for newborns with apnea/bradycardia). In newborns and infants, a fast-release oral product can be used. The total daily dose can be divided every 12 hours in newborns and every 6-8 hours in infants. In children and healthy adults, a slow-release product can be used. The total daily dose can be divided every 8-12 hours.

Use ideal body weight for obese patients

Dose should be further adjusted based on serum levels. Guidelines for drawing theophylline serum levels are shown in the table.

Guidelines for Drawing Theophylline Serum Levels

Dosage Form	Time to Draw Level*
I.V. bolus	30 min after end of 30-min infusion
I.V. continuous infusion	12-24 h after initiation of infusion
P.O. liquid, fast-release formulation	Peak: 1 h postdose after at least 1 day of therapy Trough: Just before a dose after at least 1 day of therapy
P.O. slow-release formulation	Peak: 4 h postdose after at least 1 day of therapy Trough: Just before a dose after at least 1 day of therapy

*The time to achieve steady-state serum levels is prolonged in patients with longer half-lives (eg, premature neonates, infants, and adults with cardiac or liver failure (see theophylline half-life table). In these patients, serum theophylline levels should be drawn after 48-72 hours of therapy; serum levels may need to be done prior to steady-state to assess the patients current progress or evaluate potential toxicity.

Administration

Oral: Sustained release preparations should be administered with a full glass of water, whole or cut by half only; do not crush; sustained release capsule forms may be opened and sprinkled on soft foods; do not chew or crush beads

Parenteral: Premade I.V. infusion bags for continuous infusion usage; rate of infusion dependent upon dosage; loading doses using I.V. infusion should be administered over 20-30 minutes

(Continued)

Theophylline *(Continued)*

Monitoring Parameters Respiratory rate, heart rate, serum theophylline level, arterial or capillary blood gases (if applicable); number and severity of apnea spells (apnea of prematurity)

Reference Range
Therapeutic levels:
Asthma: 10-15 µg/mL (peak level)
Apnea of prematurity: 6-14 µg/mL
Toxic concentration: >20 µg/mL

Test Interactions May elevate uric acid levels

Patient Information Contact physician whenever nausea, vomiting, persistent headache, or irregular heartbeats occur; notify physician if a new illness develops (especially if high fevers); do not alter time, dose, or frequency of administration without physician knowledge; avoid drinking or eating of large quantities of caffeine-containing beverages or food

Additional Information Due to improved theophylline clearance during the first year of life, serum concentration determinations and dosage adjustments may be needed to optimize therapy

Available also by nonproprietary name
Theophylline Immediate Release Tablet/Capsule: Bronkodyl®, Elixophyllin®, Quibron®-T, Slo-Phyllin®, Theolair™
Theophylline Liquid: Aquaphyllin®, Asmalix®, Elixophyllin®
Theophylline Timed Release Capsule: Aerolate III®, Aerolate JR®, Aerolate SR®, Elixophyllin® SR, Slo-bid™ Gyrocaps®, Slo-Phyllin® Gyrocaps®, Theobid®, Theoclear® L.A., Theospan®-SR, Theospan®-SR
Theophylline Timed Release Tablet: Quibron®-T/S, Respbid®, Sustaire®, Theochron®, Theo-Dur®, Theolair™-SR, Uniphyl®

Dosage Forms
Capsule:
Immediate release (Bronkodyl®, Elixophyllin®): 100 mg, 200 mg
Timed release:
[8-12 hours] (Aerolate®): 65 mg [III]; 130 mg [JR], 260 mg [SR]
[8-12 hours] (Slo-bid™): 50 mg, 75 mg, 100 mg, 125 mg, 200 mg, 300 mg
[8-12 hours] (Slo-Phyllin® Gyrocaps®): 60 mg, 125 mg, 250 mg
[12 hours] (Theobid® Duracaps®): 260 mg
[12 hours] (Theoclear® L.A., Theospan®-SR): 130 mg, 260 mg
[12 hours] (Theovent®): 125 mg, 250 mg
[24 hours] (Theo-24®): 100 mg, 200 mg, 300 mg
Elixir (Asmalix®, Elixomin®, Elixophyllin®, Lanophyllin® [sugar free]): 80 mg/15 mL (15 mL, 30 mL, 480 mL, 4000 mL)
Infusion, in D₅W: 0.4 mg/mL (1000 mL); 0.8 mg/mL (500 mL, 1000 mL); 1.6 mg/mL (250 mL, 500 mL); 2 mg/mL (100 mL); 3.2 mg/mL (250 mL); 4 mg/mL (50 mL, 100 mL);
Solution, oral:
Theolair™ (alcohol free): 80 mg/15 mL (15 mL, 18.75 mL, 30 mL, 480 mL)
Syrup:
Aquaphyllin® (alcohol free, dye free), Slo-Phyllin® (alcohol free, sugar free), Theoclear-80® (alcohol free, dye free), Theostat-80®: 80 mg/15 mL (15 mL, 30 mL, 500 mL)
Accurbron® (dye free): 150 mg/15 mL (480 mL)
Tablet: Immediate release:
Slo-Phyllin®: 100 mg, 200 mg
Theolair™: 125 mg, 250 mg
Quibron®-T: 300 mg
Tablet:
Controlled release (Theo-X®): 100 mg, 200 mg, 300 mg
Timed release:
[8-12 hours] (Quibron®-T/SR): 300 mg
[8-12 hours] (Respbid®): 250 mg, 500 mg
[8-12 hours] (Sustaire®): 100 mg, 300 mg
[8-12 hours] (T-Phyl®): 200 mg
[12-24 hours]: 100 mg, 200 mg, 300 mg, 450 mg
[12-24 hours] (Theochron®): 100 mg, 200 mg, 300 mg
[8-24 hours] (Theo-Dur®): 100 mg, 200 mg, 300 mg, 450 mg
[8-24 hours] (Theo-Sav®): 100 mg, 200 mg, 300 mg
[8-24 hours] (Theolair-SR®): 200 mg, 250 mg, 300 mg, 500 mg
[24 hours] (Uni-Dur®): 400 mg, 600 mg
[24 hours] (Uniphyl®): 400 mg

References

Hendeles L, Jenkins J, and Temple R, "Revised FDA Labeling Guideline for Theophylline Oral Dosage Forms," *Pharmacotherapy*, 1995, 15(4):409-427.

Kearney TE, Manoguerra AS, Curtis GP, et al, "Theophylline Toxicity and the Beta-Adrenergic System," *Ann Intern Med*, 1985, 102(6):766-9.

Kraus DM, Fischer JH, Reitz SJ, et al, "Alterations in Theophylline Metabolism During the First Year of Life," *Clin Pharmacol Ther*, 1993, 54(4):351-9.

Upton RA, "Pharmacokinetic Interactions Between Theophylline and Other Medication (Part I)," *Clin Pharmacokinet*, 1991, 20(1):66-80.

♦ **Theophylline Ethylenediamine** *see* Aminophylline *on page 61*

♦ **Theo-Sav®** *see* Theophylline *on page 910*

♦ **Theospan®-SR** *see* Theophylline *on page 910*

♦ **Theostat-80®** *see* Theophylline *on page 910*

♦ **Theovent®** *see* Theophylline *on page 910*

♦ **Theo-X®** *see* Theophylline *on page 910*

♦ **Thera-Flur®** *see* Fluoride *on page 427*

♦ **Thera-Flur-N®** *see* Fluoride *on page 427*

♦ **Thermazene®** *see* Silver Sulfadiazine *on page 867*

♦ **Theroxide® Wash [OTC]** *see* Benzoyl Peroxide *on page 126*

Thiabendazole (thye a BEN da zole)

Brand Names Mintezol®

Synonyms Tiabendazole

Therapeutic Category Anthelmintic

Generic Available No

Use Treatment of strongyloidiasis, cutaneous larva migrans, visceral larva migrans, dracunculosis, trichinosis, and mixed helminthic infections

Pregnancy Risk Factor C

Contraindications Hypersensitivity to thiabendazole or any component; pregnancy

Precautions Use with caution in patients with renal or hepatic impairment, malnutrition, anemia, or dehydration

Adverse Reactions

Cardiovascular: Flushing, hypotension, bradycardia

Central nervous system: Dizziness, drowsiness, vertigo, seizures, fever, malaise, headache, chills, hallucinations

Dermatologic: Rash, Stevens-Johnson syndrome, erythema multiforme, pruritus

Endocrine & metabolic: Hyperglycemia

Gastrointestinal: Nausea, vomiting, diarrhea, anorexia

Genitourinary: Malodor of the urine

Hematologic: Leukopenia

Hepatic: Hepatotoxicity, jaundice, cholestasis

Neuromuscular & skeletal: Paresthesia, numbness

Ocular: Blurred vision

Otic: Tinnitus

Renal: Nephrotoxicity, hematuria

Miscellaneous: Hypersensitivity reactions, lymphadenopathy

Drug Interactions Increases serum theophylline concentrations (monitor serum theophylline level in patients receiving both drugs concomitantly)

Mechanism of Action Inhibits helminth-specific mitochondrial fumarate reductase

Pharmacokinetics

Absorption: From the GI tract and through the skin

Metabolism: Extensive in the liver via hydroxylation and conjugation with sulfuric and/or glucuronic acid

Time to peak serum concentration: Within 1-2 hours

Elimination: In feces (5%) and urine (87%), primarily as conjugated metabolites

Usual Dosage

Oral:

Children and Adults: 50 mg/kg/day divided every 12 hours (maximum dose: 3 g/day)

Strongyloidiasis: For 2 consecutive days (5 days or longer for disseminated disease)

Cutaneous larva migrans: For 2-5 consecutive days

Visceral larva migrans: For 5-7 consecutive days

Trichinosis: For 2-4 consecutive days

Angiostrongylosis: 50-75 mg/kg/day divided every 8-12 hours for 3 days

Dracunculosis: 50-75 mg/kg/day divided every 12 hours for 3 days

(Continued)

Thiabendazole *(Continued)*

Topical: Cutaneous larva migrans: Instead of oral therapy, thiabendazole 10% to 15% suspension or a 10% ointment in white petrolatum has been applied topically to lesions 4-6 times/day

Administration Oral: Administer after meals; chew tablet well before swallowing; shake suspension well before use

Monitoring Parameters Periodic renal and hepatic function tests

Patient Information May cause drowsiness and impair ability to perform activities requiring mental alertness or physical coordination; avoid driving or operating machinery

Nursing Implications Purgation is not required prior to use

Dosage Forms

Suspension, oral: 500 mg/5 mL (120 mL)

Tablet, chewable (orange flavor): 500 mg

References

Walden J, "Parasitic Diseases. Other Roundworms. *Trichuris*, Hookworm, and *Strongyloides*," *Prim Care*, 1991, 18(1):53-74.

Zygmunt DJ, "*Strongyloides stearcoralis*," *Infect Control Hosp Epidemiol*, 1990, 11(9):495-7.

♦ **Thiamazole** *see* Methimazole *on page 618*

Thiamine *(THYE a min)*

Brand Names Betalin®S; Betaxin® (Canada); Bewon® (Canada)

Available Salts Thiamine Hydrochloride

Synonyms Aneurine; Thiaminium; Vitamin B$_1$

Therapeutic Category Nutritional Supplement; Vitamin, Water Soluble

Generic Available Yes

Use Treatment of thiamine deficiency including beriberi, Wernicke's encephalopathy syndrome, and peripheral neuritis associated with pellagra; alcoholic patients with altered sensorium; various genetic metabolic disorders

Pregnancy Risk Factor A (C if dose exceeds RDA recommendation)

Contraindications Hypersensitivity to thiamine or any component

Warnings Large doses should be given in divided doses for better oral absorption

Precautions Use parenteral route cautiously, see Adverse Reactions

Adverse Reactions

Cardiovascular: Cardiovascular collapse and death (primarily following repeated I.V. administration), warmth

Dermatologic: Rash, angioedema

Genitourinary: Discoloration of urine (bright yellow) with large doses

Neuromuscular & skeletal: Paresthesia

Drug Interactions I.V. dextrose solutions increase thiamine requirement; may enhance the effects of neuromuscular blocking agents

Food Interactions High carbohydrate diets may increase thiamine requirement

Stability Unstable with alkaline or neutral solutions

Mechanism of Action An essential coenzyme in carbohydrate metabolism; combines with adenosine triphosphate to form thiamine pyrophosphate

Pharmacokinetics

Absorption:

Oral: Poor

I.M.: Rapid and complete

Metabolism: In the liver

Elimination: Renally as unchanged drug only after body storage sites become saturated

Usual Dosage

Adequate intake: Infants:

<6 months: 0.2 mg (0.03 mg/kg)

6-12 months: 0.3 mg (0.03 mg/kg)

Recommended daily allowance (RDA):

1-3 years: 0.5 mg

4-8 years: 0.6 mg

9-13 years: 0.9 mg

14-18 years:

Male: 1.2 mg

Female: 1 mg

≥19 years:

Male: 1.2 mg

Female: 1.1 mg

Dietary supplement (depends on caloric or carbohydrate content of the diet)

Oral:
 Infants: 0.3-0.5 mg/day
 Children: 0.5-1 mg/day
 Adults: 1-2 mg/day
 Note: The above doses can be found in multivitamin preparations
Thiamine deficiency (beriberi):
 Children: 10-25 mg/dose I.M. or I.V. daily (if critically ill), or 10-50 mg/dose orally every day for 2 weeks, then 5-10 mg/dose orally daily for 1 month
 Adults: 5-30 mg/dose I.M. or I.V. 3 times/day (if critically ill); then orally 5-30 mg/day in single or divided doses 3 times/day for 1 month
 Wernicke's encephalopathy: Adults: Initial: 100 mg I.V., then 50-100 mg/day I.M. or I.V. until consuming a regular, balanced diet
 Metabolic disorders: Oral: Adults: 10-20 mg/day (dosages up to 4 g/day in divided doses have been used)

Administration
Oral: May administer with or without food
Parenteral: Administer by slow I.V. injection or I.M.

Reference Range Normal values: 1.6-4 mg/dL

Test Interactions False-positive for uric acid using the phosphotungstate method and for urobilinogen using the Ehrlich's reagent; large doses may interfere with the spectrophotometric determination of serum theophylline concentration

Patient Information May color urine bright yellow

Additional Information Dietary sources include legumes, pork, beef, whole grains, yeast, fresh vegetables; a deficiency state can occur in as little as 3 weeks following total dietary absence

Dosage Forms
Injection, as hydrochloride: 100 mg/mL (1 mL, 2 mL, 10 mL, 30 mL); 200 mg/mL (30 mL)
Tablet, as hydrochloride: 25 mg, 50 mg, 100 mg, 250 mg, 500 mg
Tablet, enteric coated, as hydrochloride: 20 mg

♦ **Thiamine Hydrochloride** *see* Thiamine *on page 916*

♦ **Thiaminium** *see* Thiamine *on page 916*

Thiethylperazine (thye eth il PER a zeen)

Related Information
 Overdose and Toxicology *on page 1191*

Brand Names Norzine®; Torecan®

Available Salts Thiethylperazine Maleate

Therapeutic Category Antiemetic; Phenothiazine Derivative

Generic Available No

Use Relief of nausea and vomiting

Pregnancy Risk Factor X

Contraindications Severe CNS depression, comatose states; hypersensitivity to thiethylperazine or any component; pregnancy

Warnings Safety and efficacy in children <12 years of age have not been established; postural hypotension may occur after I.M. injection; the injectable form contains sulfite which may cause allergic reactions in sensitive individuals; tablet contains yellow No.5 (tartrazine) which may cause allergic reactions in sensitive individuals; avoid use in children and adolescents whose signs and symptoms are suggestive of Reye's syndrome

Adverse Reactions
Cardiovascular: Hypotension, peripheral edema
Central nervous system: Drowsiness, extrapyramidal effects, seizures, fever, headache, neuroleptic malignant syndrome
Gastrointestinal: Xerostomia
Hepatic: Cholestatic jaundice (occasional)
Neuromuscular & skeletal: Trigeminal neuralgia
Ocular: Blurred vision
Respiratory: Dryness of mucous membranes

Drug Interactions Additive effects with anticholinergic agents and other phenothiazines; additive CNS depression with sedatives and antihistamines

Mechanism of Action Blocks postsynaptic mesolimbic dopaminergic receptors in the brain including the medullary chemoreceptor trigger zone; exhibits a strong alpha-adrenergic blocking effect and depresses the release of hypothalamic and hypophyseal hormones

Pharmacodynamics
Onset of action: Oral, I.M., rectal: Antiemetic effects occur within 30 minutes
(Continued)

Thiethylperazine *(Continued)*

Duration: ~4 hours

Usual Dosage Children >12 years and Adults: Oral, I.M., rectal: 10 mg 1-3 times/day as needed

Administration Parenteral: Inject I.M. deeply into large muscle mass, patient should be lying down and remain so for at least 1 hour; I.V. and S.C. routes of administration are not recommended

Patient Information Causes drowsiness and may impair ability to perform hazardous tasks requiring mental alertness or physical coordination; may cause photosensitivity; avoid excessive sunlight

Dosage Forms

Injection, as maleate: 5 mg/mL (2 mL)

Suppository, rectal, as maleate: 10 mg

Tablet, as maleate: 10 mg

♦ **Thiethylperazine Maleate** *see* Thiethylperazine *on page 917*

Thioguanine *(thye oh GWAH neen)*

Related Information

Emetogenic Potential of Single Chemotherapeutic Agents *on page 1095*

Brand Names Lanvis® (Canada)

Synonyms 2-Amino-6-mercaptopurine; TG; 6-TG; 6-Thioguanine; Tioguanine

Therapeutic Category Antineoplastic Agent, Antimetabolite

Generic Available No

Use Remission induction in acute myelogenous (nonlymphocytic) leukemia; treatment of chronic myelogenous leukemia and acute lymphocytic leukemia

Pregnancy Risk Factor D

Contraindications History of previous therapy resistance with thioguanine and in patients resistant to mercaptopurine; hypersensitivity to thioguanine or any component

Warnings The FDA currently recommends that procedures for proper handling and disposal of antineoplastic agents be considered; thioguanine is potentially carcinogenic and teratogenic

Precautions Use with caution and reduce dose of thioguanine in patients with renal or hepatic impairment

Adverse Reactions

Central nervous system: Neurotoxicity

Dermatologic: Skin rash, photosensitivity, staining of skin or eyes (yellow)

Endocrine & metabolic: Hyperuricemia

Gastrointestinal: Mild nausea or vomiting, anorexia, stomatitis, diarrhea

Hematologic: Myelosuppression (leukopenia, thrombocytopenia, anemia)

Hepatic: Hepatitis, jaundice, veno-occlusive hepatic disease

Neuromuscular & skeletal: Unsteady gait

Drug Interactions Busulfan (increases busulfan toxicity)

Food Interactions Enhanced absorption if administered between meals

Mechanism of Action Purine analog that is incorporated into DNA and RNA resulting in the inhibition of synthesis and utilization of purine nucleotides

Pharmacokinetics

Absorption: Oral: 30% (variable and incomplete)

Distribution: Crosses the placenta; does not appear to cross into CSF

Metabolism: Rapid and extensive hepatic metabolism by methylation of thioguanine to 2-amino-6-methylthioguanine (active) and inactive compounds

Half-life, terminal: 11 hours

Time to peak serum concentration: Within 8-12 hours

Elimination: Metabolites excreted in urine

Usual Dosage Oral (refer to individual protocols):

Infants <3 years: Combination drug therapy for ANLL: 3.3 mg/kg/day in divided doses twice daily for 4 days

Children and Adults:

Single agent chemotherapy for ANLL: 2-3 mg/kg/day once daily calculated to nearest 20 mg

Induction of remission in patients with acute leukemia (combination therapy): 75-200 mg/m²/day in 1-2 divided doses for 5-7 days or until remission is attained

Administration Oral: Administer between meals on an empty stomach

Monitoring Parameters CBC with (differential, platelet count), liver function tests, hemoglobin, hematocrit, serum uric acid

Patient Information Notify physician if fever, sore throat, bleeding, bruising, yellow discoloration of skin or eyes, or leg swelling occurs

Nursing Implications Ensure adequate patient hydration, alkalinization of the urine, and/or administration of allopurinol to prevent hyperuricemia

Additional Information Myelosuppressive effects:
WBC: Moderate
Platelets: Moderate
Onset (days): 7-10
Nadir (days): 14
Recovery (days): 21

Dosage Forms Tablet, scored: 40 mg

Extemporaneous Preparations A 40 mg/mL oral suspension compounded from tablets which were crushed, mixed with a volume of Cologel® suspending agent equal to ⅓ the final volume, and brought to the final volume with a 2:1 mixture of simple syrup and cherry syrup was stable for 84 days when stored in an amber bottle at room temperature

> Dressman JB and Poust RI, "Stability of Allopurinol and Five Antineoplastics in Suspension," *Am J Hosp Pharm*, 1983, 40:616-8.

References
Culbert SJ, Shuster JJ, Land VJ, et al, "Remission Induction and Continuation Therapy in Children With Their First Relapse of Acute Lymphoid Leukemia: A Pediatric Oncology Group Study," *Cancer*, 1991, 67(1):37-42.

Steuber CP, Civin C, Krischer J, et al, "A Comparison of Induction and Maintenance Therapy for Acute Nonlymphocytic Leukemia in Childhood: Results of a Pediatric Oncology Group Study," *J Clin Oncol*, 1991, 9(2):247-58.

♦ **6-Thioguanine** *see* Thioguanine *on page 918*

Thiopental (thye oh PEN tal)

Related Information
Preprocedure Sedatives in Children *on page 1169*

Brand Names Pentothal® Sodium

Available Salts Thiopental Sodium

Therapeutic Category Anticonvulsant, Barbiturate; Barbiturate; General Anesthetic; Hypnotic; Sedative

Generic Available Yes

Use Induction of anesthesia; adjunct for intubation in head injury patients; control of convulsive states; treatment of elevated intracranial pressure

Restrictions C-III

Pregnancy Risk Factor C

Contraindications Porphyria (variegate or acute intermittent); hypersensitivity to thiopental, pentobarbital, any component, or other barbiturates

Precautions Use with caution in patients with asthma or pharyngeal infections because cough, laryngospasm, or bronchospasms may occur; use with caution in patients with hypotension, severe cardiovascular disease, hepatic or renal dysfunction; avoid extravasation or intra-arterial injection which may cause necrosis due to pH of 10.6; ensure patient has intravenous access

Adverse Reactions
Cardiovascular: Decreased cardiac output, hypotension
Local: Necrosis with I.V. extravasation
Renal: Decreased urine output
Respiratory: Cough, laryngospasm, bronchospasm, respiratory depression, apnea
Miscellaneous: Anaphylaxis

Drug Interactions Barbiturates are enzyme inducers (monitor patients closely for decreased effect of concomitantly administered medications or increased effect when barbiturates are discontinued); CNS depressants

Stability Solutions are alkaline and incompatible with drugs with acidic pH, such as succinylcholine, atropine sulfate

Mechanism of Action Ultra-short-acting barbiturate; depresses CNS activity by binding to barbiturate site at GABA-receptor complex enhancing GABA activity; depresses reticular activating system; higher doses may be gabamimetic

Pharmacodynamics Anesthesia effects:
Onset of action: I.V.: 30-60 seconds
Duration: 5-30 minutes

Pharmacokinetics
Distribution: V_d: Adults: 1.4 L/kg
Protein binding: 72% to 86%
Metabolism: In the liver primarily to inactive metabolites but pentobarbital is also formed
(Continued)

Thiopental *(Continued)*

Half-life, adults: 3-11.5 hours (shorter half-life in children)

Usual Dosage

Induction anesthesia: I.V.:
Neonates: 3-4 mg/kg
Infants: 5-8 mg/kg
Children 1-12 years: 5-6 mg/kg
Children >12 years and Adults: 3-5 mg/kg

Maintenance anesthesia: I.V.:
Children: 1 mg/kg as needed
Adults: 25-100 mg as needed

Increased intracranial pressure: Children: I.V.: 1.5-5 mg/kg/dose; repeat as needed to control intracranial pressure; larger doses (30 mg/kg) to induce coma after hypoxic-ischemic injury do not appear to improve neurologic outcome

Seizures: I.V.:
Children: 2-3 mg/kg/dose, repeat as needed
Adults: 75-250 mg/dose, repeat as needed

Sedation: Rectal:
Children: 5-10 mg/kg/dose
Adults: 3-4 g/dose

Administration Parenteral: Avoid rapid I.V. injection (may cause hypotension or decreased cardiac output); may administer by intermittent infusion over 10-60 minutes at a maximum concentration of 50 mg/mL

Monitoring Parameters Respiratory rate, heart rate, blood pressure

Reference Range

Therapeutic:
Hypnotic: 1-5 µg/mL (SI: 4.1-20.7 µmol/L)
Coma: 30-100 µg/mL (SI: 124-413 µmol/L)
Anesthesia: 7-130 µg/mL (SI: 29-536 µmol/L)

Nursing Implications Avoid extravasation, necrosis may occur

Additional Information Accumulation may occur with chronic dosing due to lipid solubility; prolonged recovery occurs due to redistribution of thiopental from fat stores; therefore, thiopental is usually not used for procedures lasting >15-20 minutes; sodium content, injection: 4.9 mEq/g

Dosage Forms

Injection, as sodium: 250 mg, 400 mg, 500 mg, 1 g, 2.5 g, 5 g
Suspension, rectal, as sodium: 400 mg/g (2 g)

♦ **Thiopental Sodium** *see* Thiopental *on page 919*

♦ **Thioplex®** *see* Thiotepa *on page 922*

Thioridazine *(thye oh RID a zeen)*

Related Information

Overdose and Toxicology *on page 1191*

Brand Names Apo®-Thioridazine (Canada); Mellaril®; Mellaril-S®; Novo-Ridazine® (Canada); PMS-Thioridazine (Canada)

Available Salts Thioridazine Hydrochloride

Therapeutic Category Antipsychotic Agent; Phenothiazine Derivative

Generic Available Yes

Use Due to prolongation of the Q-T$_c$ interval (see Warnings), thioridazine is currently indicated only for the treatment of refractory schizophrenic patients; in the past, the drug had been used for management of psychotic disorders; depressive neurosis; dementia in elderly; severe behavioral problems in children

Pregnancy Risk Factor C

Contraindications Concurrent therapy with propranolol, pindolol, fluvoxamine, fluoxetine, paroxetine, drugs that inhibit cytochrome P-450 isoenzyme CYP2D6, drugs that prolong the Q-T$_c$ interval, and patients with reduced levels of CYP2D6, a history of cardiac arrhythmias, congenital long QT syndrome, or a Q-T$_c$ interval >450 msec (adults); severe CNS depression; hypersensitivity to thioridazine or any component; cross-sensitivity to other phenothiazines may exist; avoid use in patients with narrow-angle glaucoma, blood dyscrasias, severe liver or cardiac disease

Warnings Prolongation of the Q-T$_c$ interval may occur and may be associated with torsade de pointes arrhythmias and sudden death

Precautions Use with caution in patients with severe cardiovascular disorder or seizures

Adverse Reactions Sedation and anticholinergic effects are more pronounced than extrapyramidal effects; EKG changes and retinal pigmentation are more common than with chlorpromazine

Cardiovascular: Hypotension, orthostatic hypotension, tachycardia, arrhythmias

Central nervous system: Sedation, drowsiness, restlessness, anxiety, extrapyramidal reactions, pseudoparkinsonian signs and symptoms, tardive dyskinesia, neuroleptic malignant syndrome, seizures, altered central temperature regulation

Dermatologic: Hyperpigmentation, pruritus, rash, contact dermatitis, photosensitivity (rare)

Endocrine & metabolic: Amenorrhea, galactorrhea, gynecomastia

Gastrointestinal: GI upset, xerostomia, constipation, weight gain

Genitourinary: Urinary retention

Hematologic: Agranulocytosis, leukopenia (usually in patients with large doses for prolonged periods)

Hepatic: Cholestatic jaundice

Ocular: Retinal pigmentation, blurred vision, decreased visual acuity (may be irreversible)

Miscellaneous: Anaphylactoid reactions

Drug Interactions Cytochrome P-450 isoenzyme CYP1A2 and CYP2D6 substrate; CYP2D6 isoenzyme inhibitor

Additive effects with alcohol and other CNS depressants; concurrent use with lithium has caused acute encephalopathy-like syndrome (rare); increased cardiac arrhythmias with tricyclic antidepressants; epinephrine may cause hypotension; mixing liquid thioridazine with carbamazepine suspension will result in precipitation of an orange rubbery mass (see also Contraindications)

Food Interactions May increase dietary requirements for riboflavin; liquid thioridazine formulations may precipitate with enteral formulas

Mechanism of Action Blocks postsynaptic mesolimbic dopaminergic receptors in the brain; exhibits a strong alpha-adrenergic blocking effect and depresses the release of hypothalamic and hypophyseal hormones

Pharmacokinetics

Protein binding: 99%

Metabolism: In the liver to active and inactive metabolites

Bioavailability: 25% to 33%

Half-life: Adults: 9-30 hours

Not dialyzable: (0% to 5%)

Usual Dosage Oral:

Children >2 years: Range: 0.5-3 mg/kg/day in 2-3 divided doses; usual: 1 mg/kg/day; maximum dose: 3 mg/kg/day

Behavior problems: Initial: 10 mg 2-3 times/day, increase gradually

Severe psychoses: Initial: 25 mg 2-3 times/day, increase gradually

Children >12 years and Adults:

Psychoses: Initial: 25-100 mg 3 times/day with gradual increments as needed and tolerated; maximum daily dose: 800 mg/day in 2-4 divided doses; maintenance: 10-200 mg/dose 2-4 times/day

Depressive disorders, dementia: Initial: 25 mg 3 times/day; maintenance dose: 20-200 mg/day

Administration Oral: Administer with water, food, or milk to decrease GI upset; dilute the oral concentrate with water or juice before administration; do not administer liquid thioridazine simultaneously with carbamazepine suspension (see Drug Interactions); do not mix liquid thioridazine with enteric formulas (see Food Interactions)

Monitoring Parameters Baseline and periodic EKG and serum potassium; periodic eye exam, CBC with differential, blood pressure, liver enzyme tests

Test Interactions False-positives for phenylketonuria, urinary amylase, uroporphyrins, urobilinogen

Patient Information Avoid alcohol; may cause drowsiness and impair ability to perform activities requiring mental alertness or physical coordination; may cause dry mouth; avoid skin contact with oral suspension or solution, may cause contact dermatitis; rarely causes photosensitivity, avoid excess sun exposure, use sunscreen; do not discontinue or alter dose without physician approval

Additional Information In cases of overdoses, cardiovascular monitoring and continuous EKG monitoring should be performed; avoid drugs (such as quinidine, disopyramide, and procainamide) that may further prolong the Q-T interval

Dosage Forms

Concentrate, oral, as hydrochloride: 30 mg/mL (120 mL); 100 mg/mL (3.4 mL, 120 mL)

Suspension, oral, as hydrochloride: 25 mg/5 mL (480 mL); 100 mg/5 mL (480 mL)

(Continued)

Thioridazine *(Continued)*

Tablet, as hydrochloride: 10 mg, 15 mg, 25 mg, 50 mg, 100 mg, 150 mg, 200 mg

References
Aman MG, Marks RE, Turbott SH, et al, "Clinical Effects of Methylphenidate and Thioridazine in Intellectually Subaverage Children," *J Am Acad Child Adolesc Psychiatry*, 1991, 30(2):246-56.

♦ **Thioridazine Hydrochloride** *see* Thioridazine *on page 920*

♦ **Thiosulfuric Acid** *see* Sodium Thiosulfate *on page 875*

Thiotepa *(thye oh TEP a)*

Related Information
Emetogenic Potential of Single Chemotherapeutic Agents *on page 1095*

Brand Names Thioplex®

Synonyms TESPA; Triethylenethiophosphoramide; TSPA

Therapeutic Category Antineoplastic Agent, Alkylating Agent

Generic Available No

Use Treatment of superficial tumors of the bladder; palliative treatment of adenocarcinoma of breast or ovary; lymphomas and sarcomas; meningeal neoplasms; control of pleural, pericardial or peritoneal effusions caused by metastatic tumors; high-dose regimens with autologous bone marrow transplantation

Pregnancy Risk Factor D

Contraindications Hypersensitivity to thiotepa or any component; severe myelosuppression with leukocyte count <3000/mm^3 or platelet count <150,000 mm^3

Warnings The FDA currently recommends that procedures for proper handling and disposal of antineoplastic agents be considered. The drug is potentially mutagenic, carcinogenic, and teratogenic.

Precautions Reduce dosage in patients with hepatic, renal, or bone marrow dysfunction

Adverse Reactions

Central nervous system: Dizziness, fever, headache, confusion, somnolence

Dermatologic: Alopecia, rash, pruritus, hyperpigmentation of skin with high-dose therapy

Endocrine & metabolic: Amenorrhea, hyperuricemia

Gastrointestinal: Nausea, vomiting, stomatitis, esophagitis, anorexia

Genitourinary: Rarely hemorrhagic cystitis

Hematologic: Leukopenia (nadir: 7-10 days), anemia, thrombocytopenia (nadir: 3 weeks), granulocytopenia

Hepatic: Elevated liver transaminase and bilirubin (high-dose therapy)

Local: Pain at injection site

Renal: Hematuria

Drug Interactions Succinylcholine (thiotepa inhibits pseudocholinesterase activity; prolongs muscular paralysis); other alkylating agents (intensifies toxicity)

Stability Refrigerate, protect from light; the reconstituted 10 mg/mL solution is chemically stable for 5 days when stored in the refrigerator; since it contains no preservatives use within 8 hours; unstable in acid medium

Mechanism of Action Polyfunctional alkylating agent that reacts with DNA phosphate groups to produce cross-linking of DNA strands leading to inhibition of DNA, RNA, and protein synthesis

Pharmacokinetics

Absorption: Variable absorption through serous membranes and from I.M. injection sites; bladder mucosa: 10% to 100% and is increased with mucosal inflammation or tumor infiltration

Protein binding: 40%

Metabolism: Extensive in the liver primarily to TEPA (active metabolite)

Half-life, terminal:

Thiotepa: 109 minutes (51.6-212 minutes) with dose-dependent clearance

TEPA: 3-21 hours

Elimination: Very little thiotepa or active metabolite are excreted unchanged in urine (1.5% of thiotepa dose)

Usual Dosage Refer to individual protocols

Children: I.V.: Sarcomas: 25-65 mg/m^2 as a single dose every 3-4 weeks

High-dose thiotepa with ABMT: One regimen uses 300 mg/m^2/dose over 3 hours; repeat every 24 hours for a total of 3 doses; maximum tolerated dose over 3 days: 900-1125 mg/m^2

Adults:

I.V.: 0.3-0.4 mg/kg at 1- to 4-week intervals or 0.2 mg/kg (6 mg/m^2)/day for 4-5 days, repeat at 2- to 4-week intervals; continuous infusion: 15-35 mg/m^2 over 48 hours

Intracavitary: 0.6-0.8 mg/kg; dose should not be repeated more frequently than at a 1 week interval

Administration
Bladder instillation: Prepare with 30-60 mg diluted in 30-60 mL sterile water and instill by catheter and retain for 2 hours
Intrapleural or pericardial: Dose is further diluted to a volume of 10-20 mL in NS or D_5W;
Intraperitoneal: Administration requires dilution in larger volumes (up to 2 L)
I.V.: Filter through a 0.22 micron filter (Millex-GS) prior to administration; administer direct I.V. over 5 minutes or I.V. intermittent or continuous infusion at a final concentration for administration of 1 mg/mL (thiotepa may be further diluted in D_5W, NS, or LR)

Monitoring Parameters CBC with differential and platelet count, uric acid, urinalysis

Patient Information Notify physician if fever, sore throat, bleeding, or bruising occurs

Additional Information Myelosuppressive effects:
WBC: Moderate
Platelets: Severe
Onset (days): 7-10
Nadir (days): 14-20
Recovery (days): 28

Dosage Forms Powder for injection: 15 mg

References
Heideman R, Cole D, Balis F, et al, "Phase I and Pharmacokinetic Evaluation of Thiotepa in the Cerebrospinal Fluid and Plasma of Pediatric Patients: Evidence for Dose-Dependent Plasma Clearance of Thiotepa," Cancer Res, 1989, 49(3):736-41.
Herzig GP, "Phase I-II Studies of High-Dose Thiotepa and Autologous BMT in Patients With Refractory Malignancies," Adv Cancer Chemotherapy, 1987, 17-29 (proceedings of a symposium, Oct 1986)
Saannen UM, Hovi L, and Makipern CA, "High Dose Thiotepa With Autologous Bone Marrow Rescue in Pediatric Solid Tumors," Proc Am Soc Clin Oncol, 1989, 8:303.

Thiothixene (thye oh THIKS een)

Related Information
Overdose and Toxicology on page 1191

Brand Names Navane®
Available Salts Thiothixene Hydrochloride
Therapeutic Category Antipsychotic Agent; Phenothiazine Derivative
Generic Available Yes
Use Management of psychotic disorders
Pregnancy Risk Factor C
Contraindications Hypersensitivity to thiothixene or any component; cross-sensitivity with other phenothiazines may exist; avoid use in patients with narrow-angle glaucoma, bone marrow suppression, severe liver or cardiac disease
Precautions Use with caution in patients with cardiovascular disease or seizures
Adverse Reactions Sedation and extrapyramidal effects occur more often
Cardiovascular: Hypotension (especially with parenteral use), orthostatic hypotension, tachycardia, arrhythmias
Central nervous system: Sedation, drowsiness, restlessness, anxiety, insomnia, extrapyramidal reactions, tardive dyskinesia, neuroleptic malignant syndrome, seizures, altered central temperature regulation
Dermatologic: Rash, photosensitivity
Endocrine & metabolic: Amenorrhea, galactorrhea, gynecomastia
Gastrointestinal: GI upset, xerostomia, constipation, weight gain
Genitourinary: Urinary retention
Hematologic: Agranulocytosis, leukopenia
Ocular: Retinal pigmentation, blurred vision
Drug Interactions Cytochrome P-450 isoenzyme CYP1A2 substrate
Alcohol and other CNS depressants, anticholinergics, or hypotensive agents may increase adverse effects
Food Interactions May cause increase in dietary riboflavin requirements
Mechanism of Action Elicits antipsychotic activity by postsynaptic blockade of CNS dopamine receptors resulting in inhibition of dopamine-mediated effects; also has alpha-adrenergic blocking activity
Usual Dosage
Children ≤12 years: Oral: Not well established; 0.25 mg/kg/24 hours in divided doses
Children >12 years and Adults:
Oral: Initial: 2 mg 3 times/day, up to 20-30 mg/day; maximum dose: 60 mg/day
(Continued)

Thiothixene *(Continued)*

I.M.: 4 mg 2-4 times/day, increase dose gradually; usual: 16-20 mg/day; maximum dose: 30 mg/day; change to oral dose a soon as able

Administration
Oral: Administer with food or water
Parenteral: Injection is for I.M. use only

Monitoring Parameters Periodic eye exam, CBC with differential, blood pressure, liver enzyme tests

Patient Information Avoid alcohol; limit caffeine; may cause drowsiness and impair ability to perform activities requiring mental alertness or physical coordination; may cause dry mouth; avoid excessive sunlight, use sunscreen

Dosage Forms
Capsule: 1 mg, 2 mg, 5 mg, 10 mg, 20 mg
Concentrate, oral, as hydrochloride: 5 mg/mL (30 mL, 120 mL)
Injection, as hydrochloride: 2 mg/mL (2 mL)
Powder for injection, as hydrochloride: 5 mg/mL (2 mL)

References
Wiener JM, "Psychopharmacology in Childhood Disorders," *Psychiatr Clin North Am*, 1984, 7(4):831-43.

♦ **Thiothixene Hydrochloride** *see* Thiothixene *on page 923*
♦ **Thorazine®** *see* Chlorpromazine *on page 215*
♦ **Thrombinar®** *see* Thrombin, Topical *on page 924*

Thrombin, Topical (THROM bin, TOP i kal)

Brand Names Thrombinar®; Thrombogen®; Thrombostat®
Therapeutic Category Hemostatic Agent
Generic Available No
Use Hemostasis whenever minor bleeding from capillaries and small venules is accessible
Pregnancy Risk Factor C
Contraindications Hypersensitivity to thrombin, any component, or material of bovine origin
Warnings Do not inject - for topical use only
Adverse Reactions
Central nervous system: Fever
Miscellaneous: Allergic reactions
Stability Following reconstitution, use immediately; stable 3 hours refrigerated; stable frozen (reconstituted) for 48 hours
Mechanism of Action Catalyzes the conversion of fibrinogen to fibrin
Usual Dosage Topical: Apply powder directly to the site of bleeding or on oozing surfaces or use 1000-2000 units/mL of solution where bleeding is profuse; use 100 units/mL for bleeding from skin or mucosal surfaces
Administration Topical: May be applied directly as a powder or as reconstituted solution; the most effective hemostasis results when the thrombin mixes freely with blood as it appears; use sterile water or NS to reconstitute powder to desired concentration; **not for injection**
Additional Information One unit is amount required to clot 1 mL of standardized fibrinogen solution in 15 seconds
Dosage Forms Powder: 1000 units, 5000 units, 10,000 units, 20,000 units, 50,000 units

♦ **Thrombogen®** *see* Thrombin, Topical *on page 924*
♦ **Thrombostat®** *see* Thrombin, Topical *on page 924*
♦ **Thymocyte Stimulating Factor** *see* Aldesleukin *on page 42*
♦ **Thypinone®** *see* Protirelin *on page 821*
♦ **Thyrel® TRH** *see* Protirelin *on page 821*
♦ **Thyro-Block®** *see* Potassium Iodide *on page 785*
♦ **Tiabendazole** *see* Thiabendazole *on page 915*

Tiagabine (tye AG a bene)

Brand Names Gabitril®
Available Salts Tiagabine hydrochloride
Therapeutic Category Anticonvulsant, Miscellaneous
Generic Available No
Use Adjunctive therapy of partial epilepsy
Pregnancy Risk Factor C

Contraindications Hypersensitivity to tiagabine or any component

Warnings Do not abruptly discontinue therapy, withdraw gradually to lessen chance for increased seizure frequency (unless a more rapid withdrawal is required due to safety concerns); exacerbation of EEG abnormalities associated with CNS adverse events (cognitive and neuropsychiatric) may occur in patients with an EEG history of spike and wave discharges and may require dosage adjustment; nonconvulsant status epilepticus has also been reported and may respond to dosage reduction or discontinuation

Precautions Use with caution in patients with hepatic impairment; possible long-term ophthalmologic effects exist (more studies are needed); use with caution with alcohol or other CNS depressants

Adverse Reactions

Central nervous system: Impaired concentration, speech/language problems, confusion, somnolence, fatigue, dizziness, nervousness, depression, ataxia, insomnia, emotional lability, headache

Gastrointestinal: Nausea, abdominal pain, diarrhea

Neuromuscular & skeletal: Asthenia, tremor

Drug Interactions Cytochrome P-450 isoenzyme CYP3A substrate, may also be metabolized by CYP1A2, 2D6, or 2C19; tiagabine may decrease valproic acid concentrations by ~10%; carbamazepine, phenytoin, primidone, and phenobarbital may increase tiagabine clearance by 60%; naproxen, salicylates, and valproic acid may decrease tiagabine protein binding and increase the free concentration

Food Interactions Food may decrease the rate but not the extent of absorption

Stability Protect from moisture and light; store at room temperature

Mechanism of Action Exact mechanism unknown; thought to potentiate the action of GABA (an inhibitory neurotransmitter) by selectively binding to the GABA uptake carrier and blocking GABA uptake into presynaptic neurons. This allows more GABA to be available at its site of action to bind to postsynaptic neuronal receptors.

Pharmacokinetics

Absorption: Rapid and nearly complete (>95%)

Distribution: Mean V_d:

Children 3-10 years: 2.4 L/kg

Adults: 1.3-1.6 L/kg

V_d values are more similar between children and adults when expressed as L/m^2

Protein binding: 96%, mainly to albumin and alpha$_1$-acid glycoprotein

Metabolism: Extensive in the liver via oxidation and glucuronidation; undergoes enterohepatic recirculation

Bioavailability: 90%

Diurnal effect: Trough concentrations and AUC are lower in the evening versus morning

Half-life:

Children 3-10 years: Mean: 5.7 hours (range: 2-10 hours)

Children 3-10 years receiving enzyme-inducing AEDs: Mean: 3.2 hours (range: 2-7.8 hours)

Adults (normal volunteers): 7-9 hours

Adults receiving enzyme-inducing AEDs: 4-7 hours

Time to peak serum concentration: Fasting state: ~45 minutes

Elimination: ~2% excreted unchanged in urine; 25% excreted in urine and 63% excreted in feces as metabolites

Clearance:

Children 3-10 years: 4.2 ± 1.6 mL/minute/kg

Children 3-10 years receiving enzyme-inducing AEDs: 8.6 ± 3.3 mL/minute/kg

Adults (normal volunteers): 109 mL/minute

Adult patients: 1.9 ± 0.5 mL/minute/kg

Adults receiving enzyme-inducing AEDs: 6.3 ± 3.5 mL/minute/kg

Clearance values are more similar between children and adults when expressed as mL/minute/m^2

Hepatic impairment: Clearance of unbound drug is decreased by 60%

Usual Dosage Oral: **Note:** Doses were determined in patients receiving enzyme-inducing AEDs; lower doses or slower titration may be required in patients not receiving enzyme-inducing agents

Children <12 years: Only limited preliminary information is available; dosing guidelines are not established (see Adkins, 1998)

Children 12-18 years: Initial: 4 mg once daily for 1 week, then 8 mg/day given in 2 divided doses for 1 week, then increase weekly by 4-8 mg/day; administer in 2-4 divided doses per day; titrate dose to response; maximum dose: 32 mg/day

(Continued)

Tiagabine *(Continued)*

(doses >32 mg/day have been used in select adolescent patients for short periods of time)

Adults: Initial: 4 mg once daily for 1 week, then increase weekly by 4-8 mg/day; administer in 2-4 divided doses per day; titrate dose to response; maximum dose: 56 mg/day. **Note:** Twice daily dosing may not be well tolerated and dosing 3 times/day is the currently favored dosing frequency (see Kalviainen, 1998).

Dosing adjustment in renal impairment: None needed

Dosing adjustment in hepatic impairment: Reduced doses and longer dosing intervals may be required

Administration Oral: Administer with food (to avoid rapid increase in plasma concentrations and adverse CNS effects)

Monitoring Parameters Seizure frequency, duration, and severity

Reference Range Not established

Patient Information May cause dizziness or drowsiness and impair ability to perform activities requiring mental alertness or physical coordination

Additional Information Population pharmacokinetic analysis suggests that tiagabine may be administered at similar doses without adjustment for age, gender, or body weight in epilepsy patients ≥ 11 years of age (see Samara, et al)

Dosage Forms Tablet, as hydrochloride: 2 mg, 4 mg, 12 mg, 16 mg, 20 mg

References

Adkins JC and Noble S, "Tiagabine. A Review of Its Pharmacodynamic and Pharmacokinetic Properties and Therapeutic Potential in the Management of Epilepsy," *Drugs,* 1998, 55(3):437-60.

Gustavson LE, Boellner SW, Granneman GR, et al, "A Single-Dose Study to Define Tiagabine Pharmacokinetics in Pediatric Patients With Complex Partial Seizures," *Neurology,* 1997, 48(4):1032-7.

Kalviainen R, Brodie MJ, Duncan J, et al, "A Double-Blind, Placebo-Controlled Trial of Tiagabine Given Three-Times Daily as Add-On Therapy for Refractory Partial Seizures. Northern European Tiagabine Study Group," *Epilepsy Res,* 1998, 30(1):31-40.

Leach JP and Brodie MJ, "Tiagabine," *Lancet,* 1998, 351(9097):203-7.

Samara EE, Gustavson LE, El-Shourbagy T, et al, "Population Analysis of the Pharmacokinetics of Tiagabine in Patients With Epilepsy," *Epilepsy,* 1998, 39(8):868-73.

♦ **Tiagabine hydrochloride** *see Tiagabine on page 924*

♦ **Tiamate®** *see Diltiazem on page 323*

♦ **Tiamol® (Canada)** *see Fluocinonide on page 426*

♦ **Tiazac®** *see Diltiazem on page 323*

♦ **Ticar®** *see Ticarcillin on page 926*

Ticarcillin (tye kar SIL in)

Brand Names Ticar®

Available Salts Ticarcillin Disodium

Therapeutic Category Antibiotic, Penicillin (Antipseudomonal)

Generic Available No

Use Treatment of infections such as septicemia, acute and chronic respiratory tract infections, skin and soft tissue infections, and urinary tract infections due to susceptible strains of *Pseudomonas, Proteus, Escherichia coli,* and *Enterobacter*

Pregnancy Risk Factor B

Contraindications Hypersensitivity to ticarcillin, any component, or penicillins

Warnings Prolonged use may result in superinfection

Precautions Use with caution in patients with CHF due to ticarcillin's high sodium content; dosage modification required in patients with impaired renal and/or hepatic function

Adverse Reactions

Central nervous system: Seizures, headache, fever

Dermatologic: Rash

Endocrine & metabolic: Hypernatremia, hypokalemia, metabolic alkalosis

Gastrointestinal: Diarrhea, pseudomembranous colitis, stomatitis, nausea

Genitourinary: Cystitis, hematuria

Hematologic: Inhibition of platelet aggregation, leukopenia, neutropenia, eosinophilia, prolonged prothrombin time, bleeding diathesis, hemolytic anemia, decreased hemoglobin and hematocrit

Hepatic: Elevated AST and ALT, hepatitis

Local: Phlebitis

Renal: Elevated BUN, elevated serum creatinine

Miscellaneous: Hypersensitivity reactions including anaphylaxis; superinfection

Drug Interactions Aminoglycosides (antibacterial activity is synergistic), probenecid (increases serum concentration of ticarcillin); may alter renal elimination of lithium

Stability Reconstituted ticarcillin solution 200-300 mg/mL is stable for 24 hours at room temperature or 72 hours when refrigerated; incompatible with aminoglycosides

Mechanism of Action Inhibits bacterial cell wall synthesis by binding to one or more of the penicillin-binding proteins; inhibits the final transpeptidation step of peptidoglycan synthesis in bacterial cell walls

Pharmacokinetics

Absorption: I.M.: 86%

Distribution: V_d: Neonates: 0.42-0.76 L/kg; distributed into breast milk at low concentrations; attains high concentrations in bile; minimal concentrations attained in CSF with uninflamed meninges

Protein binding: 45% to 65%

Metabolism: 10%

Half-life, adults: 1-1.3 hours, prolonged with renal impairment and/or hepatic impairment

Neonates:

    <1 week: 3.5-5.6 hours

    1-8 weeks: 1.3-2.2 hours

Children 5-13 years: 0.9 hours

Time to peak serum concentration: I.M.: Within 30-75 minutes

Elimination: Almost entirely in urine as unchanged drug and its metabolites with small amounts excreted in feces (3.5%)

Moderately dialyzable (20% to 50%)

Usual Dosage Ticarcillin is generally only given I.M. for the treatment of uncomplicated urinary tract infections

Neonates: I.V.:

  Postnatal age ≤7 days:

    ≤2000 g: 150 mg/kg/day in divided doses every 12 hours

    >2000 g: 225 mg/kg/day in divided doses every 8 hours

  Postnatal age >7 days:

    <1200 g: 150 mg/kg/day in divided doses every 12 hours

    1200-2000 g: 225 mg/kg/day in divided doses every 8 hours

    >2000 g: 300 mg/kg/day in divided doses every 6-8 hours

Infants and Children:

  I.M.: 50-100 mg/kg/day in divided doses every 6-8 hours

  I.V.: 200-300 mg/kg/day in divided doses every 4-6 hours; doses as high as 400 mg/kg/day divided every 4-6 hours have been used in acute pulmonary exacerbations of cystic fibrosis

  Maximum dose: 24 g/day

Adults:

  I.M.: 1 g every 6 hours

  I.V.: 1-4 g every 4-6 hours; maximum dose: 24 g/day

Dosing interval in renal impairment:

Cl_{cr} 10-30 mL/minute: Administer every 8 hours

Cl_{cr} <10 mL/minute: Administer every 12 hours

Administration Parenteral:

I.M.: Reconstitute each gram of ticarcillin with 2 mL sterile water or 1% lidocaine hydrochloride injection (without epinephrine) to make a 385 mg/mL solution; administer by deep I.M. injection into a large muscle mass

I.V.: Ticarcillin may be administered I.V. push over 10-20 minutes or by I.V. intermittent infusion over 30-120 minutes at a final concentration not to exceed 100 mg/mL; concentrations ≤50 mg/mL are preferred for peripheral intermittent infusions to avoid vein irritation; if the patient is on concurrent aminoglycoside therapy, separate ticarcillin administration from the aminoglycoside by at least 30-60 minutes

Monitoring Parameters Serum electrolytes, bleeding time, and periodic tests of renal, hepatic, and hematologic function

Test Interactions False-positive urinary or serum protein, positive Coombs' [direct]

Additional Information Sodium content of 1 g: 5.2-6.5 mEq

Dosage Forms Powder for injection, as disodium: 1 g, 3 g, 6 g, 20 g, 30 g

References

Brogden RN, Heel RC, Speight TM, et al, "Ticarcillin: A Review of Its Pharmacological Properties and Therapeutic Efficacy," *Drugs*, 1980, 20(5):325-52.

Nelson JD, Kusmiesz H, Shelton S, et al, "Clinical Pharmacology and Efficacy of Ticarcillin in Infants and Children," *Pediatrics*, 1978, 61(6):858-63.

Ticarcillin and Clavulanate Potassium

(tye kar SIL in & klav yoo LAN ate poe TASS ee um)

Brand Names Timentin®

Available Salts Ticarcillin Disodium and Clavulanate Potassium

Synonyms Clavulanate Potassium and Ticarcillin

Therapeutic Category Antibiotic, Beta-lactam and Beta-lactamase Combination; Antibiotic, Penicillin (Antipseudomonal)

Generic Available No

Use Treatment of infections caused by susceptible organisms involving the lower respiratory tract, urinary tract, skin and skin structures, bone and joint, and septicemia. Clavulanate expands activity of ticarcillin to include beta-lactamase producing strains of *S. aureus*, *H. influenzae*, *Moraxella catarrhalis*, *B. fragilis*, *Klebsiella*, and *Proteus* species

Pregnancy Risk Factor B

Contraindications Hypersensitivity to ticarcillin, clavulanate, or penicillin

Warnings Abnormal platelet aggregation and prolonged bleeding have been reported in patients with renal impairment receiving high doses; prolonged use may result in superinfection

Precautions Use with caution and modify dosage in patients with renal impairment; use with caution in patients with CHF due to high sodium content of the formulation

Adverse Reactions

Central nervous system: Seizures, headache, fever

Dermatologic: Rash

Endocrine & metabolic: Hypernatremia, hypokalemia, metabolic alkalosis

Gastrointestinal: Diarrhea, stomatitis, nausea, pseudomembranous colitis

Genitourinary: Cystitis, hematuria

Hematologic: Eosinophilia, leukopenia, decreased hemoglobin and hematocrit, inhibition of platelet aggregation, prolongation of bleeding time, neutropenia, hemolytic anemia

Hepatic: Elevated ALT and AST, hepatitis

Local: Thrombophlebitis

Renal: Elevated BUN, elevated serum creatinine

Miscellaneous: Hypersensitivity reactions including anaphylaxis; superinfection

Drug Interactions Aminoglycosides (antibacterial activity is synergistic), probenecid (increases serum concentration of ticarcillin)

Stability Reconstituted 200 mg/mL solution is stable for 6 hours at room temperature and 72 hours when refrigerated; darkening of drug indicates loss of potency of clavulanate potassium; incompatible with sodium bicarbonate and aminoglycosides

Mechanism of Action Ticarcillin inhibits bacterial cell wall synthesis by binding to one or more of the penicillin-binding proteins; inhibits the final transpeptidation step of peptidoglycan synthesis in bacterial cell walls; clavulanic acid inhibits degradation of ticarcillin by binding to beta-lactamases

Pharmacokinetics

Distribution: Ticarcillin is distributed into tissue, interstitial fluid, pleural fluid, bile, and breast milk; low concentrations of ticarcillin distribute into the CSF but increase when meninges are inflamed

V_{dss} ticarcillin: 0.22 L/kg

V_{dss} clavulanic acid: 0.4 L/kg

Protein binding:

Ticarcillin: 45% to 65%

Clavulanic acid: 9% to 30%

Metabolism: Clavulanic acid is metabolized in the liver

Half-life: In patients with normal renal function

Neonates:

Clavulanic acid: 1.9 hours

Ticarcillin: 4.4 hours

Children (1 month to 9.3 years):

Clavulanic acid: 54 minutes

Ticarcillin: 66 minutes

Adults:

Clavulanic acid: 66-90 minutes

Ticarcillin: 66-72 minutes

Clavulanic acid does not affect the clearance of ticarcillin

Elimination:

Children: 71% of the ticarcillin and 50% of the clavulanic acid dose are excreted unchanged in the urine over 4 hours

Adults: 45% of clavulanate is excreted unchanged in urine, whereas 60% to 90% of ticarcillin is excreted unchanged in urine

Removed by hemodialysis

Usual Dosage I.V.:

Term neonates and Infants <3 months: 200-300 mg ticarcillin component/kg/day divided every 6-8 hours

Infants ≥3 months and Children:

Mild to moderate infection: 200 mg ticarcillin component/kg/day divided every 6 hours

Severe infections that occur outside the CNS: 300 mg ticarcillin component/kg/day in divided doses every 4-6 hours; maximum dose: 18-24 g/day

Adults: 3.1 g (ticarcillin 3 g plus clavulanic acid 0.1 g) every 4-6 hours; maximum dose: 18-24 g/day

Urinary tract infections: 3.1 g every 6-8 hours

Dosing interval in renal impairment:

Cl_{cr} 10-30 mL/minute: Administer every 8 hours

Cl_{cr} <10 mL/minute: Administer every 12 hours

Dosing interval in hepatic impairment and a Cl_{cr} <10 mL/minute: Administer every 24 hours

Administration Parenteral: Administer by I.V. intermittent infusion over 30 minutes; final concentration for administration should not exceed 100 mg/mL of ticarcillin; however, concentrations ≤50 mg/mL are preferred; if the patient is on concurrent aminoglycoside therapy, separate ticarcillin and clavulanate potassium administration from the aminoglycoside by at least 30-60 minutes

Monitoring Parameters Serum electrolytes, periodic renal, hepatic and hematologic function tests

Test Interactions Positive Coombs' [direct], false-positive urinary and serum proteins

Additional Information

Sodium content of 1 g: 4.75 mEq

Potassium content of 1 g: 0.15 mEq

Dosage Forms

Infusion, premixed (frozen): Ticarcillin disodium 3 g and clavulanic acid 0.1 (100 mL) g

Powder for injection: Ticarcillin disodium 3 g and clavulanic acid 0.1 g (3.1 g, 31 g)

References

Begue P, Quiniou F, Quinet B, "Efficacy and Pharmacokinetics of Timentin® in Paediatric Infections," *J Antimicrob Chemother*, 1986, 17(Suppl C):81-91.

Reed MD, Yamashita TS, and Blumer JL, "Pharmacokinetic-Based Ticarcillin/Clavulanic Acid Dose Recommendations for Infants and Children," *J Clin Pharmacol*, 1995, 35(7):658-65.

Stutman HR and Marks MI, "Review of Pediatric Antimicrobial Therapies," *Semin Pediatr Infect Dis*, 1991, 2:3-17.

♦ **Ticarcillin Disodium** *see* Ticarcillin *on page 926*

♦ **Ticarcillin Disodium and Clavulanate Potassium** *see* Ticarcillin and Clavulanate Potassium *on page 928*

♦ **Ticon® Injection** *see* Trimethobenzamide *on page 954*

♦ **Tigan® Injection** *see* Trimethobenzamide *on page 954*

♦ **Tigan® Oral** *see* Trimethobenzamide *on page 954*

♦ **Tigan® Rectal** *see* Trimethobenzamide *on page 954*

♦ **Tilade® Inhalation Aerosol** *see* Nedocromil *on page 674*

♦ **Tim-AK (Canada)** *see* Timolol *on page 929*

♦ **Timecelles® [OTC]** *see* Ascorbic Acid *on page 96*

♦ **Timentin®** *see* Ticarcillin and Clavulanate Potassium *on page 928*

Timolol (TYE moe lole)

Related Information

Adult ACLS Algorithm, Tachycardia *on page 1010*

Overdose and Toxicology *on page 1191*

Brand Names Apo®-Timol (Canada); Apo®-Timop (Canada); Beta-Tim® (Canada); Blocadren® Oral; Gen-Timolol® (Canada); Novo-Timol® (Canada); Nu-Timolol® (Canada); Tim-AK (Canada); Timoptic® Ophthalmic; Timoptic-XE® Ophthalmic

Available Salts Timolol Maleate

Therapeutic Category Antihypertensive Agent; Antimigraine Agent; Beta-Adrenergic Blocker; Beta-Adrenergic Blocker, Ophthalmic

Generic Available Yes

Use Ophthalmic dosage form used to treat elevated intraocular pressure such as glaucoma or ocular hypertension; orally for treatment of hypertension and angina and for prevention of MI and migraine headaches

(Continued)

Timolol *(Continued)*

Pregnancy Risk Factor C

Contraindications Uncompensated CHF, cardiogenic shock, bradycardia or heart block, bronchial asthma, severe chronic obstructive pulmonary disease or history of asthma, CHF or bradycardia

Warnings Severe CNS, cardiovascular and respiratory adverse effects have been seen following ophthalmic use; some products may contain sulfites which can cause allergic reactions

Precautions Similar to other beta-blockers; use with caution in patients with decreased renal or hepatic function (dosage adjustment required); use with a miotic in angle-closure or narrow-angle glaucoma; use with caution in patients with diabetes mellitus, may block hypoglycemia-induced tachycardia and blood pressure changes

Adverse Reactions

Cardiovascular: Bradycardia, arrhythmia, hypotension, syncope

Central nervous system: Dizziness, headache

Dermatologic: Rash

Gastrointestinal: Diarrhea, nausea

Local (ocular): Irritation, conjunctivitis, keratitis, visual disturbances

Respiratory: Bronchospasm

Drug Interactions Cytochrome P-450 isoenzyme CYP2D6 substrate

Verapamil, quinidine may increase adverse cardiac effects; drug interactions similar to other beta-blockers may occur

Mechanism of Action Blocks both $beta_1$- and $beta_2$-adrenergic receptors; reduces intraocular pressure by reducing aqueous humor production or possibly outflow; reduces blood pressure by blocking adrenergic receptors and decreasing sympathetic outflow; produces negative chronotropic and negative inotropic activity

Pharmacodynamics Hypotensive effects:

Onset of action: Oral: Within 15-45 minutes

Peak effect: 30-150 minutes

Duration:

Oral: 4 hours

Ophthalmic (intraocular effects): 24 hours

Pharmacokinetics

Protein binding: <10%

Metabolism: Extensively in the liver, extensive first-pass effect

Bioavailability: Oral: ~60%

Half-life: Adults: 2-4 hours; prolonged with reduced renal function

Elimination: Urinary excretion (15% to 20% as unchanged drug)

Not readily dialyzable

Usual Dosage

Ophthalmic: Children and Adults: Initial: 0.25% solution, instill 1 drop twice daily; increase to 0.5% solution if response not adequate; decrease to 1 drop/day if controlled; do not exceed 1 drop twice daily of 0.5% solution (see Additional Information)

Oral:

Children: No information regarding pediatric dose is currently available in literature

Adults:

Hypertension: Initial: 10 mg twice daily, increase gradually every 7 days, usual dosage: 20-40 mg/day in 2 divided doses; maximum dose: 60 mg/day

Prevention of MI: 10 mg twice daily initiated within 1-4 weeks after infarction

Migraine headache: Initial: 10 mg twice daily, increase to maximum of 30 mg/day

Administration

Ophthalmic: Apply gentle pressure to lacrimal sac during and immediately following instillation (1 minute) or instruct patient to gently close eyelid after administration, to decrease systemic absorption of ophthalmic drops; avoid contact of bottle tip with skin or eye

Oral: May be administered without regard to food

Monitoring Parameters Heart rate, blood pressure; liver enzymes, BUN, serum creatinine with long-term oral use; monitor respiratory rate, CNS status, and cardiovascular status with ophthalmic use in patients at risk for adverse effects (eg, asthmatics, CHF patients, etc)

Nursing Implications Discontinue medication if breathing difficulty occurs

Additional Information Ophthalmic: Use lowest effective dose in pediatric patients. Children had higher plasma concentrations vs adults following ophthalmic use; some achieved therapeutic levels; this may result in increased adverse systemic effects.

Dosage Forms

Gel, ophthalmic, as maleate (Timoptic-XE®): 0.25% (2.5 mL, 5 mL); 0.5% (2.5 mL, 5 mL)

Solution, ophthalmic, as maleate (Timoptic®): 0.25% (2.5 mL, 5 mL, 10 mL, 15 mL); 0.5% (2.5 mL, 5 mL, 10 mL, 15 mL)

Solution, ophthalmic, preservative free, as maleate, single use (Timoptic® OcuDose®): 0.25%, 0.5%

Tablet, as maleate (Blocadren®): 5 mg, 10 mg, 20 mg

References

Hoskins HD, Hetherington J Jr, Magee SD, et al, "Clinical Experience With Timolol in Childhood Glaucoma," *Arch Ophthalmol*, 1985, 103(8):1163-5.

Passo MS, Palmer EA, and Van Buskirk EM, "Plasma Timolol in Glaucoma Patients," *Ophthalmology*, 1984, 91(11):1361-3.

- ♦ **Timolol Maleate** *see* Timolol *on page 929*
- ♦ **Timoptic® Ophthalmic** *see* Timolol *on page 929*
- ♦ **Timoptic-XE® Ophthalmic** *see* Timolol *on page 929*
- ♦ **Tinactin® [OTC]** *see* Tolnaftate *on page 936*
- ♦ **Tincture of Opium** *see* Opium Tincture *on page 709*
- ♦ **Tinver® [OTC]** *see* Sodium Thiosulfate *on page 875*
- ♦ **Tioguanine** *see* Thioguanine *on page 918*
- ♦ **Titralac® [OTC]** *see* Calcium Supplements *on page 157*
- ♦ **TMP** *see* Trimethoprim *on page 955*
- ♦ **TMP-SMX** *see* Co-Trimoxazole *on page 258*
- ♦ **TOBI™ Inhalation Solution** *see* Tobramycin *on page 931*

Tobramycin (toe bra MYE sin)

Related Information

Blood Level Sampling Time Guidelines *on page 1189*
Overdose and Toxicology *on page 1191*

Brand Names AKTob® Ophthalmic; Nebcin® Injection; TOBI™ Inhalation Solution; Tobrex® Ophthalmic

Available Salts Tobramycin Sulfate

Therapeutic Category Antibiotic, Aminoglycoside; Antibiotic, Ophthalmic

Generic Available Yes

Use Treatment of documented or suspected infections caused by susceptible gram-negative bacilli including *Pseudomonas aeruginosa*; nonpseudomonal enteric bacillus infection which is more sensitive to tobramycin than gentamicin based on susceptibility tests; susceptible organisms in lower respiratory tract infections, septicemia; intra-abdominal, skin, bone, and urinary tract infections; empiric therapy in cystic fibrosis and immunocompromised patients; used topically to treat superficial ophthalmic infections caused by susceptible bacteria; inhalation therapy management of cystic fibrosis patients with *P. aeruginosa*

Pregnancy Risk Factor D

Contraindications Hypersensitivity to tobramycin, any component, or aminoglycosides

Warnings I.M., I.V.: Aminoglycosides are associated with significant nephrotoxicity or ototoxicity; the ototoxicity is directly proportional to the amount of drug given and the duration of treatment; tinnitus or vertigo are indications of vestibular injury and impending irreversible bilateral deafness; renal damage is usually reversible. Some formulations contain sulfites which may cause allergic reactions; transient tinnitus has been reported in tobramycin inhalation-treated patients; bronchospasm can occur with inhalation of tobramycin. Aminoglycosides can cause fetal harm when administered to a pregnant woman; aminoglycosides have been associated with several reports of total, irreversible, bilateral congenital deafness in pediatric patients exposed *in utero*

Precautions Use with caution in patients with renal impairment, pre-existing auditory or vestibular impairment, patients receiving anesthetics or neuromuscular blocking agents, and in patients with neuromuscular disorders; dosage modification required in patients with impaired renal function

Adverse Reactions

Central nervous system: Vertigo, gait instability, fever, ataxia, dizziness, headache
Dermatologic: Allergic contact dermatitis, rash
Endocrine & metabolic: Hypomagnesemia
Gastrointestinal: Nausea, vomiting
Hematologic: Granulocytopenia, thrombocytopenia, eosinophilia
(Continued)

Tobramycin *(Continued)*

Hepatic: Elevated AST and ALT

Local: Thrombophlebitis

Neuromuscular & skeletal: Neuromuscular blockade, paresthesia, tremor, weakness

Ocular: Ophthalmic use: Lacrimation, itching, edema of the eyelid, keratitis

Otic: Ototoxicity (may be associated with high serum aminoglycoside concentrations persisting for prolonged periods) with tinnitus, hearing loss; early toxicity usually affects high-pitched sound

Renal: Nephrotoxicity (high trough levels) with proteinuria, reduction in glomerular filtration rate, elevated serum creatinine, decrease in urine specific gravity, casts in urine and possible electrolyte wasting

Respiratory: With inhalation therapy: Voice alteration, bronchospasm, dyspnea, increased cough, pharyngitis, hoarseness

Drug Interactions Increased toxicity: Concurrent use of amphotericin B, cephalosporins, penicillins, loop diuretics, urea, mannitol, vancomycin, cisplatin, indomethacin; potentiates effect of neuromuscular blocking agents and botulinum toxin

Stability Incompatible with penicillins, cephalosporins, heparin

Inhalation solution: Store in refrigerator; upon removal from the refrigerator, the solution may be stored at room temperature for up to 28 days; do not use solution if it is cloudy or contains particles; a darkened yellow solution does not indicate loss of potency; protect from intense light; incompatible with dornase alfa (may precipitate)

Mechanism of Action Inhibits cellular initiation of bacterial protein synthesis by binding to 30S and 50S ribosomal subunits resulting in a defective bacterial cell membrane

Pharmacokinetics

Absorption:

Oral: Poor

I.M.: Rapid and complete

Inhalation: Low systemic bioavailability although peak tobramycin serum concentration 1 hour after inhalation ranges between 0.95-1.05 mg/mL

Distribution: Crosses the placenta; distributes primarily in the extracellular fluid volume; poor penetration into the CSF and into bronchial secretions; drug accumulates in the renal cortex; small amounts distribute into bile, sputum, saliva, tears, and breast milk

V_d: Increased by fever, edema, ascites, fluid overload, and in neonates; V_d is decreased in patients with dehydration

Neonates: 0.45 ± 0.1 L/kg

Infants: 0.4 ± 0.1 L/kg

Children: 0.35 ± 0.15 L/kg

Adolescents: 0.3 ± 0.1 L/kg

Adults: 0.2-0.3 L/kg

Protein binding: <30%

Half-life:

Neonates:

≤1200 g: 11 hours

>1200 g: 2-9 hours

Infants: 4 ± 1 hour

Children: 2 ± 1 hour

Adolescents: 1.5 ± 1 hour

Adults with normal renal function: 2-3 hours, directly dependent upon glomerular filtration rate; impaired renal function: 5-70 hours

Time to peak serum concentration:

I.M.: Within 30-60 minutes

I.V.: 30 minutes after a 30-minute infusion

Elimination: With normal renal function, ~90% to 95% of dose excreted in urine within 24 hours

Dialyzable (50% to 100%)

Usual Dosage Dosage should be based on an estimate of ideal body weight except in neonates (neonatal dosage should be based on actual weight unless the patient has hydrocephalus or hydrops fetalis)

Neonates: I.M., I.V.:

Preterm neonates <1000 g: 3.5 mg/kg/dose every 24 hours

0-4 weeks, <1200 g: 2.5 mg/kg/dose every 18 hours

Postnatal age ≤7 days:

1200-2000 g: 2.5 mg/kg/dose every 12 hours

>2000 g: 2.5 mg/kg/dose every 12 hours

Postnatal age >7 days:

1200-2000 g: 2.5 mg/kg/dose every 8-12 hours

>2000 g: 2.5 mg/kg/dose every 8 hours

Infants and Children <5 years: I.M., I.V.: 2.5 mg/kg/dose every 8 hours*

Pulmonary infection in cystic fibrosis: 2.5-3.3 mg/kg/dose every 6-8 hours

Patients on hemodialysis: 1.25-1.75 mg/kg/dose postdialysis

Children ≥5 years: I.M., I.V.: 2-2.5 mg/kg/dose every 8 hours*

Pulmonary infection in cystic fibrosis: 2.5-3.3 mg/kg/dose every 6-8 hours

Patients on hemodialysis: 1.25-1.75 mg/kg/dose postdialysis

*Note: Some patients may require larger or more frequent doses if serum levels document the need (ie, cystic fibrosis, patients undergoing continuous hemofiltration, patients with major burns, or febrile granulocytopenic patients); modify dose based on individual patient requirements as determined by renal function, serum drug concentrations, and patient-specific clinical parameters.

Children and Adults: Ophthalmic:

Ointment: Apply 0.5" ribbon into the affected eye 2-3 times/day; for severe infections, apply ointment every 3-4 hours

Solution:

Mild to moderate infections: Instill 1-2 drops every 4 hours

Severe infections: instill 2 drops every 30-60 minutes initially, then reduce to less frequent intervals

Inhalation:

Standard aerosolized tobramycin:

Children: 40-80 mg 2-3 times/day

Adults: 60-80 mg 3 times/day

High dose regimen: Children ≥6 years and Adults: 300 mg every 12 hours (do not administer doses less than 6 hours apart); administer in repeated cycles of 28 days on drug followed by 28 days off drug

Adults: I.M., I.V.: 3-6 mg/kg/day in 3 divided doses; studies of once daily dosing have used I.V. doses of 4-6.6 mg/kg once daily

Patients on hemodialysis: 0.5-0.7 mg/kg/dose postdialysis

Dosing in Renal Impairment:

Children and Adults: 2.5 mg/kg (2-3 serum level measurements should be obtained after the initial dose to measure the half-life in order to determine the frequency of subsequent doses)

Administration

Inhalation (high-dose regimen): Use a PARI LC Plus™ reusable nebulizer and a DeVilbiss Pulmo-Aide® air compressor for administration of tobramycin by inhalation; patient should be sitting or standing upright and breathing normally through the mouthpiece of the nebulizer

Parenteral: Administer by I.M., I.V. slow intermittent infusion over 30-60 minutes or by direct injection over 15 minutes; final I.V. concentration for administration should not exceed 10 mg/mL; administer other antibiotics such as penicillins and cephalosporins at least 1 hour before or after tobramycin

Monitoring Parameters Urinalysis, urine output, BUN, serum creatinine, peak and trough serum tobramycin levels; be alert to ototoxicity, audiograms

Not all pediatric patients who receive aminoglycosides require monitoring of serum aminoglycoside concentrations. Indications for use of aminoglycoside serum concentration monitoring include:

Treatment course >5 days

Patients with decreased or changing renal function

Patients with a poor therapeutic response

Infants <3 months of age

Atypical body constituency (obesity, expanded extracellular fluid volume)

Clinical need for higher doses or shorter intervals (cystic fibrosis, burns, endocarditis, meningitis, relatively resistant organism)

Patients on hemodialysis or chronic ambulatory peritoneal dialysis

Signs of nephrotoxicity or ototoxicity

Concomitant use of other nephrotoxic agents

Patients on high-dose aerosolized tobramycin: Peak tobramycin level obtained 1 hour following inhalation to identify patients who are significant absorbers

Reference Range

Peak: 4-12 µg/mL; peak values are 2-3 times greater with once daily dosing regimens

Trough: 0.5-2 µg/mL

Test Interactions Aminoglycoside serum levels measured in blood taken from Silastic® central line catheters can sometimes give falsely high readings

(Continued)

Tobramycin *(Continued)*

Patient Information Report any dizziness or sensation of ringing or fullness in ears to the physician

Nursing Implications Obtain serum concentration after the third dose except in neonates or patients with rapidly changing renal function in whom levels need to be measured sooner; peak tobramycin serum concentrations are drawn 30 minutes after the end of a 30-minute infusion, immediately on completion of a 1-hour I.V. infusion or 1 hour after an intramuscular injection; the trough is drawn just before the next dose; provide optimal patient hydration and perfusion

Dosage Forms

Injection, as sulfate: 10 mg/mL (2 mL); 40 mg/mL (1.5 mL, 2 mL)

Ointment, ophthalmic: 0.3% [3 mg/mL] (3.5 g)

Powder for injection: 40 mg/mL (1.2 g vials)

Solution for inhalation, ampul, preservative free: 300 mg/5 mL

Solution, ophthalmic: 0.3% [3 mg/mL] (5 mL)

References

Gilbert DN, "Once-Daily Aminoglycoside Therapy," *Antimicrob Agents Chemother*, 1991, 35(3):399-405.

Green TP, Mirkin BL, Peterson PK, et al, "Tobramycin Serum Level Monitoring in Young Patients With Normal Renal Function," *Clin Pharmacokinet*, 1984, 9(5):457-68.

Nahata MC, Powell DA, Durrell DE, et al, "Effect of Gestational Age and Birth Weight on Tobramycin Kinetics in Newborn Infants," *J Antimicrob Chemother*, 1984, 14(1):59-65.

Ramsey BW, Burns J, Smith A, et al, "Safety and Efficacy of Tobramycin for Inhalation in Patients With Cystic Fibrosis: The Results of Two Phase III Placebo Controlled Clinical Trials," *Pediatr Pulmonol*, 1997, (Suppl 14):137-8, S10.3.

Ramsey BW, Dorkin HL, Eisenberg JD, et al, "Efficacy of Aerosolized Tobramycin in Patients With Cystic Fibrosis," *N Engl J Med*, 1993, 328(24):1740-6.

Shaw PK, Braun TL, Liebergen A, et al, "Aerosolized Tobramycin Pharmacokinetics in Cystic Fibrosis Patients," *J Pediatr Pharm Pract*, 1997, 2(1):23-6.

♦ **Tobramycin Sulfate** *see* Tobramycin *on page 931*

♦ **Tobrex® Ophthalmic** *see* Tobramycin *on page 931*

♦ **Tofranil®** *see* Imipramine *on page 508*

♦ **Tofranil-PM®** *see* Imipramine *on page 508*

Tolazoline *(tole AZ oh leen)*

Related Information

Overdose and Toxicology *on page 1191*

Brand Names Priscoline®

Available Salts Tolazoline Hydrochloride

Synonyms Benzazoline

Therapeutic Category Alpha-Adrenergic Blocking Agent, Parenteral; Antihypertensive Agent; Vasodilator

Generic Available No

Use Persistent pulmonary hypertension of the newborn (PPHN), also known as persistent fetal circulation (PFC); peripheral vasospastic disorders

Pregnancy Risk Factor C

Contraindications Hypersensitivity to tolazoline or any component; known or suspected coronary artery disease

Warnings May activate stress ulcers via stimulation of gastric secretions

Precautions Use with caution in patients with mitral stenosis, gastritis, peptic ulcers; use with caution and decrease dose in patients with renal dysfunction

Adverse Reactions

Cardiovascular: Hypotension, flushing, tachycardia, arrhythmias

Endocrine & metabolic: Hypochloremic alkalosis

Gastrointestinal: Increased secretions, nausea, vomiting, diarrhea, epigastric discomfort, GI bleeding

Hematology: Agranulocytosis, thrombocytopenia, pancytopenia

Ocular: Mydriasis

Renal: Oliguria

Respiratory: Pulmonary hemorrhage

Miscellaneous: Increased pilomotor activity

Drug Interactions A paradoxical decrease in blood pressure followed by a significant rebound increase in blood pressure can be seen when epinephrine or norepinephrine is administered with tolazoline; a disulfiram reaction may possibly be seen with concomitant ethanol use

Stability Compatible in D_5W, $D_{10}W$ and saline solutions; do not mix with other drugs

Mechanism of Action Competitively blocks alpha-adrenergic receptors to produce brief antagonism of circulating epinephrine and norepinephrine; reduces hypertension caused by catecholamines and causes vascular smooth muscle relaxation (direct action); results in peripheral vasodilation and decreased peripheral resistance; GI adverse effects and peripheral vasodilation mediated via histamine-like action

Pharmacodynamics Peak effects: Within 30 minutes

Pharmacokinetics

Distribution: V_d: Neonates: 1.6 L/kg

Half-life, neonates: 3-10 hours; increased half-life with decreased renal function, oliguria

Elimination: Rapid in urine primarily as unchanged drug

Usual Dosage

Neonates: I.V.:

Initial: 1-2 mg/kg over 10-15 minutes via scalp vein or upper extremity

Maintenance: I.V. continuous infusion: 1-2 mg/kg/hour; **Note:** Some neonatal centers use lower maintenance doses (eg, 0.15-0.3 mg/kg/hour or 0.5-1 mg/kg/hour)

Acute vasospasm "cath toes": 0.25 mg/kg/hour (no load)

Adults: Peripheral vasospastic disorder: I.M., I.V., S.C.: 10-50 mg 4 times/day

Dosing adjustment in renal dysfunction: Neonates: Urine output <0.9 mL/kg/hour: Decrease dose by 50%

Administration Parenteral: I.V.: Usual maximum concentration: 0.1 mg/mL

Monitoring Parameters Heart rate, blood pressure, respiratory rate, blood gases, serum chloride and bicarbonate

Additional Information Little experience with infusions >48 hours; acidosis may decrease tolazoline's effects

Dosage Forms Injection, as hydrochloride: 25 mg/mL (4 mL)

References

Ward RM, Daniel CH, Kendig JW, et al, "Oliguria and Tolazoline Pharmacokinetics in the Newborn," *Pediatrics*, 1986, 77(3):307-15.

♦ **Tolazoline Hydrochloride** *see* Tolazoline *on page 934*

♦ **Tolectin®** *see* Tolmetin *on page 935*

♦ **Tolectin® DS** *see* Tolmetin *on page 935*

Tolmetin (TOLE met in)

Related Information

Overdose and Toxicology *on page 1191*

Brand Names Novo-Tolmetin® (Canada); Tolectin®; Tolectin® DS

Available Salts Tolmetin Sodium

Therapeutic Category Analgesic, Non-narcotic; Nonsteroidal Anti-inflammatory Drug (NSAID), Oral

Generic Available Yes

Use Treatment of inflammatory and rheumatoid disorders, including juvenile rheumatoid arthritis

Pregnancy Risk Factor C (D in 3rd trimester or near delivery)

Contraindications Hypersensitivity to tolmetin, any component, aspirin, or other NSAIDs

Precautions Use with caution in patients with upper GI disease, impaired renal function, CHF, hypertension, and patients receiving anticoagulants; although rare, anaphylactoid reactions occur more commonly with tolmetin than other NSAIDs

Adverse Reactions

Cardiovascular: Edema

Central nervous system: Dizziness, nervousness, drowsiness, headache

Dermatologic: Rash, urticaria

Gastrointestinal: Nausea, abdominal pain, dyspepsia, diarrhea, constipation; GI bleeding, ulcer, perforation

Hematologic: Anemia, leukopenia, prolongation of bleeding time

Hepatic: Hepatitis

Otic: Tinnitus

Renal: Acute renal failure, renal dysfunction

Drug Interactions Tolmetin may potentiate the effects of warfarin and may increase prothrombin time and bleeding; aspirin may decrease tolmetin serum concentration; tolmetin may increase serum concentrations of methotrexate; drug interactions similar to other NSAIDs may also occur

Food Interactions Food or milk may decrease the extent of oral absorption

Mechanism of Action Inhibits prostaglandin synthesis by decreasing the activity of the enzyme, cyclo-oxygenase, which results in decreased formation of prostaglandin precursors

(Continued)

Tolmetin *(Continued)*

Pharmacokinetics
Absorption: Oral: Well absorbed
Protein binding: 99%
Metabolism: In the liver via oxidation and conjugation
Half-life, elimination: 5 hours
Time to peak serum concentration: Within 30-60 minutes
Elimination: Excreted in the urine as metabolites or conjugates

Usual Dosage Oral:
Children ≥2 years:
Anti-inflammatory: Initial: 20 mg/kg/day in 3-4 divided doses, then 15-30 mg/kg/day in 3-4 divided doses; maximum dose: 30 mg/kg/day
Analgesic: 5-7 mg/kg/dose every 6-8 hours
Adults: 400 mg 3 times/day; usual dose: 600 mg to 1.8 g/day; maximum dose: 2 g/day

Administration Oral: May administer with food, milk, or antacids to decrease GI adverse effects

Monitoring Parameters CBC with differential, liver enzymes, occult blood loss, BUN, serum creatinine; periodic ophthalmologic exams

Patient Information Avoid alcohol; may cause dizziness or drowsiness and impair ability to perform activities requiring mental alertness or physical coordination

Dosage Forms
Capsule, as sodium (Tolectin® DS): 400 mg
Tablet, as sodium (Tolectin®): 200 mg, 600 mg

References
Berde C, Ablin A, Glazer J, et al, "American Academy of Pediatrics Report of the Subcommittee on Disease-Related Pain in Childhood Cancer," *Pediatrics*, 1990, 86(5 Pt 2):818-25.
Hollingworth P, "The Use of Non-Steroidal Anti-inflammatory Drugs in Paediatric Rheumatic Diseases," *Br J Rheumatol*, 1993, 32(1):73-7.
Rose CD and Doughty RA, "Pharmacological Management of Juvenile Rheumatoid Arthritis," *Drugs*, 1992, 43(6):849-63.

♦ **Tolmetin Sodium** *see* Tolmetin *on page 935*

Tolnaftate *(tole NAF tate)*

Brand Names Absorbine® Antifungal [OTC]; Absorbine® Jock Itch [OTC]; Absorbine Jr.® Antifungal [OTC]; Aftate® [OTC]; Desenex® [OTC]; Genaspor® [OTC]; NP-27® [OTC]; Pitrex® (Canada); Tinactin® [OTC]; Zeasorb-AF® [OTC]

Therapeutic Category Antifungal Agent, Topical

Generic Available Yes

Use Treatment of tinea pedis, tinea cruris, tinea corporis, tinea manuum caused by *Trichophyton rubrum*, *T. mentagrophytes*, *T. tonsurans*, *M. canis*, *M. audouinii*, and *E. floccosum*; also effective in the treatment of tinea versicolor infections due to *Malassezia furfur*

Pregnancy Risk Factor C

Contraindications Hypersensitivity to tolnaftate or any component; nail and scalp infections

Adverse Reactions
Dermatologic: Pruritus, contact dermatitis
Local: Irritation, stinging
Miscellaneous: Hypersensitivity reaction, sensitization to butylated hydroxytoluene component of cream, solution, and aerosol powder

Mechanism of Action Distorts the hyphae and stunts mycelial growth in susceptible fungi

Pharmacodynamics Onset of action: Response may be seen 24-72 hours after initiation of therapy

Usual Dosage Children and Adults: Topical: Apply 1-3 drops of solution or a small amount of cream or powder and rub into the affected areas 2-3 times/day for 2-4 weeks

Administration Topical: Wash and dry affected area before drug application; avoid contact with eyes

Monitoring Parameters Resolution of skin infection

Patient Information Avoid contact with the eyes; apply to clean dry area; consult the physician if a skin irritation develops or if the skin infection worsens or does not improve after 10 days of therapy

Additional Information Usually not effective alone for the treatment of infections involving hair follicles or nails

Dosage Forms
Aerosol, topical:
  Liquid: 1% (59.2 mL, 90 mL, 118.3 mL, 120 mL)
  Powder: 1% (90 g, 100 g, 105 g, 150 g)
Cream: 1% (15 g, 30 g)
Gel, topical: 1% (15 g)
Powder, topical: 1% (45 g, 56.7 g, 67.5 g, 70.9 g, 90 g)
Solution, topical: 1% (10 mL, 15 mL)

♦ Tolu-Sed® DM [OTC] *see* Guaifenesin and Dextromethorphan *on page 466*
♦ Topactin® (Canada) *see* Fluocinonide *on page 426*
♦ Topamax® *see* Topiramate *on page 937*
♦ Topicaine® *see* Benzocaine *on page 124*
♦ Topicycline® Topical *see* Tetracycline *on page 908*
♦ Topilene® (Canada) *see* Betamethasone *on page 130*

Topiramate (toe PYE ra mate)
Brand Names Topamax®
Therapeutic Category Anticonvulsant, Miscellaneous
Generic Available No
Use Adjunctive treatment of primary generalized tonic-clonic seizures or partial epilepsy in children 2-16 years of age and adults; also used for treatment of Lennox-Gastaut syndrome
Pregnancy Risk Factor C
Contraindications Hypersensitivity to topiramate or any component
Warnings Do not abruptly discontinue therapy, withdraw gradually to lessen chance for increased seizure frequency; CNS adverse effects are common (see Adverse Reactions); avoid use with alcohol, CNS depressants, or carbonic anhydrase inhibitors (see Drug Interactions)
Precautions Use with caution and decrease the dose in patients with renal dysfunction; use with caution in patients allergic to sulfa drugs and in patients with hepatic impairment
Adverse Reactions
  Central nervous system: Ataxia, difficulty in concentrating, dizziness, memory difficulties, fatigue, nervousness, somnolence, psychomotor slowing, speech/language problems, confusion, depression, anxiety, cognitive problems; irritability and sleep disturbances (reported in children); **Note:** Somnolence and fatigue are the most common CNS adverse effects in children
  Gastrointestinal: Weight loss, anorexia, nausea
  Hematologic: Purpura
  Neuromuscular & skeletal: Paresthesia, tremor
  Ocular: Nystagmus, diplopia, abnormal vision
  Renal: Nephrolithiasis
  Respiratory: Epistaxis
Drug Interactions Cytochrome P-450 isoenzyme CYP2C19 substrate and inhibitor Phenytoin and carbamazepine may significantly decrease topiramate serum concentrations (topiramate dosage increase may be needed); valproic acid may decrease topiramate concentrations; topiramate may decrease serum concentrations of valproic acid, digoxin, and ethinyl estradiol (may decrease the efficacy of oral contraceptives); alcohol or other CNS depressants may increase adverse CNS effects; carbonic anhydrase inhibitors may increase the risk of nephrolithiasis or paresthesia; topiramate may increase phenytoin serum concentrations by 25% in some patients
Food Interactions Food may decrease the rate but not the extent of absorption
Stability Protect from moisture; store at room temperature
Mechanism of Action Exact mechanism unknown; thought to decrease the spread of seizure activity by blockade of sodium channels, potentiation of GABA (an inhibitory neurotransmitter) and antagonism of kainate activation of glutamate (an excitatory amino acid) subtype receptors; also inhibits carbonic anhydrase (minor effect)
Pharmacokinetics Note: Sprinkle capsule is bioequivalent to tablet
  Absorption: Rapid
  Distribution: V_d: Adults: 0.6-0.8 L/kg
  Protein binding: 13% to 17%
  Metabolism: Minor amounts metabolized in liver via hydroxylation, hydrolysis, and glucuronidation; percentage of dose metabolized in liver and clearance are increased in patients receiving enzyme inducers
  Bioavailability: Tablet: 80% (relative to a prepared solution)
(Continued)

Topiramate *(Continued)*

Half-life:

Adults: 19-23 hours (mean 21 hours)

Adults with renal impairment: 59 ± 11 hours (n=7)

Time to peak serum concentration: 2 hours; range: 1.4-4.3 hours

Elimination: 70% of dose excreted unchanged in urine; may undergo renal tubular reabsorption

Clearance:

Children 4-17 years: ~50% higher than adults (per kg)

Adults: 20-30 mL/minute

Renal impairment: Reduced

Hepatic impairment: May be reduced

Dialysis: Significantly hemodialyzed; dialysis clearance: 120 mL/minute (4-6 times higher than in adults with normal renal function); supplemental doses may be required

Usual Dosage Oral:

Children 2-16 years:

Partial onset seizures: Initial: 1-3 mg/kg/day (maximum: 25 mg) given nightly for 1 week; increase at 1- to 2-week intervals by 1-3 mg/kg/day given in 2 divided doses; titrate dose to response; usual maintenance: 5-9 mg/kg/day given in 2 divided doses

Primary generalized tonic-clonic seizures: Use slower initial titration rate; titrate to 6 mg/kg/day by the end of 8 weeks

Adolescents ≥17 years and Adults:

Partial onset seizures: Initial: 50 mg/day given daily for 1 week, then 100 mg/day in 2 divided doses for 1 week; increase by 50 mg/day each week; titrate dose to response; usual maintenance: 200 mg twice daily; maximum dose: 1600 mg/day

Primary generalized tonic-clonic seizures: Use slower initial titration rate; titrate upwards to recommended dose by the end of 8 weeks

Dosing adjustment in renal impairment: Cl_{cr} <70 mL/minute/1.73 m^2: Administer 50% of the usual dose; titrate more slowly due to prolonged half-life

Dosing adjustment in hepatic impairment: Carefully adjust dose as plasma concentrations may be increased if normal dosing is used

Administration May be administered without regard to food; broken tablets have a bitter taste; tablets may be crushed, mixed with water, and administered immediately. Swallow sprinkle capsules whole or open and sprinkle contents on small amount of soft food (eg, 1 teaspoonful of applesauce); swallow sprinkle/food mixture immediately; do not chew; do not store for later use; drink fluids after dose to make sure mixture is completely swallowed

Monitoring Parameters Seizure frequency, duration, and severity; renal function

Reference Range Not applicable; plasma topiramate concentrations have not been shown to correlate with clinical efficacy

Patient Information Ensure adequate fluid intake to avoid kidney stone formation; may cause dizziness or drowsiness and impair ability to perform activities requiring mental alertness or physical coordination; avoid alcohol

Dosage Forms

Capsule: 15 mg, 25 mg

Tablet: 25 mg, 100 mg, 200 mg

References

Doose DR, Walker SA, Gisclon LG, et al, "Single-Dose Pharmacokinetics and Effect of Food on the Bioavailability of Topiramate, a Novel Antiepileptic Drug," *J Clin Pharmacol*, 1996, 36(10):884-91.

Glauser TA, "Preliminary Observations on Topiramate in Pediatric Epilepsies," *Epilepsia*, 1997, 38(Suppl 1):S37-41.

Glauser TA, "Topiramate Use in Pediatric Patients," *Can J Neurol Sci*, 1998, 25(3):S8-12.

Glauser TA, Clark PO, and Strawsburg R, "A Pilot Study of Topiramate in the Treatment of Infantile Spasms," *Epilepsia*, 1998, 39(12):1324-8.

Sachdeo RC, "Topiramate. Clinical Profile in Epilepsy," *Clin Pharmacokinet*, 1998, 34(5):335-46.

♦ **Topisone® (Canada)** *see* Betamethasone *on page 130*

♦ **Toprol XL®** *see* Metoprolol *on page 633*

♦ **Topsyn® (Canada)** *see* Fluocinonide *on page 426*

♦ **Toradol® Injection** *see* Ketorolac *on page 544*

♦ **Toradol® Oral** *see* Ketorolac *on page 544*

♦ **Torecan®** *see* Thiethylperazine *on page 917*

♦ **Tornalate®** *see* Bitolterol *on page 136*

Torsemide (TOR se mide)

Brand Names Demadex® Injection; Demadex® Oral

Therapeutic Category Antihypertensive Agent; Diuretic, Loop

Generic Available No

Use Management of edema associated with CHF and hepatic or renal disease; used alone or in combination with antihypertensives in treatment of hypertension

Pregnancy Risk Factor B

Contraindications Hypersensitivity to torsemide, any component, or other sulfonylureas; anuria

Warnings Loop diuretics are potent diuretics, excess amounts can lead to profound diuresis with fluid and electrolyte loss; close medical supervision and dose evaluation is required

Adverse Reactions

Cardiovascular: Orthostatic hypotension, EKG abnormality, chest pain, atrial fibrillation, ventricular tachycardia, syncope

Central nervous system: Headache, dizziness, insomnia, nervousness

Dermatologic: Rash, photosensitivity

Endocrine & metabolic: Hyponatremia, hypokalemia, hypochloremia, alkalosis, hypocalcemia, dehydration, hyperuricemia, gout

Gastrointestinal: Diarrhea, nausea, constipation, dyspepsia, GI hemorrhage, stomach cramps, pancreatitis

Genitourinary: Excessive urination

Hematologic: Agranulocytosis, anemia

Neuromuscular & skeletal: Myalgia, arthralgia, weakness

Otic: Ototoxicity

Renal: Prerenal azotemia, interstitial nephritis, nephrocalcinosis

Drug Interactions Increased risk of ototoxicity with aminoglycosides and cis-platinum; increased anticoagulant effects of warfarin; increased risk of digoxin toxicity when used alone or combined with other medications which cause increased potassium losses (eg, corticosteroids, amphotericin B); decreased glucose tolerance which may result in increased requirements of sulfonylureas and other antidiabetic agents; decreased diuretic effects of torsemide when combined with NSAIDs; increased lithium serum levels; increased salicylate levels with potential toxicity (with high dose salicylates)

Stability Stable for 24 hours at room temperature when mixed with D_5W or NS

Mechanism of Action Inhibits reabsorption of sodium and chloride in the ascending loop of Henle and distal renal tubule, interfering with the chloride-binding cotransport system, thus causing increased excretion of water, sodium, chloride, magnesium, and calcium

Pharmacodynamics

Onset of effect:

Oral: 60 minutes

I.V.: 10 minutes

Peak effect:

Oral: 60-120 minutes

I.V.: Within 60 minutes

Duration: Oral, I.V.: 6-8 hours

Pharmacokinetics

Absorption: Oral: Rapid

Distribution: V_d: 12-15 L (adults)

Protein binding: Plasma: ~97% to 99%

Metabolism: Hepatic by cytochrome P-450, 80%

Bioavailability: 80% to 90%

Half-life: 3.5 hours (range 2-4 hours); 7-8 hours in cirrhosis (dose modification appears unnecessary)

Elimination: 20% eliminated unchanged in urine

Usual Dosage Adults: Oral, I.V.:

Edema: 10-20 mg once daily; titrate upward as needed (maximum dose: 200 mg/day)

Hepatic cirrhosis: 5-10 mg once daily

Hypertension: Initial: 5 mg once daily; increase to 10 mg if ineffective after 4-6 weeks of therapy

Administration

Oral: May be administered with food or milk

Parenteral: May be administered undiluted direct I.V. over 3-5 minutes

Monitoring Parameters Renal function, serum electrolytes, and fluid intake and output, blood pressure

(Continued)

Torsemide *(Continued)*

Patient Information Rise slowly from a lying or sitting position to minimize dizziness, lightheadedness or fainting; also use extra care when exercising, standing for long periods of time; take last dose of day early in the evening to prevent nocturia

Additional Information 10-20 mg torsemide is approximately equivalent to:
Furosemide 40 mg
Bumetanide 1 mg

Dosage Forms
Injection: 10 mg/mL (2 mL, 5 mL)
Tablet: 5 mg, 10 mg, 20 mg, 100 mg

♦ **Totacillin®** *see* Ampicillin *on page 78*

♦ **Totacillin®-N** *see* Ampicillin *on page 78*

♦ **Touro Ex®** *see* Guaifenesin *on page 464*

♦ **T-Phyl®** *see* Theophylline *on page 910*

♦ **Trace-4®** *see* Trace Metals *on page 940*

♦ **Trace Elements** *see* Trace Metals *on page 940*

Trace Metals *(trase MET als)*

Related Information
Parenteral Nutrition (PN) *on page 1072*

Brand Names Chroma-Pak®; Iodopen®; Molypen®; M.T.E.-4®; M.T.E.-5®; M.T.E.-6®; Multe-Pak-4®; Neotrace-4®; Pedte-Pak-5®; Pedtrace-4®; P.T.E.-4®; P.T.E.-5®; Sele-Pak®; Selepen®; Trace-4®; Zinca-Pak®

Available Salts Ammonium Molybdate; Chromium Chloride; Copper Sulfate; Cupric Chloride; Iodine Sodium; Manganese Chloride; Manganese Sulfate; Zinc Chloride; Zinc Sulfate

Synonyms Multiple Trace Metals; Neonatal Trace Metals; Selenium; Trace Elements

Therapeutic Category Mineral, Parenteral; Trace Element, Parenteral; Trace Element, Multiple, Neonatal

Generic Available Yes

Use Prevent and correct trace metal deficiencies

Pregnancy Risk Factor C

Contraindications Do not give by direct injection because of potential for phlebitis, tissue irritation, and potential to increase renal loss of minerals from a bolus injection

Warnings Some of these products may contain benzyl alcohol which has been associated with fatal "gasping" syndrome in premature infants. Metals may accumulate in conditions of renal failure or biliary obstruction; consider reduction in dosage or deletion of copper and manganese in patients with biliary obstruction; avoid copper use in patients with Wilson's disease; administration of copper in the absence of zinc or zinc in the absence of copper may cause decreases in their respective plasma levels; molybdenum promotes the utilization of copper and increases its excretion; excessive amounts of molybdenum may produce copper deficiency; multiple trace metal solutions present a risk of overdosage when the need for one trace element is appreciably higher than for others in the formulation; utilization of individual trace metal solutions may be needed. Consider reduction in dosage or deletion of selenium and chromium in patients with renal dysfunction.

Adverse Reactions The following describe the symptomatology associated with excess trace metals

Chromium: Nausea, vomiting, GI ulcers, renal and hepatic dysfunction, convulsions, coma

Copper: Prostration, behavioral changes, diarrhea, progressive marasmus, hypotonia, photophobia, hepatic dysfunction, peripheral edema

Manganese: Irritability, speech disturbances, abnormal gait, headache, anorexia, apathy, impotence, cholestatic jaundice, movement disorders

Molybdenum: Gout-like syndrome with increased blood levels of uric acid and xanthine oxidase

Selenium: Alopecia, weak nails, dermatitis, dental defects, GI disorders, nervousness, mental depression, metallic taste, garlic odor of breath and sweat

Zinc: Profuse diaphoresis, decreased consciousness, blurred vision, tachycardia, hypothermia

Drug Interactions Oral zinc decreases quinolone and tetracycline absorption

Food Interactions Decreased absorption of oral zinc when given with bran products, protein, and phytates

Mechanism of Action

Chromium: Part of glucose tolerance factor, an essential activator of insulin-mediated reactions; helps maintain normal glucose metabolism and peripheral nerve function

Copper: Cofactor for serum ceruloplasmin, helps maintain normal rates of red and white cell formation

Manganese: Activator for several enzymes including manganese-dependent superoxide dismutase and pyruvate carboxylase; activates glycosyl transferases involved in mucopolysaccharide synthesis

Molybdenum: Constituent of the enzymes xanthine oxidase, sulfite oxidase, and aldehyde oxidase

Selenium: Part of glutathione peroxidase which protects cell components from oxidative damage due to peroxides produced in cellular metabolism

Zinc: A cofactor for >70 different enzymes; facilitates wound healing, helps maintain normal growth rates, normal skin hydration, and the senses of taste and smell

Pharmacokinetics

Chromium: 10% to 20% oral absorption; excretion primarily via kidneys and bile

Copper: 30% oral absorption; 80% elimination via bile; intestinal wall 16% and urine 4%

Manganese: 10% oral absorption; excretion primarily via bile; ancillary routes via pancreatic secretions or reabsorption into the intestinal lumen occur during periods of biliary obstruction

Molybdenum: 30% to 70% oral absorption; primarily renal excretion; some biliary excretion associated with an enterohepatic cycle

Selenium: Very poor oral absorption; 75% excretion via kidneys, remainder via feces, lung, and skin

Zinc: 20% to 30% oral absorption; 90% excretion in stools, remainder via urine and perspiration

Usual Dosage See table.

Trace Mineral Daily Requirements*

	Infants	Children (≥3 mo to ≤5 y)	Older Children, Adolescents, and Adults
Chromium†	0.2 mcg/kg	0.14-0.2 mcg/kg (max: 5 mcg)	5-15 mcg
Copper‡	20 mcg/kg	20 mcg/kg (max: 300 mcg)	0.2-0.5 mg
Iodide§	1 mcg/kg	1 mcg/kg	1 mcg/kg
Manganese‡	1 mcg/kg	2-10 mcg/kg (max: 50 mcg)	50-150 mcg
Selenium†¶	2-3 mcg/kg	2-3 mcg/kg (max: 30 mcg)	30-40 mcg
Zinc	400 mcg/kg (preterm) 300 mcg/kg (term <3 mo)	100 mcg/kg (max: 5 mg)	2-5 mg

*Recommended intakes of trace elements cannot be achieved through the use of a single pediatric trace element produce. Only through the use of individualized trace element products can recommended intakes be achieved.

†Omit in patients with renal dysfunction.

‡Omit in patients with obstructive jaundice.

§Percutaneous absorption from protein-bound iodine may be adequate.

¶Indicated for use in long-term parenteral nutrition patients.

Administration Parenteral: Must be diluted prior to use and infused as component of parenteral nutrition or parenteral solutions

Reference Range

Chromium: 0.18-0.47 ng/mL (SI: 35-90 nmol/L); some laboratories report much higher

*Copper: ~0.7-1.5 µg/mL (SI: 11-24 µmol/L); levels are higher in pregnant women and children

Manganese: 18-30 µg/dL (SI: 2.3-3.8 µmol/L)

Selenium: 95-165 ng/mL (SI: 120-209 nmol/L)

Zinc: 70-120 µg/dL (SI: 10-18.4 µmol/L)

*May not be a meaningful measurement of body stores

(Continued)

Trace Metals *(Continued)*

Additional Information Persistent diarrhea or excessive gastrointestinal fluid losses from ostomy sites may grossly increase zinc losses

Dosage Forms See table.

Multiple Trace Metal Parenteral Solutions

	Content per mL					
	Chromium (mcg)	Copper (mg)	Iodide (mcg)	Manganese (mg)	Selenium (mcg)	Zinc (mg)
Pedtrace-4®	0.85	0.1	—	0.025	—	0.5
Multiple trace element neonatal	0.85	0.1	—	0.025	—	1.5
Neotrace-4®	0.85	0.1	—	0.025	—	1.5
PedTE-PAK-4®	1	0.1	—	0.025	—	1
P.T.E.-4®	1	0.1	—	0.025	—	1
Multiple trace element pediatric	1	0.1	—	0.03	—	0.5
Trace metals additive in NS	2	0.2	—	0.16	—	0.8
M.T.E.-4®	4	0.4	—	0.1	—	1
MulTE-PAK-4®	4	0.4	—	0.1	—	1
Multiple trace element	4	0.4	—	0.1	—	1
Multiple trace element conc	10	1	—	0.5	—	5
ConTE-PAK-4®	10	1	—	0.5	—	5
M.T.E.-4® conc	10	1	—	0.5	—	5
PTE-5®	1	0.1	—	0.025	15	1
M.T.E.-5®	4	0.4	—	0.1	20	1
MulTE-PAK-5®	4	0.4	—	0.1	20	1
Multiple trace element w/ selenium	4	0.4	—	0.1	20	1
M.T.E.-5® conc	10	1	—	0.5	60	5
Multiple trace element w/ selenium concentrated	10	1	—	0.5	60	5
M.T.E.-6®	4	0.4	25	0.1	20	1
M.T.E.-7®*	4	0.4	25	0.1	20	1
M.T.E.-6® conc	10	1	75	0.5	60	5

*With 25 mcg molybdenum.

Injection [elemental equivalence]:

Chromium, as chromic chloride (hexahydrate): 0.0205 mg/mL [0.004 mg/mL]; 0.1025 mg/mL [0.022 mg/mL]

Copper:
  As cupric chloride: 1.07 mg/mL [0.4 mg/mL]
  As sulfate: 1.57 mg/mL [0.4 mg/mL]; 7.85 mg/mL [2 mg/mL]

Iodine, as iodine sodium: 0.118 mg/mL [0.1 mg/mL]

Manganese:
  As chloride: 0.36 mg/mL [0.1 mg/mL]
  As sulfate: 0.31 mg/mL [0.1 mg/mL]

Molybdenum, as ammonium molybdate (tetrahydrate): 46 mcg/mL [25 mcg/mL]

Selenium, as selenious acid: 0.0654 mg/mL [0.04 mg/mL]

Zinc:
  As chloride: 2.09 mg/mL [1 mg/mL]
  As sulfate: 21.95 mg/mL [5 mg/mL]
    Anhydrous: 2.46 mg/mL [1 mg/mL]
    Heptahydrate: 4.39 mg/mL [1 mg/mL]

References

Dahlstrom KA, Ament ME, Medhin MG, et al, "Serum Trace Elements in Children Receiving Long-Term Parenteral Nutrition," *J Pediatr*, 1986, 109(4):625-30.

Feil JM, Reynolds AP, Meadows N, et al, "Manganese Toxicity in Children Receiving Long-Term Parenteral Nutrition," *Lancet*, 1996, 347(9010):1218-21.

Greene HL, Hambridge KM, Schanler R, et al, "Guidelines for the Use of Vitamins, Trace Elements, Calcium, Magnesium and Phosphorus in Infants and Children Receiving Total Parenteral Nutrition: Report of the Subcommittee on Pediatric Nutrient Requirements From the Committee on Clinical Practice Issues of The American Society for Clinical Nutrition," *Am J Clin Nutr*, 1988, 48(5):1324-42.

Litov RE, and Combs GF Jr, "Selenium in Pediatric Nutrition," *Pediatrics*, 1991, 87(3):339-51.

- ♦ **Tracrium**® *see* Atracurium *on page 105*
- ♦ **Trandate**® *see* Labetalol *on page 548*

Tranexamic Acid (tran eks AM ik AS id)
Brand Names Cyklokapron®
Synonyms AMCA; CL-65336; transAMCA
Therapeutic Category Antihemophilic Agent
Generic Available No
Use Prevention of excessive bleeding after tonsillectomy; short-term use (2-8 days) in hemophilia patients during and following tooth extraction; primary menorrhagia; prevention of gastrointestinal hemorrhage and hemorrhage following ocular trauma; recurrent epistaxis; hereditary angioneurotic edema
Pregnancy Risk Factor B
Contraindications Hypersensitivity to tranexamic acid or any component; subarachnoid hemorrhage; acquired defective color vision, active intravascular clotting process
Warnings Patients receiving therapy for a long duration should have baseline and frequent ophthalmologic exams; do not administer concomitantly with factor IX complex concentrates or anti-inhibitor coagulant concentrates due to increased risk of thrombosis
Precautions Dosage modification required in patients with renal impairment; use with caution in patients with cardiovascular, renal, cerebrovascular disease, or transurethral prostatectomy
Adverse Reactions
  Cardiovascular: Hypotension (with rapid I.V. administration), thromboembolic complications
  Central nervous system: Cerebral ischemia and infarction (when used in the treatment of subarachnoid hemorrhage), headache, hydrocephalus, giddiness
  Gastrointestinal: Nausea, diarrhea, vomiting
  Hematologic: Thrombocytopenia, coagulation defects, abnormal bleeding times
  Ocular: Visual abnormalities (focal areas of retinal degeneration have been seen in animals), central venous stasis retinopathy
Drug Interactions Chlorpromazine
Stability Incompatible with solutions containing penicillin; compatible with dextrose, saline, and electrolyte solutions
Mechanism of Action Forms a reversible complex that displaces plasminogen from fibrin resulting in inhibition of fibrinolysis; it also inhibits the proteolytic activity of plasmin
Pharmacokinetics
  Distribution: Breast milk levels are 1% of serum; CSF levels are 10% of plasma
  Protein binding: 3%
  Bioavailability:
    Oral: 33% to 35%
    I.M.: 100%
  Half-life: 2 hours
  Time to peak serum concentration:
    Oral: 3 hours
    I.M.: 1 hour
    I.V.: 5 minutes
  Elimination: Elimination characteristics differ by route of administration: after I.V. administration 95% excreted as unchanged drug in urine vs 39% after oral administration
Usual Dosage Dental extraction in hemophiliacs: Children and Adults: 10 mg/kg I.V. immediately before surgery, then 25 mg/kg/dose orally 3-4 times/day for 2-8 days

  Alternatives:
    10 mg/kg/dose I.V. 3-4 times/day if unable to take orally
    25 mg/kg/dose orally 3-4 times/day beginning 1 day prior to surgery
  Menorrhagia: Oral: Adolescents and Adults: 1-1.5 g (12-25 mg/kg/dose) 3-4 times daily for 3-4 days
  Adults: Oral:
    Epistaxis: 1.5 g 3 times/day
    Ocular trauma: 1 g 3 times/day
  Dosing adjustment in renal impairment: Adults: See table on next page.
(Continued)

Tranexamic Acid *(Continued)*

Tranxemic Acid Dosage Adjustments in Renal Impairment
(Adult Data)

Serum Creatinine (mg/dL)	I.V. dose	Oral dose
1.36-2.83	10 mg/kg twice daily	15 mg/kg twice daily
>2.83-5.66	10 mg/kg once daily	15 mg/kg once daily
>5.66	10 mg/kg every 48 h or 5 mg/kg every 24 h	15 mg/kg every 48 h or 7.5 mg/kg every 24 h

Administration
Parenteral: May be administered by direct I.V. injection at a maximum rate of 100 mg/minute (1 mL/minute)
Oral: May be administered with food
Monitoring Parameters Ophthalmologic exams (baseline and at regular intervals) of chronic therapy
Reference Range 5-10 µg/mL is required to decrease fibrinolysis
Dosage Forms
Injection: 100 mg/mL (10 mL)
Tablet: 500 mg

♦ **transAMCA** *see* Tranexamic Acid *on page 943*
♦ **Transdermal-NTG® Patch** *see* Nitroglycerin *on page 690*
♦ **Transdermal-V® (Canada)** *see* Scopolamine *on page 860*
♦ **Transderm-Nitro® Patch** *see* Nitroglycerin *on page 690*
♦ **Transderm Scop®** *see* Scopolamine *on page 860*
♦ **Trans-Plantar® (Canada)** *see* Salicylic Acid *on page 854*
♦ **Trans-Plantar® Transdermal Patch [OTC]** *see* Salicylic Acid *on page 854*
♦ *trans*-**Retinoic Acid** *see* Tretinoin *on page 945*
♦ **Trans-Ver-Sal® (Canada)** *see* Salicylic Acid *on page 854*
♦ **Trans-Ver-Sal® Transdermal Patch [OTC] Verukan® Solution** *see* Salicylic Acid *on page 854*
♦ **Tranxene®** *see* Clorazepate *on page 244*
♦ **Trasylol®** *see* Aprotinin *on page 93*
♦ **Travase®** *see* Sutilains *on page 900*
♦ **Travel Aid® (Canada)** *see* Dimenhydrinate *on page 325*
♦ **Travel Tabs (Canada)** *see* Dimenhydrinate *on page 325*

Trazodone *(TRAZ oh done)*
Related Information
Comparison of Adverse Effects of Antidepressants *on page 1030*
Comparison of Usual Adult Dosage and Mechanism of Action of Antidepressants *on page 1029*
Drugs and Breast-Feeding *on page 1213*
Serotonin Syndrome *on page 1217*
Brand Names Desyrel®
Therapeutic Category Antidepressant
Generic Available Yes
Use Treatment of depression
Pregnancy Risk Factor C
Contraindications Hypersensitivity to trazodone or any component
Warnings Monitor closely and use with extreme caution in patients with cardiac disease or arrhythmias
Adverse Reactions Possesses fewer anticholinergic and cardiac adverse effects than tricyclic antidepressants
Cardiovascular: Postural hypotension (5%), arrhythmias
Central nervous system: Drowsiness (20% to 50%), sedation, dizziness, insomnia, confusion, agitation, seizures, extrapyramidal reactions, headache
Gastrointestinal: Xerostomia, constipation, nausea, vomiting
Genitourinary: Prolonged priapism (1:6000), urinary retention (rare)
Hepatic: Hepatitis
Neuromuscular & skeletal: Weakness
Ocular: Blurred vision (15% to 30%)

Drug Interactions Cytochrome P-450 isoenzyme CYP2D6 and CYP3A3/4 substrate

May antagonize the antihypertensive effects of clonidine and methyldopa; may increase the serum concentrations of phenytoin or digoxin; effects may be additive with other CNS depressants, alcohol; fluoxetine may increase trazodone serum concentration

Food Interactions Food may decrease the rate but not the extent of absorption

Mechanism of Action Inhibits reuptake of serotonin; minimal or no effect on reuptake of norepinephrine or dopamine; possesses little if any anticholinergic effects; alpha-adrenergic blockade thought to be responsible for orthostatic hypotension and dry mouth

Pharmacodynamics Maximum antidepressant effect: ~2-6 weeks

Pharmacokinetics

Protein binding: 85% to 95%

Metabolism: In the liver via hydroxylation and oxidation

Half-life, elimination: 5-9 hours, prolonged in elderly and obese patients

Elimination: Primarily in urine (74%) with ~21% excreted in feces

Usual Dosage Oral:

Children 6-18 years: Initial: 1.5-2 mg/kg/day in divided doses; increase gradually every 3-4 days as needed; maximum dose: 6 mg/kg/day in 3 divided doses

Adolescents: Initial: 25-50 mg/day; increase to 100-150 mg/day in divided doses

Adults: Initial: 150 mg/day in 3 divided doses (may increase by 50 mg/day every 3-7 days); maximum dose: 600 mg/day

Administration Oral: Administer after meals or a snack to decrease lightheadedness, sedation, and postural hypotension

Monitoring Parameters Blood pressure, mental status, liver enzymes

Reference Range

Therapeutic: 0.5-2.5 µg/mL (SI: 1-6 µmol/L)

Potentially toxic: >2.5 µg/mL (SI: >6 µmol/L)

Toxic: >4 µg/mL (SI: >10 µmol/L)

Patient Information Avoid alcohol; may cause drowsiness and impair ability to perform hazardous tasks that require mental alertness or physical coordination; may cause dry mouth

Additional Information Mean doses of ~5 mg/kg/day were used in 22 children 5-12 years of age to treat severe behavioral disorders (Zubieta, 1992). Doses of 1 mg/kg/day given in 3 divided doses were used for migraine prophylaxis in 40 patients 7-18 years of age (Battistella, 1993). Further studies are needed before trazodone can be recommended in children for these indications.

Dosage Forms Tablet: 50 mg, 100 mg, 150 mg, 300 mg

References

Battistella PA, Ruffilli R, Cernetti R, et al, "A Placebo-Controlled Crossover Trial Using Trazodone in Pediatric Migraine," *Headache*, 1993, 33(1):36-9.

Zubieta JK and Alessi NE, "Acute and Chronic Administration of Trazodone in the Treatment of Disruptive Behavior Disorders in Children," *J Clin Psychopharmacol*, 1992, 12(5):346-51.

♦ **Trecator®-SC** *see* Ethionamide *on page 392*

♦ **Tremytoine® (Canada)** *see* Phenytoin *on page 762*

♦ **Trendar® [OTC]** *see* Ibuprofen *on page 501*

♦ **Trental®** *see* Pentoxifylline *on page 750*

Tretinoin (TRET i noyn)

Brand Names Retin-A™; Retinova™ (Canada); Retisol-A® (Canada); Stieva-A® (Canada); Stieva-A® Forte (Canada); Vitinoin™ (Canada)

Synonyms Retinoic Acid; *trans*-Retinoic Acid; Vitamin A Acid

Therapeutic Category Acne Products; Retinoic Acid Derivative; Vitamin, Topical

Generic Available No

Use Treatment of acne vulgaris, photodamaged skin, and some skin cancers

Pregnancy Risk Factor C

Contraindications Hypersensitivity to tretinoin or any component; sunburn

Warnings Avoid contact with abraded skin, mucous membranes, eyes, mouth, angles of the nose; avoid excessive exposure to sunlight or sunlamps

Precautions Use with caution in patients with eczema

Adverse Reactions

Cardiovascular: Edema

Dermatologic: Excessive dryness, erythema, scaling of the skin, hyperpigmentation or hypopigmentation, photosensitivity, initial acne flare-up

Local: Stinging, blistering

(Continued)

Tretinoin *(Continued)*

Drug Interactions Sulfur, benzoyl peroxide, salicylic acid, and resorcinol potentiate adverse reactions seen with tretinoin

Food Interactions Avoid excessive intake of vitamin A

Mechanism of Action Keratinocytes in the sebaceous follicle become less adherent which allows for easy removal; inhibits microcomedone formation and eliminates lesions already present

Pharmacodynamics
Onset of therapeutic effects: 2-3 weeks
Optimal effects: May require 6 weeks or longer

Pharmacokinetics
Absorption: Topical: Minimum absorption
Metabolism: In the liver
Elimination: In bile and urine

Usual Dosage Children >12 years and Adults: Topical: Begin therapy with a weaker formulation of tretinoin (0.025% cream or 0.01% gel) and increase the concentration as tolerated; apply once daily before retiring or on alternate days; if stinging or irritation develop, decrease frequency of application

Administration Topical: Apply to dry skin (wait at least 15-30 minutes to apply after cleansing); avoid contact with eyes, mucous membranes, mouth, or open wounds

Patient Information Minimize exposure to sunlight; use of a sunscreen is recommended; avoid washing face more frequently than 2-3 times/day; avoid using topical preparations with high alcoholic content during treatment period

Additional Information Liquid preparation generally is more irritating

Dosage Forms
Cream: 0.025% (20 g, 45 g); 0.05% (20 g, 45 g); 0.1% (20 g, 45 g)
Gel, topical: 0.01% (15 g, 45 g); 0.025% (15 g, 45 g)
Liquid, topical: 0.05% (28 mL)

References
Winston MH, Shalita AR, "Acne Vulgaris, Pathogenesis and Treatment," *Pediatr Clin North Am*, 1991, 38(4):889-903.

♦ **Triacet® Topical** *see* Triamcinolone *on page 946*

♦ **Triacetyloleandomycin** *see* Troleandomycin *on page 958*

♦ **Triadapin® (Canada)** *see* Doxepin *on page 345*

♦ **Triam-A® Injection** *see* Triamcinolone *on page 946*

Triamcinolone *(trye am SIN oh lone)*

Related Information
Asthma Guidelines *on page 1178*
Corticosteroids Comparison, Topical *on page 1033*
Estimated Comparative Daily Dosages for Inhaled Corticosteroids *on page 1185*

Brand Names Amcort® Injection; Aristocort® Injection; Aristocort® A Topical; Aristocort® Forte Injection; Aristocort® Intralesional Injection; Aristocort® Oral; Aristocort® Topical; Aristospan® Intra-articular Injection; Aristospan® Intralesional Injection; Atolone® Oral; Azmacort™ Oral Inhaler; Delta-Tritex® Topical; Flutex® Topical; Kenacort® Oral; Kenaject® Injection; Kenalog® Injection; Kenalog® in Orabase®; Kenalog® Topical; Kenonel® Topical; Nasacort®; Nasacort® AQ; Tac™-3 Injection; Tac™-40 Injection; Triacet® Topical; Triam-A® Injection; Triam Forte® Injection; Triamonide® Injection; Tri-Kort® Injection; Trilog® Injection; Trilone® Injection; Trisoject® Injection

Available Salts Triamcinolone Acetonide; Triamcinolone Diacetate; Triamcinolone Hexacetonide

Therapeutic Category Adrenal Corticosteroid; Antiasthmatic; Anti-inflammatory Agent; Corticosteroid, Inhalant (Oral); Corticosteroid, Intranasal; Corticosteroid, Systemic; Corticosteroid, Topical; Glucocorticoid

Generic Available Yes

Use
Oral inhalation: Long-term (chronic) control of persistent bronchial asthma; **NOT** indicated for the relief of acute bronchospasm
Intranasal: Management of seasonal and perennial allergic rhinitis
Systemic: Immunosuppression; relief of severe inflammation
Topical: Relief of inflammation and pruritus associated with corticosteroid-responsive dermatoses

Pregnancy Risk Factor C

Contraindications Hypersensitivity to triamcinolone or any component; primary treatment of status asthmaticus; systemic fungal infections; serious infections, except septic shock or tuberculous meningitis

Warnings Fatalities have occurred due to adrenal insufficiency in asthmatic patients during and after switching from systemic corticosteroids to aerosol steroids; several months may be required for full recovery of the adrenal glands; during this period, aerosol steroids do **not** provide the systemic corticosteroid needed to treat patients requiring stress doses (ie, patients with major stress such as trauma, surgery, or infections); when used at high doses hypothalamic - pituitary - adrenal (HPA) suppression may occur; use with inhaled or systemic corticosteroids (even alternate-day dosing) may increase risk of HPA suppression; withdrawal and discontinuation of corticosteroids should be done carefully; immunosuppression may occur

Precautions Avoid using higher than recommended doses; suppression of HPA function, suppression of linear growth, or hypercorticism (Cushing's syndrome) may occur; use with extreme caution in patients with respiratory tuberculosis, untreated systemic infections, or ocular herpes simplex

Adverse Reactions

Cardiovascular: Facial edema, hypertension

Central nervous system: Fatigue

Dermatologic: Itching, hypertrichosis, skin atrophy, hyperpigmentation, hypopigmentation, acne

Endocrine & metabolic: Cushingoid state, sodium retention, pituitary-adrenal axis suppression, potential growth suppression, glucose intolerance, hypokalemia

Gastrointestinal: Oral candidiasis, dry throat, xerostomia, peptic ulcer

Local: Burning, sterile abscesses

Neuromuscular & skeletal: Osteoporosis

Ocular: Cataracts

Respiratory: Hoarseness, wheezing, cough

Drug Interactions Cytochrome P-450 isoenzyme CYP3A3/4 inducer

Barbiturates, phenytoin, rifampin increase the metabolism of triamcinolone; salicylates; NSAIDs, caffeine and alcohol may increase risk of GI ulcer; live virus vaccines (increase risk of viral infection); vaccines may have decreased effects

Food Interactions Systemic use of corticosteroids may require a diet with increased potassium, vitamins A, B_6, C, D, folate, calcium, zinc, and phosphorus and decreased sodium

Mechanism of Action Controls the rate of protein synthesis, depresses the migration of polymorphonuclear leukocytes and fibroblasts, reverses capillary permeability, and stabilizes lysosomal membranes at the cellular level to prevent or control inflammation

Pharmacokinetics

Time to peak serum concentration: I.M.: Within 8-10 hours

Half-life: 88 minutes

Usual Dosage

I.M. (as acetonide or hexacetonide): Children: 6-12 years: 0.03-0.2 mg/kg at 1- to 7-day intervals

Intra-articular (as hexacetonide): Children >12 years and Adults: 2-20 mg every 3-4 weeks

Intra-articular, intrabursal, or tendon-sheath injection: Children: 6-12 years: 2.5-15 mg, repeat as needed

Intra-articular, intrasynovial, intralesional (as diacetate or acetonide): Children >12 years and Adults: 2.5-40 mg, repeat as needed when signs and symptoms recur

Intralesional, sublesional (as diacetate or acetonide): Children >12 years and Adults: Up to 1 mg per injection site and may be repeated 1 or more times weekly; multiple sites may be injected if they are 1 cm or more apart, not to exceed 30 mg

Intranasal:

Nasacort®:

Children 6-11 years: Initial: 2 sprays in each nostril once daily; titrate to lowest effective dose once symptoms are controlled

Children >12 years and Adults: Initial: 2 sprays in each nostril once daily; may increase after 4-7 days up to 4 sprays in each nostril once daily, 2 sprays in each nostril twice daily, or 1 spray in each nostril 4 times/day

Nasacort AQ®: Children >12 years and Adults: Initial: 2 sprays in each nostril once daily; titrate to lowest effective dose once symptoms are controlled; usual maintenance dose: 1 spray in each nostril once daily

Oral: Children >12 years and Adults: 4-100 mg/day in 1-4 divided doses

Oral inhalation: Doses should be titrated to the lowest effective dose once asthma is controlled; maintenance doses may be given twice daily. Manufacturer recommendation:

Children: 6-12 years: 1-2 puffs given 3-4 times/day; maximum dose: 12 puffs/day

(Continued)

Triamcinolone *(Continued)*

Children >12 years and Adults: 2 puffs given 3-4 times/day; for severe asthma: 12-16 puffs/day divided into 3-4 doses/day; maximum dose: 16 puffs/day

NIH Guidelines (NIH, 1997) [give in divided doses 3-4 times/day]:

Children:

"Low" dose: 400-800 mcg/day (4-8 puffs/day)

"Medium" dose: 800-1200 mcg/day (8-12 puffs/day)

"High" dose: >1200 mcg/day (>12 puffs/day)

Adults:

"Low" dose: 400-1000 mcg/day (4-10 puffs/day)

"Medium" dose: 1000-2000 mcg/day (10-20 puffs/day)

"High" dose: >2000 mcg/day (>20 puffs/day)

Topical: Children and Adults: Apply a thin film 2-3 times/day

Administration

Oral: May administer with meals to decrease GI upset

Oral inhalant: Shake canister well before use; use a spacer device for children <8 years of age

Intranasal: Shake container well before use; clear nasal passages by blowing nose prior to use

Parenteral: Avoid S.C. use; do not inject I.V.; acetonide or hexacetonide may be administered I.M.; see Usual Dosage for other parenteral routes of administration

Topical: Apply sparingly to affected area, gently rub in until disappears; avoid application on face; do not occlude area unless directed; do not use on open skin; avoid contact with eyes

Patient Information Notify physician if condition being treated persists or worsens; do not decrease dose or discontinue without physicians approval

Oral inhalant: Rinse mouth with water without swallowing to decrease chance of oral candidiasis; report sore mouth or mouth lesions to physician

Nursing Implications Once daily oral doses should be given in the morning

Additional Information Oral inhalation: If bronchospasm with wheezing occurs after use, a fast-acting bronchodilator may be used; triamcinolone oral inhalation is also used to help reduce or discontinue oral corticosteroid therapy for asthma

Dosage Forms

Triamcinolone acetonide

Aerosol:

Nasal inhaler (Nasacort®): 55 mcg per actuation [100 activations] (10 g)

Nasal spray (Nasacort® AQ): 55 mcg per actuation [120 activations] (16.5 g)

Oral inhaler (Azmacort™): 100 mcg per actuation (20 g)

Topical (Kenalog®): 0.2 mg/2-second spray (23 g, 63 g)

Cream:

Aristocort®, Aristocort® A, Flutex®, Kenalog®: 0.025% (15 g, 28 g, 60 g, 80 g, 120 g, 240 g, 454 g)

Aristocort®, Aristocort® A, Delta-Tritex®, Flutex®, Kenalog®, Kenalog-H®, Kenonel®, Triacet®, Triderm®: 0.1% (15 g, 28 g, 60 g, 80 g, 120 g, 240 g, 454 g)

Aristocort®, Aristocort® A, Flutex®, Kenalog®: 0.5% (15 g, 20 g, 28 g, 57 g, 113 g, 240 g)

Injection:

Tac™-3: 3 mg/mL (5 mL)

Kenalog-10®: 10 mg/mL (5 mL)

Kenaject-40®, Kenalog-40®, Tac-40®, Triam-A®, Triamonide® 40, Tri-Kort®, Trilog®: 40 mg/mL (1 mL, 5 mL, 10 mL)

Lotion (Kenalog®): 0.025% (60 mL); 0.1% (15 mL, 60 mL)

Ointment, topical:

Flutex®, Kenalog®: 0.025% (15 g, 28 g, 57 g, 80 g, 113 g, 240 g, 454 g)

Aristocort®, Aristocort® A, Flutex®, Delta-Tritex®, Kenalog®: 0.1% (15 g, 28 g, 30 g, 57 g, 80 g, 113 g, 240 g, 454 g)

Aristocort®, Flutex®, Kenalog®: 0.5% (15 g, 20 g, 28 g, 57 g, 113 g, 240 g)

Paste, dental (Kenalog® in Orabase®): 0.1% (5 g)

Triamcinolone diacetate

Injection:

Aristocort® Intralesional: 25 mg/mL (5 mL)

Amcort®, Aristocort® Forte, Articulose® 50, Triam Forte®, Trilone®, Tristoject®: 40 mg/mL (1 mL, 5 mL)

Triamcinolone hexacetonide

Injection:

Aristospan® Intralesional: 5 mg/mL (5 mL)

Aristospan® Intra-articular: 20 mg/mL (1 mL, 5 mL)
Triamcinolone oral
Syrup (Kenacort®): 4 mg/5 mL (120 mL)
Tablet:
Aristocort®: 1 mg
Aristocort®: 2 mg
Aristocort®, Atolone®, Kenacort®: 4 mg
Aristocort®, Kenacort®: 8 mg
References
Expert Panel Report 2, "Guidelines for the Diagnosis and Management of Asthma," *Clinical Practice Guidelines*, National Institutes of Health, National Heart, Lung, and Blood Institute, NIH Publication No. 94-4051, April, 1997.

♦ **Triamcinolone Acetonide** *see* Triamcinolone *on page 946*

♦ **Triamcinolone Diacetate** *see* Triamcinolone *on page 946*

♦ **Triamcinolone Hexacetonide** *see* Triamcinolone *on page 946*

♦ **Triam Forte® Injection** *see* Triamcinolone *on page 946*

♦ **Triaminic® AM Decongestant Formula [OTC]** *see* Pseudoephedrine *on page 822*

♦ **Triaminic DM (Canada)** *see* Dextromethorphan *on page 304*

♦ **Triamonide® Injection** *see* Triamcinolone *on page 946*

Triamterene (trye AM ter een)

Brand Names Dyrenium®
Therapeutic Category Antihypertensive Agent; Diuretic, Potassium Sparing
Generic Available No
Use Used alone or in combination with other diuretics to treat edema and hypertension; decreases potassium excretion caused by kaliuretic diuretics
Pregnancy Risk Factor B (per manufacturer); D (based upon expert analysis)
Contraindications Hypersensitivity to triamterene or any component; severe renal or hepatic impairment, hyperkalemia
Precautions Use with caution in patients with impaired hepatic or renal function, history of renal calculi, diabetes mellitus; patients receiving other potassium-sparing diuretics or potassium supplements
Adverse Reactions
Cardiovascular: Hypotension
Central nervous system: Dizziness, headache
Endocrine & metabolic: Hyperkalemia, hyponatremia, hypomagnesemia, hyperchloremia, hyperuricemia, metabolic acidosis
Dermatologic: Photosensitivity
Gastrointestinal: Nausea, vomiting, diarrhea, xerostomia
Genitourinary: Slight alkalinization of urine
Hematologic: Blood dyscrasias, thrombocytopenia, megaloblastic anemia
Hepatic: Abnormal liver function
Neuromuscular & skeletal: Muscle cramps, weakness
Renal: Prerenal azotemia, nephrolithiasis (rare), reversible acute renal failure
Miscellaneous: Allergic reactions have been reported
Drug Interactions Increased risk of hyperkalemia if given together with other potassium-sparing diuretics (ie, spironolactone); may increase risk of hyperkalemia with ACE inhibitors, (ie, captopril, enalapril); concomitant administration of triamterene and indomethacin may increase nephrotoxicity; increased risk of hyperkalemia with potassium-containing preparations; may increase lithium toxicity by decreasing lithium clearance; may increase amantadine toxicity possibly by decreasing its renal excretion
Food Interactions Avoid salt substitutes and diets with increased potassium
Mechanism of Action Interferes with potassium/sodium exchange (active transport) in the distal tubule, cortical collecting tubule and collecting duct by inhibiting sodium, potassium-ATPase; decreases calcium excretion; increases magnesium loss
Pharmacodynamics
Onset of action: Diuresis occurs within 2-4 hours
Duration: 7-9 hours
Note: Maximum therapeutic effect may not occur until after several days of therapy
Pharmacokinetics
Absorption: Oral: Unreliably absorbed
Metabolism: Hepatic conjugation
Half-life: 100-150 minutes
Elimination: 21% excreted unchanged in urine
(Continued)

Triamterene *(Continued)*

Usual Dosage Oral:

Children: 2-4 mg/kg/day in 1-2 divided doses; maximum dose: 6 mg/kg/day and not to exceed 300 mg/day

Adults: 100-300 mg/day in 1-2 divided doses; maximum dose: 300 mg/day

Administration Oral: Administer with food to avoid GI upset

Monitoring Parameters Electrolytes (sodium, potassium, magnesium, HCO_3, chloride), CBC, BUN, creatinine, platelets

Test Interactions Interferes with fluorometric assay of quinidine

Additional Information Abrupt discontinuation of therapy may result in rebound kaliuresis; taper off gradually

Dosage Forms Capsule: 50 mg, 100 mg

Triazolam (trye AY zoe lam)

Related Information

Overdose and Toxicology *on page 1191*

Brand Names Apo®-Triazo (Canada); Gen-Triazolam® (Canada); Halcion®; Novo-Triolam® (Canada); Nu-Triazo® (Canada)

Therapeutic Category Benzodiazepine; Hypnotic; Sedative

Generic Available Yes

Use Short-term treatment of insomnia

Restrictions C-IV

Pregnancy Risk Factor X

Contraindications Hypersensitivity to triazolam or any component, cross-sensitivity with other benzodiazepines may occur; severe uncontrolled pain; pre-existing CNS depression; narrow-angle glaucoma; not to be used in pregnancy or lactation

Warnings Abrupt discontinuance may precipitate withdrawal or rebound insomnia

Adverse Reactions

Central nervous system: Drowsiness, anterograde amnesia, confusion, bizarre behavior, agitation, dizziness, hallucinations, nightmares, headache, ataxia

Gastrointestinal: Xerostomia, nausea, vomiting

Hepatic: Cholestatic jaundice

Miscellaneous: Physical and psychological dependence

Drug Interactions Cytochrome P-450 isoenzyme CYP3A3/4 and CYP3A5-7 substrate

CNS depressants, alcohol may increase CNS adverse effects; cimetidine, erythromycin may decrease and enzyme inducers may increase the metabolism of triazolam; protease inhibitors (indinavir, nelfinavir, ritonavir, saquinavir) and delavirdine may potentially decrease triazolam's metabolism and increase triazolam serum concentrations; concurrent use of triazolam with protease inhibitors or delavirdine is not recommended; ketoconazole, itraconazole may increase intensity and duration of triazolam effects

Food Interactions Food may decrease the rate of absorption; grapefruit juice significantly increases the bioavailability of oral triazolam

Mechanism of Action Depresses all levels of the CNS, including the limbic and reticular formation, by binding to the benzodiazepine site on the gamma-aminobutyric acid (GABA) receptor complex and modulating GABA, which is a major inhibitory neurotransmitter in the brain

Pharmacodynamics Hypnotic effects:

Onset: Within 15-30 minutes

Duration: 6-7 hours

Pharmacokinetics

Distribution: V_d: 0.8-1.8 L/kg

Protein binding: 89%

Metabolism: Extensive in the liver

Half-life: 1.7-5 hours

Elimination: In urine as unchanged drug and metabolites

Usual Dosage Oral:

Children <18 years: Dosage not established; investigational doses of 0.02 mg/kg given as an elixir have been used in children (n=20) for sedation prior to dental procedures; further studies are needed before this dose can be recommended

Adults: 0.125-0.25 mg at bedtime

Monitoring Parameters Liver enzymes with prolonged use

Patient Information Avoid alcohol; may be habit-forming with long-term use; do not discontinue abruptly; may cause drowsiness and impair ability to perform activities requiring mental alertness or physical coordination; take dose in bed at bedtime; may also cause daytime drowsiness

Additional Information Onset of action is rapid, patient should be in bed when taking medication

Dosage Forms Tablet: 0.125 mg, 0.25 mg

References

Meyer ML, Mounno AP, and Farrington FH, "Comparison of Triazolam to a Chloral Hydrate/Hydroxyzine Combination in the Sedation of Pediatric Dental Patients," *Pediatr Dent*, 1990, 12(5):283-7.

♦ **Triban®** *see* Trimethobenzamide *on page 954*
♦ **Tribavirin** *see* Ribavirin *on page 843*
♦ **Trichloroacetaldehyde Monohydrate** *see* Chloral Hydrate *on page 204*
♦ **Tricosal®** *see* Choline Magnesium Trisalicylate *on page 220*
♦ **Tridil® Injection** *see* Nitroglycerin *on page 690*

Triethanolamine Polypeptide Oleate-Condensate

(trye eth a NOLE a meen pol i PEP tide OH lee ate-KON den sate)

Brand Names Cerumenex® Otic

Therapeutic Category Otic Agent, Cerumenolytic

Generic Available No

Use Removal of ear wax (cerumen)

Pregnancy Risk Factor C

Contraindications Perforated tympanic membrane or otitis media; hypersensitivity to triethanolamine polypeptide oleate-condensate or any component

Warnings Discontinue if sensitization or irritation occurs

Precautions Avoid undue exposure to skin during administration and the flushing out of ear canal; exposure of ear canal to otic solution should be limited to 15-30 minutes

Adverse Reactions Local: Localized dermatitis, mild erythema and pruritus, severe eczematoid reactions involving the external ear and periauricular tissue

Mechanism of Action Emulsifies and disperses accumulated cerumen for easier removal

Pharmacodynamics Onset of effect: Produces slight disintegration of very hard ear wax by 24 hours

Usual Dosage Children and Adults: Otic: Fill ear canal, insert cotton plug; allow to remain 15-30 minutes; flush ear with lukewarm water as a single treatment; if a second application is needed for unusually hard impactions, repeat the procedure

Monitoring Parameters Evaluate hearing before and after instillation of medication

Patient Information For external use in the ear only; warm to body temperature before using to improve effect

Nursing Implications Avoid undue exposure of the drug to the periaural skin

Dosage Forms Solution, otic: 6 mL, 12 mL

References

Mehta AK, "An *In Vitro* Comparison of the Disintegration of Human Ear Wax by Five Cerumenolytics Commonly Used in General Practice," *Br J Clin Pract*, 1985, 39(5):200-3.

♦ **Triethylenethiophosphoramide** *see* Thiotepa *on page 922*
♦ **Trifluorothymidine** *see* Trifluridine *on page 951*

Trifluridine (trye FLURE i deen)

Brand Names Viroptic® Ophthalmic

Synonyms F_3T; Trifluorothymidine

Therapeutic Category Antiviral Agent, Ophthalmic

Generic Available No

Use Treatment of primary keratoconjunctivitis and recurrent epithelial keratitis caused by herpes simplex virus types I and II

Pregnancy Risk Factor C

Contraindications Hypersensitivity to trifluridine or any component

Adverse Reactions

Cardiovascular: Hyperemia

Local: Burning, stinging

Ocular: Palpebral edema, epithelial keratopathy, keratitis, stromal edema, increased intraocular pressure

Miscellaneous: Hypersensitivity reactions

Stability Store in refrigerator; storage at room temperature may result in a solution with altered pH which could result in ocular discomfort upon administration and/or decreased potency

(Continued)

Trifluridine *(Continued)*

Mechanism of Action Interferes with viral replication by incorporating into viral DNA in place of thymidine, inhibiting thymidylate synthetase resulting in the formation of defective proteins

Pharmacodynamics Onset of action: Response to treatment occurs within 2-7 days; epithelial healing is complete in 1-2 weeks

Pharmacokinetics Absorption: Ophthalmic: Systemic absorption is negligible, while corneal penetration is adequate

Usual Dosage Children and Adults: Ophthalmic: Instill 1 drop into affected eye every 2 hours while awake, to a maximum of 9 drops/day, until re-epithelialization of corneal ulcer occurs; then use 1 drop every 4 hours for another 7 days; do **not** exceed 21 days of treatment

Administration Ophthalmic: Avoid contact of bottle tip with skin or eye; instill drops onto the cornea of the affected eye(s)

Monitoring Parameters Ophthalmologic exam (test for corneal staining with fluorescein or rose Bengal)

Additional Information Found to be effective in 138 of 150 patients unresponsive or intolerant to idoxuridine or vidarabine

Dosage Forms Solution, ophthalmic: 1% (7.5 mL)

♦ **Triglycerides, Medium Chain** *see* Medium Chain Triglycerides *on page 598*
♦ **Trihexy®** *see* Trihexyphenidyl *on page 952*
♦ **Trihexyphen® (Canada)** *see* Trihexyphenidyl *on page 952*

Trihexyphenidyl (trye heks ee FEN i dil)

Related Information
Overdose and Toxicology *on page 1191*

Brand Names Apo®-Trihex (Canada); Artane®; Novo-Hexidyl® (Canada); PMS-Trihexyphenidyl (Canada); Trihexy®; Trihexyphen® (Canada)

Available Salts Trihexyphenidyl Hydrochloride

Synonyms Benzhexol

Therapeutic Category Anticholinergic Agent; Antidote, Drug-induced Dystonic Reactions; Anti-Parkinson's Agent

Generic Available Yes: Tablet

Use Adjunctive treatment of Parkinson's disease; also used in treatment of drug-induced extrapyramidal effects and acute dystonic reactions

Pregnancy Risk Factor C

Contraindications Hypersensitivity to trihexyphenidyl or any component; children younger than 3 years of age; patients with narrow-angle glaucoma, GI or GU obstruction; myasthenia gravis, achalasia

Precautions Use with caution in patients with hyperthyroidism, renal or hepatic dysfunction, hypertension, hiatal hernia, tachycardia, cardiac arrhythmias, peptic ulcer, esophageal reflux; use with caution in hot weather or during exercise

Adverse Reactions
Cardiovascular: Tachycardia
Central nervous system: Dizziness, nervousness, drowsiness, agitation, delirium, headache
Dermatologic: Rash
Gastrointestinal: Xerostomia, nausea, constipation
Genitourinary: Urinary hesitancy or retention
Neuromuscular & skeletal: Weakness
Ocular: Blurred vision, mydriasis, increased intraocular tension

Drug Interactions
Decreased effect: May increase gastric degradation of levodopa and decrease the amount of levodopa absorbed by delaying gastric emptying
Therapeutic effects of cholinergic agents (tacrine, donepezil) and neuroleptics may be antagonized
Increased toxicity: Central and/or peripheral anticholinergic syndrome can occur when administered with amantadine, rimantadine, narcotic analgesics, phenothiazines and other antipsychotics (especially with high anticholinergic activity), tricyclic antidepressants, quinidine and some other antiarrhythmics, and antihistamines

Mechanism of Action Presumed to act by blocking excess acetylcholine at cerebral synapses; many of its effects are due to its pharmacologic similarities with atropine

Pharmacodynamics
Onset of effect: 1 hour

Peak effect: 2-3 hours
Duration: 6-12 hours
Pharmacokinetics
Metabolism: Metabolic fate undetermined
Bioavailability: 100%
Half-life: 5.6-10.2 hours
Elimination: Some urinary excretion
Usual Dosage Adults: Oral:
Extrapyramidal: 5-15 mg/day in 3-4 divided doses
Parkinsonism: 1 mg daily; increase by 2 mg increments every 3-5 days to 6-10 mg/day (maximum daily dosage: 12-15 mg); doses >10 mg/day should be divided into 3-4 doses
Administration Oral: Administer with food or water to decrease GI irritation
Monitoring Parameters Intraocular pressure monitoring (baseline and at regular intervals)
Patient Information Causes drowsiness and may impair ability to perform hazardous duties requiring mental alertness or physical coordination
Dosage Forms
Capsule, sustained release, as hydrochloride: 5 mg
Elixir, as hydrochloride: 2 mg/5 mL (480 mL)
Tablet, as hydrochloride: 2 mg, 5 mg

♦ **Trihexyphenidyl Hydrochloride** *see* Trihexyphenidyl *on page 952*
♦ **Tri-K®** *see* Potassium Supplements *on page 786*
♦ **TriKacide® (Canada)** *see* Metronidazole *on page 636*
♦ **Trikates®** *see* Potassium Supplements *on page 786*
♦ **Tri-Kort® Injection** *see* Triamcinolone *on page 946*
♦ **Trileptal®** *see* Oxcarbazepine *on page 713*
♦ **Trilisate®** *see* Choline Magnesium Trisalicylate *on page 220*
♦ **Trilog® Injection** *see* Triamcinolone *on page 946*
♦ **Trilone® Injection** *see* Triamcinolone *on page 946*
♦ **Trimazide® Oral** *see* Trimethobenzamide *on page 954*
♦ **Trimazide® Rectal** *see* Trimethobenzamide *on page 954*
♦ **Trimethaphan Camphorsulfonate** *see* Trimethaphan Camsylate *on page 953*

Trimethaphan Camsylate (trye METH a fan KAM si late)

Brand Names Arfonad® Injection
Synonyms Trimethaphan Camphorsulfonate
Therapeutic Category Alpha-Adrenergic Blocking Agent, Parenteral; Anticholinergic Agent; Antihypertensive Agent; Ganglionic Blocking Agent
Generic Available No
Use Hypertensive emergencies; controlled hypotension during surgery
Pregnancy Risk Factor D
Contraindications Hypersensitivity to trimethaphan camsylate or any component; hypovolemia or shock; anemia; respiratory insufficiency
Precautions Use with caution in patients with allergies; cardiac, hepatic, or renal dysfunction; diabetes mellitus, Addison's disease, or glaucoma
Adverse Reactions
Cardiovascular: Hypotension (especially orthostatic), tachycardia (especially in children and young adults)
Central nervous system: Restlessness
Dermatologic: Itching, urticaria
Endocrine & metabolic: With prolonged use (>48-72 hours) sodium and water retention
Gastrointestinal: Anorexia, nausea, vomiting, xerostomia, adynamic ileus
Genitourinary: Urinary retention
Ocular: Mydriasis, cycloplegia
Neuromuscular & skeletal: Weakness
Respiratory: Apnea, respiratory arrest (especially with doses >6 mg/minute)
Drug Interactions Anesthetics, procainamide, diuretics and other hypotensive agents may increase hypotensive effects of trimethaphan; effects of tubocurarine and succinylcholine may be prolonged by trimethaphan
Stability Solution should be freshly prepared and any unused portion discarded
Mechanism of Action Blocks transmission in both adrenergic and cholinergic ganglia by blocking stimulation from presynaptic receptors to postsynaptic receptors mediated by acetylcholine; possesses direct peripheral vasodilatory activity and is a weak histamine releaser
(Continued)

Trimethaphan Camsylate *(Continued)*

Pharmacodynamics
Onset of action: I.V.: Immediate
Peak effects: 5 minutes
Duration: 10-30 minutes

Pharmacokinetics
Metabolism: Primarily by postganglionic pseudocholinesterase
Elimination: Urinary excretion

Usual Dosage I.V.:
Children: 50-150 mcg/kg/minute
Adults: Initial: 0.5-2 mg/minute; titrate to effect; usual dose: 0.3-6 mg/minute

Administration Parenteral: Must be diluted; usually administered by I.V. continuous infusion at a final concentration of 1 mg/mL in D_5W

Monitoring Parameters Blood pressure and heart rate continuously

Dosage Forms Injection: 50 mg/mL (10 mL)

Trimethobenzamide (trye meth oh BEN za mide)

Related Information
Compatibility of Medications Mixed in a Syringe *on page 1208*

Brand Names Arrestin® Injection; Tebamide® Rectal; T-Gen® Rectal; Ticon® Injection; Tigan® Injection; Tigan® Oral; Tigan® Rectal; Triban®; Trimazide® Oral; Trimazide® Rectal

Available Salts Trimethobenzamide Hydrochloride

Therapeutic Category Antiemetic

Generic Available No

Use Control of nausea and vomiting (especially for long-term antiemetic therapy)

Pregnancy Risk Factor C

Contraindications Hypersensitivity to trimethobenzamide, any component, or benzocaine (contained in suppository); suppositories are contraindicated in premature infants or neonates

Precautions Use cautiously in infants and children; may mask emesis due to Reye's syndrome or mimic CNS effects of Reye's syndrome in patients with emesis of other etiologies

Adverse Reactions
Cardiovascular: Hypotension (especially after I.M. use)
Central nervous system: Drowsiness, sedation, extrapyramidal symptoms, dizziness, seizures, coma, depression, opisthotonos
Dermatologic: Hypersensitivity skin reactions
Gastrointestinal: Diarrhea
Hematologic: Blood dyscrasias
Hepatic: Jaundice
Local: Pain, stinging, burning at I.M. injection site
Ocular: Blurred vision

Mechanism of Action Acts centrally to inhibit stimulation of the medullary chemoreceptor trigger zone

Pharmacodynamics
Onset of action:
Oral: 10-40 minutes
I.M.: 15-35 minutes
Duration:
Oral: 3-4 hours
I.M.: 2-3 hours

Pharmacokinetics
Metabolism: Not well determined
Bioavailability: Oral dose is ~60% of I.M. dose
Elimination: 20% excreted unchanged in urine in 24 hours

Usual Dosage Do not use rectally in neonates and infants
Children:
Oral, rectal: 15-20 mg/kg/day (400-500 mg/m²/day) divided into 3-4 doses; **or as an alternative**
<13.6 kg (30 lbs): 100 mg 3-4 times/day
13.6-41 kg (30-90 lbs): 100-200 mg 3-4 times/day
I.M.: Not recommended
Adults:
Oral: 250 mg 3-4 times/day
I.M., rectal: 200 mg 3-4 times/day

Administration
Oral: May administer with or without food
Parenteral: I.M. use only, **not** for I.V. use

Patient Information Causes drowsiness and may impair ability to perform activities requiring mental alertness or physical coordination

Additional Information Note: Less effective than phenothiazines but may be associated with fewer side effects

Dosage Forms
Capsule, as hydrochloride: 100 mg, 250 mg
Injection, as hydrochloride: 100 mg/mL (2 mL, 20 mL)
Suppository, rectal, as hydrochloride: 100 mg, 200 mg

♦ **Trimethobenzamide Hydrochloride** see Trimethobenzamide on page 954

Trimethoprim (trye METH oh prim)

Related Information
Blood Level Sampling Time Guidelines on page 1189
Brand Names Primsol® Solution; Proloprim®; Trimpex®
Available Salts Trimethoprim Hydrochloride
Synonyms TMP
Therapeutic Category Antibiotic, Miscellaneous
Generic Available Yes: Tablets
Use Treatment and prophylaxis of urinary tract infections; in combination with other agents for treatment of Pneumocystis carinii pneumonia; treatment of otitis media caused by susceptible Streptococcus pneumoniae and Haemophilus influenzae (not indicated for Moraxella catarrhalis due to consistent resistance); not indicated for prolonged administration or prophylaxis of otitis media
Pregnancy Risk Factor C
Contraindications Hypersensitivity to trimethoprim or any component; megaloblastic anemia due to folate deficiency
Warnings May cause folate deficiencies with subsequent bone marrow suppression and blood dyscrasias; monitor patients for fever, sore throat, purpura, or pallor; discontinue trimethoprim if bone marrow depression occurs; leucovorin (folinic acid) may be needed to restore normal hematopoiesis
Precautions Use with caution in patients with impaired renal or hepatic function or with possible folate deficiency; decrease dose in patients with renal dysfunction; safety is not established in infants <2 months of age; effectiveness for treatment of acute otitis media is not established in infants <6 months of age; oral solution contains propylene glycol and sodium benzoate
Adverse Reactions
Central nervous system: Fever, headache, aseptic meningitis
Dermatologic: Rash, pruritus, exfoliative dermatitis
Hematologic: Megaloblastic anemia, neutropenia, leukopenia, thrombocytopenia, methemoglobinemia
Hepatic: Elevated liver enzymes, cholestatic jaundice
Gastrointestinal: Nausea, vomiting, epigastric distress
Renal: Elevated BUN and serum creatinine
Drug Interactions Use with other folate antagonists (methotrexate, pyrimethamine) may increase risk of megaloblastic anemia; trimethoprim may decrease the metabolism of phenytoin resulting in increased phenytoin serum concentrations; cyclosporine, dapsone, procainamide, rifampin, warfarin
Food Interactions May cause folic acid deficiency, supplements may be needed
Mechanism of Action Binds to the enzyme dihydrofolate reductase in bacteria and inhibits conversion of dihydrofolic acid to tetrahydrofolate (functional form of folic acid). This results in depletion of folic acid, interference with bacterial biosynthesis of nucleic acids and protein production, and inhibition of microbial growth.
Pharmacokinetics
Absorption: Oral: Readily and extensively absorbed (90% to 100%)
Distribution: Penetrates into middle ear fluid with a mean peak middle ear fluid concentration in children 1-12 years of 2 mcg/mL after a single 4 mg/kg dose; crosses the placenta; excreted in breast milk
V_d:
Newborns: ~2.7 L/kg
Infants: 1.5 L/kg
Children 1-10 years: ~1 L/kg
Adults: 1.3-1.8 L/kg
Protein binding: 42% to 46%
(Continued)

Trimethoprim *(Continued)*

Metabolism: Partially (10% to 20%) metabolized in the liver via demethylation, oxidation, and hydroxylation

Bioavailbility: Similar for tablets and solution

Half-life (prolonged in renal dysfunction):

Newborns: ~19 hours

Infants 2 months to 1 year: 3-6 hours; mean: 4.6 hours

Children 1-10 years: 3-5.5 hours

Adults, normal renal function: 8-11 hours

Adults, anuric: 20-50 hours

Time to peak serum concentration: Within 1-4 hours

Elimination: Significantly excreted in urine (60% to 80%) as unchanged drug via glomerular filtration and tubular secretion; increased renal excretion with acidic urine

Moderately dialyzable (20% to 50%)

Usual Dosage Oral:

Infants and Children <12 years: Urinary tract infection: Treatment: 4-6 mg/kg/day in divided doses every 12 hours for 10 days

Infants ≥6 months and Children: Acute otitis media: 10 mg/kg/day in divided doses every 12 hours for 10 days

Children ≥12 years and Adults:

Urinary tract infection: Treatment: 100 mg every 12 hours or 200 mg every 24 hours for 10 days

Prophylaxis: 100 mg once daily

Pneumocystis carinii pneumonia treatment (given with dapsone): 15-20 mg/kg/day in 4 divided doses for 21 days

Dosing adjustment in renal impairment:

Cl_{cr} 15-30 mL/minute: Administer 50% of normal dose

Cl_{cr} <15 mL/minute: Avoid use

Administration Oral: Administer on an empty stomach; may administer with milk or food if gastrointestinal irritation occurs

Monitoring Parameters CBC with differential, platelet count, liver enzyme tests, bilirubin, serum creatinine and BUN

Reference Range Therapeutic:

Peak: 5-15 mg/L

Trough: 2-8 mg/L

Test Interactions May falsely increase creatinine determination measured by the Jaffé alkaline picrate assay; may interfere with determination of serum methotrexate when measured by methods that use a bacterial dihydrofolate reductase as the binding protein (eg, the competitive binding protein technique); does **not** interfere with RIA for methotrexate

Patient Information Report any skin rash, persistent or severe fatigue, fever, sore throat, or unusual bleeding or bruising; complete full course of therapy

Additional Information Not effective versus *Pseudomonas* or *B. fragilis*; discontinue if bone marrow suppression occurs

Dosage Forms

Solution, oral, as hydrochloride (bubble-gum flavor, dye free, alcohol free): 50 mg/5 mL (base) (473 mL)

Tablet: 100 mg, 200 mg

References

Hoppu K, "Age Differences in Trimethoprim Pharmacokinetics: Need for Revised Dosing in Children?" *Clin Pharmacol Ther*, 1987, 41(3):336-43.

Hoppu K, Koskimies O, and Vilska J, "Trimethoprim in the Treatment of Acute Urinary Tract Infections in Children," *Int J Clin Pharmacol Ther Toxicol*, 1988, 26(2):65-8.

Leff RD, Cho CT, and Reed MD, "Safety and Efficacy of Trimethoprim Hydrochloride Solution for the Treatment of Children With Otitis Media," *Journal of Pediatric Pharmacy Practice*, 1998, 3(1): 33-9.

Triprolidine and Pseudoephedrine

(trye PROE li deen & soo doe e FED rin)

Related Information

OTC Cough & Cold Preparations, Pediatric *on page 1037*

Overdose and Toxicology *on page 1191*

Brand Names Actagen® [OTC]; Actifed® [OTC]; Allercon® [OTC]; Allerfrin® [OTC]; Allerphed® [OTC]; Aprodine® [OTC]; Cenafed® Plus [OTC]; Genac® [OTC]; Silafed® [OTC]; Triofed® [OTC]; Triposed® [OTC]

Available Salts Triprolidine Hydrochloride and Pseudoephedrine Hydrochloride

Synonyms Pseudoephedrine and Triprolidine

Therapeutic Category Antihistamine/Decongestant Combination; Sympathomimetic

Generic Available Yes

Use Temporary relief of nasal congestion, running nose, sneezing, itching of nose or throat and itchy, watery eyes due to common cold, hay fever or other upper respiratory allergies

Pregnancy Risk Factor C

Contraindications Hypersensitivity to triprolidine, any component, or pseudoephedrine; severe hypertension or coronary artery disease; MAO inhibitor therapy, GI or GU obstruction, narrow-angle glaucoma

Warnings Not recommended for use in children <4 months of age

Precautions Use with caution in patients with mild to moderate high blood pressure, heart disease, diabetes mellitus, asthma, thyroid disease, or prostatic hypertrophy

Adverse Reactions

Cardiovascular: Hypertension, tachycardia

Central nervous system: Sedation, CNS stimulation, headache

Gastrointestinal: Nausea, vomiting, xerostomia, anorexia

Drug Interactions MAO inhibitors, beta-blocking agents, other sympathomimetics, methyldopa, reserpine, alpha-blocking agents, CNS depressants

Usual Dosage Oral:

Children: May dose according to **pseudoephedrine** component: 4 mg/kg/day in divided doses 3-4 times/day **or**

4 months to 2 years: 1.25 mL 3-4 times/day

2-4 years: 2.5 mL 3-4 times/day

4-6 years: 3.75 mL 3-4 times/day

6-12 years: 5 mL or ½ tablet 3-4 times/day

Children >12 years and Adults: 10 mL or 1 tablet 3-4 times/day **or** 1 extended release capsule every 12 hours

Administration Oral: Administer with food or milk to decrease GI irritation; do not crush or chew sustained release products

Patient Information May cause drowsiness and may impair ability to perform activities requiring mental alertness or physical coordination

Dosage Forms

Capsule: Triprolidine hydrochloride 2.5 mg and pseudoephedrine hydrochloride 60 mg

Capsule, extended release: Triprolidine hydrochloride 5 mg and pseudoephedrine hydrochloride 120 mg

Syrup: Triprolidine hydrochloride 1.25 mg and pseudoephedrine hydrochloride 30 mg per 5 mL

Tablet: Triprolidine hydrochloride 2.5 mg and pseudoephedrine hydrochloride 60 mg

Troleandomycin (troe lee an doe MYE sin)

Brand Names TAO®

Synonyms Triacetyloleandomycin

Therapeutic Category Antibiotic, Macrolide

Generic Available No

Use Adjunct in the treatment of severe corticosteroid-dependent asthma due to its steroid-sparing properties; obsolete antibiotic with spectrum of activity similar to erythromycin

Pregnancy Risk Factor C

Contraindications Hypersensitivity to troleandomycin or any component; concomitant administration of terfenadine, astemizole, or cisapride with troleandomycin may result in Q-T interval prolongation, ventricular tachycardia, and torsade de pointes

Warnings Cholestatic hepatitis has been reported in patients who have received troleandomycin for 2 weeks or longer and in cases where repeated courses were administered

Precautions Use with caution in patients with impaired hepatic function

Adverse Reactions

Central nervous system: Fever

Dermatologic: Urticaria, rash

Gastrointestinal: Abdominal cramping, nausea, vomiting, diarrhea, rectal burning, esophagitis

Hepatic: Cholestatic hepatitis, jaundice

Drug Interactions Troleandomycin inhibits the cytochrome P-450 microsomal enzyme system decreasing clearance of theophylline (see Additional Information), cisapride, astemizole, and terfenadine; interferes with metabolism of ergotamine and carbamazepine potentiating their action; decreases methylprednisolone clearance from a linear first order decline to a nonlinear decline in plasma concentration

Food Interactions Food delays the rate, but not the extent of absorption

Mechanism of Action Troleandomycin has an undefined action independent of its effects on steroid elimination

Pharmacokinetics

Time to peak serum concentration: Oral: Within 2 hours

Elimination: 10% to 25% excreted in urine as active drug; excreted in feces via bile

Usual Dosage Oral:

Children: 25-40 mg/kg/day divided every 6 hours

Adjunct in corticosteroid-dependent asthma: 14 mg/kg/day in divided doses every 6-12 hours not to exceed 250 mg every 6 hours; dose is tapered to once daily then alternate day dosing

Adults: 250-500 mg 4 times/day

Monitoring Parameters Hepatic function tests

Patient Information Report any prodromal symptoms of hepatitis (fatigue, weakness, nausea, vomiting, dark urine, or yellowing of eyes)

Additional Information For patients on both troleandomycin and theophylline: Troleandomycin can significantly reduce theophylline clearance resulting in higher serum theophylline concentrations; empiric reduction in theophylline dosage appears to be indicated with the initiation of troleandomycin

Dosage Forms Capsule: 250 mg

References

Brenner AM and Szefler SJ, "Troleandomycin in the Treatment of Severe Asthma," *Immunol Allergy Clin North Am*, 1991, 11(1):91-102.

Kamada AK, Hill MR, Brenner AM, et al, "Effect of Low-Dose Troleandomycin on Theophylline Clearance: Implications for Therapeutic Drug Monitoring," *Pharmacotherapy*, 1992, 12(2):98-102.

Spector SL, Katz FH, and Farr RS, "Troleandomycin: Effectiveness in Steroid-Dependent Asthma and Bronchitis," *J Allergy Clin Immunol*, 1974, 54(6):367-79.

Tromethamine (troe METH a meen)

Brand Names THAM®; THAM-E®

Synonyms Tris Buffer; Tris(hydroxymethyl)aminomethane

Therapeutic Category Alkalinizing Agent, Parenteral

Generic Available No

Use Correction of metabolic acidosis associated with cardiac bypass surgery or cardiac arrest; to correct excess acidity of stored blood that is preserved with acid citrate dextrose (ACD); to prime the pump-oxygenator during cardiac bypass surgery; indicated in severe metabolic acidosis in patients in whom sodium or carbon dioxide elimination is restricted [eg, infants needing alkalinization after receiving maximum sodium bicarbonate (8-10 mEq/kg/24 hours)]

Pregnancy Risk Factor C

Contraindications Uremia or anuria; chronic respiratory acidosis; hypersensitivity to tromethamine or any component

Precautions Reduce dose and monitor pH carefully in renal impairment

Adverse Reactions

Cardiovascular: Venospasm

Endocrine & metabolic: Hyperosmolality of serum, hyperkalemia, hypoglycemia

Hepatic: Liver cell destruction from direct contact with tromethamine, hemorrhagic hepatic necrosis (when administered through umbilical vein at concentrations ≥1.2 M)

Local: Tissue irritation, necrosis with extravasation

Respiratory: Respiratory depression, apnea

Mechanism of Action Proton acceptor, which combines with hydrogen ions to form bicarbonate and buffer

Pharmacokinetics 30% of dose is not ionized; rapidly eliminated by kidneys

Usual Dosage Infants, Children, and Adults: I.V.: Dose depends on severity and progression of acidosis:

Empiric dosage based upon base deficit: Tromethamine mL of 0.3 M solution = body weight (kg) x base deficit (mEq/L); maximum: 500 mg/kg/dose = 13.9 mL/kg/dose using 0.3 M solution

Metabolic acidosis with cardiac arrest: Tromethamine mL of 0.3 M solution: 3.5-6 mL/kg/dose (126-216 mg/kg/dose); maximum: 500 mg/kg/dose = 13.9 mL/kg/dose using 0.3 M solution

Excess acidity of acid citrate dextrose priming blood: Tromethamine mL of 0.3 M solution: 14-70 mL added added to each 500 mL of blood

Acidosis during cardiac bypass surgery: Tromethamine mL of 0.3 M solution: 9 mL/kg (324 mg/kg/dose); maximum dose: 1000 mL (36 g) as single dose

Administration Parenteral: Maximum concentration: 0.3 molar; infuse slowly over at least 1 hour (THAM-E® requires the reconstitution with 1 L sterile water before use); administer into a central venous line

Monitoring Parameters Serum electrolytes, arterial blood gases, serum pH, blood sugar, EKG monitoring, renal function tests

Nursing Implications Do not confuse THAM-E® with THAM®; THAM-E® contains electrolytes

Additional Information 1 mM = 120 mg = 3.3 mL = 1 mEq of THAM®

Dosage Forms Injection:

THAM®: 18 g [0.3 molar] (500 mL)

THAM-E®: 36 g with sodium 30 mEq, potassium 5 mEq, and chloride 35 mEq (1000 mL)

♦ **Tronolane®** *see* Hemorrhoidal Preparations *on page 470*

♦ **Tropicacyl®** *see* Tropicamide *on page 959*

Tropicamide (troe PIK a mide)

Brand Names Diotrope (Canada); I-Picamide®; Mydriacyl®; Tropicacyl®

Synonyms Bistropamide

Therapeutic Category Ophthalmic Agent, Mydriatic

Generic Available Yes

Use Short-acting mydriatic used in diagnostic procedures; as well as preoperatively and postoperatively; treatment of some cases of acute iritis, iridocyclitis, and keratitis

Pregnancy Risk Factor C

Contraindications Glaucoma, adhesions between the iris and the lens; hypersensitivity to tropicamide or any component

Warnings Tropicamide may cause an increase in intraocular pressure

Precautions Use with caution in infants and children since tropicamide may cause potentially dangerous CNS disturbances and psychotic reactions

Adverse Reactions

Cardiovascular: Tachycardia, flushing

Central nervous system: Parasympathetic stimulation, drowsiness, headache, behavioral disturbances, psychotic reactions

Gastrointestinal: Xerostomia

Local: Transient stinging

Ocular: Blurred vision, photophobia, increased intraocular pressure, follicular conjunctivitis

Miscellaneous: Allergic reactions

Stability Store at room temperature; do not refrigerate

(Continued)

Tropicamide *(Continued)*

Mechanism of Action Prevents the sphincter muscle of the iris and the muscle of the ciliary body from responding to cholinergic stimulation producing pupillary dilation and paralysis of accommodation

Pharmacodynamics
Maximum mydriatic effect: ~20-40 minutes
    Duration: ~6-7 hours
Maximum cycloplegic effect:
    Peak: 20-35 minutes
    Duration: <6 hours

Usual Dosage Children and Adults: Ophthalmic:
Cycloplegia: Instill 1-2 drops (1%); may repeat in 5 minutes. The exam must be performed within 30 minutes after the repeat dose; if the patient is not examined within 20-30 minutes, instill an additional drop. Concentrations <1% are inadequate for producing satisfactory cycloplegia.
Mydriasis: Instill 1-2 drops (0.5%) 15-20 minutes before exam; may repeat every 30 minutes as needed

Administration Ophthalmic: To minimize systemic absorption, apply finger pressure on the lacrimal sac for 1-2 minutes following instillation of the ophthalmic solution; avoid contact of bottle tip with skin or eye

Patient Information May cause blurred vision; do not drive or engage in hazardous activities while the pupils are dilated; may cause sensitivity to light

Dosage Forms Solution, ophthalmic: 0.5% (2 mL, 15 mL); 1% (2 mL, 3 mL, 15 mL)

References
Caputo AR and Schnitzer RE, "Systemic Response to Mydriatic Eyedrops in Neonates: Mydriatics in Neonates," *J Pediatr Ophthalmol Strabismus*, 1978, 15(2):109-22.

♦ **Truphylline®** *see* Aminophylline *on page 61*

♦ **TSPA** *see* Thiotepa *on page 922*

♦ **T-Stat®** *see* Erythromycin *on page 379*

Tubocurarine *(too boe kyoor AR een)*

Available Salts Tubocurarine Chloride

Synonyms *d*-Tubocurarine

Therapeutic Category Neuromuscular Blocker Agent, Nondepolarizing; Skeletal Muscle Relaxant, Paralytic

Generic Available No

Use Adjunct to anesthesia to induce skeletal muscle relaxation

Pregnancy Risk Factor C

Contraindications Hypersensitivity to tubocurarine or any component

Warnings Ventilation must be supported during neuromuscular blockade; some commercially available products may contain sulfites and benzyl alcohol; avoid products with benzyl alcohol in neonates

Precautions Use with caution in patients with renal impairment, respiratory depression, impaired hepatic or endocrine function, myasthenia gravis; several clinical conditions may antagonize or potentiate neuromuscular blockade, see table.

Clinical Conditions Affecting Neuromuscular Blockade

Potentiation	Antagonism
Electrolyte abnormalities	Alkalosis
Severe hyponatremia	Hypercalcemia
Severe hypocalcemia	Demyelinating lesions
Severe hypokalemia	Peripheral neuropathies
Hypermagnesemia	Diabetes mellitus
Neuromuscular diseases	
Acidosis	
Acute intermittent porphyria	
Renal failure	
Hepatic failure	

Adverse Reactions Most frequent adverse reactions are related to prolongation of its pharmacologic actions
Cardiovascular: Cardiac arrhythmias, hypotension, tachycardia or bradycardia
Gastrointestinal: Decreased GI motility, increased salivation
Neuromuscular & skeletal: Muscle weakness

Respiratory: Bronchospasm

Miscellaneous: Allergic reactions, hypersensitivity reactions

Drug Interactions See table.

Potential Drug Interactions

Potentiation	Antagonism
Anesthetics	Calcium
Desflurane, sevoflurane, enflurane and	Carbamazepine
isoflurane > halothane > nitrous	Phenytoin
oxide	Steroids (chronic administration)
Antibiotics	Theophylline
Aminoglycosides, polymyxins,	Anticholinesterases*
clindamycin, vancomycin	Neostigmine, pyridostigmine,
Magnesium sulfate	edrophonium, echothiophate
Antiarrhythmics	ophthalmic solution
Quinidine, procainamide, bretylium, and	Caffeine
possibly lidocaine	Azathioprine
Diuretics	
Furosemide, mannitol	
Amphotericin B (secondary to hypokalemia)	
Local anesthetics	
Dantrolene (directly depresses skeletal muscle)	
Beta blockers	
Calcium channel blockers	
Ketamine	
Lithium	
Succinylcholine (when administered prior to nondepolarizing neuromuscular-blocking agent)	
Cyclosporine	

*Can prolong the effects of acetylcholine

Stability Refrigerate; incompatible with barbiturates

Mechanism of Action Nondepolarizing neuromuscular blocking agent which blocks acetylcholine from binding to receptors on motor endplate thus inhibiting depolarization; also has histamine-releasing and ganglionic blocking properties

Pharmacodynamics

Onset of effect:

  I.M.: Unpredictable, 10-25 minutes

  I.V.: 2-5 minutes

Duration: 20-30 minutes

Pharmacokinetics Elimination: ~33% to 75% of parenteral dose excreted unchanged in urine in 24 hours; about 11% excreted in bile through a specific organic cation secretion mechanism

Usual Dosage I.V.:

Neonates <1 month: 0.3 mg/kg as a single dose; maintenance: 0.1 mg/kg/dose as needed to maintain paralysis

Children: 0.2-0.5 mg/kg as a single dose; maintenance: 0.04-0.1 mg/kg/dose as needed to maintain paralysis

Adults: 0.5-0.6 mg/kg or 0.3 mg/kg after initial dose of succinylcholine for intubation; administer maintenance doses every 40-60 minutes as needed

Dosing adjustment in renal impairment: May accumulate with multiple doses and, therefore, reduction in subsequent doses is recommended

  Cl_{cr} 50-80 mL/minute: Administer 75% of normal dose

  Cl_{cr} 10-50 mL/minute: Administer 50% of normal dose

  Cl_{cr} <10 mL/minute: Avoid use

Dosing in hepatic impairment: Larger doses may be necessary

Administration Parenteral: May infuse direct I.V. without further dilution over a period of 1-1½ minutes

Monitoring Parameters Respiratory status, heart rate, blood pressure, mechanical ventilator status, peripheral nerve stimulator measuring twitch response

(Continued)

Tuborcurarine *(Continued)*

Nursing Implications Does **not** alter the patient's state of consciousness; addition of sedation and analgesia is recommended

Dosage Forms Injection, as chloride: 3 mg/mL [3 units/mL] (5 mL, 10 mL, 20 mL)

- ♦ **Tubocurarine Chloride** see Tubocurarine *on page 960*
- ♦ **Tumor Lysis Syndrome, Management** see page 1125
- ♦ **Tums® [OTC]** see Antacid Preparations *on page 86*
- ♦ **Tums® [OTC]** see Calcium Supplements *on page 157*
- ♦ **Tums® E-X Extra Strength Tablet [OTC]** see Calcium Supplements *on page 157*
- ♦ **Tums® Extra Strength Liquid [OTC]** see Calcium Supplements *on page 157*
- ♦ **Tums® Ultra® [OTC]** see Calcium Supplements *on page 157*
- ♦ **Tusibron® [OTC]** see Guaifenesin *on page 464*
- ♦ **Tusibron-DM® [OTC]** see Guaifenesin and Dextromethorphan *on page 466*
- ♦ **Tuss-DM® [OTC]** see Guaifenesin and Dextromethorphan *on page 466*
- ♦ **Tussi-Organidin® DM NR** see Guaifenesin and Dextromethorphan *on page 466*
- ♦ **Tussi-Organidin® NR** see Guaifenesin and Codeine *on page 465*
- ♦ **Tusstat® Syrup** see Diphenhydramine *on page 327*
- ♦ **Twice-A-Day® Nasal Solution [OTC]** see Oxymetazoline *on page 718*
- ♦ **Twilite® Oral [OTC]** see Diphenhydramine *on page 327*
- ♦ **Twin-K®** see Potassium Supplements *on page 786*
- ♦ **Tylenol® [OTC]** see Acetaminophen *on page 26*
- ♦ **Tylenol® With Codeine** see Acetaminophen and Codeine *on page 27*
- ♦ **Tylox®** see Oxycodone and Acetaminophen *on page 716*
- ♦ **Ty-Pap [OTC]** see Acetaminophen *on page 26*
- ♦ **UCB-P071** see Cetirizine *on page 201*
- ♦ **U-Cort™ Topical** see Hydrocortisone *on page 486*
- ♦ **UDCA** see Ursodiol *on page 965*
- ♦ **ULR®** see Guaifenesin, Phenylpropanolamine, and Phenylephrine *on page 467*
- ♦ **Ultracef®** see Cefadroxil Monohydrate *on page 177*
- ♦ **Ultrase® MT** see Pancrelipase *on page 724*
- ♦ **Unasyn®** see Ampicillin and Sulbactam *on page 81*

Undecylenic Acid and Derivatives

(un de sil EN ik AS id & dah RIV ah tivs)

Brand Names Caldesene® Topical [OTC]; Cruex® Topical [OTC]; Desenex® (Canada); Fungoid® Topical Solution; Merlenate® Topical [OTC]; Pedi-Dri Topical; Pedi-Pro Topical [OTC]; Quinsana® Plus Topical [OTC]; Undoguent® Topical [OTC]

Available Salts Calcium Undecylenate; Zinc Undecylenate

Synonyms Zincundecate

Therapeutic Category Antifungal Agent, Topical

Generic Available Yes

Use Treatment of athlete's foot (tinea pedis), ringworm (except nails and scalp), prickly heat, jock itch (tinea cruris), diaper rash, and other minor skin irritations due to superficial dermatophytes

Contraindications Hypersensitivity to undecylenic acid and derivatives or any component; fungal infections of the scalp or nails

Warnings Do not apply to blistered, raw, or oozing areas of skin or over deep wounds or puncture wounds

Adverse Reactions
Dermatologic: Rash
Local: Skin irritation, stinging, sensitization

Mechanism of Action Undecylenic acid is a fatty acid with fungistatic activity that retards proliferation of the fungus by altering the conditions of growth; zinc undecylenate provides an astringent action that aids in the reduction of inflammation and irritation

Pharmacodynamics Onset of action: Improvement in erythema and pruritus may be seen within 1 week after initiation of therapy

Usual Dosage Children and Adults: Topical: Apply as needed twice daily for 2-4 weeks

Administration Topical: Clean and dry the affected area before topical application; if the solution is sprayed or applied onto the affected area, allow area to air dry

Monitoring Parameters Resolution of skin infection

Patient Information For external use only; avoid contact with the eye; do not inhale the powder

Additional Information Ointment or cream should be applied at night, the powder may be applied during the day or used alone when a drying effect is needed

Dosage Forms

Cream: Total undecylenate 20% (15 g, 82.5 g)

Foam, topical: Undecylenic acid 10% (42.5 g)

Liquid, topical: Undecylenic acid 10% (42.5 g)

Ointment, topical: Total undecylenate 22% (30 g, 60 g, 454 g); total undecylenate 25% (60 g, 454 g)

Powder, topical: Calcium undecylenate 10% (45 g, 60 g, 120 g); total undecylenate 22% (45 g, 54 g, 81 g, 90 g, 105 g, 165 g, 454 g)

Solution, topical: Undecylenic acid 25% (29.57 mL)

♦ **Undoguent® Topical [OTC]** *see* Undecylenic Acid and Derivatives *on page 962*

♦ **Uni-Ace® [OTC]** *see* Acetaminophen *on page 26*

♦ **Uni-Bent® Cough Syrup** *see* Diphenhydramine *on page 327*

♦ **Uni-Dur®** *see* Theophylline *on page 910*

♦ **Unipen® Injection** *see* Nafcillin *on page 666*

♦ **Unipen® Oral** *see* Nafcillin *on page 666*

♦ **Uniphyl®** *see* Theophylline *on page 910*

♦ **Uni-Pro® [OTC]** *see* Ibuprofen *on page 501*

♦ **Uni-tussin® [OTC]** *see* Guaifenesin *on page 464*

♦ **Uni-tussin® DM [OTC]** *see* Guaifenesin and Dextromethorphan *on page 466*

♦ **Urabeth®** *see* Bethanechol *on page 132*

♦ **Urasal® (Canada)** *see* Methenamine *on page 615*

♦ **Urea Peroxide** *see* Carbamide Peroxide *on page 167*

♦ **Urecholine®** *see* Bethanechol *on page 132*

♦ **Urex®** *see* Methenamine *on page 615*

♦ **Uritol® (Canada)** *see* Furosemide *on page 447*

♦ **Urobak®** *see* Sulfamethoxazole *on page 892*

♦ **Urocit®-K** *see* Citrate and Citric Acid *on page 231*

♦ **Urodine®** *see* Phenazopyridine *on page 753*

♦ **Urogesic®** *see* Phenazopyridine *on page 753*

Urokinase (yoor oh KIN ase)

Brand Names Abbokinase®

Therapeutic Category Thrombolytic Agent

Generic Available No

Use Thrombolytic agent used in treatment of recent severe or massive deep vein or arterial thrombosis, pulmonary emboli, and occluded arteriovenous cannulas

Pregnancy Risk Factor B

Contraindications Hypersensitivity to urokinase or any component; internal bleeding; CVA (within 2 months); brain carcinoma, bacterial endocarditis, anticoagulant therapy, surgery or trauma within past 10 days

Warnings Stop urokinase administration if any signs of bleeding occur. Due to problems in the manufacturing process, the FDA recommended on January 25, 1999, that Abbokinase® be reserved for critical use in specific patients after consideration has been given to alternative agents; Abbokinase® is made from kidney cell cultures that come from human neonates (post-mortem harvesting); deficiencies in the harvesting and manufacturing process may have increased the risk of transmission of an infectious agent; the FDA does not know of any cases of infectious diseases that were transmitted by the use of Abbokinase®; the manufacturer is in the process of correcting the problems and has added additional tests (but as of April, 1999, the new processes and tests have not been fully validated). For further information, see http://www.fda.gov/medwatch/safety/1999/safety99.htm

Precautions Systemic use: Use with caution in patients with severe hypertension, recent lumbar puncture, patient receiving I.M. administration of medications. If indicated, febrile patients should receive antibiotics for at least 24 hours prior to urokinase therapy; obtain an echocardiogram in febrile patients prior to therapy to rule out intracardiac vegetations; pretreatment lab studies should include platelet count, PT/PTT, fibrinogen, fibrin degradation products, plasminogen, antithrombin III, protein S, protein C.

Adverse Reactions

Central nervous system: Fever

Dermatologic: Rash

(Continued)

Urokinase *(Continued)*

Hematologic: Internal bleeding
Local: Bleeding, hematoma at I.M. or I.P. sites
Respiratory: Bronchospasm
Miscellaneous: Allergic reactions

Drug Interactions Anticoagulants, aspirin

Stability Store 250,000 unit vials in refrigerator; powder for 5000 unit/mL ("open-cath") should be stored below 77°F; avoid freezing; reconstitute by gently rolling and tilting, **do not shake**; does not contain preservative; the 5000 unit vial should be reconstituted just prior to use; discard unused portion; a reconstituted 250,000 unit vial is stable for 24 hours under refrigeration

Mechanism of Action Promotes thrombolysis by directly activating plasminogen to plasmin, which degrades fibrin, fibrinogen, and other procoagulant plasma proteins

Pharmacodynamics

Onset of action: I.V.: Fibrinolysis occurs rapidly
Duration: 4 or more hours

Pharmacokinetics

Half-life: 10-20 minutes
Elimination: Cleared by the liver with a small amount excreted in the urine and the bile

Usual Dosage

Infants, Children, and Adults:
Arterial or venous thrombosis or pulmonary emboli: I.V.: Loading dose: 4400 units/kg over 10 minutes, followed by 4400 units/kg/hour for 12-72 hours; continuous infusion doses of 4000-10,000 units/kg/hour have been used; titrate urokinase dose to bring level of plasma fibrinogen to 75% of fibrinogen measured after FFP infusion; reassess clot size every 12-24 hours
Occluded I.V. catheters:
5000 units/mL concentration; (use only Abbokinase® Open Cath), the volume to instill into the catheter is equal to the internal volume of the catheter; administer in each lumen over 1-2 minutes, leave in lumen for 1-4 hours, then **aspirate out of catheter**, flush catheter with NS; may repeat with 10,000 units in each lumen if 5000 units fails to clear the catheter; **do not infuse into the patient**
Continuous I.V. infusion: 150-200 units/kg/hour in each lumen for 8-48 hours; infuse at a rate of at least 20 mL/hour in children and adults
Dialysis patients: 5000 units is administered in each lumen over 1-2 minutes; leave urokinase in lumen for 1-2 days, then aspirate out of lumen
Adults: MI: Intracoronary: 6000 units/minute up to 2 hours

Administration Parenteral: I.V. infusion: Usual concentration: 1250-1500 units/mL; maximum concentration not yet defined
Abbokinase® Open Cath 5000 unit product is **not** for systemic administration, it must be aspirated out of the catheter; do **not** dilute Abbokinase® Open Cath for I.V. infusion

Monitoring Parameters CBC, reticulocyte, platelet count; fibrinogen level, plasminogen, fibrin/fibrinogen degradation products, D-dimer, PT, PTT, ATIII, protein C, U/A, ACT, urinalysis

Nursing Implications Use 0.22 or 0.45 micron filter during I.V. systemic therapy

Additional Information Failure of thrombolytic agents in newborns/neonates may occur due to the low plasminogen concentrations (~50% to 70% of adult levels); higher doses of urokinase may be needed, supplementing plasminogen (via administration of fresh frozen plasma) may possibly help

Dosage Forms

Powder for injection, preservative free: 250,000 units (5 mL)
Powder for injection, catheter clear, preservative free: 5000 units (1 mL, 1.8 mL)

References

Andrew M, Brooker L, Leaker M, et al, "Fibrin Clot Lysis by Thrombolytic Agents Is Impaired in Newborns Due to a Low Plasminogen Concentration," *Thromb Haemost*, 1992, 68(3):325-30.
Bagnall HA, Gomperts E, and Atkinson JB, "Continuous Infusion of Low-Dose Urokinase in the Treatment of Central Venous Catheter Thrombosis in Infants and Children," *Pediatrics*, 1989, 83(6):963-6.
David M and Andrew M, "Venous Thromboembolic Complications in Children," *J Pediatr*, 1993, 123(3):337-46.
Kothari SS, Varma S, and Wasir HS, "Thrombolytic Therapy in Infants and Children," *Am Heart J*, 1994, 127(3):651-7.
Michelson AD, Bovill E, Monagle P, et al, "Antithrombotic Therapy in Children," *Chest*, 1998, 114(5 Suppl):748S-69S.

♦ **Uro-KP-Neutral®** *see* Phosphate Supplements *on page 765*
♦ **Urolene Blue® Oral** *see* Methylene Blue *on page 626*
♦ **Uro-Mag®** *see* Magnesium Supplements *on page 588*

- ♦ **Uroplus® DS** see Co-Trimoxazole on page 258
- ♦ **Uroplus® SS** see Co-Trimoxazole on page 258
- ♦ **Urozide® (Canada)** see Hydrochlorothiazide on page 483
- ♦ **Ursacol** see Ursodiol on page 965
- ♦ **Urso®** see Ursodiol on page 965
- ♦ **Ursodeoxycholic Acid** see Ursodiol on page 965

Ursodiol (ER soe dye ole)

Brand Names Actigall™; Urso®

Synonyms UDCA; Ursacol; Ursodeoxycholic Acid

Therapeutic Category Gallstone Dissolution Agent

Generic Available No

Use Gallbladder stone dissolution; prevention of gallstone formation (obese patients experiencing rapid weight loss); primary biliary cirrhosis (Urso®); unlabeled uses: facilitate bile excretion in infants with biliary atresia; cholestasis secondary to PN; improve the hepatic metabolism of essential fatty acids in patients with cystic fibrosis

Pregnancy Risk Factor B

Contraindications Hypersensitivity to ursodiol or any component; not to be used with calcified cholesterol stones, radiopaque stones, bile pigment stones, or stones larger than 20 mm in diameter; allergy to bile acids; patients with compelling reasons for cholecystectomy (eg, unremitting acute cholecystitis, cholangitis, biliary obstruction)

Warnings Gallbladder stone dissolution may take several months of therapy; complete dissolution may not occur and recurrence of stones within 5 years has been observed in 50% of patients

Precautions Use with caution in patients with a nonvisualizing gallbladder and those with chronic liver disease

Adverse Reactions
Central nervous system: Headache, fatigue, anxiety, depression, sleep disorder
Dermatologic: Rash, pruritus, hair thinning
Gastrointestinal: Diarrhea, biliary pain, constipation, stomatitis, flatulence, nausea, vomiting, abdominal pain
Hepatic: Elevated liver enzymes
Neuromuscular & skeletal: Arthralgias, myalgia, back pain
Respiratory: Cough, rhinitis

Drug Interactions Decreased effect with aluminum-containing antacids, cholestyramine, colestipol, clofibrate, oral contraceptives (estrogens), activated charcoal

Stability Do not store above 30°C (86°F)

Mechanism of Action Decreases the cholesterol content of bile and bile stones by reducing the secretion of cholesterol from the liver and the fractional reabsorption of cholesterol by the intestines

Pharmacokinetics
Absorption: 90%
Metabolism: Undergoes extensive enterohepatic recycling; following hepatic conjugation and biliary secretion, the drug is hydrolyzed to active ursodiol, where it is recycled or transformed to lithocholic acid by colonic microbial flora
Half-life: 100 hours
Elimination: In feces via bile

Usual Dosage Oral:
Biliary atresia: Infants: 10-15 mg/kg/day once daily
Improvement in the hepatic metabolism of essential fatty acids in cystic fibrosis: Children: 30 mg/kg/day
TPN-induced cholestasis: Infants and Children: 30 mg/kg/day in 3 divided doses
Gallstone dissolution: Adults: 8-10 mg/kg/day in 2-3 divided doses; maintenance therapy: 250 mg/day at bedtime for 6 months to 1 year; use beyond 24 months is not established
Gallstone prevention: Adults: 300 mg twice daily
Primary biliary cirrhosis: Adults: 13-15 mg/kg/day in 4 divided doses

Administration Oral: Administer with food or, if a single dosage, at bedtime

Monitoring Parameters ALT, AST, sonogram, oral cholecystogram before therapy and every 6 months during therapy; obtain ultrasound images of gallbladder at 6-month intervals for the first year of therapy

Patient Information Frequent blood work necessary to follow drug effects; report any persistent nausea, vomiting, abdominal pain

Additional Information 30% to 50% of patients have stone recurrence after dissolution
(Continued)

Ursodiol *(Continued)*

Dosage Forms
Capsule: 300 mg

Tablet, film-coated: 250 mg

Extemporaneous Preparations
A 25 mg/mL ursodiol suspension may be made by opening ten 300 mg capsules; mix with 10 mL Glycerin, USP until smooth mixture is obtained. Add 60 mL Ora-Plus® and continue to levigate until a smooth mixture is achieved. Transfer mixture to a light-resistent bottle; add a small amount of Orange Syrup, NF to wash remaining drug from the mortar to bottle. Add additional syrup to make final volume of 120 mL. Label "shake well"; stable 60 days at room temperature or refrigerated. (Johnson, 1995)

A 60 mg/mL ursodiol suspension may be made in a similar method by opening twelve 300 mg capsules and wetting with sufficient glycerin and triturating to make a fine paste; gradually add simple syrup to make a final volume of 60 mL. Label "shake well"; stable 35 days in refrigerator. (Mallett, 1997)

Johnson CE and Nesbitt J, "Stability of Ursodiol in an Extemporaneously Compounded Oral Liquid," *Am J Health Syst Pharm*, 1995, 52(16):1798-800.

Mallett MS, Hagan RL, and Peters DA, "Stability of Ursodiol 25 mg/mL in an Extemporaneously Prepared Oral Liquid," *Am J Health-Syst Pharm*, 1997, 54(12):1401-4.

References
Colombo C, Setchell KD, Podda M, et al, "Effect of Ursodeoxycholic Acid Therapy for Liver Disease Associated With Cystic Fibrosis," *J Pediatr*, 1990, 117(3):482-9.

Lepage G, Paradis K, Lacaille F, et al, "Ursodeoxycholic Acid Improves the Hepatic Metabolism of Essential Fatty Acids and Retinol in Children With Cystic Fibrosis," *J Pediatr*, 1997, 130(1)52-8.

Spagnuolo MI, Iorio R, Vegnente A, et al, "Ursodeoxycholic Acid for Treatment of Cholestasis in Children on Long-Term Total Parenteral Nutrition - A Pilot Study," *Gastroenterology*, 1996, 111(3):716-9.

Ullrich D, Rating D, Schroter W, et al, "Treatment With Ursodeoxycholic Acid Renders Children With Biliary Atresia Suitable for Liver Transplantation," *Lancet*, 1987, 2(8571):1324.

♦ **Uticort® Topical** *see* Betamethasone *on page 130*

♦ **Vagifem®** *see* Estradiol *on page 386*

♦ **Valergen®** *see* Estradiol *on page 386*

♦ **Valisone® Topical** *see* Betamethasone *on page 130*

♦ **Valium® Injection** *see* Diazepam *on page 307*

♦ **Valium® Oral** *see* Diazepam *on page 307*

♦ **Valproate Sodium** *see* Valproic Acid and Derivatives *on page 966*

Valproic Acid and Derivatives *(val PROE ik AS id & dah RIV ah tivs)*

Related Information
Antiepileptic Drugs *on page 1176*

Blood Level Sampling Time Guidelines *on page 1189*

Carbohydrate and Alcohol Content of Liquid Medications for Use in Patients Receiving Ketogenic Diets *on page 1228*

Serotonin Syndrome *on page 1217*

Brand Names Depacon®; Depakene®; Depakote®

Available Salts Divalproex Sodium; Valproate Sodium

Synonyms Dipropylacetic Acid; DPA; 2-Propylpentanoic Acid; 2-Propylvaleric Acid; VPA

Therapeutic Category Anticonvulsant, Miscellaneous; Infantile Spasms, Treatment

Generic Available Yes

Use Management of simple and complex partial seizures, simple and complex absence seizures, mixed seizure types, myoclonic and generalized tonic-clonic (grand mal) seizures; may be effective in infantile spasms; divalproex sodium is also indicated for the treatment of manic episodes of bipolar disorders (manic-depressive illness) in adults and the prevention of migraine headaches

Pregnancy Risk Factor D

Contraindications Hypersensitivity to valproic acid or derivatives or any component; hepatic dysfunction

Warnings Hepatic failure resulting in death may occur; children <2 years of age (especially those on polytherapy, with congenital metabolic disorders, with seizure disorders and mental retardation, or with organic brain disease) are at considerable risk; monitor patients closely for appearance of malaise, loss of seizure control, weakness, facial edema, anorexia, jaundice and vomiting; hepatotoxicity has been reported after 3 days to 6 months of therapy. Pancreatitis resulting in death may occur; pancreatitis may be hemorrhagic and rapidly progress to death;

onset has occurred shortly after starting therapy and after several years of treatment; monitor patients closely for nausea, vomiting, anorexia, and abdominal pain and evaluate promptly; discontinue valproate if pancreatitis occurs. Dose-related thrombocytopenia may occur. I.V. valproate is not recommended for the prophylaxis of post-traumatic seizures in patients with acute head trauma

Adverse Reactions

Central nervous system: Drowsiness, irritability, confusion, restlessness, hyperactivity, malaise, headache, ataxia, dizziness, asthenia

Dermatologic: Alopecia, erythema multiforme

Endocrine & metabolic: Hyperammonemia, impaired fatty-acid oxidation, carnitine deficiency

Gastrointestinal: Nausea, vomiting, diarrhea, dyspepsia, constipation, pancreatitis (potentially fatal), weight gain, taste perversion (I.V.)

Hematologic: Thrombocytopenia (risk increases significantly with serum levels ≥110 mcg/mL (females) or ≥135 mcg/mL (males)), prolongation of bleeding time

Hepatic: Transient increased liver enzymes, liver failure (can be fatal)

Local: I.V.: Pain and local reaction at injection site

Neuromuscular & skeletal: Tremor

Ocular: Diplopia, blurred vision

Drug Interactions Cytochrome P-450 isoenzyme CYP2C19 substrate; CYP2C9 and CYP2D6 isoenzyme inhibitor, CYP3A3/4 isoenzyme inhibitor (weak)

Valproic acid may displace phenytoin and diazepam from protein binding sites. Aspirin may displace valproic acid from protein binding sites which may result in toxicity. Valproic acid may significantly increase phenobarbital serum concentrations in patients receiving phenobarbital or primidone. Valproic acid may increase zidovudine concentrations; valproic acid may inhibit the metabolism of lamotrigine and phenytoin. Phenobarbital, primidone, phenytoin, and carbamazepine may decrease serum levels of valproic acid; felbamate may increase plasma concentrations of valproic acid; antacids may increase the oral absorption of valproic acid.

Food Interactions Dietary carnitine requirements may be increased; food may decrease the rate but not the extent of absorption

Stability Injection: Stable for 24 hours at room temperature when diluted in D_5W, NS, or LR; discard unused portion of vial (does not contain preservative)

Mechanism of Action Causes increased availability of gamma-aminobutyric acid (GABA), an inhibitory neurotransmitter, to brain neurons or may enhance the action of GABA or mimic its action at postsynaptic receptor sites

Pharmacokinetics

Protein binding: 80% to 90% (dose dependent); decreased protein binding in neonates, elderly, and patients with renal impairment or chronic hepatic disease

Metabolism: Extensive in liver via glucuronide conjugation and oxidation

Bioavailability: Oral: Equivalent to I.V.

Half-life: Increased with liver disease

Newborns (exposed to VPA *in utero*): 30-60 hours

Newborns 1st week of life: 40-45 hours

Newborns <10 days: 10-67 hours

Children >2 months: 7-13 hours

Children 2-14 years: Mean: 9 hours; range: 3.5-20 hours

Adults: 8-17 hours

Time to peak serum concentration:

Oral: 1-4 hours; divalproex (enteric coated): 3-5 hours

I.V.: At the end of the infusion

Elimination: 2% to 3% excreted unchanged in urine; faster clearance in children who receive other antiepileptic drugs and those who are younger; age and polytherapy explain 80% of interpatient variability in total clearance; children >10 years of age have pharmacokinetic parameters similar to adults

Usual Dosage Children and Adults:

Oral: Initial: 10-15 mg/kg/day in 1-3 divided doses; increase by 5-10 mg/kg/day at weekly intervals until therapeutic levels are achieved; maintenance: 30-60 mg/kg/day in 2-3 divided doses; divalproex can be given twice daily

Note: Children receiving more than 1 anticonvulsant (ie, polytherapy) may require doses up to 100 mg/kg/day in 3-4 divided doses

I.V.: Total daily I.V. dose is equivalent to the total daily oral dose, however, I.V. dose should be divided with a frequency of every 6 hours; if I.V. form is administered 2-3 times/day, close monitoring of trough levels is recommended; switch patients to oral product as soon as clinically possible (I.V. use has not been studied for >14 days)

Rectal: Dilute syrup 1:1 with water for use as a retention enema; loading dose: 17-20 mg/kg one time; maintenance: 10-15 mg/kg/dose every 8 hours

(Continued)

Valproic Acid and Derivatives *(Continued)*

Dosing adjustment in renal impairment: Cl_{cr} <10 mL/minute: No dosage adjustment is needed for patients on hemodialysis (unbound clearance of valproate is reduced (27%) in these patients, but hemodialysis reduces valproate concentrations by ~20%)

Administration

Oral: May administer with food to decrease adverse GI effects; do not administer with carbonated drinks; do not administer tablet with milk; may mix contents of Depakote® Sprinkle® capsule with semisolid food (eg, applesauce, pudding, mashed potatoes) and swallow immediately, but do not crush or chew sprinkle beads; swallow delayed release tablet whole, do not crush, break, or chew

I.V.: Dilute dose with at least 50 mL of D_5W, NS, or LR; infuse over 60 minutes; maximum infusion rate: 20 mg/minute

Monitoring Parameters
Liver enzymes, bilirubin, serum ammonia, CBC with platelets, serum concentrations

Reference Range

Therapeutic: 50-100 µg/mL (SI: 350-690 µmol/L)

Toxic: >100-150 µg/mL (SI: >690-1040 µmol/L)

Seizure control may improve at levels >100 µg/mL (SI: >690 µmol/L), but toxicity may occur

Test Interactions
False-positive result for urine ketones; altered thyroid function tests

Patient Information
Avoid alcohol; may cause drowsiness and impair ability to perform activities requiring mental alertness and physical coordination; notify physician if nausea, vomiting, loss of appetite, abdominal pain, yellow skin, general feeling of weakness, or bleeding or easy bruising occurs

Nursing Implications
Instruct patients/parents to report signs or symptoms of hepatotoxicity (see Warnings); GI side effects of divalproex may be less than valproic acid

Additional Information
Acute intoxications: Naloxone may reverse the CNS depressant effects but may also block the action of other anticonvulsants; carnitine may reduce the ammonia level; multiple dosing of activated charcoal can enhance elimination

Routine prophylactic use of carnitine in children receiving valproic acid to avoid carnitine deficiency and hepatotoxicity is probably not indicated (Freeman, 1994); a case of fatal hepatotoxic reaction has been reported in a child receiving valproic acid despite carnitine supplementation (Murphy, 1993)

Sodium content of valproate sodium syrup: 5 mL = 23 mg (1 mEq of sodium); safety of I.V. form has not been well studied in children <2 years of age

Dosage Forms

Capsule, sprinkle, as divalproex sodium (Depakote® Sprinkle®): 125 mg

Capsule, as valproic acid (Depakene®): 250 mg

Injection, as sodium valproate (Depacon®): 100 mg/mL (5 mL)

Syrup, as sodium valproate (Depakene®): 250 mg/5 mL (5 mL, 50 mL, 480 mL)

Tablet, delayed release, as divalproex sodium (Depakote®): 125 mg, 250 mg, 500 mg

References

Cloyd JC, Fischer JH, Kriel RL, et al, "Valproic Acid Pharmacokinetics in Children. IV. Effects of Age and Antiepileptic Drugs on Protein Binding and Intrinsic Clearance," *Clin Pharmacol Ther*, 1993, 53(1):22-9.

Cloyd JC, Kriel RL, Fischer JH, et al, "Pharmacokinetics of Valproic Acid in Children: I. Multiple Antiepileptic Drug Therapy," *Neurology*, 1983, 33(2):185-91.

Dreifuss FE, Santilli N, Langer DH, et al, "Valproic Acid Hepatic Fatalities: A Retrospective Review," *Neurology*, 1987, 37(3):379-85.

Freeman JM, Vining EP, Cost S, et al, "Does Carnitine Administration Improve the Symptoms Attributed to Anticonvulsant Medications?: A Double-Blinded, Crossover Study," *Pediatrics*, 1994, 93(6 Pt 1):893-5.

Murphy JV, Groover RV and Hodge C, "Hepatotoxic Effects in a Child Receiving Valproate and Carnitine," *J Pediatr*, 1993, 123(2):318-20.

♦ **Vamate® Oral** *see* Hydroxyzine *on page 496*

♦ **Vancenase® AQ 84 mcg** *see* Beclomethasone *on page 122*

♦ **Vancenase® AQ Inhaler** *see* Beclomethasone *on page 122*

♦ **Vancenase® Nasal Inhaler** *see* Beclomethasone *on page 122*

♦ **Vanceril® 84 mcg Double Strength** *see* Beclomethasone *on page 122*

♦ **Vanceril® Oral Inhaler** *see* Beclomethasone *on page 122*

♦ **Vancocin® CP (Canada)** *see* Vancomycin *on page 969*

♦ **Vancocin® Injection** *see* Vancomycin *on page 969*

♦ **Vancocin® Oral** *see* Vancomycin *on page 969*

♦ **Vancoled® Injection** *see Vancomycin on page 969*

Vancomycin (van koe MYE sin)
Related Information
Blood Level Sampling Time Guidelines *on page 1189*
Carbohydrate and Alcohol Content of Liquid Medications for Use in Patients Receiving Ketogenic Diets *on page 1228*
Endocarditis Prophylaxis *on page 1127*
Brand Names Lyphocin® Injection; Vancocin® CP (Canada); Vancocin® Injection; Vancocin® Oral; Vancoled® Injection
Available Salts Vancomycin Hydrochloride
Therapeutic Category Antibiotic, Miscellaneous
Generic Available Yes
Use Treatment of patients with the following infections or conditions: Infections due to documented or suspected methicillin-resistant *S. aureus* or beta-lactam resistant coagulase negative *Staphylococcus*; serious or life-threatening infections (ie, endocarditis, meningitis, osteomyelitis) due to documented or suspected staphylococcal or streptococcal infections in patients who are allergic to penicillins and/or cephalosporins; empiric therapy of infections associated with central lines, VP shunts, hemodialysis shunts, vascular grafts, prosthetic heart valves; used orally for staphylococcal enterocolitis or for antibiotic-associated pseudomembranous colitis produced by *C. difficile*
Pregnancy Risk Factor C
Contraindications Hypersensitivity to vancomycin or any component; avoid in patients with previous hearing loss
Precautions Use with caution in patients with renal impairment or those receiving other nephrotoxic or ototoxic drugs; dosage modification required in patients with impaired renal function
Adverse Reactions Rapid infusion associated with red neck or red man syndrome: Erythema multiforme-like reaction with intense pruritus, tachycardia, hypotension, rash involving face, neck, upper trunk, back and upper arms; red man or red neck syndrome usually develops during a rapid infusion of vancomycin or with doses ≥15-20 mg/kg/hour; reaction usually dissipates in 30-60 minutes

Cardiovascular: Cardiac arrest
Central nervous system: Fever, chills
Dermatologic: Red neck or red man syndrome, urticaria, macular skin rash
Gastrointestinal: Nausea
Hematologic: Neutropenia, eosinophilia
Local: Phlebitis
Neuromuscular & skeletal: Lower back pain
Otic: Ototoxicity associated with prolonged serum concentration >40 μg/mL
Renal: Nephrotoxicity (higher incidence with trough concentrations >10 μg/mL)
Miscellaneous: Hypersensitivity reactions
Drug Interactions Anesthetic agents (erythema, hypotension, hypothermia, and facial flushing); concurrent ototoxic or nephrotoxic drugs including loop diuretics, cisplatin, and aminoglycosides
Stability After the oral or parenteral solution is reconstituted, refrigerate and use within 2 weeks; incompatible with heparin, phenobarbital, and ceftazidime
Mechanism of Action Inhibits bacterial cell wall synthesis; blocks glycopeptide polymerization of the phosphodisaccharide-pentapeptide complex in the second stage of cell wall synthesis by binding tightly to D-alanyl-D-alanine portion of cell wall precursor
Pharmacokinetics
Absorption:
Oral: Poor
I.M.: Erratic
Intraperitoneal administration can result in 38% systemic absorption
Distribution: Widely distributed in body tissues and fluids including pericardial, pleural, ascites, and synovial fluids; low concentration in CSF if meninges are inflamed
Protein binding: 55%
Metabolism: <3%
Half-life, biphasic: Prolonged significantly with reduced renal function
Terminal:
Newborns: 6-10 hours
3 months to 4 years: 4 hours
>3 years: 2.2-3 hours
Adults: 5-8 hours
(Continued)

Vancomycin *(Continued)*

Elimination: Primarily via glomerular filtration; excreted as unchanged drug in the urine (80% to 90%); oral doses are excreted primarily in the feces; presence of malignancy in children is associated with an increase in vancomycin clearance

Not dialyzable (0% to 5%)

Usual Dosage Initial dosage recommendation:

Neonates: I.V.:

Postnatal age ≤7 days:

<1200 g: 15 mg/kg/day given every 24 hours

1200-2000 g: 10-15 mg/kg/dose given every 12-18 hours

>2000 g: 10-15 mg/kg/dose given every 8-12 hours

Postnatal age >7 days:

<1200 g: 15 mg/kg/day given every 24 hours

1200-2000 g: 10-15 mg/kg/dose given every 8-12 hours

>2000 g: 15-20 mg/kg/dose given every 8 hours

Infants >1 month and Children: I.V.: 40 mg/kg/day in divided doses every 6-8 hours

Nonobese pediatric cancer patients with normal renal function (n=28, age range: 9 months to 13 years): initial dosage regimen of 60 mg/kg/day divided every 6 hours has been recommended

Staphylococcal central nervous system infection: I.V.: 60 mg/kg/day in divided doses every 6 hours; maximum dose: 1 g/dose

Adults (with normal renal function): I.V.: 0.5 g every 6 hours or 1 g every 12 hours; maximum dose: 4 g/day

Dosing interval in renal impairment:

Cl_{cr} >90 mL/minute: Administer normal dose every 6 hours

Cl_{cr} 70-89 mL/minute: Administer normal dose every 8 hours

Cl_{cr} 46-69 mL/minute: Administer normal dose every 12 hours

Cl_{cr} 30-45 mL/minute: Administer normal dose every 18 hours

Cl_{cr} 15-29 mL/minute: Administer normal dose every 24 hours

Renal dysfunction, end stage renal disease, or on dialysis: 10-20 mg/kg; subsequent dosages and frequency of administration are best determined by measurement of serum levels and assessment of renal insufficiency

Intrathecal/intraventricular:

Neonates: 5-10 mg/day

Children: 5-20 mg/day

Adults: 20 mg/day

Oral (antibiotic-associated pseudomembraneous colitis: Metronidazole is the drug of initial choice per 2000 Red Book recommendations):

Children: 40 mg/kg/day in divided doses every 6 hours for 7-10 days; not to exceed 2 g/day

Adults: 0.5-2 g/day in divided doses every 6-8 hours

Prophylaxis of endocarditis in penicillin allergic patients: I.V.:

GI or genitourinary procedures:

Children: 20 mg/kg 1 hour prior to the procedure **plus** gentamicin 1.5 mg/kg 30 minutes prior to the procedure

Adults: 1 g 1 hour prior to the procedure **plus** gentamicin 1.5 mg/kg (maximum dose: 120 mg) 30 minutes prior to the procedure

Administration

Parenteral: Administer vancomycin by I.V. intermittent infusion over 60 minutes at a final concentration not to exceed 5 mg/mL; if a maculopapular rash appears on face, neck, trunk, and upper extremities, slow the infusion rate to administer dose over 1½ to 2 hours and increase the dilution volume; the reaction usually dissipates in 30-60 minutes; administration of antihistamines just before the infusion may also prevent or minimize this reaction

Intrathecal/Intraventricular: Dilute in NS without preservatives to a final concentration between 2-5 mg/mL

Monitoring Parameters Periodic renal function tests, urinalysis, serum vancomycin concentrations, WBC; audiogram (in patients who concurrently receive ototoxic chemotherapy)

Reference Range

Peak: 25-40 µg/mL

Trough: 5-10 µg/mL

Patient Information Report pain at infusion site; dizziness, fullness or ringing in ears with I.V. use

Nursing Implications Do not administer I.M.; peak levels are drawn 30 minutes to 1 hour after the completion of a 1-hour infusion; troughs are obtained just before the next dose

Dosage Forms
Capsule, as hydrochloride: 125 mg, 250 mg
Powder for oral solution, as hydrochloride: 1 g, 10 g
Powder for injection, as hydrochloride: 500 mg, 1 g, 2 g, 5 g, 10 g

References
American Academy of Pediatrics Committee on Infectious Diseases, "Treatment of Bacterial Meningitis," *Pediatrics*, 1988, 81(6):904-7.

Chang D, "Influence of Malignancy on the Pharmacokinetics of Vancomycin in Infants and Children," *Pediatr Infect Dis J*, 1995, 14(8):667-73.

Chang D, Liem L, and Malogolowkin M, "A Prospective Study of Vancomycin Pharmacokinetics and Dosage Requirements in Pediatric Cancer Patients," *Pediatr Infect Dis J*, 1994, 13(11):969-74.

Leonard MB, Koren G, Stevenson DK, et al, "Vancomycin Pharmacokinetics in Very Low Birth Weight Neonates," *Pediatr Infect Dis J*, 1989, 8(5):282-6.

Matzke GR, Zhanel GG, and Guay DRP, "Clinical Pharmacokinetics of Vancomycin," *Clin Pharmacokinet*, 1986, 11(4):257-82.

Rodvold KA, Everett JA, Pryka RD, and Kraus DM, "Pharmacokinetics and Administration Regimens of Vancomycin in Neonates, Infants and Children," *Clin Pharmacokinet*, 1997, 33(1):32-51.

Rybak MJ, Albrecht LM, Boike SC, et al, "Nephrotoxicity of Vancomycin, Alone and With an Aminoglycoside," *J Antimicrob Chemother*, 1990, 25(4):679-87.

♦ **Vancomycin Hydrochloride** *see* Vancomycin *on page 969*

♦ **Vanoxide® [OTC]** *see* Benzoyl Peroxide *on page 126*

♦ **Vantin®** *see* Cefpodoxime *on page 187*

♦ **Vapocet® (Canada)** *see* Hydrocodone and Acetaminophen *on page 485*

♦ **Vaponefrin® [OTC]** *see* Epinephrine *on page 371*

♦ **Varicella-Zoster Immune Globulin (Human)** *see page 1138*

♦ **VasoClear® Ophthalmic [OTC]** *see* Naphazoline *on page 671*

♦ **Vasocon Regular® Ophthalmic** *see* Naphazoline *on page 671*

Vasopressin (vay soe PRES in)
Brand Names Pitressin®; Pressyn® (Canada)

Synonyms ADH; Antidiuretic Hormone; 8-Arginine Vasopressin

Therapeutic Category Antidiuretic Hormone Analog; Hormone, Posterior Pituitary

Generic Available No

Use Treatment of diabetes insipidus; prevention and treatment of postoperative abdominal distention; differential diagnosis of diabetes insipidus; adjunct in the treatment of acute massive hemorrhage of GI tract or esophageal varices

Pregnancy Risk Factor B

Contraindications Hypersensitivity to vasopressin or any component

Warnings I.V. infiltration may lead to severe vasoconstriction and localized tissue necrosis

Precautions Use with caution in patients with seizure disorders, migraine, asthma, vascular disease, renal disease, cardiac disease, goiter with cardiac complications, arteriosclerosis, chronic nephritis with nitrogen retention

Adverse Reactions
Cardiovascular: Circumoral pallor; with high doses: hypertension, bradycardia, arrhythmias, venous thrombosis, vasoconstriction, angina, heart block, cardiac arrest

Central nervous system: Vertigo, fever, headache

Dermatologic: Urticaria

Endocrine & metabolic: Water intoxication, hyponatremia

Gastrointestinal: Abdominal cramps, nausea, vomiting, flatus, diarrhea

Neuromuscular & skeletal: Tremor

Respiratory: Wheezing, bronchoconstriction

Miscellaneous: Diaphoresis

Drug Interactions
Decreased antidiuretic activity: Lithium, demeclocycline, large doses of epinephrine, heparin (therapeutic doses), alcohol

Increased antidiuretic activity: Chlorpropamide, carbamazepine, phenformin, tricyclic antidepressants, clofibrate, fludrocortisone

Mechanism of Action Increases cyclic adenosine monophosphate (cAMP) which increases water permeability at the distal convoluted tubule and collecting duct resulting in decreased urine volume and increased urine osmolality; causes peristalsis by directly stimulating the smooth muscle in the GI tract (in doses greater than those required for its antidiuretic action); causes vasoconstriction (primarily of capillaries and small arterioles)

Pharmacodynamics I.M., S.C.:
Onset of action: 1 hour
Duration of action: 2-8 hours
(Continued)

Vasopressin *(Continued)*

Pharmacokinetics Destroyed by trypsin in GI tract, must be administered parenterally

Half-life: 10-20 minutes

Metabolism: Most of dose is rapidly metabolized in liver and kidney

Usual Dosage

Diabetes insipidus:

I.M., S.C.: (Highly variable dosage; titrate dosage based upon serum and urine sodium and osmolality in addition to fluid balance and urine output)

Children: 2.5-10 units 2-4 times/day

Adults: 5-10 units 2-4 times/day as needed (range: 5-60 units/day)

Continuous infusion: Children and Adults: Initial: 0.5 milliunit/kg/hour (0.0005 unit/kg/hour); double dosage as needed every 30 minutes to a maximum of 10 milliunit/kg/hour

Abdominal distention: Adults: I.M.: 5 units initially, then repeated every 3-4 hours; dosage may be increased to 10 units if necessary

GI hemorrhage: I.V. continuous infusion (may also be infused directly into the superior mesenteric artery):

Children: Initial: 0.002-0.005 units/kg/minute; titrate dose as needed; maximum dose: 0.01 units/kg/minute; if bleeding stops for 12 hours, then taper off over 24-48 hours

Adults: Initial: I.V.: 0.2-0.4 unit/minute, then titrate dose as needed; if bleeding stops, continue at same dose for 12 hours, taper off over 24-48 hours

Dosing adjustment in hepatic impairment: Some patients with cirrhosis respond to much lower doses

Administration Parenteral: Continuous infusion: Dilute in NS or D_5W to a final concentration of 0.1-1 unit/mL; see Usual Dosage for rate of infusion

Monitoring Parameters Fluid intake and output, urine specific gravity, urine and serum osmolality, serum and urine sodium

Dosage Forms Injection, aqueous: 20 pressor units/mL (0.5 mL, 1 mL)

References

Tuggle DW, Bennett KG, Scott J, et al, "Intravenous Vasopressin and Gastrointestinal Hemorrhage in Children," *J Pediatr Surg*, 1988, 23(7):627-9.

♦ **Vasotec® I.V.** *see* Enalapril/Enalaprilat *on page 363*
♦ **Vasotec® Oral** *see* Enalapril/Enalaprilat *on page 363*
♦ **V-Cillin K®** *see* Penicillin V Potassium *on page 743*
♦ **VCR** *see* Vincristine *on page 979*

Vecuronium *(ve KYOO roe nee um)*

Brand Names Norcuron®
Available Salts Vecuronium Bromide
Synonyms ORG NC 45
Therapeutic Category Neuromuscular Blocker Agent, Nondepolarizing; Skeletal Muscle Relaxant, Paralytic
Generic Available No
Use Adjunct to anesthesia, to facilitate endotracheal intubation, and provide skeletal muscle relaxation during surgery or mechanical ventilation
Pregnancy Risk Factor C
Contraindications Hypersensitivity to vecuronium or any component

Clinical Conditions Affecting Neuromuscular Blockade

Potentiation	Antagonism
Electrolyte abnormalities	Alkalosis
Severe hyponatremia	Hypercalcemia
Severe hypocalcemia	Demyelinating lesions
Severe hypokalemia	Peripheral neuropathies
Hypermagnesemia	Diabetes mellitus
Neuromuscular diseases	
Acidosis	
Acute intermittent porphyria	
Renal failure	
Hepatic failure	

Warnings Ventilation must be supported during neuromuscular blockade; use only by individuals who are experienced in the maintenance of an adequate airway and respiratory support

Precautions Use with caution in patients with hepatic impairment, neuromuscular disease, myasthenia gravis; many clinical conditions may potentiate or antagonize neuromuscular blockade, see table on previous page.

Adverse Reactions Most frequent reactions are associated with prolongation of its pharmacologic effect
Cardiovascular: Arrhythmias, tachycardia, hypotension, hypertension
Dermatologic: Urticaria, rash
Neuromuscular & skeletal: Muscle weakness
Respiratory: Respiratory insufficiency, bronchospasm, apnea

Drug Interactions See table.

Potential Drug Interactions

Potentiation	Antagonism
Anesthetics	Calcium
Desflurane, sevoflurane, enflurane and	Carbamazepine
isoflurane > halothane > nitrous	Phenytoin
oxide	Steroids (chronic administration)
Antibiotics	Theophylline
Aminoglycosides, polymyxins,	Anticholinesterases*
clindamycin, vancomycin	Neostigmine, pyridostigmine,
Magnesium sulfate	edrophonium, echothiophate
Antiarrhythmics	ophthalmic solution
Quinidine, procainamide, bretylium, and	Caffeine
possibly lidocaine	Azathioprine
Diuretics	
Furosemide, mannitol	
Amphotericin B (secondary to hypokalemia)	
Local anesthetics	
Dantrolene (directly depresses skeletal muscle)	
Beta blockers	
Calcium channel blockers	
Ketamine	
Lithium	
Succinylcholine (when administered prior to nondepolarizing neuromuscular-blocking agent)	
Cyclosporine	

*Can prolong the effects of acetylcholine

Stability Stable for 5 days at room temperature when reconstituted with bacteriostatic water; stable for 24 hours at room temperature when reconstituted with preservative free sterile water (avoid preservatives in neonates); do not mix with alkaline drugs; compatible with dextrose, NS, or LR

Mechanism of Action Nondepolarizing neuromuscular blocker which blocks acetylcholine from binding to receptors on motor endplate thus inhibiting depolarization

Pharmacodynamics
Onset of effects: Within 1-3 minutes
Duration of effect (dose dependent): 30-40 minutes

Pharmacokinetics
Distribution: V_d: 300-400 mL/kg
Protein binding: 60% to 80%
Half-life, distribution: Adults: 4 minutes
Half-life, elimination: Adults: 65-75 minutes
Elimination: Vecuronium bromide and its metabolite(s) appear to be excreted principally in feces via biliary elimination; the drug and its metabolite(s) are also excreted in urine; the rate of elimination is appreciably reduced with hepatic dysfunction but not with renal dysfunction

(Continued)

Vecuronium (Continued)

Usual Dosage I.V.:
Neonates: 0.1 mg/kg/dose; maintenance: 0.03-0.15 mg/kg/dose every 1-2 hours as needed

Infants >7 weeks to 1 year: Initial: 0.08-0.1 mg/kg/dose; maintenance: 0.05-0.1 mg/kg/dose every hour as needed

Children >1 year and Adults: Initial: 0.08-0.1 mg/kg/dose; maintenance: 0.05-0.1 mg/kg every hour as needed; may be administered as a continuous infusion at 0.8-1.2 mcg/kg/minute (0.05-0.07 mg/kg/hour)

Note: Young children (1-9 years) may require slightly higher initial doses and slightly more frequent supplementation

Dosing adjustment in hepatic impairment: Dose reductions are necessary in patients with cirrhosis or cholestasis

Administration Parenteral: I.V.: Dilute vial to a maximum concentration of 2 mg/mL and administer by rapid direct injection; for continuous infusion, dilute to a maximum concentration of 1 mg/mL

Monitoring Parameters Assisted ventilation status, heart rate, blood pressure, peripheral nerve stimulator measuring twitch response

Nursing Implications Does not alter the patient's state of consciousness; addition of sedation and analgesia is recommended

Additional Information Produces minimal, if any, histamine release

Dosage Forms Powder for injection, as bromide: 10 mg (5 mL, 10 mL)

- **Vecuronium Bromide** see Vecuronium on page 972
- **Veetids®** see Penicillin V Potassium on page 743
- **Velban®** see Vinblastine on page 978
- **Velbe® (Canada)** see Vinblastine on page 978
- **Velosef®** see Cephradine on page 200
- **Velosulin®** see Insulin Preparations on page 518
- **Velosulin® BR Human (Buffered)** see Insulin Preparations on page 518
- **Velsar®** see Vinblastine on page 978
- **Veltane® Tablet** see Brompheniramine on page 142
- **Venoglobulin®-S** see Immune Globulin, Intravenous on page 510
- **Ventolin®** see Albuterol on page 40
- **Ventolin® Rotocaps®** see Albuterol on page 40
- **VePesid®** see Etoposide on page 397

Verapamil (ver AP a mil)

Related Information
Adult ACLS Algorithm, Tachycardia on page 1010

Brand Names Apo®-Verap (Canada); Calan®; Calan® SR; Covera-HS®; Isoptin®; Isoptin® SR; Novo-Veramil® (Canada); Nu-Verap® (Canada); Verelan®; Verelan® PM

Available Salts Verapamil Hydrochloride

Synonyms Iproveratril

Therapeutic Category Antianginal Agent; Antiarrhythmic Agent, Class IV; Antihypertensive Agent; Calcium Channel Blocker

Generic Available Yes

Use Angina, hypertension; I.V. for supraventricular tachyarrhythmias (PSVT, atrial fibrillation, atrial flutter)

Pregnancy Risk Factor C

Contraindications Sinus bradycardia; advanced heart block; ventricular tachycardia; cardiogenic shock; hypersensitivity to verapamil or any component; atrial fibrillation or flutter associated with accessory conduction pathways

Warnings Avoid I.V. use in neonates and young infants due to severe apnea, bradycardia, hypotensive reactions, and cardiac arrest; monitor EKG and blood pressure closely in patients receiving I.V. therapy; have I.V. calcium chloride 10 mg/kg available at bedside to treat hypotension

I.V. administration, hypertrophic cardiomyopathy, sick sinus syndrome, moderate to severe CHF, concomitant therapy with beta-blockers or digoxin can all increase the incidence of adverse effects

Precautions Use with caution in patients with sick sinus syndrome, severe left ventricular dysfunction, hepatic or renal impairment, hypertrophic cardiomyopathy (especially obstructive), concomitant therapy with beta-blockers or digoxin; reduce dose in patients with severe renal dysfunction

Adverse Reactions

Cardiovascular: Hypotension, bradycardia; first, second, or third degree A-V block, worsening heart failure

Central nervous system: Dizziness, fatigue, seizures (occasionally with I.V. use), headache

Gastrointestinal: Constipation, nausea, abdominal discomfort

Hepatic: Elevated hepatic enzymes

Respiratory: May precipitate insufficiency of respiratory muscle function in Duchenne muscular dystrophy

Drug Interactions Cytochrome P-450 isoenzyme CYP1A2 and CYP3A3/4 substrate; CYP3A3/4 isoenzyme inhibitor

Increased cardiovascular adverse effects with beta-adrenergic blocking agents, digoxin, quinidine, and disopyramide. Verapamil may increase serum concentrations of caffeine, ethanol, digoxin, quinidine, carbamazepine, and cyclosporine necessitating a decrease in dosage. Phenobarbital and rifampin may decrease verapamil serum concentrations by increasing hepatic metabolism. Avoid combination with disopyramide, discontinue disopyramide 48 hours before starting therapy, do not restart until 24 hours after verapamil has been discontinued.

Food Interactions Sprinkling contents of capsule onto food does not affect oral absorption

Stability Store injection at room temperature; protect from heat and from freezing; use only clear solutions; compatible in solutions of pH of 3-6, but may precipitate in solutions having a pH ≥ 6

Mechanism of Action Inhibits calcium ion from entering the "slow channels" or select voltage-sensitive areas of vascular smooth muscle and myocardium during depolarization; produces a relaxation of coronary vascular smooth muscle and coronary vasodilation; increases myocardial oxygen delivery in patients with vasospastic angina

Pharmacodynamics

Peak effects:
Oral (nonsustained tablets): 2 hours
I.V.: 1-5 minutes
Duration:
Oral: 6-8 hours
I.V.: 10-20 minutes

Pharmacokinetics

Protein binding:
Neonates: ~60%
Adults: 90%

Metabolism: Extensive first-pass effect, metabolized in the liver to several inactive dealkylated metabolites; major metabolite is norverapamil which possesses weak hemodynamic effects

Bioavailability: Oral: 20% to 30%

Half-life:
Infants: 4.4-6.9 hours
Adults (single dose): 2-8 hours, increased up to 12 hours with multiple dosing
Increased half-life with hepatic cirrhosis

Elimination: 70% of dose excreted in urine (3% to 4% as unchanged drug), and 16% in feces

Usual Dosage

Infants <1 year: I.V.: Usually not used, (see Warnings); administer with continuous EKG monitoring, have I.V. calcium available at bedside: 0.1-0.2 mg/kg (usual: 0.75-2 mg/dose) may repeat dose in 30 minutes if adequate response not achieved

Children 1-16 years: I.V.: 0.1-0.3 mg/kg/dose; maximum dose: 5 mg/dose; may repeat dose in 30 minutes if adequate response not achieved; maximum for second dose: 10 mg/dose

Children: Oral (dose not well established):
4-8 mg/kg/day in 3 divided doses
or
1-5 years: 40-80 mg every 8 hours
>5 years: 80 mg every 6-8 hours

Note: A mean daily dose of ~5 mg/kg/day (range: 2.3-8.1 mg/kg/day) was used in 22 children 15 days to 17 years of age receiving chronic oral therapy for SVT (n=20) or hypertrophic cardiomyopathy (n=2) (Piovan, 1995)

Adults:
Oral: 240-480 mg/24 hours divided 3-4 times/day or divided 1-2 times/day for extended release products

(Continued)

Verapamil *(Continued)*

I.V. (1992 ACLS guidelines): PSVT (narrow complex, unresponsive to vagal maneuvers and adenosine): 2.5-5 mg; if no response in 15-30 minutes and no adverse effects seen, give 5-10 mg every 15-30 minutes to a maximum total dose of 20 mg

I.V.: 5-10 mg (0.075-0.15 mg/kg); may repeat 10 mg (0.15 mg/kg) 15-30 minutes after the initial dose if needed and if patient tolerated initial dose

I.V. continuous infusion: Loading dose: 5-10 mg; may repeat in 30 minutes if adequate response is not achieved; follow with continuous infusion: 5 mg/hour; titrate dose to ventricular rate; usual: 5-10 mg/hour; range: 4-24 mg/hour.
Note: Previously recommended doses of 0.005 mg/kg/minute (5 mcg/kg/minute) will result in doses of ~20 mg/hour and may produce adverse effects such as hypotension; lower infusion rates (5-10 mg/hour) are effective in most adult patients.

Dosing adjustment in renal impairment: Children and Adults: Cl_{cr} <10 mL/minute: Administer 50% to 75% of normal dose

Administration

Oral: Nonsustained-release tablets can be administered with or without food; administer sustained release tablet with food or milk; swallow sustained released preparations whole, do not chew or crush

Parenteral:

I.V.: Infuse I.V. dose over 2-3 minutes; infuse I.V. over 3-4 minutes if blood pressure is in the lower range of normal: Maximum concentration: 2.5 mg/mL

I.V. continuous infusion: Final concentration for administration: 0.5-2.5 mg/mL

Monitoring Parameters EKG, blood pressure, heart rate; hepatic enzymes with long-term use

Patient Information Avoid alcohol; limit caffeine

Dosage Forms

Capsule, extended release, as hydrochloride (Verelan® PM): 100 mg, 200 mg, 300 mg

Capsule, sustained release, as hydrochloride: 120 mg, 180 mg, 240 mg
Verelan®: 120 mg, 180 mg, 240 mg, 360 mg

Injection, as hydrochloride: 2.5 mg/mL (2 mL, 4 mL)
Isoptin®: 2.5 mg/mL (2 mL, 4 mL)

Tablet, as hydrochloride: 40 mg, 80 mg, 120 mg
Calan®, Isoptin®: 40 mg, 80 mg, 120 mg

Tablet, sustained release, as hydrochloride: 120 mg, 180 mg, 240 mg
Calan® SR, Isoptin® SR: 120 mg, 180 mg, 240 mg
Covera-HS®: 180 mg, 240 mg

Extemporaneous Preparations

A 50 mg/mL oral suspension may be made using twenty 80 mg verapamil tablets (regular, not sustained release), 3 mL of purified water USP, 8 mL of methylcellulose 1% and simple syrup qs ad to 32 mL; stability is 91 days under refrigeration; shake well before use (Nahata, 1997)

A 50 mg/mL oral liquid preparation made from tablets (regular, not sustained release) and 3 different vehicles (cherry syrup, a 1:1 mixture of Ora-Sweet® and Ora-Plus®, or a 1:1 mixture of Ora-Sweet® SF and Ora-Plus®) was stable for 60 days when stored in amber plastic prescription bottles in the dark at room temperature (25°C) or under refrigeration (5°C); grind seventy-five 80 mg tablets in a mortar into a fine powder; add 40 mL of the vehicle and mix well to form a uniform paste; mix while adding the vehicle in geometric proportions to **almost** 120 mL; transfer to a calibrated bottle and qsad with vehicle to make 120 mL; label "shake well" and "protect from light" (Allen, 1996).

Allen LV and Erickson MA, "Stability of Labetalol Hydrochloride, Metoprolol Tartrate, Verapamil Hydrochloride, and Spironolactone With Hydrochlorothiazide in Extemporaneously Compounded Oral Liquids," *Am J Health Syst Pharm*, 1996, 53(19):2304-9.

Nahata MC and Hipple TF, *Pediatric Drug Formulations*, 3rd ed, Cincinnati, OH: Harvey Whitney Books Co, 1997.

References

Barbarash RA, Bauman JL, Lukazewski AA, et al, "Verapamil Infusions in the Treatment of Atrial Tachyarrhythmias," *Crit Care Med*, 1986, 14(10):886-8.

Emergency Cardiac Care Committee and Subcommittees, American Heart Association, "Guidelines for Cardiopulmonary Resuscitation and Emergency Cardiac Care, III: Adult Advanced Cardiac Life Support" and "VI: Pediatric Advanced Life Support," *JAMA*, 1992, 268(16):2199-241 and 2262-75.

Piovan D, Padrini R, Svalato Moreolo G, et al, "Verapamil and Norverapamil Plasma Levels in Infants and Children During Chronic Oral Treatment," *Ther Drug Monit*, 1995, 17(1):60-7.

Sapire DW, O'Riordan AC, and Black IF, "Safety and Efficacy of Short- and Long-Term Verapamil Therapy in Children With Tachycardia," *Am J Cardiol*, 1981, 48(6):1091-7.

Shakibi JG, "Arrhythmias in Infants and Children," *Pediatrician*, 1981, 10(1-3):117-22.

- **Verapamil Hydrochloride** *see* Verapamil *on page 974*
- **Verazinc®** [OTC] *see* Zinc Supplements *on page 994*
- **Verelan®** *see* Verapamil *on page 974*
- **Verelan® PM** *see* Verapamil *on page 974*
- **Vergogel® Gel** [OTC] *see* Salicylic Acid *on page 854*
- **Vergon®** [OTC] *see* Meclizine *on page 597*
- **Vermizine®** *see* Piperazine *on page 775*
- **Vermox®** *see* Mebendazole *on page 594*
- **Versed®** *see* Midazolam *on page 643*
- **Versel™ (Canada)** *see* Selenium Sulfide *on page 864*
- **Versiclear™** *see* Sodium Thiosulfate *on page 875*
- **Vibramycin®** *see* Doxycycline *on page 348*
- **Vibra-Tabs®** *see* Doxycycline *on page 348*
- **Vick's®** *see* Brompheniramine and Phenylpropanolamine *on page 143*
- **Vicks® 44E** [OTC] *see* Guaifenesin and Dextromethorphan *on page 466*
- **Vick's Children's Chloraseptic®** [OTC] *see* Benzocaine *on page 124*
- **Vick's Chloraseptic® Sore Throat** [OTC] *see* Benzocaine *on page 124*
- **Vicks Formula 44®** [OTC] *see* Dextromethorphan *on page 304*
- **Vicks Formula 44® Pediatric Formula** [OTC] *see* Dextromethorphan *on page 304*
- **Vicks® Pediatric Formula 44E** [OTC] *see* Guaifenesin and Dextromethorphan *on page 466*
- **Vicks® Sinex® Nasal Solution** [OTC] *see* Phenylephrine *on page 758*
- **Vicodin®** *see* Hydrocodone and Acetaminophen *on page 485*
- **Vicodin® ES** *see* Hydrocodone and Acetaminophen *on page 485*

Vidarabine (vye DARE a been)

Brand Names Vira-A®

Synonyms Adenine Arabinoside; Ara-A; Arabinofuranosyladenine

Therapeutic Category Antiviral Agent, Ophthalmic

Generic Available No

Use Treatment of acute keratoconjunctivitis and epithelial keratitis due to herpes simplex virus

Pregnancy Risk Factor C

Contraindications Hypersensitivity to vidarabine or any component; concurrent application of a corticosteroid in the treatment of herpes simplex keratitis

Warnings Vidarabine is potentially mutagenic, teratogenic, and oncogenic

Adverse Reactions Ocular: Keratitis, photophobia, lacrimation, foreign body sensation, uveitis, stromal edema, blurred vision, burning

Stability Store at room temperature; avoid freezing

Mechanism of Action Inhibits viral DNA synthesis by blocking DNA polymerase or virus-induced ribonucleotide reductase

Pharmacokinetics

Absorption: Systemic absorption is not expected to occur following ophthalmic use

Distribution: Trace amounts detected in the aqueous humor if there is an epithelial defect in the cornea

Protein binding:

Vidarabine: 20% to 30%

Ara-hypoxanthine: 0% to 3%

Elimination: Following administration, rapidly deaminated by red cell adenosine deaminase to ara-hypoxanthine (active); excreted in urine as vidarabine (1% to 3%) and the active metabolite (40% to 53%)

Usual Dosage

Children and Adults: Ophthalmic: Keratoconjunctivitis: Apply ½" of ointment in lower conjunctival sac 5 times/day every 3 hours while awake until complete re-epithelialization has occurred, then twice daily for an additional 7 days

Administration Ophthalmic: Instill 1 cm of ointment in lower conjunctival sac of the affected eye; avoid contact of tube tip with skin or eye

Patient Information Ophthalmic ointment may cause sensitivity to bright light; minimize light sensitivity by wearing sunglasses

Dosage Forms

Injection, suspension: 200 mg/mL [base 187.4 mg] (5 mL) **Withdrawn From Market**

Ointment, ophthalmic, as monohydrate: 3% [30 mg/mL = 28 mg/mL base] (3.5 g)

- **Videx® Oral** *see* Didanosine *on page 315*

Vinblastine (vin BLAS teen)

Related Information
Emetogenic Potential of Single Chemotherapeutic Agents *on page 1095*
Extravasation Treatment *on page 1050*

Brand Names Alkaban-AQ®; Velban®; Velbe® (Canada); Velsar®

Available Salts Vinblastine Sulfate

Synonyms Vincaleukoblastine; VLB

Therapeutic Category Antineoplastic Agent, Mitotic Inhibitor

Generic Available Yes

Use Palliative treatment of Hodgkin's disease; advanced testicular germinal-cell cancers; non-Hodgkin's lymphoma, histiocytosis, and choriocarcinoma

Pregnancy Risk Factor D

Contraindications Hypersensitivity to vinblastine or any component; severe leukopenia

Warnings The FDA currently recommends that procedures for proper handling and disposal of antineoplastic agents be considered; vinblastine may cause fetal toxicity when administered to pregnant women; for I.V. use only; **intrathecal administration may result in death**

Precautions Avoid extravasation; dosage modification required in patients with impaired liver function or neurotoxicity; dosage should be reduced in patients with recent exposure to radiation therapy or chemotherapy

Adverse Reactions
Cardiovascular: Tachycardia, orthostatic hypotension
Central nervous system: Depression, malaise, seizures, headache
Dermatologic: Rashes, mild alopecia, photosensitivity
Endocrine & metabolic: Hyperuricemia
Gastrointestinal: Nausea, hemorrhagic enterocolitis, vomiting, constipation, abdominal pain, paralytic ileus, stomatitis
Genitourinary: Urinary retention
Hematologic: Myelosuppression: Leukopenia (nadir: 4-10 days), thrombocytopenia
Local: Severe tissue burn if infiltrated
Neuromuscular & skeletal: Jaw pain, myalgia, peripheral neuropathy, paresthesia

Drug Interactions Concomitant administration with mitomycin has resulted in severe bronchospasm and shortness of breath; may decrease serum phenytoin concentrations

Stability Store in refrigerator; 1 mg/mL solutions prepared with preserved NS injection is stable for 30 days when refrigerated and protected from light

Mechanism of Action Binds to microtubular protein of the mitotic spindle causing metaphase arrest

Pharmacokinetics
Distribution: Poor penetration into CSF; rapidly distributed into body tissues; V_{dss}: 27.3 L/kg
Protein binding: 75%
Metabolism: Extensive in the liver to a more active metabolite
Half-life, terminal: 24 hours
Elimination: Biliary excretion (95%)

Usual Dosage Vinblastine may be administered at intervals of every 7 days or greater and only after leukocyte count has returned to at least 4000/mm³; maintenance therapy should be titrated according to leukocyte count

I.V. (refer to individual protocols):
Children:
Hodgkin's disease: 2.5-6 mg/m²/day once every 1-2 weeks for 3-6 weeks; maximum weekly dose: 12.5 mg/m²
Histiocytosis: 0.4 mg/kg once ever 7-10 days
Germ cell tumor: 0.2 mg/kg on days 1 and 2 of cycle every 3 weeks times 4 cycles
Adults: 3.7-18.5 mg/m²/day every 7-10 days or 0.1-0.5 mg/kg/day once weekly or 1.4-1.8 mg/m²/day for 5 days given as an I.V. continuous infusion

Dosing adjustment in hepatic impairment: Children and Adults: Direct serum bilirubin concentration >3 mg/dL: Reduce dose 50%

Administration Parenteral: **Do not administer intrathecally, death may occur**; do not administer I.M. or S.C. since the drug is very irritating; may be administered IVP directly into the vein or through a Y-site of a freely running I.V. over a 1-minute period at a concentration for administration of 1 mg/mL; I.V. continuous infusion: Each day's dose may be diluted in 1000 mL of D_5W or NS; administer over 24 hours

Monitoring Parameters CBC with differential and platelet count, serum uric acid, hepatic function tests

Patient Information Report to physician any fever, sore throat, bleeding, or bruising; avoid contact with the eyes since the drug is very irritating and corneal ulceration may result

Nursing Implications Maintain adequate hydration. Allopurinol may be given to prevent uric acid nephropathy; stool softeners may be helpful in preventing constipation; vinblastine is a tissue irritant and can cause sloughing upon extravasation; check vein patency before drug administration; care should be taken to avoid extravasation. If extravasation occurs, local injection of hyaluronidase into the leading edge of the extravasation site and a warm compress can be used for treatment; apply warm pack immediately for 30-60 minutes, then alternate off/on every 15 minutes for 1 day. Refer to Extravasation Treatment *on page 1050.*

Additional Information Myelosuppressive effects:
Nadir (days): 4-10
Recovery (days): 7-14

Dosage Forms
Injection, as sulfate: 1 mg/mL (10 mL)
Powder for injection, as sulfate: 10 mg

References

Balis FM, Holcenberg JS and Bleyer WA, "Clinical Pharmacokinetics of Commonly Used Anticancer Drugs," *Clin Pharmacokinet*, 1983, 8(3):202-32.

Crom WR, Glynn-Barnhart AM, Rodman JH, et al, "Pharmacokinetics of Anticancer Drugs in Children," *Clin Pharmacokinet*, 1987, 12(3):168-213.

Tannock I, Ehrlichman C, Perrault D, et al, "Failure of 5-Day Vinblastine Infusion in the Treatment of Patients With Advanced Refractory Breast Cancer," *Cancer Treat Rep*, 1982, 66(9):1783-4.

Yap HY, Blumenschein GR, Keating MJ, et al, "Vinblastine Given as a Continuous 5-Day Infusion in the Treatment of Refractory Breast Cancer," *Cancer Treat Rep*, 1980, 64(2-3):279-83.

♦ **Vinblastine Sulfate** *see* Vinblastine *on page 978*
♦ **Vincaleukoblastine** *see* Vinblastine *on page 978*
♦ **Vincasar® PFS** *see* Vincristine *on page 979*

Vincristine (vin KRIS teen)

Related Information
Emetogenic Potential of Single Chemotherapeutic Agents *on page 1095*
Extravasation Treatment *on page 1050*

Brand Names Oncovin®; Vincasar® PFS

Available Salts Vincristine Sulfate

Synonyms LCR; Leurocristine; VCR

Therapeutic Category Antineoplastic Agent, Mitotic Inhibitor

Generic Available Yes

Use Treatment of leukemias, Hodgkin's disease, neuroblastoma, malignant lymphomas, Wilms' tumor, and rhabdomyosarcoma

Pregnancy Risk Factor D

Contraindications Hypersensitivity to vincristine or any component; patients with demyelinating form of Charcot-Marie-Tooth syndrome

Warnings The FDA currently recommends that procedures for proper handling and disposal of antineoplastic agents be considered; vincristine may cause fetal toxicity when administered to pregnant women; for I.V. use only; **intrathecal administration may result in death.**

Precautions Dosage modification required in patients with impaired hepatic function, patients receiving other neurotoxic drugs, or patients with pre-existing neuromuscular disease; avoid extravasation

Adverse Reactions
Cardiovascular: Orthostatic hypotension
Central nervous system: Neurotoxicity, seizures, CNS depression, cranial nerve paralysis
Dermatologic: Alopecia, rash
Endocrine & metabolic: Hyperuricemia, SIADH
Gastrointestinal: Constipation, paralytic ileus, nausea, vomiting, diarrhea, stomatitis
Local: Pain, cellulitis and tissue necrosis if infiltrated, phlebitis
Neuromuscular & skeletal: Jaw pain, leg pain, myalgia, numbness, motor difficulties, cramping, weakness
Respiratory: Dyspnea

Drug Interactions Asparaginase may decrease vincristine clearance; acute pulmonary reactions may occur with concomitant use of mitomycin C

Stability Store in refrigerator; injectable solution is stable for 1 month at room temperature
(Continued)

Vincristine *(Continued)*

Mechanism of Action Binds to microtubular protein of the mitotic spindle causing metaphase arrest

Pharmacokinetics

Distribution: Poor penetration into the CSF; V_{dss}: 120 L/m^2

Protein binding: 75%

Metabolism: Extensive in the liver

Half-life, terminal: 24 hours

Elimination: Primarily in bile (~80%)

Clearance:

Infants: Vincristine clearance is more closely related to body weight than to body surface area

Children 2-18 years: 482 mL/minute/m^2 (faster clearance in children <10 years of age than in adolescents)

Usual Dosage I.V. (refer to individual protocols):

Children ≤10 kg or BSA <1 m^2: Initial therapy: 0.05 mg/kg once weekly then titrate dose; maximum single dose: 2 mg

Children >10 kg or BSA ≥1 m^2: 1-2 mg/m^2, may repeat once weekly for 3-6 weeks; maximum single dose: 2 mg

Neuroblastoma: I.V. continuous infusion with doxorubicin: 1 mg/m^2/day for 72 hours

Adults: 0.4-1.4 mg/m^2 up to 2 mg; may repeat every week

Dosing adjustment in hepatic impairment: Children and Adults: Direct serum bilirubin concentration >3 mg/dL: Dosage reduction of 50% is recommended

Administration Parenteral: **Do not administer intrathecally, death may occur**; do not administer I.M. or S.C. since the drug is very irritating; I.V.: Vincristine is administered IVP or through a Y-site of a freely running I.V. over a period of 1 minute at a concentration for administration of 1 mg/mL; may administer as a dilute I.V. infusion

Monitoring Parameters Serum electrolytes (sodium), hepatic function tests, neurologic examination, CBC, hemoglobin, serum uric acid

Patient Information Stool softener should be used for constipation prophylaxis; report to physician any fever, sore throat, bleeding, bruising, or shortness of breath

Nursing Implications Maintain adequate hydration. Allopurinol may be given to prevent uric acid nephropathy; vincristine is a tissue irritant; care should be taken to avoid extravasation. If extravasation occurs, local injection of hyaluronidase into the leading edge of the extravasation site and a warm compress can be used for treatment; apply warm pack immediately for 30-60 minutes, then alternate off/on every 15 minutes for 1 day; refer to Extravasation Treatment *on page 1050*. Avoid contact with the eye since vincristine is very irritating.

Dosage Forms Injection, as sulfate: 1 mg/mL (1 mL, 2 mL, 5 mL)

References

Crom WR, deGraaf SS, Synold T, et al, "Pharmacokinetics of Vincristine in Children and Adolescents With Acute Lymphocytic Leukemia," *J Pediatr*, 1994, 125(4):642-9.

Woods WG, O'Leary M, and Nesbit ME, "Life-Threatening Neuropathy and Hepatotoxicity in Infants During Induction Therapy for Acute Lymphoblastic Leukemia," *J Pediatr*, 1981, 98(4):642-5.

Vitamin A (VYE ta min aye)

Related Information
Carbohydrate and Alcohol Content of Liquid Medications for Use in Patients Receiving Ketogenic Diets *on page 1228*

Brand Names Aquasol A® [OTC]; Del-Vi-A®; Palmitate-A® 5000 [OTC]

Synonyms Oleovitamin A

Therapeutic Category Nutritional Supplement; Vitamin, Fat Soluble

Generic Available Yes

Use Treatment and prevention of vitamin A deficiency; supplementation in children 6 months to 2 years with measles

Pregnancy Risk Factor A (X if dose exceeds RDA recommendation)

Contraindications Hypervitaminosis A; hypersensitivity to vitamin A or any component

Warnings Patients receiving >25,000 units/day should be closely monitored for toxicity

Adverse Reactions Seen only with doses exceeding physiologic replacement
Central nervous system: Irritability, drowsiness, vertigo, delirium, headache, coma, increased intracranial pressure
Dermatologic: Erythema, peeling skin
Gastrointestinal: Vomiting, diarrhea
Ocular: Visual disturbances, papilledema

Drug Interactions Cholestyramine decreases absorption of vitamin A; neomycin and mineral oil may also interfere with vitamin A absorption; retinoids may have additive adverse effects; enhances hypoprothrombinemic effects of warfarin

Stability Protect injectable preparation from light

Mechanism of Action Needed for bone development, growth, visual adaptation to darkness, testicular and ovarian function, and as a cofactor in many biochemical processes

Pharmacokinetics
Absorption: Vitamin A in dosages **not** exceeding physiologic replacement is well absorbed after oral administration; water miscible preparations are absorbed more rapidly than oil preparations; large oral doses, conditions of fat malabsorption, low protein intake, or hepatic or pancreatic disease reduce oral absorption
Metabolism: Conjugated with glucuronide, undergoes enterohepatic circulation
Elimination: In feces via biliary elimination

Usual Dosage Recommended daily allowance (RDA):
<1 year: 375 mcg* (1250 units)
1-3 years: 400 mcg* (1330 units)
4-6 years: 500 mcg* (1670 units)
7-10 years: 700 mcg* (2330 units)
>10 years: Female: 800 mcg* (2670 units); Male: 1000 mcg* (3330 units)
*mcg retinol equivalent (0.3 mcg retinol = 1 unit vitamin A)
Daily dietary supplement: Oral:
Infants up to 6 months: 1500 units
Children:
6 months to 3 years: 1500-2000 units
4-6 years: 2500 units
7-10 years: 3300-3500 units
Children >10 years and Adults: 4000-5000 units
Vitamin A supplementation in measles (recommendation of the World Health Organization): Children: Oral: Give as a single dose; repeat the next day and at 4 weeks for children with ophthalmologic evidence of vitamin A deficiency:
6 months to 1 year: 100,000 units
>1 year: 200,000 units
Note: Use of vitamin A in measles is recommended only for patients 6 months to 2 years of age hospitalized with measles and its complications **or** patients >6 months of age who have any of the following risk factors and who are not already receiving vitamin A: immunodeficiency, ophthalmologic evidence of vitamin A deficiency including night blindness, Bitot's spots or evidence of xerophthalmia, impaired intestinal absorption, moderate to severe malnutrition including that associated with eating disorders, or recent immigration from areas where high mortality rates from measles have been observed
Note: Monitor patients closely; dosages >25,000 units/kg have been associated with toxicity
Vitamin A deficiency (varying recommendations available):
Severe deficiency with xerophthalmia:
Children 1-8 years: Oral: 5000 units/kg/day for 5 days or until recovery occurs; I.M.: 5000-15,000 units/day for 10 days

(Continued)

Vitamin A *(Continued)*

Children >8 years and Adults: Oral: 500,000 units/day for 3 days, then 50,000 units/day for 14 days; then 10,000-20,000 units/day for 2 months; I.M.: 50,000-100,000 units/day for 3 days; then 50,000 units/day for 14 days

Prophylactic therapy for children at risk for developing deficiency: Oral given every 4-6 months:

Infants ≤1 year: 100,000 units

Children >1 year: 200,000 units

Malabsorption syndrome (prophylaxis): Children >8 years and Adults: Oral: 10,000-50,000 units/day of water miscible product

Administration

Oral: Administer with food or milk

Parenteral: I.M. only

Additional Information 1 USP vitamin A unit = 0.3 mcg of all-*trans* isomer of retinol; 1 RE (retinol equivalent) = 1 mcg of all-*trans*-retinol

Dosage Forms

Capsule: 10,000 units, 25,000 units, 50,000 units

Drops, oral (water miscible): 5000 units/0.1 mL (30 mL)

Injection: 50,000 units/mL (2 mL)

Tablet: 5000 units

References

Committee on Infectious Diseases, "Vitamin A in the Treatment of Measles," *Pediatrics*, 1993, 91(5):1014-5.

DeMaeyer EM, "The WHO Programme of Prevention and Control of Vitamin A Deficiency, Xerophthalmia, and Nutritional Blindness," *Nutr Health*, 1986, 4(2):105-12.

Hussey GD and Klein M, "A Randomized, Controlled Trial of Vitamin A in Children With Severe Measles," *N Engl J Med*, 1990, 323(3):160-4.

♦ **Vitamin A Acid** *see* Tretinoin *on page 945*

♦ **Vitamin B₁** *see* Thiamine *on page 916*

♦ **Vitamin B₂** *see* Riboflavin *on page 844*

♦ **Vitamin B₃** *see* Niacin *on page 685*

♦ **Vitamin B₆** *see* Pyridoxine *on page 827*

♦ **Vitamin B₁₂** *see* Cyanocobalamin *on page 263*

♦ **Vitamin B₁₂** *see* Hydroxocobalamin *on page 492*

♦ **Vitamin C** *see* Ascorbic Acid *on page 96*

♦ **Vitamin C Drops [OTC]** *see* Ascorbic Acid *on page 96*

♦ **Vitamin D₂** *see* Ergocalciferol *on page 377*

Vitamin E *(VYE ta min ee)*

Related Information

Carbohydrate and Alcohol Content of Liquid Medications for Use in Patients Receiving Ketogenic Diets *on page 1228*

Brand Names Amino-Opti-E® [OTC]; Aquasol E® Oral [OTC]; E-Complex-600® [OTC]; E-Vitamin® [OTC]; Softgels® [OTC]; Vita-Plus® E; Vitec® Topical [OTC]; Vite E® Creme [OTC]

Synonyms *d*-Alpha Tocopherol; *dl*-Alpha Tocopherol

Therapeutic Category Nutritional Supplement; Vitamin, Fat Soluble; Vitamin, Topical

Generic Available Yes

Use Prevention and treatment of vitamin E deficiency

Pregnancy Risk Factor A (C if dose exceeds RDA recommendation)

Contraindications Hypersensitivity to vitamin E or any component

Warnings Necrotizing enterocolitis has been associated with oral administration of large dosages (eg, >200 units/day) of a hyperosmolar vitamin E preparation in low birth weight infants

Adverse Reactions

Central nervous system: Headache

Dermatologic: Rash

Endocrine & metabolic: Gonadal dysfunction; decreased serum thyroxine and triiodothyronine; increased cholesterol and triglycerides

Gastrointestinal: Nausea, diarrhea, intestinal cramps, necrotizing enterocolitis (see Warnings)

Neuromuscular & skeletal: Weakness

Ocular: Blurred vision

Renal: Creatinuria and increased serum creatinine kinase; increased urinary estrogens and androgens

Drug Interactions Iron, mineral oil, warfarin

Mechanism of Action Antioxidant which prevents oxidation of vitamin A and C; protects polyunsaturated fatty acids in membranes from attack by free radicals and protects red blood cells against hemolysis by oxidizing agents

Pharmacokinetics

Absorption: Oral: Depends upon the presence of bile; absorption is reduced in conditions of malabsorption, in low birth weight premature infants, and as dosage increases; water miscible preparations are better absorbed than oil preparations

Metabolism: In the liver to glucuronides

Elimination: Primarily in bile

Usual Dosage 1 unit vitamin E = 1 mg dl-alpha-tocopherol acetate. Oral:

Vitamin E - Recommended Daily Allowance (RDA) and Estimated Average Requirement (EAR)

Age	RDA (mg/day)	EAR (mg/day)
0-6 mo	–	4* (6 units)
7-12 mo	–	6* (9 units)
1-3 y	6 (9 units)	5 (7.5 units)
4-8 y	7 (10.5 units)	6 (9 units)
9-13 y	11 (16.5 units)	9 (13.5 units)
≥14 y	15 (22.5 units)	12 (18 units)

*Adequate intake (AI)

Vitamin E deficiency:

Neonates, premature, low birth weight: 25-50 units/day results in normal levels within 1 week

Children (with malabsorption syndrome): 1 unit/kg/day of water miscible vitamin E (to raise plasma tocopherol concentrations to the normal range within 2 months and to maintain normal plasma concentrations)

Adults: 60-75 units/day

Prevention of vitamin E deficiency:

Neonates:

Low birth weight: 5 units/day

Full-term: 5 units/L of formula ingested

Adults: 30 units/day

Prevention of retinopathy of prematurity or BPD secondary to O_2 therapy: Neonates and Infants: (American Academy of Pediatrics considers this use investigational and routine use is not recommended): 15-30 units/kg/day to maintain plasma levels between 1.5-2 mcg/mL (may need as high as 100 units/kg/day)

Cystic fibrosis, beta-thalassemia, sickle cell anemia may require higher daily maintenance doses: Infants, Children, and Adolescents:

Cystic fibrosis: 100-400 units/day

Beta-thalassemia: 750 units/day

Sickle cell: 450 units/day

Topical: Apply a thin layer over affected area

Administration Oral: May administer with or without food

Monitoring Parameters Plasma tocopherol concentrations

Reference Range Plasma tocopherol: 6-14 µg/mL

Dosage Forms

Capsule: 100 units, 200 units, 330 units, 400 units, 500 units, 600 units, 1000 units

Capsule, water miscible: 73.5 mg, 147 mg, 165 mg, 330 mg, 400 units

Cream: 50 mg/g (15 g, 30 g, 60 g, 75 g, 120 g, 454 g)

Drops, oral: 50 mg/mL (12 mL, 30 mL)

Liquid, topical: 10 mL, 15 mL, 30 mL, 60 mL Lotion: 120 mL

Oil: 15 mL, 30 mL, 60 mL

Ointment, topical: 30 mg/g (45 g, 60 g)

Tablet: 200 units, 400 units

References

American Academy of Pediatrics Committee on Fetus and Newborn, "Vitamin E and the Prevention of Retinopathy of Prematurity," Pediatrics, 1985, 76(2):315-6.

♦ **Vitamin G** see Riboflavin on page 844

♦ **Vitamin K₁** see Phytonadione on page 769

♦ **Vitamins, Multiple** see page 1034

♦ **Vita-Plus® E** see Vitamin E on page 982

♦ **Vitec® Topical [OTC]** see Vitamin E on page 982

- **Vite E® Creme [OTC]** *see* Vitamin E *on page 982*
- **Vitinoin™ (Canada)** *see* Tretinoin *on page 945*
- **Vito Reins® (Canada)** *see* Phenazopyridine *on page 753*
- **Vivelle® Transdermal** *see* Estradiol *on page 386*
- **Vivol® (Canada)** *see* Diazepam *on page 307*
- **V-Lax® [OTC]** *see* Psyllium *on page 823*
- **VLB** *see* Vinblastine *on page 978*
- **Volmax®** *see* Albuterol *on page 40*
- **Volmax® (Canada)** *see* Albuterol *on page 40*
- **Voltaren® Ophthalmic** *see* Diclofenac *on page 312*
- **Voltaren® Oral** *see* Diclofenac *on page 312*
- **Voltaren®-XR Oral** *see* Diclofenac *on page 312*
- **VP-16** *see* Etoposide *on page 397*
- **VP-16-213** *see* Etoposide *on page 397*
- **VPA** *see* Valproic Acid and Derivatives *on page 966*

Warfarin (WAR far in)

Related Information
Adult ACLS Algorithm, Tachycardia *on page 1010*
Overdose and Toxicology *on page 1191*

Brand Names Coumadin®; Warfilone® (Canada)

Available Salts Warfarin Sodium

Therapeutic Category Anticoagulant

Generic Available Yes

Use Prophylaxis and treatment of venous thromboembolic disorders; prevention of arterial thromboembolism in patients with prosthetic heart valves or atrial fibrillation; prevention of death, venous thromboembolism, and recurrent MI after acute MI

Pregnancy Risk Factor D

Contraindications Hypersensitivity to warfarin or any component; severe liver or kidney disease; open wounds; uncontrolled bleeding; GI ulcers; neurosurgical procedures; malignant hypertension

Warnings Concomitant use with vitamin K may decrease anticoagulant effect; monitor carefully; concomitant use with ethacrynic acid, indomethacin, NSAIDs, phenylbutazone, or aspirin increases warfarin's anticoagulant effect and may cause severe GI irritation; oral anticoagulant therapy is usually avoided in neonates due to a greater potential risk of bleeding (see Michelson, 1998)

Precautions Do not switch brands once desired therapeutic response has been achieved; use with caution in patients with active tuberculosis, diabetes mellitus, or heparin-induced thrombocytopenia with deep vein thrombosis; use with caution in patients with or at risk for hemorrhage, necrosis, or gangrene

Adverse Reactions
Central nervous system: Fever
Dermatologic: Skin lesions, skin necrosis; hair loss (rare in children)
Gastrointestinal: Anorexia, nausea, vomiting, diarrhea
Hematologic: Hemorrhage
Respiratory: Hemoptysis; tracheal calcification (rare in children)

Drug Interactions Cytochrome P-450 isoenzyme CYP1A2 substrate (minor), CYP2C8, CYP2C9, CYP2C18, CYP2C19, and CYP3A3/4 isoenzyme substrate; CYP2C9 isoenzyme inhibitor
Alcohol, amiodarone, anabolic steroids, aspirin, amoxicillin, barbiturates, carbamazepine, cefaclor, chloral hydrate, chloramphenicol, chlordiazepoxide, cholestyramine, cimetidine, clofibrate, cloxacillin, co-trimoxazole, disulfiram, erythromycin, fluconazole, griseofulvin, isoniazid, ketoconazole, metronidazole, nafcillin, omeprazole, phenylbutazone, phenytoin, phenobarbital, piroxicam, prednisone, propranolol, ranitidine, rifampin, salicylates, streptokinase, sucralfate, sulfonamides, urokinase, vitamin K, zafirlukast, zileuton; ritonavir and delavirdine may decrease warfarin metabolism; concurrent use of delavirdine and warfarin is not recommended; suspected drug interaction with nevirapine (monitor closely)

Food Interactions Vitamin K can reverse the anticoagulation effects of warfarin; large amounts of food high in vitamin K (such as green leafy vegetables) may reverse warfarin, decrease prothrombin time, and lead to therapeutic failure; a balanced diet with a consistent intake of vitamin K is essential; avoid large amounts of alfalfa, asparagus, broccoli, brussel sprouts, cabbage, cauliflower, green teas, kale, lettuce, spinach, turnip greens, watercress; avoid enteral feeds high in vitamin K. **Note:** Breast-fed infants may be more sensitive to warfarin due to low amounts of vitamin K in breast milk.

High doses of vitamin A, E, or C may alter PT; use caution with fish oils or omega 3 fatty acids; avoid fried or boiled onions as they may increase drug effect by increasing fibrinolytic activity; avoid herbal teas and remedies such as tonka beans, melilot, and woodruff as they contain natural coumarins and will increase effect of warfarin; avoid large amounts of liver, avocado, soy protein, soybean oil, papain.

Stability
Tablets and injection: Protect from light
Injection: Use within 4 hours after reconstitution, do not refrigerate, discard unused portion (does not contain preservative)

Mechanism of Action Interferes with hepatic synthesis of vitamin K-dependent coagulation factors (II, VII, IX, X)

Pharmacodynamics Anticoagulation effects:
Onset of action: Within 36-72 hours
Peak effect: Within 5-7 days

Pharmacokinetics
Absorption: Oral: Rapid
Metabolism: In the liver
Half-life: 42 hours, highly variable among individuals

Usual Dosage Oral:
Infants and Children: **To maintain an International Normalized Ratio (INR) between 2-3:**
Initial loading dose on day 1 (if baseline INR is 1-1.3): 0.2 mg/kg (maximum dose: 10 mg); use initial loading dose of 0.1 mg/kg if patient has liver dysfunction
Loading dose for days 2-4: doses are dependent upon patient's INR
if INR is 1.1-1.3, repeat the initial loading dose
if INR is 1.4-1.9, give 50% of the initial loading dose
if INR is 2-3, give 50% of the initial loading dose
if INR is 3.1-3.5, give 25% of the initial loading dose
if INR is >3.5, hold the drug until INR <3.5, then restart at 50% less than the previous dose
Maintenance dose guidelines for day 5 of therapy and beyond: doses are dependent upon patient's INR
if INR is 1.1-1.4, increase dose by 20% of previous dose
if INR is 1.5-1.9, increase dose by 10% of previous dose
if INR is 2-3, do not change the dose
if INR is 3.1-3.5, decrease dose by 10% of previous dose
if INR is >3.5, hold the drug and check INR daily until INR <3.5, then restart at 20% less than the previous dose
Usual maintenance dose: ~0.1 mg/kg/day; range: 0.05-0.34 mg/kg/day; the dose in mg/kg/day is inversely related to age; in one study (Andrew, 1994), to attain an INR of 2-3, children <12 months of age required a mean dose of 0.32 mg/kg/day, but children 11-18 years required a mean dose of 0.09 mg/kg/day; to attain an INR of 1.3-1.8, children <12 months (n=2) required 0.24 and 0.27 mg/kg/day, but children >1 year required a mean of 0.08 mg/kg/day (range: 0.03-0.17 mg/kg/day); consistent anticoagulation may be difficult to maintain in children <5 years of age
Adults: 5-15 mg/day for 2-5 days, then adjust dose according to results of INR or PT; usual maintenance dose ranges from 2-10 mg/day
I.V.: (For patients who cannot take oral form): I.V. dose is equal to oral dose

Administration
Oral: May administer on an empty or full stomach
Parenteral: I.V. use only; do not administer I.M.; reconstitute 5 mg vial with 2.7 mL sterile water for injection to produce 2 mg/mL solution; administer by slow I.V. injection over 1-2 minutes into peripheral vein

Monitoring Parameters INR (preferred) or prothrombin time; hemoglobin, hematocrit, signs and symptoms of bleeding

Reference Range The INR is now the standard test used to monitor warfarin anticoagulation; the desired INR is based upon indication; due to the lack of pediatric clinical trials assessing optimal INR ranges and clinical outcomes, the desired INR ranges for children are extrapolated from adult studies; the optimal therapeutic INR ranges may possibly be lower in children versus adults. Further pediatric studies are needed (see Michelson, 1998)

An INR of 2-3 (low-intensity regimen) is recommended for most venous thrombotic diseases including prevention and treatment of DVT, prevention of stroke after
(Continued)

Warfarin *(Continued)*

acute MI, prevention of systemic embolism with atrial fibrillation, and for cardiac valve replacement with tissue valves. An INR of 2.5-3.5 is recommended for cardiac valve replacement with mechanical prosthetic valves. An INR of 3-4.5 (high-intensity regimen) is recommended in adults who are post MI to prevent recurrent MI and reduce mortality (Hirsh, 1992)

Note: If INR is not available, prothrombin time should be 1½ to 2 times the control.

Patient Information Avoid alcohol; limit caffeine; report any signs of bleeding to physician at once (eg, gums bleeding, dark brown urine, black tar-like stools); avoid hazardous activities; use soft toothbrush; carry Medi-Alert® ID identifying drug use; be aware of other drugs and foods to avoid

Nursing Implications Be aware of drug interactions and foods that contain vitamin K which can alter anticoagulant effects; avoid I.M. injections of drugs

Additional Information Usual duration of therapy: first venous thrombotic event: treat for 3 months; mechanical prosthetic heart valves: treat for life (see Michelson, 1998)

Overdoses of warfarin may be treated with vitamin K, to reverse warfarin's anticoagulation effect

Dosage Forms

Powder for injection, as sodium, lyophilized: 2 mg, 5 mg

Tablet, as sodium: 1 mg, 2 mg, 2.5 mg, 3 mg, 4 mg, 5 mg, 6 mg, 7.5 mg, 10 mg

References

Andrew M, Marzinotto V, Brooker LA, et al, "Oral Anticoagulation Therapy in Pediatric Patients: A Prospective Study," *Thromb Haemost*, 1994, 71(3):265-9.

David M and Andrew M, "Venous Thromboembolic Complications in Children," *J Pediatr*, 1993, 123(3):337-46.

Fihn SD "Aiming for Safe Anticoagulation," *N Engl J Med*, 1995, 333(1):54-5.

Hirsh J, Dalen JE, Anderson DR, et al, "Oral Anticoagulants. Mechanism of Action, Clinical Effectiveness, and Optimal Therapeutic Range," *Chest*, 1998, 114(5 Suppl):445S-69S.

Michelson AD, Bovill E, Monagle P, et al, "Antithrombotic Therapy in Children," *Chest*, 1998, 114(Suppl 5):748S-69S.

Wells PS, Holbrook AM, Crowther NR, et al, "Interactions of Warfarin With Drugs and Food," *Ann Intern Med*, 1994, 121(9):676-83.

- ◆ **Xylocard® (Canada)** *see* Lidocaine *on page 568*
- ◆ **Xylo-Pfan® [OTC]** *see* d-Xylose *on page 354*
- ◆ **Xylose** *see* d-Xylose *on page 354*
- ◆ **Yellow Fever Vaccine** *see page 1138*
- ◆ **Yodoxin®** *see* Iodoquinol *on page 526*

Zafirlukast (za FIR loo kast)

Related Information
Asthma Guidelines *on page 1178*

Brand Names Accolate®

Therapeutic Category Antiasthmatic; Leukotriene Receptor Antagonist

Use Prophylaxis and chronic treatment of asthma

Pregnancy Risk Factor B

Contraindications Hypersensitivity to zafirlukast or any component

Warnings Zafirlukast is not indicated for use in the reversal of bronchospasm in acute asthma attacks, including status asthmaticus. Therapy with zafirlukast can be continued during acute exacerbations of asthma. An increased proportion of zafirlukast patients (>55 years of age) reported infections as compared to placebo-treated patients; these infections were mostly mild or moderate in intensity, predominantly affected the respiratory tract, were dose-proportional to the total milligrams of zafirlukast exposure, and associated with coadministration of inhaled corticosteroids.

Precautions Use with caution in patients receiving warfarin (see Drug Interactions) and patients with liver disease; dosage reduction in patients with hepatic impairment may be needed

Adverse Reactions
Central nervous system: Headache, dizziness, pain, fever, asthenia
Gastrointestinal: Nausea, diarrhea, abdominal pain, vomiting, dyspepsia, xerostomia
Hepatic: Elevated enzymes, hepatitis, hyperbilirubinemia
Neuromuscular & skeletal: Myalgia, weakness
Respiratory: Rhinitis, pharyngitis
Miscellaneous: Infections (primarily respiratory), hypersensitivity reactions

Drug Interactions Cytochrome P-450 isoenzyme CYP2C9 substrate; CYP2CP and CYP3A3/4 isoenzyme inhibitor
Erythromycin, terfenadine, and theophylline decrease zafirlukast serum levels; aspirin increases plasma levels of zafirlukast; coadministration of zafirlukast with warfarin results in a clinically significant increase in prothrombin time (PT)

Food Interactions Food decreases zafirlukast absorption by 40%

Stability Store tablets at controlled room temperature; protect from light and moisture; dispense in original airtight container

Mechanism of Action Zafirlukast is a selective and competitive leukotriene-receptor antagonist (LTRA) of cysteinyl leukotrienes C_4 (LTC$_4$), D$_4$ (LTD$_4$), and E$_4$ (LTE$_4$). This activity produces inhibition of the effects of these leukotrienes on bronchial smooth muscle resulting in the attenuation of bronchoconstriction and decreased vascular permeability, mucosal edema, and mucus production.

Pharmacodynamics Asthma symptom improvement:
Duration of effect: 12 hours
Time to maximal effects: 2-6 weeks

Pharmacokinetics
Absorption: Rapid
Distribution: Extensively excreted into breast milk; breast milk to plasma ratio: 0.15
Protein binding: 99%, predominantly albumin
Metabolism: Extensively metabolized by liver via cytochrome P-450 isoenzyme CYP2C9 pathway
Half-life, elimination: 10 hours
Time to peak serum concentration: 2-4 hours
Elimination: Fecal (90%) and urine (10%)

Usual Dosage Oral:
Children 7-11 years: 10 mg twice daily
Children ≥12 years and Adults: 20 mg twice daily
Dosing adjustment in hepatic impairment: In patients with hepatic impairment (ie, biopsy-proven cirrhosis), there is a 50% to 60% greater C_{max} and AUC compared to normal subjects; these patients should be monitored closely for adverse effects and dosage reductions made if indicated

Administration Administer at least 1 hour before or 2 hours after a meal
(Continued)

987

Zafirlukast *(Continued)*

Monitoring Parameters Pulmonary function tests (FEV-1, PEF), improvement in asthma symptoms

Reference Range Plasma levels not clinically indicated; plasma zafirlukast serum concentrations exceeding 5 ng/mL at 12-14 hours following oral doses have correlated with activity; mean trough serum levels at doses of 20 mg twice daily were 20 ng/mL

Patient Information Take regularly as prescribed, even during symptom-free periods. Do not use to treat acute episodes of asthma. Do not decrease the dose or stop taking any other asthma medications unless instructed by a physician. Nursing women should not take zafirlukast.

Dosage Forms Tablet: 10 mg, 20 mg

Zalcitabine (zal SITE a been)

Related Information
Adult and Adolescent HIV *on page 1133*
Pediatric HIV *on page 1129*

Brand Names Hivid®

Synonyms ddC; Dideoxycytidine

Therapeutic Category Antiretroviral Agent; HIV Agents (Anti-HIV Agents); Nucleoside Reverse Transcriptase Inhibitor (NRTI)

Generic Available No

Use Treatment of HIV infection in combination with other antiretroviral agents. **(Note:** HIV regimens consisting of **three** antiretroviral agents are strongly recommended)

Pregnancy Risk Factor C

Contraindications Hypersensitivity to zalcitabine or any component

Warnings An accumulative dose-related, clinically disabling peripheral neuropathy (treatment-limiting), or fatal pancreatitis may occur; discontinue therapy in patients with symptoms of pancreatitis until pancreatitis can be ruled out; cases of fatal lactic acidosis and severe hepatomegaly with steatosis may occur; hepatic failure and death (which may be related to underlying hepatitis B) have been reported (rare); discontinue therapy in patients with clinical or laboratory signs suggestive of lactic acidosis or hepatotoxicity and if liver function tests increase to >5 times the upper limit of normal

Precautions Use with extreme caution in patients with pre-existing peripheral neuropathy; avoid use in patients with moderate or severe peripheral neuropathy; zalcitabine may exacerbate existing liver dysfunction in patients with a previous history of liver disease or alcohol abuse; increased liver function tests were observed in patients on zalcitabine therapy; use with caution in patients with hepatic impairment; obtain CBC and clinical chemistry tests prior to and during therapy; obtain serum amylase and triglyceride levels and use with caution in patients with history of pancreatitis, increased amylase, ethanol abuse or patients receiving hyperalimentation; use with caution and adjust dose in patients with renal dysfunction; multiple potentially serious drug interactions exist (see Drug Interactions)

Adverse Reactions
Cardiovascular: Chest pain, edema, hypertension, palpitations, syncope, atrial fibrillation, tachycardia, CHF, heart racing

Central nervous system: Headache, dizziness, fever, malaise, fatigue, chest pain

Dermatologic: Pruritus, rash (may be erythematous, maculopapular, follicular or other)

Endocrine & metabolic: Lactic acidosis (rare, but potentially fatal), hyperglycemia, hypocalcemia

Gastrointestinal: Oral ulcers, nausea, esophageal ulcers, dysphagia, anorexia, abdominal pain, vomiting, diarrhea, constipation, pancreatitis (1.1%; can be fatal), weight loss

Hematologic: Leukopenia, absolute neutrophil count alteration, anemia, granulocytosis, neutrophilia, thrombocytopenia

Hepatic: Jaundice, hepatitis; severe hepatomegaly with steatosis (can be fatal)

Neuromuscular & skeletal: Peripheral neuropathy (22% to 35%), myalgia, arthralgia, weakness, foot pain, myositis

Respiratory: Pharyngitis, epistaxis

Miscellaneous: Anaphylactoid reactions, night sweats

Drug Interactions Magnesium- and aluminum-containing antacids and metoclopramide may decrease the bioavailability of zalcitabine; amphotericin, foscarnet,

probenecid, cimetidine, and aminoglycosides may interfere with the renal elimination of zalcitabine and potentiate the risk of peripheral neuropathy or other
zalcitabine toxicities; drugs associated with peripheral neuropathy (chloramphenicol, cisplatin, dapsone, disulfiram, ethionamide, glutethimide, gold, hydralazine,
iodoquinol, isoniazid, lithium, metronidazole, nitrofurantoin, pentamidine, phenytoin, ribavirin, and vincristine) may increase the risk for zalcitabine peripheral
neuropathy; concomitant use of zalcitabine with didanosine is not recommended
(increased risk of peripheral neuropathy); one case of fulminant pancreatitis associated with concomitant zalcitabine and pentamidine use has been reported; if I.V.
pentamidine is required to treat *Pneumocystis carinii* pneumonia, treatment with
zalcitabine should be interrupted

Food Interactions Food decreases the rate and extent of absorption (AUC
decreased by 14%)

Stability Tablets should be stored in tightly closed bottles at 59°F to 86°F

Mechanism of Action A nucleoside (pyrimidine) analogue that is converted within
cells to the active metabolite dideoxycytidine triphosphate (ddCTP) which serves
as an alternative substrate to deoxycytidine triphosphate (dCTP), a natural
substrate for cellular DNA polymerase and reverse transcriptase; inhibits HIV viral
enzyme reverse transcriptase and DNA synthesis causing chain termination

Pharmacokinetics
Distribution: V_{dss}:
Children: 9.3 L/m^2
Adults: 0.53 L/kg
CSF levels are 9% to 37% of serum levels (mean 20%)
Protein binding: Minimal, <4%
Metabolism: Converted intracellularly to active triphosphate form; minimal hepatic
metabolism; primary identified metabolite is dideoxyuridine
Bioavailability:
Children: 29% to 100% (mean: 54%)
Adults: >80%
Half-life:
Children: Mean: 1.4 hours
Adults: 1-3 hours (mean: 2 hours)
Adults with Cl_{cr} <55 mL/minute: up to 8.5 hours
Elimination: Primarily renal with 60% of dose excreted unchanged in urine within
24 hours; elimination is prolonged in patients with renal dysfunction
Hemodialysis reduces plasma levels by 50%

Usual Dosage Oral: (Use in combination with other antiretroviral agents)
Neonates: Dose unknown
Infants and Children <13 years: Usual dose: 0.01 mg/kg every 8 hours; range:
0.005-0.01 mg/kg every 8 hours
Adolescents and Adults: 0.75 mg 3 times/day
Dosing adjustment in severe renal impairment: Adults:
Cl_{cr} 10-40 mL/minute: 0.75 mg every 12 hours
Cl_{cr} <10 mL/minute: 0.75 mg every 24 hours

Administration Oral: Administer on an empty stomach 1 hour before or 2 hours
after a meal; do not administer concurrently with antacids

Monitoring Parameters Renal function, CD4 counts, viral load, CBC with differential, liver enzymes, serum chemistries, serum amylase, triglyceride, signs/symp-
toms of peripheral neuropathy

Patient Information Avoid alcohol; zalcitabine is not a cure; notify physician if
numbness, tingling, persistent severe abdominal pain, nausea, or vomiting occurs;
take zalcitabine every day as prescribed; do not change dose or discontinue
without physician's advice; if a dose is missed, take it as soon as possible, then
return to normal dosing schedule; if a dose is skipped, do **not** double the next dose

Additional Information Adverse events may be increased in patients with
decreased CD4 cell counts; an oral 0.1 mg/mL zalcitabine raspberry syrup formulation is available on an investigational basis from Roche Pharmaceuticals as part of
a U.S. pediatric compassionate use study (NV14610)

Dosage Forms Tablet: 0.375 mg, 0.75 mg

References
Adkins JC, Peters DH, and Faulds D, "Zalcitabine. An Update of Its Pharmacodynamic and Pharmaco-
kinetic Properties and Clinical Efficacy in the Management of HIV Infection," *Drugs*, 1997,
53(6):1054-80.
Bakshi SS, Britto P, Capparelli E, et al, "Evaluation of Pharmacokinetics, Safety, Tolerance, and Activity
of Combination of Zalcitabine and Zidovudine in Stable, Zidovudine-Treated Pediatric Patients With
Human Immunodeficiency Virus Infection. AIDS Clinical Trials Group Protocol 190 Team," *J Infect
Dis*, 1997, 175(5):1039-50.
Chadwick EG, Nazareno LA, Nieuwenhuis TJ, et al, "Phase I Evaluation of Zalcitabine Administered to
Human Immunodeficiency Virus-Infected Children," *J Infect Dis*, 1995, 172(6):1475-9.

(Continued)

Zalcitabine *(Continued)*

Pizzo PA, Butler K, Balis F, et al, "Dideoxycytidine Alone and in an Alternating Schedule With Zidovudine in Children With Symptomatic Human Immunodeficiency Virus Infection," *J Pediatr*, 1990, 117(5):799-808.

Spector SA, "HIV Therapy Advances. Pediatric Antiretroviral Choices," *AIDS*, 1994, 8(Suppl 3):S15-8.

Spector SA, Blanchard S, Wara DW, et al, "Comparative Trial of Two Dosages of Zalcitabine in Zidovudine-Experienced Children With Advanced Human Immunodeficiency Virus Disease. Pediatric AIDS Clinical Trials Group," *Pediatr Infect Dis J*, 1997, 16(6):623-6.

Working Group on Antiretroviral Therapy and Medical Management of HIV-Infected Children, "Guidelines for the Use of Antiretroviral Agents in Pediatric HIV Infection," January 7, 2000, http://www.hivatis.org.

- **Zantac®** *see* Ranitidine *on page 835*
- **Zantac® 75 [OTC]** *see* Ranitidine *on page 835*
- **Zarontin®** *see* Ethosuximide *on page 393*
- **Zaroxolyn®** *see* Metolazone *on page 632*
- **Zartan®** *see* Cephalexin *on page 196*
- **ZDV** *see* Zidovudine *on page 990*
- **Zeasorb-AF® [OTC]** *see* Tolnaftate *on page 936*
- **Zemuron®** *see* Rocuronium *on page 851*
- **Zemuron™ (Canada)** *see* Rocuronium *on page 851*
- **Zenapax®** *see* Daclizumab *on page 280*
- **Zerit™** *see* Stavudine *on page 879*
- **Zestril®** *see* Lisinopril *on page 575*
- **Zetar® [OTC]** *see* Coal Tar *on page 247*
- **Ziagen®** *see* Abacavir *on page 24*

Zidovudine (zye DOE vyoo deen)

Related Information
Adult and Adolescent HIV *on page 1133*
Carbohydrate and Alcohol Content of Liquid Medications for Use in Patients Receiving Ketogenic Diets *on page 1228*
Pediatric HIV *on page 1129*

Brand Names Apo®-Zidovudine (Canada); Novo-AZT® (Canada); Retrovir®

Synonyms Azidothymidine; AZT; Compound S; ZDV

Therapeutic Category Antiretroviral Agent; HIV Agents (Anti-HIV Agents); Nucleoside Reverse Transcriptase Inhibitor (NRTI)

Generic Available No

Use Treatment of HIV infection in combination with other antiretroviral agents; (**Note:** Current preferred HIV regimens consist of three antiretroviral agents); chemoprophylaxis after occupational exposure to HIV; chemoprophylaxis to reduce perinatal HIV transmission

Pregnancy Risk Factor C

Contraindications Life-threatening hypersensitivity to zidovudine or any component

Warnings Associated with hematologic toxicity including granulocytopenia and severe anemia requiring transfusions; zidovudine treatment should be stopped in children with an absolute neutrophil count <500 cells/mm^3 until marrow recovery is observed; use of erythropoietin, filgrastim, or reduced zidovudine dosage may be necessary in some patients; zidovudine has been shown to be carcinogenic in rats and mice

Precautions Use with caution in patients with bone marrow compromise or in patients with impaired renal or hepatic function; reduce dosage or interrupt therapy in patients with anemia and/or granulocytopenia, myopathy, renal or hepatic impairment

Adverse Reactions
Central nervous system: Malaise, dizziness, manic syndrome, seizures, confusion, fever, severe headache, insomnia, asthenia

Dermatologic: Rash, pigmentation of nails (blue)

Endocrine & metabolic: Lactic acidosis

Gastrointestinal: Nausea, diarrhea, vomiting, anorexia

Hematologic: Granulocytopenia, thrombocytopenia, leukopenia, anemia

Hepatic: Cholestatic hepatitis, hepatomegaly; elevation in serum AST, LDH, and alkaline phosphatase

Neuromuscular & skeletal: Myalgia, tremor, weakness; unusual: myopathy, myositis

Drug Interactions Acyclovir; coadministration with drugs that increase zidovudine concentration (acetaminophen, atovaquone, methadone, valproic acid, cimetidine, indomethacin, lorazepam, fluconazole, probenecid, aspirin) may increase toxicity of zidovudine; flucytosine, pentamidine, co-trimoxazole may increase hematologic side effects; didanosine, foscarnet, ganciclovir, zalcitabine (synergistic antiretroviral activity); ribavirin (antagonistic); coadministration with rifampin or rifabutin may increase metabolism of zidovudine; clarithromycin decreases zidovudine concentration by interfering with its absorption (administer doses 4 hours apart); do not administer in combination with stavudine (poor antiretroviral effect)

Food Interactions Folate or vitamin B_{12} deficiency increases zidovudine-associated myelosuppression

Stability Diluted I.V. zidovudine solution is stable for 24 hours when refrigerated

Mechanism of Action Zidovudine is a thymidine analog that enters the cell and is phosphorylated by cellular kinases to the active metabolite zidovudine triphosphate which serves as an alternative substrate to deoxythymidine triphosphate for incorporation by reverse transcriptase; inhibits HIV viral polymerases and DNA synthesis

Pharmacokinetics

Absorption: Oral: Well absorbed (66% to 70%)

Distribution: Significant penetration into the CSF; crosses the placenta

Protein binding: 25% to 38%

Metabolism: Extensive first-pass effect; metabolized in the liver via glucuronidation to inactive metabolites

Bioavailability:

Neonates <14 days: 89%

Infants: 60%

Half-life, terminal: 60 minutes

Premature neonate: 6.3 hours

Full-term neonates: 3.1 hours

Older infants: 1.9 hours

Time to peak serum concentration: Within 30-90 minutes

Elimination: Urinary excretion (63% to 95%)

Oral: 72% to 74% of drug excreted in urine as metabolites and 14% to 18% as unchanged drug

I.V.: 45% to 60% excreted in urine as metabolites and 18% to 29% as unchanged drug

Usual Dosage

Premature Infants: (Standard neonatal dose may be excessive in premature infants) Under investigation in PACTG 331: Oral: 1.5 mg/kg/dose every 12 hours from birth to 2 weeks of age; then increase to 2 mg/kg/dose every 8 hours after 2 weeks of age

Neonates:

Oral: 2 mg/kg/dose every 6 hours

I.V.: 1.5 mg/kg/dose every 6 hours

Children:

Oral: 160 mg/m^2/dose every 8 hours; dosage range: 90 mg/m^2/dose to 180 mg/m^2/dose every 6-8 hours; some Working Group members use a dose of 180 mg/m^2 every 12 hours when using in drug combinations with other antiretroviral compounds, but data on this dosing in children is limited

I.V. continuous infusion: 20 mg/m^2/hour

I.V. intermittent infusion: 120 mg/m^2/dose every 6 hours

Dosing adjustment in children with zidovudine toxicity:

Hemoglobin <8 g/dL: Reduce zidovudine dose by 30%

Children >12 years and Adults:

Oral: 200 mg 3 times/day or 300 mg twice daily

HIV postexposure prophylaxis: 600 mg/day in divided doses (eg, 300 mg twice daily, 200 mg 3 times/day or 100 mg every 4 hours) in combination with lamivudine 150 mg twice daily and indinavir 800 mg 3 times/day are first-line agents for HIV postexposure prophylaxis

I.V.: 1-2 mg/kg/dose every 4 hours

Administration

Oral: May administer with food (although the manufacturer recommends administration 30 minutes before or 1 hour after a meal with a glass of water); the patient should be in an upright position while taking zidovudine capsules to minimize the risk of esophageal ulceration

Parenteral: Do not administer I.M.; do not administer I.V. push or by rapid infusion; infuse I.V. zidovudine over 1 hour at a final concentration not to exceed 4 mg/mL in D_5W

Monitoring Parameters CBC with differential, hemoglobin, MCV, reticulocyte count, serum creatine kinase, CD4 cell count, HIV RNA plasma levels, renal and hepatic function tests

(Continued)

Zidovudine *(Continued)*

Patient Information Take zidovudine exactly as prescribed

Additional Information Conversion from oral to I.V. dose: I.V. dose = $^2/_3$ of the oral dose

Dosage Forms

Capsule: 100 mg

Concentration for injection (for I.V. infusion): 10 mg/mL (20 mL)

Syrup (strawberry flavor): 50 mg/5 mL (240 mL)

Tablet: 300 mg

References

Carpenter CC, Fischel MA, Hammer SM, et al, "Antiretroviral Therapy for HIV Infection in 1997. Updated Recommendations of the International AIDS Society - USA Panel," *JAMA*, 1997, 277(24):1962-9.

CDC and the National Foundation for Infectious Disease, "Public Health Service Guidelines for the Management of Health-Care Worker Exposures to HIV and Recommendations for Postexposure Prophylaxis," *MMWR Morb Mortal Wkly Rep*, May 15, 1998/47 (RR-7):29-30.

Mueller BU, Jacobsen F, Butler KM, et al, "Combination Treatment With Azidothymidine and Granulo-cyte Colony-Stimulating Factor in Children With Human Immunodeficiency Virus Infection," *J Pediatr*, 1992, 121(5 Pt 1):797-802.

Volberding PA, Lagakos SW, Koch MA, et al, "Zidovudine in Asymptomatic Human Immunodeficiency Virus Infection. A Controlled Trial in Persons With Fewer Than 500 CD4-Positive Cells Per Cubic Millimeter. The AIDS Clinical Trials Group of the National Institute of Allergy and Infectious Diseases," *N Engl J Med*, 1990, 322(14):941-9.

Working Group on Antiretroviral Therapy and Medical Management of HIV-Infected Children, "Guidelines for the Use of Antiretroviral Agents in Pediatric HIV Infection," April 15, 1999, http://www.hivatis.org.

♦ **Zidovudine and Lamivudine** *see* Lamivudine and Zidovudine *on page 553*

♦ **Zilactin-B® Medicated [OTC]** *see* Benzocaine *on page 124*

Zileuton *(zye LOO ton)*

Related Information

Asthma Guidelines *on page 1178*

Brand Names Zyflo™

Therapeutic Category Antiasthmatic; Leukotriene Receptor Antagonist

Use Prophylaxis and chronic treatment of asthma

Pregnancy Risk Factor C

Contraindications Active liver disease or transaminase elevations greater than or equal to three times the upper limit of normal; hypersensitivity to zileuton or any ingredient

Warnings Coadministration of zileuton with theophylline, propranolol, astemizole, and terfenadine is associated with significant increases in serum levels of these agents which may require reductions in dosage; elevated terfenadine and astemizole levels have been associated with severe cardiovascular effects including Q-T interval prolongation, ventricular tachycardia, ventricular fibrillation, death, cardiac arrest, hypotension, and palpitations; elevations of one or more liver function tests may occur during therapy; these laboratory abnormalities may progress, remain unchanged, or resolve with continued therapy; zileuton is **not** indicated for use in the reversal of bronchospasm in acute asthma attacks, including status asthmaticus; zileuton can be continued during acute exacerbations of asthma.

Precautions Use with caution in patients who consume substantial quantities of alcohol or have a past history of liver disease

Adverse Reactions

Cardiovascular: Chest pain

Central nervous system: Headache, pain, dizziness, fever, insomnia, fatigue, nervousness, somnolence

Gastrointestinal: Dyspepsia, nausea, abdominal pain, constipation, flatulence

Hematologic: Low white blood cell count

Hepatic: Elevated liver enzymes

Neuromuscular & skeletal: Myalgia, arthralgia, weakness, paresthesias, asthenia

Ocular: Conjunctivitis

Drug Interactions Cytochrome P-450 isoenzyme CYP1A2, CYP2CP, and CYP3A3/4 substrate; CYP1A2 and CYP3A3/4 isoenzyme inhibitor

Increased toxicity: Coadministration of zileuton with propranolol or theophylline results in an approximate doubling of serum concentrations (propranolol or theophylline); coadministration of zileuton with warfarin results in a clinically significant increase in prothrombin time (PT); coadministration of zileuton with terfenadine or astemizole results in a decrease in clearance leading to an increase in terfenadine or astemizole serum levels (elevated serum levels have been associated with severe cardiovascular effects, see Warnings)

Mechanism of Action Specific inhibitor of 5-lipoxygenase and thus inhibits leukotriene (LTB1, LTC1, LTD1, and LTE1) formation. Leukotrienes are substances that induce numerous biological effects including augmentation of neutrophil and eosinophil migration, neutrophil and monocyte aggregation, leukocyte adhesion, increased capillary permeability and smooth muscle contraction.

Pharmacodynamics After discontinuation of zileuton therapy, 5-lipoxygenase activity (eg, return of leukotriene B4 levels to baseline) occurred in approximately 7 days. See table.

Zileuton Pharmacodynamic Parameters

Parameter	Inhibition of Leukotriene B4 Production	Increased FEV-1
Onset of effect	0.5-1 h	30 min
Peak effect	2-4 h	1 h
Maximal effect	5-8 h	4 wk

Pharmacokinetics
Absorption: Rapidly absorbed
Distribution: V_d: 1.2 L/kg
Protein binding: 93%
Metabolism: Several metabolites in plasma and urine; metabolized by the cytochrome P-450 isoenzymes CYP1A2, CYP2C9, and CYP3A4
Half-life: 2 1-2.5 hours
Time to peak serum concentration: 1-3 hours
Elimination: Predominantly via metabolism; <0.5% excreted unchanged in urine
Clearance: 7 mL/minute/kg
Usual Dosage Oral: Children ≥12 years and Adults: 600 mg 4 times daily with meals and at bedtime
   Dosing adjustment in hepatic impairment: Contraindicated in patients with active liver disease
Administration Can be administered without regard to meals
Monitoring Parameters Monitor serum ALT before treatment begins, once monthly for the first 3 months, every 2-3 months for the remainder of the first year and periodically thereafter for patients receiving long-term zileuton therapy; complete blood count periodically when on long-term therapy; pulmonary function tests, improvement in asthma symptoms
Patient Information Inform patients that zileuton is indicated for the chronic treatment of asthma and to take regularly as prescribed even during symptom-free periods. Zileuton is not a bronchodilator; do not use to treat acute episodes of asthma. When taking zileuton, do not decrease the dose or stop taking any other asthma medications unless instructed by a physician.

If experiencing signs or symptoms of liver dysfunction (right upper quadrant pain, nausea, fatigue, lethargy, pruritus, jaundice, or "flu-like" symptoms), contact a physician immediately.

Zileuton can interact with other drugs. While taking zileuton, consult a physician or pharmacist before starting or stopping any prescription or nonprescription medicines.
Dosage Forms Tablet: 600 mg

♦ **Zinacef® Injection** see Cefuroxime on page 194
♦ **Zinaderm (Canada)** see Zinc Oxide on page 993
♦ **Zinca-Pak®** see Trace Metals on page 940
♦ **Zinca-Pak®** see Zinc Supplements on page 994
♦ **Zincate®** see Zinc Supplements on page 994
♦ **Zinc Carbonate** see Zinc Supplements on page 994
♦ **Zinc Chloride** see Trace Metals on page 940
♦ **Zinc Chloride** see Zinc Supplements on page 994
♦ **Zinc Gluconate** see Zinc Supplements on page 994
♦ **Zincofax® (Canada)** see Zinc Oxide on page 993

Zinc Oxide (zingk OKS ide)
   Brand Names Prevex™ Baby Diaper Rash (Canada); Zinaderm (Canada); Zincofax® (Canada)
   Synonyms Lassar's Zinc Paste
   Therapeutic Category Topical Skin Product
   (Continued)

Zinc Oxide *(Continued)*

Generic Available Yes

Use Protective coating for mild skin irritations and abrasions; soothing and protective ointment to promote healing of chapped skin, diaper rash

Contraindications Hypersensitivity to zinc oxide or any component

Stability Avoid prolonged storage at temperatures >30°C

Mechanism of Action Mild astringent, protective and weak antiseptic action

Usual Dosage Infants, Children, and Adults: Topical: Apply several times daily to affected area

Administration Topical: For external use only; do not use in the eyes

Patient Information Paste is easily removed with mineral oil

Dosage Forms

Ointment, topical: 20% in white ointment (480 g)

Paste, topical: 25% in white petrolatum (480 g)

◆ **Zinc Sulfate** *see* Trace Metals *on page 940*

◆ **Zinc Sulfate** *see* Zinc Supplements *on page 994*

Zinc Supplements *(zink SUP la ments)*

Brand Names Orazinc® [OTC]; Verazinc® [OTC]; Zinca-Pak®; Zincate®

Available Salts Zinc Carbonate; Zinc Chloride; Zinc Gluconate; Zinc Sulfate

Therapeutic Category Mineral, Oral; Mineral, Parenteral

Generic Available Yes

Use Treatment and prevention of zinc deficiency states; may improve wound healing in those who are zinc deficient

Pregnancy Risk Factor C

Contraindications Hypersensitivity to zinc salts or any component

Warnings Do not administer undiluted by direct injection into a peripheral vein due to potential for phlebitis, tissue irritation, and potential increased renal loss of minerals from a bolus injection; administration of zinc in absence of copper may decrease plasma copper levels; excessive intake in healthy persons may be deleterious as decreases in HDL (high-density lipoproteins) and impairment of immune system function have been reported

Adverse Reactions

Cardiovascular: Hypotension, tachycardia (excessive doses)

Central nervous system: Hypothermia (excessive doses)

Gastrointestinal: Indigestion, nausea, vomiting

Hematologic: Neutropenia, leukopenia

Hepatic: Jaundice (excessive doses)

Ophthalmic: Blurred vision (excessive doses)

Respiratory: Pulmonary edema (excessive doses)

Miscellaneous: Profuse diaphoresis

Drug Interactions Zinc may decrease penicillamine, tetracycline, and quinolone absorption; iron decreases zinc absorption; agents which increase gastric pH, such as H_2-blockers, may decrease zinc absorption

Food Interactions Coffee, foods high in phytate (eg, whole grain cereals & legumes), bran, and dairy products reduce zinc absorption; avoid foods high in calcium or phosphorus

Mechanism of Action A cofactor for more than 70 enzymes which are important to carbohydrate and protein metabolism, zinc helps to maintain normal growth and tissue repair, normal skin hydration, and senses of taste and smell

Pharmacokinetics

Absorption: pH dependent; poor from gastrointestinal tract (20% to 30%); solubilized by conversion to zinc chloride in the presence of gastric acid

Distribution: Storage sites are liver and skeletal muscle; serum levels do not adequately reflect whole-body zinc status

Protein binding: 55% bound to albumin; 40% bound to alpha 1-macroglobulin

Elimination: 90% in feces with only traces appearing in urine and perspiration

Usual Dosage Clinical response may not occur for up to 6-8 weeks

RDA: Oral:

Neonates and Infants <12 months: 5 mg **elemental** zinc/day

Children 1-10 years: 10 mg **elemental** zinc/day

Children ≥11 years and Adults: Male: 15 mg **elemental** zinc/day; Female: 12 mg **elemental** zinc/day

Zinc deficiency: Oral:
Infants and Children: 0.5-1 mg **elemental** zinc/kg/day divided 1-3 times/day; larger doses may be needed if impaired intestinal absorption or an excessive loss of zinc (eg, excessive, prolonged diarrhea)
Adults: 25-50 mg **elemental** zinc/dose (110-220 mg zinc sulfate) 3 times/day
Supplement to parenteral nutrition solutions (clinical response may not occur for up to 6-8 weeks): (See Trace Metals): I.V. (all doses are mcg of **elemental** zinc):
Premature Infants: 400 mcg/kg/day
Term Infants <3 months: 300 mcg/kg/day
Infants ≥3 months and Children ≤5 years: 100 mcg/kg/day (maximum: 5 mg/day)
Children >5 years and Adolescents: 2-5 mg/day
Adults:
Stable metabolically: 2.5-4 mg **elemental** zinc/day; catabolic state: Increase by an additional 2 mg/day (eg, 4.5-6 mg **elemental** zinc/day)
Stable with fluid loss from small bowel: Additional 12.2 mg **elemental** zinc/L parenteral nutrition or 17.1 mg **elemental** zinc/kg of stool or ileostomy output
Wound healing: Oral: Adults: 50 mg **elemental** zinc (220 mg zinc sulfate) 3 times daily in patients with low serum zinc levels (<110 mcg/dL)

Administration
Oral: Administer oral formulation with food if GI upset occurs
Parenteral: Dilute as component of daily parenteral nutrition or maintenance fluids; do not give undiluted by direct injection into a peripheral vein due to potential for phlebitis and tissue irritation, and potential to increase renal losses of minerals from a bolus injection

Monitoring Parameters Patients on parenteral nutrition or chronic therapy should have periodic serum copper and serum zinc levels; alkaline phosphatase, taste acuity, mental depression, wound healing (if indicated), growth (if indicated), skin integrity

Reference Range
Serum: 70-130 µg/dL

Patient Information Do not exceed recommended dose

Dosage Forms
Zinc carbonate, complex: Liquid: 15 mg/mL (30 mL)
Zinc chloride: Injection: 1 mg elemental zinc/mL (10 mL)
Zinc gluconate (14.3% zinc): Tablet: 10 mg [elemental zinc 1.4 mg]; 15 mg (elemental zinc 2 mg), 50 mg [elemental zinc 7 mg]; 78 mg [elemental zinc 11 mg]
Zinc sulfate (23% zinc):
Capsule: 110 mg [elemental zinc 25 mg]; 220 mg [elemental zinc 50 mg]
Injection: 1 mg elemental zinc/mL (10 mL, 30 mL); 4 mg elemental zinc/mL (10 mL); 5 mg elemental zinc/mL (5 mL, 10 mL)
Tablet: 66 mg [elemental zinc 15 mg]; 110 mg [elemental zinc 25 mg]; 200 mg [elemental zinc 45 mg]

APPENDIX TABLE OF CONTENTS

TABLE OF CONTENTS *(Continued)*

CPR PEDIATRIC DRUG DOSAGES

Drug and Concentration	Dose
Albumin 5%	I.V.: 5-10 mL/kg, may repeat in 15 minutes
Atropine 0.1 mg/mL	I.V.: 0.02 mg/kg every 5 minutes (minimum dose = 0.1 mg)
	Maximum single dose: Children: 0.5 mg; Adolescents: 1 mg
	Total maximum dose: Children: 1 mg; Adolescents: 2 mg
	May be administered via endotracheal tube at 2-3 times the I.V. dose. Dilute to 3-5 mL with normal saline prior to endotracheal administration.
Bretylium 50 mg/mL	I.V.: 1st dose: 5 mg/kg 2nd dose: 10 mg/kg every 15-30 minutes Maximum total dose: 30 mg/kg
Calcium chloride 100 mg/mL	I.V.: 0.2-0.25 mL/kg/dose every 10 minutes; role in resuscitation questionable, use only when hyperkalemia, hypermagnesemia, hypocalcemia, or calcium channel blocker toxicity is present
Dextrose 50% 0.5 g/mL	I.V.: 0.5-1 g/kg (or 2-4 mL/kg of dextrose 25%); dilute to a 25% solution before administration
Epinephrine injection 1:10,000 = 0.1 mg/mL 1:1000 = 1 mg/mL	Neonates: I.V.: 0.01-0.03 mg/kg (0.1-0.3 mL/kg of **1:10,000** solution) every 3-5 minutes; consider 0.1-0.2 mg/kg by E.T. if no I.V. access and neonate did not respond to standard doses.
	Pediatrics: **Bradycardia:** I.O., I.V.: 0.01 mg/kg (0.1 mL/kg of **1:10,000** solution) every 3-5 minutes E.T.: 0.1 mg/kg (0.1 mL/kg of **1:1000** solution) every 3-5 minutes. Dilute to 3-5 mL with normal saline prior to endotracheal administration.
	Pediatrics: **Asystolic or pulseless arrest**: Initial dose: I.O., I.V.: 0.01 mg/kg (0.1 mL/kg of **1:10,000** solution) E.T.: 0.1 mg/kg (0.1 mL/kg of **1:1000** solution); doses as high as 0.2 mg/kg may be effective. Dilute to 3-5 mL with normal saline prior to endotracheal administration.
	Subsequent doses: E.T., I.O., I.V.: 0.1 mg/kg (0.1 mL/kg of **1:1000** solution); doses as high as 0.2 mg/kg may be effective
Lidocaine 10 mg/mL	I.V.: 1 mg/kg loading dose, may repeat to a total dose not >3 mg/kg; may be administered via endotracheal tube. Dilute to 3-5 mL with normal saline prior to endotracheal administration. I.V. infusion: 20-50 mcg/kg/minute
Naloxone 0.4 mg/mL 1 mg/mL	Birth to 5 y or 20 kg: I.V.: 0.1 mg/kg/dose >5 y or 20 kg: 2 mg/dose May repeat doses every 2-3 minutes; may be administered via endotracheal tube. Dilute to 3-5 mL with normal saline prior to endotracheal administration.
Sodium bicarbonate 1 mEq/mL 0.5 mEq/mL	I.V.: 1 mEq/kg as a single dose, may repeat with 0.5 mEq/kg or calculate mEq = 0.3 x kg x base deficit; infuse slowly and only if ventilation is adequate. Use only the 0.5 mEq/mL solution for neonates or dilute 1 mEq/mL solution 1:1 with sterile water for injection. Sodium bicarbonate should be used based on documented metabolic acidosis. Routine use in cardiac arrest is not recommended.

Reference

American Heart Association,"Fluid Therapy and Medications" in *Textbook of Pediatric Advanced Life Support*, Chameides L and Hazinski MF, eds, American Heart Association, Dallas, TX, 1994.

EMERGENCY PEDIATRIC DRIP CALCULATIONS

Drips

Drug	Dose	Calculation*	Rate & Dose
Dobutamine	5-20 mcg/kg/min	6 x body wt (kg) is the mg added to make 100 mL	1 mL/h = 1 mcg/kg/min
Dopamine	2-20 mcg/kg/min	6 x body wt (kg) is the mg added to make 100 mL	1 mL/h = 1 mcg/kg/min
Epinephrine	0.1-1 mcg/kg/min	0.6 x body wt (kg) is the mg added to make 100 mL	1 mL/h = 0.1 mcg/kg/min
Isoproterenol	0.1-1 mcg/kg/min	0.6 x body wt (kg) is the mg added to make 100 mL	1 mL/h = 0.1 mcg/kg/min
Lidocaine	20-50 mcg/kg/min	120 mg in 100 mL of D_5W	1 mL/kg/h = 20 mcg/kg/min

Note: Patients ≥40 kg and those requiring fluid restriction may need more concentrated solutions in order to deliver less fluid per hour. In those cases, or as an alternative to the listed calculations above, use the following equation:

$$\text{Rate (mL/h)} = \frac{\text{Dose (mcg/kg/min)} \times \text{weight (kg)} \times 60 \text{ min/h}}{\text{concentration (mcg/mL)}}$$

Defibrillation/Cardioversion

	Indication/Remarks	Dose*
Pediatrics		
Defibrillation	V-fib or pulseless V-tach	2 joules/kg; repeat with 4 joules/kg thereafter
Synchronized cardioversion	Increase stepwise if needed	0.5 joules/kg
Adults		
Defibrillation	V-fib or pulseless V-tach or polymorphic V-tach	200 joules, then 200-300 joules, then 360 joules
Synchronized cardioversion		Initial†
	Atrial fibrillation	100 joules
	Atrial flutter	50 joules
	PSVT	50 joules
	monomorphic V-tach	100 joules

*1 joule = 1 watt • second.

†Increase stepwise if initial fails.

PEDIATRIC ALS ALGORITHMS

BRADYCARDIA

Fig. 1: Pediatric bradycardia decision tree. ABCs indicates airway, breathing, and circulation; ALS, advanced life support; E.T., endotracheal; I.O., intraosseous; and I.V., intravenous.

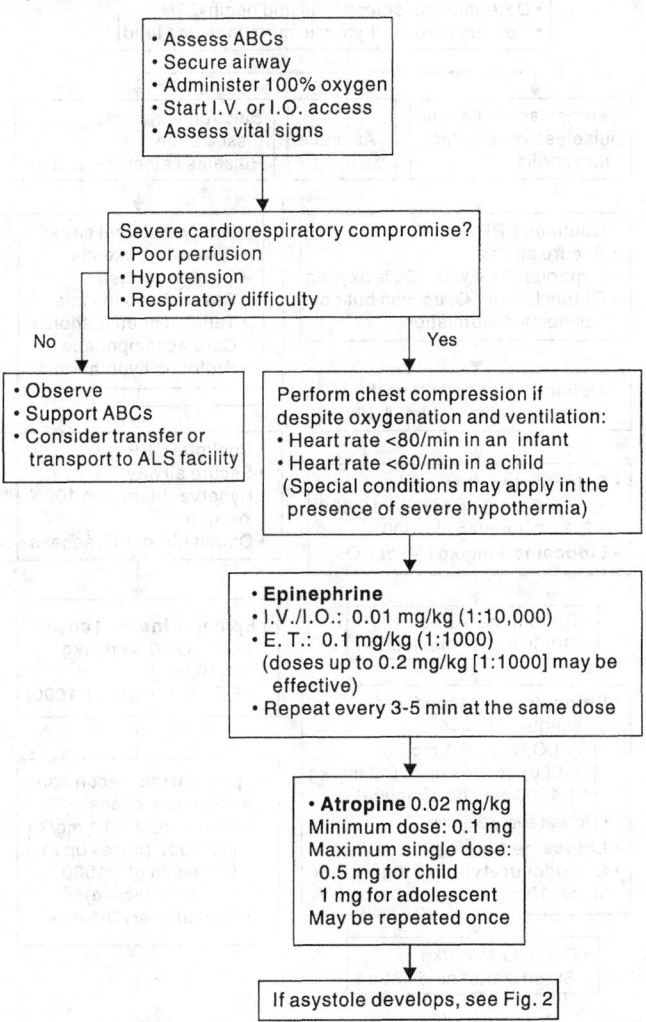

* Assess ABCs
* Secure airway
* Administer 100% oxygen
* Start I.V. or I.O. access
* Assess vital signs

Severe cardiorespiratory compromise?
* Poor perfusion
* Hypotension
* Respiratory difficulty

No

Yes

* Observe
* Support ABCs
* Consider transfer or transport to ALS facility

Perform chest compression if despite oxygenation and ventilation:
* Heart rate <80/min in an infant
* Heart rate <60/min in a child
  (Special conditions may apply in the presence of severe hypothermia)

* **Epinephrine**
* I.V./I.O.: 0.01 mg/kg (1:10,000)
* E. T.: 0.1 mg/kg (1:1000)
  (doses up to 0.2 mg/kg [1:1000] may be effective)
* Repeat every 3-5 min at the same dose

* **Atropine** 0.02 mg/kg
Minimum dose: 0.1 mg
Maximum single dose:
  0.5 mg for child
  1 mg for adolescent
May be repeated once

If asystole develops, see Fig. 2

Used with permission: Emergency Cardiac Care Committee and Subcommittees, American Heart Association, "Guidelines for Cardiopulmonary Resuscitation and Emergency Care, IV: Pediatric Advanced Life Support," *JAMA*, 1992, 268:2262-75.

PEDIATRIC ALS ALGORITHMS *(Continued)*

ASYSTOLE AND PULSELESS ARREST

Fig. 2: Pediatric asystole and pulseless arrest decision tree. CPR indicates cardiopulmonary resuscitation; E.T, endotracheal; I.O., intraosseous; and I.V., intravenous.

Used with permission: Emergency Cardiac Care Committee and Subcommittees, American Heart Association, "Guidelines for Cardiopulmonary Resuscitation and Emergency Care, IV: Pediatric Advanced Life Support," *JAMA*, 1992, 268:2262-75.

ADULT ACLS ALGORITHMS

EMERGENCY CARDIAC CARE

Fig. 1: Universal algorithm for adult emergency cardiac care (ECC)

Used with permission: Emergency Cardiac Care Committee and Subcommittees, American Heart Association, "Guidelines for Cardiopulmonary Resuscitation and Emergency Care, III: Adult Advanced Cardiac Life Support," *JAMA*, 1992, 268:2199-2241.

ADULT ACLS ALGORITHMS *(Continued)*

V. FIB AND PULSELESS V. TACH

Fig. 2: Adult algorithm for ventricular fibrillation and pulseless ventricular tachycardia (VF/VT)

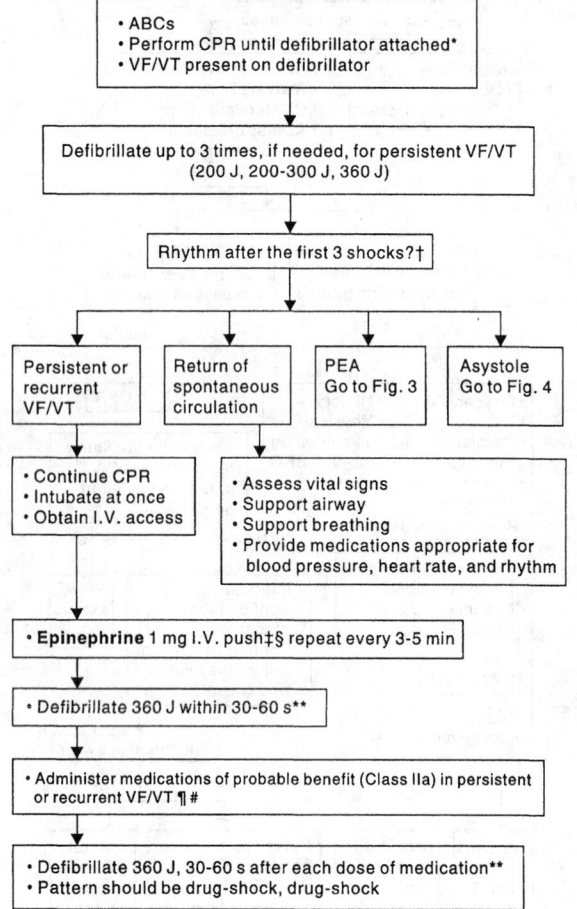

Class I: Definitely helpful
Class IIa: Acceptable, probably helpful
Class IIb: Acceptable, possibly helpful
Class III: Not indicated, may be harmful
* Precordial thump is a Class IIb action in witnessed arrest, no pulse, and no defibrillator immediately available.
† Hypothermic cardiac arrest is treated differently after this point.
‡ The recommended dose of **epinephrine** is 1 mg I.V. push every 3-5 min. If this approach fails, several Class IIb dosing regimens can be considered:
 • Intermediate: **Epinephrine** 2-5 mg I.V. push, every 3-5 min
 • Escalating: **Epinephrine** 1 mg-3 mg-5 mg I.V. push (3 min apart)
 • High: **Epinephrine**: 0.1 mg/kg I.V. push, every 3-5 min
§ **Sodium bicarbonate (1 mEq/kg)** is Class I if patient has known pre-existing hyperkalemia
** Multiple sequenced shock (200 J, 200-300 J, 360 J) are acceptable here (Class I), especially when medications are delayed
¶ **Lidocaine** 1.5 mg/kg I.V. push. Repeat in 3-5 min to total loading dose of 3 mg/kg; then use
 • **Bretylium** 5 mg/kg I.V. push. Repeat in 5 min at 10 mg/kg
 • **Magnesium sulfate** 1-2 g I.V. in torsade de pointes or suspected hypo-magnesemic state or severe refractory VF
 • **Procainamide** 30 mg/min in refractory VF (maximum total: 17 mg/kg)
Sodium bicarbonate (1 mEq/kg I.V.): Class IIa
 • If known pre-existing bicarbonate-responsive acidosis
 • If overdose with tricyclic antidepressants
 • To alkalinize the urine in drug overdoses
 Class IIb
 • If intubated and continued long arrest interval
 • Upon return of spontaneous circulation after long arrest interval
 Class III
 • Hypoxic lactic acidosis

Used with permission: Emergency Cardiac Care Committee and Subcommittees, American Heart Association, "Guidelines for Cardiopulmonary Resuscitation and Emergency Care, III: Adult Advanced Cardiac Life Support," *JAMA*, 1992, 268:2199-2241.

ADULT ACLS ALGORITHMS *(Continued)*

PULSELESS ELECTRICAL ACTIVITY

Fig. 3: Adult algorithm for pulseless electrical activity (PEA) (electromechanical dissociation [EMD]).

PEA includes:

- Electromechanical dissociation (EMD)
- Pseudo-EMD
- Idioventricular rhythms
- Ventricular escape rhythms
- Bradyasystolic rhythms
- Postdefibrillation idioventricular rhythms

- Continue CPR
- Intubate at once
- Obtain I.V. access
- Assess blood flow using Doppler ultrasound

↓

Consider possible causes (Parentheses = possible therapies and treatments)
- Hypovolemia (volume infusion)
- Hypoxia (ventilation)
- Cardiac tamponade (pericardiocentesis)
- Tension pneumothorax (needle decompression)
- Hypothermia
- Massive pulmonary embolism (surgery, **thrombolytics**)
- Drug overdoses such as tricyclics, digitalis, beta blockers, calcium channel blockers
- Hyperkalemia*
- Acidosis†
- Massive acute myocardial infarction

↓

Epinephrine 1 mg I.V. push*‡, repeat every 3-5 min

↓

- If absolute bradycardia (<60 beats/min) or relative bradycardia, give **atropine** 1 mg I.V.
- Repeat every 3-5 min up to a total of 0.04 mg/kg§

Class I: Definitely helpful
Class IIa: Acceptable, probably helpful
Class IIb: Acceptable, possibly helpful
Class III: Not indicated, may be harmful
* **Sodium bicarbonate** 1 mEq/kg is Class I if patient has known pre-existing hyperkalemia
† **Sodium bicarbonate** 1 mEq/kg:
  Class IIa
  • If known pre-existing bicarbonate-responsive acidosis
  • If overdose with tricyclic antidepressants
  • To alkalinize the urine in drug overdoses
  Class IIb
  • If intubated and long arrest interval
  • Upon return of spontaneous circulation after long arrest interval
  Class III
  • Hypoxic lactic acidosis
‡ The recommended dose of **epinephrine** is 1 mg I.V. push every 3-5 min. If this approach fails, several Class IIb dosing regimens can be considered.
  • Intermediate: **Epinephrine** 2-5 mg I.V. push every 3-5 min
  • Escalating: **Epinephrine** 1 mg-3 mg-5 mg I.V. push (3 min apart)
  • High: **Epinephrine** 0.1 mg/kg I.V. push every 3-5 min
§ Shorter **atropine** dosing intervals are possibly helpful in cardiac arrest (Class IIb)

Used with permission: Emergency Cardiac Care Committee and Subcommittees, American Heart Association, "Guidelines for Cardiopulmonary Resuscitation and Emergency Care, III: Adult Advanced Cardiac Life Support," *JAMA*, 1992, 268:2199-2241.

ADULT ACLS ALGORITHMS *(Continued)*

ASYSTOLE

Fig. 4: Adult asystole treatment algorithm.

- Continue CPR
- Intubation at once
- Obtain I.V. access
- Confirm asystole in more than one lead

Consider possible causes
- Hypoxia
- Hyperkalemia
- Hypokalemia
- Pre-existing acidosis
- Drug overdose
- Hypothermia

Consider immediate transcutaneous pacing (TCP)*

- **Epinephrine** 1 mg I.V. push†‡, repeat every 3-5 min

- **Atropine** 1 mg I.V., repeat every 3-5 min up to a total of 0.04 mg/kg§**

Consider
- Termination of efforts¶

Class I: Definitely helpful
Class IIa: Acceptable, probably helpful
Class IIb: Acceptable, possibly helpful
Class III: Not indicated, may be harmful

* TCP is a Class IIb intervention. Lack of success may be due to delays in pacing. To be effective, TCP must be performed early, simultaneously with drugs. Evidence does not support routine use of TCP for asystole.

† The recommended dose of **epinephrine** is 1 mg I.V. push every 3-5 min. If this approach fails, several Class IIb dosing regimens can be considered:
  - Intermediate: **Epinephrine** 2-5 mg I.V. push every 3-5 min
  - Escalating: **Epinephrine** 1 mg-3 mg-5 mg I.V. push (3 min apart)
  - High: **Epinephrine** 0.1 mg/kg I.V. push every 3-5 mim

‡ **Sodium bicarbonate** 1 mEq/kg is Class I if patient has known pre-existing hyperkalemia

§ Shorter **atropine** dosing intervals are Class IIb in asystolic arrest

****Sodium bicarbonate** 1 mEq/kg:
  Class IIa
  - If known pre-existing bicarbonate responsive acidosis
  - If overdose with tricyclic antidepressants
  - To alkalinize the urine in drug overdoses
  Class IIb
  - If intubated and continued long arrest interval
  - Upon return of spontaneous circulation after long arrest interval
  Class III
  - Hypoxic lactic acidosis

¶ If patient remains in asystole or other agonal rhythms after successful intubation and initial medications and no reversible causes are identified, consider termination of resuscitative efforts by a physician. Consider interval since arrest.

Used with permission: Emergency Cardiac Care Committee and Subcommittees, American Heart Association, "Guidelines for Cardiopulmonary Resuscitation and Emergency Care, III: Adult Advanced Cardiac Life Support," *JAMA*, 1992, 268:2199-2241.

ADULT ACLS ALGORITHMS *(Continued)*

TACHYCARDIA

Fig. 5: Adult tachycardia algorithm.

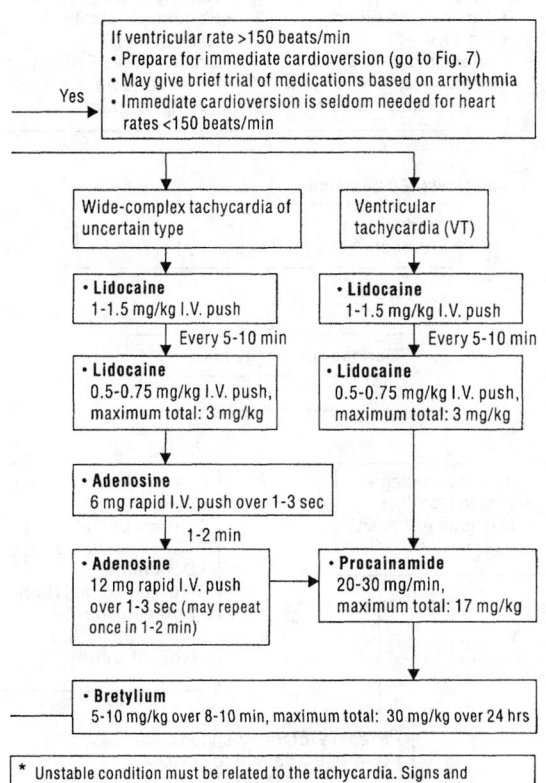

If ventricular rate >150 beats/min
- Prepare for immediate cardioversion (go to Fig. 7)
- May give brief trial of medications based on arrhythmia
- Immediate cardioversion is seldom needed for heart rates <150 beats/min

Yes

Wide-complex tachycardia of uncertain type

Ventricular tachycardia (VT)

- **Lidocaine**
1-1.5 mg/kg I.V. push
Every 5-10 min

- **Lidocaine**
1-1.5 mg/kg I.V. push
Every 5-10 min

- **Lidocaine**
0.5-0.75 mg/kg I.V. push, maximum total: 3 mg/kg

- **Lidocaine**
0.5-0.75 mg/kg I.V. push, maximum total: 3 mg/kg

- **Adenosine**
6 mg rapid I.V. push over 1-3 sec
1-2 min

- **Adenosine**
12 mg rapid I.V. push over 1-3 sec (may repeat once in 1-2 min)

- **Procainamide**
20-30 mg/min, maximum total: 17 mg/kg

- **Bretylium**
5-10 mg/kg over 8-10 min, maximum total: 30 mg/kg over 24 hrs

* Unstable condition must be related to the tachycardia. Signs and symptoms may include chest pain, shortness of breath, decreased level of consciousness, low blood pressure (BP), shock, pulmonary congestion, congestive heart failure, acute myocardial infarction.
† Carotid sinus pressure is contraindicated in patients with carotid bruits; avoid ice water immersion in patients with ischemic heart disease.
‡ If the wide-complex tachycardia is known with certainty to be PSVT and BP is normal/elevated, sequence can include **verapamil.**

Used with permission: Emergency Cardiac Care Committee and Subcommittees, American Heart Association, "Guidelines for Cardiopulmonary Resuscitation and Emergency Care, III: Adult Advanced Cardiac Life Support," *JAMA*, 1992, 268:2199-2241.

ADULT ACLS ALGORITHMS *(Continued)*

BRADYCARDIA

Fig. 6: Adult bradycardia algorithm (with the patient not in cardiac arrest).

* Serious signs or symptoms must be related to the slow rate. Clinical manifestations include:
  Symptoms (chest pain, shortness of breath, decreased level of consciousness), and
  Signs (low BP, shock, pulmonary congestion, CHF, acute MI)

† Do not delay TCP while awaiting I.V. access or for **atropine** to take effect if patient is symptomatic.

‡ Denervated transplanted hearts will not respond to **atropine**. Go at once to pacing, **catecholamine** infusion, or both.

§ **Atropine** should be given in repeat doses in 3-5 min up to a total of 0.04 mg/kg. Consider shorter dosing intervals in severe clinical conditions. It has been suggested that atropine should be used with caution in atrioventricular (A-V) block at the His-Purkinje level (type II A-V block and new third degree block with wide QRS complexes) (Class IIb).

** Never treat third degree heart block plus ventricular escape beats with **lidocaine.**

¶ **Isoproterenol** should be used, if at all, with extreme caution. At low doses it is Class IIb (possibly helpful); at higher doses it is Class III (harmful).

Verify patient tolerance and mechanical capture. Use analgesia and sedation as needed.

Used with permission: Emergency Cardiac Care Committee and Subcommittees, American Heart Association, "Guidelines for Cardiopulmonary Resuscitation and Emergency Care, III: Adult Advanced Cardiac Life Support," *JAMA*, 1992, 268:2199-2241.

ADULT ACLS ALGORITHMS *(Continued)*

ELECTRICAL CONVERSION

Fig. 7: Adult electrical cardioversion algorithm (with the patient not in cardiac arrest).

* Effective regimens have included a sedative (eg, **diazepam, midazolam, barbiturates, etomidate, ketamine, methohexital**) with or without an analgesic agent (eg, **fentanyl, morphine, meperidine**). Many experts recommend anesthesia if service is readily available.
† Note possible need to resynchronize after each cardioversion.
‡ If delays in synchronization occur and clinical conditions are critical, go to immediate unsynchronized shocks.
§ Treat polymorphic VT (irregular form and rate) like VF: 200 J, 200-300 J, 360 J.
**PSVT and atrial flutter often respond to lower energy levels (start with 50 J).

Used with permission: Emergency Cardiac Care Committee and Subcommittees, American Heart Association, "Guidelines for Cardiopulmonary Resuscitation and Emergency Care, III: Adult Advanced Cardiac Life Support," *JAMA*, 1992, 268:2199-2241.

ADULT ACLS ALGORITHMS *(Continued)*

HYPOTENSION, SHOCK

Fig. 8: Adult algorithm for hypotension, shock, and acute pulmonary edema.

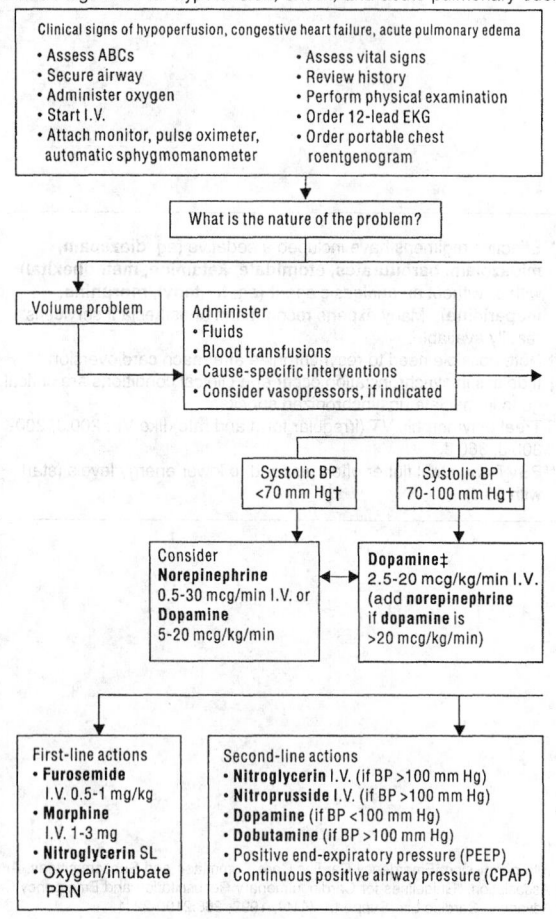

Clinical signs of hypoperfusion, congestive heart failure, acute pulmonary edema

- Assess ABCs
- Secure airway
- Administer oxygen
- Start I.V.
- Attach monitor, pulse oximeter, automatic sphygmomanometer

- Assess vital signs
- Review history
- Perform physical examination
- Order 12-lead EKG
- Order portable chest roentgenogram

What is the nature of the problem?

Volume problem

Administer
- Fluids
- Blood transfusions
- Cause-specific interventions
- Consider vasopressors, if indicated

Systolic BP <70 mm Hg†

Systolic BP 70-100 mm Hg†

Consider **Norepinephrine** 0.5-30 mcg/min I.V. or **Dopamine** 5-20 mcg/kg/min

Dopamine‡ 2.5-20 mcg/kg/min I.V. (add **norepinephrine** if **dopamine** is >20 mcg/kg/min)

First-line actions
- **Furosemide** I.V. 0.5-1 mg/kg
- **Morphine** I.V. 1-3 mg
- **Nitroglycerin** SL
- Oxygen/intubate PRN

Second-line actions
- **Nitroglycerin** I.V. (if BP >100 mm Hg)
- **Nitroprusside** I.V. (if BP >100 mm Hg)
- **Dopamine** (if BP <100 mm Hg)
- **Dobutamine** (if BP >100 mm Hg)
- Positive end-expiratory pressure (PEEP)
- Continuous positive airway pressure (CPAP)

NORMAL HEART RATES

Age	Mean Heart Rate (beats/minute)	Heart Rate Range (2nd – 98th percentile)
<1 d	123	93-154
1-2 d	123	91-159
3-6 d	129	91-166
1-3 wk	148	107-182
1-2 mo	149	121-179
3-5 mo	141	106-186
6-11 mo	134	109-169
1-2 y	119	89-151
3-4 y	108	73-137
5-7 y	100	65-133
8-11 y	91	62-130
12-15 y	85	60-119

Adapted from *The Harriet Lane Handbook*, 12th ed, Greene MG, ed, St Louis, MO: Mosby Yearbook, 1991.

NORMAL QRS AXES (in degrees)

Age	Mean	Range
1 wk – 1 mo	+110	+30 to +180
1–3 mo	+70	+10 to +125
3 mo – 3 y	+60	+10 to +110
>3 y	+60	+20 to +120
Adults	+50	−30 to +105

INTERVALS AND SEGMENTS
OF AN EKG CYCLE

HEXAXIAL REFERENCE
SYSTEM

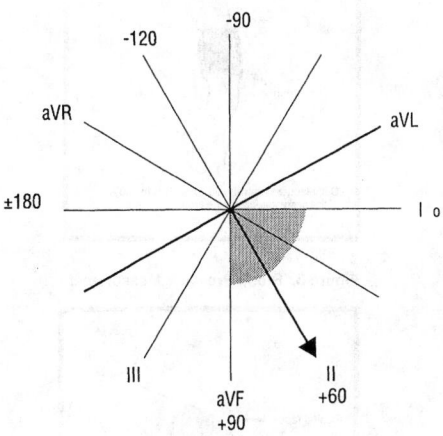

MEASURING PEDIATRIC BLOOD PRESSURE

Figure 1. Determine of Proper Cuff Size, Step 1

The cuff bladder width should be approximately 40% of the circumference of the arm measured at a point midway between the olecranon and acromion.

Figure 2. Determination of Proper Cuff Size, Step 2

Cuff bladder length should cover 80% to 100% of the circumference of the arm.

Figure 3. Blood Pressure Measurement

Blood pressure should be measured with cubital fossa at heart level. The arm should be supported. The stethoscope bell is placed over the brachial artery pulse, proximal and medial to the cubital fossa, and below the bottom edge of the cuff.

Used with permission: Perloff D, Grim C, Flack J, et al, "Human Blood Pressure Determination by Sphygmomanometry," *Circulation*, 1993, 88:2460-7.

HYPERTENSION, CLASSIFICATION BY AGE GROUP*

Age Group	Significant Hypertension (mm Hg)	Severe Hypertension (mm Hg)
Newborn (7 d)		
systolic BP	≥96	≥106
Newborn (8-30 d)		
systolic BP	≥104	≥110
Infant (<2 y)		
systolic BP	≥112	≥118
diastolic BP	≥74	≥82
Children (3-5 y)		
systolic BP	≥116	≥124
diastolic BP	≥76	≥84
Children (6-9 y)		
systolic BP	≥122	≥130
diastolic BP	≥78	≥86
Children (10-12 y)		
systolic BP	≥126	≥134
diastolic BP	≥82	≥90
Adolescents (13-15 y)		
systolic BP	≥136	≥144
diastolic BP	≥86	≥92
Adolescents (16-18 y)		
systolic BP	≥142	≥150
diastolic BP	≥92	≥98

Adapted from Horan MJ, *Pediatrics*, 1987, 79:1-25.

*See also Blood Pressure Measurement, Age Specific Percentiles *on page 1022* and 90th and 95th Percentiles of Blood Pressure by Percentiles of Height *on page 1024*

BLOOD PRESSURE IN PREMATURE INFANTS, NORMAL

(Birth weight 600-1750 g)*

Day	600-999 g		1000-1249 g	
	S (± 2SD)	D (± 2SD)	S (± 2SD)	D (± 2SD)
1	37.9 (17.4)	23.2 (10.3)	44 (22.8)	22.5 (13.5)
3	44.9 (15.7)	30.6 (12.3)	48 (15.4)	36.5 (9.6)
7	50 (14.8)	30.4 (12.4)	57 (14)	42.5 (16.5)
14	50.2 (14.8)	37.4 (12)	53 (30)	
28	61 (23.5)	45.8 (27.4)	57 (30)	

Day	1250-1499 g		1500-1750 g	
	S (± 2SD)	D (± 2SD)	S (± 2SD)	D (± 2SD)
1	48 (18)	27 (12.4)	47 (15.8)	26 (15.6)
3	59 (21.1)	40 (13.7)	51 (18.2)	35 (10)
7	68 (14.8)	40 (11.3)	66 (23)	41 (24)
14	64 (21.2)	36 (24.2)	76 (34.8)	42 (20.3)
28	69 (31.4)	44 (26.2)	73 (5.6)	50 (9.9)

*Blood pressure was obtained by the Dinamap method.

S = systolic; D = diastolic; SD = standard deviation.

Modified from Ingelfinger JR, Powers L, and Epstein MF, "Blood Pressure Norms in Low-Weight Infants: Birth Through Four Weeks", *Pediatr Res*, 1983, 17:319A.

BLOOD PRESSURE MEASUREMENTS, AGE-SPECIFIC PERCENTILES

Blood Pressure Measurements: Ages 0-12 Months, Boys

Korotkoff phase IV (K4) used for diastolic BP. Reproduced with permission from Horan MJ, *Pediatrics*, 1987, 79:11-25.

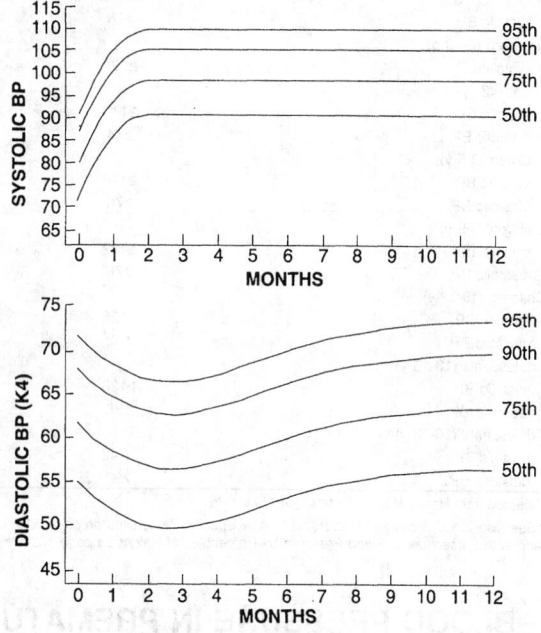

90th PERCENTILE												
SYSTOLIC BP	87	101	106	106	106	105	105	105	105	105	105	105	105
DIASTOLIC BP	68	65	63	63	63	65	66	67	68	68	69	69	69
HEIGHT CM	51	59	63	66	68	70	72	73	74	76	77	78	80
WEIGHT KG	4	4	5	5	6	7	8	9	9	10	10	11	11

Blood Pressure Measurements: Ages 0-12 Months, Girls

Korotkoff phase IV (K4) used for diastolic BP. Reproduced with permission from Horan MJ, *Pediatrics*, 1987, 79:11-25.

90th PERCENTILE													
SYSTOLIC BP	76	98	101	104	105	106	106	106	106	106	106	105	105
DIASTOLIC BP	68	65	64	64	65	65	66	66	66	67	67	67	67
HEIGHT CM	54	55	56	58	61	63	66	68	70	72	74	75	77
WEIGHT KG	4	4	4	5	5	6	7	8	9	9	10	10	11

BLOOD PRESSURE MEASUREMENTS, AGE-SPECIFIC PERCENTILES (Continued)

90th AND 95th PERCENTILES
OF BLOOD PRESSURE BY PERCENTILES OF HEIGHT

BOYS AGE 1-9 YEARS

Height Percentiles* →		Systolic BP (mm Hg)							Diastolic BP (mm Hg)‡						
Age (y)	BP Percentiles† ↓	5%	10%	25%	50%	75%	90%	95%	5%	10%	25%	50%	75%	90%	95%
1	90th	94	95	97	98	100	102	102	50	51	52	53	54	54	55
	95th	98	99	101	102	104	106	106	55	55	56	57	58	59	59
2	90th	98	99	100	102	104	105	106	55	55	56	57	58	59	59
	95th	101	102	104	106	108	109	110	59	59	60	61	62	63	63
3	90th	100	101	103	105	107	108	109	59	59	60	61	62	63	63
	95th	104	105	107	109	111	112	113	63	63	64	65	66	67	67
4	90th	102	103	105	107	109	110	111	62	62	63	64	65	66	66
	95th	106	107	109	111	113	114	115	66	67	67	68	69	70	71
5	90th	104	105	106	108	110	112	112	65	65	66	67	68	69	69
	95th	108	109	110	112	114	115	116	69	70	70	71	72	73	74
6	90th	105	106	108	110	111	113	114	67	68	69	70	70	71	72
	95th	109	110	112	114	115	117	117	72	72	73	74	75	76	76
7	90th	106	107	109	111	113	114	115	69	70	71	72	72	73	74
	95th	110	111	113	115	116	118	119	74	74	75	76	77	78	78
8	90th	107	108	110	112	114	115	116	71	71	72	73	74	75	75
	95th	111	112	114	116	118	119	120	75	76	76	77	78	79	80
9	90th	109	110	112	113	115	117	117	72	73	73	74	75	76	77
	95th	113	114	116	117	119	121	121	76	77	78	79	80	80	81

*Height percentile determined by standard growth curves.

† Blood pressure percentile determined by a single measurement

‡Korotkoff phase V (K5) used for diastolic BP

Source: National Institutes of Health, National Heart, Lung, and Blood Institute, "Update on the Task Force Report (1987) on High Blood Pressure in Children and Adolescents: A Working Group Report from the National High Blood Pressure Education Program," NIH No. 96-3790, 1996.

BOYS AGE 10-17 YEARS

Systolic BP (mm Hg)

Age (y)	BP Percentiles†	Height Percentiles* 5%	10%	25%	50%	75%	90%	95%
10	90th	110	112	113	115	117	118	119
	95th	114	115	117	119	121	122	123
11	90th	112	113	115	117	119	120	121
	95th	116	117	119	121	123	124	125
12	90th	115	116	117	119	121	123	123
	95th	119	120	121	123	125	126	127
13	90th	117	118	120	122	124	125	126
	95th	121	122	124	126	128	129	130
14	90th	120	121	123	125	126	128	128
	95th	124	125	127	128	130	132	132
15	90th	123	124	125	127	129	131	131
	95th	127	128	129	131	133	134	135
16	90th	125	126	128	130	132	133	134
	95th	129	130	132	134	136	137	138
17	90th	128	129	131	133	134	136	136
	95th	132	133	135	136	138	140	140

Diastolic BP (mm Hg)‡

Age (y)	BP Percentiles†	Height Percentiles* 5%	10%	25%	50%	75%	90%	95%
10	90th	73	74	74	75	76	77	78
	95th	77	78	79	80	80	81	82
11	90th	74	74	75	76	77	78	78
	95th	78	79	79	80	81	82	83
12	90th	75	75	76	77	78	78	79
	95th	79	79	80	81	82	83	83
13	90th	75	76	76	77	78	79	80
	95th	79	80	81	82	83	83	84
14	90th	76	76	77	78	79	80	80
	95th	80	81	81	82	83	84	85
15	90th	77	77	78	79	80	81	81
	95th	81	82	83	83	84	85	86
16	90th	79	79	80	81	82	82	83
	95th	83	83	84	85	86	87	87
17	90th	81	81	82	83	84	85	85
	95th	85	85	86	87	88	89	89

*Height percentile determined by standard growth curves.

† Blood pressure percentile determined by a single measurement

‡Korotkoff phase V (K5) used for diastolic BP

Source: National Institutes of Health, National Heart, Lung, and Blood Institute, "Update on the Task Force Report (1987) on High Blood Pressure in Children and Adolescents: A Working Group Report from the National High Blood Pressure Education Program," NIH No, 96-3790, 1996.

BLOOD PRESSURE MEASUREMENTS, AGE-SPECIFIC PERCENTILES *(Continued)*

GIRLS 1 TO 9 YEARS

Age (y)	BP Percentile†	Systolic BP (mm Hg)							Diastolic BP (mm Hg)‡						
	Height Percentiles* →	5%	10%	25%	50%	75%	90%	95%	5%	10%	25%	50%	75%	90%	95%
1	90th	97	98	99	100	102	103	104	53	53	53	54	55	56	56
	95th	101	102	103	104	105	107	107	57	57	57	58	59	60	60
2	90th	99	99	100	102	103	104	105	57	57	58	58	59	60	61
	95th	102	103	104	105	107	108	109	61	61	62	62	63	64	65
3	90th	100	100	102	103	104	105	106	61	61	61	62	63	63	64
	95th	104	104	105	107	108	109	110	65	65	65	66	67	67	68
4	90th	101	102	103	104	106	107	108	63	63	64	65	65	66	67
	95th	105	106	107	108	109	111	111	67	67	68	69	69	70	71
5	90th	103	103	104	106	107	108	109	65	66	66	67	68	68	69
	95th	107	107	108	110	111	112	113	69	70	70	71	72	72	73
6	90th	104	105	106	107	109	110	111	67	67	68	69	69	70	71
	95th	108	109	110	111	112	114	114	71	71	72	73	73	74	75
7	90th	106	107	108	109	110	112	112	69	69	69	70	71	72	72
	95th	110	110	112	113	114	115	116	73	73	73	74	75	76	76
8	90th	108	109	110	111	112	113	114	70	70	71	71	72	73	74
	95th	112	112	113	115	116	117	118	74	74	75	75	76	77	78
9	90th	110	110	112	113	114	115	116	71	72	72	73	74	74	75
	95th	114	114	115	117	118	119	120	75	76	76	77	78	78	79

*Height percentile determined by standard growth curves.

† Blood pressure percentile determined by a single measurement

‡Korotkoff phase V (K5) used for diastolic BP

Source: National Institutes of Health, National Heart, Lung, and Blood Institute, "Update on the Task Force Report (1987) on High Blood Pressure in Children and Adolescents: A Working Group Report from the National High Blood Pressure Education Program," NIH No, 96-3790, 1996.

GIRLS AGE 10-17 YEARS

Age (y)	BP Percentiles†	Systolic BP (mm Hg) 5%	10%	25%	50%	75%	90%	95%	Diastolic BP (mm Hg)‡ 5%	10%	25%	50%	75%	90%	95%
10	90th	112	112	114	115	116	117	118	73	73	73	74	75	76	76
	95th	116	116	117	119	120	121	122	77	77	77	78	79	80	80
11	90th	114	114	116	117	118	119	120	74	74	75	75	76	77	77
	95th	118	118	119	121	122	123	124	78	78	79	79	80	81	81
12	90th	116	116	118	117	118	121	120	75	75	76	76	77	78	78
	95th	120	120	121	123	124	125	126	79	79	79	80	81	82	82
13	90th	118	118	119	121	122	123	124	76	76	77	78	79	79	80
	95th	121	122	123	125	126	127	128	80	80	81	82	83	83	84
14	90th	119	120	121	122	124	125	126	77	77	78	79	79	80	81
	95th	123	124	125	126	128	129	130	81	81	82	83	83	84	85
15	90th	121	121	122	124	125	126	127	78	78	79	79	80	81	82
	95th	124	125	126	128	129	130	131	82	82	83	83	84	85	86
16	90th	122	122	123	125	126	127	128	79	79	79	80	81	82	82
	95th	125	126	127	128	130	131	132	83	83	83	84	85	86	86
17	90th	122	123	124	125	126	128	128	79	79	79	80	81	82	82
	95th	126	126	127	129	130	131	132	83	83	83	84	85	86	86

*Height percentile determined by standard growth curves.
† Blood pressure percentile determined by a single measurement
‡Korotkoff phase V (K5) used for diastolic BP

Source: National Institutes of Health, National Heart, Lung, and Blood Institute, "Update on the Task Force Report (1987) on High Blood Pressure in Children and Adolescents: A Working Group Report from the National High Blood Pressure Education Program," NIH No. 96-3790, 1996.

ANTIHYPERTENSIVE AGENTS BY CLASS

Alpha 2 Agonists
Clonidine
Methyldopa

Alpha 1 Antagonists
Prazosin

Beta Antagonists
Atenolol
Esmolol
Nadolol
Propranolol
Timolol

Mixed Alpha/Beta Antagonists
Labetalol

Calcium Channel Blockers
Diltiazem
Nifedipine
Verapamil

Angiotensin Converting Enzyme Inhibitors
Captopril
Enalapril/Enalaprilat
Lisinopril

Nitrates
Isosorbide dinitrate
Nitroglycerin

Ganglionic Blockers
Trimethaphan

Diuretics
Amiloride
Bumetanide
Chlorothiazide
Ethacrynic acid
Furosemide
Hydrochlorothiazide
Mannitol
Metolazone
Spironolactone
Torsemide
Triamterene

Vasodilators (Direct-acting)
Diazoxide
Hydralazine
Minoxidil
Nitroprusside

ANTIDEPRESSANT AGENTS

Comparison of Usual Adult Dosage and Mechanism of Action

Drug	Usual Adult Dosage (mg/d)	Reuptake Inhibition	
		Norepinephrine	Serotonin
First-Generation Antidepressants *Tricyclic Antidepressants*			
Amitriptyline (Elavil®, Endep®)	100-300	Moderate	High
Clomipramine† (Anafranil®)	100-250	Moderate	High
Desipramine (Norpramin®, Pertofrane®)	100-300	High	Low
Doxepin (Adapin®, Sinequan®)	100-300	Low	Moderate
Imipramine (Janimine®, Tofranil®)	100-300	Moderate	Moderate
Nortriptyline (Aventyl®, Pamelor®)	50-200	Moderate	Low
Protriptyline (Vivactil®)	15-60	Moderate	Low
Trimipramine (Surmontil®)	100-300	Low	Low
Monoamine Oxidase Inhibitors			
Phenelzine (Nardil®)	15-90	—	—
Tranylcypromine (Parnate®)	10-40	—	—
Second-Generation Antidepressants *Older Second-Generation Antidepressants*			
Amoxapine (Asendin®)	100-400	Moderate	Low
Maprotiline (Ludiomil®)	100-225	Moderate	Low
Trazodone (Desyrel®)	150-500	Very low	Moderate
Newer Second-Generation Antidepressants			
Bupropion (Wellbutrin®)	300-450‡	Very low§	Very low§
Third-Generation Antidepressants *Selective Serotonin Reuptake Inhibitors*			
Fluoxetine (Prozac®)	10-40	Very low	High
Fluvoxamine (Luvox®)	100-300	Very low	Very high
Paroxetine (Paxil®)	20-50	Very low	Very high
Sertraline (Zoloft®)	50-150	Very low	Very high
Serotonin/Norepinephrine Reuptake Inhibitors			
Venlafaxine (Effexor®)	75-375	Very high	Very high
Atypical Antidepressants with 5HT2 Receptor Antagonist Properties			
Mirtazapine (Remeron®)**	15-45	Very low	Very low
Nefazodone (Serzone®)**	300-600	Very low	High

†Not approved by FDA for depression

‡Not to exceed 150 mg/dose to minimize seizure risk

§Norepinephrine and serotonin reuptake inhibition is minimal, but inhibits dopamine reuptake

**These agents work primarily through antagonizing the postsynaptic 5HT2 receptor.

ANTIDEPRESSANT AGENTS *(Continued)*

Comparison of Adverse Effects

Drug	ACH	Drowsiness	Orthostatic Hypotension	Cardiac Arrhythmias	GI Distress	Weight Gain
Adverse Effects						
First-Generation Antidepressants *Tricyclic Antidepressants*						
Amitriptyline (Elavil®, Endep®)	4+	4+	4+	3+	0	4+
Clomipramine† (Anafranil®)	4+	4+	2+	3+	1+	4+
Desipramine (Norpramin®, Pertofrane®)	1+	2+	2+	2+	0	1+
Doxepin (Adapin®, Sinequan®)	3+	4+	2+	2+	0	4+
Imipramine (Janimine®, Tofranil®)	3+	3+	4+	3+	1+	4+
Nortriptyline (Aventyl®, Pamelor®)	2+	2+	1+	2+	0	1+
Protriptyline (Vivactil®)	2+	1+	2+	3+	0	0
Trimipramine (Surmontil®)	4+	4+	3+	3+	0	4+
Monoamine Oxidase Inhibitors						
Phenelzine (Nardil®)	2+	2+	2+	1+	1+	3+
Tranylcypromine (Parnate®)	2+	1+	2+	1+	1+	2+
Second-Generation Antidepressants *Older Second-Generation Antidepressants*						
Amoxapine (Asendin®)	2+	2+	2+	2+	0	2+
Maprotiline (Ludiomil®)	2+	3+	2+	2+	0	2+
Trazodone (Desyrel®)	0	4+	3+	1+	1+	2+
Newer Second-Generation Antidepressants						
Bupropion (Wellbutrin®)	0	0	0	1+	1+	0
Third-Generation Antidepressants *Selective Serotonin Reuptake Inhibitors*						
Fluoxetine (Prozac®)	0	0	0	0	3+¶	0
Fluvoxamine (Luvox®)	0	0	0	0	3+¶	0
Paroxetine (Paxil®)	1+	1+	0	0	3+¶	1+
Sertraline (Zoloft®)	0	0	0	0	3+¶	0
Serotonin/Norepinephrine Reuptake Inhibitors						
Venlafaxine# (Effexor®)	1+	1+	0	1+	3+¶	0

Comparison of Adverse Effects *(continued)*

			Adverse Effects			
Drug	ACH	Drowsiness	Orthostatic Hypotension	Cardiac Arrhythmias	GI Distress	Weight Gain
Atypical Antidepressants with 5HT2 Receptor Antagonist Properties						
Mirtazapine (Remeron®)	1+	2+	0	0	3+	0
Nefazodone (Serzone®)	1+	1+	0	0	1+	0

Key: ACH = anticholinergic effects (dry mouth, blurred vision, urinary retention, constipation); 0 - 4+ = absent or rare - relatively common.

†Not approved by FDA for depression

¶Nausea is usually mild and transient

#Comparative studies evaluating the adverse effects of venlafaxine in relation to other antidepressants have not been performed

CORTICOSTEROIDS, SYSTEMIC

Relative Potencies and Equivalent Doses of Corticosteroids

(Glucocorticoid potency compared to hydrocortisone "mg" for "mg" basis)

Compound	Gluco-corticoid Potency	Mineralo-corticoid Potency	Equivalent Dose (mg)	Duration* of Action
Cortisone (Cortone®)	0.8	++	25	S
Injection: 50 mg/mL suspension				
Tablet: 5 mg				
Dexamethasone (Decadron®, Dexone®, Hexadrol®)	25-30	0	0.75	L
Elixir: 0.5 mg/5 mL				
Injection: 4 mg/mL				
Intensol: 1 mg/mL				
Tablet: 0.25 mg, 0.5 mg, 0.75 mg, 1 mg, 1.5 mg, 2 mg, 4 mg				
Fludrocortisone (Florinef®)	10	+++++		I
Tablet: 0.1 mg				
Hydrocortisone (Cortef®)	1	++	20	S
Injection: 50 mg/mL				
Suspension: 10 mg/5 mL				
Tablet: 5 mg, 10 mg, 20 mg				
Methylprednisolone (Medrol®, Solu-Medrol®, Depo-Medrol®)	5	0	4	I
Injection: 40 mg, 125 mg, 500 mg, 1 g				
Injection, susp: 80 mg/mL				
Tablet: 2 mg, 4 mg, 16 mg, 24 mg				
Prednisolone (Delta-Cortef®, Prelone® Syrup, Pediapred®)	4	+	5	I
Liquid: 5 mg/5 mL				
Syrup: 15 mg/5 mL				
Tablet: 5 mg				
Prednisone (Deltasone®, Liquid Pred®, Orasone®)	4	+	5	I
Liquid: 5 mg/5 mL				
Tablet: 1 mg, 2.5 mg, 5 mg, 10 mg, 20 mg, 50 mg				

*S = Short, 8-12 hours biologic activity

I = Intermediate, 12-36 hours biologic activity

L = Long, 36-54 hours biologic activity

Reference

Knoben JE, and Anderson PO, *Handbook of Clinical Drug Data*, 6th ed, Drug Intelligence Pub, Inc, 1988.

CORTICOSTEROIDS, TOPICAL

The following topical corticosteroid preparations are grouped according to relative anti-inflammatory activity. Preparations in each group are approximately equivalent.

Drug	Dosage Form
Lowest Potency	
Hydrocortisone	0.5% cream, ointment
Hydrocortisone	1% cream, ointment
Hydrocortisone	2.5% cream, ointment
Hydrocortisone	1% solution
Hydrocortisone	1% lotion
Low Potency	
Alclometasone Dipropionate (Aclovate®)	0.05% cream, ointment
Desonide (Tridesilon®)	0.05% cream, ointment
Fluocinolone Acetonide	
(Fluonid®)	0.01% solution
(Synalar®)	0.01% cream
Low Intermediate Potency	
Betamethasone Valerate (Valisone®)	0.01% cream
Flurandrenolide (Cordran®)*	0.025% cream, ointment
Hydrocortisone Valerate (Westcort®)	0.2% cream, ointment
Triamcinolone Acetonide (Kenalog®)	0.025% cream, ointment, lotion
High Intermediate Potency	
Betamethasone Valerate (Valisone®)	0.1% cream, ointment, lotion
Desoximetasone (Topicort®)	0.05% gel
Fluocinolone Acetonide (Synalar®)*	0.025% cream, ointment
Flurandrenolide (Cordran®)*	0.05% cream, ointment, lotion
Halcinonide (Halog®)	0.025% cream
Triamcinolone Acetonide (Aristocort®, Kenalog®)	0.1% cream, ointment, lotion
High Potency	
Amcinonide (Cyclocort®)*	0.1% ointment
Betamethasone Dipropionate (Diprosone®)	0.05% cream, ointment, lotion
Desoximetasone (Topicort®)	0.25% cream, ointment
Diflorasone Diacetate (Florone®)	0.05% cream, ointment
Fluocinolone Acetonide (Synalar®-HP)	0.2% cream
Fluocinonide (Lidex®)	0.05% cream, ointment, solution
Halcinonide (Halog®)	0.1% cream, ointment, solution
Triamcinolone Acetonide (Aristocort®, Kenalog®)	0.5% cream, ointment

*Does not contain propylene glycol.

Reference
Cornell RC and Stoughton RB, "The Use of Topical Steroids in Psoriasis," *Dermatol Clin*, 1984, 2:397-407.

MULTIPLE VITAMIN PRODUCTS

Product	Content Given Per	A IU	D IU	E IU	C mg	FA mg	B₁ mg	B₂ mg	B₃ mg	B₅ mg	B₆ mg	B₁₂ mcg	Elemental Fe mg	Fluoride mg	Other
Drops															
Poly-Vi-Sol®	1 mL	1500	400	5	35		0.5	0.6	8		0.4	2			
Poly-Vi-Sol® with Iron	1 mL	1500	400	5	35		0.5	0.6	8		0.4	2	10		
Tri-Vi-Sol®	1 mL	1500	400		35										
Tri-Vi-Flor® 0.25 mg	1 mL	1500	400		35									0.25	
Adek®	1 mL	1500	400	40	45		0.5	0.6	6	3	0.6	4			Biotin 15 mcg, vitamin K 0.1 mg, zinc 5 mg, beta carotene 1 mg
Liquid															
Theragran®	5 mL	5000	400		200		10	10	300	21.4	4.1	5			
Vi-Daylin® Multivitamin	5 mL	2500	400	15	60		1.05	1.2	13.5		1.05	4.5			
B Complex	5 mL						2.3	1	6.7		0.3				
Tablet															
Adek®	1 tablet	4000	400	150	60	0.2	1.2	1.3	10	10	1.5	12			Zinc 1.1 mg, beta carotene 3 mg, vitamin K, biotin 50 mcg
Centrum Jr® with Iron	1 tablet	5000	400	30	60	0.4	1.5	1.7	20	10	2	6	18		Biotin 45 mcg, zinc 15 mg, Ca, Cu 1, Mg, Mn, Mo, P, vitamin K
Nephro-Vite®	1 tablet				100	1	1.5	1.7	20	5	10	6			Biotin 150 mcg
Poly-Vi-Flor® 1 mg	1 tablet	2500	400	15	60	0.3	1.05	1.2	13.5		1.05	4.5		1	
Poly-Vi-Sol®	1 tablet	2500	400	15	60	0.3	1.05	1.2	13.5		1.05	4.5			
Vi-Daylin® with Iron	1 tablet	2500	400	15	60	0.3	1.05	1.2	13.5		1.05	4.5	12		
Capsule															
Nephrocaps®	1 capsule				100	1	1.5	1.7	20	5	10	6			Biotin 150 mcg

NARCOTIC ANALGESICS COMPARISON

Drug	Dosage Form	Onset (min)	Duration (h)	Equi-analgesic I.M. Dose (mg)	Equi-analgesic P.O. Dose (mg)	Parenteral Oral Ratio	Partial Antagonist
Alfentanil hydrochloride	Inj: 500 mcg/mL 5 mL amp	Immediate (I.V.)	ND	ND	—	—	No
Codeine	Inj: 30 mg/mL as phosphate Tab: 15 mg, 30 mg as sulfate, 60 mg as phosphate	10-30 (I.M.)	4-6 (I.M.)	120	200	1/2-2/3	No
Fentanyl citrate (Sublimaze®)	Inj: 50 mcg/mL 2 mL, 10 mL amp	7-8 (I.M.)	1-2 (I.M.); 0.5-1 (I.V.)	0.1-0.2	—	—	No
Hydrocodone and acetaminophen	Tab: 5 mg hydrocodone + 500 mg acetaminophen (Vicodin®)	ND	4-6 (P.O.)	—	ND	ND	No
Hydromorphone hydrochloride (Dilaudid®)	Inj: 2 mg/mL amp Tab: 2 mg	15-30 (I.M.)	4-5 (I.M.)	1.5	7.5	1/5	No
Meperidine hydrochloride (Demerol®)	Inj: 25 mg/0.5 mL, 50 mg/mL, 100 mg/mL amp Syrup: 10 mg/mL Tab: 50 mg	10-45 (I.M.)	2-4 (I.M.)	75-100	300	1/3-1/2	No
Methadone hydrochloride (Dolophine®)	Inj: 10 mg/mL amp Solution: 1 mg/mL Tab: 5 mg, 10 mg	30-60 (I.M.)	4-6 (I.M.); duration increases with repeated use due to cumulative effects	10	20	1/2	No

NARCOTIC ANALGESICS COMPARISON *(Continued)*

Drug	Dosage Form	Onset (min)	Duration (h)	Equi-analgesic I.M. Dose (mg)	Equi-analgesic P.O. Dose (mg)	Parenteral Oral Ratio	Partial Antagonist
Morphine sulfate	Inj: 10 mg/mL, 15 mg/mL amp, 2 mg/mL Carbuject®, 1 mg/mL 30 mL PCA syringe, Inj, preservative free: 1 mg/mL 10 mL vial, 5 mg/10 mL amp (Duramorph® PF), Solution: 10 mg/5 mL, 20 mg/5 mL, Tab (soluble): 10 mg, 30 mg, Tab (controlled release): 30 mg (MS Contin®)	15-60 (epidural or I.T.), 15-30 (S.C.)	4-5 (I.M.) (S.C.)	10	60	1/6; ratio decreases to 1/1.5-2.5 upon chronic dosing	No
Oxycodone hydrochloride and acetaminophen (P.O.) (Percodan®, Tylox®)	Cap: Oxycodone 5 mg + acetaminophen 500 mg, Tab: Oxycodone (~5 mg) + acetaminophen 325 mg	15-30 (P.O.)	4-6 (P.O.)	—	30	—	No
Pentazocine (Talwin® NX)	Inj: 30 mg/mL as lactate, 1 mL, 1.5 mL, 2 mL uni-amp or Carbuject®, 10 mL vial, Tab: 50 mg with 0.5 mg naloxone (Talwin® NX)	15-30 (I.M.) (P.O.)	2-3 (I.M) 4-5 (P.O.)	50	150	1/3	Yes
Propoxyphene and acetaminophen (P.O.) (Darvocet-N® 50, Darvocet-N® 100, Darvon®)	Cap: Propoxyphene HCl (Darvon®) 32 mg, 65 mg, Tab: Propoxyphene napsylate 50 mg + acetaminophen 325 mg (Darvocet-N® 50); Propoxyphene napsylate 100 mg + acetaminophen 650 mg (Darvocet-N® 100)	30-60 (P.O.)	4-6 (P.O.)	—	HCl salt: 130 Napsylate salt: 200	—	No

ND = no data.

*These values are based on adult studies. Duration may be shorter in children due to faster elimination (in general) compared to adults.

OTC COUGH AND COLD PREPARATIONS, PEDIATRIC

Commonly Used Pediatric OTC Cough & Cold Preparations

Brand Name	Type of Preparation
Actifed®	Antihistamine/Decongestant
Benadryl® Allergy Decongestant Elixir	Antihistamine/Decongestant
Chlor-Trimeton® Allergy 4-Hour	Antihistamine
Dimetane®	Antihistamine/Decongestant
Dimetapp® Elixir	Antihistamine/Decongestant
Dimetapp® DM Elixir	Antihistamine/Antitussive/Decongestant
Dorcol® Children's Cough Syrup	Antitussive/Decongestant/Expectorant
Naldecon® DX Children's Syrup	Antihistamine/Antitussive/Decongestant
Naldecon® DX Pediatric Drops	Antihistamine/Antitussive/Decongestant
Neosynephrine® 2-Hour Children's Nose Drops	Decongestant
Neosynephrine® Nose Drops/Nasal Spray	Decongestant
Organidin® NR	Expectorant
Pediacare® Infant Oral Drops	Decongestant
Pediacare® Cough-Cold Formula	Antihistamine/Antitussive/Decongestant
Pediacare® "Night Rest"	Antihistamine/Antitussive/Decongestant
Robitussin®	Expectorant
Robitussin-CF®	Antitussive/Decongestant/Expectorant
Robitussin-DM®	Antitussive/Expectorant
Robitussin-PE®	Decongestant/Expectorant
Robitussin® Pediatric Cough Suppressant	Antitussive
St. Joseph® Cold Tablets	Decongestant
Sudafed®	Decongestant
Sudafed Plus	Antihistamine/Decongestant
Triaminic-DM® Syrup (dark red)	Antitussive/Decongestant
Triaminic® Expectorant (yellow)	Decongestant/Expectorant
Triaminic® Nite Light	Antihistamine/Antitussive/Decongestant
Triaminic Syrup® (orange)	Antihistamine/Decongestant
Triaminicol® Multi-System Relief (red)	Antihistamine/Antitussive/Decongestant
Tylenol® Cold, Children's	Antihistamine/Decongestant
Vick's Nyquil®, Children's	Antihistamine/Antitussive/Decongestant
Vick's Pediatric Formula 44® Cough and Cold	Antihistamine/Antitussive/Decongestant
Vick's Pediatric Formula 44® Cough and Congestion	Antitussive/Decongestant

OTC COUGH AND COLD PREPARATIONS, PEDIATRIC
(Continued)

Content of Commonly Used Pediatric Cough & Cold Preparations

The following chart lists the contents of the more common OTC cough and cold preparations. Products are grouped by preparation type. For specific recommendations, see individual drug monographs.

Brand Name	Generic(s)	Strength	Other Information
Decongestants			
Neosynephrine® 12-Hour Children's Nose Drops	Oxymethazoline	0.025%	Benzalkonium chloride, phenylmercuric acetate 0.002% as preservative
Neosynephrine® Nose Drops/Nasal Spray	Phenylephrine	0.16% 0.125% 0.25% 0.25%-0.5%	Infants >6 mo 1-6 y >6-12 y >12 y to adult
Pediacare® Infant Oral Drops	Pseudoephedrine	7.5 mg/0.8 mL	–
St. Joseph® Cold Tablets	Phenylpropanolamine	3.125 mg/tab	Acetaminophen 80 mg/chew tab
Sudafed®	Pseudoephedrine	15 mg/5 mL 30 mg/5 mL 30 mg/tab 60 mg/tab 120 mg/tab or cap (timed release) 240 mg/tab (timed release)	–
Antihistamines			
Chlor-Trimeton® Allergy 4-Hour	Chlorpheniramine	2 mg/5 mL	5% EtOH
Expectorants			
Organidin® NR Robitussin®	Guaifenesin	100 mg/5 mL	–
Antitussives			
Robitussin® Pediatric Cough Suppressant	Dextromethorphan HBr	7.5 mg/5 mL	–
Antihistamine/Decongestants			
Actifed®	Triprolidine	1.25 mg/5 mL 2.5 mg/tab	–
	Pseudoephedrine	30 mg/5 mL 60 mg/tab	
Benadryl®Allergy Decongestant Liquid	Diphenhydramine Pseudoephedrine	12.5 mg/5 mL 30 mg/5 mL	
Dimetane®	Phenylephrine Brompheniramine	5 mg/5 mL 2 mg/5 mL	2.3% EtOH
Dimetapp®	Brompheniramine	2 mg/5 mL 4 mg/tab 1 mg/chew tab	2.3% EtOH
	Phenylpropanolamine	12.5 mg/5 mL 25 mg/tab 6.25 mg/chew tab	
Sudafed Plus	Chlorpheniramine	2 mg/5 mL 4 mg/tab	–
	Pseudoephedrine	30 mg/5 mL 60 mg/tab	
Triaminic® Syrup (orange)	Chlorpheniramine	1 mg/5 mL 0.5 mg/chew tab	–
	Phenylpropanolamine	6.25 mg/5 mL 6.25 mg/chew tab	
Tylenol® Cold, Children's	Chlorpheniramine	1 mg/5 mL 0.5 mg/tab	Acetaminophen, 160 mg/5 mL, 80 mg/tab
	Pseudoephedrine	15 mg/5 mL 7.5 mg/tab	

Brand Name	Generic(s)	Strength	Other Information
Antitussive/Decongestant			
Triaminic-DM® Syrup (dark red)	Dextromethorphan Phenylpropanolamine	5 mg/5 mL 6.25 mg/5 mL	–
Vick's® Pediatric Formula 44 Cough & Congestion	Dextromethorphan Pseudoephedrine	5 mg/5 mL 10 mg/5 mL	–
Antitussive/Expectorant			
Robitussin-DM®	Dextromethorphan Guaifenesin	10 mg/5 mL 100 mg/5 mL	1.4% EtOH
Decongestant/Expectorant			
Robitussin-PE®	Pseudoephedrine Guaifenesin	30 mg/5 mL 100 mg/5 mL	1.4% EtOH
Triaminic® Expectorant (yellow)	Phenylpropanolamine Guaifenesin	6.25 mg/5 mL 50 mg/5 mL	–
Antihistamine/Antitussive/Decongestant			
Dimetapp® DM Elixir	Brompheniramine Dextromethorphan Phenylpropanolamine	2 mg/5 mL 10 mg/5 mL 12.5 mg/5 mL	–
Pediacare® Cough-Cold Formula	Chlorpheniramine Dextromethorphan Pseudoephedrine	1 mg/5 mL 0.5 mg/tab 1 mg/chew tab 5 mg/5 mL 2.5 mg/tab 5 mg/chew tab 15 mg/5 mL 7.5 mg/tab 15 mg/chew tab	–
Pediacare® "Night Rest"	Chlorpheniramine Dextromethorphan Pseudoephedrine	1 mg/5 mL 7.5 mg/5 mL 15 mg/5 mL	–
Triaminic® Nite Light	Chlorpheniramine Dextromethorphan Pseudoephedrine	1 mg/5 mL 7.5 mg/5 mL 15 mg/5 mL	–
Triaminicol® Multi-System Relief (red)	Chlorpheniramine Dextromethorphan Phenylpropanolamine	2 mg/5 mL 10 mg/5 mL 12.5 mg/5 mL	–
Vick's Nyquil®, Children's	Chlorpheniramine Dextromethorphan Pseudoephedrine	0.67 mg/5 mL 5 mg/5 mL 10 mg/5 mL	–
Vick's Pediatric Formula 44® Cough & Cold	Chlorpheniramine Dextromethorphan Pseudoephedrine	0.67 mg/5 mL 5 mg/5 mL 10 mg/5 mL	–
Antitussive/Decongestant/Expectorant			
Dorcol® Children's Cough Syrup	Dextromethorphan Pseudoephedrine Guaifenesin	5 mg/5 mL 15 mg/5 mL 50 mg/5 mL	–
Naldecon® DX Children's Syrup	Dextromethorphan Phenylpropanolamine Guaifenesin	5 mg/5 mL 6.25 mg/5 mL 100 mg/5 mL	–
Naldecon® DX Pediatric Drops	Dextromethorphan Phenylpropanolamine Guaifenesin	5 mg/1 mL 6.25 mg/1 mL 50 mg/1 mL	–
Robitussin-CF®	Dextromethorphan Phenylpropanolamine Guaifenesin	10 mg/5 mL 12.5 mg/5 mL 100 mg/5 mL	4.75% EtOH

CONVERSIONS

Apothecary-Metric Exact Equivalents

1 gram (g)	=	15.43 grains	0.1 mg	=	1/600 gr
1 milliliter (mL)	=	16.23 minims	0.12 mg	=	1/500 gr
1 minim	=	0.06 mL	0.15 mg	=	1/400 gr
1 grain (gr)	=	64.8 milligrams	0.2 mg	=	1/300 gr
1 fluid ounce (fl. oz)	=	29.57 mL	0.3 mg	=	1/200 gr
1 pint (pt)	=	473.2 mL	0.4 mg	=	1/150 gr
1 ounce (oz)	=	28.35 grams	0.5 mg	=	1/120 gr
1 pound (lb)	=	453.6 grams	0.6 mg	=	1/100 gr
1 kilogram (kg)	=	2.2 pounds	0.8 mg	=	1/80 gr
1 quart (qt)	=	946.4 mL	1 mg	=	1/65 gr

Apothecary-Metric Approximate Equivalents*

Liquids			Solids		

*Use exact equivalents for compounding and calculations requiring a high degree of accuracy.

1 teaspoonful	=	5 mL	¼ grain	=	15 mg
1 tablespoonful	=	15 mL	½ grain	=	30 mg
			1 grain	=	60 mg
			1½ grain	=	100 mg
			5 grains	=	300 mg
			10 grains	=	600 mg

Pounds-Kilograms

1 pound = 0.45359 kilograms
1 kilogram = 2.2 pounds

Temperature Conversion

Celsius to Fahrenheit = (°C x 9/5) + 32 = °F
Fahrenheit to Celsius = (°F - 32) x 5/9 = °C

CYTOCHROME P-450 ENZYMES AND DRUG METABOLISM

Background

The cytochrome P-450 enzymes are a "superfamily" of enzymes that catalyze the biotransformation (metabolism) of endogenous and exogenous lipophilic substances. These enzymes are considered to be the most important of the phase I enzymes and account for the majority of drug metabolism in humans. Enzyme "families," known as isoenzymes, are located primarily in the liver. The nomenclature of this system has been standardized. Isoenzyme "families" are identified using a CYP prefix, followed by an Arabic number (eg, CYP1). Subfamilies are designated by a letter following the number (eg, CYP1A) and individual isoenzymes are numbered sequentially within the subfamily (eg, CYP1A2). Cytochrome P-450 isoenzymes that are important in the metabolism of drugs in humans are primarily found in the CYP1, CYP2, and CYP3 families.

Enzymes may be inhibited (slowing metabolism through this pathway) or induced (increased in activity or number). Individual drugs metabolized by a specific enzyme are identified as substrates for the isoenzyme. Considerable effort has been expended in recent years to classify drugs metabolized by this system as either an inhibitor, inducer, or substrate of a specific isoenzyme. It should be noted that a drug may demonstrate complex activity within this scheme, acting as an inhibitor of one isoenzyme while serving as a substrate for another.

By recognizing that a substrate's metabolism may be dramatically altered by concurrent therapy with either an inducer or inhibitor, potential interactions may be identified and addressed. For example, a drug which inhibits CYP1A2 is likely to block metabolism of theophylline (a substrate for this isoenzyme). Because of this interaction, the dose of theophylline required to maintain a consistent level in the patient should be reduced when an inhibitor is added. Failure to make this adjustment may lead to supratherapeutic theophylline concentrations and potential toxicity.

This approach does have limitations. For example, the metabolism of specific drugs may have primary and secondary pathways. The contribution of secondary pathways to the overall metabolism may limit the impact of any given inhibitor. In addition, there may be up to a tenfold variation in the concentration of an isoenzyme across the broad population. In fact, a complete absence of an isoenzyme may occur in some genetic subgroups. Finally, the relative potency of inhibition, relative to the affinity of the enzyme for its substrate, demonstrates a high degree of variability. These issues make it difficult to anticipate whether a theoretical interaction will have a clinically relevant impact in a specific patient.

The details of this enzyme system continue to be investigated, and information is expanding daily. However, to be complete, it should be noted that other enzyme systems also influence a drug's pharmacokinetic profile. For example, a key enzyme system regulating the absorption of drugs is the p-glycoprotein system. Recent evidence suggests that some interactions originally attributed to the cytochrome system may, in fact, have been the result of inhibition of this enzyme.

The following tables represent an attempt to detail the available information with respect to isoenzyme activities. Within certain limits, they may be used to identify potential interactions. Of particular note, an effort has been made in each drug monograph to identify involvement of a particular isoenzyme in the drug's metabolism. These tables are intended to supplement the limited space available to list drug interactions in the monograph. Consequently, they may be used to define a greater range of both actual and potential drug interactions.

CYTOCHROME P-450 ENZYMES AND DRUG METABOLISM *(Continued)*

DRUGS CAUSING INHIBITORY AND INDUCTIVE INTERACTION

INHIBITORY (Enhancement of Interacting Drug Effect)	INDUCTIVE (Impairment of Interacting Drug Effect)
Amiodarone (Cordarone®)	Anticonvulsants
Cimetidine (Tagamet®)	Chronic ethanol use
Contraceptives, oral	Cigarette smoking
Erythromycin	Rifampin (Rifadin®, Rimactane®)
Ethanol intoxication	
Fluconazole	
Isoniazid (Laniazid®, Nydrazid®)	
Itraconazole	
Ketoconazole	
Neuroleptics	
Psoralen dermatologics	
Quinidine	
Quinolone antibiotics	
SSRIs	
Tricyclic antidepressants	

LOW THERAPEUTIC INDEX DRUGS

Hepatic Oxidation (Cytochrome P-450 Mediated Clearance)
Antiarrhythmic drugs
Anticoagulants, oral
Anticonvulsants
Antineoplastic/immunosuppressive drugs
Theophylline

CYTOCHROME P-450 ENZYMES AND RESPECTIVE METABOLIZED DRUGS

CYP1A2

Substrates

Acetaminophen	Metoclopramide
Acetanilid	Mirtazapine (hydroxylation)
Alosetron	Nortriptyline
Aminophylline	Olanzapine (demethylation, hydroxylation)
Amitriptyline (demethylation)	Ondansetron
Antipyrine	Phenacetin
Betaxolol	Phenothiazines
Caffeine	Propafenone
Chlorpromazine	Propranolol
Clomipramine (demethylation)	Riluzole
Clozapine	Ritonavir
Cyclobenzaprine (demethylation)	Ropinirole
Desipramine (demethylation)	Ropivacaine
Diazepam	Tacrine
Estradiol	Tamoxifen
Fluvoxamine	Theophylline
Grepafloxacin	Thioridazine
Haloperidol	Thiothixene
Imipramine (demethylation)	Trifluoperazine
Levobupivacaine	Verapamil
Levopromazine	Warfarin (R-warfarin, minor pathway)
Maprotiline	Zileuton
Methadone	Zopiclone

Inducers

Carbamazepine	Omeprazole
Charbroiled foods	Phenobarbital
Cigarette smoke	Phenytoin
Cruciferous vegetables (cabbage, brussels sprouts, broccoli, cauliflower)	Primidone
	Rifampin
Moricizine	Ritonavir
Nicotine	

Inhibitors

Anastrozole	Grapefruit juice
Cimetidine	Isoniazid
Ciprofloxacin	Levofloxacin
Citalopram (weak)	Mexiletine
Clarithromycin	Mibefradil
Diethyldithiocarbamate	Norfloxacin
Diltiazem	Paroxetine (high dose)(weak)
Enoxacin	Ritonavir
Entacapone (high dose)	Sertraline (weak)
Erythromycin	Tacrine
Ethinyl estradiol	Tertiary TCAs
Fluvoxamine	Zileuton
Fluoxetine (high dose)	

CYP2A6

Substrates

Dexmedetomidine	Nicotine
Letrozole	Ritonavir
Montelukast	Tamoxifen

Inducers

Barbiturates	

Inhibitors

Diethyldithiocarbamate	Ritonavir
Entacapone (high dose)	Tranylcypromine
Letrozole	

CYP2B6

Substrates

Antipyrine	Nicotine
Bupropion (hydroxylation)	Orphenadrine
Cyclophosphamide	
Ifosfamide	Tamoxifen

Inducers

Phenobarbital	Primidone
Phenytoin	

Inhibitors

Diethyldithiocarbamate	Orphenadrine

CYP2C
(Specific isozyme has not been identified)

Substrates

Antipyrine	Mephobarbital
Carvedilol	
Clozapine (minor)	Tamoxifen
Mestranol	Ticrynafen

Inducers

Carbamazepine	Primidone
Phenobarbital	Rifampin
Phenytoin	Sulfinpyrazone

CYTOCHROME P-450 ENZYMES AND DRUG METABOLISM *(Continued)*

Inhibitors

Isoniazid
Ketoconazole

Ketoprofen

CYP2C8

Substrates

Carbamazepine	Paclitaxel
Diazepam	Pioglitazone
Diclofenac	Retinoic acid
Ibuprofen	Rosiglitazone
Mephobarbital	Tolbutamide
Naproxen (5-hydroxylation)	Warfarin (S-warfarin)
Omeprazole	

Inducers

Carbamazepine	Primidone
Phenobarbital	Rifampin
Phenytoin	

Inhibitors

Anastrozole	Omeprazole

CYP2C9

Substrates

Alosetron	Mirtazapine
Amitriptyline (demethylation)	Montelukast
Celecoxib	Naproxen (5-hydroxylation)
Dapsone	Phenytoin
Diclofenac	Piroxicam
Flurbiprofen	Quetiapine (minor pathway)
Fluvastatin	Ritonavir
Glimepiride	Rosiglitazone (minor)
Hexobarbital	Sildenafil citrate
Ibuprofen	Tenoxicam
Imipramine (demethylation)	Tetrahydrocannabinol
Indomethacin	Tolbutamide
Irbesartan	Torsemide
Losartan	Warfarin (S-warfarin)
Mefenamic acid	Zafirlukast (hydroxylation)
Metronidazole	Zileuton

Inducers

Carbamazepine	Phenytoin
Fluconazole	
Fluoxetine	Rifampin
Phenobarbital	Secobarbital

Inhibitors

Amiodarone	Metronidazole
Anastrozole	Omeprazole
Chloramphenicol	Phenylbutazone
Cimetidine	Ritonavir
Diclofenac	Sertraline
Disulfiram	Sulfamethoxazole-trimethoprim
Entacapone (high dose)	Sulfaphenazole
Flurbiprofen	Sulfinpyrazone
Fluoxetine	Sulfonamides
Fluvastatin	Troglitazone
Fluvoxamine (potent)	Valproic acid
Isoniazid	Warfarin (R-warfarin)
Ketoprofen	Zafirlukast

CYP2C18

Substrates

Dronabinol
Naproxen
Omeprazole
Piroxicam

Proguanil
Propranolol
Retinoic acid
Warfarin

Inducers

Carbamazepine
Phenobarbital

Phenytoin
Rifampin

Inhibitors

Cimetidine

CYP2C19

Substrates

Amitriptyline (demethylation)
Barbiturates
Carisoprodol
Citalopram
Clomipramine (demethylation)
Desmethyldiazepam
Diazepam (N-demethylation, minor pathway)
Divalproex sodium
Hexobarbital
Imipramine (demethylation)
Lansoprazole
Mephenytoin
Mephobarbital

Moclobemide
Olanzapine (minor)
Omeprazole
Pantoprazole
Pentamidine
Phenytoin
Proguanil
Propranolol
Ritonavir
Tolbutamide
Topiramate
Valproic acid
Warfarin (R-warfarin)

Inducers

Carbamazepine
Phenobarbital

Phenytoin
Rifampin

Inhibitors

Cimetidine
Citalopram (weak)
Felbamate
Fluconazole
Fluoxetine
Fluvoxamine
Isoniazid
Ketoconazole (weak)
Letrozole
Omeprazole

Oxcarbazepine
Proguanil
Ritonavir
Sertraline
Teniposide
Tolbutamide
Topiramate
Tranylcypromine
Troglitazone

CYP2D6

Substrates

Amitriptyline (hydroxylation)
Amphetamine
Betaxolol
Bisoprolol
Brofaromine
Bufurolol
Bupropion
Captopril
Carvedilol
Cevimeline
Chlorpheniramine
Chlorpromazine
Cinnarizine
Clomipramine (hydroxylation)
Clozapine (minor pathway)
Codeine (hydroxylation, o-demethylation)
Cyclobenzaprine (hydroxylation)

Cyclophosphamide
Debrisoquin
Delavirdine
Desipramine
Dexfenfluramine
Dextromethorphan (o-demethylation)
Dihydrocodeine
Diphenhydramine
Dolasetron
Donepezil
Doxepin
Encainide
Fenfluramine
Flecainide
Fluoxetine (minor pathway)
Fluphenazine
Halofantrine

CYTOCHROME P-450 ENZYMES AND DRUG METABOLISM *(Continued)*

Haloperidol (minor pathway)
Hydrocodone
Hydrocortisone
Hydroxyamphetamine
Imipramine (hydroxylation)
Labetalol
Loratadine
Maprotiline
m-Chlorophenylpiperazine (m-CPP)
Meperidine
Methadone
Methamphetamine
Metoclopramide
Metoprolol
Mexiletine
Mianserin
Mirtazapine (hydroxylation)
Molindone
Morphine
Nortriptyline (hydroxylation)
Olanzapine (minor, hydroxymethylation)
Ondansetron
Orphenadrine
Oxycodone
Papaverine
Paroxetine (minor pathway)
Penbutolol
Pentazocine

Perhexiline
Perphenazine
Phenformin
Pindolol
Promethazine
Propafenone
Propranolol
Quetiapine
Remoxipride
Risperidone
Ritonavir (minor)
Ropivacaine
Selegiline
Sertindole
Sertraline (minor pathway)
Sparteine
Tamoxifen
Thioridazine
Tiagabine
Timolol
Tolterodine
Tramadol
Trazodone
Trimipramine
Tropisetron
Venlafaxine (o-desmethylation)
Yohimbine

Inhibitors

Amiodarone
Celecoxib
Chloroquine
Chlorpromazine
Cimetidine
Citalopram
Clomipramine
Codeine
Delavirdine
Desipramine
Dextropropoxyphene
Diltiazem
Doxorubicin
Entacapone (high dose)
Fluoxetine
Fluphenazine
Fluvoxamine
Haloperidol
Labetalol
Lobeline
Lomustine

Methadone
Mibefradil
Moclobemide
Norfluoxetine
Paroxetine
Perphenazine
Propafenone
Quinacrine
Quinidine
Ranitidine
Risperidone (weak)
Ritonavir
Sertindole
Sertraline (weak)
Thioridazine
Valproic acid
Venlafaxine (weak)
Vinblastine
Vincristine
Vinorelbine
Yohimbine

CYP2E1

Substrates

Acetaminophen
Acetone
Aniline
Benzene
Caffeine
Chlorzoxazone
Clozapine
Dapsone
Dextromethorphan
Enflurane
Ethanol
Halothane

Isoflurane
Isoniazid
Methoxyflurane
Nitrosamine
Ondansetron
Phenol
Ritonavir
Sevoflurane
Styrene
Tamoxifen
Theophylline
Venlafaxine

Inducers

Ethanol

Isoniazid

Inhibitors

Diethyldithiocarbamate (disulfiram metabolite)
Dimethyl sulfoxide
Disulfiram

Entacapone (high dose)
Ritonavir

CYP3A3/4

Substrates

Acetaminophen
Alfentanil
Alosetron
Alprazolam**
Amiodarone
Amitriptyline (minor)
Amlodipine
Anastrozole
Androsterone
Antipyrine
Astemizole**
Atorvastatin
Benzphetamine
Bepridil
Bexarotene
Bromazepam
Bromocriptine
Budesonide
Bupropion (minor)
Buspirone
Busulfan
Caffeine
Cannabinoids
Carbamazepine
Cevimeline
Cerivastatin
Chlorpromazine
Cimetidine
Cisapride**
Citalopram
Clarithromycin
Clindamycin
Clomipramine
Clonazepam
Clozapine
Cocaine
Codeine (demethylation)
Cortisol
Cortisone
Cyclobenzaprine (demethylation)
Cyclophosphamide
Cyclosporine
Dapsone
Dehydroepiandrostendione
Delavirdine
Desmethyldiazepam
Dexamethasone
Dextromethorphan (minor, N-demethylation)
Diazepam (minor; hydroxylation,
    N-demethylation)
Digitoxin
Diltiazem
Disopyramide
Docetaxel
Dolasetron
Donepezil
Doxorubicin
Doxycycline
Dronabinol
Enalapril
Erythromycin
Estradiol
Ethinyl estradiol
Ethosuximide
Etoposide

Exemestene
Dofetilide (minor)
Felodipine
Fentanyl
Fexofenadine
Finasteride
Fluoxetine
Flutamide
Glyburide
Granisetron
Haloperidol
Halofantrine
Hydrocortisone
Hydroxyarginine
Ifosfamide
Imipramine
Indinavir
Isradipine
Itraconazole
Ketoconazole
Lansoprazole (minor)
Letrozole
Levobupivicaine
Lidocaine
Loratadine
Losartan
Lovastatin
Methadone
Mibefradil
Miconazole
Midazolam
Mifepristone
Mirtazapine (N-demethylation)
Montelukast
Navelbine
Nefazodone
Nelfinavir**
Nevirapine
Nicardipine
Nifedipine
Niludipine
Nimodipine
Nisoldipine
Nitrendipine
Omeprazole (sulfonation)
Ondansetron
Oral contraceptives
Orphenadrine
Paclitaxel
Pantoprazole
Pimozide**
Pioglitazone
Pravastatin
Prednisone
Progesterone
Proguanil
Propafenone
Quercetin
Quetiapine
Quinidine
Quinine
Repaglinide
Retinoic acid
Rifampin
Risperidone

CYTOCHROME P-450 ENZYMES AND DRUG METABOLISM (Continued)

Ritonavir**
Salmeterol
Saquinavir
Sertindole
Sertraline
Sibutramine##
Sildenafil citrate
Simvastatin
Sirolimus
Sufentanil
Tacrolimus
Tamoxifen
Temazepam
Teniposide
Terfenadine**
Testosterone
Tetrahydrocannabinol
Theophylline
Tiagabine

Tolterodine
Toremifene
Trazodone
Tretinoin
Triazolam**
Troglitazone
Troleandomycin
Venlafaxine (N-demethylation)
Verapamil
Vinblastine
Vincristine
Warfarin (R-warfarin)
Yohimbine
Zaleplon (minor pathway)
Zatoestron
Zileuton
Ziprasidone
Zolpidem**
Zonisamide

Inducers

Carbamazepine
Dexamethasone
Glucocorticoids
Griseofulvin
Nafcillin
Nelfinavir
Nevirapine
Oxcarbazepine
Phenobarbital
Phenylbutazone
Phenytoin

Primidone
Progesterone
Rifabutin
Rifampin
Rofecoxib (mild)
Secobarbital
St John's wort
Sulfadimidine
Sulfinpyrazone
Troglitazone

Inhibitors

Amiodarone
Anastrozole
Azithromycin
Cannabinoids
Cimetidine
Clarithromycin**
Clotrimazole
Cyclosporine
Danazol
Delavirdine
Dexamethasone
Diethyldithiocarbamate
Diltiazem
Dirithromycin
Disulfiram
Entacapone (high dose)
Erythromycin**
Ethinyl estradiol
Fluconazole (weak)
Fluoxetine
Fluvoxamine**
Gestodene
Grapefruit juice
Haloperidol
Indinavir
Isoniazid
Itraconazole**

Ketoconazole**
Metronidazole
Mibefradil**
Miconazole (moderate)
Nefazodone**
Nelfinavir
Nevirapine
Norfloxacin
Norfluoxetine
Omeprazole (weak)
Oxiconazole
Paroxetine (weak)
Propoxyphene
Quinidine
Quinine**
Quinupristin and dalfopristin
Ranitidine
Ritonavir**
Saquinavir
Sertindole
Sertraline
Troglitazone
Troleandomycin
Valproic acid (weak)
Verapamil
Zafirlukast
Zileuton

CYP3A5-7

Substrates

Cortisol
Ethinyl estradiol
Lovastatin
Nifedipine
Quinidine

Terfenadine
Testosterone
Triazolam
Vinblastine
Vincristine

Inducers

Phenobarbital
Phenytoin
Primidone

Rifampin
Secobarbital

Inhibitors

Clotrimazole
Ketoconazole
Metronidazole

Miconazole
Troleandomycin

**Contraindications:
Terfenadine, astemizole, cisapride, and triazolam contraindicated with nefazodone
Pimozide contraindicated with macrolide antibiotics
Alprazolam and triazolam contraindicated with ketoconazole and itraconazole
Terfenadine, astemizole, and cisapride contraindicated with fluvoxamine
Terfenadine contraindicated with mibefradil, ketoconazole, erythromycin, clarithromycin, troleandomycin
Ritonavir contraindicated with triazolam, zolpidem, astemizole, rifabutin, quinine, clarithromycin, troleandomycin
Mibefradil contraindicated with astemizole
Nelfinavir contraindicated with rifabutin

\#\#Do not use with SSRIs, sumatriptan, lithium, meperidine, fentanyl, dextromethorphan, or pentazocine within 2 weeks of an MAOI.

References
Baker GB, Urichuk CJ, and Coutts RT, "Drug Metabolism and Metabolic Drug-Drug Interactions in Psychiatry," *Child Adolescent Psychopharm News (Suppl)*.
DeVane CL, "Pharmacogenetics and Drug Metabolism of Newer Antidepressant Agents," *J Clin Psychiatry*, 1994, 55(Suppl 12):38-45.
Drug Interactions Analysis and Management. Cytochrome (CYP) 450 Isozyme Drug Interactions, Vancouver, WA: Applied Therapeutics, Inc, 523-7.
Ereshefsky L, "Drug-Drug Interactions Involving Antidepressants: Focus on Venlafaxine," *J Clin Psychopharmacol*, 1996, 16(3 Suppl 2):375-535.
Ereshefsky L, *Psychiatr Annal*, 1996, 26:342-50.
Fleishaker JC and Hulst LK, "A Pharmacokinetic and Pharmacodynamic Evaluation of the Combined Administration of Alprazolam and Fluvoxamine," *Eur J Clin Pharmacol*, 1994, 46(1):35-9.
Flockhart DA, et al, *Clin Pharmacol Ther*, 1996, 59:189.
Ketter TA, Flockhart DA, Post RM, et al, "The Emerging Role of Cytochrome P-450 3A in Psychopharmacology," *J Clin Psychopharmacol*, 1995, 15(6):387-98.
Leeder JS and Kearns GL, "Pharmacogenetics in Pediatrics. Implications for Practice," *Pediatr Clin North Am*, 1997, 44(1):55-77.
Michalets EL, "Update: Clinically Significant Cytochrome P-450 Drug Interactions," *Pharmacotherapy*, 1998, 18(1):84-112.
Nemeroff CB, DeVane CL, and Pollock BG, "Newer Antidepressants and the Cytochrome P450 System," *Am J Psychiatry*, 1996, 153(3):311-20.
Pollock BG, "Recent Developments in Drug Metabolism of Relevance to Psychiatrists," *Harv Rev Psychiatry*, 1994, 2(4):204-13.
Richelson E, "Pharmacokinetic Drug Interactions of New Antidepressants: A Review of the Effects on the Metabolism of Other Drugs," *Mayo Clin Proc*, 1997, 72(9):835-47.
Riesenman C, "Antidepressant Drug Interactions and the Cytochrome P450 System: A Critical Appraisal," *Pharmacotherapy*, 1995, 15(6 Pt 2):84S-99S.
Schmider J, Greenblatt DJ, von Moltke LL, et al, "Relationship of *In Vitro* Data on Drug Metabolism to *In Vivo* Pharmacokinetics and Drug Interactions: Implications for Diazepam Disposition in Humans," *J Clin Psychopharmacol*, 1996, 16(4):267-72.
Slaughter RL, *Pharm Times*, 1996, 7.6-16.
Watkins PB, "Role of Cytochrome P450 in Drug Metabolism and Hepatotoxicity," *Semin Liver Dis*, 1990, 10(4):235-50.

EXTRAVASATION TREATMENT

Medication Extravasated	Cold/Warm Pack	Antidote
Chemotherapeutic agents		
DNA Intercalators		
Amsacrine Daunorubicin Doxorubicin	Cold	None
Vinca alkaloids		
Paclitaxel Vinblastine Vincristine Vindesine Vinorelbine	Warm	Hyaluronidase (Wydase®) 1. Add 1 mL NS to 150 units vial to make 150 units/mL concentration 2. Administer 0.2 mL injection subcutaneously or intradermally into the extravasation site at the leading edge; **Note:** Some institutions utilize a 1:10 dilution in infants and children; prepare by mixing 0.1 mL of 150 units/mL solution with 0.9 mL NS in 1 mL syringe to make final concentration = 15 units/mL
Alkylating agents		
Cisplatin Mechlorethamine (Nitrogen mustard)	Cold	Sodium thiosulfate 1/6 molar solution: mix 4 mL of 10% sodium thiosulfate with 6 mL of sterile water; inject 2 mL for each mg mechlorethamine or 100 mg cisplatinum (use only for large cisplatinum infiltrates >20 mL and when using cisplatinum concentrations >0.5 mg/mL; no data for use in cisplatinum infusions in children)
Other vesicant chemotherapeutic agents	Cold	None
Vasopressors		
Dobutamine Dopamine Epinephrine Metaraminol Norepinephrine Phenylephrine	None	Phentolamine (Regitine®) Mix 5 mg with 9 mL of NS Inject a small amount of this dilution into extravasated area. Blanching should reverse immediately. Monitor site. If blanching should recur, additional injections of phentolamine may be needed.
I.V. fluids and other medications		
Nafcillin Calcium	Cold	Hyaluronidase (Wydase®) As described above

BURN MANAGEMENT

Modified Lund-Browder Burn Assessment Chart
Estimation of Total Body Surface Area of Burn Involvement*
(% by site and age)

Site†	0-1 years	1-4 years	5-9 years	10-14 years	15 years	Adult
Head	9.5	8.5	6.5	5.5	4.5	3.5
Neck	0.5	0.5	0.5	0.5	0.5	0.5
Trunk	13	13	13	13	13	13
Upper arm	2	2	2	2	2	2
Forearm	1.5	1.5	1.5	1.5	1.5	1.5
Hand	1.5	1.5	1.5	1.5	1.5	1.5
Perineum	1	1	1	1	1	1
Buttock (each)	2.5	2.5	2.5	2.5	2.5	2.5
Thigh	2.75	3.25	4	4.25	4.5	4.75
Leg	2.5	2.5	2.75	3	3.25	3.5
Foot	1.75	1.75	1.75	1.75	1.75	1.75

*Applies only to second- and third-degree burns

†Percentage for each site is only for **a single extremity with** anterior **OR** posterior involvement. Percentage should be **doubled if both anterior and posterior** involvement of a single extremity.

The total body surface area of burn involvement is determined by the sum of the percentages of each site.

Adapted from Coren CV, "Burn Injuries in Children," *Pediatric Annals*, 1987, 16(4):328-39.

Parkland Fluid Replacement Formula

A guideline for replacement of deficits and ongoing losses (**Note:** For infants, maintenance fluids may need to be added to this): Administer 4 mL/kg/% burn of Ringer's lactate (glucose may be added but beware of stress hyperglycemia) over the first 24 hours; half of this total is given over the first 8 hours **calculated from the time of injury**; the remaining half is given over the next 16 hours. The second 24-hour fluid requirements average 50% to 75% of first day's requirement. Concentrations and rates best determined by monitoring weight, serum electrolytes, urine output, NG losses, etc.

Colloid may be added after 18-24 hours (1 g/kg/day of albumin) to maintain serum albumin >2 g/100 mL.

Potassium is generally withheld for the first 48 hours due to the large amount of potassium that is released from damaged tissues. To manage serum electrolytes, monitor urine electrolytes twice weekly and replace calculated urine losses.

ORAL CONTRACEPTIVES

Brand Name	Type	Progestin	Estrogen	Availability
Brevicon® Genora®0.5/35 Modicon® Nelova®0.5/35E	Combo	Norethindrone 0.5 mg	Ethinyl estradiol 35 mcg	21, 28
Demulen®1/35	Combo	Ethynodiol diacetate 1 mg	Ethinyl estradiol 35 mcg	21, 28
Demulen®1/50	Combo	Ethynodiol diacetate 1 mg	Ethinyl estradiol 50 mcg	21, 28
Desogen®	Combo	Desogestrel 0.15 mg	Ethinyl estradiol 30 mcg	28
Jenest™-28	Biphasic			
	1-7 d	Norethindrone 0.5 mg	Ethinyl estradiol 35 mcg	28
	8-21 d	Norethindrone 1 mg	Ethinyl estradiol 35 mcg	
	22-28 d	Inert	—	
Lo/Ovral®	Combo	Norgestrel 0.3 mg	Ethinyl estradiol 30 mcg	21, 28
Loestrin 21®1.5/30	Combo	Norethindrone acetate 1.5 mg	Ethinyl estradiol 30 mcg	21
Loestrin® Fe 1.5/30	Combo/Iron 21-28 d	Norethindrone acetate 1.5 mg	Ethinyl estradiol 30 mcg	28
Loestrin 21® 1/20	Combo	Norethindrone acetate 1 mg	Ethinyl estradiol 20 mcg	21
Loestrin® Fe 1/20	Combo/Iron 21-28 d	Norethindrone acetate 1 mg	Ethinyl estradiol 20 mcg	28
Genora® 1/35 N.E.E.® 1/35 Nelova®1/35 E Noriryl®1+35 Ortho-Novum™1/35	Combo	Norethindrone 1 mg	Ethinyl estradiol 35 mcg	21, 28
Genora® 1/50 Nelova®1/50M Norethin® 1/50M Noriryl®1+50 Ortho-Novum™1/50	Combo	Norethindrone 1 mg	Mestranol 50 mcg	21, 28
Levlen® Levora® Nordette®	Combo	Levonorgestrel 0.15 mg	Ethinyl estradiol 20 mcg	21, 28
Micronor®	Progestin only	Norethindrone 0.35 mg	—	28
Norlestrin® 2.5/50	Combo	Norethindrone acetate 2.5 mg	Ethinyl estradiol 30 mcg	21
Nor-QD®	Progestin only	Norethindrone 0.35 mg	—	42
Ortho-Cept®	Combo	Desogestrel 0.15 mg	Ethinyl estradiol 30 mcg	21, 28
Ortho-Cyclen®	Combo	Norgestimate 0.25 mg	Ethinyl estradiol 35 mcg	21, 28
Nelova™ 10/11	Biphasic			
	1-10 d	Norethindrone 0.5 mg	Ethinyl estradiol 35 mcg	21, 28
	11-21 d	Norethindrone 1 mg	Ethinyl estradiol 35 mcg	
	22-28 d	Inert	—	
Ortho-Novum™10/11	Biphasic			
	1-10 d	Norethindrone 0.5 mg	Ethinyl estradiol 35 mcg	21, 28
	11-21 d	Norethindrone 1 mg	Ethinyl estradiol 35 mcg	
	22-28 d	Inert	—	
Ortho-Novum™ 7/7/7	Triphasic			
	1-7 d	Norethindrone 0.5 mg	Ethinyl estradiol 35 mcg	21, 28
	8-14 d	Norethindrone 0.75 mg	Ethinyl estradiol 35 mcg	
	15-21 d	Norethindrone 1 mg	Ethinyl estradiol 35 mcg	
	22-28 d	Inert	—	

Brand Name	Type	Progestin	Estrogen	Availability
Ortho Tri-Cyclen®	Triphasic			
	1-7 d	Norgestimate 0.18 mg	Ethinyl estradiol 35 mcg	21, 28
	8-14 d	Norgestimate 0.215 mg	Ethinyl estradiol 35 mcg	
	15-21 d	Norgestimate 0.25 mg	Ethinyl estradiol 35 mcg	
	22-28 d	Inert	—	
Ovcon® 35	Combo	Norethindrone 0.4 mg	Ethinyl estradiol 35 mcg	21, 28
Ovcon® 50	Combo	Norethindrone 1 mg	Ethinyl estradiol 50 mcg	21, 28
Ovral®	Combo	Norgestrel 0.5 mg	Ethinyl estradiol 50 mcg	21, 28
Ovrette®	Progestin only	Norgestrel 0.075 mg	—	28
Tri-Norinyl®	Triphasic			
	1-7 d	Norethindrone 0.5 mg	Ethinyl estradiol 35 mcg	21, 28
	8-16 d	Norethindrone 1 mg	Ethinyl estradiol 35 mcg	
	17-21 d	Norethindrone 0.5 mg	Ethinyl estradiol 35 mcg	
	22-28 d	Inert	—	
Tri-Phasil® Tri-Levlen®	Triphasic			
	1-6 d	Levonorgestrel 0.05 mg	Ethinyl estradiol 30 mcg	21, 28
	7-11 d	Levonorgestrel 0.075 mg	Ethinyl estradiol 40 mcg	
	12-21 d	Levonorgestrel 0.125 mg	Ethinyl estradiol 30 mcg	
	22-28 d	Inert	—	

Combo = Monophasic combination

Monophasic Oral Contraceptives
In Order of Decreasing Estrogen Content

Estrogen	Brand Name (Progestin Content)
Mestranol 50 mcg	Genora®1/50, Nelova®1/50M, Norethin®1/50M, Norinyl®1+50, Ortho-Novum®1/50 (Norethindrone 1 mg)
Ethinyl estradiol 50 mcg	Ovcon®-50 (Norethindrone 1 mg)
	Demulen ®1/50 (Ethynodiol diacetate 1 mg)
	Ovral® (Norgestrel 0.5 mg)
Ethinyl estradiol 35 mcg	Genora ®1/35, N.E.E ®1/35, Nelova®1/35E, Norethin®1/35E, Norinyl®1+35, Ortho-Novum®1/35 (Norethindrone 1 mg)
	Brevicon ®, Genora ®0.5/35, Modicon®, Nelova ®0.5/35E (Norethindrone 0.5 mg)
	Ovcon®-35 (Norethindrone 0.4 mg)
	Ortho-Cyclen® (Norgestimate 0.25 mg)
	Demulen® 1/35 (Ethynodiol diacetate 1 mg)
Ethinyl estradiol 30 mcg	Loestrin 21® 1.5/30, Loestrin®Fe 1.5/30 (Norethindrone acetate 1.5 mg)
	Lo/Ovral® (Norgestrel 0.3 mg)
	Desogen®, Ortho-Cept® (Desogestrel 0.15 mg)
Ethinyl estradiol 20 mcg	Levlen®, Levora®, Nordette® (Levonorgestrel 0.15 mg)
	Loestrin 21® 1/20, Loestrin®Fe 1/20 (Norethindrone acetate 1 mg)

ORAL CONTRACEPTIVES *(Continued)*

Hormonal Effects of Progestins

	Progestin Effect	Estrogen Effect	Antiestrogen Effect	Androgen Effect
Norethynodrel	+1	+3	0	0
Norethindrone	+1	+1 (Low dose)	+1 (Higher doses)	+2
Norethindrone acetate	+1	+1	+3	+2
Ethynodiol diacetate	+2	+1 (Low dose)	+1 (Higher doses)	+2
Norgestimate	+3	0	+3	0
Desogestrel	+3	0/+1	+3	0/+1
Norgestrel/ levonorgestrel	+3	0	+2	+3

0=No effect; +1=Slight effect; +2=Moderate effect; +3=Pronounced effect

Adapted from *Facts and Comparisons*, St Louis, MO; Facts and Comparisons, Inc, 1996.

Signs/Symptoms of Hormonal Imbalance With Oral Contraceptives

Estrogen Excess	Fluid retention, edema, cyclic weight gain, "bloating," hypertension, breast fullness/tenderness, nausea, migraine headache, melasma, telangiectasia, cervical mucorrhea, and polyposis
Estrogen Deficiency	Increased spotting, early or midcycle breakthrough bleeding, hypomenorrhea
Progestin Excess	Fatigue, lethargy, depression, decreased libido, increased appetite, weight gain, breast regression, monilial vaginitis, hypomenorrhea, hair loss, hirsutism, acne, oily scalp. **Note:** Hair loss, hirsutism, acne, and oily scalp are effects of the androgenic activity of progestins.
Progestin Deficiency	Amenorrhea, late breakthrough bleeding, hypermenorrhea

FLUIDS, ELECTROLYTES, & NUTRITION

ENTERAL NUTRITIONAL PRODUCT FORMULARY, INFANTS

Milk Based Formulas*
(Indications: Feeding normal term infants or sick infants without special nutritional requirements)

	Human Milk	Enfamil® With Iron	Similac® With Iron
Calories /100 mL	67	67.6	67.6
Protein g/100 mL	1.0	1.42	1.45
Protein source	Mature Term human milk	60% whey 40% casein	Nonfat milk
Carbohydrate g/100 mL	6.8	7.4	7.23
Carbohydrate source	Lactose	Lactose	Lactose
Fat g/100 mL	4.0	3.6	3.65
Fat source	Human milk, fat	45% palm oil† 20% coconut oil 20% soy oil 15% high oleic sunflower oil	Soy and coconut oils§
Osmolality mOsm/kg	300	300	300
Sodium mEq/L (mg/L)	7.8 (180)	8 (183)	8.0 (183)
Potassium mEq/L (mg/L)	13.5 (525)	18.7 (730)	18.2 (710)
Chloride mEq/L (mg/L)	11.9 (420)	12 (426)	12.2 (433)
Calcium mEq/L (mg/L)	14 (280)	26.4 (528)	24.6 (492)
Phosphorus mEq/L (mg/L)	9 (140)	20.5 (358)	25.2 (380)
Iron mg/L	0.3	12.2 (4.7)¶	12.2 (1.49)¶

*Information based on manufacturer's literature as of 1999 and is subject to change.

†Enfamil® with iron powder: 45% corn oil, 55% coconut oil.

§Similac® with iron powder: coconut and corn oil.

¶Low iron formulation in parenthesis.

FLUIDS, ELECTROLYTES, & NUTRITION *(Continued)*

Hypercaloric Milk Based Formulas - 24*†
(Indications: Fluid restriction, increased caloric demands)

	Enfamil® 24	Similac® 24
Calories /100 mL	81.1	81.2
Protein g/100 mL	1.8	2.2
Protein source	Nonfat milk and whey	Nonfat milk
Carbohydrate g/100 mL	8.3	8.53
Carbohydrate source	Lactose	Lactose
Fat g/100 mL	4.5	4.28
Fat source	45% palm oil 20% coconut oil 20% soy oil 15% high oleic sunflower oil	Soy and coconut oils
Osmolality mOsm/kg	360	380
Sodium mEq/L (mg/L)	9.6 (220)	12.2 (280)
Potassium mEq/L (mg/L)	22.3 (870)	27.4 (1070)
Chloride mEq/L (mg/L)	14.4 (510)	18.6 (660)
Calcium mEq/L (mg/L)	31.4 (628)	36.4 (730)
Phosphorus mEq/L (mg/L)	27.6 (427)	36.8 (570)
Iron mg/L	14.6 (5.7)¶	15 (14.5)¶

*Information based on manufacturer's literature as of 1999 and is subject to change; 24 calories/oz

†To approximate values for the content of a 30 cal/oz formula (made by dilution of a powder formulation) multiply the value desired, found in a 20 cal/oz formula, by 1.5 (20 cal/oz formula contents for Enfamil® and Similac® are listed in preceding Milk Based Formula chart). For example, the fat in a 30 cal/oz Enfamil® formula = 1.5 x 3.6 = 5.4 g/100 mL.

¶Low iron formulation in parentheses

Soy Formulas*
(Indications: Lactose deficiency, milk intolerance, or galactosemia)

	Prosobee®	Isomil®
Calories /100 mL	67.6	67.6
Protein g/100 mL	2	1.8
Protein source	Soy protein isolate	Soy protein isolate
Carbohydrate g/100 mL	6.8	6.83
Carbohydrate source	Corn syrup solids	Corn syrup and sucrose
Fat g/100 mL	3.6	3.69
Fat source	45% palm oil† 20% coconut oil 20% soy oil 15% high oleic sunflower oil	Soy and coconut oils
Osmolality mOsm/kg	200	230
Sodium mEq/L (mg/L)	10.6 (243)	13 (300)
Potassium mEq/L (mg/L)	21 (825)	18.7 (730)
Chloride mEq/L (mg/L)	15.3 (561)	11.9 (420)
Calcium mEq (mg/L)	31.8 (636)	35.5 (710)
Phosphorus mEq/L (mg/L)	32.4 (500)	32.9 (510)
Iron mg/L	12.8	12

*Information based on manufacturer's literature as of 1999 and is subject to change.
†Prosobee® powder: 45% corn oil, 55% coconut oil.

FLUIDS, ELECTROLYTES, & NUTRITION *(Continued)*

Hypercaloric Soy Formulas - 24*†
(Indications: Fluid restriction, increased caloric demands)

	Prosobee® 24
Calories /100 mL	81.1
Protein g/100 mL	2.4
Protein source	Soy protein isolate
Carbohydrate g/100 mL	8.2
Carbohydrate source	Corn syrup solids
Fat g/100 mL	4.3
Fat source	45% palm oil 20% coconut oil 20% soy oil 15% high oleic sunflower oil
Osmolality mOsm/kg	240
Sodium mEq/L (mg/L)	12.7 (292)
Potassium mEq/L (mg/L)	25.2 (990)
Chloride mEq/L (mg/L)	19 (672)
Calcium mEq/L (mg/L)	38 (761)
Phosphorus mEq/L (mg/L)	38.9 (602)
Iron mg/L	15.2

*Information based on manufacturer's literature as of 1999 and is subject to change.

†To approximate values for the content of a 27 or 30 cal/oz formula (made by dilution of a powder based formulation), multiply the value desired, found in the 20 cal/oz formula (20 cal/oz formula contents for Prosobee® are listed in the preceding Soy Formulas chart), by the following factors: 1.35 (27 cal/oz) or 1.5 (30 cal/oz).

Casein Hydrolysate Formulas*
(Indications: For infants whose renal or cardiovascular
functions would benefit from lowered mineral levels)

	Similac® PM 60/40
Calories /100 mL	67.6
Protein g/100 mL	1.58
Protein source	Whey and caseinate
Carbohydrate g/100 mL	6.9
Carbohydrate source	Lactose
Fat g/100 mL	3.78
Fat source	Soy and coconut oils†
Osmolality mOsm/kg	280
Sodium mEq/L (mg/L)	7 (160)
Potassium mEq/L (mg/L)	14.9 (580)
Chloride mEq/L (mg/L)	11.3 (400)
Calcium mEq/L (mg/L)	19 (380)
Phosphorus mEq/L (mg/L)	12.3 (190)
Iron mg/L	1.5
Special uses	Renal and cardiovascular disease

*Information based on manufacturer's literature as of 1999 and is subject to change.

†Similac® PM 60/40 powder: corn and coconut oil.

FLUIDS, ELECTROLYTES, & NUTRITION *(Continued)*

Casein Hydrolysate Formulas*
(Indications: For infants requiring low molecular weight peptides or amino acids)

	Nutramigen®	Pregestimil®
Calories /100 mL	67.6	68
Protein g/100 mL	1.9	1.9
Protein source	Casein hydrolysate, L-cystine, L-tyrosine, and L-tryptophan	Casein hydrolysate, L-cystine, L-tyrosine, and L-tryptophan
Carbohydrate g/100 mL	7.4	6.8
Carbohydrate source	Corn syrup solids and modified corn starch	Corn syrup solids, dextrose, and modified corn starch
Fat g/100 mL	3.4	3.8
Fat source	Palm olein, soy, coconut, high-oleic sunflower oils	60% MCT oil 20% corn oil 20% high oleic sunflower oil
Osmolality mOsm/kg	320	320
Sodium mEq/L (mg/L)	13.8 (318)	11.5 (264)
Potassium mEq/L (mg/L)	19 (744)	18.9 (737)
Chloride mEq/L (mg/L)	16.4 (582)	16.4 (581)
Calcium mEq/L (mg/L)	31.8 (636)	31.8 (636)
Phosphorus mEq/L (mg/L)	27.3 (426)	27.3 (423)
Iron mg/L	12.2	12.8
Special uses	Sensitivity to intact proteins, galactosemia	Malabsorption, cystic fibrosis

*Information based on manufacturer's literature as of 1999 and is subject to change.

To approximate values for the content of a 24, 27, or 30 cal/oz formula (made by dilution of a powder based formulation), multiply the value desired, found in the above 20 cal/oz formula, by the following factors: 1.2 (24 cal/oz), 1.35 (27 cal/oz), or 1.5 (30 cal/oz).

Other Infant and Pediatric Formulas* - Special Care
(Indications: Premature infant formulas designed for rapidly growing LBW infants)

	Human Milk Fortifier	Special Care 20 With Fe	Special Care 24 With Fe	Neosure
Calories /100 mL	80.6	67.6	81.2	74.6
Protein g/100 mL	2.2	1.83	2.2	2
Protein source	Nonfat milk and whey protein concentrate	Nonfat milk and whey protein concentrate	Nonfat milk and whey protein concentrate	Nonfat milk and whey protein concentrate
Carbohydrate g/100 mL	8.55	7.17	8.61	7.7
Carbohydrate source	Corn syrup solids and lactose	Hydrolyzed cornstarch and lactose	Hydrolyzed cornstarch and lactose	Corn syrup solids and lactose
Fat g/100 mL	4.37	3.67	4.41	4
Fat source	Medium chain triglycerides and coconut oils	Medium chain triglycerides, soy, and coconut oils	Medium chain triglycerides, soy, and coconut oils	Medium chain triglycerides, soy, and coconut oils
Osmolality mOsm/kg	280	210	252	250
Sodium mEq/L (mg/L)	15.3 (350)	12.6 (290)	15.2 (350)	10.4 (246)
Potassium mEq/L (mg/L)	26.6 (1040)	22.3 (870)	26.9 (1050)	27 (1060)
Chloride mEq/L (mg/L)	18.6 (660)	15.5 (550)	18.6 (660)	15.7 (560)

Other Infant and Pediatric Formulas* - Special Care

(Indications: Premature infant formulas designed for rapidly growing LBW infants) *(continued)*

	Human Milk Fortifier	Special Care 20 With Fe	Special Care 24 With Fe	Neosure
Calcium mEq/L (mg/L)	84.7 (1694)	60.8 (1220)	72.8 (1460)	39 (784)
Phosphorus mEq/L (mg/L)	60.2 (935)	39.4 (610)	47 (730)	29.6 (460)
Iron mg/L	3	12.2 (2.5)†	14.6 (3.0)†	13.4

*Information based on manufacturer's literature as of 1999 and is subject to change.

†Low iron formulation in parentheses.

ENTERAL FORMULAS– PEDIATRIC
(A selection of the commonly used enteral feedings for children 1-10 years of age)

	Pediasure®	Peptamen Junior®	Vivonex® Pediatric	Boost®	Carnation Instant Breakfast®*	Ensure®	Ensure® HN	Sustacal® Liquid
Calories/oz	30	30	24	30	28	30	30	30
Calories/mL	1.06	1.06	0.8	1.01	0.94	1.06	1.06	1.0
Carbohydrate g/100 mL	11	13.8	12.6	17.4	14.6	14	14	14.0
Carbohydrate source	Corn syrup solids, sucrose	Maltodextrin, corn starch	Maltodextrin, modified starch	Sucrose, corn syrup solids	Maltodextrin, sucrose, lactose	Corn syrup solids, sucrose	Corn syrup solids, sucrose	Corn syrup solids, sucrose
Protein g/100 mL	3.0	3.0	2.4	4.3	4.5	3.7	4.4	6.1
Protein source	Caseinate, whey protein conc	Hydrolyzed whey protein	L-amino acids	Milk protein conc	Nonfat milk	Caseinates, soy protein isolate	Caseinates, soy protein isolate	Casein, soy protein isolate
Fat g/100 mL	5.0	3.8	2.4	1.7	1.9	3.7	3.5	2.3
Fat source	High-oleic safflower, soy, and MCT oils	MCT, soy, and canola oils	MCT and soy solids	Canola, sunflower, and corn oils	Butterfat	Corn oil	Corn oil	Partially hydrogenated soy oil
Osmolality mOsm/kg	310	260 unflavored 360 vanilla	360	590-620	661-747	470	470	650
Sodium mg/100 mL (mEq/100 mL)	38 (1.7)	46 (2)	40 (1.7)	55 (2.4)	90 (3.9)	83 (3.6)	79.1 (3.4)	93 (4.0)
Potassium mg/100 mL (mEq/100 mL)	131 (3.4)	132 (3.4)	120 (3.1)	169 (4.3)	250 (6.4)	154 (3.9)	154 (3.9)	204 (5.2)
Iron (mg/100 mL)	1.4	1.4	1.0	—	—	—	—	—

*Mixed with 2% milk as directed.

FLUIDS, ELECTROLYTES, & NUTRITION *(Continued)*

ENTERAL FORMULAS – ADOLESCENTS - ADULTS

	Isocal®	Osmolite®	Osmolite HN®	Jevity®*
Calories/mL	1.06	1.06	1.06	1.06
Carbohydrate g/100 mL	13.5	15.1	14.4	15.0
Carbohydrate source	Maltodextrin	Corn syrup solids	Corn syrup solids	Corn syrup solids
Protein g/100 mL	3.4	3.7	4.4	4.4
Protein source	Caseinate, soy protein isolate	Caseinate, soy protein isolate	Caseinate, soy protein isolate	Caseinates
Fat g/100 mL	4.4	3.5	3.5	3.5
Fat source	Soy oil, MCT oil	High-oleic safflower, canola, and MCT oils	High-oleic safflower, canola, and MCT oils	High-oleic safflower, canola, and MCT oils
Osmolality mOsm/kg	270	300	300	300
Sodium mg/100 mL (mEq/100 mL)	53 (2.3)	63 (2.7)	92 (4.0)	91.6 (4.0)
Potassium mg/100 mL (mEq/100 mL)	132 (3.4)	100 (2.6)	154 (3.9)	154 (3.9)

*Contains 13.6 g/L soy fiber.

ENTERAL FORMULAS WITH HIGH CALORIC DENSITY

	Ensure Plus®	Ensure Plus HN®	Sustacal Plus®	Sustagen®	TraumaCal®
Calories/mL	1.5	1.5	1.5	1.9	1.5
Carbohydrate g/100 mL	20	20	19	31.6	14.5
Carbohydrate source	Corn syrup solids, sucrose	Corn syrup solids, sucrose	Corn syrup solids, sucrose	Corn syrup solids, lactose, dextrose	Corn syrup solids, sucrose
Protein g/100 mL	5.4	6.2	6.1	11.5	8.3
Protein source	Caseinate, soy protein isolate	Caseinate, soy protein isolate	Caseinates	Cow's milk, caseinates	Caseinates
Fat g/100 mL	5.3	5.0	5.8	1.7	6.8
Fat source	Corn oil	Corn oil	Corn oil	Butterfat	Soy oil, MCT oil
Osmolality mOsm/kg	690	650	630	1130	490
Sodium mg/100 mL (mEq/100 mL)	104 (4.5)	117 (5.1)	85 (3.7)	92 (4.0)	120 (5.2)
Potassium mg/100 mL (mEq/100 mL)	192 (4.9)	179 (4.6)	148 (3.8)	296 (7.6)	140 (3.6)

ENTERAL FORMULAS WITH MODIFIED PROTEIN - "ELEMENTAL"
Adolescents and Adults

	Criticare HN®	Peptamen®	Tolerex®	Vivonex Plus®
Calories/mL	1.06	1.0	1.0	1.0
Carbohydrate g/100 mL	22	12.7	22.6	19.0
Carbohydrate source	Maltodextrin, modified corn starch	Maltodextrin, corn starch	Maltodextrin	Maltodextrin, modified starch
Protein g/100 mL	3.8	4.0	2.1	4.5
Protein source	Hydrolyzed casein, L-amino acids	Hydrolyzed whey	L-amino acids	L-amino acids
Fat g/100 mL	0.53	3.9	0.1	0.7
Fat source	Safflower oil	Sunflower and MCT oils	Safflower oil	Soy oil
Osmolality mOsm/kg	650	270 unflavored 380 vanilla	550 unflavored 617-678 flavored	650
Sodium mg/100 mL (mEq/100 mL)	63 (2.7)	50 (2.2)	46 (2.0)	61 (2.7)
Potassium mg/ 100 mL (mEq/100 mL)	132 (3.4)	125 (3.2)	117 (3.0)	110 (2.8)

FLUIDS, ELECTROLYTES, & NUTRITION *(Continued)*

Nutritional Modules*

	Polycose® Liquid	Polycose® Powder	Promod® Powder†
Indication	Carbohydrate additive for use as a caloric supplement which is readily mixable in most foods, enteral formulas or beverages without appreciably altering their taste	Carbohydrate additive for use as a caloric supplement which is readily mixable in most foods, enteral formulas or beverages without appreciably altering their taste	Protein supplement which mixes readily in enteral formulas, most foods, or beverages without appreciably altering their taste
Calories	2/mL	3.8/g‡	4.2/g
Protein (g)	—	—	0.76/g
Protein source	—	—	Whey protein concentrate
Carbohydrate (g)	0.5/mL	0.94/g	<0.1/g
Carbohydrate source	Glucose polymers	Glucose polymers	Lactose
Fat (g)	—	—	<0.09/g
Fat source	—	—	Soy lecithin
Osmolality mOsm/kg	900	900 in solution	—
Sodium mEq/L (mg/L)	<0.03/mL (<0.7/mL)	<0.05/g (<1.1/g)	<0.099/g (<2.3/g)
Potassium mEq/L (mg/L)	<0.002/mL (<0.06/mL)	<0.003/g (<0.1/g)	<0.25/g (<9.85/g)
Chloride mEq/L (mg/L)	<0.04/mL (<1.4/mL)	<0.06/g (<2.23/g)	—
Calcium mEq/L (mg/L)	<0.01/mL (<0.2/mL)	<0.02/g (<0.3/g)	<0.33/g (<6.67/g)
Phosphorus mEq/L (mg/L)	(<0.03/mL)	(<0.05/g)	(<5/g)
Iron mg/L	—	—	—

*These products are not complete formulations and should not be used as a sole source of nutrition.

†1 scoop = 6.6 g, 1 tsp = 1.3 g, 1 tbsp = 4 g.

‡1 tsp (2 g) = 8 calories, 1 tbsp (6 g) = 23 calories, ¼ cup (24 g) = 95 calories.

Nutritional Modules*

	Vegetable Oil†	Microlipid®	MCT Oil®‡	Whole Milk
Indications	Inexpensive fat source for calories and essential fatty acids	50% fat emulsion for use as a source of calories or essential fatty acids; it mixes easily and stays in emulsion	Fat supplement for use for patients who cannot efficiently digest and absorb long-chain fats	
Calories	8/mL	4.5/mL	7.67/mL	157/8 oz
Protein (g)	—	—	—	8/8 oz
Protein source	—	—	—	82% casein, 18% whey
Carbohydrate (g)	—	—	—	11/8 oz
Carbohydrate source	—	—	—	Lactose
Fat (g)	0.93/mL	0.5/mL•	0.93/mL	8.9/8 oz
Fat source	Corn, soybean, sunflower or safflower oils♦	Safflower oil, polyglycerol esters, soy lecithin	Lipid fraction of coconut oil (consists primarily of C_8 and C_{10} saturated fatty acids)	Butter fat
Osmolality mOsm/kg	—	60	—	288
Sodium mEq/L (mg/L)	—	—	—	5.3/8 oz (122/8 oz)
Potassium mEq/L (mg/L)	—	—	—	9/8 oz (351/8 oz)
Chloride mEq/L (mg/L)	—	—	—	7/8 oz (247/8 oz)
Calcium mEq/L (mg/L)	—	—	—	14.4/8 oz (288/8 oz)
Phosphorus mEq/L (mg/L)	—	—	—	14.6/8 oz (227/8 oz)
Iron mg/L	—	—	—	0.12/8 oz

*These products are not complete formulations and should not be used as a sole source of nutrition.

†1 tbsp = 14 g.

‡Does not contain essential fatty acids.

•1 tbsp = 5.5 g linoleic.

♦% of linoleic from fat: soybean oil 51%, corn oil 58%, sunflower oil 65%, safflower oil 77%.

FLUID AND ELECTROLYTE
REQUIREMENTS IN CHILDREN

Maintenance Fluids (Two methods)

Surface area method (most commonly used in children >10 kg): 1500-2000 mL/m^2/day

Body weight method

<10 kg	100 mL/kg/day
11-20 kg	1000 mL + 50 mL/kg (for each kg >10)
>20 kg	1500 mL + 20 mL/kg (for each kg >20)

Maintenance Electrolytes (See specific electrolyte in Alphabetical Listing of Drugs for more detailed information)

Sodium: 3-4 mEq/kg/day **or** 30-50 mEq/m^2/day
Potassium: 2-3 mEq/kg/day **or** 20-40 mEq/m^2/day

Dehydration Fluid Therapy

Goals of therapy:

- Restore circulatory volume to prevent shock (10% to 15% dehydration)
- Restore combined intracellular and extracellular deficits of water and electrolytes within 24 hours
- Maintain adequate water and electrolytes
- Resolve homeostatic distortions (eg, acidosis)
- Replace ongoing losses

Analysis of the Severity of Dehydration by Physical Signs

Clinical Sign	Mild*	Moderate*	Severe*
Pre-illness body weight	5% loss	10% loss	15% loss
Skin turgor	↓	Tenting	Tenting
Mucous membranes	Dry	Very dry	Parched
Skin color	Pale	Grey	Mottled
Urine output	↓	↓↓	Azotemic
Blood pressure	Normal	Normal, ↓	↓↓
Heart rate	Normal, ↑	↑	↑↑
Fontanelle (<7 mo)	Flat	Soft	Sunken
CNS	Consolable	Irritable	Lethargic/coma

*Postpubertal children and adults experience the same symptoms with mild, moderate, and severe dehydration associated with 3%, 6%, and 9% losses in body weight respectively.

Restoration of Circulatory Volume (10% to 15% dehydration estimate)

Fluid boluses of 20 mL/kg using crystalloid (eg, normal saline) or 10 mL/kg colloid (eg, 5% albumin) administered as rapidly as possible; repeat until improved circulation (eg, warm skin, decreased heart rate (towards normal), improved capillary refill time, urine output restored).

Classification of Dehydration (based upon the serum sodium concentration)

Isotonic	130-150 mEq/L
Hypotonic	<130 mEq/L
Hypertonic	>150 mEq/L

Estimated Water & Electrolyte Deficits in Dehydration
(moderate to severe)

Type of Dehydration	Water (mL/kg)	Na+ (mEq/kg)	K+ (mEq/kg)	Cl⁻ and HCO₃⁻ (mEq/kg)
Isotonic	100-150	8-10	8-10	16-20
Hypotonic	50-100	10-14	10-14	20-28
Hypertonic	120-180	2-5	2-5	4-10

Current Pediatric Diagnosis & Treatment, 10th ed, 1991.

Water deficit may also be calculated (in isotonic dehydration):

$$\text{Water deficit (mL)} = \frac{\% \text{ dehydration} \times \text{wt (kg)} \times 1000 \text{ g/kg}}{100}$$

Assessment of Water Loss in Relation to Serum Na⁺ Concentrations
Degree of Dehydration as % Body Weight

Serum Na⁺	Mild	Moderate	Severe
Isotonic	5%	10%	15%
Hypotonic (Na⁺< 130)	4%	6%	8%
Hypertonic (Na⁺ >150)	7%	12%	17%

Example of Fluid Replacement
(assume 10 kg infant with 10% isotonic dehydration)

	Water	Sodium (mEq)	Potassium (mEq)
Maintenance	1000 mL	40	20
Deficit*	1000 mL	80	80
Total	2000 mL	120	100

*Reduce this total by any fluid boluses given initially.

First 8 hours: Replace ⅓ maintenance water   = 330 mL

Replace ½ deficit water   = <u>500 mL</u>

Total   830 mL/8 h = 103 mL/h

Replace ½ of Na⁺ & K⁺ = 60 mEq sodium/803 mL; 50 mEq potassium/803 mL (It is suggested that the maximum potassium initially used is 40 mEq/L and is **not** started until urine output has been established.)

The actual order would appear as: D₅½NS at 103 mL/hour for 8 hours; add 40 mEq/L KCl after patient voids.

Second 16 hours: Replace ⅔ maintenance water   = 670 mL

Replace ½ deficit water   = <u>500 mL</u>

Total   1260 mL/16 h = 79 mL/h

Replace remainder of sodium and potassium.

The actual order would appear as: D₅⅓NS with KCl 40 mEq/L at 79 mL/hour for 16 hours. (Use of ¼NS may be more desirable for convenience.)

FLUID AND ELECTROLYTE REQUIREMENTS IN CHILDREN *(Continued)*

Analysis of Ongoing Losses

Electrolyte Composition of Biological Fluids (mEq/L)

Fluid Type	Sodium	Potassium	Chloride	Total HCO$_3^-$
Stomach	20-120	5-25	90-160	0-5
Duodenal drainage	20-140	3-30	30-120	10-50
Biliary tract	120-160	3-12	70-130	30-50
Small intestine Initial drainage	100-140	4-40	60-100	30-100
Small intestine Established drainage	4-20	4-10	10-100	40-120
Pancreatic	110-160	4-15	30-80	70-130
Diarrheal stool	10-25	10-30	30-120	10-50

Current Pediatric Diagnosis & Treatment, 9th ed, Appleton & Lange, 1987.

Because of the wide range of normal values, specific analyses are suggested in individual cases.

Alterations of Maintenance Fluid Requirements

Fever	Increase maintenance fluids by 12% per degree centigrade above 37°C (eg, do **not** correct for 38°C, but increase fluids by 24% for fever of 39°C)
Hyperventilation	Increase maintenance fluids by 10-60 mL/100 kcal BEE (basal energy expenditure)
Sweating	Increase maintenance fluids by 10-25 mL/100 kcal BEE (basal energy expenditure)
Hyperthyroidism	Variable increase in maintenance fluids: 25%-50%
GI loss and renal disease	Monitor and analyze output; adjust therapy accordingly
Renal failure	Maintenance fluids are equal to insensible losses (300 mL/m^3) + urine replacement (mL for mL)

Oral Rehydration

Due to the high worldwide incidence of dehydration from infantile diarrhea, effective, inexpensive oral rehydration solutions have been developed. In the U.S., a typical effective solution for rehydration contains 50-60 mEq/L sodium, 20-30 mEq/L potassium, 30 mEq/L bicarbonate or its equivalent, and sufficient chloride to provide electroneutrality. Two percent to 3% glucose facilitates electrolyte absorption and short-term calories. The following table describes the electrolyte/sugar content of commonly used oral rehydration solutions.

Composition of Frequently Used
Oral Electrolyte Replacement Solutions

Solutions	% CHO	Na⁺ (mEq/L)	K⁺ (mEq/L)	Cl⁻ (mEq/L)	HCO⁻ (mEq/L)
Normal saline		154		154	
Ringer's lactate		130	4	109	28
Dextrose 5% in 0.25% NaCl	5% glucose	38		38	
WHO solution	2% glucose or 4% sucrose	90	20	80	30 citrate
WHO solution, modified	2% glucose	55	25	30	50
Rehydralyte®	2.5% glucose	75	20	65	30 citrate
Ricelyte®	3% carbohydrate	50	25	45	34 citrate
Resol®	2% glucose	50	20	50	34 citrate
Rice water	2.5% carbohydrate	90	20	30	80
Pedialyte® (Ross)	2.5% glucose	45	20	35	30 citrate
Infalyte® (Penwalt)	3% glucose	50	25	45	34
Gatorade®	2.6% glucose, 2% fructose	23.5	<1	17	
Apple juice	3.2% glucose, 1.3% sucrose, 7.5% fructose	<1	25		
Orange juice 1:3 (dilution with water)	1% glucose, 1.2% fructose	<1	50		50 citrate
Grape juice	1.6% glucose, 2.1% fructose	0.2-0.7	8-11		8
One package cherry gelatin dissolved in 4 cups water		24	Needs added K⁺		
Coca-Cola®		1.6	<1		13.4 citrate
Pepsi-Coal®		6.5	0.8		
Beef broth		120	10		
Chicken broth		250	8		

Adapted from Aranda-Michel, J and Giannella RA, "Acute Diarrhea" A Practical Review," *Am J of Med,* 1999, 106:670-6.

PARENTERAL NUTRITION (PN)

The following information is intended as a brief overview of the use of parenteral nutrition in infants and children.

General Indications for Use

Parenteral nutrition is the provision of required nutrients by the intravenous route to replenish, optimize, or maintain nutritional status.

Specific Indications

Parenteral nutrition of **all** required nutrients (total parenteral nutrition) is indicated in patients for whom it is expected that it would be impossible or dangerous to enterally administer nutrition. Parenteral nutrition in combination with enteral nutrition is indicated in patients who are expected to be unable to meet their nutritional needs by the enteral route alone within 5 days.

1. Patients with an inability to absorb nutrients via the gastrointestinal tract which may include the following: severe diarrhea, short bowel syndrome, developmental anomalies of the GI tract, inflammatory bowel disease, cystic fibrosis, or anatomic or functional loss of GI integrity.

2. Severe malnutrition.

3. Severe catabolic states such as: burns, trauma, or sepsis.

4. Patients undergoing high dose chemotherapy, radiation, and bone marrow transplantation.

5. Patients whose clinical condition may necessitate complete bowel rest (eg, necrotizing enterocolitis, pancreatitis, GI fistulas, or recent GI surgery).

6. Intensive care low-birth-weight infants.

7. Neonatal asphyxia.

8. Meconium ileus.

9. Respiratory distress syndrome (RDS).

Nutritional Assessment

As many as 33% of hospitalized pediatric patients are malnourished and require nutritional therapy. The type of nutritional support indicated depends on the underlying disease, the degree of gastrointestinal function, and the severity of malnutrition. Acutely malnourished patients have an increased risk for serious infection, postoperative complications, and death. Indicators of acute protein-calorie malnutrition include low weight for height, low serum albumin, lymphopenia, decreased body fat folds, and decreased arm muscle area. Nutritional screening may be done by the dietitian. Those patients who are at nutritional risk should receive a complete nutritional assessment.

Nutritional Requirements

Approximate requirements for energy and protein at various ages for normal subjects are listed in the first table at the end of this section. Patients who are severely malnourished or markedly catabolic may require higher levels to achieve catch-up growth or meet increased requirements. Patients who are well-nourished and/or inactive may require less.

During parenteral nutrition, 10% to 16% of calories should be in the form of amino acids to achieve optimal benefit (approximately 2-3 g/kg/day in infants and 1.5-2.5 g/kg/day ideal body weight in older patients). Exceptions include patients with renal or hepatic failure (where less protein is indicated), or in the treatment of severe trauma, head injury, or sepsis (where more protein may be indicated).

PN ORDERING

Fluid Intake

The patient should be given a total volume of fluid reasonable for his/her age and cardiovascular status. It is generally safe to start with the fluid maintenance level of 1500 mL/m^2/day in children. The fluid requirements in preterm infants are extremely variable due to much greater insensible water losses from radiant warmers and bili-lights. While the standard fluid maintenance of 100 mL/kg/day may be sufficient for term infants, intakes of up to 150 mL/kg/day may be necessary in the very low birth weight infants. Be sure to consider significant fluid intake from medications or other I.V. fluids and enteral diets in planning the fluids available for parenteral nutrition.

Dextrose

For central PN, dextrose is usually begun with a 10% to 12.5% solution or a solution providing dextrose at no more than 5 mg/kg/minute (in neonates and premature infants). The concentration is advanced, if tolerated, by 2.5% to 5% per day (2-2.5 mg/kg/minute increments in neonates and premature infants) to the desired caloric density, usually 20% to 25% dextrose. Fluid restricted patients often need 30% to 35% dextrose to meet their energy needs. For peripheral PN, 5% to 12.5% dextrose is utilized.

Dextrose calculations:

% Dextrose = Dextrose (g)/100 mL

Dextrose calorie value = 3.4 kcal/g

$$\text{Dextrose infusion rate (mg/kg/minute)} = \frac{\text{rate (mL/h) x \% dextrose x 0.166}}{\text{weight (kg)}}$$

$$\text{\% Dextrose desired*} = \frac{\text{desired rate (mg/kg/min) x weight (kg)}}{0.166 \text{ x rate (mL/h)}}$$

*Do not use dextrose concentrations <5% due to hypotonicity.

Amino Acids

Amino acids may be described as either a "standard" mixture of essential and nonessential amino acids or "specialized" mixtures. Specialized mixtures are intended for use in patients whose physiologic or metabolic needs may not be met with the "standard" amino acid compositions. Examples of specialized solutions include:

Trophamine®, Aminosyn® PF	Indicated for use in premature infants and young children due to addition of taurine, L-glutamic acid, L-aspartic acid, increased amounts of histidine, and reduction in amounts of methionine, alanine, phenylalanine, and glycine. Supplementation with a cysteine additive has been recommended.
Hepatamine®	Indicated for treatment in patients with hepatic encephalopathy due to cirrhosis or hepatitis or in patients with liver disease who are intolerant of standard amino acid solutions. Contains higher percentage of branched-chain amino acids and a lower percentage of aromatic amino acids than standard mixtures.
Nephramine®, Aminosyn® RF	Indicated for use in patients with compromised renal function who are intolerant of standard amino acid solutions. Contains a mixture of essential amino acids and histidine.

PARENTERAL NUTRITION (PN) *(Continued)*

Amino acid calculations:

% amino acid	=	amino acid (g)/100mL
Grams of protein	=	grams of nitrogen x 6.25
% amino acid desired	=	(g amino acid/kg) x weight (kg) x 100
		total PN fluid volume (mL)

Fat Emulsion (FE)

There are three roles for intravenous fat in parenteral nutrition:

1. to provide nonprotein calories
2. to provide essential fatty acids and a "balanced" calorie source
3. to provide calories in catabolic patients with limited ability to excrete CO_2

The FE dosage is increased as tolerated daily (see General Guidelines for Initiation and Advancement for PN following). The maximum fat intake is 4 g/kg/day and no more than 60% of the total daily caloric intake. It is administered as a continuous infusion over 24 hours or at a rate no greater than 0.15-0.2 g/kg/hour via a Y-connector with the dextrose-amino acid I.V. line. In patients receiving cyclic PN, the FE should be administered over the duration of the PN infusion. The triglyceride concentration should be checked before the first infusion and daily as the dose is increased. Subsequently, it should be monitored at least weekly. Triglyceride concentrations should be maintained at <150 mg/dL in neonates, <350 mg/dL in renal patients, and <250 mg/dL in other patients. FE should be used cautiously in neonates with hyperbilirubinemia due to displacement of bilirubin from albumin by the free fatty acids. An increase in free bilirubin may increase the risk of kernicterus. Significant displacement occurs when the free fatty acid to serum albumin molar ratio (FFA/SA) >6. For example, infants with a total bilirubin >8-10 mg/dL (assuming an albumin concentration of 2.5-3 g/dL) should not receive more parenteral FE than required to meet the essential fatty acid requirement of 0.5-1 g/kg/day.

Note: Avoid use of 10% FE in preterm infants because a greater accumulation of plasma lipids occurs due to the greater phospholipid load of the 10% concentration.

Fat emulsion calculations:

20% FE = 20 g fat/100 mL = 2 kcal/mL

Desired 20% FE (mL)	=	(% total kcal as fat) x (total kcal)
		2 kcal/mL

or as an alternative

Desired 20% FE (mL)	=	FE (g/kg) x weight (kg) x 5 mL/g

General Guidelines for Initiation and Advancement of PN*

Age	Initiation and Advancement	Dextrose	Protein (g/kg/ day)	Fat (g/kg/ day)
Premature infant	Initial	4-6 mg/kg/min	0.5-1.5	0.5
	Daily Increase	1-2.5 mg/kg/min	0.5-1	0.5
	Maximum	18 mg/kg/min	2.5-3	3
Term infant to 1 year	Initial	7-9 mg/kg/min	1-1.5	0.5-1
	Daily Increase	1-2.5 mg/kg/min	1	0.5-1
	Maximum	21 mg/kg/min	2.5-3	4
Children 1-10 years	Initial Dextrose Concentration	10% to 12.5%	1-1.5	1
	Daily Increase	5% increments	1	1
	Maximum	15 mg/kg/min	2-2.5	3
>10 years	Initial Dextrose Concentration	10% to 15%	1-1.5	1
	Daily Increase	5% increments	1	1
	Maximum	8.5 mg/kg/min	1.5-2	3

*Rate of advancement may be limited by metabolic tolerance (eg, hyperglycemia, azotemia, hypertriglyceridemia)

Reference

National Advisory Group on Standards and Practice Guidelines for Parenteral Nutrition, "Safe Practices for Parenteral Nutrition Formulation," *JPEN*, 1998, 22(2):49-66.

MINERALS, TRACE ELEMENTS, AND VITAMINS

Guideline for Daily Electrolyte Requirements

	Neonates (mEq/kg)	Infants/Children (mEq/kg)	Adolescents
Sodium	2-5	2-6	60-150 mEq/d
Potassium	2-4	2-4	60-150 mEq/d
Calcium gluconate*	3-4	1-2.5	10-20 mEq/d
Magnesium	0.3-0.5	0.3-0.5	10-30 mEq/d
Phosphate*	1-2 mmol/kg	0.5-1 mmol/kg	10-40 mmol/d

*Calcium-phosphate stability in parenteral nutrition solutions is dependent upon the pH of the solution, temperature, and relative concentration of each ion. The pH of the solution is primarily dependent upon the amino acid concentration. The higher the percentage amino acids the lower the pH, the more soluble the calcium and phosphate. Individual commercially available amino acid solutions vary significantly with respect to pH lowering potential and consequent calcium phosphate compatibility. See the pharmacist for specific calcium phosphate stability information.

Vitamins

A pediatric parenteral multivitamin product is indicated for children <11 years of age. Children >11 years of age may receive adult multivitamin formulations.

Dosage:

    Pediatric MVI:
        Neonates: 2 mL/kg/d; maximum 5 mL/d
        Infants and children ≤11 y: 5 mL
        Children >11 y and adults: Use adult formulation 10 mL/d

PARENTERAL NUTRITION (PN) *(Continued)*

Trace Mineral Daily Requirements*

	Infants	Children (≥3 mo to ≤5 y)	Older Children and Adolescents
Chromium†	0.2 mcg/kg	0.14-0.2 mcg/kg (max: 5 mcg)	5-15 mcg
Copper‡	20 mcg/kg	20 mcg/kg (max: 300 mcg)	0.2-0.5 mg
Iodide§	1 mcg/kg	1 mcg/kg	1 mcg/kg
Manganese‡	1 mcg/kg	2-10 mcg/kg (max: 50 mcg)	50-150 mcg
Selenium†¶	2-3 mcg/kg	2-3 mcg/kg (max: 30 mcg)	30-40 mcg
Zinc	400 mcg/kg (preterm) 300 mcg/kg (term <3 mo)	100 mcg/kg (max: 5 mg)	2-5 mg

*Recommended intakes of trace elements cannot be achieved through the use of a single pediatric trace element produce. Only through the use of individualized trace element products can recommended intakes be achieved.

†Omit in patients with renal dysfunction.

‡Omit in patients with obstructive jaundice.

§Percutaneous absorption from protein-bound iodine may be adequate.

¶Indicated for use in long-term parenteral nutrition patients.

These are recommended daily trace mineral requirements. Additional supplementation may be indicated in clinical conditions resulting in excessive losses. For example, additional zinc may be needed in situations of excessive gastrointestinal losses.

Developing the PN Goal Regimen

The purpose of this example is to illustrate the thought process in determining what dextrose and amino acid solution and fat emulsion intake would provide the desired daily fluid calorie and protein goals.

1. Calculate the fluid, protein, and caloric goals. Example:

   Weight = 10 kg
   Fluids = 100 mL/kg/day = 1000 mL
   Calories = 100 kcal/kg/day = 1000 kcal
   Protein = 2.5 g/kg/day = 25 g

2. If fat emulsion (FE) comprises 40% to 60% of the total daily calories, using the above example: 40% of 1000 kcal = 400 kcal.

   400 kcal ÷ 2 kcal/mL (20% FE) = 200 mL

3. To determine the goal dextrose concentration calculate the total daily calories remaining. Example:

1000 kcal	(total daily calories)	
-400 kcal	(daily calories from fats)	
600 kcal	(total daily calories remaining)	

4. Determine the concentration of dextrose to achieve the total daily calories remaining. Example:

   600 kcal ÷ 3.4 kcal/g x [100 ÷ 800 mL*] = 22%

   *Total daily fluids desired minus that from fats.

5. Calculate percent amino acid solution to achieve goal protein intake. Example:

$$[25 \text{ g (total protein)} \div 800 \text{ mL (total fluid)}] \times 100 = 3.1\%$$

This patient's goal regimen would be: dextrose 22%, amino acid 3.1%, 800 mL/day plus fat emulsion 20% 200 mL/day.

Parenteral Nutrition Monitoring Guidelines

	Frequency	
Parameter	Initial	Maintenance
Body weight	Daily	Daily
Height or length	Weekly	Weekly
Triceps Skin Fold (TSF)/ Midarm Circumference (MAC)	PRN	PRN
Calories/protein intakes	Daily	PRN
Intake/output	Every 8 hours	Every 8 hours
Urine glucose	Every 4 hours	Every 8 hours
Urine specific gravity	Every 8 hours	Every 8 hours
Urine protein	Every 8 hours	Every 8 hours
Electrolytes	Daily	1-2 times weekly
Ca, Mg, PO_4	Daily	Weekly
BUN/Cr	Daily	Weekly
Serum glucose	Daily	Weekly
Albumin	Weekly	Weekly
Triglycerides	Daily	Weekly
Transferrin or prealbumin	Weekly	Weekly
Bilirubin, direct	Once	PRN (after 2 weeks minimum PN)
Liver function tests	Once	PRN

Nutritional Guidelines for Pediatric Patients*

Age	kcal/kg/d	Protein g/kg/d
Preterm neonate	120-140	2.5-3
Term infant - 1 y	90-120	2-2.5
1-7 y	75-90	1.5-2
12 y	60-75	1.5-2
12-18 y	30-60	0.8-2

*Kerner JA, Manual of Pediatric Parenteral Nutrition, Wiley & Sons, Inc, 1983.

PN kcal/mL*

Dextrose Concentration						
5%	10%	15%	20%	25%	30%	35%
0.17	0.34	0.51	0.68	0.85	1.02	1.19

Dextrose provides 3.4 kcal/g.

Intralipid 10% provides 1.1 kcal/mL.

Intralipid 20% provides 2 kcal/mL.

*Calories derived from amino acids are not included.

PARENTERAL NUTRITION (PN) *(Continued)*

Y-Site Compatibility of Medications With TPN and Lipid
(Administered in D_5W or NS via Y-connector into PN line)

Medication	PN	Lipid	Comments
Acetazolamide	I	—	
Acyclovir	I	—	Visual precipitate forms
Albumin	C	I	May crack emulsion
Aldesleukin	C	C	
Alprostadil	—	—	
Amikacin	C	I	Causes oiling out of fat emulsion
Aminophylline	C	C	Incompatible with insulin; caution with high concentration of Ca/Phos
Amphotericin B	I	I	Formation of fine yellow particles
Ampicillin	I	I	
Ampicillin/sulbactam	I	—	
Atracurium	C	—	
Azlocillin	C	C	
Aztreonam	C	—	
Bicarbonate	I	I	Incompatible with many electrolytes; precipitate forms
Cefamandole	C	C	
Cefazolin	C	C	
Cefepime	C	—	
Cefonicid	—	—	
Cefoperazone	C	—	
Cefotaxime	C	C	
Cefotetan	—	—	
Cefoxitin	C	C	
Ceftazidime	C	—	
Ceftizoxime	—	—	
Ceftriaxone	C	—	
Cefuroxime	C	—	
Cephalothin	C	C	
Cephapirin	C	C	
Cephradine	I	—	Heavy precipitate of Ca/Phos due to increased pH
Chloramphenicol	C	C	
Cimetidine	C	C	
Ciprofloxacin	C	C	
Chlorothiazide	I	—	Precipitate forms
Clindamycin	C	C	
Co-trimoxazole	I	—	Precipitate forms
Cyanocobalamin	C	C	
Cyclophosphamide	C	—	
Cyclosporine	C	C	
Cytarabine	C	—	
Dexamethasone (sodium phosphate)	C	—	
Digoxin	C	C	
Diphenhydramine	C	C	
Dobutamine	C	—	
Dopamine	C	C	

Y-Site Compatibility of Medications With TPN and Lipid
(Administered in D₅W or NS via Y-connector into PN line)
(continued)

Medication	PN	Lipid	Comments
Doxycycline	C	—	
Droperidol	—	—	
Epinephrine	C	—	
Epoetin alfa	C	—	
Erythromycin	C	C	
Famotidine	C	C	
Fentanyl	C	—	
Filgrastim	I	C	Incompatible with salt solutions
Fluconazole	C	—	
Fluorouracil	C	—	
Folic acid	C	C	
Foscarnet	C	—	
Fosphenytoin	C	—	
Furosemide	C	C	
Ganciclovir	I	—	Precipitate forms
Gentamicin	C	C	
Granisetron	C	—	
Haloperidol (lactate)	C	—	
Heparin	C	C	
Hydralazine	C	—	
Hydrocortisone	C	C	
Hydromorphone	C	—	
Idarubicin	C	—	
IL-2	C	C	
Imipenem/cilastatin	I	—	Significant loss of activity noted after 15 minutes
Indomethacin	I	—	
Insulin, regular	C	C	
Iron dextran	C	I	Causes oiling out of fat emulsion
Isoproterenol	C	C	
Kanamycin	C	C	
Levofloxacin	—	—	
Levorphanol	—	—	
Lidocaine	C	C	
Meperidine	C	—	
Meropenem	—	—	
Metaraminol	—	—	
Methicillin	C	I	Microscopic globule coalescence noted in 24 hours
Methotrexate	C	—	
Methyldopa	C	I	May crack emulsion
Methylprednisolone	C	—	
Metoclopramide	C	—	
Metronidazole	C	—	
Mezlocillin	C	C	
Miconazole	C	—	
Midazolam	I	—	Precipitate forms
Morphine	C	C	

PARENTERAL NUTRITION (PN) *(Continued)*

Y-Site Compatibility of Medications With TPN and Lipid (Administered in D₅W or NS via Y-connector into PN line) *(continued)*

Medication	PN	Lipid	Comments
Moxalactam	C	—	
Nafcillin	C	C	
Netilmicin	C	—	
Norepinephrine	C	C	
Octreotide	I	C	
Ondansetron	C	—	
Oxacillin	C	C	
Penicillin G Na/K	C	C	
Pentamidine	—	—	
Phenytoin	I	I	Immediate precipitate
Phytonadione	C	C	
Piperacillin	C	C	
Propofol	C	—	
Ranitidine	C	I	Loss of 10% of ranitidine activity after 24 hours
Sargramostim	C	—	
Sodium bicarbonate	I	I	Incompatible with many electrolytes; precipitate forms
Tetracycline	C	I	Highly acidic pH may disrupt emulsion
Thiamine	C	C	
Ticarcillin	C	C	
Ticarcillin/clavulanate	—	—	
Trimethoprim/ sulfamethoxazole	I	—	Precipitate forms
Tobramycin	C	C	
Urokinase	C	—	
Vancomycin	C	—	
Verapamil	—	—	
Vitamin K	C	—	

C = Compatible, may simultaneously infuse drug and TPN/lipid.

I = Incompatible, drug should be given through a **separate** I.V. line or turn off the TPN/liquid during drug administration. Flush I.V. line with normal saline **before** and **after** drug administration.

— = Information on compatibility not available. Give drug through a **separate** I.V. line or turn off TPN infusion during drug administration. Flush line with normal saline **before** and **after** drug administration.

Reference
Trissel LA, "Handbook on Injectable Drugs," 10th ed, Bethesda, MD: American Society of Health-System Pharmacists, Inc, 1998.

Pharmacologic considerations of mixing medications with PN solutions include:

Adsorption — bag, bottle, tubing, filter
Blood levels
Site of injection/administration
Flush
Amino acid-dextrose concentrations

pH factors
Temperature
Additives in solution
Heparin dose

GROWTH CHARTS

CDC Growth Charts: United States

Weight-for-age percentiles:
Boys, birth to 36 months

SOURCE: Developed by the National Center for Health Statistics in collaboration with the National Center for Chronic Disease Prevention and Health Promotion (2000).
Available at http://www.cdc.gov/growthcharts

CDC

GROWTH CHARTS (Continued)

CDC Growth Charts: United States

Weight-for-age percentiles: Girls, birth to 36 months

SOURCE: Developed by the National Center for Health Statistics in collaboration with the National Center for Chronic Disease Prevention and Health Promotion (2000).
Available at http://www.cdc.gov/growthcharts

CDC Growth Charts: United States

**Weight-for-age percentiles:
Boys, 2 to 20 years**

Age (years)

SOURCE: Developed by the National Center for Health Statistics in collaboration with the
National Center for Chronic Disease Prevention and Health Promotion (2000).
Available at http://www.cdc.gov/growthcharts

CDC Growth Charts: United States

**Weight-for-age percentiles:
Girls, 2 to 20 years**

SOURCE: Developed by the National Center for Health Statistics in collaboration with the
National Center for Chronic Disease Prevention and Health Promotion (2000).
Available at http://www.cdc.gov/growthcharts

CDC Growth Charts: United States

Length-for-age percentiles: Boys, birth to 36 months

Chart axes: Vertical axis labeled in cm (45–105) and in (17–42). Horizontal axis labeled Age (months): Birth, 3, 6, 9, 12, 15, 18, 21, 24, 27, 30, 33, 36.

Percentile curves labeled: 97th, 95th, 90th, 75th, 50th, 25th, 10th, 5th, 3rd.

SOURCE: Developed by the National Center for Health Statistics in collaboration with the National Center for Chronic Disease Prevention and Health Promotion (2000).
Available at http://www.cdc.gov/growthcharts

GROWTH CHARTS *(Continued)*

CDC Growth Charts: United States

Length-for-age percentiles:: Girls, birth to 36 months

SOURCE: Developed by the National Center for Health Statistics in collaboration with the
National Center for Chronic Disease Prevention and Health Promotion (2000).
Available at http://www.cdc.gov/growthcharts

CDC Growth Charts: United States

Stature-for-age percentiles: Boys, 2 to 20 years

(Growth chart plotting stature-for-age percentiles for boys from 2 to 20 years. Left and right vertical axes show stature in cm and inches; horizontal axis shows Age (months) from 2 to 20. Percentile curves shown: 97th, 95th, 90th, 75th, 50th, 25th, 10th, 5th, 3rd.)

cm — in axes: 200/79, 195/78, 190/74, 185/72, 180/70, 175/68, 170/66, 165/64, 160/62, 155/60, 150/58, 145/56, 140/54, 135/52, 130/50, 125/48, 120/46, 115/44, 110/42, 105/40, 100/38, 95/36, 90/34, 85/32, 80/30, 75

Age (months): 2 3 4 5 6 7 8 9 10 11 12 13 14 15 16 17 18 19 20

SOURCE: Developed by the National Center for Health Statistics in collaboration with the National Center for Chronic Disease Prevention and Health Promotion (2000).
Available at http://www.cdc.gov/growthcharts

CDC

GROWTH CHARTS *(Continued)*

CDC Growth Charts: United States

**Stature-for-age percentiles:
Girls, 2 to 20 years**

(Chart with vertical axis labeled cm/in on the left and in on the right, ranging from 75 cm/in at the bottom to 200 cm/78 in at the top. Percentile curves labeled 97th, 95th, 90th, 75th, 50th, 25th, 10th, 5th, 3rd. Horizontal axis labeled Age (months) from 2 to 20.)

Age (months)

SOURCE: Developed by the National Center for Health Statistics in collaboration with the
National Center for Chronic Disease Prevention and Health Promotion (2000).
Available at http://www.cdc.gov/growthcharts

CDC

CDC Growth Charts: United States

Head circumference-for-age percentiles: Boys, birth to 36 months

SOURCE: Developed by the National Center for Health Statistics in collaboration with the National Center for Chronic Disease Prevention and Health Promotion (2000).
Available at http://www.cdc.gov/growthcharts

GROWTH CHARTS *(Continued)*

CDC Growth Charts: United States

Head circumference-for-age percentiles: Girls, birth to 36 months

SOURCE: Developed by the National Center for Health Statistics in collaboration with the National Center for Chronic Disease Prevention and Health Promotion (2000).
Available at http://www.cdc.gov/growthcharts

IDEAL BODY WEIGHT CALCULATION

Adults (18 years and older)

IBW (male) = 50 + (2.3 x height in inches over 5 feet)
IBW (female) = 45.5 + (2.3 x height in inches over 5 feet)

IBW is in kg.

Children

a. 1-18 years (Traub and Johnson, 1980)

$$IBW = \frac{(height^2 \times 1.65)}{1000}$$

IBW is in kg.
Height is in cm.

b. 5 feet and taller (Traub and Johnson, 1980)

IBW (male) = 39 + (2.27 x height in inches over 5 feet)
IBW (female) = 42.2 + (2.27 x height in inches over 5 feet)

IBW is in kg.

c. 1-17 years (Traub and Kichen, 1983)

$$IBW = 2.396e^{0.01883 \,(height)}$$

IBW is in kg.
Height is in cm.

References

Traub SL and Johnson CE, "Comparison of Methods of Estimating Creatinine Clearance in Children," *Am J Hosp Pharm*, 1980, 37(2):195-201.
Traub SL and Kichen L, "Estimating Ideal Body Mass in Children," *Am J Hosp Pharm*, 1983, 40(1):107-10.

BODY SURFACE AREA OF CHILDREN AND ADULTS

Calculating Body Surface Area in Children

In a child of average size, find weight and corresponding surface area on the boxed scale to the left; or, use the nomogram to the right. Lay a straightedge on the correct height and weight points for the child, then read the intersecting point on the surface area scale.

FOR CHILDREN OF NORMAL HEIGHT AND WEIGHT

NOMOGRAM

BODY SURFACE AREA FORMULA
(Adult and Pediatric)

$$BSA\ (m^2) = \sqrt{\frac{Ht\ (in)\ x\ Wt\ (lb)}{3131}} \quad \text{or, in metric: } BSA\ (m^2) = \sqrt{\frac{Ht\ (cm)\ x\ Wt\ (kg)}{3600}}$$

References

Lam TK and Leung DT, "More on Simplified Calculation of Body Surface Area," *N Engl J Med*, 1988, 318(17):1130 (Letter).

Mosteller RD, "Simplified Calculation of Body Surface Area", *N Engl J Med*, 1987, 317(17):1098 (Letter).

AVERAGE WEIGHTS AND SURFACE AREAS

Average Weight and Surface Area of Preterm Infants, Term Infants, and Children

Age	Average Weight (kg)*	Approximate Surface Area (m²)
Weeks Gestation		
26	0.9-1	0.1
30	1.3-1.5	0.12
32	1.6-2	0.15
38	2.9-3	0.2
40 (term infant at birth)	3.1-4	0.25
Months		
3	5	0.29
6	7	0.38
9	8	0.42
Year		
1	10	0.49
2	12	0.55
3	15	0.64
4	17	0.74
5	18	0.76
6	20	0.82
7	23	0.90
8	25	0.95
9	28	1.06
10	33	1.18
11	35	1.23
12	40	1.34
Adults	70	1.73

*Weights from age 3 months and over are rounded off to the nearest kilogram.

PHYSICAL DEVELOPMENT

Weight gain first 6 weeks
20 g/day

Birth weight
regained by day 14
doubles by age 4 mo
triples by age 12 mo
quadruples by age 2 y

Teeth
1st tooth 6-18 mo
teeth = age (mo) − 6
(until 30 mo)

Head circumference
35 cm at birth
44 cm by 6 mo
47 cm by 1 y
1 cm/mo for 1st y
3 cm/mo 2nd y

Length
increases 50% by age 1 y
doubles by age 4 y
triples by age 13 y

Tanner Stages of Sexual Development

Stage	Characteristics	Age at onset (mean ± SD)
Genital stages: Male		
1	Prepubertal	
2	Scrotum and testes enlarge; skin of scrotum reddens and rugations appear	11.4 ± 1.1 y
3	Penis lengthens; testes enlarge further	12.9 ± 1 y
4	Penis growth continues in length and width; glans develops adult form	13.8 ± 1 y
5	Development completed; adult appearance	14.9 ± 1.1 y
Breast development: Female		
1	Prepubertal	
2	Breast buds appear; areolae enlarge	11.2 ± 1.1 y
3	Elevation of breast contour; areolae enlarge	12.2 ± 1.1 y
4	Areolae and papilla form a secondary mound on breast	13.1 ± 1.2 y
5	Adult form	15.3 ± 1.7 y
Menarche		
Pubic hair: Both sexes		13.5 ± 1 y
1	Prepubertal, no coarse hair	
2	Longer, silky hair appears at base of penis or along labia	F: 11.7 ± 1.2 y M: 12 ± 1 y
3	Hair coarse, kinky, spreads over pubic bone	F: 12.4 ± 1.1 y M: 13.9 ± 1 y
4	Hair of adult quality but not spread to junction of medial thigh with perineum	F: 13 ± 1 y M: 14.4 ± 1.1 y
5	Spread to medial thigh	F: 14.4 ± 1.1 y M: 15.2 ± 1.1 y
6	"Male escutcheon"	Variable if occurs

Maximum growth rate
Male at 14.1±0.9 y
Female at 12.1±0.9 y

EMETOGENIC POTENTIAL OF SINGLE CHEMOTHERAPEUTIC AGENTS

Class I — Low (<10%)

Asparaginase/Pegaspargase

Bleomycin

Busulfan

Chlorambucil (oral)

Cladribine

Corticosteroids

Cyclophosphamide (oral)

Fludarabine

Hydroxyurea

Melphalan (oral)

Mercaptopurine

Methotrexate <50 mg/m^2

Thioguanine (oral)

Vinblastine

Vincristine

Class II — Moderately Low (10% to 30%)

Cytarabine <500 mg/m^2

Doxorubicin ≤20 mg/m^2

Etoposide

Fluorouracil <1000 mg/m^2

Gemcitabine

Interferon-beta

Lomustine

Methotrexate ≥50-250 mg/m^2

Mitomycin <8 mg/m^2

Paclitaxel

Raltitrexed

Thiotepa

Class III — Moderate (30% to 60%)

Amsacrine

Azacitidine

Cyclophosphamide <750 mg/m^2

Cytarabine 500-1000 mg/m^2

Daunorubicin

Docetaxel

Doxorubicin >20 mg to <60 mg/m^2

Fluorouracil ≥1000 mg/m^2

Idarubicin

Ifosfamide

Irinotecan

Methotrexate >250 mg/m^2 to ≤1000 mg/m^2

Mitomycin ≥8 mg/m^2

Mitoxantrone

Teniposide

Topotecan

Tretinoin

Vinorelbine

Class IV — Moderately High (60% to 90%)

Actinomycin D

Aldesleukin

Carboplatin 200-400 mg/m^2

Carmustine <250 mg

Cisplatin <50 mg/m^2

Cyclophosphamide 750-1500 mg/m^2

Cytarabine >1000 mg/m^2

Dacarbazine <500 mg/m^2

Doxorubicin ≥60 mg/m^2

Melphalan 20-80 mg/m^2

Methotrexate >1000 mg/m^2

Procarbazine (oral)

Class V — High (>90%)

Busulfan (as part of BMT regimen)

Carboplatin >500 mg/m^2

Carmustine ≥250 mg/m^2

Cisplatin ≥50 mg/m^2

Cyclophosphamide ≥1500 mg/m^2

Dacarbazine ≥500 mg/m^2

Mechlorethamine

Melphalan >80 mg/m^2

Pentostatin

COMPATIBILITY OF CHEMOTHERAPY AND RELATED SUPPORTIVE CARE MEDICATIONS

Compatible: The drugs are physically compatible when mixed in the same container or infused through the same I.V. line simultaneously.

Y-site compatible: The drugs are physically compatible when infused through the same I.V. line simultaneously.

Incompatible: The drugs are physically incompatible when mixed in the same container, or infused through the same I.V. line simultaneously.

Variable compatibility: The compatibility of the drugs varies according to the concentration and/or diluent of the drugs. Please refer to the table at the end of this section for more information on variable compatibility.

Abbreviations

AA	Amino acid solution
BNS	Bacteriostatic normal saline
BWI	Bacteriostatic water for injection
D_5W	5% dextrose in water
D_5/NS	5% dextrose in 0.9% sodium chloride
D_5/$^1/_4$NS	5% dextrose in 0.225% sodium chloride
D_5/$^1/_2$NS	5% dextrose in 0.45% sodium chloride
D_5LR	5% dextrose in lactated Ringer's injection
$D_{10}W$	10% dextrose in water
$D_{10}W$/0.01% albumin	10% dextrose in water with 0.01% albumin
$D_{10}W$/0.05% albumin	10% dextrose in water with 0.05% albumin
$D_{10}W$/0.1% albumin	10% dextrose in water with 0.1% albumin
D_{10}/NS	10% dextrose in water in 0.9% sodium chloride
LR	Lactated Ringer's injection
NS	0.9% sodium chloride (normal saline)
SWI	Sterile water for injection
TPN	Total parenteral nutrition solution

Reported Compatibilities and Incompatibilities
of Parenteral Dosage Forms

Aldesleukin

Compatible:

D$_5$W   SWI

Y-Site Compatible:

Amikacin	Fluconazole	Ondansetron
Amphotericin	Foscarnet	Piperacillin
Calcium gluconate	Gentamicin	Potassium chloride
Cotrimoxazole	Heparin	Ranitidine
Diphenhydramine	Magnesium sulfate	Thiethylperazine
Dopamine	Metoclopramide	Ticarcillin
Fat emulsion	Morphine	Tobramycin

Incompatible:

Ganciclovir	Pentamidine	Promethazine
Heparin	Prochlorperazine	

Amifostine

Compatible:

NS

Y-Site Compatible:

Amikacin	Diphenhydramine	Mannitol
Aminophylline	Dobutamine	Mechlorethamine
Ampicillin	Dopamine	Meperidine
Ampicillin/sulbactam	Doxorubicin	Mesna
Aztreonam	Doxycycline	Methotrexate
Bleomycin	Droperidol	Methylprednisolone
Bumetanide	Enalaprilat	Metoclopramide
Buprenophine	Etoposide	Metronidazole
Butorphanol	Famotidine	Mezlocillin
Calcium gluconate	Floxuridine	Mitomycin
Carboplatin	Fluconazole	Mitoxantrone
Carmustine	Fludarabine	Morphine
Cefamdole	Fluorouracil	Nalbuphine
Cefepime	Furosemide	Netilmicin
Cefotaxime	Galium nitrate	Ondansetron
Cefotetan	Gemcitabine	Piperacillin
Cefoxitin	Gentamicin	Plicamycin
Ceftazidime	Granisetron	Potassium chloride
Ceftizoxime	Haloperidol	Promethazine
Ceftriaxone	Heparin	Ranitidine
Cefuroxime	Hydrocortisone sodium	Sodium bicarbonate
Cimetidine	phosphate	Streptozocin
Ciprofloxacin	Hydrocortisone sodium	Teniposide
Clindamycin	succinate	Thiotepa
Cotrimoxazole	Hydromorphone	Ticarcillin
Cyclophosphamide	Idarubicin	Ticarcillin/clavulanate
Cytarabine	Ifosfamide	Tobramycin
Dacarbazine	Imipenem/cilastatin	Trimetrexate
Dactinomycin	Leucovorin	Vancomycin
Daunomycin	Lorazepam	Vinblastine
Dexamethasone	Magnesium sulfate	Vincristine

Incompatible:

Acyclovir	Cisplatin	Minocycline
Amphotericin	Ganciclovir	Prochlorperazine
Chlorpromazine	Hydroxyzine	

COMPATIBILITY OF CHEMOTHERAPY AND RELATED SUPPORTIVE CARE MEDICATIONS *(Continued)*

Asparaginase

Compatible:

D_5W	NS	SWI

Y-Site Compatible:

Methotrexate	Sodium bicarbonate

Bleomycin

Compatible:

BNS	Dexamethasone	Leucovorin
BWI	Diphenhydramine	Metoclopramide
SWI	Droperidol	Phenytoin
Amikacin	Fluorouracil	Streptomycin
Amsacrine	Furosemide	Tobramycin
Ceftazidime	Gentamicin	Vinblastine
Cephapirin	Heparin	Vincristine
Cimetidine	Hydrocortisone sodium	
Dacarbazine	phosphate	

Y-Site Compatible:

Allopurinol	Doxorubicin, liposomal	Paclitaxel
Amifostine	Filgrastim	Piperacillin
Aztreonam	Fludarabine	Sargramostim
Cefepime	Gemcitabine	Teniposide
Cisplatin	Methotrexate	Thiotepa
Cyclophosphamide	Mitomycin	Vinorelbine
Doxorubicin	Ondansetron	

Incompatible:

Aminophylline	Diazepam	Nafcillin
Ascorbic acid	Doxapram	Penicillin G
Cefazolin	Hydrocortisone sodium	Terbutaline
Cephalothin	succinate	

Variable Compatibility:

D_5W	NS

Busulfan

Compatible:

D_5W	NS

Carboplatin

Compatible:

D_5W	Etoposide	Ifosfamide
SWI	Floxuridine	

Y-Site Compatible:

Allopurinol	Fludarabine	Propofol
Amifostine	Gemcitabine	Sargramostim
Aztreonam	Granisetron	Teniposide
Cefazolin	Ondansetron	Thiotepa
Doxorubicin, liposomal	Piperacillin	TPN
Filgrastim	Piperacillin/tazobactam	Vinorelbine

Incompatible:

Fluorouracil	Mesna	Sodium bicarbonate

Variable Compatibility:†

D_5/NS	$D_5/^1/_2NS$	NS
$D_5/^1/_4NS$		

Carmustine

Compatible:

D₅W	SWI	Dacarbazine
NS		

Y-Site Compatible:

Amifostine	Gemcitabine	Sargramostim
Aztreonam	Ondansetron	Teniposide
Cefepime	Piperacillin	Thiotepa
Filgrastim	Piperacillin/tazobactam	Vinorelbine
Fludarabine		

Incompatible:

Allopurinol	Sodium bicarbonate

Cisplatin

Compatible:

D₅/NS	Cephalothin	Ifosfamide
D₅/¼NS	Cyclophosphamide	Leucovorin
D₅/½NS	Floxuridine	Mannitol
NS	Hydroxyzine	Mechlorethamine
Cefazolin	Hydroxyurea	Ondansetron

Y-Site Compatible:

Allopurinol	Filgrastim	Mitomycin
Aztreonam	Fludarabine	Morphine
Bleomycin	Fluorouracil	Paclitaxel
Bumetanide	Furosemide	Potassium chloride
Chlorpromazine	Ganciclovir	Prochlorperazine
Cimetidine	Gemcitabine	Promethazine
Dexamethasone	Granisetron	Propofol
Diphenhydramine	Heparin	Ranitidine
Doxapram	Hydromorphone	Sargramostim
Doxorubicin	Lorazepam	Teniposide
Doxorubicin, liposomal	Methotrexate	Thiotepa
Droperidol	Methylprednisolone	Vinorelbine
Famotidine	Metoclopramide	

Incompatible:

Amifostine	Gallium nitrate	Piperacillin
Amsacrine	Mesna	Piperacillin/tazobactam
Cefepime	Oxacillin	Sodium bicarbonate

Variable Compatibility:†

D₅W	SWI	Etoposide

Cladribine

Compatible:

NS

Cyclophosphamide

Compatible:

D₅W	AA 4.25%/D₂₅W	Hydroxyzine
D₅/NS	Cisplatin	Mesna
D₅/LR	Dacarbazine	Methotrexate
NS	Etoposide	Mitoxantrone
LR	Fluorouracil	Ondansetron
SWI		

Y-Site Compatible:

Allopurinol	Ceftriaxone	Doxycycline
Amifostine	Cephalothin	Droperidol
Amikacin	Cephapirin	Erythromycin
Ampicillin	Chloramphenicol	Famotidine
Azlocillin	Chlorpromazine	Filgrastim
Aztreonam	Cimetidine	Fludarabine
Bleomycin	Clindamycin	Furosemide
Cefamandole	Cotrimoxazole	Gallium nitrate
Cefazolin	Dexamethasone	Ganciclovir
Cefepime	Diphenhydramine	Gemcitabine
Cefoperazone	Doxapram	Gentamicin
Cefotaxime	Doxorubicin	Granisetron
Cefoxitin	Doxorubicin, liposomal	Heparin

COMPATIBILITY OF CHEMOTHERAPY AND RELATED SUPPORTIVE CARE MEDICATIONS *(Continued)*

Hydromorphone	Moxalactam	Sodium bicarbonate
Idarubicin	Nafcillin	Teniposide
Kanamycin	Oxacillin	Thiotepa
Leucovorin	Paclitaxel	Ticarcillin
Lorazepam	Penicillin G	Ticarcillin/clavulanate
Methylprednisolone	Piperacillin	Tobramycin
Metoclopramide	Piperacillin/tazobactam	TPN
Metronidazole	Prochlorperazine	Vancomycin
Mezlocillin	Promethazine	Vinblastine
Minocycline	Propofol	Vincristine
Mitomycin	Ranitidine	Vinorelbine
Morphine	Sargramostim	

Cytarabine

Compatible:

BNS	NS	Hydroxyurea
BWI	LR	Lincomycin
D₅W	AA 4.25%/D₂₅W	Mitoxantrone
D₅/NS	Corticotropin	Ondansetron
D₅/¼NS	Dacarbazine	Potassium chloride
D₅/½NS	Daunomycin	Prednisolone
D₅/LR	Etoposide	Sodium bicarbonate
D₁₀/NS	Hydroxyzine	Vincristine

Y-Site Compatible:

Amifostine	Filgrastim	Piperacillin
Amsacrine	Fludarabine	Piperacillin/tazobactam
Aztreonam	Furosemide	Prochlorperazine
Cefepime	Gemcitabine	Promethazine
Chlorpromazine	Granisetron	Propofol
Cimetidine	Heparin	Ranitidine
Dexamethasone	Idarubicin	Sargramostim
Diphenhydramine	Lorazepam	Teniposide
Doxorubicin, liposomal	Metoclopramide	Thiotepa
Droperidol	Morphine	TPN
Famotidine	Paclitaxel	Vinorelbine

Incompatible:

Allopurinol	Gallium nitrate	Nafcillin
Ceftazidime	Ganciclovir	Oxacillin
Fluorouracil	Insulin	Penicillin G

Variable Compatibility:

Cephalothin	Hydrocortisone sodium	Methylprednisolone
Gentamicin	phosphate	

Dacarbazine

Compatible:

NS	Cyclophosphamide	Mercaptopurine
SWI	Cytarabine	Methotrexate
Bleomycin	Dactinomycin	Ondansetron
Carmustine	Doxorubicin	Vinblastine
Cimetidine	Fluorouracil	

Y-Site Compatible:

Amifostine	Granisetron	Sargramostim
Aztreonam	Hydrocortisone sodium	Teniposide
Doxorubicin, liposomal	phosphate	Thiotepa
Filgrastim	Lidocaine	Vinorelbine
Fludarabine	Paclitaxel	

Incompatible:

D₅W	Hydrocortisone sodium	Piperacillin
Allopurinol	succinate	Piperacillin/tazobactam
Cefepime		

Variable Compatibility:†

Heparin

Dactinomycin

Compatible:

D₅W	SWI	Dacarbazine
NS		

Y-Site Compatible:

Allopurinol	Fludarabine	Teniposide
Amifostine	Gemcitabine	Thiotepa
Aztreonam	Ondansetron	Vinorelbine
Cefepime	Sargramostim	

Incompatible:

BNS	BWI	Filgrastim

Daunomycin

Compatible:

D₅W	SWI	Hydrocortisone sodium
NS	Cytarabine	succinate
LR	Etoposide	

Y-Site Compatible:

Amifostine	Methotrexate	Teniposide
Filgrastim	Ondansetron	Thiotepa
Gemcitabine	Sodium bicarbonate	Vinorelbine

Incompatible:

Allopurinol	Dexamethasone	Piperacillin
Aztreonam	Fludarabine	Piperacillin/tazobactam
Cefepime		

Dexrazoxane

Compatible:

D₅W

Y-Site Compatible:

Gemcitabine

Diphenhydramine

Compatible:

Amikacin	Glycopyrrolate	Penicillin G (sodium
Aminophylline	Hydrocortisone sodium	and potassium)
Ascorbic acid	succinate	Pentazocine
Atropine	Hydromorphone	Perphenazine
Bleomycin	Hydroxyzine	Prochlorperazine
Butorphanol	Lidocaine	Promazine
Cephapirin	Meperidine	Promethazine
Chlorpromazine	Methicillin	Ranitidine
Cimetidine	Methyldopate	Scopolamine
Colistimethate	Metoclopramide	Sufentanil
Dimenhydrinate	Midazolam	Thiothixene
Droperidol	Morphine	Polymyxin B
Erythromycin	Nalbuphine	Vitamin B complex
Fentanyl	Nafcillin	with C
Fluphenazine	Netilmicin	

Y-Site Compatible:

Acyclovir	Filgrastim	Methotrexate
Aldesleukin	Fluconazole	Ondansetron
Amifostine	Fludarabine	Paclitaxel
Amsacrine	Gallium nitrate	Piperacillin/tazobactam
Aztreonam	Gemcitabine	Potassium chloride
Ciprofloxacin	Granisetron	Sargramostim
Cisplatin	Heparin	Tacrolimus
Cyclophosphamide	Idarubicin	Teniposide
Cytarabine	Melphalan	Thiotepa
Doxorubicin	Meperidine	Vinorelbine

COMPATIBILITY OF CHEMOTHERAPY AND RELATED SUPPORTIVE CARE MEDICATIONS *(Continued)*

Incompatible:

Allopurinol	Cephalothin	Pentobarbital
Amobarbital	Dexamethasone	Secobarbital
Amphotericin	Foscarnet	Thiopental
Cefepime	Haloperidol	

Variable Compatibility:

Diatrizoate	Iodipamide

Docetaxel

Compatible:

D$_5$W	NS

Y-Site Compatible:

Gemcitabine

Incompatible:

Doxorubicin, liposomal

Doxorubicin

Compatible:

D$_5$W	LR	Ondansetron
NS	Dacarbazine	Vincristine

Y-Site Compatible:

Amifostine	Fludarabine	Paclitaxel
Aztreonam	Gemcitabine	Prochlorperazine
Bleomycin	Granisetron	Promethazine
Chlorpromazine	Hydromorphone	Propofol
Cimetidine	Leucovorin	Ranitidine
Cisplatin	Lorazepam	Sargramostim
Cyclophosphamide	Methotrexate	Sodium bicarbonate
Dexamethasone	Methylprednisolone	Teniposide
Diphenhydramine	Metoclopramide	Thiotepa
Famotidine	Mitomycin	Vinorelbine
Filgrastim	Morphine	

Incompatible:

Allopurinol	Gallium nitrate	Piperacillin/tazobactam
Aminophylline	Ganciclovir	
Cefepime	Heparin	TPN
Cephalothin	Hydrocortisone sodium	
Diazepam	succinate	Paclitaxel
Furosemide		Tobramycin

Variable Compatibility:

Fluorouracil	Vinblastine

Doxorubin, Liposomal

Compatible:

D$_5$W

Y-Site Compatible:

Allopurinol	Ciprofloxacin	Fluorouracil
Aldesleukin	Cisplatin	Furosemide
Aminophylline	Clindamycin	Ganciclovir
Ampicillin	Cotrimoxazole	Gentamicin
Aztreonam	Cyclophosphamide	Granisetron
Bleomycin	Cytarabine	Haloperidol
Calcium chloride	Dacarbazine	Heparin
Calcium gluconate	Dexamethasone	Hydrocortisone sodium
Cefazolin	Diphenhydramine	succinate
Cefepime	Dobutamine	Hydromorphone
Cefoperazone	Dopamine	Ifosfamide
Cefoxitin	Droperidol	Leucovorin
Ceftizoxime	Enalaprilat	Lorazepam
Ceftriaxone	Etoposide	Magnesium sulfate
Chlorpromazine	Famotidine	Mesna
Cimetidine	Fluconazole	Methotrexate

Methylprednisolone	Potassium chloride	Tobramycin
Metronidazole	Prochlorperazine	Vancomycin
Mezlocillin	Ranitidine	Vinblastine
Netilmicin	Ticarcillin	Vincristine
Ondansetron	Ticarcillin/clavulanate	Vinorelbine
Piperacillin		

Incompatible:

Amphotericin	Mannitol	Morphine
Buprenorphine	Meperidine	Ofloxacin
Ceftazidime	Metoclopramide	Piperacillin/tazobactam
Docetaxel	Miconazole	Promethazine
Gallium nitrate	Mitoxantrone	Sodium bicarbonate
Hydroxyzine		

Droperidol

Compatible:

Atropine	Doxorubicin	Nalbuphine
Bleomycin	Fentanyl	Pentazocine
Butorphanol	Glycopyrrolate	Perphenazine
Chlorpromazine	Hydroxyzine	Prochlorperazine
Cimetidine	Meperidine	Promazine
Cisplatin	Metoclopramide	Promethazine
Cyclophosphamide	Midazolam	Scopolamine
Dimenhydrinate	Mitomycin	Vinblastine
Diphenhydramine	Morphine	Vincristine

Y-Site Compatible:

Amifostine	Idarubicin	Teniposide
Aztreonam	Melphalan	Thiotepa
Filgrastim	Ondansetron	Vinorelbine
Fluconazole	Paclitaxel	Vitamin B complex
Fludarabine	Potassium chloride	with C
Gemcitabine	Sargramostim	
Hydrocortisone sodium succinate		

Incompatible:

Allopurinol	Furosemide	Nafcillin
Cefepime	Heparin	Pentobarbital
Fluorouracil	Leucovorin	Piperacillin/tazobactam
Foscarnet	Methotrexate	

Erythropoietin

Compatible:

BNS	D_{10}/0.05% albumin	D_{10}/0.1% albumin

Incompatible:

D_{10}W	NS	SWI
D_{10}/0.01% albumin		

Etoposide

Compatible:

D_5W	Cyclophosphamide	Fluorouracil
NS	Cytarabine	Hydroxyzine
LR	Daunomycin	Ifosfamide
Carboplatin	Floxuridine	Ondansetron

Y-Site Compatible:

Allopurinol	Granisetron	Piperacillin/tazobactam
Amifostine	Haloperidol	Sargramostim
Aztreonam	Methotrexate	Sodium bicarbonate
Doxorubicin, liposomal	Paclitaxel	Teniposide
Fludarabine	Piperacillin	Vinorelbine
Gemcitabine		

Incompatible:

Cefoperazone	Cefepime	Gallium nitrate
Ceftazidime	Filgrastim	Idarubicin

Variable Compatibility:

Cisplatin	Mannitol	Potassium chloride

COMPATIBILITY OF CHEMOTHERAPY AND RELATED SUPPORTIVE CARE MEDICATIONS *(Continued)*

Filgrastim

Compatible:

D_5W SWI

Y-Site Compatible:

Acyclovir	Dexamethasone	Mechlorethamine
Allopurinol	Diphenhydramine	Meperidine
Amikacin	Doxorubicin	Mesna
Aminophylline	Doxycycline	Methotrexate
Ampicillin	Droperidol	Metoclopramide
Ampicillin/sulbactam	Enalaprilat	Miconazole
Aztreonam	Fat emulsion	Minocycline
Bleomycin	Floxuridine	Mitoxantrone
Bumetanide	Fluconazole	Morphine
Buprenorphine	Fludarabine	Nalbuphine
Butorphanol	Gallium nitrate	Netilmicin
Calcium gluconate	Ganciclovir	Ondansetron
Carboplatin	Gentamicin	Plicamycin
Carmustine	Haloperidol	Potassium chloride
Cefazolin	Hydrocortisone sodium	Promethazine
Cefotetan	phosphate	Ranitidine
Ceftazidime	Hydrocortisone sodium	Sodium bicarbonate
Chlorpromazine	succinate	Streptozocin
Cimetidine	Hydromorphone	Ticarcillin
Cisplatin	Hydroxyzine	Ticarcillin/clavulanate
Cotrimoxazole	Idarubicin	Tobramycin
Cyclophosphamide	Ifosfamide	Vancomycin
Cytarabine	Imipenem/cilastatin	Vinblastine
Dacarbazine	Leucovorin	Vincristine
Daunomycin	Lorazepam	Vinorelbine

Incompatible:

NS	Ceftizoxime	Mannitol
Amphotericin	Ceftriaxone	Methylprednisolone
Amsacrine	Cefuroxime	Metronidazole
Cefepime	Dactinomycin	Mezlocillin
Cefonicid	Etoposide	Mitomycin
Cefoperazone	Fluorouracil	Piperacillin
Cefotaxime	Furosemide	Prochlorperazine
Cefoxitin	Heparin	Thiotepa

Floxuridine

Compatible:

D_5W	Carboplatin	Fluorouracil
NS	Cisplatin	Heparin
SWI	Etoposide	Leucovorin

Y-Site Compatible:

Amifostine	Gemcitabine	Sargramostim
Aztreonam	Ondansetron	Teniposide
Filgrastim	Paclitaxel	Thiotepa
Fludarabine	Piperacillin/tazobactam	Vinorelbine

Incompatible:

Allopurinol	Cefepime

Fludarabine

Compatible:

D_5W NS   SWI

Y-Site Compatible:

Allopurinol	Butorphanol	Ceftizoxime
Amifostine	Carboplatin	Ceftriaxone
Amikacin	Carmustine	Cefuroxime
Aminophylline	Cefazolin	Cimetidine
Ampicillin	Cefepime	Cisplatin
Ampicillin/sulbactam	Cefoperazone	Cotrimoxazole
Amsacrine	Cefotaxime	Cyclophosphamide
Aztreonam	Cefotetan	Cytarabine
Bleomycin	Ceftazidime	Dacarbazine

1104

Dactinomycin	Hydrocortisone sodium	Nalbuphine
Dexamethasone	succinate	Netilmicin
Diphenhydramine	Hydromorphone	Ondansetron
Doxorubicin	Ifosfamide	Pentostatin
Doxycycline	Imipenem/cilastatin	Piperacillin
Droperidol	Lorazepam	Piperacillin/tazobactam
Etoposide	Magnesium sulfate	Potassium chloride
Famotidine	Mannitol	Promethazine
Filgrastim	Mechlorethamine	Ranitidine
Floxuridine	Meperidine	Sodium bicarbonate
Fluconazole	Mesna	Teniposide
Fluorouracil	Methotrexate	Tetracycline
Furosemide	Methylprednisolone	Ticarcillin
Gemcitabine	Metoclopramide	Ticarcillin/clavulanate
Gentamicin	Mezlocillin	Tobramycin
Haloperidol	Minocylcine	Vancomycin
Heparin	Mitoxantrone	Vinblastine
Hydrocortisone sodium	Morphine	Vincristine
phosphate	Multivitamins	Vinorelbine

Incompatible:

Acyclovir	Daunomycin	Miconazole
Amphotericin	Ganciclovir	Prochlorperazine
Chlorpromazine	Hydroxyzine	

Fluorouracil

Compatible:

D$_5$W	Cyclophosphamide	Magnesium sulfate
D$_5$/LR	Dacarbazine	Methotrexate
NS	Etoposide	Mitoxantrone
Bleomycin	Floxuridine	Prednisolone
Cephalothin	Ifosfamide	Vincristine

Y-Site Compatible:

Allopurinol	Granisetron	Piperacillin/tazobactam
Amifostine	Heparin	Potassium chloride
Aztreonam	Hydrocortisone sodium	Propofol
Cefepime	succinate	Sargramostim
Cisplatin	Mannitol	Teniposide
Doxorubicin, liposomal	Metoclopramide	Thiotepa
Fludarabine	Mitomycin	Vinblastine
Furosemide	Paclitaxel	Vitamin B complex
Gemcitabine	Piperacillin	

Incompatible:

Carboplatin	Epirubicin	Ondansetron
Cytarabine	Filgrastim	TPN
Diazepam		
Droperidol	Gallium nitrate	Vinorelbine

Variable Compatibility:†

Doxorubicin	Leucovorin

Gemcitabine

Compatible:
NS

Y-Site Compatible:

Amifostine	Ceftizoxime	Doxorubicin
Amikacin	Ceftriaxone	Doxycycline
Aminophylline	Cefuroxime	Droperidol
Ampicillin	Chlorpromazine	Enalaprilat
Ampicillin/sulbactam	Cimetidine	Etoposide
Aztreonam	Ciprofloxacin	Etoposide phosphate
Bleomycin	Cisplatin	Famotidine
Bumetanide	Clindamycin	Floxuridine
Buprenorphine	Cyclophosphamide	Fludarabine
Butorphanol	Cytarabine	Fluorouracil
Calcium gluconate	Dactinomycin	Fluconazole
Carboplatin	Daunomycin	Gallium nitrate
Carmustine	Dexamethasone	Gentamicin
Cefazolin	Dexrazoxane	Granisetron
Cefonicid	Diphenhydramine	Haloperidol
Cefotetan	Dobutamine	Heparin
Cefoxitin	Docetaxel	Hydrocortisone sodium
Ceftazidime	Dopamine	phosphate

COMPATIBILITY OF CHEMOTHERAPY AND RELATED SUPPORTIVE CARE MEDICATIONS *(Continued)*

Hydrocortisone sodium succinate
Hydromorphone
Hydroxyzine
Idarubicin
Ifosfamide
Leucovorin
Lorazepam
Mannitol
Meperidine
Mesna
Metoclopramide
Metronidazole
Miconazole

Minocycline
Mitoxantrone
Morphine
Nalbuphine
Netilmicin
Ofloxacin
Ondansetron
Paclitaxel
Plicamycin
Potassium chloride
Promethazine
Ranitidine
Sodium bicarbonate

Streptozocin
Teniposide
Thiotepa
Ticarcillin
Ticarcillin/clavulanate
Tobramycin
Topotecan
Trimethoprim
Vancomycin
Vinblastine
Vincristine
Vinorelbine
Zidovudine

Incompatible:

Acyclovir
Amphotericin
Cefoperazone
Cefotaxime
Furosemide

Ganciclovir
Imipenem/cilastatin
Irinotecan
Methotrexate
Methylprednisolone

Mezlocillin
Mitomycin
Piperacillin
Piperacillin/tazobactam
Prochlorperazine

Granisetron

Compatible:

BWI
D5W
D5/NS

D5/½NS
NS

Dexamethasone
Methylprednisolone

Y-Site Compatible:

Acyclovir
Allopurinol
Amifostine
Amikacin
Aminophylline
Ampicillin
Ampicillin/sulbactam
Amsacrine
Aztreonam
Bleomycin
Bumetanide
Buprenorphine
Butorphanol
Calcium gluconate
Carboplatin
Carmustine
Cefazolin
Cefepime
Cefonicid
Cefoperazone
Cefotaxime
Cefotetan
Cefoxitin
Ceftazidime
Ceftizoxime
Ceftriaxone
Cefuroxime
Chlorpromazine
Cimetidine
Ciprofloxacin
Cisplatin
Cotrimoxazole
Cyclophosphamide
Cytarabine
Dacarbazine

Dactinomycin
Daunomycin
Diphenhydramine
Dobutamine
Dopamine
Doxorubicin
Doxorubicin, liposomal
Doxycycline
Droperidol
Enalaprilat
Etoposide
Famotidine
Filgrastim
Floxuridine
Fluconazole
Fludarabine
Fluorouracil
Gemcitabine
Haloperidol
Heparin
Hydrocortisone sodium phosphate
Hydrocortisone sodium succinate
Hydromorphone
Hydroxyzine
Idarubicin
Ifosfamide
Imipenem/cilastatin
Leucovorin
Levoleucovorin
Lorazepam
Magnesium sulfate
Mechlorethamine

Meperidine
Mesna
Methotrexate
Metoclopramide
Metronidazole
Mezlocillin
Minocycline
Mitomycin
Mitoxantrone
Morphine
Nalbuphine
Netilmicin
Ofloxacin
Paclitaxel
Piperacillin
Piperacillin/tazobactam
Plicamycin
Potassium chloride
Prochlorperazine
Promethazine
Propofol
Ranitidine
Sargramostim
Sodium bicarbonate
Streptozocin
Teniposide
Ticarcillin
Ticarcillin/clavulanate
Tobramycin
TPN
Vancomycin
Vinblastine
Vincristine
Vinorelbine

Incompatible:

Amphotericin

Haloperidol

Compatible:

Hydromorphone

Sufentanil

Y-Site Compatible:

Amifostine
Amsacrine
Aztreonam
Cimetidine
Dobutamine
Dopamine
Famotidine
Filgrastim
Fludarabine

Gemcitabine
Lidocaine
Lorazepam
Melphalan
Midazolam
Nitroglycerin
Norepinephrine bitartrate
Ondansetron

Paclitaxel
Phenylephrine
Tacrolimus
Teniposide
Theophylline
Thiotepa
TPN
Vinorelbine

Incompatible:

Allopurinol
Cefepime
Diphenhydramine
Fluconazole

Foscarnet
Gallium nitrate
Heparin
Hydroxyzine

Ketorolac
Piperacillin/tazobactam
Sargramostim

Variable Compatibility:

Benztropine
Cyclizine

Diamorphine

Sodium nitroprusside

Heparin

Compatible:

Aminophylline
Amphotericin
Ascorbic acid
Bleomycin
Calcium gluconate
Cefepime
Cephapirin
Chloramphenicol
Cibenzoline
Clindamycin
Cloxacillin
Colistimethate
Dimenhydrinate

Dopamine
Enalaprilat
Erythromycin
Esmolol
Floxacillin
Fluconazole
Flumazenil
Furosemide
Isoproterenol
Lidocaine
Lincomycin
Methyldopa
Methylprednisolone

Metronidazole
Nafcillin
Norepinephrine
Octreotide
Potassium chloride
Prednisolone
Promazine
Ranitidine
Sodium bicarbonate
Verapamil
Vitamin B complex
with C

Y-Site Compatible:

Acyclovir
Aldesleukin
Allopurinol
Amifostine
Ampicillin
Ampicillin/sulbactam
Atracurium
Atropine
Aztreonam
Betamethasone sodium
phosphate
Cefazolin
Cefotetan
Ceftazidime
Ceftriaxone
Cephalothin
Chlordiazepoxide
Chlorpromazine
Cimetidine
Cisplatin
Cyanocobalamin
Cyclophosphamide
Cytarabine
Digoxin
Diphenhydramine
Edrophonium
Epinephrine
Erythromycin
Esmolol
Estrogens, conjugated
Ethacrynate
Famotidine

Fentanyl
Fludarabine
Fluorouracil
Foscarnet
Gallium nitrate
Gemcitabine
Hydralazine
Hydrocortisone sodium
succinate
Insulin
Kanamycin
Leucovorin
Lorazepam
Magnesium sulfate
Melphalan
Menadiol sodium
dipshosphate
Methicillin
Methotrexate
Methoxamine
Methyldopa
Metoclopramide
Metronidazole
Midazolam
Minocycline
Mitomycin
Morphine
Neostigmine
Nitroglycerin
Ondansetron
Oxacillin

Oxytocin
Paclitaxel
Pancuronium
Penicillin G potassium
Pentazocine
Phytonadione
Piperacillin
Piperacillin/tazobactam
Procainamide
Prochlorperazine
Propranolol
Pyridostigmine
Sargramostim
Scopolamine
Sodium nitroprusside
Streptokinase
Succinylcholine
Tacrolimus
Teniposide
Theophylline
Thiotepa
Ticarcillin
Ticarcillin/clavulanate
TPN
Trimethobenzamide
Trimethaphan
Vercuronium
Vinblastine
Vincristine
Vinorelbine
Zidovudine

Incompatible:

Alteplase
Amikacin
Amiodarone
Amsacrine
Ciprofloxacin
Codeine phosphate
Daunomycin

Diazepam
Dobutamine
Doxorubicin
Doxycycline
Ergotamine
Filgrastim
Gentamicin

Haloperidol
Hyaluronidase
Idarubicin
Labetalol
Levorphanol
Methadone
Methotrimeprazine

COMPATIBILITY OF CHEMOTHERAPY AND RELATED SUPPORTIVE CARE MEDICATIONS (Continued)

Phenytoin
Polymyxin B

Streptomycin
Tobramycin

Triflupromazine

Variable Compatibility:

Cephalothin
Dacarbazine
Diltiazem
Droperidol

Hydrocortisone sodium
  succinate
Methylprednisolone
Penicillin G sodium

Promethazine
Quinidine gluconate
Vancomycin

Hydroxyzine

Compatible:

Atropine
Benzquinamide
Bupivicaine
Butorphanol
Chlorpromazine
Cimetidine
Cisplatin
Codeine
Cyclophosphamide
Cytarabine
Diphenhydramine
Doxapram
Droperidol

Etoposide
Fentanyl
Fluphenazine
Glycopyrrolate
Hydromorphone
Lidocaine
Meperidine
Methotrimeprazine
Metoclopramide
Midazolam
Morphine
Nalbuphine
Oxymorphone

Pentazocine
Mesna
Methotrexate
Nafcillin
Perphenazine
Procaine
Prochlorperazine
Promazine
Promethazine
Scopolamine
Sufentanil
Thiothixene

Y-Site Compatible:

Aztreonam
Ciprofloxacin
Filgrastim
Foscarnet

Gemcitabine
Melphalan
Ondansetron
Sufentanil

Teniposide
Thiotepa
Vinorelbine

Incompatible:

Allopurinol
Amifostine
Aminophylline
Amobarbital
Cefepime
Chloramphenicol
Diphenhydramine

Fluconazole
Fludarabine
Haloperidol
Ketorolac
Paclitaxel
Penicillin G (sodium
  and potassium)

Pentobarbital
Phenobarbital
Piperacillin/tazobactam
Ranitidine
Sargramostim

Idarubicin

Compatible:

D5W
D5/NS

NS

LR

Y-Site Compatible:

Amifostine
Amikacin
Aztreonam
Ciprofloxacin
Cyclophosphamide
Cytarabine
Diphenhydramine

Droperidol
Erythromycin
Filgrastim
Gemcitabine
Imipenem/cilastatin
Magnesium sulfate
Mannitol

Metoclopramide
Potassium chloride
Ranitidine
Sargramostim
Thiotepa
Vinorelbine

Incompatible:

Acyclovir
Allopurinol
Ampicillin/sulbactam
Cefazolin
Cefepime
Ceftazidime
Dexamethasone
Etoposide

Furosemide
Gentamicin
Heparin
Hydrocortisone sodium
  succinate
Lorazepam
Meperidine

Methotrexate
Mezlocillin
Piperacillin/tazobactam
Sodium bicarbonate
Teniposide
Vancomycin
Vincristine

Ifosfamide

Compatible:

D5W
D5/NS
D5/¼NS
D5/LR

NS
LR
SWI
Carboplatin

Cisplatin
Etoposide
Fluorouracil

Y-Site Compatible:

Allopurinol
Amifostine
Aztreonam
Doxorubicin, liposomal
Filgrastim
Fludarabine
Gallium nitrate

Gemcitabine
Granisetron
Ondansetron
Paclitaxel
Piperacillin
Piperacillin/tazobactam
Propofol

Sargramostim
Sodium bicarbonate
Teniposide
Thiotepa
TPN
Vinorelbine

Incompatible:

Cefepime

Methotrexate

Variable Compatibility:

Epirubicin

Mesna

Irinotecan

Compatible:

D_5W

Incompatible:

Gemcitabine

Leucovorin

Compatible:

BWI
D_5W
D_{10}/NS

NS
LR
SWI

Bleomycin
Cisplatin
Floxuridine

Y-Site Compatible:

Amifostine
Aztreonam
Cefepime
Cyclophosphamide
Doxorubicin
Doxorubicin, liposomal
Filgrastim
Fluconazole

Furosemide
Gemcitabine
Heparin
Methotrexate
Metoclopramide
Mitomycin
Piperacillin
Piperacillin/tazobactam

Sodium bicarbonate
Tacrolimus
Teniposide
Thiotepa
TPN
Vinblastine
Vincristine

Incompatible:

Droperidol

Foscarnet

Trimetrexate

Variable Compatibility:†

Fluorouracil

Lorazepam

Compatible:

Cimetidine

Hydromorphone

Y-Site Compatible:

Acyclovir
Albumin
Amifostine
Amikacin
Amoxicillin
Amoxicillin/clavulanate
Amsacrine
Atracurium
Bumetanide
Cefepime
Cefotaxime
Ciprofloxacin
Cisplatin
Cotrimoxazole
Cyclophosphamide
Cytarabine
Dexamethasone

Diltiazem
Doxorubicin
Erythromycin
Etomidate
Fentanyl
Filgrastim
Fluconazole
Fludarabine
Furosemide
Gemcitabine
Gentamicin
Granisetron
Haloperidol
Heparin
Hydrocortisone sodium
  succinate
Kantaserin

Melphalan
Methotrexate
Metronidazole
Morphine
Paclitaxel
Pancuronium
Piperacillin
Piperacillin/tazobactam
Potassium chloride
Ranitidine
Tacrolimus
Teniposide
Thiotepa
Vancomycin
Vercuronium
Vinorelbine
Zidovudine

COMPATIBILITY OF CHEMOTHERAPY AND RELATED SUPPORTIVE CARE MEDICATIONS *(Continued)*

Incompatible:

Aldesleukin	Gallium nitrate	Sargramostim
Aztreonam	Idarubicin	Sufentanil
Buprenorphine	Imipenem/cilastatin	
Floxacillin	Ondansetron	Thiopental

Variable Compatibility:

Foscarnet

Mechlorethamine

Compatible:

NS   SWI

Y-Site Compatible:

Amifostine	Fludarabine	Sargramostim
Aztreonam	Granisetron	Teniposide
Filgrastiim	Ondansetron	Vinorelbine

Incompatible:

D_5W	Cefepime	Methohexital
Allopurinol		

Melphalan

Compatible:

NS

Y-Site Compatible:

Acyclovir	Doxycycline	Methotrexate
Amikacin	Droperidol	Methylprednisolone
Aminophylline	Enalaprilat	Metoclopramide
Ampicillin	Etoposide	Metronidazole
Aztreonam	Famotidine	Miconazole
Bleomycin	Filgrastim	Minocycline
Bumetanide	Floxuridine	Mitomycin
Buprenorphine	Fluconazole	Mitoxantrone
Butorphanol	Fludarabine	Morphine
Calcium gluconate	Fluorouracil	Nalbuphine
Carboplatin	Furosemide	Netilmicin
Carmustine	Gallium nitrate	Ondansetron
Cefazolin	Ganciclovir	Pentostatin
Cefepime	Gentamicin	Piperacillin
Cefoperazone	Haloperidol	Plicamycin
Cefotaxime	Heparin	Potassium chloride
Cefotetan	Hydrocortisone sodium	Prochlorperazine
Ceftazidime	phosphate	Promethazine
Ceftriaxone	Hydrocortisone sodium	Ranitidine
Cefuroxime	succinate	Sodium bicarbonate
Cimetidine	Hydromorphone	Streptozocin
Cisplatin	Hydroxyzine	Teniposide
Cotrimoxazole	Idarubicin	Thiotepa
Cyclophosphamide	Ifosfamide	Ticarcillin
Cytarabine	Imipenem/cilastatin	Ticarcillin/clavulanate
Dacarbazine	Lorazepam	Tobramycin
Dactinomycin	Mannitol	Vancomycin
Daunomycin	Mechlorethamine	Vinblastine
Diazepam	Meperidine	Vincristine
Doxorubicin	Mesna	Vinorelbine

Incompatible:

D_5W	SWI	Chlorpromazine
LR	Amphotericin	

Mesna

Compatible:

BWI	LR	Hydroxyzine
D₅W	Cyclophosphamide	Ifosfamide
NS		

Y-Site Compatible:

Allopurinol	Gallium nitrate	Sargramostim
Amifostine	Gemcitabine	Sodium acetate
Aztreonam	Granisetron	Teniposide
Cefepime	Methotrexate	Thiotepa
Doxorubicin, liposomal	Ondansetron	TPN
Filgrastim	Paclitaxel	Vinorelbine
Fludarabine	Piperacillin/tazobactam	

Incompatible:

Carboplatin	Cisplatin	Chlorpromazine

Methadone

Incompatible:

Aminophylline	Phenytoin	Pentobarbital
Ammonium chloride	Heparin	Sodium bicarbonate
Amobarbital	Methicillin	
Chlorothiazide	Nitrofurantoin	Thiopental

Methotrexate

Compatible:

D₅W	Cyclophosphamide	Imipenem/cilastatin
NS	Cytarabine	Mercaptopurine
LR	Dacarbazine	Ondansetron
SWI	Fluorouracil	Sodium bicarbonate
Amino acid 4.25%/D₂₅W	Hydroxyzine	Vincristine
Cephalothin		

Y-Site Compatible:

Allopurinol	Doxorubicin, liposomal	Methylprednisolone
Amifostine	Etoposide	Mitomycin
Asparaginase	Famotidine	Morphine
Aztreonam	Filgrastim	Oxacillin
Bleomycin	Fludarabine	Paclitaxel
Cefepime	Furosemide	Piperacillin/tazobactam
Ceftriaxone	Gallium nitrate	Prochlorperazine
Cimetidine	Ganciclovir	Ranitidine
Cisplatin	Granisetron	Sargramostim
Daunomycin	Heparin	Teniposide
Dexchlorpheniramine	Hydromorphone	Thiotepa
Diphenhydramine	Leucovorin	Vinblastine
Doxapram	Lorazepam	Vindesine
Doxorubicin	Mesna	Vinorelbine

Incompatible:

Dexamethasone	Midazolam	Promethazine
Gemcitabine	Nalbuphine	Propofol
Idarubicin		
Ifosfamide	Prednisolone	TPN

Variable Compatibility:

Droperidol	Metoclopramide	Vancomycin

COMPATIBILITY OF CHEMOTHERAPY AND RELATED SUPPORTIVE CARE MEDICATIONS *(Continued)*

Metoclopramide

Compatible:

D_5W	Multivitamins	Potassium phosphate
NS	Potassium acetate	Verapamil
Clindamycin	Potassium chloride	TPN
Mannitol		

Y-Site Compatible:

Acyclovir	Fluconazole	Morphine
Aldesleukin	Fludarabine	Ondansetron
Amifostine	Fluorouracil	Paclitaxel
Aztreonam	Foscarnet	Piperacillin/tazobactam
Bleomycin	Gallium nitrate	Sargramostim
Ciprofloxacin	Gemcitabine	Sufentanil
Cisplatin	Heparin	Tacrolimus
Cyclophosphamide	Idarubicin	Teniposide
Cytarabine	Leucovorin	Thiotepa
Diltiazem	Melphalan	Vinblastine
Doxorubicin	Meperidine	Vincristine
Droperidol	Methotrexate	Vinorelbine
Famotidine	Mitomycin	Zidovudine
Filgrastim		

Incompatible:

Allopurinol	Cephalothin	Floxacillin
Ampicillin	Chloramphenicol	Furosemide
Calcium gluconate	Dexamethasone	Penicillin G potassium
Cefepime	Erythromycin	Sodium bicarbonate

Metronidazole

Compatible:

Amikacin	Cefuroxime	Heparin
Aminophylline	Cephalothin	Hydrocortisone
Cefazolin	Chloramphenicol	Moxalactam
Cefotaxime	Ciprofloxacin	Multielectrolyte concentrate
Cefotetan	Clindamycin	Multivitamins
Cefoxitin	Disopyramide	Netilmicin
Ceftazidime	Floxacillin	Penicillin G potassium
Ceftizoxime	Fluconazole	Tobramycin
Ceftriaxone	Gentamicin	

Y-Site Compatible:

Acyclovir	Gemcitabine	Perphenazine
Allopurinol	Heparin	Piperacillin/tazobactam
Amifostine	Hydromorphone	Sargramostim
Cefepime	Labetalol	Tacrolimus
Cyclophosphamide	Lorazepam	Teniposide
Diltiazem	Magnesium sulfate	Theophylline
Enalaprilat	Melphalan	Thiotepa
Esmolol	Meperidine	TPN
Fluconazole	Midazolam	Vinorelbine
Foscarnet	Morphine	

Incompatible:

Aztreonam	Dopamine	Filgrastim

Variable Compatibility:

Ampicillin	Cefamandole

Mitomycin

Compatible:

NS	Hydrocortisone sodium
LR	succinate
Dexamethasone	

Y-Site Compatible:

Allopurinol	Droperidol	Ondansetron
Amifostine	Fluorouracil	Teniposide
Bleomycin	Furosemide	Thiotepa
Cisplatin	Leucovorin	Vinblastine
Cyclophosphamide	Methotrexate	Vincristine
Doxorubicin	Metoclopramide	

Incompatible:

Aztreonam	Gemcitabine	Sargramostim
Cefepime	Piperacillin/tazobactam	Vinorelbine
Filgrastim		

Variable Compatibility:†

D₅W	SWI	Heparin

Mitoxantrone

Compatible:

D₅W	Cyclophosphamide	Fluorouracil
D₅/NS	Cytarabine	Potassium chloride
NS		

Y-Site Compatible:

Allopurinol	Gemcitabine	Teniposide
Amifostine	Ondansetron	Thiotepa
Filgrastim	Sargramostim	Vinorelbine
Fludarabine		

Incompatible:

Aztreonam	Heparin	Piperacillin/tazobactam
Cefepime	Paclitaxel	Propofol
Doxorubicin, liposomal	Piperacillin	

Variable Compatibility:

Hydrocortisone sodium	Hydrocortisone sodium	TPN
phosphate	succinate	

Ondansetron

Compatible:

D₅W	Dexamethasone	Mannitol
NS	Doxorubicin	Meperidine
LR	Etoposide	Methotrexate
Cisplatin	Fluconazole	Morphine
Cyclophosphamide	Hydrocortisone sodium	Ranitidine
Cytarabine	succinate	
Dacarbazine		

Y-Site Compatible:

Aldesleukin	Droperidol	Miconazole
Amifostine	Famotidine	Mitomycin
Amikacin	Filgrastim	Mitoxantrone
Aztreonam	Floxuridine	Paclitaxel
Bleomycin	Fludarabine	Pentostatin
Carboplatin	Gallium nitrate	Piperacillin/tazobactam
Carmustine	Gemcitabine	Potassium chloride
Cefazolin	Gentamicin	Prochlorperazine
Cefotaxime	Haloperidol	Promethazine
Cefoxitin	Heparin	Sodium acetate
Ceftazidime	Hydrocortisone sodium	Streptozocin
Ceftizoxime	phosphate	Teniposide
Cefuroxime	Hydromorphone	Thiotepa
Chlorpromazine	Hydroxyzine	Ticarcillin
Cimetidine	Ifosfamide	Ticarcillin/clavulanate
Dactinomycin	Imipenem/cilastatin	TPN
Daunomycin	Magnesium sulfate	Vancomycin
Diphenhydramine	Mechlorethamine	Vinblastine
Doxorubicin, liposomal	Mesna	Vincristine
Doxycycline	Metoclopramide	Vinorelbine

COMPATIBILITY OF CHEMOTHERAPY AND RELATED SUPPORTIVE CARE MEDICATIONS *(Continued)*

Incompatible:

Acyclovir	Amsacrine	Methylprednisolone
Allopurinol	Cefepime	Mezlocillin
Aminophylline	Cefoperazone	Piperacillin
Amphotericin	Furosemide	Sargramostim
Ampicillin	Ganciclovir	Sodium bicarbonate
Ampicillin/sulbactam	Lorazepam	

Variable Compatibility:

Fluorouracil

Paclitaxel

Compatible:

NS

Y-Site Compatible:

Acyclovir	Etoposide	Mannitol
Amikacin	Famotidine	Meperidine
Aminophylline	Floxuridine	Mesna
Ampicillin/sulbactam	Fluconazole	Methotrexate
Bleomycin	Fluorouracil	Metoclopramide
Butorphanol	Furosemide	Morphine
Calcium chloride	Ganciclovir	Nalbuphine
Carboplatin	Gemcitabine	Ondansetron
Cefepime	Gentamicin	Pentostatin
Cefotetan	Granisetron	Potassium chloride
Ceftazidime	Haloperidol	Prochlorperazine
Cefuroxime	Heparin	Propofol
Cimetidine	Hydrocortisone sodium phosphate	Ranitidine
Cyclophosphamide		Sodium bicarbonate
Cytarabine	Hydrocortisone sodium succinate	Thiotepa
Dacarbazine		TPN
Dexamethasone	Hydromorphone	Vancomycin
Diphenhydramine	Ifosfamide	Vinblastine
Doxorubicin	Lorazepam	Vincristine
Droperidol	Magnesium sulfate	

Incompatible:

Amphotercin	Doxorubicin, liposomal	Methylprednisolone
Chlorpromazine	Hydroxyzine	Mitoxantrone

Variable Compatibility:

D$_5$W	Cisplatin

Pentostatin

Compatible:

NS	LR

Y-Site Compatible:

Fludarabine	Paclitaxel	Sargramostim
Ondansetron		

Variable Compatibility:†

D$_5$W

Phytonadione

Compatible:

Amikacin	Chloramphenicol	Doxapram
Calcium gluceptate	Cimetidine	Sodium bicarbonate
Cefapirin	Netilmicin	TPN

Y-Site Compatible:

Ampicillin	Hydrocortisone sodium	Tolazoline
Epinephrine	succinate	Vitamin B complex
Famotidine	Potassium chloride	with C
Heparin		

Incompatible:

Dobutamine	Ranitidine

Plicamycin

Compatible:

D$_5$W	SWI	Piperacillin
NS		

Y-Site Compatible:

Allopurinol	Filgrastim	Teniposide
Amifostine	Gemcitabine	Vinorelbine
Aztreonam	Piperacillin/tazobactam	

Incompatible:

Cefonicid

Prochlorperazine

Compatible:

Amikacin	Erythromycin	Sodium bicarbonate
Ascorbic acid	Ethacrinate	Vitamin B complex
Dexamethasone	Lidocaine	with C
Dimenhydrinate	Nafcillin	

Y-Site Compatible:

Amsacrine	Hydrocortisone sodium	Potassium chloride
Cisplatin	succinate	Sargramostim
Cyclophosphamide	Melphalan	Sufentanil
Cytarabine	Methotrexate	Teniposide
Doxorubicin	Ondansetron	Thiotepa
Fluconazole	Paclitaxel	Vinorelbine
Heparin		

Incompatible:

Aldesleukin	Cefepime	Gallium nitrate
Allopurinol	Cephalothin	Gemcitabine
Amifostine	Chloramphenicol	Methohexital
Aminophylline	Floxacillin	Penicillin G sodium
Amphotericin	Fludarabine	Piperacillin/tazobactam
Ampicillin	Foscarnet	Phenobarbital
Aztreonam	Filgrastim	Thiopental
Calcium gluceptate	Furosemide	

Variable Compatibility:

Calcium gluconate	Penicillin G potassium

COMPATIBILITY OF CHEMOTHERAPY AND RELATED SUPPORTIVE CARE MEDICATIONS *(Continued)*

Promethazine

Compatible:

Amikacin	Chloroquine	Vitamin B complex
Ascorbic acid	Netilmicin	with C

Y-Site Compatible:

Amifostine	Cytarabine	Melphalan
Amsacrine	Doxorubicin	Ondansetron
Aztreonam	Filgrastim	Sargramostim
Ciprofloxacin	Fluconazole	Teniposide
Cisplatin	Fludarabine	Thiotepa
Cyclophosphamide	Gemcitabine	Vinorelbine

Incompatible:

Aldesleukin	Chlorothiazide	Methohexital
Allopurinol	Floxacillin	Methotrexate
Aminophylline	Foscarnet	Penicillin G (sodium
Cefepime	Furosemide	and potassium)
Cefoperazone	Heparin	Pentobarbital
Cefotetan	Hydrocortisone sodium	Piperacillin/tazobactam
Ceftizoxime	succinate	Thiopental
Chloramphenicol	Methicillin	

Variable Compatibility:

Potassium chloride

Sargramostim

Compatible:

BWI	NS	SWI
D5W		

Y-Site Compatible:

Allopurinol	Dacarbazine	Mechlorethamine
Amikacin	Dactinomycin	Meperidine
Aminophylline	Dexamethasone	Mesna
Aztreonam	Diphenhydramine	Methotrexate
Bleomycin	Dobutamine	Metoclopramide
Butorphanol	Doxorubicin	Metronidazole
Calcium gluconate	Doxycycline	Mezlocillin
Carboplatin	Droperidol	Miconazole
Carmustine	Etoposide	Minocycline
Cefazolin	Famotidine	Mitoxantrone
Cefepime	Fentanyl	Netilmicin
Cefotetan	Floxuridine	Pentostatin
Cefoxitin	Fluconazole	Piperacillin/tazobactam
Ceftizoxime	Fluorouracil	Potassium chloride
Ceftriaxone	Furosemide	Prochlorperazine
Cefuroxime	Gentamicin	Promethazine
Cimetidine	Heparin	Ranitidine
Cisplatin	Human immune globulin	Teniposide
Cotrimoxazole	Idarubicin	Ticarcillin
Cyclophosphamide	Ifosfamide	Ticarcillin/clavulanate
Cyclosporine	Magnesium sulfate	Vinblastine
Cytarabine	Mannitol	Vincristine

Incompatible:

Acyclovir	Hydrocortisone sodium	Mitomycin
Ampicillin	phosphate	Morphine
Ampicillin/sulbactam	Hydrocortisone sodium	Nalbuphine
Cefonicid	succinate	Ondansetron
Cefoperazone	Hydromorphone	Piperacillin
Chlorpromazine	Hydroxyzine	Sodium bicarbonate
Ganciclovir	Imipenem/cilastatin	Tobramycin
Haloperidol	Methylprednisolone	

Variable Compatibility:†

Amphotericin	Ceftazidime	Vancomycin
Amsacrine		

Streptozocin

Compatible:

D₅W	NS	SWI

Y-Site Compatible:

Filgrastim	Ondansetron	Thiotepa
Gemcitabine	Teniposide	Vinorelbine
Granisetron		

Incompatible:

Allopurinol	Cefepime	Piperacillin/tazobactam
Aztreonam	Piperacillin	

Teniposide

Compatible:

D₅W	NS	LR

Y-Site Compatible:

Acyclovir	Dacarbazine	Mechlorethamine
Allopurinol	Dactinomycin	Meperidine
Amifostine	Daunomycin	Mesna
Amikacin	Dexamethasone	Methotrexate
Aminophylline	Diphenhydramine	Methylprednisolone
Amphotericin	Doxorubicin	Metoclopramide
Ampicillin	Doxycycline	Metronidazole
Ampicillin/sulbactam	Droperidol	Mezlocillin
Aztreonam	Enalaprilat	Miconazole
Bleomycin	Etoposide	Midazolam
Bumetanide	Famotidine	Mitomycin
Buprenorphine	Floxuridine	Mitoxantrone
Butorphanol	Fluconazole	Morphine
Calcium gluconate	Fludarabine	Nalbuphine
Carboplatin	Fluorouracil	Netilmicin
Carmustine	Furosemide	Ondansetron
Cefazolin	Gallium nitrate	Piperacillin
Cefonicid	Ganciclovir	Plicamycin
Cefoperazone	Gemcitabine	Potassium chloride
Cefotaxime	Gentamicin	Prochlorperazine
Cefotetan	Haloperidol	Promethazine
Cefoxitin	Heparin	Ranitidine
Ceftazidime	Hydrocortisone sodium phosphate	Sargramostim
Ceftizoxime		Sodium bicarbonate
Ceftriaxone	Hydrocortisone sodium succinate	Streptozocin
Cefuroxime		Thiotepa
Chlorpromazine	Hydromorphone	Ticarcillin
Cimetidine	Hydroxyzine	Ticarcillin/clavulanate
Cisplatin	Ifosfamide	Tobramycin
Corticotropin	Imipenem/cilastatin	Vancomycin
Cotrimoxazole	Leucovorin	Vinblastine
Cyclophosphamide	Lorazepam	Vincristine
Cytarabine	Mannitol	Vinorelbine

Incompatible:

Idarubicin

COMPATIBILITY OF CHEMOTHERAPY AND RELATED SUPPORTIVE CARE MEDICATIONS *(Continued)*

Thiethylperazine

Compatible:

NS	Hydromorphone	Ranitidine
Butorphanol	Midazolam	

Y-Site Compatible:
   Aldesleukin

Incompatible:

Ketorolac	Perphenazine

Variable Compatibility:
   Nalbuphine

Thiotepa

Compatible:

NS	SWI

Y-Site Compatible:

Acyclovir	Daunomycin	Mannitol
Allopurinol	Dexamethasone	Meperidine
Amifostine	Diphenhydramine	Mesna
Amikacin	Dobutamine	Methotrexate
Aminophylline	Dopamine	Methylprednisolone
Amphotericin	Doxorubicin	Metoclopramide
Ampicillin	Doxycycline	Metronidazole
Ampicillin/sulbactam	Droperidol	Mezlocillin
Aztreonam	Enalaprilat	Miconazole
Bleomycin	Etoposide	Mitomycin
Bumetanide	Famotidine	Mitoxantrone
Buprenorphine	Floxuridine	Morphine
Butorphanol	Fluconazole	Nalbuphine
Calcium gluconate	Fludarabine	Netilmicin
Carboplatin	Fluorouracil	Ofloxacin
Carmustine	Furosemide	Ondansetron
Cefazolin	Gallium nitrate	Paclitaxel
Cefepime	Ganciclovir	Piperacillin
Cefonicid	Gemcitabine	Piperacillin/tazobactam
Cefoperazone	Gentamicin	Plicamycin
Cefotaxime	Granisetron	Potassium chloride
Cefotetan	Haloperidol	Prochlorperazine
Cefoxitin	Heparin	Promethazine
Ceftazidime	Hydrocortisone sodium	Ranitidine
Ceftizoxime	phosphate	Sodium bicarbonate
Ceftriaxone	Hydrocortisone sodium	Streptozocin
Cefuroxime	succinate	Teniposide
Chlorpromazine	Hydromorphone	Ticarcillin
Cimetidine	Hydroxyzine	Ticarcillin/clavulanate
Ciprofloxacin	Idarubicin	Tobramycin
Cotrimoxazole	Ifosfamide	TPN
Cyclophosphamide	Imipenem/cilastatin	Vancomycin
Cytarabine	Leucovorin	Vinblastine
Dacarbazine	Lorazepam	Vincristine
Dactinomycin	Magnesium sulfate	

Incompatible:

Cisplatin	Filgrastim	Minocycline

Topotecan

Compatible:

D₅W	NS	LR

Y-Site Compatible:
   Gemcitabine

Trimetrexate

Compatible:

D₅W

Y-Site Compatible:

Amifostine

Incompatible:

BNS	D₅/LR	Calcium chloride
D₅/NS	D₁₀/NS	Chloride ion
D₅/¹/₄NS	NS	Leucovorin
D₅/¹/₂NS	LR	Potassium chloride

Vinblastine

Compatible:

BNS	NS	Bleomycin
D₅W	LR	Dacarbazine

Y-Site Compatible:

Allopurinol	Fludarabine	Paclitaxel
Amifostine	Fluorouracil	Piperacillin
Aztreonam	Gemcitabine	Piperacillin/tazobactam
Cisplatin	Leucovorin	Sargramostim
Cyclophosphamide	Methotrexate	Teniposide
Doxorubicin, liposomal	Metoclopramide	Vincristine
Droperidol	Mitomycin	Vinorelbine
Filgrastim	Ondansetron	

Incompatible:

Cefazolin	Furosemide

Variable Compatibility:†

Doxorubicin	Heparin

Vincristine

Compatible:

D₅W	Bleomycin	Fluorouracil
NS	Cytarabine	Methotrexate
LR	Doxorubicin	

Y-Site Compatible:

Allopurinol	Filgrastim	Ondansetron
Amifostine	Fludarabine	Paclitaxel
Aztreonam	Gemcitabine	Piperacillin/tazobactam
Cisplatin	Granisetron	Sargramostim
Cyclophosphamide	Heparin	Teniposide
Doxapram	Leucovorin	Vinblastine
Doxorubicin, liposomal	Metoclopramide	Vinorelbine
Droperidol	Mitomycin	

Incompatible:

Cefepime	Idarubicin	Sodium bicarbonate
Furosemide		

COMPATIBILITY OF CHEMOTHERAPY AND RELATED SUPPORTIVE CARE MEDICATIONS *(Continued)*

Vinorelbine

Compatible:

D_5W NS   LR

$D_5/\frac{1}{2}NS$

Y-Site Compatible:

Amikacin	Doxycycline	Lorazepam
Aztreonam	Droperidol	Mannitol
Bleomycin	Enalaprilat	Mechlorethamine
Bumetanide	Etoposide	Meperidine
Buprenorphine	Famotidine	Mesna
Butorphanol	Filgrastim	Methotrexate
Calcium gluconate	Fluconazole	Metoclopramide
Carboplatin	Fludarabine	Metronidazole
Carmustine	Fluorouracil	Minocycline
Cefotaxime	Gallium nitrate	Mitoxantrone
Ceftazidime	Gemcitabine	Morphine
Ceftizoxime	Gentamicin	Nalbuphine
Chlorpromazine	Haloperidol	Netilmicin
Cimetidine	Heparin	Ondansetron
Cisplatin	Hydrocortisone sodium	Plicamycin
Cyclophosphamide	phosphate	Streptozocin
Cytarabine	Hydrocortisone sodium	Teniposide
Dacarbazine	succinate	Ticarcillin
Dactinomycin	Hydromorphone	Ticarcillin/clavulanate
Daunomycin	Hydroxyzine	Tobramycin
Dexamethasone	Idarubicin	Vinblastine
Diphenhydramine	Ifosfamide	Vincristine
Doxorubicin	Imipenem/cilastatin	Vindesine
Doxorubicin, liposomal		

Incompatible:

Acyclovir	Cefoperazone	Furosemide
Allopurinol	Cefotetan	Ganciclovir
Aminophylline	Ceftriaxone	Methylprednisolone
Amphotericin	Cefuroxime	Mitomycin
Ampicillin	Cotrimoxazole	Sodium bicarbonate
Cefazolin	Fluorouracil	Thiotepa

Drug	Variable Compatibility
Carboplatin	Solutions in saline are less stable than in dextrose.
Carmustine	Solutions should be dispensed in glass and protected from light. Solutions are stable for <8 hours under most circumstances.
Cisplatin	Must have a chloride concentration of at least 0.2% in the final solution. The commercial product has a NS concentration. Etoposide + mannitol + potassium chloride in normal saline precipitates within 24 hours; when in $D_5/\frac{1}{2}NS$, it is stable for 24 hours.
Dacarbazine	Heparin 100 units/mL with dacarbazine 25 mg/mL is **incompatible**. Heparin 100 units/mL with dacarbazine 10 mg/mL is **compatible**.
Filgrastime	Gentamicin is reported to be physically **compatible** for Y-site injection, but with a decrease in biologic activity. Imipenem/cilastatin with filgrastim 40 mcg/mL is reported to be physically **compatible** for Y-site injection, but with a decrease in biologic activity.
Fluorouracil	Doxorubicin 2 mg/mL with fluorouracil 50 mg/mL is **compatible** for 13 minutes. Doxorubicin 0.5-1 mg/mL with fluorouracil 50 mg/mL is **incompatible**. Fluorouracil with doxorubicin is **Y-site compatible**. Variable compatibility with leucovorin.
Mesna	**Compatible** with ifosfamide. **Incompatible** with ifosfamide and epinephrine.
Leucovorin	Variable compatibility with fluorouracil.
Mitomycin	Mitomycin 50 mg/L in NS has a color change and 10% loss of drug concentration in 12 hours. Mitomycin 1 g/L in SWI precipitates in 24 hours under refrigeration. Other temperatures and concentrations are reported to be stable. Mitomycin in D_5W is **incompatible** in 20 mg/L; **compatible** in 40 mg/L. Mitomycin 500 mg/L with heparin 33,300 units/L in NS is **compatible**. PVC containers of mitomycin 167 mg/L with heparin 33,300 units/L in NS is **compatible**. Glass containers of mitomycin 167 mg/L with heparin 33,300 units/L in NS are **incompatible**.
Pentostatin	Pentostatin 20 mg/mL in D_5W at room temperature: a 2% loss of drug in 24 hours; 8% to 10% loss in 48 hours; and a 10% loss in 54 hours. Under refrigeration, there is no loss in 96 hours. There is a 10% loss in 23 hours at room temperature of pentostatin 2 mg/mL in D_5W
Sargramostim	Amphotericin B 0.6 mg/mL in D_5W with sargramostim 10 mcg/mL in NS forms immediate precipitate. Amphotericin B 0.6 mg/mL in D_5W with sargramostim 10 mcg/mL in D_5W is **Y-site compatible**. Amsacrine with sargramostim in NS forms immediate precipitate. Amsacrine with sargramostim in D_5W is **Y-site compatible**. Ceftazidime 40 mg/mL in NS with sargramostim 10 mcg/mL in NS is **incompatible**, with particle formation within 4 hours. Ceftazidime 40 mg/mL with sargramostim 6 or 15 mcg/mL is **compatible** for 2 hours (Y-site **compatible**). Vancomycin 20 mg/mL and sargramostim 6 mcg/mL is **incompatible**. Vancomycin 10 mg/mL and sargramostim 10 mcg/mL is **Y-site compatible**. Vancomycin 20 mg/mL and sargramostim 15 mcg/mL is **Y-site compatible**.
Vancomycin	Vancomycin 5 mg/mL with methotrexate 30 mg/mL is **compatible** for 2 hours, precipitates within 4 hours. Other concentrations tested were **compatible** for 1 hour. Vancomycin with methotrexate is **Y-site compatible**.
Vinblastine	In various volumes, doxorubicin 2 mg/mL with vinblastine 1 mg/mL yields erratic assay results. Vinblastine with doxorubicin is **Y-site compatible**. Heparin 200 units/mL with vinblastine 1 mg/mL is **incompatible** in a syringe for 13 minutes. Heparin 500 units/mL with vinblastine 0.5 mg/mL is **compatible** in a syringe for 13 minutes.

COMPATIBILITY OF CHEMOTHERAPY AND RELATED SUPPORTIVE CARE MEDICATIONS *(Continued)*

Suggested Readings

Hall PD, Yui D, Lyons S, et al, "Compatibility of Filgrastim With Selected Antimicrobial Drugs During Simulated Y-Site Administration," *Am J Health-System Pharm*, 1997, 54:184-9.

McGuire TR, Narducci WA, and Fox JL, "Compatibility and Stability of Ondansetron Hydrochloride, Dexamethasone and Lorazepam in Injectable Solutions," *Am J Health-System Pharm*, 1993, 50:1410-4.

Najari Z and Rucho WJ, "Compatibility of Commonly Used Bone Marrow Drugs During Y-Site Delivery," *Am J Health-System Pharm*, 1997, 54:181-4.

Trissel LA, Chandler SW, and Folstad JT, "Visual Compatibility of Amsacrine With Selected Drugs During Simulated Y-Site Injection," *Am J Hospital Pharm*, 1990, 47:2525-8.

Trissel LA, Bready BB, Kwan JW, et al, "Visual Compatibility of Sargramostim With Selected Antineoplastic Agents, Anti-infectives, or Other Drugs During Simulated Y-Site Injection," *Am J Hospital Pharm*, 1992, 49:402-6.

Trissel LA and Martinez JF, "Physical Compatibility of Melphalan With Selected Drugs During Simulated Y-Site Administration," *Am J Hospital Pharm*, 1993, 50:2359-63.

Trissel LA and Martinez JF, Visual, "Turbidimetric and Particle-Content Assessment of Compatibility of Vinorelbine Tartrate With Selected Drugs During Simulated Y-Site Injection," *Am J Hospital Pharm*, 1994, 51:495-9.

Trissel LA and Martinez JF, "Physical Compatibility of Allopurinol Sodium With Selected Drugs During Simulated Y-Site Administration," *Am J Hospital Pharm*, 1994, 51:1792-9.

Trissel LA and Martinez JF, "Compatibility of Filgrastim With Selected Drugs During Simulated Y-Site Administration," *Am J Hospital Pharm*, 1994, 51:1907-13.

Trissel LA and Martinez JF, "Screening Teniposide For Y-Site Compatibility," *Hospital Pharm*, 1994, 29:1010, 1012-4, 1017.

Trissel LA, *Handbook on Injectable Drugs*, 9th Ed. Bethesda, MD: *Am Society Health-Systems Pharmacists*, 1996.

Trissel LA, *Supplement to Handbook on Injectable Drugs*, 9th Ed. Bethesda, MD: *Am Society of Health-Systems Pharmacists*, 1997.

Trissel LA, Gilbert DL, and Martinez JF, "Compatibility of Granisetron Hydrochloride With Selected Drugs During Simulated Y-Site Administration," *Am J Health-System Pharm*, 1997, 54:56-60.

Trissel LA, Gilbert DL, and Martinez JF, "Compatibility of Propofol With Selected Drugs During Simulated Y-Site Administration," *Am J Health-System Pharm*, 1997, 54:1287-92.

Trissel LA, Gilbert DL, Martinez JF, et al, "Compatibility of Parenteral Nutrient Solutions With Selected Drugs During Simulated Y-Site Administration," *Am J Health-System Pharm*, 1997, 54:1295-300.

Trissel LA, Gilbert DL, and Martinez JF, "Compatibility of Doxorubicin Hydrochloride Liposome With Selected Other Drugs During Simulated Y-Site Administration," *Am J Health-System Pharm*, 1997; 54:2708-13.

Trissel LA, Martinez JF, and Gilbert DL, "Compatibility of Gemcitabine Hydrochloride With 107 Selected Drugs During Simulated Y-Site Administration," *J Am Pharmaceutical Association*, 1999, 39 (4):514-18.

Zhang Y, Xu QA, Trissel LA, et al, "Compatibility and Stability of Paclitaxel Combined With Cisplatin and With Carboplatin in Infusion Solutions," *Ann Pharmacother*, 1997, 31 (12):1465-70.

HEMATOLOGIC ADVERSE EFFECTS OF DRUGS

Drug	Red Cell Aplasia	Thrombo-cytopenia	Neutrope-nia	Pancytope-nia	Hemoly-sis
Acetazolamide		+	+	+	
Allopurinol			+		
Amiodarone	+				
Amphotericin B				+	
Amrinone		++			
Asparaginase		+++	+++	+++	++
Barbiturates		+		+	
Benzocaine					++
Captopril			++		+
Carbamazepine		++	+		
Cephalosporins			+		++
Chloramphenicol		+	++	+++	
Chlordiazepoxide			+	+	
Chloroquine		+			
Chlorothiazides		++			
Chlorpropamide	+	++	+	++	+
Chlortetracycline				+	
Chlorthalidone			+		
Cimetidine		+	++	+	
Codeine		+			
Colchicine				+	
Cyclophosphamide		+++	+++	+++	+
Dapsone					+++
Desipramine		++			
Digitalis		+			
Digitoxin		++			
Erythromycin		+			
Estrogen		+		+	
Ethacrynic acid			+		
Fluorouracil		+++	+++	+++	+
Furosemide		+	+		
Gold salts	+	+++	+++	+++	
Heparin		++		+	
Ibuprofen			+		+
Imipramine			++		
Indomethacin		+	++	+	
Isoniazid		+		+	
Isosorbide dinitrate					+
Levodopa					++
Meperidine		+			
Meprobamate		+	+	+	
Methimazole			++		
Methyldopa		++			+++
Methotrexate		+++	+++	+++	++
Methylene blue					+
Metronidazole			+		
Nalidixic acid					+
Naproxen				+	
Nitrofurantoin			++		+
Nitroglycerine		+			
Penicillamine		++	+		
Penicillins		+	++	+	+++
Phenazopyridine					+++

HEMATOLOGIC ADVERSE EFFECTS OF DRUGS *(Continued)*

Drug	Red Cell Aplasia	Thrombo-cytopenia	Neutrope-nia	Pancytope-nia	Hemoly-sis
Phenothiazines		+	++	+++	+
Phenylbutazone		+	++	+++	+
Phenytoin		++	++	++	+
Potassium iodide		+			
Prednisone		+			
Primaquine					+++
Procainamide			+		
Procarbazine		+	++	++	+
Propylthiouracil		+	++	+	+
Quinidine		+++	+		
Quinine		+++	+		
Reserpine		+			
Rifampicin		++	+		+++
Spironolactone			+		
Streptomycin		+		+	
Sulfamethoxazole with trimethoprim			+		
Sulfonamides	+	++	++	++	++
Sulindac	+	+	+	+	
Tetracyclines		+			+
Thioridazine			++		
Tolbutamide		++	+	++	
Triamterene					+
Valproate	+				
Vancomycin			+		

+ = rare or single reports.

++ = occasional reports.

+++ = substantial number of reports.

Adapted from D'Arcy PF and Griffin JP, eds, *Iatrogenic Diseases*, New York, NY: Oxford University Press, 1986, 128-30.

TUMOR LYSIS SYNDROME, MANAGEMENT

Tumor lysis syndrome (TLS) may be seen with any tumor that is undergoing rapid cell turnover as a result of high growth fraction or high cell death due to therapy. It occurs most often in Burkitt's lymphoma and T-cell ALL, both of which have large tumor burdens and high sensitivity to chemotherapy. Acute lysis of tumor cells results in the rapid release of potassium, phosphates, and nucleic acids into the circulation. Hypocalcemia, hyperuricemia, and renal failure may result. Secondary acute precipitation of calcium and urates in the kidney, tumor infiltration of the kidney, obstructive uropathy, and dehydration may increase the primary metabolic disturbances. The following chart reviews the management of TLS.

Therapy	Infants & Children	Adolescents & Adults
Hydration (patients typically present with dehydration; I.V. fluids should be started immediately)	3000-6000 mL/m^2/day D_5W 1/4 NS (+ sodium bicarbonate) Maintain urine output at ≥1 mL/kg/hour Maintain urine specific gravity at ≤1.010 Strict monitoring of I & O	3000-6000 mL/m^2/day D_5W 1/4 NS (+ sodium bicarbonate) Maintain urine output at 100-150 mL/hour Maintain urine specific gravity at ≤1.010 Strict monitoring of I & O
Alkalinization	50-100 mEq/L sodium bicarbonate in I.V. fluid Maintain urine pH at 7.0-7.5 Reduce bicarbonate if serum bicarbonate >30 mEq/L or urine pH >7.5	50-100 mEq/L sodium bicarbonate in I.V. fluid Maintain urine pH at 7.0-7.5 Reduce bicarbonate if serum bicarbonate >30 mEq/L or urine pH >7.5
Uric acid reduction	Allopurinol: I.V., oral: 200-400 mg/m^2/day in 1-3 divided doses (maximum: 600 mg/day) Urate oxidase: I.V. (investigational, see protocol): 0.2 mg/kg/dose once or twice daily	Allopurinol: I.V.: 200-400 mg/m^2/day in 1-3 divided doses (maximum: 600 mg/day) Oral: 600-800 mg/day in 1-2 doses
Diuretics (avoid if hypovolemic)	Furosemide: I.V.: 1 mg/kg/dose as needed Mannitol: I.V.: 0.25-0.5 g/kg/dose as needed	Furosemide: I.V.: 20-40 mg/dose as needed Mannitol: I.V.: 0.25-0.5 g/kg/dose as needed
Phosphate reduction	Aluminum hydroxide: Oral: 50 mg/kg/dose every 8 hours	Aluminum hydroxide: Oral: 30-40 mL/dose every 6-8 hours
Dialysis indications (peritoneal dialysis is much less efficient for reducing uric acid than other modalities, and is contraindicated in patients with abdominal tumors.)	Potassium level >6 mEq/L Uric acid level >10 mg/dL Creatinine >10 times normal Uremia Phosphorus >10 mg/dL or rapidly rising Symptomatic hypocalcemia Severe, unmanageable hypertension Volume overload	

Kelly KM and Lange B, "Oncologic Emergencies," *Pediatr Clin North Am*, 1997, 44(4):809-30.

HOTLINE PHONE NUMBERS

AIDS Hotline	800-590-2437
AMA Foreign Drug	312-464-4575
AMA Library Answer Center	312-464-4818
American Association of Poison Control Centers (AAPCC) Poison Prevention	202-625-3333
American College of Clinical Pharmacy (ACCP)	816-531-2177
American Dental Association (ADA)	800-621-8099
American Medical Association (AMA)	312-464-5000
American Pharmaceutical Association (APhA)	202-628-4410
American Association of Health-System Pharmacists	301-657-3000
Animal Poison Care Hotline (24-hours)	800-548-2423
Canadian Pharmaceutical Association	613-523-7877
Center for Disease Control	1-800-311-3435

Use this number for the following departments also:

- CDC Disease Information
- CDC Epidemiology Program
- CDC Immunity Division
- CDC Influenza Branch
- CDC International Travelers Information
- CDC Parasitic Division
- CDC STDs
- CDC Tuberculosis Section

FDA (Rare Diseases/Orphan Drugs)	800-300-7469
National Cancer Institute	301-496-1196
Asthma and Allergy Foundation of America	1-800-7-ASTHMA
Cancer Treatment (of NCI)	1-800-4-CANCER
Epilepsy Foundation of America	301-459-3700
National Council on Patient Information & Education	301-656-8565
National Institute of Health	301-496-4000
National Poison Center	202-362-3867
Emergency	202-625-3333
Parental Stress	800-632-8188
Pediatric Pharmacy Advocacy Group (PPAG) Membership and Drug Information	720-981-7356
Pesticides (Mon-Fri, 6:30 AM - 4:30 PM Pacific)	800-858-7378
Rocky Mountain Poison Control Information	800-525-6115

ENDOCARDITIS PROPHYLAXIS*

	Dosage for Adults	Dosage for Children†
DENTAL AND UPPER RESPIRATORY PROCEDURES		
Oral§		
Amoxicillin¶	2 g 1 h before procedure	50 mg/kg 1 h before procedure
Penicillin allergy:		
Clindamycin or	600 mg 1 h before procedure	20 mg/kg 1 h before procedure
Cephalexin or	2 g 1 h before procedure	50 mg/kg 1 h before procedure
Azithromycin or Clarithromycin	500 mg 1 h before procedure	15 mg/kg 1 h before procedure
Parenteral§		
Ampicillin	2 g I.M. or I.V. 30 minutes before procedure	50 mg/kg I.M. or I.V. 30 minutes before procedure
Penicillin allergy:		
Clindamycin or	600 mg I.V. 30 minutes before procedure	20 mg/kg I.V. 30 minutes before procedure
Cefazolin (not to be used in individuals with immediate-type hypersensitivity reaction to penicillins)	1 g I.M. or I.V. 30 minutes before procedure	25 mg/kg I.M. or I.V. 30 minutes before procedure
GASTROINTESTINAL AND GENITOURINARY PROCEDURES‡		
Oral§		
Amoxicillin for moderate risk patients	2 g 1 h before procedure	50 mg/kg 1 h before procedure
Parenteral§		
Ampicillin for moderate risk patients	2 g I.M. or I.V. 30 minutes before procedure	50 mg/kg I.M. or I.V. 30 minutes before procedure
Ampicillin **plus**	2 g I.M. or I.V. 30 minutes before procedure; ampicillin 1 g I.M./I.V. or amoxicillin 1 g P.O. 6 h later	50 mg/kg I.M. or I.V. 30 minutes before procedure and 25 mg/kg I.M./I.V. or amoxicillin 25 mg/kg P.O. 6 h later
Gentamicin for high-risk patients	1.5 mg/kg (max: 120 mg) I.M. or I.V. 30 minutes before procedure	1.5 mg/kg I.M. or I.V. 30 minutes before procedure

ENDOCARDITIS PROPHYLAXIS* *(Continued)*

	Dosage for Adults	Dosage for Children†
Penicillin allergy:		
Vancomycin for moderate-risk patients	1 g I.V. infused **slowly over 1 h**; complete infusion within 30 minutes before procedure	20 mg/kg I.V. infused **slowly over 1 h**; complete infusion within 30 minutes before procedure
Vancomycin **plus**	1 g I.V. infused slowly over 1 h; complete infusion within 30 minutes before procedure	20 mg/kg I.V. infused slowly over 1 h; complete infusion within 30 minutes before procedure
Gentamicin for high-risk patients	1.5 mg/kg (max: 120 mg) I.M. or I.V. 30 minutes before procedure	1.5 mg/kg I.M. or I.V. 30 minutes before procedure

*Endocarditis prophylaxis recommended

  High-risk category:

    Prosthetic cardiac valves

    Previous bacterial endocarditis

    Complex cyanotic congenital heart disease (eg, single ventricle states, transposition of the great arteries, tetralogy of Fallot)

    Surgically constructed systemic pulmonary shunts or conduits

  Moderate-risk category:

    Most other congenital cardiac malformations (other than high-risk category)

    Acquired valvar dysfunction (eg, rheumatic heart disease)

    Hypertrophic cardiomyopathy

    Mitral valve prolapse with valvar regurgitation and/or thickened leaflets

†Children's dose should not exceed adult dosage.

‡For a review of the risk of bacteremia and endocarditis with various procedures, see Mandell GL, Bennett JE, Dolin R, eds, *Principles and Practice of Infectious Diseases*, 4th ed, New York, NY: Churchill Livingstone, 1995, 794.

§Oral regimens are more convenient and safer. Parenteral regimens are more likely to be effective; they are recommended especially for patients with prosthetic heart valves, those who have had endocarditis previously, or those taking continuous oral penicillin for rheumatic fever prophylaxis.

¶Amoxicillin is recommended because of its excellent bioavailability and good activity against streptococci and enterococci.

References
Dajani AS, Taubert KA, Wilson W, et al, "Prevention of Bacterial Endocarditis. Recommendations by the American Heart Association," *JAMA*, 1997, 277(22):1794-1801.

PEDIATRIC HIV

Selected tables from the Centers for Disease Control and Prevention, "Guidelines for the Use of Antiretroviral Agents in Pediatric HIV Infection," first published in *MMWR*, 1998:47(No.RR-4), April 17, 1998, updated as a "Living Document", January 7, 2000, located at (URL) http://www.hivatis.org.

Table 1. 1994 Revised Human Immunodeficiency Virus Pediatric Classification System: Immune Categories Based on Age-specific CD4+ T-lymphocyte and Percentage*

Immune Category	<12 mo		1-5 y		6-12 y	
	No./μL	%	No./μL	%	No./μL	%
Category 1 no suppression	≥1500	≥25	≥1000	≥25	≥500	≥25
Category 2 moderate suppression	750-1499	15-24	500-999	15-24	200-499	15-24
Category 3 severe suppression	<750	<15	<500	<15	<200	<15

*Modified from: "1994 Revised Classification System for Human Immunodeficiency Virus Infection in Children Less Than 13 Years of Age," *MMWR*, 1994, 43(RR-12):1-10.

Table 2. 1994 Revised Human Immunodeficiency Virus Pediatric Classification System: Clinical Categories*

Category N: Not Symptomatic
Children who have no signs or symptoms considered to be the result of HIV infection or who have only **one** of the conditions listed in category A

Category A: Mildly Symptomatic
Children with **two** or more of the following conditions, but none of the conditions listed in categories B and C:
- Lymphadenopathy (≥0.5 cm at more than two sites; bilateral = one site)
- Hepatomegaly
- Splenomegaly
- Dermatitis
- Parotitis
- Recurrent or persistent upper respiratory infection, sinusitis, or otitis media

Category B: Moderately Symptomatic
Children who have symptomatic conditions other than those listed for category A or category C that are attributed to HIV infection. Examples of conditions in clinical category B include, but are not limited to, the following:
- Anemia (<8 g/dL), neutropenia (<1000/mm³), or thrombocytopenia (<100,000/mm³) persisting ≥30 days
- Bacterial meningitis, pneumonia, or sepsis (single episode)
- Candidiasis, oropharyngeal (ie, thrush) persisting for >2 months in children aged >6 months
- Cardiomyopathy
- Cytomegalovirus infection with onset before age 1 month
- Diarrhea, recurrent or chronic
- Hepatitis
- Herpes simplex virus (HSV) stomatitis, recurrent (ie, more than two episodes within 1 year)
- HSV bronchitis, pneumonitis, or esophagitis with onset before age 1 month
- Herpes zoster (ie, shingles) involving at least two distinct episodes or more than one dermatome
- Leiomyosarcoma
- Lymphoid interstitial pneumonia (LIP) or pulmonary lymphoid hyperplasia complex

PEDIATRIC HIV *(Continued)*

- Nephropathy
- Nocardiosis
- Fever lasting >1 month
- Toxoplasmosis with onset before age 1 month
- Varicella, disseminated (ie, complicated chickenpox)

Category C: Severely Symptomatic

Children who have any condition listed in the 1987 surveillance case definition for acquired immunodeficiency syndrome, with the exception of LIP (which is a category B condition).

*Modified from: "1994 Revised Classification System for Human Immunodeficiency Virus Infection in Children Less Than 13 Years of Age," *MMWR*, 1994, 43(RR-12):1-10.

Table 3. Indications for Initiation of Antiretroviral Therapy in Children With Human Immunodeficiency Virus (HIV) Infection*

- Clinical symptoms associated with HIV infection (ie, clinical categories A, B, or C [Table 2])
- Evidence of immune suppression, indicated by CD4$^+$ T-lymphocyte absolute number or percentage (ie, immune category 2 or 3 [Table 1])
- Age <12 months - regardless of clinical, immunologic, or virologic status
- For asymptomatic children ≥1 year of age with normal immune status, two options can be considered:

  1. Preferred approach: Initiate therapy regardless of age or symptom status

  2. Alternative approach: Defer treatment in situations in which the risk for clinical disease progression is low and other factors (eg, concern for the durability of response, safety, and adherence) favor postponing treatment. In such cases, the healthcare provider should regularly monitor virologic, immunologic, and clinical status. Factors to be considered in deciding to initiate therapy include the following:

     - High or increasing HIV RNA copy number
     - Rapidly declining CD4$^+$ T-lymphocyte number or percentage to values approaching those indicative of moderate immune suppression (ie, immune category 2 [Table 1])
     - Development of clinical symptoms

---

*Indications for initiation of antiretroviral therapy in postpubertal HIV-infected adolescents should follow the adult guidelines. (Office of Public Health and Science, Department of Health and Human Services. Availability of report of NIH panel to define principles of therapy of HIV infection and guidelines for the use of antiretroviral agents in HIV-infected adults. Federal Register, 1997, 62:33417-8 and updated as "Guidelines for the Use of Antiretroviral Agents in HIV-Infected Adults and Adolescents," January 28, 2000, http://www.hivatis.org. See page 1133).

Table 4. Recommended Antiretroviral Regimens for Initial Therapy for Human Immunodeficiency Virus (HIV) Infection in Children

Strongly Recommended

Clinical trial evidence of clinical benefit and/or sustained suppression of HIV replication in adults and/or children.

- One highly active protease inhibitor plus two nucleoside analogue reverse transcriptase inhibitors (NRTIs)
  - Preferred protease inhibitor for infants and children who cannot swallow pills or capsules: nelfinavir or ritonavir; alternative for children who can swallow pills or capsules: indinavir
  - Recommended dual NRTI combinations: the most data on use in children are available for the combinations of zidovudine (ZDV) and dideoxyinosine (ddI) and for ZDV and lamivudine (3TC); more limited data is available for the combinations of stavudine (d4T) and ddI, d4T and 3TC, and ZDV and zalcitabine (ddC)*
- Alternative for children who can swallow capsules: Efavirenz (Sustiva®)** plus 2 NRTIs (see above) or efavirenz (Sustiva®) plus nelfinavir and 1 NRTI

Recommended as an Alternative

Clinical trial evidence of suppression of HIV replication, but 1) durability may be less in adults and/or children than with strongly recommended regimens; or 2) the durability of suppression is not yet defined; or 3) evidence of efficacy may not outweigh potential adverse consequences (eg, toxicity, drug interactions, cost, etc).

- Nevirapine and two NRTIs
- Abacavir in combination with ZDV and 3TC

Offer Only in Special Circumstances

Clinical trial evidence of 1) limited benefit for patients, or 2) data are inconclusive, but may be reasonably offered in special circumstances.

- Two NRTIs
- Amprenavir in combination with 2 NRTIs or abacavir

Not Recommended

Evidence against use because of 1) overlapping toxicity, and/or 2) because use may be virologically undesirable

- Any monotherapy†
- d4T and ZDV
- ddC and ddI
- ddC and d4T
- ddC and 3TC

*ddC is not available in a liquid preparation commercially, although a liquid formulation is available through a compassionate use program of the manufacturer (Hoffman-LaRoche Inc, Nutley, New Jersey). ZDV and ddC is a less preferred choice for use in combination with a protease inhibitor.

Efavirenz is currently available only in capsule form, but liquid preparation is currently being evaluated. There are currently no data on appropriate dosage of efavirenz in children <3 years of age. **Note: A liquid efavirenz preparation is available from the manufacturer (DuPont Pharmaceuticals Company, Wilmington, Delaware) through an expanded access program for HIV-infected children and adolescents 3-16 years of age.

†Except for ZDV chemoprophylaxis administered to HIV-exposed infants during the first 6 weeks of life to prevent perinatal HIV transmission; if an infant is identified as HIV-infected while receiving ZDV prophylaxis, therapy should be changed to a combination antiretroviral drug regimen.

PEDIATRIC HIV (Continued)

Table 5. Considerations for Changing Antiretroviral Therapy for Human Immunodeficiency Virus (HIV)-Infected Children

Virologic Considerations*

- Less than a minimally acceptable virologic response after 8-12 weeks of therapy; for children receiving antiretroviral therapy with two nucleoside analogue reverse transcriptase inhibitors (NRTIs) and a protease inhibitor, such a response is defined as a <10-fold (1.0 log_{10}) decrease from baseline HIV RNA levels; for children who are receiving less potent antiretroviral therapy (ie, dual NRTI combinations), an insufficient response is defined as a <5-fold (0.7 log_{10}) decrease in HIV RNA levels from baseline
- HIV RNA not suppressed to undetectable levels after 4-6 months of antiretroviral therapy†
- Repeated detection of HIV RNA in children who initially responded to antiretroviral therapy with undetectable levels‡
- A reproducible increase in HIV RNA copy number among children who have had a substantial HIV RNA response, but still have low levels of detectable HIV RNA; such an increase would warrant change in therapy if, after initiation of the therapeutic regimen, a >3-fold (0.5 log_{10}) increase in copy number for children ≥2 years of age and a >5-fold (0.7 log_{10}) increase is observed for children <2 years of age

Immunologic Considerations*

- Change in immunologic classification (Table 1)§
- For children with CD4⁺ T-lymphocyte percentages of <15% (ie, those in immune category 3), a persistent decline of five percentiles or more in CD4⁺ cell percentage (eg, from 15% to 10%)
- A rapid and substantial decrease in absolute CD4⁺ T-lymphocyte count (eg, a >30% decline in <6 months)

Clinical Considerations

- Progressive neurodevelopmental deterioration
- Growth failure defined as persistent decline in weight-growth velocity despite adequate nutritional support and without other explanation
- Disease progression defined as advancement from one pediatric clinical category to another (eg, from clinical category A to clinical category B)**

*At least two measurements (taken 1 week apart) should be performed before considering a change in therapy.

†The initial HIV RNA level of the child at the start of therapy and the level achieved with therapy should be considered when contemplating potential drug changes. For example, an immediate change in therapy may not be warranted if there is a sustained 1.5-2.0 log_{10} decrease in HIV RNA copy number, even if RNA remains detectable at low levels.

‡More frequent evaluation of HIV RNA levels should be considered if the HIV RNA increase is limited (eg, if when using an HIV RNA assay with a lower limit of detection of 1000 copies/mL, there is a ≤0.7 log_{10} increase from undetectable to approximately 5000 copies/mL in an infant <2 years of age).

§Minimal changes in CD4⁺ T-lymphocyte percentile that may result in change in immunologic category (eg, from 26% to 24%, or 16% to 14%) may not be as concerning as a rapid substantial change in CD4⁺ percentile within the same immunologic category (eg, a drop from 35% to 25%).

**In patients with stable immunologic and virologic parameters, progression from one clinical category to another may not represent an indication to change therapy. Thus, in patients whose disease progression is not associated with neurologic deterioration or growth failure, virologic and immunologic considerations are important in deciding whether to change therapy.

ADULT AND ADOLESCENT HIV

Selected tables from the Centers for Disease Control and Prevention, "Report of the NIH Panel to Define Principles of Therapy of HIV Infection and Guidelines for the Use of Antiretroviral Agents in HIV-Infected Adults and Adolescents," first published in *MMWR*, 1998:47(No. RR-5), April 24, 1998, updated as a "Living Document," January 28, 2000, located at (URL) http://www.hivatis.org.

Indications for Plasma HIV RNA Testing*

Clinical Indication	Information	Use
Syndrome consistent with acute HIV infection	Establishes diagnosis when HIV antibody test is negative or indeterminate	Diagnosis†
Initial evaluation of newly diagnosed HIV infection	Baseline viral load "set point"	Decision to start or defer therapy
Every 3-4 months in patients not on therapy	Changes in viral load	Decision to start therapy
2-8 weeks after initiation of antiretroviral therapy	Initial assessment of drug efficacy	Decision to continue or change therapy
3-4 months after start of therapy	Maximal effect of therapy	Decision to continue or change therapy
Every 3-4 months in patients on therapy	Durability of antiretroviral effect	Decision to continue or change therapy
Clinical event or significant decline in CD4+ T cells	Association with changing or stable viral load	Decision to continue, initiate, or change therapy

*Acute illness (eg, bacterial pneumonia, tuberculosis, HSV, PCP, etc) and immunizations can cause increases in plasma HIV RNA for 2-4 weeks; viral load testing should not be performed during this time. Plasma HIV RNA results should usually be verified with a repeat determination before starting or making changes in therapy.

†Diagnosis of HIV infection determined by HIV RNA testing should be confirmed by standard methods (such as Western blot serology) performed 2-4 months after the initial indeterminate or negative test.

Recommendations for the Use of Drug Resistance Assays

Clinical Setting / Recommendation	Rationale
Recommended	
Virologic failure during HAART*	Determine the role of resistance in drug failure and maximize the number of active drugs in the new regimen, if indicated.
Suboptimal suppression of viral load after initiation of antiretroviral therapy	Determine the role of resistance and maximize the number of active drugs in the new regimen, if indicated.
Consider	
Acute HIV infection	Determine if drug-resistant virus was transmitted and change regimen accordingly.
Not Generally Recommended	
Chronic HIV infection prior to initiation of therapy	Uncertain prevalence of resistant virus. Current assays may not detect minor drug-resistant species.
After discontinuation of drugs	Drug-resistant mutations may become minor species in the absence of selective drug pressure. Current assays may not detect minor drug-resistant species.
Plasma viral load <1000 HIV RNA copies/mL	Resistance assays cannot be reliably performed because of low copy number of HIV RNA.

*HAART: Highly active antiretroviral therapy

ADULT AND ADOLESCENT HIV *(Continued)*

Risks and Benefits of Early Initiation of Antiretroviral Therapy in the Asymptomatic HIV-infected Patient

Potential Benefits

Control of viral replication and mutation; reduction of viral burden

Prevention of progressive immunodeficiency; potential maintenance or reconstitution of a normal immune system

Delayed progression to AIDS and prolongation of life

Decreased risk of selection of resistant virus

Decreased risk of drug toxicity

Possible decreased risk of viral transmission

Potential Risks

Reduction in quality of life from adverse drug effects and inconvenience of current maximally suppressive regimens

Earlier development of drug resistance

Transmission of drug-resistant virus

Limitation in future choices of antiretroviral agents due to development of resistance

Unknown long-term toxicity of antiretroviral drugs

Unknown duration of effectiveness of current antiretroviral therapies

Goals of HIV Therapy and Tools to Achieve Them

Goals of Therapy

Maximal and durable suppression of viral load

Restoration and/or preservation of immunologic function

Improvement of quality of life

Reduction of HIV-related morbidity and mortality

Tools to Achieve Goals of Therapy

Maximize adherence to the antiretroviral regimen

Rational sequencing of drugs

Preservation of future treatment options

Use of resistance testing in selected clinical settings

Indications for the Initiation of Antiretroviral Therapy in the Chronically HIV-Infected Patient

Clinical Category	CD4+ T-cell Count and HIV RNA	Recommendation
Symptomatic (AIDS, thrush, unexplained fever)	Any value	Treat
Asymptomatic	CD4+ T cells <500/mm^3 **or** HIV RNA >10,000 (bDNA) or >20,000 (RT-PCR)	Treatment should be offered. Strength of recommendation is based on prognosis for disease-free survival and willingness of the patient to accept therapy*
Asymptomatic	CD4+ T cells >500/mm^3 **and** HIV RNA <10,000 (bDNA) or <20,000 (RT-PCR)	Many experts would delay therapy and observe; however, some experts would treat

*Some experts would observe patients whose CD4+ T cell counts are between 350-500/mm^3 and HIV RNA levels <10,000 (bDNA) or <20,000 (RT-PCR).

Recommended Antiretroviral Agents for Initial Treatment of Established HIV Infection

This table provides a guide to the use of available treatment regimens for individuals with no prior or limited experience on HIV therapy. In accordance with the established goals of HIV therapy, priority is given to regimens in which clinical trials data suggest the following: Sustained suppression of HIV plasma RNA (particularly in patients with high baseline viral load) and sustained increase in CD4+ T cell count (in most cases over 48 weeks), and favorable clinical outcome (ie, delayed progression to AIDS and death). Particular emphasis is given to regimens that have been compared directly with other regimens that perform sufficiently well with regard to these parameters to be included in the "Strongly Recommended" category. Additional consideration is given to the regimen's pill burden, dosing frequency, food requirements, convenience, toxicity, and drug interaction profile compared with other regimens.

It is important to note that all antiretroviral agents, including those in the "Strongly Recommended" category, have potentially serious toxic and adverse events associated with their use (see individual drug monographs).

Antiretroviral drug regimens are comprised of one choice each from column A and column B. Drugs are listed in alphabetical, not priority order:

	Column A	Column B
Strongly Recommended	Efavirenz Indinavir Nelfinavir Ritonavir + Saquinavir (SGC* or HGC*)	Stavudine + Didanosine Stavudine + Lamivudine Zidovudine + Didanosine Zidovudine + Lamivudine
Recommended as an Alternative	Abacavir Amprenavir Delavirdine Nelfinavir + Saquinavir - SGC Nevirapine Ritonavir Saquinavir - SGC	Didanosine + Lamivudine Zidovudine + Zalcitabine
No Recommendation; Insufficient Data†	Hydroxyurea in combination with other antiretroviral drugs Ritonavir + Indinavir Ritonavir + Nelfinavir	
Not Recommended; Should Not be Offered (All monotherapies, whether from column A or B‡)	Saquinavir - HGC§	Stavudine + Zidovudine Zalcitabine + Didanosine Zalcitabine + Lamivudine Zalcitabine + Stavudine

*Saquinavir-SGC, soft-gel capsule (Fortovase®); Saquinavir-HGC, hard-gel capsule (Invirase®).

†This category includes drugs or combinations for which information is too limited to allow a recommendation for or against use.

‡Zidovudine monotherapy may be considered for prophylactic use in pregnant women with low viral load and high CD4+ T cell counts to prevent perinatal transmission.

§Use of saquinavir-HGC (Invirase®) is not recommended, except in combination with ritonavir.

ADULT AND ADOLESCENT HIV *(Continued)*

Guidelines for Changing an Antiretroviral Regimen for Suspected Drug Failure

- Criteria for changing therapy include a suboptimal reduction in plasma viremia after initiation of therapy, reappearance of viremia after suppression to undetectable, significant increases in plasma viremia from the nadir of suppression, and declining CD4+ T cell numbers.

- When the decision to change therapy is based on viral load determination, it is preferable to confirm with a second viral load test.

- Distinguish between the need to change a regimen due to drug intolerance or inability to comply with the regimen versus failure to achieve the goal of sustained viral suppression; single agents can be changed in the event of drug intolerance.

- In general, do not change a single drug or add a single drug to a failing regimen; it is important to use at least two new drugs and preferably to use an entirely new regimen with at least three new drugs. If susceptibility testing indicates resistance to only one agent in a combination regimen, it may be possible to replace only that drug; however, this approach requires clinical validation.

- Many patients have limited options for new regimens of desired potency; in some of these cases, it is rational to continue the prior regimen if partial viral suppression was achieved.

- In some cases, regimens identified as suboptimal for initial therapy are rational due to limitations imposed by toxicity, intolerance, or nonadherence. This especially applies in late-stage disease. For patients with no rational alternative options who have virologic failure with return of viral load to baseline (pretreatment levels) and a declining CD4+ T cell count, there should be consideration for discontinuation of antiretroviral therapy.

- Experience is limited with regimens using combinations of two protease inhibitors or combinations of protease inhibitors with NNRTIs; for patients with limited options due to drug intolerance or suspected resistance, these regimens provide possible alternative treatment options.

- There is limited information about the value of restarting a drug that the patient has previously received. Susceptibility testing may be useful in this situation if clinical evidence suggestive of the emergence of resistance is observed. However, testing for phenotypic or genotypic resistance in peripheral blood virus may fail to detect minor resistant variants. Thus, the presence of resistance is more useful information in altering treatment strategies than the absence of detectable resistance.

- Avoid changing from ritonavir to indinavir, or vice versa, for drug failure, since high-level cross-resistance is likely.

- Avoid changing among NNRTIs for drug failure, since high-level cross-resistance is likely.

- The decision to change therapy and the choice of a new regimen requires that the clinician have considerable expertise in the care of persons living with HIV. Physicians who are less experienced in the care of persons with HIV infection are strongly encouraged to obtain assistance through consultation with or referral to a clinician with considerable expertise in the care of HIV-infected patients.

Acute Retroviral Syndrome: Associated Signs and Symptoms (Expected Frequency)

- Fever (96%)
- Lymphadenopathy (74%)
- Pharyngitis (70%)
- Rash (70%)
    - Erythematous maculopapular with lesions on face and trunk and sometimes extremities, including palms and soles
    - Mucocutaneous ulceration involving mouth, esophagus, or genitals
- Myalgia or arthralgia (54%)
- Diarrhea (32%)
- Headache (32%)
- Nausea and vomiting (27%)
- Hepatosplenomegaly (14%)
- Weight loss (13%)
- Thrush (12%)
- Neurologic symptoms (12%)
    - Meningoencephalitis or aseptic meningitis
    - Peripheral neuropathy or radiculopathy
    - Facial palsy
    - Guillain-Barré syndrome
    - Brachial neuritis
    - Cognitive impairment or psychosis

Zidovudine (ZDV) Perinatal Transmission Prophylaxis Regimen

Antepartum	Initiation at 14-34 weeks gestation and continued throughout pregnancy:
	  A. PACTG 076 regimen: ZDV 100 mg 5 times daily
	  B. Acceptable alternative regimen:
	    ZDV 200 mg 3 times daily
	    or
	    ZDV 300 mg 2 times daily

Intrapartum	During labor, ZDV 2 mg/kg I.V. over 1 hour, followed by a continuous infusion of 1 mg/kg/hour I.V. until delivery
Postpartum	Oral administration of ZDV to the newborn (ZDV syrup, 2 mg/kg every 6 hours) for the first 6 weeks of life, beginning at 8-12 hours after birth

IMMUNIZATION GUIDELINES
Standards for Pediatric Immunization Practices

Standard 1. Immunization services are readily available.

Standard 2. There are no barriers or unnecessary prerequisites to the receipt of vaccines.

Standard 3. Immunization services are available free or for a minimal fee.

Standard 4. Providers utilize all clinical encounters to screen and, when indicated, immunize children.

Standard 5. Providers educate parents and guardians about immunizations in general terms.

Standard 6. Providers question parents or guardians about contraindications and, before immunizing a child, inform them in specific terms about the risks and benefits of the immunizations their child is to receive.

Standard 7. Providers follow only true contraindications.

Standard 8. Providers administer simultaneously all vaccine doses for which a child is eligible at the time of each visit.

Standard 9. Providers use accurate and complete recording procedures.

Standard 10. Providers co-schedule immunization appointments in conjunction with appointments for other child health services.

Standard 11. Providers report adverse events following immunization promptly, accurately, and completely.

Standard 12. Providers operate a tracking system.

Standard 13. Providers adhere to appropriate procedures for vaccine management.

Standard 14. Providers conduct semiannual audits to assess immunization coverage levels and to review immunization records in the patient populations they serve.

Standard 15. Providers maintain up-to-date, easily retrievable medical protocols at all locations where vaccines are administered.

Standard 16. Providers operate with patient-oriented and community-based approaches.

Standard 17. Vaccines are administered by properly trained individuals.

Standard 18. Providers receive ongoing education and training on current immunization recommendations.

Recommended by the National Vaccine Advisory Committee, April 1992.
Approved by the United States Public Health Service, May 1992.
Endorsed by the American Academy of Pediatrics, May 1992.

The Standards represent the consensus of the National Vaccine Advisory Committee (NVAC) and of a broad group of medical and public health experts about what constitutes the most desirable immunization practices. It is recognized by the NVAC that not all of the current immunization practices of public and private providers are in compliance with the Standards. Nevertheless, the Standards are expected to be useful as a means of helping providers to identify needed changes, to obtain resources if necessary, and to actually implement the desirable immunization practices in the future.

Table 1. Dosage and Administration Guidelines for Vaccines Available in the United States

Vaccine	Dosage	Route of Administration	Type
DT*	0.5 mL	I.M.	Toxoids
Td*	0.5 mL	I.M.	Toxoids
DTP*	0.5 mL	I.M.	Diphtheria and tetanus toxoids with killed *B. pertussis* organisms
DTaP (Acel-Imune®)†††	0.5 mL	I.M.	Diphtheria and tetanus toxoids with acellular pertussis
DTP-HbOC (Tetramune®)⁺	0.5 mL	I.M.	Diphtheria and tetanus toxoids with killed *B. pertussis* organisms and *Haemophilus* b conjugate (diphtheria CRM_{197} protein conjugate)
Haemophilus B conjugate vaccine	0.5 mL	I.M.	
ProHIBit® (PRP-D), manufactured by Connaught Laboratories	0.5 mL	I.M.	Polysaccharide (diphtheria toxoid conjugate)
HibTITER® (HbOC)†, manufactured by Praxis Biologicals	0.5 mL	I.M.	Oligosaccharide (diphtheria CRM_{197} protein conjugate)
PedvaxHIB® (PRP-OMP)‡, manufactured by MSD	0.5 mL	I.M.	Polysaccharide (meningococcal protein conjugate)
Hepatitis A vaccine, inactivated (Havrix®)		I.M.	Inactivated virus
Children 2-18 y:	Primary 0.5 mL (360 units) immunization consists of 2 doses given 1 month apart		
Children >18 y and adults:	Primary 1 mL (1440 units) immunization consists of a single dose		
Children and adults:	Booster dose is recommended between 6 and 12 months after the primary dose		
Hepatitis B§ Infants born to HB_sAg-negative mothers and children <11 y‖		I.M. in the anterolateral thigh or in the upper arm; S.C. in individuals at risk of hemorrhage	Yeast recombinant-derived inactivated viral antigen
Recombivax HB® (MSD)	5 mcg (0.5 mL)		
Engerix-B® (SKF)	10 mcg (0.5 mL)		

Infants born to HB_sAg-positive mothers (immunization and administration of 0.5 mL hepatitis B immune globulin is recommended for **infants** born to HB_sAg^+ mothers using different administration sites) within 12 hours of birth; administer vaccine at birth; repeat vaccine dose at 1 and 6 months following the initial dose

IMMUNIZATION GUIDELINES *(Continued)*

Table 1. Dosage and Administration Guidelines for Vaccines Available in the United States *(continued)*

Vaccine	Dosage	Route of Administration	Type
Recombivax HB® (MSD)	5 mcg (0.5 mL)		
Engerix-B® (SKF)	10 mcg (0.5 mL)		
Children 11-19 y			
Recombivax HB® (MSD)	5 mcg (0.5 mL)		
Engerix-B® (SKF)	20 mcg (1 mL)		
Adults >19 y			
Recombivax HB® (MSD)	10 mcg (1 mL)		
Engerix-B® (SKF)	20 mcg (1 mL)		
Dialysis patients and immunosuppressed patients			
Recombivax HB® (MSD)	<11 y, 20 mcg (0.5 mL); ≥11 y, 40 mcg (1 mL) using special dialysis formulation		
Engerix-B® (SKF)¶	<11 y, 20 mcg (1 mL); ≥11 y, 40 mcg (2 mL), give as two 1 mL doses at different sites		
Influenza		I.M. (2 doses 4+ weeks apart in children <9 years of age not previously immunized; only 1 dose needed for annual updates)	Inactivated virus subvirion (split) (contraindicated in patients allergic to chicken eggs)
split virus only in pediatric patients			
6-35 mo	0.25 mL (1 or 2 doses)		
3-8 y	0.5 mL (1 or 2 doses)		
≥9 y	0.5 mL (1 dose)		
Measles	0.5 mL	S.C.	Live virus (contraindicated in patients with anaphylactic allergy to neomycin)

Most areas: Two doses (1st dose at 15 months with MMR; 2nd dose at 4-6 years or 11-12 years, depending on local school entry requirements)

High-risk area: Two doses (1st dose at 12 months with MMR; 2nd dose as above)

Children 6-15 months in epidemic situations: Dose is given at the time of first contact with a health care provider; children <1 year of age should receive single antigen measles vaccine. If vaccinated before 1 year, revaccinate at 15 months with MMR. A 3rd dose is administered at 4-6 years or 11-12 years, depending on local school entry requirements.

Meningococcal	0.5 mL#	S.C.	Polysaccharide
MMR•	0.5 mL	S.C.	Live virus
MR	0.5 mL	S.C.	Live virus
Mumps	0.5 mL	S.C.	Live virus
Pneumococcal polyvalent ♦	0.5 mL (≥2 y)	I.M. or S.C. (I.M. preferred)	Polysaccharide
Poliovirus (OPV) trivalent	0.5 mL	Oral	Live virus
Poliovirus (IPV)** trivalent	0.5 mL	S.C.	Inactivated virus
Rabies	1 mL	I.M.‡‡, ID§§	Inactivated virus

Table 1. Dosage and Administration Guidelines for Vaccines Available in the United States *(continued)*

Vaccine	Dosage	Route of Administration	Type
Rotavirus	2.5 mL	Oral	Live virus
Rubella	0.5 mL (≥12 mo)¶¶	S.C.	Live virus
Tetanus (adsorbed)##	0.5 mL	I.M.	Toxoid
Tetanus (fluid)	0.5 mL	I.M., S.C.	Toxoid
Varicella (Varivax®)	0.5 mL	S.C.	Live virus
Children 12 mo - 12 y: Single 0.5 mL dose			
Adolescents ≥13 y and adults: 0.5 mL dose x 2 (second 0.5 mL dose is administered 4 to 8 weeks later)			
Yellow fever	0.5 mL••	S.C.	Live attenuated virus

See footnotes on the following page.

IMMUNIZATION GUIDELINES (Continued)

*DT & DTP for use in children <7 years of age. Td contains same amount of tetanus toxoid as DT & DTP, but a reduced dose of diphtheria toxoid. Td for use in children ≥7 years of age.

†††DTaP (Acel-Imune®) is the recommended vaccine for primary vaccination against diphtheria, tetanus, and pertussis; including completion of the series in children who have received 1 or more doses of whole-cell DTP. The occurrence of fever and local reactions is lower with acellular pertussis vaccine than with whole-cell DTP.

⁺DTP-HbOC may be substituted for DTP and *Haemophilus* b conjugate vaccines which are administered separately, whenever recommended schedules for use of these 2 vaccines coincide. Initiate at 2 months of age for 3 doses (2 months, 4 months, and 6 months), followed by a 4th dose at 15-18 months of age. DTaP and *Haemophilus* b conjugate vaccine may be administered separately as an alternative to DTP-HbOC at 15-18 months of age.

†The conjugate (HbCV) vaccine is preferred over the polysaccharide (HbPV) vaccine. In children with a high risk for *Haemophilus influenzae* type b disease and HbCV is unavailable, an acceptable alternate is to give HbPV at 18 months of age with a 2nd dose at 24 months of age. Children <5 years of age who were previously vaccinated with HbPV between 18-23 months of age should be revaccinated with a single dose of HbCV at least 2 months after the initial dose of HbPV. Either HbCV or HbPV can be administered up to the 5th birthday. However, they are generally not recommended for children >5 years of age.

‡PRP-OMP (PedvaxHIB®) manufactured by Merck, Sharp & Dohme is initiated at 2 months of age for 3 doses (2 months, 4 months and 12 months). If initiated at 7-11 months of age, 3 doses are administered (initial 2 doses at 2-month intervals, 3rd dose at 15-18 months of age); initiated at 12-14 months of age, 2 doses are administered at 2- to 3-month intervals between doses; initiated at 15-59 months of age, 1 dose is administered.

§Hepatitis B vaccine can be given at the same time with DTP, HbOC, polio, and/or MMR; administer 3 doses at 0, 1, and 6 months).

[]Administer to newborns at 0-2 days of age before hospital discharge; repeat at 1-2 months and 6-18 months following the initial dose. If not vaccinated at birth, administer at 2, 4, and 6-18 months of age.

¶Engerix-B® — an alternate schedule for postexposure prophylaxis or more rapid induction using 4 doses at 0, 1, 2, and 12 months of age is recommended.

#Indicated in children ≥2 years of age at risk in epidemic or highly endemic areas.

•See measles.

♦Indicated for children with sickle cell disease; asplenia; nephrotic syndrome or chronic renal failure; conditions associated with immunosuppression; CSF leaks; HIV infection.

**The primary series consists of 3 doses. The first 2 doses should be administered at an interval of 8 weeks. The 3rd dose should be given at least 6 and preferably 12 months after the 2nd dose. A booster dose of 0.5 mL should be given to all children who have completed the primary series, before entering school. However, if the 3rd dose of the primary series is given on or after the 4th birthday, a 4th dose is not required before entering school. When polio vaccine is given to persons >18 years of age, IPV should be given.

‡‡In infants and small children, I.M. injection can be given into the midlateral aspect of the thigh; in older children and adults, I.M. injection can be given into the deltoid muscle. Repeat doses are given on days 3, 7, 14, and 28 postexposure.

§§For pre-exposure prophylaxis against rabies for high-risk individuals, 1 mL I.M. or 0.1 mL intradermal is administered on days 0, 7, and 21 (or 28). Both I.M. and I.D. dosage forms are available.

¶¶As MMR in a 2-dose schedule.

##Adsorbed preferred to fluid toxoid because of longer lasting immunity.

••≥9 months of age living in or traveling to endemic areas. Contraindicated in infants <4 months of age and in patients who have had an anaphylactic reaction to eggs. Increased risk of encephalitis associated with use of yellow fever vaccine in infants <9 months of age.

Note: For each vaccine, check the manufacturer's package insert for specific product information since preparations may change from time to time.

References

ACIP, Measles Prevention, Recommendations of the Immunization Practices Advisory Committee, *MMWR* 1989, 38(5-9):1-18.

American Academy of Pediatrics, Report of the Committee on Infectious Diseases (Red Book), 24th ed, 1997.

American Academy of Pediatrics, Committee on Infectious Diseases, "Acellular Pertussis Vaccines: Recommendations for Use as the Fourth and Fifth Doses," *Pediatrics*, 1992, 90:121-3.

American Academy of Pediatrics, Committee on Infectious Diseases, "Universal Hepatitis B Immunization," *Pediatrics*, 1992, 89:795-800.

American Academy of Pediatrics, Committee on Infectious Diseases, "Recommendations for the Use of Live Attenuated Varicella Vaccine," *Pediatrics*, 1995, 95(5):791-6.

American Academy of Pediatrics, Committee on Infectious Diseases, "*Haemophilus influenzae* Type B Conjugate Vaccines: Recommendations for Immunization of Infants and Children 2 Months of Age and Older," *Pediatrics*, 1991, 88(1):169-72.

American Academy of Pediatrics, Committee on Infectious Diseases, "Recommended Childhood Immunization Schedule," *Pediatrics*, 1996, 97(1):143-45.

Pope A, "The Recommended Childhood Immunization Schedule of the United States," *Pediatrics*, 1995, 95:135-7.

Table 2. High-Risk Groups Who Should Receive Hepatitis B Immunization Regardless of Age*

- Hemophiliac patients and other recipients of certain blood products

- Intravenous drug abusers

- Heterosexual persons who have had more than one sex partner in the previous 6 months and/or those with a recent episode of a sexually transmitted disease

- Sexually active homosexual and bisexual males

- Household and sexual contacts of hepatitis B virus (HBV) carriers

- Members of households with adoptees from HBV-endemic, high-risk countries who are hepatitis B surface antigen-positive

- Children and other household contacts in populations of high HBV endemicity

- Staff and residents of institutions for the developmentally disabled

- Staff of nonresidential day care and school programs for developmentally disabled if attended by known HBV carrier; other attendees in certain circumstances

- Hemodialysis patients

- Healthcare workers and others with occupational risk

- International travelers who will live for more than 6 months in areas of high HBV endemicity and who otherwise will be at risk

- Inmates of long-term correctional facilities

*Adapted from Report of the Committee on Infectious Disease, 1991, 246-9.

See **Table 3** for recommended Hepatitis B immunization schedule.

IMMUNIZATION GUIDELINES *(Continued)*

Table 3. Childhood Immunization Schedule

Recommended Childhood Immunization Schedule
United States, January - December 2000

Vaccines [1] are listed under the routinely recommended ages. ⬚Bars⬚ indicate range of recommended ages for immunization. Any dose not given at the recommended age should be given as a "catch up" immunization at any subsequent visit when indicated and feasible.

🔵Ovals🔵 indicate vaccines to be given if previously recommended doses were missed or given earlier than the recommended minimum age.

Age ▶ Vaccine ▼	Birth	1 mo	2 mo	4 mo	6 mo	12 mo	15 mo	18 mo	24 mo	4-6 y	11-12 y	14-16 y
Hepatitis B [2]	Hep B											
		Hep B			Hep B						(Hep B)	
Diphtheria, Tetanus, Pertussis [3]			DTaP	DTaP	DTaP		DTaP [3]			DTaP	Td	
H. influenzae type b [4]			Hib	Hib	Hib	Hib						
Polio [5]			IPV	IPV		IPV [5]				IPV [5]		
Measles, Mumps, Rubella [6]						MMR				MMR [6]	(MMR [6])	
Varicella [7]						Var					(Var [7])	
Hepatitis A [8]										Hep A [8] in selected areas		

[1] This schedule indicates the recommended ages for routine administration of currently licensed childhood vaccines as of 11/1/99. Additional vaccines may be licensed and recommended during the year. Licensed combination vaccines may be used whenever any components of the combinations are indicated and its other components are not contraindicated. Providers should consult the manufacturers' package inserts for detailed recommendations.

[2] Infants born to HBsAg-negative mothers should receive the 1st dose of hepatitis B (Hep B) vaccine by age 2 months. The 2nd dose should be at least one month after the 1st dose. The 3rd dose should be administered at least 4 months after the 1st dose and at least 2 months after the 2nd dose, but not before 6 months of age for infants.

Infants born to HBsAg-positive mothers should receive hepatitis B vaccine and 0.5 mL hepatitis B immune globulin (HBIG) within 12 hours of birth at separate sites. The 2nd dose is recommended at 1 month of age and the 3rd dose at 6 months of age.

Infants born to mothers whose HBsAg status is unknown should receive hepatitis B vaccine within 12 hours of birth. Maternal blood should be drawn at the time of delivery to determine the mother's HBsAg status; if the HBsAg test is positive, the infant should receive HBIG as soon as possible (no later than 1 week of age).

All children and adolescents (through 18 years of age) who have not been immunized against hepatitis B may begin the series during any visit. Special efforts should be made to immunize children who were born in or whose parents were born in areas of the world with moderate or high endemicity of hepatitis B virus infection.

[3] The 4th dose of DTaP (diphtheria and tetanus toxoids and acellular pertussis vaccine) may be administered as early as 12 months of age, provided 6 months have elapsed since the 3rd dose and the child is unlikely to return to at age 15-18 months. Td (tetanus and diphtheria toxoids) is recommended at 11-12 years of age if at least 5 years have elapsed since the last dose of DTP, DTaP or DT. Subsequent routine Td boosters are recommended every 10 years.

[4] Three *Haemophilus influenzae* type b (Hib) conjugate vaccines are licensed for infant use. If PRP-OMP (PedvaxHIB® and ComVax® [Merck]) is administered at 2 and 4 months of age, a dose at 6 months is not required. Because clinical studies in infants have demonstrated that using some combination products may induce a lower immune response to the Hib vaccine component, DTaP/Hib combination products should not be used for primary immunization in infants at 2, 4, or 6 months of age, unless FDA-approved for these ages.

[5] To eliminate the risk of vaccine-associated paralytic polio (VAPP), an all-IPV schedule is now recommended for routine childhood polio vaccination in the United States. All children should receive four doses of IPV at 2 months, 4 months, 6-18 months, and 4-6 years. OPV (if available) may be used only for the following special circumstances: **1)** Mass vaccination campaigns to control outbreaks of paralytic polio. **2)** Unvaccinated children who will be traveling in <4 weeks to areas where polio is endemic or epidemic. **3)** Children of parents who do not accept the recommended number of vaccine injections. These children may receive OPV only for the third or fourth dose or both; in this situation, healthcare providers should administer OPV only after discussing the risk for VAPP with parents or caregivers. **4)** During the transition to an all-IPV schedule, recommendations for the use of remaining OPV supplies in physicians' offices and clinics have been issued by the American Academy of Pediatrics (see *Pediatrics*, December 1999).

[6] The 2nd dose of measles, mumps, and rubella vaccine (MMR) is recommended routinely at 4-6 years of age but may be administered during any visit, provided at least 4 weeks have elapsed since receipt of the 1st dose and that both doses are administered beginning at or after 12 months of age. Those who have not previously received the second dose should complete the schedule by the 11 to 12-year-old visit.

[7] Varicella (Var) vaccine is recommended at any visit on or after the first birthday for susceptible children, ie, those who lack a reliable history of chickenpox (as judged by a healthcare provider) and who have not been immunized. Susceptible persons 13 years of age or older should receive 2 doses, given at least 4 weeks apart.

[8] Hepatitis A (Hep A) is shaded to indicate its recommended use in selected states and/or regions; consult your local public health authority. (Also see *MMWR*, Oct. 01, 1999/48(RR12); 1-37).

Adapted from the Advisory Committee on Immunization Practices (ACIP), the American Academy of Pediatrics (AAP), and the American Academy of Family Physicians (AAFP).

Table 4. Recommended Schedule for Active Immunization of Normal Infants and Children**

Recommended Age	Vaccine(s)	Comments
Birth	Hep B-1	
2 mo	DTP1*, OPV1, HbOC1,† Hep B-2	OPV and DTP can be given earlier in areas of high endemicity†
4 mo	DTP2, OPV2, HbOC2	6 weeks to 2 months interval desired between OPV doses†
6 mo	DTP3, HbOC3, Hep B-3	An additional dose of OPV at this time is optional in areas with a high risk of poliovirus infection†
12 mo	MMR, Var§	MMR may be given from 12-15 months of age
15 mo	DTP4,‡ OPV3, HbOC4	Completion of primary series of DTP and OPV†; OPV3 may be given any time between 6 and 18 months of age
4-6 y	DTP5,‡ OPV4, MMR	At or before school entry; the second dose of MMR may be given at 4-6 years or at 11-12 years
11-12 y	Td, Var§	Td may be given at age 11-12 years or at 14-16 years; repeat every 10 years throughout life

**Please also refer to Hepatitis B Vaccine Guidelines in Table 2.

*DTP may be used up to the 7th birthday. The 1st dose can be given at 6 weeks of age, and the 2nd and 3rd doses given 4-8 weeks after the preceding dose.

†DTP-HbOC may be given in place of DTP and HbOC

‡DTaP may be used in place of whole cell DTP only for the 4th and 5th doses for children >15 months and <7 years of age. DTaP can be given at the same time with OPV, IPV, MMR, *Haemophilus influenzae* type b conjugate vaccine, and/or hepatitis B vaccine.

§Varicella vaccine may be administered to susceptible children any time after 12 months of age. Unvaccinated children who lack a reliable history of chickenpox should be vaccinated at the 11-12 year old visit; those patients immunized after >13 years of age should be given 2 doses, with the second dose administered 4-8 weeks later.

Table 5. Recommended Immunization Schedule for Infants and Children up to the 7th Birthday Not Immunized at the Recommended Time in Early Infancy

Timing	Vaccine(s)	Comments
First visit	DTaP1, IPV1, MMR* (if child ≥15 months)†	DTaP, IPV, and MMR should be administered simultaneously to children ≥15 months of age
	HbOC1	DTaP, IPV, MMR, and HbOC may be given simultaneously to children aged 18 months to 5 years
2 mo after DTaP1, IPV1	DTaP2, IPV2, (HbOC2)†	HbOC2 if first dose was received when child <15 months of age
2 mo after DTaP2	DTaP3	An additional dose of OPV at this time is optional in areas with a high risk of poliovirus infection
6-12 mo after DTaP3	DTaP4,‡ (OPV1)	OPV is given if third dose was not given earlier.
Preschool (4-6 y)	DTP5,‡ OPV2 (MMR2)	Preferably at or before school entry. The preschool doses are not needed if DTP4 and OPV3 are give after the 4th birthday. Local public health regulations may require MMR2 at school entry.
14-16 y	Td	Repeat every 10 years throughout life

*Can be given at 12 months of age to children residing in areas at high-risk for measles transmission. The second dose of measles vaccine can be given at 4-6 years of age or 11-12 years of age.

†DTP-HbOC may be given in place of DTP and HbOC.

‡DTaP may be used in place of whole cell DTP. DTaP can be given at the same time with OPV, IPV, MMR, *Haemophilus influenzae* type b conjugate vaccine, and/or hepatitis B vaccine.

IMMUNIZATION GUIDELINES *(Continued)*

Table 6. Recommended Immunization Schedule for Children >7 Years of Age Not Immunized at the Recommended Time in Early Infancy

Timing	Vaccine(s)	Comments
First visit	Td1, OPV1, MMR, HbOC*	OPV not routinely recommended for persons ≥18 years of age
2 mo after Td1, OPV1	Td2, OPV2	OPV may be given as soon as 6 weeks after OPV1
6-12 mo after Td2, OPV2	Td3, OPV3	OPV3 may be given as soon as 6 weeks after OPV2
10 y after Td3	Td	Repeat every 10 years throughout life
11-12 y	MMR2	MMR2 is given if 2nd dose was not given earlier

*Indicated only in children with a chronic illness associated with increased risk of *Haemophilus influenzae* type b disease.

Table 7. Spacing Live and Killed Antigen Administration Guidelines

Antigen Combinations	Recommended Minimum Interval Between Doses
≥2 killed antigens	None; may give simultaneously or at any interval between doses.
Killed and live antigens	None. May be given simultaneously or at any interval between doses. (**Exception:** Concurrent administration of cholera and yellow fever vaccines should be avoided. Separate these vaccines by at least 3 weeks.)
≥2 live antigens	4 weeks minimum interval if not administered simultaneously. (Recent receipt of OPV is not a contraindication to MMR.) Vaccines associated with systemic reactions (cholera and parenteral typhoid or influenza and DTP in young children) should be given on separate occasions.

Table 8. Passive Immunization Agents — Immune Globulins

Immune Globulin	Dosage	Route
Hepatitis B (H-BIG®)		I.M.
percutaneous inoculation	0.06 mL/kg/dose (within 24 hours) (5 mL max)	
perinatal	0.5 mL/dose (within 12 hours of birth)	
sexual exposure	0.06 mL/kg/dose (within 14 days of contact) (5 mL max)	
Immune globulin (IG)		I.M.*
hepatitis A prophylaxis	0.02 mL/kg/dose (as soon as possible or within 2 weeks after exposure) (single exposure)	
	0.06 mL/kg/dose (>3 months or continuous exposure) repeat every 4-6 months	
hepatitis B	0.06 mL/kg/dose (H-BIG® should be used)	
hepatitis C	0.06 mL/kg/dose (percutaneous exposure)	
measles†	0.25 mL/kg/dose (max: 15 mL/dose) (within 6 days of exposure)	
	0.5 mL/kg/dose (max: 15 mL/dose) (immunocompromised children)	
Rabies‡	20 IU/kg/dose (within 3 days)	
Tetanus (serious, contaminated wounds; <3 previous tetanus vaccine doses)	250-500 units/dose	I.M.
Varicella-zoster§ (VZIG)	Within 48 hours but not later than 96 hours after exposure	I.M.¶
	0-10 kg — 125 units = 1 vial	
	10.1-20 kg — 250 units = 2 vials	
	20.1-30 kg — 375 units = 3 vials	
	30.1-40 kg — 500 units = 4 vials	
	>40 kg — 625 units = 5 vials	

*Deep I.M. in the gluteal region for large doses only. Deltoid muscle or the anterolateral aspect of the thigh are preferred sites for injection. No greater than 5 mL/site in adults or large children; 1-3 mL/site in small children and infants. Max: 20 mL at one time.

†IG prophylaxis may not be indicated in a patient who has received IGIV within 3 weeks of exposure.

‡½ of dose used to infiltrate the wound with the remaining ½ of dose given I.M. Rabies immune globulin is not recommended in previously HDCV immunized patients.

§Infants born to women who develop varicella within 5 days before or 48 hours after delivery should receive 125 units I.M. as a single dose.

¶No greater than 2.5 mL of VZIG/one injection site. Doses >2.5 mL should be divided and administered at different sites.

Table 9. Guidelines for Spacing the Administration of Immune Globulin (IG) - Preparations and Vaccines

Immunobiologic Combinations	Recommended Minimum Interval Between Doses
Simultaneous Administration	
IG and killed antigen	None. May be given simultaneously at different sites or at any time between doses.
IG and live antigen	Should generally not be given simultaneously. If unavoidable to do so, give at different sites and revaccinate or test for seroconversion in 3 months. **Example:** MMR should not be given to patients who have received immune globulin within the previous 3 months.

Nonsimultaneous Administration		
First	Second	
IG	Killed antigen	None
Killed antigen	IG	None
IG	Live antigen	6 weeks, and preferably 3 months
Live antigen	IG	2 weeks

*The live virus vaccines, OPV, and yellow fever are exceptions to these recommendations. Either vaccine may be administered simultaneously or any time before or after IG without significantly decreasing antibody response.

IMMUNIZATION GUIDELINES *(Continued)*

Table 10. Recommended for Routine Immunization of HIV-Infected Children — United States

Vaccine	Known HIV Infection	
	Asymptomatic	Symptomatic
DTP	Yes	Yes
OPV	No	No
IPV	Yes	Yes
MMR	Yes	Yes
HbCV	Yes	Yes
Pneumococcal	Yes	Yes
Influenza	No*	Yes

*Not contraindicated.

IMMUNIZATION SIDE EFFECTS

Vaccine	Side Effect	Incidence/Dose
DPT	Slight fever and irritability (within 2 days of immunization)	"Most"
	Pain and swelling at immunization site	1/2
	Continuous crying >3 hours	1/100
	Fever >105°F	1/330
	Unusual, high pitched crying	1/900
	Seizures or episodes of limpness/pallor	1/1750
	Acute encephalopathy (within 3 days of immunization)	1/110,000
	Permanent neurological sequelae*	1/310,000
DT, Td	Pain at immunization site, slight fever	"Not common"
OPV	Paralytic polio in patient immunized	1/8.1 million
	Paralytic polio in close contact of patient immunized	1/5 million
Hib	Swelling and warmth at immunization site	1/100
	Fever >101°F	2/100
	Redness at immunization site	2/100
MMR	Rash or slight fever lasting a few days 1-2 weeks following immunization	1/5
	Rash or lymphadenopathy lasting a few days 1-2 weeks following immunization	1/7
	Arthralgias, joint swelling lasting 2-3 days 1-3 weeks following immunization	1/20 (higher in adults)
	Encephalitis, seizure with fever, nerve deafness	"Very rarely"

*Red Book (1991, p 355) states "The committee concludes, based on currently available data, that pertussis vaccine has not been proven to be a cause of brain damage. Although the data does not prove that pertussis vaccine will never cause brain damage, it does indicate that such occurrences are exceedingly rare."

IMMUNIZATION SIDE EFFECTS *(Continued)*

REPORTABLE VACCINE SIDE EFFECTS

Vaccine/Toxoid	Event	Interval From Vaccination
DTP, P, DTP/ poliovirus combined	Anaphylaxis or anaphylactic shock	24 hours
	Encephalopathy (or encephalitis)	7 days
	Shock-collapse or hypotonic-hyporesponsive collapse	7 days
	Residual seizure disorder	
	Any acute complication or sequela (including death) of above events	No limit
	See package insert	See package insert
Measles, mumps, and rubella; DT, Td, T toxoid	Anaphylaxis or anaphylactic shock	24 hours
	Encephalopathy (or encephalitis)	15 days for measles, mumps, and rubella vaccines; 7 days for DT, Td, and toxoids
	Residual seizure disorder	
	Any acute complication or sequela (including death) of above events	No limit
	See package insert	See package insert
Oral poliovirus vaccine	Paralytic poliomyelitis	
	– in a nonimmunodeficient recipient	30 days
	– in an immunodeficient recipient	6 months
	– in a vaccine-associated community case	No limit
	Any acute complication or sequela (including death) of above events	No limit
	See package insert	See package insert
Inactivated poliovirus vaccine	Anaphylaxis or anaphylactic shock	24 hours
	Any acute complication or sequela (including death) of above events	No limit
	See package insert	See package insert

CONTRAINDICATIONS TO IMMUNIZATION

Minor illness is not a contraindication to vaccination, especially if the patient has a minor upper respiratory infection or allergic rhinitis. Delay of immunization should be considered if expected or potential vaccine side effects may accentuate or be accentuated by an underlying illness. Note that fever is not itself a contraindication to vaccination, however, if fever is associated with other signs of serious underlying illness, vaccination should be deferred until the patient has recovered. Moderate or severe illness, with or without fever, is considered a contraindication to DPT administration, as signs and symptoms associated with the underlying illness may be incorrectly attributed to the DPT vaccine.

The following conditions should be evaluated as possible contraindications to vaccination:

Vaccine	Possible Contraindications
DPT	Previous serious reaction to DPT, TD, or dT
	Serious immunosuppressive therapy
	Thimerosal allergy
	Progressive neurological disorder or uncontrolled seizure disorder
	Disorders associated with conditions that predispose to either seizures or neurological deterioration
	Age 7 years or older (dT recommended)
OPV	Immunosuppression
	Immunosuppressive household contacts
	Age 18 years and older (IPV recommended)
	Pregnancy
Hib	Serious thimerosal allergy
	Serious allergic reaction to vaccine containing diphtheria toxoid
	Age 5 years and older
MMR	Serious egg allergy
	Immunosuppression
	Gamma globulin therapy within preceding 3 months
	Serious neomycin or streptomycin allergy
	Pregnancy

CONTRAINDICATIONS TO IMMUNIZATION *(Continued)*

Conditions Not Considered to Be Contraindications to Vaccinations

- Reaction to a previous DTP dose that involved only soreness, redness, or swelling in the area of the vaccination site or temperature of less than 105°F (40.5°C)

- Mild acute illness with low-grade fever or mild diarrheal illness in an otherwise well child

- Current antimicrobial therapy or the convalescent phase of illness

- Prematurity

- Pregnancy of mother or other household contact

- Recent exposure to an infectious disease

- Breast-feeding

- A history of nonspecific allergies or relatives with allergies

- Allergies to penicillin or any other antibiotic, except anaphylactic reactions to neomycin or streptomycin

- Allergies to duck meat or duck feathers

- Family history of convulsions in persons considered for pertussis or measles vaccination

- Family history of sudden infant death syndrome in children considered for DTP vaccination

- Family history of an adverse event, unrelated to immunosuppression, following vaccination

SKIN TESTS FOR DELAYED HYPERSENSITIVITY

Skin tests for delayed hypersensitivity are used diagnostically to assess previous infection (ie, PPD, histoplasmin, and coccidioidin) or used to evaluate cellular immune function by testing for anergy (ie, mumps, *Candida*, tetanus toxoid, trichophyton, PPD). Anergy, a defect in cell-mediated immunity, is characterized by a depressed response or lack of response to skin testing with injected antigens. Anergy has been associated with congenital and acquired immunodeficiencies, and malnutrition.

Candida 1:100

Dose = 0.1 mL intradermally (30% of children younger than 18 months of age and 50% older than 18 months of age respond)

Can be used as a control antigen

Coccidioidin 1:100

Dose = 0.1 mL intradermally (apply with PPD **and** a control antigen)
Mercury derivative used as a preservative for spherulin.

Histoplasmin 1:100

Dose = 0.1 mL intradermally (yeast derived)

Multitest CMI (*Candida,* diphtheria toxoid, tetanus toxoid, *Streptococcus,* old tuberculin, *Trichophyton, Proteus* antigen, and negative control)

Press loaded unit into the skin with sufficient pressure to puncture the skin and allow adequate penetration of all points.

Mumps 40 cfu per mL

Dose = 0.1 mL intradermally (contraindicated in patients allergic to eggs, egg products, or thimerosal)

Purified Protein Derivative 5 TU (PPD* Mantoux Tuberculin)

Screening for tuberculosis:

Children who have no risk factors but who reside in high-prevalence regions: skin test at 4-6 years and 11-16 years of age

Children exposed to HIV-infected individuals, homeless, residents of nursing homes, institutionalized adolescents, users of illicit drugs, incarcerated adolescents and migrant farm workers: skin test every 2-3 years

Children at high risk (children infected with HIV, incarcerated adolescents): annual skin testing

Dose = 0.1 mL intradermally

Definition of positive Mantoux skin test (regardless of previous BCG administration):

Reaction ≥5 mm for high-risk group (children in close contact with known or suspected infectious cases of tuberculosis; children suspected to have disease based on clinical and/or roentgenographic evidence; and children with underlying host factors (immunosuppressive conditions, receiving immunosuppressive therapy, and HIV infection).

Reaction ≥10 mm for children <4 years; those with medical diseases who are at increased risk for dissemination or for those at increased risk because of environmental exposure.

Reaction ≥15 mm for children ≥4 years of age including those with no risk factors.

*PPD 1 TU (first strength) is only used in individuals suspected of being highly sensitive. PPD 250 TU (second strength) is used only for individuals

SKIN TESTS FOR DELAYED HYPERSENSITIVITY
(Continued)

who fail to respond to a previous injection of 5 TU, or anergic patients in whom TB is suspected.

Tetanus Toxoid 1:5

Dose = 0.1 mL intradermally (29% of children younger than 2 years of age and 78% older than 2 years of age respond if they have received 3 immunizing doses)

Can be used as a control antigen.

Tine Test

Indication: survey and screen for exposure to tuberculosis (grasp forearm firmly; stretch the skin of the volar surface tightly; apply the tines to the selected site; press for at least one second so that a circular halo impression is left on the skin)

General Information

1. Intradermal skin tests should be injected in the flexor surface of the forearm.

2. A pale wheal 6-10 mm in diameter should form over the needle tip as soon as the injection is administered. If no bleb forms, the injection must be repeated.

3. Space skin tests at least 2 inches apart to prevent reactions from overlapping.

4. Read skin tests for diameter of induration and presence of erythema at 24, 48, and 72 hours. Reactions occurring before 24 hours are indicative of an immediate rather than a delayed hypersensitivity reaction.

5. False-negative results may occur in patients with malnutrition, viral infections, febrile illnesses, immunodeficiency disorders, severe disseminated infections, uremia, patients who have received immunosuppressive therapy (steroids, antineoplastic agents), patients who have received a recent live attenuated virus vaccine (MMR, measles).

6. False-positive results may occur in patients sensitive to ingredients in the skin test solution such as thimerosal; cross-sensitivity between similar antigens; or with improper interpretation of skin test.

7. Side effects are pain, blisters, extensive erythema and necrosis at the injection site.

   *Emergency equipment and epinephrine should be readily available to treat severe allergic reactions that may occur.

Recommended Interpretation of Skin Test Reactions

Reaction	Local Reaction	
	After Intradermal Injections of Antigens	After Dinitrochlorobenzene
1+	Erythema >10 mm and/or induration >1-5 mm	Erythema and/or induration covering <1/2 area of dosing site
2+	Induration 6-10 mm	Induration covering >1/2 area of dose site
3+	Induration 11-20 mm	Vesiculation and induration at dose site or spontaneous flare at days 7-14 at the site
4+	Induration >20 mm	Bulla or ulceration at dose site or spontaneous flare at days 7-14 at the site

References

American Academy of Pediatrics Committee on Infectious Diseases, "Screening for Tuberculosis in Infants and Children," *Pediatrics*, 1994, 93(1):131-4.
American Academy of Pediatrics Committee on Infectious Diseases, "Update on Tuberculosis Skin Testing of Children," *Pediatrics*, 1996, 97(2):282-4.

NORMAL LABORATORY VALUES FOR CHILDREN

Normal Values

CHEMISTRY

Albumin	0-1 y	2.0-4.0 g/dL
	1 y to adult	3.5-5.5 g/dL
Ammonia	Newborns	90-150 µg/dL
	Children	40-120 µg/dL
	Adults	18-54 µg/dL
Amylase	Newborns	0-60 units/L
	Adults	30-110 units/L
Bilirubin, conjugated, direct	Newborns	<1.5 mg/dL
	1 mo to adult	0-0.5 mg/dL
Bilirubin, total	0-3 d	2.0-10.0 mg/dL
	1 mo to adult	0-1.5 mg/dL
Bilirubin, unconjugated, indirect		0.6-10.5 mg/dL
Calcium	Newborns	7.0-12.0 mg/dL
	0-2 y	8.8-11.2 mg/dL
	2 y to adult	9.0-11.0 mg/dL
Calcium, ionized, whole blood		4.4-5.4 mg/dL
Carbon dioxide, total		23-33 mEq/L
Chloride		95-105 mEq/L
Cholesterol	Newborns	45-170 mg/dL
	0-1 y	65-175 mg/dL
	1-20 y	120-230 mg/dL
Creatinine	0-1 y	≤0.6 mg/dL
	1 y to adult	0.5-1.5 mg/dL
Glucose	Newborns	30-90 mg/dL
	0-2 y	60-105 mg/dL
	Children to Adults	70-110 mg/dL
Iron		
	Newborns	110-270 µg/dL
	Infants	30-70 µg/dL
	Children	55-120 µg/dL
	Adults	70-180 µg/dL
Iron binding	Newborns	59-175 µg/dL
	Infants	100-400 µg/dL
	Adults	250-400 µg/dL
Lactic acid, lactate		2-20 mg/dL
Lead, whole blood		<30 µg/dL
Lipase		
	Children	20-140 units/L
	Adults	0-190 units/L
Magnesium		1.5-2.5 mEq/L
Osmolality, serum		275-296 mOsm/kg
Osmolality, urine		50-1400 mOsm/kg
Phosphorus	Newborns	4.2-9.0 mg/dL
	6 wk to 19 mo	3.8-6.7 mg/dL
	19 mo to 3 y	2.9-5.9 mg/dL
	3-15 y	3.6-5.6 mg/dL
	>15 y	2.5-5.0 mg/dL

NORMAL LABORATORY VALUES FOR CHILDREN
(Continued)

Normal Values

CHEMISTRY

Potassium, plasma	Newborns	4.5-7.2 mEq/L
	2 d to 3 mo	4.0-6.2 mEq/L
	3 mo to 1 y	3.7-5.6 mEq/L
	1-16 y	3.5-5.0 mEq/L
Protein, total	0-2 y	4.2-7.4 g/dL
	>2 y	6.0-8.0 g/dL
Sodium		136-145 mEq/L
Triglycerides	Infants	0-171 mg/dL
	Children	20-130 mg/dL
	Adults	30-200 mg/dL
Urea nitrogen, blood	0-2 y	4-15 mg/dL
	2 y to Adult	5-20 mg/dL
Uric acid	Male	3.0-7.0 mg/dL
	Female	2.0-6.0 mg/dL

ENZYMES

Alanine aminotransferase (ALT) (SGPT)	0-2 mo	8-78 units/L
	>2 mo	8-36 units/L
Alkaline phosphatase (ALKP)	Newborns	60-130 units/L
	0-16 y	85-400 units/L
	>16 y	30-115 units/L
Aspartate aminotransferase (AST) (SGOT)	Infants	18-74 units/L
	Children	15-46 units/L
	Adults	5-35 units/L
Creatine kinase (CK)	Infants	20-200 units/L
	Children	10-90 units/L
	Adult male	0-206 units/L
	Adult female	0-175 units/L
Lactate dehydrogenase (LDH)	Newborns	290-501 units/L
	1 mo to 2 y	110-144 units/L
	>16 y	60-170 units/L

Blood Gases

	Arterial	Capillary	Venous
pH	7.35-7.45	7.35-7.45	7.32-7.42
pCO$_2$ (mm Hg)	35-45	35-45	38-52
pO$_2$ (mm Hg)	70-100	60-80	24-48
HCO$_3$ (mEq/L)	19-25	19-25	19-25
TCO$_2$ (mEq/L)	19-29	19-29	23-33
O$_2$ saturation (%)	90-95	90-95	40-70
Base excess (mEq/L)	-5 to +5	-5 to +5	-5 to +5

Thyroid Function Tests

T$_4$ (thyroxine)	1-7 d	10.1-20.9 µg/dL
	8-14 d	9.8-16.6 µg/dL
	1 mo to 1 y	5.5-16.0 µg/dL
	>1 y	4.0-12.0 µg/dL
FTI	1-3 d	9.3-26.6
	1-4 wk	7.6-20.8
	1-4 mo	7.4-17.9
	4-12 mo	5.1-14.5
	1-6 y	5.7-13.3
	>6 y	4.8-14.0
T$_3$	Newborns	100-470 ng/dL
	1-5 y	100-260 ng/dL
	5-10 y	90-240 ng/dL
	10 y to Adult	70-210 ng/dL
T$_3$ uptake		35%-45%
TSH	Cord	3-22 µlU/mL
	1-3 d	<40 µlU/mL
	3-7 d	<25 µlU/mL
	>7 d	0-10 µlU/mL

NORMAL LABORATORY
VALUES FOR CHILDREN (Continued)

Hematology Values

Age	Hgb (g/dL)	Hct (%)	RBC (mill/mm³)	RDW	MCV (fL)	MCH (pg)	MCHC (%)	PLTS (x 10³/mm³)
0-3 d	15.0-20.0	45-61	4.0-5.9	<18	95-115	31-37	29-37	250-450
1-2 wk	12.5-18.5	39-57	3.6-6.5	<17	86-110	28-36	28-38	250-450
1-6 mo	10.0-13.0	29-42	3.1-4.3	<16.5	74-96	25-35	30-36	300-700
7 mo to 2 y	10.5-13.0	33-38	3.7-4.9	<16	70-84	23-30	31-37	250-600
2-5 y	11.5-13.0	34-39	3.9-5.0	<15	75-87	24-30	31-37	250-550
5-8 y	11.5-14.5	35-42	4.0-4.9	<15	77-95	25-33	31-37	250-550
13-18 y	12.0-15.2	36-47	4.5-5.1	<14.5	78-96	25-35	31-37	150-450
Adult male	13.5-16.5	41-50	4.5-5.5	<14.5	80-100	26-34	31-37	150-450
Adult female	12.0-15.0	36-44	4.0-4.9	<14.5	80-100	26-34	31-37	150-450

WBC and Diff

Age	WBC (x 10³/mm³)	Segs	Bands	Lymphs	Monos	Eosinophils	Basophils	Atypical Lymphs	No. of NRBCs
0-3 d	9.0-35.0	32-62	10-18	19-29	5-7	0-2	0-1	0-8	0-2
1-2 wk	5.0-20.0	14-34	6-14	36-45	6-10	0-2	0-1	0-8	0
1-6 mo	6.0-17.5	13-33	4-12	41-71	4-7	0-3	0-1	0-8	0
7 mo to 2 y	6.0-17.0	15-35	5-11	45-76	3-6	0-3	0-1	0-8	0
2-5 y	5.5-15.5	23-45	5-11	35-65	3-6	0-3	0-1	0-8	0
5-8 y	5.0-14.5	32-54	5-11	28-48	3-6	0-3	0-1	0-8	0
13-18 y	4.5-13.0	34-64	5-11	25-45	3-6	0-3	0-1	0-8	0
Adults	4.5-11.0	35-66	5-11	24-44	3-6	0-3	0-1	0-8	0

Segs = segmented neutrophils

Bands = band neutrophils

Lymphs = lymphocytes

Monos = monocytes

NORMAL LABORATORY
VALUES FOR CHILDREN *(Continued)*

Erythrocyte Sedimentation Rates and Reticulocyte Counts

Sedimentation rate, Westergren	Children	0-20 mm/hour
	Adult male	0-15 mm/hour
	Adult female	0-20 mm/hour
Sedimentation rate, Wintrobe	Children	0-13 mm/hour
	Adult male	0-10 mm/hour
	Adult female	0-15 mm/hour
Reticulocyte count	Newborns	2%-6%
	1-6 mo	0%-2.8%
	Adults	0.5%-1.5%

Cerebrospinal Fluid Values, Normal

		% PMNs
Cell count		
Preterm mean	9 (0-25.4 WBC/mm^3)	57%
Term mean	8.2 (0-22.4 WBC/mm^3)	61%
>1 mo	0.7	0
Glucose		
Preterm	24-63 mg/dL	mean 50
Term	34-119 mg/dL	mean 52
Children	40-80 mg/dL	
CSF glucose/blood glucose		
Preterm	55-105%	
Term	44-128%	
Children	50%	
Lactic acid dehydrogenase	5-30 units/mL	mean 20 units/mL
Myelin basic protein	<4 ng/mL	
Pressure: Initial LP (mm H$_2$O)		
Newborns	80-110 (<110)	
Infants/children	<200 (lateral recumbent position)	
Respiratory movements	5-10	
Protein		
Preterm	65-150 mg/dL	mean 115
Term	20-170 mg/dL	mean 90
Children		
Ventricular	5-15 mg/dL	
Cisternal	5-25 mg/dL	
Lumbar	5-40 mg/dL	

APGAR SCORING SYSTEM

Sign	Score		
	0	1	2
Heart rate	Absent	Under 100 beats per minute	Over 100 beats per minute
Respiratory effort	Absent	Slow (irregular)	Good crying
Muscle tone	Limp	Some flexion of extremities	Active motion
Reflex irritability	No response	Grimace	Cough or sneeze
Color	Blue, pale	Pink body, blue extremities	All pink

From Apgar V, "A Proposal for a New Method of Evaluation of the Newborn Infant," *Anesth Analg*, 1953, 32:260.

FETAL HEART RATE MONITORING

Normal Heart Rates

Fetal heart rate (FHR) 120-160 bpm. Isolated accelerations are normal and considered reassuring. Mild (100-120 bpm) and transient bradycardias may be normal. Normal fetal heart rate tracings show beat-to-beat variability of 5-10 bpm (poor beat-to-beat variability suggests fetal hypoxia).

Abnormal Heart Rates

Bradycardia (FHR <120 bpm): Potential causes include fetal distress, drugs, congenital heart block (associated with maternal SLE, congenital cardiac defects).

Tachycardia (FHR >160 bpm): Potential causes include maternal fever, chorioamnionitis, drugs, fetal dysrhythmias, eg, SVT (with or without fetal CHF).

Decreased Beat-to-Beat Variability

Results from fetal CNS depression. Potential causes include fetal hypoxia, fetal sleep, fetal immaturity, and maternal narcotic/sedative administration.

Fetal Heart Rate Decelerations

Type 1 (early decelerations)

- Seen most commonly in late labor
- Mirror uterine contractions in time of onset, duration, and resolution
- Uniform shape
- Usually associated with good beat-to-beat variability
- Heart rate may dip to 60-80 bpm
- Associated with fetal head compression (increases vagal tone)
- Considered benign, and not representative of fetal hypoxia

APGAR SCORING SYSTEM *(Continued)*

Type 2 (late decelerations)

- Deceleration 10-30 seconds after onset of uterine contraction
- Heart rate fails to return to baseline after contraction is completed
- Asymmetrical shape (longer deceleration, shorter acceleration)
- Late decelerations of 10-20 bpm may be significant
- Probably associated with fetal CNS and myocardial depression

Type 3 (variable decelerations)

- Heart rate variations do not correlate with uterine contractions
- Variable shape and duration
- Occur occasionally in many normal labors
- Concerning if severe (HR <60 bpm), prolonged (duration >60 seconds), associated with poor beat-to-beat variability, or combined with late decelerations
- Associated with cord compression (including nuchal cord)

Reference
Manual of Neonatal Care, Joint Program in Neonatology, 1991.

CREATININE CLEARANCE ESTIMATING METHODS IN PATIENTS WITH STABLE RENAL FUNCTION

The following formulas provide an acceptable estimate of the patient's creatinine clearance except when:

    a.   The patient's serum creatinine is changing rapidly (either up or down).

    b.   Patients are markedly emaciated.

In these situations (a and b above), certain assumptions have to be made:

    a.   In patients with rapidly rising serum creatinines (ie, increasing by >0.5-0.7 mg/dL/day), it is best to assume that the patient's creatinine clearance is probably less than 10 mL/minute.

    b.   In emaciated patients, although their actual creatinine clearance is less than their calculated creatinine clearance (because of decreased creatinine production), it is not possible to predict easily how much less.

Estimation of creatinine clearance using serum creatinine and body length (to be used when an adequate timed urine specimen cannot be obtained). **Note:** This formula may not provide an accurate estimation of creatinine clearance for infants <6 months of age or for patients with severe starvation or muscle wasting.

$$CL_{cr} = K \times L/S_{cr}$$

where:

Cl_{cr} = Creatinine clearance in mL/minute/1.73 m^2

K = Constant of proportionality that is age specific

Age	K
Low birth weight ≤1 y	0.33
Full-term ≤1 y	0.45
2-12 y	0.55
13-21 y female	0.55
13-21 y male	0.70

L = Length in cm

S_{Cr} = Serum creatinine concentration in mg/dL

Reference

Schwartz GJ, Brion LP, and Spitzer A, "The Use of Plasma Creatinine Concentration for Estimating Glomerular Filtration Rate in Infants, Children and Adolescents," *Ped Clin N Amer*, 1987, 34:571-90.

Children 1-18 years

Method 1: (Traub SL, Johnson CE, *Am J Hosp Pharm*, 1980, 37:195-201)

Equation:

$$Cl_{cr} = \frac{0.48 \times (height)}{S_{cr}}$$

where

Cl_{cr} =   creatinine clearance in mL/min/1.73 m^2

S_{cr} =   serum creatinine in mg/dL

Height   =   height in cm

Method 2: See the following nomogram.

CREATININE CLEARANCE ESTIMATING METHODS IN PATIENTS WITH STABLE RENAL FUNCTION *(Continued)*

Children 1-18 Years

The nomogram below is for rapid evaluation of endogenous creatinine clearance (Cl_{cr}) in pediatric patients (aged 1-18 years).

To predict Cl_{cr}, connect the child's Scr (serum creatinine) and Ht (height) with a ruler and read the Cl_{cr} where the ruler intersects the center line.

Adults 18 years and older

Method 1: (Cockroft DW and Gault MH, *Nephron*, 1976, 16:31-41)

Estimated creatinine clearance (Cl_{cr}) (mL/min):

$$\text{Male} = \frac{(140 - \text{age}) \text{ IBW (kg)}}{72 \times \text{serum creatinine}}$$

$$\text{Female} = \text{Estimated } Cl_{cr} \text{ male} \times 0.85$$

Note: The use of the patient's ideal body weight (IBW) is recommended for the above formula except when the patient's actual body weight is less than ideal. Use of the IBW is especially important in obese patients. See appendix Growth & Development section for Ideal Body Weight Calculation.

Method 2: (Jelliffe RW, *Ann Intern Med*, 1973, 79:604)

Estimated creatinine clearance (Cl_{cr}) (mL/min/1.73 m²):

$$\text{Male} = \frac{98 - 0.8 (\text{age} - 20)}{\text{serum creatinine}}$$

$$\text{Female} = \text{Estimated } Cl_{cr} \text{ male} \times 0.90$$

RENAL FUNCTION TESTS

Endogenous creatinine clearance vs age (timed collection)

Creatinine clearance (mL/min/1.73 m^2) = (Cr$_u$V/S$_{cr}$T) (1.73/A)

where:

Cr$_u$	=	Urine creatinine concentration (mg/dL)
V	=	Total urine volume collected during sampling period (mL)
S$_{Cr}$	=	Serum creatinine concentration (mg/dL)
T	=	Duration of sampling period (min) (24 h = 1440 min)
A	=	Body surface area (m^2)

Age-specific normal values

5-7 d	50.6±5.8 mL/min/1.73 m^2
1-2 mo	64.6±5.8 mL/min/1.73 m^2
5-8 mo	87.7±11.9 mL/min/1.73 m^2
9-12 mo	86.9±8.4 mL/min/1.73 m^2
≥18 mo	
male	124±26 mL/min/1.73 m^2
female	109±13.5 mL/min/1.73 m^2
Adults	
male	105±14 mL/min/1.73 m^2
female	95±18 mL/min/1.73 m^2

Note: In patients with renal failure (creatinine clearance <25 mL/min), creatinine clearance may be elevated over GFR because of tubular secretion of creatinine.

Serum BUN/Serum Creatinine Ratio

Serum BUN (mg/dL):serum creatinine (mg/dL)

Normal BUN:creatinine ratio is 10-15.

BUN:creatinine ratio >20 suggests prerenal azotemia (also seen with high urea-generation states such as GI bleeding).

BUN:creatinine ratio <5 may be seen with disorders affecting urea biosynthesis such as urea cycle enzyme deficiencies and with hepatitis.

Fractional Sodium Excretion

Fractional sodium secretion (FENa) = Na$_u$S$_{cr}$ /Na$_s$Cr$_u$ x 100%

where:

Na$_u$	=	Urine sodium (mEq/L)
Na$_s$	=	Serum sodium (mEq/L)
Cr$_u$	=	Urine creatinine (mg/dL)
S$_{Cr}$	=	Serum creatinine (mg/dL)

FENa <1% suggests prerenal failure
FENa >2% suggest intrinsic renal failure
(for newborns, normal FENa is approximately 2.5%)

Note: Disease states associated with a falsely elevated FENa include severe volume depletion (>10%), early acute tubular necrosis and volume depletion in chronic renal disease. Disorders associated with a lowered FENa include acute glomerulonephritis, hemoglobinuric or myoglobinuric renal failure, nonoliguric acute tubular necrosis, and acute urinary tract obstruction. In addition, FENa may be <1% in patients with acute renal failure **and** a second condition predisposing to sodium retention (eg, burns, congestive heart failure, nephrotic syndrome).

RENAL FUNCTION TESTS *(Continued)*

Urine Calcium/Urine Creatinine Ratio (spot sample)

Urine calcium (mg/dL): urine creatinine (mg/dL)

Normal values <0.21 (mean values 0.08 males, 0.06 females)

Premature infants show wide variability of calcium:creatinine ratio, and tend to have lower thresholds for calcium loss than older children. Prematures without nephrolithiasis had mean Ca:Cr ratio of 0.75±0.76. Infants with nephrolithiasis had mean Ca:Cr ratio of 1.32±1.03 (Jacinto, et al, *Pediatrics*, vol 81, p 31).

Urine Protein/Urine Creatinine Ratio (spot sample)

P_u/Cr_u	Total Protein Excretion (mg/m^2/day)
0.1	80
1	800
10	8000

where:

P_u =   Urine protein concentration (mg/dL)

Cr_u =   Urine creatinine concentration (mg/dL)

Serum Osmolality

Predicted serum osmolality =

$$2 \times Na \ (mEq/L) + BUN \ (mg/dL) / 2.8 + glucose \ (mg/dL) / 18$$

High Anion Gap (see Toxicology section)

ACID/BASE ASSESSMENT

Henderson-Hasselbalch Equation

$pH = 6.1 + \log (HCO_3^- / (0.03) (pCO_2))$

Alveolar Gas Equation

P_iO_2 = f_iO_2 x (total atmospheric pressure – vapor pressure of H_2O at 37°C)

= f_iO_2 x (760 mm Hg – 47 mm Hg)

PAO_2 = $P_iO_2 – PACO_2 / R$

Alveolar/arterial oxygen gradient = $PAO_2 – PaO_2$

Normal ranges:

Children	15-20 mm Hg
Adults	20-25 mm Hg

Where:

P_iO_2	=	Oxygen partial pressure of inspired gas (mm Hg) (150 mm Hg in room air at sea level)
f_iO_2	=	Fractional pressure of oxygen in inspired gas (0.21 in room air)
PAO_2	=	Alveolar oxygen partial pressure
$PACO_2$	=	Alveolar carbon dioxide partial pressure
PaO_2	=	Arterial oxygen partial pressure
R	=	Respiratory exchange quotient (typically 0.8, increases with high carbohydrate diet, decreases with high fat diet)

Acid/Base Disorders

Acute metabolic acidosis (<12 h duration)

$PaCO_2$ expected = 1.5 (HCO_3^-) + 8±2

or

expected change in pCO = (1-1.5) x change in HCO_3^-

Acute metabolic alkalosis (<12 h duration)

expected change in pCO_2 = (0.5-1) x change in HCO_3^-

Acute respiratory acidosis (<6 h duration)

expected change in HCO_3^- = 0.1 x pCO_2

Acute respiratory acidosis (>6 h duration)

expected change in HCO_3^- = 0.4 x change in pCO_2

Acute respiratory alkalosis (<6 h duration)

expected change in HCO_3^- = 0.2 x change in pCO_2

Acute respiratory alkalosis (>6 h duration)

expected change in HCO_3^- = 0.5 x change in pCO_2

ACUTE DYSTONIC REACTIONS, MANAGEMENT

1. Confirm that patient has stable airway and adequate respiratory activity.

2. Administer **one** of the following:

   Diphenhydramine 0.7-1 mg/kg/dose I.V./P.O. q4-6h prn **or**

   Hydroxyzine 0.5-1 mg/kg/dose I.M./P.O. q4-6h prn
   (adult dose: 25-100 mg I.M./P.O. q6h) **or**

   Children >3 years: Benztropine 0.02-0.05 mg/kg/dose or maximum of 1-2 mg I.V./P.O. (avoid use in children <3 years of age except in cases of extreme emergency)

Agents which predispose patients to acute dystonic reactions, such as phenothiazine neuroleptics or antiemetics, often have long therapeutic half-lives. Anticholinergic administration should therefore be continued for 6-24 hours after discontinuation of phenothiazine therapy.

PREPROCEDURE SEDATIVES IN CHILDREN

Purpose: The following table is a guide to aid the clinician in the selection of the most appropriate sedative to sedate a child for a procedure. One must also consider:

- Not all patients require sedation. It is dependent on the procedure and age of the child.

- When sedation is desired, one must consider the time of onset, the duration of action, and the route of administration.

- Each of the following drugs is well absorbed when given by the suggested routes and doses.

- Each drug was assigned an "intensity" based upon the class of drug, dose, and route.[1]

    - Conscious sedation: A medically controlled state of depressed consciousness that retains the patient's ability to independently and continuously maintain a patent airway, respond appropriately to physical stimulation and/or verbal commands. The protective reflexes are maintained.

    - Deep sedation: A medically controlled state of depressed consciousness associated with partial or complete loss of protective reflexes and inability to respond appropriately to physical stimulation and/or verbal commands.

- Those drugs classified as producing deep sedation require more frequent monitoring postprocedure.

- For painful procedures, an analgesic agent needs to be administered.

Sedatives Used to Produce Conscious Sedation

Drug	Route	Dose (mg/kg)	Onset (min)	Duration (h)	Comments
Chloral hydrate	P.O./P.R.	25-100	10-20	4-8	May cause hepatic neoplasms in rats; maximum single dose: infants: 1 g; children: 2 g
Diazepam[2,3] (Valium®)	P.O.	0.2-0.3 90 min prior	60-90	6-8	Maximum oral dose: 10 mg
	I.V.	0.1-0.2	1-3	6-8	Maximum dose I.V.: 5 mg; due to poor absorption and tissue irritation, I.M. route **not** recommended
	P.R.	0.2-0.4	2-10	6-8	May use I.V. solution rectally
"DPT" cocktail[4] (Demerol®, Phenergan®, Thorazine®)	I.M.	Demerol® 1-2, Phenergan® 0.5-1, Thorazine® 0.5-1	30	2-14	May be mixed in single syringe; I.M. only. This combination of agents may have a higher rate of adverse effects compared with alternative sedative/ analgesics.
Fentanyl	Trans-mucosal	5-15 mcg/kg	5-15	1-2	Maximum trans-mucosal dose: 400 mcg
	I.M.	1-3 mcg/kg	7-15	1-2	
	I.V.	1-3 mcg/kg	Immediate	30-60 min	
Lorazepam[5] (Ativan®)	P.O.	0.05; 90-120 min prior	60	8-12	
	Deep I.M.	0.05; 90-120 min prior	30-60	8-12	
	I.V.	0.05; over 5-10 min	15-30	8-12	

PREPROCEDURE SEDATIVES
IN CHILDREN (Continued)

Sedatives Used to Produce Conscious Sedation (continued)

Drug	Route	Dose (mg/kg)	Onset (min)	Duration (h)	Comments
Meperidine (Demerol®)	P.O.	2-4	10-15	2-4	Doses I.M./I.V. >2 mg/kg are considered deep sedation
	I.M.	0.5-2	10-15	2-4	
	I.V.	0.5-2	5	2-3	
Midazolam[6,7] (Versed®)	P.O.	0.2-0.4; 30-45 min prior	20-30	1-2	Maximum oral dose: 15 mg
	Deep I.M.	0.1-0.15; 30-60 min prior	15	1-2	Maximum total dose: 10 mg
	I.V.	6 mo - 5 y: 0.05-0.1; 6-12 y: 0.025-0.05; >12 y - Adult: 2.5-5 mg (total dose); give over 10-20 min	1-5	1-2	Maximum concentration: 1 mg/mL; maximum I.M./I.V. dose: 6 mo - 5 y: 6 mg 6 y - Adult: 10 mg
	P.R.	0.3	20-30	1-2	Dilute injection in 5 mL NS; administer rectally
	Intranasal	0.2-0.3	5	30-60 min	Administer nasally: Use a 1 mL needle-less syringe into the nares over 15 seconds; use 5 mg/mL concentration; ½ dose may be administered into each nare
Morphine	P.O.	0.2-0.5	20-30	3-5	
	I.M.	0.05-0.2	20-30	3-5	
	I.V.	0.05-0.2	10-15	2-5	

Note: See individual drug monographs for further information.

Sedatives Used to Produce Deep Sedation

Drug	Route	Dose (mg/kg)	Onset (min)	Duration (h)	Comments
Methohexital[8,9] (Brevital®)	I.M.	5-10	5	1-1.5	Maximum concentration for I.M./I.V.: 50 mg/mL; maximum I.M./I.V. dose: 200 mg. Greater incidence of adverse effects with I.V. use.
	I.V.	0.75-2	1	7-10 min	
	P.R.	20-35	5-10	1-1.5	Shorter duration of action than thiopental; rectal given as a 10% solution in sterile water; maximum dose rectal: 500 mg
Pentobarbital	P.O./ I.M./P.R.	2-6	10-25	1-4	Maximum I.M./I.V./P.O./P.R. dose: 100 mg
	I.V.	1-3	1	15 min	
Thiopental[10,4] (Pentothal)	I.V.	4-6	0.5-1	5-10 min	Variable rectal absorption; may use additional 12.5 mg/kg if necessary; maximum rectal dose: 1-1.5 g
	P.R.	25; immediately prior to procedure	10	1-5	

Note: See individual drug monographs for further information.

Sedatives Used to Produce Dissociative Anesthesia
(Monitor as if deep sedation)

Drug	Route	Dose (mg/kg)	Onset (min)	Duration	Comments
Ketamine	P.O.	6-10; 30 min prior	30-45	10-30	Use only under direct supervision of physicians experienced in administering general anesthetics; has analgesic effects; may use injectable product orally diluted in a beverage of the patient's choice
	I.M.	3-7	7	12-25	
	I.V.	0.5-2	1	5-10	

Note: See individual drug monographs for further information.

Footnotes

1. Committee on Drugs, Section of Anesthesiology, American Academy of Pediatrics, "Guidelines for Monitoring and Management of Pediatric Patient During and After Sedation for Diagnostic and Therapeutic Procedures," *Pediatrics*, 1992, 89:1110-5.
2. Yager JY and Seshia SS, "Sublingual Lorazepam in Childhood Serial Seizures," *Am J Dis Child*, 1988, 142(9):931-2.
3. Fell D, Gough MB, Northan AA, et al, "Diazepam Premedication in Children," *Anaesthesia*, 1985, 40:12-7.
4. Burckart GJ, White III TJ, Siegle RL, et al, "Rectal Thiopental Versus an Intramuscular Cocktail for Sedating Children Before Computer Tomography," *Am J Hosp Pharm*, 1980, 37:222-4.
5. Burtles R and Astley B, "Lorazepam in Children," *Br J Anaesth*, 1983, 55:275-9.
6. Roelofse JA, van der Bijl P, Stegmann DH, et al, "Preanesthetic Medication With Rectal Midazolam in Children Undergoing Dental Extractions," *J Oral Maxillofac Surg*, 1990, 48(8):791-7.
7. Wilton NC, Leigh J, Rosen DR, et al, "Preanesthetic Sedation of Preschool Children Using Intranasal Midazolam," *Anesthesiology*, 1988, 60(6):972-5.
8. Elman DS and Denson JS, "Preanesthetic Sedation of Children With Intramuscular Methohexital Sodium," *Anesth Analg*, 1965, 44(5):494-8.
9. Miller JR, Grayson M, and Stoelting VK, "Sedation With Intramuscular Methohexital Sodium," *Am J Ophthalmol*, 1966, 62(1):38-43.
10. "Drug Evaluations," *AMA*, 1980.

FEBRILE SEIZURES

A febrile seizure is defined as a seizure occurring for no reason other than an elevated temperature. It does not have an infectious or metabolic origin within the CNS (ie, it is not caused by meningitis or encephalitis). Fever is usually >102°F rectally, but the more rapid the rise in temperature, the more likely a febrile seizure may occur. About 4% of children develop febrile seizures at one time of their life, usually occurring between 3 months and 5 years of age with the majority occurring at 6 months to 3 years of age. There are three types of febrile seizures:

1. **Simple** febrile seizures are nonfocal febrile seizures of less than 15 minutes duration. They do not occur in multiples.

2. **Complex** febrile seizures are febrile seizures that are either focal, have a focal component, are longer than 15 minutes in duration, or are multiple febrile seizures that occur within 30 minutes.

3. **Febrile status epilepticus** is a febrile seizure that is a generalized tonic clonic seizure lasting longer than 30 minutes.

Note: Febrile seizures should not be confused with true epileptic seizures associated with fever or "seizure with fever." "Seizure with fever" includes seizures associated with acute neurologic illnesses (ie, meningitis, encephalitis).

Long-term prophylaxis with phenobarbital may reduce the risk of subsequent febrile seizures. The 1980 NIH Consensus paper stated that after the first febrile seizure, long-term prophylaxis should be considered under any of the following:

1. Presence of abnormal neurological development or abnormal neurological exam

2. Febrile seizure was complex in nature:

   duration >15 minutes

   focal febrile seizure

   followed by transient or persistent neurological abnormalities

3. Positive family history of afebrile seizures (epilepsy)

Also consider long-term prophylaxis in certain cases if:

1. the child has multiple febrile seizures

2. the child is <12 months of age

Anticonvulsant prophylaxis is usually continued for 2 years or 1 year after the last seizure, whichever is longer. With the identification of phenobarbital's adverse effects on learning and cognitive function, many physicians will not start long-term phenobarbital prophylaxis after the first febrile seizure unless the patient has more than one of the above risk factors. Most physicians would start long-term prophylaxis if the patient has a second febrile seizure.

Daily administration of phenobarbital and therapeutic phenobarbital serum concentrations ≥15 mcg/mL decrease recurrence rates of febrile seizures. Valproic acid is also effective in preventing recurrences of febrile seizures, but is usually reserved for patients who have significant adverse effects to phenobarbital. The administration of rectal diazepam (as a solution or suppository) at the time of the febrile illness has been shown to be as effective as daily phenobarbital in preventing recurrences of febrile seizures. These rectal dosage forms are just now available in the United States. Some centers in the USA are still using the injectable form of diazepam rectally. The solution for injection is filtered prior to use if drawn from an ampul. A recent study suggests that oral diazepam, 0.33 mg/kg/dose given every 8 hours only when the child has a fever, may reduce the risk of recurrent febrile seizures (see Rosman, et al). (**Note:** A more recent study by Uhari (1995) showed that lower doses of diazepam, 0.2 mg/kg/dose, were not effective.) Carbamazepine and phenytoin are **not** effective in preventing febrile seizures.

References

Berg AT, Shinnar S, Hauser WA, et al, "Predictors of Recurrent Febrile Seizures: A Meta-Analytic Review," *J Pediatr*, 1990, 116(3):329-37.

Camfield PR, Camfield CS, Gordon K, et al, "Prevention of Recurrent Febrile Seizures," *J Pediatr*, 1995, 126(6):929-30.

NIH Consensus Statement, "Febrile Seizures: A Consensus of Their Significance, Evaluation and Treatment," *Pediatrics*, 1980, 66(6):1009-12.

Rosman NP, Colton T, Labazzo J, et al, "A Controlled Trial of Diazepam Administration During Febrile Illnesses to Prevent Recurrence of Febrile Seizures," *N Engl J Med*, 1993, 329(2):79-84.

Uhari M, Rantala H, Vainionpää L, et al, "Effect of Acetaminophen and of Low Intermittent Doses of Diazepam on Prevention of Recurrences of Febrile Seizures," *J Pediatr*, 1995, 126(6):991-5.

CAUSES OF NEONATAL SEIZURES

1. Trauma
   a. subdural hematoma
   b. intracortical hemorrhage
   c. cortical vein thrombosis

2. Asphyxia — subependymal hemorrhage

3. Congenital abnormalities (cerebral dysgenesis)
   a. lissencephaly
   b. schizencephaly

4. Hypertension

5. Metabolic
   a. hypocalcemia
      - hypomagnesemia
      - high phosphate load
      - IDM (infants of diabetic mothers)
      - hypoparathyroidism
      - maternal hyperparathyroidism
      - idiopathic
      - DiGeorge's syndrome
   b. hypoglycemia
      - galactosemia
      - IUGR (intrauterine growth retardation)
      - IDM (infants of diabetic mothers)
      - glycogen storage disease
      - idiopathic
      - methylmalonic acidemia
      - propionic acidemia
      - maple syrup urine disease
      - asphyxia
   c. electrolyte imbalance
      - hypernatremia
      - hypomagnesemia
      - hyponatremia

6. Infections
   a. bacterial meningitis
   b. cerebral abscess
   c. herpes encephalitis
   d. Coxsackie meningoencephalitis
   e. cytomegalovirus
   f. toxoplasmosis
   g. syphilis

7. Drug withdrawal
   a. methadone
   b. heroin
   c. barbiturate (short-acting, such as secobarbital and butalbital)
   d. propoxyphene
   e. benzodiazepines (chlordiazepoxide, diazepam)
   f. cocaine
   g. ethanol
   h. codeine

8. Pyridoxine dependency

9. Amino acid disturbances
   a. maple syrup urine disease
   b. urea cycle abnormalities
   c. nonketotic hyperglycinemia
   d. ketotic hyperglycinemia
   e. Leigh disease
   f. isovaleric acidemia

10. Toxins
    a. local anesthetics
    b. isoniazid
    c. lead
    d. indomethacin (from breast feeding)
    e. fentanyl

11. Familial seizures
    a. neurocutaneous syndromes
       • tuberous sclerosis
       • incontinentia pigmenti
    b. genetic syndromes
       • Zellweger's
       • Smith Lemli Opitz
       • neonatal adrenoleukodystrophy
    c. benign familial epilepsy

12. Cerebral hemorrhage
    a. intraventricular
    b. subarachnoid
    c. subdural

Adapted from Painter MJ, Bergman I, and Crumrie P, "Neonatal Seizures," *Pediatr Clin North Am*, 1986, 33:91-107.

ANTIEPILEPTIC DRUGS

Antiepileptic Drugs for Children and Adolescents by Seizure Type and Epilepsy Syndrome

Seizure Type or Epilepsy Syndrome	First Line Therapy	Alternatives
Partial seizures (with or without secondary generalization)	Carbamazepine	Valproate, phenytoin, gabapentin, lamotrigine, vigabatrin, phenobarbital, primidone; consider clonazepam, clorazepate, acetazolamide
Generalized tonic-clonic seizures	Valproate or carbamazepine	Phenytoin, phenobarbital, primidone; consider clonazepam
Childhood absence epilepsy		
Before 10 years of age	Ethosuximide or valproate	Methsuximide, acetazolamide, clonazepam, lamotrigine
After 10 years of age	Valproate	Ethosuximide, methsuximide, acetazolamide, clonazepam, lamotrigine; consider adding carbamazepine, phenytoin, or phenobarbital for generalized tonic-clonic seizures if valproate not tolerated
Juvenile myoclonic epilepsy	Valproate	Phenobarbital, primidone, clonazepam; consider carbamazepine, phenytoin, methsuximide, acetazolamide
Progressive myoclonic epilepsy	Valproate	Valproate plus clonazepam, phenobarbital
Lennox-Gastaut and related syndromes	Valproate	Clonazepam, phenobarbital, lamotrigine, ethosuximide, felbamate; consider methsuximide, ACTH or steroids, pyridoxine, ketogenic diet
Infantile spasms	ACTH or steroids	Valproate; consider clonazepam, vigabatrin (especially with tuberous sclerosis), pyridoxine
Benign epilepsy of childhood with centrotemporal spikes	Carbamazepine or valproate	Phenytoin; consider phenobarbital, primidone
Neonatal seizures	Phenobarbital	Phenytoin; consider clonazepam, primidone, valproate, pyridoxine

Adapted from Bourgeois BFD, "Antiepileptic Drugs in Pediatric Practice," *Epilepsia*, 1995, 36(Suppl 2):S34-S45.

COMA SCALES

Glasgow Coma Scale

Activity	Best Response	Score
Eye opening	Spontaneous	4
	Responds to voice	3
	Responds to pain	2
	No response	1
Verbal Response	Oriented and appropriate	5
	Confused / disoriented conversation	4
	Inappropriate words	3
	Nonspecific sounds (incomprehensible)	2
	No response	1
Motor Response	Follows commands	6
	Localizes pain	5
	Withdraws to pain	4
	Abnormal flexion (decorticate posturing)	3
	Abnormal extension (decerebrate posturing)	2
	No response	1

Modified Coma Scale for Infants

Activity	Best Response	Score
Eye opening	Spontaneous	4
	Responds to voice	3
	Responds to pain	2
	No response	1
Verbal Response	Coos, babbles	5
	Irritable	4
	Cries to pain	3
	Moans to pain	2
	No response	1
Motor Response	Normal spontaneous movements	6
	Withdraws to touch	5
	Withdraws to pain	4
	Abnormal flexion (decorticate posturing)	3
	Abnormal extension (decerebrate posturing)	2
	No response	1

Interpretation of Coma Scale Scores
Maximum Score: 15; Minimum Score: 3
(low score indicates greater severity of coma)

Range of Score	Interpretation
3- 8	Coma. Severe brain injury. Immediate action needed. Notify ICU staff STAT. Will require intubation regardless of respiratory status.
9-12	Lethargic. Needs close observation in special care unit. Frequent neuro checks. Notify ICU staff.
13-14	Needs observation
15	Normal

References
James HE, "Neurologic Evaluation and Support in the Child With an Acute Brain Insult," *Pediatr Ann*, 1986, 15(1):16-22.
Jennett B and Teasdale G, "Aspects of Coma After Severe Head Injury," *Lancet*, 1977, 1(8017): 878-81.

ASTHMA

Expert Panel Report II: Guidelines for the Diagnosis and Management of Asthma

Stepwise Approach for Managing Asthma in Adults and Children >5 Years of Age: Classify Severity

Goals of Asthma Treatment

- Prevent chronic and troublesome symptoms (eg, coughing or breathlessness in the night, in the early morning, or after exertion)
- Maintain (near) "normal" pulmonary function
- Maintain normal activity levels (ie, exercise and other physical activity)
- Prevent recurrent exacerbations of asthma and minimize the need for emergency department visits or hospitalizations
- Provide optimal pharmacotherapy with minimal or no adverse effects
- Meet patients' and families' expectations of and satisfaction with asthma care

Clinical Features Before Treatment*

Symptoms**	Night-time Symptoms	Lung Function
STEP 4: Severe Persistent		
• Continual symptoms • Limited physical activity • Frequent exacerbations	Frequent	• FEV_1/PEF ≤60% predicted • PEF variability >30%
STEP 3: Moderate Persistent		
• Daily symptoms • Daily use of inhaled short-acting beta$_2$-agonist • Exacerbations affect activity • Exacerbations ≥2 times/week may last days	>1 time/week	• FEV_1/PEF >60% - <80% predicted • PEF variability >30%
STEP 2: Mild Persistent		
• Symptoms >2 times/week but <1 time/day • Exacerbations may affect activity	>2 times/month	• FEV_1/PEF ≥80% predicted • PEF variability 20% - 30%
STEP 1: Mild Intermittent		
• Symptoms ≤2 times/week • Asymptomatic and normal PEF between exacerbations • Exacerbations brief (from a few hours to a few days); intensity may vary	≤2 times/month	• FEV_1/PEF ≥80% predicted • PEF variability ≤20%

*The presence of one of the features of severity is sufficient to place a patient in that category. An individual should be assigned to the most severe grade in which any feature occurs. The characteristics noted in this figure are general and may overlap because asthma is highly variable. Furthermore, an individual's classification may change over time.

**Patients at any level of severity can have mild, moderate, or severe exacerbations. Some patients with intermittent asthma experience severe and life-threatening exacerbations separated by long periods of normal lung function and no symptoms.

Stepwise Approach for Managing Infants and Young Children (≤5 Years of Age) With Acute or Chronic Asthma Symptoms

Long-Term Control	Quick Relief
STEP 4: Severe Persistent	
Daily anti-inflammatory medicine • High-dose inhaled corticosteroid with spacer/holding chamber and face mask • If needed, add systemic corticosteroids 2 mg/kg/day and reduce to lowest daily or alternate-day dose that stabilizes symptoms	• Bronchodilator as needed for symptoms (see step 1) up to 3 times/day
STEP 3: Moderate Persistent	
Daily anti-inflammatory medication. Either: • Medium-dose inhaled corticosteroid with spacer/holding chamber and face mask **or** Once control is established: • Medium-dose inhaled corticosteroid and nedocromil **or** • Medium-dose inhaled corticosteroid and long-acting bronchodilator (theophylline)	• Bronchodilator as needed for symptoms (see step 1) up to 3 times/day
STEP 2: Mild Persistent	
Daily anti-inflammatory medication. Either: • Cromolyn (nebulizer is preferred; or MDI) or nedocromil (MDI only) tid-qid • Infants and young children usually begin with a trial of cromolyn or nedocromil **or** • Low-dose inhaled corticosteroid with spacer/holding chamber and face mask	• Bronchodilator as needed for symptoms (see step 1)
STEP 1: Mild Intermittent	
No daily medication needed	• Bronchodilator as needed for symptoms <2 times/week. Intensity of treatment will depend upon severity of exacerbation (see "Managing Exacerbations"). Either: – Inhaled short-acting beta$_2$-agonist by nebulizer or face mask and spacer/holding chamber **or** – Oral beta$_2$-agonist for symptoms • With viral respiratory infection: – Bronchodilator q4-6h up to 24 hours (longer with physician consult) but, in general, repeat no more than once every 6 weeks – Consider systemic corticosteroid if current exacerbation is severe **or** Patient has history of previous severe exacerbations

↓ **Step Down**
Review treatment every 1-6 months. If control is sustained for at least 3 months, a gradual stepwise reduction in treatment may be possible.

↑ **Step Up**
If control is not achieved, consider step up. First: review patient medication technique, adherence, and environmental control (avoidance of allergens or other precipitant factors)

ASTHMA *(Continued)*

Notes:

- **The stepwise approach presents guidelines to assist clinical decision making. Asthma is highly variable; clinicians should tailor specific medication plans to the needs and circumstances of individual patients.**

- Gain control as quickly as possible; then decrease treatment to the least medication necessary to maintain control. Gaining control may be accomplished by either starting treatment at the step most appropriate to the initial severity of their condition or by starting at a higher level of therapy (eg, a course of systemic corticosteroids or higher dose of inhaled corticosteroids).

- A rescue course of systemic corticosteroid (prednisolone) may be needed at any time and step.

- In general, use of short-acting beta$_2$-agonist on a daily basis indicates the need for additional long-term control therapy.

- It is important to remember that there are very few studies on asthma therapy for infants.

- Consultation with an asthma specialist is recommended for patients with moderate or severe persistent asthma in this age group. Consider consultation for all patients with mild persistent asthma.

Stepwise Approach for Managing Asthma in Adults and Children >5 Years of Age: Treatment

(Preferred treatments are in **bold** print)

Long-Term Control	Quick Relief	Education
STEP 4: Severe Persistent		
Daily medications: • **Anti-inflammatory: Inhaled corticosteroid (high dose)** **and** • Long-acting bronchodilator: Either **long-acting inhaled beta$_2$-agonist**, sustained-release theophylline, or long-acting beta$_2$-agonist tablets **and** • Corticosteroid tablets or syrup long term (2 mg/kg/day, generally do not exceed 60 mg per day).	• Short-acting bronchodilator: **Inhaled beta$_2$-agonists** as needed for symptoms. • Intensity of treatment will depend on severity of exacerbation; see "Managing Exacerbations" • Use of short-acting inhaled beta$_2$-agonists on a daily basis, or increasing use, indicates the need for additional long-term control therapy.	Steps 2 and 3 actions plus: • Refer to individual education/counseling

STEP 3: Moderate Persistent

Long-Term Control	Quick Relief	Education
Daily medication: • Either – **Anti-inflammatory: Inhaled corticosteroid (medium dose) or** – **Inhaled corticosteroid (low-medium dose)** and add a long-acting bronchodilator, especially for night-time symptoms: Either **long-acting inhaled beta$_2$-agonist**, sustained-release theophylline, or long-acting beta$_2$-agonist tablets. • If needed – **Anti-inflammatory: Inhaled corticosteroids (medium-high dose) and** – **Long-acting bronchodilator**, especially for nighttime symptoms; either **long-acting inhaled beta$_2$-agonist**, sustained release theophylline, or long-acting beta$_2$-agonist tablets.	• Short-acting bronchodilator: **Inhaled beta$_2$-agonists** as needed for symptoms. • Intensity of treatment will depend on severity of exacerbation; see "Managing Exacerbations." • Use of short-acting inhaled beta$_2$-agonists on a daily basis, or increasing use, indicates the need for additional long-term control therapy.	Step 1 actions plus: • Teach self-monitoring • Refer to group education if available • Review and update self-management plan

Long-Term Control	Quick Relief	Education

STEP 2: Mild Persistent

Long-Term Control	Quick Relief	Education
One daily medication: • **Anti-inflammatory:** Either **inhaled corticosteroid** (low doses) or **cromolyn or nedocromil** (children usually begin with a trial of cromolyn or nedocromil). • Sustained-release theophylline to serum concentration of 5-15 mcg/mL is an alternative, but not preferred, therapy. Zafirlukast or zileuton may also be considered for patients ≥12 years of age, although their position in therapy is not fully established.	• Short-acting bronchodilator: **Inhaled beta$_2$-agonists** as needed for symptoms. • Intensity of treatment will depend on severity of exacerbation; see "Managing Exacerbations." •Use of short-acting inhaled beta$_2$-agonists on a daily basis, or increasing use, indicates the need for additional long-term control therapy.	Step 1 actions plus: • Teach self-monitoring • Refer to group education if available • Review and update self-management plan

STEP 1: Mild Intermittent

Long-Term Control	Quick Relief	Education
No daily medication needed.	• Short-acting bronchodilator: **Inhaled beta$_2$-agonists** as needed for symptoms. • Intensity of treatment will depend on severity of exacerbation; see "Managing Exacerbations" • Use of short-acting inhaled beta$_2$-agonists more than 2 times/week may indicate the need to initiate long-term control therapy	• Teach basic facts about asthma • Teach inhaler/spacer/holding chamber technique • Discuss roles of medications •Develop self-management plan • Develop action plan for when and how to take rescue actions, especially for patients with a history of severe exacerbations • Discuss appropriate environmental control measures to avoid exposure to known allergens and irritants

ASTHMA *(Continued)*

↓ Step down
Review treatment every 1-6 months; a gradual stepwise reduction in treatment may be possible.

↑Step up
If control is not maintained, consider step up. First, review patient medication technique, adherence, and environmental control (avoidance of allergens or other factors that contribute to asthma severity.)

Notes:

- **The stepwise approach presents general guidelines to assist clinical decision making; it is not intended to be a specific prescription. Asthma is highly variable; clinicians should tailor specific medication plans to the needs and circumstances of individual patients.**

- Gain control as quickly as possible; then decrease treatment to the least medication necessary to maintain control. Gaining control may be accomplished by either starting treatment at the step most appropriate to the initial severity of the condition or starting at a higher level of therapy (eg, a course of systemic corticosteroids or higher dose of inhaled corticosteroids).

- A rescue course of systemic corticosteroids may be needed at any time and at any step.

- Some patients with intermittent asthma experience severe and life-threatening exacerbations separated by long periods of normal lung function and no symptoms. This may be especially common with exacerbations provoked by respiratory infections. A short course of systemic corticosteroids is recommended.

- At each step, patients should control their environment to avoid or control factors that make their asthma worse (eg, allergens, irritants); this requires specific diagnosis and education.

Management of Asthma Exacerbations: Home Treatment*

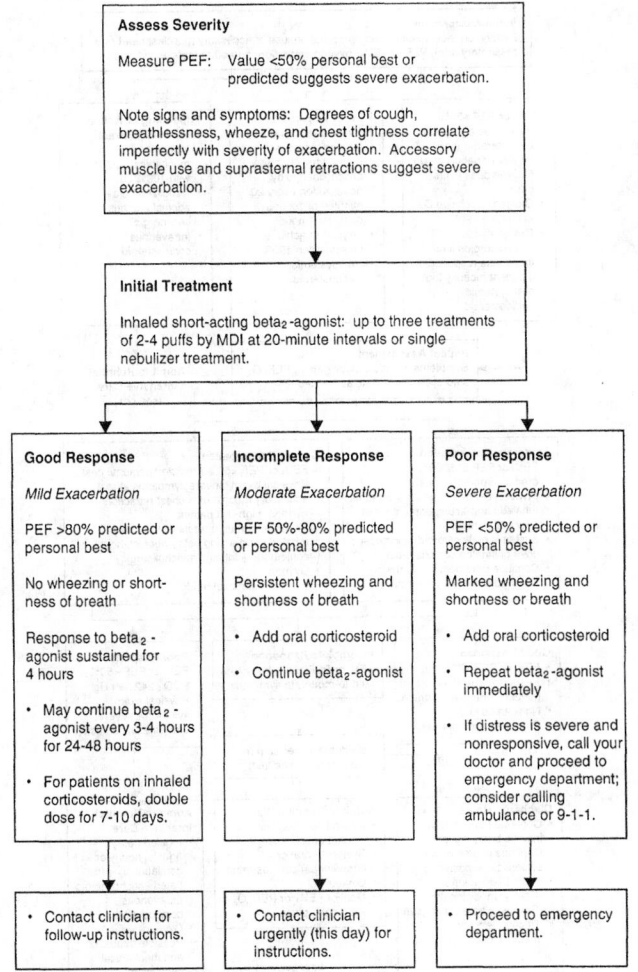

Assess Severity

Measure PEF: Value <50% personal best or predicted suggests severe exacerbation.

Note signs and symptoms: Degrees of cough, breathlessness, wheeze, and chest tightness correlate imperfectly with severity of exacerbation. Accessory muscle use and suprasternal retractions suggest severe exacerbation.

Initial Treatment

Inhaled short-acting beta₂-agonist: up to three treatments of 2-4 puffs by MDI at 20-minute intervals or single nebulizer treatment.

Good Response

Mild Exacerbation

PEF >80% predicted or personal best

No wheezing or shortness of breath

Response to beta₂-agonist sustained for 4 hours

- May continue beta₂-agonist every 3-4 hours for 24-48 hours

- For patients on inhaled corticosteroids, double dose for 7-10 days.

- Contact clinician for follow-up instructions.

Incomplete Response

Moderate Exacerbation

PEF 50%-80% predicted or personal best

Persistent wheezing and shortness of breath

- Add oral corticosteroid

- Continue beta₂-agonist

- Contact clinician urgently (this day) for instructions.

Poor Response

Severe Exacerbation

PEF <50% predicted or personal best

Marked wheezing and shortness or breath

- Add oral corticosteroid

- Repeat beta₂-agonist immediately

- If distress is severe and nonresponsive, call your doctor and proceed to emergency department; consider calling ambulance or 9-1-1.

- Proceed to emergency department.

*Patients at high risk of asthma-related death should receive immediate clinical attention after initial treatment. Additional therapy may be required.

ASTHMA (Continued)

Management of Asthma Exacerbations: Emergency Department and Hospital-Based Care

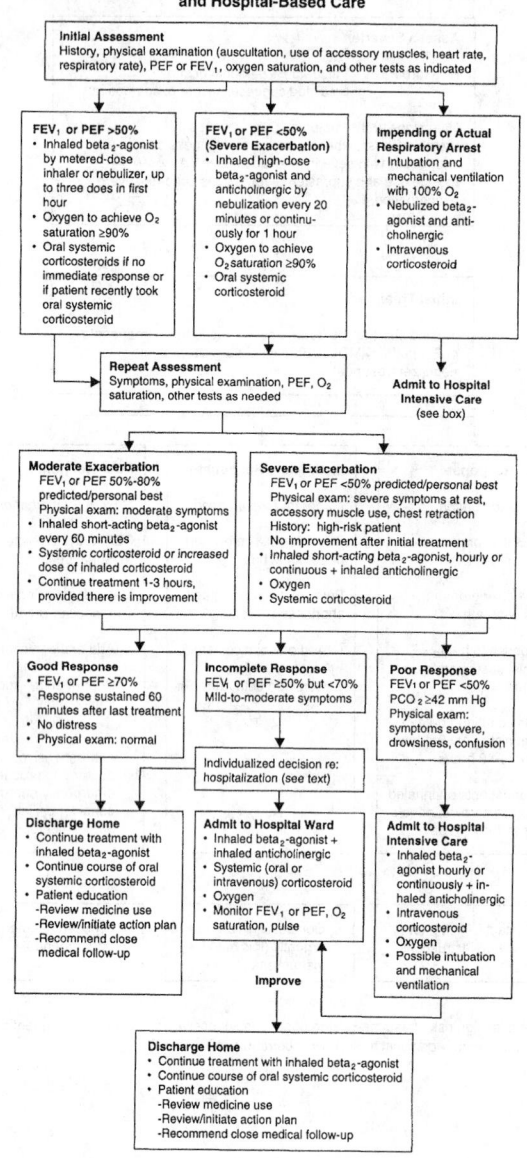

Initial Assessment
History, physical examination (auscultation, use of accessory muscles, heart rate, respiratory rate), PEF or FEV_1, oxygen saturation, and other tests as indicated

FEV_1 or PEF >50%
- Inhaled beta$_2$-agonist by metered-dose inhaler or nebulizer, up to three does in first hour
- Oxygen to achieve O_2 saturation ≥90%
- Oral systemic corticosteroids if no immediate response or if patient recently took oral systemic corticosteroid

FEV_1 or PEF <50% (Severe Exacerbation)
- Inhaled high-dose beta$_2$-agonist and anticholinergic by nebulization every 20 minutes or continuously for 1 hour
- Oxygen to achieve O_2 saturation ≥90%
- Oral systemic corticosteroid

Impending or Actual Respiratory Arrest
- Intubation and mechanical ventilation with 100% O_2
- Nebulized beta$_2$-agonist and anticholinergic
- Intravenous corticosteroid

Repeat Assessment
Symptoms, physical examination, PEF, O_2 saturation, other tests as needed

Admit to Hospital Intensive Care (see box)

Moderate Exacerbation
FEV_1 or PEF 50%-80% predicted/personal best
Physical exam: moderate symptoms
- Inhaled short-acting beta$_2$-agonist every 60 minutes
- Systemic corticosteroid or increased dose of inhaled corticosteroid
- Continue treatment 1-3 hours, provided there is improvement

Severe Exacerbation
FEV_1 or PEF <50% predicted/personal best
Physical exam: severe symptoms at rest, accessory muscle use, chest retraction
History: high-risk patient
No improvement after initial treatment
- Inhaled short-acting beta$_2$-agonist, hourly or continuous + inhaled anticholinergic
- Oxygen
- Systemic corticosteroid

Good Response
- FEV_1 or PEF ≥70%
- Response sustained 60 minutes after last treatment
- No distress
- Physical exam: normal

Incomplete Response
FEV_1 or PEF ≥50% but <70%
Mild-to-moderate symptoms

Individualized decision re: hospitalization (see text)

Poor Response
FEV_1 or PEF <50%
PCO_2 ≥42 mm Hg
Physical exam: symptoms severe, drowsiness, confusion

Discharge Home
- Continue treatment with inhaled beta$_2$-agonist
- Continue course of oral systemic corticosteroid
- Patient education
  -Review medicine use
  -Review/initiate action plan
  -Recommend close medical follow-up

Admit to Hospital Ward
- Inhaled beta$_2$-agonist + inhaled anticholinergic
- Systemic (oral or intravenous) corticosteroid
- Oxygen
- Monitor FEV_1 or PEF, O_2 saturation, pulse

Admit to Hospital Intensive Care
- Inhaled beta$_2$-agonist hourly or continuously + inhaled anticholinergic
- Intravenous corticosteroid
- Oxygen
- Possible intubation and mechanical ventilation

Improve

Discharge Home
- Continue treatment with inhaled beta$_2$-agonist
- Continue course of oral systemic corticosteroid
- Patient education
  -Review medicine use
  -Review/initiate action plan
  -Recommend close medical follow-up

ESTIMATED COMPARATIVE DAILY DOSAGES FOR INHALED CORTICOSTEROIDS

Children

Drug	Low Dose	Medium Dose	High Dose
Beclomethasone dipropionate 42 mcg/puff 84 mcg/puff	84-336 mcg (2-8 puffs)	336-672 mcg (8-16 puffs)	>672 mcg (>16 puffs)
Budesonide Turbuhaler 200 mcg/dose	100-200 mcg	200-400 mcg (1-2 inhalations – 200 mcg)	>400 mcg (>2 inhalations – 200 mcg)
Flunisolide 250 mcg/puff	500-750 mcg (2-3 puffs)	1000-1250 mcg (4-5 puffs)	>1250 mcg (>5 puffs)
Fluticasone Metered dose inhaler: 44, 110, 220 mcg/puff	88-176 mcg (2-4 puffs – 44 mcg)	176-440 mcg (4-10 puffs – 44 mcg) or (2-4 puffs – 110 mcg)	>440 mcg (>4 puffs – 110 mcg)
Dry powder inhaler: 50, 100, 250 mcg/dose	(2-4 inhalations – 50 mcg)	(2-4 inhalations – 100 mcg)	(>4 inhalations – 100 mcg)
Triamcinolone acetonide 100 mcg/puff	400-800 mcg (4-8 puffs)	800-1200 mcg (8-12 puffs)	>1200 mcg (>12 puffs)

Adults

Drug	Low Dose	Medium Dose	High Dose
Beclomethasone dipropionate 42 mcg/puff 84 mcg/puff	168-504 mcg (4-12 puffs – 42 mcg) (2-6 puffs – 84 mcg)	504-840 mcg (12-20 puffs – 42 mcg) (6-10 puffs – 84 mcg)	>840 mcg (>20 puffs – 42 mcg) (>10 puffs – 84 mcg)
Budesonide Turbuhaler 200 mcg/dose	200-400 mcg (1-2 inhalations)	400-600 mcg (2-3 inhalations)	>600 mcg (>3 inhalations)
Flunisolide 250 mcg/puff	500-1000 mcg (2-4 puffs)	1000-2000 mcg (4-8 puffs)	>2000 mcg (>8 puffs)
Fluticasone Metered dose inhaler: 44, 110, 220 mcg/puff	88-264 mcg (2-6 puffs – 44 mcg) or (2 puffs – 110 mcg)	264-660 mcg (2-6 puffs – 110 mcg)	>660 mcg (>6 puffs – 110 mcg) or (>3 puffs – 220 mcg)
Dry powder inhaler: 50, 100, 250 mcg/dose	(2-6 inhalations – 50 mcg)	(3-6 inhalations – 100 mcg)	(>6 inhalations – 100 mcg)
Triamcinolone acetonide 100 mcg/puff	400-1000 mcg (4-10 puffs)	1000-2000 mcg (10-20 puffs)	>2000 mcg (>20 puffs)

ASTHMA *(Continued)*

Notes:

- **The most important determinant of appropriate dosing is the clinician's judgment of the patient's response to therapy.** The clinician must monitor the patient's response on several clinical parameters and adjust the dose accordingly. The stepwise approach to therapy emphasizes that once control of asthma is achieved, the dose of mediation should be carefully titrated to the minimum dose required to maintain control, thus reducing the potential for adverse effect.

- The reference point for the range in the dosages for children is data on the safety on inhaled corticosteroids in children, which, in general, suggest that the dose ranges are equivalent to beclomethasone dipropionate 200-400 mcg/day (low dose), 400-800 mcg/day (medium dose), and >800 mcg/day (high dose).

- Some dosages may be outside package labeling.

- Metered-dose inhaler (MDI) dosages are expressed as the actuator dose (the amount of drug leaving the actuator and delivered to the patient), which is the labeling required in the United States. This is different from the dosage expressed as the valve dose (the amount of drug leaving the valve, all of which is not available to the patient), which is used in many European countries and in some of the scientific literature. Dry powder inhaler (DPI) doses (eg, Turbuhaler) are expressed as the amount of drug in the inhaler following activation.

ESTIMATED CLINICAL COMPARABILITY OF DOSES FOR INHALED CORTICOSTEROIDS

Data from *in vitro* and in clinical trials suggest that the different inhaled corticosteroid preparations are not equivalent on a per puff or microgram basis. However, it is not entirely clear what implications these differences have for dosing recommendations in clinical practice because there are few data directly comparing the preparations. Relative dosing for clinical comparability is affected by differences in topical potency, clinical effects at different doses, delivery device, and bioavailability. The Expert Panel developed recommended dose ranges for different preparations based on available data and the following assumptions and cautions about estimating relative doses needed to achieve comparable clinical effect.

- **Relative topical potency using human skin blanching**

  - Standard test for determining relative topical anti-inflammatory potency is the topical vasoconstriction (MacKenzie skin blanching) test.

  - The MacKenzie topical skin blanching test correlates with binding affinities and binding half-lives for human lung corticosteroid receptors (see following table) (Dahlberg, et al, 1984; Hogger and Rohdewald 1994).

  - The relationship between relative topical anti-inflammatory effect and clinical comparability in asthma management is not certain. However, recent clinical trials suggest that different *in vitro* measures of anti-inflammatory effect is not certain. However, recent clinical trials suggest that different in vitro measures of anti-inflammatory effect correlate with clinical efficacy (Barnes and Pedersen 1993; Johnson 1996; Kamada, et al, 1996; Ebden, et al, 1986; Leblanc, et al, 1994; Gustaffson, et al, 1993; Lundback, et al, 1993; Barnes, et al, 1993; Fabbri, et al, 1993; Langdon and Capsey, 1994; Ayres, et al, 1995; Rafferty, et al, 1985; Bjorkander, et al, 1982, Stiksa, et al, 1982; Willey, et al, 1982.)

Medication	Topical Potency (Skin Blanching)*	Corticosteroid Receptor Binding Half-Life	Receptor Binding Affinity
Beclomethasone dipropionate (BDP)	600	7.5 hours	13.5
Budesonide (BUD)	980	5.1 hours	9.4
Flunisolide (FLU)	330	3.5 hours	1.8
Fluticasone propionate (FP)	1200	10.5 hours	18.0
Triamcinolone acetonide (TAA)	330	3.9 hours	3.6

*Numbers are assigned in reference to dexamethasone, which has a value of "1" in the MacKenzie test.

- **Relative doses to achieve similar clinical effects**

  - Clinical effects are evaluated by a number of outcome parameters (eg, changes in spirometry, peak flow rates, symptom scores, quick-relief $beta_2$-agonist use, frequency of exacerbations, airway responsiveness).

  - The daily dose and duration of treatment may affect these outcome parameters differently (eg, symptoms and peak flow may improve at lower doses and over a shorter treatment time than bronchial reactivity) (van Essen-Zandvliet, et al, 1992; Haahtela, et al, 1991)

  - Delivery systems influence comparability. For example, the delivery device for budesonide (Turbuhaler) delivers approximately twice the amount of drug to the airway as the MDI, thus enhancing the clinical effect (Thorsson, et al, 1994); Agertoft and Pedersen, 1993).

  - Individual patients may respond differently to different preparations, as noted by clinical experience.

  - Clinical trials comparing effects in reducing symptoms and improving peak expiratory flow demonstrate:

  - BDP amd BUD achieved comparable effects at similar microgram doses by MDI (Bjorkander, et al, 1982; Ebden, et al, 1986; Rafferty, et al, 1985).

  - BDP achieved effects similar to twice the dose of TAA on a microgram basis.

Reference
National Asthma Education and Prevention Program, February 1997

NORMAL RESPIRATORY RATES

Hour After Birth	Average Respiratory Rate	Range
1st hour	60 breaths per minute	20-100
2-6 hours	50 breaths per minute	20-80
>6 hours	30-40 breaths per minute	20-60

Age (years)	Mean RR (breaths/minute)
0-2	25-30
3-9	20-25
10-18	16-20

BLOOD LEVEL SAMPLING TIME GUIDELINES

Drug	Infusion Time	Therapeutic Range	When to Draw Levels
Amikacin sulfate			
I.V.	30 min	Peak: 20-30 µg/mL	Peak: 30 min after end of 30 min infusion
		Trough: <10 µg/mL	Trough: Within 30 min before next dose
I.M.			Peak: 1 h after I.M. injection
			Trough: Within 30 min before next dose
Carbamazepine		4-12 µg/mL	Just before next dose
Chloramphenicol			
I.V.	30 min	Peak: 15-25 µg/mL	Peak: 90 min after end of 30 min infusion
			Trough: Just before next dose
P.O.			Peak: 2 h post-P.O. dose
Cyclosporine			
I.V./P.O.		BMT 100-200 ng/mL	Just before next dose
		Liver transplant 200-300 ng/mL	
		Renal transplant 100-200 ng/mL	
Digoxin			
I.V./P.O.		Age and disease related: 0.8-2 ng/mL	6 h postdose to just before next dose
Ethosuximide			
P.O.		40-100 µg/mL	Just before next dose
Flucytosine			
P.O.		25-100 µg/mL	Peak: 2 h postdose after at least 4 d of therapy
Fosphenytoin (measure phenytoin levels)			
I.V.		Phenytoin: 10-20 µg/mL	Peak: 2 h after end of an infusion
I.M.			Peak: 4 h after I.M. injection
Gentamicin			
I.V.	30 min	Peak: 4-10 µg/mL	Peak: 30 min after end of 30 min infusion
		Trough: 0.5-2 µg/mL	Trough: Within 30 min before next dose
I.M.			Peak: 1 h after I.M. injection
			Trough: Within 30 min before next dose
Phenobarbital		15-40 µg/mL	Trough: Just before next dose
Phenytoin			
P.O., I.V.		10-20 µg/mL	Trough: Just before next dose
I.V.			Post-load/Peak: 1 h after end of infusion
Theophylline			
I.V. bolus	30 min	10-20 µg/mL	Peak: 30 min after end of 30 min infusion
Continuous infusion			16-24 h after the start or change in a constant I.V. infusion

BLOOD LEVEL SAMPLING TIME GUIDELINES
(Continued)

Drug	Infusion Time	Therapeutic Range	When to Draw Levels
P.O. liquid, fast-release tablet (Somophyllin®, Slo-Phyllin® liquid & tablet)			Peak: 1 h postdose Trough: Just before next dose
P.O. slow-release (Theo-Dur®, Slo-Phyllin® GC, Slo-bid®)			Peak: 4 h postdose Trough: Just before next dose
Tobramycin			
I.V.	30 min	Peak: 4-10 µg/mL	Peak: 30 min after end of 30 min infusion
		Trough: 0.5-2 µg/mL	Trough: Within 30 min before next dose
I.M.			Peak: 1 h post-I.M. injection
			Trough: Within 30 min before next dose
Trimethoprim			
I.V., dose 20 mg/kg	60 min	Peak: 5-10 µg/mL	Peak: 30 min after end of 60 min infusion
I.V., dose 8-10 mg/kg		Peak 1-3 µg/mL	
P.O.			Peak: 1 h postdose
Valproic acid			
P.O.		50-100 µg/mL	Trough: Just before next dose
Vancomycin	60 min	Peak: 25-40 µg/mL	Peak: 20-30 min after end of 60 min infusion*
		Trough: 5-15 µg/mL	Trough: Within 30 min before next dose

*Some institutions may draw vancomycin peak 1 hour after 1-hour infusion and accept the lower range of therapeutic.

OVERDOSE AND TOXICOLOGY*

Drug or Drug Class	Signs/Symptoms	Treatment/Comments
Acetaminophen	Nausea, vomiting, diaphoresis, delirium, fever, coma, vascular collapse, hepatic necrosis, transient azotemia, renal tubular necrosis	Assess severity of ingestion; doses ≥150 mg/kg for children and 7.5 g for adults are thought to be toxic. Obtain serum concentration ≥4 hours postingestion and use acetaminophen nomogram to evaluate need for acetylcysteine. Empty stomach with ipecac (if <1 hour postingestion) or gastric lavage. May administer activated charcoal for one dose, this may decrease absorption of acetylcysteine if given within 1 hour of acetylcysteine. For unknown ingested quantities and for significant ingestion, give acetylcysteine orally (diluted 1:4 with juice or carbonated beverage); initial: 140 mg/kg then give 70 mg/kg every 4 hours for 17 doses.
Alpha-adrenergic blocking agents	Hypotension, drowsiness	Induce emesis, give activated charcoal, additional treatment is symptomatic; use I.V. fluids, dopamine, or ephedrine to treat hypotension. Epinephrine may worsen hypotension due to beta effects.
Aminoglycosides	Ototoxicity, nephrotoxicity, neuromuscular toxicity	Hemodialysis or peritoneal dialysis may be useful in patients with decreased renal function.
Anticholinergics, antihistamines	Coma, hallucinations, delirium, tachycardia, dry skin, urinary retention, dilated pupils	For life-threatening arrhythmias or seizures physostigmine may be used. See Physostigmine monograph on page 768 for dosage recommendation.
Anticholinesterase agents	Nausea, vomiting, diarrhea, miosis, CNS depression, excessive salivation, excessive sweating, muscle weakness	Suction oral secretions, decontaminate skin, atropinize patient; atropine dose must be individualized. Infants and children: Initial dose: 0.01-0.02 mg/kg/dose; may need to increase as high as 0.05 mg/kg. Adults: Initial atropine dose: 1 mg; may need to increase to 2-5 mg/dose; pralidoxime (2-PAM) may need to be added for severe intoxications.
Barbiturates	Respiratory depression, circulatory collapse, bradycardia, hypotension, hypothermia, slurred speech, confusion	Repeated oral doses of activated charcoal given every 3-6 hours will increase clearance: Children: 1-2 g/kg/dose; adults: 30-60 g. Assure GI motility, adequate hydration, and renal function. Urinary alkalinization with I.V. sodium bicarbonate will increase renal elimination of longer-acting barbiturates (eg, phenobarbital).
Benzodiazepines	Respiratory depression, apnea, hypoactive reflexes, hypotension, slurred speech, unsteady gait, coma	For comatose patient, use gastric lavage with endotracheal tube in place to prevent aspiration; flumazenil, a benzodiazepine antagonist, can be used to reverse the effects of benzodiazepines. See Flumazenil monograph on page 421 for dose. Action of flumazenil may be shorter than duration of benzodiazepine; repeat doses as needed. Norepinephrine, phenylephrine, or dopamine may be used to treat hypotension; dialysis is of limited value; support blood pressure and respiration.

OVERDOSE AND TOXICOLOGY* *(Continued)*

Drug or Drug Class	Signs/Symptoms	Treatment/Comments
Beta-adrenergic blockers	Hypotension, bronchospasm, bradycardia, hyperglycemia, or hypoglycemia	Induce emesis, followed by activated charcoal; treat symptomatically; glucagon, atropine, isoproterenol, or cardiac pacing may be needed to treat bradycardia, conduction defects, or hypotension
Carbamazepine	Dizziness, drowsiness, ataxia, involuntary movements, opisthotonos, seizures, nausea, vomiting, agitation, nystagmus, coma, urinary retention, respiratory depression, tachycardia	Use supportive therapy, general poisoning management as needed; use repeated oral doses of activated charcoal given every 3-6 hours to decrease serum concentrations; children 1-2 g/kg/dose, adults: 30-60 g/dose; charcoal hemoperfusion may be needed; treat hypotension with I.V. fluids, dopamine, or norepinephrine; monitor EKG; diazepam may control convulsions but may exacerbate respiratory depression
Cardiac glycosides	Hyperkalemia may develop rapidly and result in life-threatening cardiac arrhythmias, progressive bradyarrhythmias, 2nd or 3rd degree heart block unresponsive to atropine, ventricular fibrillation, asystole	Obtain serum drug level, induce emesis or perform gastric lavage; give activated charcoal to reduce further absorption; atropine may reverse heart block, phenytoin will improve A-V conduction; digoxin immune Fab (digoxin specific antibody fragments) is used in life-threatening cases, each 38 mg of digoxin immune Fab binds with 0.5 mg of digoxin or digitoxin; see Digoxin Immune Fab monograph *on page 320* for dosing recommendations
Heparin	Severe hemorrhage	1 mg of protamine sulfate will neutralize approximately 90 units of heparin sodium (bovine) or 115 units of heparin sodium (porcine) or 100 units of heparin calcium (porcine)
Hydantoin derivatives	Nausea, vomiting, nystagmus, slurred speech, ataxia, coma	Gastric lavage or emesis; repeated oral doses of activated charcoal may increase clearance of phenytoin. Children: 1-2 g/kg/dose, adults: 30-60 g/dose activated charcoal every 3-6 hours until nontoxic serum concentration is obtained; assure adequate GI motility, supportive therapy; dialysis may be helpful.
Iron	Lethargy, nausea, vomiting, green or tarry stools, hypotension, weak rapid pulse, metabolic acidosis, shock, coma, hepatic necrosis, renal failure, local GI erosions	Induce emesis if awake or lavage with saline solution; give deferoxamine mesylate I.V. at 15 mg/kg/hour in cases of severe poisoning (serum Fe >350 mcg/mL) and continue chelation therapy for 24 hours after child is excreting normal color urine; urine output should be maintained at >2 mL/kg/hour to avoid hypovolemic shock
Isoniazid	Nausea, vomiting, blurred vision, CNS depression, intractable seizures, coma, metabolic acidosis	Control seizures with diazepam; if suspected ingestion of >80 mg/kg, give pyridoxine I.V. equal dose to the suspected overdose of isoniazid; lavage after seizure control is reached; force diuresis with I.V. fluids; hemo- or peritoneal dialysis may be beneficial in severe cases
Nonsteroidal anti-inflammatory drugs	Dizziness, abdominal pain, sweating, apnea, nystagmus, cyanosis, hypotension, coma	Induce emesis; give activated charcoal via NG tube; provide symptomatic and supportive care.

Drug or Drug Class	Signs/Symptoms	Treatment/Comments
Opiates and morphine analogs	Respiratory depression, miosis, hypothermia, bradycardia, circulatory collapse, pulmonary edema, apnea	Establish airway and adequate ventilation; give naloxone 0.1 mg/kg for children up to 5 years of age or 20 kg; for those >5 years or 20 kg give 2 mg naloxone; repeat doses every 2-3 minutes if needed; additional doses may be needed every 20-60 minutes. May need to institute continuous infusion, as duration of action of opiates can be longer than duration of action of naloxone.
Phenothiazines	Deep, unarousable sleep, anticholinergic symptoms, extrapyramidal signs, diaphoresis, rigidity, tachycardia, cardiac dysrhythmias, hypotension, or hypertension	Emesis or gastric lavage; do **not** dialyze; use I.V. benztropine mesylate 0.02-0.05 mg/kg/dose or for adults 1-2 mg/dose slowly over 3-6 minutes for extrapyramidal signs; use loading dose of phenytoin 10-15 mg/kg slow I.V. push for ventricular dysrhythmias; use I.V. fluids and norepinephrine or phenylephrine to treat hypotension; avoid epinephrine which may cause hypotension due to phenothiazine-induced alpha-adrenergic blockade and unopposed epinephrine B_2 action; dantrolene orally 0.5 mg/kg/dose every 12 hours may help with the rigidity
Salicylates	Nausea, vomiting, respiratory alkalosis, hyperthermia, dehydration, hyperapnea, tinnitus, headache, dizziness, metabolic acidosis, coma	Induce emesis or gastric lavage immediately; give charcoal with cathartic via NG tube; correct fluid imbalance by giving D_5LR at 10-20 mL/kg/hour for 1-2 hours, more rapid fluid resuscitation may be needed for patients in shock; use sodium bicarbonate to correct metabolic acidosis and enhance renal elimination by alkalinizing the urine; give supplemental potassium after renal function has been determined to be adequate. Monitor electrolytes; obtain serum salicylate level ≥6 hours postingestion; use poisoning nomogram to assess the significance of the ingestion and the need for more aggressive measures.
Tricyclic antidepressants	Agitation, confusion, hallucinations, urinary retention, hypothermia, hypotension, tachycardia, arrhythmias, widened QRS complex, prolonged PR intervals	Maintain normal temperature; correct acidosis with sodium bicarbonate to *increase protein binding and decrease free fraction*; correction of acidosis may decrease cardiovascular toxicities; avoid disopyramide, procainamide, and quinidine; lidocaine, phenytoin or propranolol may be necessary; reserve physostigmine for refractory life-treating anticholinergic toxicities. For life-threatening arrhythmias or seizures: Children: I.V., slow: Physostigmine 0.01-0.03 mg/kg/dose up to 0.5 mg/dose over 2-3 minutes, repeat in 5 minutes (maximum total dose is 2 mg). Adolescents and adults: 2 mg/dose physostigmine, may repeat 1-2 mg in 20 minutes and give 1-4 mg slow I.V. over 5-10 minutes if signs and symptoms recur.
Warfarin	Internal or external hemorrhage, hematuria	For moderate overdoses, give oral or I.V. phytonadione; for severe hemorrhage, give fresh frozen plasma or whole blood

OVERDOSE AND TOXICOLOGY* *(Continued)*

Drug or Drug Class	Signs/Symptoms	Treatment/Comments
Xanthine derivatives	Vomiting, abdominal pain, bloody diarrhea, tachycardia, extrasystoles, tachypnea, tonic/clonic seizures	Induce emesis, except in a convulsive patient; give activated charcoal orally; repeated oral doses of activated charcoal may increase clearance; children: 1-2 g/kg/dose, adults: 30-60 g/dose of activated charcoal every 3-6 hours until nontoxic serum concentrations are obtained. Assure adequate GI motility, supportive therapy; charcoal hemoperfusion can also be effective in decreasing serum concentrations.

*As for all overdoses and toxic ingestions, provide airway, breathing, and cardiac support; use appropriate general poisoning management and give general supportive therapy when needed (eg, I.V. fluids, blood pressure support, control seizures, etc). Consult more specific toxicology references (eg, Leikin JB and Paloucek FP, *Poisoning & Toxicology Handbook*, Hudson, OH: Lexi-Comp Inc, 1998, and Poisondex®) for further information.

COMMONLY USED ANTIDOTES FOR ACUTE OVERDOSES

While certain drugs may modify symptoms produced by a toxin, only a relatively few toxins have specific antidotes. The purpose of this chart is to identify those drugs, non-medicinal chemicals, plants, snakes, and spiders to which specific antidotes exist. Please refer to the specific monograph for dosing information. This information does not preclude the use of "conventional" therapeutic modalities for the treatment of intoxication (eg, emesis, lavage, charcoal, etc).

Poisoning Agent	Antidote(s)	Indications	Comments
Chemicals, Nonmedicinal			
Arsenic	Dimercaprol (BAL in Oil®)	• Symptomatic arsenic exposure	• Monitor for hypertension, tachycardia, hyperpyrexia, and urticaria • Pretreatment with diphenhydramine may diminish side effects
Calcium oxide	Edetate calcium disodium (EDTA) (Calcium Disodium Versenate®)	• Eye exposure from calcium oxide	• Immediate irrigation with saline followed by an irrigation with 0.01-0.05 M EDTA solution for at least 15 minutes
Carbon monoxide	Oxygen	• Any suspected carbon monoxide intoxication • Hyperbaric oxygen for any patient with signs and symptoms of severe intoxication regardless of the carboxyhemoglobin concentration • Patients with ischemic heart disease, acute ECG changes, anemia, seizure history, or pregnancy should receive hyperbaric oxygen if the carboxy hemoglobin (COHB) >20% or if any acute symptoms are present	
Carbamate insecticides	Atropine	• Symptomatic bradycardia • Myoclonic seizures, severe hallucinations, weakness, arrhythmias, excessive salivation, involuntary urination and defecation	• Caution should be used in patients with narrow-angle glaucoma, cardiovascular disease, or pregnancy • Plasma and/or erythrocyte cholinesterase levels will be depressed from normal
Copper	Penicillamine (Cuprimine®, Depen®)	• Symptomatic copper intoxication	• Little experience with chelation therapy in the setting of acute ingestion
Cyanide	Amyl nitrite, sodium nitrite, sodium thiosulfate (cyanide antidote kit)	• Begin treatment at the first sign of toxicity if exposure is known or strongly expected	• Do not use methylene blue to reduce elevated methemoglobin levels • Oxygen therapy may be useful when combined with sodium thiosulfate therapy

COMMONLY USED ANTIDOTES FOR ACUTE OVERDOSES *(Continued)*

Poisoning Agent	Antidote(s)	Indications	Comments
Ethylene glycol	Ethanol **OR** Fomepizole (Antizol®)	• Ingestion of >0.25 mL/kg ethylene glycol • Ethylene glycol serum level >20 mg/dL • History or strong clinical suspicion of ingestion and at least two of the following criteria: Arterial pH <7.3 Serum bicarbonate <20 mEq/L Osmolality gap >10 mosm/L Urinary oxalate crystals present	• Goal: Blood ethanol concentration at least 100 mg/dL (22 mmol/L) • Indications for use of fomepizole over ethanol: Ingestion of multiple substances resulting in depressed level of consciousness, altered consciousness, lack of adequate intensive care staffing or laboratory support to monitor ethanol, critically-ill patient with anion gap metabolic acidosis of unknown origin and potential exposure to ethylene glycol, or patients with active hepatic disease • Continue therapy until ethylene glycol level <10 mg/dL • Monitor blood glucose especially in children as ethanol may cause hypoglycemia
Hydrazine	Pyridoxine (Vitamin B_6)	• Antidote for seizures and coma	
Hydrofluoric acid (HF)	Calcium gluconate	• Dermal burns (topical treatment with calcium gluconate gel for dermal exposures of HF <20% concentration) •S.C. injections of calcium gluconate for dermal exposures of HF >20% concentration or failure to respond to calcium gluconate gel	• Oral calcium also used as fluoride-binding agent following oral ingestion • Hypocalcemia occurs frequently following oral ingestion and dermal exposure • Topical calcium gels are not available commercially in U.S.; may be compounded; see Extemporaneous Preparations, Calcium Supplements *on page 157* •Injections of calcium gluconate should not be used in digital area
Hydrogen sulfide	Amyl nitrite **AND** Sodium nitrite	• Severe anoxia, if therapy can be started early – within one hour of exposure	• Do **NOT** use sodium thiosulfate

Poisoning Agent	Antidote(s)	Indications	Comments
Lead	Edetate calcium disodium (EDTA) (Calcium Disodium Versenate®) **with or without** Dimercaprol (BAL in Oil®)	Use both calcium EDTA and BAL: • Symptoms of lead encephalopathy and/or blood lead level >70 mcg/dL • Symptomatic without encephalopathy or asymptomatic with blood lead level >70 µg/dL Use only EDTA for: • Asymptomatic with blood lead level 45-69 µg/dL	• Do not confuse or interchange therapy of **calcium** disodium edetate with disodium edetate (Chealamide®, Disotate®, Endrate®) – tetany and possibly fatal hypocalcemia may occur • Calcium EDTA should only be administered after adequate urine flow is established • If urine flow is not established, hemodialysis must accompany calcium EDTA dosing
	Succimer (Chemet®)	• Lead level >45 µg/dL in patients without encephalopathy or protracted vomiting	• Do not use with calcium disodium edetate or BAL
Manganese	Edetate calcium disodium (EDTA) (Calcium Disodium Versenate®)		• Do not confuse or interchange therapy of **calcium** disodium edetate with disodium edetate (Chealamide®, Disotate®, Endrate®) – tetany and possibly fatal hypocalcemia may occur • Calcium EDTA should only be administered after adequate urine flow is established
Methanol	Ethanol **OR** Fomepizole (Antizol®)	• Anion gap metabolic acidosis associated with a history of methanol ingestion • Methanol blood level >20 mg/dL (6.2 mmoles/L) • Any symptomatic patient with a history of methanol ingestion	• Goal: Ethanol blood level 100-130 mg/dL (22-28 mmoles/L) • Continue therapy until methanol blood level <10 mg/dL • Fomepizole therapy is considered investigational
Organophosphate insecticides	Atropine Pralidoxime (2-PAM, Protopam®)	• Symptomatic bradycardia • Myoclonic seizures, severe hallucinations, weakness, arrhythmias, excessive salivation, involuntary urination and defecation	• Caution should be used in patients with narrow-angle glaucoma, cardiovascular disease, or pregnancy •Most effective when used in initial 24-36 hours after exposure • Plasma and/or erythrocyte cholinesterase levels will be depressed from normal

COMMONLY USED ANTIDOTES FOR ACUTE OVERDOSES *(Continued)*

Poisoning Agent	Antidote(s)	Indications	Comments
Drug / Drug Class			
Acetaminophen	Acetylcysteine (Mucomyst®)	• Serum acetaminophen level >150 µg/mL at 4 hours postingestion (see Acetaminophen *on page 26*) • Acute ingestion with dose ≥150 mg/kg (child) or 7.5 g (adolescent/adult) within 24 hours of presentation if results of plasma levels cannot be obtained within 8-10 hours of ingestion • Unknown quantity ingested and <24 hours have elapsed since the time of ingestion or unable to obtain serum acetaminophen levels within 12 hours of ingestion • Consider repeating an acetaminophen level 4-6 hours after an initial 4-hour level that is under the treatment range if extended release actaminophen was ingested • Patients presenting >24 hours postacute ingestion who have measurable levels or biochemical evidence of hepatic injury	• Activated charcoal has been shown to adsorb acetylcysteine; therefore, administer activated charcoal before 4-hour acetaminophen level is drawn • If patient vomits within 1 hour of acetylcysteine dose, readminister the dose • I.V. N-acetylcysteine is available in the U.S. by investigational use only; contact a poison control center for further information
Anticholinergics	Physostigmine (Antilirium®)	• Refractory seizures or arrhythmias unresponsive to conventional therapy • Symptoms should be life-threatening	• Due to potential for producing severe adverse effects, (eg, seizures, bradycardia) routine use of physostigmine is controversial • Atropine should be available to reverse life-threatening cholinergic effects of physostigmine
Baclofen	Physostigmine (Antilirium®)	• Distinguish anticholinergic delirium from other causes of altered mental status	• Long-lasting reversal of anticholinergic signs and symptoms is generally not achieved due to the relatively short duration of action of physostigmine • Atropine should be available to reverse life-threatening cholinergic effects of physostigmine

Poisoning Agent	Antidote(s)	Indications	Comments
Benzodiazepines	Flumazenil (Romazicon®)	• Reverses sedative effects of benzodiazepines	• May precipitate benzodiazepine withdrawal in dependent patients • Not indicated for ethanol, barbiturate, general anesthetic, or narcotic overdose • Mixed drug overdose patients who have ingested drugs that increase the likelihood of seizures (eg, cocaine, lithium, cyclic antidepressants) are at extremely high risk for seizures when flumazenil is used • Action of flumazenil may be shorter than duration of benzodiazepines; repeat doses of flumazenil may be needed • Contraindicated in patients given benzodiazepines for potentially life-threatening conditions (eg, increased intracranial pressure, seizures) and patients with signs of serious cyclic-antidepressant overdosage
Beta-blockers	Isoproterenol (Isuprel®)	• Reversal of bradycardia and hypotension	
	Glucagon	• Reversal of bradycardia unresponsive to isoproterenol	• Glucagon activates adenyl cyclase system at a different site than isoproterenol • Requires liver glycogen stores for hyperglycemic response • I.V. glucose must also be given in treatment of hypoglycemia
Calcium channel blockers	Calcium chloride **OR** Calcium gluconate	• Reversal of cardiovascular effects of calcium channel blockers (calcium antagonists)	• Monitor serum calcium levels • Calcium is most effective in mild to moderate intoxications • May not be effective in correcting symptomatic bradyarrhythmias

COMMONLY USED ANTIDOTES FOR ACUTE OVERDOSES *(Continued)*

Poisoning Agent	Antidote(s)	Indications	Comments
Digitalis glycosides	Digoxin immune Fab (Digibind®)	• Treatment of potentially life-threatening digoxin or digitoxin intoxication in carefully selected patients [serum digoxin level >10 ng/mL or ingestion of >4 mg (child) or >10 mg (adult)] • Life-threatening ventricular arrhythmias secondary to digoxin or digitoxin • Hyperkalemia (K^+ >5 mEq/L) in the setting of digitalis toxicity • Life-threatening cardiac arrhythmias, progressive bradyarrhythmias, second or third degree heart block unresponsive to atropine	• Monitor potassium levels and continuous EKG • Digibind® interferes with the interpretation of serum digoxin/digitoxin levels
Heparin, Enoxaparin, Dalteparin	Protamine	• Severe hemorrhage	• Effect can be immediate and last for 2 hours • Protamine dosage related to anticoagulant dosage and time of anticoagulant administration • Monitor PTT • Monitor for hypotension
Insulin	Dextrose (25%-50%)	• Severe, symptomatic hypoglycemia	• Very hypertonic solutions; dilute with sterile water prior to I.V. administration
Iron	Deferoxamine (Desferal®)	• Serum iron level >350 µg/mL • Inability to obtain serum iron level within a reasonable time and patient is symptomatic	• Passing of vin rose colored urine indicates free iron was present • Discontinue therapy when urine returns to normal color • Monitor for hypotension during treatment
Isoniazid	Pyridoxine (Vitamin B_6)	• Ingestion of >80 mg/kg isoniazid	
Neuromuscular blocking agents, nondepolarizing (eg, pancuronium)	Edrophonium OR Neostigmine OR Pyridostigmine	• Reversal of neuromuscular blockade	• Atropine should be available to treat acute cholinergic crisis • Not effective for reversal of **depolarizing** neuromuscular blocking agents (eg, succinylcholine)

Poisoning Agent	Antidote(s)	Indications	Comments
Opiates	Naloxone (Narcan®)	• Reversal of symptoms associated with severe toxicity	• May precipitate withdrawal symptoms in patients with physical dependence to opiates • For prolonged intoxication, a continuous infusion may be used
Phenothiazines	Diphenhydramine (Benadryl®) OR Benztropine (Cogentin®)	• Reversal of phenothiazine-induced dystonic reactions	
	Sodium bicarbonate	• Reversal of "quinidine-like" cardiovascular effects (eg, prolonged QRS complex) – QRS duration >100 msec – Ventricular dysrhythmias and hypotension	• Goal is arterial pH of 7.45-7.55 and urine pH of 7.5-8 • Attempts at urine alkalinization may be dangerous in patients with renal dysfunction or where sodium and fluid overload may compromise respiratory or cardiac status
Tricyclic antidepressants	Sodium bicarbonate	• Reversal of "quinidine-like" cardiovascular effects (eg, prolonged QRS complex) – QRS duration >100 msec – Ventricular dysrhythmias and hypotension	• Goal is arterial pH of 7.45-7.55 and urine pH of 7.5-8 • Attempts at urine alkalinization may be dangerous in patients with renal dysfunction or where sodium and fluid overload may compromise respiratory or cardiac status
Warfarin	Phytonadione (Vitamin K_1)	• Large, acute ingestion • Prothrombin time greater than normal	• Vitamin K is relatively contraindicated in patients with prosthetic heart valves unless toxicity is life-threatening
Zinc	Edetate calcium disodium (EDTA) and/or Dimercaprol (BAL in Oil®)	• Symptomatic zinc ingestion	• Few case reports • Monitor zinc levels
Plants			
Foxglove Oleander	Digoxin immune Fab (Digibind®)	• Severely intoxicated patients who fail to respond to conventional therapy • Life-threatening ventricular arrhythmias, progressive bradyarrhythmias, or second- or third degree heart block not responsive to atropine • Hyperkalemia (K^+ >5 mEq/L) in the setting of digitalis toxicity	• Monitor potassium levels and continuous EKG
Mushroom (genus *Gyomitra*)	Pyridoxine (Vitamin B_6)		
Mushrooms containing muscarine (inocybe or clitocybe)	Atropine	•Myoclonic seizures, severe hallucinations, weakness, arrhythmias, excessive salivation, involuntary urination and defecation	•Atropine should only be used when indicated; otherwise use may result in anticholinergic poisoning

COMMONLY USED ANTIDOTES FOR ACUTE OVERDOSES *(Continued)*

Poisoning Agent	Antidote(s)	Indications	Comments
Snake Bites			
Coral snakes (Eastern and Texas coral snakes only)	Antivenin *(Micrurus fulvius)*		• Not effective for Arizona or Sonoran coral snakes • Skin testing is recommended • Treatment for hypersensitivity reactions, including anaphylaxis, should be available
Pit vipers (Rattlesnakes, cottonmouths, copperheads)	Antivenin *(Crotalidae)* Polyvalent (equine origin)	• Administration within 4 hours of envenomation is ideal; however, administer within 30 hours in all severe cases of poisoning	• Skin testing is recommended • Treatment for hypersensitivity reactions, including anaphylaxis, should be available
Spiders, Scorpions			
Black widow spider	Antivenin *(Lactrodectus mactans)*	• Severe symptoms including respiratory failure, seizures, or pain and spasms not relieved by calcium, muscle relaxants, or analgesics • Symptomatic pregnant patients • Children <5 years or adults >60 years (at greatest risk for severe toxicity)	• Either dermal or conjunctival sensitivity testing should be done prior to administration of antivenin
Scorpion	Antivenin *(Centruroides)*		• No FDA-approved *Centruroides* antivenin in U.S.; only a *Centruroides exilicauda (sculpturatus)*-specific antivenin is available in Arizona (for intrastate use only)

Leikin JR and Paloucek FP, "Poisoning & Toxicology Compendium," Hudson, OH: Lexi-Comp, Inc, 1998.

Mowry JB, Furbee RB, and Chyka PA, "Poisoning," *Essentials of Critical Care Pharmacology,* 3rd ed, Baltimore, MD: Williams & Wilkens, 1994, 501-29.

Zed PJ and Krenzelok EP, "Treatment of Acetaminophen Overdose,"*Am J Health Syst Pharm,* 1999, 56(11):1081-91.

ANION GAP

Definition: The difference in concentration between unmeasured cation and anion equivalents in serum.

Anion gap = $Na^+ - Cl^- - HCO_3^-$
(The normal anion gap is 10-14 mEq/L.)

Differential diagnosis of increased anion gap

Organic anions
Lactate (sepsis, hypovolemia, large tumor burden)
Pyruvate
Uremia
Ketoacidosis (β-hydroxybutyrate and acetoacetate)
Amino acids and their metabolites
Other organic acids (eg, formate from methanol, glycolate from ethylene glycol)

Inorganic anions
Hyperphosphatemia
Sulfates
Nitrates

Medications and toxins
Penicillins and cephalosporins
Salicylates (including aspirin)
Cyanide
Carbon monoxide

Differential diagnosis of decreased anion gap
Organic cations
Hypergammaglobulinemia

Inorganic cations
Hyperkalemia
Hypercalcemia
Hypermagnesemia

Medications and toxins
Lithium

Hypoalbuminemia

LABORATORY DETECTION OF DRUGS IN URINE

Agent	Time Detectable in Urine*
Alcohol	12-24 h
Amobarbital	2-4 d
Amphetamine	2-4 d
Butalbital	2-4 d
Cannabinoids	
Occasional use	2-7 d
Regular use	30 d
Cocaine (benzoylecgonine)	12-72 h
Codeine	2-4 d
Chlordiazepoxide	30 d
Diazepam	30 d
Ethanol	12-24 h
Heroin (morphine)	2-4 d
Hydromorphone	2-4 d
Marijuana	
Occasional use	2-7 d
Regular use	30 d
Methamphetamine	2-4 d
Methaqualone	2-4 d
Morphine	2-4 d
Pentobarbital	2-4 d
Phencyclidine (PCP)	
Occasional use	2-7 d
Regular use	30 d
Phenobarbital	30 d
Secobarbital	2-4 d

*The periods of detection for the various abused drugs listed above should be taken as estimates since the actual figures will vary due to metabolism, user, laboratory, and excretion.

Adapted from Chang JY, "Drug Testing and Interpretation of Results," *Pharmchem Newsletter*, 1989, 17:1.

OSMOLALITY

Definition: The summed concentrations of all osmotically active solute particles.

Predicted serum osmolality =

2 Na$^+$ (mEq/L) + glucose (mg/dL) / 18 + BUN (mg/dL) / 2.8

The normal range of serum osmolality is 285-295 mOsm/L.

Differential diagnosis of increased serum osmolal gap
(increased by >10 mOsm/L)

Medications and toxins
Alcohols (ethanol, methanol, isopropanol, glycerol, ethylene glycol)
Mannitol
Paraldehyde

SALICYLATE INTOXICATION

SERUM SALICYLATE LEVEL AND
SEVERITY OF INTOXICATION SINGLE DOSE
ACUTE INGESTION NOMOGRAM

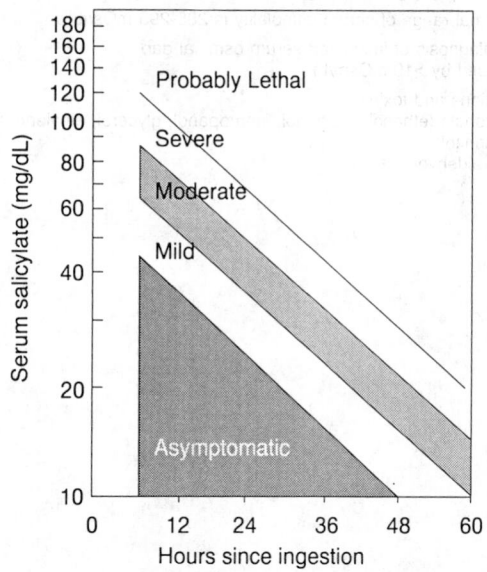

Nomogram relating serum salicylate concentration and expected severity of intoxication at varying intervals following the ingestion of a single dose of salicylate.

From Done AK, "Aspirin Overdosage: Incidence, Diagnosis, and Management," *Pediatrics*, 1978, 62:890-7 with permission.

ACETAMINOPHEN

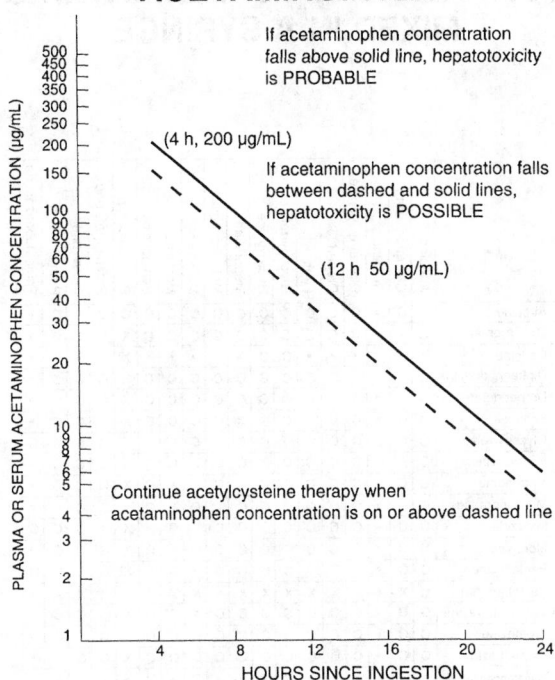

Nomogram relating plasma or serum acetaminophen concentration and probability of hepatotoxicity at varying intervals following ingestion of a single toxic dose of acetaminophen. Modified from Rumack BH, Matthew H, "Acetaminophen Poisoning and Toxicity", Pediatrics, 1975, 55:871-6,
© American Academy of Pediatrics, 1975, and from Rumack BH, et al, "Acetaminophen Overdose", Arch Intern Med, 1981, 141:380-5,
© American Medical Association.

COMPATIBILITY OF MEDICATIONS MIXED IN A SYRINGE

	Atropine	Chlorpromazine	Codeine	Diphenhydramine	Droperidol	Fentanyl	Glycopyrrolate	Hydroxyzine	Meperidine	Metoclopramide	Midazolam	Morphine	Pentazocine	Pentobarbital†	Prochlorperazine	Promazine	Promethazine	Trimethobenzamide
Atropine		C	•	C	C	C	C	C	C	C	C	C	C	C	C	C	C	•
Chlorpromazine	C		•	C	C	C	C	C	C	C	C	C	C	X	C	C	C	•
Codeine	•	•		•	•	•	C	C	•	•	•	•	•	X	•	•	•	•
Diphenhydramine	C	C	•		C	C	C	C	C	C	C	C	C	X	C	C	C	•
Droperidol	C	C	•	C		C	C	C	C	C	C	C	C	X	C	C	C	•
Fentanyl	C	C	•	C	C		C	C	C	C	C	C	C	X	C	C	C	•
Glycopyrrolate	C	C	C	C	C	C		C	C	•	C	C	X	X	C	C	C	C
Hydroxyzine	C	C	C	C	C	C	C		C	C	C	C	C	X	C	C	C	•
Meperidine	C	C	•	C	C	C	C	C		C	C	C	C	X	C	C	C	•
Metoclopramide	C	C	•	C	C	C	•	C	C		C	C	C	•	C	C	C	•
Midazolam	C	C	•	C	C	C	C	C	C	C		C	•	X	X	C	C	C
Morphine	C	C	•	C	C	C	C	C	C	C	C		C	X	C*	C	C	•
Pentazocine	C	C	•	C	C	C	X	C	C	C	•	C		X	C	C	C	C
Pentobarbital†	C	X	X	X	X	X	X	X	X	•	X	X	X		X	X	X	•
Prochlorperazine	C	C	•	C	C	C	C	C	C	C	X	C*	C	X		C	C	C
Promazine	C	C	•	C	C	C	C	C	C	C	C	C	C	X	C		C	•
Promethazine	C	C	•	C	C	C	C	C	C	C	C	C	C	X	C	C		•
Trimethobenzamide	•	•	•	•	•	•	C	•	•	•	C	•	C	•	C	•	•	

C = Physically compatible if used within 15 minutes after mixing in a syringe
X = Incompatible
• = No documented information
C* = Potential incompatibility produced by certain manufacturers
† = Compatibility profile is characteristic of most barbiturate salts, such as phenobarbital and secobarbital

The following combinations have been found to be compatible:
    atropine / meperidine / promethazine
    atropine / meperidine / hydroxyzine
    meperidine / promethazine / chlorpromazine

The following drugs should *not* be mixed with any other drugs in the same syringe:
    diazepam, chlordiazepoxide

References

Forman JK and Sourney PF, "Visual Compatibility of Midazolam Hydrochloride With Common Preoperative Injectable Medications," *Am J Hosp Pharm*, 1987, 44(10):2298-9.

King JC, "Guide to Parenteral Admixtures," St Louis, MO: Cutter Laboratories, 1986.

Parker WA, *Hosp Pharm*, 1984, 19:475-8.

Trissel LA, "Handbook on Injectable Drugs," 5th ed, Bethesda, MD: American Society of Health System Pharmacists, Inc, 1988.

Stevenson JG and Patriarca C, "Incompatibility of Morphine Sulfate and Prochlorperazine Edisylate in Syringes," *Am J Hosp Pharm*, 1985, 42:2651.

CONTROLLED SUBSTANCES

Note: These are federal classifications. Your individual state may place a substance into a more restricted category. When this occurs, the more restricted category applies. Consult your state law.

Schedule I = C-I

The drugs and other substances in this schedule have no legal medical uses except research. They have a **high** potential for abuse. They include opiates, opium derivatives, and hallucinogens.

Schedule II = C-II

The drugs and other substances in this schedule have legal medical uses and a **high** abuse potential which may lead to severe dependence. They include former "Class A" narcotics, amphetamines, barbiturates, and other drugs.

Schedule III = C-III

The drugs and other substances in this schedule have legal medical uses and a **lesser** degree of abuse potential which may lead to **moderate** dependence. They include former "Class B" narcotics and other drugs.

Schedule IV = C-IV

The drugs and other substances in this schedule have legal medical uses and **low** abuse potential which may lead to **moderate** dependence. They include barbiturates, benzodiazepines, propoxyphenes and other drugs.

Schedule V = C-V

The drugs and other substances in this schedule have legal medical uses and **low** abuse potential which may lead to **moderate** dependence. They include narcotic cough preparations, diarrhea, preparations, and other drugs.

FEVER DUE TO DRUGS

Aminosalicylic acid
Antihistamines
Asparaginase
Barbiturates
Bleomycin
Cephalosporins
Iodides
Methyldopa
Penicillins
Phenolphthalein
Phenytoin
Procainamide
Quinidine
Sulfonamides
Thiouracil

Abstracted from Harrison's *Principles of Internal Medicine*, 12th ed, Wilson JD, ed, New York, NY: McGraw-Hill Book Co, 1991 and Tabor PA, "Drug-Induced Fever," *Drug Intell Clin Pharm*, 1986, 20:413-20.

DISCOLORATION OF FECES DUE TO DRUGS

Black
Acetazolamide
Alcohols
Alkalies
Aminophylline
Amphetamine
Amphotericin
Antacids
Anticoagulants
Aspirin
Betamethasone
Charcoal
Chloramphenicol
Chlorpropamide
Clindamycin
Corticosteroids
Cortisone
Cyclophosphamide
Cytarabine
Dicumarol
Digitalis
Ethacrynic acid
Ferrous salts
Floxuridine
Fluorouracil
Halothane
Heparin
Hydralazine
Hydrocortisone
Ibuprofen
Indomethacin
Iodine drugs
Iron salts
Levarterenol
Levodopa
Manganese
Melphalan
Methylprednisolone
Methotrexate
Methylene blue
Oxyphenbutazone

Paraldehyde
Phenacetin
Phenolphthalein
Phenylbutazone
Phenylephrine
Phosphorous
Potassium salts
Prednisolone
Procarbazine
Pyrvinium
Reserpine
Salicylates
Sulfonamides
Tetracycline
Theophylline
Thiotepa
Triamcinolone
Warfarin

Blue
Chloramphenicol
Methylene blue

Dark Brown
Dexamethasone

Gray
Colchicine

Green
Indomethacin
Iron
Medroxyprogesterone

Greenish Gray
Oral antibiotics
Oxyphenbutazone
Phenylbutazone

Light Brown
Anticoagulants

Orange-Red
Phenazopyridine
Rifampin

Pink
Anticoagulants
Aspirin
Heparin
Oxyphenbutazone
Phenylbutazone
Salicylates

Red
Anticoagulants
Aspirin
Heparin
Oxyphenbutazone
Phenolphthalein
Phenylbutazone
Pyrvinium
Salicylates
Tetracycline syrup

Red-Brown
Oxyphenbutazone
Phenylbutazone
Rifampin

Tarry
Ergot preparations
Ibuprofen
Salicylates
Warfarin

White/Speckling
Aluminum hydroxide
Antibiotics (oral)
Indocyanine green

Yellow
Senna

Yellow-Green
Senna

Adapted from Drugdex® — Drug Consults, Micromedex, vol 62, Rocky Mountain Drug Consultation Center, Denver, CO: January, 1995.

DISCOLORATION OF URINE DUE TO DRUGS

Black
Cascara
Ferrous salts
Iron dextran
Levodopa
Methocarbamol
Methyldopa
Naphthalene
Phenacetin
Phenols
Quinine
Sulfonamides

Blue
Anthraquinone
Indigo blue
Indigo carmine
Methocarbamol
Methylene blue
Nitrofurans
Resorcinol
Triamterene

Blue-Green
Amitriptyline
Anthraquinone
DeWitt's pills
Doan's® pills
Indigo blue
Indigo carmine
Methylene blue

Brown
Anthraquinone dyes
Cascara
Levodopa
Methocarbamol
Methyldopa
Metronidazole
Nitrofurans
Nitrofurantoin
Phenacetin
Primaquine
Quinine
Rifampin
Senna
Sodium diatrizoate
Sulfonamides

Brown-Black
Quinine

Dark
Aminosalicylic acid
Cascara
Levodopa
Metronidazole
Nitrites
Phenacetin
Phenol
Primaquine
Quinine
Resorcinol

Riboflavin
Senna

Green
Anthraquinone
DeWitt's pills
Indigo blue
Indigo carmine
Indomethacin
Methocarbamol
Methylene blue
Nitrofurans
Phenols
Resorcinol
Suprofen

Green-Yellow
DeWitt's pills
Methylene blue

Milky
Phosphates

Orange
Chlorzoxazone
Dihydroergotamine mesylate
Heparin sodium
Phenazopyridine
Phenindione
Rifampin
Sulfasalazine
Warfarin

Orange-Red
Chlorzoxazone
Doxidan
Phenazopyridine
Rifampin

Orange-Yellow
Fluorescein sodium
Rifampin
Sulfasalazine

Pink
Aminopyrine
Anthraquinone dyes
Danthron
Deferoxamine
Merbromin
Phenolphthalein
Phenothiazines
Phenytoin
Salicylates

Red
Anthraquinone
Cascara
Daunorubicin
Dimethyl sulfoxide
DMSO
Doxorubicin
Heparin

Ibuprofen
Methyldopa
Oxyphenbutazone
Phenacetin
Phenazopyridine
Phenolphthalein
Phenothiazines
Phensuximide
Phenylbutazone
Phenytoin
Rifampin
Senna

Red-Brown
Cascara
Methyldopa
Oxyphenbutazone
Phenacetin
Phenolphthalein
Phenothiazines
Phenylbutazone
Phenytoin
Quinine

Red-Purple
Chlorzoxazone
Ibuprofen
Phenacetin
Senna

Rust
Cascara
Chloroquine
Metronidazole
Nitrofurantoin
Phenacetin
Riboflavin
Senna
Sulfonamides

Yellow
Nitrofurantoin
Phenacetin
Riboflavin
Sulfasalazine

Yellow-Brown
Cascara
Chloroquine
DeWitt's pills
Methylene blue
Metronidazole
Nitrofurantoin
Primaquine
Quinacrine
Senna
Sulfonamides

Yellow-Pink
Cascara
Senna

Adapted from Drugdex® — Drug Consults, Micromedex, vol 62, Rocky Mountain Drug Consultation Center, Denver, CO: January, 1995.

DRUGS AND BREAST-FEEDING

The following question and options should be considered when prescribing drug therapy to lactating women. 1) Is the drug therapy really necessary? Consultation between the pediatrician and the mother's physician can be most useful. 2) Use the safest drug, for example, acetaminophen rather than aspirin, for analgesia. 3) If there is a possibility that a drug may present a risk to the infant, consideration should be given to measurement of blood concentrations in the nursing infant. 4) Drug exposure to the nursing infant may be minimized by having the mother take the medication just after she has breast-fed the infant and/or just before the infant is due to have a lengthy sleep period.

In tables 1-6, the fact that a pharmacologic or chemical agent does not appear on the lists is not meant to imply that it is not transferred into human milk or that it does not have an effect on the infant; it only indicates that there were no reports found in the literature.

Table 1. Drugs That Are Contraindicated During Breast-Feeding

Bromocriptine	Ergotamine
Cocaine	Lithium
Cyclophosphamide	Methotrexate
Cyclosporine	Phencyclidine (PCP)
Doxorubicin*	Phenindione

*Drug is concentrated in human milk.

Table 2. Drugs of Abuse: Contraindicated During Breast-Feeding*

Amphetamine†	Marijuana
Cocaine	Nicotine (smoking)
Heroin	Phencyclidine

*The Committee on Drugs strongly believes that nursing mothers should not ingest any compounds listed in Table 2. Not only are they hazardous to the nursing infant, but they are also detrimental to the physical and emotional health of the mother. This list is obviously not complete; no drug of abuse should be ingested by nursing mothers even though adverse reports are not in the literature.

†Drug is concentrated in human milk.

Table 3. Radioactive Compounds That Require Temporary Cessation of Breast-Feeding*

Drug	Recommended Time for Cessation of Breast-Feeding
Copper-64 (^{64}Cu)	Radioactivity in milk present at 50 h
Gallium-67 (^{67}Ga)	Radioactivity in milk present for 2 wk
Indium-111 (^{111}In)	Very small amount present at 20 h
Iodine-123 (^{123}I)	Radioactivity in milk present up to 36 h
Iodine-125 (^{125}I)	Radioactivity in milk present for 12 d
Iodine-131 (^{131}I)	Radioactivity in milk present 2-14 d, depending on study
Radioactive sodium	Radioactivity in milk present 96 h
Technetium-99m (^{99m}Tc), ^{99m}Rc macroaggregates, ^{99m}Tc O4	Radioactivity in milk present 15 h to 3 d

*Consult nuclear medicine physician before performing diagnostic study so that radionuclide that has shortest excretion time in breast milk can be used. Before study, the mother should pump her breast and store enough milk in freezer for feeding the infant; after study, the mother should pump her breast to maintain milk production but discard all milk pumped for the required time that radioactivity is present in milk. Milk samples can be screened by radiology departments for radioactivity before resumption of nursing.

DRUGS AND BREAST-FEEDING *(Continued)*

Table 4. Drugs Whose Effect on Nursing Infants Is Unknown But May Be of Concern

Psychotropic drugs, the compounds listed under antianxiety, antidepressant, and antipsychotic categories, are of special concern when given to nursing mothers for long periods. Although there are no case reports of adverse effects in breast-feeding infants, these drugs do appear in human milk and thus could conceivably alter short-term and long-term central nervous system function.

Antianxiety
 Diazepam
 Lorazepam
 Midazolam
 Perphenazine
 Prazepam*
 Quazepam
 Temazepam

Antidepressant
 Amitriptyline
 Amoxapine
 Desipramine
 Dothiepin
 Doxepin
 Fluoxetine
 Fluvoxamine
 Imipramine
 Trazodone

Antipsychotic
 Chlorpromazine
 Chlorprothixene
 Haloperidol
 Mesoridazine

Miscellaneous
 Chloramphenicol
 Metoclopramide*
 Metronidazole
 Tinidazole

*Drug is concentrated in human milk.

Table 5. Drugs That Have Been Associated With Significant Effects on Some Nursing Infants and Should Be Given to Nursing Mothers With Caution*

Aspirin (salicylates)
Clemastine
Mesalamine
Phenobarbital

Primidone
Sulfasalazine (salicylazosulfapyridine)

*Measure blood concentration in the infant when possible.

Table 6. Maternal Medications Usually Compatible With Breast-Feeding

Acebutolol	Dapsone	Morphine
Acetaminophen	Dexbrompheniramine	Moxalactam
Acetazolamide	maleate with d-	Nadolol†
Acitretin	isoephedrine*	Nalidixic acid*
Acyclovir†	Digoxin	Naproxen
Alcohol (ethanol)*#	Diltiazem	Nefopam
Allopurinol	Dipyrone	Nifedipine
Amoxicillin	Disopyramide	Nitrofurantoin*
Antimony	Domperidone	Norethynodrel
Atenolol	Dyphylline†	Norsteroids
Atropine	Enalapril	Noscapine
Azapropazone	Erythromycin†	Oxprenolol
(apazone)	Estradiol*	Phenylbutazone
Aztreonam	Ethambutol	Phenytoin*
B₁ (thiamine)	Ethanol (cf. alcohol)	Piroxicam
B₆ (pyridoxine)	Ethosuximide	Prednisone
B₁₂ (vitamin)	Fentanyl	Procainamide
Baclofen	Flecainide	Progesterone
Barbiturate*	Flufenamic acid	Propoxyphene
Bendroflumethiazide#	Fluorescein	Propranolol
Bishydroxycoumarin	Folic acid	Propylthiouracil
(dicumarol)	Gold salts	Pseudoephedrine†
Bromide*	Halothane	Pyridostigmine
Butorphanol	Hydralazine	Pyrimethamine
Caffeine*	Hydrochlorothiazide	Quinidine
Captopril	Hydroxychloroquine†	Quinine
Carbamazepine	Ibuprofen	Riboflavin
Carbimazole*	Indomethacin*	Rifampin
Cascara	Iodides*	Scopolamine
Cefadroxil	Iodine (povidone-iodine/	Secobarbital
Cefazolin	vaginal douche)*	Senna
Cefotaxime	Iodine*	Sotalol
Cefoxitin	Iopanoic acid	Spironolactone
Cefprozil	Isoniazid	Streptomycin
Ceftazidime	K₁ (vitamin)	Sulbactam
Ceftriaxone	Kanamycin	Sulfapyridine*
Chloral hydrate*	Ketorolac	Sulfisoxazole*
Chloroform	Labetalol	Suprofen
Chloroquine	Levonorgestrel	Terbutaline
Chlorothiazide	Lidocaine	Tetracycline
Chlorthalidone*	Loperamide	Theophylline*
Cimetidine†	Magnesium sulfate	Thiopental
Cisapride	Medroxyprogesterone	Thiouracil
Cisplatin	Mefenamic acid	Ticarcillin
Clindamycin	Methadone	Timolol
Clogestone	Methimazole (active	Tolbutamide*
Clomipramine	metabolite of carbi-	Tolmetin
Codeine	mazole)	Trimethoprim/sulfameth-
Colchicine	Methocarbamol	oxazole
Contraceptive pill with	Methyldopa	Triprolidine
estrogen/proges-	Methyprylon*	Valproic acid
terone#	Metoprolol†	Verapamil
Cycloserine	Metrizamide	Warfarin
D (vitamin)	Mexiletine	Zolpidem
Danthron*	Minoxidil	

*Effects in infants have been reported in the literature.
†Drug is concentrated in human milk.
#Reported effect on lactation.
From "American Academy of Pediatrics Committee on Drugs: The Transfer of Drugs and Other Chemicals Into Human Milk," *Pediatrics*, 1994, 93(1):137-50, with permission.

MILLIEQUIVALENT
FOR SELECTED IONS

Approximate Milliequivalents — Weights of Selected Ions

Salt	mEq/g Salt	mg Salt/mEq
Calcium carbonate ($CaCO_3$)	20	50
Calcium chloride ($CaCl_2 \bullet 2H_2O$)	14	73
Calcium gluconate (Ca gluconate$_2 \bullet 1H_2O$)	4	224
Calcium lactate (Ca lactate$_2 \bullet 5H_2O$)	6	154
Magnesium sulfate ($MgSO_4$)	16	60
Magnesium sulfate ($MgSO_4 \bullet 7H_2O$)	8	123
Potassium acetate (K acetate)	10	98
Potassium chloride (KCl)	13	75
Potassium citrate (K_3 citrate$\bullet 1H_2O$)	9	108
Potassium iodide (KI)	6	166
Sodium bicarbonate ($NaHCO_3$)	12	84
Sodium chloride (NaCl)	17	58
Sodium citrate (Na_3 citrate$\bullet 2H_2O$)	10	98
Sodium iodide (NaI)	7	150
Sodium lactate (Na lactate)	9	112
Zinc sulfate ($ZnSO_4 \bullet 7H_2O$)	7	144

Valences and Approximate Weights of Selected Ions

Substance	Electrolyte	Valence	Ionic Wt
Calcium	Ca^{++}	2	40
Chloride	Cl^-	1	35.5
Magnesium	Mg^{++}	2	24
Phosphate	PO_4^{3-}	3	95*
	HPO_4^{2-}	2	96
	$H_2PO_4^-$	1	97
Potassium	K^+	1	39
Sodium	Na^+	1	23
Sulfate	SO_4^{2-}	2	96*

*The atomic weight of phosphorus is 31, and of sulfur is 32.

SEROTONIN SYNDROME

Diagnostic Criteria for Serotonin Syndrome

- Recent addition or dosage increase of any agent increasing serotonin activity or availability (usually within 1 day).
- Absence of abused substances, metabolic infectious etiology, or withdrawal.
- No recent addition or dosage increase of a neuroleptic agent prior to onset of signs and symptoms.
- Presence of three or more of the following:
  - Altered mental status (seen in 40% of patients, primarily confusion or hypomania)
  - Agitation
  - Tremor (50% incidence)
  - Shivering
  - Diarrhea
  - Hyperreflexia (pronounced in lower extremities)
  - Myoclonus (50% incidence)
  - Ataxia or incoordination
  - Fever (50% incidence; temperature >105°F associated with grave prognosis)
  - Diaphoresis

Drugs (as Single Causative Agent) Which Can Induce Serotonin Syndrome

Specific serotonin reuptake inhibitors (SSRI)
MDMA (Ecstasy)
Clomipramine

Drug Combinations Which Can Induce Serotonin Syndrome*

Alprazolam – Clomipramine
Bromocriptine – Levodopa/carbidopa
Buspirone – Trazodone
Citalopram – Moclobemide
Clomipramine – Clorgiline
Clomipramine – Lithium
Dihydroergotamine – Sertraline
Dihydroergotamine – Amitriptyline
Fentanyl – Sertraline
Fluoxetine – Carbamazepine
Fluoxetine – Lithium
Fluoxetine – Remoxipide
Fluoxetine – Tryptophan
Lithium – Fluvoxamine
Lithium – Paroxetine
Lysergic acid diethylamide (LSD) – Fluoxetine
Moclobemide – Citalopram
Moclobemide – Clomipramine
Moclobemide – Fluoxetine
Moclobemide – Pethidine
Monoamine oxidase inhibitor – Fluoxetine
Monoamine oxidase inhibitor – Fluvoxamine
Monoamine oxidase inhibitor – Meperidine
Monoamine oxidase inhibitor – Sertraline
Monoamine oxidase inhibitor – Tricyclic antidepressants
Monoamine oxidase inhibitor – Tryptophan
Monoamine oxidase inhibitor – Venlafaxine

SEROTONIN SYNDROME *(Continued)*

Nefazodone – Paroxetine
Nortriptyline – Trazodone
Paroxetine – Dextromethorphan
Paroxetine – Dihydroergotamine
Paroxetine – Trazodone
Phenelzine, Trazodone – Dextropropoxyphene
S-adenosylmethionine – Clomipramine
Sertraline – Amitriptyline
Sumatriptan – Sertraline
Tranylcypromine – Clomipramine
Tramadol – Sertraline
Trazodone– Lithium – Amitriptyline
Trazodone – Fluoxetine
Valproic acid – Nefazodone
Venlafaxine – Tranylcypromine
Venlafaxine – Selegiline

*When administered within 2 weeks of each other

TREATMENT OF SEROTONIN SYNDROME

Therapy is primarily supportive with intravenous crystalloid solutions utilized for hypotension and cooling blankets for mild hyperthermia. Norepinephrine is the preferred vasopressor. Chlorpromazine or dantrolene sodium may have a role in controlling fevers, although there is no proven benefit. Benzodiazepines are the first-line treatment in controlling rigors and thus, limiting fever and rhabdomyolysis, while clonazepam may be specifically useful in treating myoclonus. Endotracheal intubation and paralysis may be required to treat refractory muscular contractions. Tachycardia or tremor can be treated with beta-blocking agents; although due to its blockade of 5-HTIA receptors, the syndrome may worsen. Serotonin blockers such as diphenhydramine, cyproheptadine, or chlorpromazine have been used with variable efficacy. Methysergide and nitroglycerin (with lorazepam) also have been utilized with variable efficacy in case reports. It appears that cyproheptadine is most consistently beneficial.

Recovery seen within 1 day in 70% of cases; mortality rate is about 11%.

References

Gitlin MJ, "Venlafaxine, Monoamine Oxidase Inhibitors, and the Serotonin Syndrome," *J Clin Psychopharmacol*, 1997, 17:66-7.

Heisler MA, Guidery JR, and Arnecke B, "Serotonin Syndrome Induced by Administration of Venlafaxine and Phenelzine," *Ann Pharmacother*, 1996, 30:84.

Hodgman MJ, Martin TG, and Krenzelok EP, "Serotonin Syndrome Due to Venlafaxine and Maintenance Tranylcypromine Therapy," *Hum Exp Toxicol*, 1997, 16:14-7.

John L, Perreault MM, Tao T, et al, "Serotonin Syndrome Associated With Nefazodone and Paroxetine," *Ann Emerg Med*, 1997, 29:287-9.

LoCurto MJ, "The Serotonin Syndrome," *Emerg Clin North Am*, 1997, 15(3):665-75.

Martin TG, "Serotonin Syndrome," *Ann Emerg Med*, 1996, 28:520-6.

Mills K, "Serotonin Toxicity: A Comprehensive Review for Emergency Medicine," *Top Emerg Med*, 1993, 15:54-73.

Mills KC, "Serotonin Syndrome: A Clinical Update," *Crit Care Clin*, 1997, 13(4):763-83.

Nisijima K, Shimizu M, Abe T, et al, "A Case of Serotonin Syndrome Induced by Concomitant Treatment With Low-Dose Trazodone, and Amitriptyline and Lithium," *Int Clin Psychopharmacol*, 1996, 11:289-90.

Sobanski T, Bagli M, Laux G, et al, "Serotonin Syndrome After Lithium Add-On Medication to Paroxetine," *Pharmacopsychiatry*, 1997, 30:106-7.

Sporer, "The Serotonin Syndrome: Implicated Drugs, Pathophysiology and Management," *Drug Safety*, 1995, 13(2):94-104.

Sternbach H, "The Serotonin Syndrome," *Am J Psychiatry*, 1991, 146:705-7.

Van Berkum MM, Thiel J, Leikin JB, et al, "A Fatality Due to Serotonin Syndrome," *Medical Update for Psychiatrists*, 1997, 2:55-7.

SODIUM CONTENT
OF SELECTED MEDICINALS

Name and Dosage Unit*	Sodium	
	mg	mEq
Antibiotics		
Amikacin sulfate, 1 g	29.9	1.3
Aminosalicylate sodium, 1 g	109	4.7
Ampicillin, suspension, 250 mg/5 mL, 5 mL	10	0.4
Ampicillin sodium, 1 g	66.7	3
Azlocillin sodium, 1 g	50	2.2
Carbenicillin disodium, 382 mg (tablet)	22	1
Cefazolin sodium, 1 g	47	2
Cefotaxime sodium, 1 g	30.5	2.2
Cefoxitin sodium, 1 g	53	2.3
Ceftriaxone sodium, 1 g	83	3.6
Cefuroxime, 1 g	54.2	2.4
Chloramphenicol sodium succinate, 1 g	51.8	2.3
Dicloxacillin, 250 mg (capsule)	13	0.6
Dicloxacillin, suspension 65 mg/5 mL	27	1.2
Erythromycin ethyl succinate, suspension 200 mg/5 mL	29	1.3
Erythromycin Base Filmtab®, 250 mg	70	3
Methicillin sodium, 1 g	66.7	2.9
Metronidazole, 500 mg I.V.	322	14
Mezlocillin sodium, 1 g	42.6	1.9
Moxalactam sodium, 1 g	88	3.8
Nafcillin sodium, 1 g	66.7	2.9
Nitrofurantoin, suspension, 25 mg/5 mL	7	0.3
Penicillin G potassium, 1,000,000 units I.V.	7.6	0.3
Penicillin G sodium, 1,000,000 units I.V.	46	2
Penicillin V potassium, suspension, 250 mg/5 mL	38	1.7
Piperacillin sodium, 1 g	42.6	1.8
Ticarcillin disodium, 1 g	119.6	5.2
Antacids, Liquid (content per 5 mL)		
Amphojel®	<2.3	<0.1
ALternaGEL®	2	0.1
Basaljel®	2.4	0.1
Extra Strength Maalox®-Plus	0.65	≅0.05
Gaviscon®	13	0.57
Maalox®	1.3	0.06
Tums E-X™	<4.8	<0.2
Sodium Content of Miscellaneous Medicinals		
Acetazolamide sodium, 500 mg	47.2	2.05
Chlorothiazide sodium, 500 mg	57.5	2
Cisplatin, 10 mg	35.4	1.54
Edetate calcium disodium, 1 g	122	5.3
Fleet® Enema, 4.5 oz	5000†	218
Fleet® Phospho®-Soda, 20 mL	2217	96.4
Hydrocortisone sodium succinate, 1 g	47.5	2.07

SODIUM CONTENT
OF SELECTED MEDICINALS *(Continued)*

Name and Dosage Unit*	Sodium	
	mg	mEq
Hypaque® M 75%, injection, 20 mL	200	8.7
Hypaque® M 90%, injection, 20 mL	220	9.6
Metamucil® Instant Mix (orange)	6	0.27
Methotrexate sodium, 100 mg vial	20	0.86
Methotrexate sodium, 100 mg vial (low sodium)	15	0.65
Naproxen sodium, 250 mg (tablet)	23	1
Neutra-Phos®, capsule and 75 mL reconstituted solution	164	7.13
Oragrafin® (capsule)	19	0.8
Pentobarbital sodium, 50 mg/mL, 1 mL vial	5	0.2
Phenobarbital sodium, 65 mg, 1 mL vial	6	0.3
Phenytoin sodium, 1 g	88	3.8
Promethazine expectorant, 5 mL	53	2.3
Shohl's solution modified, 1 mL	23	1
Sodium ascorbate, 500 mg acid equivalent	65.3	2.84
Sodium bicarbonate, 50 mL 8.4%	1150	50
Sodium nitroprusside, 50 mg	7.8	0.34
Sodium polystyrene sulfonate, 1 g	94.3‡	4.1
Thiopental sodium, 1 g	86.8	3.8
Valproate sodium, 250 mg/5 mL, 5 mL	23	1

*Product formulations and hence sodium content are subject to change by the manufacturer.
†Average systemic absorption 250-300 mg.
‡Total sodium content. Only about 33% is liberated in clinical use.

SUGAR-FREE LIQUID PHARMACEUTICALS

The following sugar-free liquid preparations are listed by therapeutic category and alphabetically within each category. Please note that product formulations are subject to change by the manufacturer. Some of these products may contain sorbitol, xylitol, or other sweeteners which may be partially metabolized to provide calories.

Analgesics
Acetaminophen Elixir (various)
APAP/APAP Plus
Aspirin/Buffered Aspirin (Medique®)
Bufferin® A/F Nite Time
Children's Anacin-3® Infants Drops
Children's Myapap® Elixir
Children's Panadol® Drops, Liquid, and Chewable Tablets
Children's Tylenol® Chewable Tablets
Conex® Liquid
Cone® With Codeine Liquid
Dolanex® Elixir
Extra Strength Tylenol® PM
Febrol® and Febrol® EX
Methadone Hydrochloride Intensol
MS-Ai®
Myapap® Drops
No Drowsiness Tylenol®
Pain-Off®
Paregoric USP (Abbott)
Sep-A-Soothe® II
St Joseph® Aspirin-Free Liquid and Drops
Tempra® Chewable Tablets
Tylenol® Drops

Antacids/Antiflatulents
Alcalak®
Aldroxicon®
Almag® Suspension
Aludrox® Suspension
Aluminum Hydroxide Suspension
Calglycine® Tablets
Camalox® Suspension
Citrocarbonate® Granules
Creamalin® Suspension
Delcid®
Di-Gel® Liquid (mint, lemon & orange flavored)
Digestamic®
Dimacid®
Gaviscon® Liquid
Gelusil® II
Gelusil® Liquid
Gelusil® Liquid Flavor Pack
Gelusil-M® Liquid
Kolantyl® Gel
Maalox® Plus Suspension
Maalox® Suspension
Maalox® Therapeutic Concentrate
Magnatril® Suspension
Magnesia and Alumina Oral Suspension USP (Abbott, Phillips Roxane)
Mallamint® Chewable Tablets
Marblen® Suspension and Tablets
Medi-Seltzer®/Plus
Milk of Bismuth
Milk of Magnesia USP
Mylanta® Liquid

SUGAR-FREE LIQUID PHARMACEUTICALS *(Continued)*

Mylanta®-II Liquid
Mylicon® Drops
Nephrox® Suspension
Nutrajel®
Nutramag®
Pepto-Bismol® Liquid and Tablets
Phosphaljel® Suspension
Riopan Plus®
Riopan® Suspension
Silain-Gel® Liquid
Trisogel®
Titralac® Liquid
Titralac® Plus Liquid
WinGel® Liquid and Tablets

Antiasthmatics

Aerolate® Liquid
Alupent® Syrup
Choledyl® Pediatric Syrup
Droxine®
Elixophyllin® Elixir
Elixophyllin®-GG Liquid
Lanophyllin® Elixir
Lixolin® Liquid
Lufyllin® Elixir
Metaprel® Syrup
Mucomyst®-10
Mucomyst®-20
Mudrane® GG Elixir
Neothylline® Elixir
Neothylline® G
Organidin® NR
Slo-Phyllin® 80 Syrup
Somophyllin® Oral Liquid
Somophyllin®-DF Oral Liquid
Tedral® Elixir and Suspension
Theolair™ 80 Syrup
Theolixir®
Theon® Syrup
Theo-Organidin® Elixir
Theophylline Elixir (Phillips Roxane)

Antidepressants

Sinequan® Oral Concentrate

Antidiarrheals

Corrective Mixture With Paregoric
Diasorb® Liquid and Tablets
Di-Gon® II
Diotame®
Donnagel®
Infantol® Pink
Kalicon® Suspension
Kaolin Mixture With Pectin NF (Abbott)
Kaolin-Pectin Suspension (Phillips Roxane)
Konsyl® Powder
Lomanate®
Lomotil® Liquid
Paregoric USP (various)
Parepectolin® (various)
Pepto-Bismol®
St Joseph® Antidiarrheal

Antiepileptics
Mysoline® Suspension
Paradione® Solution

Antihistamine-Decongestants
Actifed® With Codeine
Actifed® Syrup
Actidil® Syrup
Bromphen® Elixir
Dimetane® Decongestant Elixir
Dimetapp® Elixir
Hay-Febrol® Liquid
Isoclor® Liquid and Capsules
Naldecon® Pediatric Drops and Syrup
Naldecon® Syrup
Novahistine® Elixir
Phenergan® Fortis Syrup
Phenergan® Syrup
Rondec® DM Drops
Ryna® Liquid
S-T® Forte® Liquid
Tavist® Syrup
Trind® Liquid
Veltap® Elixir
Vistaril® Oral Suspension

Anti-infectives
Augmentin® Suspension
Furadantin® Oral Suspension
Furoxone® Suspension
Humatin®
Mandelamine® Suspension/Forte®
Minocin® Suspension
Mycifradin® Sulfate Oral Solution
NegGram® Suspension
Proklar® Suspension
Sulfamethoxazole and Trimethoprim Suspension (Biocraft, Beecham, Burroughs Wellcome)
Vibramycin® Syrup

Antiparkinsonism Agents
Artane® Elixir

Antispasmodics
Antrocol® Elixir
Spasmophen® Elixir

Corticosteroids
Decadron® Elixir
Dexamethasone Solution (Roxane)
Dexamethasone Intensol Solution
Pediapred® Oral Liquid

Cough Medicines
Anatuss® With Codeine Syrup
Anatuss® Syrup
Brown Mixture NF (Lannett)
CCP® Caffeine Free
CCP® Cough/Cold Tablets
Cerose-DM®
Chlorgest-HD®
Codegest® Expectorant
Codiclear® DH Syrup
Codimal® DM
Colrex® Compound Elixir
Colrex® Expectorant
Conar® Syrup

SUGAR-FREE LIQUID PHARMACEUTICALS *(Continued)*

Conar® Expectorant Syrup
Conex® Liquid
Conex® With Codeine Syrup
Contac Jr® Liquid
Day-Night Comtrex®
Decoral® Forte®
Dexafed® Cough Syrup
Dimetane®-DC Cough Syrup
Dimetane®-DX Cough Syrup
Entuss® Expectorant Liquid
Fedahist® Expectorant Syrup and Pediatric Drops
Guaificon®-DMS
Histafed® Pediatric Liquid
Hycomine® Syrup and Pediatric Syrup
Lanatuss® Expectorant
Medicon® D
Medi-Synal®
Naldecon-DX® Pediatric Drops and Syrup
Naldecon-DX® Adult Liquid
Non-Drowsy Comtrex®
Noratuss®-II Expectorant and Liquid
Organidin® NR
Potassium Iodide Solution (various)
Prunicodeine®
Queltuss® Tablets
Robitussin-CF® Liquid
Robitussin® Night Relief Liquid
Rondec®-DM Drops
Rondec®-DM Syrup
Ryna® Liquid
Ryna-C® Liquid
Ryna-CX® Liquid
Scot-Tussin® DM Syrup
Scot-Tussin® Expectorant
Scot-Tussin® DM Cough Chasers
Silexin® Cough Syrup
Sorbutuss®
S-T® Expectorant, SF/D-F
S-T® Forte®, Sugar-Free
Sudodrin®/Sudodrin® Forte®
Terpin® Hydrate With Codeine Elixir (various)
Toclonol® Expectorant
Toclonol® Expectorant With Codeine
Tolu-Sed® Cough Syrup
Tolu-Sed® DM
Tricodene® Liquid
Trind-DM® Liquid
Tuss-Ornade®
Tussar® SF
Tuss-Organidin® DM NR
Tussirex® Sugar-Free

Dental Preparations and Fluoride Preparations

Cepacol® Mouthwash
Cepastat® Mouthwash and Gargle
Chloraseptic® Mouthwash and Gargle
Fluorigard® Mouthrinse
Fluorinse®
Flura-Drops®
Flura-Loz®
Flura® Tablets
Gel-Kam®
Karigel®
Karigel® N

Luride® Drops
Luride® SF Lozi-Tabs
Luride® 0.25 and 0.5 Lozi-Tabs
Luride® Lozi-Tabs
Pediaflor® Drops
Phos-Flur® Rinse/Supplement
Point-Two® Mouthrinse
Prevident® Disclosing Drops
Thera-Flur® Gel and Drops

Diagnostic Agents
Gastrografin®

Dietary Substitutes
Co-Salt®

Iron Preparations/Blood Modifiers
Amicar® Syrup
Beminal® Stress Plus With Iron
Chel-Iron® Drops
Chel-Iron® Liquid
Geritol® Complete Tablets
Geritonic™ Liquid
Hemo-Vite® Liquid
Iberet® Liquid
Iberet®-500 Liquid
Incremin® With Iron Syrup
Kovitonic® Liquid
Niferex®
Nu-Iron® Elixir
Vita-Plus H® Half Strength, Sugar-Free
Vita-Plus H®, Sugar-Free

Laxatives
Agoral® (plain, marshmallow, and raspberry)
Aromatic Cascara Fluidextract USP
Castor Oil
Castor Oil (flavored)
Castor Oil USP
Colace®, Liquid
Cologel®
Disonate™ Liquid
Doxinate® Solution
Emulsoil®
Fiberall® Powder
Haley's MO®
Hydrocil® Instant Powder
Hypaque® Oral Powder
Kondremul®
Kondremul® With Cascara
Kondremul® With Phenolphthalein
Konsyl® Powder
Liqui-Doss®
Magnesium Citrate Solution NF
Metamucil® Instant Mix (lemon-lime or orange)
Metamucil® SF Powder
Milk of Magnesia
Milk of Magnesia/Cascara Suspension
Milk of Magnesia/Mineral Oil Emulsion (various)
Milkinol® Liquid
Mineral Oil (various)
Neoloid® Liquid
NuLYTELY®
Phospho-Soda®
Sodium Phosphate & Biphosphate Oral Solution USP (Phillips Roxane)
Zymenol® Emulsion

SUGAR-FREE LIQUID PHARMACEUTICALS *(Continued)*

Potassium Products
Cena-K® Solution
EM-K®-10% Liquid
K-G® Elixir
Kaochlor-Eff® Tablets for Solution
Kaochlor® S-F Solution
Kaon® Elixir (grape and lemon-lime flavor)
Kaon-Cl® 20% Liquid
Kay Ciel® Elixir
Kay Ciel® Powder
Kaylixir®
Klor-Con®/25 Powder
Klor-Con® EF Tablets
Klor-Con® Liquid 20%
Klor-Con® Powder
Klorvess® Effervescent Tablets
Klorvess® Granules
Kolyum® Liquid and Powder
Potachlor® 10% and 20% Liquid
Potasalan® Elixir
Potassine® Liquid
Potassium Chloride Oral Solution USP 5%, 10%, and 20% (various)
Potassium Gluconate Elixir NF
Rum-K® Solution
Tri-K® Liquid
Trikates® Solution

Sedatives-Tranquilizers-Antipsychotics
Butabarbital Sodium Elixir
Butisol Sodium® Elixir
Haldol® Concentrate
Loxitane® C Drops
Mellaril® Concentrate
Serentil® Concentrate
Thorazine® Concentrate

Vitamin Preparations-Nutritionals
Aquasol A® Drops
BioCal® Tablets
Bugs Bunny™ Chewable Tablets
Bugs Bunny™ Plus Iron Chewable Tablets
Bugs Bunny™ With Extra C Chewable Tablets
Bugs Bunny™ Plus Minerals Chewable Tablets
Calciferol™ Drops
Caltrate® 600 Tablets
Ce-Vi-Sol® Drops
Cod Liver Oil (various)
Decagen® Tablets
DHT™ Intensol Solution (Roxane)
Drisdol® in Propylene Glycol
Flintstones™ Complete Chewable Tablets
Flintstones™ With Extra C Chewable Tablets
Flintstones™ Plus Iron Chewable Tablets
Incremin® With Iron Liquid
Kandium® Drops Tablets
Lanoplex® Elixir
Lycolan® Elixir
Oyst-Cal® 500 Tablets
Pediaflor®
PMS® Relief
Poly-Vi-Flor® Drops
Poly-Vi-Flor®/Iron Drops
Poly-Vi-Sol® Drops
Poly-Vi-Sol®/Iron Drops

Posture® Tablets
Spiderman™ Children's Chewable Vitamin Tablets
Spiderman™ Children's Plus Iron Tablets
Theragran® Jr Children's Chewable Tablets
Tri-Vi-Flor® Drops
Tri-Vi-Sol® Drops
Tri-Vi-Sol®/Iron Drops
Vi-Daylin® ADC Drops
Vi-Daylin® ADC/Fluoride Drops
Vi-Daylin® ADC Plus Iron Drops
Vi-Daylin® Drops
Vi-Daylin®/Fluoride Drops
Vi-Daylin® Plus Iron Drops
Vitalize®

Miscellaneous

Altace™ Capsules
Bicitra® Solution
Cibalith-S® Syrup
Colestid® Granules
Dayto® Himbin® Liquid
Digoxin® Elixir (Roxane)
Duvoid®
Glandosane®
Lipomul®
Lithium Citrate Syrup
Nicorette® Chewing Gum
Polycitra®-K Solution
Polycitra®-LC Solution
Tagamet® Liquid

References

Hill EM, Flaitz CM, and Frost GR, "Sweetener Content of Common Pediatric Oral Liquid Medications," *Am J Hosp Pharm*, 1988, 45:135-42.

Kumar A, Rawlings RD, and Beaman DC, "The Mystery Ingredients: Sweeteners, Flavorings, Dyes, and Preservatives in Analgesic/Antipyretic, Antihistamine/Decongestant, Cough and Cold, Antidiarrheal, and Liquid Theophylline Preparations," *Pediatrics*, 1993, 91:927-33.

"Sugar Free Products," *Drug Topics Red Book*, 1992, 17-8.

CARBOHYDRATE AND ALCOHOL CONTENT OF LIQUID MEDICATIONS FOR USE IN PATIENTS RECEIVING KETOGENIC DIETS

Generic Name	Carbohydrate g/5 mL				Ethyl Alcohol g/5 mL
	Sucrose	Sorbitol	Glycerin	Total	
Acetaminophen					
Tylenol® children's drops	0	0	0.43	0.43	0
Tylenol® children's elixir	1.6	1	0.43	3.03	0
Tylenol® children's suspension	3.7*	1	0.43	5.13	0
Tylenol® maximum strength liquid	5.49*	1	0	6.49	0
Acetaminophen/codeine					
Tylenol® elixir with codeine	3	0	0	3.0	0.35
Acyclovir					
Zovirax® suspension	0	0.3	0	0.3	0
Albuterol					
Ventolin® syrup	0	0	0	0	0
Proventil® syrup	0	0	0	0	0
AlOH/MgOH					
Maalox® Extra Strength Plus	0	0.5	0	0.5	0
Maalox® suspension	0	0.225	0	0.225	0
AlOH/MgOH/simethicone					
Mylanta® cherry cream liquid	0	0.6	0	0.6	0
Mylanta® double strength liquid	0	0.8	0	0.8	0
Mylanta® liquid	0	0.8	0	0.8	0
Mylanta® mint cream liquid	0	0.6	0	0.6	0
AlOH					
Alternagel®	0	0.6	0	0.6	0
Gaviscon® liquid	5.55§	0.36	0.51	6.42	0
AlOH gel (Roxane)					
Conc aluminum hydroxide gel	0	0.52	0	0.52	0
Alprazolam					
Alprazolam Intensol®	0	0	0	0	0
Aminocaproic acid					
Amicar® syrup	0	0.7	0	0.7	0
Amoxicillin					
Amoxicillin 125 suspension (Biocraft)	2	0	0	2	0
Amoxicillin 250 suspension (Biocraft)	3	0	0	3	0
Trimox® suspension	3.3	0	0	3.3	0
Amoxicillin 125 suspension (Lederle)	2.08	0	0	2.08	0
Amoxicillin 250 suspension (Lederle)	1.923	0	0	1.923	
Amoxicillin/clavulanate					
Augmentin® 125 suspension	0	0	0	0	0
Augmentin® 250 suspension	0	0	0	0	0
Ampicillin					
Ampicillin 125 suspension (Lederle)	4.021	0	0	4.021	0
Ampicillin 250 suspension (Lederle)	4.024	0	0	4.024	0
Ampicillin 125 suspension (Biocraft)	2.6	0	0	2.6	0
Ampicillin 250 suspension (Biocraft)	2.6	0	0	2.6	0
Azithromycin					
Zithromax® 100 suspension	3.86	0	0	3.86	0
Zithromax® 200 suspension	3.87	0	0	3.87	0
Calcium carbonate (Roxane)					
CaCO₃ oral suspension	0	1.4	0	1.4	0
Calcium glubionate					
Neo-Calglucon®	0	0.45	0	0.45	0
Carbamazepine					
Tegretol® suspension	2	0.6	0	2.6	0

(continued)

Generic Name	Carbohydrate g/5 mL				Ethyl Alcohol g/5 mL
	Sucrose	Sorbitol	Glycerin	Total	
Cefaclor					
Ceclor® suspension	3	0	0	3	0
Cefadroxil					
Duricef® 125 suspension	2.55	0	0	2.55	0
Duricef® 250 suspension	2.43	0	0	2.43	0
Cefpodoxime					
Vantin® 50 suspension	2.94	0	0	2.94	0
Vantin® 100 suspension	2.94	0	0	2.94	0
Cefprozil					
Cefzil® suspension	2.03	0	0	2.03	0
Cefuroxime					
Ceftin® 125 suspension	3.214	0	0	3.214	0
Cephalexin					
Cephalexin 125 suspension (Lederle)	1.4	0	0	1.4	0
Cephalexin 250 suspension (Lederle)	1.2	0	0	1.2	0
Cephalexin 125 suspension (Biocraft)	2.6	0	0	2.6	0
Keflex® oral suspension	3	0	0	3	0
Cephradine					
Velosef® suspension	3.3	0	0	3.3	0
Chloral hydrate					
Chloral hydrate syrup (Geneva)	0	0	0.2	0.2	0
Chloral hydrate syrup (UDL Labs)	2.5	1.4	0	3.9	0
Chlorothiazide					
Diuril® oral suspension	2	0	0	2.0	0.025
Chlorpromazine					
Thorazine® concentrate	4.22	0	0	4.22	0
Cimetidine					
Tagamet® liquid	0	2.8	0	2.8	0.5
Cisapride					
Propulsid® suspension	0	3.85	0	3.85	0
Clarithromycin					
Biaxin® 125 suspension	3	0	0	3	0
Biaxin® 250 suspension	2.28	0	0	2.28	0
Clemastine					
Tavist® syrup	0	2.5	0	2.5	0
Clindamycin					
Cleocin® pediatric oral solution	1.825	0	0	1.825	0
Cloxacillin (Biocraft)					
Cloxacillin 250 suspension	2.4	0	0	2.4	0
Cyclosporine					
Sandimmune® oral solution	0	0	0	0	0.6
Dexamethasone (Roxane)					
Dexamethasone oral solution	0	1.2	0.5	1.7	0
Dexamethasone Intensol®	0	0	0	0	1.5
Diazepam					
Diazepam Intensol®	0	0	0	0	0.95
Diazepam solution	0	1	0	1	0
Dicyclomine					
Bentyl® liquid	0	0	0	4	0
Digoxin					
Lanoxin® elixir	1.5	0	0	1.5	0.5
Digoxin elixir (Roxane)	0	1	1	2.0	0.5
Diphenhydramine					
Benadryl® elixir cherry	0	0	0.3	0.3	0
Benadryl® elixir diet	0	2.25	0.6	2.85	0
EES					
EES	3.5	0	0	3.5	0

CARBOHYDRATE AND ALCOHOL CONTENT OF LIQUID MEDICATIONS FOR USE IN PATIENTS RECEIVING KETOGENIC DIETS *(Continued)*

Generic Name	Carbohydrate g/5 mL				Ethyl Alcohol g/5 mL
	Sucrose	Sorbitol	Glycerin	Total	
EES/Sulfisoxazole					
EES/Sulfisoxazole (Lederle)	2	0	0	2	0
Pediazole®	1.95	0	0	1.95	0
Ethosuximide					
Zarontin® syrup	3	0	0.625	3.625	0
Famotidine					
Pepcid® oral suspension	1.186	0	0	1.186	0
Felbamate					
Felbatol® suspension	0	1.5	0	1.5	0
Ferrous gluconate					
Fergon®	2	0	0	2.0	0.436
Ferrous sulfate					
Fer-in-Sol® drops	1.9	1.55	0	3.45	0
Fer-in-Sol® syrup	3	0.325	0	3.325	0
Fer-Gen-Sol®	2	0	0	2.0	0.436
Fluconazole					
Diflucan® 50 suspension	2.88	0	0	2.88	0
Diflucan® 200 suspension	2.73	0	0	2.73	0
Fluoxetine					
Furazolidone					
Furoxone® oral solution	0	0	0.1893	0.1893	0
Furosemide					
Lasix® oral solution	1.75	0	0	1.75	0.25
Furosemide solution (10 mg/5 mL)	0	2.4	0	2.4	0
Furosemide solution (40 mg/5 mL)	0	2.4	0	2.4	0
Griseofulvin					
Grifulvin V® oral suspension	3.5	0	0	3.5	0
Haloperidol					
Haldol® concentrate	3.9¶	0	0	3.9	0
Haldoperidol Intensol®	0	0	0	0	0
Hydrochlorothiazide					
Hydrochlorothiazide solution	0	0	2	2	0
Hydrocortisone cypionate					
Cortef® oral suspension	0.4	0	0	0.4	0
Hydroxyzine					
Vistaril® suspension	0	5	0	5	0
Ibuprofen					
Pedia-Profen® suspension	0	1.55	0	1.55	0
Kaolin/pectin (Roxane)					
Kaolin Pectin suspension	0	0	0.1	0.1	0
Kaopectin					
Kaopectate® concentrated antidiarrheal regular	0.6	0	0	0.6	0
L-carnitine					
Carnitor® oral solution	0.2385	0	0	0.2385	0
Lactulose					
Cephulac® syrup	4.67¶	0	0	4.67	0
Chronulac® syrup	4.67¶	0	0	4.67	0
Lithium citrate					
Lithium citrate USP	0	2.7	0	2.7	0
Loperamide					
Imodium A-D®	3.7¶	0	0.43	4.13	0.26
Loperamide oral solution	0	0	3	3	0

(continued)

Generic Name	Carbohydrate g/5 mL				Ethyl Alcohol g/5 mL
	Sucrose	Sorbitol	Glycerin	Total	
Loracarbef					
Lorabid®	3	0	0	3	0
Lorazepam					
Lorazepam Intensol®	0	0	0	0	0
Metaproterenol (Biocraft)					
Metaproterenol syrup	0	1.7	0	1.7	0
Metaproterenol sulfate					
Alupent® syrup	0	1.4	0	1.4	0
Metaprel® syrup	0	1.4	0	1.4	0
Metoclopramide					
Metoclopramide syrup (Biocraft)	0	2.1	0	2.1	0
Metoclopramide Intensol®	0	1.4	0.5	1.9	0
Metoclopramide oral solution (Roxane)	0	1.4	0.5	1.9	0
Milk of Magnesia					
Concentrated Milk of Magnesia	0.4	1	0.2	1.6	0
Multivitamins					
Iberet® 250 liquid	0	3.61	0	3.61	0
Iberet® 500 liquid	0.62	2.1	0	2.72	0
Theragran® liquid	1.75	0	0	1.75	0
Poly-Vi-Sol® drops	0	0	4.25	4.25	0
Vi-Daylin® liquid	0.778	0	0.025	6.053	0
Vi-Daylin® multivitamin drops	0	0	4.8	4.8	0
Multivitamins with fluoride drops					
Poly-Vi-Flor® drops	0	0	4.25	4.25	0
Multivitamins with fluoride drops					
Tri-Vi-Flor® drops	0	0	4.25	4.25	0
Multivitamins with iron					
Poly-Vi-Flor® With Iron drops	0	0	3.9	3.9	0
Multivitamins with iron					
Tri-Vi-Flor® With Iron drops	0	0	3.9	3.9	0
Multivitamins with minerals					
Advanced Formula Centrum® liquid	1.67	0	0	1.67	0.335
Multivitamins/fluoride					
Vi-Daylin®/f	0	0	4.8	4.8	0
Naproxen					
Naprosyn® oral suspension	1.275	0.45	0	1.725	0
Nitrofurantoin					
Furadantin® suspension	0	0.7	0.7	1.4	0
Nystatin					
Nystatin oral suspension (Biocraft)	2.5	0	0.75	3.25	0.05
Nilstat® oral suspension	3	0	0	3	0
Oxybutynin					
Ditropan® syrup	4#	1.3	1.74	7.04	0
Paregoric					
Paregoric	0	0	0.25	0.25	2.25
PE/Triprolidine					
Children's Actifed® liquid	2.6	2.5	0	5.1	0
PE/PPA/chlorpheniramine/phenyltoloxamine					
Naldecon Ped® drops	0	1.14	0	1.14	0
Naldecon Ped® syrup	0	2	0	2	0
Naldecon syrup	0	2	0	2	0
Penicillin VK					
VeeTids®	3.5	0	0	3.5	0
Penicillin V Potassium (Biocraft)					
Penicillin VK 125® suspension	2.4	0	0	2.4	0
Phenobarbital (Lilly)					
Phenobarbital elixir	0.65	0	2.8	3.45	0.7125

CARBOHYDRATE AND ALCOHOL CONTENT OF LIQUID MEDICATIONS FOR USE IN PATIENTS RECEIVING KETOGENIC DIETS *(Continued)*

Generic Name	Carbohydrate g/5 mL				Ethyl Alcohol g/5 mL
	Sucrose	Sorbitol	Glycerin	Total	
Phenytoin					
Dilantin® suspension 125	1	0	0.385	1.385	0
Potassium chloride					
Rum-K®	0	0.54	1.72	2.26	0
Kay Ciel® liquid	0	0	0	0	0.14
Potassium chloride oral solution 10% (Roxane)	0	0	0.25	0.25	0.25
Potassium chloride oral solution 20%	0	0	0.25	0.25	0.25
Kaochlor S-F®	0	0	0	0	0.25
Kaon® elixir (potassium gluconate)	0	0	0	0	0.25
Kaon-Cl® 20%	0	0	0	0	0.25
Klor-Con® powder	0	0	0	0	0
Klor-Con/25® powder	0	0	0	0	0
Potassium citrate					
Polycitra-K®	0	0	0	0	0
Potassium citrate/sodium citrate					
Polycitra®	0	0	0	0	0
Potassium iodide					
SSKI®	0	0	0	0	0
Prednisolone					
Pediapred®	0	1.53	0	1.53	0
Prelone® syrup	1.84	0	0	1.84	0.18
Prednisone					
Prednisone Intensol®	0	0	0	1.5	1.5
Prednisone solution (Roxane)	1.8•	0	0	1.8	0.25
Primadone					
Mysoline® suspension	0	0	0	0	0
Prochlorperazine					
Compazine® syrup	3.15	0	0	3.15	0
Propranolol (Roxane)					
Propranolol oral solution (20 mg/5 mL)	0	3.2	0	3.2	0
Propranolol oral solution (40 mg/5 mL)	0	3.2	0	3.2	0
Ranitidine					
Zantac® syrup	0	0.5	0	0.5	0.375
Senokot					
Senokot® syrup	3.3	0	0	3.3	0.35
Simethicone					
Mylicon® drops	0	0	0	0	0
Phazyme® liquid	0	0	0	0	0
Sodium citrate/citric acid					
Bicitra®	0	0	0	0	0
Sodium polystyrene sulfonate (Roxane)					
Sodium polystyrene sulfonate suspension	0	1.2	0	1.2	0.1
Sucralfate					
Carafate® suspension	0	0.7	0.77	1.47	0
Sulfisoxazole					
Gantrisin® pediatric suspension	2.77	0	0	2.77	0.14
Tetracyline					
Sumycin®	2.2	1.5	0	3.7	0

(continued)

Generic Name	Carbohydrate g/5 mL				Ethyl Alcohol g/5 mL
	Sucrose	Sorbitol	Glycerin	Total	
Theophylline					
Theolair® liquid	2.5	0.48	0	2.98	0
Theoclear-80® syrup	0	4	3.5	7.5	0
Elixophylline® elixir	0	0	0.312	0.312	0.86
Elixophylline GG® elixir	0	2.3	1.625	3.925	0
Slo-Phyllin® 80 syrup	0	2.87	0	2.87	0
Slo-Phyllin GG® syrup	0.93	0.6	0.83	2.36	0
Aminophylline oral solution (105 mg/5 mL)	0	0.7	1	1.7	0
Theophylline oral solution (Roxane)	0	2.3	0.5	2.8	0.4
Trimethoprim/Sulfamethoxazole					
Sulfamethoxazole/trimethoprim (Biocraft)	0	0.35	0.7	1.05	0
Septra® suspension	0	2.25	0	2.25	0
Bactrim® pediatric suspension	2.5	0.35	0.75	3.6	0
Valproic acid					
Depakene® syrup	3	0.75	0.75	4.5	0
Vancomycin					
Vancocin® oral solution	0	0	0	0	0
Vitamin A					
Aquasol A® drops	0	0	0	0	0
Vitamin D					
Drisdol®	0	0	0	0	0
Vitamin E					
Aquasol E® drops	0	1	0	1	0
Zidovudine					
Retrovir® syrup	3	0	0	3	0

Generic name abbreviations: DM: dextromethorphan; APAP: acetaminophen; PE: phenylephrine; Pyril: pyrilamine; PPA: phenylpropanolamine; EES: erythromycin ethylsuccinate

*Corn syrup

§Lactulose

•Fructose

¶Lactulose, galactose, lactose, and other sugars

#Glucose

Reference
Adapted from Feldstein TJ, "Carbohydrate and Alcohol Content of 200 Oral Liquid Medications for Use in Patients Receiving Ketogenic Diets," *Pediatrics*, 1996, 97:506-11.

TABLETS THAT CANNOT BE CRUSHED OR ALTERED

There are a variety of reasons for crushing tablets or capsule contents prior to administering to the patient. Patients may have nasogastric tubes which do not permit the administration of tablets or capsules; an oral solution for a particular medication may not be available from the manufacturer or readily prepared by pharmacy; patients may have difficulty swallowing capsules or tablets; or mixing of powdered medication with food or drink may make the drug more palatable.

Generally, medications which should not be crushed fall into one of the following categories.

- **Extended-Release Products.** The formulation of some tablets is specialized as to allow the medication within it to be slowly released into the body. This is sometimes accomplished by centering the drug within the core of the tablet, with a subsequent shedding of multiple layers around the core. Wax melts in the GI tract. Slow-K® is an example of this. Capsules may contain beads which have multiple layers which are slowly dissolved with time.

Common Abbreviations for Extended-Release Products

CR	Controlled release
CRT	Controlled-release tablet
LA	Long-acting
SR	Sustained release
TR	Timed release
TD	Time delay
SA	Sustained action
XL	Extended length
XR	Extended release

- **Medications Which Are Irritating to the Stomach**. Tablets which are irritating to the stomach may be enteric-coated which delays release of the drug until the time when it reaches the small intestine. Enteric-coated aspirin is an example of this.

- **Foul-Tasting Medication**. Some drugs are quite unpleasant to taste so the manufacturer coats the tablet in a sugar coating to increase its palatability. By crushing the tablet, this sugar coating is lost and the patient tastes the unpleasant tasting medication.

- **Sublingual Medication**. Medication intended for use under the tongue should not be crushed. While it appears to be obvious, it is not always easy to determine if a medication is to be used sublingually. Sublingual medications should indicate on the package that they are intended for sublingual use.

- **Effervescent Tablets.** These are tablets which, when dropped into a liquid, quickly dissolve to yield a solution. Many effervescent tablets, when crushed, lose their ability to quickly dissolve.

Recommendations

1. It is not advisable to crush certain medications.

2. Consult individual monographs prior to crushing capsule or tablet.

3. If crushing a tablet or capsule is contraindicated, consult with your pharmacist to determine whether an oral solution exists or can be compounded.

Drug Product	Dosage Forms	Reasons/Comments
Accutane®	Capsule	Mucous membrane irritant
Actifed 12® Hour	Capsule	Slow release†
Acutrim®	Tablet	Slow release
Adalat® CC	Tablet	Slow release
Aerolate® SR, JR, III	Capsule	Slow release*†
Afrinol® Repetabs®	Tablet	Slow release
Allerest® 12-Hour	Capsule	Slow release
Anaplex SR	Capsule	Slow release
Ansaid®	Tablet	Taste††
Artane® Sequels®	Capsule	Slow release*†
Arthritis Bayer® Time Release	Capsule	Slow release
Asacol®	Tablet	Slow release
A.S.A.® Enseals®	Tablet	Enteric-coated
Asbron G® Inlay	Tablet	Multiple compressed tablet†
Atrohist® LA	Tablet	Slow release
Atrohist® Plus	Tablet	Slow release
Atrohist® Sprinkle	Capsule	Slow release*
Azulfidine® EN-tabs®	Tablet	Enteric-coated
Baros	Tablet	Effervescent tablet¶
Bayer® Aspirin, low adult 81 mg strength	Tablet	Enteric-coated
Bayer® Aspirin, regular strength 325 mg caplet	Tablet	Enteric-coated
Bayer® Aspirin, regular strength EC caplet	Tablet	Enteric-coated
Betachron E-R®	Capsule	Slow release
Betapen®-VK	Tablet	Taste††
Biohist® LA	Tablet	Slow release♦
Bisacodyl	Tablet	Enteric-coated‡
Bisco-Lax®	Tablet	Enteric-coated‡
Bontril® Slow-Release	Capsule	Slow release
Breonesin®	Capsule	Liquid filled§
Brexin® L.A.	Capsule	Slow release†
Bromfed®	Capsule	Slow release†
Bromfed-PD®	Capsule	Slow release†
Calan® SR	Tablet	Slow release♦
Cama® Arthritis Pain Reliever	Tablet	Multiple compressed tablet
Carbiset-TR®	Tablet	Slow release
Cardizem®	Tablet	Slow release
Cardizem® CD	Capsule	Slow release*
Cardizem® SR	Capsule	Slow release*
Carter's Little Pills®	Tablet	Enteric-coated
Ceftin®	Tablet	Taste **Note:** Use suspension for children
Charcoal Plus®	Tablet	Enteric-coated
Chloral Hydrate	Capsule	**Note:** Product is in liquid form within a special capsule†
Chlorpheniramine Maleate Time Release	Capsule	Slow release
Chlor-Trimeton® Repetab®	Tablet	Slow release†
Choledyl® SA	Tablet	Slow release†
Cipro™	Tablet	Taste††
Claritin-D®	Tablet	Slow release
Cleocin®	Capsule	Taste††
Codimal-L.A.®	Capsule	Slow release
Codimal-L.A.® Half	Capsule	Slow release

TABLETS THAT CANNOT BE CRUSHED OR ALTERED
(Continued)

Drug Product	Dosage Forms	Reasons/Comments
Colace®	Capsule	Taste††
Comhist® LA	Capsule	Slow release*
Compazine® Spansule®	Capsule	Slow release†
Congess SR, JR	Capsule	Slow release
Contac®	Capsule	Slow release*
Cotazym-S®	Capsule	Enteric-coated*
Covera-HS™	Tablet	Slow release
Creon®	Capsule	Enteric-coated*
Creon® 10 Minimicrospheres™	Capsule	Enteric-coated*
Creon® 20	Capsule	Enteric-coated*
Cytospaz-M®	Capsule	Slow release
Cytoxan®	Tablet	**Note:** Drug may be crushed, but maker recommends using injection
Dallergy®	Capsule	Slow release†
Dallergy-D®	Capsule	Slow release
Dallergy-JR®	Capsule	Slow release
Deconamine® SR	Capsule	Slow release†
Deconsal® II	Tablet	Slow release
Deconsal® Sprinkle®	Capsule	Slow release*
Defen L.A.®	Tablet	Slow release
Demazin® Repetabs®	Tablet	Slow release†
Depakene®	Capsule	Slow-release-mucous membrane irritant††
Depakote®	Capsule	Enteric-coated
Desoxyn® Gradumets®	Tablet	Slow release
Desyrel®	Tablet	Taste††
Dexatrim® Max Strength	Tablet	Slow release
Dexedrine® Spansule®	Capsule	Slow release
Diamox® Sequels®	Capsule	Slow release
Dilatrate-SR®	Capsule	Slow release
Dimetane® Extentab®	Tablet	Slow release†
Disobrom®	Tablet	Slow release
Disophrol® Chronotab®	Tablet	Slow release
Ital®	Capsule	Slow release
Docusate	Capsule	Liquid filled§
Docusate with Casanthranol	Capsule	Liquid filled§
Donnatal® Extentab®	Tablet	Slow release†
Donnazyme®	Tablet	Enteric-coated
Doxidan® Liquigels	Capsule	Liquid filled§
Drisdol®	Capsule	Liquid filled§
Drixoral®	Tablet	Slow release†
Drixoral® Sinus	Tablet	Slow release
Dulcolax®	Tablet	Enteric-coated‡
Dynabac®	Tablet	Enteric-coated
Easprin®	Tablet	Enteric-coated
Ecotrin®	Tablet	Enteric-coated
E.E.S.® 400	Tablet	Enteric-coated†
Efidac/24®	Tablet	Slow release
Efidac® 24 Chlorpheniramine	Tablet	Slow release
Elixophyllin® SR	Capsule	Slow release*†
E-Mycin®	Tablet	Enteric-coated
Endafed®	Capsule	Slow release

Drug Product	Dosage Forms	Reasons/Comments
Entex® LA	Tablet	Slow release†
Entex® PSE	Tablet	Slow release†
Equanil®	Tablet	Taste††
Eryc®	Capsule	Enteric-coated*
Ergostat®	Tablet	Sublingual form•
Ery-Tab®	Tablet	Enteric-coated
Erythrocin Stearate	Tablet	Enteric-coated
Erythromycin Base	Tablet	Enteric-coated
Eskalith CR®	Tablet	Slow release
Exgest® LA	Tablet	Slow release
Fedahist® Timecaps®	Capsule	Slow release†
Feldene®	Capsule	Mucous membrane irritant
Feocyte	Tablet	Slow release
Feosol®	Tablet	Enteric-coated†
Feosol® Spansule®	Capsule	Slow release*†
Feratab®	Tablet	Enteric-coated†
Fergon®	Tablet	May cause excessive GI upset
Fero-Grad 500®	Tablet	Slow release
Fero-Gradumet®	Tablet	Slow release
Ferralet S.R.®	Tablet	Slow release
Ferrous Gluconate	Tablet	Film-coated
Feverall™ Sprinkle Caps	Capsule	Taste* **Note:** Capsule contents intended to be placed in a teaspoonful of water or soft food.
Fumatinic®	Capsule	Slow release
Gastrocrom®	Capsule	**Note:** Contents should be dissolved in water for administration.
Geocillin®	Tablet	Taste
Glucotrol® XL	Tablet	Slow release
Gris-PEG®	Tablet	**Note:** Crushing may result in precipitation of larger particles.
Guaifed®	Capsule	Slow release
Guaifed®-PD	Capsule	Slow release
Guaifenex® LA	Tablet	Slow release♦
Guaifenex® PSE	Tablet	Slow release♦
GuaiMAX-D®	Tablet	Slow release
Humibid® DM	Tablet	Slow release
Humibid® DM Sprinkle	Capsule	Slow release*
Humibid® LA	Tablet	Slow release
Humibid® Sprinkle	Capsule	Slow release*
Hydergine® LC	Capsule	**Note:** Product is in liquid form within a special capsule††
Hydergine® Sublingual	Tablet	Sublingual route†
Hytakerol®	Capsule	Liquid filled§†
Iberet®	Tablet	Slow release†
Iberet-500®	Tablet	Slow release†
ICAPS® Plus	Tablet	Slow release
ICAPS® Time Release	Tablet	Slow release
Ilotycin®	Tablet	Enteric-coated
Imdur™	Tablet	Slow release♦
Inderal® LA	Capsule	Slow release
Inderide® LA	Capsule	Slow release
Indocin® SR	Capsule	Slow release*†
Ionamin®	Capsule	Slow release

TABLETS THAT CANNOT BE CRUSHED OR ALTERED
(Continued)

Drug Product	Dosage Forms	Reasons/Comments
Isoptin® SR	Tablet	Slow release
Isordil® Sublingual	Tablet	Sublingual form•
Isordil® Tembid®	Tablet	Slow release
Isosorbide Dinitrate Sublingual	Tablet	Sublingual form•
Isosorbide Dinitrate SR	Tablet	Slow release
K+ 8®	Tablet	Slow release†
K+ 10®	Tablet	Slow release†
Kaon-Cl® 6.7	Tablet	Slow release†
Kaon-Cl® 10	Tablet	Slow release†
K+ Care® ET	Tablet	Effervescent tablet†¶
K-Dur®	Tablet	Slow release♦
K-Lease®	Capsule	Slow release*†
Klor-Con®	Tablet	Slow release†
Klor-Con/EF®	Tablet	Effervescent tablet†¶
Klorvess®	Tablet	Effervescent tablet†¶
Klotrix®	Tablet	Slow release†
K-Lyte®	Tablet	Effervescent tablet¶
K-Lyte®/Cl	Tablet	Effervescent tablet¶
K-Lyte DS®	Tablet	Effervescent tablet¶
K-Tab®	Tablet	Slow release†
Levsinex® Timecaps®	Capsule	Slow release
Lexxel®	Tablet	Slow release
Lodrane LD®	Capsule	Slow release*
Mag-Tab® SR	Tablet	Slow release
Meprospan®	Capsule	Slow release*
Mestinon® Timespan®	Tablet	Slow release†
Mi-Cebrin®	Tablet	Enteric-coated
Mi-Cebrin® T	Tablet	Enteric-coated
Micro-K®	Capsule	Slow release*†
Monafed®	Tablet	Slow release
Monafed® DM	Tablet	Slow release
Motrin®	Tablet	Taste†††
Motrin® IB	Tablet	Taste†††
Motrin® IB-Sinus	Tablet	Taste††
MS Contin®	Tablet	Slow release†
Muco-Fen-LA®	Tablet	Slow release
Naldecon®	Tablet	Slow release
Naprelan®	Tablet	Slow release
Nasatab LA®	Tablet	Slow release
Niaspan®	Tablet	Slow release
Nico-400®	Capsule	Slow release
Nicobid®	Capsule	Slow release
Nitro-Bid®	Capsule	Slow release*
Nitroglyn®	Capsule	Slow release*
Nitrong®	Tablet	Slow release
Nitrostat®	Tablet	Sublingual route•
Nitro-Time®	Capsule	Slow release
Noctec®	Capsule	**Note:** Product is in liquid form within a special capsule
Nolamine®	Tablet	Slow release
Nolex® LA	Tablet	Slow release
Norflex®	Tablet	Slow release

Drug Product	Dosage Forms	Reasons/Comments
Norpace CR®	Capsule	Slow release form within a special capsule
Novafed® A	Capsule	Slow release
Ondrox®	Tablet	Slow release
Optilets-500® Filmtab®	Tablet	Enteric-coated
Optilets-M-500® Filmtab®	Tablet	Enteric-coated
Oragrafin®	Capsule	**Note:** Product is in liquid form within a special capsule
Oramorph SR™	Tablet	Slow release†
Ornade® Spansule®	Capsule	Slow release
OxyContin®	Tablet	Slow release
Pabalate®	Tablet	Enteric-coated
Pabalate-SF®	Tablet	Enteric-coated
Pancrease®	Capsule	Enteric-coated*
Pancrease® MT	Capsule	Enteric-coated*
Panmycin®	Capsule	Taste
Papaverine Sustained Action	Capsule	Slow release
Pathilon® Sequels®	Capsule	Slow release*
Pavabid® Plateau®	Capsule	Slow release*
PBZ-SR®	Tablet	Slow release†
Pentasa®	Capsule	Slow release
Perdiem®	Granules	Wax coated
Peritrate® SA	Tablet	Slow release♦
Permitil® Chronotab®	Tablet	Slow release†
Phazyme®	Tablet	Slow release
Phazyme® 95	Tablet	Slow release
Phenergan®	Tablet	Taste†††
Phyllocontin®	Tablet	Slow release
Plendil®	Tablet	Slow release
Pneumomist®	Tablet	Slow release♦
Polaramine® Repetabs®	Tablet	Slow release†
Prelu-2®	Capsule	Slow release
Prevacid®	Capsule	Slow release
Prilosec™	Capsule	Slow release
Pro-Banthine®	Tablet	Taste
Procainamide HCl SR	Tablet	Slow release
Procan® SR	Tablet	Slow release
Procanbid®	Tablet	Slow release
Procardia®	Capsule	Delays absorption§#
Procardia XL®	Tablet	Slow release **Note:** AUC is unaffected.
Profen® II	Tablet	Slow release♦
Profen LA®	Tablet	Slow release♦
Pronestyl-SR®	Tablet	Slow release
Proscar®	Tablet	**Note:** Crushed tablets should not be handled by women who are pregnant or who may become pregnant
Proventil® Repetabs®	Tablet	Slow release†
Prozac®	Capsule	Slow release*
Quibron-T/ SR®	Tablet	Slow release†
Quinaglute® Dura-Tabs®	Tablet	Slow release
Quinidex® Extentabs®	Tablet	Slow release
Quin-Release®	Tablet	Slow release
Respa-1st®	Tablet	Slow release♦
Respa-DM®	Tablet	Slow release♦

TABLETS THAT CANNOT BE CRUSHED OR ALTERED
(Continued)

Drug Product	Dosage Forms	Reasons/Comments
Respa-GF®	Tablet	Slow release♦
Respahist®	Capsule	Slow release*
Respaire® SR	Capsule	Slow release
Respbid®	Tablet	Slow release
Ritalin-SR®	Tablet	Slow release
Robimycin®	Tablet	Enteric-coated
Rondec-TR®	Tablet	Slow release†
Roxanol SR™	Tablet	Slow release†
Ru-Tuss® DE	Tablet	Slow release
Sinemet CR®	Tablet	Slow release♦
Singlet for Adults®	Tablet	Slow release
Slo-bid™ Gyrocaps®	Capsule	Slow release*
Slo-Niacin®	Tablet	Slow release
Slo-Phyllin GG®	Capsule	Slow release†
Slo-Phyllin® Gyrocaps®	Capsule	Slow release*†
Slow FE®	Tablet	Slow release†
Slow FE® With Folic Acid	Tablet	Slow release
Slow-K®	Tablet	Slow release†
Slow-Mag®	Tablet	Slow release
Sorbitrate SA®	Tablet	Slow release
Sorbitrate® Sublingual	Tablet	Sublingual route
Sparine®	Tablet	Taste††
S-P-T	Capsule	**Note:** Liquid gelatin thyroid suspension.
Sudafed® 12-Hour	Caplet	Slow release†
Sudal® 60/500	Tablet	Slow release
Sudal® 120/600	Tablet	Slow release
Sudex®	Tablet	Slow release♦
Surfak® Liquigels	Capsule	Liquid filled§
Sustaire®	Tablet	Slow release†
Syn™-Rx	Tablet	Slow release
Syn™-Rx DM	Tablet	Slow release
Tavist-D®	Tablet	Multiple compressed tablet
Teczam®	Tablet	Slow release
Tedrol® SA	Tablet	Slow release
Tegretol XR®	Tablet	Slow release
Teldrin®	Capsule	Slow release*
Temaril® Spansule®	Capsule	Slow release†
Tepanil® Tentab®	Capsule	Slow release
Tessalon® Perles	Capsule	Slow release
Theo-24®	Tablet	Slow release†
Theoclear® L.A	Capsule	Slow release†
Theochron®	Tablet	Slow release
Theobid®	Capsule	Slow release*†
Theobid® Jr	Capsule	Slow release*†
Theo-Dur®	Tablet	Slow release†
Theo-Dur® Sprinkles	Capsule	Slow release*†
Theolair SR®	Tablet	Slow release†
Theo-Sav®	Tablet	Slow release♦
Theo-Time® SR	Tablet	Slow release
Theovent®	Capsule	Slow release†
Theo-X®	Tablet	Slow release

Drug Product	Dosage Forms	Reasons/Comments
Thorazine® Spansule®	Capsule	Slow release
Toprol XL®	Tablet	Slow release ♦
Touro A&H®	Capsule	Slow release
Touro DM®	Tablet	Slow release
Touro EX®	Tablet	Slow release
Touro LA®	Tablet	Slow release
T-Phyl®	Tablet	Slow release
Trental®	Tablet	Slow release
Triaminic®	Tablet	Enteric-coated†
Triaminic®-12	Tablet	Slow release†
Triaminic® TR	Tablet	Multiple compressed tablet†
Trilafon® Repetabs®	Tablet	Slow release†
Tri-Phen-Chlor® Time Release	Tablet	Slow release
Tri-Phen-Mine® SR	Tablet	Slow release
Triptone® Caplets	Tablet	Slow release
Tuss-LA®	Tablet	Slow release
Tuss-Ornade® Spansule®	Capsule	Slow release
Tylenol® Extended Relief	Capsule	Slow release
ULR-LA®	Tablet	Slow release
Uni-Dur®	Tablet	Slow release
Uniphyl®	Tablet	Slow release
Valrelease®	Capsule	Slow release
Vanex® Forte	Caplet	Slow release
Vantin®	Tablet	Taste†††
Verelan®	Capsule	Slow release*
Volmax®	Tablet	Slow release†
Wellbutrin®	Tablet	Anesthetize mucous membrane
Wygesic®	Tablet	Taste
Zephrex LA®	Tablet	Slow release
ZORprin®	Tablet	Slow release
Zyban®	Tablet	Slow release
Zymase®	Capsule	Enteric-coated

*Capsule may be opened and the contents taken without crushing or chewing; soft food such as applesauce or pudding may facilitate administration; contents may generally be administered via nasogastric tube using an appropriate fluid, provided entire contents are washed down the tube.

†Liquid dosage forms of the product are available; however, dose, frequency of administration, and manufacturers may differ from that of the solid dosage form.

‡Antacids and/or milk may prematurely dissolve the coating of the tablet.

§Capsule may be opened and the liquid contents removed for administration.

††The taste of this product in a liquid form would likely be unacceptable to the patient; administration via nasogastric tube should be acceptable.

¶Effervescent tablets must be dissolved in the amount of diluent recommended by the manufacturer.

#If the liquid capsule is crushed or the contents expressed, the active ingredient will be, in part, absorbed sublingually.

•Tablets are made to disintegrate under the tongue.

♦Tablet is scored and may be broken in half without affecting release characteristics.

Adapted from Mitchell JF and Pawlicki KS, "Oral Solid Dosage Forms That Should Not Be Crushed: 1998 Update," *Hosp Pharm*, 1998, 33(4):399-415.

THERAPEUTIC CATEGORY & KEY WORD INDEX

ANTIASTHMATIC *(Continued)*

ANTIBACTERIAL, OTIC

ANTIBACTERIAL, TOPICAL

ANTIBIOTIC, AMINOGLYCOSIDE

ANTIBIOTIC, ANAEROBIC

ANTIBIOTIC, BETA-LACTAM AND BETA-LACTAMASE COMBINATION

ANTIBIOTIC, CARBACEPHEM

ANTIBIOTIC, CARBAPENEM

ANTIBIOTIC, PENICILLIN *(Continued)*

ANTIBIOTIC, PENICILLIN (ANTIPSEUDOMONAL)

ANTIBIOTIC, PENICILLIN (ANTISTAPHYLOCOCCAL)

ANTIBIOTIC, QUINOLONE

ANTIBIOTIC, STREPTOGRAMIN

ANTIBIOTIC, SULFONAMIDE DERIVATIVE

ANTIBIOTIC, SULFONE

ANTIBIOTIC, TETRACYCLINE DERIVATIVE

ANTIBIOTIC, TOPICAL

ANTIBIOTIC, URINARY IRRIGATION

ANTI-INFLAMMATORY AGENT

ANTI-INFLAMMATORY AGENT, OPHTHALMIC

ANTI-INFLAMMATORY AGENT, RECTAL

ANTILIPEMIC AGENT

ANTIMALARIAL AGENT

ANTIMANIC AGENT

ANTIMIGRAINE AGENT

(Continued)

(Continued)

BETA₂-ADRENERGIC AGONIST AGENT *(Continued)*
Salmeterol 855
Terbutaline 903

BIOLOGICAL RESPONSE MODULATOR
Aldesleukin 42
Interferon Alfa-2a 522
Interferon Alfa-2b 524

BIOTINIDASE DEFICIENCY, TREATMENT AGENT
Biotin 133

BISPHOSPHONATE DERIVATIVE
Etidronate Disodium 396
Pamidronate 722

BLOOD PRODUCT DERIVATIVE
Albumin 39
Antihemophilic Factor (Human) 89
Factor IX Complex (Human) 399

BLOOD VISCOSITY REDUCER AGENT
Pentoxifylline 750

BRONCHODILATOR
Albuterol 40
Aminophylline 61
Atropine 107
Bitolterol 136
Ephedrine 369
Epinephrine 371
Ipratropium 527
Isoetharine 533
Isoproterenol 536
Levalbuterol 563
Metaproterenol 611
Pirbuterol 776
Salmeterol 855
Terbutaline 903
Theophylline 910

CALCIUM CHANNEL BLOCKER
Diltiazem 323
Nifedipine 687
Verapamil 974

CALCIUM SALT
Calcium Supplements 157

CALORIC AGENT
Fat Emulsion 403
Medium Chain Triglycerides 598

CARBONIC ANHYDRASE INHIBITOR
Acetazolamide 29

CARDIAC GLYCOSIDE
Digoxin 318

CENTRAL NERVOUS SYSTEM STIMULANT, AMPHETAMINE
Dextroamphetamine 300
Dextroamphetamine and Amphetamine 302

HYPNOTIC *(Continued)*

IMMUNE GLOBULIN

IMMUNOSUPPRESSANT AGENT

INFANTILE SPASMS, TREATMENT

INHALATION, MISCELLANEOUS

INTERFERON

INTRAVENOUS NUTRITIONAL THERAPY

IRON SALT

IRON SALT, PARENTERAL

KERATOLYTIC AGENT

LAXATIVE, BOWEL EVACUANT

LAXATIVE, BULK-PRODUCING

LAXATIVE, HYPEROSMOLAR

LAXATIVE, LUBRICANT

NOTES

NOTES

NOTES

NOTES

NOTES

NOTES

NOTES

NOTES

NOTES

NOTES

NOTES

NOTES

NOTES

NOTES

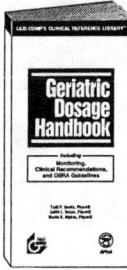

INFECTIOUS DISEASES HANDBOOK (International edition available)

by Carlos M. Isada MD; Bernard L. Kasten Jr. MD; Morton P. Goldman PharmD; Larry D. Gray PhD; and Judith A. Aberg MD

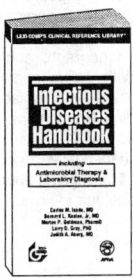

This four-in-one quick reference is concerned with the identification and treatment of infectious diseases. Each of the four sections of the book (166 disease syndromes, 152 organisms, 238 laboratory tests, and 295 antimicrobials) contain related information and cross-referencing to one or more of the other three sections.

The disease syndrome section provides the clinical presentation, differential diagnosis, diagnostic tests, and drug therapy recommended for treatment of more common infectious diseases. The organism section presents the microbiology, epidemiology, diagnosis, and treatment of each organism. The laboratory diagnosis section describes performance of specific tests and procedures. The antimicrobial therapy section presents important facts and considerations regarding each drug recommended for specific diseases of organisms.

DRUG-INDUCED NUTRIENT DEPLETION HANDBOOK

by Ross Pelton, RPh, PhD, CCN; James B. LaValle, RPh, DHM, NMD, CCN; Ernest B. Hawkins, RPh, MS; Daniel L. Krinsky, RPh, MS

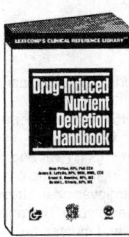

A complete and up-to-date listing of all drugs known to deplete the body of nutritional compounds.

This book is alphabetically organized and provides extensive cross-referencing to related information in the various sections of the book. Nearly 150 generic drugs that cause nutrient depletion are identified and are cross-referenced to more detailed descriptions of the nutrients depleted and their actions. Symptoms of deficiencies, and sources of repletion are also included. This book also contains a Studies and Abstracts section, a valuable Appendix, and Alphabetical & Pharma-cological Indices.

NATURAL THERAPEUTICS POCKET GUIDE

by James B. LaValle, RPh, DHM, NMD, CCN; Daniel L. Krinsky, RPh, MS; Ernest B. Hawkins, RPh, MS; Ross Pelton, RPh, PhD, CCN; Nancy Ashbrook Willis, BA, JD

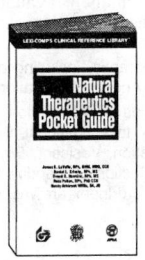

Provides condition-specific information on common uses of natural therapies.

Containing information on over 70 conditions, each including the following: review of condition, decision tree, list of commonly recommended herbals, nutritional supplements, homeopathic remedies, lifestyle modifications, and contraindications & warnings. Provides herbal/nutritional/nutraceutical monographs with over 10 fields including references, reported uses, dosage, pharmacology, toxicity, warnings & interactions, and cautions & contraindications.

Appendix: drug-nutrient depletion, herb-drug interactions, drug-nutrient interaction, herbal medicine use in pediatrics, unsafe herbs, and reference of top herbals.

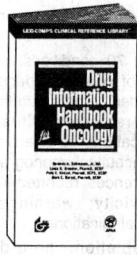

DRUG INFORMATION HANDBOOK FOR ADVANCED PRACTICE NURSING
by Beatrice B. Turkoski, RN, PhD; Brenda R. Lance, RN, MSN; Mark F. Bonfiglio, PharmD

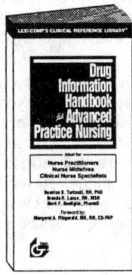

This handbook was designed specifically to meet the needs of Nurse Practitioners, Clinical Nurse Specialists, Nurse Midwives and graduate nursing students. The handbook is a unique resource for detailed, accurate information, which is vital to support the advanced practice nurse's role in patient drug therapy management.

A concise introductory section reviews topics related to Pharmacotherapeutics.

Over 4750 U.S., Canadian, and Mexican medications are covered in the 1055 monographs. Drug data is presented in an easy-to-use, alphabetically organized format covering up to 46 key points of information. Monographs are cross-referenced to an Appendix of over 230 pages of valuable comparison tables and additional information. Also included are two indices, Pharmacologic Category and Controlled Substance, which facilitate comparison between agents.

DRUG INFORMATION HANDBOOK FOR NURSING
by Beatrice B. Turkoski, RN, PhD; Brenda R. Lance, RN, MSN; Mark F. Bonfiglio, PharmD

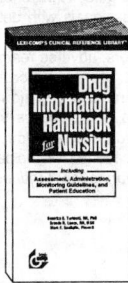

Registered Professional Nurses and upper-division nursing students involved with drug therapy will find this handbook provides quick access to drug data in a concise easy-to-use format.

Over 4750 U.S., Canadian, and Mexican medications are covered with up to 43 key points of information in each monograph. The handbook contains basic pharmacology concepts and nursing issues such as patient factors that influence drug therapy (ie, pregnancy, age, weight, etc) and general nursing issues (ie, assess-ment, administration, monitoring, and patient education). The Appendix contains over 220 pages of valuable information.

ANESTHESIOLOGY & CRITICAL CARE DRUG HANDBOOK
by Andrew J. Donnelly, PharmD; Francesca E. Cunningham, PharmD; and Verna L. Baughman, MD

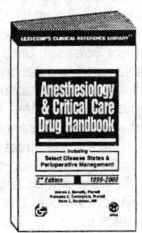

Contains over 512 generic medications with up to 25 fields of information presented in each monograph. It also contains the following Special Issues and Topics: Allergic Reaction, Anesthesia for Cardiac Patients in Noncardiac Surgery, Anesthesia for Obstetric Patients in Nonobstetric Surgery, Anesthesia for Patients With Liver Disease, Chronic Pain Management, Chronic Renal Failure, Conscious Sedation, Perioperative Management of Patients on Antiseizure Medication, Substance Abuse and Anesthesia.

The Appendix includes Abbreviations & Measurements, Anesthesiology Information, Assessment of Liver & Renal Function, Comparative Drug Charts, Infectious Disease-Prophylaxis & Treatment, Laboratory Values, Therapy Recommendation, Toxicology, *and much more . . .*

To order call toll free anywhere in the U.S.: 1-800-837-LEXI (5394)
Outside of the U.S. call: 330-650-6506 or online at www.lexi.com

DRUG INFORMATION HANDBOOK FOR PSYCHIATRY
(International edition available) by Matthew A. Fuller, PharmD; Martha Sajatovic, MD

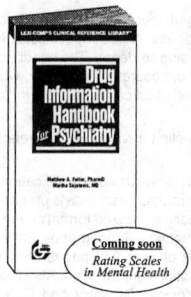

Coming soon
*Rating Scales
in Mental Health*

As a source for comprehensive and clinically relevant drug information for the mental health professional, this handbook is alphabetically arranged by generic and brand name for ease-of-use. It covers over 4,000 brand names and up to 32 key fields of information including effect on mental status and effect on psychiatric treatment.

A special topics/issues section includes psychiatric assessment, overview of selected major psychiatric disorders, clinical issues in the use of major classes of psychotropic medications, psychiatric emergencies, special populations, diagnostic and statistical manual of mental disorders (DSM-IV), and suggested readings. Also contains a valuable Appendix section, as well as, a Therapeutic Category Index and an Alphabetical Index.

PSYCHOTROPIC DRUG INFORMATION HANDBOOK
by Matthew A. Fuller, PharmD; Martha Sajatovic, MD

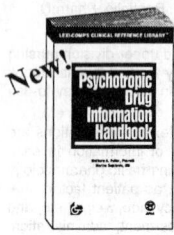

This portable, yet comprehensive guide to psychotropic drugs provides healthcare professionals with detailed information on use, warnings/precautions, drug interactions, pregnancy risk factors, adverse reactions, mechanism of action, and contraindications. Alphabetically organized by brand and generic name this concise handbook provides quick access to the information you need and includes patient education sheets on the psychotropic medications. It is the perfect pocket companion to the *Drug Information Handbook for Psychiatry*.

DRUG INFORMATION HANDBOOK FOR THE CRIMINAL JUSTICE PROFESSIONAL
by Marcelline Burns, PhD; Thomas E. Page, MA; and Jerrold B. Leikin, MD

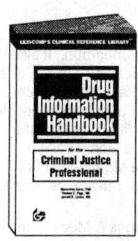

Compiled and designed for police officers, law enforcement officials, and legal professionals who are in need of a reference which relates to information on drugs, chemical substances, and other agents that have abuse and/or impairment potential. This handbook covers over 450 medications, agents, and substances. Each monograph is presented in a consistent format and contains up to 33 fields of information including Scientific Name, Commonly Found In, Abuse Potential, Impairment Potential, Use, When to Admit to Hospital, Mechanism of Toxic Action, Signs & Symptoms of Acute Overdose, Drug Interactions, Warnings/Precautions, and Reference Range. There are many diverse chapter inclusions as well as a glossary of medical terms for the layman along with a slang street drug listing. The Appendix contains Chemical, Bacteriologic, and Radiologic Agents - Effects and Treatment; Controlled Substances - Uses and Effects; Medical Examiner Data; Federal Trafficking Penalties, *and much more.*

DRUG INFORMATION HANDBOOK FOR DENTISTRY
by Richard L. Wynn, BSPharm, PhD; Timothy F. Meiller, DDS, PhD; and Harold L. Crossley, DDS, PhD

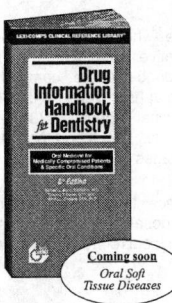

Coming soon
Oral Soft
Tissue Diseases

This handbook presents dental management and therapeutic considerations in medically compromised patients. Issues covered include oral manifestations of drugs, pertinent dental drug interactions, and dosing of drugs in dental treatment.

Selected oral medicine topics requiring therapeutic intervention include managing the patient with acute or chronic pain including TMD, managing the patient with oral bacterial or fungal infections, current therapeutics in periodontal patients, managing the patient receiving chemotherapy or radiation for the treatment of cancer, managing the anxious patient, managing dental office emergencies, and treatment of common oral lesions.

DENTAL OFFICE MEDICAL EMERGENCIES
by Timothy F. Meiller, DDS, PhD; Richard L. Wynn, BSPharm, PhD; Ann Marie McMullin, MD; Cynthia Biron, RDH, EMT, MA; Harold L. Crossley, DDS, PhD

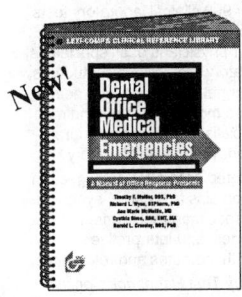

Designed specifically for general dentists during times of emergency. A tabbed paging system allows for quick access to specific crisis events. Created with urgency in mind, it is spiral bound and drilled with a hole for hanging purposes.

- Basic Action Plan for Stabilization
- Loss of Consciousness / Respiratory Distress / Chest Pain
- Allergic / Drug Reactions
- Altered Sensation / Changes in Affect
- Management of Acute Bleeding
- Office Preparedness / Procedures and Protocols

CLINICIAN'S ENDODONTIC HANDBOOK
by Thom C. Dumsha, MS, DDS; James L. Gutmann, DDS, FACD, FICD

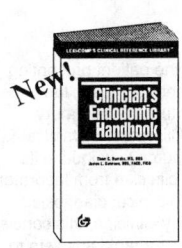

Designed for all general practice dentists.

- A quick reference addressing current endodontics
- Easy to use format and alphabetical index
- Latest techniques, procedures, and materials
- Root canal therapy: Why's and Why Nots
- A guide to diagnosis and treatment of endodontic emergencies
- Facts and rationale behind treating endodontically-involved teeth
- Straight-forward dental trauma management information
- Pulpal Histology, Access Openings, Bleaching, Resorption, Radiology, Restoration, and Periodontal / Endodontic Complications
- Frequently Asked Questions (FAQ) section and "Clinical Note" sections throughout.

LEXI-COMP, INC
1100 Terex Road · Hudson, OH 44236

Thank you!

for purchasing Lexi-Comp's *Pediatric Dosage Handbook*, 7th Edition

Return this postage-paid card so we can keep you up-to-date on all the latest products, promotions and upgrades.

☐ Please put me on your **"Mailing List"**.

☐ Please put me on your **"Standing Order List"** to automatically receive the new edition each year.

Please print the title of the book here that you would like to receive a new edition of automatically each year.

☐ Please send me information on **quantity discounts.**

Name (First): _____ (Last): _____

Title / Occupation: _____

Institution / Company: _____

Address: _____

City: _____ State/Province: _____

Zip/Postal Code: _____ Country: _____

Telephone: (___) _____ Fax: (___) _____

E-Mail Address: _____

OTHER AREAS OF INTEREST (listed alphabetically by topic):

☐ Advanced Practice Nursing Drug Information
☐ Allied Health Professional Drug Information
☐ Anesthesiology & Critical Care Drug Information
☐ Cardiology Drug Information
☐ Criminal Justice Professional Drug Information
☐ Dental Office Medical Emergencies
☐ Dentistry Drug Information
☐ Diagnostic Procedures
☐ Drug-Induced Nutrient Depletion
☐ Drug Information
☐ Endodontic Handbook, Clinician's
☐ Geriatric Dosage Information

☐ Infectious Diseases
☐ Laboratory Tests
☐ Lab Medicine, Clinician's Guide to
☐ Mental Health Prof. Drug Information
☐ Natural Therapeutics
☐ Nursing Drug Information
☐ Oncology Drug Information
☐ Pediatric Dosage
☐ Physician Assistants Drug Information
☐ Poisoning & Toxicology
☐ Psychotropic Drug Information
☐ Rating Scales in Psychiatry

ALSO INTERESTED IN THE FOLLOWING:

☐ Formulary or Laboratory Custom Publishing Service
☐ Lexi-Comp's CRL™ on CD-ROM ___ Academic ___ Personal ___ Institutional
☐ Lexi-Comp database on a hand-held device ___ Palm Pilot ___ Windows CE™ ___ Other